D0161587

VOLUME TWO

DIAGNOSTIC ULTRASOUND

SECOND EDITION

VOLUME TWO

DIAGNOSTIC ULTRASOUND

SECOND EDITION

Carol M. Rumack, M.D.
Professor of Radiology and Pediatrics
University of Colorado Health Sciences Center
Denver, Colorado

Stephanie R. Wilson, M.D.
Professor of Radiology and Obstetrics and Gynecology
University of Toronto
Head, Division of Ultrasound
The Toronto Hospital
Toronto, Ontario, Canada

J. William Charboneau, M.D.
Professor of Radiology
Mayo Clinic
Rochester, Minnesota

with 3698 illustrations, including 461 in color

Mosby

St. Louis Baltimore Boston Carlsbad Chicago Minneapolis New York Philadelphia Portland
London Milan Sydney Tokyo Toronto

Mosby
Dedicated to Publishing Excellence

A Times Mirror
Company

Executive Editor: Robert A. Hurley
Managing Editor: Elizabeth Corra
Associate Developmental Editor: Mia Cariño
Project Manager: Christopher J. Baumle
Project Specialist: David Orzechowski
Manufacturing Manager: William A. Winneberger, Jr.
Designer: Carolyn O' Brien

Copyright © 1998 Mosby–Year Book, Inc.

All rights reserved. No part of this publication may be reproduced, stored in a retrieval system, or transmitted, in any form or by any means, electronic, mechanical, photocopying, recording, or otherwise, without prior written permission from the publisher.

Permission to photocopy or reproduce solely for internal or personal use is permitted for libraries or other users registered with the Copyright Clearance Center, provided that the base fee of $4.00 per chapter plus $.10 per page is paid directly to the Copyright Clearance Center, 222 Rosewood Drive, Danvers, MA 01923. This consent does not extend to other kinds of copying, such as copying for general distribution, for advertising or promotional purposes, for creating new collected works, or for resale.

Composition by Accu-Color Inc.
Printing/binding by Von Hoffman Press, Inc.
Printed in the United States of America

Mosby–Year Book, Inc.
11830 Westline Industrial Drive
St. Louis, Missouri 63146

Library of Congress Cataloging-in-Publication Data

Diagnostic ultrasound / [edited by] Carol M. Rumack, Stephanie R.
Wilson, J. William Charboneau. — 2nd ed.
p. cm.
Includes bibliographical references and index.
ISBN 0-8151-8683-5
1. Diagnosis, Ultrasonic. I. Rumack, Carol M. II. Wilson,
Stephanie R. III. Charboneau, J. William.
[DNLM: 1. Ultrasonography. WN 208 D5357 1997]
RC78.7.U4D514 1997
616.07'543—dc21
DNLM/DLC 97-41915
for Library of Congress CIP

98 99 00 01 02 / 9 8 7 6 5 4 3 2

EDITORS

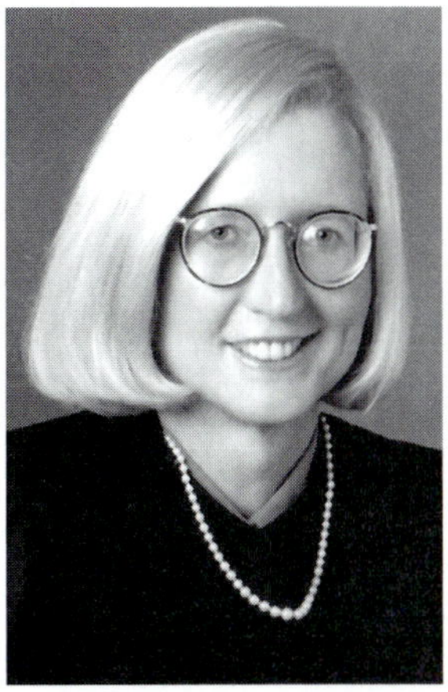

CAROL M. RUMACK, M.D., is Professor of Radiology and Pediatrics at the University of Colorado School of Medicine in Denver, Colorado. Her clinical practice is based at The Children's Hospital and University Hospital in Denver. Her main research focus has been on neonatal sonography in the high-risk perinatal nursery and in newborns referred for complex imaging. Dr. Rumack has published widely in this field and has lectured frequently on pediatric ultrasound. She was the Founding President of the American Association for Women Radiologists and has been a member of the Board of Directors of the American Institute of Ultrasound in Medicine and the Society for Pediatric Radiology. She and her husband, Barry, have two children, Becky and Marc.

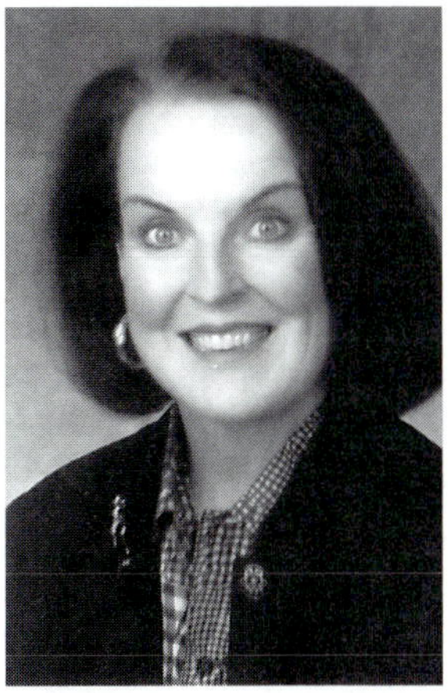

STEPHANIE R. WILSON, M.D., is Professor of Radiology and Obstetrics and Gynecology at the University of Toronto and Head of the Division of Ultrasound at The Toronto Hospital. Her current research endeavors with Dr. Peter N. Burns are focused on oral and intravascular ultrasound contrast agents. An authority on ultrasound of the gastrointestinal tract and abdominal and pelvic viscera, she is the recipient of many university awards and is a frequent international speaker and author. Dr. Wilson also was the first woman President of the Canadian Association of Radiologists and a past Vice President of the Radiological Society of North America. A golf enthusiast, she and her husband, Ken, have two children, Jessica and Jordan.

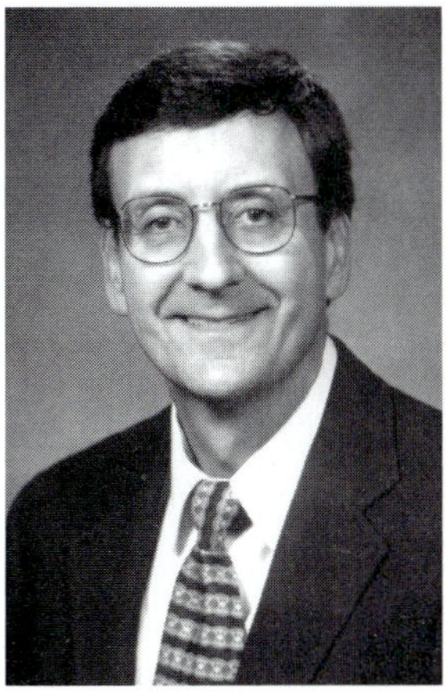

J. WILLIAM CHARBONEAU, M.D., is Professor of Radiology at the Mayo Clinic at Rochester, Minnesota. His current research interests are in small-parts imaging and ultrasound-guided interventional procedures. He is a coauthor of approximately 100 publications, assistant editor of the *Mayo Clinic Family Health Book*, and an active lecturer nationally and internationally. He and his wife, Cathy, have three children, Nick, Ben, and Laurie.

CONTRIBUTORS

Mostafa Atri, M.D., F.R.C.P.(C)
Associate Professor of Radiology
McGill University
Director, Division of Ultrasound
Montreal General Hospital
Montreal, Quebec, Canada

E. Michel Azouz, M.D., F.R.C.P.C.
Professor of Radiology
McGill University
Assistant Director, Department of Medical Imaging
Montreal Children's Hospital
Montreal, Quebec, Canada

Diane S. Babcock, M.D., F.A.C.R.
Professor of Radiology and Pediatrics
University of Cincinnati College of Medicine
University Hospital
Children's Hospital Medical Center
Cincinnati, Ohio

Carol B. Benson, M.D.
Associate Professor of Radiology
Harvard Medical School
Co-Director of Ultrasound
Brigham & Women's Hospital
Boston, Massachusetts

William E. Brant, M.D.
Associate Professor of Radiology
University of California, Davis, School of Medicine
Department of Radiology
University of California, Davis, Medical Center
Sacramento, California

Robert L. Bree, M.D.
Professor of Radiology
University of Michigan Medical School
University of Michigan Medical Center
Ann Arbor, Michigan

Linda K. Brown, M.D.
Staff Radiologist
Quantum Radiology Northwest
Atlanta, Georgia

Peter N. Burns, Ph.D.
Professor of Medical Biophysics and Radiology
University of Toronto
Senior Scientist, Imaging Research
Sunnybrook Health Science Centre
Toronto, Ontario, Canada

Barbara A. Carroll, M.D.
Professor of Radiology
Chief, Section of Ultrasound
Duke University Medical Center
Durham, North Carolina

John M. Caspers, M.D.
Abdominal Imaging Fellow
Mayo Clinic
Rochester, Minnesota
Staff Radiologist
St. Paul Radiology
United Hospital
St. Paul, Minnesota

Daniel E. Challis, M.B., B.S., F.R.A.C.O.G., D.D.U.
Clinical Fellow
University of Toronto
Mount Sinai Hospital
Toronto, Ontario, Canada

William F. Chandler, M.D.
Professor of Neurosurgery
University of Michigan Medical Center
Ann Arbor, Michigan

J. William Charboneau, M.D.
Professor of Radiology
Mayo Clinic
Rochester, Minnesota

David Chitayat, M.D., F.C.C.M.G., F.A.B.M.G., F.R.C.P.C.
Associate Professor
University of Toronto
Head, Prenatal Diagnosis Program
The Toronto Hospital General Division
Toronto, Ontario, Canada

Christine H. Comstock, M.D.
Assistant Professor
Wayne State University
Detroit, Michigan
Director, Fetal Imaging
William Beaumont Hospital
Royal Oak, Michigan

Peter L. Cooperberg, M.D., F.R.C.P.C.
Professor and Vice Chairman of Radiology
University of British Columbia
Chairman of Radiology
St. Paul's Hospital
Vancouver, British Columbia, Canada

Jeanne A. Cullinan, M.D.
Assistant Professor of Radiology
and Radiological Sciences
Assistant Professor of Obstetrics and Gynecology
Vanderbilt University Medical Center
Nashville, Tennessee

Timothy J. Dambro, M.D.
Hospital of the University of Pennsylvania
Philadelphia, Pennsylvania

Sidney M. Dashefsky, M.D., F.R.C.P.
Assistant Professor of Radiology
University of Manitoba
Radiologist
Health Sciences Centre
Winnipeg, Manitoba, Canada

Michael A. DiPietro, M.D.
Associate Professor of Radiology
University of Michigan
Pediatric Radiologist
C.S. Mott Children's Hospital
Ann Arbor, Michigan

Peter M. Doubilet, M.D., Ph.D.
Associate Professor of Radiology
Harvard Medical School
Co-Director of Ultrasound
Brigham & Women's Hospital
Boston, Massachusetts

Dónal B. Downey, M.B., B.Ch., F.R.C.P.C.
Assistant Professor, Department of Diagnostic
Radiology and Nuclear Medicine
Associate Scientist, The John P. Robarts
Research Institute
University of Western Ontario
Director of Diagnostic Ultrasound
London Health Sciences Centre
London, Ontario, Canada

Julia A. Drose, B.A., R.D.M.S., R.D.C.S.
Senior Instructor
University of Colorado School of Medicine
Chief Diagnostic Medical Sonographer
University of Colorado Health Sciences Center
Denver, Colorado

Steven Falcone, M.D.
Assistant Professor of Clinical Radiology and
Neurological Surgery
University of Miami School of Medicine
University of Miami/Jackson Memorial
Medical Center
Attending Neuroradiologist
MRI Center
Miami, Florida

Dan Farine, M.D., F.R.C.S.C.
Associate Professor, Department of Obstetrics
and Gynecology
University of Toronto
Staff Perinatologist and Director of Obstetrics
Mount Sinai Hospital
Toronto, Ontario, Canada

Paul W. Finnegan, M.D., C.M., F.R.C.P.(C)
MBA Program
University of Chicago, Graduate School of Business
Chicago, Illinois
Private Practice
Toronto, Ontario, Canada, and Chicago, Illinois

Katherine W. Fong, M.B., B.S., F.R.C.P.(C)
Assistant Professor of Medical Imaging
University of Toronto
Head, Division of Ultrasound
Women's College Hospital
Toronto, Ontario, Canada

Bruno D. Fornage, M.D.
Professor of Radiology
Chief, Section of Ultrasound
University of Texas, M.D. Anderson Cancer Center
Houston, Texas

J. Brian Fowlkes, Ph.D.
Assistant Research Scientist
University of Michigan Medical Center
Ann Arbor, Michigan

Margaret A. Fraser-Hill, M.D., F.R.C.P.C.
Assistant Professor
Faculty of Medicine
McGill University
Department of Radiology
Montreal General Hospital
Montreal, Quebec, Canada

Kelly S. Freed, M.D.
Clinical Associate
Duke University Medical Center
Durham, North Carolina

Phyllis Glanc, M.D., F.R.C.P.C.
Assistant Professor
University of Toronto
Women's College Hospital
Toronto, Ontario, Canada

Charles M. Glasier, M.D.
Professor of Radiology and Pediatrics
University of Arkansas for Medical Sciences
Chief, Magnetic Resonance Imaging
Arkansas Children's Hospital
Little Rock, Arkansas

Lawrence P. Gordon, M.D.
Associate Pathologist
Crouse Hospital
Associate Professor of Pathology
State University of New York Health Science Center
Syracuse, New York

Calvin A. Greene, M.D., F.R.S.C.(C)
Assistant Clinical Professor
University of Calgary
Division Chief, Reproductive Endocrinology
and Infertility
Director, Regional Fertility Program
Foothills Hospital
Calgary, Alberta, Canada

Leslie E. Grissom, M.D.
Assistant Professor of Radiology and Pediatrics
Jefferson Medical College
Philadelphia, Pennsylvania
Attending Radiologist
Chief of Diagnostic Imaging
Alfred I. duPont Institute
Wilmington, Delaware

H. Theodore Harcke, M.D.
Professor of Radiology and Pediatrics
Jefferson Medical College
Philadelphia, Pennsylvania
Attending Radiologist
Chief of Imaging Research
Alfred I. duPont Institute
Wilmington, Delaware

Curtis L. Harlow, M.D.
Assistant Clinical Professor
University of Colorado
Chief of Radiology
St. Thomas More Hospital
Cañon City, Colorado

Christopher R. Harman, M.D., F.R.C.S.C.
Associate Professor, Department of Obstetrics
and Gynecology
University of Manitoba
Director, Fetal Assessment Unit
Women's Hospital
Winnipeg, Manitoba, Canada

**Ian D. Hay, M.B., Ph.D., F.A.C.E.,
F.A.C.P., F.R.C.P.**
Professor of Medicine
Mayo Medical School
Consultant in Endocrinology and Internal Medicine
Mayo Clinic
Rochester, Minnesota

Christy K. Holland, Ph.D.
Associate Professor, Department of Radiology
University of Cincinnati College of Medicine
Cincinnati, Ohio

Susan C. Holt, M.D., F.R.C.P.(C)
Assistant Professor, Department of Radiology
Health Sciences Centre
Winnipeg, Manitoba, Canada

C. Richard Hopkins, M.D.
Associate in Radiology
Ogden Regional Medical Center
Ogden, Utah
Davis North Hospital
Layton, Utah

E. Meredith James, M.D., F.A.C.R.
Associate Professor of Radiology
Mayo Clinic
Rochester, Minnesota

Ann Jefferies, M.D., F.R.C.P.C.
Assistant Professor
University of Toronto
Neonatologist
Mount Sinai Hospital
Toronto, Ontario, Canada

Susan D. John, M.D.
Associate Professor of Radiology and Pediatrics
University of Texas Medical Branch
Galveston, Texas

Jo-Ann M. Johnson, M.D., F.R.C.S.C.
Assistant Professor
University of Toronto
Division of Maternal Fetal Medicine
The Toronto Hospital
Toronto, Ontario, Canada

Neil D. Johnson, M.B., B.S., F.R.A.C.R., M.Med.
Assistant Professor
University of Cincinnati
Associate Director, Department of Radiology
Children's Hospital Medical Center
Cincinnati, Ohio

Robert A. Kane, M.D., F.A.C.R.
Vice Chairman, Department of Radiological Sciences
Director, Ultrasonography
Associate Professor of Radiology
Harvard Medical School
Beth Israel Deaconess Medical Center
Boston, Massachusetts

Terese I. Kaske, M.D.
Radiology Resident
University of Colorado Health Sciences Center
Denver, Colorado

Bernard F. King, Jr., M.D.
Associate Professor, Department of
Diagnostic Radiology
Mayo Graduate School
Mayo Clinic and Affiliated Hospitals
Rochester, Minnesota

Cheryl L. Kirby, M.D.
Assistant Professor of Diagnostic Imaging
Temple University School of Medicine
Attending Radiologist
Albert Einstein Medical Center
Philadelphia, Pennsylvania

Janet S. Kirk, M.D.
Assistant Director, Fetal Imaging
William Beaumont Hospital
Royal Oak, Michigan

Faye C. Laing, M.D.
Professor of Radiology
Harvard University
Director, Resident Education and Training
Brigham & Women's Hospital
Boston, Massachusetts

Eric J. Lantz, M.D.
Assistant Professor
Mayo Medical School
Staff Radiologist
Mayo Clinic
Rochester, Minnesota

Robert A. Lee, M.D.
Assistant Professor of Radiology
Consultant in Diagnostic Radiology
Mayo Foundation
Rochester, Minnesota

Richard E. Leithiser, Jr., M.D.
Associate Professor of Radiology
University of Arkansas for Medical Sciences
Arkansas Children's Hospital
Little Rock, Arkansas

Clifford S. Levi, M.D., F.R.C.P.(C)
Professor of Radiology
University of Manitoba
Section Head, Diagnostic Ultrasound
Health Sciences Centre
Winnipeg, Manitoba, Canada

Bernard J. Lewandowski, M.D., C.M., R.V.T., M.B.A.
Clinical Associate Professor
University of Ottawa
Head, Ultrasound (Radiology)
Ottawa Civic Hospital
Ottawa, Ontario, Canada

Bradley D. Lewis, M.D.
Assistant Professor
Mayo Medical School
Mayo Graduate School of Medicine
Consultant in Diagnostic Imaging
Mayo Clinic
Rochester, Minnesota

Edward A. Lyons, M.D., F.R.C.P.(C), F.A.C.R.
Professor of Radiology and Obstetrics and Gynecology
University of Manitoba
Health Sciences Centre
Winnipeg, Manitoba, Canada

†Laurence A. Mack, M.D.
Professor of Radiology, Obstetrics and Gynecology, and Orthopaedics
Director of Ultrasound
University of Washington School of Medicine
Seattle, Washington

Marie-Jocelyne Martel, M.D.
Fellow, Maternal Fetal Medicine
University of Manitoba
Winnipeg, Manitoba, Canada

John R. Mathieson, M.D., F.R.C.P.C.
Head, Section of Radiology
Department of Medical Imaging
Capital Health Region
Royal Jubilee Hospital
Victoria, British Columbia, Canada

Frederick A. Matsen, III, M.D.
Professor and Chairman, Department of Orthopaedics
University of Washington Medical Center
Seattle, Washington

John P. McGahan, M.D.
Professor of Radiology
Professor and Director of Abdominal Imaging
University of California, Davis, Medical Center
Sacramento, California

Ellen B. Mendelson, M.D.
Clinical Associate Professor of Diagnostic Radiology
University of Pittsburgh School of Medicine
Director, Mammography and Women's Imaging
Western Pennsylvania Hospital
Pittsburgh, Pennsylvania

Christopher R.B. Merritt, M.D.
Chairman, Department of Radiology
Ochsner Clinic and the Alton Ochsner Medical Foundation
New Orleans, Louisiana

Berta Maria Montalvo, M.D.
Associate Professor of Radiology
University of Miami School of Medicine
Medical Director, Vascular Diagnostic Center
University of Miami Hospitals and Clinics
University of Miami/Jackson Memorial Medical Center
Miami, Florida

Khanh T. Nguyen, M.Sc., M.D., F.R.C.P.C.
Associate Professor
Queen's University
Kingston General Hospital
Hotel Dieu Hospital
Kingston, Ontario, Canada

Stuart F. Nicholson, M.D., F.R.C.P.C.
Clinical Associate Professor
University of Calgary
Foothills Hospital
Calgary, Alberta, Canada

Carl A. Nimrod, M.B., F.R.C.S.C.
Professor of Obstetrics and Gynecology and Radiology
University of Ottawa
Chief of Obstetrics and Gynecology
Ottawa General Hospital
Ottawa, Ontario, Canada

† Deceased

Robert L. Nolan, B.Sc., M.D., F.R.C.P.C.
Professor and Head, Department of
Diagnostic Radiology
Queen's University
Head, Imaging Services
Kingston General Hospital
Hotel Dieu Hospital
St. Mary's of the Lake Hospital
Kingston, Ontario, Canada

David A. Nyberg, M.D.
Associate Clinical Professor of Radiology and
Obstetrics and Gynecology
University of Washington Medical Center
Co-Director of Obstetric Ultrasound
Swedish Medical Center
Seattle, Washington

Heidi B. Patriquin, M.D., F.R.C.P.(C)
Clinical Professor of Radiology
University of Montreal
Hopital Ste. Justine
Montreal, Quebec, Canada

Roger A. Pierson, M.S., Ph.D.
Professor, Department of Obstetrics and Gynecology
University of Saskatchewan College of Medicine
Royal University Hospital
Saskatoon, Saskatchewan, Canada

Joseph F. Polak, M.D., M.P.H.
Associate Professor of Radiology
Harvard Medical School
Director of Noninvasive Vascular Imaging
Brigham & Women's Hospital
Boston, Massachusetts

Carl C. Reading, M.D.
Professor of Diagnostic Radiology
Mayo Medical School
Consultant, Diagnostic Radiology
Mayo Clinic
Rochester, Minnesota

Henrietta Kotlus Rosenberg, M.D., F.A.C.R., F.A.A.P.
Professor of Diagnostic Imaging
Temple University School of Medicine
Chairman, Department of Radiology
Albert Einstein Medical Center
Philadelphia, Pennsylvania

Jonathan M. Rubin, M.D., Ph.D.
Professor of Radiology
University of Michigan
Ann Arbor, Michigan

Carol M. Rumack, M.D., F.A.C.R.
Professor of Radiology and Pediatrics
University of Colorado School of Medicine
Denver, Colorado

Greg Ryan, M.B., M.R.C.O.G., F.R.C.S.C.
Assistant Professor, Department of Obstetrics
and Gynecology
Faculty of Medicine
University of Toronto
Director of the Fetal Assessment Unit
Staff Perinatologist
Mount Sinai Hospital
Toronto, Ontario, Canada

Shia Salem, M.D., F.R.C.P.C.
Associate Professor, Medical Imaging
University of Toronto
Head, Division of Ultrasound
Mount Sinai Hospital
Toronto, Ontario, Canada

Eric E. Sauerbrei, B.Sc., M.Sc., M.D., F.R.C.P.C.
Professor of Radiology
Queen's University
Director of Ultrasound
Kingston General Hospital
Hotel Dieu Hospital
Kingston, Ontario, Canada

Joanna J. Seibert, M.D.
Professor of Radiology and Pediatrics
University of Arkansas for Medical Sciences
Director of Radiology
Arkansas Children's Hospital
Little Rock, Arkansas

Robert W. Seibert, M.D.
Professor, Department of Otolaryngology-Head and
Neck Surgery
University of Arkansas for Medical Sciences
Chief, Pediatric Otolaryngology
Arkansas Children's Hospital
Little Rock, Arkansas

†Nancy H. Sherman, M.D.
Assistant Professor of Radiology
Jefferson Medical College
Philadelphia, Pennsylvania
Director of Ultrasound
Alfred I. duPont Institute
Wilmington, Delaware

Luigi Solbiati, M.D.
Vice Chairman and Radiologist
Department of Radiology
General Hospital
Busto Arsizio, Varese, Italy

Beverly A. Spirt, M.D., F.A.C.R.
Professor of Radiology and Obstetrics
and Gynecology
Chief of Women's Imaging Section
State University of New York Health Science Center
Syracuse, New York

Elizabeth R. Stamm, M.D.
Associate Professor
University of Colorado Health Sciences Center
Administrative Co-Director of Body CT
University Hospital
Denver, Colorado

Rhonda R. Stewart, M.D.
Diagnostic Radiologist
Director of CT
Alexandria Hospital
Alexandria, Virginia

Leonard E. Swischuk, M.D.
Professor of Radiology and Pediatrics
University of Texas Medical Branch
Director of Pediatric Radiology
Children's Hospital
Galveston, Texas

George A. Taylor, M.D.
Associate Professor of Radiology and Pediatrics
Harvard Medical School
Director, Body Imaging Division
Children's Hospital
Boston, Massachusetts

Wendy Thurston, M.D., B.Sc., F.R.C.P.C.
Assistant Professor
Division Head, Genitourinary Radiology
University of Toronto
Staff Radiologist
The Toronto Hospital
Toronto, Ontario, Canada

Ants Toi, M.D., F.R.C.P.C.
Associate Professor
University of Toronto
Radiologist
The Toronto Hospital
Toronto, Ontario, Canada

Marnix T. van Holsbeeck, M.D.
Associate Professor of Radiology
Case Western Reserve University
Director, Musculoskeletal and ER Radiology
Henry Ford Hospital
Detroit, Michigan

Keith Y. Wang, Ph.D., M.D.
Clinical Assistant Professor, Department
of Radiology
University of Washington
Swedish Medical Center
Seattle, Washington

Stephanie R. Wilson, M.D., F.R.C.P.C.
Professor of Radiology and Obstetrics and
Gynecology
University of Toronto
Head, Division of Ultrasound
The Toronto Hospital
Toronto, Ontario, Canada

David A. Wiseman, M.D., F.R.C.P.(C)
Associate Professor
Faculty of Medicine
University of Calgary School of Medicine
Radiologist
Foothills Hospital
Calgary, Alberta, Canada

Cynthia E. Withers, M.D., F.R.C.P.C.
Staff Radiologist
Sansum Medical Clinic
Santa Barbara, California

† Deceased

To Barry, Becky, and Marc, for their love and wonderful support through an extremely intense year. To my parents, for their love and their belief in me. And to all my students, for responding to the challenge and joy of studying medicine, in particular ultrasound.

CMR

To Ken, Jessica, and Jordan, who generously lived without me for the many months required for this endeavor. Your independence and continuous encouragement were my inspiration.

SRW

To Cathy, Nicholas, Ben, and Laurie, for all the love and joy you bring to my life. You are all I could ever hope for.

JWC

PREFACE TO THE SECOND EDITION

The First Edition of *Diagnostic Ultrasound*, released at the RSNA in 1991, has become the most commonly used reference textbook at ultrasound practices worldwide. Because sonography has so expanded its frontiers in the past 6 years, we believed that a major revision was required for *Diagnostic Ultrasound* to remain the definitive reference work for this specialty. In particular, greater use of color and power Doppler imaging and improved high-resolution transducers have required the introduction of new chapters and new authors, as well as the expansion and enhancement of the First Edition's original material.

Approximately 100 outstanding authors, all recognized experts in the field of ultrasound, bring you the latest state-of-the-art concepts on ultrasound performance, imaging, diagnosis, and expanded applications, including hysterosonography, laparoscopic sonography, and ultrasound-guided biopsy and drainage techniques.

There has been a 25% increase in the size of the two volumes, the major space reallocation applied to obstetrics and gynecology. Thousands of the original images have been replaced, and new images have been added. The Second Edition also includes more than 450 images in full color. The layout has been exhaustively revamped and now includes multiple-picture "Key Feature Collages." These reflect the spectrum of sonographic changes that may occur in a given disease instead of just the most common manifestation.

Many improvements in the book's format have been designed to facilitate reading and review. Color-enhanced boxes highlight the important or critical features of sonographic diagnoses. Key terms and concepts are emphasized in boldface type. To direct the reader to other research and literature of interest, the comprehensive reference lists are well organized by topic.

The book is again divided into two volumes. Volume I consists of Parts I–IV. Part I contains chapters on physics and biologic effects of ultrasound, as well as the latest developments in ultrasound contrast agents. Part II covers abdominal, pelvic, and thoracic sonography, including interventional procedures. Part III presents intraoperative and laparoscopic sonography. Part IV contains many chapters on small-parts imaging, including carotid and peripheral artery and vein evaluation. Volume II begins with Part V, a greatly expanded section on obstetric and fetal sonography. Part VI comprehensively covers pediatric sonography. Two new chapters on pediatric brain Doppler and pediatric interventional sonography have been added to Part VI.

This book is for practicing physicians, residents, medical students, sonographers, and others interested in understanding the vast applications of diagnostic sonography in patient care. As with the First Edition, *it is our goal to present to you the most comprehensive reference book available on diagnostic ultrasound.*

PREFACE TO THE FIRST EDITION

Sonography has expanded rapidly over the last two decades on a world-wide basis. Despite the explosive growth of this field and the extensive applications of sonographic techniques, few comprehensive reference texts are available. To this end, we undertook the task of producing a state-of-the-art text on ultrasonography.

The authors who have contributed chapters to this book are recognized experts in their fields. We believe that they have provided the most up-to-date information available, making the book current and comprehensive. We hope that it will become a trusted primary reference for all who are interested in this exciting field of medical imaging.

This book is intended for practicing physicians, residents, medical students, and sonographers. It is organized into six parts, covering all aspects of sonography except cardiac and opthalmologic applications. The information in Volume One, Part I, covers the physics of sonography; Part II, abdominal, pelvic, and thoracic imaging; Part III, intraoperative imaging; and Part IV, small parts imaging, including carotid and peripheral vessels. The contents of Volume Two include Part V, obstetric and fetal topics and Part VI, pediatric applications. Every effort was made to cover the broad scope of ultrasound practice without redundancy.

We greatly appreciate the efforts of the contributing authors. Without their experience, expertise, and commitment, we could not have achieved the goal of a comprehensive and authoritative textbook. We are indebted to them.

The high-quality images are the product of many talented sonographers, and to them we offer our sincere thanks. Their dedication to sonography has contributed substantially to its rapid growth and acceptance.

We also thank Janine Jacobson, our talented manuscript coordinator, whose patience and care with multiple manuscript revisions has led to a first-class product. Further, we acknowledge the support of Elaine Steinborn, Jo Salway, Jim Ryan, and Anne Patterson of Mosby–Year Book for encouraging us in this endeavor.

ACKNOWLEDGMENTS

Our deepest appreciation and sincerest gratitude:

To all of our outstanding authors who have contributed extensive, newly updated, and authoritative text and images. We cannot thank them enough for their efforts on this project.

To Lisa Wolfe in Denver, Colorado, whose outstanding secretarial skills and smooth coordination supported the review and final revision of the entire manuscript between editors and authors. Her speed and organization are greatly appreciated.

To Mark Sawyer of Science Imaging Group in Toronto, Canada for excellent photographic assistance, and Jenny Tomash, also in Toronto, for her beautiful illustrations.

To Nick Charboneau, our digital image editor, for his outstanding work in the production of the "Key Image Collages" and other image enhancements.

To Rose Baldwin and Lori Kulas, our secretaries, for their expert and energetic assistance in the preparation of the manuscripts.

To Mia Cariño and Dave Orzechowski at Mosby who have been dedicated and enthusiastic coordinators of the project through development and production.

To Liz Corra at Mosby, an outstanding managing editor, who has guided the project with patient and untiring encouragement.

To Anne Patterson at Mosby who guided this project through its First Edition and has encouraged us to climb this steep mountain of effort again.

CONTENTS

VOLUME ONE

PART V

Obstetric and Fetal Sonography

CHAPTER 31

Overview of Obstetric Sonography

Jo-Ann M. Johnson, M.D., F.R.C.S.C.

CHAPTER OUTLINE

The introduction of sonography to obstetrics by Ian Donald and colleagues in 1958 is now regarded as one of the major milestones of modern medicine. For the first time it became possible to obtain information about the fetus and its environment directly with a noninvasive diagnostic procedure considered safe even when used repeatedly. Initially, acceptance of the technique was slow because it was new and unfamiliar and because the equipment was large and cumbersome to use. With the advent of small, mobile, high-resolution, real-time scanners in the mid to late 1970s, the ease of use together with increased physician awareness of the capabilities of ultrasound accelerated its application to an ever-expanding number of pregnancies. At present, between 60% and 100% of mothers in North America, Great Britain, and Western Europe have a sonographic examination in the antenatal period.[1] The benefits in terms of accurate assessment of gestational age, verification of fetal viability, documentation of multiple pregnancy, placental localization, diagnosis of intrauterine growth retardation (IUGR), and the detection of fetal abnormalities are widely accepted. In addition, more recent advances in technology and expertise have enhanced image quality and allowed for considerable insight into fetal physiology. This has resulted in the development of more specific and accurate tests for the evaluation of fetal well-being, including the biophysical profile score. Sonography has also become an essential aid in the safe performance of invasive obstetric techniques, including chorionic villus sampling (CVS), amniocentesis, percutaneous umbilical blood sampling (PUBS), and intrauterine transfusions.

Although this ability to collect precise structural and functional information about the fetus is exciting, it has raised a new series of questions and problems, including how best to use this technology in pregnancy. Although there are standards regarding obstetric ultrasound, controversies regarding its use in pregnancy, including its safety, indications, and accuracy, as well as the risks, benefits, and limitations of the "routine obstetric scan," remain.

IS ULTRASOUND SAFE?

Diagnostic ultrasound uses sound energy with wave frequencies that exceed 20,000 Hz, the audible range in humans. When a sound beam crosses an interface between objects of different densities, some of the energy is reflected and some is transmitted, the amount of each proportional to the difference in density. Reflected waves are detected by a transducer that creates an image of the scanned object.

Theoretic safety risks from ultrasound energy include **thermal** damage (due to a rise in temperature) and **cavitation** (production and collapse of gas-filled bubbles) with subsequent tissue injury.[2] Fortunately, there is **no evidence** that diagnostic ultrasound is associated with these or any other deleterious biologic effects. In the last 30 years, more than 50 million women have had diagnostic ultrasound *in utero*, and several epidemiologic studies have reported no increase in the incidence of fetal death, abnormality, IUGR, or childhood malignancy with as much as 12 years follow-up.[2,3,4] Similarly, no adverse behavioral or neurologic consequences attributable to diagnostic ultrasound have been demonstrated.[5] In a study by Salvesen et al. comparing 8- and 9-year-old children, half of whose mothers had screening ultrasounds while pregnant and half of whose mothers did not, there was no difference between the two groups with respect to reading, writing, mathematics, incidence of dyslexia, or overall school performance.[6] The study suggested a possible association with left-handedness in infants exposed to ultrasound; however, the significance of this is unclear.[7] Newnham et al. reported an increase in growth-retarded neonates exposed to serial *in utero* ultrasound examinations (five or more)[8]; however, other studies have not shown an association with birth weight after limited ultrasound exposure.[5,9] The general consensus as stated by The American Institute of Ultrasound in Medicine (AIUM) Bioeffects Committee is that **"no confirmed biological effects on patients or instrument operators caused by exposure at intensities typical of present diagnostic ultrasound instruments have ever been reported.** Although the possibility exists that such biological effects may be identified in the future, current data indicate that the benefits to patients with the prudent use of diagnostic ultrasound outweigh the risks, if any, that may be present."[10]

THE OBSTETRIC ULTRASOUND EXAMINATION

With the increasing use of ultrasound in pregnancy, **standards and practice** guidelines have gradually emerged to ensure a **"minimum standard of care."** The American College of Obstetricians and Gynecologists (ACOG) describes three types of ultrasound examinations: the basic, limited, and comprehensive scans. The **basic** examination varies with gestational age but should include confirming the presence or absence of cardiac activity, the number of fetuses, an evaluation of the uterus and adnexae, placental location, amniotic fluid volume (AFv), estimate of fetal age, fetal presentation, and survey of fetal anatomy for "gross" malformations.[11] A **limited** examination may include the assessment of AFv, biophysical profile testing, amniocentesis, external cephalic version, confirmation of fetal viability, placental localization, and fetal presentation. The limited study is appropriate only in urgent clinical situations or when very specific information is required. The **comprehensive** examination is reserved for patients whose history, clinical evaluation, or basic ultrasound study puts them at increased risk of carrying an abnormal fetus. The comprehensive examination should be performed by a "more experienced operator," although ACOG does not specify the training qualifications.

The AIUM, on the other hand, does not differentiate between the basic, limited, and comprehensive examinations but rather defines the examinations according to the **gestational** age of the patient. Their guidelines for the **first trimester ultrasound examination** include confirmation of the location of the gestational sac, the presence or absence of fetal life, fetal number, and evaluation of the uterus and adnexae.[12] The **second** and **third trimester examinations** include these parameters as well as documentation of fetal presentation, AFv, location of the placenta, assessment of gestational age using biparietal diameter (BPD), femur length (FL), and abdominal circumference (AC), and fetal anatomy. The fetal anatomic assessment includes the evaluation of intracranial anatomy, heart, spine, abdomen (including kidneys, bladder, and stomach), and cord insertion. It specifies that evaluation of fetal anatomy is "not necessarily limited to these organ systems" and suspected defects "require further investigation with additional and more specialized study."

In 1993 the Society of Obstetricians and Gynaecologists of Canada (SOGC) **recommended** that all patients be offered a mid-trimester fetal ultrasound examination.[13] They suggested that **18 weeks is the ideal time** to perform the scan that should combine an evaluation of dates, biometry, number of fetuses, and assessment for fetal abnormalities, and gave specific recommended images and measurements (see first box on p. 963).

GUIDELINES FOR SCREENING MID-TRIMESTER OBSTETRIC SCAN

Key images
Fetal viability and number
Placenta and cervix
Umbilical cord
Amniotic fluid volume

Fetal anatomy
Intracranial anatomy (BPD, ventricles, transcerebellar diameter)
Fetal spine
Heart (4 chambers)
Stomach
Kidneys
Abdominal wall
Bladder
Limbs

Measurements
Biparietal diameter (BPD)
Head circumference (HC)
Transcerebellar diameters (TCD)
Ventricular plane (posterior horns ≤10mm)
Abdominal circumference (AC)
Femur length (FL)

Multiple pregnancy
Placental number
Comparison of size
Number of sacs
Genitalia
Presence/nature of separating membrane

Developed by the Society of Obstetricians and Gynaecologists of Canada (SOGC).

Level I Versus Level II Examination

The concept of the "level I" and "level II" ultrasound examination was initially introduced in the context of alpha-fetoprotein (AFP) screening where an initial scan only confirming dates or common causes for AFP elevations (twins, wrong dates, fetal demise) was performed as a "level I" scan (box, right column).[14] If the AFP levels in the amniotic fluid were truly elevated, the patient was referred to an "expert" sonographer for a more detailed study of fetal anatomy as a "level II" scan.[15] While these distinctions are no longer appropriate in the context of current standards of care as well as current technology and operator expertise, the terminology remains in widespread use. Now, the term **"level I scan,"** for example, in our own institution, is used synonymously with **"complete scan"** and indicates that a comprehensive examination of fetal and extra-fetal structures has been performed. If an abnormality is suspected or confirmed at the level I scan,

PREGNANCY CRITERIA CONSTITUTING "STANDARD" LEVEL I ULTRASOUND EXAMINATION

Assigning dates
Assessment of growth
Amniotic fluid volume
Single versus multiple pregnancy
Fetal heart motion
Fetal presentation at term
Placental position and texture
Review of fetal anatomy
Presence of adnexal masses or uterine myomas

the patient undergoes a **"level II scan."** The level II scan, also known as the **"specialized" or targeted imaging for fetal anomaly** (TIFFA) scan,[14] should be performed in a center with individuals experienced in the diagnosis and management of fetal abnormalities.

How and By Whom Should Obstetric Ultrasound Be Performed?

All obstetric ultrasound examinations should be carried out by individuals **trained and accredited in obstetric ultrasound.** These usually include registered ultrasound technologists, nurse technologists, obstetricians (usually maternal fetal medicine specialists) or radiologists. The AIUM has recently approved "training guidelines for physicians who evaluate and interpret diagnostic ultrasound examinations" in the hope of ensuring the consistent performance of quality ultrasound examinations and interpretation.[16]

The particular equipment used for obstetric ultrasound is determined by operator preference and the availability of hardware. In general, a 3.5- to 5-MHz transducer frequency should be used as these provide high resolution with adequate depth penetration in all but the most extremely obese patient. Some form of video or hard copy documentation is necessary to prove the examination was carried out in a systematic and competent manner and to allow for auditing of the examination should medicolegal concerns arise. Good visualization is essential if the operator is to avoid missing fetal structural abnormalities; however, the clarity of results may be compounded by factors such as maternal obesity, uterine abnormalities, fetal position, and amniotic fluid volume. These limitations should be recorded.

Indications for Obstetric Ultrasound

Existing evidence shows that the use of ultrasound in the presence of certain risk factors and clinical signs and symptoms contributes to improved maternal and fetal outcome (**"the selective or indicated scan"**). Indications for the selective scan as defined by the

SELECTIVE ULTRASOUND

The Consensus Development Conference, sponsored by the National Institute of Child Health and Human Development, has supported ultrasound examinations in the following clinical situations:

1. Estimation of gestational age for patients with uncertain clinical dates, or verification of dates for patients who are to undergo scheduled elective repeat cesarean delivery, indicated induction of labor, or other elective termination of pregnancy
2. Evaluation of fetal growth
3. Vaginal bleeding of undetermined etiology in pregnancy
4. Determination of fetal presentation
5. Suspected multiple gestation
6. Adjunct to amniocentesis
7. Significant uterine size/clinical date discrepancy
8. Pelvic mass
9. Suspected hydatidiform mole
10. Adjunct to cervical cerclage placement
11. Suspected ectopic pregnancy
12. Adjunct to special procedures such as fetoscopy, intrauterine transfusion, shunt placement, in vitro fertilization, embryo transfer, or chorionic villi sampling
13. Suspected fetal death
14. Suspected uterine abnormality
15. Intrauterine contraceptive device localization
16. Ovarian follicle development surveillance
17. Biophysical evaluation for fetal well-being
18. Observation of intrapartum events
19. Suspected polyhydramnios or oligohydramnios
20. Suspected abruptio placenta
21. Adjunct to external version from breech to vertex presentation
22. Estimation of fetal weight and/or presentation in premature rupture of membranes and/or vertex presentation
23. Abnormal serum alpha-fetoprotein value
24. Follow-up observation of identified fetal anomaly
25. Follow-up evaluation of placenta localization for identified placenta previa
26. History of previous congenital anomaly
27. Evaluation of fetal condition in late registrants for prenatal care
28. Serial evaluation of fetal growth in multiple gestation

From U.S. Dept. of Health and Human Services. *Diagnostic Ultrasound in Pregnancy*. NIH Publ. No. 84-667. Washington, DC: National Institutes of Health; 1984.

National Institute of Child Health and Human Development (NIH) in the United States are listed in the box in the left column.[17]

On the other hand, the value of routine ultrasound screening ("the routine or screening scan") in apparently normal pregnancies to identify those at high risk for unsuspected problems is controversial. At present, such screening scans at 16-20 weeks gestation are recommended as a standard of care in Canada,[18] Britain,[19] Finland,[20] and Norway.[21] In France[22] and Germany,[23] at least two scans are common: one in the second trimester (18 to 22 weeks) and another in the third trimester (31 to 33 weeks). In the United States, however, none of the professional associations, including ACOG, the NIH, and the AIUM, endorse routine ultrasound screening. This is mainly because they believe there is a lack of evidence that it benefits the low-risk fetus.

Evidence For and Against the "Routine Scan"

Between 1980 and 1984, four randomized clinical trials (RCTs) addressed the issue of routine ultrasound screening in pregnancy.[24-27] In all four trials, it was shown there was more accurate pregnancy dating and a higher rate of detection of twins in the ultrasound-screened groups, but an improvement in overall pregnancy outcome was not demonstrated (Table 31-1). The extent of the ultrasound examination performed in these trials was, however, often limited to a single measurement of BPD, which is not the standard of practice today.[31] Furthermore, advances in ultrasound technology make the results from these previous studies outdated.

More recently, five RCTs have addressed the sensitivity and specificity of routine ultrasound screening[28-30,32] (see Table 31-1). Secher et al. performed serial ultrasound screening on 2771 low-risk women; one scan was performed prior to 22 weeks gestation followed by two more scans in the third trimester.[28] There was a statistically significant increase in the rate of induction of labor in women found to have IUGR fetuses, along with a trend toward higher 1-minute Apgar scores and cord pH. However, there was no difference in gestational age at delivery, birth weight, incidence of operative delivery, or admission to the neonatal intensive care unit. Waldenstrom et al. obtained a single screening scan on 2482 women between 13 and 19 weeks gestation.[29] He reported a decrease in the number of labor inductions and IUGR infants and earlier detection of twin pregnancies; however, no effect on perinatal mortality was observed. Ewigman et al. also found no difference in poor perinatal outcomes in a group of women undergoing single-stage scanning (between 10 and 12 weeks gestation) compared with a control group having ultrasound examinations only as

TABLE 31-1
COMPARISON OF RANDOMIZED CLINICAL TRIALS

Author	No. of Inductions	Detection of Twins	Detection of SGA Infants	No. of SGA Infants	No. or Length of Antepartum Admissions	Perinatal Morbidity and/or Mortality
Bakketeig et al.[24]	↓(NS)	↑	↑+	↓ NS	↑	No difference
Eik-Nes et al.[25]	↓	↑+	↑	Unclear	↓	↓
Bennett et al.[26]	↑+	—	—	No difference	—	No difference
Neilson et al.[27]	No difference	—	↑	—	—	No difference
Secher et al.[28]	↑	—	↑	No difference	—	No difference
Waldenstrom et al.[29]	↓	↑+	—	↓	No difference	↓ (NS)
Ewigman et al.[30]	No difference	↑+	—	—	—	No difference
Saari-Kemppainen et al.[20]	No difference	↑	—	No difference	↓ (NS)	↓$^{+}$
RADIUS Trial[32]	No difference	↑	—	No difference	No difference	No difference

NS, Not significant; —, not addressed; +, statistical significance unclear; $^{+}$, not significant if elective terminations secondary to malformations are counted as deaths.
Modified from Garmel SH, D'Alton EM. Diagnostic ultrasound in pregnancy. *Semin Perinatal* 1994;18:117-132.

clinically indicated.[30] There was, however, earlier detection of twins in the routine ultrasound group. Saari-Kemppainen et al. screened 4691 women between 10 and 20 weeks gestation. His study, known as the "Helsinki Trial," reported no difference in birth weights when compared with controls; however, 58% of major malformations were detected.[20] This early detection of anomalies allowed parents the option of preparing for the delivery of a child with an abnormality or terminating the pregnancy. A significant decrease in perinatal mortality was reported in this study (from 9 per 1000 to 4.6 per 1000) due to the subsequent termination of fetuses with anomalies.

The "Routine Antenatal Diagnostic Imaging with Ultrasound" (RADIUS) trial, a multicentered randomized study of screening ultrasound, studied more than 15,000 low-risk women.[32] The study group underwent two screening ultrasound examinations at 15 to 22 weeks gestation and 31 to 35 weeks gestation. The control group underwent ultrasonography only for medical indications as identified by their physician (45% of patients in the control group had an ultrasound examination). Their findings were similar to those reported in other RCTs and included an increased rate of detection of congenital anomalies and a lower incidence of tocolysis in the scanned group. In addition, there was earlier diagnosis of multiple gestation and a lower rate of postdate pregnancy due to more accurate pregnancy dating. Unlike the Helsinki Trial, however, the investigators did not find a significant difference in adverse perinatal outcome (defined as fetal death, neonatal death, or neonatal morbidity) in the screened versus control groups. The most likely explanation for this was the limited sensitivity of routine sonography in the detection of congenital abnormalities in the RADIUS trial (16.6% before 24 weeks) coupled with a low rate of pregnancy termination once the diagnosis had been made.[32] Although they concluded, on this basis, that routine ultrasound screening offered "no significant benefits to low-risk pregnant women," we believe this low sensitivity does not truly represent the current diagnostic capability of ultrasound. In a recent review of 52,295 patients screened in six different European centers, for example, the overall sensitivity of ultrasound in the detection of abnormalities before 24 weeks gestation was 52.9% (range 20.8% to 84.3%).[33-39]

Bucher et al. recently reported a metaanalysis of four RCTs that included data on 15,935 women; 7992 allocated to routine sonography versus 7943 to selective scanning.[39] The detection rate of IUGR infants, multiple pregnancy, and severe malformations was higher in patients undergoing routine sonography than in the control groups. In addition, the **perinatal mortality rate** was significantly **lower** in patients allocated to **routine scanning.**[39] This effect was largely due to the contribution of the Helsinki Trial, which reported a 49.2% reduction in perinatal mortality in women undergoing routine sonography due to the improved early detection of fetal abnormalities that lead to induced abortions.[20] In both the RADIUS study and the metaanalysis by Bucher et al., however, routine sonography **did not reduce perinatal morbidity** as measured by an Apgar score of less than 7 at 1 minute and the rate of labor induction, nor did it appear to improve the "clinical management" of the pregnancy. One explanation for this finding is that the outcome parameter of perinatal morbidity and mortality is not necessarily a measure of the test being performed. This is particularly true in the RADIUS study, given the wide variation in ultrasound expertise and clinical management among the various participating centers. Basically, it is unreasonable to expect a **diagnostic** tool such as ultrasound to improve perinatal outcome unless effective management protocols are available and consistent changes incorporating these protocols are made based on the examination results. In addition, many of the benefits of ultrasound may be nonquantifiable. For example, prenatal adjustment to information about an anomaly has the potential to improve both the clinician's and the parent's approach to the pregnancy and birth as well as their abilities to make decisions about prenatal and/or postnatal treatment. This preparation will not appear in estimations of perinatal morbidity. In addition, for many women, routine ultrasound offers the benefit of reduced anxiety of giving birth to a malformed baby. Again the value of this in terms of perinatal outcome may not be quantifiable.

Finally, all of the trials described above are limited by their sample size and low statistical power. Although some are able to detect differences in more common outcomes such as the incidence of postdate (postterm) induction, larger trials are necessary to prove the statistical significance of infrequent outcomes such as perinatal mortality. In addition, the ability of these studies to detect any impact of ultrasound on pregnancy outcome is substantially diminished by the high frequency of indicated scans in the control groups, which ranged from 20% to 77%.

In summary, the results of these RCTs show that routine ultrasound scanning in the second trimester in the low-risk patient does not improve the outcome of pregnancy in terms of live birth rate and Apgar score. The studies do show, however, that the **perinatal mortality rate** is reduced because fetuses with severe malformations are aborted in the early stage of pregnancy rather than dying perinatally. The question remains, therefore, **is the detection of severe malformations through ultrasonography in itself sufficient reason to justify its general use?** Advocates for routine ultrasonography would argue yes and suggest there are

TABLE 31-2
ACCURACY OF ULTRASOUND IN DETECTION OF CONGENITAL MALFORMATIONS IN LOW-RISK POPULATIONS

Author	No. of Pts.	Years of Study	Sensitivity	Specificity
Lys et al.[37]	8,316	1986	14%	98%
Li et al.[38]	678	1980-1981	38%	98%
Levi et al.[40]	13,309	1986-1987	34%-55%	>99%
Rosendahl et al.[41]	9,012	1980-1988	58%	>99%
Shirley et al.[42]	6,183	1989-1990	67%	>99%
Chitty et al.[43]	8,432	1988-1989	74%	>99%
Luck[44]	8,523	1988-1991	85%	>99%
RADIUS Trial[32]	15,151	1987-1991	35%	—

From Garmel SH, D'Alton ME. Diagnostic ultrasound in pregnancy. *Semin Perinatol* 1994;18:117-132.

TABLE 31-3
ACCURACY OF ULTRASOUND IN DETECTION OF CONGENITAL MALFORMATIONS IN SELECTED POPULATIONS

Author	No. of Pts.	Years of Study	Sensitivity	Specificity
Hill et al.[45]	5,420	1979-1983	27%	—
Sollie et al.[46]	481	1980-1985	86%	100%
Sabbagha et al.[47]	596	1980-1983	95%	99%
Campbell et al.[48]	2,372	1978-1983	95%	>99%
Manchester et al.[49]	257	1983-1985	99%	91%

From Garmel SH, D'Alton ME. Diagnostic ultrasound in pregnancy. *Semin Perinatol* 1994;18:117-132.

many additional benefits that we are unable to quantitate by current means. Others would caution that the **substantial cost** involved in providing **quality ultrasound studies** to every pregnant woman would preclude their widespread use. All would argue, however, that the advantages of routine scanning must be weighed against the risks. While there are no apparent adverse biologic effects, the potential for these must always be kept in mind. In addition, there are the risks of **false-positive** and **false-negative** diagnoses. Fetal anomalies can be missed, and misleading information (e.g., false-positive diagnoses and findings with uncertain prognosis) is not uncommon.[32]

Accuracy in Diagnosing Fetal Malformations

The incidence of major congenital abnormalities at birth in the general population is approximately 2% to 3%, yet they are responsible for 20% to 25% of perinatal deaths and an even higher percentage of perinatal morbidity. Although some congenital abnormalities are specifically sought because of a known pattern of inheritance or because obstetric conditions leading to sonography are associated with underlying fetal malformations (e.g., amniotic fluid volume abnormalities), most occur sporadically in fetuses **without** known risk factors. For these reasons, routine ultrasound as a screening tool for congenital abnormalities is an attractive concept. Its sensitivity and specificity in the **low-risk** population are, however, variable, with sensitivities ranging from 14% to 85%, and specificities from 93% to over 99% (Table 31-2). This indicates that although ultrasound may be useful in ruling out abnormalities in the **low-risk** population, it is not particularly reliable in their detection. Although targeted studies performed on high-risk patients are significantly more accurate (Table 31-3), it is important to counsel patients that prenatal ultrasound may miss abnormalities. Reported **false-negative** diagnoses involve virtually all organ systems, but the majority affect the craniofacial, cardiac, and genitourinary structures. **False-positive** diagnoses are infrequent but worrisome as they may increase parental anxiety and lead to unnecessary invasive testing and obstetric intervention with its attendant risks.

Cost-Effectiveness of Routine Ultrasound Screening

The cost involved in providing quality ultrasound examinations (time, space, personnel, training, equipment) is the main argument against the widespread use of ultrasound. It has been estimated that with approximately 4 million deliveries in the United States per year, the cost of screening every woman, with a conservative estimate of $200 per scan, would be approximately $800 million. If the additional cost for multiple examinations is included, the health care cost would be over $1 billion.[32]

There is evidence, however, that the introduction of routine scanning actually results in an overall reduction in the number of scans per patient and potentially saves money. The National Institute of Hospital Research in Norway evaluated the extent of use of ultrasound prior to and following the introduction of one routine scan between 16 and 19 weeks gestation as part of routine prenatal care. Prior to the introduction of routine scanning, an average of 2.46 scans were done per pregnant woman in Norway; this decreased to 2.24 scans per patient 2 years afterward.[35] The institutions that practiced routine screening did an average of 2.1 examinations per pregnancy versus 2.75 for those that did not perform routine ultrasound.

There are two main reasons for this reduction in the number of scans following the introduction of routine scanning. One is the effect of **experience**. With more experience, the need for repeated scans is decreased. The other reason is related to the **time** in pregnancy when the first scan is performed. A scan performed between 16 and 19 weeks gestation will accurately date the pregnancy, confirm the number of fetuses, the location of the placenta, and the structural integrity of the fetus. If questions of growth deviation come up later, proper information can usually be obtained with one or two further scans. The questions of multiple gestation, fetal age, or placental location will usually never be raised because the answers are already known and, therefore, fewer scans for suspect abnormalities and suspect placenta previa will be done.

Supporting this potential cost-effectiveness of routine ultrasound is a recently published report based on the Helsinki ultrasound trial.[36] In this study, a trial population of 9310 pregnant women was randomly allocated to undergo routine ultrasound screening between 16 and 20 weeks of gestation or to a control group. All patients received similar antenatal care. When screened patients were compared with controls, a significant decrease in perinatal mortality and an increased rate of detection of fetal malformations occurred.

Although the health care system in Finland is different from that of the United States, De Vore et al. extrapolated in a subsequent editorial that by subtracting the cost of the ultrasound examination from the savings resulting from its use, a net savings of approximately $80 (United States) per patient could result. With 3.5 million annual births in the United States per year, this would result in savings of approximately $280 million because of fewer inpatient and outpatient visits and fewer unnecessary ultrasound scans.

De Vore et al. also compared the financial impact of ultrasound screening versus maternal serum screening (MSS). Based on the high rate of detection of congenital abnormalities before 24 weeks in the Helsinki Trial (over 50%), they found that screening ultrasound was as cost-effective as MSS because of the termination of abnormal pregnancies before viability and, secondly, better neonatal management of continuing pregnancies with abnormalities. Both of these factors were associated with an overall reduction in health care costs. Thus, while further evaluation is needed, it appears that the second trimester screening ultrasound may be cost-effective when all significant costs and benefits are taken into account.

First Trimester Ultrasound Screening for Fetal Anomalies

With the introduction of high-resolution ultrasound, in particular, transvaginal ultrasound, reports describing the prenatal diagnosis of congenital abnormalities in the **first trimester** are emerging. Anomalies of virtually every organ system have been described, including craniospinal (e.g., anencephaly, meningomyelocele), genitourinary tract (enlarged fetal bladder, multicystic dysplastic kidneys), abdominal wall defects (omphalocele, gastroschisis), and skeletal abnormalities (caudal regression syndrome, conjoined twins).[40-50] There are, however, obvious limitations when scanning for abnormalities in the first trimester because of the developmental stage of the fetus. It is important, for example, to know that at 10 to 11 weeks, herniation of the midgut into the umbilical cord is normal, and that omphalocele cannot be diagnosed until the crown rump length (CRL) is at least 43 mm (11.2 weeks gestation). However, if the liver is herniated with the midgut into the cord, this can be called an omphalocele even before 11 weeks because the liver does not normally migrate out of the abdominal cavity throughout development as does the bowel.[50] Thus, a good knowledge of basic embryology is essential when interpreting a first trimester sonogram.

In addition, the recognition that **first trimester nuchal abnormalities** have an association with fetal aneuploidy has created a new level of interest in first trimester sonography. The **nuchal translucency** (also called the **nuchal membrane**) refers to a collection of fluid in the cervical spine region of the fetus between 10 and 14 weeks gestation. Its role as a nonspecific marker for autosomal trisomies (21, 18, and 13), as well as Turner's syndrome and triploidy, is currently the subject of intense scrutiny to determine its usefulness as a **noninvasive screening tool** for chromosome disorders in the **first trimester.**

The first trimester ultrasound examination also allows for **accurate dating** of the pregnancy. This is important in screening for chromosomal defects because both the fetal nuchal thickness and the concentration of **maternal serum biochemical markers** change with gestational age. In fetuses with chromosomal defects, the median CRL is **not significantly different** from normal except for trisomy 18 where there is evidence of early-onset IUGR. A policy of routine pregnancy dating by measuring the CRL thus allows for more accurate interpretation of results from nuchal translucency and biochemical screening.

BIOCHEMICAL SCREENING

In recent years, the implementation of biochemical screening programs, including **maternal serum alpha-fetoprotein screening** (MSAFP) and, more recently, **multiple marker screening, including AFP, human chorionic gonadotropin** (hCG), and **estriol** (uE3), also known as the "triple test," has resulted in the increased detection of open neural tube defects (ONTDs) and Down's syndrome (DS) in developing fetuses.

Alpha-fetoprotein

Alpha-fetoprotein (AFP) is the major serum protein of early fetal life and is a marker for ONTDs and other open fetal defects when it is present in excessive amounts in the amniotic fluid. In recent years it has become possible to measure the tiny fraction of this substance that leaks into the maternal circulation, and it is now clear that high concentrations of AFP in the maternal serum also indicate an increased risk of ONTDS or other fetal defects (see box below). Although the specificity of this test may be low, the sensitivity approaches 100% when the AFP measurement is combined with a detailed ultrasound examination and the selective use of amniocentesis for the measurement of amniotic fluid AFP and acetylcholinesterase (ACHe).[51,52] As a result, **maternal serum AFP screening** between 15 and 22 weeks of gestation has become a **standard of care** in the United States and in many parts of the world.

Ultrasound evaluation in the presence of an abnormal result is the key aspect of all MSAFP screening programs. In the past, amniocentesis was recommended for all pregnancies in which the results of the ultrasound examination did not explain the elevated MSAFP; with better equipment and increasing operator expertise, the ultrasound sensitivity in the detection of NTDs now approaches 100%. Open NTDs are typically associated with abnormal intracranial anatomy, including ventriculomegaly, scalloped frontal bones (the "lemon" sign), and anterior curvature of the cerebellar hemispheres with obliteration of the cisterna magna (the "banana" sign).[52,53] Because of the sensitivity of these ultrasound markers in the detection of ONTDs, revised risks (based on the MSAFP value and normal ultrasound) have been published.[54-56]

At our institution amniocentesis is offered to women with an unexplained elevated maternal serum AFP but only after the revised risk estimate, based on a normal ultrasound examination, is discussed. Usually with a normal ultrasound examination, women decline the amniocentesis.

CAUSES OF ELEVATED MATERNAL SERUM ALPHA-FETOPROTEIN LEVELS

- Neural tube defects (NTDs)
- Ventral abdominal wall defects
- Gastrointestinal obstruction
- Cystic hygroma
- Congenital nephrosis
- Some chromosomal abnormalities
- Rh-sensitization
- Potter's syndrome
- Other minor abnormalities
- Fetal death
- Placental abnormalities (abruption, pilonidal sinus, hydrocele)

The Maternal Serum Marker Screen

Following the introduction of AFP screening for ONTDs, it became apparent that **very low levels of AFP were associated with an increased risk of fetal trisomy,** in particular Down's syndrome or trisomy 21.[56,57] Subsequently, **two additional markers** (human chorionic gonadotropin [hCG] and unconjugated estriol [uE3]) were also found to be **effective in screening for fetal DS.**[58,59] The levels of hCG tend to be higher (about two times the median value) and the uE3 levels lower (0.75 times the median) in DS fetuses compared with normal control subjects (Table 31-4). Following the discovery of these markers, it was confirmed that all three were independent predictors of DS, and they could be combined with maternal age to increase the effectiveness of antenatal screening for DS.[60]

With **maternal serum marker (MSS) screening, all pregnant women** are offered a blood test in the second trimester (15 to 22 weeks) and provided with an estimate of their fetus being affected with an ONTD, DS, or trisomy 18. The risk estimate is derived from the individual tests of the three markers, which are combined with maternal age-specific risks to produce a summary probability that the fetus has DS or trisomy 18. Women with a calculated probability exceeding a predetermined cut-off (i.e., usually 1:200 to 1:385 for fetal DS) are offered a fetal ultrasound ex-

TABLE 31-4
PATTERN OF BIOCHEMICAL MARKERS IN ONTDS, TRISOMY 21, AND TRISOMY 18

	Fetal Abnormality		
	ONTD*	**Trisomy 21 (DS)**	**Trisomy 18**
Alpha-fetoprotein (AFP)	↑	↓ (0.75×)	↓
Human chorionic gonadotropin (hCG)	—	↑ (2×)	↓
Unconjugated estriol (uE3)	—	↑ (0.75×)	↓

TABLE 31-5
PRENATAL SCREENING FOR DOWN'S SYNDROME: DETECTION RATE, FALSE-POSITIVE RATE FOR DIFFERENT SCREENING PARAMETERS

Screening Parameters Risk cutoff = 1:385	Down's Syndrome Detection Rate	False-Positive Rate (%)	No. Down's Syndrome Detected per No. Amniocenteses Performed
MA (≥35 years)	39.8	11.9	1:202
MA and MSAFP	49.8	12.2	1:166
MA and MSAFP, hCG, uE3 (triple test)	73.5	9.5	1:87

MA, Maternal age; *MSAFP*, maternal serum alpha-fetoprotein; *hCG*, human chorionic gonadotropin; *uE3*, unconjugated estriol.

From Summers A, Farrell S. Prenatal screening for and diagnosis of Down syndrome, Letter to the Editor. *J Can Med Assoc* 1996; in press.

amination to verify the gestational age of the pregnancy. If, on the basis of accurate dating, the risks still exceed the cut-off, the woman is offered genetic counseling and amniocentesis.

Table 31-5 describes the performance of these various screening parameters in the detection of trisomy 21. As can be seen, at a risk cut-off of 1:385, the detection rate is higher and false-positive rate lower when all three markers are combined with maternal age, meaning fewer amniocenteses need to be performed per case of fetal DS detected, compared with using maternal age alone or maternal age plus AFP.

Role of Ultrasound in MSS Screening

The concentration of the three markers is highly dependent on gestational age; therefore, an error in gestational dating can result in a large discrepancy in risk calculation. Haddow et al. showed in a large prospective study that the use of ultrasound to establish gestational age prior to maternal serum screening decreased the false-positive rate from 6.6% to 3.8%, leading to a major reduction in the need for amniocentesis.[60] Accurate dating using ultrasound also allows diagnostic tests to be undertaken more expeditiously and helps avoid missing the occasional case of fetal DS following reclassification of risk after follow-up ultrasound.

In the Province of Ontario, a dating ultrasound before screening is recommended. The results of the serum screen are then interpreted using the ultrasound measurements, including crown rump length (CRL) before 12 weeks and BPD after 12 weeks. If both ultrasound and clinical data are available (e.g., last menstrual period), the ultrasound data are used preferentially to interpret the screen. If ultrasound data are not available, the gestational age based on last menstrual period is used.

Use of MSS as a Screen for Other Chromosome Disorders

In trisomy 18, the maternal serum levels of **AFP, hCG, and uE3** are **all depressed.**[61] Using these markers, approximately 60% to 80% of cases of trisomy 18 can be detected with a false-positive rate of 0.4%. It is thus possible to add trisomy 18 screening to the DS and the ONTD protocol without significantly altering the false-positive rate.

Trisomy 13, 47,XXY, or 47,XYY are not detected more with multiple marker screening. Turner's syndrome (45,XO) detection is, however, enhanced from 8% based on maternal age alone to as high as 50% when the three markers are combined with maternal age.

MSS Screening in the First Trimester

The optimal time to perform MSS screening at present is **16 weeks** gestation. By the time the patient receives the results of the assay, undergoes counseling and/or amniocentesis, if indicated, and receives the results of a fetal karyotype, she is often approaching 20 weeks of gestation. For many couples, this prolonged waiting period is unacceptable. Thus there has been great impetus to develop markers that will be effective in screening for chromosome disorders in the **first trimester.** Recent data suggest that the concentrations of **free beta-human chorionic gonadotropin (free beta-hCG)** are **higher** and **pregnancy associated plasma protein-A** (PAPP-A) concentrations are **lower** in DS fetuses than in chromosomally normal pregnancies. Snijders et al. has reported that using a combination of maternal serum PAPP-A, free beta-hCG, and fetal nuchal translucency in the first trimester, they were able to identify approximately 90% of trisomy 21 fetuses at a 5% screen positive rate.[62] The sensitivities and specificities of these markers remain, however, to be determined in prospective trials.

Can Ultrasound Modify an Abnormal Screen Result?

A common clinical question is whether ultrasound can be used to modify a woman's risk for fetal DS as determined by her multiple marker screening test. For example, if a woman is determined to be "screen positive" (her calculated risk for DS is greater than the specified cut-off for offering amniocentesis), can a normal ultrasound examination alter her "biochemical risk"? In general, second trimester ultrasonography is not sensitive or specific enough to be used alone for DS. However, ultrasound assessment of **nuchal fold thickness, fetal biometry,** and other **subtle sonographic findings** may **complement** the maternal age and biochemical markers in the assignment of the DS risk. In a study by Bahado-Singh et al. of 1034 cases at risk for trisomy 18 or 21 on the basis of abnormal MSS results, normal ultrasonographic anatomy and biometry reduced the risk of a significant chromosome defect from 1:270 to 1:2,100.[63] Abnormal nuchal thickness and observed/expected humerus length of <0.92 were the most sensitive parameters for DS detection. While this study supports that **a normal ultrasound** scan significantly **reduces the risk** of a chromosome abnormality as determined by the patient's biochemical profile, a multicentered trial is necessary to determine whether this information can be used in a wider epidemiologic setting.

IMPACT

The diagnostic capability of ultrasonography has increased dramatically in recent years. The ability of ultrasound to determine gestational age, detect multiple gestations, and assess fetal well-being by diagnosing growth and fluid abnormalities in a safe, accurate, and noninvasive fashion has had a significant impact on the practice of obstetrics. In addition, the role of ultrasound in detecting fetal malformations, both major and minor, and subtle abnormalities associated with chromosomal and syndromic disorders, is increasingly being recognized. This, combined with the introduction of biochemical screening tests such as maternal serum screening, which are intimately dependent on ultrasound for their accuracy and interpretation, has led to even more widespread use of ultrasound. It can be expected this will continue to increase as newer techniques, such as nuchal translucency measurements, gain their way into clinical practice. Given all the options now available, it is incumbent on us to develop a rational and responsible approach to the use of ultrasound in pregnancy that will allow for maximum information to be obtained while minimizing exposure with its attendant potential risks.

In our center we support offering all low-risk patients a second trimester screening scan between 16 and 20 weeks gestation. For patients who choose biochemical screening (e.g., MSS) as well, we recommend a dating ultrasound prior to screening being performed. While nuchal translucency screening in combination with first trimester biochemical markers appears to be an attractive and exciting new option, we currently believe introduction to clinical practice must await further evaluation in prospective trials.

REFERENCES

1. Nicolaides K, Campbell S. Diagnosis of fetal abnormalities by ultrasound. In: Milunsky A, ed. *Genetic Disorders and the Fetus: Diagnosis, Prevention and Treatment.* 2nd ed. New York: Plenum Press; 1986;521-570.

Is Ultrasound Safe?

2. Kremkau WF. Biologic effects and possible hazards. *Clin Obstet Gynecol* 1983;10:395.
3. Graber P. Biologic actions of ultrasonic waves. In: Laurence JH, Tobias CA, eds. *Advances in Biology and Physics.* 1984; 3:191.
4. Stark CR, Orelans, M, Haverrkamp AD et al. Short and long term risk after exposure to diagnostic ultrasound *in utero. Obstet Gynecol* 1984;63:194-200.
5. Lyons EA, Dyke C, Toms M et al. *In utero* exposure to diagnostic ultrasound: a 6-year follow-up. *Radiology* 1988;166: 687-690.
6. Salvesen KA, Bakketeig LS, Eik-Nes SH et al. Routine ultrasonography *in utero* and school performance at age 8-9. *Lancet* 1992;339:85-89.
7. Salvesen KA, Vatten LJ, Eik-Nes SH et al. Routine ultrasonography *in utero* and subsequent handedness and neurological development, *Br Med J* 1993;307:159-164.
8. Newnham JP, Evans SF, Michael CA et al. Effects of frequent ultrasound during pregnancy: a randomised controlled trial. *Lancet* 1993;3421:887-891.
9. U.S. Dept. of Health and Human Services. Diagnostic ultrasound in pregnancy. Publ. no. 84-667. Bethesda, MD: 1984;161.

The Obstetric Ultrasound Examination

10. AIUM official statements. *AIUM Reporter* November 1993;6.
11. Ultrasonography in pregnancy. *ACOG Technical Bulletin* Publ. no. 187. Washington, DC: 1993.

12. AIUM. Guidelines for performance of the antepartum ultrasound examination. *J Ultrasound Med* 1991;10:576-578.
13. SOGC Policy Statement. No. 24, October 1993.
14. Sabbagha RG, Tamura RK. Some controversial issues. *Clin Diagn Ultrasound* 1987;20:319-325.
15. Haddow JE, Wald NJ, eds. Alpha-fetoprotein screening: the current issues, a report of the Third Scarborough Conference. Scarborough ME: The Foundation for Blood Research; 1981.
16. Training guidelines for physicians who evaluate and interpret diagnostic ultrasound examination. *AIUM Reporter* Rockville, MD; May 1993.
17. Diagnostic ultrasound imaging in pregnancy. Bethesda, MD: U.S. Dept. of Health and Human Services; Publ. no. 84-667; 1984.
18. Canadian Task Force Periodic Health Examination 1992 Update: 2. Routine prenatal ultrasound screening. *Can Med Assoc J* 1992;147:627-633.
19. Routine ultrasound examination in pregnancy. London: Royal College of Obstetricians and Gynaecologists; 1984.
20. Saari-Kemppainen A, Karjalainen O, Ylostalo P et al. Ultrasound screening and perinatal mortality: controlled trial of systematic one-stage screening in pregnancy. *Lancet* 1990;336: 387-339.
21. Neisheim B. Ultrasound in pregnancy. *J Technol Assess Health Care* 1987;32:463-470.
22. Blondel B, Ringa V, Breart G. The use of ultrasound examination intrapartum fetal heart rate monitoring and beta-mimetic drugs in France. *Br J Obstet Gynecol* 1989;96:44-51.
23. Hansman, M. Ultrasound screening in pregnancy: warning about overutilization. *Geburtshilfe Frauenheilk* 1981;41:725.
24. Bakketeig LS, Jacobsen G, Brodtkorb CJ et al. Randomized controlled trial of ultrasonographic screening in pregnancy. *Lancet* 1984;2:207-211.
25. Eik-Nes SH, Okland O, Aure JC et al. Ultrasound screening in pregnancy: A randomized controlled trial. *Lancet* 1984; 1:1347.
26. Bennett MJ, Little GH, Dewhurst J et al. Predictive value of ultrasound measurement in early pregnancy: a randomised controlled trial. *Br J Obstet Gynaecol* 1988;89:338-341.
27. Neilson JP, Munjana SP, Whitfield CR. Screening for small dates fetuses: a controlled trial. *Br Med J* 1984;289:1179-1182.
28. Secher NJ, Hansen PK, Lenstrup C et al. A randomized study of fetal abdominal diameter and fetal weight estimation for detection of light-for-gestation infants in low-risk pregnancies. *Br J Obstet Gynaecol* 1987;94:105-109.
29. Waldenstrom U, Nilsson S, Fall O et al. Effects of routine one-stage ultrasound screening in pregnancy: a randomized controlled trial. *Lancet* 1988;2:585-588.
30. Ewigman B, LeFebre M, Hesser J. A randomized trial of routine prenatal ultrasound. *Obstet Gynecol* 1990;76:189-194.
31. Wladimiroff JW, Laar J. Ultrasonic measurement of fetal body size. *Acta Obstet Gynecol Scand* 1980;59:177-179.
32. Ewigman BG, Crane JP, Frigoletto FD et al. and the RADIUS Study Group. Effect of prenatal ultrasound screening on perinatal outcome *N Engl J Med* 1993;329:821-827.
33. Saari-Kemppainen A, Karjalainen O, Ylostalo P et al. Ultrasound screening and perinatal mortality: controlled trial of systematic one-stage screening in pregnancy. The Helsinki Ultrasound Trial. *Lancet* 1990;336:387-91.
34. Eik-Nes SH. An overview of routine versus selective use of ultrasound. In: Chervenak F, Isaacson GC, Campbell S, eds. *Ultrasound in Obstetrics and Gynecology*. Boston: Little, Brown and Co; 1993:(2)229-238.
35. Leivo T, Tuominen R, Saari-Kemppainen A et al. Cost-effectiveness of one-stage ultrasound screening in pregnancy: a report from the Helskini ultrasound trial. *Ultrasound Obstet Gynecol* 1996;7:309-314.
36. DeVore GR. Opinion: financial implications of routine screening ultrasound. *Ultrasound Obstet Gynecol* 1996;7:307-308.
37. Lys F, DeWals P, Borlee-Grimee I et al. Evaluation of routine ultrasound examination for the prenatal diagnosis of malformation. *Eur J Obstet Gynecol Reprod Biol* 1989;30:101-109.
38. Li TM, Greenes RA, Weisburg M et al. Data assessing the usefulness of screening obstetrical ultrasonography for detecting fetal and placental abnormalities in uncomplicated pregnancy: effects of screening a low-risk population. *Med Decision Making* 1988;8:48-54.
39. Bucher HC, Schmidt, JG. Does routine ultrasound scanning improve outcome in pregnancy? Meta-analysis of various outcome measures. *Br Med J* 1993;307:13-17.
40. Levi S, Crouzet P, Schapps JP et al. Ultrasound screening for fetal malformations. *Lancet* 1989;1:678.
41. Rosendahl H, Kivinen S. Antenatal detection of congenital malformations by routine ultrasonography. *Obstet Gynecol* 1989;3:947-950.
42. Shirley IM, Bottomley F, Robinson VP. Routine radiographer screening for fetal abnormalities by ultrasound in an unselected low risk population. *Br J Radiol* 1992;65:564-569.
43. Chitty LS, Hunt GH, Moore J et al. Effectiveness of routine ultrasonography in detecting fetal structural abnormalities in a low risk population. *Br Med J* 1992;303:1165-1169.
44. Luck C. Value of routine ultrasound scanning at 19 weeks: a four year study of 8849 deliveries. *Br Med J* 1992;304:1474-1478.
45. Hill LM, Breckle R, Gehrking WC. Prenatal detection of congenital malformations by ultrasonography. *Am J Obstet Gynecol* 1985;151:44-50.
46. Sollie JE, Van Geijn HP, Arts NFT. Validity of a selective policy for ultrasound examination of fetal congenital anomalies. *Eur J Obstet Gynecol Reprod Biol* 1988;27:125-132.
47. Sabbagha RE, Sheikh Z, Tamura RK. Predictive value, sensitivity, and specificity of ultrasonic targeted imaging for fetal anomalies in gravid women at high risk for birth defects. *Am J Obstet Gynecol* 1985;152:822-827.
48. Campbell S, Pearce JM. The prenatal diagnosis of fetal structural anomalies by ultrasound. *Clin Obstet Gynaecol* 1983; 10:475-506.
49. Manchester DK, Pretorius DH, Avery C et al. Accuracy of ultrasound diagnoses in pregnancies complicated by suspected fetal anomalies. *Prenat Diagn* 1988;8:109-117.
50. Bronshtein M, Timor-Tritsch IE, Rottem S. Early detection of fetal anomalies. In: Timor-Tritsch IE, Rottem S, eds. *Transvaginal Sonography*. 2nd ed. New York: Elsevier Science Publishing Co; 1991;327-372.

Biochemical Screening

51. Macri JN, Weiss RR. Prenatal serum alpha-fetoprotein screening for neural tube defects. *Obstet Gynecol* 1982;59: 663-639.
52. Aitken DA, Morrison NM, Ferguson-Smith MA. Predictive values of amniotic acetycholinesterase analysis in the diagnosis of fetal abnormality in 3,700 pregnancies. *Prenat Diagn* 1984;4:329-340.
53. Nicolaides KH, Gabbe SG, Campbell S et al. Ultrasound screening for spina bifida: cranial and cerebellar signs. *Lancet* 1986;2:72-74.
54. Schell DL, Drugin A, Brindley BA et al. Combined ultrasonography and amniocentesis for pregnant women with elevated serum α-fetoprotein: revising the risk estimate. *J Reprod Med* 1990;35:543-546.

55. Nadel AS, Green JK, Holmes LB et al. Absence of need for amniocentesis in patients with elevated levels of maternal serum alpha-fetoprotein and normal ultrasonographic examinations. *N Engl J Med* 1990;323:557-561.
56. Richards DS, Seeds JW, Katz VL et al. Elevated maternal serum alpha-fetoprotein with normal ultrasound: is amniocentesis always appropriate? A review of 26,069 screened patients. *Obstet Gynecol* 1988;71:203-207.
57. Cuckle HS, Wald NJ, Lindenbasum RH. Maternal serum alpha-fetoprotein measurement: a screening test for Down syndrome. *Lancet* 1984;1:926-929.
58. Bogart MH, Pandian MR, Jones OW. Abnormal maternal serum chorionic gonadotropin levels in pregnancies with fetal chromosome abnormalities. *Prenat Diagn* 1987;7:623-30.
59. Canick JA, Knight GJ, Palomaki GE et al. Low second trimester maternal serum unconjugated estriol pregnancies with Down syndrome. *Br J Obstet Gynecol* 1988;95(4):330-333.
60. Haddow JE, Palomaki GE, Knight GJ et al. Prenatal screening for Down syndrome with the use of maternal serum markers. *N Engl J Med* 1992;327:588-593.
61. Canick JA, Palomaki GE, Osathanondh R. Prenatal screening for trisomy 18 in the second trimester. *Prenat Diagn* 1990; 10:546.
62. Snijders RJM, Nicolaides KH. *Ultrasound Markers for Fetal Chromosomal Defects.* New York: The Parthenon Publishing Group; 1996.
63. Bahado-Singh RO, Tan A, Deredn O et al. Risk of Down syndrome and any clinically significant chromosome defect in pregnancies with abnormal triple-screen and normal target ultrasonographic results. *Am J Obstet Gynecol* Oct 1996;824-829.

CHAPTER 32

The First Trimester

Edward A. Lyons, M.D., F.R.C.P.(C), F.A.C.R.
Clifford S. Levi, M.D., F.R.C.P.(C)
Sidney M. Dashefsky, M.D., F.R.C.P

CHAPTER OUTLINE

The first trimester of pregnancy is a period of rapid change that spans fertilization, formation of the blastocyst, implantation, gastrulation, neurulation, the embryonic period (weeks 6 to 10), and early fetal life.[1-5] First-trimester sonographic diagnosis traditionally has centered around evaluation of growth by serial examination to differentiate normal from abnormal gestations. This has changed radically since the advent of endovaginal sonography (EVS), which affords enhanced resolution over transvesical sonography (TVS) with resultant earlier visualization of the gestational sac and its contents,[6] earlier identification of embryonic cardiac activity,[7] and improved visualization of embryonic and fetal structures. As investigators have gained experience with high-resolution TVS and EVS, reliable indicators of early pregnancy failure have been identified, making serial examination necessary in a minority of patients, resulting in decreased morbidity and patient anxiety.

Despite these technologic improvements, it is important to set clinically relevant and realistic goals for first-trimester sonographic diagnosis. Most examinations are requested because the patient has presented with vaginal bleeding or pain or a palpable mass has been identified on physical examination. The referring physician usually requests the ultrasound examination to exclude early embryonic demise, an anembryonic gestation, or an ectopic pregnancy.

The **goals of first trimester sonography** include: visualization and localization of the gestational sac (intrauterine or ectopic pregnancy); early identification of embryonic demise and anembryonic gestation; identification of those embryos that are still alive but at increased risk for embryonic or fetal demise; determination of the number of embryos and the chorionicity and amnionicity in multifetal pregnancies; estimation of the duration or menstrual age of the pregnancy; and early diagnosis of fetal abnormalities, including identification of those embryos that are more likely to be abnormal, based on secondary criteria (abnormal yolk sac).

GOALS OF FIRST TRIMESTER SONOGRAPHY

Localization of the gestational sac
- Intrauterine or ectopic

Identification of:
- Embryonic demise
- Anembryonic gestation
- Embryos at increased risk for demise

Estimation of menstrual age of the pregnancy

Assessment of multifetal pregnancy
- Number of embryos
- Chorionicity and amnionicity

FORMATION OF THE EMBRYO

Herein, all dates are presented in menstrual age (in keeping with the radiologic and obstetric literature) rather than in embryologic age or gestational age as is used by embryologists (Table 32-1).[1-5,8,9]

Weeks 1 to 2

Early in the menstrual cycle, the pituitary secretes rising levels of follicle-stimulating hormone (FSH) and luteinizing hormone (LH), which cause the enlargement and differentiation of multiple primary ovarian follicles (Fig. 32-1).[1,8] When a fluid-filled cavity or antrum forms in the follicle, it is referred to as a secondary follicle. One follicle becomes dominant and continues to enlarge until ovulation, with the remainder of the follicles becoming atretic.[1,8] The developing follicles produce estrogen.[8] The estrogen level remains relatively low until 4 days before ovulation when the dominant or active follicle produces an estrogen surge. Following this surge, there is an LH and prostaglandin surge, resulting in ovulation.

Weeks 3 to 4

Ovulation occurs on approximately day 14 of the menstrual cycle with expulsion of the secondary oocyte from the surface of the ovary. After ovulation, the follicle collapses to form the **corpus luteum,** which secretes progesterone and, to a lesser degree, estrogen.[1,10] If a pregnancy does not occur, the corpus luteum involutes. In pregnancy, involution of the corpus luteum is prevented by human chorionic gonadotropin (hCG), which is produced by the outer layer of cells of the gestational sac (syncytiotrophoblast).[1]

Before ovulation, endometrial proliferation occurs in response to estrogen secretion. After ovulation, the endometrium becomes thickened, soft, and edematous under the influence of progesterone.[9] The glandular epithelium secretes a glycogen-rich fluid. If pregnancy occurs, continued production of progesterone results in more marked hypertrophic changes in the endometrial cells and glands to provide nourishment to the blastocyst. These hypertrophic changes are referred to as the **decidual reaction** and occur as a hormonal response regardless of the site of implantation, intrauterine or ectopic.

Fertilization occurs on or about day 14 as the mature ovum and sperm unite to form the **zygote** in the outer third of the fallopian tube (Fig. 32-1). Cellular division of the zygote occurs during transit through

TABLE 32-1
CHRONOLOGY OF EMBRYOLOGIC DEVELOPMENT

Menstrual Age	Embryologic Event
Day 14	Fertilization
Day 18	Morula (12–16 cell) enters uterus
Day 20	Blastocyst implants
Day 23	Implantation complete
Day 23	Primary yolk sac forms
Day 27–28	Secondary yolk sac forms (MSD = 3 mm)
Cardiovascular system	
Fifth week	Paired cardiac tubes form, begin pumping by week's end
Eighth week	Heart has definite form
Tenth week	Peripheral vascular system completed
Gut	
Sixth week	Primitive gut forms
8-12 weeks	Midgut herniation into base of umbilical cord
Eighth week	Rectum separates from urogenital sinus
Tenth week	Anal membrane perforates
Kidneys	
Eighth week	Primitive kidneys (metanephros) ascend from pelvis
Eleventh week	Kidneys in adult position
Genitalia	
Tenth week	External genitalia still sexless
Fourteenth week	External genitalia mature fetal form
Central nervous system	
Sixth week	Primary brain vesicles form
Ninth week	Third and lateral ventricles identified
Limbs	
Fifth week	Limb buds form
Ninth week	Upper limbs—bent at elbow Fingers are distinct

Seven to 10 weeks: embryologic period; 11 to 40 weeks: fetal period.

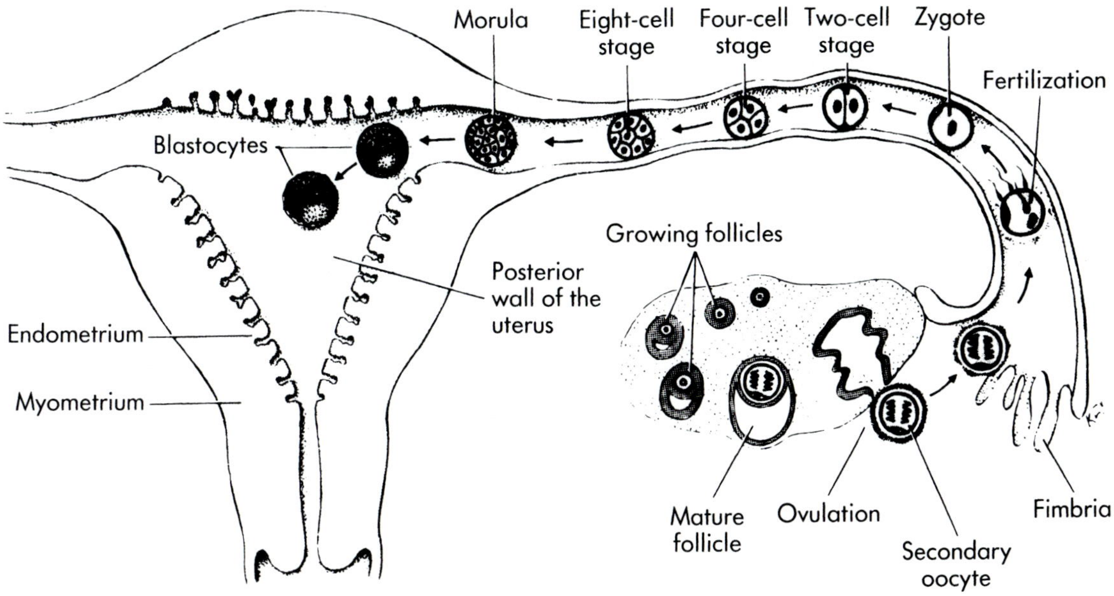

FIG. 32-1. Diagram of ovarian cycle, fertilization, and human development to the blastocyst stage. (From Moore KL, ed. *The Developing Human: Clinically Oriented Embryology*, 4th ed. Philadelphia: WB Saunders, 1988.)

the fallopian tube. By the time the conceptus enters the uterus (approximately day 18) it is at the 12- to 16-cell stage (**morula**).[1] By day 20, the conceptus has matured to the **blastocyst stage.** The blastocyst is a fluid-filled cyst lined with trophoblastic cells that contain a cluster of cells at one side called the **inner cell mass.** On day 20 the blastocyst at the site of the inner cell mass burrows through the endometrial membrane into the hyperplastic endometrium and implantation begins (Fig. 32-2, *A*).[1]

Implantation is completed by day 23 as the endometrial membrane reforms over the blastocyst (Fig. 32-2, *B*). The **primary (primitive) yolk sac** forms at approximately 23 days of menstrual age as the blastocyst cavity becomes lined by the exocelomic membrane and hypoblast (Fig. 32-2). As the extraembryonic celom forms (Fig. 32-3, *A*), the primary yolk sac is pinched off and extruded, resulting in the formation of the **secondary yolk sac** (Fig. 32-3, *B* and *C*). Standard embryology texts indicate that the secondary yolk sac actually forms at approximately 27 to 28 days of menstrual age, when the mean diameter of the gestational sac is approximately 3 mm. It is the secondary yolk sac, rather than the primary yolk sac, that is visible with ultrasound. Hereafter, the term **yolk sac** is used to refer to the secondary yolk sac. Later, because of differential growth, the yolk sac comes to lie between the amnion and chorion.[1] During week 4, there is rapid proliferation and differentiation of the syncytiotrophoblast, forming primary **chorionic villi** by the end of the fourth week.[1] Traditional thinking had the syncytiotrophoblastic cells invade the maternal endometrial vessels leaving maternal blood to bathe the trophoblastic ring. This has been challenged by Hustin et al.[10] who compared endovaginal imaging, hysteroscopy of the placenta, chorionic villous sampling tissue, and hysterectomy specimens with an early pregnancy *in situ*. They found that before 12 weeks, the intervillous space contained no blood, only clear fluid, and that on histological examination, the villous tissue is separated from the maternal circulation by a continuous layer of trophoblastic cells. Only after the third month does the trophoblastic shell become broken and the maternal circulation become continuous with the intervillous space. Further, at weeks 8 and 9 of gestation, the trophoblastic shell forms plugs within the spiral arteries allowing only filtered plasma to permeate the placenta.[11] It was also noted that in two thirds of abnormal pregnancies, the trophoblastic shell is thinner and fragmented and the trophoblastic invasion of the spiral arteries is reduced or absent.[12]

Week 5

During the fifth week, the embryo is converted by the process of **gastrulation** from a bilaminar disk to a trilaminar disk with the three primary germ-cell layers: ectoderm, mesoderm, and endoderm. During gastrulation, the primitive streak and notochord form. The primitive streak gives rise to the mesenchyme, which forms the connective tissue of the embryo and stromal components of all glands.

The formation of the neural plate and its closure to form the neural tube is referred to as the process of **neurulation.** This process begins in the fifth week in the thoracic region and extends caudally and cranially, resulting in complete closure by the end of the sixth week (day 42 of menstrual age). Failure of closure of the neural tube results in neural tube defects.

During the fifth week, two cardiac tubes (the primitive heart) develop from splanchnic mesodermal cells. By the end of the fifth week, these tubes begin to pump into a primitive paired vascular system. By the end of the fifth week, a vascular network develops in the chorionic villi that connects through the umbilical arteries and vein to the primitive embryonic vascular network.

Weeks 6 to 10

Essentially all internal and external structures are present in the adult form during the **embryonic period.** By the end of the sixth week, blood flow is unidirectional, and by the end of the eighth week, the heart attains its definitive form. The peripheral vascular system develops slightly later and is completed by the end of the tenth week. The primitive gut forms during week 6. The midgut herniates into the umbilical cord from week 8 through the end of week 12. The rectum separates from the urogenital sinus by the end of week 8, and the anal membrane perforates by the end of week 10. The metanephros, or primitive kidneys, ascend from the pelvis, starting at approximately week 8, but do not reach their adult position until week 11. Limbs are formed with separate fingers and toes. **Nearly all congenital malformations** except abnormalities of the genitalia **originate before or during the embryonic period**. External genitalia are still in a sexless state at the end of week 10 and do not reach mature fetal form until the end of week 14.

Week 11 and After

Early in the **fetal period,** body growth is rapid and head growth is relatively slower, with the crown-rump length doubling between weeks 11 and 14.

SONOGRAPHY OF NORMAL INTRAUTERINE GESTATION

Gestational Sac

Implantation usually occurs in the fundal region of the uterus between day 20 and day 23.[1] In a study

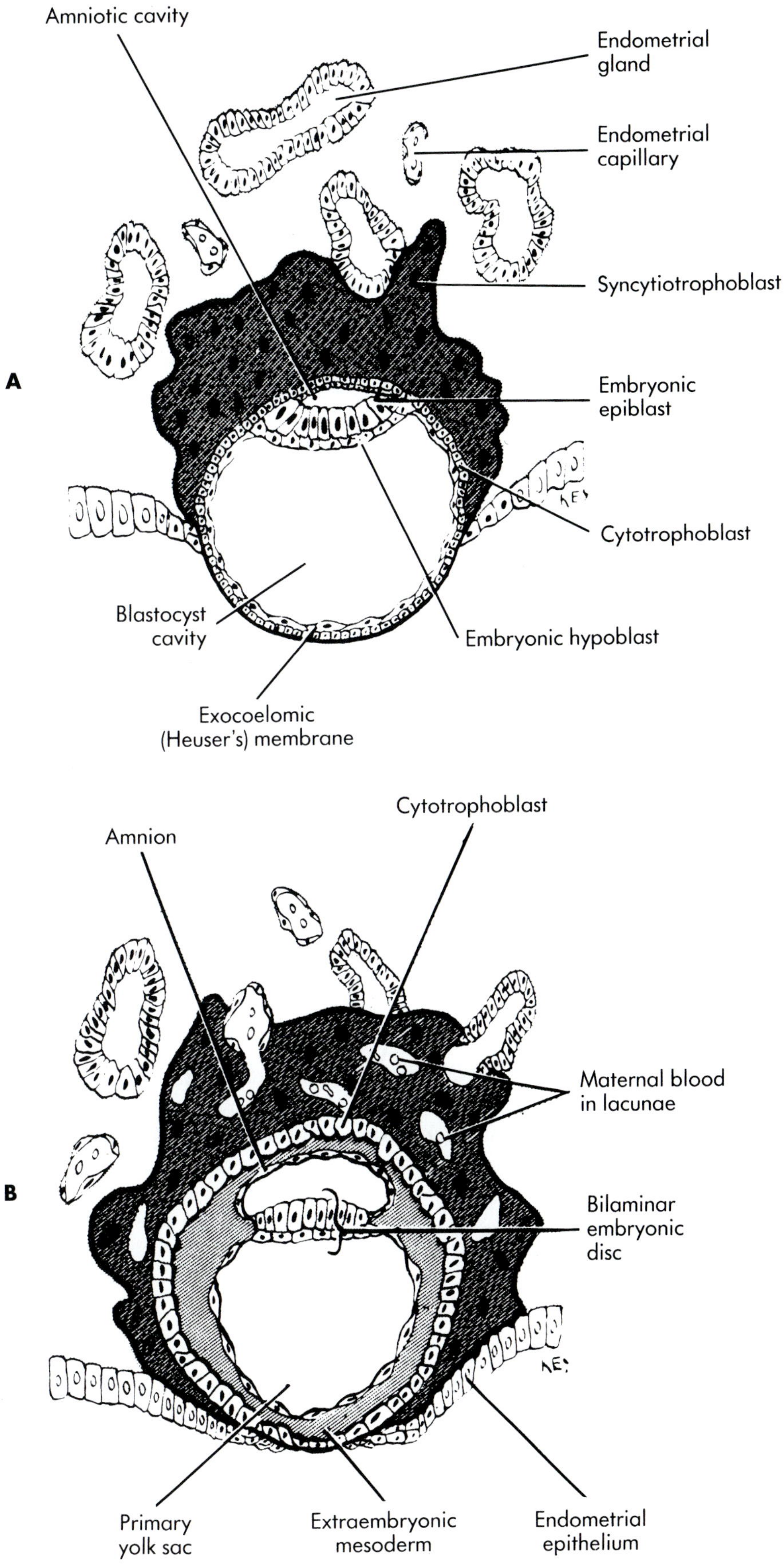

FIG. 32-2. Implantation of the blastocyst into endometrium. Entire conceptus is approximately 0.1 mm at this stage. **A**, Partially implanted blastocyst at approximately 22 days of menstrual age. **B**, Almost completely implanted blastocyst at approximately 23 days. (From Moore KL, ed. *The Developing Human: Clinically Oriented Embryology*, 4th ed. Philadelphia: WB Saunders, 1988.)

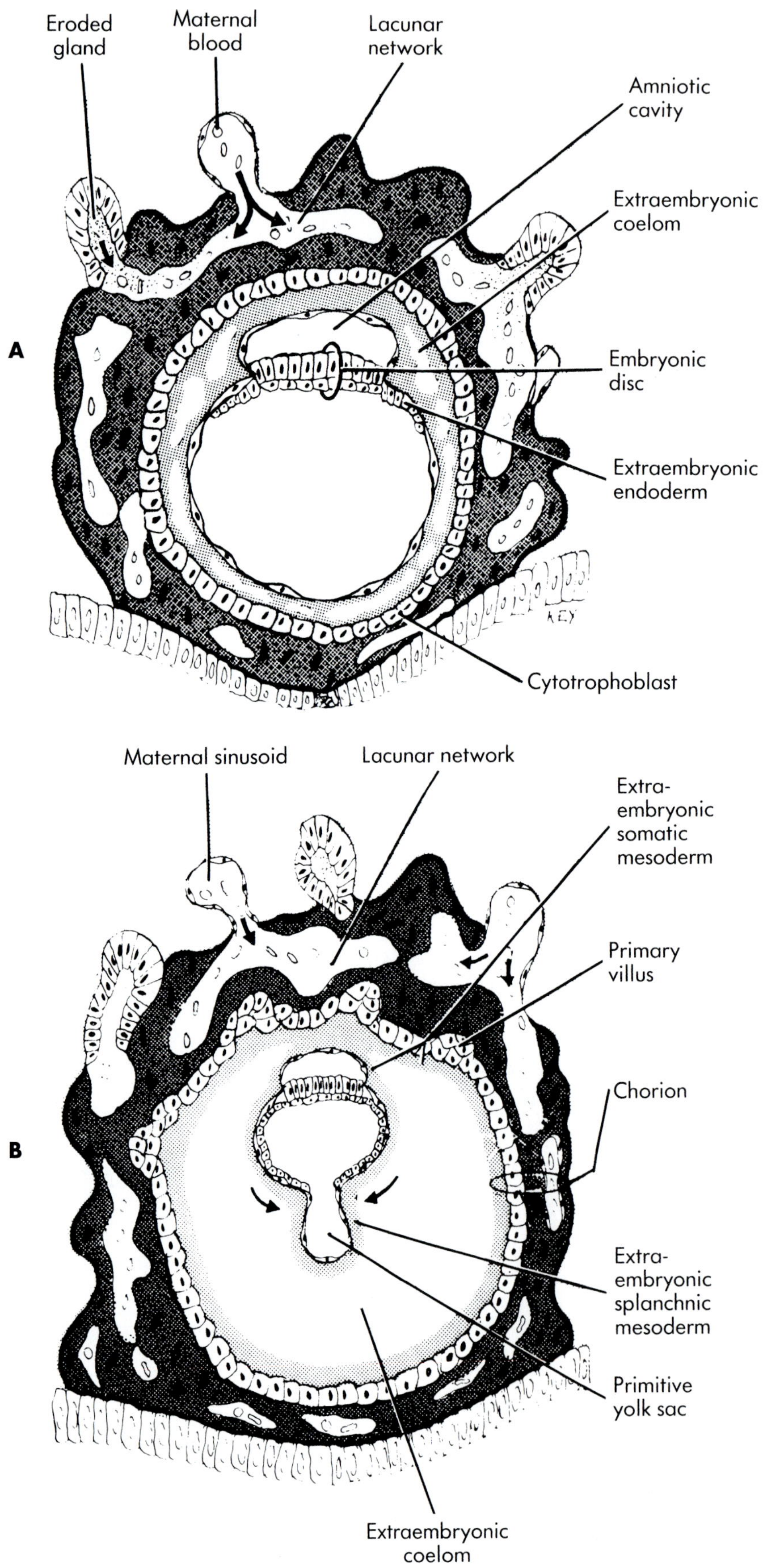

FIG. 32-3. Formation of secondary yolk sac. **A,** Approximately 26 days of menstrual age: formation of cavities within extraembryonic mesoderm. These cavities will enlarge to form extraembryonic celom. **B,** 27 days and **C,** 28 days of menstrual age: formation of secondary yolk sac with extrusion of primary yolk sac. Extraembryonic celom will become chorionic cavity. (From Moore KL, ed. *The Developing Human: Clinically Oriented Embryology*, 4th ed. Philadelphia: WB Saunders, 1988.)

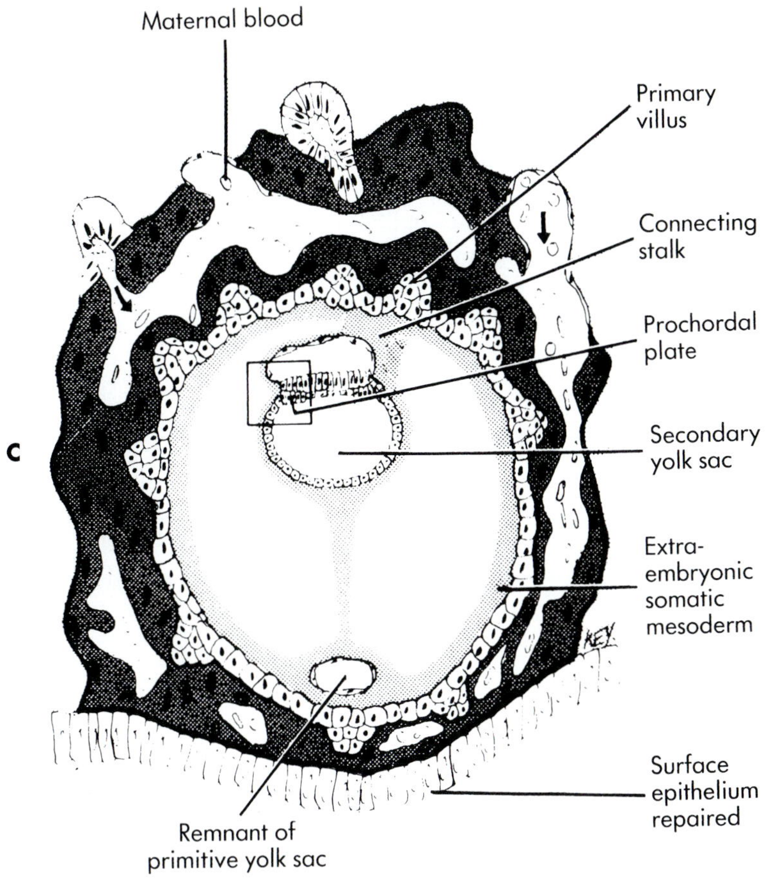

FIG. 32-3, cont'd. For legend see opposite page.

of early implantation sites in 21 patients, it was found that implantation occurs most frequently on the uterine wall ipsilateral to the ovulating ovary and least often on the contralateral wall.[13] At 23 days, the entire conceptus measures approximately 0.1 mm in diameter and cannot be imaged by transvesical or endovaginal techniques. Yeh et al.[14] reported the earliest consistent demonstration of intrauterine gestational sacs on transvesical sonography at approximately 3.5 weeks of menstrual age, at about the time that the serum β-hCG results are positive (Table 32-2).[14] They described a small gestational sac within the decidua and referred to this finding as the **intradecidual sign.** They also described focal echogenic thickening of the endometrium at the site of implantation within the decidua between 25 and 29 days of menstrual age (Fig. 32-4).[14]

In a study of pregnancies achieved through *in vivo* (intrauterine insemination by husband or donor) or *in vitro* fertilization (IVF), Pellicer et al.[15] found no difference in the timing, serum beta-hCG levels and endovaginal sonographic detection of implantation and early embryonic development of human embryos. An embryonic sac was detected 23 to 24 days (37 to 38 days or 5 weeks MA) after hCG administration in pregnancies achieved by assisted reproductive techniques.[15,16]

In a series of 60 patients whose ovulation was timed by ultrasonic follicle monitoring, Sengoku et al.[17] assessed sac appearance, size and levels of β-hCG. They identified a gestational sac less than 6 mm in 57.9% of cases at 4 weeks gestation. The mean number of cycle days was 34.1 ± 2.5. Fetal cardiac activity was detected as early as ± 43 days. Only 10 of the sacs were seen with a β-hCG of less than 1000 mIU/ml (FIRP) in five of six cases with levels of 1000 to 2000 mIU/ml and all patients with levels above 2000 mIU/ml.

As a general rule, it is possible to demonstrate an early intrauterine pregnancy as a small intradecidual sac between 4.5 to 5 weeks of menstrual age using EVS. Using most high-resolution scanners and the transvesical approach, it should be possible to identify a normal gestational sac at 5 weeks of menstrual age (Fig. 32-5, *A* and *B*).[18]

The mean level of β-hCG at the time of gestational sac appearance was 1771 mIU/ml (FIRP) for intrauterine insemination and 920 mIU/ml for IVF. Keith et al.[19] found that the β-hCG level **above which** a singleton sac was always seen with EVS was 1161 mIU/ml Third International Standard (TIS). This increased to 1556 in twins and 3372 in triplets in patients fertilized by gamete intrafallopian transfer (GIFT) or IVF. The level of hCG at the time fetal heart visualization in a singleton was 25,237 ± 8756 (1 SD) and occurred 31± 1.8 days after ovulation or 45 days' menstrual age.

The threshold values for sac diameter, serum hCG level, and gestational age below which the yolk sac was not visible were 3.7 mm, 1900 IU/L, and 36 days, respectively.[20]

When the serum β-hCG level is low, a normal intrauterine gestational sac may be too small to image either by TVS or EVS. Nyberg et al.[21] identified a β-hCG threshold level of 1800 mIU/ml (Second International Standard). Using TVS, they demonstrated gestational sacs in all of 36 patients with normal intrauterine pregnancies in whom the serum β-hCG was greater than 1800 mIU/ml.

In a subsequent article by Nyberg et al.,[22] endovaginal sonography correctly identified intrauterine gestational sacs in 20% of patients with β-hCG levels below 500 mIU/ml (Second International Standard), four of five with β-hCG levels between 500 and 1000 mIU/ml, and all 17 with β-hCG levels greater than 1000 mIU/ml.

The relation of maternal serum β-hCG to gestational sac size from a series of normal pregnancies is presented in Figure 32-6. A disproportionately low β-hCG is considered to be an indicator of a poor prognosis.[23] Although many of the earlier published studies from the 1970s use the SIS for serum β-hCG, the World Health Organization's First International Reference Preparation (FIRP) has been developed more recently and is in

TABLE 32-2
TIMING OF EVENTS IN EARLY PREGNANCY

Event	Timing	References
β-hCG first positive	23 days	
Intradecidual sac sign	25-29 days	
Double decidual sac sign	Only in 50% of early pregnancies	24, 27
Gestational sac seen	Earliest 34 days, usually 37-38 days	14, 15
Yolk sac seen	Earliest 36 days, usually 42 days	16
Embryo	Earliest 43 days, usually 45 days	
Embryonic cardiac activity	Earliest 43 days, usually 45 days	18
	CRL > 5 mm	
	β-hCG is above 25,237 ± 8756 (1SD)	18

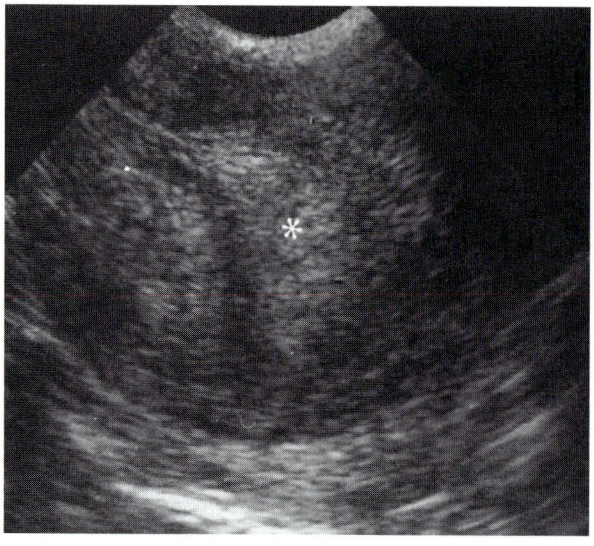

FIG. 32-4. Implantation site seen as focal thickening of posterior fundal endometrium (asterisk). Endovaginal sonography: sagittal plane at 4 weeks of menstrual age.

common usage. The preparations differ by a factor of approximately 2, however, this ratio varies from lab to lab. To convert from the SIS to the FIRP, the following simple formula can be used:

$$\frac{\beta\text{-hCG (1st IRP)}}{\beta\text{-hCG (2nd IS)}} = 2$$

The FIRP is now synonymous with the newly developed TIS, which uses the same units and values as the SIS and therefore requires no conversion factor.

The **double-decidual sign** was described previously by Nyberg et al.[24] as a method of differentiation between an early intrauterine pregnancy and the decidual cast of an ectopic pregnancy. The double-decidual sign was based on sonographic visualization of the three layers of decidua in early pregnancy (Fig. 32-7).[25] A ring formed by the chorion frondosum and decidua basalis at the site of implantation and the chorion laeve and decidua capsularis is surrounded, except at the chorion frondosum and decidua basalis

A

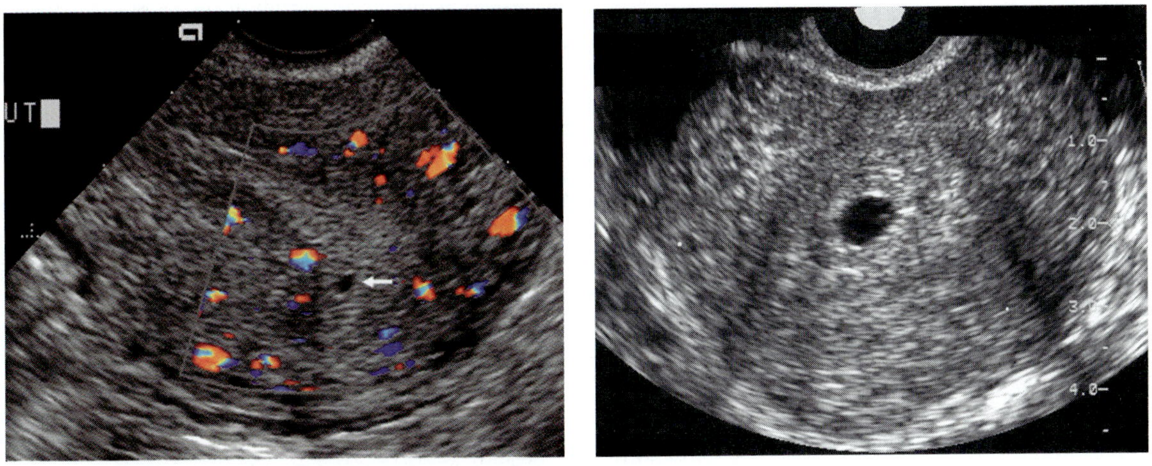

B

FIG. 32-5. Intradecidual gestational sac. **A,** Endovaginal sonography at 33 days (4 weeks and 5 days) of menstrual age shows sac (*arrow*). **B,** Follow-up 6 days later shows normal sac growth with a small yolk sac.

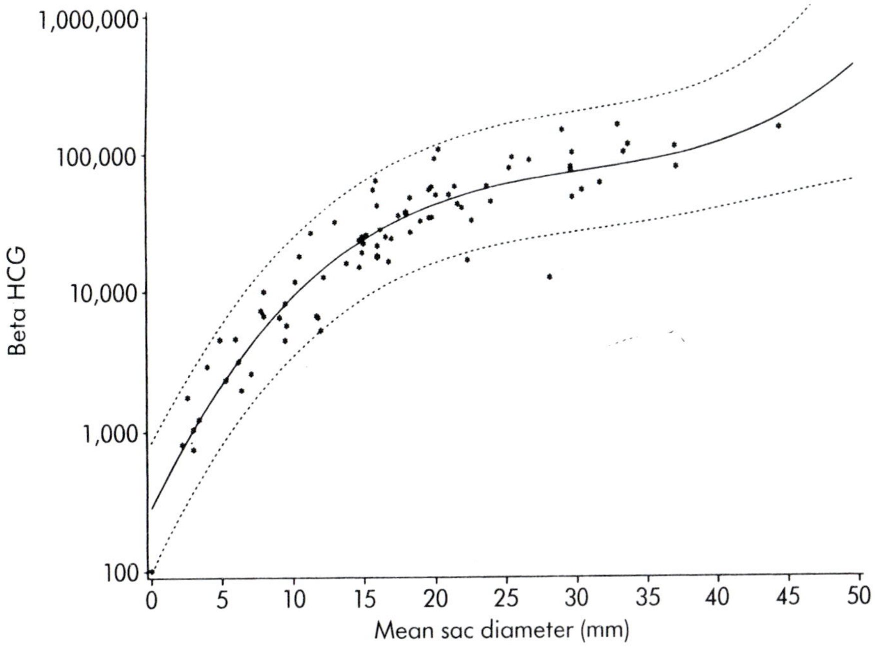

FIG. 32-6. Mean gestational sac diameter (mm) relation to maternal serum β-hCG (IU/L, First International Reference Preparation). Solid line indicates mean; dotted lines, 5% and 95% confidence limits.

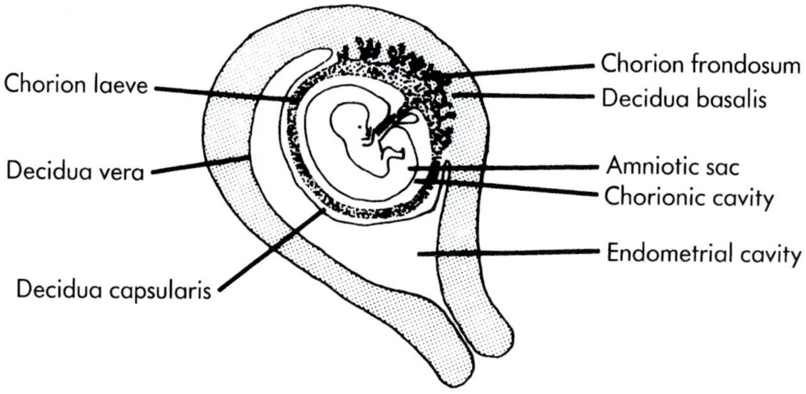

FIG. 32-7. Double-decidual sign. Diagram of anatomic basis showing three layers of decidual and endometrial cavity. (From Lyons EA, Levi CS: The first trimester. *Radiol Clin North Am* 1982;20:259.)

complex, by the echogenic decidua vera (Fig. 32-8). This finding was originally described as specific for an early intrauterine pregnancy. In the study by Yeh et al.,[14] the double-decidual sign was seen clearly in 30.6%, vaguely in 33.3%, and not at all in 36.1% of intrauterine pregnancies studied between 3.5 and 7 weeks of menstrual age. Yeh et al.[14] identified a double-decidual sign in two of five ectopic pregnancies, casting doubt on the usefulness of this sign. In our experience, a clear double-decidual sign is of use in predicting the presence of an intrauterine pregnancy. A vague or absent double-decidual sign is considered nondiagnostic. Parvey et al.[26] found a double-decidual sac in only 53% of early pregnancies with no yolk sac or embryo present. They also assessed visualization of the echogenic chorionic rim alone as a sign of an intrauterine gestation and found it present in 64% of cases. It was more clearly defined in later pregnancies with a higher β-hCG (mean 16,082 ± 16,972) and thin, less clearly defined or even absent in the earliest pregnancies. The "pseudogestational sac" of ectopic pregnancy may occasionally appear as a double-decidual sac or chorionic rim sign, but with further scanning, it should be possible to differentiate the two.

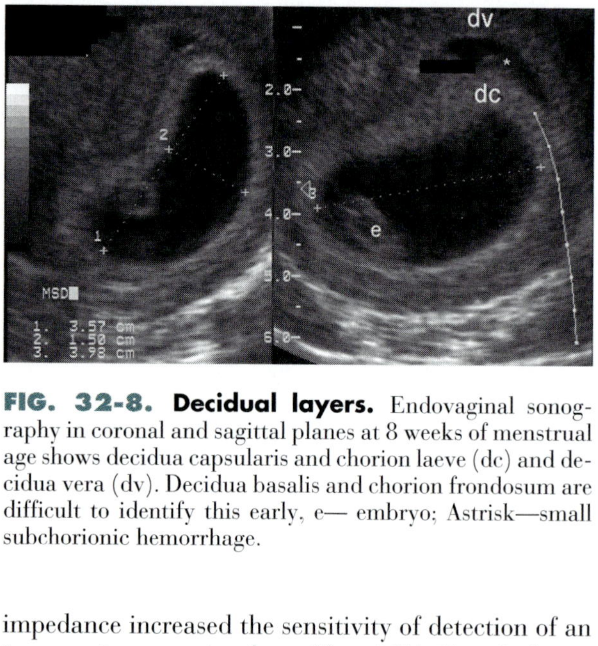

FIG. 32-8. Decidual layers. Endovaginal sonography in coronal and sagittal planes at 8 weeks of menstrual age shows decidua capsularis and chorion laeve (dc) and decidua vera (dv). Decidua basalis and chorion frondosum are difficult to identify this early, e— embryo; Astrisk—small subchorionic hemorrhage.

The extracoelomic or **chorionic sac fluid** is normally weakly reflective and more echogenic than the amniotic fluid. If the system gain is increased, one normally sees low level echoes within the chorionic fluid and not usually within the amniotic fluid.[27]

Endovaginal color-flow Doppler (EVCFD) may be helpful in identifying the presence of an early intrauterine gestational sac. It also has been proven helpful in distinguishing a normal from a failed intrauterine gestation and in the detection of an ectopic pregnancy through the exclusion of an intrauterine gestation.[28] Emerson et al.[28] has found that the detection of peritrophoblast flow of high velocity and low impedance increased the sensitivity of detection of an intrauterine gestation from 90 to 99%. Even before a sac is seen flows of 8 to 30 cm/sec were found in the endometrium at the implantation site. Parvey et al.[26] found that 15% of their intrauterine pregnancies without the presence of a sac had high-velocity, low-impedance intradecidual arterial-type flow. A specificity and positive predictive value of 95% could be achieved in diagnosing an intrauterine gestation by using a peak systolic intradecidual flow velocity of 15 cm/sec or more and a resistive index of less than or equal to 0.55.

The use of EVCFD to assess early pregnancies is not widely used. Recent work on first-trimester intervillous circulation by Jauniaux[11] hypothesizes that the gestational sac and lacunae are isolated from the maternal circulation by a layer of trophoblastic cells which line the lacunae and plug the spiral arteries. In

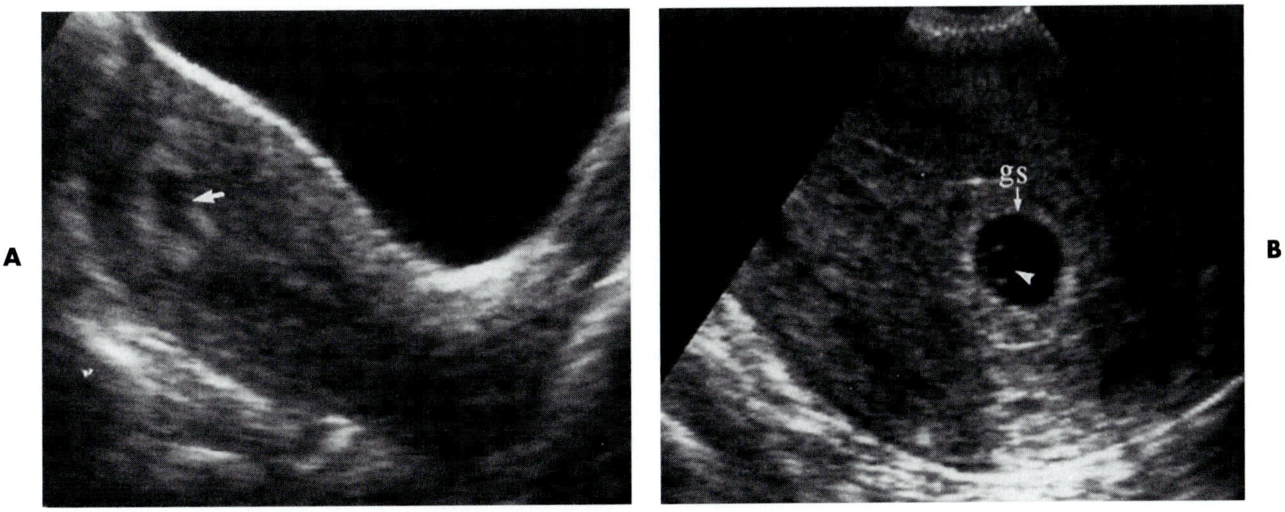

FIG. 32-9. Normal early gestation. **A,** Transvesical sonography in sagittal plane at 5 weeks of menstrual age shows saclike structure (*arrow*) in endometrial canal. **B,** Endovaginal sonography of same patient shows gestational sac (gs) and clearly identifiable yolk sac (*arrowhead*).

fact, if there is a breech of the barrier, maternal blood floods the intervillous spaces and this may be the final event prior to spontaneous abortion. This is especially true up until weeks nine to ten when the definitive placenta is formed. This is also the time after which the rate of spontaneous abortion drops to its steady state of approximately 2%.[11]

Yolk Sac

The yolk sac is the **first structure** to be seen normally within the gestational sac. Using TVS, it is often seen when the mean gestational sac diameter (MSD) is approximately 10 to 15 mm[18] and should always be visualized by an MSD of 20 mm.[29] Endovaginal techniques allow earlier visualization of the yolk sac (Fig. 32-9), which should always be visualized by an MSD of 8 mm.[6]

The demonstration of a yolk sac may be critical in differentiating an early intrauterine gestational sac from a decidual cast.[30] Although the double-decidual sign is not 100% specific for the presence of an intrauterine pregnancy, the identification of a yolk sac within the early gestational sac is diagnostic of an intrauterine pregnancy (Fig. 32-10).

The yolk sac plays an important role in human embryonic development. While the placental circulation is developing, the yolk sac has a role in **transfer of nutrients** to the developing embryo in the third and fourth weeks. **Hematopoiesis** occurs in the wall of the yolk sac in the fifth week before a takeover of hematopoiesis by the liver in the eighth week. The dorsal part of the yolk sac is incorporated into the embryo as **primitive gut** in the sixth week. The yolk sac remains connected to the midgut by a stock called the vitelline duct. Not infrequently, the vitelline duct can be demonstrated sonographically (Fig. 32-11).

Lindsay et al.[31] reported that the yolk sac **grows** at a rate of approximately 0.1 mm per millimeter of growth of the MSD when the MSD is less than 15 mm, and then it slows to 0.03 mm per millimeter of growth of the MSD. The upper limit of normal for **yolk sac diameter** between 5 and 10 weeks of menstrual age is 5.6 mm.

The **number** of yolk sacs present can be helpful in determining amnionicity of the pregnancy. In general, if the embryos are alive, the number of yolk sacs and the number of amniotic sacs are the same. In a monochorionic monoamniotic (MCMA) twin gestation, there will be two embryos, one chorionic sac, one amniotic sac, and one yolk sac. Levi et al.[32] looked at four MCMA pregnancies, all of which had a single yolk sac. One was a conjoined and one a twin ectopic which were both terminated. The other two delivered normally at 34 weeks. Of the four cases, two had a larger than normal yolk sac ($>$ 5.6 mm), and in two the yolk sacs were normal. Therefore, a single, large- or normal-sized yolk sac with two live embryos can result in a normal twin delivery. All embryos in the four cases had cardiac activity. It is not uncommon to see a dead embryo with no yolk sac. This is probably a normal sequela of embryonic demise with reabsorption of the amnion, then the yolk sac, and lastly the embryo itself. This is largely anecdotal as no published reports of the exact order of reabsorption have been found.

Visualization of the vitelline arteries and/or veins is possible on the vitelline duct and should be possible

A 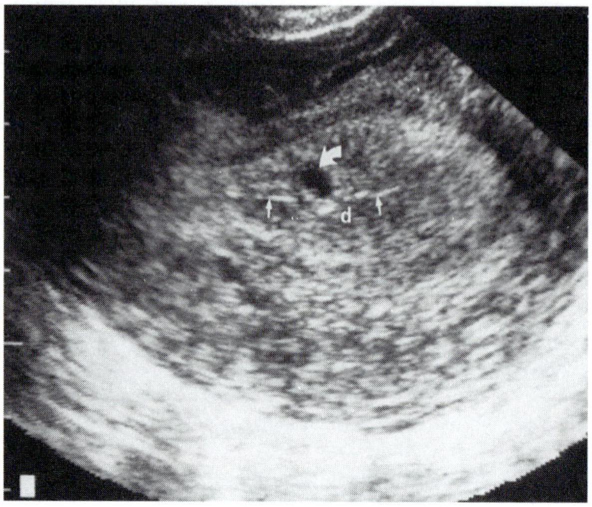

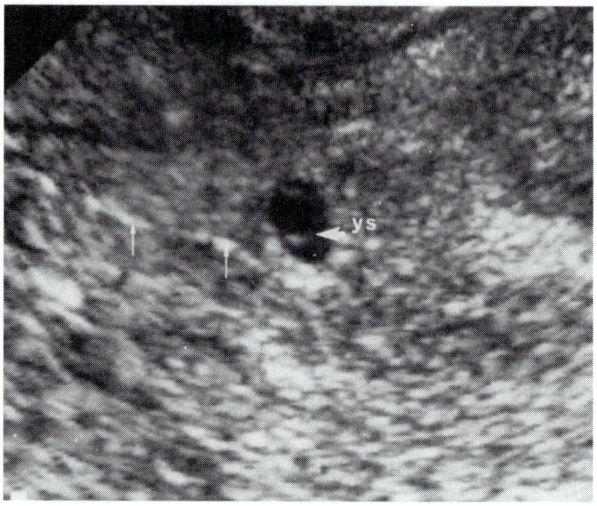 B

FIG. 32-10. Normal early gestation. **A,** Endovaginal sonography in sagittal plane at 5 weeks and 2 days gestation shows small sac (*curved arrow*) within decidua (d). **B,** Magnified image shows yolk sac (ys) within the gestational sac. Small arrows indicate endometrial canal. (From Levi CS, Lyons EA, Lindsay DJ: Ultrasound in the first trimester of pregnancy. *Radiol Clin North Am* 1990;28:19-38.)

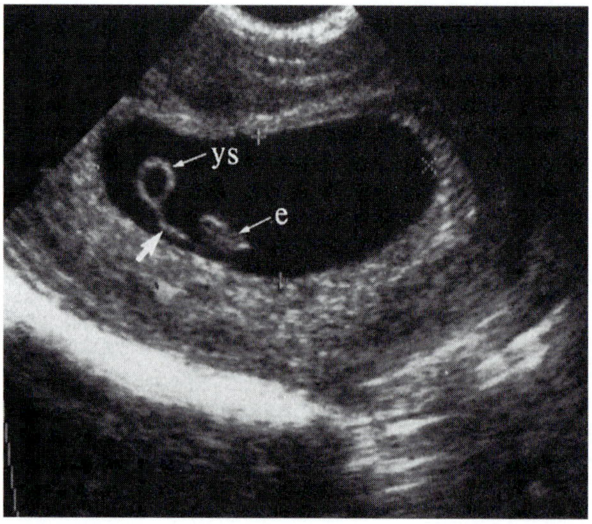

FIG. 32-11. Normal embryo at 8 weeks of menstrual age. Endovaginal sonography shows vitelline duct (*arrow*), yolk sac (ys), and embryo (e).

on the periphery of the yolk sac itself. With the 7 to 8 weeks MA sac magnified, one can see irregularities in the wall which correspond to the arteries (Fig. 32-12). Using power mode of color Doppler which is the most sensitive, one can see flow in these vessels. The flow must be confirmed with spectral Doppler, because it is equally as simple to create a false color image on power Doppler by virtue of the fact that the yolk sac is a strong specular reflector. This usually gives rise to color around the entirety of the sac rather than just at discrete locations of the vessels. Kurjak et al.[33] have described the patterns of color flow of the yolk sac vessels and have shown an overall visualization rate of 72.3% with the highest rate in the seventh and eighth weeks MA. The typical waveform was one of low velocity (5.8 ± 1.7 cm/sec) with no diastolic flow. A pulsatility index showed a mean value of 3.24 ± 0.94.[33]

Embryo and Amnion

Yeh and Rabinowitz[34] have described the **double-bleb sign** as the earliest demonstration of the amnion. The two blebs represent the amnion and yolk sac and can be identified by TVS as early as 5.5 weeks when the crown-rump length (CRL) is 2 mm. At that point, the embryonic disk is situated between the yolk sac and amnion.[3,34] It should be noted, however, that although visualization of the tiny, less than 2-mm bleb of amnion may occur before visualization of the embryo, this is a transient phenomenon. Visualization of the amnion in the absence of an embryo usually occurs in intrauterine embryonic death with resorption of the embryo (Fig. 32-13).

Amniotic fluid is a colorless, fetal dermal transudate initially and then, as the skin cornifies and the kidneys begin to function at approximately 11 weeks, it becomes pale yellow.[27] The amnion becomes barely visible when the embryo has a CRL of 2 mm at 6 weeks. The cavity becomes almost spherical by approximately 7 weeks likely caused by the more rapid increase in fluid volume relative to the growth of the sac membrane to accommodate it. The actual rate of fluid increase is more rapid after approximately 9 weeks, when fetal urine is produced. It is estimated

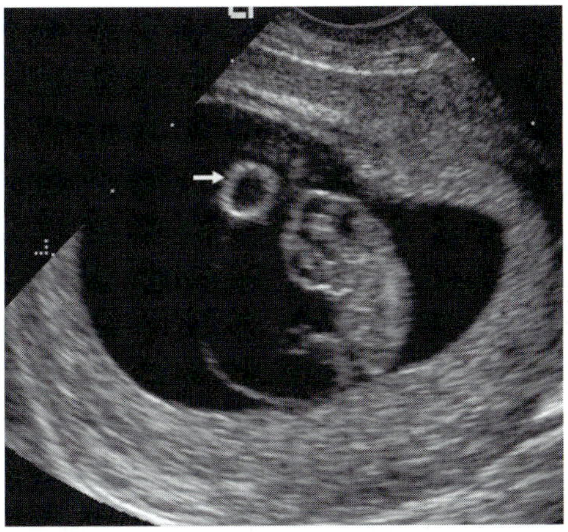

FIG. 32-12. Normal yolk sac in a 9-week gestation. Note the irregularities of the yolk sac wall (*arrow*) which represent the small vitelline arteries.

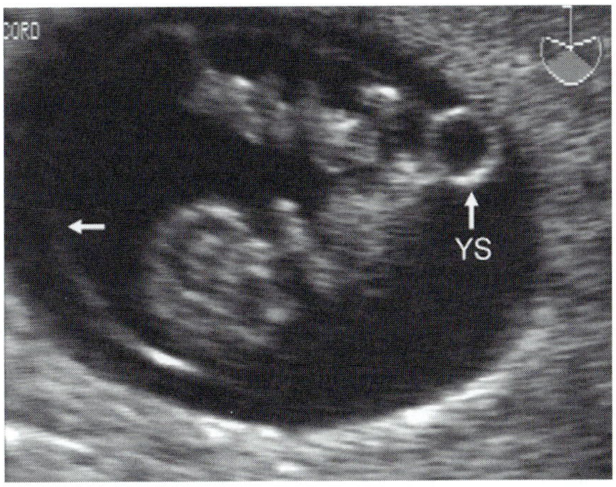

FIG. 32-14. Normal separation of amnion (*arrow*) and chorionic sacs at 10 weeks of menstrual age. Endovaginal sonography shows the yolk sac (YS) and embryo.

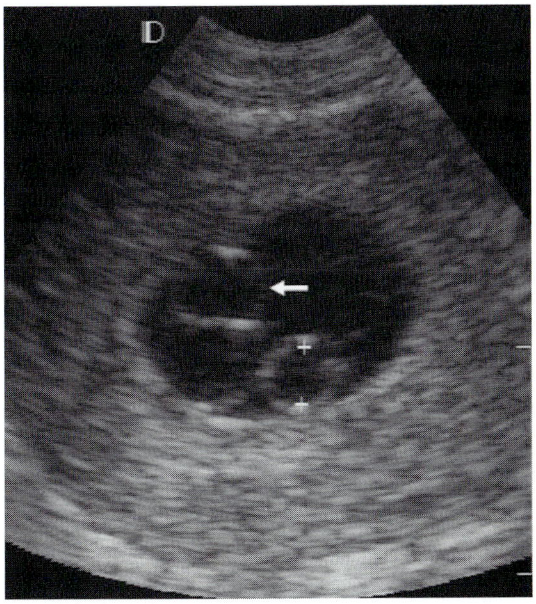

FIG. 32-13. Twins (MCMA) with one intrauterine embryonic death and one alive. Endovaginal sonography at 10 weeks of menstrual age. On the left, the arrow is pointing to one of two adjacent sacs, one is the amnion and the other the yolk sac. To the right is a single yolk sac (calipers) with the live embryo not in the scan plane. Both pregnancies went on to abort.

that fluid accumulates at about 5 cc per day at 12 weeks MA. The amniotic cavity expands to fill the chorionic cavity completely by week 14 to 16. It is normal to identify the amnion as a separate membrane or sac within the chorionic cavity before 14 to 16 weeks of menstrual age (Fig. 32-14).[35] Occasionally, the amnion and chorionic membranes may fail to fuse at week 16, and separation of these membranes may persist for a short time.[36]

Iatrogenic or spontaneous rupture of the amniotic membrane is a rare occurrence and even more rarely results in the **amniotic band syndrome.** This rupture may result in retraction of the amnion in part or in whole, up to the base of the umbilical cord where the two membranes are adherent. More often, the floating amniotic membranes **do not** adhere to the fetus and no fetal anomalies occur. Zimmer[37] studied 30 cases and Wehbeh[38] 25 cases at the end of the first trimester, and there were no fetal anomalies seen in any at birth. In the amniotic band syndrome, portions of the embryo may extend into the space between the amniotic band and the chorion. The embryo may become adherent to or swallow parts of the band, giving rise to a wide variety of anomalies that range from digital amputation to the limb body wall complex and that are collectively known as the amniotic band syndrome. This form of chorioamnionic separation can be differentiated from simple developmental chorioamnionic separation because normally the fetus is completely contained by the amniotic sac but is not adherent to it.[39]

Using EVS, an embryo with a CRL of as small as 1 to 2 mm may be identified immediately adjacent to the yolk sac (Fig. 32-15). **Embryonic cardiac activity** can be identified routinely by EVS when the **CRL is greater than 5 mm.** EVS can often demonstrate cardiac activity in embryos with a CRL of 2 to 4 mm. Cadkin and McAlpin[40] described cardiac activity using TVS adjacent to the yolk sac before visualization of the embryo at the end of the fifth week. Ragavendra[41] used a 12.5-MHz endoluminal catheter transducer placed into the endometrial canal adjacent to the gestational sac. He identified cardiac activity in an embryo with a CRL of 1.5 mm and resolved the two walls of the heart, seen only as a tube.

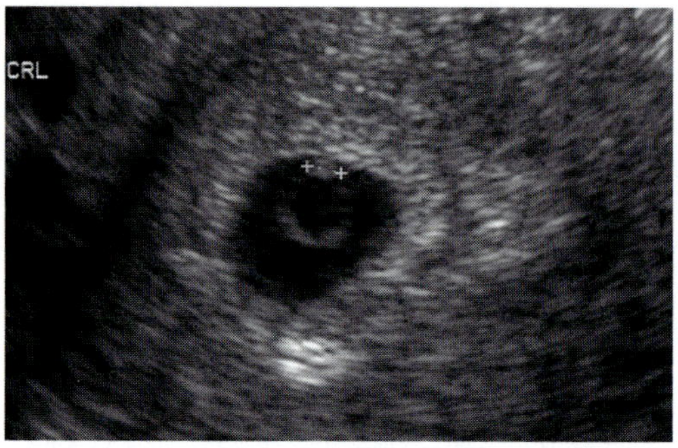

FIG. 32-15. Small embryo (CRL 2.3 mm) adjacent to the yolk sac at 5 weeks menstrual age.

UMBILICAL CORD AND CORD CYST

The umbilical cord is formed at the end of the sixth week of menstrual age (CRL = 4.0 mm) as the amnion expands and envelops the connecting stalk, the yolk stalk, and the allantois. The cord contains two umbilical **arteries,** a single umbilical **vein,** the **allantois, and yolk stalk (also called the omphalomesenteric or vitelline duct),** all of which are imbedded in **Wharton's jelly.** The umbilical arteries arise from the fetal internal iliac arteries and in the newborn become the superior vesical arteries and the medial umbilical ligaments. The umbilical vein carries oxygenated blood from the placenta to the fetus through the ductus venosus into the inferior vena cava (IVC) and the heart. The single left umbilical vein in the newborn becomes the ligamentum teres, left main portal vein, and the ligamentum venosum.

The allantois is associated with bladder development and becomes the urachus and the median umbilical ligament. It extends into the proximal portion of the umbilical cord. The yolk stalk connects the primitive gut to the yolk sac.

The paired vitelline arteries and veins accompany the stalk to provide blood supply to the yolk sac. The arteries arise from the dorsal aorta to initially supply the yolk sac and then the primitive gut. The arteries remain as the celiac axis, superior and inferior mesenteric arteries supplying the foregut, midgut, and hindgut, respectively. The vitelline veins drain directly into the sinus venosus of the heart. The right vein is later incorporated into the right hepatic vein. The portal vein is also formed by an anastomotic network of vitelline veins.

The length of the umbilical cord has a close linear relationship with menstrual age in normal pregnancies.[42] Hill et al.[42] found they could reliably measure the cord lengths in 53 fetuses from 6 to 11 weeks' menstrual age. They also found that the cord lengths in 60% of dead fetuses were more than 2 SD below the value for that expected menstrual age.

Cysts within the cord have been described to occur in the first trimester.[43] They are usually seen in the eighth week of menstrual age and disappear by the twelfth week. The cyst is singular and closer to the fetus than the placenta with a mean size of 5.2 mm. Although umbilical cord cysts have been associated with chromosomal abnormalities if seen in the second and third trimesters, those seen in the first trimester have been normal at delivery. Based on one pathological case, it is hypothesized that the cyst is an amnion inclusion cyst that likely occurred as the amnion was enveloping the umbilical cord. This explanation of a transient developmental aberration makes sense given the normal outcome at delivery (Fig. 32-16, *A* and *B*).

ESTIMATION OF MENSTRUAL AGE IN THE FIRST TRIMESTER

Within the first trimester, menstrual age may be estimated sonographically with greater accuracy than at any other stage. As pregnancy progresses, biologic variation results in wider variation about the mean for sonographic parameters at a given menstrual age. In order of appearance, the following structures can be measured as indicators of menstrual age.

Gestational Sac Size

It is possible to estimate menstrual age from weeks 5 to 10 on the basis of gestational sac size. Dating on this basis is clinically relevant before visualization of the embryo. The pregnancy should be followed, however, until the embryonic pole with cardiac activity is identified as a reliable indicator of embryonic life. Gestational sac measurement is accurate to within approximately 1 week of menstrual age.[44]

The MSD is measured using the sum of three orthogonal dimensions of the fluid-sac wall interface divided by three. The measurements are most accurate when obtained by a high-frequency endovaginal probe in the sagittal and transverse planes at right angles to one another. Normally, the MSD will be 8 mm or more with a yolk sac present and 16 mm or more with an embryo. Sacs larger than 8 mm or 16 mm without a yolk sac or embryo, respectively, should be watched carefully for impending early pregnancy failure. Occasionally, one will see a sac up to 20 mm without an embryo and the outcome will be a normal pregnancy. Although this is most uncommon, one must always give the fetus the benefit of the doubt and use not only the sac signs but clinical presentation as well.

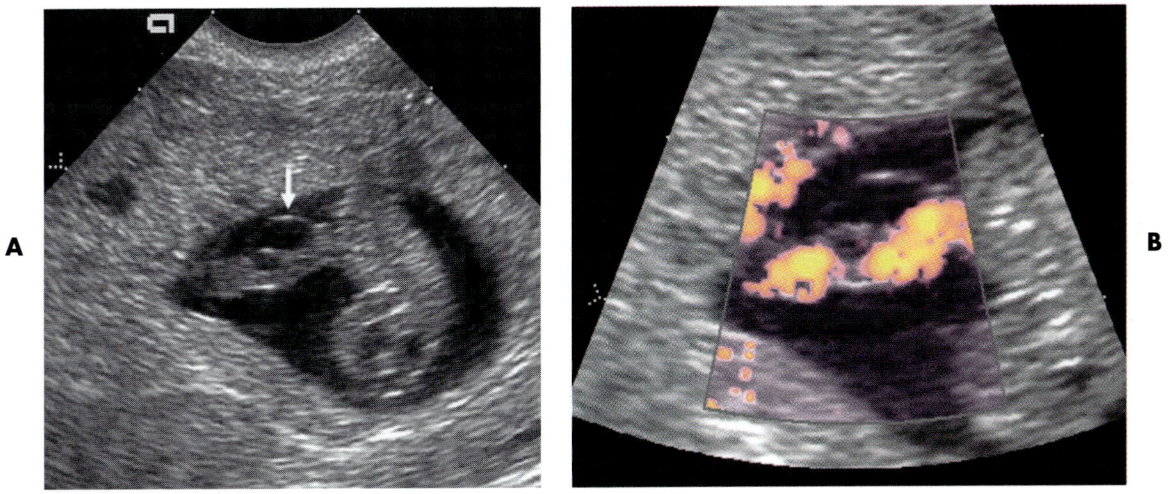

FIG. 32-16. Umbilical cord cyst. **A,** Live embryo at 9 weeks' menstrual age with a cyst on the cord (*arrow*) close to the embryonic end. On subsequent examination, the cyst was no longer seen. **B,** A power Doppler image of the cord and cyst with flow in the vessels of the cord and no flow in the cyst.

Crown-Rump Length

Using EVS, the embryo can be visualized from the fifth menstrual week onward. Conventional CRL charts derived from TVS data are available beginning from 6 weeks and 2 days of menstrual age. A well-performed CRL measurement in the first trimester of pregnancy is accurate to 5 to 7 days and is equivalent to or greater in accuracy than the biparietal diameter measured early in the second trimester.[43]

Biparietal Diameter, Head Circumference, Abdominal Circumference, and Femoral Length

By the end of the first trimester, measurement of the biparietal diameter (BPD) becomes more accurate than the CRL, which by that time reflects errors associated with fetal flexion and extension.[44] In the second and third trimesters, the mean menstrual age—defined as the mean of the menstrual ages predicted by the BPD, head circumference (HC), abdominal circumference (AC), and femoral length (FL)—may be used to eliminate errors caused by inaccuracy of any one parameter.[45-46] Late in the first trimester, however, the BPD remains a highly accurate measurement when used alone.

If the patient is to receive only **one ultrasound examination** during pregnancy, a single, first-trimester sonographic examination solely for the purpose of assessing menstrual age is not recommended.[47] Although this is the most accurate time for estimation of menstrual age, there is inadequate embryonic development to confidently identify anomalies that could be seen in the second trimester. The mean menstrual age—as predicted by BPD, HC, AC, and FL—between weeks 16 to 18 is equal to or only slightly less accurate than a first-trimester CRL. The second trimester is the most appropriate period to assess patients for routine dating, because of the added clinically relevant fetal information that can be obtained.

EMBRYONIC DEMISE

One of the most important roles of ultrasound in the first trimester is to diagnose early pregnancy failure and embryonic demise. Wilcox et al.[48] and others[49] have demonstrated a 20% to 31% rate of early pregnancy loss after implantation in normal healthy volunteers. Overall, approximately 75% of all pregnancies will fail. Approximately 15% of fertilized ova fail to divide, 15% are lost prior to implantation, 30% during implantation, 13% to 16% after implantation and before the first missed period[50] and 9% to 10% following the first missed period. The rate of unrecognized or **preclinical** pregnancy loss was 22%; many pregnancies aborted before the time when a gestational sac would be demonstrable by EVS. The higher numbers of preclinical loses reported more recently likely reflect the use of a more sensitive pregnancy tests.

Cytogenetic abnormalities have also recently been documented in 20% of ostensibly normal *in vitro* fertilization embryos.[49]

All the above are consistent with the early pathological studies of Hertig and Rock[50,51] who showed high frequencies of morphological abnormalities in preimplantation embryos. Loss rates are increased with increased maternal age and the use of tobacco and alcohol.

Sorokin et al.[52] performed chorionic villous samplings (CVS) in 795 first-trimester pregnancies. Of

TABLE 32-3
FIRST TRIMESTER—NUMBERS TO REMEMBER***

Event	Number	Reference
β-hCG level above which a sac should be seen (EVS)	1000–2000 mIU/mL, FIRP	16,18,20
Minimal threshold of MSD for determination of pregnancy failure:		
Yolk sac	EVS 8 mm	
	TVS 20 mm	
Embryo	EVS 16 mm	
	TVS 25 mm	
Fetal heart beat always present	CRL > 5	
Normal growth rate of MSD	1.1 mm/day	
Normal growth rate of embryo	1 mm/day	
MSD-CRL (5.5 to 9 weeks MA)	Must be > 5 mm or 94% loss rate	
Fetal heart rate	Mean 140 bpm	
Significant bradyarrhythmia		69
CRL < 5 mm	< 80 bpm	
CRL 5–9 mm	< 100 bpm	
CRL 10–15 mm	< 110 bpm	

***Remember—use these numbers in conjunction with other information (sonographic and clinical). If the sonographic data suggest early pregnancy failure, *always* give the fetus the benefit of the doubt and follow the patient until it is clear that the pregnancy will not continue (i.e., other signs become apparent—bleeding, inadequate sac growth, loss of cardiac activity, etc.)

these, 35 were found to have a blighted ovum or missed abortion prior to the procedure. Nineteen women had subsequent CVS and all of them had documented aneuploidy. Ten cases had chromosome abnormalities virtually always lethal in the embryonic period and nine had defects with moderate potential for fetal viability. Gestations with low viability potential had a larger discrepancy (23.4 ± 8.3 days) in estimated minus observed menstrual age and were significantly greater than gestations with moderate viability potential (8.9 ± 4.3 days) ($p < .001$). The absence of a fetal pole was more common in the first group. They conclude that the more severe the anomaly, the more likely there will be very early fetal demise or intrauterine growth retardation.

Another cause of early pregnancy failure is due to **"luteal phase defect."** It is believed to be failure of the corpus luteum to adequately support the conceptus once implantation has occurred. This may be the result of a shortened luteal phase in cases of ovulation induction and IVF, or luteal dysfunction more commonly seen in obese women or women over 37 years of age.[53]

Blumenfeld and Ruach[53] were successful in treating luteal phase defect in a group undergoing ovulation induction and in patients with previous abortions, using hCG administration two times weekly in the sixth and tenth weeks of menstrual age. This reduced the rate of miscarriage from 49% to 17.8% ($p < 0.01$).[53]

The etiology of first-trimester pregnancy loss is still not fully understood. There are a multitude of known and suspected causes. In a study of 232 first-trimester patients with an endovaginal scan at the first visit, Goldstein[54] determined the incidence of subsequent pregnancy loss by following all of them to delivery or spontaneous abortion. All patients had a positive urinary pregnancy test and none had vaginal bleeding. The overall loss rate was 11.5% in the embryonic period (i.e., < 70 days from last menstrual period) and 1.7% in the fetal period. The loss rate diminished as the pregnancy progressed and more structures were identifiable. The loss rate was 8.5% when a yolk sac was seen, 7.2% with an embryo of a CRL less than 5 mm, 3.3% with a CRL of 6 to 10 mm and 0.5% with a CRL greater than 10 mm. The loss rate leveled off at 2% from 14 to 20 weeks, the fetal period.

In patients who present with a closed cervical os and uterine bleeding in the first trimester, 50% will eventually abort.[55,56] These patients are clearly at an increased risk over the general population for pregnancy loss.

Falco et al.[57] reported on a group of 270 patients with transvaginal ultrasound between 5 and 12 weeks' gestation with first-trimester bleeding. Forty-five percent were diagnosed initially as a nonviable pregnancy or anembryonic sac. Those with multiple gestation were excluded. Of the 149 remaining with demonstrable fetal cardiac activity, 15% (23 of 149) subsequently aborted.

Table 32-4 summarizes the rate of spontaneous abortion in a number of studies of women with and without bleeding in early pregnancy.

A B

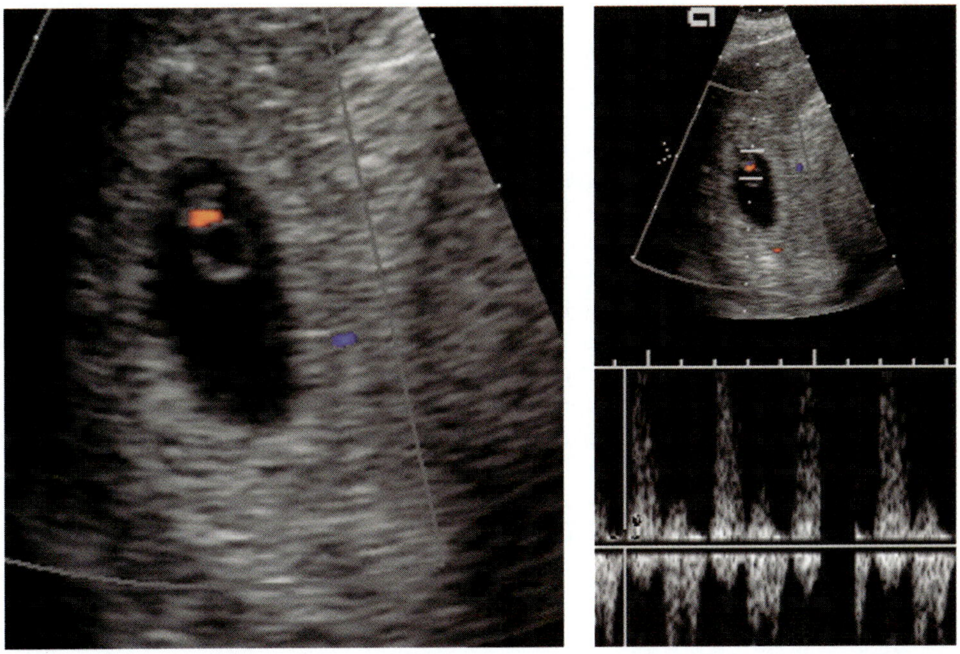

FIG. 32-17. Contribution of Doppler. **A,** This 6-week embryo was examined just prior to therapeutic abortion. Color and spectral Doppler are **not** recommended at this stage unless indicated. Cardiac activity was demonstrated by color Doppler in an embryo just anterior to the yolk sac. **B,** The cardiac activity is demonstrated by color and spectral Doppler.

TABLE 32-4
RATE OF SPONTANEOUS ABORTION IN EARLY PREGNANCY

Author	Age (wks)	Number	Indication	Abortion Rate (%)
Goldstein (1994)	5–10	232	Routine	11.5
Pandya (1996)	10–13	17,870	Routine	2.8
Stabile (1987)	5–16	624	Bleeding	45
Falco (1996)	5–12	270	Bleeding	51.5
Falco (1996)	5–12	149	Bleeding + live fetus	15
Pandya (1996)[58]	10–13	17,870	Bleeding	15.6

Modern clinical management centers on whether or not the embryo is present and alive. In our laboratory, we have found that in normal pregnancies, an embryo with cardiac activity can always be identified with EVS by 45 days of menstrual age.[56-59] The menstrual history, however, may be unreliable, and sonographic diagnosis of embryonic demise based on the menstrual history may be incorrect. It is more appropriate to predict outcome by comparing sonographic findings to quantifiable parameters, including other sonographic measurements (MSD) or quantitative serum β-hCG. Menstrual age can be used if there is corroboration with a previous positive β-hCG test result. For example, if a patient had a positive serum β-hCG test result 5 weeks ago, the current menstrual age must be at least 8 weeks.

After the gestational sac becomes demonstrable by ultrasound, the diagnosis of early pregnancy failure can be made reliably using sonographic criteria.

Embryonic Cardiac Activity

The single most important feature for the confirmation of embryonic and fetal life is the identification of cardiac activity. Using TVS, cardiac activity is always present when the embryo is visualized—that is, with TVS, it is abnormal to visualize the embryo without demonstrating cardiac activity. The caveat is that the examination must be of high quality, using modern equipment, and the entire embryo must be visualized. It is essential to use a high-frame rate and the frame-averaging mode must be turned off.

Using EVS, the embryo and embryonic cardiac activity can be reliably and consistently identified earlier than with TVS (Fig. 32-17, *A* and *B*). Whereas it is abnormal to identify an embryo without cardiac activity with TVS, **EVS can identify a normal embryo without cardiac activity.** In a study by Pennell et al., 16 to 18 patients with a CRL of less than 5 mm had no cardiac activity on initial endovaginal assessment and demonstrated cardiac activity on follow-up EVS.

We reviewed a series of 96 patients with CRLs of less than 5 mm to assess the predictive value of the presence or absence of cardiac activity using EVS. The data from this series are reproduced from the original article as Tables 32-5 through 32-7.[7] Of the 71 patients available for follow-up, 46 embryos had cardiac activity; 35 progressed to at least the late second trimester; and 11 ended as first-trimester embryonic or fetal deaths. Of the 25 embryos without demonstrable cardiac activity, 5 were normal. Only 20 ended as first-trimester embryonic deaths. Of the five normal embryos without demonstrable cardiac activity on initial EVS, three had initial CRL of less than 1.9 mm. Standard embryology texts indicate that the embryonic heart begins to beat at the beginning of the sixth week when the CRL is 1.5 to 3 mm. Thus, it is not surprising that we were unable to identify cardiac activity in normal embryos with less than 2-mm CRL. Of note is the finding that the only embryo with less than a 2-mm CRL in which cardiac activity could be demonstrated by EVS had a subsequent spontaneous abortion in the first trimester. Initial endovaginal sonographic assessment failed to identify cardiac activity in 2 of 25 normal embryos with CRL of 2 to 4 mm. EVS enabled correct identification of cardiac activity in 100% of normal embryos with CRL of 4 to 4.9 mm. As a result, in our practice, follow-up sonography is performed in patients with embryos of less than 5-mm CRL with no cardiac activity, unless the yolk sac is absent.

In patients with a sonographically demonstrable embryo, absent cardiac activity is clearly the most important factor in predicting the pregnancy outcome. It is also important to know the predictive value of the presence of cardiac activity in an embryo with respect to its ultimate viability. After 7 weeks' menstrual age the pregnancy loss rate is 2% to 2.3%.[60,61] and after 16 weeks, the rate is only 1%.[62] In our series of predominantly symptomatic patients with embryos of less than 5-mm CRL, identification of cardiac activity with EVS was associated with a 24% risk of spontaneous abortion.[7] In the series of Falco[57] they had a 15% abortion rate in pregnancies from 5 to 12 weeks where cardiac activity was recognized using endovaginal sonography.

Other secondary findings may also be helpful in predicting the outcome of a pregnancy. In our series, the combination of absent cardiac activity and vaginal bleeding was associated with 100% embryonic mortality.[7] Subchorionic hemorrhage and absent cardiac activity were associated with 88% embryonic mortality.

TABLE 32-5
PRESENCE OR ABSENCE OF CARDIAC ACTIVITY IN NORMAL EMBRYOS—BASED ON CROWN-RUMP LENGTH (n = 40)

	Cardiac Activity at EVS	
CRL (mm)	**Present**	**Absent**
0-0.9	0	0
1-1.9	0	3
2-2.9	12	0
3-3.9	11	2
4-4.9	12	0
Total	35	5

From Levi CS, Lyons EA, Zheng XA, et al. Endovaginal ultrasound: demonstration of cardiac activity in embryos of less than 5.0 mm in crown-rump length. *Radiology* 1990;176(1):71-74.

TABLE 32-6
PRESENCE OR ABSENCE OF CARDIAC ACTIVITY IN EMBRYOS THAT SUBSEQUENTLY ABORTED IN FIRST TRIMESTER—BASED ON CROWN-RUMP LENGTH (n = 31)

	Cardiac Activity at EVS	
CRL (mm)	**Present**	**Absent**
0-0.9	0	0
1-1.9	1	0
2-2.9	1	8
3-3.9	6	6
4-4.9	3	6
Total	11	20

From Levi CS, Lyons EA, Zheng XA, et al. Endovaginal ultrasound: demonstration of cardiac activity in embryos of less than 5.0 mm in crown-rump length. *Radiology* 1990;176(1):71-74.

TABLE 32-7
PERCENTAGE OF EMBRYOS THAT ABORTED SUBSEQUENT TO SONOGRAPHIC DEMONSTRATION OF CARDIAC ACTIVITY AT SPECIFIC CROWN-RUMP LENGTHS

CRL (mm)	Spontaneous Abortions/Total	Percentage Aborted
0-0.9	0/0	0%
1-1.9	1/1	100%
2-2.9	1/1	38%
3-3.9	6/17	35%
4-4.9	3/15	20%
Total	11/46	24%

From Levi CS, Lyons EA, Zheng XA, et al. Endovaginal ultrasound: demonstration of cardiac activity in embryos of less than 5.0 mm in crown-rump length. *Radiology* 1990;176(1):71-74.

Gestational Sac Features

In many patients, the embryo is not visualized on the initial sonogram and the diagnosis of demise cannot be made on the basis of abnormal cardiac activity. In those cases, it may be possible to make the diagnosis of pregnancy failure based on gestational sac characteristics.

The most reliable indicator of abnormal outcome based on gestational sac characteristics is abnormal gestational sac size.[6,29] In 1985, Bernard and Cooperberg,[63] using an TVS, observed that a gestational sac with an MSD greater than 2 cm diameter and no embryo had a poor outcome. In 1986, also using TVS, Nyberg et al.[29] refined the definition of an abnormal gestational sac as one with an MSD of 25 mm or more without an embryo, or an MSD of 20 mm or more without a yolk sac.

These criteria were re-evaluated for EVS with the result that an MSD of 8 mm or more without a demonstrable yolk sac or 16 mm with no demonstrable embryo is abnormal and indicates pregnancy failure.[31] Furthermore, these parameters only apply to high-resolution EVS and cannot be used for examinations performed with a 5-MHz endovaginal probe.[64] Our practice and the practice of others is to repeat a suspicious study in 3 to 4 days. With an expected growth rate of 1 mm/day, one should see an appropriate increase in sac size and, if normal, the appearance of a yolk sac or an embryo. If the growth is less than expected, it gives one confidence of the diagnosis of early pregnancy failure. It is also important to view the pregnancy in light of the clinical condition. A patient who is in the process of a spontaneous abortion will often present with brownish spotting, a decrease in the symptoms of pregnancy (breast tenderness and nausea) and on examination, a uterus smaller than expected. The latter is very subjective and not very reliable in early gestation (Fig. 32-18, *A* and *B*).

Other **gestational sac criteria for poor outcome** are less reliable alone but together or with an abnormally large sac give additional support for the diagnosis of early pregnancy failure. These criteria include:[29] a distorted gestational sac shape (Fig. 32-19), a thin trophoblastic reaction (< 2 mm), weakly echogenic trophoblast, or an abnormally low position of the gestational sac within the endometrial cavity (Fig. 32-20).

Normal **gestational sac growth** is 1.1 mm per day. Nyberg et al.[64] found that patients with early pregnancy failure had MSD growth rates of less than 0.7 mm per day. This growth rate is useful informa-

POOR OUTCOME: GESTATIONAL SAC CRITERIA

Most valuable—abnormal gestational sac size
Distorted sac shape
Thin, weakly echogenic trophoblast
Low position in endometrial cavity

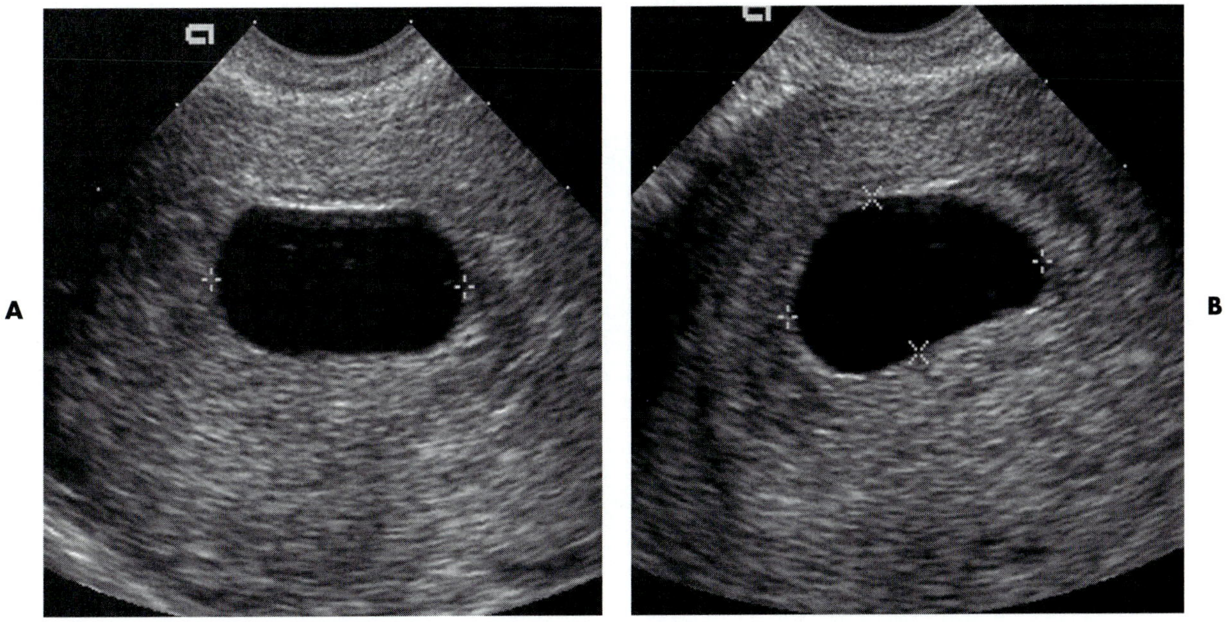

FIG. 32-18. Intrauterine embryonic death or anembryonic gestation on endovaginal sonography. **A,** Coronal scan and **B,** sagittal scan show mean gestational sac diameter is 18 mm. No yolk sac is identified.

tion in assessing the normalcy of development in serial examinations.

Amnion and Yolk Sac Criteria

Visualization of the amnion in the absence of a sonographically demonstrable embryo after 7 weeks MA is abnormal and is diagnostic of an anembryonic gestation or embryonic demise with resorption of the embryo.

Other findings which can be useful in the diagnosis of embryonic demise include a collapsing irregularly marginated amnion, visualization of the amnion in the absence of a visible embryo, and yolk sac calcification. In general, however, other signs of embryonic demise are present when these findings are positive.

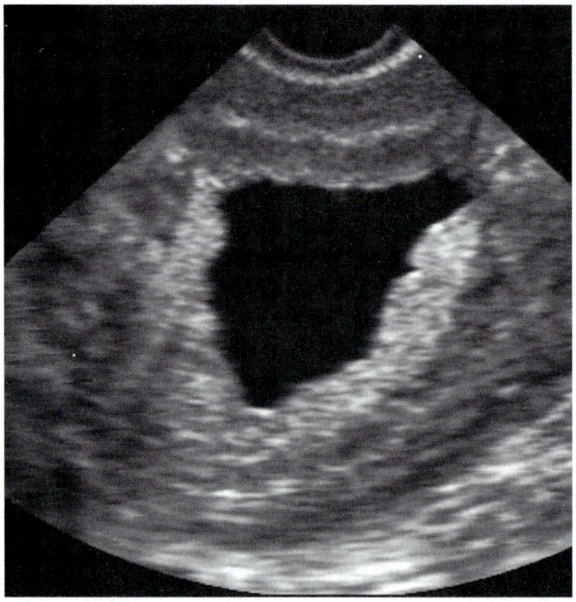

FIG. 32-19. Abnormal gestational sac feature. A coronal sac shows a large irregular and empty gestational sac with irregular trophoblast.

Sonographic Predictors of Abnormal Outcome

Sonographic findings may be used to predict abnormal outcome in the presence of a live embryo or prior to visualization of the embryo. These findings can be used to identify a high-risk subgroup of embryos which are at risk for embryonic demise or subsequent diagnosis of fetal anomaly and require close follow-up.

Embryonic Bradycardia

Although embryonic cardiac activity indicates that the embryo is alive at the time of the examination, an abnormally slow heart rate may predict impending demise. In a study by Doubilet and Benson,[65] a heart rate of less than 80 bpm in embryos with a CRL of less than 5 mm was universally associated with subsequent embryonic demise (Fig. 32-21), a rate of 80 to 90 bpm had a 64% risk of demise, a rate of 90 to 99 bpm a 32% risk, and a heart rate of 100 bpm was associated with an 11% risk. Heart rates above 100 bpm are considered normal in embryos of CRL of less than 5 mm.

In embryos of CRL 5 to 9 mm, a heart rate less than 100 bpm was always associated with abnormal outcome with the normal heart rate being 120 bpm or more. In embryos 10 to 15 mm CRL, a heart rate of less than 110 bpm appears to be associated with a very poor prognosis.

A

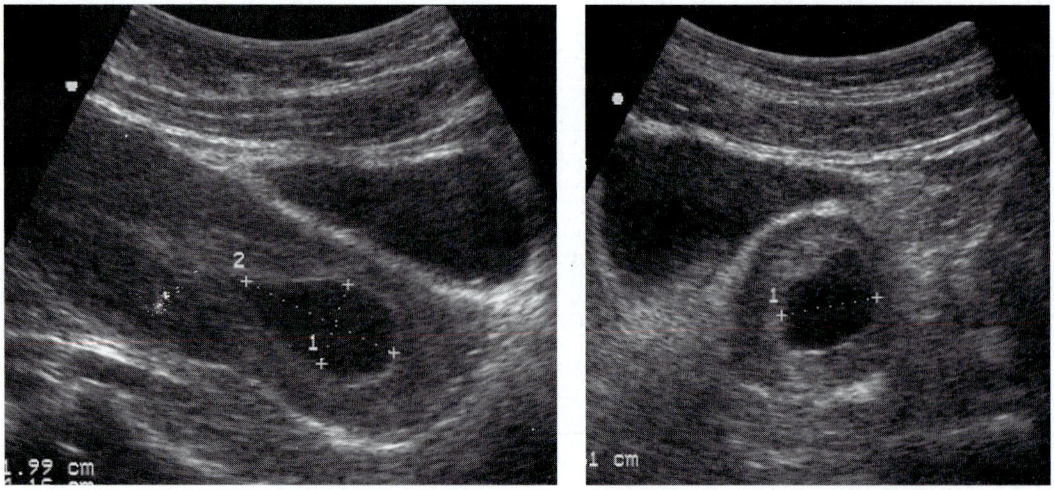

B

FIG. 32-20. Abnormal gestational sac location. **A,** A sagittal scan of a uterus with a gestational sac in the lower uterine segment or upper cervix. This gestation aborted 2 hours later. **B,** Coronal scan of the sac within the upper cervix.

MSD and CRL Less Than 5 mm

Bromley et al. found that in 16 patients between 5.5 and 9 weeks' menstrual age in whom the MSD was less than 5 mm greater than the CRL (i.e., MSD and CRL < 5 mm) 15 of 16 patients had spontaneous first-trimester abortions (Fig. 32-22).

Yolk Sac Size and Shape

Although the subject is still controversial,[66] in our experience, yolk sac size is a very useful predictor of abnormal outcome.[31] Perhaps the most important consideration is that yolk sac abnormalities may predict abnormal outcome in pregnancies which appear otherwise **completely normal** by all other ultrasound criteria.

Currently, the **major sonographic applications** of the evaluation of the yolk sac are diagnosis of embryonic demise, confirmation of the presence of an intrauterine pregnancy, and an indicator of increased risk of fetal abnormality.

Rat embryo experiments demonstrate defects in the yolk sac structure and ultrastructure in response to hyperglycemia. Human data indicate that yolk sac malformations occur in embryos of diabetic mothers in the first trimester of pregnancy before 9 weeks of menstrual age.[67] Several authors have hypothesized that sonographic detection of abnormal yolk sac morphologic features may predict abnormal fetal outcome. Attempts have been made to characterize the normal sonographic appearance of the yolk sac and to identify abnormal parameters.

In a study by Green and Hobbins[68] in patients between 8 and 12 weeks of menstrual age, yolk sacs less than or equal to 2 mm were associated with a poor outcome. A solid echodense yolk sac was associated with fetal death or an anomalous fetus. In our experience, an echogenic yolk sac is not always associated with anomalies or impending demise and may revert to a more normal appearance.

Lindsay et al.[31] reviewed the normal and abnormal EVS appearances of the yolk sac in pregnancies between 5 and 10 weeks of menstrual age.[31] As noted previously, **nonvisualization of the yolk sac by EVS** in patients with an MSD of greater than **8 mm** is abnormal.[32] **Nonvisualization of the yolk sac in the presence of an embryo** demonstrated by EVS has been associated with embryonic demise in 100% of patients, either at the time of the examination or on follow-up sonographic assessment.[31] It is essential to use an endovaginal transducer of high enough frequency (6.0 MHz or higher) to confidently detect a yolk sac in a gestational sac of less than 10 mm. We

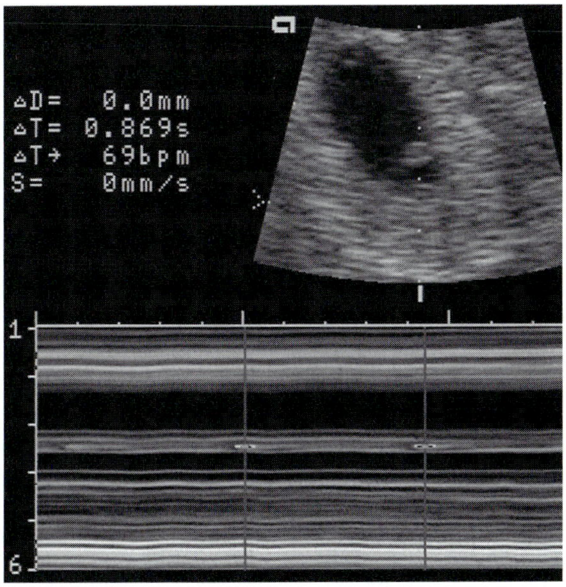

FIG. 32-21. Embryonic bradycardia. A 6-week embryo with a crown-rump length of 4 mm and a fetal heart rate of 69 bpm. This embryo died 1 week later.

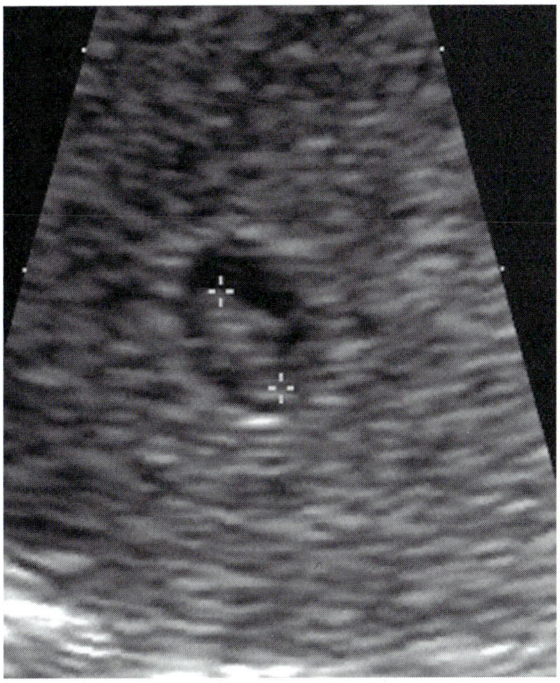

FIG. 32-22. Mean gestational sac diameter (MSD) and crown-rump length (CRL) less than 5 mm. A small embryo (crown-rump length 4 mm) at 7 weeks' menstrual age within a small gestational sac. The MSD-CRL was less than 5 mm and the embryo succumbed within 2 weeks.

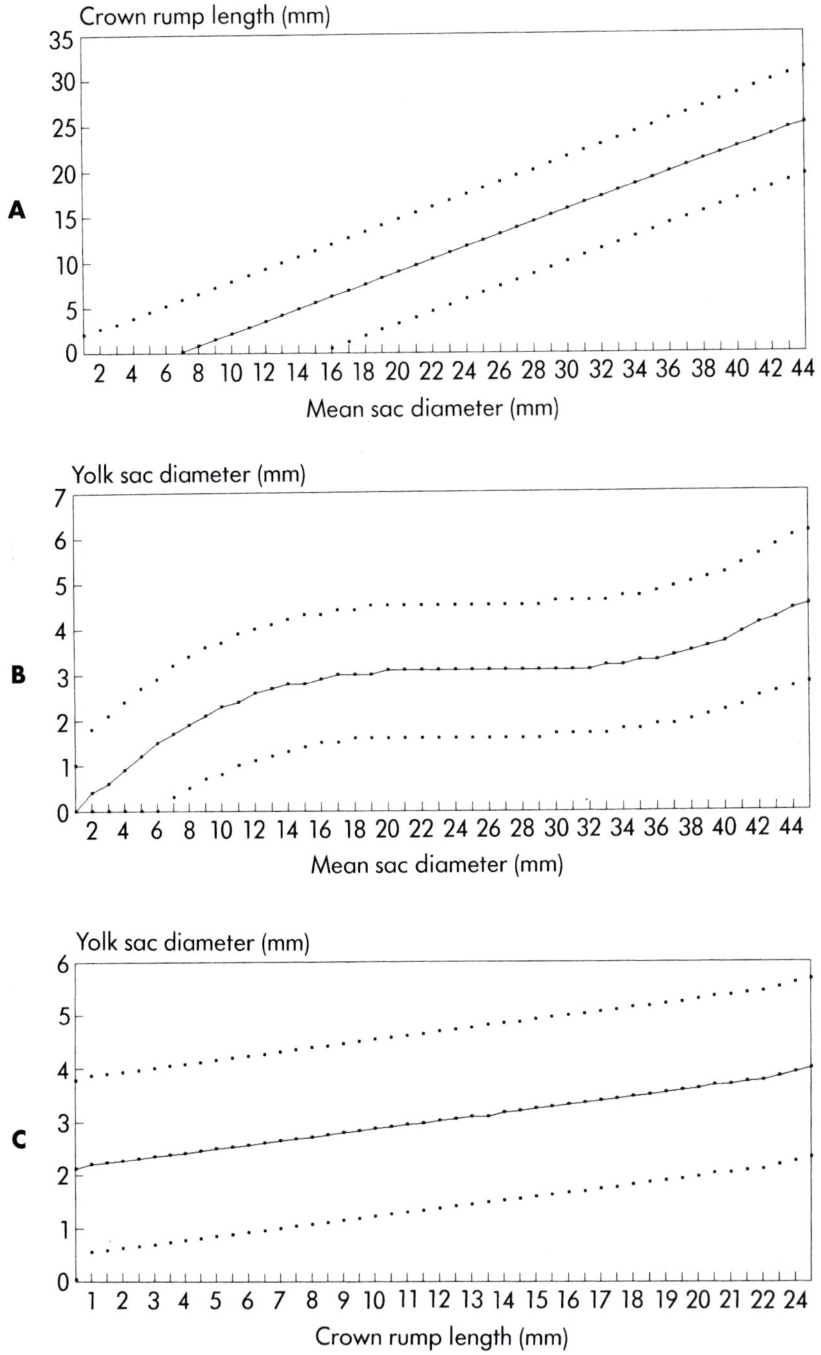

FIG. 32-23. Normal obstetric data. **A,** Mean gestational sac diameter (MSD) versus crown-rump length (CRL). **B,** Yolk sac versus MSD. **C,** CRL versus yolk sac.

have recently reported[64] two cases where no yolk sac was demonstrated in a gestational sac of 9 and 10 mm and a live embryo was subsequently identified. Our original data had been based on work performed with a 6.5-MHz probe. Our policy is to now repeat the study with a probe of at least 6.5 MHz if the initial examination fails to demonstrate a yolk sac with a gestational sac in excess of 8 mm.

Lindsay et al.[31] also compared yolk sac internal diameter with menstrual age, CRL, and MSD (Fig. 32-23). A yolk sac diameter that is outside the 95% confidence limits for these other parameters is a relative indicator of **increased risk** of embryonic demise or fetal abnormality (see box on p. 997). The sensitivity of yolk sac size as a predictor of outcome is, however, only 15.6% because 50% of abnormal preg-

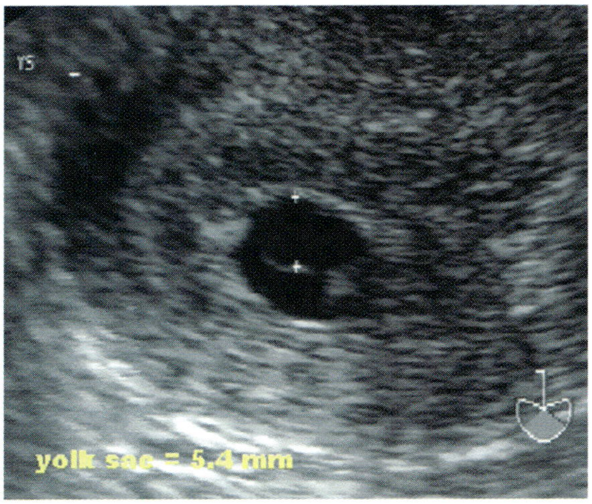

FIG. 32-24. Large yolk sac. EVS at 5.5 weeks shows gestational sac with live embryo (only partially included in this scan plane) and large yolk sac with mean internal diameter of 5.4 mm. Cardiac activity was demonstrated. On follow-up examination 7 days later, no cardiac activity was identified, indicating embryonic demise.

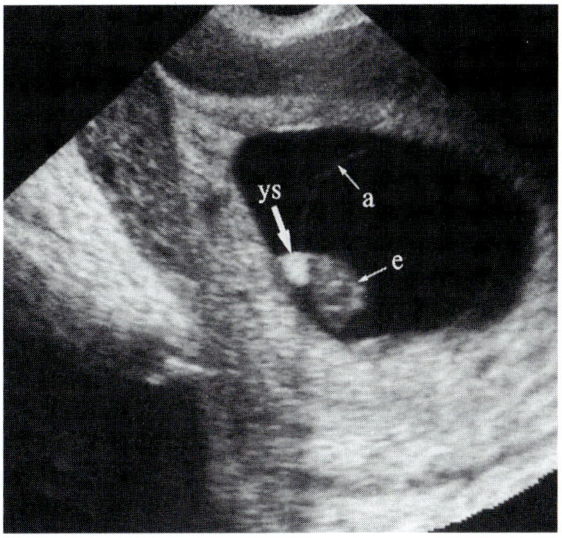

FIG. 32-25. Intrauterine embryonic death with yolk sac calcification (endovaginal sonography, sagittal plane). Yolk sac (ys) is calcified. No cardiac activity is identified. Crown-rump length is 17.8 mm. a—Amnion; e—embryo.

YOLK SAC

Confirmation of pregnancy:
- First structure seen in gestational sac

Diagnosis of embryonic demise:
- Threshold MSD—must see yolk sac
  - EVS 8 mm
  - TVS 20 mm

Prediction of abnormal outcome
- Yolk sac size
  - D>5.6 mm (5 to 10 wk MA)
  - Abnormal outcome
- Yolk sac shape not predictive
- Calcified yolk sac—dead embryo

nancies have a sonographically normal yolk sac. Although the 5% and 95% confidence limits can be used to predict increased risk, **a yolk sac diameter greater than 5.6 mm** between 5 and 10 weeks is always associated with an abnormal outcome (Fig. 32-24). Further, a thick symmetric yolk sac has a predictive value of 93.3% for normal outcome (Fig. 32-14).[45] A thin yolk sac has a predictive value of 53.8% for abnormal outcome. Yolk sac shape is **not** predictive of outcome. In a recent, unpublished study we found that a yolk sac that had an irregular shape that persisted or ones that converted to a normal appearance had a normal outcome in virtually all cases. Yolk sac shape and any subsequent change is therefore **not** predictive of outcome. Size, on the other hand, was always predictive if above the 95% confidence limit regardless of whether there was a live embryo or no embryo. They all went on to die. In spite of these findings, always correlate with the clinical findings and give the fetus the benefit of the doubt.

An **abnormally large yolk sac** is often the first sonographic indicator of pathologic condition(s) and is invariably associated with subsequent embryonic demise. Even if the pregnancy survives the first trimester, however, the fetus may still be abnormal. In our experience, although the number of cases is small, large yolk sacs have been associated with fetal pathologic states, including chromosomal abnormalities (trisomy 21, partial molar pregnancy) and omphalocele.

A **calcified yolk sac** appears as a shadowing echogenic mass in the absence of any other identifiable yolk sac. It has not been reported to be associated with a live embryo before 12 weeks' menstrual age. In fact, a calcified yolk sac will only be seen with a dead embryo and may calcify within 36 hours after demise. One must differentiate between an echogenic and a calcified yolk sac, the former being seen with a live embryo. Harris et al.[69] demonstrated yolk sac calcification in two cases of long-standing (possibly 2 weeks or more), first-trimester intrauterine embryonic demise (Fig. 32-25).

β-hCG/Mean Gestational Sac Diameter. Nyberg et al.[70] found that 65% of abnormal pregnancies had a disproportionately low serum β-hCG for gestational sac size. This had a positive predictive value and specificity of 100%.

Subchorionic Hemorrhage. Subchorionic hemorrhage or a hematoma resulting from abruption of the placental margin or marginal sinus rupture[71] causes elevation of the chorionic membrane. This is a

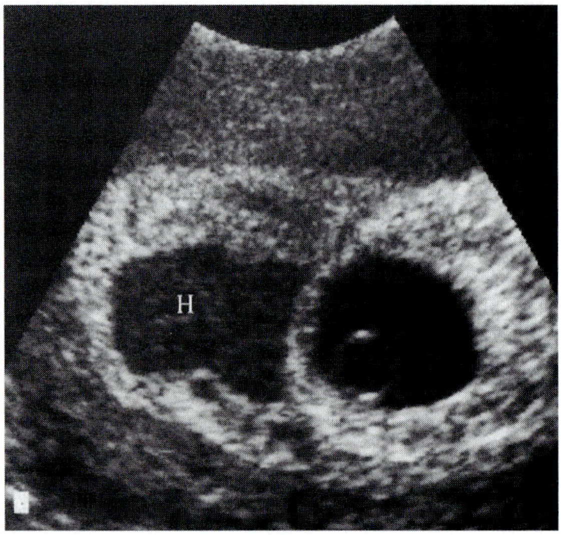

FIG. 32-26. Subchorionic hemorrhage at 6 weeks of menstrual age. Endovaginal sonography shows echogenic collection of blood (H) in endometrial canal. (From Levi CS, Lyons EA, Lindsay DJ: Ultrasound in the first trimester of pregnancy. *Radiol Clin North Am* 1990;28:19-38.)

common finding late in the first trimester and may be associated with vaginal bleeding. The chorionic membrane is stripped from the endometrium (decidua vera) and elevated by the hematoma (Fig. 32-26). These hemorrhages have been shown to be contiguous with the placental edge, but the predominant hemorrhage is often remote from the placenta.[72] **Acute hemorrhage** is usually hyperechoic or isoechoic relative to the placenta. The hemorrhage gradually becomes sonolucent in 1 to 2 weeks. Often the cause of membrane elevation is obvious as a result of the presence of fluid deep to the membrane, which is more echoic than the amniotic fluid, indicating a subchorionic hemorrhage. In a group of patients presenting with vaginal bleeding between 10 and 20 weeks of menstrual age, identification of a subchorionic hemorrhage was associated with a 50% fetal loss rate.[71] Bennet et al.[72] found, in a retrospective study of 516 patients with first-trimester bleeding, an overall pregnancy loss rate of 9.3%. This increases with increasing maternal age and decreasing menstrual age. For women over 35 years of age the rate is 13.8% versus 7.3 for those younger and for those presenting at or before 8 weeks, it is 13.7% compared with only 5.9% for those later in gestation.

Their most important criterion was the **size** of the bleed.[73] The small or medium sized ones (i.e., less than one third or one half of the sac circumference) have a miscarriage rate of 9% compared with 18.8% for the large ones.

EVCFD Predictors of Pregnancy Failure. Normally, prior to 12 weeks gestation, no flow is detectable within the trophoblastic ring which is comprised of the intervillous space, chorionic villi, and their fetal vessels.[73] As noted previously, low resistance arterial flow is present normally in the decidual spiral arteries.[74]

The decidual spiral arteries are invaded by extravillous trophoblastic cells. Inadequate trophoblastic invasion of the spiral arteries may be seen in early pregnancy failure and may be associated with increased resistance to flow in the spiral arteries. A recent study suggests that an abnormal resistive index (>0.55) in the decidual spiral arteries and active arterial blood flow in the intervillous space may be associated with an increased incidence of early pregnancy failure. The authors speculate that abnormal high pressure blood flow in the spiral arteries may result in significant increased pressure to the immature villi causing detachment of the early villi and subsequent miscarriage.

Amniotic Sac Abnormalities. A larger than **normal or "floppy" amniotic sac** has been described with early pregnancy failure caused by embryonic demise.[79] The explanation for the larger than normal sac may be a relatively small embryo after death or failure of resorption of the amniotic fluid through the embryonic skin surface. Horrow[75] has determined that in normal embryos, the difference between the CRL and the amniotic sac diameter is 1.1 ± 2.0 mm, whereas it is 8.6 ± 3.8 mm in abnormal pregnancies. He also found that the chorionic cavity remains appropriate in size relative to the embryonic CRL.

ECTOPIC PREGNANCY

Ectopic pregnancy remains one of the leading causes of maternal death in the United States. It accounts for 1.4% of all pregnancies and approximately 15% of maternal deaths. Although the incidence of the disease is increasing, the mortality has declined (the risk of death from ectopic pregnancy is now well below 1 of 1000 cases compared with 3.5 of 1000 in 1970).[76,77] The increase in ectopic pregnancies likely is the result of an increase in the prevalence of the risk factors, whereas heightened awareness and improved diagnostic capabilities have played a role in the decreased mortality.

Clinical Presentation

The **classical clinical triad** of pain—abnormal vaginal bleeding—and a palpable adnexal mass is only present in approximately 45% of patients with ectopic pregnancy.[78] In addition, the positive predictive value of this triad is only 14%. Other presenting signs and symptoms include any combination of the classic triad, as well as amenorrhea, adnexal tenderness, and cervical excitation pain. In a study by

> **SONOGRAPHY: SUSPECT ECTOPIC GESTATION**
>
> **Specific feature**
> - Live embryo in the adnexa
>
> **Nonspecific features** (correlate with β-hCG)
> - Empty uterus
> - Pseudogestational sac of ectopic pregnancy
> - Particulate ascites
> - Adnexal mass
> - Ectopic tubal ring
>
> **Nonsupportive features**
> - Live intrauterine pregnancy
> - Intradecidual sign and double decidual sign of early intrauterine pregnancy
> - Peritrophoblastic blood flow

Schwartz and Di Pietro[78] only 9% of patients with clinically suspected ectopic pregnancy actually had an ectopic pregnancy, 17% had symptomatic ovarian cysts, 13% had pelvic inflammatory disease (PID), 8% had dysfunctional uterine bleeding, and 7% had spontaneous abortions. These data demonstrate that the clinical presentation is by no means specific.

Of major significance is that even in the 1990s, 5% of proven ectopics bypass all imaging and go directly to surgery.[79] In addition, even in retrospect, 8.7% of proven ectopics are sonographically normal.[79]

Several factors increase the **risk of ectopic pregnancy** such as (1) any tubal abnormality that may prevent passage of the zygote or result in delayed transit; (2) previous tubal pregnancy;[80,81] (3) previous history of tubal reconstructive surgery; (4) pelvic inflammatory disease, chlamydia salpingitis,[82] intrauterine contraceptive devices (IUCD); and (5) other maternal factors, including increased age and parity.

There is a strong association between infertility and ectopic pregnancy. This is likely because of the shared tubal abnormalities in both conditions. The risk factors for ectopic pregnancy are therefore present in patients who undergo ovulation induction or IVF and embryo transfer. The increased incidence of multiple pregnancy with ovulation induction and IVF further increases the risk for both ectopic and **heterotopic** (coexistent intrauterine and ectopic) gestation. The hydrostatic forces generated during embryo transfer may also contribute to the increased risk.[83] The frequency of heterotopic pregnancy was originally estimated on a theoretic basis to be 1 in 30,000 pregnancies. More recent data indicate that the rate is approximately 1 in 7000.[84,85]

The **prevalence of ectopic pregnancy** varies according to the patient population and their inherent risk factors (approximately 10% to 40%). Nevertheless, all patients in the reproductive age group are at risk for ectopic pregnancy.

Sonographic Diagnosis

When patients present with a positive pregnancy test or a history suggestive of ectopic (a missed period, pain, unprotected intercourse), it is critical to identify the presence and location of the gestational sac. Pelvic ultrasound and especially an endovaginal examination must be the first line of imaging investigation. The endovaginal study allows for a more detailed evaluation of the endometrium, the endometrial canal, and the adnexa. The imaging component must be augmented by the clinical findings of tenderness elicited by the endovaginal probe. Uterine tenderness is uncommon but adnexal tenderness may be important in leading one to the site of the ectopic or less commonly a ruptured or leaking corpus luteum cyst.

It is our practice to begin the examination with a transvesical examination through a full bladder if possible. If the patient arrives from emergency without a full bladder, we proceed anyway. We are looking for a large mass which may be outside of the pelvis and therefore outside of the range of the endovaginal probe. The mass may be the extrauterine gestational sac or a large hematoma. At the end of the examination we always look for free fluid in the hepatorenal space (Fig. 32-27, *A* through *D*). This will give a sense of how much blood has been lost. The critical issue is actually not how much, but how fast it has been lost. The patient may be hemodynamically stable with a large volume of fluid loss if it has been gradual with some volume replacement either naturally or with IV fluids. If fluid is seen in the hepatorenal space, it should impart a greater sense of urgency to the surgeon.

Finally, a good point to remember is that if the ovary cannot be seen on one side, in a suspected ectopic pregnancy, it is a very helpful maneuver to try and push the ovary down toward the endovaginal probe by pressing firmly on the anterior abdominal wall and "milking" the adnexa down when watching the screen carefully during the endovaginal examination.

In early intrauterine pregnancy, incomplete abortion, or ectopic pregnancy, it is not always possible to identify the gestational sac. Several nonspecific sonographic findings may help in localization of the gestational sac; however, ectopic pregnancy is excluded with the demonstration of an intrauterine pregnancy (which reduces the likelihood of coexistent ectopic pregnancy to 1 in 7000) or is confirmed with demonstration of a live embryo in the adnexa.

Specific Sonographic Findings

Diagnosis of Early Intrauterine Pregnancy.

The earlier demonstration of an intrauterine pregnancy is the single most important contribution of EVS

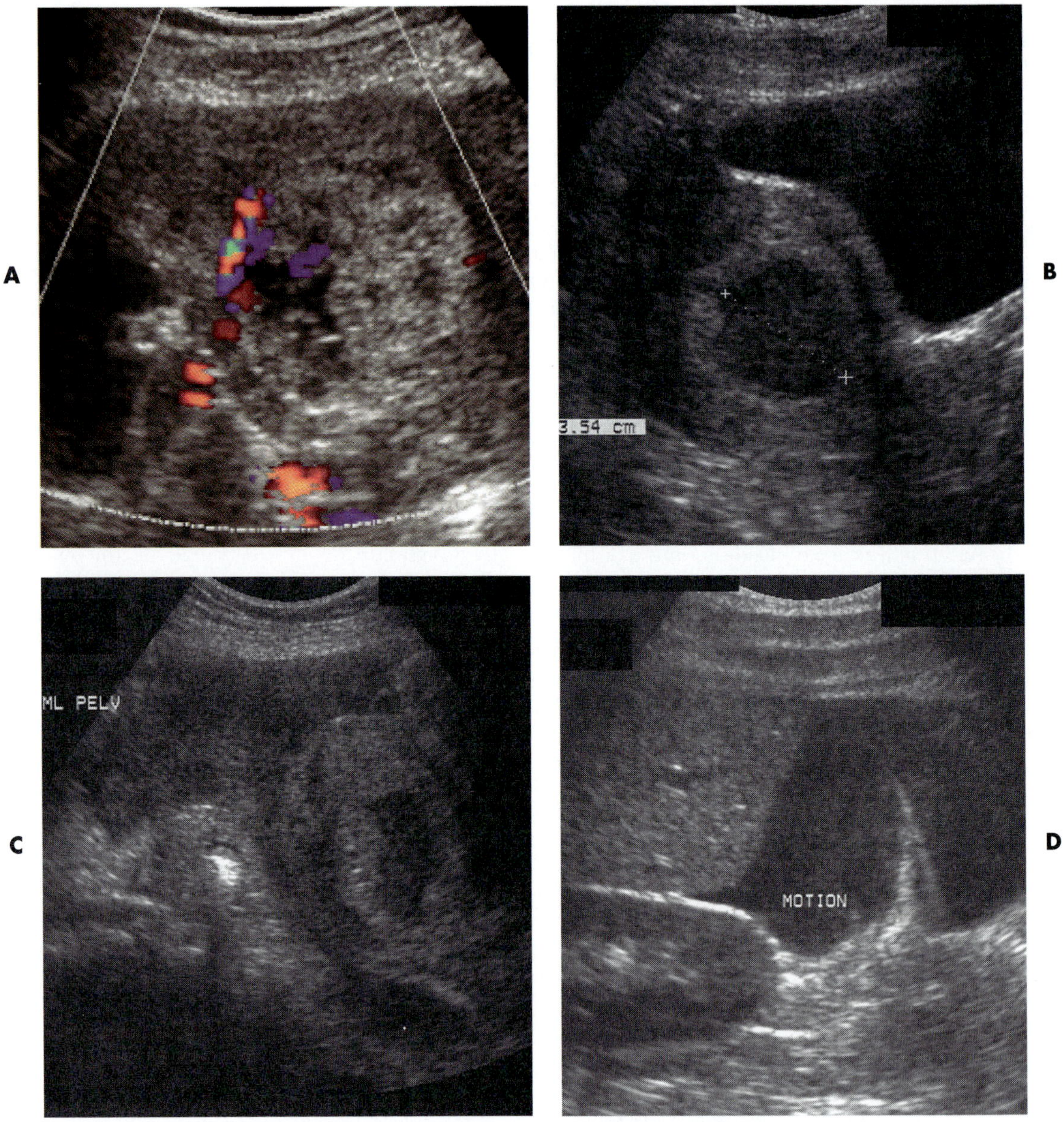

FIG. 32-27. Ectopic pregnancy with pseudogestational sac in the uterus. A scan of an ectopic with a right adnexal mass, a large decidual cast, and free echogenic fluid around the uterus and in the hepatorenal space. **A,** An endovaginal sonographic scan of the right adnexa showing a heterogeneous mass with possibly an irregular sac and blood flow. This is the hemorrhagic ectopic mass. **B,** A transvesical sonographic sagittal scan of the enlarged uterus with a large 3.5-cm decidual cast that almost resembles a gestational sac. **C,** A transvesical sonography sagittal scan of the uterus and pelvis with echogenic blood around the uterine body and fundus. **D,** A sagittal scan of the right upper quadrant with echogenic blood seen moving in the hepatorenal space.

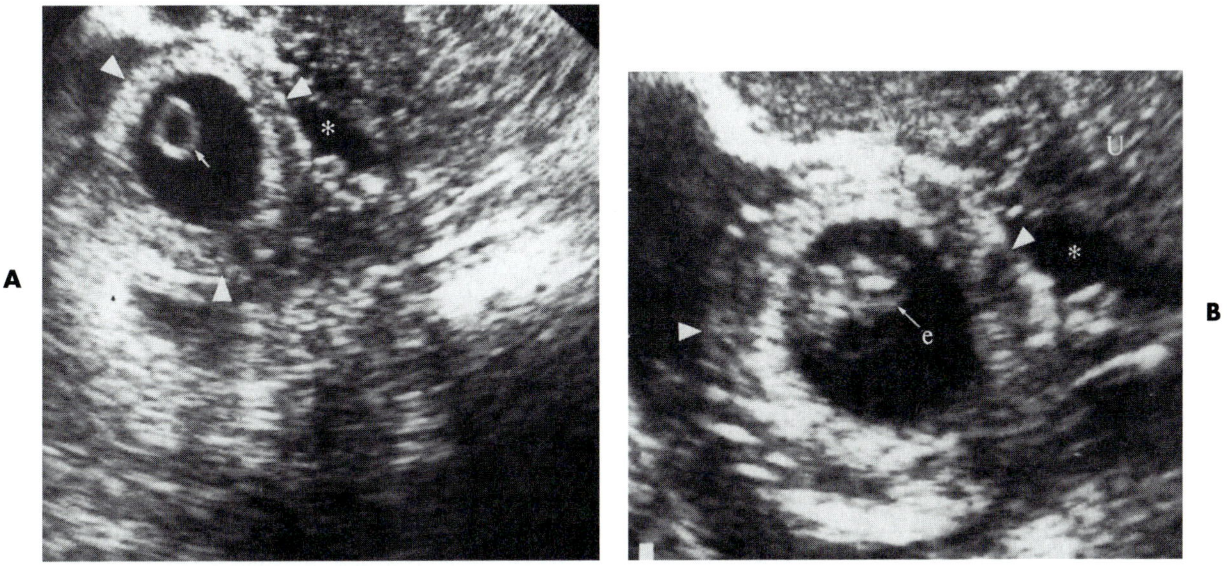

FIG. 32-28. Ectopic pregnancy with live embryo in adnexa. A and B, endovaginal sonography shows tubal ring (*arrowheads*) and gestational sac, containing yolk sac (ys) and live embryo (e). Asterisk indicates free fluid; U—uterus.

(compared with TVS) in the evaluation of patients presenting with suspected ectopic pregnancy. In a series of suspected ectopics by Dashefsky et al.,[86] all 19 normal intrauterine pregnancies were identified by endovaginal sonography compared with only 11 of 19 for TVS. In addition, endovaginal sonography identified 7 of 16 abnormal intrauterine pregnancies compared with 3 of 16 for TVS.[86]

As described in the section on the normal gestational sac, the intradecidual sign and the double-decidual sign can be used to identify an intrauterine pregnancy before visualization of the yolk sac or embryo. The double-decidual sign is to be distinguished from the **decidual cast or pseudogestational sac of ectopic pregnancy.** A decidual cast is an intrauterine-fluid collection surrounded by a single-decidual layer (Fig. 32-27) as opposed to the two concentric rings of the double-decidual sign. EVS improves differentiation of the decidua, which produces the pseudogestational sac, from the choriodecidual reaction of the double-decidual sign of intrauterine pregnancy.[87]

Doppler ultrasound and in particular color-flow Doppler imaging may further help distinguish a gestational sac from decidual cast. **Peritrophoblastic flow** is high-velocity, low-resistance flow with a low-resistive index and low-pulsatility index. Dillon et al.[88] studied a series of 40 patients with an empty saclike structure in the uterus. They defined peritrophoblastic flow as a peak systolic frequency of 0.8 kHz or greater (corresponding to 21 cm/sec with no angle correction) and correctly classified 26 of 31 intrauterine pregnancies and 9 of 9 pseudogestational sacs.[88]

When the presence of an intrauterine pregnancy is demonstrated with ultrasound, the extremely low frequency of heterotopic pregnancy effectively excludes the diagnosis of an ectopic gestation. However, heterotopic pregnancy should be suspected in the appropriate clinical setting, for instance, in patients undergoing ovulatory induction or IVF. In IVF patients, the rate of heterotopic pregnancy can be as high as 1%. Clearly, if a live embryo is demonstrated in the adnexa in a patient with an intrauterine gestational sac, a specific diagnosis can be made. In our experience, of about one heterotopic pregnancy per year with approximately 6000 obstetric scans, one may see an intrauterine gestation but only a complex echogenic adnexal mass which may have a sac only or a sac and an embryo. The complex mass is usually a large hematoma or hematosalpinx as a result of the ectopic.

When there is no sonographic evidence of an intrauterine pregnancy, the pregnant patient is more likely to harbor an extrauterine gestation. Because EVS allows for the earlier identification of an intrauterine pregnancy, it significantly increases the accuracy of diagnosis in patients with suspected ectopic gestation.[86,88]

Live Embryo in the Adnexa. The sonographic demonstration of a live embryo in the adnexa is specific for the diagnosis of ectopic pregnancy (Fig. 32-28). A live extrauterine fetus has been detected with EVS in approximately 17% to 28% of patients with ectopic pregnancies[86,87,89-91] compared with only 10% with TVS (Fig. 32-29).[92]

We have reported three cases of twin ectopics seen on the same side. All had pathology confirmation. In one case, only the gestational sacs were seen; in another, a yolk sac was also present and in the last one, two live embryos were detected.[93]

Nonspecific Findings

When the sonographic findings are nonspecific, correlation with **serum β-hCG** levels improves the ability of sonography to distinguish between intrauterine and ectopic pregnancy. **A negative β-hCG essentially excludes the presence of a live pregnancy.** The serum β-hCG test yields positive results at approximately 23 days of menstrual age.[94] This is before a normal intrauterine gestational sac may be imaged with either TVS or EVS. Different types of sonographic techniques and equipment have different hCG threshold levels or discriminatory zones above which gestational sacs are large enough to be imaged routinely. Nyberg et al.[23] identified a β-hCG threshold level of 1800 mIU/ml (Second International Standard) greater than which it was always possible to identify a normal intrauterine gestational sac by TVS. Threshold levels of 500 to 1000 mIU/ml (Second International Standard) have been proposed for EVS.[22] Some further refinement of a threshold level is recommended for the equipment and expertise in each individual institution. **If the hCG level is above the threshold level and an intrauterine gestational sac is not identified, the patient is presumed to have an ectopic pregnancy.** An early complete or incomplete abortion may, however, give a similar clinical and sonographic appearance. If the β-hCG level is below the threshold level the sonogram is less likely to identify an ectopic pregnancy. EVS should be performed even when the β-hCG levels are low because some patients may have suggestive or diagnostic findings. In indeterminate cases in which the patient is clinically stable, **serial quantitative serum hCG levels** may be helpful in distinguishing ectopic pregnancy, abortion, and early intrauterine pregnancy. The β-hCG level in a normal pregnancy has a doubling time of approximately 2 days, whereas patients with a dead or dying gestation have a falling β-hCG level. Patients with ectopic pregnancy usually have a slower increase in hCG levels, although they occasionally show patterns similar to a normal pregnancy or spontaneous abortion.

The presence of **nonspecific adnexal findings** improves the ability of sonography to predict an ectopic pregnancy. An adnexal mass can be found in conditions other than ectopic pregnancy (hemorrhagic corpus luteum cyst, endometriosis, abscess) and is therefore not diagnostic. However, the presence of an adnexal mass, in patients without sonographic evidence of an intrauterine pregnancy and a positive β-hCG test result, strongly suggests the presence of an ectopic pregnancy.

EVS has improved demonstration of nonspecific findings in patients with ectopic gestations.[87,95] Fleischer et al.[87] report finding an **ectopic tubal ring** in 49% of patients with ectopic pregnancy and in 68% of unruptured tubal pregnancies, using EVS (Fig. 32-30). The tubal ring can usually be differentiated from a corpus luteum cyst because the corpus luteum cyst is eccentrically located with a rim of ovarian tissue. A tubal ring is a concentric ring created by the

A

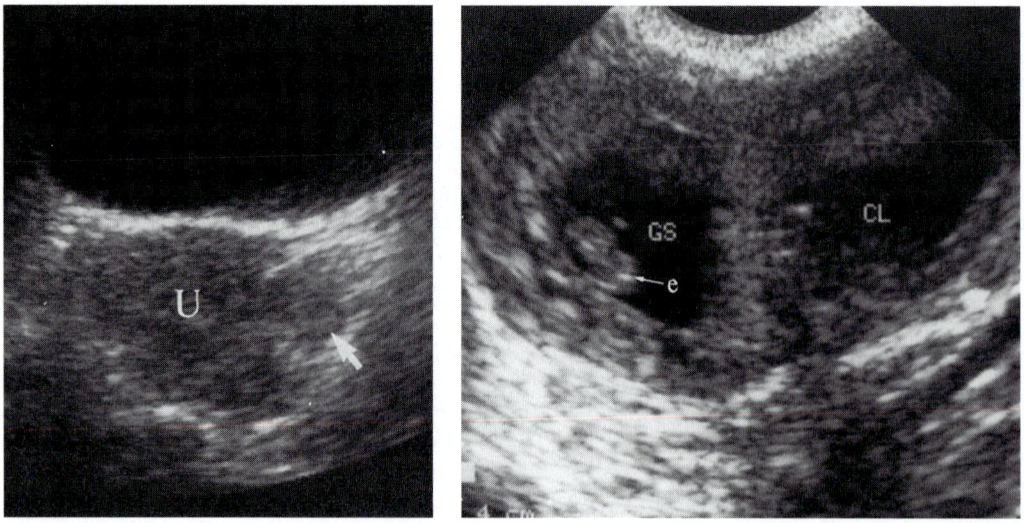

B

FIG. 32-29. Left ectopic pregnancy. A, Transvesical sonography in transverse plane shows ill-defined mass (*arrow*) in left adnexa. U—Uterus. **B,** Endovaginal sonography through left adnexa clearly shows gestational sac (GS) and live embryo (e) adjacent to corpus luteum cyst (CL). (From Dashefsky SM, Lyons EA, Levi CS, et al. Suspected ectopic pregnancy: endovaginal and transvesical ultrasound. *Radiology* 1988;169:181-184.)

trophoblast of the ectopic pregnancy surrounding the chorionic sac.

EVS is extremely sensitive in its ability to detect **free pelvic fluid.** The presence of echogenic free fluid (hemoperitoneum) or blood clots in the posterior cul-de-sac in pregnant patients, without sonographic evidence of an intrauterine pregnancy, should strongly suggest the presence of an ectopic pregnancy. The presence of small amounts of free, nonechogenic fluid is nonspecific and is seen in normal patients.

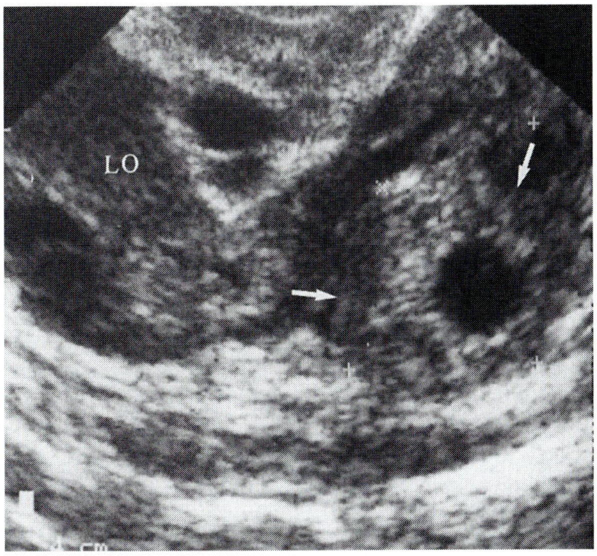

FIG. 32-30. Ectopic pregnancy. Sonogram shows a tubal ring (*arrows*). LO—left ovary.

Frates et al.,[96] in a group of 132 consecutive patients with surgical confirmation, found that the presence or the amount of intraperitoneal fluid was not a reliable indicator of rupture. Rupture was present in 21% of patients with no fluid and increasingly up to 63% with large amounts. Interestingly, 37% of patients with a large amount of fluid had intact tubes and no evidence of rupture. This is possible if the blood escapes through the fimbriated end of the intact fallopian tube.[97]

Ectopic pregnancy may occur in several sites. Approximately 95% of ectopic pregnancies occur in the ampullary or isthmic portions of the fallopian tube.[98] The second most common site—approximately 2% to 3% of all ectopics—is an interstitial pregnancy occurring in the intramural portion of the tube where it traverses the wall of the uterus to enter the endometrial canal. Ovarian, cervical, and abdominal sites of ectopic pregnancy are extremely rare.

Because of their intramural location, **interstitial ectopic pregnancies** (cornual) rupture later than other tubal gestations, often causing massive intraperitoneal hemorrhage from the dilated arcuate arteries and veins which lie in the outer third of the myometrium between the thin outer myometrium and the thick intermediate layer. The mortality of interstitial pregnancy is twice that of other tubal ectopics. Ackerman et al.[99] found that the two currently used signs are unreliable and then described a more useful **interstitial line sign** (Fig. 32-31). The interstitial line is a thin echogenic line extending from the endometrial canal up to the cornual sac or hemorrhagic

A

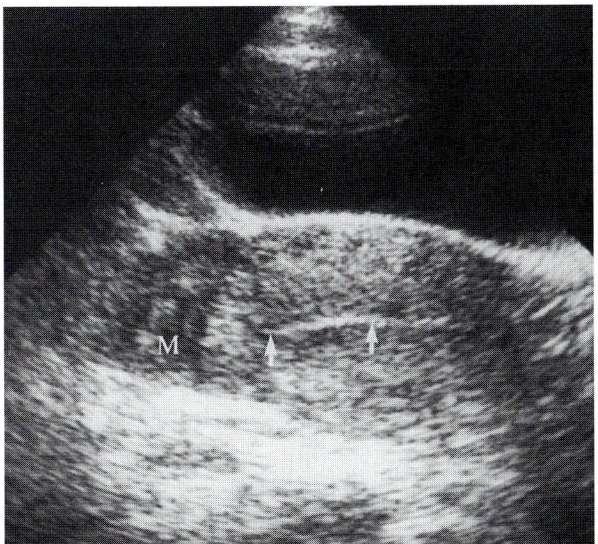

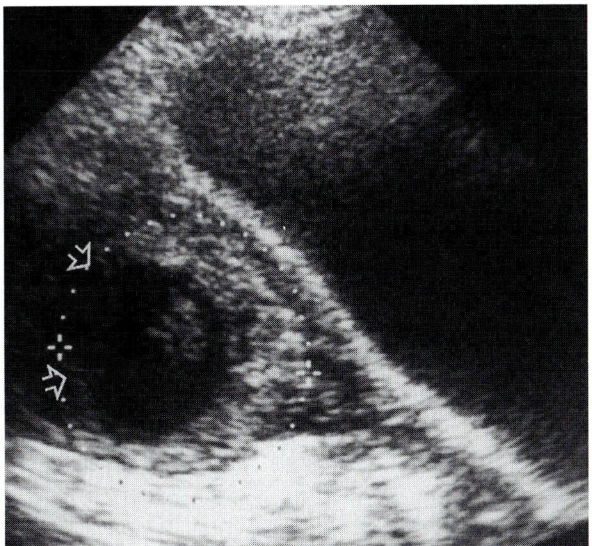

B

FIG. 32-31. Right interstitial pregnancy. A, Transvesical sonography in transverse plane shows eccentrically located gestational sac. Echogenic trophoblastic ring (M) abuts endometrial canal (*arrows*), indicating its interstitial location. **B,** Transvesical sonography through gestational sac (calipers) shows thin mantle of myometrium (*open arrows*).

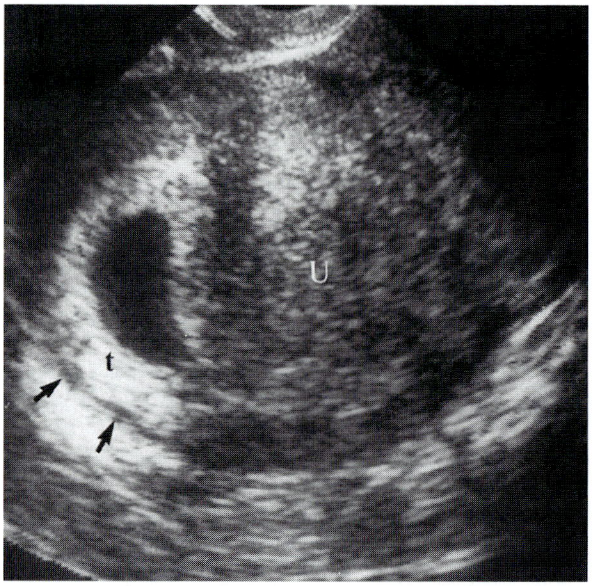

FIG. 32-32. Right interstitial pregnancy. Endovaginal sonography shows eccentrically located sac with thin mantle of myometrium (*arrows*) surrounding trophoblast (t). U—uterus.

mass. It was seen in 92% of interstitial ectopics in a retrospective 7-year study. Thinning of the myometrial mantle (Fig. 32-32) was seen in 3 of 4 interstitial sacs, however, 8 additional patients only had a mass with no sac, and therefore, no mantle thinning or eccentricity of the sac. All of these had an interstitial line. The line is thin because it does not contain any thick echogenic decidual tissue which is confined to the endometrial canal and does not extend out into the intramural portion of the fallopian tube.

Taylor et al.[100] demonstrated **trophoblastic Doppler flow signals** (high velocity, low impedance) in 54% of ectopic pregnancies. The peak-systolic frequencies were in the range of 2 to 4 KHz with diastolic frequencies in the range of 1 to 2.5 KHz. Although there is overlap, they distinguished this pattern from corpus luteal signals, which have a lower-velocity, low-impedance ovarian waveform and from the high-impedance pattern of the nonfunctioning ovary. The addition of EVS and color-flow Doppler imaging should improve Doppler diagnosis of ectopic pregnancy by further characterizing the trophoblastic flow in ectopic and intrauterine gestations.

Achiron et al.[101] studied 42 consecutive ectopics and 19 intrauterine gestations all of which were suspected ectopics. All were stable with a positive β-hCG. They compared standard two-dimensional imaging with transvaginal color Doppler. Trophoblastic flow (high velocity, low impedance) seen outside the uterus had a sensitivity of only 48% although their presence within the uterus or absence outside, excluded an ectopic with a specificity of 89%. The positive predictive value for ectopics was 91% and for two-dimensional imaging was 95%, whereas the negative predictive values were 89% for imaging and 44% for Doppler. These data suggest that Doppler has a significantly lower sensitivity and negative predictive value and do not provide more useful diagnostic information than two-dimensional imaging alone for a stable patient with a suspected ectopic pregnancy.

Management and Future Applications

The conventional management of ectopic pregnancy has been **surgical,** with resection of the diseased tube. Improved diagnostic capabilities, including EVS, allow for earlier diagnosis and the potential of a more conservative approach to treatment. The ultimate goal is to diagnose the ectopic pregnancy before tubal rupture and to treat it in such a manner as to minimize tubal scarring while maintaining tubal patency.

Laparoscopy is often used for definitive diagnosis in ectopic pregnancy. More recently, it has been used for the more conservative surgical procedures such as salpingotomy.[102] The diseased tube is incised and microdissection is used to remove the gestational sac; the incision is then left to heal by secondary intention. The rate of subsequent intrauterine pregnancy in these surgical patients is 61.4% with a 15% rate of recurrent ectopic.[103]

Medical management has also been successful in the treatment of early ectopic pregnancy. Cell-growth inhibitors, such as methotrexate, are injected systemically (IV or IM or oral administration) and the serum β-hCG levels are followed closely. The methotrexate kills the rapidly dividing trophoblastic cells, which are then reabsorbed, resulting in falling β-hCG levels and, ideally, preservation of the tubal lumen.[104] Success rates are generally in the range of 92% with 21% rate of side effects with parenteral administration and 70% to 95% success with local injection under ultrasonic guidance.[103] The rate of side effects with local injection was only 2%—significantly lower than with parenteral administration. The success rates of conception in this group were 58% for an intrauterine gestation and a 9% recurrent ectopic rate. Conservative management is becoming more common for the stable patient with low or declining levels of β-hCG. Success rates of up to 69.2% have been reported.[103]

EVALUATION OF THE EMBRYO

As the resolution of ultrasound equipment improves, visualization of embryologic anatomic structures becomes possible. Although the possibility of early diagnosis of fetal anomalies appears to be the natural progression, it is critical that incorrect decisions are not made on the basis of incomplete understanding of normal and abnormal anatomy in the first trimester. Therefore, a

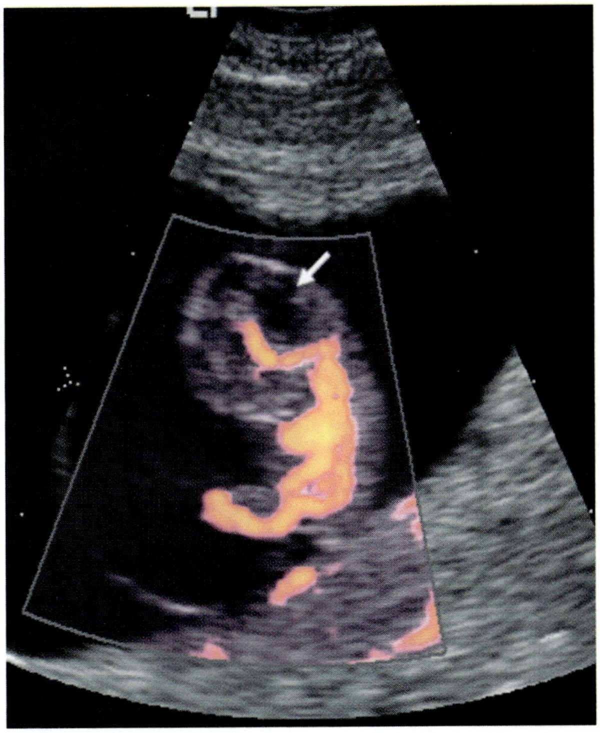

FIG. 32-33. Normal embryonic intracranial anatomy and intra- and extracranial power Doppler flow in a 9-week embryo going for therapeutic abortion. The arrow is pointing to the fourth ventricle.

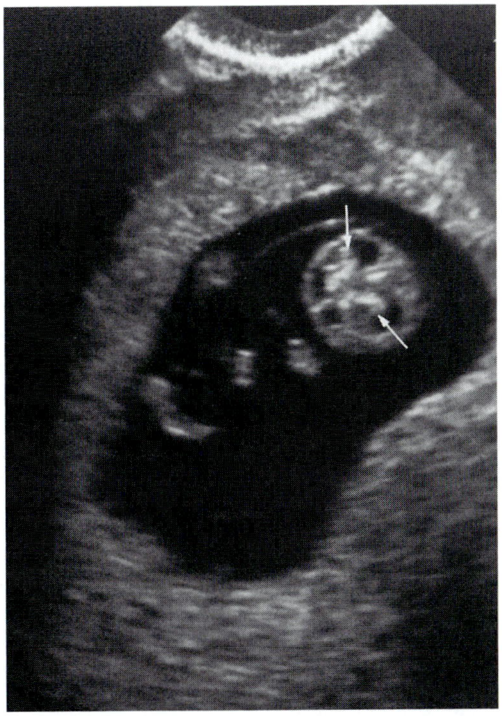

FIG. 32-34. Normal embryonic intracranial anatomy at 10 weeks of menstrual age. Endovaginal sonography shows axial view of lateral ventricles and choroid plexus (*arrows*).

follow-up sonographic examination may be indicated for evaluation of fetal morphologic characteristics in the second trimester between 16 to 19 weeks.

Three major points should be considered: (1) normal embryologic development; (2) normal-appearing abnormal embryos; and (3) discrepancies between dates and embryo size.

Normal Embryologic Development

Normal embryologic development in the first trimester **may mimic pathologic changes** more commonly seen in the second and third trimester.

Intracranial Cystic Structures in the First Trimester

During the sixth week, three primary brain vesicles form the **prosencephalon** (forebrain), the **mesencephalon** (midbrain), and the **rhombencephalon** (hindbrain).[105] Small cystic structures can be seen normally in the posterior aspect of the embryonic head. The earliest cystic structure seen at 6 to 8 weeks represents the normal embryonic **rhombencephalon,** which later forms the normal fourth ventricle and should not be mistaken for a posterior fossa cyst of pathologic significance (Fig. 32-33).[106] The prosencephalon divides into an anterior portion known as the **telencephalon** and a posterior **diencephalon.** The telencephalic vesicles later form the lateral ventricles, and the diencephalon (and to a lesser degree the telencephalon) forms the third ventricle. After approximately 9 weeks, the third ventricle and lateral ventricles can be identified sonographically as three small cystic spaces in the embryonic head (Fig. 32-34).

By 12 weeks of menstrual age, the lateral ventricles extend almost to the inner table of the skull, and on sonography, only a small rim of cerebral cortex can be demonstrated to surround them. The choroid plexus is echogenic and fills the lateral ventricles completely except for the frontal horns.

Physiologic Anterior Abdominal Wall Herniation

During embryogenesis, the midgut normally herniates into the umbilical cord at the beginning of the eighth week. The midgut rotates 90° counterclockwise and then returns to the abdomen during the twelfth week. As the midgut returns to the abdomen, further rotation occurs, completing the normal rotation of the midgut.

Schmidt et al.[107] described the normal physiologic appearance of the anterior abdominal wall during this period. The herniated bowel appeared as a small echogenic mass (6 to 9 mm) protruding into the cord

A

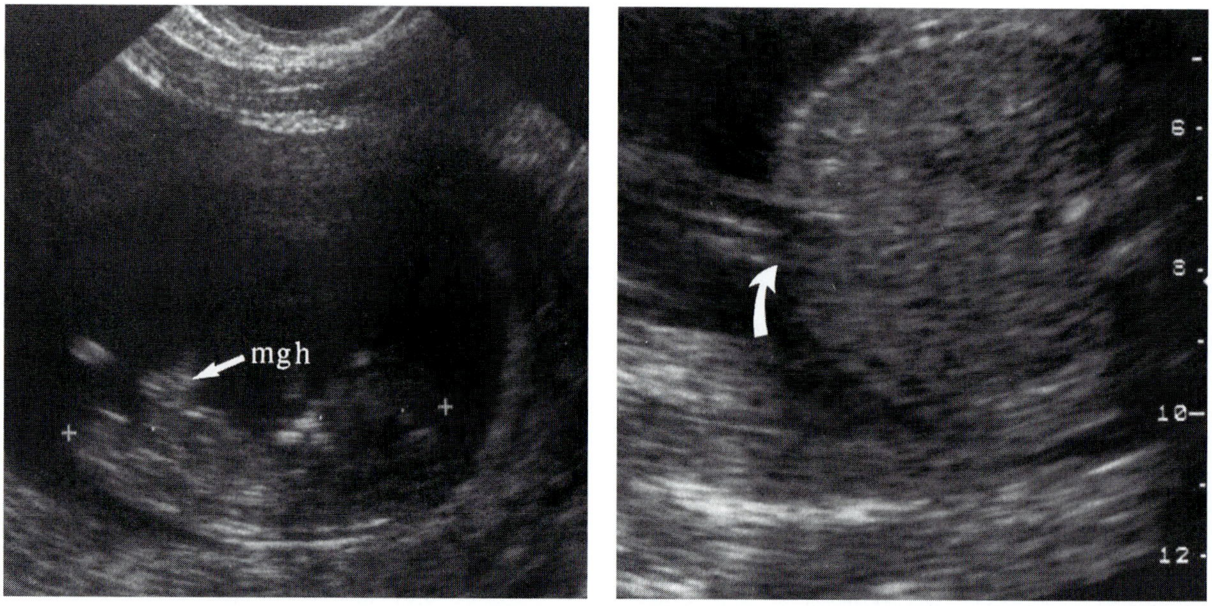

B

FIG. 32-35. Physiologic midgut herniation into umbilical cord. **A,** Transvesical sonography at 11.5 weeks menstrual age. mgh—Physiologic midgut hernia. **B,** At 24 weeks, cord insertion (*curved arrow*) is normal with no evidence of bowel herniation.

at approximately 8 weeks of menstrual age (CRL approximately 17 to 20 mm). The echogenic mass decreased to a size of approximately 5 to 6 mm at 9 weeks (CRL 23 to 26 mm). The size of the mass of herniated bowel varied considerably from one embryo to another. Follow-up examinations revealed reduction of the hernia between 10 and 12 weeks. In up to 20% of normal pregnancies, the herniated bowel may still be found outside the fetal abdomen at 12 weeks (Fig. 32-35).

Normal-Appearing Abnormal Embryos

Many grossly **abnormal embryos may appear normal** in the first trimester.

Anencephaly. Anencephaly results from failure of the rostral neuropore to close (normal closure occurs at approximately 42 days of menstrual age). The resultant abnormality is absence of the bony calvarium. The sonographic diagnosis depends on the absence of the cranial vault superior to the level of the skull base and the orbits. A variable amount of neural tissue (usually grossly deformed) may be present superior to the orbital line, but with time, it is usually eroded away. In classic anencephaly, the neural tissue superior to the orbital line should be absent. This finding, however, is seen in the second trimester of pregnancy. The diagnosis of anencephaly should be made with 100% accuracy after 14 weeks of menstrual age. In a series by Goldstein and Filly,[108] one case of anencephaly was missed at 12.5 weeks. In our own experience, we have missed a case of anencephaly at 8 weeks. The cranial vault does not appear as an echogenic line until late in the first trimester, and failure of the cranial vault to form cannot be demonstrated with certainty before that time (Fig. 32-36).

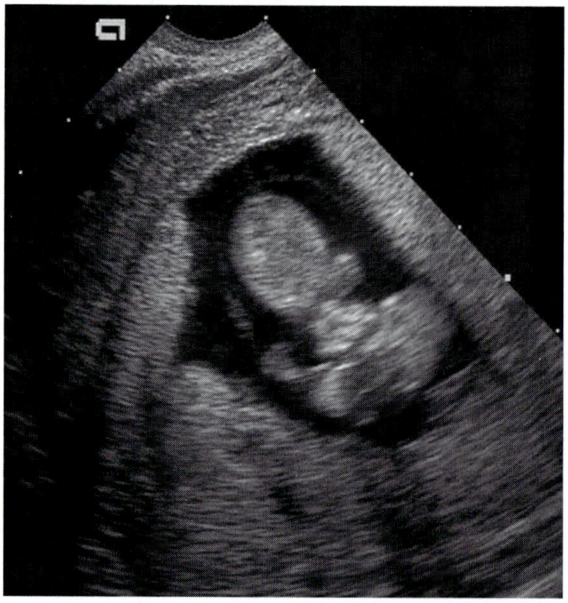

FIG. 32-36. Anencephalic fetus at 11 weeks menstrual age. This coronal scan shows a large irregular cranial end inferiorly with no visible echogenic calvarium. Calvarial echogenicity might not be seen this early in gestation.

Other Fetal Abnormalities

Nuchal Thickening. The appearance of a lucency in the nuchal region has been used recently in the diagnosis of fetal aneuploidy. Van Vugt et al.[109] studied 102 fetuses in the first trimester with a nuchal translucency of greater than 3 mm and found an abnormal karyotype in 46% overall. Septated translucencies in women under 35 years of age had the highest risk for aneuploidy. There was a two hundredfold increased risk for an abnormal karyotype in women under 34 years of age with a septated lucency and a twentyfold increase in women 35 years of age and older. For a nonseptated lucency, the risk was increased twenty-sevenfold and ninefold, respectively. These compared the rate of aneuploidy in women with no lucency who were going for chorionic villus sampling.[109] They also found a 27% incidence of associated anomalies, although there was a higher than normal prevalence of anomalies in their selected population.

In a subsequent article, Reynders et al.[110] looked at first-trimester fetuses with no identifiable anomalies other than an isolated localized nuchal lucency of 3 mm or more. Five of 41 (12%) had abnormal karyotypes and an additional 6 had a poor outcome.

Although it is possible to visualize many normal fetal structures in the first trimester, it is currently necessary to wait until the mid-second trimester to diagnose most sonographically detectable fetal anomalies. The fetal stomach can be seen in 93% of fetuses by 12 weeks.[69] The fetal kidneys and adrenals can be demonstrated by approximately 9 weeks of menstrual age. By 12 weeks, the bladder can be seen in 50% of fetuses. The limbs form as buds at approximately 40 days (5 weeks and 5 days) of menstrual age and are paddle shaped from approximately 46 to 55 days of menstrual age. By 64 days (9 weeks and 1 day), the upper limbs are bent at the elbows and the fingers are distinct.[5] With the advent of high-resolution EVS, earlier (first-trimester) diagnosis of some fetal anomalies may be possible. It is likely, however, that many or most anomalies may still be second-trimester diagnoses for anatomic and physiologic reasons. For example, nonvisualization of the kidneys and bladder may suggest renal agenesis in the first trimester; however, it is not until the second trimester that associated oligohydramnios will demonstrate the lack of renal function. In our zeal to make earlier diagnoses, we should not lose sight of the embryologic and physiologic changes that normally occur in this period of rapid change.

Discrepancy Between Dates and Embryo Size

A major discrepancy between dates and embryologic size may be the only sonographic indicator of an embryonic abnormality in the first trimester. Although discrepancy between the estimated menstrual age by sonographic CRL and menstrual history is common, a major discrepancy in dates may result from growth retardation in the first trimester.[111] First-trimester intrauterine growth retardation is usually related to gross fetal abnormality (often genetic), or the result of viral infection. In a recent article, Benacerraf described a patient with first-trimester growth retardation associated with triploidy.

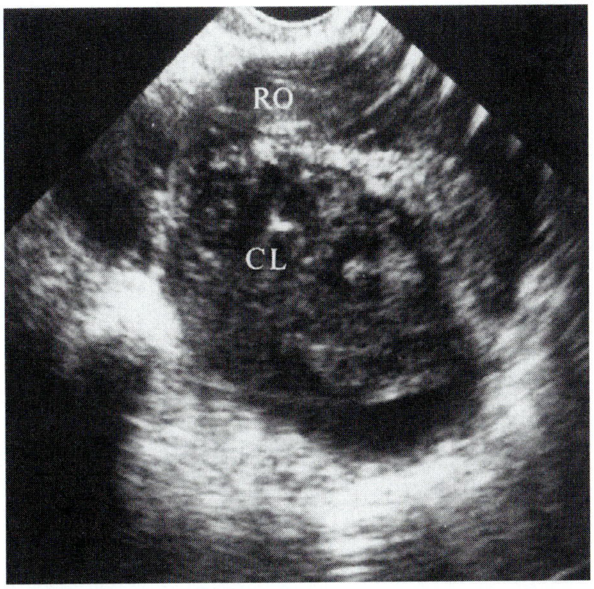

FIG. 32-37. Hemorrhagic corpus luteum cyst at 6 weeks of menstrual age. Endovaginal sonography parasagittal plane to right of midline shows oval echogenic cystic mass (CL) with internal debris (arising from right ovary [RO]). (From Levi CS, Lyons EA, Lindsay DJ. Ultrasound in the first trimester of pregnancy. *Radiol Clin North Am* 1990;28:19-38.)

FIRST TRIMESTER MASSES

Ovarian Masses

The most common mass seen in the first trimester of pregnancy is the **corpus luteum cyst.**[112] The corpus luteum cyst secretes progesterone to support the pregnancy until the placenta can take over its hormonal function. The corpus luteum forms in the secretory phase of the menstrual cycle and increases in size if a pregnancy occurs. The corpus luteum of pregnancy is usually less than 5 cm in diameter and most commonly appears as a thin-walled, unilocular cyst.[112] The appearance of the corpus luteum cyst, however, may vary considerably. Corpus luteum cysts may be much larger, occasionally attaining a size of greater than 10 cm. Internal septation and echogenic debris may be present secondary to internal hemorrhage (Fig. 32-37). The cyst wall and septation may be markedly thick.[113] Clearly, a

A

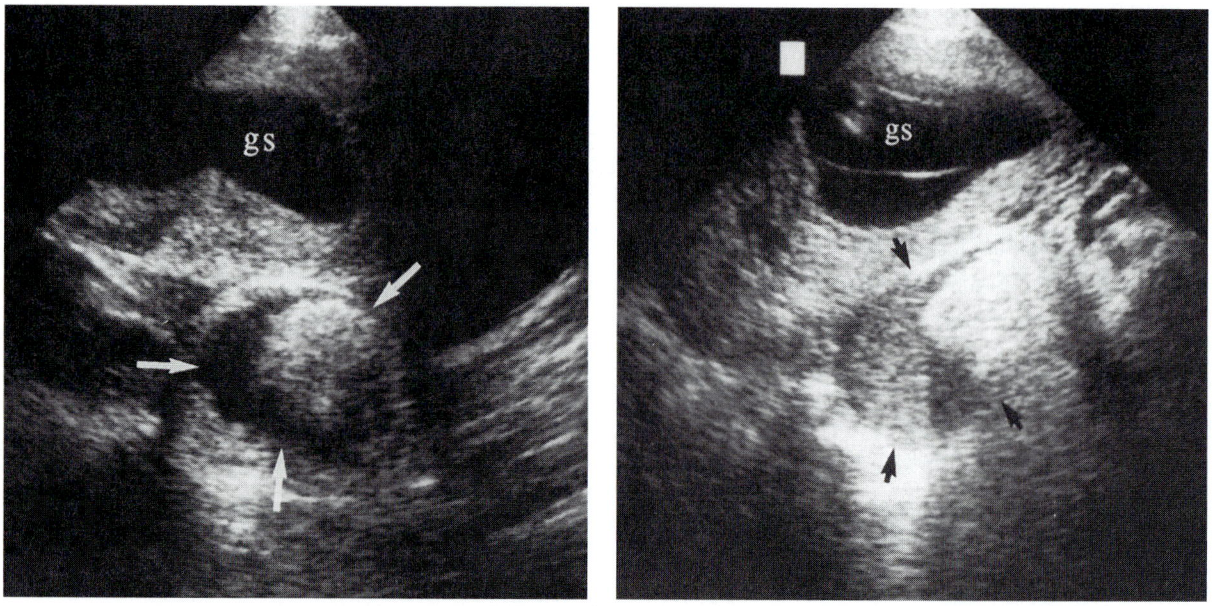

B

FIG. 32-38. Dermoid cyst (*arrows*) at 12 weeks of menstrual age associated with single live fetus. Transvesical sonography in longitudinal (**A**) and transverse (**B**) planes. Dermoid cyst ruptured at 20 weeks, resulting in surgical intervention. gs—Gestational sac. (From Levi CS, Lyons EA, Lindsay DJ. Ultrasound in the first trimester of pregnancy. *Radiol Clin North Am* 1990;28:19-38.)

hemorrhagic corpus luteum cyst may be impossible to differentiate from a pathologic cyst on the basis of a single ultrasound examination. Corpus luteum cysts usually regress or have decreased in size on follow-up sonographic examination at 16 to 18 weeks of menstrual age. Cystic masses that persist should be followed up. Surgical intervention is often indicated in large cysts that do not regress by the mid-second trimester. It should be noted, however, that not all corpus luteum cysts regress, and differentiation from a pathologic cyst may be impossible on sonography.

Other cystic masses may present for the first time in the first trimester of pregnancy because of displacement by the enlarged uterus. Torsion, rupture, and dystocia have all been described as complications of ovarian cystic masses associated with pregnancy. Malignant ovarian neoplasm associated with pregnancy is rare. When elective surgical intervention is indicated, it is usually performed in the second trimester when the likelihood of inducing premature labor is considered to be lowest. Dermoid cysts may present the characteristic appearance of a cystic mass with focal calcification and a fluid-fluid level (Fig. 32-38). Other cystic masses may be more difficult to differentiate from corpus luteum cysts. All cysts should be observed carefully to assess change in size.

Uterine Masses

Uterine fibroids are a common pelvic mass often identified during pregnancy. Most fibroids do not change in size during pregnancy. Some fibroids, however, may enlarge rapidly as a result of stimulation by estrogen. Infarction and necrosis may occur because of rapid growth.[69] These patients often experience pain. Sonographically, uterine fibroids appear as solid uterine masses that attenuate sound to a variable degree, may or may not be calcified, and may have focal cystic areas related to necrosis. Fibroids may be differentiated from focal myometrial contractions by the transient nature of myometrial contractions. A repeat examination 20 to 30 minutes after the initial examination reveals disappearance of a focal myometrial contraction, whereas a fibroid will still be present. Fibroids also may distort the uterine contour (serosal surface), whereas focal myometrial contractions usually do not.

ACKNOWLEDGMENT

We wish to acknowledge the following author's participation in the successful accomplishment of this chapter: Susan C. Holt, MD, FRCP(C), Lecturer, Diagnostic Radiology; Health Sciences Centre, Winnipeg, Manitoba, Canada.

REFERENCES

1. Moore KL. The beginning of development: the first week. In: Moore KL, editor. *The Developing Human: Clinically Oriented Embryology.* ed 4. Philadelphia: WB Saunders; 1988:13-37.
2. Moore KL. Formation of the bilaminar embryo: the second week. In: Moore KL, editor. *The Developing Human: Clinically Oriented Embryology.* ed 4. Philadelphia: WB Saunders; 1988:38-49.
3. Moore KL. Formation of the trilaminar embryo: the third week, In: Moore KL, editor. *The Developing Human: Clinically Oriented Embryology.* ed 4. Philadelphia: WB Saunders; 1988:50-64.
4. Moore KL. Formation of basic organs and systems: the fourth to eighth weeks. In: Moore KL, editor. *The Developing Human: Clinically Oriented Embryology.* ed 4. Philadelphia: WB Saunders; 1988:65-86.
5. Moore KL. The fetal period: the ninth week to birth. In: Moore KL, editor. *The Developing Human: Clinically Oriented Embryology.* ed 4. Philadelphia: WB Saunders; 1988:87-103.
6. Levi CS, Lyons EA, Lindsay DJ. Early diagnosis of nonviable pregnancy with endovaginal ultrasound. *Radiology* 1988; 167:383-385.
7. Levi CS, Lyons EA, Zheng XH et al. Endovaginal ultrasound: demonstration of cardiac activity in embryos of less than 5.0 mm in crown-rump length. *Radiology* 1990;176(1):71-74.

Formation of the Embryo

8. Jones GS, Jones HW. Physiology of menstruation and pregnancy. In: Jones GS, Jones HW, editors. *Gynecology.* ed 3. Baltimore: Williams & Wilkins; 1982:9-45.
9. Jones GS, Jones HW. Cyclical cytology and histology. In: Jones GS, Jones HW, editors. *Gynecology.* ed 3. Baltimore: Williams & Wilkins; 1982:46-68.
10. Hustin J: Vascular physiology and pathophysiology of early pregnancy. In Bourne T, Jauniaux E, and Jurkovic D, editors. *Transvaginal Color Doppler,* Heidelberg: Springer-Verlag, 47-56.
11. Jauniaux E: Intervillous circulation in the first trimester: the phantom of the Doppler obstetric opera. editorial. *Ultras Obstet Gynecol* 1996;8:73-76.
12. Hustin J, Jauniaux E, Schaaps JP. Histological study of the materno-embryonic interface in spontaneous abortion. *Placenta* 1990;11:477-486.

Sonography of Normal Uterine Gestation

13. Kawakami-Y; Andoh-K; Mizunuma-H; et al: Assessment of the implantation site by transvaginal ultrasonography. *Fertil Steril* 1993;59:1003-1006.
14. Yeh H-C, Goodman JD, Carr L et al. Intradecidual sign: a ultrasound criterion of early intrauterine pregnancy. *Radiology* 1986;161:463-467.
15. Pellicer A, Calatayud C, Miro F et al. Comparison of implantation and early development of human embryos fertilized *in vitro* versus *in vivo* using transvaginal ultrasound. *J Ultras Med* 1991 Jan; 10(1):31-35.
16. Keith SC, O'Brien TJ, London SN et al. Serial transvaginal ultrasound scans and B-human chorionic gonadotropin levels in early singleton and multiple pregnancies *Fertil Steril* 1993;59:1007-1010.
17. Sengoku K, Tamate K, Ishikawa M et al. Transvaginal ultrasonographic findings and hCG levels in early intrauterine pregnancies. *Nippon-Sanka-Fujinka-Gakkai-Zasshi* 1991; 43:535-540.
18. Filly RA. The first trimester. In: Callen PW, editor. *Ultrasonography in Obstetrics and Gynecology.* ed 2. Philadelphia: WB Saunders, 1988:19-46.
19. Keith SC, London SN, Weitzman GA et al. Serial transvaginal ultrasound scans and beta-human chorionic gonadotropin levels in early singleton and multiple pregnancies. *Fertil Steril* 1993;59:1007-1010.
20. Daya S, Woods S, Ward S, Lappalainen R, Caco C. Early pregnancy assessment with transvaginal ultrasound scanning. *Can Med Assoc J* 1991;144:441-446.
21. Nyberg DA, Filly RA, Mahony BS et al. Early gestation: correlation of HCG levels and sonographic identification. *AJR* 1985;144:951-954.
22. Nyberg DA, Mack LA, Laing FC et al. Early pregnancy complications: endovaginal sonographic findings correlated with human chorionic gonadotropin levels. *Radiology* 1988;167: 619-622.
23. Nyberg DA, Filly RA, Laing FC et al: Ectopic pregnancy: diagnosis by sonography correlated with quantitative HCG levels. *J Ultra Med* 1987;6(3):145-150.
24. Nyberg DA, Laing FC, Filly RA et al. Ultrasonographic differentiation of the gestational sac of early intrauterine pregnancy from the pseudogestational sac of ectopic pregnancy. *Radiology* 1983;146:755-759.
25. Lyons EA, Levi CS. The first trimester. *Radiol Clin North Am* 1982:20:259.
26. Parvey RH, Dubinsky TJ, Johnston DA, Maklad NF. The chorionic rim and low-impedance intrauterine arterial flow in the diagnosis of early intrauterine pregnancy: Evaluation of efficacy. *AJR* 1996;167:1479-1485.
27. Birnholz JC, Madanes AE. Amniotic fluid accumulation in the first trimester. *J Ultra Med* 1995;14:597-602.
28. Emerson DS, Carter MS, Altieri LA et al: Diagnostic efficacy of endovaginal color flow imaging in an ectopic pregnancy screening program. *Radiology* 183:413, 1992.
29. Nyberg DA, Laing FA, Filly RA: Threatened abortion: sonographic distinction of normal and abnormal gestation sacs. *Radiology* 1986;158:397-400.
30. Nyberg DA, Mack LA, Harvey D et al. Value of the yolk sac in evaluating early pregnancies. *J Ultrasound Med* 1988; 7(3):129-135.
31. Lindsay DJ, Lovett IS, Lyons EA, Levi CS et al: Yolk sac diameter and shape at endovaginal US: predictors of pregnancy outcome in the first trimester. *Radiology* 1992;183:115-118.
32. Levi CS, Lyons EA, Dashefsky SM et al. Yolk sac number, size and morphologic features in monochorionic monoamniotic twin pregnancy. *Can Assoc Radiol J* 1996;47:98-100.
33. Kurjak A, Kupesic S, Kostovic L. Vascularization of yolk sac and vitelline duct in normal pregnancies studied by transvaginal color and pulsed Doppler. *J Perinat Med* 1994; 22:433-440.
34. Yeh H-C, Rabinowitz JG. Amniotic sac development: ultrasound features of early pregnancy—the double bleb sign. *Radiology* 1988;166(1):97-103.
35. Levi CS, Lyons EA, Lindsay DJ. Ultrasound in the first trimester of pregnancy. *Radiol Clin North Am* 1990;28:19-38.
36. Kaufman AJ, Fleischer AC, Thieme GA et al. Separated chorioamnion and elevated chorion: sonographic features and clinical significance. *J Ultrasound Med* 1985;4(3):119-125.
37. Zimmer EZ, Bronshtein M. Ultrasound observation of amnion dysmorphism at 14.5-16 weeks. *Prenat Diagn* 1995; 15:447-449.
38. Wehbeh H, Fleisher J, Karimi A, et al. The relationship between the ultrasonographic diagnosis of innocent amniotic band development and pregnancy outcomes. *Obstet Gynecol* 1993;81:565-568.
39. Mahony BS, Filly RA, Callen PW. Amnionicity & chorionicity in twin pregnancies: using ultrasound. *Radiology* 1985;155: 205-209.

40. Cadkin AV, McAlpin J. Detection of fetal cardiac activity between 41 and 43 days of gestation. *J Ultrasound Med* 1984; 3(11):499-503.
41. Ragavendra N, McMahon JT, Perrella RR et al. Endoluminal catheter-assisted transcervical US of the human embryo. Work in progress. *Radiology* 1991;181:779-783.

Umbilical Cord and Cord Cyst

42. Hill LM, DiNofrio DM, Guzick-D. Sonographic determination of first trimester umbilical cord length. *J Clin Ultra* 1994; 22:435-438.
43. Skibo LK, Lyons EA, Levi CS. First trimester umbilical cord cysts. *Radiology* 1992;182:719-722.

Estimation of Menstrual Age in the First Trimester

44. Kurtz AB, Needleman L. Ultrasound assessment of fetal age. In: Callen PW, editor. *Ultrasonography in Obstetrics and Gynecology*. ed 2. Philadelphia: WB Saunders, 1988:47-64.
45. Hadlock FP, Deter RL, Harrist RB et al. Estimating fetal age: computer-assisted analysis of multiple fetal growth parameters. *Radiology* 1984;152:497-501.
46. Hadlock FP, Harrist RB, Shah YP et al. Estimating fetal age using multiple parameters: a prospective evaluation in a racially mixed population. *Am J Obstet Gynecol* 1987;156: 955-957.
47. Filly RA. Appropriate use of ultrasound in early pregnancy. *Radiology* 1988;166:274-275.

Embryonic Demise

48. Wilcox AJ, Weinberg CR, O'Connor JF et al. Incidence of early loss of pregnancy. *N Engl J Med* 1988;319:189-194.
49. Bateman BG, Felder R, Kolp LA. et al. Subclinical pregnancy loss in clomiphene citrate treated women. *Fertil Steril* 1992; 57:25-27.
50. Hertig AT, Rock J. A series of potentially abortive ova recovered from fertile women prior to the first missed menstrual period. *Am J Obstet Gynecol* 1949;58:968-993.
51. Hertig AT, Rock J, Adams BC, Menkin MC. Thirty-four fertilized human ova, good, bad and indifferent, recovered from 210 women of known fertility: a study of biologic wastage in early human pregnancy. *Pediatrics* 1959;23:202-211.
52. Sorokin Y, Johnson MP, Uhlmann WR et al. Postmortem chorionic villus sampling: correlation of cytogenetic and ultrasound findings. *Am J Med Genet* 1991;39:314-316.
53. Blumenfeld Z, Ruach M. Early pregnancy wastage: the role of repetitive human chorionic gonadotrophin supplementation during the first 8 weeks of gestation. *Fertil Steril* 1992;58:19-23.
54. Goldstein SR. Embryonic death in early pregnancy: a new look at the first trimester. *Obstet Gynecol* 1994;84:294-297.
55. Filly RA. Ultrasound evaluation during the first trimester. In: Callen PW (editor): *Ultrasonography in Obstetrics and Gynecology*, ed 3, Philadelphia: WB Saunders, 1994;63-85.
56. Scott JR. Early pregnancy loss. In Scott JR, DiSaia PJ, Hammond CB, et al editors: *Danforth's Obstetrics and Gynecology*, ed 7. Philadelphia, JB Lippincott, 1994, p 175.
57. Falco P, Milano V, Pilu G, et al. Sonography of pregnancies with first trimester bleeding and a viable embryo: a study of prognostic indicators by logistic regression analysis. *Ultra Obstet Gynecol* 1996;7:165-169.
58. Pandya PP, Snijders RJM, Psara N, et al. The prevalence of non-viable pregnancy at 10-13 weeks of gestation. *Ultra Obstet Gynecol* 1996;7:170-173.
59. Zheng XH. Early diagnosis of nonviable pregnancy with endovaginal ultrasound CRL versus menstrual age. Unpublished data.
60. Cashner KA, Christopher CR, Dysert GA. Spontaneous fetal loss after demonstration of a live fetus in the first trimester. *Obstet Gynecol* 1987;70:827-830.
61. Wilson RD, Kendrick V, Wittmann BK, McGillivray B. Spontaneous abortion and pregnancy outcome after normal first-trimester ultrasound examination. *Obstet Gynecol* 1986; 67:352-355.
62. Simpson JL. Incidence and timing of pregnancy losses: relevance to evaluating safety of early prenatal diagnosis. *Am J Med Genet* 1990;35:165-173.
63. Bernard KG, Cooperberg PL. Sonographic differentiation between blighted ovum and early viable pregnancy. *AJR* 1985;144:597-602.
64. Nyberg DA, Mack LA, Laing FC et al. Distinguishing normal from abnormal gestational sac growth in early pregnancy. *J Ultra Med* 1987;6:23-26.
65. Doubilet PM, Benson CB. Embryonic heart rate in the early first trimester; What rate is normal? *J Ultra Med* 1995; 14:431-434.
66. Kurtz AB, Needleman L, Pennell RG, et al. Can detection of the yolk sac in the first trimester be used to predict the outcome of pregnancy? A prospective sonographic study. *AJR* 1992;158:843-847.
67. Pedersen JF, Molsted-Pedersen L, Mortensen HB. Fetal growth delay and maternal hemoglobin A 1 c in early diabetic pregnancy. *Obstet Gynecol* 1984;64:351-352.
68. Green JJ, Hobbins JC. Abdominal ultrasound examination of the first trimester fetus. *Am J Obstet Gynecol* 1988;159:165-175.
69. Harris RD, Vincent LM, Askin FB. Yolk sac calcification: a sonographic finding associated with intrauterine embryonic demise in the first trimester. *Radiology* 1988;166:109-110.
70. Nyberg DA, Filly RA, Filho DRD et al. Abnormal pregnancy: early diagnosis by US and serum chorionic gonadotropin levels. *Radiology* 1986;158:393-396.
71. Nyberg DA, Cyr DR, Mack LA et al. Sonographic spectrum of placental abruption. *AJR* 1987;148:161-164.
72. Bennet GL, Bromley B, Lieberman E, Benacerraf BR. Subchorionic hemorrhage in first trimester pregnancies: Prediction of pregnancy outcome with sonography. *Radiology* 1996;200:803-806.
73. Jaffe R, Dorgan A, Abramowicz JS. Color Doppler imaging of the uteroplacental circulation in the first trimester: value in predicting pregnancy failure or complication. *AJR* 1995; 164:1255-1258.
74. Taylor KJW, Ramos IM, Feycock AL et al. Ectopic pregnancy: duplex Doppler evaluation. *Radiology* 1989;173:93-97.
75. Horrow MM: Enlarged amniotic cavity: a new sonographic sign of early embryonic death. *Am J Roentgenol* 1992; 158:359-362.

Ectopic Pregnancy

76. Atrash HK, Friede A, Hogue CJR. Ectopic pregnancy mortality in the Unites States, 1970-1983. *Obstet Gynecol* 1987;70:817-822.
77. Lawson HW, Atrash HK, Saftlas AF et al. Ectopic pregnancy surveillance, Unites States, 1970-1985. *MMWR CDC Surveill Summ* 1988;37:9-18.
78. Schwartz RO, Di Pietro DL. β-hCG as a diagnostic aid for suspected ectopic pregnancy. *Obstet Gynecol* 1980;56(2): 197-203.
79. Ackerman TE, Levi CS, Lyons EA et al. Decidual cyst: Endovaginal sonographic sign of ectopic pregnancy. *Radiology* 1993;189:727-731.
80. Nagamani M, London S, St. Amand P. Factors influencing fertility after ectopic pregnancy. *Am J Obstet Gynecol* 1984; 149:533-535.

81. Schoen JA, Nowak RJ. Repeat ectopic pregnancy: a 16 year clinical survey. *Obstet Gynecol* 1975;45:542-546.
82. Couplet E. Ectopic pregnancy: the surgical epidemic. *J Natl Med Assoc* 1989;81(5):567-572.
83. Rein MS, Di Salvo DN, Friedman AJ. Heterotopic pregnancy associated with *in vitro* fertilization and embryo transfer: a possible role for routine vaginal ultrasound. *Fertil Steril* 1989;51(6):1057-1058.
84. Hann LE, Bachman DM, McArdle CR. Coexistent intrauterine and ectopic pregnancy: a reevaluation. *Radiology* 1984;152:151-154.
85. Wong WSF, Mao K. Combined intrauterine and tubal ectopic pregnancy. *Aust NZ J Obstet Gynecol* 1989;29:76-77.
86. Dashefsky SM, Lyons EA, Levi CS et al. Suspected ectopic pregnancy: endovaginal and transvesical ultrasound. *Radiology* 1988;169:181-184.
87. Fleischer AC, Pennell RG, McKee MS et al. Ectopic pregnancy: features at transvaginal sonography. *Radiology* 1990; 174:375-378.
88. Dillon EH, Feycock AL, Taylor KJW. Pseudogestational sacs: Doppler ultrasound differentiation from normal or abnormal intrauterine pregnancies. *Radiology* 1990;176(2):359-364.
89. Timor-Tritsch IE, Yeh MN, Peisner DB et al. The use of transvaginal ultrasonography in the diagnosis of ectopic pregnancy. *Obstet Gynecol* 1989;161:157-161.
90. Thorsen MK, Lawson TL, Aiman EJ et al. Diagnosis of ectopic pregnancy: endovaginal vs transabdominal sonography. *AJR* 1990;155:307-310.
91. Cacciatore B, Stenman UH, Ylostalo P. Comparison of abdominal and vaginal sonography in suspected ectopic pregnancy. *Obstet Gynecol* 1989;73:770-774.
92. Mahony BS, Filly RA, Nyberg DA et al. Sonographic evaluation of ectopic pregnancy. *J Ultra Med* 1985;4:221-228.
93. Ash KM, Lyons EA, Levi CS, Lindsay DJ. Endovaginal sonographic diagnosis of ectopic twin gestation. *J Ultra Med* 1991;10:497-500.
94. Golstein DP, Koaca TS. The subunit radioimmunoassay for hCG—clinical application. In Taymar M, Green TH, editors. *Progress in Gynecology*, vol 6. New York: Grune & Stratton; 1975:145-184.
95. Nyberg DA, Mack LA, Jeffery RB Jr, et al. Endovaginal sonographic evaluation of ectopic pregnancy: a prospective study. *AJR* 1987;149:1181-1186.
96. Frates MC, Brown DL, Doubilet PM, Hornstein MD. Tubal rupture in patients with ectopic pregnancy: diagnosis with transvaginal US. *Radiology* 1994;191:769-772.
97. Cartwright PS. Ectopic pregnancy. In: Jones HW III, Wentz AC, Burnett LC, editors. *Novak's Textbook of Gynecology*, ed 11. Baltimore: Williams & Wilkins; 1988:479-506.
98. Cartwright PS. Ectopic pregnancy. In: Jones HW III, Wentz AC, Burnett LC, editors. *Novak's Textbook of Gynecology*, ed 11. Baltimore: Williams & Wilkins; 1988:479-506.
99. Ackerman TE, Levi CS, Dashefsky SM, et al. Interstitial line: Sonographic finding in interstitial (cornual) ectopic pregnancy. *Radiology* 1993;189:83-87.
100. Taylor KW, Ramos IM, Feycock AL, et al. Ectopic pregnancy: duplex Doppler evaluation. *Radiology* 1989;173:93-97.
101. Achiron R, Goldenberg M, Lipitz S et al. Transvaginal Doppler sonography for detecting ectopic pregnancy: is it really necessary. *Isr J Med Sci* 1994;30:820-825.
102. Stangel JJ. Recent techniques for the conservative management of tubal pregnancy. *J Reprod Med* 1986;31(2):98-101.
103. Yao M, Tulandi T. Current status of surgical and nonsurgical management of ectopic pregnancy. *Fertil Steril* 1997;67:421-433.
104. Ory SJ, Villanueva AL, Sand PK et al. Conservative treatment of ectopic pregnancy with methotrexate. *Am J Obstet Gynecol* 1986;154:1299-1306.

Evaluation of the Embryo

105. Moore KL. The nervous system. In: Moore KL, editor. *The Developing Human: Clinically Oriented Embryology*. ed 4. Philadelphia: WB Saunders 1988:364-401.
106. Cyr DR, Mack LA, Nyberg DA et al. Fetal rhombencephalon: normal ultrasound findings. *Radiology* 1988;166:691-692.
107. Schmidt W, Yarkoni S, Crelin ES et al. Sonographic visualization of physiologic anterior abdominal wall hernia in the first trimester. *Obstet Gynecol* 1987;69:911-915.
108. Goldstein RB, Filly RA. Prenatal diagnosis of anencephaly: spectrum of sonographic appearances and distinction from the amniotic band syndrome. *AJR* 1988;151:547-550.
109. van Vugt JMG, van Zalen-Sprock RM, Kostense PJ. First-trimester nuchal translucency: A risk analysis on fetal chromosome abnormality. *Radiology* 1996;200:537-540.
110. Reynders CS, Pauker SP, Benacerraf BR. First trimester isolated fetal nuchal lucency: Significance and outcome. *JUM* 1997;16:101-105.
111. Benacerraf BR. Intrauterine growth retardation in the first trimester associated with triploidy. *J Ultra Med* 1988; 7(3):153-154.

First Trimester Masses

112. Fleischer AC, Boehm FH, James AE Jr. Sonographic evaluation of pelvic masses and maternal disorders occurring during pregnancy. In: Sanders RC, James AE Jr, editors. *The Principles and Practice of Ultrasonography in Obstetrics and Gynecology*, ed 3. Norwalk, CT: Appleton-Century-Crofts; 1985;435-447.
113. Pennes DR, Bowerman RA, Silver TM. Echogenic adnexal masses associated with first-trimester pregnancy: sonographic appearance and clinical significance. *J Clin Ultra* 1985;13: 391-396.

CHAPTER 33

Fetal Measurements—Normal and Abnormal Fetal Growth

Carol B. Benson, M.D.
Peter M. Doubilet, M.D., Ph.D.

CHAPTER OUTLINE

Sonographic measurements of the fetus provide information about fetal age and growth. They are used to assign gestational age, estimate fetal weight, and diagnose growth disturbances. Another use of fetal measurements, discussed in other chapters, is their contribution to the diagnosis of a number of fetal anomalies such as skeletal dysplasias[1] and microcephaly.[2] Each of these abnormalities can be diagnosed or suspected on the basis of measurements that deviate from the normal for dates.

By convention, pregnancies are dated beginning from the first day of the last menstrual period (LMP). In women with regular 28-day cycles, conception occurs approximately two weeks after the LMP. **Gestational age,** the term commonly used to date the pregnancy, is thus defined as conceptual age plus two weeks. In women with regular 28-day cycles, gestational age and **menstrual age** are the same.

Accurate knowledge of gestational age is important for a number of reasons. The timings of chorionic villous sampling in the first trimester, genetic amniocentesis in the second trimester, and elective induction or cesarean delivery in the third trimester are all based on the gestational age. The differentiation between term and preterm labor and the characterization of a fetus as postdates depend on gestational age. Knowledge of the gestational age can be critical in distinguishing normal from pathologic fetal development. Midgut herniation, for example, is normal up to 11 to 12 weeks of gestation[3] but signifies omphalocele thereafter. The normal size of a variety of fetal body parts depends on gestational age, as do levels of maternal serum alpha-fetoprotein,[4] human chorionic gonadotropin,[5] and estriol.[6]

Estimation of the fetal weight, on its own and in relation to the gestational age, can influence obstetric management decisions concerning the timing and route of delivery. Early delivery may benefit a fetus that is small for dates. Such a fetus may be inadequately supplied by its placenta with oxygen and nutrients and may therefore do better in the care of a neonatologist than in utero. When the fetus is large, cesarean section may be the preferred route of delivery, particularly in pregnancies complicated by maternal diabetes. In view of these considerations, fetal measurements should be a component of every obstetric sonogram.[7]

GESTATIONAL AGE DETERMINATION

Clinical dating of a pregnancy is usually based on the patient's recollection of the first day of her last menstrual period and on physical examination of uterine size. Unfortunately, both these methods are subject to imprecision, leading to inaccuracies in gestational age assignment. Dating by last menstrual period may be inaccurate because of variability in length of menstrual cycles, faulty memory, or bleeding during early pregnancy.[8] Determining gestational age from the palpated dimension of the uterus may be affected by uterine fibroids and maternal body habitus.

Clinical dating is accurate only if one of the following two conditions applies: first, the patient is a good historian with regular menstrual cycles and the uterine size correlates closely with the last menstrual period; second, information is available specifying the time of conception, such as a basal body temperature chart or in vitro fertilization. In cases where the pregnancy cannot be dated accurately by clinical evaluation, sonography is a useful and accurate tool for estimating gestational age.

First Trimester Gestational Dating

Sonographic milestones of early pregnancy and measurement of the embryo once it can be visualized by ultrasound allow highly accurate dating from 5 weeks' gestation until the end of the first trimester. The earliest sign of an intrauterine pregnancy is identification of a gestational sac in the uterine cavity. This appears as a round or oval fluid collection surrounded by two echogenic rings. It is first seen at approximately 5 weeks' gestation by transvaginal scanning, and at 5 to 5.5 weeks transabdominally.[9-11] A yolk sac within the gestational sac is first seen at 5.5 weeks transvaginally (Fig. 33-1), and at 5.5 to 6 weeks transabdominally. The embryonic heartbeat, which is sometimes identified even before a measurable embryo is seen, is identified at 6 weeks transvaginally (Fig. 33-2) and at 6 to 6.5 weeks transabdominally.[12] From 6.3 weeks onward, ultrasound will visualize an embryo 5 mm or greater in length, by which time a heartbeat should always be seen if the embryo is alive. The timing of these milestones is subject to some variability, but they usually are seen within 0.5 week of the stated gestational ages. Gestational age can be assigned based on these milestones (Table 33-1).

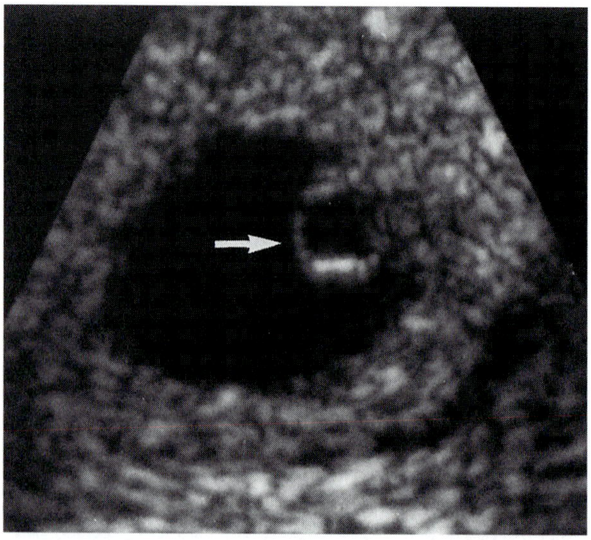

FIG. 33-1. Gestational sac contains yolk sac *(arrow)*. Transvaginal sonogram at 5.5 weeks gestation. No embryo is seen.

TABLE 33-1
GESTATIONAL DATING BY ULTRASOUND IN THE FIRST TRIMESTER

Sonographic Findings	Gestational Age (weeks)
Gestational sac, no yolk sac, embryo, or heartbeat	5.0
Gestational sac with yolk sac, no embryo or heartbeat	5.5
Gestational sac with heartbeat and embryo <5 mm in length	6.0
Embryo/fetus ≥5 mm in length	Age based on crown-rump length (see Table 33-2)

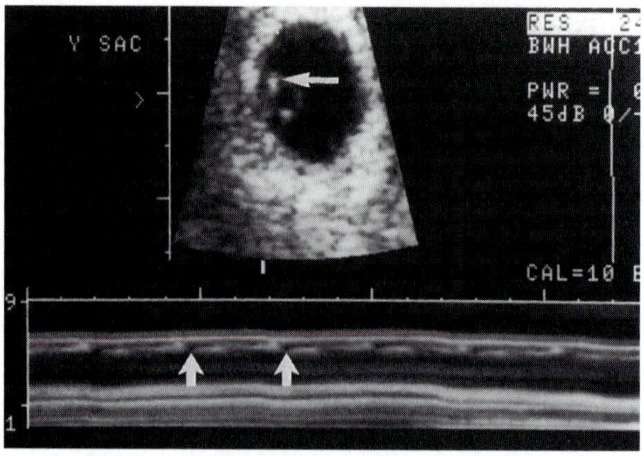

FIG. 33-2. Embryonic heartbeat at 6 weeks. Transvaginal sonogram and M-mode demonstrate cardiac activity *(short arrows)* originating from tiny embryo *(long arrow)* adjacent to the yolk sac.

From 6 weeks until the end of the first trimester, gestational age correlates closely with the crown-rump length (CRL) of the embryo or fetus.[13,14] The term **embryo** applies up to the end of organogenesis at 10 weeks' gestation; the term **fetus** applies thereafter.[15] The CRL is the length of the embryo or fetus from the top of its head to the bottom of its torso. It is measured as the longest dimension of the embryo, excluding the yolk sac and extremities (Fig. 33-3). The CRL can be used to assign gestational age accurately (Table 33-2). After 12 to 13 weeks' gestation, the CRL of the longer, more developed fetus becomes less reliable. At this later stage, the CRL is affected by the fetal position, measuring shorter in a fetus whose spine is flexed and longer in a fetus whose spine is straight.

The accuracy of gestational age determination by ultrasound, as measured by the width of the 95% confidence range, is approximately ± 0.5 week throughout the first trimester.[13,14] The sonographic estimation of gestational age will be within 0.5 week of the actual age in 95% of cases.

Second and Third Trimester Gestational Dating

Many sonographic parameters have been proposed for estimating gestational age in the second and third trimesters. These include several fetal measurements: biparietal diameter (BPD),[16,17] head circumference (HC),[18] abdominal circumference (AC),[19] femur length (FL),[17,20,21] length of other long bones,[21] and binocular distance;[22] and combinations of two or more fetal measurements—the corrected-BPD (BPDc)[23] and composite age formulas.[19,24] Measurements of structurally abnormal fetal body parts should not be used in the assignment of gestational age.

Fetal Head Measurements. Three measurements or parameters involve the fetal head: BPD, corrected-BPD, and HC. All three measurements are taken from transaxial sonograms of the fetal head at the level of the paired thalami and cavum septi pellucidi (Fig. 33-4).[25] The BPD is measured from the outer edge of the cranium nearest the transducer to the inner edge of the cranium farthest from the transducer (Fig. 33-4). The occipitofrontal diameter (OFD) is obtained from the same transaxial image as the BPD and is measured from midskull to midskull along the long axis of the fetal head (Fig. 33-4). This latter measurement is used in conjunction with the BPD to calculate the corrected-BPD via the formula:[23]

$$\text{Corrected-BPD} = \text{square root of } [(\text{BPD} \times \text{OFD})/1.265]$$

The rationale for the corrected-BPD is that it represents the BPD of the standard-shaped head (one with an OFD/BPD ratio of 1.265) of the same cross-sectional area.[23] The same tables or formulas used to determine gestational age from the BPD are used to determine gestational age from the corrected-BPD.

The HC is the length of the outer perimeter of the cranium, made on the same transaxial image of the fetal head. It can be measured by using an electronic ellipse available on most ultrasound scanners.[26] Alternatively, it can be calculated from the outer-edge-to-outer-edge analogs of the BPD and OFD:

$$\text{HC} = 1.57 \times [(\text{outer-to-outer BPD}) + (\text{outer-to-outer OFD})]$$

Although the BPD is simpler to measure than the corrected-BPD or HC, it has the disadvantage of being the only one of the three measurements that disregards head shape. This means that two heads of equal

A

B

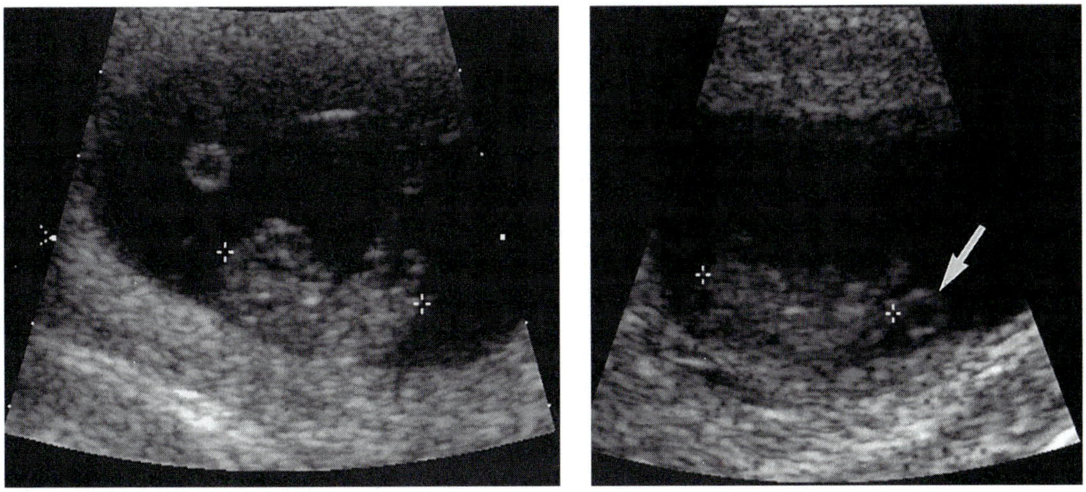

FIG. 33-3. Crown-rump length measurement. A, Cursors delineate the length of the fetus from the top of its head to the bottom of its torso. **B,** The yolk sac *(arrow)* should not be included in the fetal crown-rump length measurements.

TABLE 33-2
GESTATIONAL AGE ESTIMATION BY CROWN-RUMP LENGTH

CRL* (mm)	Gestational Age (weeks)**	CRL (mm)	Gestational Age (weeks)
5	6.0	45	11.1
6	6.2	46	11.2
7	6.4	47	11.3
8	6.6	48	11.4
9	6.8	49	11.4
10	7.0	50	11.5
11	7.2	51	11.6
12	7.4	52	11.7
13	7.5	53	11.8
14	7.7	54	11.8
15	7.8	55	11.9
16	8.0	56	12.0
17	8.1	57	12.1
18	8.3	58	12.2
19	8.4	59	12.2
20	8.5	60	12.3
21	8.7	61	12.4
22	8.8	62	12.4
23	8.9	63	12.5
24	9.0	64	12.6
25	9.1	65	12.7
26	9.3	66	12.7
27	9.4	67	12.8
28	9.5	68	12.9
29	9.6	69	12.9
30	9.7	70	13.0
31	9.8	71	13.1
32	9.9	72	13.2
33	10.0	73	13.2
34	10.1	74	13.3
35	10.2	75	13.4
36	10.3	76	13.4
37	10.4	77	13.5
38	10.5	78	13.5
39	10.6	79	13.6
40	10.7	80	13.7
41	10.8		
42	10.8		
43	10.9		
44	11.0		

*CRL, crown-rump length.

**Values derived from formula in reference 13.

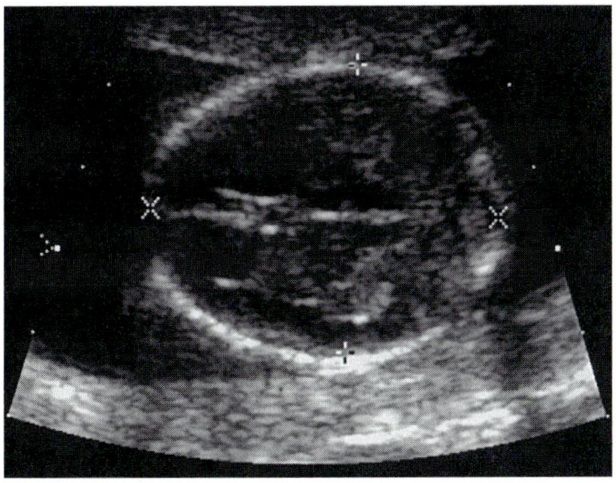

FIG. 33-4. Biparietal diameter and occipitofrontal diameter measurements. Transaxial sonogram of the fetal head at the level of the paired thalami *(arrow)*, with BPD (+ . . . +) and OFD (× . . . ×).

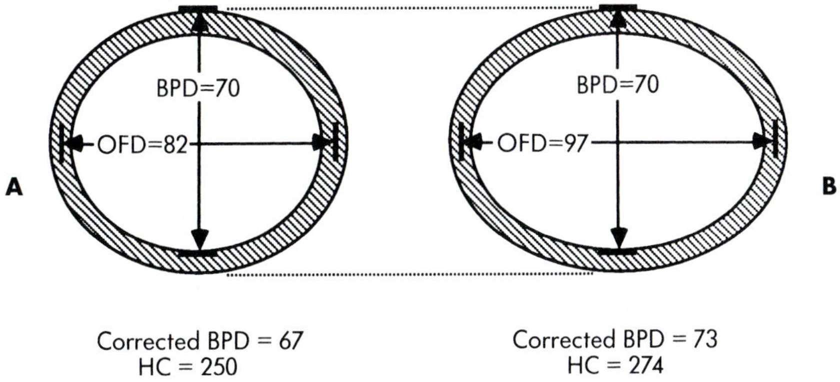

FIG. 33-5. Effect of head shape on corrected-BPD and HC. Heads **A** and **B** have equal BPDs, but **A** has a smaller OFD than **B.** Therefore, the corrected-BPD and HC are smaller for **A** than **B.** Based on BPD, fetuses **A** and **B** would be assigned the same gestational age. Based on corrected-BPD or HC, however, fetus **A** would be assigned a lower gestational age than fetus **B.**

widths but different lengths will have the same BPDs, but the longer head will have a greater corrected-BPD and HC than the shorter head (Fig. 33-5). The fetus with the longer head will, therefore, be assigned a greater GA based on the corrected-BPD or HC; however, both fetuses will be assigned the same GA if the BPD is used as the basis for age assignment.

Femoral Length (FL). The length of the diaphysis of the fetal femur is often used for gestational age prediction.[17,20,21] Careful measurement of the ossified diaphysis of the femur is necessary in order to obtain an accurate estimate of gestational age by FL (Fig. 33-6). The entire femur should be imaged and the thin bright reflection of the cartilaginous epiphysis should not be included in the measurement.[27]

Abdominal Circumference. The fetal **abdominal circumference** (AC) is the length of the outer perimeter of the fetal abdomen, measured on transverse scan at the level of the stomach and intrahepatic portion of the umbilical vein (Fig. 33-7).

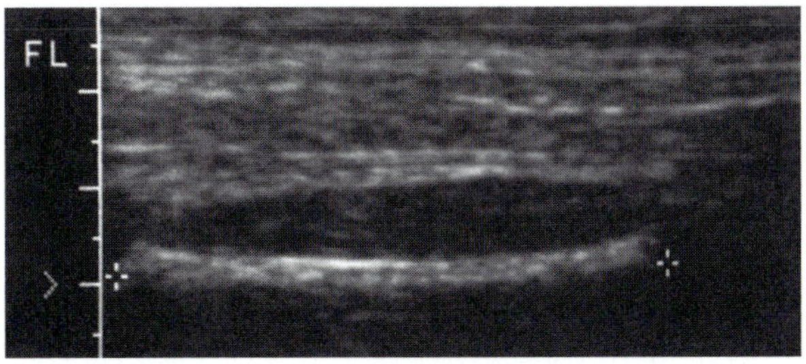

FIG. 33-6. Femur length measurement. Electronic calipers measure the ossified diaphysis of the femur.

Alternatively, the AC may be calculated with equivalent results from two orthogonal abdominal diameters (AD), one anteroposterior and the other transverse, measured on the same image, as follows:[26]

$$AC = 1.57 \times (AD_1 + AD_2)$$

Gestational age can be estimated from measurements of the head, abdomen, or femur by means of ta-

TABLE 33-3
GESTATIONAL AGE ESTIMATION BY BIPARIETAL DIAMETER

BPD or BPDc* (mm)	Gestational Age (weeks)**	BPD or BPDc (mm)	Gestational Age (weeks)
20	13.2	60	24.2
21	13.4	61	24.5
22	13.6	62	24.9
23	13.8	63	25.3
24	14.0	64	25.7
25	14.3	65	26.1
26	14.5	66	26.5
27	14.7	67	26.9
28	14.9	68	27.3
29	15.1	69	27.7
30	15.4	70	28.1
31	15.6	71	28.5
32	15.8	72	29.0
33	16.1	73	29.4
34	16.3	74	29.9
35	16.6	75	30.3
36	16.8	76	30.8
37	17.1	77	31.2
38	17.3	78	31.7
39	17.6	79	32.2
40	17.9	80	32.7
41	18.1	81	33.2
42	18.4	82	33.7
43	18.7	83	34.2
44	19.0	84	34.7
45	19.3	85	35.2
46	19.6	86	35.8
47	19.9	87	36.3
48	20.2	88	36.9
49	20.5	89	37.4
50	20.8	90	38.0
51	21.1	91	38.6
52	21.4	92	39.2
53	21.7	93	39.8
54	22.1	94	40.4
55	22.4	95	41.0
56	22.8	96	41.6
57	23.1	≥97	42.0
58	23.5		
59	23.8		

*BPD, biparietal diameter; BPDc, corrected-BPD

**Calculated from a formula in reference 17

bles or formulas that present the mean value of each measurement for a given gestational age (Tables 33-3 to 33-5). Composite age formulas that combine several fetal measurements can also be used to predict gestational age.[20,24]

The accuracy of gestational age determination ranges from 1.2 weeks for the HC and corrected-BPD between 14 and 20 weeks to 3.5 weeks in the late third trimester for the FL. As pregnancy progresses, each parameter becomes less accurate. The two fetal head measurements that take head shape into account, corrected-BPD and HC, are equivalent in accuracy to each other and more accurate than the BPD throughout gestation. In the second trimester, these two head measurements are the best predictors of gestational age. In the third trimester, these two head measurements, the FL, and the composite age formulas all predict gestational age with similar accuracy.[17,28]

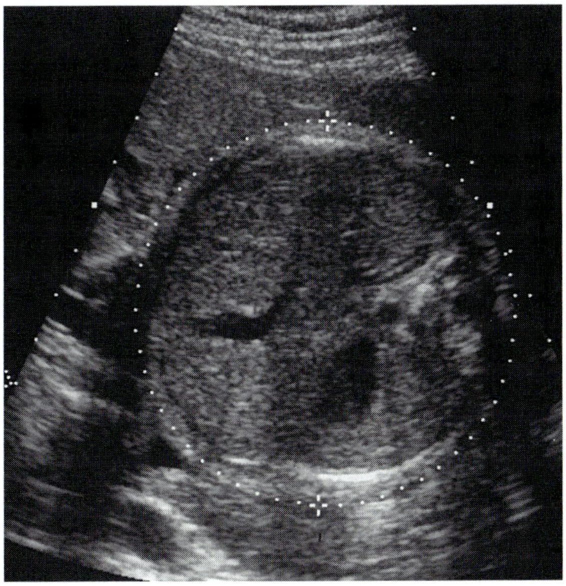

FIG. 33-7. Abdominal circumference measurement. Electronic ellipse cursor measures the perimeter of the fetal abdomen.

TABLE 33-4
GESTATIONAL AGE ESTIMATION BY HEAD CIRCUMFERENCE

HC (mm)*	Gestational Age (weeks)**	HC (mm)	Gestational Age (weeks)
80	13.4	225	24.5
85	13.7	230	25.0
90	14.0	235	25.5
95	14.3	240	26.1
100	14.7	245	26.6
105	15.0	250	27.1
110	15.3	255	27.7
115	15.6	260	28.3
120	16.0	265	28.9
125	16.3	270	29.4
130	16.6	275	30.0
135	17.0	280	30.7
140	17.3	285	31.3
145	17.7	290	31.9
150	18.1	295	32.6
155	18.4	300	33.3
160	18.8	305	33.9
165	19.2	310	34.6
170	19.6	315	35.3
175	20.0	320	36.1
180	20.4	325	36.8
185	20.8	330	37.6
190	21.3	335	38.3
195	21.7	340	39.1
200	22.2	345	39.9
205	22.6	350	40.7
210	23.1	355	41.6
215	23.6	360	42.4
220	24.0		

*HC, head circumference

**Values derived from formula in reference 19.

TABLE 33-5
GESTATIONAL AGE ESTIMATION BY FEMUR LENGTH

FL (mm)*	Gestational Age (weeks)**	FL (mm)	Gestational Age (weeks)
10	13.7	45	24.5
11	13.9	46	24.9
12	14.2	47	25.3
13	14.4	48	25.7
14	14.6	49	26.2
15	14.9	50	26.6
16	15.1	51	27.0
17	15.4	52	27.5
18	15.6	53	28.0
19	15.9	54	28.4
20	16.2	55	28.9
21	16.4	56	29.4
22	16.7	57	29.9
23	17.0	58	30.4
24	17.3	59	30.9
25	17.6	60	31.4
26	17.9	61	31.9
27	18.2	62	32.5
28	18.5	63	33.0
29	18.8	64	33.6
30	19.1	65	34.1
31	19.4	66	34.7
32	19.7	67	35.3
33	20.1	68	35.9
34	20.4	69	36.5
35	20.7	70	37.1
36	21.1	71	37.7
37	21.4	72	38.3
38	21.8	73	39.0
39	22.2	74	39.6
40	22.5	75	40.3
41	22.9	76	40.9
42	23.3	77	41.6
43	23.7	≥78	42.0
44	24.1		

*FL, femur length.

**Values derived from formula in reference 17.

Composite age formulas use two or more measurements in conjunction to estimate gestational age. A potential disadvantage of using such formulas is that an abnormal measurement or anomaly might be obscured. For example, in a fetus with a skeletal dysplasia manifested by shortened long bones and a normal head size, the gestational age based on the composite formula will be an underestimation, falling between that predicted by the corrected-BPD and that predicted by the short FL. As a result, the FL might not appear to be abnormally small when compared to this gestational age.

Assignment of Gestational Age

The recommended approach to gestational age assignment at the time of the first sonogram is presented in Table 33-6. In the second and third trimesters, the choice depends on which measurements are available, because two or more parameters may be equivalent in accuracy. In some cases, especially when the initial scan occurs late in pregnancy, judgment must be applied to decide whether to use clinical or sonographic criteria to determine the gestational age. As a general rule, we recommend using ultrasound criteria up to 26 weeks of gestation and the LMP (if clearly recalled) thereafter.

TABLE 33-6
APPROACH TO GESTATIONAL AGE ASSIGNMENT BY ULTRASOUND ON INITIAL SCAN

Stage of Pregnancy	Basis for GA	Table	Accuracy (weeks)*
First trimester			
Early (5–6 weeks)	Sonographic milestones	33-1	±0.5
Mid-to-late (6–13 weeks)	CRL	33-2	±0.5
Second trimester			
If OFD measurable	BPDc or HC	33-3 and 33-4	±1.2 (14–20 weeks) ±1.9 (20–26 weeks)
If OFD not measurable	BPD or FL	33-3 and 33-5	±1.4 (14–20 weeks) ±2.1–2.5 (20–26 weeks)
Third trimester			
If OFD measurable	BPDc, HC, or FL	33-3, 33-4, and 33-5	±3.1–3.4 (26–32 weeks) ±3.5–3.8 (32–42 weeks)
If OFD not measurable	FL	33-5	±3.1 (26–32 weeks) ±3.5 (36–42 weeks)

*Two standard deviations, or 95% confidence interval.
CRL, crown-rump length; OFD, occipitofrontal diameter; BPD, biparietal diameter; BPDc, corrected BPD; HC, head circumference; FL, femur length.

Because fetal measurements become progressively less accurate predictors of gestational age as pregnancy progresses, the age assigned at the time of the first scan should not be changed thereafter. The age at any time later in pregnancy should be based on the initial sonographic study, calculated by taking the gestational age assigned at the time of the first scan and adding the number of weeks that have elapsed since that scan. On subsequent examinations, standard fetal measurements (BPD, OFD, AC, and FL) should be obtained and should be compared to the normal standards for the gestational age, based on the initial sonogram, to determine whether the fetus is appropriate in size.

WEIGHT ESTIMATION AND ASSESSMENT

Estimation of Fetal Weight

Prior to the availability of ultrasound, manual examination of the maternal abdomen was the only approach that could be used to estimate fetal size. The physical examination, however, provides only a rough approximation of fetal weight because the palpated dimensions of the uterus are affected by several factors other than fetal size. These include amniotic fluid volume, placental bulk, presence of fibroids, and maternal obesity.

Sonographic measurements of fetal body parts provide a direct way of assessing fetal size. Numerous formulas have been published for estimating fetal weight from one or more of the following fetal body measurements: head (BPD or HC), abdomen (AD or AC), and femur (FL).[29-38] Other measurements, such as thigh circumference, have been used as well.[38]

The accuracy of a weight-prediction formula is determined by assessing how well the formula works in a group of fetuses scanned close to delivery. An important measure of a formula's performance is its 95% confidence range. If the 95% confidence range is ±18%, for example, then the estimated weight will fall within 18% of the actual weight in 95% of cases, and the error will be greater than 18% in only 5% of cases. The narrower the confidence range, the more reliable the formula.

Many published studies provide information that allows one to estimate this measure of a formula's accuracy (Table 33-7).[31,32,35,36,38-40]

The following points are noteworthy:

- The accuracy of weight-prediction formulas improves as the number of measured body parts increases up to three, achieving greatest accuracy when measurements of the head, abdomen, and femur are used. There is no apparent benefit from adding the thigh circumference as a fourth measurement.
- Even when based on measurements of the head, abdomen, and femur, sonographic weight prediction has a rather wide 95% confidence range of at least ±15%. Based on the abdomen and either the head or femur, the range is at least ±16–18%. Precision is considerably worse when only the abdomen is used.

A number of factors have been studied to determine their effect on accuracy of weight prediction.

TABLE 33-7
ACCURACY OF FETAL WEIGHT-PREDICTION FORMULAS

Body Part(s) Included in Formula	Formula*	95% Confidence Range (%)**
Abdomen	Campbell[29]	±17.1–23.8[35,39]
	Higginbottom[30]	±23.8[35]
	Hadlock[35]	±22.2[35]
	Vintzileos[38]	±22.8[38]
Head and abdomen	Warsof[31]	±17.4–21.2[31,35,39]
	Shepard[32]	±18.2–18.3[32,39]
	Thurneau[33]	±19.8[35]
	Jordaan[34]	±25.8[35]
	Hadlock[35]	±18.2[35]
	Hadlock[36]	±18.2[36]
	Birnholz[37]	±17.7[40]***
	Vintzileos[38]	±21.2[38]
Abdomen and femur	Hadlock[35]	±16.4[35]
	Hadlock[36]	±16.0[36]
Head, abdomen, and femur	Hadlock[35]	±15.0–15.4[35]
	Hadlock[36]	±14.8–15.0[36]
	Vintzileos[38]	±17.6[38]
Head, abdomen, femur, and thigh	Vintzileos[38]	±15.6–17.8[38]

*First author and reference number of the study in which formula was developed.
**Computed as two standard deviations of the relative error, as reported in the study(ies) referenced, unless otherwise indicated.
***Based on the fraction of cases in which the estimated weight falls within 10% of the actual weight.

Accuracy appears to be worse in fetuses that weigh under 1000 grams than in larger fetuses.[40] Over the rest of the birth-weight range, however, accuracy is fairly constant.[35,36,39,41] Weight prediction is less accurate in diabetic than in nondiabetic mothers. In diabetics, formulas that use measurements of the head, abdomen, and femur have a 95% confidence range of ±24%,[42] wider than the range of ±15% in the general population.[35,36] The presence of oligohydramnios or polyhydramnios has no impact on accuracy.[39,40] Scan quality may have an effect on accuracy; in one study there was a trend toward greater accuracy in scans that were rated "good" as compared with those rated "poor" based on ability to visualize anatomic landmarks, although the difference was not statistically significant.[40]

Recommended Approach to Fetal Weight Estimation. An attempt should be made to image all three of the **key anatomic regions,** that is, the head, abdomen, and femur, at the appropriate anatomic levels (Table 33-8). If measurements of all three structures can be obtained, then Formula 1 should be used to estimate fetal weight. This formula should be used with the corrected-BPD when the OFD is available, and with the BPD itself if not. An alternative approach, equally accurate but more cumbersome, would be to use Formula 1 when the OFD is unavailable, and a formula based on HC, AC, and FL when the OFD is available. If the abdomen and only the head or the femur can be appropriately imaged, then Formula 2 or 3 should be used. If the abdomen cannot be measured, or both the head and femur cannot be measured, then a weight estimate should not be calculated. Using the approach outlined in Table 33-8, an accuracy of ±15% to 18% can be achieved for weight estimation.

Assessment of Weight in Relation to Gestational Age

When an ultrasound is performed in the third trimester, best estimates of gestational age and fetal weight should be established. The gestational age may be based on a prior ultrasound, clinical dating criteria, or current measurements; fetal weight is always calculated from current measurements. The two values should be assessed in relation to one another to determine whether the fetus is appropriate in size for dates. This can be accomplished by using a table that provides norms of values for fetal weight as a function of gestational age (Table 33-9), several of which appear in the literature.[43-48]

As an example, suppose that an obstetric sonogram is performed and the best estimated gestational age is 34 weeks. According to Table 33-9 a weight of 2146

TABLE 33-8
APPROACH TO FETAL WEIGHT ESTIMATION

Body Parts Imaged	Formula Used for Weight Estimate
Head, abdomen, and femur	
OFD measurable	Formula 1, using corrected-BPD in place of BPD
OFD not measurable	Formula 1
Head and abdomen	
OFD measurable	Formula 2, using corrected-BPD in place of BPD
OFD not measurable	Formula 2
Abdomen and femur	Formula 3

Formula 1:[36] Log_{10} (EFW) = 1.4787 − 0.003343 AC × FL + 0.001837 BPD^2 + 0.0458 AC + 0.158FL

Formula 2:[36] Log_{10} (EFW) = 1.1134 + 0.05845 AC − 0.000604 AC^2 − 0.007365 BPD^2 + 0.00595 BPD × AC + 0.1694 BPD

Formula 3:[36] Log_{10} (EFW) = 1.3598 + 0.051 AC + 0.1844 FL − 0.0037 AC × FL

EFW, estimated fetal weight, in gm; BPD, biparietal diameter, in cm; AC, abdominal circumference, in cm; FL, femur length, in cm; OFD, occipitofrontal diameter, in cm.

TABLE 33-9
FETAL WEIGHT PERCENTILES IN THE THIRD TRIMESTER[43]

	Weight Percentiles (g)		
Gestational Age (weeks)	10th	50th	90th
25	490	660	889
26	568	760	1016
27	660	875	1160
28	765	1005	1322
29	884	1153	1504
30	1020	1319	1706
31	1171	1502	1928
32	1338	1702	2167
33	1519	1918	2421
34	1714	2146	2687
35	1919	2383	2959
36	2129	2622	3230
37	2340	2859	3493
38	2544	3083	3736
39	2735	3288	3952
40	2904	3462	4127
41	3042	3597	4254
42	3142	3685	4322
43	3195	3717	4324

corresponds to the 50th percentile, and weights of 1714 and 2687 correspond to the 10th and 90th percentiles, respectively. A weight between the 10th and 90th percentiles is generally considered to be appropriate for gestational age. When the estimated weight falls outside this range, the diagnosis of a small- or large-for-gestational-age fetus is suggested.

The weight gain between two ultrasound examinations can be estimated as the difference between the two estimated weights. Adequacy of weight gain can be assessed by comparing this difference to established normal fetal growth rate as a function of gestational age. These data indicate that median fetal weight gain per week increases progressively until 37 weeks of gestation, reaching a maximum rate of 240 per week.[43] After 37 weeks, the rate of weight gain steadily decreases in the normal fetus. The longer the time between scans, the more accurate is the sonographic estimate of interval weight gain. When two scans are performed within 1 week of each other, weight gain cannot be determined reliably, so that there is little or no value in computing an estimated weight at the time of the second scan.

When several examinations have been performed, fetal growth can be depicted graphically by means of a trend plot, or growth curve. One form of growth curve plots the **estimated fetal weight versus gestational age,** with the curve for the fetus being examined superimposed on lines depicting the 1st, 10th, 50th, 90th, and 99th percentiles (Fig. 33-8, *A*). An alternative mode of display plots the **estimated weight percentile versus gestational age** (Fig. 33-8, *B*). In this latter format, the graph for a normally growing fetus will be a horizontal line, indicating maintenance of a particular weight percentile throughout gestation. A downsloping line indicates a subnormal growth rate, and an upsloping line indicates accelerated growth.

Calculation of weight percentiles and plotting of growth curves are most easily accomplished via computer, using an obstetric ultrasound software package that performs these tasks.[49-51] Alternatively, similar results can be achieved by means of a calculator and manual plotting of data.

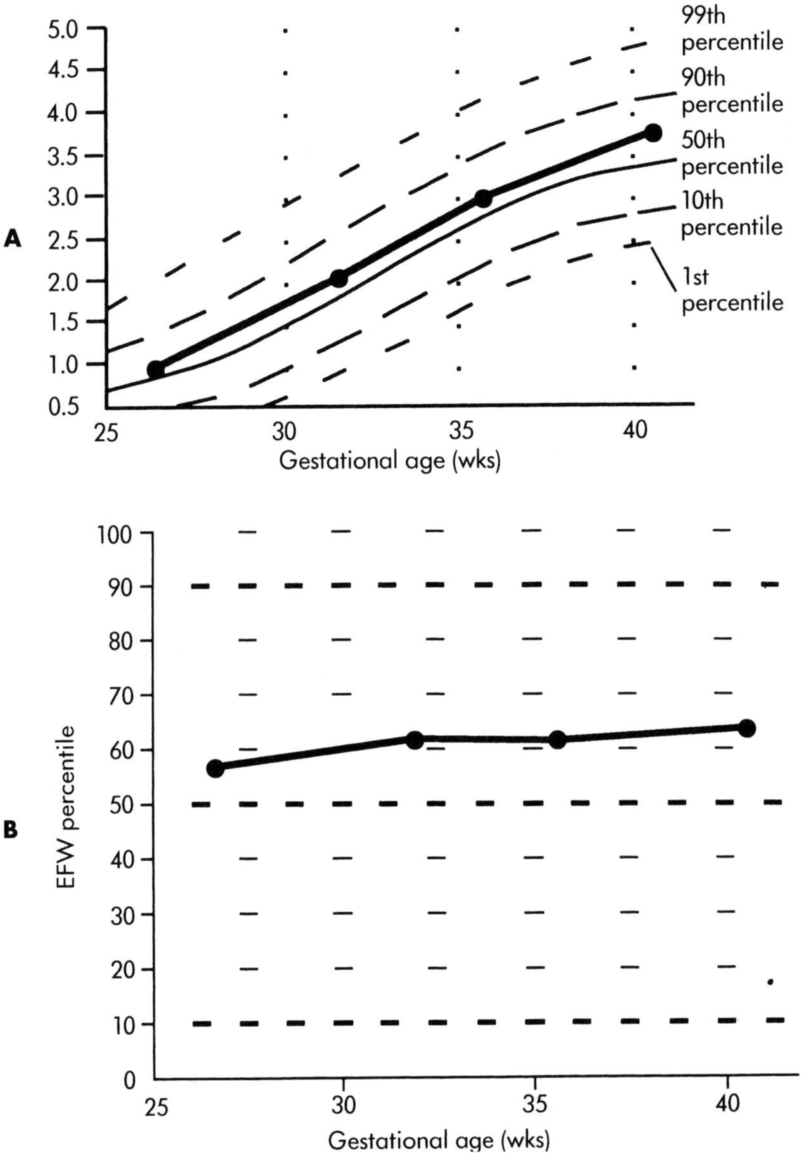

FIG. 33-8. Fetal growth curves. A, Estimated fetal weight plotted against gestational age, superimposed on 1st, 10th, 50th, 90th, and 99th percentile curves. The fetus depicted here has a normal growth pattern, with estimated fetal weights between the 50th and 90th percentiles over four sonograms. **B,** Estimated fetal weight percentile against gestational age.

FETAL GROWTH ABNORMALITIES

The Large Fetus

The large-for-gestational-age (LGA) neonate (or fetus) is defined as one whose weight is above the 90th percentile for gestational age.[43,52-54] Macrosomia, a related entity, is most often defined on the basis of a weight above 4000 g. Other weight cutoffs (4100 g, 4500 g) are occasionally used.[53,55-57] These growth disturbances occur with different frequencies and are associated with different morbidities and mortalities in diabetic mothers as compared to the general population. We will therefore consider these two patient populations separately.

General Population. Ten percent (10%) of all infants have birth weights above the 90th percentile for gestational age and are considered LGA infants. Of all newborns, 8% to 10% have birth weights over 4000 g and are thus classified as macrosomic.[53,55-57] Risk factors for LGA and macrosomia include maternal obesity, diabetes, history of a previous LGA infant, prolonged pregnancy (more than 40 weeks), excess pregnancy weight gain, multiparity, and advanced maternal age.[52,53,55,58-60]

Large fetuses have an increased incidence of perinatal morbidity and mortality, in large part because of obstetric complications. Shoulder dystocia, fractures, and facial and brachial plexus palsies occur more frequently as a result of traumatic delivery.[58,61,62] The incidence of perinatal asphyxia, meconium aspiration, neonatal hypoglycemia, and other metabolic complications is significantly increased in these pregnancies.[52,55,58]

The most straightforward approach to diagnosing LGA and macrosomia is to use the estimated fetal weight computed from sonographic measurements. An estimated weight above the 90th percentile for gestational age suggests LGA, and a weight estimate above 4000 g suggests macrosomia. Although weight estimation is less accurate in large than in average-sized fetuses,[39,63-65] this approach has been demonstrated to be moderately good for diagnosing LGA and macrosomia. It has positive predictive values of up to 51% for LGA and 67% for macrosomia. Other proposed sonographic parameters have either lower sensitivities and/or lower positive predictive values than does the estimated fetal weight (see Table 33-10).[39,52,63,66-70]

Diabetic Mothers. Fetuses of insulin-dependent and gestational diabetic mothers are exposed to high levels of glucose throughout pregnancy and, as a result, produce excess insulin. This leads to overgrowth of the fetal trunk and abdominal organs, while the head and brain grow at a normal rate.[53,54] Therefore, these fetuses tend to have different body proportions than do those of nondiabetic mothers. Sonographic measurements of fetuses of diabetic mothers demonstrate accelerated growth of the fetal thorax and abdomen beginning between 28 and 32 weeks' gestation.[53,54,71]

TABLE 33-10

SONOGRAPHIC CRITERIA FOR LARGE-FOR-GESTATIONAL-AGE (LGA) AND MACROSOMIA IN THE GENERAL POPULATION: PERFORMANCE CHARACTERISTICS[66]

			Predictive Values (%)[66]	
	Sensitivity (%)	Specificity (%)	Positive	Negative
Criterion to predict LGA*				
Elevated AD-BPD[67]	46	79	19	93
Low FL/AC[52,67]	24–75	44–93	13–26	92–94
Elevated AFV[68,69]	12–17	92–98	19–35	91
Elevated ponderal index[52,67]	13–15	85–98	13–36	91–94
High EFW[52,69]	20–74	93–96	6–51	88–94
Elevated growth score[52]	14	91	10	90
Elevated AFV and high EFW[69]	11	99	54	99
Criterion to predict macrosomia				
Elevated FL[70]	24	96	52	88
Elevated AC[70]	53	94	63	89
High EFW[40,65,70]	11–65	89–96	38–67	83–91
Elevated BPD[70]	29	98	71	92

*Predictive values for criteria for LGA computed using Bayes' theorem[89] assuming an LGA prevalence rate of 10%.

AD, abdominal diameter; BPD, biparietal diameter; FL, femur length; AC, abdominal circumference; AFV, amniotic fluid volume; EFW, estimated fetal weight.

LGA occurs in 25% to 42% and macrosomia in 10% to 50% of infants of diabetic mothers.[53,54,72] As many as 12% weigh more than 4500 g at birth. Perinatal complications are more frequent in macrosomic fetuses of diabetic mothers than in those of nondiabetic mothers.[57,61,62,73,74] Shoulder dystocia, for example, occurs in 31% of macrosomic fetuses of diabetic mothers and in only 3% to 10% of macrosomic fetuses of nondiabetic mothers.[58,61]

Many sonographic parameters, involving a variety of measurements, formulas, and ratios, have been proposed for diagnosing LGA and macrosomia in the diabetic mother (Table 33-11).[42,54,66,72,73,75-77] As a group, these have higher sensitivities and positive predictive values than do sonographic criteria in the general population, in part because of the higher prevalence of large fetuses in diabetic mothers.

As in the general population, the most straightforward approach to diagnosing LGA and macrosomia in the fetuses of diabetic mothers is by means of the sonographically estimated fetal weight.[42,66,75] A fetus whose estimated weight falls above the 90th percentile for gestational age has a 74% likelihood of being LGA, as compared to 19% if the estimated weight lies below the 90th percentile.[75] A weight estimate above 4000 g is associated with a 77% chance of macrosomia, and one above 4500 g with an 86% chance. The chance of macrosomia is only 16% when the weight estimate is less than 4000 g.[42] It follows that if vaginal delivery is believed to be contraindicated for the macrosomic fetuses of diabetic mothers, the estimated fetal weight should be taken into account when selecting the route of delivery.

Intrauterine Growth Retardation

Intrauterine growth retardation (IUGR) is a fetal growth disorder most commonly defined on the basis of a weight below the 10th percentile for gestational age.[78-82] This disorder is sometimes termed small-for-gestational-age (SGA). Most cases of growth retardation are caused by placental insufficiency, either primary or secondary to a maternal etiology such as hypertension, collagen vascular disease, poor nutrition, or substance abuse. IUGR may also result from a chromosomal anomaly (e.g., trisomy 18) or intrauterine infection (e.g., cytomegalovirus).[79,82,83]

In many cases, the specific cause of IUGR cannot be determined prenatally. As a group, regardless of the etiology, growth-retarded fetuses have a poor prognosis, with increased perinatal morbidity and mortality. Their mortality rate is four to eight times that of non-IUGR fetuses.[83,84] One half of surviving growth-retarded infants suffer serious short- or long-term morbidity, including meconium aspiration pneumonia and metabolic disorders.[82,83-85]

TABLE 33-11
SONOGRAPHIC CRITERIA FOR LARGE-FOR-GESTATIONAL-AGE (LGA) AND MACROSOMIA IN DIABETIC MOTHERS: PERFORMANCE CHARACTERISTICS[66]

			Predictive Values (%)	
	Sensitivity (%)	Specificity (%)	Positive	Negative
Criterion to predict LGA				
Elevated HC[75]	50	80	64	70
Elevated AC/BPD[76]	83	60	71	75
High EFW[75]	78	78	74	81
Elevated BPD[75]	13	86	75	57
Elevated AC[54,73,75]	71–88	81–85	56-78	81–96
Elevated AC growth[54]	84	85	79	89
Low FL/AC[54,76]	58–79	75–80	68-83	75–76
Elevated AC and high EFW[75]	72	71	89	89
Criterion to predict macrosomia				
Elevated AC[73]	84	78	41	96
Low FL/AC[77]	48–64	60–74	36–42	80–83
Elevated TD-BPD[72]	87	72	61	92
High EFW[42]	48	95	77	84

HC, head circumference; AC, abdominal circumference; BPD, biparietal diameter; EFW, estimated fetal weight; FL, femur length; TD, thoracic diameter.

IUGR has been categorized as **symmetric** or **asymmetric.** Symmetric growth-retarded fetuses are proportionately reduced in size, whereas in asymmetric IUGR the fetal abdomen is disproportionately small in relation to the head and limbs. There is, however, considerable overlap between these two groups, so this categorization is probably not useful clinically.[86]

Numerous sonographic parameters, using both conventional and Doppler ultrasound, have been proposed for antenatal diagnosis of IUGR.[87,88] To be clinically useful for diagnosis, a criterion must detect a substantial fraction of cases of growth retardation (i.e., its **sensitivity** must be high), and a positive result must be associated with a high likelihood of IUGR (i.e., its **positive predictive value** must be high). Similarly, to be valuable for excluding IUGR, a criterion must have high specificity and negative predictive value.[89]

The performance characteristics of conventional sonographic criteria for IUGR are presented in Table 33-12, listed in order of increasing positive predictive value.[87] The best criterion is the HC/AC ratio, with a positive predictive value of 62%. It should be noted that even when based on this criterion, IUGR cannot be diagnosed with confidence because more than one third (38%) of fetuses with an abnormal HC/AC ratio will not be growth retarded. Other parameters have even lower positive predictive values, with seven of the nine parameters listed having positive predictive values that are under 50%.

Doppler criteria for IUGR assess blood flow in the feto-placental or utero-placental circulations, both of which are essential for fetal nourishment and oxygenation. These criteria, however, are no better than conventional criteria at predicting IUGR.[88] In particular, the positive predictive values of well-studied Doppler criteria for IUGR fall in the range of 11% to 57%. Therefore, Doppler criteria do not permit confident diagnosis of that disorder. Doppler may, however, play a useful role in determining the prognosis of fetuses with IUGR.[90-93] In growth-retarded fetuses, reversed diastolic flow in the umbilical artery carries a grave prognosis, and absent diastolic flow or an elevated systolic-to-diastolic ratio is associated with increased likelihood of fetal distress in labor, admission to the intensive care unit, and mortality.[91,94-99]

Although no single criterion permits confident **diagnosis of IUGR,** there are three key parameters that can be used in combination to establish the diagnosis with greater certainty:[100]

- estimated fetal weight;
- amniotic fluid volume; and
- maternal blood pressure status (normal versus hypertensive).

Other proposed parameters for diagnosing IUGR can be safely ignored because they add no significant information.[101,102]

The three key parameters can be combined into an IUGR score or a table that permits the confident diagnosis or exclusion of growth retardation in most cases (Table 33-13).[100,101] For any gestational age, amniotic

TABLE 33-12
CONVENTIONAL SONOGRAPHIC CRITERIA FOR INTRAUTERINE GROWTH RETARDATION (IUGR): PERFORMANCE CHARACTERISTICS[87]

			Predictive Values (%)*	
	Sensitivity (%)	**Specificity (%)**	**Positive**	**Negative**
Advanced placental grade	62	64	16	94
Elevated FL/AC	34–49	78–83	18–20	92–93
Low TIUV	57–80	72–76	21–24	92–97
Small BPD	24–88	62–94	21–44	92–98
Small BPD and advanced placental grade	59	86	32	95
Slow rate of BPD growth	75	84	35	97
Low EFW	89	88	45	99
Decreased AFV	24	98	55	92
Elevated HC/AC	82	94	62	98

*Computed using Bayes' theorem,[89] assuming an IUGR prevalence rate of 10%. A range of values is given for a criterion when different studies apply that criterion in two or more ways.

FL/AC, femur length/abdominal circumference ratio; TIUV, total intrauterine volume; BPD, biparietal diameter; EFW, estimated fetal weight; AFV, amniotic fluid volume; HC/AC, head circumference/abdominal circumference ratio.

TABLE 33-13

CRITICAL VALUES* FOR ESTIMATED FETAL WEIGHT (IN GRAMS) FOR DIAGNOSING OR EXCLUDING GROWTH RETARDATION[101]

	Status of Maternal Blood Pressure and Amniotic Fluid Volume*					
GA	Nl BP Nl/Poly	Nl BP M-M Oligo	Nl BP Sev Oligo	Htn Nl/Poly	Htn M-M Oligo	Htn Sev Oligo
26	516–660	646–826	743–950	610–780	763–976	878–1123
27	597–761	745–949	855–1090	704–898	878–1119	1009–1285
28	693–877	859–1087	982–1244	813–1030	1008–1276	1153–1460
29	803–1008	988–1239	1124–1410	937–1176	1152–1446	1312–1646
30	931–1155	1132–1405	1281–1589	1078–1337	1311–1627	1483–1840
31	1075–1317	1293–1584	1452–1779	1234–1512	1484–1819	1667–2042
32	1235–1493	1468–1774	1635–1976	1405–1698	1670–2018	1860–2248
33	1411–1682	1656–1973	1830–2180	1590–1895	1865–2223	2061–2456
34	1600–1880	1853–2177	2031–2386	1785–2098	2067–2429	2266–2662
35	1798–2083	2055–2382	2236–2590	1987–2302	2272–2633	2471–2863
36	1997–2285	2257–2583	2437–2789	2189–2504	2474–2830	2671–3056
37	2192–2479	2452–2774	2631–2976	2383–2696	2666–3016	2861–3236
38	2371–2658	2631–2949	2807–3147	2563–2872	2843–3186	3034–3400
39	2526–2812	2785–3101	2961–3296	2717–3025	2996–3335	3185–3545
40	2645–2933	2906–3223	3083–3419	2838–3147	3118–3458	3307–3668
41	2717–3013	2985–3310	3166–3511	2915–3232	3202–3551	3396–3766
42	2736–3045	3016–3356	3205–3567	2942–3274	3243–3609	3447–3836

*For each pair, estimated weight less than the lower value allows confident diagnosis of IUGR (positive predictive value, 74%). Estimated weight greater than the upper value virtually excludes IUGR (negative predictive value, 97%). Estimated weight between the two values is indeterminate for IUGR (likelihood of IUGR, 13%).

GA, gestational age; Nl BP, normal blood pressure; Htn, hypertension; Nl, normal fluid; Poly, polyhydramnios; M-M, mild to moderate; Oligo, oligohydramnios; Sev, severe

fluid volume (subjectively assessed), and maternal blood pressure status, the table presents two values. When a fetus has an estimated weight below the smaller value, IUGR can be diagnosed with confidence. If the estimated weight is above the larger value, growth retardation can be excluded with near certainty. An estimated weight between the two values is indeterminate for IUGR.

When accurate dating by an ultrasound performed prior to 20 weeks' gestation is available, a simpler rule applies, using only the lower value in the appropriate column. IUGR can be diagnosed if the estimated fetal weight falls below this value and can be excluded if the weight estimate falls above this same value.

To illustrate the use of this table in the diagnosis of IUGR, consider a case in which the gestational age is 34 weeks (based on a 24-week ultrasound), there is moderate oligohydramnios, and the mother is normotensive. On the basis of Table 33-13, if the estimated fetal weight is below 1853 g, IUGR can be diagnosed with confidence, and if it is above 2177 g, growth retardation can be ruled out. A weight estimate between these two values is indeterminate for IUGR. If the age of 34 weeks has been based on a 12-week ultrasound, then IUGR can be diagnosed if the estimated weight is below 1853 g and excluded if the weight estimate is above 1853 g.

This table provides a rational and reliable means for prenatal diagnosis of IUGR. When growth retardation is diagnosed, further evaluation using Doppler velocimetry can help to determine the prognosis.

Once IUGR has been diagnosed, an attempt should be made to determine its etiology, via evaluation of both the mother and the fetus. Maternal assessment should include physical examination and blood tests directed toward diagnosis of hypertension, renal disease, and other maternal conditions that can cause IUGR. Fetal assessment begins with a careful sonographic examination, looking especially for findings suggestive of a chromosomal or viral etiology (e.g., holoprosencephaly, clenched hands, rocker-bottom feet, intracranial calcifications). If such a finding is present, amniocentesis or umbilical blood sampling can confirm the diagnosis of a chromosomal abnormality. A viral etiology of IUGR may also be diagnosed by these procedures, in some cases.[102]

Growth-retarded fetuses, other than those with a lethal condition such as trisomy 13 or 18, should be carefully monitored for the remainder of the pregnancy. The monitoring is usually performed at weekly or semiweekly intervals. Sonographic features to be followed include amniotic fluid volume, biophysical profile score, estimated fetal weight percentile, and umbilical artery Doppler. A worsening trend in one or more of these features should prompt consideration of early delivery.

REFERENCES

1. Filly RA, Golbus MS, Carey JC et al. Short-limbed dwarfism: ultrasonographic diagnosis by mensuration of fetal femoral length. *Radiology* 1981;138:653-656.
2. Chervenak FA, Rosenberg J, Brightman RC et al. A prospective study of the accuracy of ultrasound in predicting fetal microcephaly. *Obstet Gynecol* 1987;69:908-910.
3. Bowerman RA. Sonography of fetal midgut herniation: normal size criteria and correlation with crown-rump length. *J Ultrasound Med* 1993;12:251-254.
4. Wald NJ, Cuckle HS, Densem JW et al. Maternal serum screening for Down's syndrome in early pregnancy. *Br Med J* 1988;8:883-887.
5. Osathanondh R, Canick JA, Abell KB et al. Second trimester screening for Trisomy 21. *Lancet* 1989;2:52.
6. Canick JA, Knight GJ, Palomaki GE et al. Low second trimester maternal serum unconjugated oestriol in pregnancies with Down's syndrome. *Br J Obstet Gynaecol* 1988;95: 330-333.
7. Guidelines for performance of the antepartum obstetrical ultrasound examination. American Institute of Ultrasound in Medicine; 1994.

Gestational Age Determination

8. Campbell S, Warsof SL, Little D et al. Routine ultrasound screening for the prediction of gestational age. *Obstet Gynecol* 1985;65:613-620.
9. Bradley WF, Fiske CE, Filly RA. The double sac sign in early intrauterine pregnancy: use in exclusion of ectopic pregnancy. *Radiology* 1982;148:223-226.
10. Fossum GT, Davajan V, Kletzky OA. Early detection of pregnancy with transvaginal ultrasound. *Fertile Steril* 1988;49: 788-791.
11. Bree RL, Edwards M, Bohm-Velez M et al. Transvaginal sonography in the evaluation of normal early pregnancy: correlation with HCG level. *AJR* 1989;153:75-79.
12. Jain KA, Hamper UM, Sanders RC. Comparison of transvaginal and transabdominal sonography in the detection of early pregnancy and its complications. *AJR* 1988;151: 1139-1143.
13. Robinson HP, Fleming JEE. A critical evaluation of sonar "crown-rump length" measurements. *Br J Obstet Gynecol* 1975;82:702-710.
14. MacGregor SN, Tamara RK, Sabbagha RE et al. Underestimation of gestational age by conventional crown-rump length dating curves. *Obstet Gynecol* 1987;70:344-348.
15. Moore KL, Persaud TVN. *The Developing Human*. 5th ed. Philadelphia: WB Saunders Co; 1993.
16. Kurtz AB, Wapner RJ, Kurtz RJ et al. Analysis of biparietal diameter as an accurate indicator of gestational age. *J Clin Ultrasound* 1980;8:319-326.
17. Doubilet PM, Benson CB. Improved prediction of gestational age in the late third trimester. *J Ultrasound Med* 1993; 12:647-653.
18. Law RG, MacRae KD. Head circumference as an index of fetal age. *J Ultrasound Med* 1982;1:281-288.
19. Hadlock FP, Deter RL, Harrist RB et al. Fetal abdominal circumference as a predictor of menstrual age. *AJR* 1982;139: 367-370.
20. Hadlock FP, Deter RL, Harrist RB et al. Estimating fetal age: computer-assisted analysis of multiple fetal growth parameters. *Radiology* 1984;152:497-501.
21. Jeanty PJ, Rodesch F, Delbeke D et al. Estimation of gestational age from measurements of fetal long bones. *J Ultrasound Med* 1984;3:75-79.
22. Jeanty P, Cantraine F, Cousaert E et al. The binocular distance: a new way to estimate fetal age. *J Ultrasound Med* 1984;3:241-243.
23. Doubilet PM, Greenes RA. Improved prediction of gestational age from fetal head measurements. *AJR* 1984;142:797-800.
24. Hadlock FP, Deter RL, Harrist RB et al. Computer assisted analysis of fetal age in the third trimester using multiple fetal growth parameters. *J Clin Ultrasound* 1983;11:313-316.
25. Hadlock FP, Deter RL, Harrist RB et al. Fetal biparietal diameter: rational choice of plane of section for sonographic measurement. *AJR* 1982;138:871-874.
26. Hadlock FP, Kent WR, Loyd JL et al. An evaluation of two methods for measuring fetal head and body circumferences. *J Ultrasound Med* 1982;1:359-360.
27. Goldstein RB, Filly RA, Simpson G. Pitfalls in femur length measurements. *J Ultrasound Med* 1987;6:203-207.
28. Benson CB, Doubilet PM. Fetal measurements for predicting gestational age in the second and third trimesters: a reappraisal with a more reliable gold standard. *Radiology* 1988; 169(P):210.

Weight Estimation and Assessment

29. Campbell S, Wilkin D. Ultrasonic measurements of fetal abdominal circumference in the estimation of fetal weight. *Br J Obstet Gynecol* 1975;82:689-697.
30. Higginbottom J, Slater J, Porter G et al. Estimation of fetal weight from ultrasonic measurement of trunk circumference. *Br J Obstet Gynecol* 1975;82:698-701.
31. Warsof SL, Gohari P, Berkowitz RL et al. The estimation of fetal weight by computer-assisted analysis. *Am J Obstet Gynecol* 1977;128:881-892.
32. Shepard MJ, Richards VA, Berkowitz RL et al. An evaluation of two equations for predicting fetal weight by ultrasound. *Am J Obstet Gynecol* 1982;142:47-54.
33. Thurneau GR, Tamura RK, Sabbagha R et al. A simple estimated fetal weight equation based on real-time ultrasound measurements of fetuses less than thirty-four weeks' gestation. *Am J Obstet Gynecol* 1983;145:557-561.
34. Jordaan HVF. Estimation of fetal weight by ultrasound. *J Clin Ultrasound* 1983;11:59-66.
35. Hadlock FP, Harrist RB, Carpenter RJ et al. Sonographic estimation of fetal weight: the value of femur length in addition to head and abdomen measurements. *Radiology* 1984;150: 535-540.
36. Hadlock FP, Harrist RB, Sharman RS et al. Estimation of fetal weight with the use of head, body, and femur measurements: a prospective study. *Am J Obstet Gynecol* 1985;151: 333-337.
37. Birnholz JC. An algorithmic approach to accurate ultrasonic fetal weight estimation. *Invest Radiol* 1986;21:571-576.
38. Vintzileos AM, Campbell WA, Rodis JF et al. Fetal weight estimation formulas with head, abdominal, femur, and thigh circumference measurements. *Am J Obstet Gynecol* 1987; 157:410-414.
39. Benacerraf BR, Gelman R, Frigoletto FD. Sonographically estimated fetal weights: accuracy and limitation. *Am J Obstet Gynecol* 1988;159:1118-1121.

40. Townsend RR, Filly RA, Callen PW et al. Factors affecting prenatal sonographic estimation of weight in extremely low birthweight infants. *J Ultrasound Med* 1988;7:183-187.
41. Hill LM, Breckle R, Wolfgram KR et al. Evaluation of three methods for estimating fetal weight. *J Clin Ultrasound* 1986;14:171-178.
42. Benson CB, Doubilet PM, Saltzman DH. Sonographic determination of fetal weights in diabetic pregnancies. *Am J Obstet Gynecol* 1987;156:441-444.
43. Doubilet PM, Benson CB, Nadel AS, Ringer SA. Improved birth weight table for neonates developed from gestations dated by early ultrasonography. *J Ultrasound Med* 1997; 16:241-249.
44. Brenner WE, Edelman DA, Hendricks CH. A standard of fetal growth for the United States of America. *Am J Obstet Gynecol* 1976;126:555-564.
45. Lubchenco LO, Hansman C, Dressler M et al. Intrauterine growth as estimated from liveborn birth-weight data at 24 to 42 weeks of gestation. *Pediatrics*. 1963;32:793-800.
46. Gruenwald P. Fetus and newborn: growth of the human fetus. I. Normal growth and its variation. *Am J Obstet Gynecol* 1966;94:1112-1119.
47. Thomson AM, Billewicz WZ, Hytten FE. The assessment of fetal growth. *J Obstet Gynecol Br Commonw* 1968;75:903-916.
48. Hutchins CJ. Delivery of the growth-retarded infant. *Obstet Gynecol* 1980;56:683-686.
49. Greenes RA. OBUS: a microcomputer system for measurement, calculation, reporting, and retrieval of obstetric ultrasound examinations. *Radiology* 1982;144:879-883.
50. Jeanty P. A simple reporting system for obstetrical ultrasonography. *J Ultrasound Med* 1985;4:591-593.
51. Ott WJ. The design and implementation of a computer-based ultrasound data system. *J Ultrasound Med* 1986;5:25-32.

Fetal Growth Abnormalities

52. Ott WJ. The diagnosis of altered fetal growth. *Obstet Gynecol Clin North Am* 1988;15:237-263.
53. Mintz MC, Landon MB. Sonographic diagnosis of fetal growth disorders. *Clin Obstet Gynecol* 1988;31:44-52.
54. Landon MB, Mintz MC, Gabbe SG. Sonographic evaluation of fetal abdominal growth: predictor of the large-for-gestational-age infant in pregnancies complicated by diabetes mellitus. *Am J Obstet Gynecol* 1989;160:115-121.
55. Boyd ME, Usher RH, McLean FH. Fetal macrosomia: prediction, risks, proposed management. *Obstet Gynecol* 1983;61: 715-722.
56. Modanlou HD, Dorchester WL, Thorosian A et al. Macrosomia: maternal, fetal, and neonatal implications. *Obstet Gynecol* 1980;55:420-424.
57. Deter RL, Hadlock FP. Use of ultrasound in the detection of macrosomia: a review. *J Clin Ultrasound* 1985;13:519-524.
58. Golditch IM, Kirkman K. The large fetus: management and outcome. *Obstet Gynecol* 1978;52:26-30.
59. Rodriguez MH. Ultrasound evaluation of the postdate pregnancy. *Clin Obstet Gynecol* 1989;32:257-261.
60. Arias F. Predictability of complications associated with prolongation of pregnancy. *Obstet Gynecol* 1987;70:101-106.
61. Acker DB, Sachs BP, Friedman EA. Risk factors for shoulder dystocia. *Obstet Gynecol* 1985;66:762-768.
62. Gross SJ, Shime J, Farine D. Shoulder dystocia: predictors and outcome. A five-year review. *Am J Obstet Gynecol* 1987; 156:334-336.
63. Miller JM, Korndorffer FA, Gabert HA. Fetal weight estimates in late pregnancy with emphasis on macrosomia. *J Clin Ultrasound* 1986;14:437-442.
64. Sabbagha RE, Minogue J, Tamura RK et al. Estimation of birthweight by use of ultrasonographic formulas targeted to large-, appropriate-, and small-for-gestational-age fetuses? *Am J Obstet Gynecol* 1989;160:854-862.
65. Miller JM, Kissling GA, Brown HL et al. Estimated fetal weight: applicability to small- and large-for-gestational-age fetus. *J Clin Ultrasound* 1988;16:95-97.
66. Doubilet PM, Benson CB. Fetal growth disturbances. *Semin Roentgenol* 1990;25:309-316.
67. Miller JM, Korndorffer FA, Kissling GE et al. Recognition of the overgrown fetus: in utero ponderal indices. *Am J Perinatol* 1987;4:86-89.
68. Chamberlain PF, Manning FA, Morrison I. Ultrasound evaluation of amniotic fluid volume. II. The relationship of increased amniotic fluid volume to perinatal outcome. *Am J Obstet Gynecol* 1984;150:250-254.
69. Benson CB, Doubilet PM. Amniotic fluid volume in the large-for-gestational-age fetus. *Radiology* 1989;173(P):248.
70. Miller JM, Brown HL, Khawli OF et al. Ultrasonographic identification of the macrosomic fetus. *Am J Obstet Gynecol* 1988;159:1110-1114.
71. Basel D, Lederer R, Diamant YZ. Longitudinal ultrasonic biometry of various parameters in fetuses with abnormal growth rate. *Acta Obstet Gynecol Scand* 1987;66:143-149.
72. Elliott JP, Garite TJ, Freeman RK et al. Ultrasonic prediction of fetal macrosomia in diabetic patients. *Obstet Gynecol* 1982;60:159-162.
73. Bochner CJ, Medearis AL, William J et al. Early third-trimester ultrasound screening in gestational diabetes to determine the risk of macrosomia and labor dystocia at term. *Am J Obstet Gynecol* 1987;157:703-708.
74. Sandmire HF, O'Halloin TJ. Shoulder dystocia: its incidence and associated risk factors. *Int J Gynaecol Obstet* 1988; 26:65-73.
75. Tamura RK, Sabbagha RE, Depp R et al. Diabetic macrosomia: accuracy of third-trimester ultrasound. *Obstet Gynecol* 1986;67:828-832.
76. Bracero LA, Baxi LV, Rey HR et al. Use of ultrasound in antenatal diagnosis of large-for-gestational-age infants in diabetic gravid patients. *Am J Obstet Gynecol* 1985;152:43-47.
77. Benson CB, Doubilet PM, Saltzman DH et al. Femur length/abdominal circumference ratio: poor predictor of macrosomic fetuses in diabetic mothers. *J Ultrasound Med* 1986;5:141-144.
78. Lugo G, Cassady G. Intrauterine growth retardation: clinicopathologic findings in 233 consecutive infants. *Am J Obstet Gynecol* 1971;109:615-622.
79. Galbraith RS, Karchmar EJ, Piercy WN et al. The clinical prediction of intrauterine growth retardation. *Am J Obstet Gynecol* 1979;133:281-286.
80. Divon MY, Chamberlain PF, Sipos L et al. Identification of the small-for-gestational-age fetus with the use of gestational-age-independent indices of fetal growth. *Am J Obstet Gynecol* 1986;155:1197-1201.
81. Sabbagha RE. Intrauterine growth retardation: avenues of future research in diagnosis and management by ultrasound. *Semin Perinatol* 1984;8:31-36.
82. Reed K, Droegmueller W. Intrauterine growth retardation. In: Centrullo CL, Sbarra AJ, eds. *The Problem-oriented Medical Record*. New York: Plenum; 1984:175-194.
83. Lockwood CJ, Weiner S. Assessment of fetal growth. *Clin Perinatol* 1986;13:3-35.
84. Seeds JW. Impaired fetal growth: definition and clinical diagnosis. *Obstet Gynecol* 1984;64:303-310.
85. Dodson PC, Abell DA, Beischer NA. Mortality and morbidity of fetal growth retardation. *Aust NZ J Obstet Gynecol* 1981;21:69-72.
86. Benson CB, Doubilet PM. Head-sparing in fetuses with intrauterine growth retardation: does it really occur? *Radiology* 1986;161(P):75.

87. Benson CB, Doubilet PM, Saltzman DH. Intrauterine growth retardation: predictive value of ultrasound criteria for antenatal diagnosis. *Radiology* 1986;160:415-417.
88. Benson CB, Doubilet PM. Doppler criteria for intrauterine growth retardation: predictive values. *J Ultrasound Med* 1988;7:655-659.
89. Weinstein MC, Fineberg HV, Elstein AS et al. *Clinical Decision Analysis*. Philadelphia: WB Saunders Co, 1980.
90. McCowan LM, Erskine LA, Ritchie K. Umbilical artery Doppler blood flow studies in the preterm, small-for-gestational-age fetus. *Am J Obstet Gynecol* 1987;156:655-659.
91. Reuwer PJH, Sijmons EA, Reitman GW et al. Intrauterine growth retardation: prediction of perinatal distress by Doppler ultrasound. *Lancet* 1987;2:415-418.
92. Rochelson BL, Schulman H, Fleischer A et al. The clinical significance of Doppler umbilical artery velocimetry in the small-for-gestational-age fetus. *Am J Obstet Gynecol* 1987;156:1223-1226.
93. Berkowitz GS, Mehalek KE, Chitkara U et al. Doppler umbilical velocimetry in the prediction of adverse outcome in pregnancies at risk for intrauterine growth retardation. *Obstet Gynecol* 1988;71:742-746.
94. Illyes M, Gati I. Reverse flow in the human fetal descending aorta as a sign of severe fetal asphyxia preceding intrauterine death. *J Clin Ultrasound* 1988;16:403-407.
95. Brar HS, Platt LD. Reverse end-diastolic flow velocity on umbilical artery velocimetry in high-risk pregnancies: an ominous finding with adverse pregnancy outcome. *Am J Obstet Gynecol* 1988;159:559-561.
96. Woo JSK, Liang ST, Lo RLS. Significance of an absent or reversed end diastolic flow in Doppler umbilical artery waveforms. *J Ultrasound Med* 1987;6:291-297.
97. Rochelson BL, Schulman H, Fleischer A et al. The clinical significance of Doppler umbilical artery velocimetry in the small-for-gestational-age fetus. *Am J Obstet Gynecol* 1987; 256:1223-1226.
98. Berkowitz GS, Mehalek KE, Chitkara U et al. Doppler umbilical velocimetry in the prediction of adverse outcome in pregnancies at risk for intrauterine growth retardation. *Obstet Gynecol* 1988;71:742-746.
99. Trudinger BJ, Giles WB, Cook CM. Flow velocity waveforms in the maternal uteroplacental and fetal umbilical placental circulations. *Am J Obstet Gynecol* 1985;152:155-163.
100. Benson CB, Boswell SB, Brown DL et al. Improved prediction of intrauterine growth retardation with use of multiple parameters. *Radiology* 1988;168:7-12.
101. Benson CB, Belville JS, Lentini JF et al. Diagnosis of intrauterine growth retardation using multiple parameters: a prospective study. *Radiology* 1990;177:499-502.
102. Doubilet PM, Benson CB. Sonographic evaluation of intrauterine growth retardation. *AJR* 1995;164:709-717.

CHAPTER 34

Fetal Biophysical Profile Scoring

Jo-Ann M. Johnson, M.D., F.R.C.S.C.
Christopher R. Harman, M.D., F.R.C.S.C.

CHAPTER OUTLINE

In recent years there has been a dramatic improvement in perinatal outcome, with most centers reporting perinatal mortality rates of less than 12 per 1000.[1] This is a decrease to half the rate of the previous decade (Fig. 34-1).[2] This trend may reflect, in part, the application of specific fetal evaluation techniques. In this context, high-resolution sonography has increasingly facilitated the accurate diagnosis of not only acute and chronic asphyxia, but also potential fetal disease and congenital anomalies. In modern management of high-risk pregnancy, therefore, real-time ultrasound "fetal assessment" has a central essential role. **Biophysical profile scoring (BPS)** is a method of **antepartum evaluation** using **dynamic ultrasound assessment** of multiple fetal biophysical variables to **identify the fetus at risk** for death or damage in utero and to facilitate management of the high-risk pregnancy.

Biophysical profile scoring is designed to **detect fetal asphyxia.** The use of **five** fetal behaviors that have different cyclicity and different time periods improves test sensitivity and specificity compared with single-variable testing, such as the nonstress test.[3] Fetal health can be assessed accordingly, and this has influenced clinical practice. Accurate recognition of fetal risk, when combined with maternal obstetric assessment, permits a selective approach to intervention. For example, in a postdates patient with an unfavorable cervix and a normal biophysical profile score, intervention can be safely deferred until maternal obstetric factors improve, thereby reducing the induction rate and the concomitant cesarean section rate.[4] In contrast, identification of fetal asphyxia would precipitate aggressive obstetric intervention; this has improved perinatal outcome. The method has evolved as more information on fetal physiology and pathology has become available. While research continues to evaluate the potential addition of further variables (e.g., Doppler information) or refinement of existing variables, increasing numbers of perinatal units regard the biophysical profile score (BPS) as the gold standard for determination of fetal health.

FETAL BIOPHYSICAL ACTIVITIES

Normal Patterns of Behavior

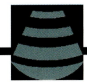

The developing fetus exhibits a wide range of biophysical activities, ranging from **gross motor activities,** such as body, limb, and breathing movements, to **fine motor activities,** such as eye movements, pur-

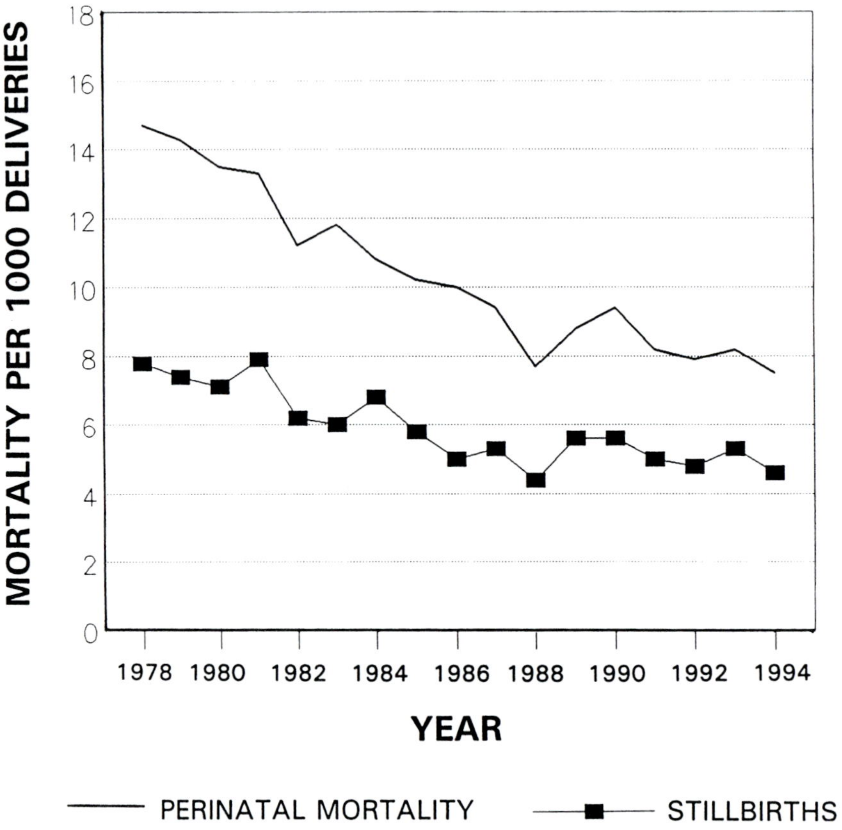

FIG. 34-1. Declining perinatal mortality and stillbirth rates in Manitoba since 1978.

poseful limb movements, sucking, and swallowing. With real-time ultrasound, fetal movements can be seen **as early as 6 weeks gestation,** and they become increasingly organized as gestation advances, progressing from total body clonic motion to discrete fine movements of fingers and lips. **Fetal respiratory activity** begins with diaphragmatic contractions ("hiccups") with more rhythmic fetal breathing movements becoming dominant in the second half of pregnancy. **Fetal heart rate changes,** in response to fetal movement, may be recognized by 12 to 14 weeks gestation. Transient bradycardia appears to be a primary cardiac response to fetal movement in early gestation, but with advancing maturity of the central nervous system (CNS) (e.g., 24 weeks gestation), fetal heart rate (FHR) accelerations become the primary response with fetal movement. This coupling of FHR with movement is the basis for the **nonstress test** (NST), one element of the biophysical profile.

These biophysical activities are not random events but rather highly specific movements regulated by complex central neurologic pathways. Fetal activity becomes increasingly organized and patterned as pregnancy progresses, with grouping of behaviors as term approaches. Thus, by **the end of the pregnancy,** the fetus has defined periods of active and quiet sleep, responds to maternal glucose levels (increased fetal breathing about an hour after meals), has circadian rhythms in swallowing, micturition, and most movements, and demonstrates behavior states directly analogous to those illustrated by healthy newborns.[5]

Responses to Asphyxia

Because the fetal brain and spinal cord (CNS) are exquisitely oxygen sensitive, it follows that if these biophysical activities are present, then functioning and well-oxygenated neurologic pathways are operating. Thus, the presence of **normal activity** is a powerful **predictor** of a **normal and intact CNS.**

Abnormal or normal fetuses challenged by inadequate placental provisions (oxygen, nutrients, or both) may **alter their activity**—first subtly, later dramatically—in response to progressive compromise. Such changes are usually conservative—reduced activity results in reduced oxygen utilization, allowing conservation for "essential" central functions.[6] **Prolonged cessation of all activity,** for example, is strongly suggestive of **severe fetal compromise.** The partial or short-term absence of a specific activity is considerably more difficult to interpret since, in a normal fetus, **periodicity** is characteristic of biophysical activities. Periodicity is markedly influenced by sleep-wake cycles, and the absence of one or more activities for short periods is often observed during quiet sleep. For example, periods of fetal breathing alternate with periods of apnea, and although fetal breathing occupies up to 40% of any hour, apnea can be as long as 120 minutes in a normal fetus.[7,8] Similarly, episodes of nonreactivity of the fetal heart rate may be observed for up to 108 minutes in the normal fetus.[9] In the term fetus, coincident episodes of low activity, nonbreathing, and reduced FHR variation may leave the fetus with only repetitive small jaw motions to signify **normal** behavior state.[10]

To differentiate the normal fetus in quiet sleep from the asphyxiated fetus, it may be necessary to observe a variety of fetal activities over an extended period. This premise is the foundation of fetal biophysical profile scoring. In addition, by using a **"binary approach"** to document fetal biophysical activity (**minimum criteria present or absent**) rather than a proportional approach (**the incidence of the given activity per unit of time**), the problem of intrinsic rhythm may largely be circumvented.[11]

Finally, factors other than CNS rhythm or asphyxia may alter biophysical response.[7,11,12] Smoking, administration of medication that may suppress biophysical activity (narcotics), fetal CNS injury, or a variety of congenital abnormalities must always be considered as potential causes of an absent biophysical variable.

Acute Versus Chronic Fetal Asphyxia

The effects of asphyxia on fetal biophysical behavior depend on the extent, duration, chronicity, and frequency of the insult. Fetal asphyxia may be transient without acidosis. If prolonged, with associated metabolic or respiratory acidosis, multiple organ systems may be affected.

Acute fetal asphyxia produces a decrease or abolition of short-term variables—fetal breathing movements[13,14] and fetal heart rate reactivity[15]—and, when severe, may result in reduced or absent fetal movement and tone.[16] There is strong circumstantial evidence that these biophysical changes reflect fetal compromise at the time of the test (Fig. 34-2).[17]

Chronic fetal asphyxia is usually a gradual process associated with primary uteroplacental insufficiency. In the **early** stages, no alteration in fetal biophysical behavior may be observed. However, **repeated episodes** of transient hypoxemia may result in a dramatic redistribution of fetal cardiac output such that cerebral blood flow is maintained while renal, pulmonary, and splanchnic blood flow falls dramatically.[18] Because fetal urine and pulmonary fluid are the major sources of amniotic fluid after 14 to 16 weeks of gestation, a decrease in the production of these fluids will result in progressive reduction of amniotic fluid volume, ultimately leading to **oligohydramnios.**[19] Therefore, estimation of amniotic fluid volume, an integral part of the biophysical profile score, may be viewed as a marker of repetitive, intermittent fetal asphyxia if low, and a valuable indirect marker of fetal health[20] with an intermediate time frame as compared with short-term behaviors.

In general, the fetus with normal renal tissue and bladder filling, in association with oligohydramnios and intact membranes, should be considered as having evidence of chronic asphyxia until proven otherwise. In a prospective study, this principle has proven clinically effective when oligohydramnios is a "mandatory" indication for delivery.[21]

Nonasphyxic Assessment

The chance detection of clinically unsuspected conditions that contribute to perinatal morbidity and mortality (other than fetal asphyxia resulting from inadequate placental perfusion) is an additional advantage of using ultrasound for fetal assessment. For example, gestational diabetes may be suspected, disorders of fetal growth detected, and nonimmune hydrops discovered.[11,22] Antepartum detection of major fetal anomalies, which may have a significant effect on ultimate obstetric management, is also an integral part of fetal biophysical examination. Abnormal placentation, fetal malpresentation, and potentially lethal cord presentation (Fig. 34-3)[23] are all readily noted during BPS performance. Thus, although profile scoring is the primary intent, it is artificial to separate a biophysical profile examination from a complete fetal assessment.

FETAL BIOPHYSICAL PROFILE SCORING

The Method

Fetal biophysical profile scoring (BPS) is a **sonographic-based** method of fetal assessment first described by Manning and Platt in 1980.[24] The score consists of **five parameters:** fetal movement (FM), fetal posture and tone (FPT), fetal breathing movements (FBM), quantitative amniotic fluid volume (qAFV), and cardiotocogram or nonstress test (NST).

BIOPHYSICAL PROFILE SCORING

Fetal movement (FM)
Fetal posture and tone (FPT)
Fetal breathing movements (FBM)
Quantitative amniotic fluid volume (qAFV)
Cardiotocogram or nonstress test (NST)

As noted, the first three ultrasound variables (FM, FPT, and FBM) are considered "acute" CNS markers, and the fourth ultrasound variable (AFV) is of a more chronic time frame. Initially, these ultrasound variables are evaluated in real time and are assessed as normal or abnormal, according to fixed criteria (Table 34-1).[11] If necessary, **observation time** is **extended to 30 minutes,** at which point the variable is classified as absent (abnormal). The observations are assigned a score of 2 if normal/present and 0 if abnormal/absent. If all ultrasound variables are present (BPS 8/8), the test is concluded as normal. If not all ultrasound variables are normal, the **nonstress test (cardiotocogram)** is added. This evaluates **FHR response to activity** and is also an "acute" variable. With hypoxia, coupling of FHR accelerations with FM is reduced or absent ("nonreactive NST") (Fig. 34-4). **Any score** that is persistently **less than or equal to 6** is considered **abnormal** and an **indication for delivery.** The general guide for management based on the fetal BPS is given in Table 34-2. It is important to emphasize that the clinical situation is always taken into consideration when interpreting the score and advising management. For example, we consider a dete-

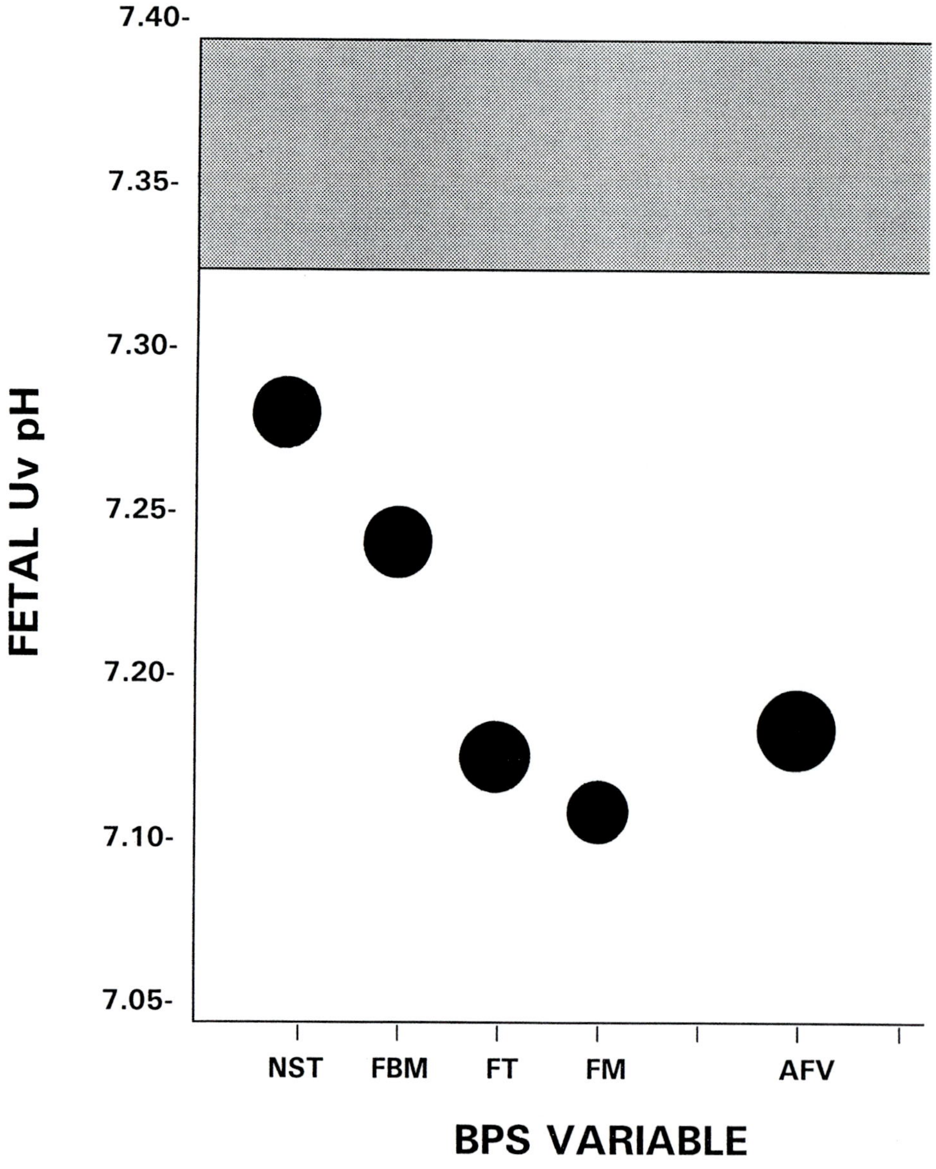

FIG. 34-2. Sequential loss of behaviors with declining fetal pH. Closed circles indicate mean pH ±2 SD at which the individual variable was lost (abnormal). Shaded area indicates pH for population who had umbilical venous blood sampling, normal behaviors. (From Manning FA, Snijders R, Harman CR et al. The relationship between fetal biophysical profile score and fetal pH. In: *Proceedings of the Society of Perinatal Obstetricians' Annual Meeting* (abstract). Feb. 1993.)

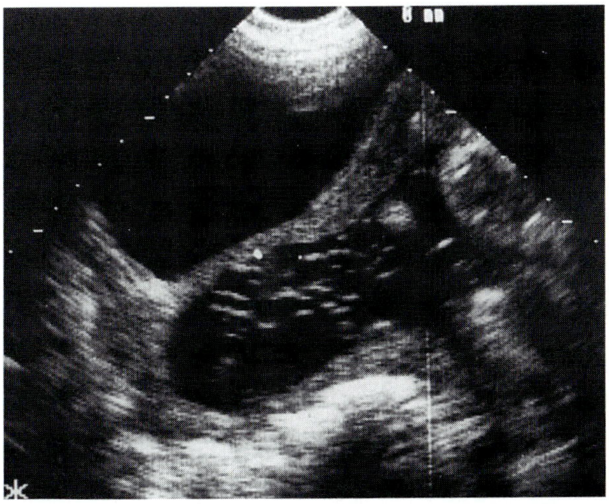

FIG. 34-3. Potentially lethal cord presentation. Sonogram at term shows marked cervical effacement and funneling of the lower segment in an asymptomatic mother. Cord accidents account for 10% to 20% of perinatal mortality in fetuses > 1000 g. (From College of Physicians and Surgeons of Manitoba. Perinatal and Maternal Welfare Committee. *1993 Annual Report.* Winnipeg, Manitoba; 1995.)

rioration in maternal condition (e.g., severe proteinuric preeclampsia) as an indication for delivery even in the presence of a normal fetal BPS. The emphasis is to respond to both maternal and fetal problems and not to treat the test.

In general, fetal BPS is reserved for patients referred with recognized high-risk factors. **Testing begins** at a gestational age at which results will modify management (**approximately 26 weeks**) and is done in a **serial fashion.** Most referred patients are tested **weekly.** Those with severe or unstable conditions (e.g., proteinuric preeclampsia, fetal macrosomia, and hydramnios due to insulin-dependent diabetes) and those with postdates pregnancies are tested twice weekly.[11,25] Testing is continued until the initial risk factor resolves (e.g., suspected intrauterine growth retardation with proven normal growth), until delivery occurs, or until the test becomes abnormal.

In clinical practice, the NST is included only about 10% to 15% of the time (when one or more of the dynamic ultrasound variables are abnormal) or when clinical severity warrants. This modification has been studied prospectively and has not been shown to alter

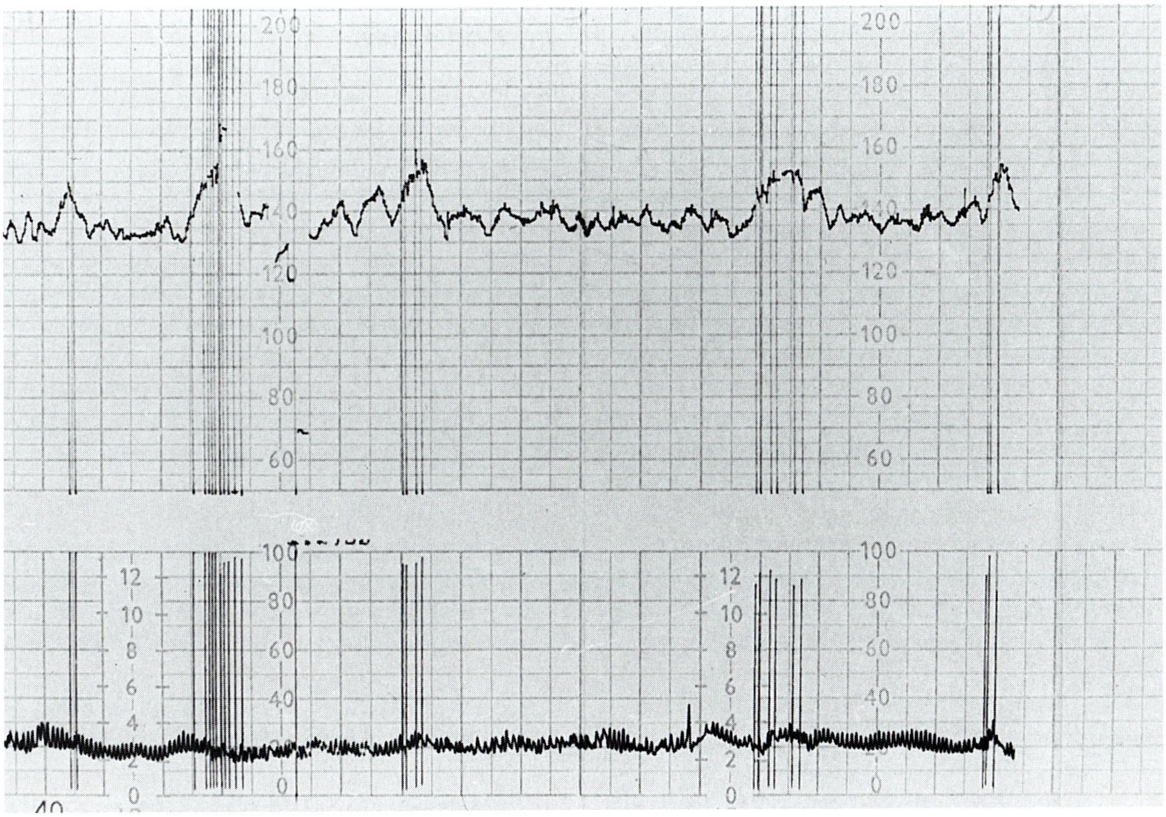

FIG. 34-4. Normal or reactive nonstress test (NST). The fetal heart rate is recorded from an autoregulating multiheaded Doppler array. Maternal perception of fetal activity is used to correlate activity (marks on lower portion of graph) with accelerations, clearly evident on upper trace.

TABLE 34-1
BIOPHYSICAL PROFILE SCORING: TECHNIQUE AND INTERPRETATION

Biophysical Variable	Normal (score = 2)	Abnormal (score = 0)
Fetal breathing movements (FBM)	≥ 1 episode of ≥ 30 s of FBM in 30 min or less	Absent or no episode of ≥ 30 s in full 30 min
Fetal movements (FM)	≥ 3 discrete body/limb movements in 30 min or less (episodes of active continuous movement considered as single movement)	< 2 episodes of body/limb movements in full 30 min
Fetal posture and tone (FPT)	≥ 1 episode of active extension with return to flexion of fetal limb(s) or trunk; opening and closing of hand considered normal tone	Slow extension with return to partial flexion, movement of limb in full extension, or absent fetal movement
Reactive fetal heart rate (the NST)	≥ 2 episodes of acceleration of ≥ 15 bpm and of > 15 s associated with fetal movement in 20 min	< 2 episodes of acceleration of fetal heart rate or acceleration of < 15 bpm in 20 min
Qualitative amniotic fluid volume (qAFV)	≥ 1 pocket of fluid measuring 2 cm in vertical axis	Either no pockets or largest pocket < 2 cm in vertical axis

bpm, Beats per minute.
Adapted from Manning FA, Platt LD, Sipos L et al. Fetal breathing movements and the non-stress test in high-risk pregnancies. *Am J Obstet Gynecol* 1979;135:511-515.

the predictive accuracy of the method.[26] Reduced use of the nonstress test saves approximately 30 minutes of time per patient per test, noting that the normal BPS (8/8) takes an average of 11 minutes to document. (In other words, it is not necessary to extend the BPS beyond the time when all four ultrasound criteria have been met—BPS 8/8.)

Clinical Results

The concept of fetal biophysical profile scoring was first tested by Manning et al. in a prospective single-blinded study of 216 high-risk patients.[24] These patients were managed primarily by the NST, and the results of the other biophysical variables were not disclosed and, therefore, did not influence management or outcome. There was a significant correlation between abnormal BPS and low 5-minute Apgar scores, fetal distress in labor, and perinatal death rate. The combination of the individual parameters of the profile resulted in a significant change in both the false-negative and false-positive result rates as compared with any single test. The **most accurate** differentiation of the normal from the compromised fetus was obtained when **all five** biophysical variables were studied. When all variables were normal (score of 10/10), the perinatal death rate was 0, and when all were abnormal (score of 0/10), the perinatal death rate was 600 per 1000 and the fetal death rate was 400 per 1000. The results of this study were used as the basis for the development of the **management protocol** (see Table 34-2).

This protocol was tested prospectively by the same investigators in a study involving 1184 consecutive high-risk patients who had 2238 fetal biophysical profiles performed.[27] There were 6 perinatal deaths in this study group (perinatal mortality 0.5 per 1000). This perinatal mortality rate was significantly less than the predicted rate for a similar high-risk population (65 per 1000) or the general population (14.3 per 1000) in their province of Manitoba, Canada, at the time. Only 1 fetus suffered an unpredicted death, giving a true false-negative rate of 0.8 per 1000. In addition, 13 of 19 (69%) fetuses with major congenital anomalies were detected as a result of ultrasound scanning. With the higher-resolution equipment now available, this detection rate currently approaches 95%.

Data from several centers are now available to evaluate the **relationship between BPS** and the **perinatal mortality rate.**[16,28-31] Three large series were performed in an identical manner by nurse-ultrasonographers and perinatologists on high-risk referred patient groups, totaling 62,500 fetuses.[16,28,29] The perinatal mortality rate (corrected for lethal anomalies) was 1.98 per 1000 overall (range 3.1 to 1.86). In all cases, these rates were much lower than those of the unmonitored, lower-risk pregnancies, and statistically significant impacts of this approach were apparent in as little as 2 years. Although they do not constitute a randomized controlled trial, these collected data strongly suggest that the **application of the fetal BPS to the high-risk pregnant population** results in **an improvement in perinatal mortality.**

TABLE 34-2
RECOMMENDED CLINICAL MANAGEMENT BY FETAL BIOPHYSICAL PROFILE SCORE

Test Score	Interpretation	Recommended Management
10/10 8/8 (NST not done) 8/10 (N-AVF)	No evidence of acute or chronic asphyxia	Conservative management Serial testing as per protocol
8/10 (ABN-AFV)	No evidence of acute asphyxia Chronic asphyxia likely	Deliver if > 36 wks*; if < 36 wks, serial testing
6/10 (N-AFV)	Acute asphyxia possible	Deliver if > 36 wks; if < 36 wks, repeat test within 24 hrs
6/10 (ABN-AFV)	Acute/chronic asphyxia possible	Deliver if > 26 wks
4/10 (N-AFV)	Acute asphyxia likely	Deliver if > 32 wks; if < 32 wks, repeat test same day; if repeat test < 6, deliver
4/10 (ABN-AFV)	Acute/chronic asphyxia likely	Deliver if > 26 wks
2/10	Acute/chronic asphyxia very likely	Extend test to 60 min; deliver if score remains < 6 and gestational age > 26 wks
0/10	Acute/chronic asphyxia nearly certain	Deliver if > 26 wks

N, Normal; *ABN*, abnormal; *AFV*, amniotic fluid volume; *NST*, nonstress test.
*Gestational age in weeks.
From Manning FA. Fetal biophysical profile scoring: theoretical considerations and practical application. In: Fleischer AC, Manning FM, Jeanty P et al, eds. *Sonography in Obstetrics and Gynecology*. 5th ed. Stamford, Conn: Appleton & Lange; 1996.

The probability of fetal death within 1 week of a normal test is reported to range from 0.65 to 0.7 per 1000.[16,28-33] These "false-negative deaths" have been analyzed in detail in the Canadian studies monitoring more than 58,000 high-risk fetuses, with 35 reported fetal deaths (0.60 per 1000).[16,29] There was no definable pattern to these unexpected losses, that is, they appear to be random rather than a specific failure of the system. These figures are of clinical importance because they allow conservative management of high-risk pregnancies when the known risks of premature delivery are balanced against the low probability of fetal death with a normal BPS.

As might be expected, there is a strong statistical relationship between the last test score and perinatal mortality (Fig. 34-5). Perinatal mortality is an absolute end point by which test performance can be measured. It is not the ideal. A method of fetal assessment in which an abnormal test correlates with perinatal mortality is too late to be of clinical value. Therefore, early intervention for an abnormal score should not only reduce mortality but should also reduce perinatal morbidity. The two largest studies to address this[16,29] have, in fact, shown a strong relationship between the last test score and various markers of perinatal morbidity (Fig. 34-6). New information from the University of Manitoba, which is now able to access a BPS database of more than 90,000 high-risk referred cases, addresses issues surrounding cerebral palsy. Among fetuses followed for various defined risk factors, 27 subsequently developed cerebral palsy. These

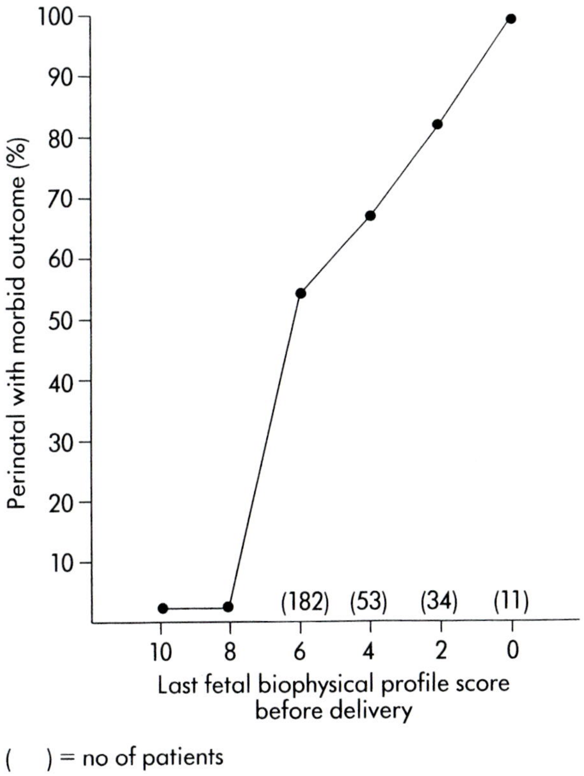

FIG. 34-5. Perinatal morbidity: outcome variables (five) versus biophysical profile score (before delivery). A significant inverse linear correlation is observed for each variable. (From Manning FA, Morrison I, Lange IR et al. Fetal biophysical profile scoring: a prospective study of 1,184 high-risk patients. *Am J Obstet Gynecol* 1981;140:289-294.)

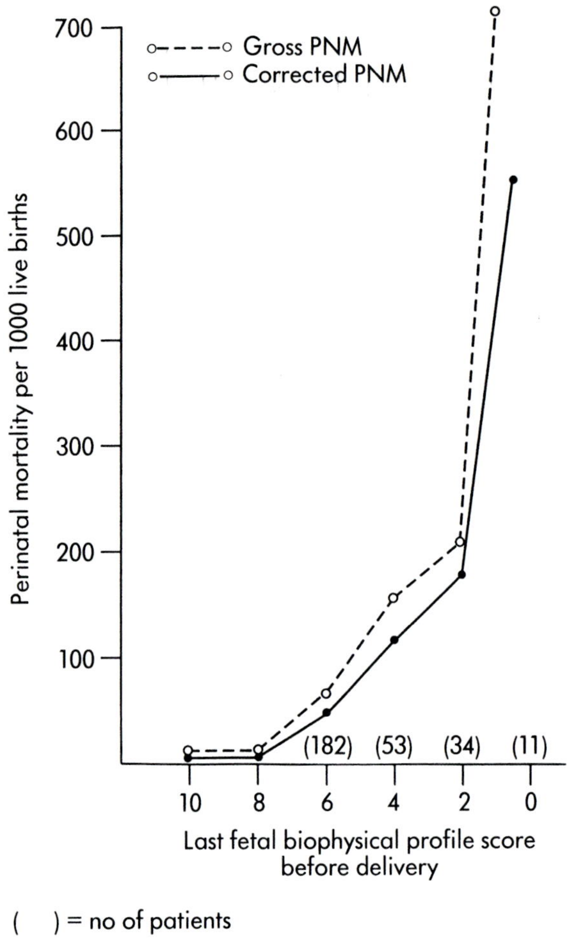

FIG. 34-6. Perinatal mortality (either total or corrected for major anomaly) versus the last biophysical profile score. This relationship is exponential, yielding a highly significant inverse correlation using *log*10 conversion. (From Manning FA, Morrison I, Lange IR et al. Fetal biophysical profile scoring: a prospective study of 1,184 high-risk patients. *Am J Obstet Gynecol* 1981; 140:289-294.)

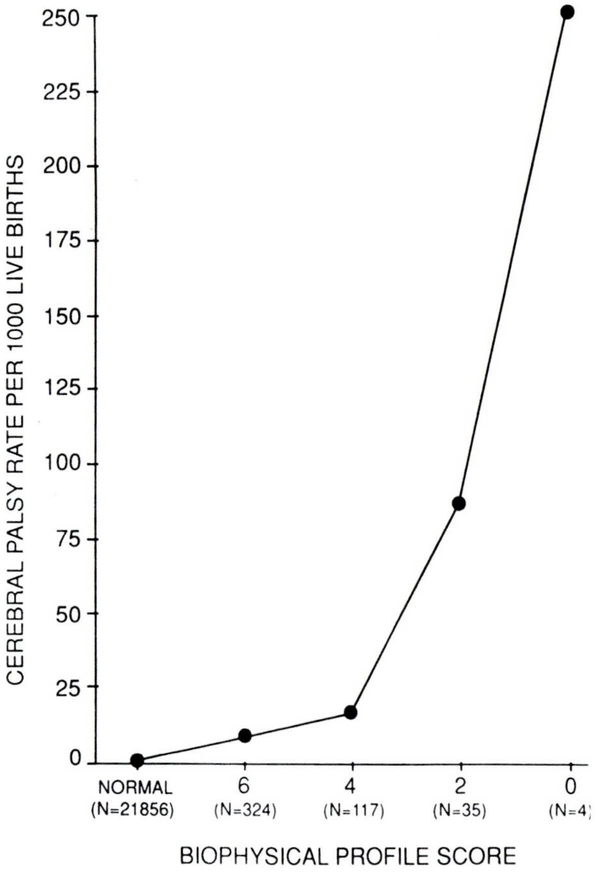

FIG. 34-7. Cerebral palsy by age 3 years versus last biophysical profile score before delivery. (A total of 22,000 fetuses assessed in 1989-1992, for whom detailed follow-up is available). (From Manning F, Bondagji N, Harman C et al. Fetal assessment based on the fetal biophysical profile score. VIII. Relationship of last BPS result to subsequent cerebral palsy. *Am J Obstet Gynecol.* In press.)

cases, again, follow the exponentially accelerating course of increasing cerebral palsy with progressively lower BPS (Fig. 34-7).[34] Further, with management according to the BPS protocol, a lower rate of cerebral palsy was observed. In the low-risk unreferred population of Manitoba, the cerebral palsy rate was 5.36 per 1000 deliveries, while in the high-risk population referred to fetal assessment units and managed per protocol, the rate of cerebral palsy diagnosed by age 3 was only 1.2 per 1000.[35]

Other Considerations

Many aspects of BPS continue to evolve. The minimum criterion for **normal amniotic fluid** has been elevated from 1 to 2 cm; the nonstress test is used only selectively; the frequency of evaluations in insulin-dependent diabetics has been reduced to weekly, and so on. Doppler velocimetry (especially in fetuses with intrauterine growth restriction) is now integrated in management. **Markedly diminished or absent end diastolic velocity** requires a minimum of 2 BPS scored "out of 10" be performed per week (i.e., NST is always done even if ultrasound parameters are 8/8). **Reverse end diastolic flow** calls for **daily BPS** in most circumstances.

The subjective nature of the assessment and the flexible attitude to frequency of testing (such as with Doppler) may be seen as limitations of the method. The decision on **test frequency** (more tests if maternal or fetal condition is unstable) is a matter of individual judgment based on **clinical** assessment. Obstetric training and experience greatly influence BPS application; it may be that the **perinatal team** is important in producing the advantages rather than the method by itself. Another limitation is that the test is designed to detect fetuses at increased risk of death or morbidity because of hypoxemia related to placental dysfunction. Its role in other situations in which fetal jeopardy has a different cause has not been fully addressed. For example, the cause of fetal death in the diabetic mother may not necessarily be asphyxia. Therefore, the heterogeneity of the underlying pregnancy complication must be a consideration in the interpretation of the test, particularly with normal results, particularly at term (when delivery and neonatal care may be a more certain situation).

An additional source of controversy has been the nature of some of the measurements (e.g., amniotic fluid volume, fetal tone). Although measurement of an amniotic fluid pocket in two perpendicular planes of greater than 2 cm is normal by definition, it may also be interpreted as subjectively reduced and an indication for delivery, depending on the overall subjective impression (e.g., cramped fetus, no other measurable pockets).[11] Overly strict adherence by an inexperienced examiner to criteria printed in a table may provide false reassurance. We have found no difference in amniotic fluid evaluation, comparing maximum fluid pocket depth with amniotic fluid index (AFI). The subjective interpretation of fetal tone is an inherent part of BPS. An experienced observer can place the velocity and recoil of fetal movement in context for the stated gestation. Individual factor analysis supports the continued inclusion of these parameters in the BPS while reinforcing the principle of multiple parameter evaluation.

BPS represents a recognition of the patterns of fetal behavior and provides precision in fetal evaluation. Fetal health is accurately depicted, allowing the pregnancy to continue with low risk of fetal loss, even in complicated maternal situations. Fetal compromise is detected with accuracy, allowing timely intervention to lower perinatal mortality and perinatal morbidity. As an ultrasound-based modality, BPS offers additional opportunities to enhance perinatal care for fetal anomalies and nonasphyxial problems. In many centers, BPS represents the standard of practice for surveillance of the high-risk fetus.

REFERENCES

1. Morrison I. Perinatal mortality: basic considerations. *Semin Perinatol* 1985;9:144-150.
2. College of Physicians and Surgeons of Manitoba. Perinatal and Maternal Welfare Committee. *1993 Annual Report*. Winnipeg, Ontario; 1995.
3. Morrison I, Menticoglou S, Manning FA et al. Comparison of antepartum tests and the relationship of multiple test results to perinatal outcome. *J Mat-Fet Med* 1994;3:75-83.
4. Johnson JM, Harman CR, Lange IR et al. Biophysical profile scoring in the management of the post-term pregnancy: an analysis of 307 cases. *Am J Obstet Gynecol* 1987;154:269-273.

Fetal Biophysical Activities

5. Pillai M, James D. Development of human fetal behavior: a review. *Fet Diagn Ther* 1990;5:15-32.
6. Rurak DW, Selke P, Fisher M et al. Fetal oxygen extraction: comparison of the human and sheep. *Am J Obstet Gynecol* 1987;156:360-366.
7. Boddy K, Dawes ES. Fetal breathing. *Br Med J* 1975;31:3.
8. Patrick JE, Campbell K, Carmicheal L. Patterns of gross fetal body movements in 24 hour observation intervals during the last 10 weeks of pregnancy. *Am J Obstet Gynecol* 1982; 142:363-371.
9. Brown R, Patrick JE. The non-stress test: how long is enough. *Am J Obstet Gynecol* 1981;141:646-650.
10. Pillai M, James D. Human fetal mouthing movements: a potential biophysical variable for distinguishing state IF from abnormal fetal behavior. Report of 4 cases. *Eur J Obstet Gynecol Reprod Sci* 1991;38:151-156.
11. Harman C, Menticoglou S, Manning F et al. Prenatal fetal monitoring: abnormalities of fetal behavior. In: James DK, Steer PJ, Weiner CP et al, eds. *High Risk Pregnancy Management Options*. London: WB Saunders; 1994.
12. Manning FA. Fetal biophysical profile scoring: theoretical considerations and practical application. In: Fleischer AC, Manning FM, Jeanty P et al, eds. *Sonography in Obstetrics and Gynecology*. 5th ed. Stamford, Conn: Appleton & Lange; 1996.
13. Manning FA, Platt LD. Human fetal breathing movements and maternal hypoxemia. *Obstet Gynecol* 1979;53:758-760.
14. Body K, Dawes GS, Fisher R. Fetal respiratory movement electrocortical and cardiovascular responses to hypoxemia and hypercapnia. *J Physiol* 1974;243:599.
15. Manning FA, Platt LD, Sipos L et al. Fetal breathing movements and the non-stress test in high-risk pregnancies. *Am J Obstet Gynecol* 1979;135:511-515.
16. Manning FA. Fetal biophysical profile scoring. In: Manning FA, ed. *Fetal Medicine: Principles and Practice*. Norwalk, Conn: Appleton & Lange; 1995.
17. Manning FA, Snijders R, Harman CR et al. The relationship between fetal biophysical profile score and fetal pH. In: *Proceedings of the Society of Perinatal Obstetricians' Annual Meeting* (abstract). Feb. 1993.
18. Cohn HE, Sacks GT. Cardiovascular responses to hypoxemia and acidemia in fetal lambs. *Am J Obstet Gynecol* 1974;120:817-824.
19. Seeds AE. Current concepts of amniotic fluid dynamics. *Am J Obstet Gynecol* 1980;138:575-586.
20. Chamberlain PF, Manning FA, Morrison I et al. Ultrasound evaluation of amniotic fluid volume. I. The relationship of marginal and decreased amniotic fluid volumes to perinatal outcome. *Am J Obstet Gynecol* 1984;150:245-249.
21. Bastide A, Manning F, Harman CR et al. Ultrasound evaluation of amniotic fluid: outcome of pregnancies with severe oligohydramnios. *Am J Obstet Gynecol* 1986;154:895-900.
22. Johnson JM, Lange IR, Harman CR et al. Biophysical profile scoring in the management of the diabetic pregnancy. *Obstet Gynecol* 1988;72:841-846.
23. Lange IR, Manning FA, Morrison I et al. Cord prolapse: is antenatal diagnosis possible? *Am J Obstet Gynecol* 1985; 151:1083-1085.

Fetal Biophysical Profile Scoring

24. Manning FA, Platt LD, Sipos L. Antepartum fetal evaluation: development of fetal biophysical profile score. *Am J Obstet Gynecol* 1980;136:787-795.
25. Manning FA, Harman CR, Morrison I. Fetal biophysical profile scoring: selective use of the NST. *Am J Obstet Gynecol* 1987;156:709-712.

26. Manning FA, Lange IR, Morrison I et al. Fetal biophysical profile score and the nonstress test: a comparative trial. *Obstet Gynecol* 1984;64:326-331.
27. Manning FA, Morrison I, Lange IR et al. Fetal biophysical profile scoring: a prospective study of 1,184 high-risk patients. *Am J Obstet Gynecol* 1981;140:289-294.
28. Chamberlain PF. Later fetal death—has ultrasound a role to play in its prevention? *Irish J Med Sci* 1991;160:251-254.
29. Baskett TF, Allen AC, Gray JH et al. Fetal biophysical profile and perinatal death. *Obstet Gynecol* 1987;70:357-360.
30. Vintzileos AM, Campbell WA et al. Fetal biophysical profile scoring: current status. *Clin Perinatol* 1989;16:661-689.
31. Jackson GM, Forouzan I, Cohen AW. Fetal well-being: nonimaging assessment and the biophysical profile. *Semin Roentgenol* 1991;26:21-31.
32. Platt LD, Eglington GS, Sipos L et al. Further experience with the fetal biophysical profile. *Obstet Gynecol* 1983;61:480-485.
33. Shime J, Gare JD, Andrews J et al. Prolonged pregnancy: surveillance of the fetus and the neonate and the course of labor and delivery. *Am J Obstet Gynecol* 1984;148:547-552.
34. Manning F, Bondagji N, Harman C et al. Fetal assessment based on the fetal biophysical profile score. VII. Relationship of last BPS result to subsequent cerebral palsy. *Am J Obstet Gynecol* (in press).
35. Manning F, Harman C, Menticoglou S. Fetal biophysical profile score and cerebral palsy at age 3 years. *Am J Obstet Gynecol* 1996;174:319.

CHAPTER 35

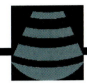

Sonography in the Diagnosis and Management of Multifetal Pregnancy

•

Clifford S. Levi, M.D., F.R.C.P.(C)
Edward A. Lyons, M.D., F.R.C.P.(C), F.A.C.R.
Marie-Jocelyne Martel, M.D.
Sidney M. Dashefsky, M.D., F.R.C.P.
Susan C. Holt, M.D., F.R.C.P.(C)

CHAPTER OUTLINE

The incidence of twins in North America is approximately 1.1% to 1.5% or approximately 1 per 80 live births.[1-5] Despite the relatively low incidence of twinning, 12% of all perinatal deaths occur in multifetal pregnancies.[4,6] The **perinatal death rate** for twins is 5 to 10 times greater than that for singletons.[3,7-9] A study by Spellacy et al.[7] demonstrated a perinatal mortality rate of 54 per 1000 live births compared with 10.4 per 1000 live births in singletons. Multifetal pregnancy is also associated with an increased incidence of spontaneous abortion and a wide range of fetal and maternal pregnancy complications.[10]

Multifetal pregnancies are **high-risk pregnancies** that require increased surveillance in the antepartum period[4,5,10] and may require delivery at a high-risk center. Based on clinical findings alone, up to 50% of multifetal pregnancies may be unsuspected until the time of delivery.[5,11] In 1979, based on data accumulated between 1973 and 1977, Persson and co-workers reported a twin detection rate of 98% with ultrasound.[11] Using current equipment, the sonographic detection rate of live twins should be 100%. In addition, many anomalies and complications of multifetal pregnancy can be diagnosed early in pregnancy with ultrasound, allowing for change in obstetric management.

INCIDENCE

Twins may arise from the fertilization of two separate ova (dizygotic or "fraternal" twins) or a single fertilized ovum that subsequently divides (monozygotic or "identical" twins). The relative frequency of **monozygotic (MZ) twins** is approximately 1 per 250 live births and is relatively constant worldwide.[1,3,5,12] Although the relative frequency of MZ twinning was thought to be constant and independent of influencing factors,[13] it has recently been shown that the incidence of MZ twinning is affected by ovulation induction agents[14] and may be as high as 3.2%[15] in patients undergoing assisted reproductive techniques. In North America, MZ twins represent approximately 30% of all twin births.[3,5,12,16]

Dizygotic (DZ) twins represent 70% of all twin births in North America.[3,5,12,16] The relative frequency of DZ twinning is variable in different populations and is influenced by many factors, including:

- **Maternal age and parity.** The incidence of twinning increases with advancing maternal age up to 35 to 40 years old and increases with parity up to 7.
- **Ethnic origin.** There is significant variation in the rates of DZ twinning between different populations and racial groups. In North America, the incidence of DZ twinning in Caucasians is approximately 7.1 per 1000 live births whereas the incidence in blacks is approximately 11.1 per 1000. In Nigeria, the incidence is 49 per 1000. In Japan, the incidence is approximately 1.3 per 1000.[5]
- **Heredity.** A maternal family history of DZ twinning is associated with a higher incidence of twins. In a study by White and Wyshak,[17] the incidence of DZ twin births in women who themselves were a DZ twin was 1 per 58. No similar effect was associated with a paternal history of DZ twinning.
- **Ovulation induction agents.** Clomiphene therapy is associated with a 7% to 9% incidence of twinning, and human menopausal gonadotropin (hMG) is associated with an 18% incidence.[1,3,5]

FACTORS INCREASING FREQUENCY OF DIZYGOTIC TWINS

Maternal age and parity
Ethnic origin
Heredity
Ovulation induction agents
Endogenous gonadotropin
Assisted reproductive technology

A

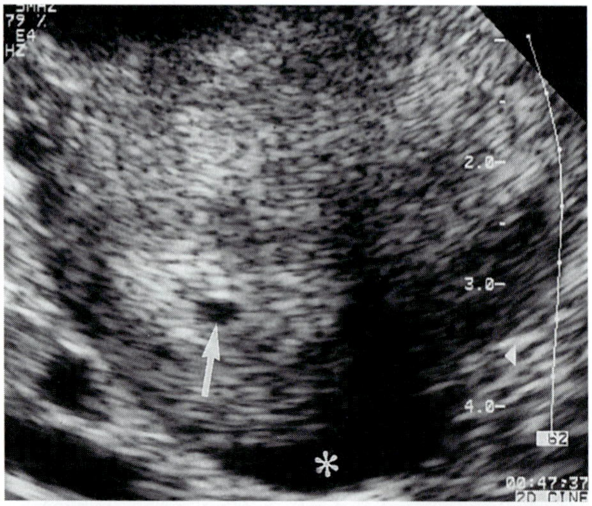

B

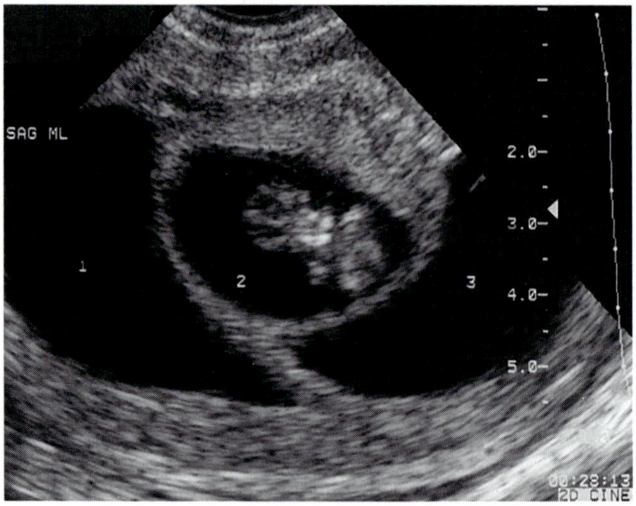

C

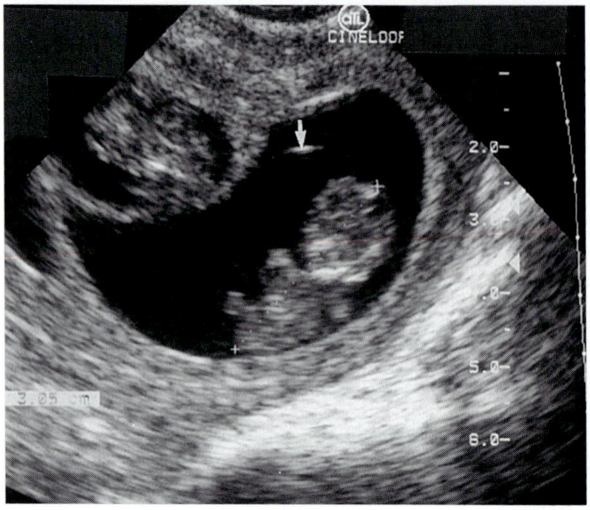

FIG. 35-1. Trichorionic triamniotic triplets after ovulation induction. **A,** Endovaginal sonogram shows a small intrauterine gestational sac *(arrow)*. The uterus is retroverted, and there is a small amount of fluid in the posterior cul de sac *(asterisk)*. **B,** Follow-up examination 5 weeks later shows three chorionic sacs with a live embryo in each. **C,** The crown rump length is 30.5 mm, corresponding to a gestational age of 10 weeks. Follow-up is necessary in all patients until the number of gestational sacs and live embryos can be demonstrated with certainty. *Small arrow*, Amnion. (From Levi CS, Dashefsky SM, Lyons EA et al. First-trimester ultrasound: a practical approach. In: McGahan JP, Porto M, eds. *Diagnostic Obstetrical Ultrasound.* Philadelphia: JB Lippincott Co; 1994.)

- **Endogenous gonadotropin.** The incidence of DZ twins in the first cycle after cessation of oral contraceptives is increased possibly on the basis of increased levels of endogenous follicle stimulating hormone (FSH).[1,18]
- **Assisted reproductive technology.** Multiple gametes or embryos are routinely transferred using these techniques, resulting in increased potential for multifetal pregnancy.[19] In one study, the incidence of multiple fetuses was 37% at 12 weeks, but decreased to 22% at the time of delivery.[20]

The incidence of triplets and higher-order multifetal pregnancies has increased dramatically with the use of ovulation induction agents and assisted reproductive techniques (Fig. 35-1). Spontaneous reduction of the number of fetuses is common in the first trimester. In a study of 116 women with multiple gestations who conceived using ovulation induction drugs, spontaneous reduction occurred in 88 of the 116 patients prior to 13 weeks.[21]

EMBRYOLOGY AND PLACENTATION

Dizygotic twins arise from two separate fertilized ova (zygotes) (Fig. 35-2). The two zygotes develop into

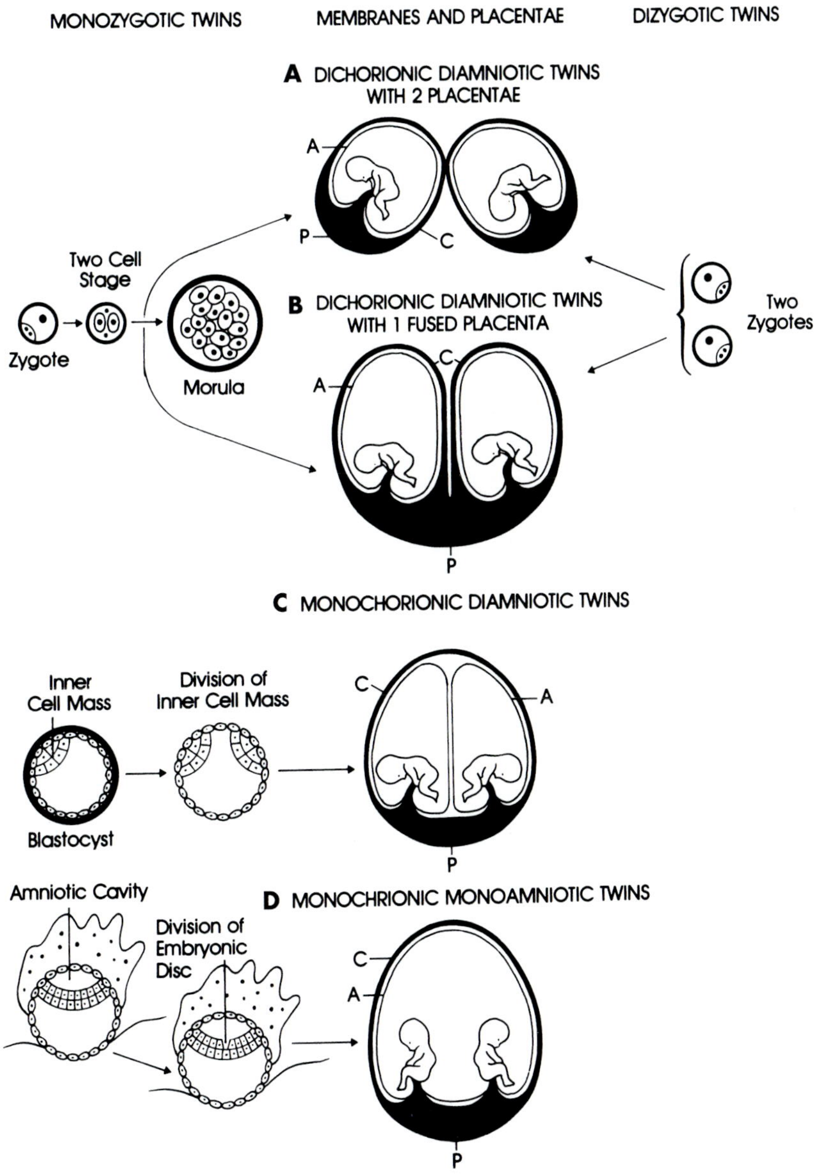

FIG. 35-2. Diagram depicting the formation of membranes and placentas in monozygotic and dizygotic twins. Monozygotic twins may show any pattern, but most commonly show **C** and least often **D.** (From Levi CS, Lyons EA, Lindsay DJ et al. The sonographic evaluation of multiple gestation pregnancy. In Fleischer AC, Romero R, Manning FA et al, eds. *The Principles and Practice of Ultrasonography in Obstetrics and Gynecology.* 4th ed. East Norwalk, Conn: Appleton & Lange; 1991.)

blastocysts that implant independently, each forming an embryo with its own amnion, chorion, and yolk sac, resulting in a **dichorionic diamniotic** (DC/DA) twin pregnancy. The chorion frondosum and the decidua basalis combine to form the placenta. DC/DA twins have two placentas unless implantation of the two blastocysts is close enough to result in the formation of one fused placenta.

Monozygotic twins arise from the division of a single zygote. The chorionicity and amnionicity of MZ twins depend on the stage at which division occurs[5,12] and may be categorized as follows (see Fig. 35-2):

- **Dichorionic diamniotic (DC/DA)** twins. Division of the zygote between the two-cell stage (blastomere) and morula stage (i.e., during the first 3 days postconception) results in the formation of two embryos with two amnions and two chorions. DC/DA twins comprise 18% to 36% of MZ twins. As with DZ twins, MZ DC/DA twins have two placentas or one fused placenta.
- **Monochorionic diamniotic (MC/DA)** twins. MD/DA twins are the most common form of MZ twinning, accounting for approximately 70%. Division of the inner cell mass between the 4th and 8th days postconception results in division after the cells destined to become the chorion have already differentiated. Consequently, two embryos, two amnions, and two yolk sacs will be formed within a single chorion. MC/DA twins have a single placenta.
- **Monochorionic monoamniotic (MC/MA)** twins. Division of the embryonic disk after day 8 postconception results in the formation of two embryos within a single amnion and a single chorion. A single yolk sac may be present,[22] however, there are insufficient data in the literature regarding the number of yolk sacs in MC/MA twins to know if two yolk sacs may also occur normally in MC/MA twins. MC/MA twins account for approximately 4% of MZ twins.[12] Incomplete division of the embryonic disk results in **conjoined twins.** Division of the embryonic disk after day 13 postconception is usually incomplete, resulting in varying degrees of fusion of the embryos. It has been estimated that the prevalence of conjoined twins is approximately 1 per 50,000 to 1 per 100,000 births.[23]

SONOGRAPHIC DETERMINATION OF AMNIONICITY AND CHORIONICITY

Chorionicity and amnionicity have important **prognostic** and **diagnostic significance.** The placentas in MC/DA twin pregnancies usually have vascular anastomoses between the circulations of the two fetuses. These anastomoses may be artery-to-artery, artery-to-vein, or vein-to-vein and result in twin transfusion syndrome, twin embolization syndrome, and the acardiac parabiotic twin syndrome. Although DC/DA twins may have fused placentas, vascular anastomoses do not develop between the circulations of these fetuses.[5] The perinatal mortality rate is higher for MC/DA twins than for DC/DA twins, partially related to the vascular anastomoses within the placenta.[10,24] The diagnosis of the etiology of discordant growth depends on the chorionicity of the twin pregnancy. DC/DA twins would be unlikely to have twin transfusion syndrome and more likely to have intrauterine growth retardation (IUGR) of one fetus.

Obstetric management may also be affected by knowledge of the chorionicity and amnionicity of the pregnancy. Timing of delivery in MC/MA twins may prevent cord entanglement, which was responsible for a mortality rate of 30% to 50% in this group.

In the first trimester, sonographic determination of chorionicity should not be a problem. From approximately 4.5 to 5.5 weeks gestational age, the chorion is visualized as an echogenic ring within the thickened decidua (intradecidual sign)[25] (Fig. 35-3). After approximately 5.5 weeks gestational age, the chorion laeve/decidua capsularis is visualized as the thick-walled, echogenic ring situated eccentrically within the thick ring of the decidua vera, which constitutes the double decidual sign[26] (Fig. 35-4). Later in the first trimester, as the decidua basalis/chorion frondosum form the placenta, the decidua capsularis/chorion laeve can still be visualized as a thick, echogenic membrane (Figs. 35-5 to 35-7). Based on the presence of a thick membrane or two placentas, Kurtz et al. were able to diagnose 96% of 85 twin pairs correctly as DC/DA.[27]

In the first trimester, the amnion is thin and filamentous. The amnion can first be visualized as a 2 mm bleb adjacent to the yolk sac at approximately 5.5 weeks menstrual age.[28] The amnion then becomes difficult to visualize (see Fig. 35-4) until the CRL is 8 to 12 mm (Fig. 35-8) at which point it has the sonographic appearance of a thin, filamentous, rounded membrane surrounding the embryo.[29] Early in the first trimester, the amnions can be visualized as a membrane surrounding each embryo in MC/DA twins (see Fig. 35-8). By approximately 10 weeks gestation, the amnions have grown enough to contact each other, resulting in the sonographic appearance of a single, thin membrane separating the two fetuses[24] (Figs. 35-9 and 35-10). The amnion remains thin and filamentous in appearance throughout the first trimester and is surrounded by the thick, echogenic chorion. The yolk sac is situated between the amnion and chorion.

In general, in the first trimester, chorionicity and amnionicity can be determined simply by counting the number of chorionic sacs, the number of amnions within each chorion, and the number of embryos

A

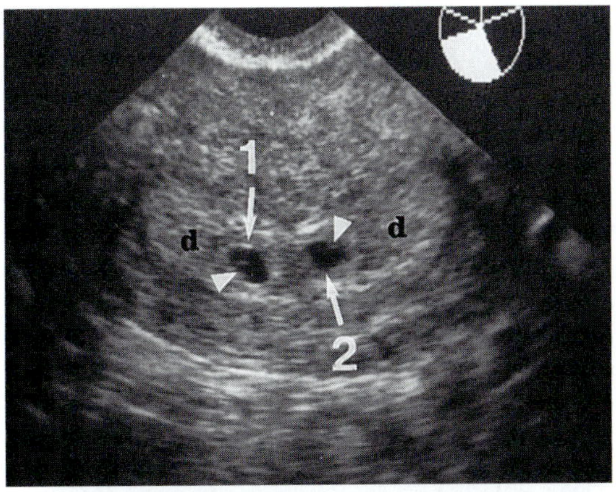

B

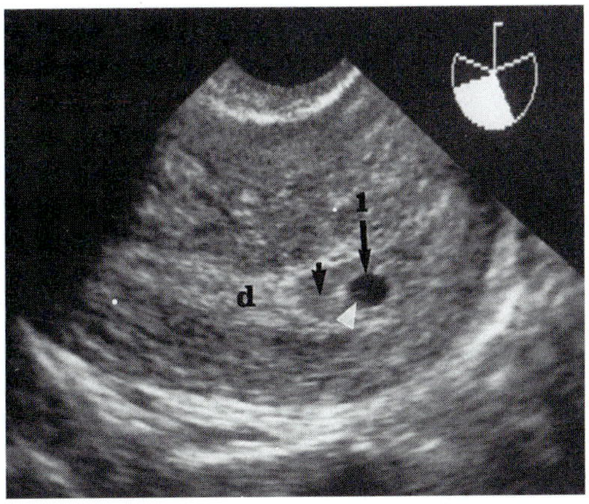

C

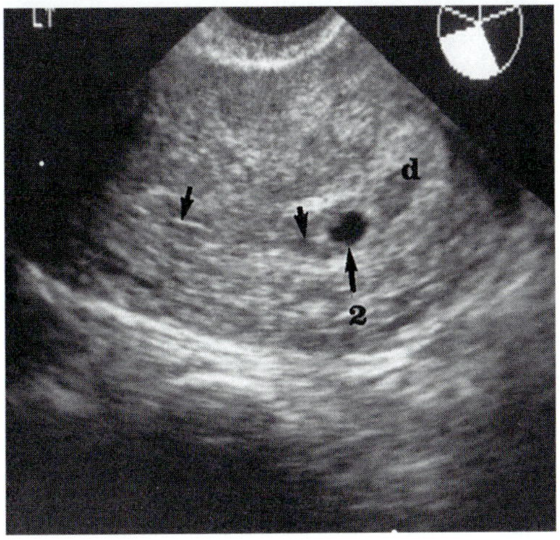

FIG. 35-3. DC/DA twins at 5 weeks gestational age (intradecidual sign). Endovaginal images in the, **A**, coronal and, **B** and **C**, sagittal planes. Two gestational sacs are present, *1* and *2*, within the echogenic decidua, *d*. The mean gestational sac diameters are approximately 5 mm, corresponding to a gestational age of 5 weeks. A tiny yolk sac *(arrowhead)* is present within each gestational sac. The uterus is retroverted. *Small black arrows*, Endometrial canal.

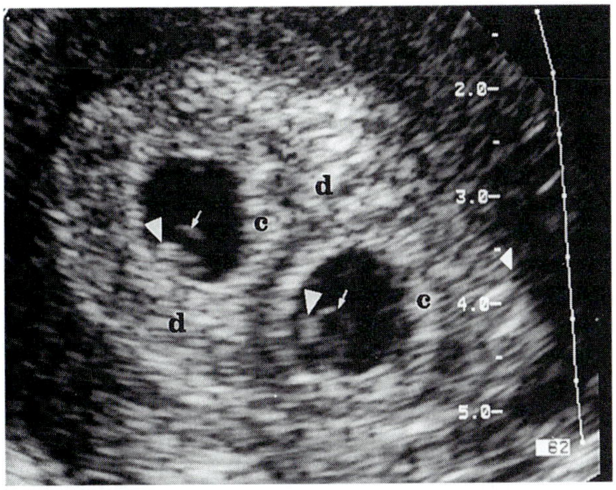

FIG. 35-4. DC/DA twins at 6.5 weeks gestational age (double decidual sign). Endovaginal sonogram shows two gestational sacs surrounded by the echogenic chorionic ring, *c*, comprised of the decidua capsularis/chorion laeve within the decidua vera, *d*. A yolk sac *(small arrow)* and live embryo *(arrowhead)* are present within each gestational sac. The CRLs measure 5.4 mm and 4.7 mm, corresponding to a gestational age of 6.5 weeks.

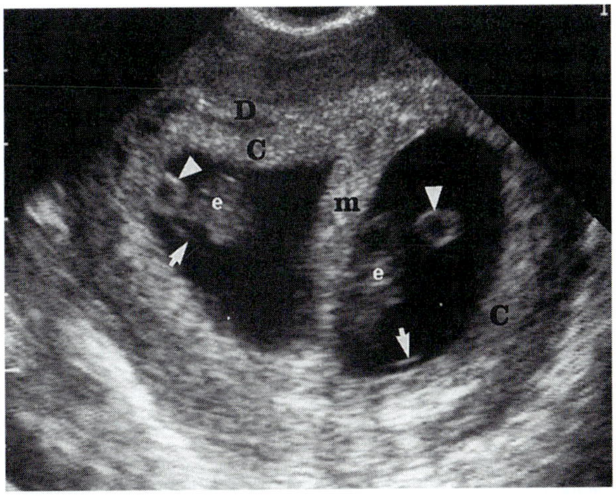

FIG. 35-5. Intertwin membrane thickness in DC/DA twins at 8 weeks gestational age. Endovaginal sonogram demonstrating two gestational sacs each with a yolk sac *(arrowhead)* and live embryo, *e*. The gestational sacs are separated by a thick membrane, *m*, comprised of the two opposed layers of decidua capsularis/chorion laeve, *c*. The amnion is thin and filamentous *(small arrows)*. *D*, Decidua vera.

A

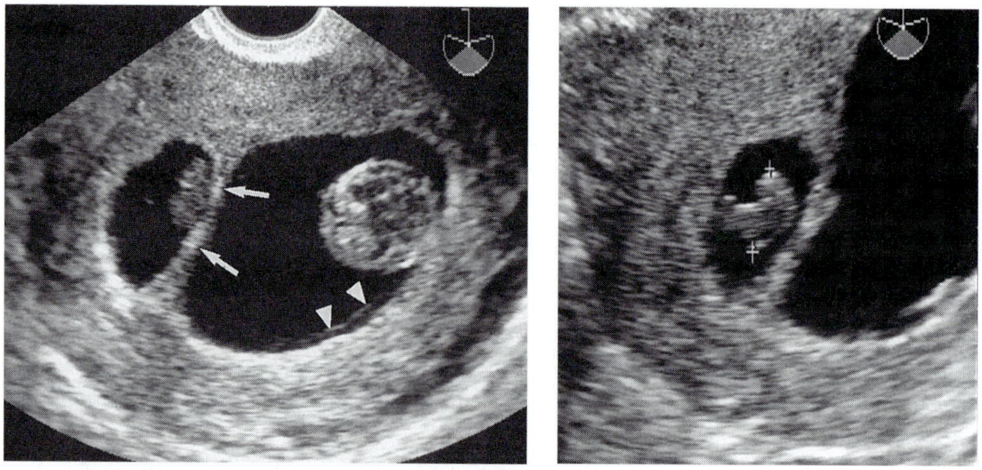

B

C

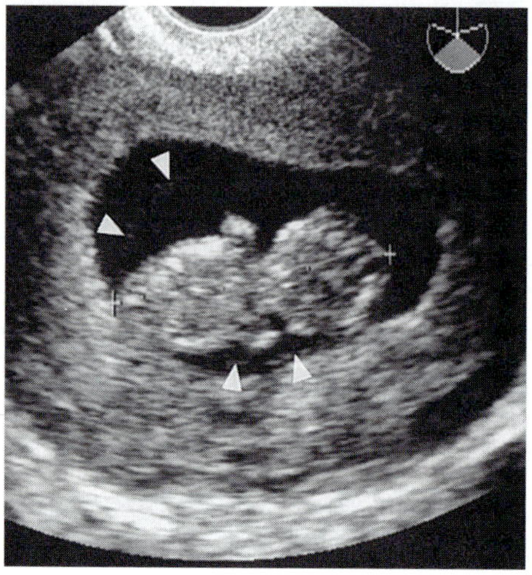

FIG. 35-6. Intertwin membrane thickness in DC/DA twins at 11 weeks gestational age with cotwin demise. **A,** Endovaginal sonogram in the coronal plane shows two gestational (chorionic) sacs separated by a thick membrane *(arrows)*. The amnion is thin and filamentous *(arrowheads)*. The gestational sac to the maternal right is small. **B,** The fetus to the maternal right is dead. The CRL measures 11 mm. **C,** The CRL of the fetus to the maternal left is 34 mm, corresponding to a gestational age of 11 weeks. *Arrowheads*, Amnion.

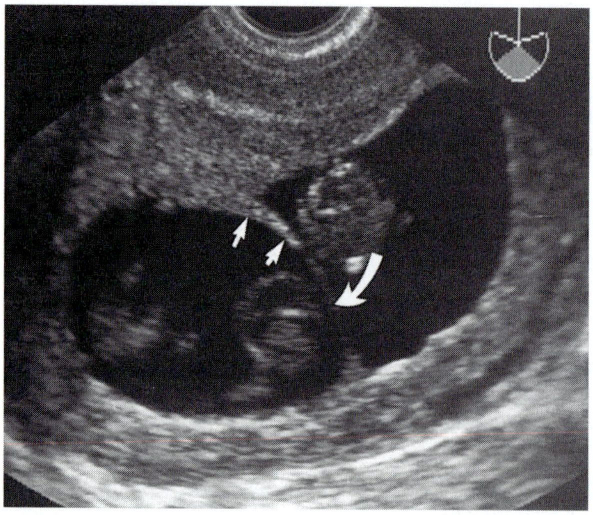

FIG. 35-7. Intertwin membrane thickness in DC/DA twins at 11 weeks gestational age: chorionic peak. Endovaginal sonogram shows a thick membrane *(curved arrow)* separating two live fetuses (CRL = 37 mm). A chorionic peak is present *(small arrows)*.

within each amnion. Occasionally, differentiation between MC/DA and MC/MA twins can be difficult, necessitating careful evaluation of the amnion(s) to determine whether the embryos are surrounded by a single amnion or if each embryo is surrounded by its own amnion. The presence of a thin membrane between the embryos should indicate a MC/DA twin pregnancy. In the series by Kurtz et al., a membrane was identified separating the fetuses in 88% of MC/DA twins and in 0 of 4 MC/MA twins.[27] In early pregnancy, with embryonic CRLs measuring only a few millimeters, the ability of sonography to differentiate between singleton embryos, MC/MA twins, and conjoined twins has not been demonstrated and may not be possible with current technology.

After the first trimester, determination of amnionicity and chorionicity is more difficult.[23,24,30,31] Because the placenta is derived from the chorion frondosum/decidua basalis, the presence of two placentas is indicative of a DC/DA twin pregnancy[23] (Fig. 35-11). In rare circumstances, two placentas may be

A

C

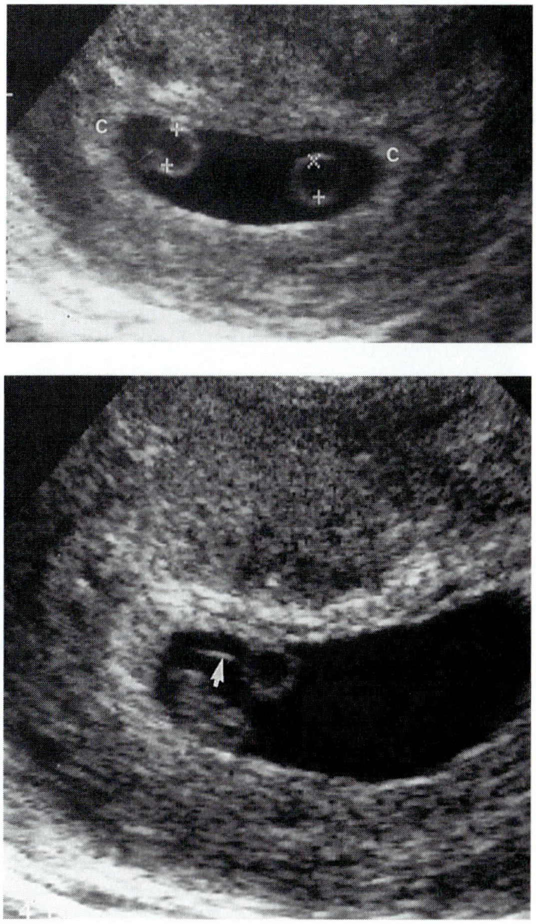

B

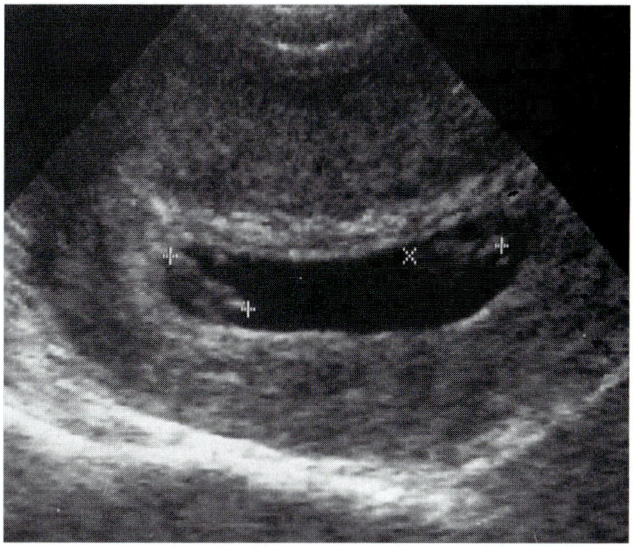

FIG. 35-8. MC/DA twins at 7 weeks gestational age. **A,** Endovaginal sonogram demonstrating two yolk sacs and, **B,** two live embryos within a single chorionic sac. **C,** The CRLs are 8.3 and 8.8 mm. Both embryos are surrounded by a thin and filamentous amnion, one of which is shown in C *(small arrow)*. (From Levi CS, Lyons EA, Lindsay DJ et al. The sonographic evaluation of multiple gestation pregnancy. In: Fleischer AC, Romero R, Manning FA et al, eds. *The Principles and Practice of Ultrasonography in Obstetrics and Gynecology*. 4th ed. East Norwalk, Conn: Appleton & Lange; 1991.)

A

B

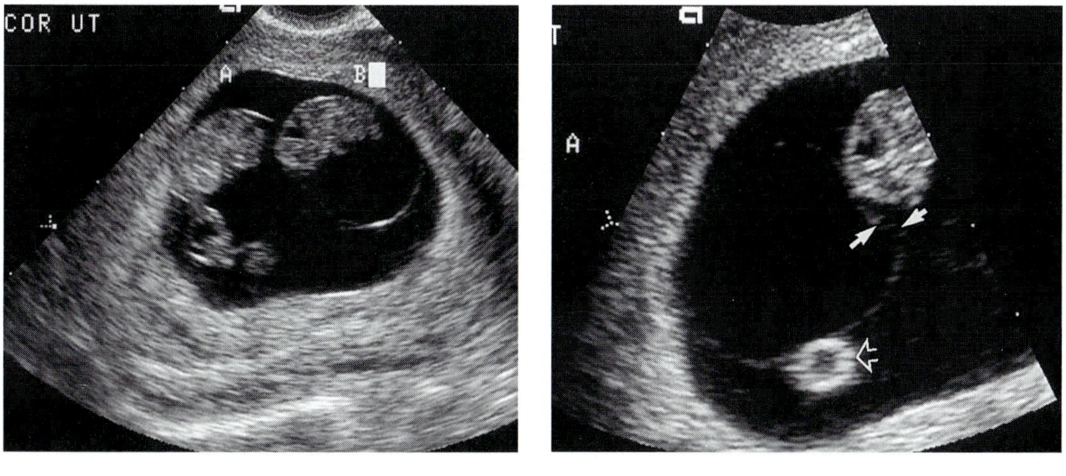

FIG. 35-9. MC/DA twins at 9 weeks gestational age: growth of the amnions. **A,** Endovaginal sonogram shows a MC/DA twin pregnancy. Two live embryos are present. The CRLs are 18.6 mm, corresponding to a gestational age of 9 weeks. **B,** Endovaginal sonogram shows contact of the amnions *(arrows)*. *Open arrow*, yolk sac.

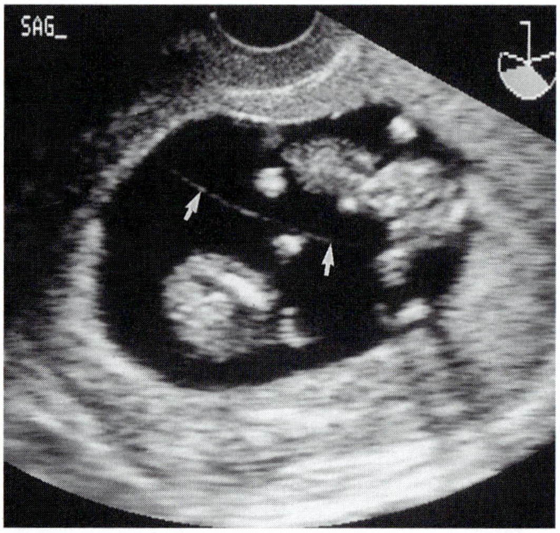

FIG. 35-10. MC/DA twins at 12 weeks gestational age: intertwin membrane. Endovaginal sonogram shows a thin membrane *(arrows)* comprised of the two amnions separating the fetuses. The CRLs are 46 mm and 48 mm, corresponding to a gestational age of 12 weeks.

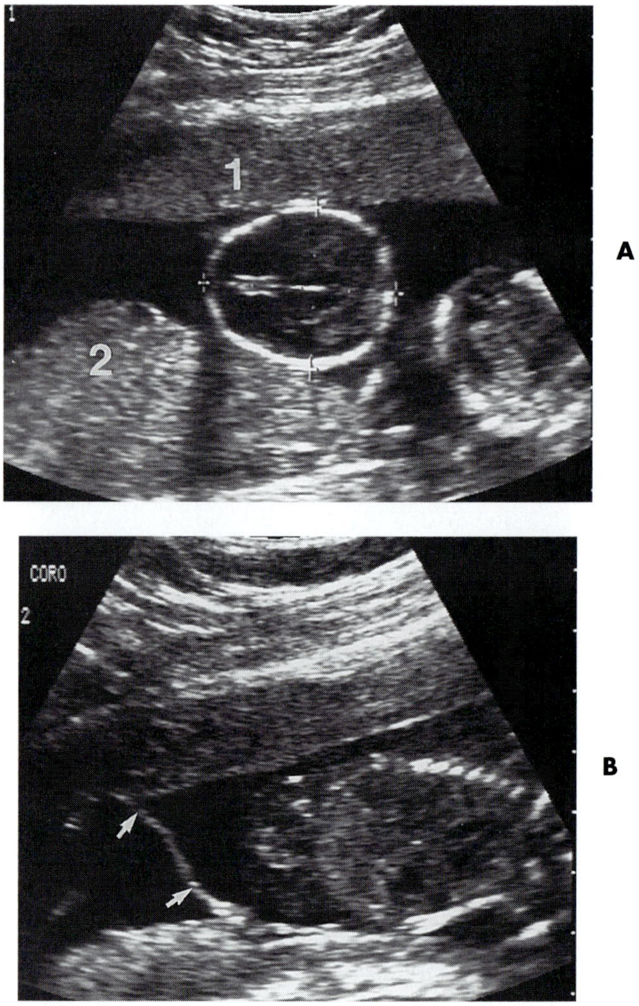

FIG. 35-11. Two placentas in a DC/DA twin pregnancy at 15.5 weeks gestational age. **A,** Twin pregnancy with two placentas (*1, 2*). The biometric measurements correspond to a gestational age of 15.5 weeks. Sonogram in a sagittal plane shows that the placentas are separate. **B,** The twins are separated by a thick membrane *(arrows)* that extends from the edge of one placenta to the edge of the other.

CHORIONICITY AND AMNIONICITY

Determine **number** of placentas
Two placentas indicate DC/DA twins
If a **single placental mass** is present:
- a membrane separating fetuses excludes MC/MA
- different sexes are diagnostic of DC/DA
- chorionic or "twin peak" is diagnostic of DC/DA
- thick membrane, <22 weeks, is diagnostic of DC/DA
- absence of a membrane may mean (1) MC/MA twins, or (2) closely applied membrane to stuck twin of MC/DA twin gestation

present in monochorionic twins due to a succenturiate lobe of the placenta; however, the presence of a cord insertion in each placental mass should differentiate between DC/DA twins and a monochorionic pregnancy with a succenturiate lobe.[23] Although the presence of two placentas is indicative of a dichorionic pregnancy, in approximately 50% of DC/DA twin pregnancies, the placentas are fused and appear as a single placental mass.[23] The presence of a single placenta in a twin pregnancy, therefore, is not necessarily indicative of a monochorionic twin pregnancy. After determining that **one placental mass** is present (which could be two fused placentas or a single placenta), the following steps may be used to **determine chorionicity** and **amnionicity** (see box):

- Step 1. **Identification of a membrane separating the fetuses.** The presence of a membrane indicates that the pregnancy is not a MC/MA twin pregnancy. Nonvisualization of a membrane between the fetuses occurs in up to 10% of diamniotic (either DC/DA or MC/DA) twin pregnancies and cannot be used as the sole indicator of a MC/MA pregnancy.[23,32] Although identification of a membrane is a useful step in determining chorionicity and amnionicity in twin pregnancies with a single placental mass, identification of an intervening membrane, evaluation of its thickness, and its relationship to both fetuses should be performed in all twin pregnancies.
- Step 2. **Fetal sex determination.** Examination of the fetal genitalia is part of a complete sonographic examination and can be used as an indicator of chorionicity and amnionicity. If examination of the

fetal genitalia indicates clearly that **one fetus is male** and the **other female**, it can be inferred that the pregnancy is a **dizygotic** twin pregnancy and, therefore, DC/DA. If the fetuses are of the **same sex, zygosity cannot be inferred**, and a pregnancy with a single placenta could be either monochorionic or dichorionic.

- Step 3. **Assess the presence of a chorionic or "twin peak" sign** (see Fig. 35-7; Fig. 35-12). The chorionic peak is defined as a projection of tissue of similar appearance and echogenicity to the placenta, extending into the intertwin membrane and tapering to a point within this membrane.[30] According to Finberg,[30] the presence of the chorionic peak sign is indicative of extension of placental villi into the potential interchorionic space at the site where the placenta abuts the placenta and chorion of its cotwin. The chorionic peak cannot occur in a monochorionic twin pregnancy because the single chorion serves as a barrier to the growth of placental villi into the intertwin membrane. The **presence of a chorionic peak** is diagnostic of a **DC/DA twin pregnancy**. Nonvisualization of a chorionic peak cannot be used as a predictor of chorionicity.
- Step 4. **Membrane thickness, in the absence of other diagnostic features, may be used as an indicator of chorionicity.**[23,24] In theory, the thickness of the two opposing layers of amnion in a MC/DA twin pregnancy should be thinner than the thickness of the two layers of chorion and two layers of amnion that make up the intertwin membrane in DC/DA twins. In a study by Townsend et al.,[33] a thick membrane had a predictive value of 83% and was present in 89% of the first sonograms in DC/DA twins. In the third trimester, however, a thick membrane was demonstrated in only 52% of DC/DA twins. A thin membrane had a predictive value of 83% for MC/DA twins but was seen in only 54% of MC/DA twins. Prior to 22 weeks gestation, membrane thickness is an accurate predictor of chorionicity; after 22 weeks it is far less reliable.[23]
- Step 5. **In the absence of a visible intertwin membrane, two causes are likely. If the two umbilical cords can be followed to a common tangle,** the diagnosis is a MC/MA twin pregnancy (Fig. 35-13). The membrane may be difficult to visualize in MC/DA twins. An extreme example is that of the **"stuck twin" syndrome in which the intertwin membrane is closely applied to the smaller twin**, which has severe oligohydramnios, resulting in restriction of movement of the stuck fetus. The cotwin usually has marked polyhydramnios. Close inspection of the smaller, stuck twin will identify the intertwin membrane that restricts its movement (Fig. 35-14).

Chorionicity and amnionicity of **higher-order multifetal pregnancies** can be inferred by applying the same principles as those used for twins (Fig. 35-15). Early in the first trimester, however, the diagnosis of dichorionic and higher-order polychorionic pregnancies should be made only on the basis of strict sonographic criteria. In the mid 1970s, several reports were published describing a high incidence of concomitant blighted ovum and normal intrauterine pregnancy.[34-36] In one study[34] using bistable technology, the authors identified a high incidence of twins based on visualization of one or more gestational sacs, 71.4% of which did not result in a twin birth. This finding was referred to as the **disappearing or vanishing twin.** The high incidence of twins may have in fact been based partially on the erroneous interpretation of either a subchorionic hemorrhage or the decidua vera as a second gestational (chorionic) sac. Using current equipment and diagnostic criteria, differentiation between a subchorionic hemorrhage and a gestational sac should not present a problem, and the decidua

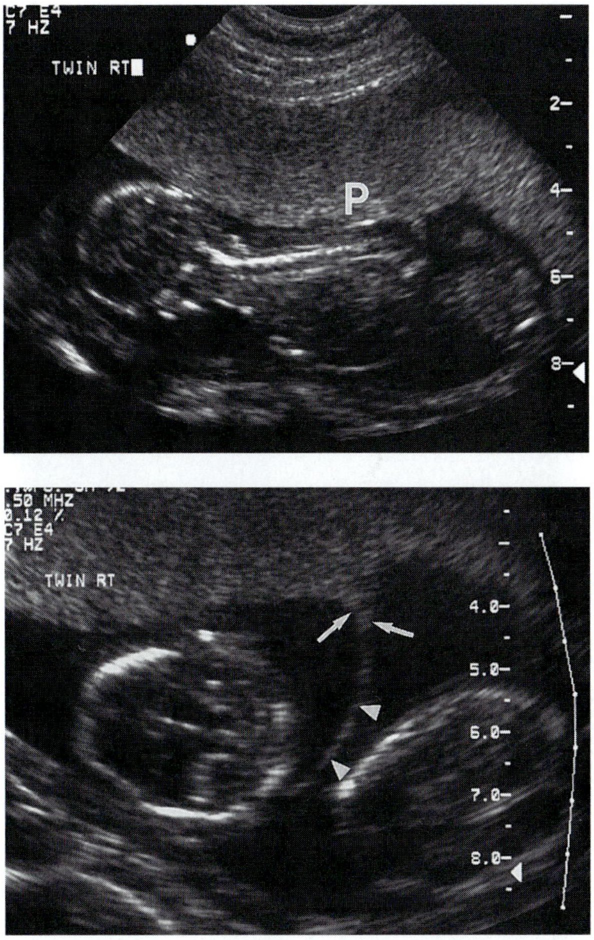

A

B

FIG. 35-12. Chorionic peak in a DC/DA twin pregnancy at 15 weeks gestational age. **A**, Twin pregnancy with a single placental mass, *P*. **B**, A chorionic peak *(arrows)* is present, indicative of a DC/DA twin pregnancy. *Arrowheads*, Intertwin membrane.

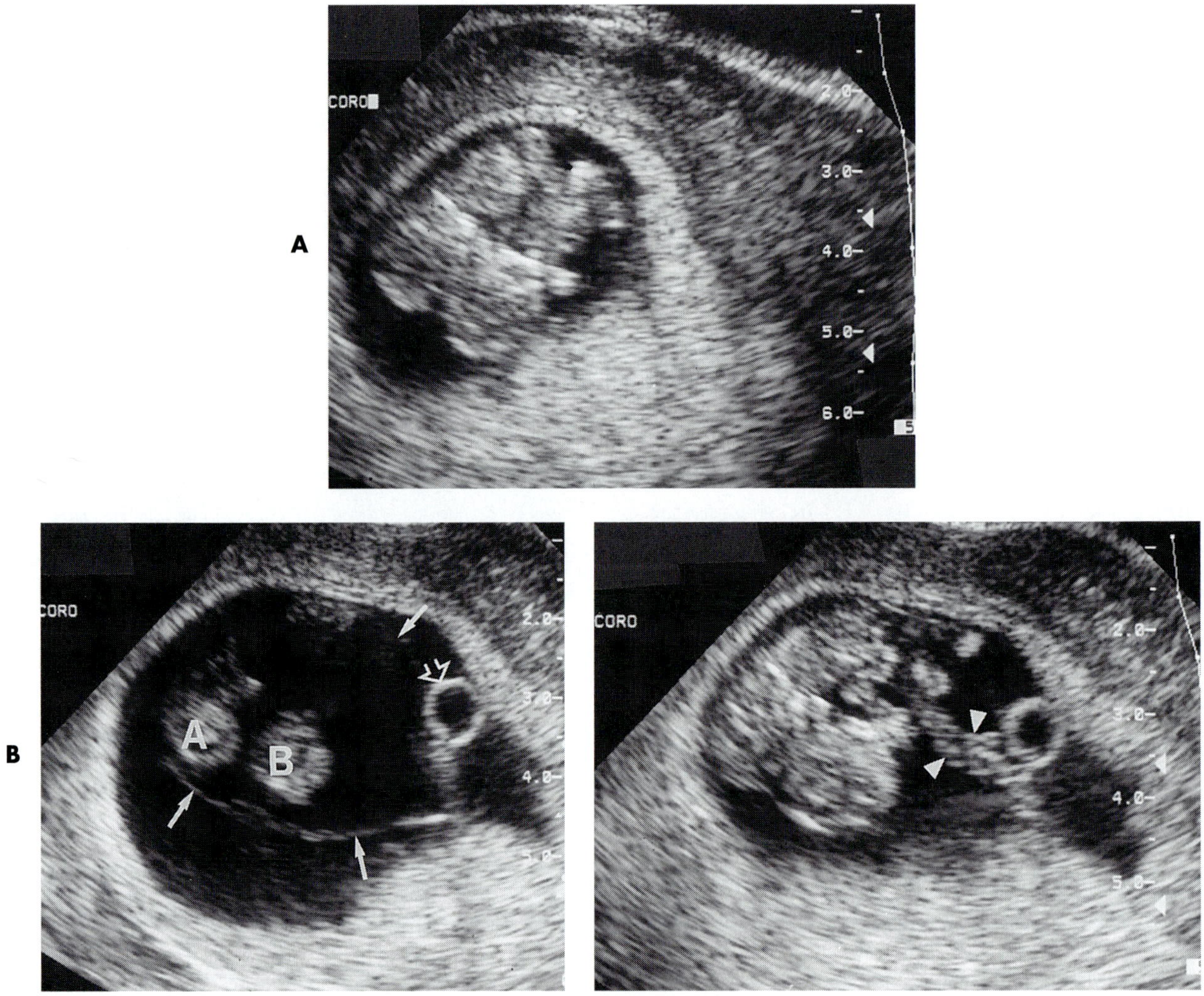

FIG. 35-13. MC/MA twins at 10.5 weeks gestational age. **A**, The two fetuses are in contact but move separately with no evidence of fusion. **B**, The fetuses (*A*, *B*) are surrounded by a single amnion *(arrows)*. A single large yolk sac is present *(open arrow)*. **C**, The umbilical cords form a common tangle *(arrowheads)*.

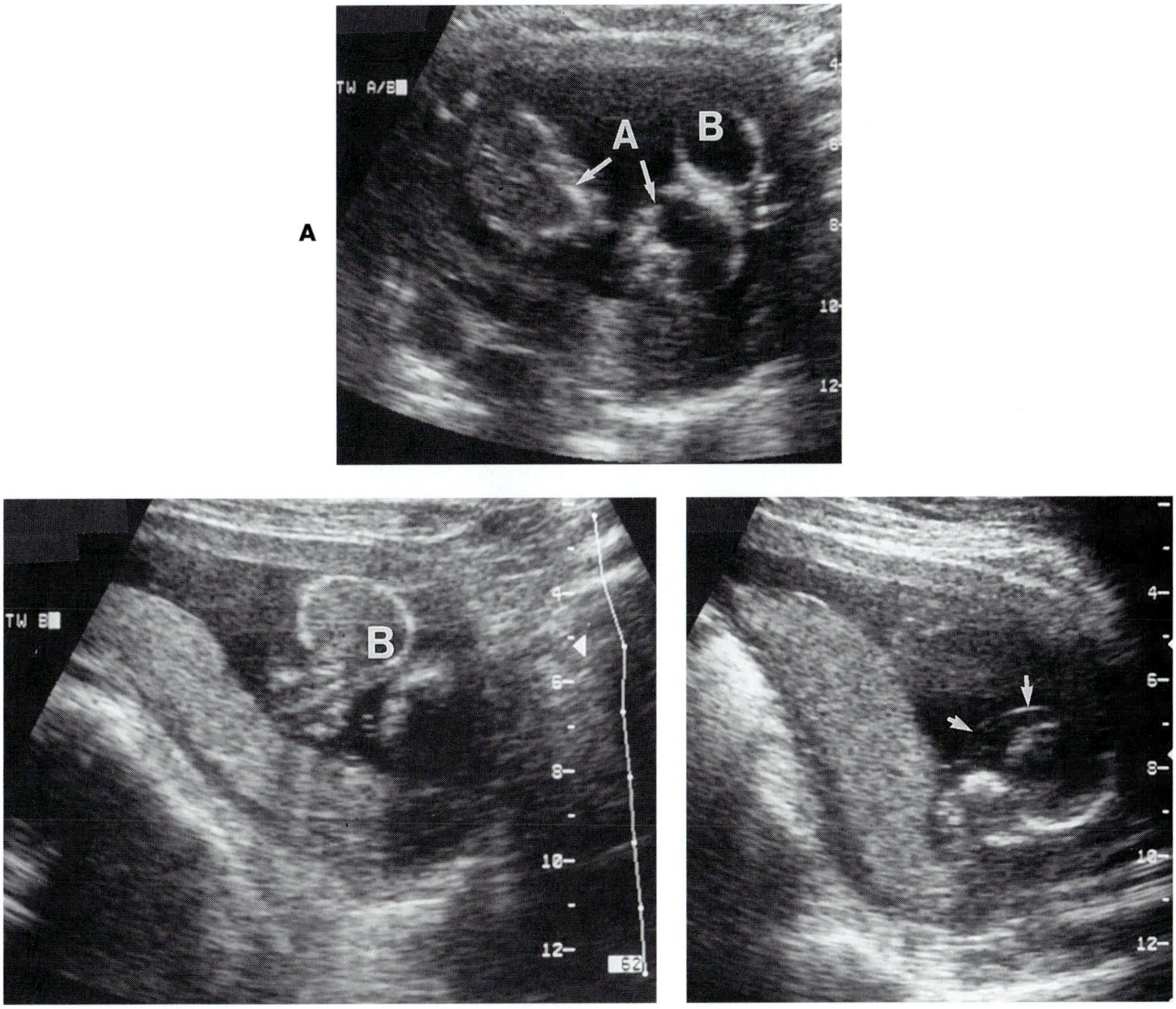

FIG. 35-14. "Stuck twin" syndrome. MC/DA twins at 14.5 weeks gestational age. **A** and **B**, The larger fetus, *A*, is alive and moves normally. Twin *B* is small, dead. **C**, Twin *B* has marked oligohydramnios or anhydramnios and is held in an "antigravitational" position by the intertwin membrane *(arrows)*.

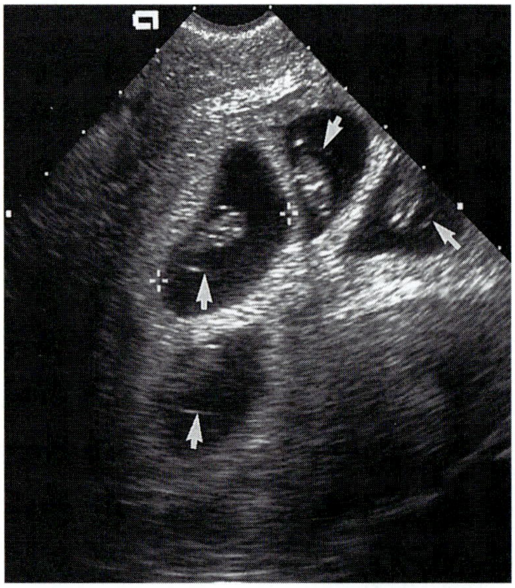

FIG. 35-15. Quadrachorionic quadraamniotic quadruplet pregnancy at 8 weeks gestational age. Four separate chorionic sacs, each with a live embryo, amnion *(arrows)*, and yolk sac, are present. The yolk sacs are not in the plane of scan. The CRLs are 15 mm, 13.8 mm, 14.8 mm, and 14 mm.

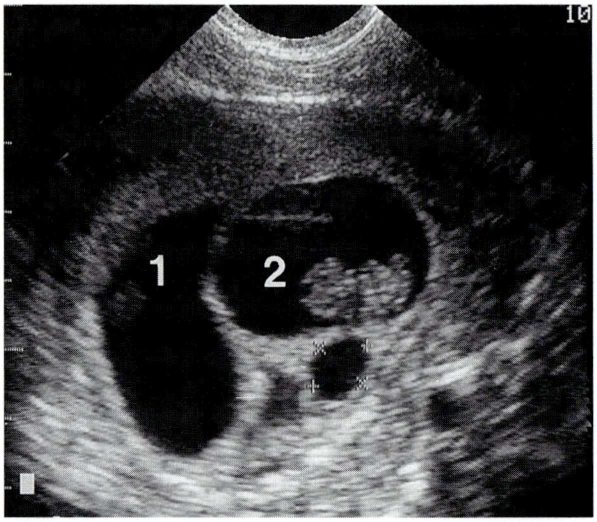

FIG. 35-16. Trichorionic triamniotic triplets at 9 weeks gestational age with demise of one embryo. Endovaginal sonogram shows three chorionic sacs. A live embryo is present in both chorionic sacs labeled *1* and *2* (the embryo in chorionic sac *1* is not in the plane of scan). The CRLs are 21 and 19 mm. The electronic calipers outline the third chorionic sac, which is small (mean diameter = 9 mm). The third chorionic sac is "empty," consistent with an embryonic demise with resorption of the embryo.

vera is well recognized as the basis for the double decidual sign. However, as noted in the section **"First Trimester Pregnancy Loss," the vanishing twin syndrome** does exist and is not uncommon in the first trimester of pregnancy. Published reports are based on the disappearance or spontaneous loss of one of two or more live embryos or on the basis of a discrepancy between the number of documented gestational sacs and outcome. Although early embryonic demise of one embryo in a DC/DA twin pregnancy may result in a sonographically "empty sac" (Figs. 35-16 and 35-17), this diagnosis should be made with caution.

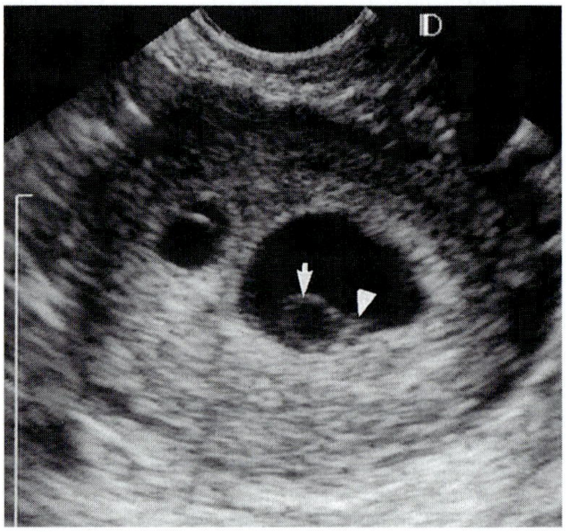

FIG. 35-17. DC/DA twins at 6.5 weeks gestational age with demise of one embryo. Endovaginal sonogram in the sagittal plane, demonstrating two chorionic sacs. The larger sac contains a live embryo *(arrowhead)* with a CRL of 5.8 mm and a yolk sac *(arrow)*. The smaller sac contains a yolk sac but no embryo. The smaller sac failed to grow on follow-up sonography.

PERINATAL MORBIDITY AND MORTALITY IN TWINS

The perinatal mortality rate is disproportionately high for twins compared with singleton pregnancies. **Prematurity**[4-7,10,24] and **growth retardation**[4,5,10,24] are the leading causes of perinatal mortality in twin and higher-order multifetal pregnancies (see box).

The **mean duration of gestation** for twins is approximately 37 weeks.[4,5] Twin pregnancies deliver earlier than singletons, have lower birth weights and Apgar scores, and are more likely to have anomalies. The intrauterine growth pattern for twins is similar to that of singletons until 30 to 34 weeks,[6,37] after which growth of twin fetuses slows, resulting in comparatively lower birth weights.[6] Ghai and Vidyasager[6] also noted an increased perinatal mortality in twins near term and postulated postmaturity due to relative uteroplacental insufficiency occurring earlier than in singleton pregnancies as the cause. In Spellacy's series,[7] in twin pregnancies with intrapair birth weight differences of 25% or greater, the perinatal mortality

TWIN PERINATAL LOSS

Prematurity
IUGR
Problems of **monochorionicity**
- vascular anastomoses in a shared placenta; twin transfusion syndrome (TTS); twin embolism syndrome (TES); acardiac twin syndrome

Problems of **MC/MA twins**
- cord knots; wrapping of cord around cotwin; locking of twins at delivery

rate was 103 per 1000 births. In pregnancies with the intrapair birth weight differences of less than 25%, the perinatal mortality rate was 46 per 1000.

These problems are compounded in **triplet pregnancy.** Compared with twins, triplets have a higher incidence of preterm delivery (87% in triplets, 26.7% in twins)[38] and a lower mean birth weight and gestational age at delivery. In a series by Sassoon et al.,[38] IUGR occurred in 53.3% of triplets compared with 6.7% of twins, and discordancy occurred in 66.7% of triplets compared with 13.3% of twins.

The **perinatal morbidity rate** is also higher for twins than for singletons. In Ghai and Vidyasagar's series,[6] the perinatal morbidity rate for twins was 47% compared with 26.6% for singletons. When respiratory-related morbidity was excluded, there was no significant difference in morbidity between twins and singletons, implicating prematurity as the etiologic factor. Morbidity, as determined by length of neonatal hospital stay and the requirement of neonatal intensive care, is higher in triplets than in twins.[38]

Although all twins are at increased risk in pregnancy, **monochorionic twins** have a **mortality rate** of two to three times that of dichorionic twins.[39] The perinatal mortality rate is only slightly higher for MZ dichorionic twins than for DZ dichorionic twins whereas the mortality rate for monochorionic (MZ) twins is more than twice that of dichorionic (MZ or DZ) twins,[39] suggesting that the increased mortality rate in monochorionic twins is due to the **vascular anastomoses in the shared placenta.**[23,39] MC/MA twins have an even higher mortality rate (approximately 30% to 50%) that is related to cord problems, including cord knots and wrapping of the cord around the cotwin and locking of the twins at the time of delivery.[39]

The sonographic assessment of **IUGR** in twin pregnancy is a controversial issue. Some studies have shown that the growth of the BPD and AC decrease in twins relative to singletons after 30 to 32 weeks gestational age, and twin growth charts have been generated based on this data.[37] More recent prospective studies have failed to show a significant difference in BPD or HC between singleton and twin pregnancies.[40] The femur lengths and other biometric parameters, including humerus length, ulna length, and tibia length, show no difference in growth rate between singletons and twins.[37,41] These data suggest that the use of twin growth charts is unwarranted and that biometric data in twins should be compared with standard singleton growth charts to identify twin fetuses that are small for gestational age.[10,24,40,41]

Discordant growth may also be associated with fetal morbidity and mortality in twins. In one series, a first trimester intrapair difference of 5 days or more gestational age as predicted by the CRL was associated with major congenital anomalies in the smaller twin in 5 out of 5 twin pairs.[42] Later in pregnancy, growth discordancy is associated with an increased risk for perinatal mortality and morbidity. Discordant growth, as defined as an intrapair birth weight discrepancy of 20% to 25%, occurs in 15% to 29% of twin gestations and may be associated with a perinatal mortality rate of 20%, or 2.5 times greater than twins without discordant growth.[43] In a study by Storlazzi et al.,[43] the estimated fetal weight was predictive of discordancy in 100% of cases when discordancy was defined as a birth weight difference of >25%. For prediction of an intrapair birth weight difference of >20%, the estimated fetal weight and an intrapair AC difference of 20 mm or more (Fig. 35-18) had similar sensitivities (80%) and negative predictive values (93%). An intrapair AC difference of 20 mm or more may have a higher positive predictive value than estimated fetal weight.[44] In some studies, the estimated fetal weight has had a low sensitivity in predicting discordant birth weight.[45] To provide a margin of error, some authors advocate the use of an intrapair estimated fetal weight discrepancy of 15% as a predictor of discordancy.[24] Others suggest that discordancy is not a risk factor if the lighter twin weighs more than 2500 g[46] and assess significant growth discordance only when one twin meets the singleton criteria for IUGR and the other does not.[10]

Doppler velocimetry of the umbilical artery may also provide information that can be used to identify twin fetuses at increased risk for morbidity and mortality in the perinatal period. In twins, the **systolic diastolic ratio (A/B ratio)** correlates closely with singleton data.[47-49] In twins with abnormal A/B ratios compared with normal singleton data, there is a high incidence of mortality and significant perinatal morbidity.[50] Studies have shown that an abnormal A/B ratio in twins has a sensitivity of approximately 80% and a positive predictive value of 70% to 90% for identification of discordancy or small-for-gestational-age fetuses[47,51] (Fig. 35-19).

A

B

C

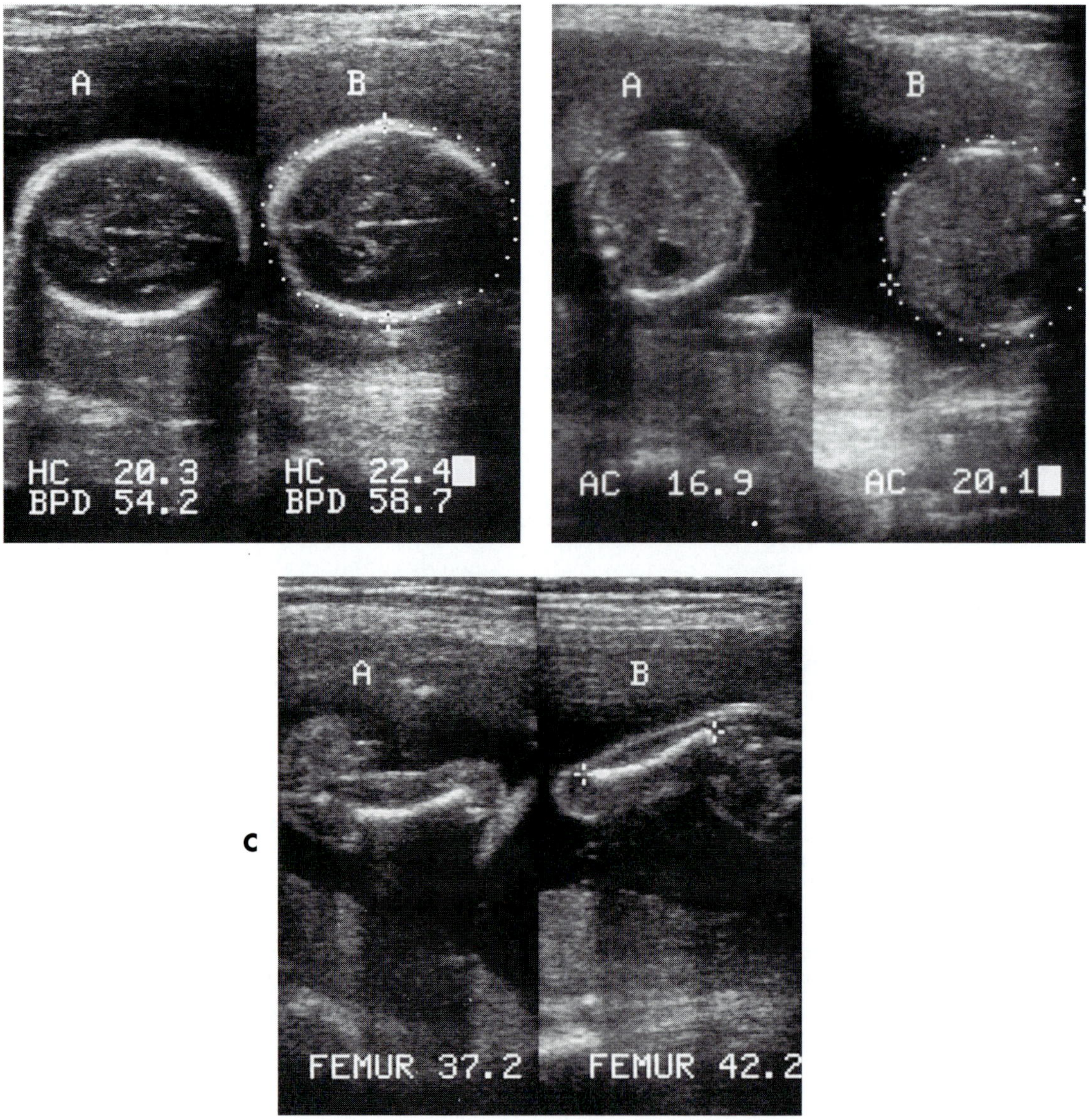

FIG. 35-18. Discordant growth at 24 weeks gestational age. **A**, The head circumference, **B**, abdominal circumference, *AC*, and, **C**, femoral length measurements in twins with discordant growth. There is a 32 mm intrapair AC difference. (From Levi CS, Lyons EA, Lindsay DJ et al. The sonographic evaluation of multiple gestation pregnancy. In: Fleischer AC, Romero R, Manning FA et al, eds. *The Principles and Practice of Ultrasonography in Obstetrics and Gynecology*. 4th ed. East Norwalk, Conn: Appleton & Lange; 1991.)

A

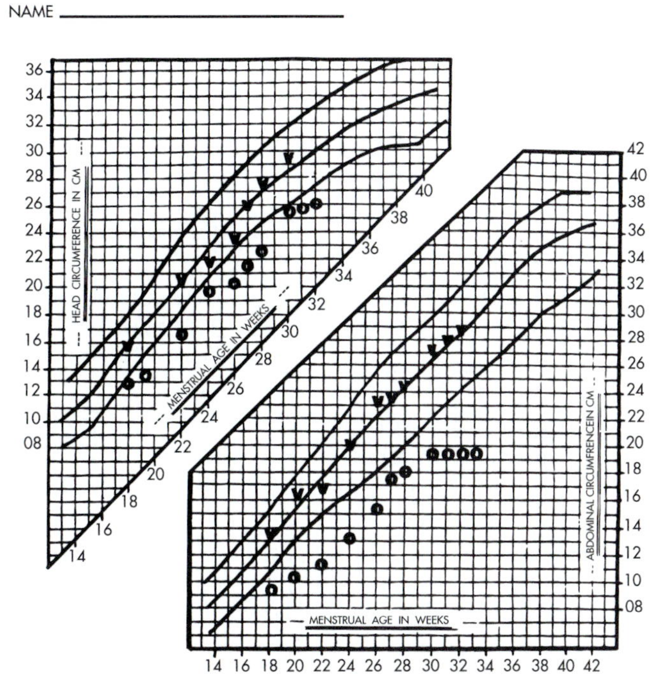

B

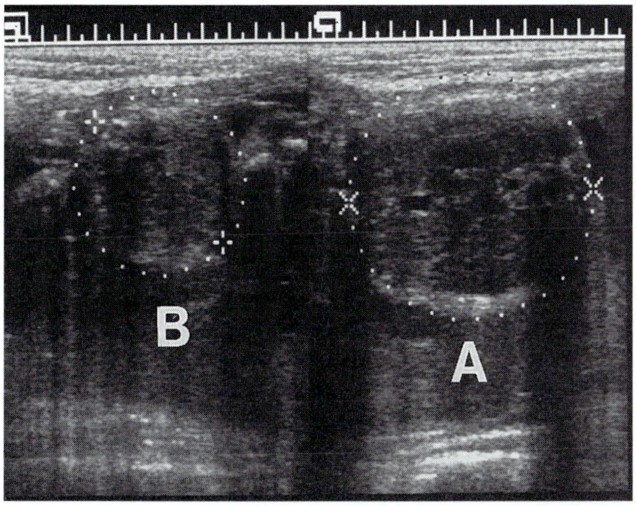

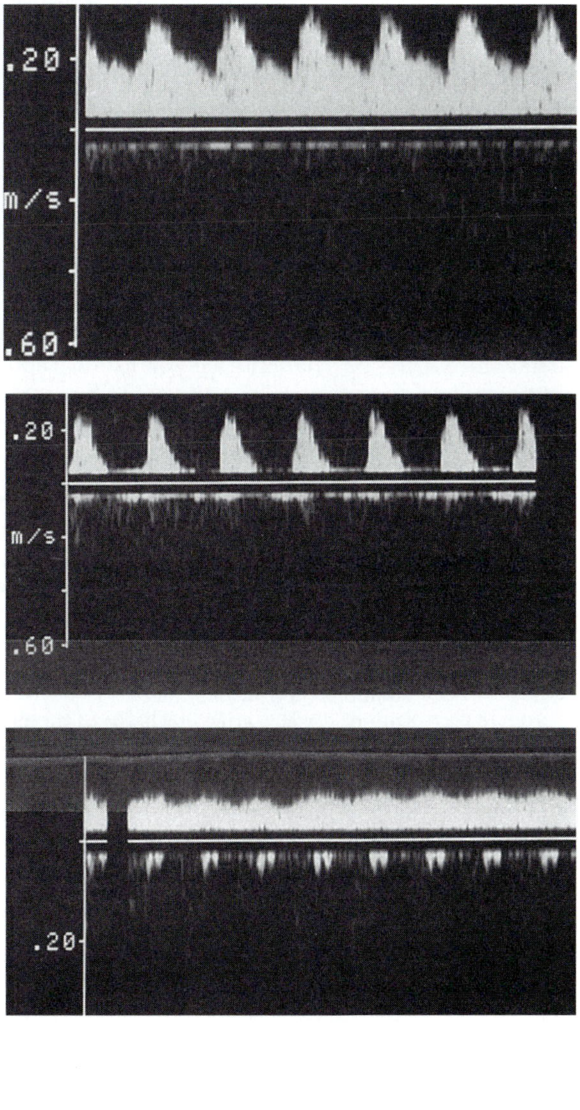

C

D

E

FIG. 35-19. Discordant growth: serial measurements, abnormal A/B ratio. The patient presented at 18 weeks with an elevated serum alpha-fetoprotein. Sonography showed structurally normal twins of the same sex. **A,** Graph demonstrating serial measurements of head and abdominal circumference. *V*, twin A; *O*, twin B. **B,** Abdominal circumference at 30 weeks gestational age of both twins (AC = 278 for twin A, 201 for twin B). **C,** Umbilical artery velocimetry of twin A at 30 weeks: normal. **D,** Umbilical artery velocimetry of twin B at 30 weeks: absent arterial diastolic flow and, **E,** venous pulsation.

In patients with evidence of **IUGR,** discordant growth, abnormal Doppler velocimetry, oligohydramnios, or triplets (or higher-order multifetal pregnancy), the pregnancy should be considered to be high risk, and frequent monitoring of the biophysical profile should be performed after potential viability. According to Finberg, it may be appropriate to perform routine, twice-weekly assessment of the biophysical profile in all twin pregnancies from 26 weeks on.[24]

SONOGRAPHIC DIAGNOSIS OF COMPLICATIONS OF TWIN AND MULTIFETAL PREGNANCY

After determining the number of embryos or fetuses and the chorionicity and amnionicity of the pregnancy, complete sonographic assessment of the fetuses and placentas should be performed. While the examination and technique are similar to the sonographic assessment of singleton pregnancies, some complications are more common or specific to twin or multifetal pregnancies.

First Trimester Pregnancy Loss

Twins and higher-order multifetal pregnancies are at increased risk for spontaneous loss of one or more embryos (or fetuses) early in pregnancy. The frequency of spontaneous loss varies from one study to another and depends on study populations, sonographic criteria, and the study design. Dickey et al.[52] reviewed a series of 2873 patients who had become pregnant as a result of treatment for infertility and who had ultrasound examinations at 7 weeks gestational age. Of the 227 patients who had sonographic evidence of two gestational sacs, the probability of delivering twins was 63% for maternal age <30 and 52% for maternal age >30. In patients with two live embryos, the probability of a twin birth was 90% for women <30 years old and 84% for maternal age >30. Using endovaginal ultrasound, Blumenfeld et al.[21] reviewed a series of 116 women with multifetal pregnancies due to assisted reproductive techniques, 88 of whom had spontaneous disappearance of one or more gestational sacs or embryos.

In a prospective series of 137 twin pregnancies with documented cardiac activity in both embryos or fetuses in the first trimester, Benson et al.[53] used a polychotomous logistic regression analysis to determine the prognosis of first trimester twin pregnancies (Table 35-1). They found that gestational age at the time of sonography, chorionicity, and sonographic findings were independent, statistically significant, prognostic factors. In their series, maternal age, method of conception, and indication for sonography were not predictive of outcome. Abnormal sonographic findings included **gestational sac size discrepancy, fibroids,** or a **subchorionic hemorrhage.** Of the 137 patients with twin pregnancies, 80.3% had viable twins (born at or beyond 25 weeks gestation), 8.8% had one infant, and 10.9% had none.

For **monochorionic twins,** the probability of two live infants based on a normal ultrasound scan at 6 weeks was 39.8%, the probability of one live infant was 30.4%, and the probability of zero live infants was 29.8%. If the scan was abnormal, these probabilities changed to 11.3%, 45.4%, and 43.3%, respectively. At 12 weeks, if the scan was normal, the probabilities were 74.4% for two live infants, 0.5% for one live infant, and 25.1% for zero live infants; the probabilities changed to 36%, 1.3%, and 62.7%, respectively, for an abnormal scan.

For **dichorionic twins,** the probability of two live infants based on a normal scan at 6 weeks was 75.8%, the probability of one live infant was 17.1%, and the probability of zero live infants was 7.1%. The probabilities changed to 37.4%, 44.7%, and 17.9%, respectively, if the scan was abnormal. At 12 weeks, if the scan was normal, the probabilities were 95.8% for two live infants, 0.2% for one live infant, and 4.3% for zero live infants; the probabilities changed to 81.4%, 0.9%, and 17.7%, respectively, for an abnormal scan.

The authors noted that the probabilities were based on the gestational age at the time of the patient's most recent scan and not on the gestational age of the original scan. As a result, the probabilities can be upgraded at the time of follow-up examination.

Monochorionic Twin Syndromes

Vascular anastomoses in the shared placenta of monochorionic twins are frequent, occurring in 85% to 100% of patients.[23] Although dichorionic placentas may fuse, vascular anastomoses do not occur. As a result of the vascular anastomoses in the placentas of monochorionic twins, **three syndromes** have been identified, which are specific to **monochorionic twins.**

Twin Transfusion Syndrome. Twin transfusion syndrome (TTS) (see box on p. 1060) occurs as a result of shunting of blood between the circulatory systems in approximately 5% to 30% of monochorionic twins.[54] The intraplacental anastomosis is usually situated in a single shared cotyledon of the common placenta[23,24] and is usually arteriovenous but may be arterial-arterial.[10] The clinical findings depend on the volume of blood shunted from one fetus to the other; however, the **classic findings** are that of a hypovolemic, anemic donor and a fluid-overloaded recipient. The donor is usually small, hypotensive, and has oligohydramnios whereas the recipient is often edematous, hypertensive, polycythemic, and has polyhydramnios.

TABLE 35-1

PROBABILITY VALUES (%) FOR PREDICTING THE OUTCOME OF A TWIN GESTATION AT THE TIME OF FIRST TRIMESTER SONOGRAPHY DEMONSTRATING TWO HEARTBEATS

Gestational Age (wk)	Monochorionic Gestation						Dichorionic Gestation					
	Normal US Scan			Abnormal US Scan			Normal US Scan			Abnormal US Scan		
	2 LI	1 LI	0 LI	2 LI	1 LI	0 LI	2 LI	1 LI	0 LI	2 LI	1 LI	0 LI
6.0	39.8	30.4	29.8	11.3	45.4	43.3	75.8	17.1	7.1	37.4	44.7	17.9
6.5	45.2	23.3	31.6	13.6	37.2	49.2	80.7	12.3	7.0	44.3	35.8	19.9
7.0	49.9	17.4	32.7	16.1	29.6	54.3	84.4	8.7	6.9	50.9	27.7	21.4
7.5	54.1	12.7	33.2	18.5	23.0	58.5	87.3	6.1	6.7	56.8	20.9	22.3
8.0	57.7	9.2	33.1	20.9	17.5	61.6	89.4	4.2	6.4	61.8	15.4	22.8
8.5	60.8	6.5	32.7	23.1	13.1	63.8	91.0	2.9	6.1	66.1	11.1	22.8
9.0	63.5	4.6	31.9	25.2	9.6	65.2	92.2	2.0	5.8	69.6	7.9	22.5
9.5	65.8	3.2	31.0	27.2	7.0	65.8	93.2	1.4	5.5	72.5	5.6	21.9
10.0	67.9	2.2	29.9	29.0	5.1	65.9	93.9	0.9	5.2	74.9	3.9	21.2
10.5	69.7	1.6	28.7	30.9	3.6	65.5	94.5	0.6	4.9	76.9	2.7	20.4
11.0	71.4	1.1	27.5	32.6	2.6	64.8	95.0	0.4	4.6	78.6	1.9	19.5
11.5	72.9	0.7	26.3	34.3	1.8	63.8	95.4	0.3	4.3	80.1	1.3	18.6
12.0	74.4	0.5	25.1	36.0	1.3	62.7	95.8	0.2	4.0	81.4	0.9	17.7
12.5	75.7	0.4	24.0	37.7	0.9	61.4	96.1	0.1	3.8	82.6	0.6	16.8
13.0	77.0	0.2	22.8	39.3	0.7	60.0	96.4	0.1	3.6	83.7	0.4	15.9

LI, Liveborn infant(s).

From Benson CB, Doubilet PM, David V. Prognosis of first-trimester twin pregnancies: polychotomous logistic regression analysis. *Radiology* 1994;192:765-768.

TWIN TRANSFUSION SYNDROME

Monochorionic twins
Discordant fetal growth
 Large twin - normal or macrosomic
 Small twin - symmetrically growth retarded
Disparity of amniotic fluid volume
 Polyhydramnios - large twin
 Oligohydramnios - small twin
May have "stuck twin" syndrome
S/D ratio difference of greater than 0.4

The **sonographic diagnosis** depends on:

- The presence of a **monochorionic** twin pregnancy.
- A significant **discrepancy in size** between the two fetuses. The larger fetus is usually normal in size but may be macrosomic. The smaller fetus is usually symmetrically growth retarded. The smaller fetus may not satisfy the criteria for IUGR, but there should be evidence of discordancy between the two fetuses. **Discordant growth** may be defined as a 20% to 25% intrapair birth weight discrepancy. Predictors of discordant growth include a difference in AC of greater than or equal to 18 to 20 mm,[43,55] an estimated fetal weight disparity of 15% (providing a margin of error),[55-57] or a second trimester BPD difference of 5 mm.
- **A disparity in amniotic fluid volume** (Fig. 35-20). The growth-retarded fetus usually has oligohydramnios, and the recipient usually has polyhydramnios. The disparity in amniotic fluid volume is often progressive and may result in the stuck twin syndrome in which the donor twin is stuck to the uterine wall by a nonvisualized membrane that restricts movement of the donor twin and may hold the fetus in an apparently antigravitational position. Close inspection will identify the amnion applied closely to the stuck twin, indicating severe oligohydramnios of the donor and severe polyhydramnios of the recipient. The stuck twin syndrome **is not** synonymous with TTS and may occur in dichorionic twins.

Other findings include:

- **Nonimmune hydrops** in one of the fetuses (usually the larger or recipient fetus).
- A **disparity** in the size or number of **vessels within the umbilical cord.**
- An umbilical artery **systolic/diastolic ratio difference of greater than 0.4**[54,55] (see Fig. 35-20). Doppler has not been shown to be effective in differentiating donor from recipient nor in providing prognostic data regarding outcome. Increased flow resistance may be present in both the donor and recipient.[54,58] Hecher et al. noted that absent or reversed diastolic flow occurs only in the donor fetus.[58]
- In some patients with TTS, a superficial communicating vessel with an arterial waveform may be demonstrated at the placental insertion of the intertwin membrane using color flow Doppler ultrasound.[59]

The **mortality rate of TTS** is high, ranging from 40% to 70%.[60] In a series by Patten et al.[61] in 25 patients with TTS and the stuck twin syndrome, perinatal mortality was 88% for the larger twin with polyhydramnios and 96% for the smaller twin with oligohydramnios. Premature labor and perinatal morbidity occurred in all cases. Some studies suggest that aggressive amniocentesis to reduce the amniotic fluid volume in the fetus with polyhydramnios and maintain the amniotic fluid volume at normal levels may improve outcome[62-64] (see Fig. 35-20). Survival rates after aggressive amniocentesis range from 32% to 79%.[62-64] In the pregnancies with poor outcomes, the disparity in fetal size and mean volume of amniotic fluid drained at each amniocentesis were greater than in pregnancies in which one or both twins survived.[63] As an alternative to aggressive amniocentesis, fetoscopic laser coagulation of the communicating vessel in the intertwin membrane in patients with TTS has been associated with a survival rate of 53%.[64]

Velamentous cord insertion occurs more commonly in twins than in singletons. In a series by Fries et al., velamentous cord insertions occurred in 63.6% of twins with TTS as compared with 18.5% of MC/DA twins without TTS.[65] The authors postulate that the velamentous cord insertion may result in compression of the cord, resulting in increased resistance in the placental circulation and shunting of blood to the recipient. The resultant mild polyhydramnios in the recipient would further compress the velamentous cord of the donor, resulting in progressive changes. Aggressive amniocentesis may reduce the compressive force, accounting for the relative success of this technique.[65] Aggressive amniocentesis has also been shown to increase uterine artery blood flow and may improve uteroplacental perfusion.[66]

Twin Embolization Syndrome. In **demise of the cotwin in DC/DA pregnancies,** the surviving twin is not at significant risk.[4,67] If cotwin demise occurs in the second trimester, as the surviving twin grows, the water content and most of the soft tissue of the dead fetus may be reabsorbed, resulting in a small, flattened fetus surrounded by minimal or no amniotic fluid, referred to as fetus papyraceus[5] (Fig. 35-21). Fetus papyraceus may occur in DC/DA or MC/DA twins.

In **monoamniotic twins,** demise of the cotwin may result in renal, hepatic, and cerebral damage in the surviving twin.[13,68,69] Benirschke originally postulated that demise of the cotwin may result in transfusion of

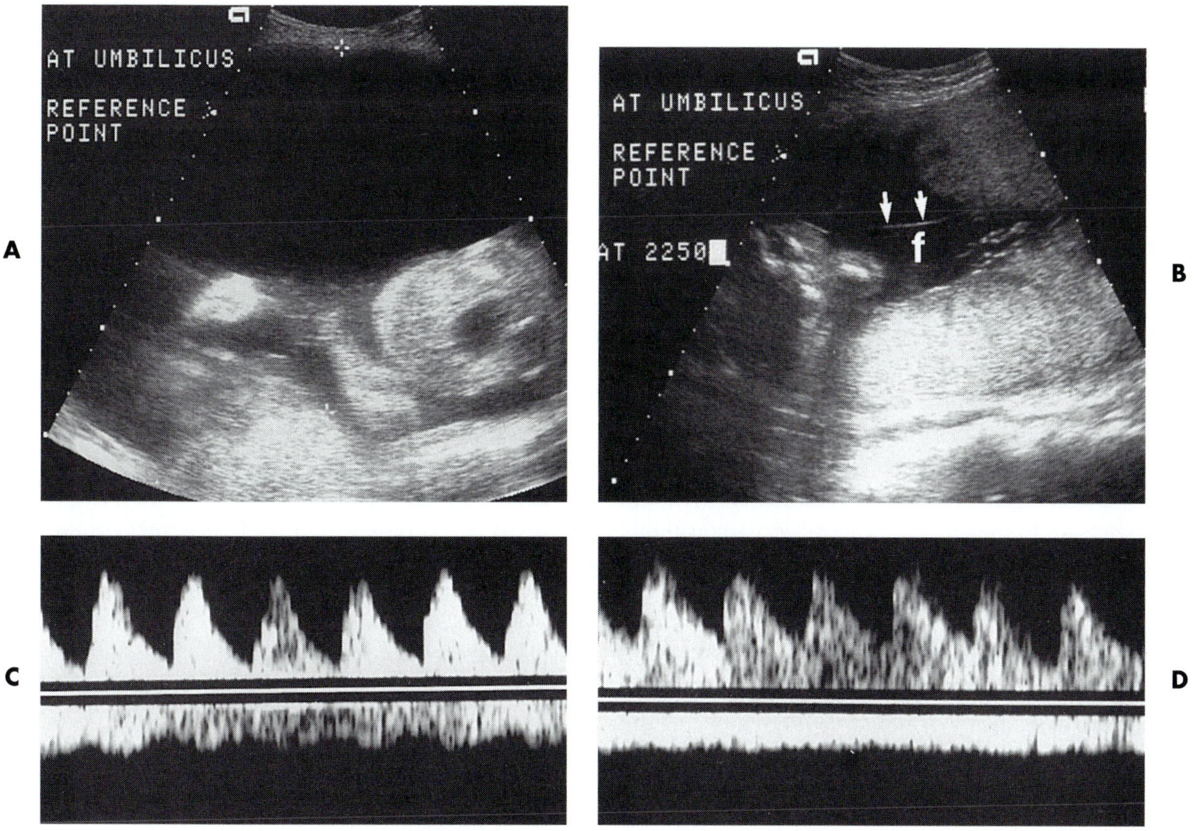

FIG. 35-20. Twin transfusion syndrome (TTS). The patient presented at 26 weeks gestational age with discordant MC/DA twins. The smaller fetus had no measurable amniotic fluid and the larger had polyhydramnios. Fetal anatomy was normal. **A,** Polyhydramnios of the larger twin at 27 weeks gestational age. **B,** After reduction amniocentesis of 2250 cc from the amniotic cavity of the larger twin, the intertwin membrane *(arrows)* becomes visible, and fluid, *f*, is demonstrated around the smaller fetus. **C,** Umbilical artery velocimetry of the smaller fetus at 31.5 weeks, demonstrating an abnormal A/B ratio of 6.2 and venous pulsation. **D,** Umbilical artery velocimetry of the larger fetus, demonstrating a normal A/B ratio of 2.2. The twins were delivered at 33 weeks after spontaneous rupture of the membranes.

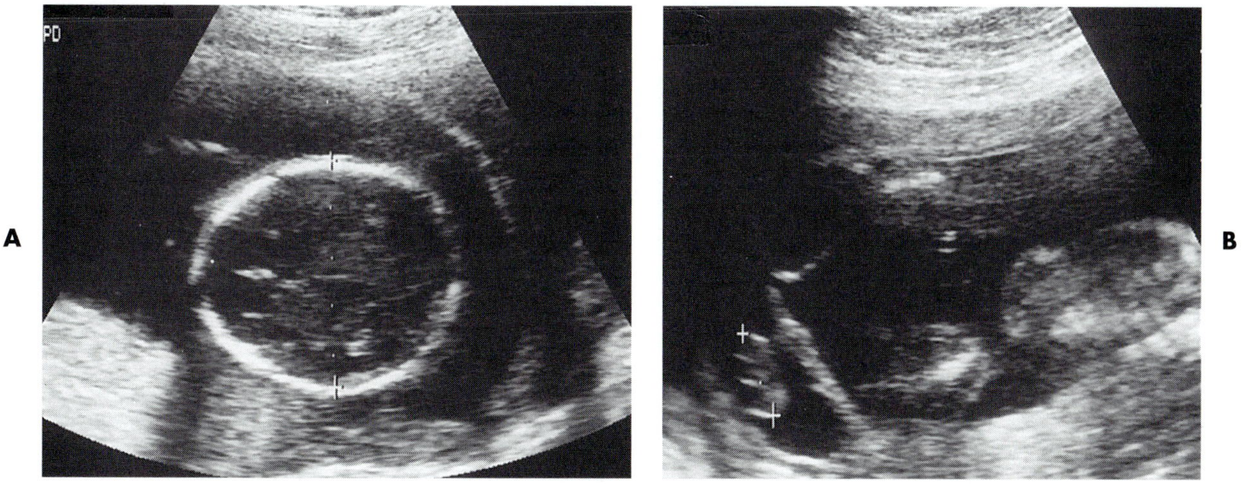

FIG. 35-21. Fetus papyraceus in DC/DA twins at 20 weeks gestational age. **A,** Biparietal diameter of the normal fetus. **B,** Transverse sonogram showing a second gestational sac separated from the larger sac by a thick membrane. A small fetus (CRL 16 mm) with no evidence of cardiac activity or movement is present.

thromboplastin-rich blood or embolization of clot and debris across the placental vascular anastomoses to the surviving twin. More recently, Benirschke has suggested that the degenerative change in these organs may be related to acute exsanguination of the surviving twin into the twin that died *in utero* rather than thromboplastin infusion from the dead twin to the survivor. The transplacental exsanguination of the survivor is thought to result in an acute hypotensive event.[69] Common intracranial manifestations of the twin embolization syndrome (TES) include ventriculomegaly, porencephalic cysts, diffuse cerebral atrophy, and microcephaly.[68] Gastrointestinal manifestations include hepatic and splenic infarcts and gut atresias.[68] Other anomalies, including renal cortical necrosis, pulmonary infarcts, facial anomalies, and terminal limb defects, may also occur. In pregnancies where selective termination is considered, termination of one fetus of a monochorionic twin pair should not be performed because of risk of TES for the surviving fetus.[23,24,68]

Acardiac Parabiotic Twin. Acardiac parabiotic twinning (Fig. 35-22) is a rare occurrence in which there is shunting of blood through arterial-to-arterial and venous-to-venous anastomoses within the placenta. Flow direction in the umbilical arteries and vein of the recipient fetus is reversed. Because the acardiac twin receives poorly oxygenated blood through the umbilical arteries, structures supplied by the iliac arteries and distal abdominal aorta are relatively well perfused whereas the upper body and head receive essentially no oxygenated blood. As a result, the acardiac twin has limited development of the upper half of the body characterized by anencephaly or a small rudimentary head with holoprosencephaly, absent or hypoplastic upper torso and limbs, and absent or anomalous two-chambered heart.[10,23,24] A multiloculated dorsal cystic hygroma is usually present.[24] The acardiac twin usually has severe oligohydramnios.

Mortality of the acardiac twin is universal either *in utero* or at the time of delivery. The normal or "pump" twin is at increased risk because of high cardiac output and polyhydramnios. The overall perinatal mortality of the pump twin is approximately 50% to 55%.[10,23,24]

Problems Specific to Monoamniotic Twinning (MC/MA Twins)

Conjoined Twins. Conjoined twins are rare, occurring in approximately 1 per 50,000 to 1 per 100,000 births.[10,23] Conjoined twinning occurs only in MC/MA twins and is sporadic with no known associations. Conjoined twinning results from incomplete division of the embryonic disk and resultant fusion with shared body parts, the site and extent of which vary (Fig. 35-23). The most common form of conjoined twinning is fusion of the anterior thorax and/or abdomen (referred to as thoracopagus, omphalopagus, and thoracoomphalopagus) (Fig. 35-24), which together constitute 70% of conjoined twins.[2,10,23] Sacral (pygopagus), pelvic (ischiopagus), and cranial (craniopagus) fusions are less common.[5] When duplication is less complete, the site of attachment is more commonly lateral, as in diprosopus with lateral fusion of the head and body with two faces.

A

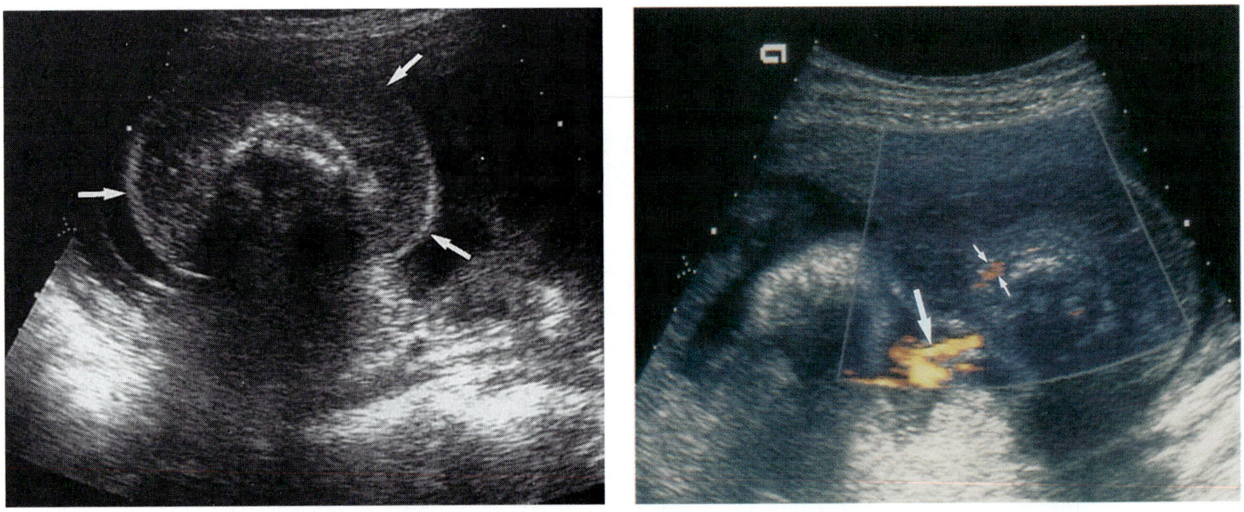

B

FIG. 35-22. Acardiac parabiotic twinning—twin reversed arterial perfusion sequence. The patient presented at 23 weeks with elevated maternal serum alpha-fetoprotein. **A,** Sonography shows a normal twin and an ill-formed mass *(arrows)*, with skin and muscular and skeletal structures, that moved throughout pregnancy. **B,** Power mode Doppler ultrasound shows the arterial anastomosis feeding the acardiac twin *(large arrow)* and low flow vessels in the abnormal mass *(small arrows)*.

A B C

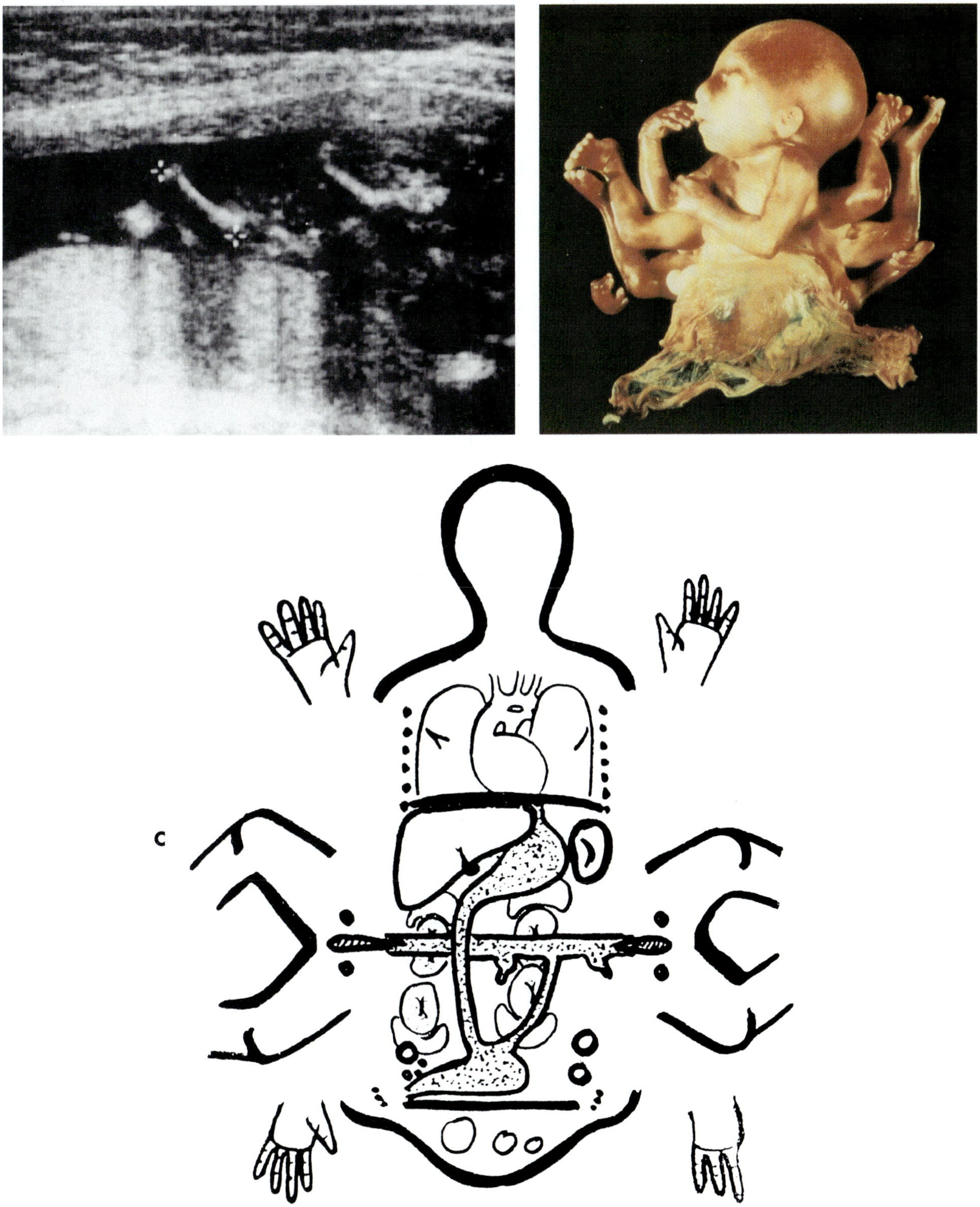

FIG. 35-23. Conjoined twins. The patient presented at 18 weeks gestational age with a grossly elevated maternal serum alpha-fetoprotein. **A,** Sonogram shows a grossly malformed mass with multiple limbs. The mass was adherent to the placenta. **B,** The gross specimen. **C,** Diagram of the extent of fusion.

A 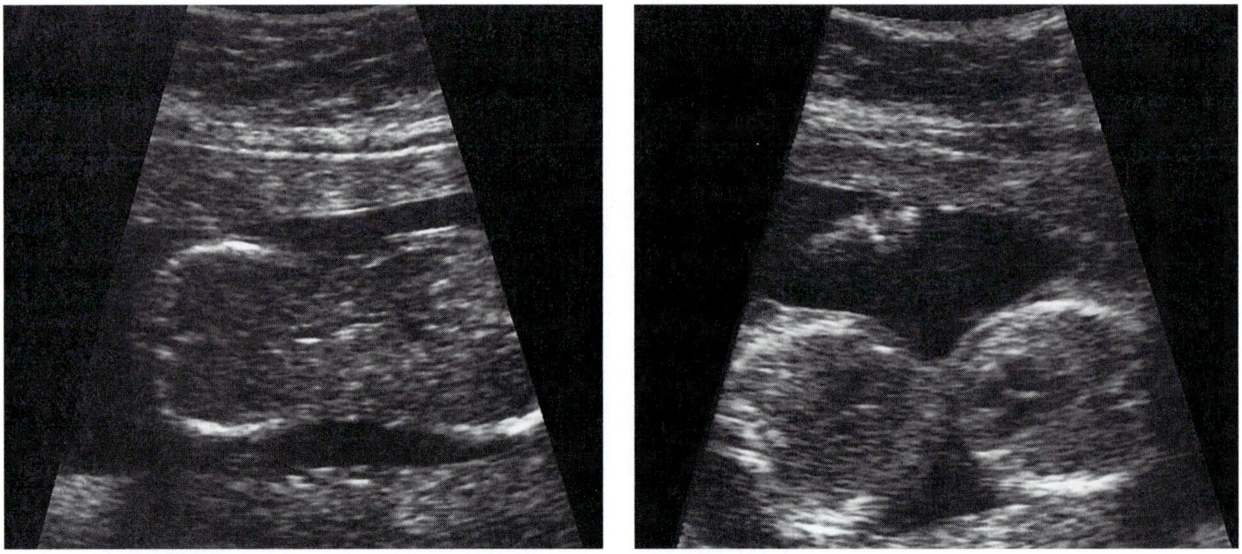 B

FIG. 35-24. Conjoined twins—omphalopagus. **A,** Sonogram shows a cross-sectional view through the fetal abdomen, which shows the liver. **B,** A scan at a slightly more cephalad level shows the thoraces are touching but separate. The fetal hearts are seen. (Courtesy Ants Toi, M.D., University of Toronto.)

A 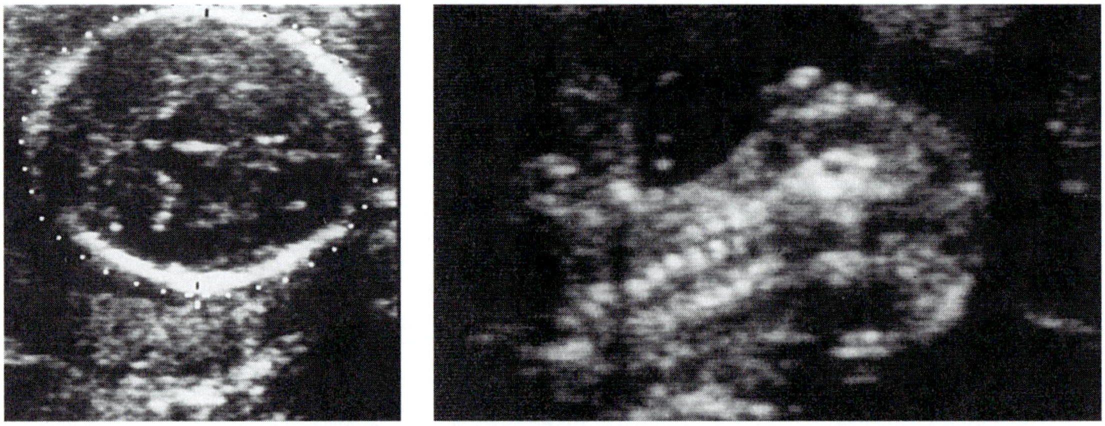 B

FIG. 35-25. Discordance for anomalies: anencephaly. **A,** Twins at 19 weeks gestational age. The fetal head of twin B is normal. **B,** No fetal head is identified for twin A. Only the base of skull and disorganized neural tissue are present.

Conjoined twins should be suspected in all MC/MA twin pregnancies, and careful sonographic assessment should be performed to identify the presence of shared fetal organs. The index of suspicion of conjoined twinning should increase if the twins maintain a constant and often unusual relative position and move together, and if the neck and head are constantly hyperextended. In thoracopagus the heart is often conjoined with associated cardiac anomalies, and in omphalopagus the liver is often conjoined. Prognosis, obstetric management, and treatment planning are contingent on careful sonographic mapping of the degree of fusion and the extent of joining of fetal organs.[2,10,23]

Morbidity and Mortality in Nonconjoined MC/MA Twins. In addition to the potential complications associated with monochorionic twinning, nonconjoined MC/MA twins have the additional risk of **cord entanglement** and **cord knotting** with resultant demise of both fetuses. Cord entanglement is a sign of MC/MA twins and is not necessarily associated with unfavorable outcome.[70]

The antepartum management of MC/MA twins is a controversial issue. Because of the risk of fetal death due to knotting of the entangled cord late in pregnancy, prophylactic preterm delivery by elective cesarean section has been advocated[71,72] at 32 weeks gestational age. Aisenbrey et al.[72] recommend the use of color flow Doppler ultrasound to identify the presence or absence of cord entanglement in MC/MA twins at 25 to 26 weeks in order to direct management in these patients.

STRUCTURAL DEFECTS IN MONOZYGOTIC TWINS

Malformations due to limited intrauterine space
Anomalies related to TTS, TES, and acardiac twinning
Early defects of morphogenesis
- Conjoined twins
- Neural tube defects
- Holoprosencephaly
- VACTERL association
- Congenital heart disease
- Cloacal exstrophy
- Sirenomelia
- Gonadal dysgenesis

In patients with cord entanglement, they recommend close follow-up and frequent fetal monitoring with amniocentesis for both groups at 32 weeks with delivery as soon as lung maturity is demonstrated.

Congenital Anomalies in Twins

The incidence of congenital anomalies appears to be approximately twice as common in the infants of a twin gestation than in a singleton.[13] Major malformations occur in approximately 2.12% of infants of a twins gestation as opposed to 1.05% of singletons. Minor malformations occur in 4.13% of twins as opposed to 2.45% of singletons.[13] The increased prevalence of anomalies in twins has been shown to be due **entirely to the increased rate of anomalies in MZ twins.**[39] DZ twins are not at increased risk for anomalies as compared with singletons.

The **structural defects** in MZ twins have been categorized as follows[2,10,39]:

- Malformations occurring late in pregnancy due to limited intrauterine space, including torticollis, talipes, and hip dislocation.
- Anomalies related to TTS, TES, and acardiac twinning.
- Early defects of morphogenesis. The etiology of these anomalies is thought to be related to the etiology of MZ twinning. Structural defects commonly associated with MZ twins include conjoined twins, neural tube defects, holoprosencephaly, the VACTERL association, congenital heart disease, cloacal exstrophy, sirenomelia, and gonadal dysgenesis.

The concordance rate of congenital anomalies in MZ twins is 5% to 50%, with the majority having a concordance rate of 10% to 20%.[73] Of note, anencephaly (Fig. 35-25) and hydrocephaly are rarely concordant.[74]

REFERENCES

1. Benirschke K, Kim CK. Multiple pregnancy. Pt 1. *N Engl J Med* 1973;288:1276-1284.
2. Benacerraf BR. Pregnancy with multiple fetuses. In: Rumack CR, Wilson SR, Charboneau JW, eds. *Diagnostic Ultrasound.* St Louis: Mosby-Year Book; 1991:745-758.
3. Crane JP. Sonographic evaluation of multiple pregnancy. *Semin US CT MR* 1984;5:144-156.
4. Spellacy WN. Multiple pregnancies. In: Scott JR, DiSaia PJ, Hammond CB et al, eds. *Danforth's Obstetrics and Gynecology.* 7th ed. Philadelphia: JB Lippincott Co; 1994:333-341.
5. Multifetal pregnancy. In: Cunningham FG, MacDonald PC, Gant NF et al, eds. *Williams Obstetrics.* 19th ed. Norwalk, Conn: Appleton & Lange; 1993:891-918.
6. Ghai V, Vidyasagar D. Morbidity and mortality factors in twins: an epidemiologic approach. *Clin Perinatal* 1988;15:123-140.
7. Spellacy WN, Handler A, Ferre CD. A case-control study of 1,253 twin pregnancies from a 1982-1987 perinatal data base. *Obstet Gynecol* 1990;75:168-171.
8. Naeye RL, Tafari N, Judge D et al. Twins: causes of perinatal death in twelve United States cities and one African city. *Am J Obstet Gynecol* 1978;131:267-272.
9. Hawrylyshyn PA, Barkin M, Berstein A et al. Twin pregnancies—a continuing perinatal challenge. *Obstet Gynecol* 1982;59:463-466.
10. Pretorius DH, Mahony BS. Twin gestations. In: Nyberg DA, Mahony BS, Pretorius DH, eds. *Diagnostic Ultrasound of Fetal Anomalies: Text and Atlas.* Chicago: Year Book Medical Publishers, Inc; 1990:592-622.
11. Persson P-H, Grennert L, Gennser G et al. On improved outcome of twin pregnancies. *Acta Obstet Gynecol Scand* 1979;58:3-7.

Incidence

12. Moore KL. The placenta and fetal membranes. In: Moore KL, ed. *The Developing Human: Clinically Oriented Embryology.* 4th ed. Philadelphia: WB Saunders Co; 1988:104-130.
13. Levi CS, Lyons EA, Lindsay DJ et al. The sonographic evaluation of multiple gestation pregnancy. In: Fleischer AC, Romero R, Manning FA et al, eds. *The Principles and Practice of Ultrasonography in Obstetrics and Gynecology.* 4th ed. East Norwalk, Conn: Appleton & Lange; 1991:359-380.
14. Derom C, Vlietinck R, Derom R et al. Increased monozygotic twinning rate after ovulation induction. *Lancet* 1987;1(8544):1236-1238.
15. Wenstrom KD, Syrop CH, Hammett DG et al. Increased risk of monochorionic twinning associated with assisted reproduction. *Fertil Steril* 1993;60:510-514.
16. Benson CB, Doubilet PM. Twin pregnancy. In: McGahan JP, Porto M, eds. *Diagnostic Obstetrical Ultrasound.* Philadelphia: JB Lippincott Co; 1994:434-448.
17. White C, Wyshak G. Inheritance in human dizygotic twinning. *N Engl J Med* 1964;271:1003-1005.
18. Rothman KJ. Fetal loss, twinning and birthweight after oral-contraceptive use. *N Engl J Med* 1977;297:468-471.
19. Medical Research International. The Society for Assisted Reproductive Technology. *In vitro* fertilization/embryo transfer in the United States: 1990 results from the national IVF-ET Registry. *Fertil Steril* 1992;57:15-24.
20. Andrews MC, Muasher SJ, Levy DL et al. An analysis of the obstetric outcome of 125 consecutive pregnancies conceived *in vitro* and resulting in 100 deliveries. *Am J Obstet Gynecol* 1986;154:848-854.

Embryology and Placentation

21. Blumenfeld Z, Dirnfeld M, Abramovici H et al. Spontaneous fetal reduction in multiple gestations assessed by transvaginal ultrasound. *Br J Obstet Gynaecol* 1992;99:333-337.
22. Levi CS, Lyons EA, Dashefsky SM et al. Yolk sac number, size and morphologic features in monochorionic monoamniotic twin pregnancy. *Can Assoc Radiol J* 1996;47:98-100.
23. Filly RA, Goldstein RB, Callen PW. Monochorionic twinning: sonographic assessment. *AJR* 1990;154:459-469.

Sonographic Determination of Amnionicity and Chorionicity

24. Finberg HJ. Ultrasound evaluation in multiple gestation. In: Callen PW, ed. *Ultrasonography in Obstetrics and Gynecology*. 3rd ed. Philadelphia: WB Saunders Co.; 1994:102-128.
25. Yeh H-C, Goodman JD, Carr L et al. Intradecidual sign: a US criterion of early intrauterine pregnancy. *Radiology* 1986; 161:463-467.
26. Nyberg DA, Laing FC, Filly RA et al. Ultrasonographic differentiation of the gestational sac of early intrauterine pregnancy from the pseudogestational sac of ectopic pregnancy. *Radiology* 1983;146:755-759.
27. Kurtz AB, Wapner RJ, Mata J et al. Twin pregnancies: accuracy of first-trimester abdominal US in predicting chorionicity and amnionicity. *Radiology* 1992;185:759-762.
28. Yeh H-C, Rabinowitz JG. Amniotic sac development: ultrasound features of early pregnancy. The double bleb sign. *Radiology* 1988;166:97-103.
29. Filly RA. Ultrasound evaluation during the first trimester. In: Callen PW, ed. *Ultrasonography in Obstetrics and Gynecology*. 3rd ed. Philadelphia: WB Saunders Co; 1994:63-85.
30. Finberg HJ. The "twin peak" sign: reliable evidence of dichorionic twinning. *J Ultrasound Med* 1992;11:571-577.
31. Mahony BS, Filly RA, Callen PW. Amnionicity and chorionicity in twin pregnancies: prediction using ultrasound. *Radiology* 1985;155:205-209.
32. Hertzberg BS, Kurtz AB, Choi HY et al. Significance of membrane thickness in the sonographic evaluation of twin gestations. *AJR* 1987;148:151-153.
33. Townsend RR, Simpson GF, Filly RA. Membrane thickness in ultrasound prediction of chorionicity of twin gestations. *J Ultrasound Med* 1988;7:327-332.
34. Levi S. Ultrasonic assessment of the high rate of human multiple pregnancy in the first trimester. *J Clin Ultrasound* 1976;4:3-5.
35. Varma TR. Ultrasound evidence of early pregnancy failure in patients with multiple conceptions. *Br J Obstet Gynaecol* 1979;86:290-292.

Perinatal Morbidity and Mortality in Twins

36. Robinson HP, Caines JS. Sonar evidence of early pregnancy failure in patients with twin conceptions. *Br J Obstet Gynaecol* 1977;84:22-25.
37. Grumbach K, Coleman BG, Arger PH et al. Twin and singleton growth patterns compared using US. *Radiology* 1986; 158:237-241.
38. Sassoon DA, Castro LC, Davis JL et al. Perinatal outcome in triplet versus twin gestations. *Obstet Gynecol* 1990;75:817-820.
39. McCulloch K. Neonatal problems in twins. *Clin Perinatal* 1988;15:141-158.
40. Reece EA, Yarkoni S, Abdalla M et al. A prospective longitudinal study of growth in twin gestations compared with growth in singleton pregnancies: I. The fetal head. *J Ultrasound Med* 1991;10:439-443.
41. Reece EA, Yarkoni S, Abdalla M et al. A prospective longitudinal study of growth in twin gestations compared with growth in singleton pregnancies: II. The fetal limbs. *J Ultrasound Med* 1991;10:445-450.

Sonographic Diagnosis of Complications of Twin and Multifetal Pregnancy

42. Weissman A, Achiron R, Lipitz S et al. The first trimester growth-discordant twin: an ominous prenatal finding. *Obstet Gynecol* 1994;84:110-114.
43. Storlazzi E, Vintzileos AM, Campbell WA et al. Ultrasonic diagnosis of discordant fetal growth in twin gestations. *Obstet Gynecol* 1987;69:363-367.
44. Hill LM, Guzick D, Chenevey P et al. The sonographic assessment of twin growth discordancy. *Obstet Gynecol* 1994; 84:501-504.
45. Chamberlain P, Murphy M, Comerford FR. How accurate is antenatal identification of discordant birthweight in twins? *Eur J Obstet Gynecol Reprod Biol* 1991;40:91-96.
46. Blickstein I, Shoham-Schwartz Z, Lancet M. Growth discordancy in appropriate for gestational age, term twins. *Obstet Gynecol* 1988;72:582-584.
47. Giles WB, Trudinger BJ, Cook CM. Fetal umbilical artery flow velocity-time waveforms in twin pregnancies. *Br J Obstet Gynaecol* 1985;92:490-497.
48. Trudinger BJ, Giles WB, Cook CM et al. Fetal umbilical artery waveforms and placental resistance: clinical significance. *Br J Obstet Gynaecol* 1985;92:23-30.
49. Divon MY, Boldes R, McGahan JP. Assessment of intrauterine growth retardation. In: McGahan JP, Porto M, eds. *Diagnostic Obstetrical Ultrasound*. Philadelphia JB Lippincott Co; 1994:67-82.
50. Gaziano EP, Knox GE, Bendel RP et al. Is pulsed Doppler velocimetry useful in the management of multiple-gestation pregnancies? *Am J Obstet Gynecol* 1991;164:1426-31.
51. Gerson AG, Wallace DM, Bridgens NK et al. Duplex Doppler ultrasound in the evaluation of growth in twin pregnancies. *Obstet Gynecol* 1987;70:419-420.
52. Dickey RP, Olar TT, Curole DN et al. The probability of multiple births when multiple gestational sacs or viable embryos are diagnosed at first trimester ultrasound. *Hum Reprod* 1990;5:880-882.
53. Benson CB, Doubilet PM, David V. Prognosis of first-trimester twin pregnancies: polychotomous logistic regression analysis. *Radiology* 1994;192:765-768.
54. Pretorius DH, Manchester D, Barkin S et al. Doppler ultrasound of twin transfusion syndrome. *J Ultrasound Med* 1988;7:117-124.
55. Blickstein I. The twin-twin transfusion syndrome. *Obstet Gynecol* 1990;76:714-722.
56. O'Brien WF, Knuppel RA, Scerbo JC et al. Birth weight in twins: an analysis of discordancy and growth retardation. *Obstet Gynecol* 1986;67:483-486.
57. Blickstein I, Shoham-Schwartz Z, Lancet M et al. Characterization of the growth discordant twin. *Obstet Gynecol* 1987;70:11-15.
58. Hecher K, Ville Y, Nicolaides KH. Fetal arterial Doppler studies in twin-twin transfusion syndrome. *J Ultrasound Med* 1995;14:101-108.
59. Hecher K, Ville Y, Nicolaides KH. Color Doppler ultrasonography in the identification of communicating vessels in twin-twin transfusion syndrome and acardiac twins. *J Ultrasound Med* 1995;14:37-40.
60. Brown DL, Benson CB, Driscoll SG et al. Twin-twin transfusion syndrome: sonographic findings. *Radiology* 1989; 170: 61-63.
61. Patten RM, Mack LA, Harvey D et al. Disparity of amniotic fluid volume and fetal size: problem of the stuck twin-US studies. *Radiology* 1989;172:153-157.

62. Elliott JP, Urig MA, Clewell WH. Aggressive therapeutic amniocentesis for treatment of twin-twin transfusion syndrome. *Obstet Gynecol* 1991;77:537-540.
63. Saunders NJ, Snijders RJM, Nicolaides KH. Therapeutic amniocentesis in twin-twin transfusion syndrome appearing in the second trimester of pregnancy. *Am J Obstet Gynecol* 1992;166:820-824.
64. Ville Y, Hyett J, Hecher K et al. Preliminary experience with laser surgery for severe twin-twin transfusion syndrome. *N Engl J Med* 1995;332:224-227.
65. Fries MH, Goldstein RB, Kilpatrick SJ et al. The role of velamentous cord insertion in the etiology of twin-twin transfusion syndrome. *Obstet Gynecol* 1993;81:569-574.
66. Bower SJ, Flack NJ, Sepulveda W et al. Uterine artery blood flow response to correction of amniotic fluid volume. *Am J Obstet Gynecol* 1995;173:502-507.
67. Hagay ZJ, Mazor M, Leiberman JR et al. Management and outcome of multiple pregnancies complicated by the antenatal death of one fetus. *J Reprod Med* 1986;31:717-720.
68. Patten RM, Mack LA, Nyberg DA et al. Twin embolization syndrome: prenatal sonographic detection and significance. *Radiology* 1989;173:685-689.
69. Beminschle K. The contribution of placental anastomoses to prenatal twin damage. *Hum Pathol* 1992;23:1319-1320.
70. Townsend RR, Filly RA. Sonography of nonconjoined monoamniotic twin pregnancies. *J Ultrasound Med* 1988; 7:665-670.
71. Rodis JF, Vintzileos AM, Campbell WA et al. Antenatal diagnosis and management of monoamniotic twins. *Am J Obstet Gynecol* 1987;157:1255-1257.
72. Aisenbrey GA, Catanzarite VA, Hurley TJ et al. Monoamniotic and pseudomonoamniotic twins: sonographic diagnosis, detection of cord entanglement, and obstetric management. *Obstet Gynecol* 1995;86:218-222.
73. Schinzel AAGL, Smith DW, Miller JR. Monozygotic twinning and structural defects. *J Pediatr* 1979;95:921-930.
74. Hay S, Wehrung DA. Congenital malformations in twins. *Am J Hum Genet* 1970;22:662-678.

CHAPTER 36

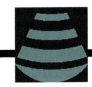

The Fetal Chest and Abdomen

Christine H. Comstock, M.D.
Janet S. Kirk, M.D.

CHAPTER OUTLINE

THE FETAL CHEST

Only the lungs and heart are visible to the ultrasonographer when examining the chest of a normal fetus. When an abnormality is detected, however, the diverse differential diagnosis reflects all the other "invisible" structures of the chest: the pleura and pleural spaces, the pericardium, and the contents of the three compartments of the mediastinum. The origin of an abnormality of the thorax may not always be clear. However, the traditional compartmental approach used in examining a chest radiograph can be useful when approaching the sonogram of the fetal chest. If the source of a mass can be assigned to a particular compartment, the differential diagnostic list itself becomes shorter and clearer. Characterization of the mass as cystic or solid narrows the differential further (Table 36-1).

The Pleural Space

Pleural Effusions. Pleural effusions, or fluid collected in the space between the parietal and visceral pleura, can be associated with ascites or skin thickening; they are then described as part of the appearance of fetal hydrops, the differential diagnosis of which is discussed in Chapter 45. Pleural effusions often precede the other fluid collections of hydrops, or they may be a persistent and isolated finding.

Pleural effusions appear as a rim of fluid around the lungs, the tips of which produce a "bat-wing" appearance (Fig. 36-1). If fluid does not form a crescent-shaped rim around the lung, the fluid is either loculated or not pleural in origin.

Pleural effusions have been associated with fetal infection, congestive heart failure, Turner's and Down syndromes and, in a rare case, with pulmonary lymphangiectasia.[1] Unilateral effusions are often related to a unilateral process such as a right diaphragmatic hernia, sequestration, cystic adenomatoid malformation, or (rarely) segmental pulmonary hypoplasia.[2] Chylous effusions are also often unilateral.

Isolated pleural effusions in fetuses without an underlying chest mass, subsequent hydrops, or chromosomal abnormality usually have a good outcome[3,4] and can even be quite transient (Fig. 36-2).[4,5] Larger, long-standing effusions raise the fear that the underlying lung will not develop. Therefore, intrauterine thoracentesis has been performed in an attempt to allow lung expansion,[6,7-9] but, unfortunately, fluid usually reaccumulates within hours. Consequently, permanent shunts have been attempted.[7,9] However, the outcome of these fetuses might have been satisfactory despite the shunt. A review of outcomes of all reported *isolated* pleural effusions concludes that not enough data exist to support either conservative or aggressive management.[10] Another review (of all reported cases of pleural effusion, both isolated and not isolated) concludes that intervention is worthwhile if hydrops is present and the gestational age is less than 32 weeks.[11]

TABLE 36-1
ULTRASOUND APPEARANCE OF THORACIC MASSES

Appearance	Types of Masses
Cystic	Bronchogenic cyst
	Dilated esophagus
	Dilated bronchus
	Diaphragmatic hernia
	Enteric cyst
	Mediastinal meningo
	Pericardial cyst
Solid and cystic	Diaphragmatic hernia
	Cystic adenomatoid malformation: macrocystic
	Teratoma
	Cystic hygroma
	Eventration
	Neuroblastoma
Solid masses	Diaphragmatic hernia
	Sequestration: intralobar or extralobar
	Cystic adenomatoid malformation: microcystic
	Teratoma
	Bronchial obstruction
	Eventration
	Hamartoma
	Ectopic kidney
	Spleen-intrathoracic (Fairhurst)

Congenital Diaphragmatic Hernias

Foramen of Bochdalek Hernias. Congenital diaphragmatic hernias (CDH) occur in two locations. The more common type involves the foramen of Bochdalek, which is located in the posterolateral corners of the chest. If this portion of the diaphragm fails to close completely during fetal development, abdominal viscera herniate into the chest. In an evaluation of newborn autopsies, Butler found that stomach herniated into the chest in 60% of cases, colon in 56%,

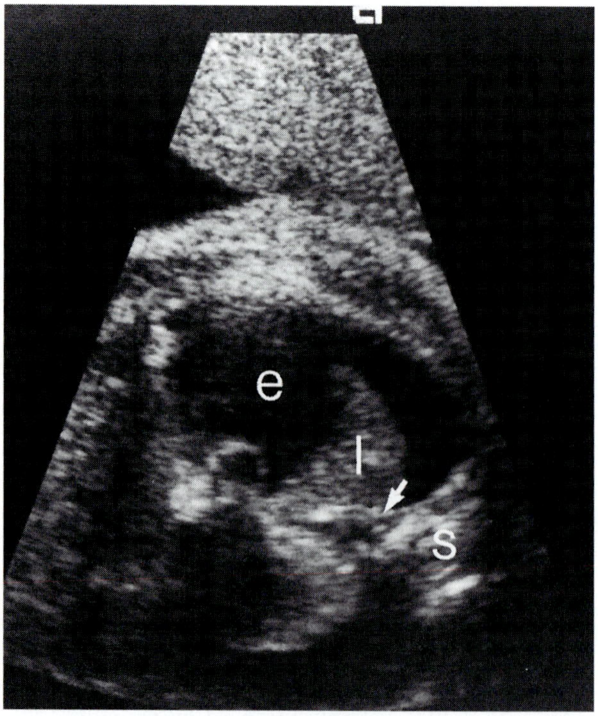

FIG. 36-1. Large pleural effusion, *e*, outlines lung, *l*, which has a bat-wing appearance. *s* indicates spine; *arrow*, posterior mediastinum.

small intestine in 88%, spleen in 45%, liver in 51%, pancreas in 24%, and a kidney in 22%.[12] Liver and gallbladder usually herniate through the right foramen of Bochdalek.[13] Butler also found intestine in the right thorax in three out of four cases.[12] Malrotation of the herniated bowel is very frequent.[14]

Left-sided hernias are much more frequent than right-sided ones[12,15-17] and, consequently, there is considerably less information about the prenatal diagnosis of right-sided hernias. Fortunately, bilateral congenital diaphragmatic hernias are rare; the outcome is uniformly poor.

On **sonography**, CDHs have been detected as early as 17 weeks of gestation.[18] Mediastinal deviation is often seen first and is the most obvious ultrasound sign of a CDH.[13,16] In the normal fetus the apex of the heart touches the interior wall of the left anterior chest, and the intersection of the atrial septum with the posterior heart border lies just to the right of the center of the chest (Fig. 36-3). In CDH the entire

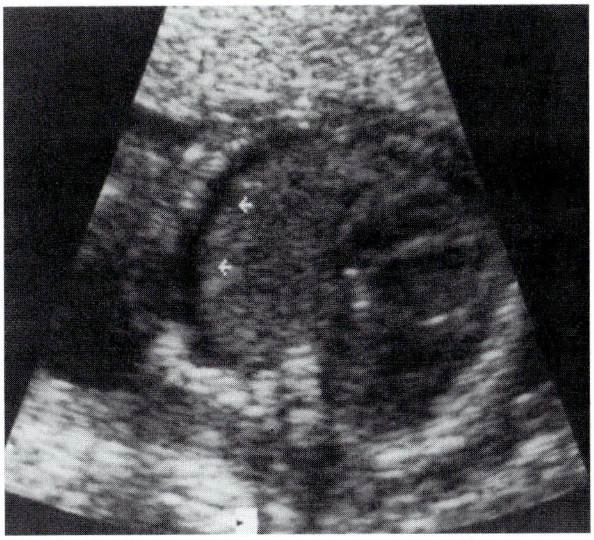

FIG. 36-2. Transient pleural effusion, seen as small crescent effusion (*arrows*), disappeared by time of next examination. Neonate was normal.

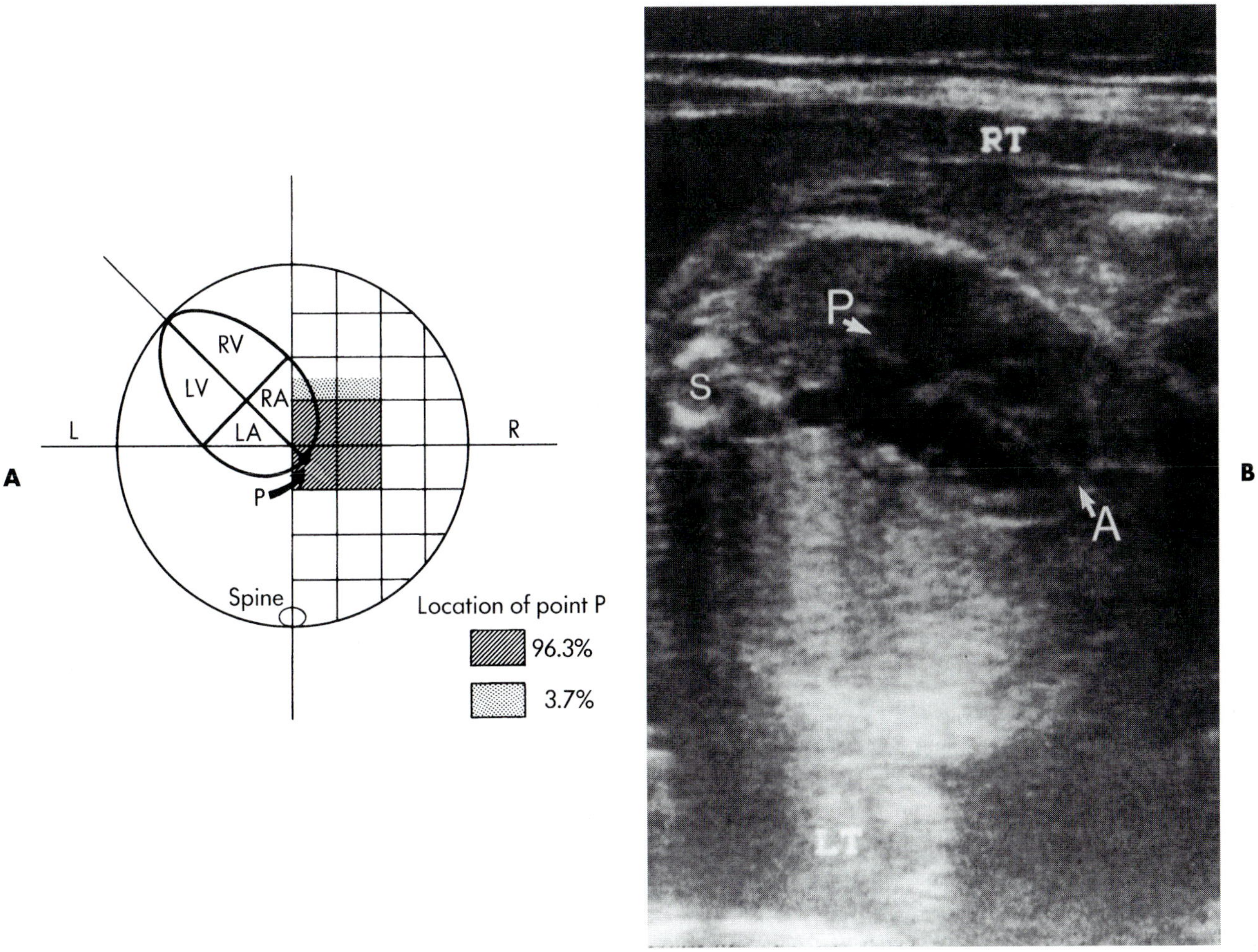

FIG. 36-3. Normal position of fetal heart. **A,** Point of intersection of atrial septum with back of heart, *P*, lies to right of midline. Apex of heart touches anterior chest wall. **B,** Shift of heart to right in fetus at 24 weeks of gestation. Point *P* lies far to right and posterior to its normal location. *S*, Spine; *A*, heart apex. (From Comstock CH. Normal fetal heart axis and position. *Obstet Gynecol* 1987;70:255-259.)

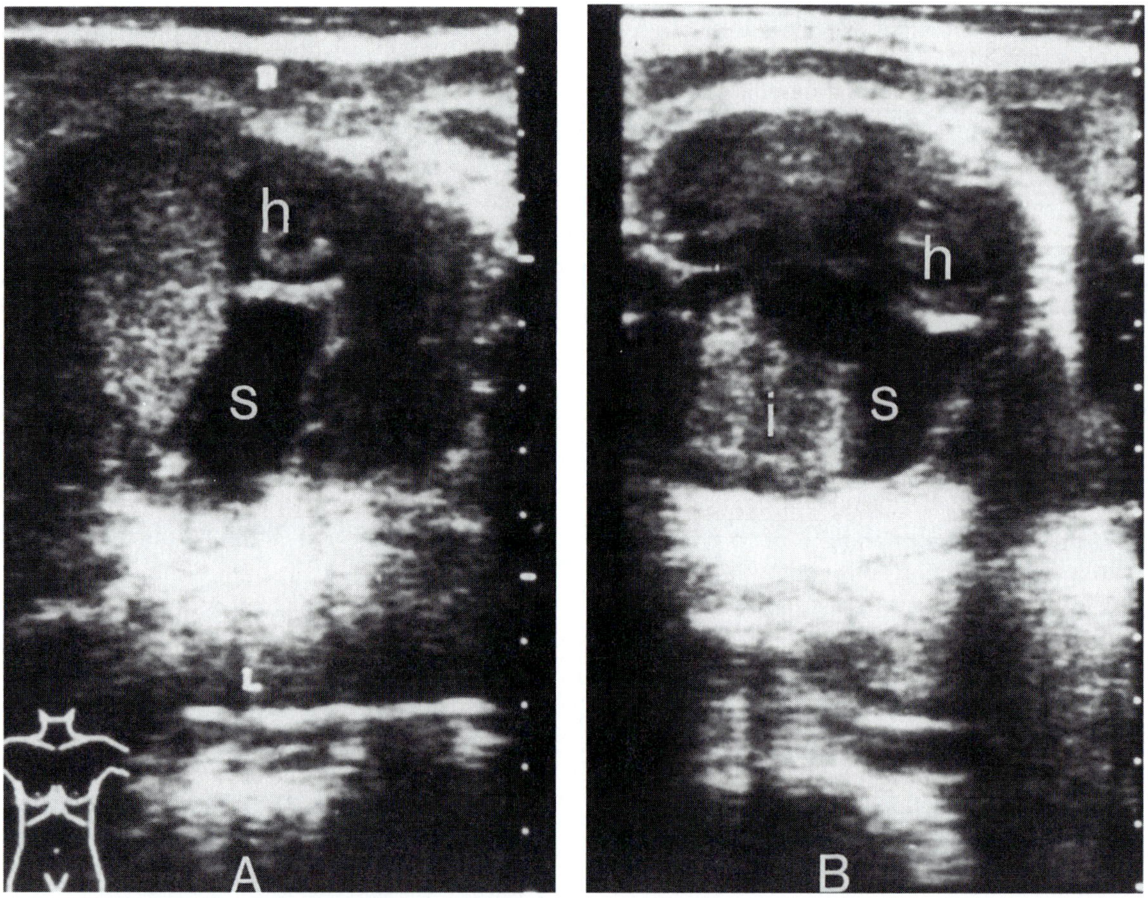

FIG. 36-4. Foramen of Bochdalek diaphragmatic hernia. **A,** Left coronal, and **B,** right transverse views show that stomach, *s*, lies at level of the heart, *h*, which is displaced to right. *i* indicates intestine. (From Comstock CH. The antenatal diagnosis of diaphragmatic anomalies. *J Ultrasound Med* 1986;4:391-396.)

heart is usually displaced to the side of the thorax opposite the herniation, but sometimes the heart axis also is changed (Fig. 36-4).[16] In cases in which no hollow viscera lie in the chest, mediastinal deviation, as evidenced by a shift in heart position, may be the only detectable abnormality by all but very close scrutiny.

If the stomach lies in the chest, it is certain that the fetus has a CDH. However, care must be taken to obtain a true transverse scan so that the stomach is not artificially projected at the level of the heart. The abdominal circumference is usually lower than the fifth percentile for gestational age because the abdominal organs are displaced upwardly.[13,16,19] Because most fetuses with CDH (and with no other major anomalies or chromosomal defects) are not growth-retarded, a small abdominal circumference is a reliable supportive finding.[17] In our experience, the umbilical vein can also be displaced upwardly. Polyhydramnios is usually not seen early or is very mild, but it can increase dramatically in the third trimester.[20]

These are all supportive signs, but they are not absolutely diagnostic. However, visualization of peristalsis in the chest is diagnostic, as is paradoxical motion of the abdominal contents on fetal inspiration. As the fetus inspires, the abdominal organs rise into the chest on the side of the defect and move down as they normally would on the normal side, giving a rocking motion in the coronal view.[16] As useful as these latter two signs are, however, they may not allow the examiner to distinguish a CDH from eventration of the diaphragm.

Because the liver can so closely resemble the lungs, **right-sided hernias** are more difficult to detect. Displacement of the mediastinum to the left is sometimes more difficult to appreciate than displacement to the right. Absence of the gallbladder in the abdomen is usual.[13] A small abdominal circumference is suggestive, as is a unilateral pleural effusion.[13] In two reported cases, fluid in a right-sided hernia sac exactly simulated a right pleural effusion.[18,21] In one series, three out of four fetuses with right diaphragmatic hernias also had hydrops.[22]

Pressure on the left ventricle or redirected blood flow from the inferior vena cava have been suggested as possible causes of a relatively hypoplastic left ventricle. Unlike the true hypoplastic heart, the mitral and aortic valves are normal.[23,24] Lack of growth of the left ventricle over the course of gestation is a poor prognostic factor.[25]

It is important to examine carefully the fetus with a CDH. There is an increase in accompanying abnormalities, the majority of which are of central nervous system (CNS) origin. **Anencephaly** is the most frequent of these, followed by **hydrocephaly, encephalocele**, and **spina bifida**.[17] The very rare **iniencephaly** appears to have a higher incidence in fetuses with diaphragmatic hernias.[13,17,26]

The likelihood of survival is 55% in the absence of other major anomalies,[27] but it may be greater if extracorporeal oxygenation is used on the neonate. Although the size of both lungs, including the one on the side opposite the defect, is usually decreased, the greatly thickened musculature around the pulmonary arterioles is probably responsible for at least some, if not the major part, of the poor clinical course. These infants maintain a fetal circulation that cannot be explained by lack of lung mass alone.[28]

The **prognosis** is thought to be related to the size of the defect, but this is difficult to assess in the fetus. Herniation of the liver generally signifies a larger defect and one much more difficult to repair. If the stomach can be seen in the posterior or midchest, this signifies that the liver has herniated. The presence of the vessels leading to the left lobe of the liver in the chest is very predictive as well. Curvature of the umbilical vein to the left (instead of its usual straight course) is also suggestive.[29]

Foramen of Morgagni Hernias. Partial or complete absence of the central diaphragm behind the sternum can allow liver or bowel to herniate into the anterior mediastinum. If only muscle is missing, the hernia will be covered by peritoneum and parietal pleura. However, occasionally there is no peritoneum at all—and in other cases there is not even pericardium—which allows for herniation of bowel or liver directly into the pericardial space (Fig. 36-5).[16,30,31] Most foramen of Morgagni hernias occur to the right of the sternum because the heart and pericardium lie to the left; or they may occur bilaterally.[32] Omentum and colon are the most frequent hernial contents, but liver, stomach, and small intestine have also been reported.[32]

Accompanying defects are even more frequent in this type of hernia than in those of the foramen of Bochdalek.[30,31] **Abnormal rotation of the gut** with a right gastroduodenal loop has been reported.[31] This type of hernia has been associated with trisomy 13-15 and 22 short-arm translocation.[30]

Eventration of the Diaphragm. When there is a relative lack of muscle in the dome of the diaphragm, the involved leaf (fibrous material) and underlying abdominal contents rise up into the chest.

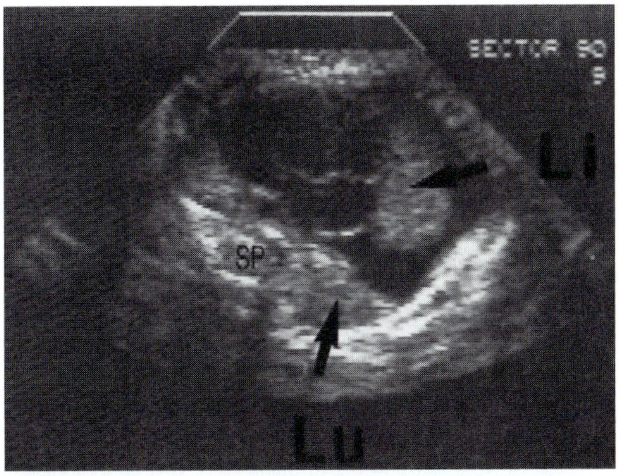

FIG. 36-5. Foramen of Morgagni hernia, transverse view through the heart. Liver, *Li*, has herniated into pericardial sac, producing large pericardial effusion. Lung, *Lu*, is displaced posteriorly toward spine, *SP*. (From Comstock CH. The antenatal diagnosis of diaphragmatic anomalies. *J Ultrasound Med* 1986;4:391-396.)

Eventrations may be partial or complete, located on the right or left or bilateral. If the eventration is on the left, the stomach can be seen at the level of the heart, which is then displaced to the right.[16] Because diaphragmatic motion may be impaired, it may be difficult or impossible to distinguish a left eventration from a congenital diaphragmatic hernia.[16]

On the right, however, the liver usually rises into the thorax. Although it may simulate a chest mass on a transverse scan, continuity in the configuration of the diaphragm above the chest mass may suggest the diagnosis (Fig. 36-6).[33] In addition, the mass appears to be anterior and lateral, a location not characteristic of either Bochdalek's or Morgagni's foramens.

Unilateral eventration is usually asymptomatic but, if severe, may produce a mild degree of pulmonary hypoplasia.[34]

Bilateral eventration has been reported in trisomies 13 and 18,[35] congenital cytomegalovirus infection,[34] congenital rubella,[36] and arthrogryposis multiplex.[37] Pulmonary hypoplasia, or at least some respiratory distress, appears to be more frequent in bilateral eventration.[37]

The Lungs

Pulmonary Hypoplasia. One or both lungs may not develop completely or at all. When lung weight in relation to body weight is low at autopsy, a diagnosis of pulmonary hypoplasia can be made. Clinically, the spectrum of outcomes ranges from neonatal death to mild respiratory insufficiency.

Unilateral pulmonary hypoplasia is quite rare and is presumed to be developmental in origin. It pro-

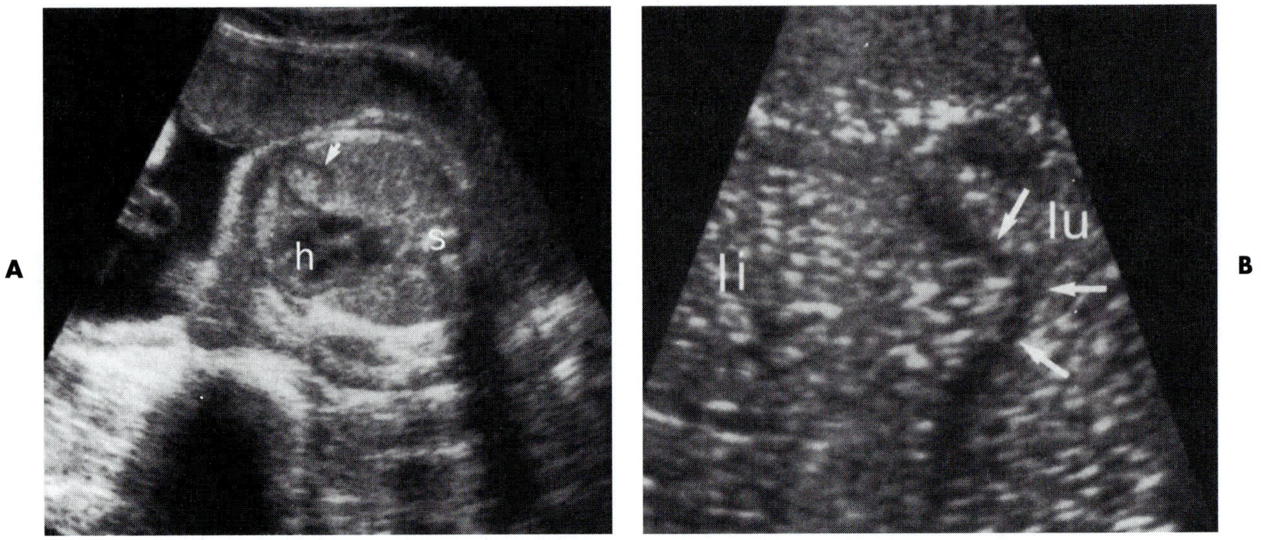

FIG. 36-6. Eventration of diaphragm presenting as chest mass. **A,** Transverse view. Elliptical mass with sonolucent border lies in anterior right chest (*arrow*). *h* indicates heart; *s*, spine. **B,** Coronal view. Arrows indicate eventration; *lu*, lungs; *li*, liver. (From Jurcak-Zaleski C, Comstock CH, Kirk JS. Eventration of the diaphragm: prenatal diagnosis. *J Ultrasound Med* 1990;9:351-354.)

duces a mediastinal shift in the absence of a thoracic mass. The remaining lung has been reported to be echogenic.[38] Occasionally the right and left lungs may develop at discrepant rates, suggesting unilateral hypoplasia. We have seen one fetus in whom the heart lay in the right thorax at 18 weeks of gestation but gradually returned to its usual midline position by full term; the neonate was normal.[39] Presumably the shift was a result of more rapid growth of one lung than the other. Unilateral pulmonary hypoplasia may also be produced by space-occupying lesions such as a cystic adenomatoid malformation, diaphragmatic hernia, or hydrothorax. If there is significant mediastinal displacement, there is usually also pulmonary hypoplasia of the contralateral lung, although this occurs to a lesser degree.

Bilateral pulmonary hypoplasia may be caused by the restricted chest cage found in such severe skeletal dysplasias as thanatophoric dwarfism, Jeune's asphyxiating dystrophy (Jeune's syndrome), achondrogenesis and, rarely, as an isolated anomaly. More frequently it is caused by a lack of amniotic fluid, either because of lack of production or loss (premature rupture of membranes, renal agenesis, or posterior urethral valves).

It would be useful clinically to be able to predict which fetuses will prove to have lethal pulmonary hypoplasia and which will not.[40-43] Evaluation of the prediction is complicated by the varying criteria used in measurement and in different study populations. Chest circumference measurements at the level of the heart have been quite predictive in some studies,[42-44] but these measurements may not apply to other populations because chest circumference can be reduced in growth-retarded infants and in premature rupture of the membranes.[43] Comparing chest circumference to abdominal circumference is not useful in obstructive uropathies, asymmetric intrauterine growth rate, or anterior abdominal wall defects. DeVore has developed tables that compare chest circumference with femur length, but these cannot be used to evaluate fetuses with skeletal dysplasias.[40] In Vintzileos' series, the following formula,

$$[\text{chest area} - \text{heart area}] \times 100/\text{chest area},$$

was the most accurate (85% sensitivity, 85% specificity). This formula is gestational-age-independent and was not altered by premature rupture of membranes. However, its predictive value was used only in separating lethal from nonlethal hypoplasia.[43] Unfortunately, most of the available studies reflect cross-sectional data. In one study, comparison of measurements of individual fetuses over time (longitudinal data) appeared to be the most useful.[45] In a review of all methods of prediction,[46] none was found to be useful in clinical decisions—with one exception: the gestational age at which membranes ruptured. Interestingly, rupture of membranes in twins is infrequently associated with pulmonary hypoplasia. The fluid in the other sac or less compression seems to be protective.[47]

Cystic Adenomatoid Malformations. Cystic adenomatoid malformations (CAM) are actually hamartomas that usually involve just one lobe of the lung. Stocker has suggested three types, based on cyst size,[48] but outcome and antenatal ultrasound appearance correlate best with the two groups proposed by Adzich.[49] The **macroscopic type** contains cysts that are larger than 5 mm (Fig. 36-7) and encompasses Stocker's types I and II (Fig. 36-8). The **microscopic cyst type** contains smaller cysts that cannot be distinguished individually but that produce a solid echogenic mass (Stocker's type III). There have been many descriptions of the prenatal diagnosis of CAM, the findings and outcome of which are tabulated by Nyberg.[50]

Although both types may produce a mediastinal shift and can be associated with hydrops, the macroscopic type is less frequently accompanied by hydrops and has a better prognosis. Currently, there is only one reported case of the microscopic type identified in the fetus that has been associated with newborn survival.[49] Interestingly, it is also the only reported case of the microscopic type without hydrops. It is not clear if it is hydrops or the type that determines the prognosis. The prognosis for fetuses with the microscopic type is difficult to determine because many of those pregnancies have been terminated based on the poor outcome of neonates with microscopic CAM and hydrops. Roelofsen et al. in their review of all reported cases to date, evaluated hydrops using logistic regression. Hydrops has occurred in 47% of reported cases, with 13% of those surviving. On the other hand, survival rate was 91% if no hydrops existed. Hydrops is strongly predictive of a poor outcome; echogenicity was not predictive if hydrops was present.[51]

The size of the mass is not necessarily predictive of outcome because size may decrease markedly over the prenatal period[52,53] or the mass may even disappear entirely; in some instances a neonate has survived despite a CAM occupying over half the thorax.[49] Withdrawal of cyst fluid has been reported to be followed by rapid reaccumulation.[54] Placement of a shunt in a large cyst has been followed by rupture of membranes or displacement of the catheter.[54] Resection has been performed in fetuses with hydrops and, although the hydrops resolved, premature delivery was a problem.

Diagnostic possibilities are limited. A **cystic adenomatoid malformation** may be difficult to distinguish from a congenital diaphragmatic hernia. The large cysts of the macroscopic type, unlike bowel, do not show peristalsis. The abdomen of the fetus with a CAM is not small, as is that of a fetus with a congenital diaphragmatic hernia. The abdominal organs are in their usual position, and there is no upward motion of abdominal contents into the chest on fetal inspiration, as there is in a diaphragmatic hernia.[16] **Bronchial cysts** are usually single, although the occasional multicystic type is difficult to distinguish from a CAM. A rare case of **cystic dilation of the bronchus** with hydrops was difficult to distinguish from CAM.[55] A **pericardial teratoma** may contain large cysts, but it is usually surrounded by pericardial fluid. The microscopic or dense type of CAM may be simulated by a **diaphragmatic hernia involving liver or spleen** only, by a **pulmonary sequestration**, or even by the echogenic lung distal to **bronchial atresia**.[56] A large cystic adenomatoid malformation has been associated with echogenic skin lesions, linear nevus sebaceus, which are a form of hamartomas.[57]

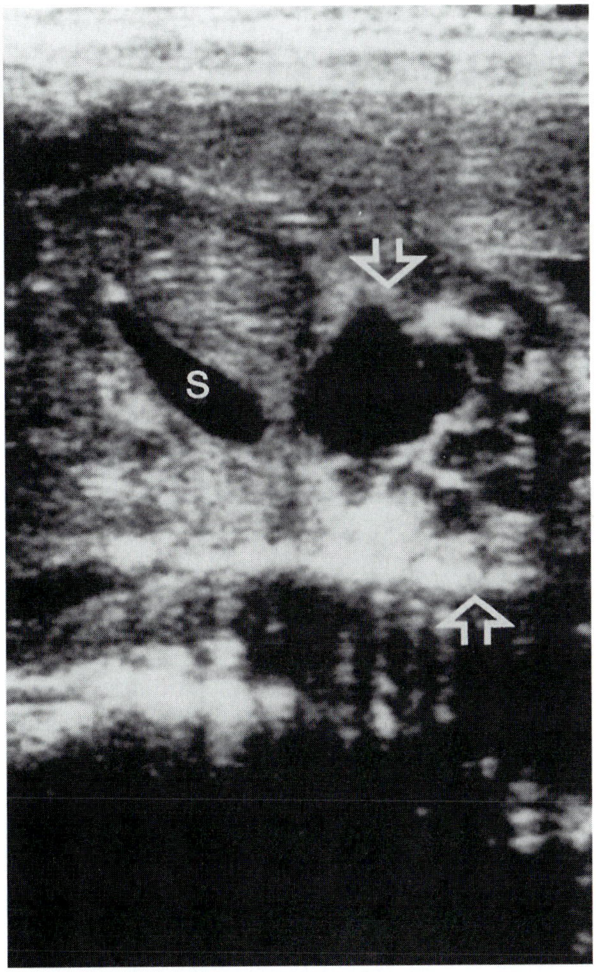

FIG. 36-7. Cystic adenomatoid malformation of lung (macrocystic type) with large cysts of varying sizes *(arrows)*. Sagittal scan of fetal chest and abdomen (head to right). *s* indicates stomach. (From Comstock CH. Sagittal scan of fetal chest and abdomen. *Ultrasound Q* 1988;6:229-256.)

Pulmonary Sequestration. These are congenital lesions consisting of normal pulmonary tissue that has no connection with the bronchial tree and is supplied by arteries arising from the aorta. **Intralobar** sequestrations share the pleural covering of the surrounding normal lung and drain into the pulmonary veins, whereas **extralobar** sequestrations have a separate pleural covering and drain into the systemic circulation. Both types are much more frequent on the left side. Recent cases have been described in which an apparent sequestration disappeared over several months in a neonate[58] and a fetus.[59]

An **intralobar sequestration** has been described once in a fetus.[60] It appeared as a dense, round mass at the base of the lung without hydrops or mediastinal shift. This type of sequestration almost always involves the posterior basal segments of a lower lobe but is not truly segmental and may involve part of an adjacent segment as well. Only occasionally has an intralobar sequestration been seen in an apical segment.[61] Accompanying anomalies are rare. Eventration, segmental bronchial obstruction, or a thoracic kidney should be included in the differential diagnosis.[62]

Extralobar sequestrations are also usually basal in origin but have been reported in more varied locations, such as within the substance of the diaphragm, in the mediastinum, in the pericardial or pleural spaces, in the hilum, or within lung substance.[63] In the fetus they appear as dense round or conical masses, always with accompanying hydrops.[55,64-69] Pleural effusion may outline the margin of the mass, separating the mass from surrounding lung. The primary **differential diagnosis** includes a diaphragmatic hernia (of liver or spleen), cystic adenomatoid malformation, or congenital lobar emphysema. An aberrant vessel arising from the aorta and coursing into the mass has been demonstrated in the fetus by ultrasound.[71] Presumably, demonstration of the supplying vessels and their origin in the aorta could be attempted with color Doppler imaging in the fetus.

Although outcome of infants and children with pulmonary sequestrations is excellent, the outcome of fetuses who also have hydrops has been uniformly poor, with death occurring in the early neonatal period. **Accompanying malformations** have been reported in up to 50% of infants with extralobar sequestrations (often involving the sternum or diaphragm), but none of the reported fetuses have had anomalies.

Congenital Bronchogenic Cysts. These cysts probably arise from the primitive foregut early in embryogenesis, are lined with ciliated columnar epithelium, and may contain cartilage in their walls. They may be intrapulmonary[72] or may lie in the posterior mediastinum. They are occasionally connected to the tracheobronchial tree, allowing air to pass into them at birth. The **simple intrapulmonary cysts,** which are usually 1.5 to 2.0 cm in diameter, do not displace the mediastinum.[55,66,72,73] Hydrops has been reported in one case.[63] They are rarely associated with anomalies and are usually not symptomatic.

On the other hand, close association of **mediastinal bronchogenic cysts** with the trachea or bronchi may cause narrowing of those structures, with distal trapping of fluid within the lungs. The distal lung may be expanded and dense, simulating the solid form of cystic adenomatoid malformation.[74]

Bronchial/laryngeal Atresia. Laryngeal atresia causes fetal lung secretions to accumulate in the tracheobronchial tree, resulting in an echogenic appearance of the lungs (Fig. 36-9) and can cause

A

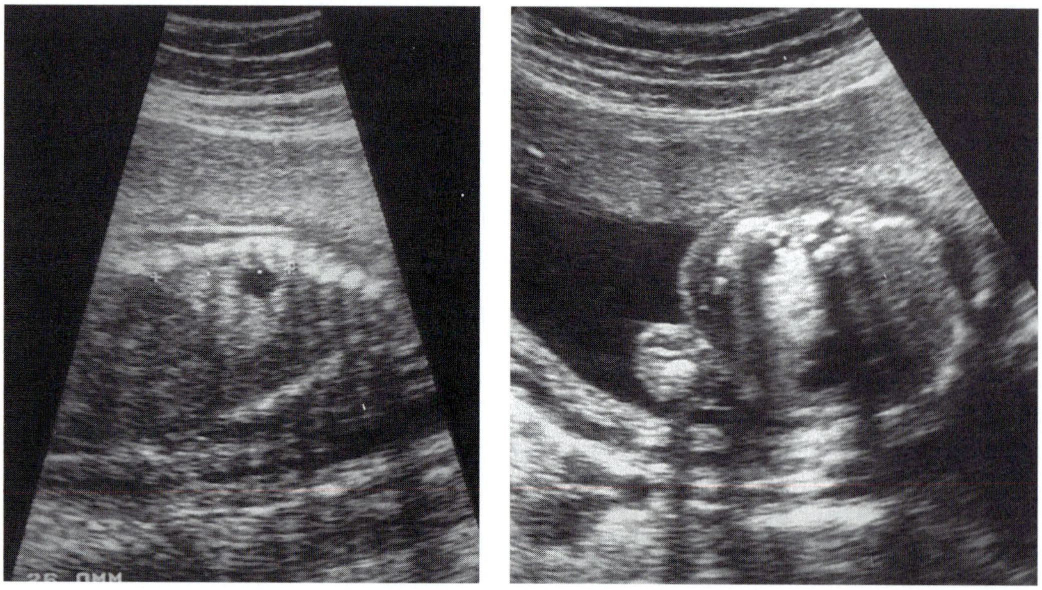

B

FIG. 36-8. Cystic adenomatoid malformation of the lung, type I, at 22 weeks gestation. **A,** Long axis sonogram shows a triangular area of increased echogenicity with a single cyst at the posterior base of the right lung. **B,** Transverse image with the spine up shows the mass is posterior and paraspinal. The heart is partially seen in the anterior chest. (Courtesy of Stephanie R. Wilson, M.D., University of Toronto) hydrops.[75,76,77,78,79] The trachea has been dilated in some cases.[77] Normal measurements of the trachea and pharynx are available, against which measurements of possibly dilated ones can be compared (Fig. 36-10).[80]

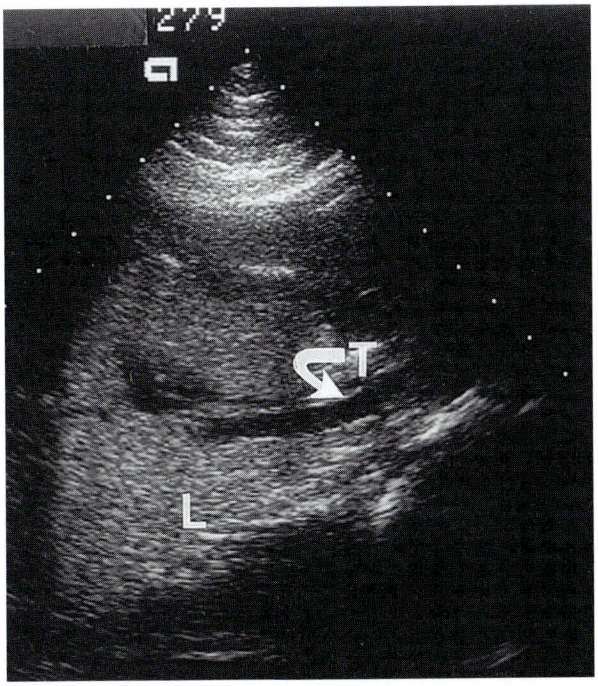

FIG. 36-9. Bilateral laryngeal atresia. Coronal sonogram with the fetal head to the right shows the lungs, *L*, are echogenic. The trachea, *T*, is dilated.

The Mediastinum

Thymus. The anterior mediastinum of the fetus lies between the heart and sternum. The thymus occupies most of the upper part of this space and can best be identified on transverse sections of the thorax at the level of the great vessels. It enlarges linearly with age. The majority of normal thymuses are hyperechoic before 27 weeks and hypoechoic after 27 weeks of gestational age. They can be identified as early as 14 weeks of gestational age. Thymic cysts[81] have been identified in the neonate, but they have not yet been reported in the fetus.

Cystic Hygroma. Because these have occasionally been reported in the newborn,[82,83] they probably will also eventually be reported *in utero*. These primarily cystic masses may contain solid elements that are usually lymphangiomas. They can extend into the neck (as can thymic cysts), but this extension is difficult to demonstrate *in utero*. They have been reported to be dumbbell-shaped, extending into both thoraces in a neonate.[82]

Teratomas. Teratomas are tumors that contain elements of more than one of the three germ cell layers. Teratomas may arise from the pericardial sac, in which case they are usually attached to the great vessels by a pedicle. They are predominantly solid, sometimes with some cystic areas, and can contain foci of calcification.[84] They can resemble other thoracic masses such as a cystic adenomatoid malformation or sequestration. The key to the diagnosis of a pericardial teratoma is that the mass and heart are

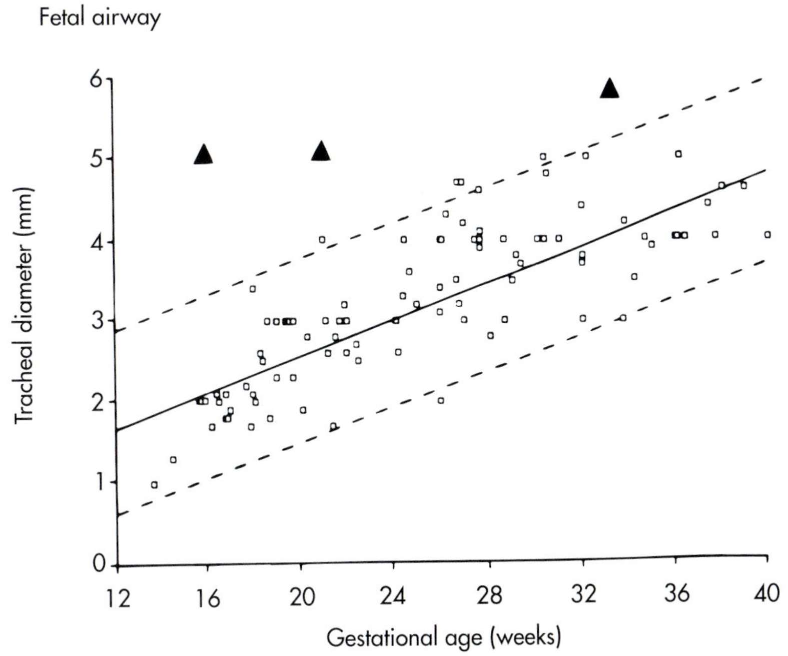

FIG. 36-10. Normal measurements of the trachea vs gestational age. (From Richards DS, Farah LA. Sonographic visualization of the fetal upper airway. *Ultrasound Obstet Gynecol* 1994;4:21-23.)

surrounded by pericardial fluid. At least three cases have been reported in the antenatal period,[84-86] all of which were associated with moderate or large pericardial effusions and appeared to be almost entirely solid. The **differential diagnosis** includes a **foramen of Morgagni hernia** or a **hemangioepithelioma**.[87]

Teratomas can arise in the neck and are thought, in these cases, to be related to the thyroid. A single report described a cystic and solid mass in the anterior superior mediastinum, which actually originated in the superior thyroid. It deviated the trachea, esophagus, and aortic arch on a long pedicle from the neck into the chest. Although there was nonimmune hydrops, there was no pericardial effusion.[88]

Posterior Mediastinum

The posterior mediastinum lies in the midline behind the heart and is covered on both sides by visceral pleura. Neural tissue and the esophagus are the main components of this part of the mediastinum. In the neonate **neurogenic tumors** are the most common cause of a posterior mediastinal mass; **neuroblastomas** appear in the paravertebral areas as echogenic masses with echolucent centers.[89]

Enteric cysts are the second most common posterior mediastinal mass in the neonate (Fig 36-11). Several enteric cysts have also been described in the fetus.[90-92] In one case a cyst occupied an entire hemithorax at 31 weeks of gestational age, and yet there was no mediastinal shift. The cystic fluid was removed but reaccumulated rapidly, and hydrops was evident by 33 weeks of gestational age. The fetus died in the newborn period; at autopsy the cyst measured 8.5 × 4.4 × 4.4 cm and was attached by a broad pedicle to the posterior mediastinum. It was lined with mucosa that resembled that of the small bowel. In another fetus a large tubular cyst exhibited septae and deviated the mediastinum. At surgery in the newborn period, there was evidence of peptic ulceration of this cyst, which can be life-threatening.[92]

Duplication cysts originating from the jejunum and traversing the diaphragm into the chest have been reported[93] and are often accompanied by vertebral anomalies.[92,93]

THE FETAL ABDOMEN

Ultrasonic evaluation of the fetal abdomen consists primarily of assessment of the fetal gastrointestinal tract. Because abnormalities of the gastrointestinal tract may not be clinically apparent in the newborn, prenatal diagnosis facilitates prompt treatment and prevents or minimizes subsequent complications.

Esophagus and Stomach

The **normal fetal stomach** (Fig. 36-12) is visualized as a fluid-filled structure in the left upper abdomen as early as 9 weeks[94] and reliably by 13 weeks of gestational age. The presence of echogenic linear rugae distinguishes it from other fluid-filled structures. Echogenic areas within the fetal stomach may represent blood from abruption or previous amniocentesis,[95,96] prominent rugae, or clumps of vernix.

A

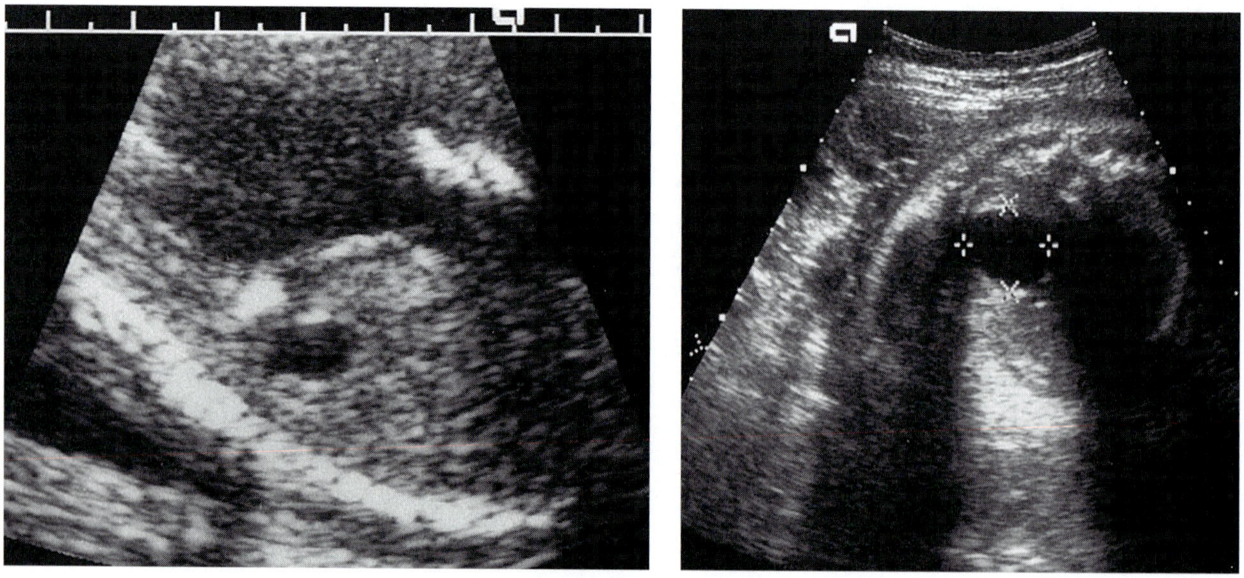

B

FIG. 36-11. Esophageal duplication cyst. **A,** A cystic mass is seen in apex of the chest in the middle mediastinum in this sagittal view with the fetal head on the left and the spine at the back. **B,** Transverse view. Spine at 12 o'clock.

The stomach cannot be assumed to be on the left. Fetal lie must be determined, followed by identification of the right and left sides of the fetus. When the fetal stomach is found in the right upper abdomen, there may be **total situs inversus** if there is a right-sided stomach and right-sided heart or **partial situs inversus** if there is a right-sided stomach and a left-sided heart. When the stomach and heart are on opposite sides, there is a higher incidence of **associated serious defects** than when the situs inversus is total. When the fetal stomach is found in the right upper abdomen, the possibilities include total situs inversus without associated malformations, **Kartagener's syndrome** (total situs inversus, bronchiectasis, and sinusitis),[97] **defects in laterality**, or **polysplenia syndrome** and **asplenia**. Consequently, when the fetal stomach is found on the right side, fetal echocardiography is indicated, as is an attempt to visualize the fetal spleen.

A

B

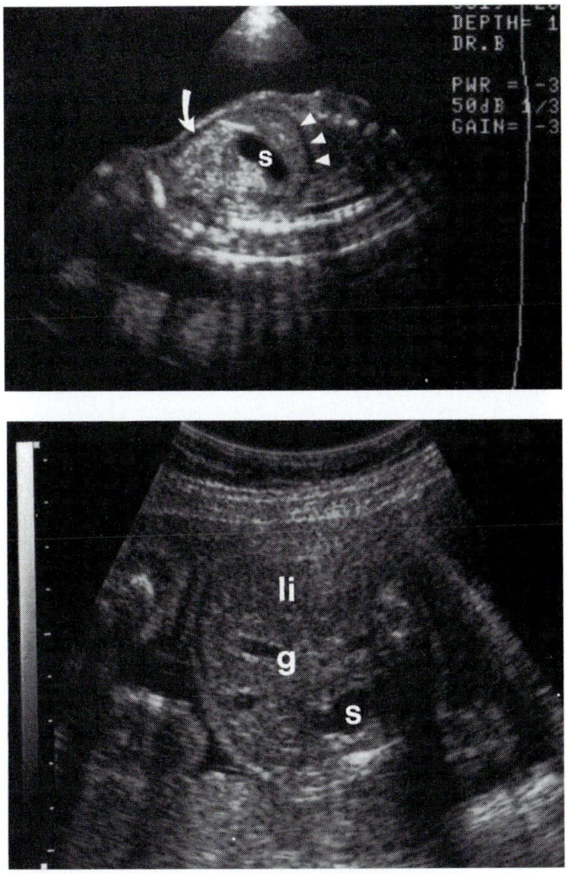

FIG. 36-12. Normal fetal abdomen. **A,** Sagittal view with head to right. Diaphragm (*arrowheads*) is echolucent, as is stomach, *s*. Small bowel is quite echogenic (*curved arrow*). Left lobe of liver lies between diaphragm and stomach. **B,** Transverse with spine at 3-o'clock position. Stomach lies on left, *s*; gallbladder, *g*, is usually midline or slightly to right and more anterior than stomach. Right lobe of liver, *li*, occupies large part of fetal abdomen and is homogeneous.

Stomach size has been measured at different gestations[94]; these measurements have been used to diagnose an enlarged stomach secondary to pyloric atresia.[98]

Esophageal Atresia. Visualization of the fetal stomach is an essential part of the second or third trimester ultrasound examination. If the stomach cannot be visualized over the course of several hours, a repeat scan is indicated. In a study series of 995 patients, 11 of the 20 patients in whom the fetal stomach was not visualized had an abnormal pregnancy outcome.[99]

Failure to visualize the stomach in the left upper quadrant may be due to:

- Normal stomach that has just emptied;
- Displacement of the stomach into the chest or into the umbilical cord;
- Nonproduction of amniotic fluid or failure to reach the amniotic cavity (renal agenesis, posterior ureteral valves);
- Esophageal atresia; or
- Microgastria.[100]

If the remainder of the fetus is normal, failure to visualize the fetal stomach over several hours strongly suggests esophageal atresia.

There are **five types of tracheoesophageal anomalies:**[101-103]

- Type A: esophageal atresia without tracheoesophageal fistula (Fig. 36-13);
- Type B: esophageal atresia with tracheoesophageal fistula to the proximal esophageal segment;
- Type C: Esophageal atresia with tracheoesophageal fistula to the distal esophageal segment;
- Type D: Esophageal atresia with tracheoesophageal fistula to both the proximal and distal esophageal segments; and
- Type E: Tracheoesophageal fistula without esophageal atresia.

Type C is the most common type in neonates, accounting for 87% of cases.[99] Many fetuses with esophageal atresia and a distal tracheoesophageal fistula (type C) have a normal-appearing stomach, since

FAILURE TO VISUALIZE THE STOMACH IN THE LEFT UPPER QUADRANT

Normal stomach that has just emptied
Displacement of the stomach into the chest or into the umbilical cord
Nonproduction of amniotic fluid or failure to reach the amniotic cavity (renal agenesis, posterior urethral valves)
Esophageal atresia
Microgastria[100]

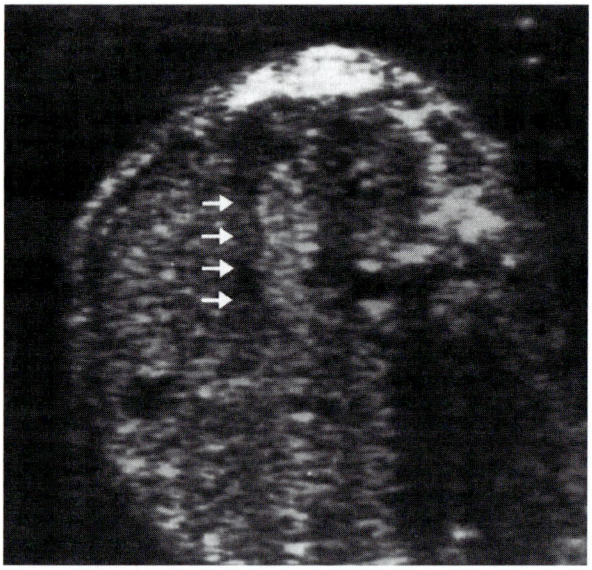

FIG. 36-13. Esophageal atresia without fistula. Transverse view of abdomen shows the walls of the empty stomach (*arrows*) as parallel dense white lines.

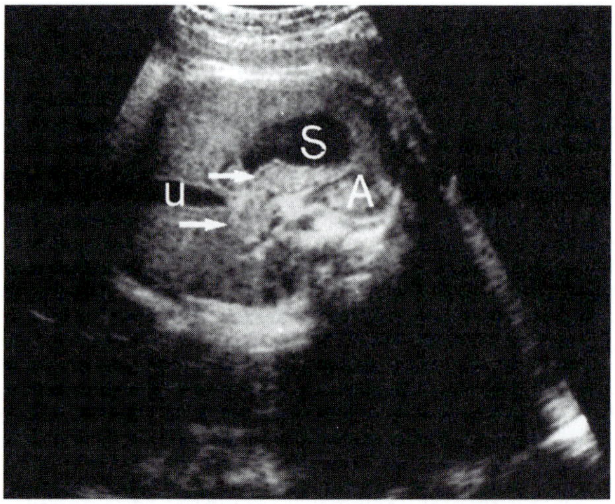

FIG. 36-14. Normal fetal pancreas (*arrows*) is between left adrenal gland, *A*, and stomach, *S*. *u* indicates umbilical vein.

some fluid may be passing through the fistula into the stomach. Often, however, there is polyhydramnios. In fact, marked polyhydramnios with a visualized stomach and no other obvious findings is suggestive of this diagnosis. Interestingly, sometimes no fluid passes across this fistula and the stomach is never filled.[101]

Nonvisualization of, or only slight filling (from gastric juices) of the fetal stomach is always the case in pure esophageal atresia (type A) (Fig. 36-13). The collapsed stomach can often be seen as two parallel, dense, white lines in the upper abdomen. It is worthwhile to look in the upper mediastinum in these cases for a dilated proximal esophageal pouch.

There is an increased incidence of **other anomalies** in fetuses with esophageal atresia, most with type C.[99,102,103] The most common organ systems involved are cardiovascular, musculoskeletal, and gastrointestinal.[102,103] When the diagnosis of esophageal atresia is suspected, a detailed ultrasound examination including fetal echocardiography is indicated.

Pancreas

The head of the fetal pancreas can be visualized between the left kidney and stomach and is slightly more echogenic than the liver (Fig. 36-14).[104] The pancreas has been visualized in 74% of cases between 14 and 20 weeks of gestational age.[105]

Gallbladder and Biliary Ducts

The fetal gallbladder appears as an elongated fluid-filled structure to the right and inferior to the umbilical vein. As might be expected, its width and length increase with gestational age. Visualization in normal fetuses peaks in the 20- to 32-week range.[106,107] Nonvisualization does not carry the import of nonvisualization of other organs such as the stomach and bladder. Hertzberg et al. were not able to visualize the gallbladder in 17.5%[107] of 576 fetuses. Five of the 86 in whom the exam was free of technical limiting factors had very minor abnormalities such as pyelectasis or mild hypospadias.[107]

Fetal **gallstones** have been reported as echogenic foci with acoustic shadowing.[108-111] Sludge, the precursor of gallstones, appears to be a more frequent finding; it is echogenic but does not show acoustic shadowing.[110] In almost all reported cases there has been spontaneous resolution of sludge and gallstones in the neonatal period by the age of 6 weeks.

In **biliary atresia** the gallbladder is often tiny or absent.[112] However, if there is extrahepatic biliary obstruction of the distal portion of the common bile duct, the gallbladder may be enlarged.[113]

Choledochal cysts, or congenital cysts of the biliary system, can be of one of four types, the most common of which is cystic dilation of the common bile duct.[114] It is imaged as a cystic structure inferior to the umbilical vein and anterior to the right kidney (Fig. 36-15). The location just inferior to the liver and the presence of dilated ducts distinguish choledochal cysts from the dilated proximal duodenum seen in duodenal atresia.

Choledochal cysts may first be visualized in the late second and third trimesters,[115-119] despite a previously normal scan.[116,118] The earliest reported cysts were de-

A

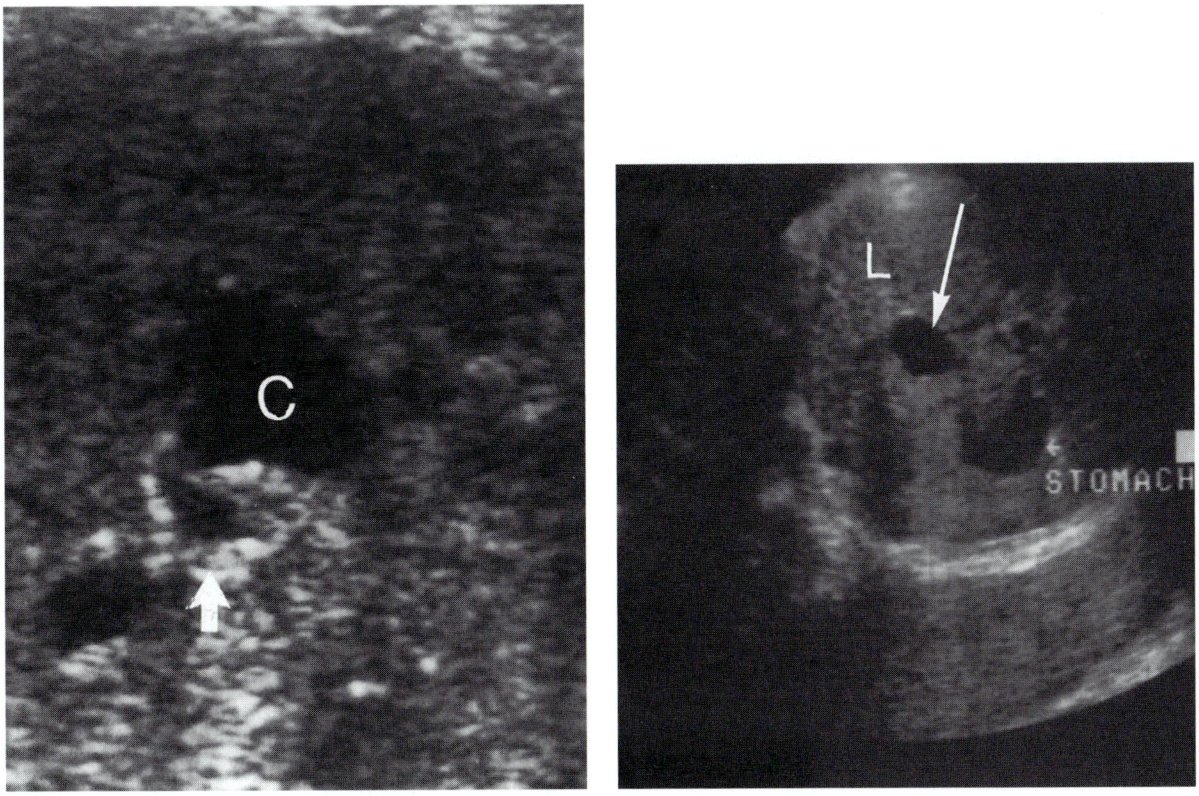

B

FIG. 36-15. Choledochal cyst *(C)*. **A,** Transverse scan shows gallbladder (*arrow*) adjacent to cyst. **B,** Choledochal cyst (*arrow*) is cystic mass separate from stomach. *L* indicates liver.

tected at 25 weeks of gestational age.[117] Because these cysts may initially be asymptomatic, prenatal diagnosis facilitates early treatment and may prevent the potential complications of recurrent cholangitis, biliary obstruction and cirrhosis, biliary calculi, and carcinoma.

Liver

Unlike that of an adult, the left lobe of the fetal liver is larger than the right lobe.[120] Normal liver-length measurements have been determined for fetuses after 20 weeks of gestational age.[121] **Hepatomegaly** has been seen in fetuses with severe hemolytic disease in isoimmunized pregnancies, in congenital infection, and in Beckwith-Wiedemann and Zellweger syndromes. The fetal liver is normally quite homogeneous in appearance; diffuse echogenic foci suggest possible **hepatitis.**

A **mesenchymal hamartoma, hemangioendothelioma,** and **hemangioma** have each appeared as a hypoechoic mass in the fetal liver.[122-124] Hemangioendotheliomas and hepatoblastomas may be accompanied by hydrops.[125,126] One author reported a fetal liver adenoma present in the third trimester as a solid mass with irregular borders within the liver.[127] A solitary nonparasitic hepatic cyst has also been reported prenatally.[128] It may be impossible to make an accurate diagnosis of a liver mass from appearance alone, although vascularity can be characterized by color Doppler imaging.

Liver calcifications (Fig. 36-16) may be seen not only in hepatic tumors but also in cases of intrauterine infection or vascular insult.[129] More commonly, however, they are of unexplained origin in fetuses who appear normal at birth.[130]

Spleen

The spleen is visualized as an echogenic organ in the left upper abdomen lateral to the spine and either inferior or posterior to the fluid-filled stomach, depending on fetal position (Fig. 36-17). Normal measurements have been determined for 18 to 40 weeks of gestational age.[131] Fetal splenomegaly has also been recognized in a case of cytomegalovirus infection.[132]

A simple splenic cyst has been diagnosed prenatally,[133,134] as have multiple splenic cysts in congenital lymphangiomatosis.[135] An absent spleen has been reported in two cases of asplenia and polysplenia syndrome.[136] Currently, the multiple accessory spleens in polysplenia have not been identified *in utero*; the additional spleens are often very small.

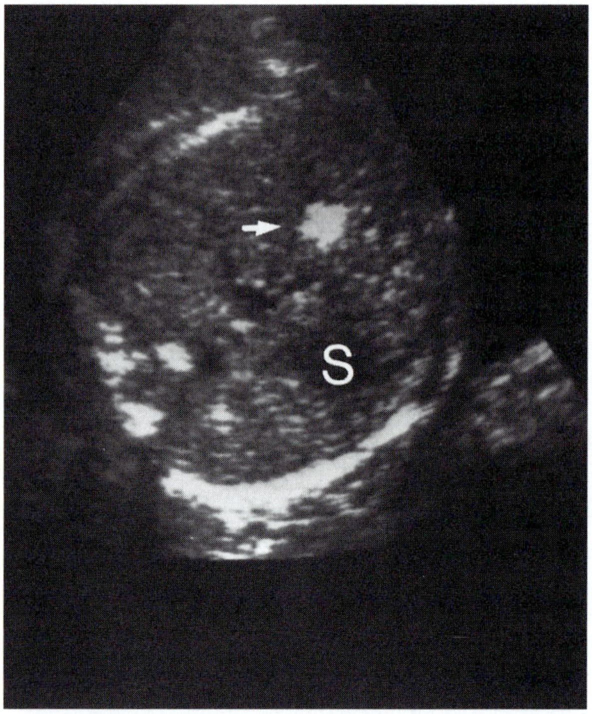

FIG. 36-16. Liver calcifications *(arrow)* of unknown cause. *S* indicates stomach.

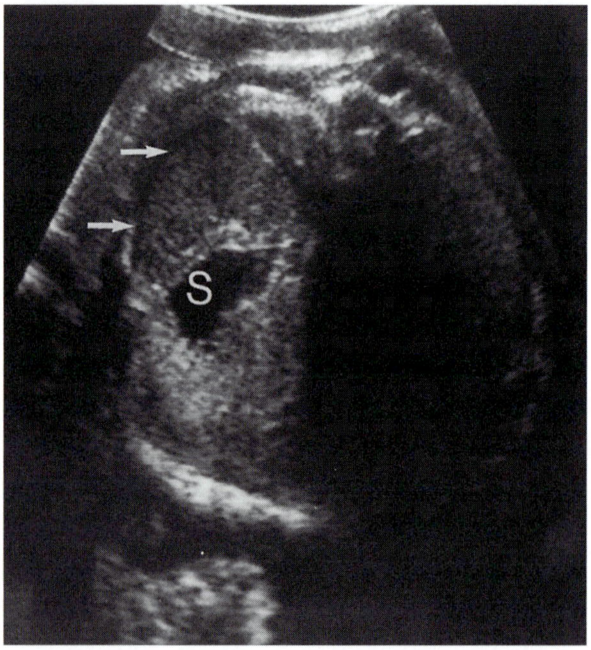

FIG. 36-17. Normal fetal spleen *(arrows)*. *S* indicates stomach.

The Fetal Adrenal Glands

The fetal adrenal glands can be reliably visualized after 20 or 30 weeks of gestational age.[137,138] They lie superior and medial to the corresponding kidney, with the medial border adjacent to the aorta or inferior vena cava. In the longitudinal plane they are oval-shaped (Fig. 36-18, *A*), and in the transverse plane, they have been compared with radially oriented rice grains (Fig. 36-18, *B*). They have a hypoechoic periphery and echogenic center. The internal band can be quite bright in two-thirds of fetuses and seems to become more so in the last 5 weeks of pregnancy.[137,138] Length increases with age, maintaining a constant relation to kidney length of 0.48 to 0.66 to 1. The anteroposterior diameter is equal to that of the kidney from 30 to 39 weeks of gestational age.[138]

The adrenal glands enlarge to fill the renal fossa in some cases of bilateral renal agenesis. Because the adrenal glands may so closely resemble the kidneys, particularly when the image is degraded by lack of fluid, other signs such as oligohydramnios and nonvisualization of the bladder may need to be used in making a diagnosis of nonfunctioning or absent kidneys.

The adrenal glands should be evaluated if ambiguous genitalia are present because all types of adrenal hyperplasia cause this finding. Adrenal hypoplasia occurs in many cases of anencephaly.

Neuroblastoma, the most common neonatal tumor, is a malignant tumor of the adrenal glands. It is usually unilateral and hyperechogenic or of mixed appearance and may be diagnosed in the antenatal period.[139-142] It often metastasizes to the placenta, liver, or subcutaneous tissues, causing hydrops.[143] Neuroblastoma needs to be distinguished from recent hemorrhage that can also be echogenic in its early stage.

Small Bowel and Colon

Normal Appearance. Physiologic midgut herniation into the umbilical cord can be seen with transvaginal scanning as early as 8 weeks of gestation, with the gut normally returning to the abdomen by 11 weeks. In fetuses from 10 to 14 weeks (intravaginal probe), the intra-abdominal small bowel can have an echogenic appearance in some (but not all) fetuses. The fluid-filled lumen cannot be seen until 13 weeks but is much easier to see after 20 weeks.[144] In the older fetus, the small bowel appears as a central amorphous echogenic area in the abdomen (Fig. 36-19). Discrete small-bowel segments are difficult to visualize and are seen in only 30% of fetuses after 34 weeks of gestation.[145] Occasionally, discrete, very dense segments of small bowel are identified, particularly close to full term. These may be found in normal fetuses but have also been identified occasionally in Down syndrome and cystic fibrosis. Currently, there is no consensus about how the parent should be counseled in these instances.

The colon can be seen in 44% of 18- to 20-week fetuses, 89% of 20- to 25-week fetuses, and 100% after 25 weeks. As gestation progresses, larger segments of

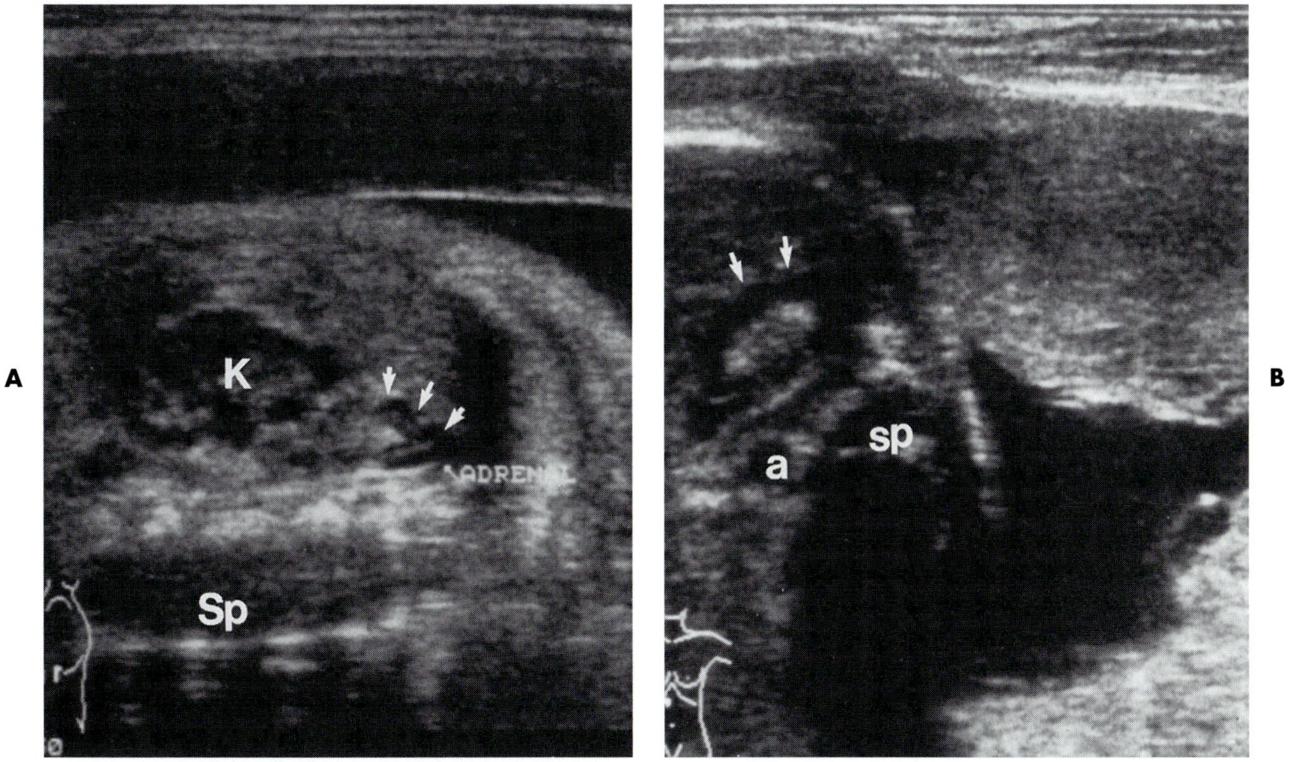

FIG. 36-18. Adrenal gland. **A,** In this view adrenal gland (*arrows*) lies superior to kidney, *K*. Note peripheral echolucency and central echogenicity. **B,** In transverse view one edge of adrenal gland (*arrows*) can be found anterior to aorta or inferior vena cava. Note central echogenic area. *SP* indicates spine; *a* indicates aorta.

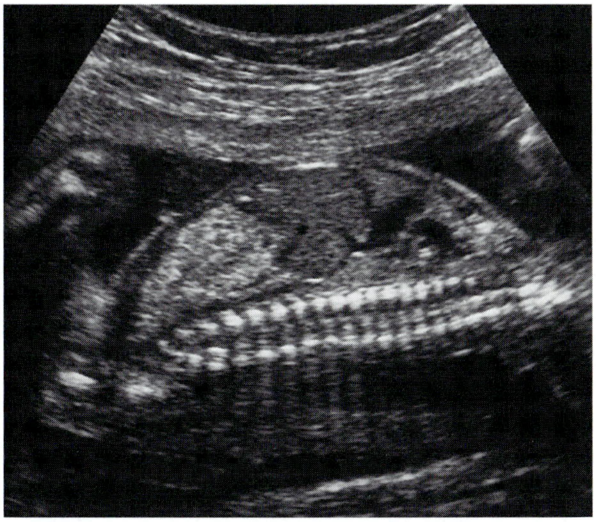

FIG. 36-19. Normal fetal gut echogenicity at 18 weeks gestation. A sagittal midline sonogram shows the contour of the fetal body with the head to the right. The gut is seen as an amorphous area of increased echogenicity relative to both the liver and the lung. The echogenicity is not as bright as that of the spine. (Courtesy of Stephanie R. Wilson, M.D., University of Toronto)

colon and haustra can be identified in most fetuses after 30 weeks.[146] Peristalsis is often seen in the small bowel but not in the colon. The appearance of the fetal bowel throughout gestation can be used to help determine gestational age based on echolucency, peristalsis, and presence of haustra.[147,148,149] Toward full term, the colon becomes larger (up to 28 mm in diameter) and the meconium within it gradually develops a density approaching that of the liver. Detection rate, lumen diameters, and average length of visible segments at varying gestational ages are summarized in Table 36-2.[144]

Duodenal Atresia. The classic "double-bubble" radiographic appearance of duodenal atresia in the neonate is produced by a large, obstructed stomach and a distended proximal duodenal segment. On prenatal ultrasound examination, two echolucent structures, corresponding to the **double-bubble,** can be seen as side-to-side sonolucent areas (Fig. 36-20, *A*). The stomach bubble is distinguished by its rugae. It is important to demonstrate contiguity of the dilated duodenal segment with the stomach (Fig. 36-20, *B*) to exclude other cystic structures, such as choledochal cysts. Care must be taken to avoid the diagnosis of duodenal atresia in a stomach with a prominent incisura angularis.[150] If the stomach is imaged in its longitudinal axis, as well as in

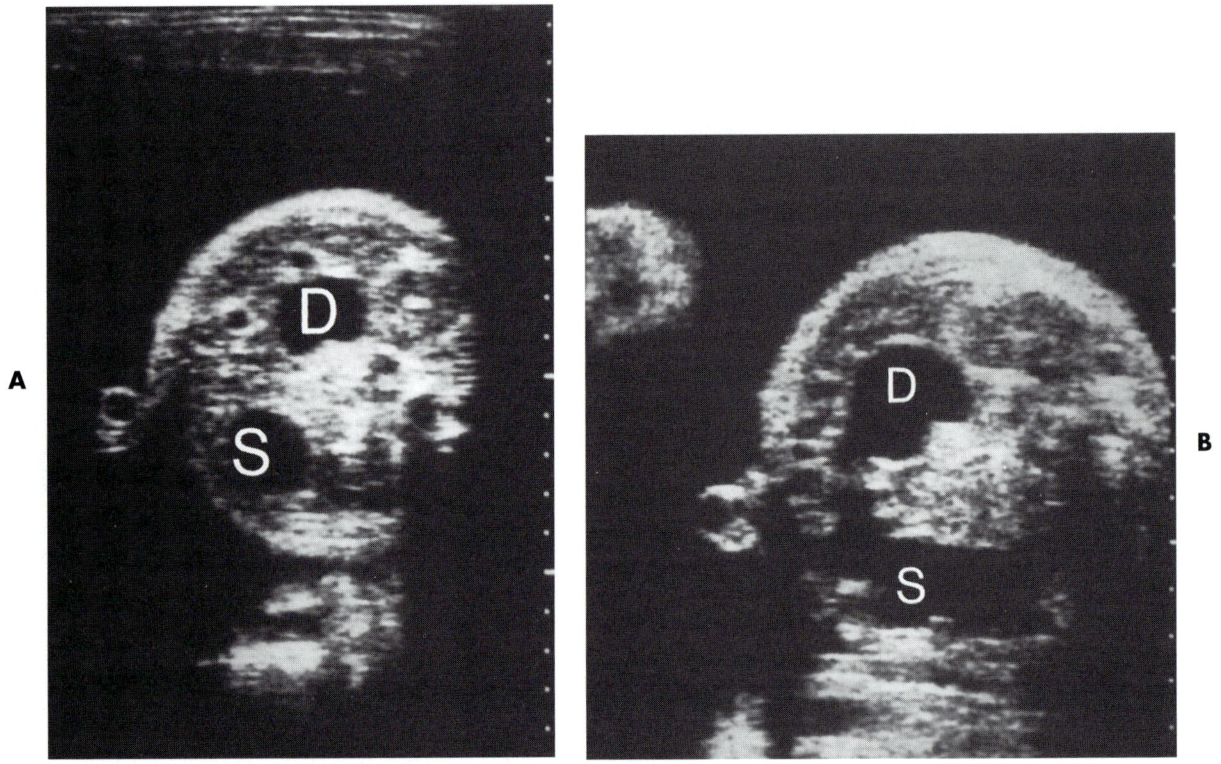

FIG. 36-20. Duodenal atresia. **A**, Transverse view of double-bubble. **B**, Oblique view shows stomach is continuous with duodenum. *S* indicates stomach; *D*, duodenum.

TABLE 36-2
FETAL BOWEL, LUMEN DIAMETER, AND LENGTH OF CONTIGUOUS BOWEL SEGMENT

Gestational Age (weeks)	Small Bowel Lumen Size (mm)		Colon Lumen Size (mm)		Average Length (mm)	
	Average	Largest	Average	Largest	Small Bowel	Colon
>40	4.4	6	18.7	28	11.3	63.0
35-40	3.7	8	16.8	26	11.0	70.0
30-35	2.9	6	11.4	16	9.8	55.0
25-30	1.8	3	8.0	13	7.9	37.0
20-25	1.4	2	4.4	6	4.5	19.0
15-20	1.2	2	3.6	5	4.5	9.8
10-15	1.0	1	1.5	2	2.4	10.0

Adapted from Parulekar SG: Sonography of normal fetal bowel. *J Ultrasound Med* 1991;10:211-220.

the transverse, this error will be avoided. Although the prenatal ultrasound diagnosis of duodenal atresia has been made as early as 22 weeks of gestational age, it is usually not apparent until 29 to 32 weeks.[151-153]

In contrast to more distal atresias, duodenal atresia is associated with a 30% incidence of **trisomy 21** and a high incidence of other anomalies.[154,155] **Esophageal atresia** has been found in about 10% of cases of duodenal obstruction.[156] An **annular pancreas** is often found coincidentally and is not considered to be a true cause of obstruction. **Cardiac anomalies** occur in about 20% of cases.[154,155] In addition, there is an association between duodenal atresia and the **VACTERL complex** (Vertebral defects, Anal atresia, Cardiac defects, Tracheoesophageal fistula with Esophageal atresia, and Renal and Limb defects [radial dysplasia]).[157,158] Consequently, when duodenal atresia is diagnosed prenatally, a detailed scan including fetal echocardiography is indicated. In addition, fetal karyotype determination should be offered.

Atresia of the Small Bowel. The most usual sites are the proximal jejunum (31%), distal jejunum (20%), proximal ileum (13%), and distal ileum (36%). The ultrasound findings are primarily those of dilated small bowel segments that are undistinguishable from those resulting from meconium ileus. It can also be difficult to distinguish dilated small bowel loops from a dilated colon or even redundant megaureters. Vascular impairment is probably the cause. Other system anomalies are rare, but anomalies of the remainder of the bowel are frequent (volvulus, malrotation, and duplications). Polyhydramnios is seen in half of fetuses with obstruction at or above the level of the proximal jejunum and rarely with more distal obstruction.[159]

Meconium Ileus. Meconium ileus refers to the obstruction and subsequent dilation of the ileum that occurs from impaction of the abnormally sticky and thick meconium of fetuses with cystic fibrosis. The ileum dilates above the obstruction, and volvulus or perforation may result. The distal colon is unused and small. Although usually apparent only in the third trimester, meconium ileus has been reported as early as 22 weeks of gestational age. The sonographic picture cannot be distinguished from that caused by atresia of the jejunum or ileum.

Occasionally, inspissated meconium may obstruct the colon rather than the ileum, causing the **mucous plug syndrome,** or transient colonic obstruction. Far fewer of these fetuses will prove to have cystic fibrosis than will those with meconium ileus.

Meconium Peritonitis. Volvulus, jejunal or ileal atresia, or meconium ileus can cause perforation of the small intestine. The meconium that exits into the abdominal cavity produces a sterile chemical peritonitis.

There is usually immediate ascites. The intense inflammation from meconium peritonitis may incite calcification along the surface of the bowel or peritoneum; it can be linear and difficult to see. Calcification is thought to occur less frequently in fetuses with cystic fibrosis, perhaps because of lack of pancreatic enzymes. In time, the inflammatory response may seal over the perforation or, alternatively, may form a **pseudocyst** of walled-off meconium. The pseudocyst has thin, often calcified walls (Fig. 36-21). The prognosis of meconium peritonitis depends on the underlying etiologic factors. The majority of fetuses with meconium peritonitis do not have cystic fibrosis.[160]

Hirschsprung's Disease. Hirschsprung's disease, or congenital aganglionosis of a segment of the colon, is a cause of functional bowel obstruction (Fig. 36-22). Three cases have been reported in which prenatal ultrasound examinations were performed. In one confirmed case with a family history of the disease, serial ultrasound examination findings were negative.[161] In the other two cases, polyhydramnios and multiple dilated loops of fetal bowel were noted.[162,163] Intraluminal

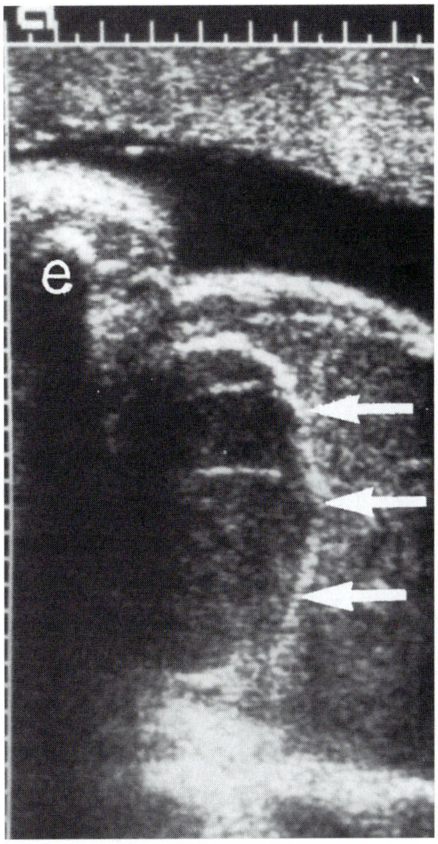

FIG. 36-21. Meconium pseudocyst (*arrows*). *e* indicates lower extremity.

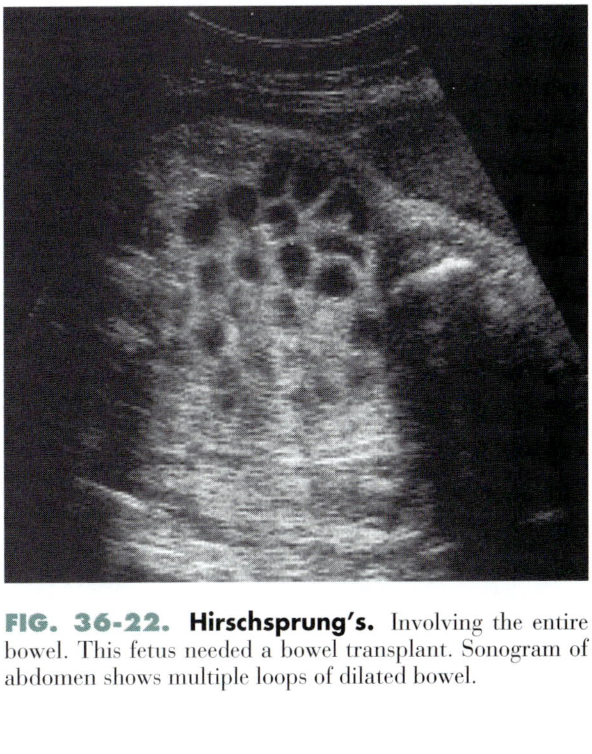

FIG. 36-22. Hirschsprung's. Involving the entire bowel. This fetus needed a bowel transplant. Sonogram of abdomen shows multiple loops of dilated bowel.

calcifications have been seen in the newborn[164] and presumably might be seen in third trimester fetuses.

Echogenic Bowel. Occasionally, the fetal bowel appears more echogenic than normal so that individual segments are prominent (Fig. 36-23). The contents of the bowel, rather than the walls, create this appearance. There has been considerable discussion regarding the significance of this finding. To summarize: to be considered echogenic, the bowel needs to be as echogenic or more echogenic than the iliac crest.[165-168] In large studies with controls, fetuses with echogenic bowel had an increased incidence of **cystic fibrosis, perinatal death, cytomegalovirus** (CMV), **subsequent growth retardation,** and **trisomy 21** (Fig. 36-23). Meconium in the colon of a normal fetus may appear echogenic close to term (Fig. 36-24).[165-167,168a] Bloody amniotic fluid at the time of amniocentesis has also been found to be associated with a 15.6% incidence of hyperechogenic bowel 2 to 4 weeks later.[169] Risk of an abnormal outcome is elevated with increased echogenicity.[166,170] Echogenicity may be a later finding in fetuses with trisomy 21 who had had earlier normal scans[171] (see box below).

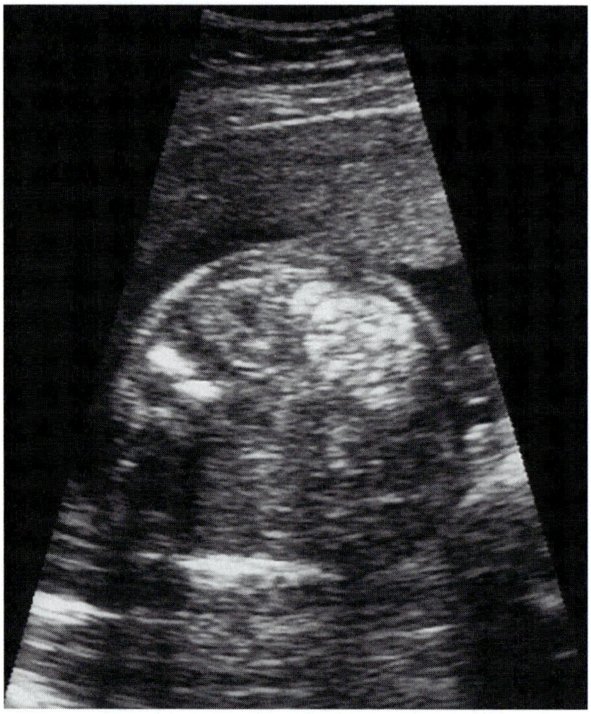

FIG. 36-23. Echogenic bowel. Echogenic gut, 18-week fetus with abdominal MSS and Down syndrome. Transverse sonogram through fetal abdomen shows that the gut is as white as the fetal spine, on the left of the image. (Courtesy of Stephanie R. Wilson, M.D., University of Toronto)

FETUSES WITH ECHOGENIC BOWEL ARE AT RISK FOR:

Cystic fibrosis
Trisomy 21
Cytomegalovirus (CMV)
Parvovirus
Intra-amniotic blood
Gastrointestinal obstruction
Severe IUGR
Unexplained intrauterine demise

A

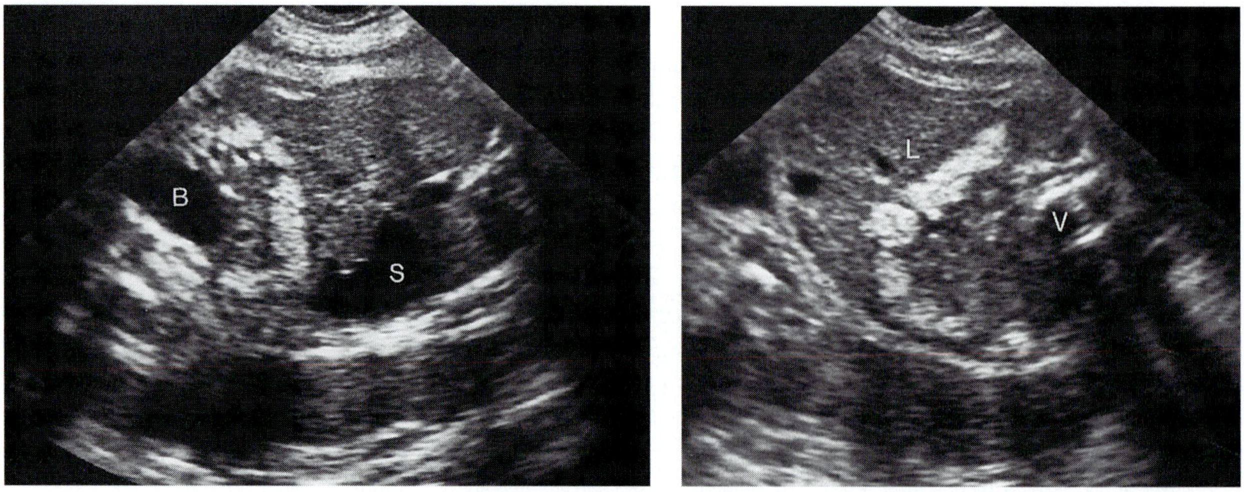

B

FIG. 36-24. Normal fetus with echogenic colon. **A,** Coronal and **B,** oblique sonograms of a 30.9 week fetus show highly echogenic meconium filling the colon. *B,* bladder; *S,* stomach; *L,* liver; *V,* vertebra. (From Fung A, Wilson SW, Toi A, et al. Echogenic colonic meconium in the third trimester: a normal sonographic finding. *J Ultrasound Med* 1992;11:676-678.)

Anorectal Atresia. The normal fetal rectum is visualized directly posterior to the fetal bladder (Fig. 36-25). In about half of patients with anorectal atresia, the distal colon may be dilated. Many cases have other anomalies, particularly of the VACTERL complex.[172,173] Round calcifications representing **intraluminal calcified meconium** can sometimes be visualized (Fig. 36-26).[159] However, these calcifications are not diagnostic of an imperforate anus; they can also be found in **cloacal dysgenesis and total colonic aganglionosis.**[174] The differential diagnosis of a dilated colon includes all causes of bowel obstruction, including the small bowel, because the latter can simulate colon when dilated. Colonic obstruction is less often associated with polyhydramnios than is obstruction of the small bowel.

A 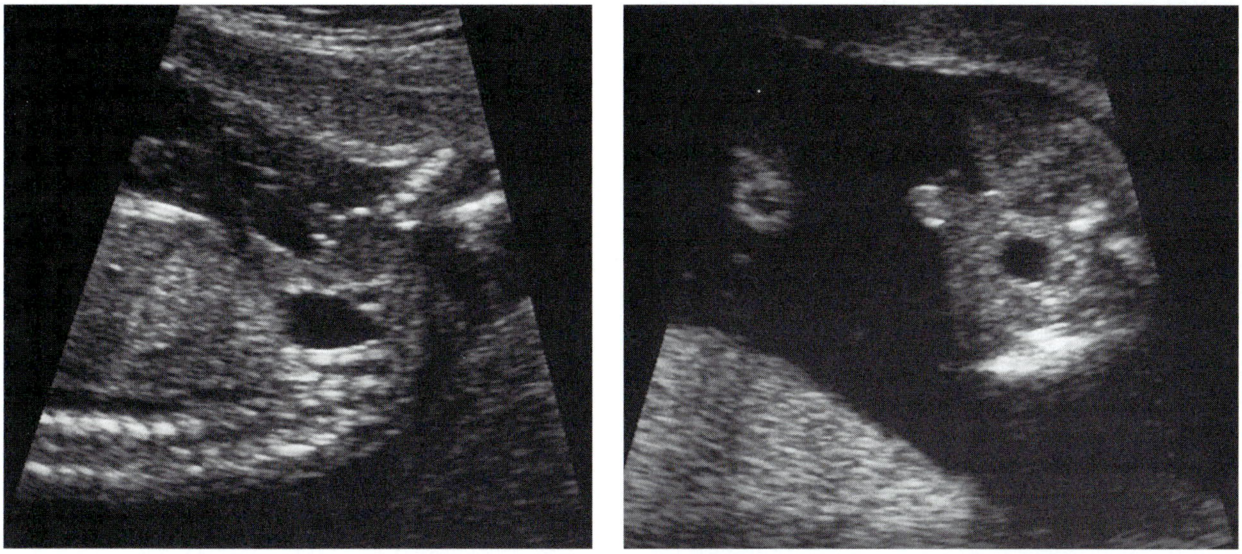 B

FIG. 36-25. Fetal rectum at 18 weeks gestation. **A,** Sagittal midline scan and **B,** transverse pelvic scan show the rectum as a small hypoechoic tubular structure posterior to the bladder. (Courtesy of Stephanie R. Wilson, M.D., University of Toronto.)

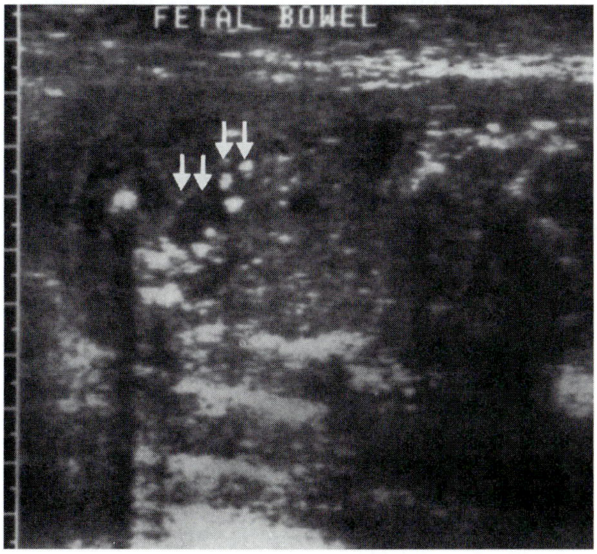

FIG. 36-26. Inspissated meconium *(arrows)* in rectum of fetus with anal atresia.

A

B

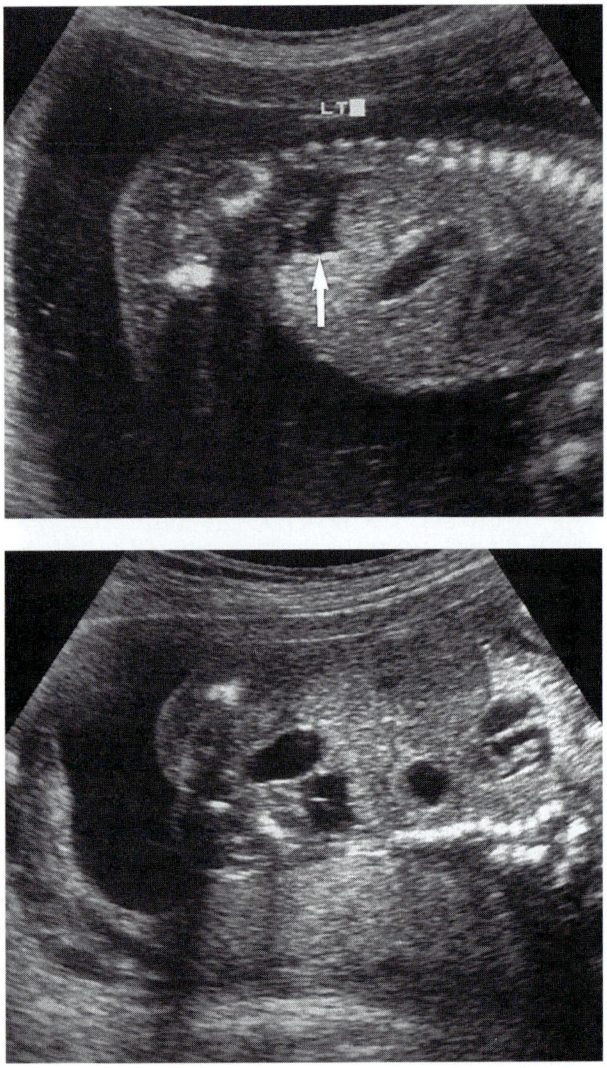

FIG. 36-27. Retroperitoneal lymphangioma at 18 weeks gestation. **A,** Sagittal sonogram of the fetal body shows the spine is up. In the left retroperitoneum there is a fluid of cystic collection (*arrows*) at the inferior aspect of the kidney. The stomach and heart are also seen cephalad to the mass. **B,** Coronal sonogram shows the mass lies beside the bladder. (Courtesy of Stephanie R. Wilson, M.D., University of Toronto.)

The anus can be visualized in the transverse plane as a hypoechoic circle around a central linear echo. The absence of this structure has been used to suggest imperforate anus,[175] but the sensitivity and specificity of this finding have not been described.

Miscellaneous Masses

A variety of rare masses may be seen in the fetal abdomen, including tumors of mesenchymal origin, mesenteric cysts, and lymphangiomas (Fig. 36-27).

REFERENCES

The Fetal Chest

1. Jouppila P, Kirkinen P, Herva R et al. Prenatal diagnosis of pleural effusions by ultrasound. *J Clin Ultrasound* 1983;11: 516-519.
2. Murayama K, Jimbo T, Matsumoto Y et al. Fetal pulmonary hypoplasia with hydrothorax. *Am J Obstet Gynecol* 1987; 157:119-120.
3. Lange IR, Manning FA. Antenatal diagnosis of congenital pleural effusions. *Am J Obstet Gynecol* 1981;140:839-840.
4. Pijpers L, Reuss A, Stewart PA et al. Noninvasive management of isolated bilateral fetal hydrothorax. *Am J Obstet Gynecol* 1989;161:330-332.
5. Yaghoobian J, Comrie M. Transitory bilateral isolated fetal pleural effusions. *J Ultrasound Med* 1988;7:231-232.
6. Petres RE, Redwine FO, Cruikshank DP. Congenital bilateral chylothorax: antepartum diagnosis and successful intrauterine management. *JAMA* 1982;248:1360-1361.
7. Radix CH, Fisk NM, Fraser DI et al. Long-term *in utero* drainage of fetal hydrothorax. *N Engl J Med* 1988;319:1135-1138.
8. Schmidt W, Harms E, Wold D. Successful prenatal treatment of non-immune hydrops fetalis due to congenital chylothorax: case report. *Br J Obstet Gynaecol* 1985;92:685-687.
9. Seeds JW, Bowes WA. Results of treatment of severe hydrothorax with bilateral pleuramniotic catheters. *Obstet Gynecol* 1986;68:577-579.
10. Hagay Z, Reece EA, Roberts A et al. Isolated pleural effusion: a prenatal management dilemma. *Obstet Gynecol* 1993; 81:147-152.
11. Weber AM, Philipson EH. Fetal pleural effusion: a review and meta-analysis for prognostic indicators. *Obstet Gynecol* 1992;79:281-286.
12. Butler N, Claireaux AE. Congenital diaphragmatic hernia as a cause of perinatal mortality. *Lancet* 1962;1:659-663.
13. Chinn DH, Filly RA, Callen PW et al. Congenital diaphragmatic hernia diagnosed prenatally by ultrasound. *Radiology* 1983;148:199-203.
14. Marshall A, Sumner E. Improved prognosis in congenital diaphragmatic hernia: experience of 62 cases over 2-year period. *J Roy Soc Med* 1982;75:607-612.
15. Adzick NS, Harrison MR, Glick PL et al. Diaphragmatic hernia in the fetus: prenatal diagnosis and outcome in 94 cases. *J Pediatr Surg* 1985;20:357-361.
16. Comstock CH. The antenatal diagnosis of diaphragmatic anomalies. *J Ultrasound Med* 1986;5:391-396.
17. David TJ, Illingworth CA. Diaphragmatic hernia in the southwest of England. *J Med Genet* 1976;13:253-262.
18. Benacerraf BR, Greene MF. Congenital diaphragmatic hernia: ultrasound diagnosis prior to 22 weeks gestation. *Radiology* 1986;158:809-810.
19. Stiller RJ, Roberts NS, Weiner S et al. Congenital diaphragmatic hernia: antenatal diagnosis and obstetrical management. *J Clin Ultrasound* 1985;13:212-215.
20. Benacerraf BR, Adzick NS. Fetal diaphragmatic hernia: ultrasound diagnosis and clinical outcome in 19 cases. *Am J Obstet Gynecol* 1987;156:573-576.
21. Whittle MJ, Gilmore DH, McNay MB et al. Diaphragmatic hernia presenting *in utero* as a unilateral hydrothorax. *Prenat Diagn* 1989;9:115-118.
22. Nakayama DK, Harrison MR, Chinn DH. Prenatal diagnosis and natural history of the fetus with a congenital diaphragmatic hernia: initial clinical experience. *J Pediatr Surg* 1985;20:118-124.
23. Crawford DC, Drake DP, Kwaitkowski D et al. Prenatal diagnosis of reversible cardiac hypoplasia associated with congen-

ital diaphragmatic hernia: implications for postnatal management. *J Clin Ultrasound* 1986;14:718-721.
24. Siebert JR, Hass JE, Beckwith JB. Left ventricular hypoplasia in congenital diaphragmatic hernia. *J Pediatr Surg* 1984; 19:567-571.
25. Sharland GK, Lockhart SM, Heward AJ et al. Prognosis in fetal diaphragmatic hernia. *Am J Obstet Gynecol* 1992;166: 9-13.
26. Puri P, Gorman F. Lethal nonpulmonary anomalies associated with congenital diaphragmatic hernia: implications for early intrauterine surgery. *J Pediatr Surg* 1984;19:29-32.
27. Wenstrom KD, Weiner CP, Manson JW. A five-year statewide experience with congenital diaphragmatic hernia. *Am J Obstet Gynecol* 1991;165:838-842.
28. Shochat SJ, Naeye RL, Ford WDA et al. Congenital diaphragmatic hernia. *Ann Surg* 1979;190:332-341.
29. Bootstaylor FS, Filly RA, Harrison MR et al. Prenatal sonographic predictors of liver herniation in congenital diaphragmatic hernias. *J Ultrasound Med* 1995;14:515-520.
30. Merten DF, Bowie JD, Kirks DR et al. Anteromedial diaphragmatic defects in infancy: current approaches to diagnostic imaging. *Radiology* 1982;142:361-365.
31. Wesselhoeft CW, DeLuca FG. Neonatal septum transversum diaphragmatic defects. *Am J Surg* 1984;147:481-485.
32. Baran EM, Houston HE, Lynn HB et al. Foramen of Morgagni hernias in children. *Surgery* 1967;62:1076-1081.
33. Jurcak-Zaleski S, Comstock CH, Kirk JS. Eventration of the diaphragm: prenatal diagnosis. *J Ultrasound Med* 1990; 9:351-354.
34. Wayne ER, Campbell JB, Burrington JD et al. Eventration of the diaphragm. *J Pediatr Surg* 1974;9:643-650.
35. Wexler HA, Poole CA. Neonatal diaphragmatic dysfunction. *AJR* 1976;127:617-622.
36. Briggs VA, Reilly BJ, Loewig K. Lung hypoplasia and membranous diaphragm in the congenital rubella syndrome: a rare case. *J Can Assoc Radiol* 1973;24:126-127.
37. Weller MH. Bilateral eventration of the diaphragm. *West J Med* 1976;124:415-419.
38. Yancey MF, Richards DS. Antenatal sonographic findings associated with unilateral pulmonary agenesis. *Obstet Gynecol* 1993;81:847-849.
39. Comstock CH. Normal fetal heart axis and position. *Obstet Gynecol* 1987;70:255-259.
40. DeVore GR, Horenstein J, Platt LD. Fetal echocardiography, VI; assessment of cardiothorax disproportion: a new technique for the diagnosis of thoracic dysplasia. *Am J Obstet Gynecol* 1986;155:1066-1071.
41. Johnson A, Callan NA, Bhutani VK et al. Ultrasonic ratio of fetal thoracic to abdominal circumference: an association with fetal pulmonary hypoplasia. *Am J Obstet Gynecol* 1987;157:764-769.
42. Nimrod C, Nicholson S, Davies D et al. Pulmonary hypoplasia testing in clinical obstetrics. *Am J Obstet Gynecol* 1988; 158:277-280.
43. Vintzileos AM, Campbell WA, Rodis JR et al. Comparison of six different ultrasonographic methods for predicting lethal fetal pulmonary hypoplasia. *Am J Obstet Gynecol* 1989; 161:606-612.
44. Fong K, Ohlsson A, Zalev A. Fetal thoracic circumference: a prospective cross-sectional study with real-time ultrasound. *Am J Obstet Gynecol* 1988;158:277-280.
45. Songster GS, Gray DL, Crane JP. Prenatal prediction of lethal pulmonary hypoplasia using ultrasound fetal chest circumference. *Obstet Gynecol* 1989;73:261-266.
46. Lauria MR, Gonik B, Romero R. Pulmonary hypoplasia: pathogenesis, diagnosis, and antenatal detection. *Obstet Gynecol* 1995;86:466-475.
47. McNamara MF, McCurdy CM, Reed KL et al. The relation between pulmonary hypoplasia and amniotic fluid volume: lessons learned from discordant urinary tract anomalies in monoamniotic twins. *Obstet Gynecol* 1995;85:867-869.
48. Stocker JT, Madewell JE, Drake RM. Congenital cystic adenomatoid malformation of the lung classification and morphologic spectrum. *Hum Pathol* 1977;8:155-171.
49. Adzick NS, Harrison MR, Glick PL et al. Fetal cystic adenomatoid malformation: prenatal diagnosis and natural history. *J Pediatr Surg* 1985;20:483-488.
50. Nyberg DA, Mahony BS, Pretorius DH. Diagnostic ultrasound of fetal anomalies: text and atlas. Chicago: Year Book; 1990.
51. Roelofsen J, Oostendorp R, Volovics A et al. Prenatal diagnosis and fetal outcome of cystic adenomatoid malformation of the lung: case report and historical survey. *Ultrasound in Obstet & Gynecol* 1994;4:78-82.
52. Fine C, Adzick NS, Doubilet PM. Decreasing size of a congenital cystic adenomatoid malformation *in utero*. *J Ultrasound Med* 1988;7:405-408.
53. Saltzman DH, Adzick NS, Benacerraf BR. Fetal cystic adenomatoid malformation of the lung: apparent improvement *in utero*. *Obstet Gynecol* 1988;71:1000-1002.
54. Adzick NS, Harrison MR, Flake AW et al. Fetal surgery for cystic adenomatoid malformation of the lung. *J Ped Surg* 1993;28:806-812.
55. Mayden KL, Tortora M, Chervenak FA et al. The antenatal sonographic detection of lung masses. *Am J Obstet Gynecol* 1984;148:349-351.
56. McAlister WH, Wright JR, Crane JP. Main-stem bronchial atresia: intrauterine sonographic diagnosis. *AJR* 1987; 148:364-366.
57. Sweeney WJ, Kuller JA, Chescheir NC et al. Prenatal ultrasound findings of linear nevus sebaceous and its association with cystic adenomatoid malformation of the lung. *Obstet Gynecol* 1994;83:860-862.
58. Sintzoff SA, Avni EF, Rocmans P et al. Pulmonary sequestration-like anomaly presenting as a spontaneously resolving mass. *Ped Radiol* 1991;21:143-144.
59. Meizner I, Rosenak D. The vanishing fetal intrathoracic mass: consider an obstructing mucous plug. *Ultrasound Obstet Gynecol* 1995;5:275-277.
60. Maulik D, Robinson L, Daily DK et al. Prenatal sonographic depiction of intralobar pulmonary sequestration. *J Ultrasound Med* 1987;6:703-706.
61. Buntain WL, Woolley MM, Mahour GH et al. Pulmonary sequestration in children: a twenty-five year experience. *Surgery* 1977;81:413-420.
62. Liddell RM, Rosenbaum DM, Blumhagen JD. Delayed radiologic appearance of bilateral thoracic ectopic kidneys. *AJR* 1989;152:120-122.
63. O'Mara CS, Baker RR, Jeyasingham K. Pulmonary sequestration. *Surg Gynecol Obstet* 1978;147:609-616.
64. Knochel JQ, Lee TG, Melendez MG et al. Fetal anomalies involving the thorax and abdomen. *Radiol Clin North Am* 1982;20:297-310.
65. Kristofferson SE, Ipsen L. Ultrasonic real time diagnosis of hydrothorax before delivery in an infant with extralobar lung sequestration. *Acta Obstet Gynecol Scand* 1984;63:723-725.
66. Reece EA, Lockwood CJ, Rizzo N et al. Intrinsic intrathoracic malformations of the fetus: sonographic detection and clinical presentation. *Obstet Gynecol* 1987;70:627-632.
67. Romero R, Chervenak FA, Kotzen J et al. Antenatal sonographic findings of extralobar pulmonary sequestration. *J Ultrasound Med* 1982;1:131-132.
68. Siffring PA, Forrest TS, Hill WC et al. Prenatal sonographic diagnosis of bronchopulmonary foregut malformation. *J Ultrasound Med* 1989;8:277-280.

69. Thomas CS, Leopold GR, Hilton S et al. Fetal hydrops associated with extralobar pulmonary sequestration. *J Ultrasound Med* 1986;5:668-671.
70. West MS, Donaldson JS, Shkolnik A. Pulmonary sequestration: diagnosis by ultrasound. *J Ultrasound Med* 1989;8:125-129.
71. Sauerbrei E. Lung sequestration: Duplex Doppler diagnosis at 19 weeks gestation. *J Ultrasound Med* 1991;10:101-105.
72. Albright EB, Crane JP, Shackelford GD. Prenatal diagnosis of a bronchogenic cyst. *J Ultrasound Med* 1988;7:91-95.
73. Avni EF, Vanderelst A, VanGansbeke D et al. Antenatal diagnosis of pulmonary tumors: report of two cases. *Pediatr Radiol* 1986;16:190-192.
74. Young G, L'Heureux PR, Krueckeberg S et al. Mediastinal bronchogenic cyst: prenatal sonographic diagnosis. *AJR* 1989;152:125-127.
75. Watson WJ, Thorp JK, Miller RC et al. Prenatal diagnosis of laryngeal atresia. *Am J Obstet Gynecol* 1990;163:1456-1457.
76. Choong KKL, Trudinger B, Chow C et al. Fetal laryngeal obstruction: sonographic detection. *Ultrasound Obstet Gynecol* 1992;2:357-359.
77. Dolkart LA, Reimers FT, Wertheimer IS. Prenatal diagnosis of laryngeal atresia. *J Ultrasound Med* 1992;11:496-498.
78. Weston MJ, Rorter HJ, Berry PJ et al. Ultrasonographic prenatal diagnosis of upper respiratory tract atresia. *J Ultrasound Med* 1992;11:673-675.
79. deHullu JA, Kornman LH, Beekhuis JR et al. The hyperechogenic lungs of laryngotracheal obstruction. *Ultrasound Obstet Gynecol* 1995;5:271-274.
80. Richards DS, Farah LA. Sonographic visualization of the fetal upper airway. *Ultrasound Obstet Gynecol* 1994;4:21-23.
81. Felker RE, Cartier MS, Emerson DS et al. Ultrasound of the fetal thymus. *J Ultrasound Med* 1989;8:669-673.
82. Bratu M, Brown M, Carter M et al. Cystic hygroma of the mediastinum in children. *Am J Dis Child* 1970;119:348-351.
83. King RM, Telander RL, Smithson WA et al. Primary mediastinal tumors in children. *J Pediatr Surg* 1982;17:512-520.
84. Cyr DR, Guntheroth WG, Nyberg DA et al. Prenatal diagnosis of an intrapericardial teratoma: a cause for nonimmune hydrops. *J Ultrasound Med* 1988;7:87-90.
85. DeGeeter B, Kretz JG, Nisand I et al. Intrapericardial teratoma in a newborn infant: use of fetal echocardiology. *Ann Thorac Surg* 1983;35:664-666.
86. Rasmussen SL, Hwang WS, Harder J et al. Intrapericardial teratoma: ultrasonic and pathological features. *J Ultrasound Med* 1987;6:159-162.
87. Riggs T, Sholl JS, Ilbawi M et al. *In utero* diagnosis of pericardial tumor with successful surgical repair. *Pediatr Cardiol* 1984;5:23-26.
88. Weinraub Z, Gembruch U, Forisch HJ et al. Intrauterine mediastinal teratoma associated with non-immune hydrops fetalis. *Prenat Diagn* 1989;9:369-372.
89. De Filippi G, Caustri G, Bosio U et al. Thoracic neuroblastoma: antenatal demonstration in a case with unusual postnatal findings. *Br J Radiol* 1986;59:704-706.
90. Franzek DA, Strayer SA, Hull MT et al. Enteric cyst as a cause of nonimmune hydrops fetalis: fetal thoracentesis with fluid analysis. *J Clin Ultrasound* 1989;17:275-279.
91. Hobbins JC, Grannum PAT, Berkowitz RL et al. Ultrasound in the diagnosis of congenital anomalies. *Am J Obstet Gynecol* 1979;134:331-345.
92. Newnham JP, Crues JV, Vinstein AL et al. Sonographic diagnosis of thoracic gastroenteric cyst *in utero*. *Prenat Diagn* 1984;4:467-471.
93. Grosfeld JL, O'Neill JA, Clatworthy HW. Enteric duplications in infancy and childhood: an 18-year review. *Ann Surg* 1970;172:83-90.

The Fetal Abdomen

94. Goldstein I, Reese EA, Yarkoni S et al. Growth of the fetal stomach in normal pregnancies. *Obstet Gynecol* 1987;70:641-644.
95. Walker JM, Ferguson DD. The sonographic appearance of blood in the fetal stomach and its association with placental abruption. *J Ultrasound Med* 1988;7:155-161.
96. Daly-Jones E, Sepulveda W, Hollingsworth J, Fisk NM. Fetal intraluminal gastric masses after second trimester amniocentesis. *J Ultrasound Med* 1994;13:963-966.
97. Bergsma D. *Birth Defects Compendium*. 2nd ed. New York: Alan R Liss; 1979.
98. Hasegawa T, Kubota A, Imura K et al. Prenatal diagnosis of congenital pyloric atresia. *J Clin Ultrasound* 1993;21:278-281.
99. Pretorius DH, Gosink BB, Clautice-Engle T et al. Sonographic evaluation of the fetal stomach: significance of nonvisualization. *AJR* 1988;151:987-989.
100. Hill LM. Congenital microgastria: absence of the fetal stomach and normal third trimester amniotic fluid volume. *J Ultrasound Med* 1994;13:894-896.
101. Pretorius DH, Drose JA, Dennis MA et al. Tracheoesophageal fistula *in utero*. *J Ultrasound Med* 1987;6:509-513.
102. German JC, Mahour GH, Woolley MM. Esophageal atresia and associated anomalies. *J Pediatr Surg* 1976;1:299-306.
103. Holder TM, Cloud DT, Lewis JE Jr et al. Esophageal atresia and tracheoesophageal fistula: a survey of its members by the surgical section of the American Academy of Pediatrics. *Pediatrics* 1964;34:542-549.
104. Hata K, Hata T, Kitao M. Ultrasonographic identification and measurement of the human fetal pancreas *in utero*. *Int J Gynecol Obstet* 1988;26:61-64.
105. Hill LM, Peterson C, Rivello D et al. Sonographic detection of the fetal pancreas. *J Clin Ultrasound* 1989;17:475-479.
106. Goldstein I, Tamir A, Weisman A et al. Growth of the fetal gallbladder in normal pregnancies. *Ultrasound Obstet Gynecol* 1994;4:289-293.
107. Hertzberg BS, Kliewer MA, Maynor C et al. Nonvisualization of the fetal gallbladder: frequency and prognostic importance. *Radiology* 1996;199:679-682.
108. Beretsky I, Lankin DH. Diagnosis of fetal cholelithiasis using real-time high-resolution imaging employing digital detection. *J Ultrasound Med* 1983;2:381-383.
109. Klingensmith WC III, Cioffi-Ragan DT. Fetal gallstones. *Radiology* 1988;167:143-144.
110. Devonald KJ, Ellwood DA, Colditz PB. The variable appearance of fetal gallstones. *J Ultrasound Med* 1992;11:579-585.
111. Brown DL, Teele RL, Doubilet PM et al. Echogenic material in the fetal gallbladder: sonographic and clinical observations. *Radiology* 1992;182:73-76.
112. Lilly JR, Karrer FM. Contemporary surgery on biliary atresia. *Pediatr Clin North Am* 1985;32:1233-1246.
113. Schwartz SI, Shires GT, Spencer FC et al. *Principles of Surgery*. 4th ed. New York: McGraw-Hill; 1984.
114. Olbourne NA. Choledochal cysts: a review of the cystic anomalies of the biliary tree. *Ann R Coll Surg Engl* 1975;56:26-32.
115. Dewbury KC, Aluwihari APR, Birch SJ et al. Prenatal ultrasound demonstration of a choledochal cyst. *Br J Radiol* 1980;53:906-907.
116. Elrad H, Mayden KL, Ahart S et al. Prenatal ultrasound diagnosis of choledochal cyst. *J Ultrasound Med* 1985;4:553-555.
117. Frank JL, Hill MC, Chirathivat S et al. Antenatal observation of a choledochal cyst by sonography. *AJR* 1981;137:166-168.

118. Howell, CG, Templeton JM, Weiner S et al. Antenatal diagnosis and early surgery for choledochal cyst. *J Pediatr Surg* 1983;18:387-393.
119. Wiedman MA, Tan A, Martinez CJ. Fetal sonography and neonatal scintigraphy of a choledochal cyst. *J Nucl Med* 1985;26:893-896.
120. Gross BH, Harter LP, Filly RA. Disproportionate left hepatic lobe size in the fetus: ultrasonic demonstration. *J Ultrasound Med* 1982;1:79-81.
121. Vintzileos AM, Neckles S, Campbell WA et al. Fetal liver ultrasound measurements in isoimmunized pregnancies. *Obstet Gynecol* 1986;68:162-167.
122. Foucar E, Williamson RA, Yiu-Chiu V et al. Mesenchymal hamartoma of the liver identified by fetal sonography. *AJR* 1983;140:970-972.
123. Horgan JG, King DL, Taylor KJW. Sonographic detection of prenatal liver mass. *J Clin Gastroenterol* 1984;6:277-280.
124. Platt LD, De Vore GR, Benner P et al. Antenatal diagnosis of a fetal liver mass. *J Ultrasound Med* 1983;2:521-522.
125. Gonen R, Fong K. Chiasson DA. Prenatal sonographic diagnosis of hepatic hemangioendothelioma with secondary nonimmune hydrops fetalis. *Obstet Gynecol* 1989;73:485-487.
126. Kazzi NJ, Chang C-H, Roberts EC et al. Fetal hepatoblastoma presenting as nonimmune hydrops. *Am J Perinatol* 1989; 6:278-280.
127. Marks F, Thomas P, Lustig I et al. *In utero* sonographic description of a fetal liver adenoma. *J Ultrasound Med* 1990; 9:119-122.
128. Chung W-M. Antenatal detection of hepatic cyst. *J Clin Ultrasound* 1986;14:217-219.
129. Richards DS, Cruz AC, Dowdy KA. Prenatal diagnosis of fetal liver calcifications. *J Ultrasound Med* 1988;7:691-694.
130. Bronshtein M, Blazer S. Prenatal diagnosis of liver calcifications. *Obstet Gynecol* 1995;86:739-743.
131. Schmidt W, Yarkoni S, Jeanty P et al. Sonographic measurements in the fetal spleen: clinical implications. *J Ultrasound Med* 1985;4:667-672.
132. Eliezer S, Feldman E, Ehud W et al. Fetal splenomegaly, ultrasound diagnosis of cytomegalovirus infection: a case report. *J Clin Ultrasound* 1984;12:520-521.
133. Lichman JP, Miller EJ. Prenatal ultrasonic diagnosis of splenic cyst. *J Ultrasound Med* 1988;7:637-638.
134. Hertzberg BS. Sonography of the fetal gastrointestinal tract: anatomic variants, diagnostic pitfalls, and abnormalities. *AJR* 1994;162:1175-1182.
135. Dembner AG, Taylor KJ. Gray scale sonographic diagnosis: multiple congenital splenic cysts. *J Clin Ultrasound* 1978; 6:173-174.
136. Chitayat D, Lao A, Wilson, RD et al. Prenatal diagnosis of asplenia/polysplenia syndrome. *Am J Obstet Gynecol* 1988; 158:1085-1087.
137. Jeanty P, Chervenak F, Grannum P et al. Normal ultrasonic size and characteristics of the fetal adrenal glands. *Prenat Diagn* 1984;4:21.
138. Lewis E, Kurtz A, Dubbins P et al. Real-time ultrasonographic evaluation of normal fetal adrenal glands. *J Ultrasound Med* 1982;1:265.
139. Janetschek G, Weizel D, Stein W et al. Prenatal diagnosis of neuroblastoma by sonography. *Urology* 1984;24:397.
140. Guillian BB, Chang CCN, Yoss BS. Prenatal ultrasonographic diagnosis of fetal neuroblastoma. *J Clin Ultrasound* 1986; 14:225.
141. Fowlie F, Griacomantonia M, McKenzie E et al. Antenatal sonographic diagnosis of adrenal neuroblastoma. *J Can Assoc Radiol* 1987;37:50.
142. Ferraro EM, Fakhry J, Aruny JE et al. Prenatal adrenal neuroblastoma. *J Ultrasound Med* 1988;7:275.
143. VanderSlikke JW, Bulk AG. Hydramnios with hydrops fetalis and disseminated fetal neuroblastoma. *Obstet Gynecol* 1980; 55:250.
144. Parulekar SG. Sonography of normal fetal bowel. *J Ultrasound Med* 1991;10:211-220.
145. Nyberg DA, Mack LA, Patten RM et al. Fetal bowel: normal sonographic findings. *J Ultrasound Med* 1987;6:3-6.
146. Goldstein I, Lockwood C, Hobbins JC. Ultrasound assessment of fetal intestinal development in the evaluation of gestational age. *Obstet Gynecol* 1987;70:682-686.
147. Fakhry J, Reiser M, Shapiro LR. Increased echogenicity in the lower fetal abdomen: a common normal variant in the second trimester. *J Ultrasound Med* 1986;5:489-492.
148. Muller F, Aubry MC, Gasser B et al. Prenatal diagnosis of cystic fibrosis II: meconium ileus in affected fetuses. *Prenat Diagn* 1985;5:109-117.
149. Zilianti M, Fernandez S. Correlation of ultrasonic images of fetal intestine with gestational age and fetal maturity. *Obstet Gynecol* 1983;62:569-573.
150. Gross BH, Filly RA. Potential for a normal fetal stomach to simulate the sonographic "double-bubble" sign. *J Can Assoc Radiol* 1982;33:39-40.
151. Balcar I, Grand DC, Miller WA et al. Antenatal detection of Down syndrome by sonography. *AJR* 1984;143:29-30.
152. Romero R, Ghidini A, Costigan K et al. Prenatal diagnosis of duodenal atresia: does it make any difference? *Obstet Gynecol* 1988;71:739-741.
153. Nelson LH, Clark CE, Fishburne JI et al. Value of serial sonography in the *in utero* detection of duodenal atresia. *Obstet Gynecol* 1982;59:657-660.
154. Fonkalsrud EW, deLorimier AA, Hays DM. Congenital atresia and stenosis of the duodenum: a review compiled from the members of the surgical section of the American Academy of Pediatrics. *Pediatrics* 1969;43:79-83.
155. Nixon HH, Tawes R. Etiology and treatment of small intestinal atresia: analysis of a series of 127 jejunoileal atresias and comparison with 62 duodenal atresias. *Surgery* 1971; 69:49-51.
156. Young DG, Wilkinson AW. Abnormalities associated with neonatal duodenal obstruction. *Surgery* 1968;63:832-836.
157. Quan L, Smith DW. The VATER association: vertebral defects, anal atresia, T-E fistula with esophageal atresia, radial and renal dysplasia: a spectrum of associated defects. *J Pediatr* 1973;82:104-107.
158. Touloukian RJ. Intestinal atresia. *Clin Perinatol* 1978;5:3-18.
159. Pierro A, Cozzi F, Colarossi G et al. Does fetal gut obstruction cause hydramnios and growth retardation? *J Pediatr Surg* 1987;22:454-457.
160. Foster MA, Nyberg DA, Mahoney BS et al. Meconium peritonitis: prenatal sonographic findings and their clinical significance. *Radiology* 1987;165:661-665.
161. Jarmas AL, Weaver DD, Padilla LM et al. Hirschsprung disease: etiologic implications of unsuccessful prenatal diagnosis. *Am J Med Genet* 1983;16:163-167.
162. Vermesh M, Mayden K, Confino E et al. Prenatal sonographic diagnosis of Hirschsprung's Disease. *J Ultrasound Med* 1986; 5:37-39.
163. Wrobleski D, Wesselhoeft C. Ultrasonic diagnosis of prenatal intestinal obstruction. *J Pediatr Surg* 1979;14:598-660.
164. Fletcher BD, Yulish BS. Intraluminal calcifications in the small bowel of newborn infants with total colonic aganglionosis. *Radiology* 1978;126:451-453.
165. Dicke JM, Crane JP. Sonographically detected hyperechoic fetal bowel: significance and implications for pregnancy management. *Obstet Gynecol* 1992;80:778-782.

166. Nyberg DA, Dubinsky T, Resta RG et al. Echogenic fetal bowel during the second trimester: clinical importance. *Radiology* 1993;188:527-531.
167. Muller F, Dommergues M, Aubry MC et al. Hyperechogenic fetal bowel: an ultrasonographic marker for adverse fetal and neonatal outcome. *Am J Obstet Gynecol* 1995;173:508-513.
168. Slotnick RN, Abuhamad AZ. Prognostic implications of fetal echogenic bowel. *Lancet* 1996;347:85-87.
168a. Fung A, Wilson SW, Toi A, et al. Echogenic colonic meconium in the third trimester: a normal sonographic finding. *J Ultrasound Med* 1992;11:676-678.
169. Sepulveda W, Hollingsworth J, Bower S et al. Fetal hyperechogenic bowel following intra-amniotic bleeding. *Obstet Gynecol* 1994;83:947-950.
170. Scioscia AL, Pretorius DH, Budorick NE et al. Second trimester echogenic bowel and chromosome abnormalities. *Am J Obstet Gynecol* 1992;167:889-894.
171. Sepulveda W, Bower S, Fish NM. Mid-trimester hyperechogenic bowel in Down syndrome. *Am J Obstet Gynecol* 1995;172:210-211.
172. Nora AH, Nora JJ. A syndrome of multiple congenital anomalies associated with teratogenic exposure. *Arch Environ Health* 1975;30:17-21.
173. Shalev E, Weiner E, Zuckerman H. Prenatal ultrasound diagnosis of intestinal calcifications with imperforate anus. *Acta Obstet Gynecol Scand* 1983;62:95-96.
174. Sepulveda W, Romero R, Qureshi F et al. Prenatal diagnosis of enterolithiasis: a sign of fetal large bowel obstruction. *J Ultrasound Med* 1994;13:581-585.
175. Guzman ER, Ranzini A, Day-Salvatore D et al. The prenatal ultrasonographic visualization of imperforate anus in monoamniotic twins. *J Ultrasound Med* 1995;14:547-555.

CHAPTER 37

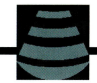

The Fetal Urogenital Tract

Katherine W. Fong, M.B., B.S., F.R.C.P. (C)
Greg Ryan, M.B., M.R.C.O.G., F.R.C.S.C.

CHAPTER OUTLINE

Evaluation of the fetal genitourinary tract is an integral part of the obstetric ultrasound examination. Sonography depicts normal developmental anatomy and allows detection and characterization of many genitourinary abnormalities. In addition, assessment of the amniotic fluid volume often provides important prognostic information regarding fetal renal function. Accurate and early prenatal diagnosis is important, because this may influence obstetric and neonatal management.

The urogenital tract is the most common site (30%) of all antenatally detected anomalies. A systematic sonographic approach is proposed, which includes a search for associated anomalies, as well as detailed evaluation of both renal structure and function.

THE NORMAL URINARY TRACT

Embryology

The permanent kidney (metanephros) is the third in a series of excretory organs in the human embryo, forming after the pronephros and mesonephros.[1] In the seventh menstrual week, the metanephros begins to develop from two sources: the ureteric bud and the metanephric mesoderm (Fig. 37-1). The ureteric bud is an outgrowth from the mesonephric duct, near its entry into the cloaca. It elongates and branches in a dichotomous pattern, giving rise to the ureter, renal pelvis, calyces, and collecting tubules. Through interaction with the metanephric mesoderm, the ureteric bud induces the formation of nephrons. In early embryonic life, the kidneys are located in the pelvis, but they "ascend" to their adult position by the eleventh menstrual week. They begin to produce urine by the end of the first trimester.

By the ninth menstrual week, the cloaca (the caudal part of the hind gut) is divided by the urorectal septum into the rectum posteriorly and urogenital sinus anteriorly (Fig. 37-1). The urinary bladder develops from the urogenital sinus and the surrounding splanchnic mesenchyme. The female urethra and almost all of the male urethra have a similar origin. Initially, the dome of the bladder is continuous with the allantois, but this connection soon constricts and becomes a fibrous cord, called the urachus, which extends from the apex of the bladder to the umbilicus.

Sonographic Appearance

On transvaginal sonography, the **fetal kidneys** may be identified late in the first trimester as hyperechoic structures, distinguishable from the hypoechoic adrenal glands.[2,3] With transabdominal sonography, they can be demonstrated by 14 to 16 menstrual weeks as hypoechoic structures adjacent to the fetal spine (Fig. 37-2, *A*). As the fetus matures, the kidneys become better delineated because of fat deposition in the perinephric and renal sinus regions.[4] An echogenic border develops, and there is increased echogenicity of the central renal sinus. In the third trimester, corticomedullary distinction becomes apparent (Fig. 37-2, *B* and *C*). The renal pyramids orient in anterior and posterior rows and are hypoechoic relative to the renal cortex. Normal fetal lobations are often visible and give the kidneys an undulating contour.[5]

The kidneys grow throughout pregnancy. An often-quoted rule of thumb is that "renal length in millimeters approximates gestational age in weeks."[6] However, a recent study and our own experience show that renal lengths are longer than previously reported.[7] Mean renal lengths, their standard deviations, and 95% confidence intervals for various gestational ages are shown in Table 37-1. Sometimes, it is difficult to define the exact renal borders, especially at the upper pole, because of shadowing from ribs or poor distinction from the adrenal gland. Fetal breathing can aid in renal visualization. It is also important to avoid using an oblique section through the kidney for measurement. The ratio of renal to abdominal circumference remains constant at 0.27 to 0.30 throughout pregnancy.[8]

Although the calyces are not normally visualized, it is common to see some fluid in the renal pelvis. The highly characteristic renal pelvic echo is often the key to finding the kidneys in the second trimester. Measurements of the renal pelvis will be discussed in the section on hydronephrosis. The normal ureter is 1 to 2 mm in diameter and is not normally visible.

Using transvaginal sonography, the **bladder** can be seen as early as 10 weeks, and in all cases by 13 weeks of gestation.[3] With transabdominal sonography, it should be seen routinely by 14 weeks. It is thin walled and is situated anteriorly in the pelvis. The umbilical (superior vesical) arteries run lateral to the bladder as they course toward the umbilicus (Fig. 37-3). The hourly fetal urine production increases with advancing gestation, from a mean value of 5 ml/hr at 20 weeks to 56 ml/hr at 41 weeks.[9] The maximum bladder volume increases from a mean value of 1 ml at 20 weeks to 36 ml at 41 weeks. The normal bladder fills and empties (either partially or completely) approximately every 25 minutes (range, 7 to 43 minutes).[9] Therefore, changes in bladder volume should be observed during the course of the obstetric sonogram.

Amniotic Fluid Volume

Evaluation of amniotic fluid volume (AFV) provides important information about fetal renal and placental function. Evaluation of AFV is a key component of fetal biophysical assessment (see Chapter 34). After 16 weeks, fetal urine production becomes the major source of amniotic fluid.[10] There are several methods to assess AFV. One can combine subjective assessment with semiquantitative techniques such as measurement of the largest single (cord-free) pocket and/or amniotic fluid index (AFI). Intra- and interobserver studies have shown that the subjective assessment of AFV by experienced sonographers is reliable.[11,12] Significant oligohydramnios results in compression of the fetus, marked crowding of fetal parts, and poor definition of fetal interfaces. The following classification has been proposed for the largest single-pocket method: vertical depth of the pocket less than 2 cm indicates moderate-to-severe oligohydramnios, 2 to 8 cm is normal, and greater than 8 cm indicates polyhydramnios.[13]

Amniotic Fluid Index. The AFI is obtained by measuring the vertical depth (mm) of the largest cord-free amniotic fluid pocket in the four quadrants of the

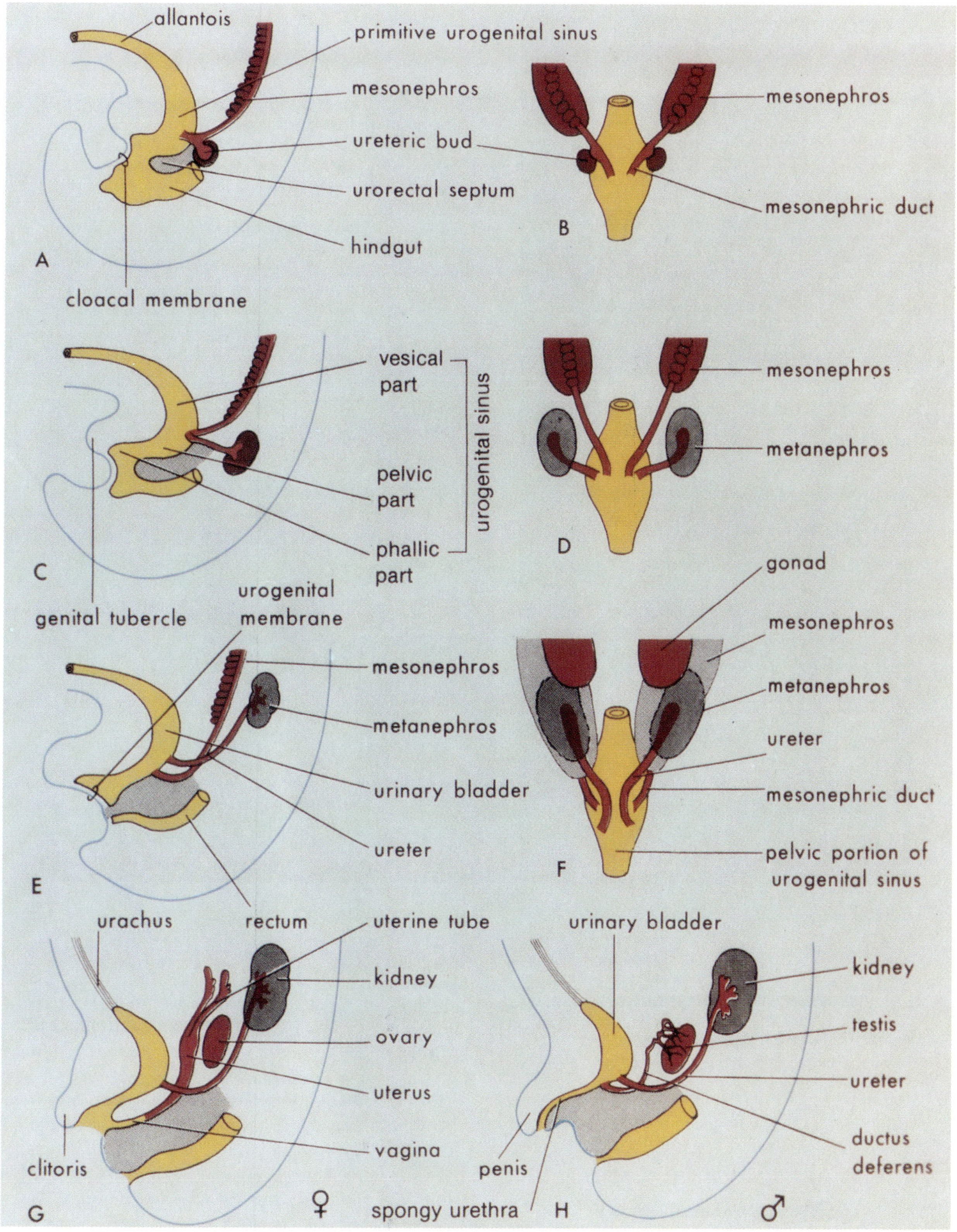

FIG. 37-1. Embryology of the urinary tract. Diagrams showing: (1) division of the cloaca into the urogenital sinus and rectum; (2) absorption of the mesonephric ducts: (3) development of the urinary bladder, urethra, and urachus; and (4) changes in the location of the ureters. **A,** Lateral view of the caudal half of a 5-week-old embryo. **B, D,** and **F,** Dorsal views. **C, E, G,** and **H,** Lateral views. The stages shown in **G** and **H** are reached by the twelfth week. (From Moore KL, Persaud TVN: *The Developing Human: Clinically Oriented Embryology*, 5th ed. Philadelphia: WB Saunders; 1993.)

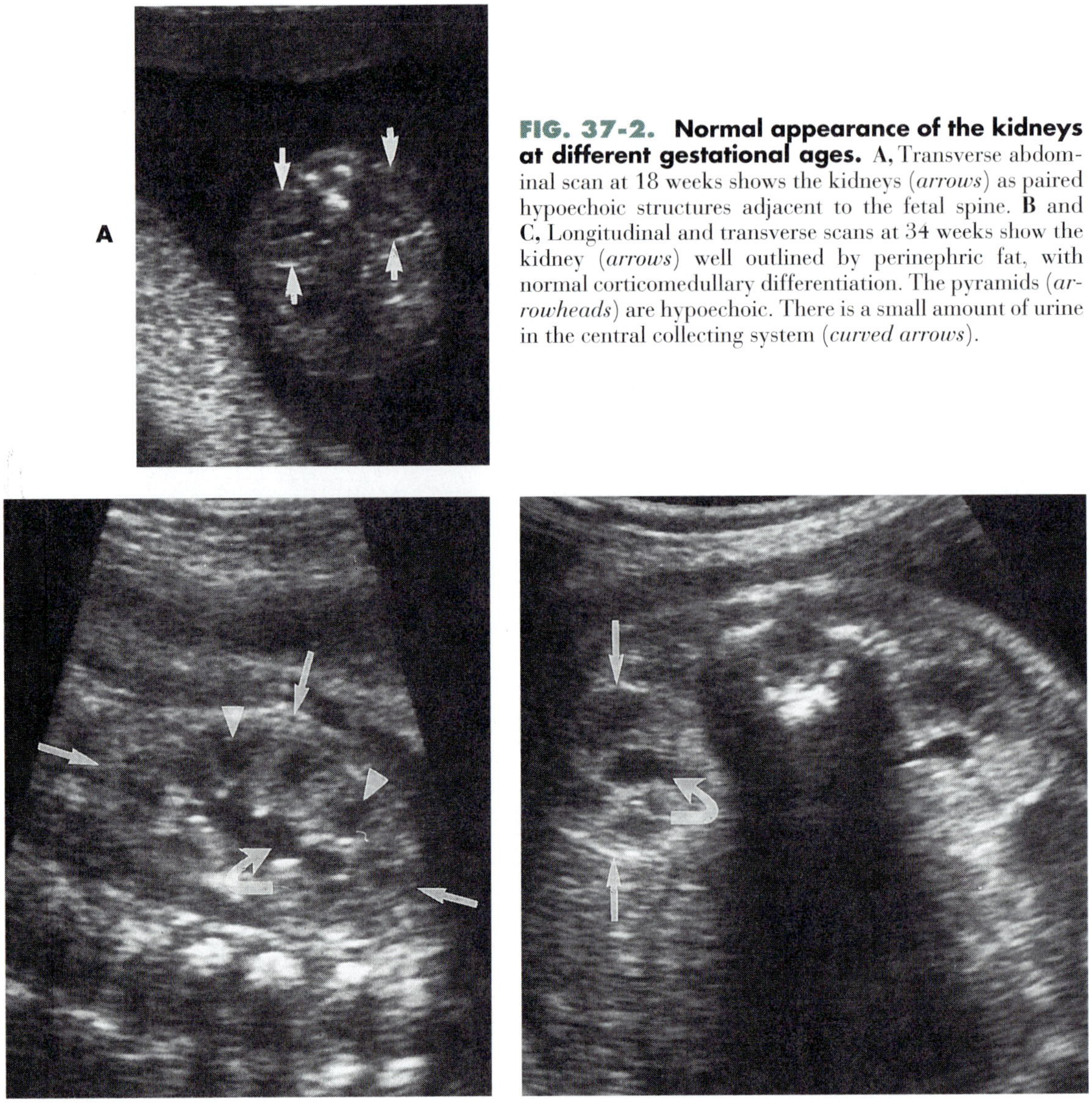

FIG. 37-2. Normal appearance of the kidneys at different gestational ages. A, Transverse abdominal scan at 18 weeks shows the kidneys (*arrows*) as paired hypoechoic structures adjacent to the fetal spine. B and C, Longitudinal and transverse scans at 34 weeks show the kidney (*arrows*) well outlined by perinephric fat, with normal corticomedullary differentiation. The pyramids (*arrowheads*) are hypoechoic. There is a small amount of urine in the central collecting system (*curved arrows*).

AMNIOTIC FLUID ASSESSMENT (LARGEST SINGLE-POCKET METHOD)

Vertical depth:

< 2 cm	Oligohydramnios
2–8 cm	Normal
> 8 cm	Polyhydramnios

uterus, and the sum of the four measurements is the index.[14,15] It varies with gestational age (Table 37-2). Oligohydramnios should be defined as more than two standard deviations below the mean for the specific gestational age, although the fifth percentile value is recommended for screening. The AFI is a reproducible, objective method for amniotic fluid measurement[15] and is useful for serial examinations of patients by multiple examiners of varying experience. However, there are several technical and interpretative limitations to the semiquantitative methods.[16] If the fetus is active, fetal movement may rapidly change the size of pockets. A large pocket may be replaced by multiple small pockets between extremities. Measuring pockets filled with cord or pockets with large vertical dimensions but with small widths (< 1 cm) would lead to overestimation. It has been recommended that when the index is below 100 mm, three AFI measurements should be averaged.[15] The AFI is not a substitute for experience in assessment of amniotic fluid volume.

A

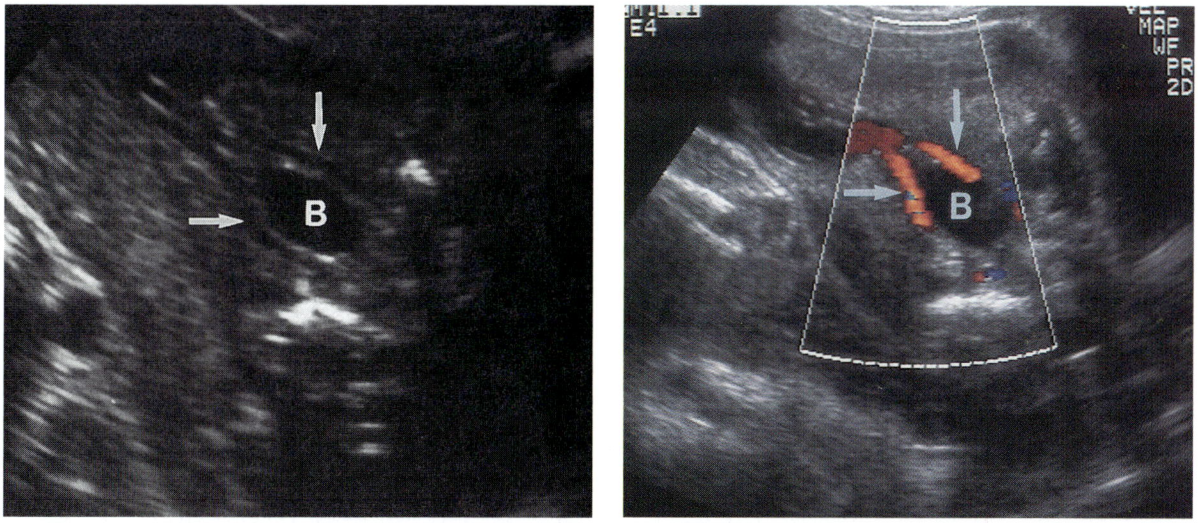

B

FIG. 37-3. Normal urinary bladder. **A,** The umbilical arteries (*arrows*) are seen adjacent to the urinary bladder (B). **B,** Color Doppler imaging of the umbilical arteries (*arrows*) helps in the definitive identification of any questionable fluid-filled structure in the pelvis as the urinary bladder (B).

TABLE 37-1

MEAN RENAL LENGTHS, STANDARD DEVIATION (SD), AND 95% CONFIDENCE INTERVAL (CI) FOR VARIOUS GESTATIONAL AGES

Gestational Age (weeks)	Mean Length (cm)	SD	95% CI	*n*
18	2.2	0.3	1.6-2.8	14
19	2.3	0.4	1.5-3.1	23
20	2.6	0.4	1.8-3.4	22
21	2.7	0.3	2.1-3.2	20
22	2.7	0.3	2.0-3.4	18
23	3.0	0.4	2.2-3.7	13
24	3.1	0.6	1.9-4.4	13
25	3.3	0.4	2.5-4.2	9
26	3.4	0.4	2.4-4.4	9
27	3.5	0.4	2.7-4.4	15
28	3.4	0.4	2.6-4.2	19
29	3.6	0.7	2.3-4.8	12
30	3.8	0.4	2.9-4.6	24
31	3.7	0.5	2.8-4.6	23
32	4.1	0.5	3.1-5.1	23
33	4.0	0.3	3.3-4.7	28
34	4.2	0.4	3.3-5.0	36
35	4.2	0.5	3.2-5.2	17
36	4.2	0.4	3.3-5.0	36
37	4.2	0.4	3.3-5.1	40
38	4.4	0.6	3.2-5.6	32
39	4.2	0.3	3.5-4.8	17
40	4.3	0.5	3.2-5.3	10
41	4.5	0.3	3.9-5.1	4

SD = standard deviation; 95% CI = 95% confidence interval
From Cohen HL, Cooper J, Eisenberg P, et al. Normal length of fetal kidneys: sonographic study in 397 obstetric patients. *AJR* 1991;157:545-548.

TABLE 37-2
AMNIOTIC FLUID INDEX VALUES (mm) IN NORMAL PREGNANCY

	Amniotic Fluid Index Percentile Values				
Week	**2.5th**	**5th**	**50th**	**95th**	**97.5th**
16	73	79	121	185	201
17	77	83	127	194	211
18	80	87	133	202	220
19	83	90	137	207	225
20	86	93	141	212	230
21	88	95	143	214	233
22	89	97	145	216	235
23	90	98	146	218	237
24	90	98	147	219	238
25	89	97	147	221	240
26	89	97	147	223	242
27	85	95	146	226	245
28	86	94	146	228	249
29	84	92	145	231	254
30	82	90	145	234	258
31	79	88	144	238	263
32	77	86	144	242	269
33	74	83	143	245	274
34	72	81	142	248	278
35	70	79	140	249	279
36	68	77	138	249	279
37	66	75	135	244	275
38	65	73	132	239	269
39	64	72	127	226	255
40	63	71	123	214	240
41	63	70	116	194	216
42	63	69	110	175	192

Modified from Moore TR, Cayle JE: The amniotic fluid index in normal human pregnancy. *Am J Obstet Gynecol* 1990;162:1168-1173.

URINARY TRACT ABNORMALITIES

Congenital abnormalities of the kidneys and ureters are quite common and found in 3% to 4% of the population.[1] Abnormalities of the urogenital tract account for 30% of all malformations detected *in utero* by ultrasonography.[17]

A **systematic approach** to the prenatal diagnosis of urinary tract abnormalities includes: assessment of amniotic fluid volume, localization and characterization of urinary tract abnormalities, and search for associated abnormalities.

PRENATAL DIAGNOSIS OF URINARY TRACT ABNORMALITIES

Assessment of amniotic fluid volume
Localization and characterization of urinary tract abnormalities
Search for associated abnormalities

Normal AFV in the second half of pregnancy implies at least one functioning kidney. If **oligohydramnios** is present (without a history of ruptured membranes or evidence of intrauterine growth restriction), **urinary tract anomalies must be strongly suspected.** In the setting of a urinary tract abnormality, normal AFV indicates a good prognosis. Oligohydramnios in the early second trimester carries a very poor prognosis because of the associated pulmonary hypoplasia.[18] Occasionally and paradoxically, polyhydramnios may occur, especially with unilateral obstructive uropathy, mesoblastic nephroma, or when there are concomitant abnormalities of the central nervous system or gastrointestinal tract.

The following five questions are helpful in defining and characterizing the urinary tract abnormality:

EVALUATION OF THE URINARY TRACT

Bladder	Presence
	Appearance and size
Kidneys	Presence
	Number
	Position
	Appearance (echogenicity, cysts)
	Unilateral or bilateral
Collecting system	Dilatation
	Level of obstruction
	Cause of obstruction
	Unilateral or bilateral
Fetal gender	

1. Is the bladder identified and normal in appearance? 2. Are kidneys present? Are they normal in position, size, and echogenicity? Are renal cysts identified? 3. Is the urinary tract dilated? If so, to what degree, at which level, and what is the cause? 4. Is the involvement unilateral or bilateral, symmetric, or asymmetric? 5. What is the fetal gender?

Prenatal detection of a genitourinary anomaly may indicate the presence of associated abnormalities, a syndrome, or chromosomal abnormality. Hence, a thorough sonographic search is necessary. Renal anomalies may be part of the VACTERL syndrome (*v*ertebral, *a*nal, *c*ardiac, *t*racheosophageal, *r*enal and *l*imb). When there are additional malformations, the risk for chromosomal abnormalities is significantly increased: **× 30 for multiple defects versus × 3 for isolated renal defects.**[19]

In addition, renal ultrasound is recommended for parents (and siblings) of fetuses suspected to have certain renal abnormalities (polycystic kidney disease, bilateral renal agenesis), because it may help to diagnose the type of polycystic kidney disease in the fetus and/or detect asymptomatic renal pathology in parents and siblings.[20]

Bilateral Renal Agenesis

Bilateral renal agenesis (BRA) is a lethal congenital anomaly, with an incidence of approximately 1 in 4000 births, and a male preponderance of 2.5 to 1.[21] The ureteric bud fails to develop, nephrons do not form, no urine is produced, and severe oligohydramnios results. Pulmonary hypoplasia is the major cause of neonatal death. Other features of "Potter's sequence" include typical facies (flattened nose, low-set ears, prominent epicanthic folds, and hypertelorism), limb deformities, and growth restriction.

The ultrasound findings include **severe oligohydramnios** and **non-visualization of the kidneys and bladder.** Prior to 16 weeks' gestation, AFV is not dependent on urine production and may be normal despite absent renal function. The absence of fetal kidneys should be the most specific finding, but this may be difficult to document because of poor image quality associated with oligohydramnios. In addition, bowel or adrenal glands in the renal fossae may be mistaken for kidneys.[22,23] However, recognition of the distinctive, flattened appearance of the adrenal gland on longitudinal sonogram (**"lying down" adrenal sign**) helps to confirm that the kidney did not develop in the flank (Fig. 37-4).[24]

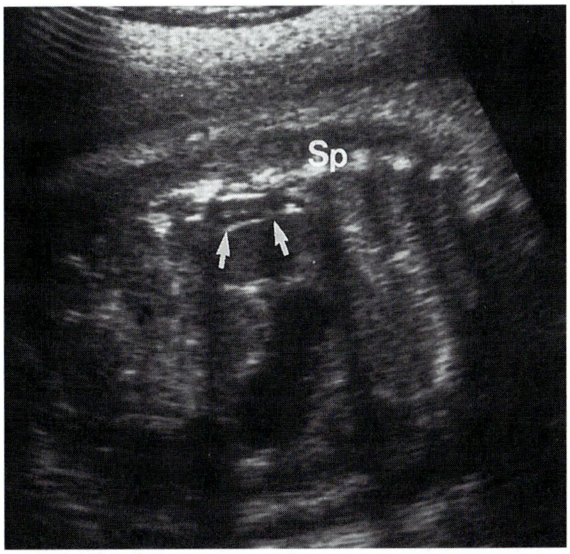

FIG. 37-4. The "lying down" adrenal sign—an indicator of renal agenesis or ectopia. Longitudinal scan of the renal fossa shows the flattened adrenal gland (*arrows*) in a fetus with bilateral renal agenesis. Sp—spine.

Repeated and consistent nonvisualization of the urinary bladder (over 1-hour period) is a secondary sign of bilateral renal agenesis. Conversely, identification of a normal bladder excludes this diagnosis. A small urachal diverticulum may mimic the bladder, but its lack of filling and emptying distinguishes it from the bladder. Furosemide challenge is not a useful test, because it does not reliably distinguish between fetuses with renal agenesis and those with impaired renal function from other causes (e.g., intrauterine growth restriction).[25,26]

Other techniques have been proposed to improve visualization of fetal structures: intra-amniotic and intraperitoneal infusion of isotonic saline,[27] transvaginal ultrasound[28] and recently, color Doppler imaging.[29-31] The transvaginal probe is particularly useful in the second trimester and with breech presentation. Color Doppler imaging can be used to diagnose absent renal arteries, providing further evidence for the diagnosis of bilateral renal agenesis. More importantly, it helps to map out the renal arteries in difficult cases of oligo-

BILATERAL RENAL AGENESIS

Sonographic findings:
- Severe oligohydramnios
- Absent kidneys
- "Lying down" adrenal sign
- Absent renal arteries on color Doppler imaging
- Non-visualization of the bladder (over 1 hour period)

Technical limitations:
- Poor image quality due to oligohydramnios
- Fetal position (breech presentation)

Pitfalls:
- AFV may be normal prior to 16 weeks' gestation
- Bowel or adrenal glands can be mistaken for kidneys
- Urachal diverticulum may mimic the bladder
- Empty bladder may be due to impaired renal function from other causes

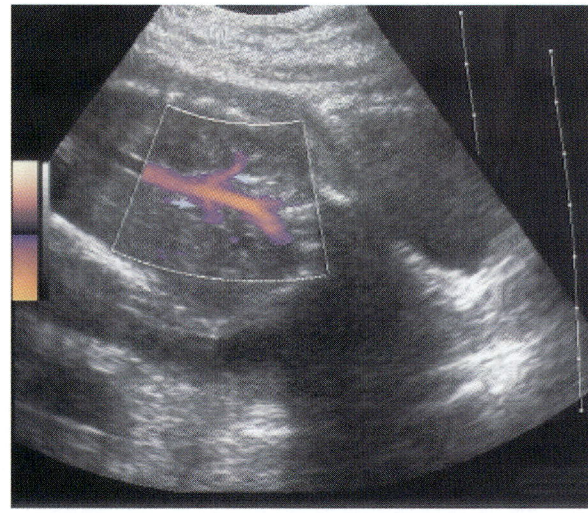

FIG. 37-5. Normal renal arteries. Power Doppler maps out the renal arteries bilaterally (*arrows*) in a growth-restricted fetus with oligohydramnios, confirming the presence of kidneys which are poorly visualized.

hydramnios, thereby confirming the presence of kidneys and avoiding confusion (Fig. 37-5).

Associated anomalies are quite common, involving the musculoskeletal (40%) (especially sirenomelia), cardiovascular (15%), gastrointestinal, and central nervous systems.

Obstetrical management includes the option of pregnancy termination, early delivery, and nonintervention in labor.

In the majority of cases, BRA is a multifactorial disorder. Parents should be counseled about two risks. Firstly, the recurrence risk of having another child with BRA is approximately 4%.[20,32] Secondly, parents and "unaffected" siblings have an increased risk of having silent genitourinary malformations. It has been shown that 9% of first-degree relatives have asymptomatic renal malformations, most often unilateral renal agenesis. Therefore, screening family members with renal ultrasound is recommended.[20]

Unilateral Renal Agenesis

Unilateral renal agenesis is three to four times more common than bilateral renal agenesis, occurring once in every 1000 births. It may be difficult to diagnose prenatally. There is a normal volume of amniotic fluid, the bladder appears normal, and the prognosis is good. A common pitfall is failure to image the renal fossa in the far field owing to acoustic shadowing from the spine, especially in the transverse plane. Meticulous attention to technique is necessary (rotating the transducer, changing the maternal position or repeated observations), otherwise the diagnosis may be missed. The contralateral kidney tends to be enlarged because of compensatory hypertrophy.[33] There may be additional genitourinary anomalies which are rarely life threatening.

Renal Ectopia

The reported incidence of renal ectopia varies between 1:500 and 1:1,200, **pelvic kidney** being the most common form.[34] When the renal fossa is empty, careful scanning may demonstrate the ectopic kidney adjacent to the bladder or iliac wing.[35] It may be associated with skeletal, cardiovascular, gastrointestinal, and gynecological abnormalities. Less commonly, crossed renal ectopia with or without fusion is identified. In this condition, the kidney is located on the opposite side from its ureter. Typically, the crossed-fused kidney is enlarged and bilobed, often with findings of obstructive uropathy.[36]

Horseshoe Kidney

Horseshoe kidney occurs once in 400 to 500 births.[1,34] Usually, the inferior poles of the kidneys are fused. Despite its relative frequency, the prenatal diagnosis of this disorder is rarely reported, presumably because the findings are subtle and often missed on routine sonography.[37] Multiple transverse and coronal images may be necessary to **demonstrate the bridge of renal tissue connecting the kidneys** (Fig. 37-6). A horseshoe kidney is frequently associated with other anomalies, including urogenital, central nervous system, cardiac and chromosomal abnormalities such as **Turner syndrome and trisomy 18.** Isolated horseshoe kidney is a relatively benign disorder that requires postnatal urologic follow-up because of higher prevalence of renal calculi, urinary tract infections, and hydronephrosis.

Bladder Exstrophy

This severe anomaly occurs once in 10,000 to 40,000 births, predominantly in males. It is caused by incomplete median closure of the inferior portion of the anterior abdominal wall, and the anterior wall of the urinary bladder. As a result, exposure and protrusion of the posterior wall of the bladder occur. Epispadias and wide separation of the pubic bones are associated with complete exstrophy of the bladder.

Sonographically, the amniotic fluid volume and kidneys are normal, but **a fluid-filled bladder is not identified.** Instead, the everted bladder with heaped-up mucosa may be seen as an irregular mass on the anterior abdominal wall, inferior to the umbilicus (Fig. 37-7). A low umbilical cord insertion site into the abdomen also suggests the diagnosis.[38,39]

Upper Urinary Tract Dilatation

Dilatation of the urinary tract can be **obstructive or nonobstructive.** In a review of 400 neonates with hydronephrosis, the various causes were ureteropelvic junction obstruction (44%), ureterovesical junction

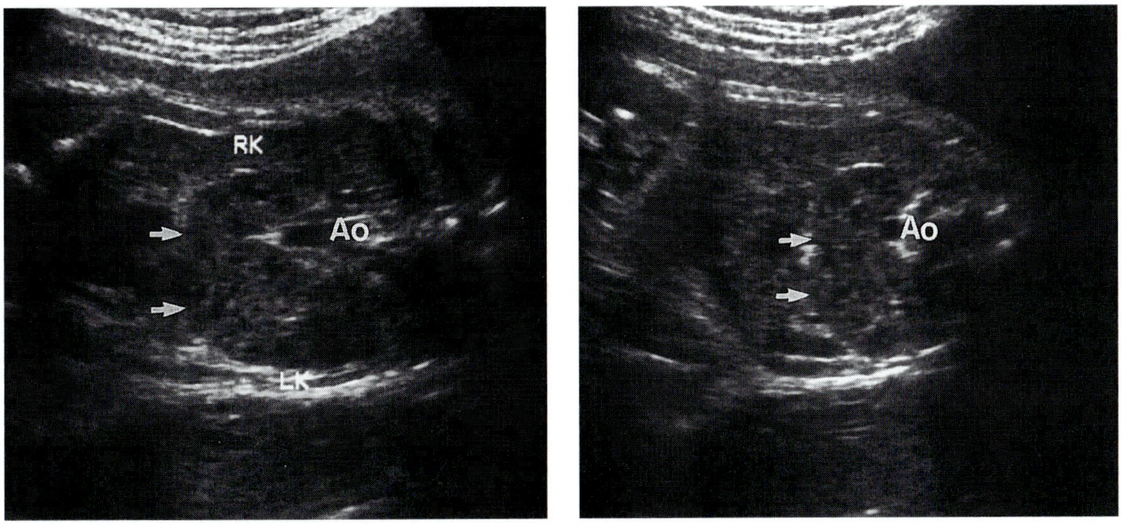

FIG. 37-6. Horseshoe kidney. A, Coronal and **B,** transverse images show the bridge of renal parenchyma (*arrows*) connecting the lower poles of the kidneys (RK, LK), anterior to the aorta (Ao).

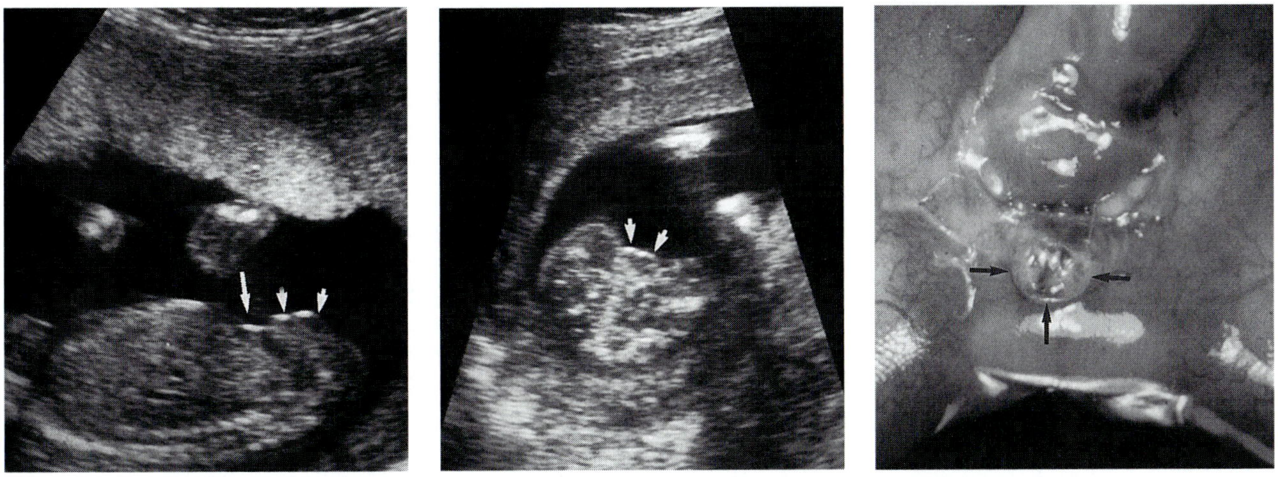

FIG. 37-7. Bladder exstrophy. A, Longitudinal scan of the lower fetal abdomen shows an irregular mass on the anterior abdominal wall (*small arrows*), below the umbilical cord insertion (*large arrow*), which is more caudal than usual. No bladder can be identified. **B,** Transverse view of the perineum showing two small excresences (*arrows*) which represent the everted bladder with heaped-up mucosa. **C,** Corresponding photograph of the everted bladder with heaped-up mucosa (*arrows*). (Courtesy of Ants Toi, MD, Toronto Hospital, Toronto).

NONVISUALIZATION OF FETAL BLADDER DIFFERENTIAL DIAGNOSIS

Renal abnormality
Bilateral renal agenesis
Bilateral multicystic dysplastic kidneys
Bilateral ureteropelvic junction obstruction
Bilateral combinations of any of the above
Autosomal recessive (infantile) polycystic kidney disease

Bladder abnormality
Bladder (or cloacal) exstrophy

Systemic cause
Severe intrauterine growth restriction

obstruction (21%), vesicoureteric reflux (14%), duplex collecting system (12%), and posterior urethral valves (9%).[40] However, this distribution may not reflect the situation before birth. Lethal malformations may be detected by prenatal sonography, but may lead to stillbirth or early neonatal death.

Diagnosis of Hydronephrosis. Hydronephrosis is the most common abnormality reported on prenatal sonography.[41] The objectives of antenatal diagnosis are to define those criteria which best correlate with either postnatal renal function or need for surgery (which is itself controversial).[42] Measurement of the anteroposterior (intra) renal pelvic diameter (RPD) in the transverse plane is the simplest and most commonly used technique (Fig. 37-8). **Prior to 20 weeks' gestation,** it has been suggested that an **RPD of 4 mm** or greater should be considered **abnormal**.[43,44] However, **after 20 weeks,** the exact RPD that indicates significant hydronephrosis remains **controversial.** A proposed classification for fetal hydronephrosis (detected after 20 weeks) is based on the RPD and the absence or presence of caliectasis in sonograms obtained with an empty fetal bladder (Table 37-3).[45] When correlated with postnatal outcome, grade IV and V (RPD > 15mm, with moderate or severe caliectasis) were clearly pathologic and required postnatal urologic surgery in 100% of cases. Grade II (RPD 10 to 15 mm) and III (RPD > 15 mm, with mild caliectasis) required surgery in nearly 50% of cases. However, if the renal pelvis measured between 5 to 9 mm (grade I), 97% of the kidneys were normal. It was concluded that for fetuses greater than 20 weeks' gestation, an RPD of 1 cm or greater was abnormal and predicted abnormal outcome. A 5- to 9-mm renal pelvis was likely physiological dilatation. At least three other groups of investigators supported this conclusion.[46-48]

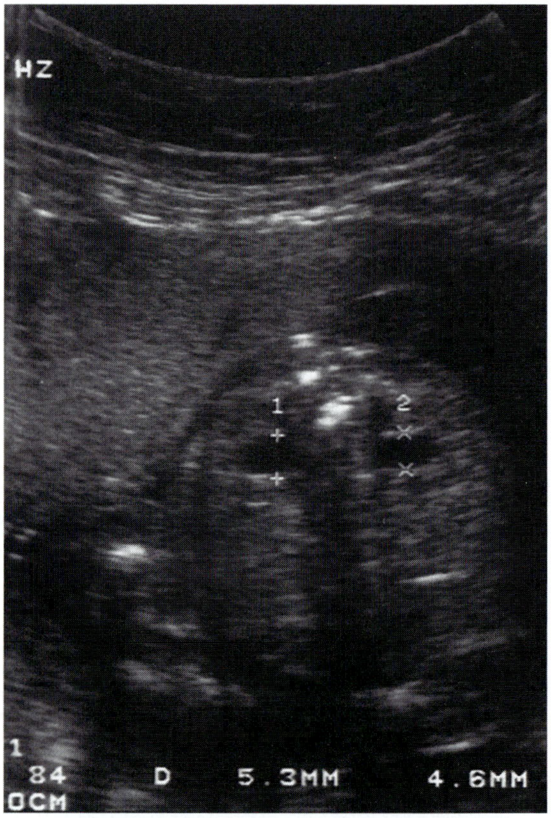

FIG. 37-8. Measurement of renal pelvis. Transverse scan of the abdomen in a 22-week-old fetus shows prominent renal pelves (calipers), measuring 5 mm in anteroposterior diameter.

On the other hand, data from several studies indicate that a threshold of 10 mm may be too high,[43,44,49-52] and using a cut-off of 10 mm for fetuses 24 weeks of age or older, the sensitivity for diagnosing congenital hydronephrosis was only 74%–82% (Table 37-4). If the RPD measured 7 to 9 mm after 24 weeks, a significant number of cases had hydronephrosis confirmed postnatally, with abnormal renal function and/or required surgery (Table 37-5). Corteville et al.[43] have proposed an RPD of 4 mm or greater before 33 weeks or 7 mm or greater after 33 weeks as being abnormal.[43] Their recommendations would lead to a high false-positive rate (Table 37-4), perhaps generating unnecessary anxiety. However, if the goal is to identify all "at-risk" fetuses, their proposed thresholds may be justified. In our study of 642 kidneys in 328 fetuses, the ninety-fifth percentile values for renal pelvic diameter at 20 weeks and 33 weeks were 4 mm and 6 mm, respectively.[53]

A ratio of the anteroposterior diameters of the renal pelvis and kidney greater than 50% has also been used to indicate significant fetal hydronephrosis.[46] Others consider the presence of caliectasis, *per se*, a significant abnormality, independent of the pelvic size.[54]

TABLE 37-3
PRENATAL GRADING AND POSTNATAL OUTCOME FETAL HYDRONEPHROSIS AFTER 20 MENSTRUAL WEEKS

Grade	AP Pelvic Diameter	Caliectasis	Normal	Medical Management	Surgery
I	5-9 mm	None	97%	3%	0%
II	10-15 mm	None	48%	13%	39%
III	>15 mm	Slight	13%	25%	62%
IV	>15 mm	Moderate	0%	0%	100%
V	>15 mm	Severe	0%	0%	100%

Modified from Grignon A, Filion R, Filiatrault D, et al. Urinary tract dilatation *in utero:* classification and clinical applications. *Radiology* 1986;160:645-647.

TABLE 37-4
ANTEROPOSTERIOR RENAL PELVIC DIAMETER (AT DIFFERENT STAGES OF GESTATION) VERSUS RISK OF POSTNATAL CONGENITAL HYDRONEPHROSIS

Anteroposterior Pelvic Diameter (mm)	14-23 wk		24-32 wk		33-42 wk	
	Sensitivity (%)	False-Positive Rate (%)	Sensitivity (%)	False-Positive Rate (%)	Sensitivity (%)	False-Positive Rate (%)
≥ 4	100	55	100	42	100	24
≥ 7	61	35	91	34	100	21
≥ 10	32	18	74	14	82	18

From Corteville JE, Gray DL, Crane JP. Congenital hydronephrosis: correlation of fetal ultrasonographic findings with infant outcome. *Am J Obstet Gynecol* 1991;165:384-388.

TABLE 37-5
ANTEROPOSTERIOR RENAL PELVIC DIAMETER (AT DIFFERENT STAGES OF GESTATION) CORRELATED WITH POSTNATAL CONGENITAL HYDRONEPHROSIS AND UROLOGIC SURGERY OR RENAL COMPROMISE

Anteroposterior Pelvic Diameter (mm)	14-23 wk		24-32 wk		33-42 wk	
	CH (%)	S/C (%)	CH (%)	S/C (%)	CH (%)	S/C (%)
< 3	0	0	0	0	0	0
4-6	41	19	38	13	0	0
7-9	53	40	33	6	67	50
> 10	82	73	86	72	82	59

CH, Congenital hydronephrosis confirmed postnatally; *S/C,* postnatal surgery and/or renal compromise.

From Corteville JE, Gray DL, Crane JP. Congenital hydronephrosis: correlation of fetal ultrasonographic findings with infant outcome. *Am J Obstet Gynecol* 1991;165:384-388.

Renal pelvic dilatation may be the first manifestation of a urinary tract abnormality. On serial ultrasound examinations, the RPD may show progression, regression, or no change. *In utero* progression increases the likelihood that postnatal corrective surgery will be required.[51] So far, all the published studies reported only a small number of postnatally confirmed hydronephrosis (< 100 in each). There was also a lack of standardization in the definition of obstructive uropathy, and different postnatal outcomes were used as endpoints, so that exact comparison is difficult. Further studies involving a large number of patients are necessary to determine the significance of the renal pelvis that measures 4 to 9 mm, particularly after 20 weeks' gestation. The important message is: if the renal pelvis appears to be abnormal, follow-up ultrasound in 6 to 8 weeks is warranted. If renal pelvic dilatation persists, postnatal follow-up studies should be carried out.

The timing of postnatal ultrasound depends on the severity of prenatal hydronephrosis.[55] If there is severe dilatation of the renal pelvis, early ultrasound evaluation should be performed to permit early intervention. Otherwise, ultrasound examination should be postponed for 3 to 7 days. In the first 48 hours of life, a relative state of dehydration and physiologic oliguria can cause an underestimation of the degree of hydronephrosis, and may result in a false-negative renal sonogram.[56] If the initial postnatal ultrasound is normal, a repeat ultrasound in 4 to 6 weeks is necessary to exclude obstruction.[55,57] Ultrasound is a poor screening test for reflux in the neonate with prenatally detected hydronephrosis. Therefore, routine screening for reflux with voiding cystourethrography is recommended, although the postnatal ultrasound may be normal.[57,58] A radionuclide (DTPA) renal scan is a useful test to distinguish between obstructive and nonobstructive hydronephrosis. It is also the most widely used technique to assess renal function and drainage in the presence of hydronephrosis.

Pyelectasis and Aneuploidy. Pyelectasis (mild hydronephrosis) is found in 2% of normal fetuses.[59] However, the incidence is increased to 17% to 25% in fetuses with trisomy 21.[59,60] In a referral population of 1177 fetuses with mild hydronephrosis detected at 16 to 26 weeks' gestation, the **frequency of chromosomal abnormalities** was **1.1%** in fetuses with **isolated hydronephrosis**, compared with 5.4%, 22.9%, and 63.3% in those with 1, 2, or 3 additional abnormalities, respectively.[61] The risk for trisomy 21 in fetuses with isolated mild hydronephrosis was 1.6 times higher than the maternal age–and gestational age–related risk *(observed frequency 0.62% versus expected frequency 0.4%)*.[61] Larger studies are necessary to determine whether such a difference is significant. It has been suggested that parents be counselled that isolated mild hydronephrosis is not associated with significantly increased risk for trisomy 21.[59,61] Our policy is to interpret this finding in conjunction with maternal serum screen results and discuss amniocentesis accordingly.

Ureteropelvic Junction Obstruction. Obstruction at the ureteropelvic junction (UPJ) is the **most common cause of neonatal hydronephrosis.**[40] Most cases of UPJ obstruction are functional (caused by a muscular abnormality) rather than the result of fixed anatomic lesions such as fibrous adhesions, kinks, valves, or aberrant vessels. UPJ obstruction is often unilateral.[62] In 10% to 30% of cases, it is bilateral.

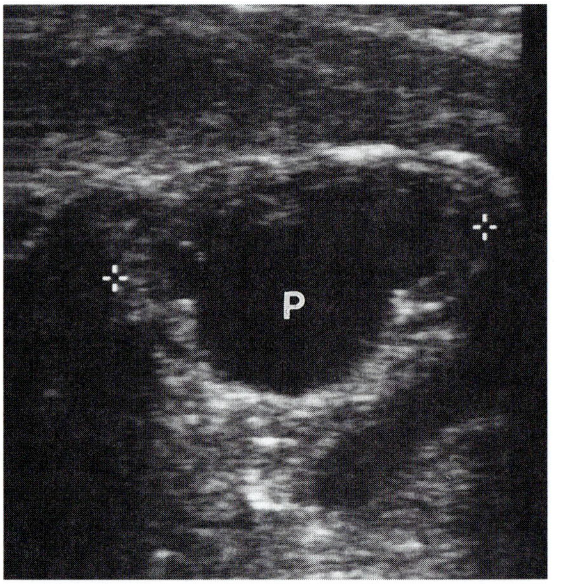

FIG. 37-9. Ureteropelvic junction obstruction. Longitudinal scan shows moderate caliectasis with dilated renal pelvis (P). Calipers indicate renal margin.

Sonographically, a dilated renal pelvis with or without caliectasis is identified (Fig. 37-9). The ureter is not visualized. The AFV is usually normal but may be increased paradoxically. When unilateral hydronephrosis is accompanied by oligohydramnios, a search for contralateral renal pathology is warranted (e.g., agenesis, multicystic dysplasia, etc). With severe chronic obstruction, there may be marked dilatation of the renal pelvis, with a thin rim of cortex, presenting as a large, unilocular cystic mass.[63] A perirenal urinoma from rupture of the collecting system correlates with severe obstruction and poor residual function of the ipsilateral kidney (Fig. 37-10).[64]

When the contralateral kidney is normal, the prenatal detection of unilateral UPJ obstruction should not alter obstetric management, because the prognosis is good. With bilateral UPJ obstruction, the prognosis depends on the severity and duration of obstruction, and the AFV. Serial ultrasound evaluations are necessary to assess the AFV and any progression of hydronephrosis. Early delivery is rarely indicated and only if there is marked progressive bilateral obstruction with severe oligohydramnios.

Ureterovesical Junction Obstruction. This is the second most common cause for hydronephrosis.[40] Ureteral obstruction is almost always caused by an aperistaltic distal ureteral segment, so-called **primary megaureter**. Rarely, it is caused by a distal ureteral stricture or valve. Bilateral distal ureteral obstruction is uncommon. However, coexisting anomalies

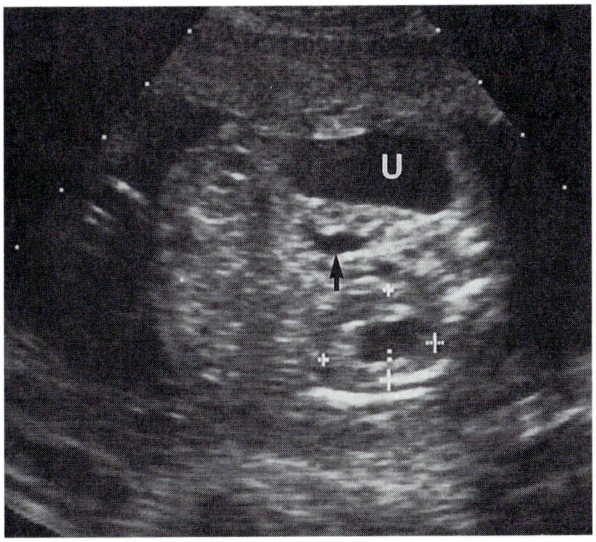

FIG. 37-10. Perinephric urinoma. Transverse scan of the abdomen shows decompressed renal pelvis (*arrow*) and large perinephric urinoma (U). Note dilated renal pelvis in the contralateral kidney, marked by calipers. Ureteropelvic junction obstruction is bilateral in 10% to 30% of cases.

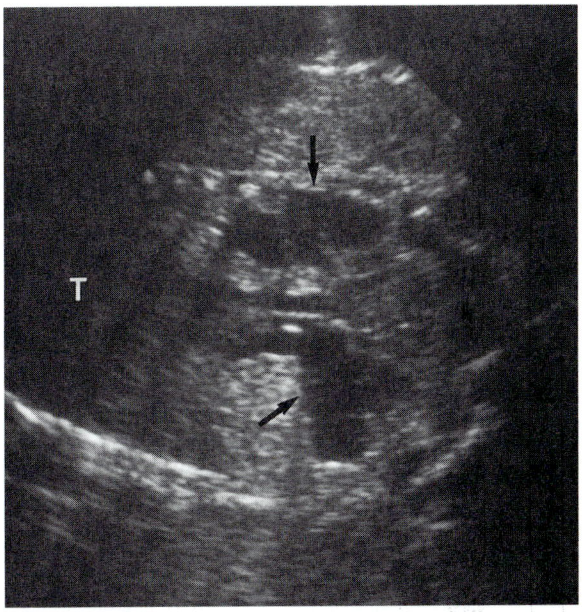

FIG. 37-11. Bilateral hydroureters/primary megaureters. Coronal scan shows bilateral serpiginous, markedly dilated ureters (*arrows*) on either side of the spine. T—thorax.

of the urinary tract (vesicoureteral reflux, UPJ obstruction, multicystic dysplasia) are frequently present.

Sonographically, hydroureter with variable degree of hydronephrosis is seen (Fig. 37-11). Sometimes, a slightly dilated ureter can be difficult to recognize or can be mistaken for bowel, although bowel contents are usually more echogenic than urine. Identification of peristalsis in a fluid-filled tubular structure does not confirm bowel; it is often seen with hydroureter as well. To be sure, the serpiginous cystic segments must be traced to the renal pelvis and/or bladder. In addition, the ureter generally comes into close contact with the spine, but the small bowel does not. Because the dilatation can be severe, size alone does not preclude megaureter as a possible diagnosis.

Nonobstructive causes such as vesicoureteral reflux usually cannot be differentiated from ureterovesical junction obstruction on a prenatal sonogram. Definitive diagnosis requires postnatal investigations.

Duplication Anomalies. Unlike most urinary tract disorders, duplication of the renal collecting system is more common in females. Two ureteral buds arise from the mesonephric duct to grow into the metanephric blastema. Classically, the **upper pole moiety obstructs** (with or without an ectopic ureterocele), whereas the **lower pole moiety refluxes**. Hydronephrosis of the upper pole, with a normal lower pole is the key to sonographic diagnosis of an obstructed duplex kidney (Fig. 37-12, *A*). Identification of two separate collecting systems, or the nondilated lower pole of a duplex kidney may be difficult, because of its small size and displacement by the dilated upper renal pelvis and ureter.[65] The ectopic ureter may be markedly dilated and tortuous, and can mimic multiseptated, cystic, abdominal masses. A careful evaluation of the urinary bladder is necessary to detect the **ureterocele**, which is seen as a thin-walled, cystlike structure within the bladder (Fig. 37-12, *B*). The diagnosis is easy when the bladder is partially full but can be overlooked if the bladder is empty or only minimally distended. Also, a full bladder can result in non-visualization of the ureterocele.[65] Ureteroceles are bilateral in 15% of cases. If ureteroceles become sufficiently large, they may cause bladder outlet obstruction. Prenatal detection of upper-pole hydronephrosis in a duplex kidney allows the use of prophylactic antibiotics at birth, and this has decreased the proportion of affected neonates presenting with urinary tract infection and urosepsis.[66]

DETECTION OF A URETEROCELE

Thin-walled, cystlike structure in bladder
Overlooked if the bladder is empty
Full bladder can compress ureterocele
May cause bladder outlet obstruction

Lower Urinary Tract Obstruction

Urethral Obstruction. The effect of urinary obstruction upon subsequent renal development

A

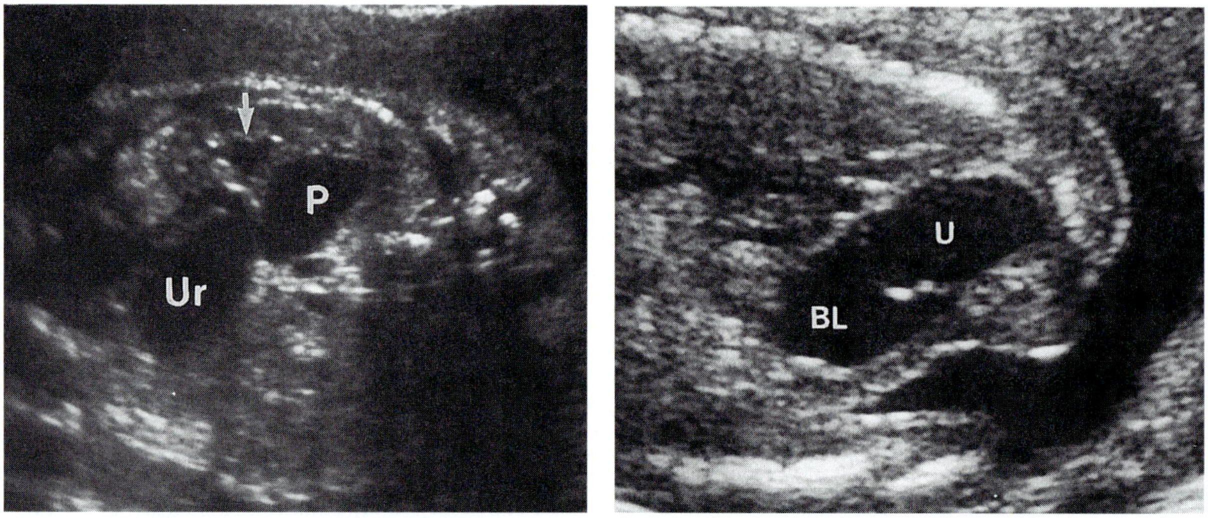

B

FIG. 37-12. Duplication anomalies. **A,** Longitudinal scan showing the hydronephrotic, upper-pole renal pelvis (P) continuous with the dilated ectopic ureter (Ur). No ureterocele is identified. The lower-pole collecting system is not dilated (*arrow*). **B,** Longitudinal scan of the pelvis in another fetus. The ureterocele (U) is separated from the lumen of the bladder (BL) by a thin curvilinear rim of echoes.

depends on the time of onset and severity of the obstruction. The fetal urinary tract responds to chronic obstruction differently from adults. In adults with chronic urethral obstruction, the pelvicalyceal system is usually markedly dilated; in the fetus, there may be relative lack of pelvicalyceal dilatation and possible development of macroscopic renal cysts. Experimental work in lambs has shown that ureteral obstruction originating in the last half of gestation causes simple hydronephrosis and parenchymal atrophy.[67] However, if it originates during the first half of gestation, renal dysplasia and sometimes cyst formation will occur (Fig. 37-13).[68]

Posterior urethral valves are the most common cause of lower urinary tract obstruction (LUTO), followed by urethral atresia or stricture, and persistent cloaca (see box). Posterior urethral valves (PUV) are seen exclusively in males and may cause either total, intermittent, or partial obstruction, with variable prognosis. Most cases are sporadic, and the recurrence risk is small. Back pressure causes a persistently dilated urinary bladder, with a dilated proximal urethra (**"keyhole" sign**) (Fig. 37-14, *A*). There may be thickening of the bladder wall (>2 mm), bilateral tortuous hydroureters, and hydronephrosis (Fig. 37-14, *B*). If the obstruction is severe and long standing, progressive renal parenchymal fibrosis and dysplasia develop, resulting in severe oligohydramnios, pulmonary hypoplasia, and compression deformities. There may be evidence of spontaneous rupture: urinary ascites (Fig. 37-15) or a perirenal urinoma (Fig. 37-10).[69] If spontaneous decompression occurs, this "safety valve" may protect the kidneys from further prenatal damage and may diminish the degree of hydronephrosis in some cases. Fetal lamb studies have shown that recovery of renal function is inversely proportional to the duration of urinary tract obstruction and is directly proportional to the duration of *in utero* decompression.[70]

CAUSES OF FETAL MEGACYSTIS

Posterior urethral valves
Urethral atresia/stricture
Prune belly syndrome
Primary megacystis
Megacystis-microcolon-intestinal hypoperistalsis syndrome (MMIHS)
Cloacal malformation

Urethral atresia causes the most severe form of obstructive uropathy. This is often detected in the early second trimester, with anhydramnios and a markedly distended bladder (Fig. 37-16). In the absence of antenatal treatment, this condition is almost always fatal, because of associated renal dysplasia and pulmonary hypoplasia.[71]

Fetal megacystis has been reported as early as 10 to 14 weeks' gestation when the longitudinal bladder diameter is ≥ 8 mm.[72] In some cases, there was spontaneous resolution by 20 weeks, whereas in others, there was progressive obstructive uropathy.[72] Therefore, follow-up ultrasound is necessary to correctly interpret the significance of megacystis detected in the first trimester.

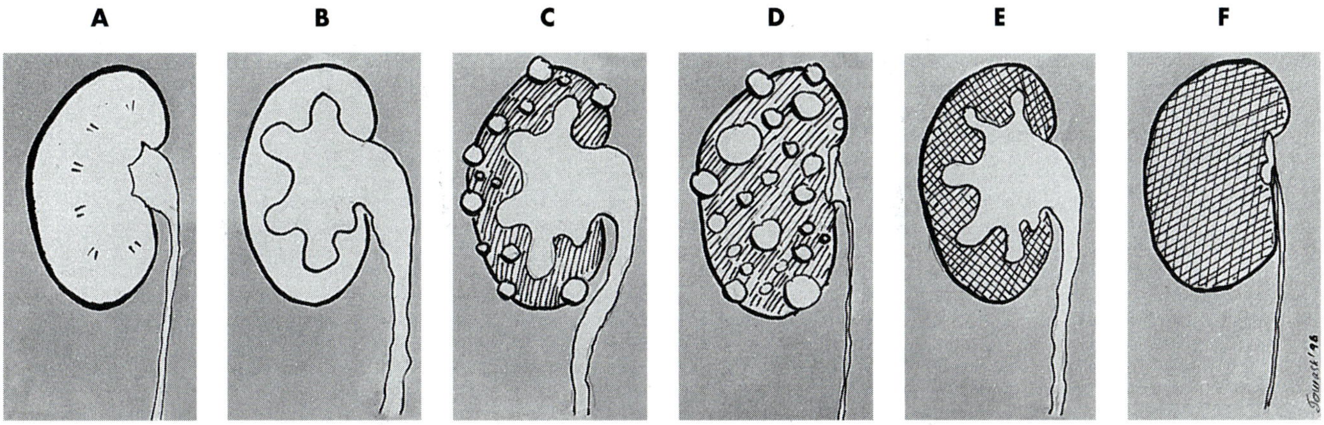

FIG. 37-13. Urinary tract obstruction produces a varied response from the kidneys. **A,** Normal kidney. **B,** Pelvocaliectasis, with or without parenchymal atrophy. **C,** Renal cystic dysplasia, with parenchymal cysts. **D,** The dysplastic kidney may cease to function (lack of pelvocaliectasis). **E,** Alternatively, the kidney may show increased echogenicity, with no visible cysts, but with pelvocaliectasis or **F,** without pelvocaliectasis. In the case of E and F, dysplasia is probably, but not invariably, present.

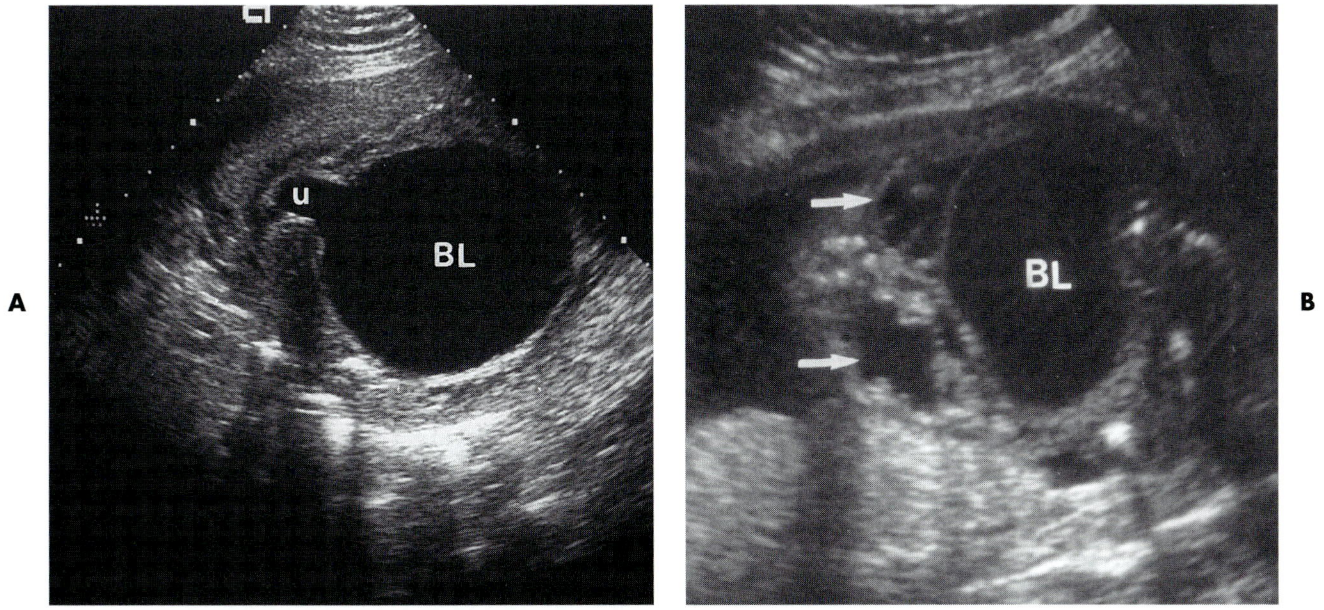

FIG. 37-14. Posterior urethral valves causing urethral level obstruction. **A,** The dilated urinary bladder (BL) and proximal urethra (u) give the appearance of a keyhole characteristic of urethral obstruction. **B,** Transverse scan shows dilated bladder (BL) and bilateral hydronephrosis (*arrows*).

Cloacal malformation (persistent cloaca) results from failure of the urorectal septum to reach the perineum. It occurs exclusively in phenotypic females, with an incidence of 1 in 50,000 births. The typical patient has a single perineal opening that serves as the outlet for urine, genital secretions, and meconium. Lower urinary tract abnormalities (reflux, ureteral ectopia, duplication of bladder) and genital abnormalities (duplication or atresia of uterus and vagina) are frequent, as well as abnormalities of the bony pelvis and kidneys. Additional complications are related to urinary tract obstruction, hydrometrocolpos, and bowel obstruction. Prenatal sonographic findings include: normal or diminished AFV, normal, distended or nonvisualized bladder, a retrovesical cystic mass, ascites, hydronephrosis, ambiguous genitalia, and vertebral anomalies.[73,74]

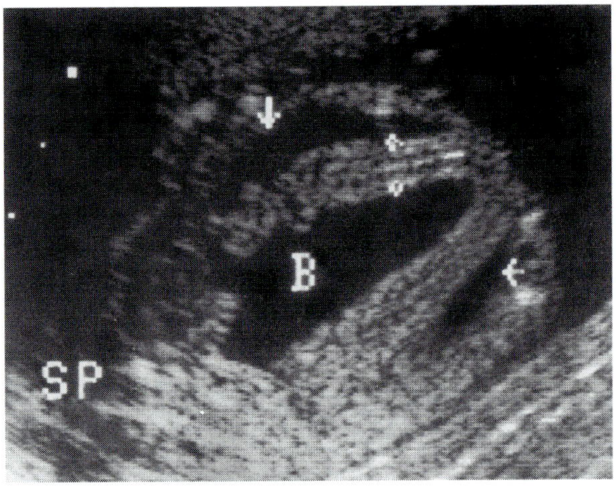

FIG. 37-15. Urinary ascites. Transverse scan at 18 weeks' gestation shows ascites (*arrows*) and a thick-walled urinary bladder (calipers) caused by spontaneous rupture of severe megacystis. SP—spine; B—bladder.

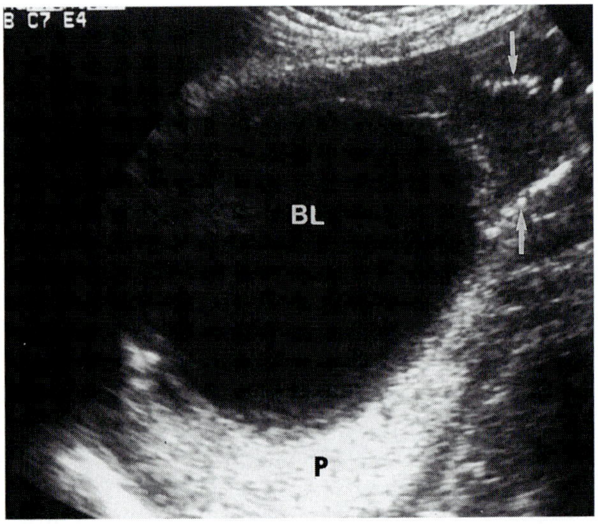

FIG. 37-16. Urethral atresia. Coronal scan of a 17-week-old fetus, showing a very distended bladder (BL) which occupies the entire abdomen. The thorax (*arrows*) is compressed and bell-shaped. There is profound oligohydramnios. P—placenta.

Prune belly syndrome is characterized by the classic triad of absent abdominal musculature, undescended testes, and urinary tract abnormalities (megacystis, ureterectasis). Although some authors believe that the syndrome results from a primary mesodermal defect, others explain the pathogenesis as a urethral obstruction malformation complex (the muscular defect is secondary to the distended urinary system).[75] The bladder is typically very large. The prostatic urethra is dilated, and the appearance resembles posterior urethral valves. The ureters tend to be tortuous and dilated. The kidneys may be normal, hydronephrotic, or dysplastic. Other abnormalities may be present, including intestinal malrotation, congenital heart disease and musculoskeletal deformities. Although not all infants have urethral obstruction at birth, it is believed that transient *in utero* obstruction may initiate the sequence responsible for this syndrome.[76]

Megacystis-microcolon-intestinal hypoperistalsis syndrome (MMIHS) is a rare, **nonobstructive** cause for megacystis, with a strong female predominance (4:1). The syndrome involves not only a distended bladder, but also functional small bowel obstruction and microcolon. Because it carries a dismal prognosis and fetal bladder shunting is of no benefit, it is important to differentiate this syndrome from the more common posterior urethral valves. The key features are: (1) the amniotic fluid is usually normal or increased; (2) the fetus is usually female; and (3) rarely, a dilated small bowel may be present.[77]

PRUNE BELLY SYNDROME

Absent abdominal musculature
Undescended testes
Very large bladder
Prostatic urethra dilated
Ureters tortuous and dilated
Kidneys normal, hydronephrotic, or dysplastic

In Utero Intervention

Vesicoamniotic Shunting. For a carefully selected group of fetuses with severe LUTO, permanent *in utero* bladder drainage may be a therapeutic option. The object of vesicoamniotic shunting is to allow free drainage of urine from the bladder into the amniotic cavity. This relieves back pressure on the urinary tract and should prevent or stabilize renal dysplastic change, correct oligohydramnios, and allow unimpeded lung development. This approach presumes that renal dysfunction has not been predetermined by whatever insult originally resulted in the anatomical obstruction. Careful selection of suitable cases is critical and the identification and rigorous evaluation of reliable predictors of postnatal renal function continue to be the goal of many investigators.[78-85]

A detailed sonographic evaluation of the fetus is a prerequisite, including a diligent search for associated structural or chromosomal abnormalities.[19] The sonographic appearances and clinical sequelae of severe LUTO are discussed elsewhere in this chapter. A thorough assessment of the urinary tract is necessary to define the probable cause and evaluate prognosis. Intervention is not indicated if the ultrasound is suggestive of either MMIHS or severe cloacal dysgenesis.

TABLE 37-6
PREDICTIVE VALUE OF FETAL URINALYSIS FOR POSTNATAL RENAL FUNCTION

	Author	Threshold	Sensitivity	Specificity	PPV	NPV
Sodium	Muller[80]	> 50 mmol/L	0.82	0.64	0.6	
	Nicolini[78]	> 95th centile** (mmol/L)	0.87	0.8		
	Johnson[82]*	> 100 mg/dl	1.0	0.79	0.7	1.0
	Nicolaides[81]	> 95th centile** (mmol/L)			0.9	0.7
β_2 microglobulin	Muller[80]	> 2 mg/L	0.8	0.83	0.8	
	Johnson[82]*	> 4 mg/L	0.22	1.0	1.0	0.68
Calcium	Muller[80]	> 0.95 mmol/L	0.53	0.84	0.6	
	Nicolini[78]	> 95th centile** (mmol/L)	1.0	0.6		
	Johnson[82]*	> 8 mg/dl	0.88	0.47	0.47	0.88
	Nicolaides[81]	> 95th centile* (mmol/L)			1.0	0.7
Osmolality	Johnson[82]*	> 200 mOsm/L	1.0	0.84	0.77	1.0
Creatinine	Nicolaides[81]	> 95th centile** (mmol/L)			1.0	0.4
	Muller[80]	< 200 mmol/L	0.64	0.89	0.85	
Total protein	Muller[80]	> 0.04 g/L	0.65	0.89	1.0	
	Johnson[82]*	> 20 mg/dl	0.88	0.71	0.64	0.91

*Results from 3rd of 3 sequential samples; ** for gestational age
PPV = positive predictive value; NPV = negative predictive value
Definitions of "normal" renal function: Muller[80]—serum creatinine ≥50 mmol/L at 1 year of age; Johnson[82]—urine creatinine < 1.0 mg/dl at 2 years of age; Nicolaides[81]—serum creatinine < 70 mmol/L at 1–6 years of age; Nicolini[78]—not stated.

Fluid instillation may aid in visualization if there is anhydramnios,[27] although we have rarely found this to be necessary.

Fine-needle aspiration under ultrasound guidance (vesicocentesis) temporarily relieves the megacystis and allows urine to be analyzed for **assessment of renal function**[78-81] and karyotype.[86] If the urine reaccumulates rapidly (which itself is indicative of function) and the other prognostic factors (see box) are favorable, placement of a permanent shunt may be considered. Fetal urinary sodium (Na^+), calcium (Ca^{++}), osmolality, and β_2 microglobulin (in combination) appear to be the most predictive of outcome[78-84] and form the mainstay of biochemical evaluation at present (Table 37-6). Initially, fixed cutoff values were suggested for each variable as predictors of poor prognosis.[70] However, it is now clear that the normal levels of many parameters vary with gestational age and must be interpreted accordingly. Specifically, sodium and β_2 microglobulin levels decrease throughout gestation, whereas calcium and creatinine rise.[78,81,85] In general, more hypotonic fetal urine correlates with a more favorable outcome. Some groups advocate that the last of three sequential urine samplings at 48- to 72-hr intervals is most reflective of true renal function.[82,87,90] Recently, it has been suggested that fetal blood levels of β_2 microglobulin may better assess glomerular filtration rate, as opposed to urinary markers which generally reflect tubular function.[88] As yet, this has not been shown to hold any advantages over the simpler urinalysis.[89] A "urinary function profile," which combines a number of biochemical *and* sonographic predictors, appears to be of most clinical value. Only carefully selected fetuses, with adequate renal function, despite significant oligohydramnios, are likely to benefit from *in utero* intervention, and in our center, only a handful of the fetuses who are referred with LUTO go on to such treatment.

ANTENATAL PREDICTORS OF POOR POSTNATAL RENAL FUNCTION

Ultrasound	Severe oligohydramnios—especially if early onset
	Increased renal echogenicity
	Renal cortical cysts
	Slow bladder refilling after vesicocentesis
Fetal urine	↑Na^+, ↑Ca^{++}, ↑osmolality, ↑β_2 microglobulin
Fetal blood	↑β_2 microglobulin

Our approach is to **counsel the parents** extensively beforehand, with input from perinatology, pediatrics, urology, nephrology, and social work. Parents are also given the opportunity to speak to others who have faced similar dilemmas. Before any decision is made, we try to ensure that they have an unbiased and complete account of the situation, and are fully aware that, despite successful shunt placement, renal failure or pulmonary hypoplasia may still ensue.

The **technique** involves the insertion of a small plastic double coiled silastic "pigtail" catheter (see Chapter 50 and Fig. 50-8) into the bladder under continuous ultrasound guidance. To facilitate insertion, amnioinfusion is always undertaken beforehand. Antibiotic prophylaxis (cefazolin) and tocolysis (indomethacin) are used for 24 hours. We aim to place the shunt anteriorly in the midline well below the umbilical cord insertion (Fig. 37-17).[90] Color Doppler is used to help avoid maternal and fetal blood vessels. Early intervention is probably necessary for this procedure to be successful in the prevention of pulmonary hypoplasia and preservation of renal function. Usually, significant oligohydramnios is a prerequisite for shunting. Occasionally, intervention may be considered in light of documented worsening renal function on urinalysis or progressively abnormal renal appearance on ultrasound, despite a normal volume of amniotic fluid. Rarely, it may be warranted to place the shunt directly into a dilated renal pelvis rather than the bladder. Shunts may become blocked or dislodged and require replacement in up to 25% of cases.

Antenatal management of LUTO is difficult because: the natural history is unclear; comparison with postnatal series is misleading; patients present at varying stages of progression; and postnatal management and follow up are very variable. To date, no formal randomized evaluation of antenatal vesicoamniotic shunting has been attempted. This assessment must be undertaken if this procedure is to find its true clinical role.

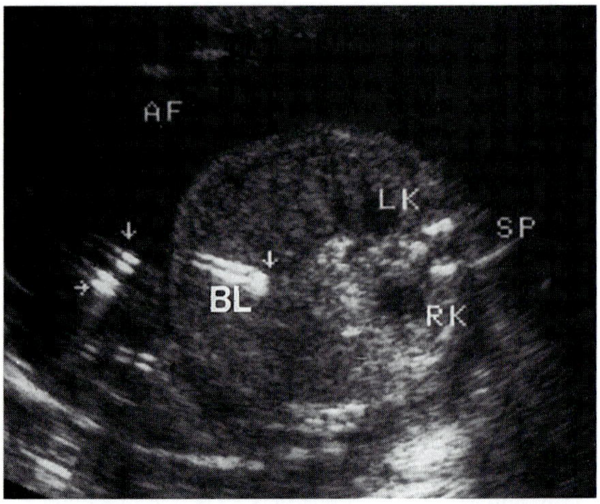

FIG. 37-17. Vesicoamniotic shunt. Arrows indicate catheter in the decompressed bladder (BL) and amniotic fluid (AF). LK—left kidney; RK—right kidney; SP—spine. Note normal amniotic fluid volume.

Renal Cystic Disease

Multicystic Dysplastic Kidney. The classic multicystic dysplastic kidney (MCDK) results from an early, severe urinary obstruction, usually before 8 to 10 weeks. There is atresia of the proximal third of the ureter, with pelvinfundibular atresia.[91,92] This interferes with ureteral branching, resulting in decreased division of collecting tubules and inhibition of induction and maturation of nephrons. Few nephrons develop, and the collecting tubules become cystically enlarged, such that the renal parenchyma is replaced by cysts of varying sizes. Renal function is absent or markedly deficient.

The **sonographic findings** correlate with the gross pathologic appearance. The malformed kidney is usually enlarged but may be normal or small. There are multiple cysts of varying sizes, which do not communicate with each other and are randomly distributed (Fig. 37-18). Large peripheral cysts distort the reniform contour. No normal renal parenchyma exists. The renal pelvis and ureter are usually atretic and not visible.

The appearance and size of MCDK may change markedly over time. On serial examinations, the MCDK and its cysts may either increase or decrease in size or may initially enlarge and later involute.[93,94] This variable appearance is probably caused by minimal residual capacity for glomerular filtration and/or progressive fibrosis.

Assessment of the contralateral kidney is very important. If it is normal, if the bladder is visualized, and if the amniotic fluid volume is normal, then the prognosis is good. However, up to 40% of cases are associated with contralateral renal abnormalities, including **UPJ obstruction, renal agenesis, renal hypoplasia, and bilateral MCDK** (Fig. 37-19).[95] In fetuses with MCDK, severe oligohydramnios and nonvisualization of the urinary bladder imply lethal renal disease, either bilateral MCDK (20%) or contralateral renal agenesis (10%). Contralateral hydronephrosis is present in approximately 7% of cases, usually from UPJ obstruction. Although the prognosis may be favorable in this situation, follow-up ultrasound is necessary to monitor any progressive dilatation or oligohydramnios that may affect obstetric management.

Atypical hydronephrotic form of MCDK is rare. It results from *in utero* obstruction later in development, between the tenth and thirty-sixth week. There is atresia of the proximal third of the ureter, without atresia of the renal pelvis and infundibula.[96] Pathologically, the cystic changes are similar to the classic form. However, because the renal pelvis is dilated, differentiation of this entity from hydronephrosis with predominant calyceal dilatation may be difficult. In hydronephrosis, the dilated calyces are of uniform size, anatomically aligned, and communicate with the dilated renal pelvis. As well, the kidney usually maintains the reniform contour, with renal parenchyma present peripherally.[97]

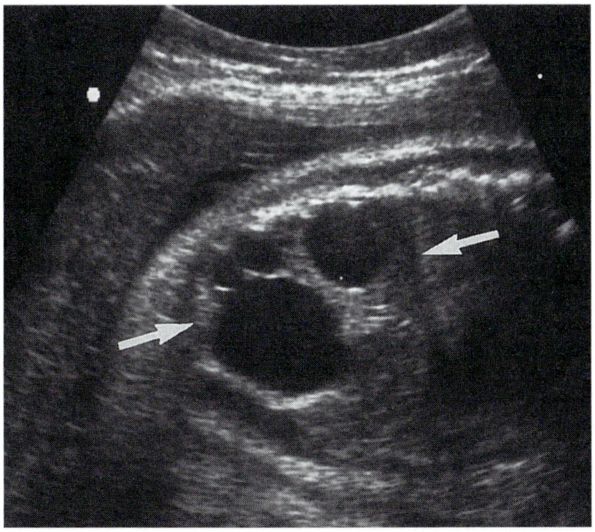

FIG. 37-18. Unilateral multicystic dysplastic kidney. The kidney (*arrows*) is enlarged with multiple cysts of varying sizes which do not communicate with each other and are randomly distributed.

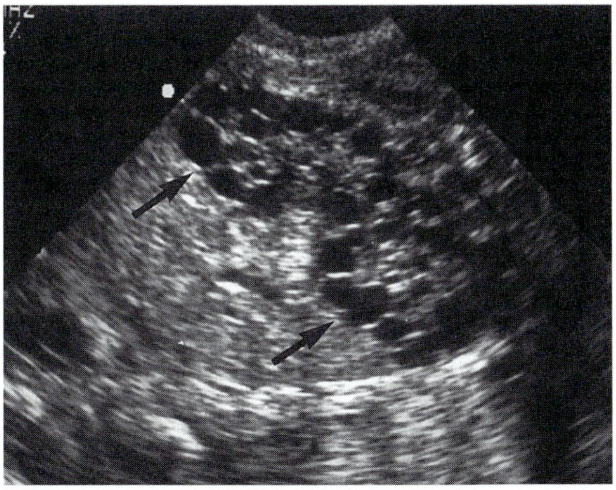

FIG. 37-19. Bilateral multicystic dysplastic kidneys. Transvaginal ultrasound demonstrates numerous small bilateral cysts (*arrows*) and no normal renal parenchyma. There is severe oligohydramnios.

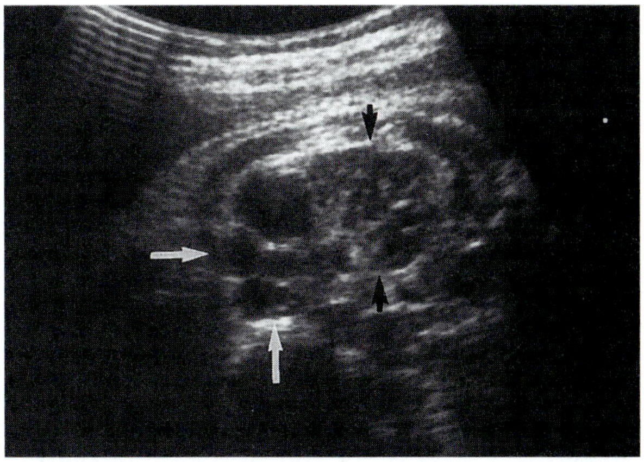

FIG. 37-20. Segmental multicystic dysplasia. Cystic dysplasia (*white arrows*) isolated to the lower pole of a duplex kidney. The upper-pole moiety is normal (*black arrows*).

Segmental multicystic dysplasia occurs in the portion of the duplex kidney supplied by the atretic ureter (Fig. 37-20).

The tendency for MCDK to **involute** in time has been well documented, both before and after birth.[93,98] Complications in MCDK, such as hypertension, sepsis, and malignancy, are extremely rare.[99] Therefore, most urologists currently advocate close follow-up with serial ultrasound, rather than prophylactic nephrectomy.[99] Most cases of MCDK are sporadic, with a low recurrence risk.

Obstructive Cystic Renal Dysplasia. Experimental work in lambs has shown that urinary obstruction in the first half of gestation produces renal dysplasia, defined as disturbed differentiation of nephrogenic tissue.[67,70] The pathogenesis of renal dysplasia associated with obstructive uropathy remains unclear. Osathanondh and Potter[91] theorized that the changes seen are a result of ampullary injury caused by increased back pressure secondary to interference with urinary outflow.[91] They found the kidneys to be variable in size, from small, normal, to greatly enlarged. In some cases, the enlargement is due partly to the presence of cysts and partly to hydronephrosis. Cysts are usually present in the subcapsular area of the cortex. In a fetus with obstructive uropathy, the sonographic identification of **cortical cysts** is indicative of **renal dysplasia** (i.e., irreversible renal damage) (Fig. 37-21).[100] Dysplastic kidneys may also demonstrate increased echogenicity relative to the surrounding fetal structures, presumably from abundant fibrous tissue (Fig. 37-22). However, **increased cortical echogenicity is not a specific finding,**[100,101] and a diagnosis of renal dysplasia cannot be made on the basis of increased parenchymal echogenicity alone. Further, it is important to recognize that not all dysplastic kidneys have sonographically visible cysts or increased cortical echogenicity, so one cannot accurately predict the absence of renal dysplasia. The functional capacity of an affected kidney depends on the severity of renal dysplasia, which varies with the timing and degree of obstruction and determines the prognosis of patients surviving the perinatal period.

In general, if the obstruction is early and complete, the renal parenchymal findings will be predominantly macroscopic cysts, and simulate multicystic dysplasia. Distinction between MCDK and obstructive cystic renal dysplasia may be difficult, especially in the absence of hydronephrosis. In cystic renal dysplasia,

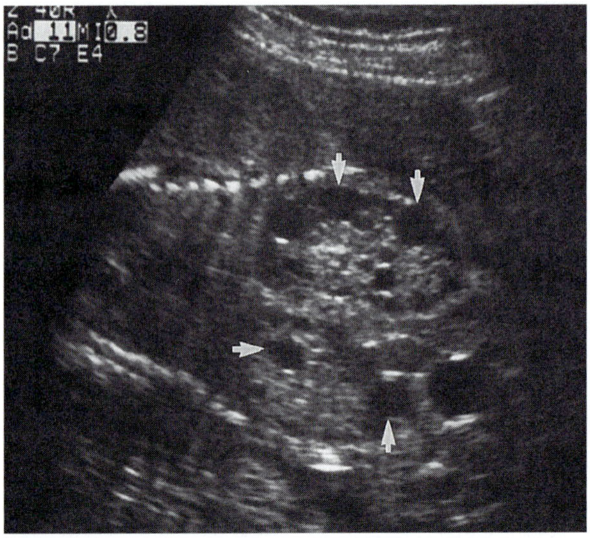

FIG. 37-21. Obstructive cystic dysplasia. Coronal scan in a fetus with posterior urethral valves shows diffuse cortical cysts in both kidneys (*arrows*), indicative of irreversible renal damage.

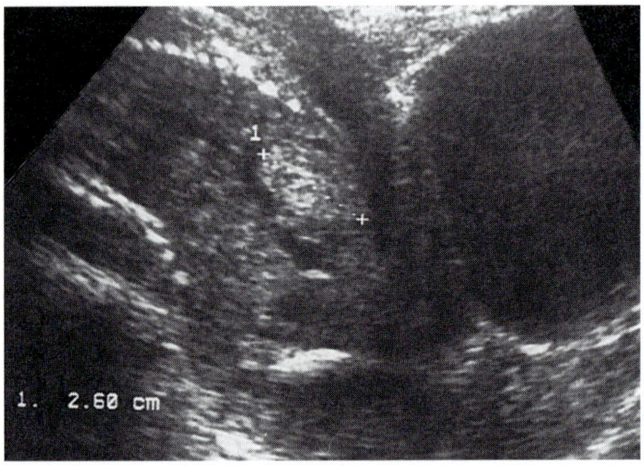

FIG. 37-22. Echogenic, dysplastic kidney. The kidney (marked by calipers) is intensely echogenic in a fetus with urethral obstruction. Note the absence of hydronephrosis.

recognizable parenchyma surrounds the relatively small cysts, whereas in MCDK, no normal renal parenchyma can be identified between cysts. Cystic renal dysplasia most commonly occurs with urethral obstruction. Therefore, sonographic evidence of urethral obstruction would be helpful. In addition, cystic renal dysplasia from LUTO frequently involves both kidneys, but bilateral MCDK occurs in only 20% of cases.

Autosomal Recessive (Infantile) Polycystic Kidney Disease (ARPKD). ARPKD involves both the kidneys and liver. There is a wide clinical spectrum, which varies from the **perinatal form** (with severe renal disease, minimal hepatic fibrosis, and early death from pulmonary hypoplasia), to the **juvenile form** (with minimal renal disease, marked hepatic fibrosis and longer survival). Diffuse saccular dilatation of the renal collecting tubules produces numerous 1- to 2-mm cysts. Both kidneys are enlarged, but a smooth contour is maintained. The cut surface has a spongelike appearance with linear cysts present throughout the renal cortex and medulla.

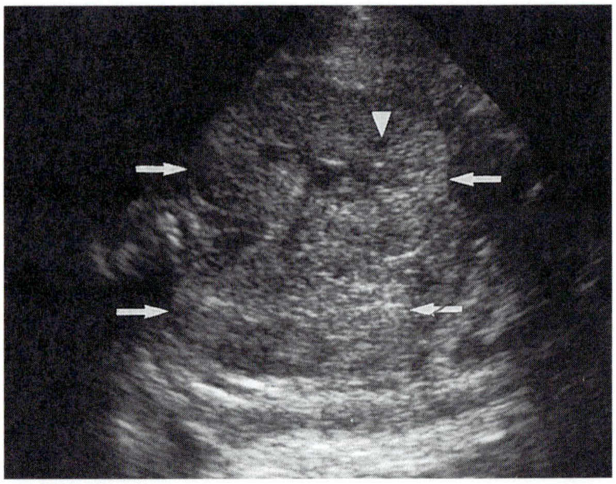

FIG. 37-23. Autosomal recessive polycystic kidney disease. Coronal scan shows enlarged kidneys with increased echogenicity (*arrows*). Occasionally, small 1- to 2-mm cysts (*arrowhead*) may be detected.

Sonography reveals **bilateral reniform enlargement** of the kidneys (Fig. 37-23). There is poor delineation of the intrarenal structures. The numerous tiny cysts are usually smaller than the limit of sonographic resolution, but they create multiple acoustic interfaces accounting for the characteristic **increased renal echogenicity.**[102] Sometimes, a peripheral hypoechoic rim may be seen, surrounding the centrally increased echogenicity. With high-resolution equipment, scattered small cysts may be identified. When renal function is abnormal, there is oligohydramnios and the bladder may not be seen. The size of the kidneys and cyst size do not correlate with renal function.

ARPKD may be diagnosed as early as 16 weeks on the basis of oligohydramnios and the characteristic renal abnormalities, especially if the fetus is at risk.[102] Because of the variability in expression and gestational age at onset, the kidneys may appear normal initially and only become abnormal later on.[103-105] **Thus, a normal sonogram in a fetus at risk for ARPKD does not exclude this disease, and early prenatal diagnosis is not always possible.** Couples who have a child with ARPKD have a 25% risk of having another affected child with each subsequent pregnancy. Usually, but not always, ultrasound shows evidence of recurrence by 24 to 26 weeks.[103,105]

A

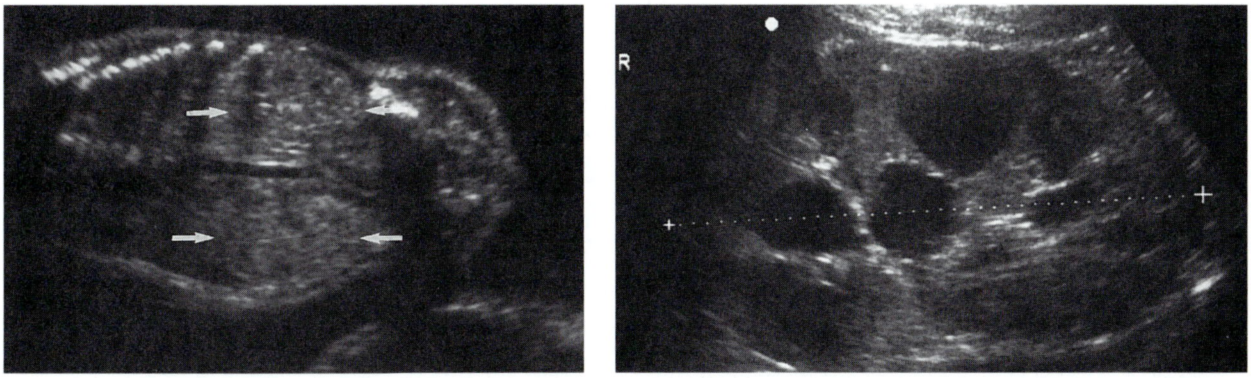

B

FIG. 37-24. Autosomal dominant polycystic kidney disease. **A,** Coronal scan of fetal abdomen shows enlarged, echogenic kidneys (*arrows*). No cysts were seen. **B, Maternal** autosomal dominant polycystic kidney disease. Classic ultrasound appearance of large kidney (15 cm) with multiple cysts.

Even in the absence of a family history, sonographic demonstration of bilaterally enlarged echogenic kidneys most likely indicates ARPKD, although other rare possibilities would include early manifestation of autosomal dominant polycystic kidney disease (ADPKD), congenital nephrotic syndrome (Finnish nephrosis), medullary cystic disease, bilateral renal tumors, congenital metabolic diseases, etc. Ultrasound of the parents' kidneys may help to distinguish between ARPKD and ADPKD suspected in the fetus. Because ADPKD is transmitted by a do minant gene, one parent has the disease, and sonography usually establishes the diagnosis.

Autosomal Dominant (Adult) Polycystic Kidney Disease (ADPKD). This disease occasionally presents *in utero*. The sonographic appearance of the kidneys is variable in the reported cases. Renal enlargement is the most common finding.[106] Often, there is increased renal echogenicity (Fig. 37-24, *A*). Cysts may or may not be present. Amniotic fluid volume is usually normal. Although antenatal diagnosis by ultrasound has been made at 14 weeks, the kidneys may appear normal in the second trimester, and only become abnormal in the third trimester.[107] ADPKD can be difficult or impossible to distinguish sonographically from ARPKD. A family history of ADPKD is critical in making the diagnosis of ADPKD in the fetus, as the recurrence risk is 50%. However, in one review, only 38% of the affected parents were aware of their disease prior to the diagnosis in the affected child.[106] Therefore, ultrasound of the parents' kidneys is necessary (Fig. 37-24, *B*). When there is a positive family history, prenatal diagnosis is now possible with DNA studies after chorionic villus sampling.[107]

The outcome of the fetus with ADPKD diagnosed by ultrasound is variable.[108] If the AFV is normal, the prognosis is reasonably favorable.

CONDITIONS ASSOCIATED WITH RENAL CYSTS (PARTIAL LIST)

Autosomal dominant
Autosomal dominant (adult) polycystic kidney disease
Tuberous sclerosis
Von Hippel-Lindau disease

Autosomal recessive
Autosomal recessive (infantile) polycystic kidney disease
Jeune syndrome (asphyxiating thoracic dystrophy)
Laurence-Moon-Bardet-Biedl syndrome
Meckel-Gruber syndrome
Short-rib polydactyly syndromes
Zellweger (cerebro-hepato-renal) syndrome

X-Linked
Orofaciodigital syndrome type 1

Chromosomal
Trisomy 13
Trisomy 18
Turner syndrome
Triploidy

Other Conditions Associated With Renal Cysts

A wide variety of rare inherited syndromes, genetic and chromosomal disorders are associated with cystic kidneys (see box above).[109] Approximately 30% of fetuses with trisomy 13 and 10% of fetuses with trisomy 18 have cystic kidneys.

Meckel-Gruber syndrome. This is a lethal autosomal recessive disorder that carries a 25% risk of recurrence. Sonographic diagnosis requires identification

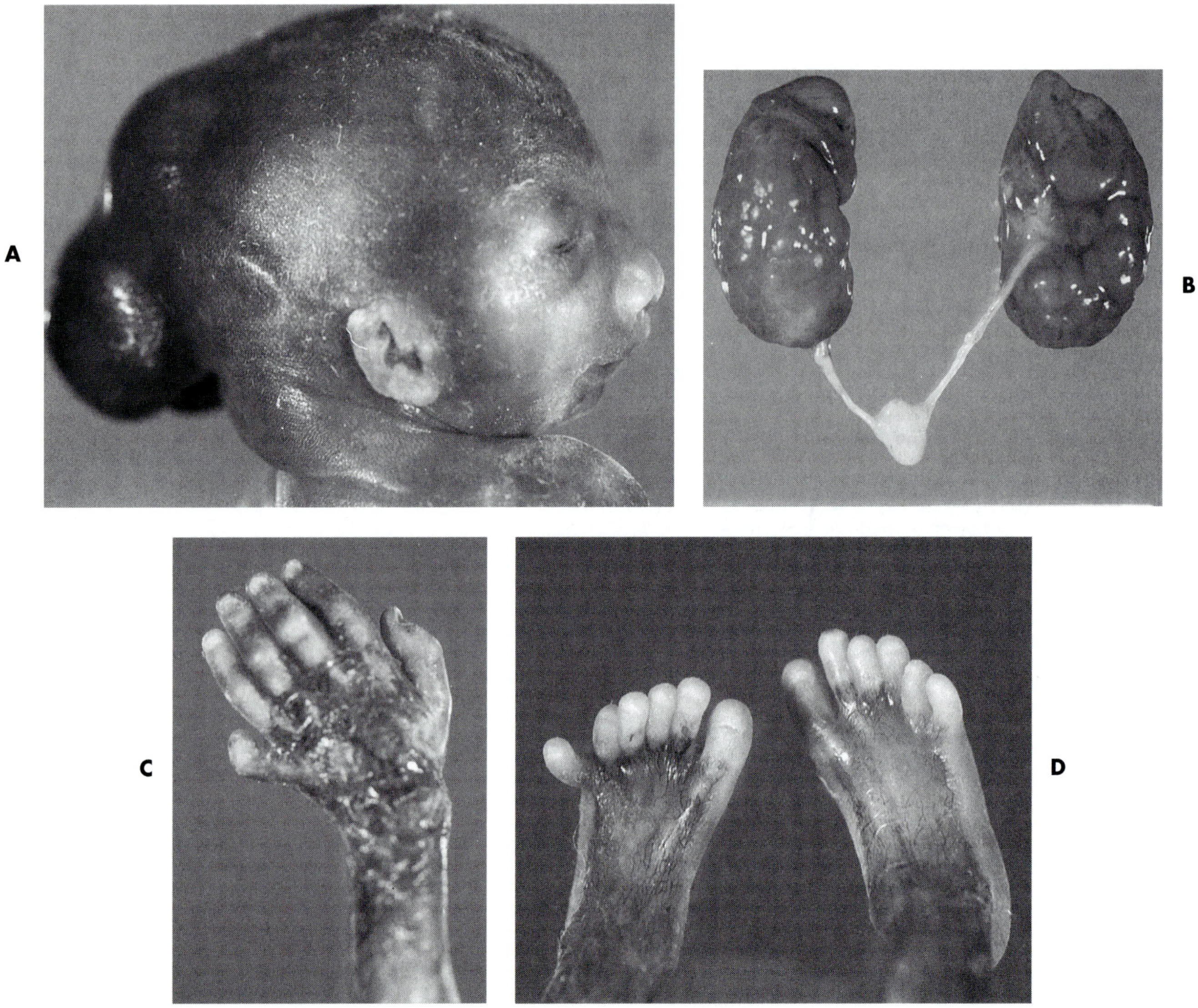

FIG. 37-25. Meckel-Gruber syndrome. Eighteen-week-old fetus with classic features of Meckel-Gruber syndrome. **A,** Occipital encephalocele. **B,** Large polycystic kidneys. **C and D,** Polydactyly.

of at least two features of the **classic triad: polycystic kidneys** (present in nearly 100% of cases), occipital **cephalocele** (60% to 85%), and postaxial **polydactyly** (55%) (Fig. 37-25).[110] The kidneys are usually large and echogenic. Often, small discrete cysts are visible. The cephalocele is variable in size and can be difficult to detect in the presence of marked oligohydramnios. Microcephaly can be a useful clue to the presence of a cephalocele. Early prenatal diagnosis of Meckel-Gruber syndrome is possible, especially if there is a positive family history. Detection of bilateral renal cystic dysplasia should initiate a search for an occipital cephalocele. The diagnosis of Meckel-Gruber syndrome is particularly important for counselling future pregnancies in families not previously known to be at risk.

Renal Neoplasm

Congenital renal tumors are rare. The most common tumor is **mesoblastic nephroma**, also known as leiomyomatous hamartoma or fetal renal hamartoma. Histologically, it is composed of mesenchymal tissue (spindle cells), as opposed to the epithelial tissue of Wilms' tumor. Mesoblastic nephroma typically presents in the first year of life, has a benign course, and nephrectomy is usually curative. Wilms' tumor is a malignant lesion which is extremely uncommon in the neonate.

Sonographically, mesoblastic nephroma is indistinguishable from Wilms' tumor.[111-113] Mesoblastic nephroma is unilateral and may be seen as a solid mass completely replacing the kidney or localized to part of the kidney (Fig. 37-26). It may contain cystic areas,

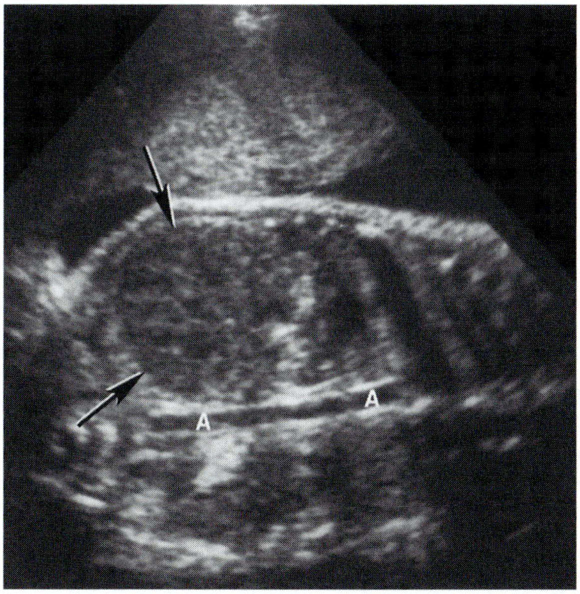

FIG. 37-26. Congenital mesoblastic nephroma. Longitudinal scan shows a large solid mass (*arrows*) replacing the lower pole of the kidney. A—fetal aorta. (Courtesy of Randall M. Pattern, MD; Laurence A. Mack, MD; Keith Y. Wang, MD, PhD; Dale R. Cyr, RDMS.)

caused by hemorrhage and cystic degeneration. **Polyhydramnios** is a frequent association (for unknown reasons), and may lead to premature labor, premature rupture of membranes, and premature birth.

Adrenal Mass

The adrenal glands are normally quite prominent *in utero*. They are seen as disclike paraspinal structures on transverse view and as Y- or V-shaped structures at the superior border of the kidneys on longitudinal sonogram (Fig. 37-27). The echogenicity of the adrenal glands is similar to that of the kidneys, with a hyperechoic center (medulla) and a hypoechoic periphery (cortex). **The differential diagnosis for fetal suprarenal masses** includes: neuroblastoma or hemorrhage in the adrenal, pulmonary sequestration, enteric duplication cysts, and renal masses including mesoblastic nephroma, upper-pole cystic dysplasia, or hydronephrosis in a duplex kidney.[114]

Neuroblastoma is the most common neonatal malignancy, and the adrenal gland is the most common primary site. The sonographic appearance is variable, and can be solid, cystic, or mixed.[114,115] Occasionally, there may be maternal symptoms related to increased catecholamines in late pregnancy. Patients with neuroblastoma detected by prenatal sonography generally follow a clinically favorable course in which surgical resection is curative.[116]

Adrenal hemorrhage can have a sonographic appearance similar to that of an adrenal or renal neoplasm. The key to the diagnosis is evolution of the lesion over time, serial sonograms demonstrating a change in echogenicity (from solid to cystic), and a decrease in size of the mass (Fig. 37-28).[117,118]

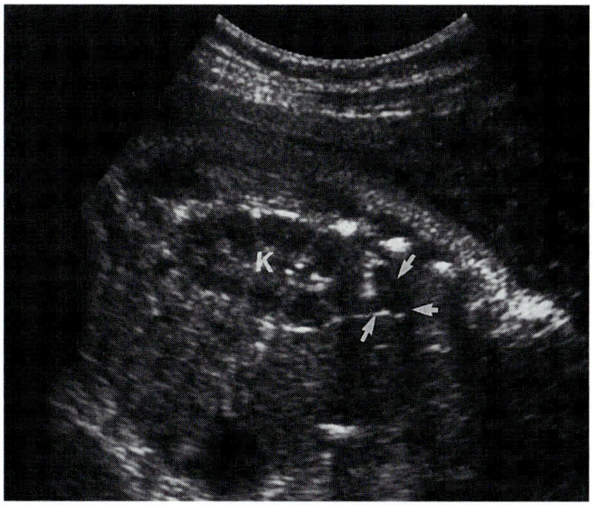

FIG. 37-27. Normal adrenal gland. Longitudinal scan demonstrates the Y- or V-shaped adrenal gland (*arrows*) at the superior border of the kidney (K).

THE GENITAL TRACT

Normal Genitalia

There are medical (as well as social) implications for documentation of fetal gender. These include identification of male fetuses at risk for severe X-linked disorders, and in twin pregnancies, documentation of different sexes proves zygosity and thus excludes the possibility of complications seen only in monozygotic twins. Accurate sonographic determination of fetal gender depends on the gestational age, fetal position, and operator experience. Between 16 and 20 weeks of gestation, the external genitalia can be visualized in 84% of fetuses, and fetal gender can be correctly assigned in 93% of these cases (Fig. 37-29, *A*).[119] The rate of sonographic visualization of the genitalia and the accuracy of fetal gender determination improve after 24 weeks.[120,121] Inopportune fetal position, early gestation, oligohydramnios, and maternal obesity represent the major limitations in fetal gender assessment. Errors may occur when the rounded, apposed labia are mistaken for a small, empty scrotum or when the umbilical cord is confused with a phallus. Using transvaginal sonography, Bronshtein et al.[122] reported that fetal sex can be correctly diagnosed in the majority (> 90%) of fetuses between 13 and 16 weeks of gestation. The testicles normally descend into the scrotum between 26 and 34 menstrual weeks.[120] When testicles are identified within the scrotum, the diagnosis of a male fetus is certain. Small hydroceles are common in

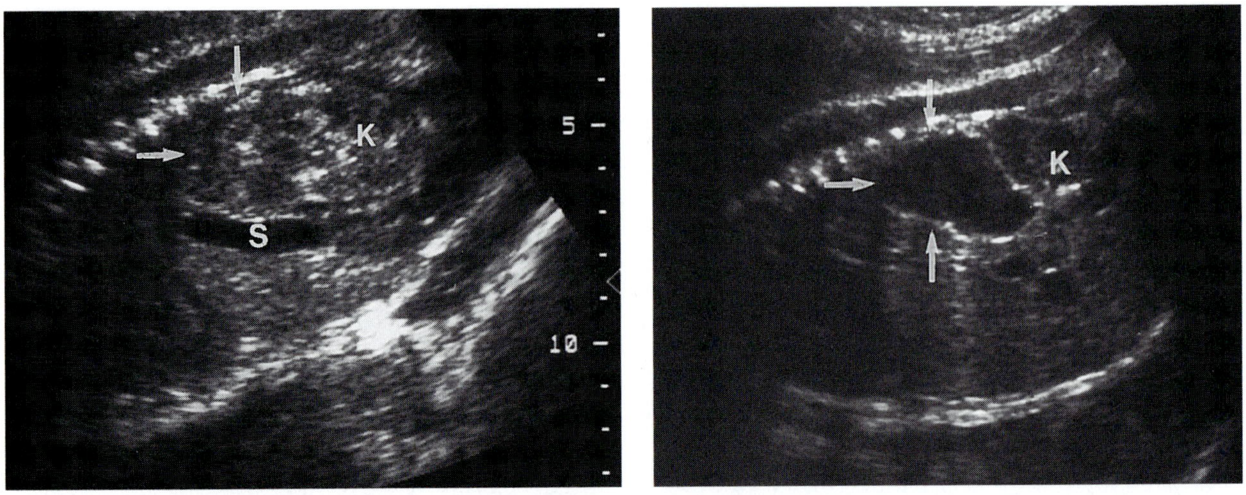

FIG. 37-28. Adrenal hemorrhage. A, Longitudinal scan shows a solid mass (*arrows*) adjacent to the upper pole of the kidney (K). S—stomach. **B,** Four days later, the mass (*arrows*) has a mixed echo pattern, with a predominant cystic component. Ultrasound scan of patient at 2 months of age (not shown) showed complete resolution of the mass.

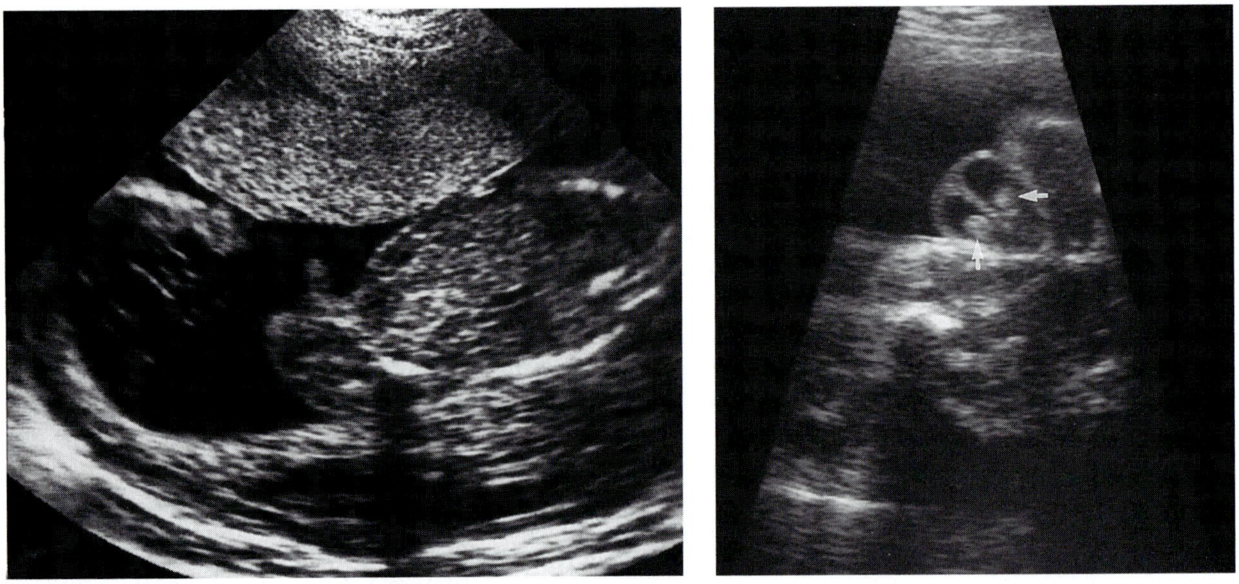

FIG. 37-29. Male fetus. A, Normal 20-week-old fetus, midsagittal scan showing the typical erect position of the normal phallus. **B,** Scan of the scrotal sac (in a 36-week-old fetus) demonstrates testicles (*arrows*) and bilateral hydroceles.

third-trimester male fetuses and are usually of no clinical significance (Fig. 37-29, *B*). However, large hydroceles, especially if they increase in size over time, suggest an open communication between the processus vaginalis and peritoneal cavity. In such cases, postnatal evaluation for inguinal hernia should be performed.[123]

Abnormal Genitalia

With careful examination of the fetal perineum, abnormalities of the phallus (hypospadias, micropenis) and ambiguous genitalia can be diagnosed.[124-126] In cases of hypospadias, a ventral curvature of the penis (chordee) may be observed (Fig. 37-30). Making this diagnosis in some families may be important because hypospadias can be associated with certain diseases such as Opitz syndrome (hypertelorism and hypospadias).[127] A male fetus with micropenis and undescended testes cannot be distinguished from the virilized female who has labioscrotal fusion and clitoral hypertrophy.

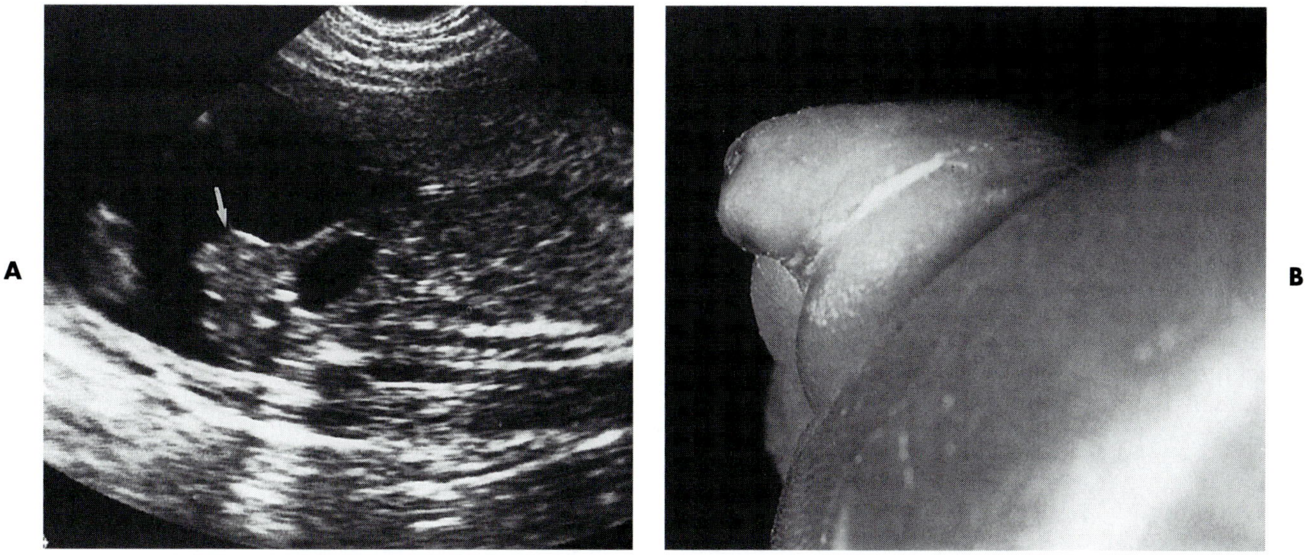

FIG. 37-30. Hypospadias. **A,** Fetus with Opitz syndrome, midsagittal scan showing ventral curvature of the penis (*arrow*). **B,** Lateral view of affected phallus with hypospadias. (From Hogdall C, Siegel-Bartelt J, Toi A, et al. Prenatal diagnosis of Opitz syndrome in the second trimester by ultrasound detection of hypospadias and hypertelorism. *Prenat Diagn* 1989;9:783-793. Reprinted by permission of John Wiley & Sons, Ltd.)

Intersex states may be divided into hormonally and nonhormonally mediated abnormalities. The former includes **congenital adrenal hyperplasia,** the most common cause of virilization of the newborn female. Intersex states that are not hormonally mediated often have associated caudal or urinary tract anomalies, chromosomal aberrations, or may conform to one of numerous multiple malformation syndromes.

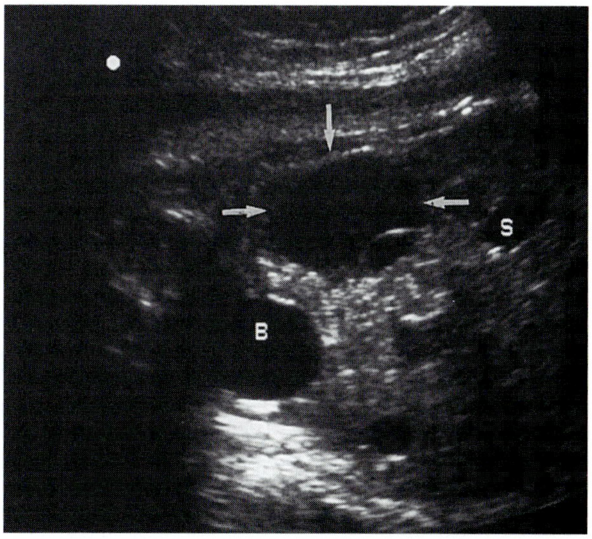

FIG. 37-31. Ovarian cyst. Cystic mass (*arrows*) in the lower abdomen of a female fetus, separate from the kidneys (not shown), bladder (B), and stomach (S). Subsequent postnatal ultrasound showed spontaneous resolution.

Hydrometrocolpos

Hydrometrocolpos, enlargement of the obstructed uterus and vagina from retained secretions, may be the result of a number of causes including vaginal or cervical atresia, imperforate hymen, and vaginal membranes. Sonographically, an ovoid mass, either cystic or complex, is seen posterior to the bladder.[128] This should be differentiated from the rectosigmoid colon (either normally filled with meconium or obstructed) which is seen as a tubular structure. The enlarged uterus may compress the urinary tract and cause hydronephrosis or hydroureter.

Ovarian Cysts

The vast majority (97%) of fetal ovarian cysts are **benign functional cysts.**[129] They probably result from maternal and placental hormonal stimulation; and simple cysts usually resolve spontaneously within 6 months of birth.[129,130]

The main criteria for diagnosis are: the presence of a cystic mass, usually located on one side of the pelvis or lower abdomen; normal urinary and gastrointestinal tracts; and female gender.[131] The diagnosis is always presumptive, since rare lesions such as **enteric duplications, mesenteric cysts, or urachal cysts** cannot be ruled out with absolute certainty. Most ovarian cysts are small and simple by ultrasound criteria. Sometimes, internal septae can be seen (Fig. 37-31). The presence of fluid-debris level, retracting clot, and/or solid components correlates with torsion or hemorrhage of the cyst.[132,133] In most cases, identification of an ovarian cyst does not alter obstetric care. Large ovarian cysts may cause intestinal obstruction, polyhydramnios, and/or dystocia.

Postnatal management depends on the cyst size and sonographic patterns. Simple cysts that are smaller than **4 cm** are managed conservatively with serial ultrasound. Complex cystic masses, symptomatic cysts, and cysts that do not resolve require surgery. With cysts larger than 4 cm, there is a significant risk of complications, such as torsion and rupture. Early surgery has been advocated, but this remains controversial.[129,134]

CONCLUSION

The most common antenatally detected fetal anomalies are genitourinary in origin. A thorough sonographic evaluation of renal structure, function, and associated anomalies will improve the accuracy of antenatal diagnosis, thus enabling optimal obstetric and neonatal management.

REFERENCES

The Normal Urinary Tract

1. Moore KL, Persaud TVN. The urogenital system. In: *The Developing Human: Clinically Oriented Embryology*, ed 5. Philadelphia: WB Saunders, 1993:265-303.
2. Bronshtein M, Kushnir O, Ben-Rafael Z et al. Transvaginal sonographic measurement of fetal kidneys in the first trimester of pregnancy. *J Clin Ultrasound* 1990;18:299-301.
3. Bronshtein M, Yoffe N, Brandes JN et al. First and early second trimester diagnosis of fetal urinary tract anomalies using transvaginal sonography. *Prenat Diagn* 1990;10:653-666.
4. Bowie JD, Rosenberg ER, Andreotti RF et al. The changing sonographic appearance of fetal kidneys during pregnancy. *J Ultrasound Med* 1983;2:505-507.
5. Patriquin H, Lefaivre J, Lafortune M et al. Fetal lobation: an anatomo-ultrasonographic correlation. *J Ultrasound Med* 1990;9:191-197.
6. Bertagnoli L, Lalatta F, Gallicchio MD et al. Quantitative characterization of the growth of the fetal kidney. *J Clin Ultrasound* 1983;11:349-356.
7. Cohen HL, Cooper J, Eisenberg P et al. Normal length of fetal kidneys: sonographic study in 397 obstetric patients. *AJR* 1991;157:545-548.
8. Grannum P, Bracken M, Silverman R et al. Assessment of fetal kidney size in normal gestation by comparison of ratio of kidney circumference. *Am J Obstet Gynecol* 1980;136:249-254.
9. Rabinowitz R, Peters MT, Vya S et al. Measurements of fetal urine production in normal pregnancy by real-time ultrasonography. *Am J Obstet Gynecol* 1989;161:1264-1266.
10. Abramovich DR. The volume of amniotic fluid and its regulating factors. In Fairweather DVI, Eskers TKA editors: *Amniotic Fluid Research and Clinical Application*, ed 2. Amsterdam: Excerpta Medica, 1978:31-49.
11. Halpern ME, Fong KW, Zalev AH et al. Reliability of amniotic fluid volume estimation from ultrasonograms: intraobserver and interobserver variation before and after the establishment of criteria. *Am J Obstet Gynecol* 1985;153:264-267.
12. Goldstein RB, Filly RA. Sonographic estimation of amniotic fluid volume: subjective assessment versus pocket measurements. *J Ultrasound Med* 1988;7:363-369.
13. Chamberlain PF, Manning FA, Morrison I et al. Ultrasound evaluation of amniotic fluid volume. *Am J Obstet Gynecol* 1984;150:245-249.
14. Rutherford SE, Smith CV, Phelan JP et al. Four-quadrant assessment of amniotic fluid volume. Interobserver and intraobserver variation. *J Reprod Med* 1987;32:587-589.
15. Moore TR, Cayle JE. The amniotic fluid index in normal human pregnancy. *Am J Obstet Gynecol* 1990;162:1168-1173.
16. Hashimoto BE, Kramer DJ, Brennan L. Amniotic fluid volume: fluid dynamics and measurement technique. *Semin US CT MR* 1993;14:40-55.

Urinary Tract Abnormalities

17. Levi S, Schaaps JP, De Havay P et al. End-result of routine ultrasound screening for congenital anomalies: the Belgian multicentric study 1984-92. *Ultrasound Obstet Gynecol* 1995;5:366-371.
18. Barss VA, Benacerraf BR, Frigoletto FD. Second trimester oligohydramnios, a predictor of poor fetal outcome. *Obstet Gynecol* 1984;64:608-610.
19. Nicolaides KH, Cheng HH, Abbas A et al. Fetal renal defects: associated malformations and chromosomal defects. *Fetal Diagn Ther* 1992;7:1-11.
20. Roodhooft AM, Birnholz JC, Holmes LB. Familial nature of congenital absence and severe dysgenesis of both kidneys. *N Engl J Med* 1984;310:1341-1345.
21. Potter EL. Bilateral absence of ureters and kidneys. A report of 50 cases. *Obstet Gynecol* 1965;25:3-12.
22. Dubbins P, Curt A, Rappner R et al. Renal agenesis: spectrum of *in utero* findings. *J Clin Ultrasound* 1981;9:189-193.
23. McGahan JP, Myracle MR. Adrenal hypertrophy: possible pitfall in the sonographic diagnosis of renal agenesis. *J Ultrasound Med* 1986;5:265-268.
24. Hoffman CK, Filly RA, Callen PW. The "lying down" adrenal sign: a sonographic indicator of renal agenesis or ectopia in fetuses and neonates. *J Ultrasound Med* 1992;11:533-536.
25. Harman CR. Maternal furosemide may not provoke urine production in the compromised fetus. *Am J Obstet Gynecol* 1984;150:322-323.
26. Raghavendra BN, Young BK, Greco MA et al. Use of furosemide in pregnancies complicated by oligohydramnios. *Radiology* 1987;165:455-458.
27. Haeusler MCH, Ryan G, Robson SC et al. The use of saline solution as a contrast medium in suspected diaphragmatic hernia and renal agenesis. *Am J Obstet Gynecol* 1993;168:1486-1492.
28. Benacerraf BR. Examination of the second trimester fetus with severe oligohydramnios using transvaginal scanning. *Obstet Gynecol* 1990;175:491-493.
29. Wladimiroff JW, Heydanus R, Stewart PA et al. Fetal renal artery flow velocity waveforms in the presence of congenital renal tract anomalies. *Prenat Diagn* 1993;13:545-548.
30. DeVore GR. The value of color Doppler sonography in the diagnosis of renal agenesis. *J Ultrasound Med* 1995;14:443-449.
31. Sepulveda W, Stagiannis KD, Flack NJ et al. Accuracy of prenatal diagnosis of renal agenesis with color flow imaging in severe second-trimester oligohydramnios. *Am J Obstet Gynecol* 1995;173:1788-1792.
32. Carter CO, Evans K, Pescia G. A family study of renal agenesis. *J Med Genet* 1979;16:176-188.
33. Glazebrook KN, McGrath FP, Steele BT. Prenatal compensatory renal growth: documentation with US. *Radiology* 1993;189:733-735.

34. Dunnick NR, McCallum RW, Sandler CM. Congenital anomalies. In: *Textbook of Uroradiology*, Baltimore, Williams and Wilkins, 1991, pp 15-18.
35. Hill LM, Peterson CS. Antenatal diagnosis of fetal pelvic kidneys. *J Ultrasound Med* 1987;6:393-396.
36. Greenblatt AM, Beretsky I, Lankin DH et al. *In utero* diagnosis of crossed renal ectopia using high resolution real-time ultrasound. *J Ultrasound Med* 1985;4:105-107.
37. King KL, Kofinas AD, Simon NV et al. Antenatal ultrasound diagnosis of fetal horseshoe kidney. *J Ultrasound Med* 1991;10:643-644.
38. Barth RAD, Filly RA, Sondheimer FK. Prenatal sonographic findings in bladder exstrophy. *J Ultrasound Med* 1990;9:359-361.
39. Gearhart JP, Ben-Chaim J, Jeffs RD et al. Criteria for the prenatal diagnosis of classic bladder exstrophy. *Obstet Gynecol* 1995;85:961-964.
40. Preston A, Lebowitz RL. What's new in pediatric uroradiology? *Urol Radiol* 1989;11:217-220.
41. Crane JP, LeFevre ML, Winborn RC et al. A randomized trial of prenatal ultrasonographic screening: impact on the detection, management, and outcome of anomalous fetuses. *Am J Obstet Gynecol* 1994;171:392-399.
42. Woodward JR. Hydronephrosis in the neonate. *Urology* 1993;42:620-621.
43. Corteville JE, Gray DL, Crane JP. Congenital hydronephrosis: Correlation of fetal ultrasonographic findings with infant outcome. *Am J Obstet Gynecol* 1991;165:384-388.
44. Anderson NG, Clautice-Engle T, Allan RB et al. Detection of obstructive uropathy in the fetus: predictive value of sonographic measurements of renal pelvic diameter at various gestational ages. *AJR* 1995;164:719-723.
45. Grignon A, Filion R, Filiatrault D et al. Urinary tract dilatation *in utero:* classification and clinical applications. *Radiology* 1986;160:645-647.
46. Arger PH, Coleman BG, Mintz MC et al. Routine fetal genitourinary tract screening. *Radiology* 1985;156:485-489.
47. Ghidini A, Sirtori M, Vergani P et al. Ureteropelvic junction obstruction in utero and ex utero. *Obstet Gynecol* 1990;75:805-808.
48. Lam BC, Wong SN, Yeung CY et al. Outcome and management of babies with prenatal ultrasonographic renal abnormalities. *Am J Perinatol* 1993;(10)4:263-268.
49. Mandell J, Blyth BR, Peters CA et al. Structural genitourinary defects *in utero. Radiology* 1991;178:193-196.
50. Adra AM, Mejides AA, Dennaoui MS et al. Fetal pyelectasis: is it always "physiologic"? *Am J Obstet Gynecol* 1995;173:1263-1266.
51. Wickstrom E, Maizels M, Sabbagha R et al. Isolated fetal pyelectasis: assessment of risk for postnatal uropathy and Down syndrome. *Ultrasound Obstet Gynecol* 1996;8:236-240.
52. Podevin G, Mandelbrot L, Vuillard E et al. Outcome of urological abnormalities prenatally diagnosed by ultrasound. *Fetal Diagn Ther* 1996;11:181-190.
53. Toi A, Fong KW, Salem S et al. Preliminary results of the anteroposterior measurement of the fetal renal pelvis in 328 normal fetuses. Unpublished data.
54. Kleiner B, Callen PW, Filly RA. Sonographic analysis of the fetus with ureteropelvic junction obstruction. *AJR* 1987;148:359-365.
55. Dejter SW, Gibbons MD. The fate of infant kidneys with fetal hydronephrosis but initially normal postnatal sonography. *J Urol* 1989;142:661-663.
56. Laing FC, Burke VD, Wing VW et al. Postpartum evaluation of fetal hydronephrosis: optimal timing for follow-up sonography. *Radiology* 1984;152:423-424.
57. Clautice-Engle T, Anderson NG, Allan RB et al. Diagnosis of obstructive hydronephrosis in infants: comparison sonograms performed 6 days and 6 weeks after birth. *AJR* 1995;164:963-967.
58. Zerin JM, Ritchey ML, Chang ACH: Incidental vesicoureteral reflux in neonates with antenatally detected hydronephrosis and other renal abnormalities. *Radiology* 1993;187:157-160.
59. Corteville JE, Dicke JM, Crane JP. Fetal pyelectasis and Down syndrome: is genetic amniocentesis warranted? *Obstet Gynecol* 1992;79:770-772.
60. Benacerraf BR, Mandell J, Estroff JA et al. Fetal pyelectasis: A possible association with Down syndrome. *Obstet Gynecol* 1990;76:58-60.
61. Snijders RJM, Sebire NJ, Faria M et al. Fetal mild hydronephrosis and chromosomal defects: relation to maternal age and gestation. *Fetal Diagn Ther* 1995;10:349-355.
62. Grignon A, Filiatrault D, Homsy Y et al. Ureteropelvic junction stenosis: antegrade ultrasonographic diagnosis, postnatal investigation, and follow-up. *Radiology* 1986;160:649-651.
63. Jaffe R, Abramowicz J, Feigin M et al. Giant fetal abdominal cyst: ultrasonic diagnosis and management. *J Ultrasound Med* 1987;6:45-47.
64. Ghidini A, Strobelt N, Lynch L et al. Fetal urinoma: a case report and review of its clinical significance. *J Ultrasound Med* 1994;13:989-991.
65. Nussbaum AR, Dorst JP, Jeffs RD et al. Ectopic ureter and ureterocele: Their varied sonographic manifestations. *Radiology* 1986;159:227-235.
66. Winters WD, Lebowitz RL. Importance of prenatal detection of hydronephrosis of the upper pole. *AJR* 1990;155:125-129.
67. Beck AD. The effect of intrauterine urinary obstruction upon the development of the fetal kidney. *J Urol* 1971;105:784-789.
68. Glazer GM, Filly RA, Callen PW. The varied sonographic appearance of the urinary tract in the fetus and newborn with ureteral obstruction. *Radiology* 1982;144:563-568.
69. Mahony BS, Callen PW, Filly RA. Fetal urethral obstruction: ultrasound evaluation. *Radiology* 1985;157:221-224.
70. Harrison MR, Filly RA. The fetus with obstructive uropathy: Pathophysiology, natural history, selection and treatment, in Harrison MR, Golbus MS, Filly RA (editors): *The Unborn Patient: Prenatal Diagnosis and Treatment*, ed 2. Philadelphia, WB Saunders, 1991:328-393.
71. Bierkens AF, Feitz WFJ, Nijhuis JG et al. Early urethral obstruction sequence: a lethal entity? *Fetal Diagn Ther* 1996;11:137-145.
72. Sebire NJ, von Kaisenberg C, Rubio C et al. Fetal megacystis at 10-14 weeks of gestation. *Ultrasound Obstet Gynecol* 1996;8:387-390.
73. Jaramillo D, Lebowitz RL, Hendren WH. The cloacal malformation: radiologic findings and imaging recommendations. *Radiology* 1990;177:441-448.
74. Cilento BG, Benacerraf BR, Mandell J. Prenatal diagnosis of cloacal malformation. *Urology* 1994;43:386-388.
75. Greskovich FJ, Nyberg LM. The prune belly syndrome: a review of its etiology, defects, treatment and prognosis. *J Urol* 1988;140:707-712.
76. Fitzsimons RB, Keohane C, Galvin J. Prune-belly syndrome with ultrasound demonstration of reduction of megacystis *in utero. Br J Radiol* 1985;58:374.
77. Stamm E, King G, Thickman D. Megacystis-microcolon-intestinal hypoperistalsis syndrome: prenatal identification in siblings and review of the literature. *J Ultrasound Med* 1991;10:599-602.

In utero Intervention

78. Nicolini U, Fisk MN, Rodeck CH. Fetal urine biochemistry: an index of renal maturation and dysfunction. *Br J Obstet Gynecol* 1992;99:46-50.

79. Lipitz S, Ryan G, Samuell C et al. Fetal urine analysis for the assessment of renal function in obstructive uropathy. *Am J Obstet Gynecol* 1993;1:174-179.
80. Muller F, Dommergues M, Mandelbrot L, et al. Fetal Urinary Biochemistry Predicts Postnatal Renal Function in Children With Bilateral Obstructive Uropathies. *Obstet Gynecol* 1993; 2:813-820.
81. Nicolaides KH, Cheng HH, Snijders RJM et al. Fetal urine biochemistry in the assessment of obstructive uropathy. *Am J Obstet Gynecol* 1992;166:932-937.
82. Johnson MP, Corsi P, Bradfield W et al. Sequential urinalysis improves evaluation of fetal renal function in obstructive uropathy. *Am J Obstet Gynecol* 1995;173:59-65.
83. Crombleholme TM, Harrison MR, Golbus MS et al. Fetal intervention in obstructive uropathy: Prognostic indicators and efficacy of intervention. *Am J Obstet Gynecol* 1990;162: 1239-1244.
84. Qureshi F, Jacques SM, Seifman et al. *In utero* Fetal Urine Analysis and Renal Histology Correlate with the Outcome in Fetal Obstructive Uropathies. *Fetal Diagn Ther* 1996;11: 306-312.
85. Muller F, Dommergues M, Bussieres L et al. Development of human renal function: reference intervals for 10 biochemical markers in fetal urine. *Clinical Chemistry* 1996;42(11):1855-1860.
86. Teoh TG, Ryan G, Johnson JA, Winsor E. The role of fetal karyotyping from unconventional sources. *Am J Obstet Gynecol* 1996;175:873-877.
87. Johnson MP, Bukowski TP, Reitleman C et al. *In utero* surgical treatment of fetal obstructive uropathy: A new comprehensive approach to identify appropriate candidates for vesicoamniotic shunt therapy. *Am J Obstet Gynecol* 1994;170: 1770-1779.
88. Berry SM, Lecolier B, Smith RS et al. Predictive value of fetal serum β_2-microglobulin for neonatal renal function. *Lancet* 1995;345:1277.
89. Tassis BMG, Trespidi L, Tirelli AS et al. Serum β_2 microglobulin in fetuses with urinary tract abnomalies. *Am J Obstet Gynecol* 1997;1:54-57.
90. Freedman AL, Johnson MP, Evans MI et al. Advances in Fetal Therapy for Obstructive Uropathy. *Dialog Pediatr Urol* 1996;19(4):1-8.

Fetal Renal Cystic Disease

91. Osathanondh V, Potter EL. Pathogenesis of polycystic kidneys, historical survey. *Arch Pathol* 1964;77:459-512.
92. Griscom NT, Vawter GF, Fellers FX. Pelvoinfundibular atresia: the usual form of multicystic kidney: 44 unilateral and 2 bilateral cases. *Semin Roentgenol* 1975;10:125-131.
93. Hashimoto BE, Filly RA, Callen PW. Multicystic dysplastic kidney *in utero:* changing appearance on ultrasound. *Radiology* 1986;159:107-109.
94. Dungan JS, Fernandez MT, Abbitt PL et al. Multicystic dysplastic kidney: natural history of prenatally detected cases. *Prenat Diagn* 1990;10:175-182.
95. Kleiner B, Filly RA, Mack LA et al. Multicystic dysplastic kidney: observations of contralateral disease in the fetal population. *Radiology* 1986;161:27-29.
96. Felson B, Cussen LJ. The hydronephrotic type of unilateral congenital multicystic disease of the kidney. *Semin Roentgenol* 1975;10:113-123.
97. Sanders RC, Hartman DS. The sonographic distinction between neonatal multicystic kidney and hydronephrosis. *Radiology* 1984;151:621-625.
98. Avni EF, Thoua Y, Lalmand B et al. Multicystic dysplastic kidney: natural history from in utero diagnosis and postnatal follow-up. *J Urol* 1987;138:1420-1424.
99. Gordon AC, Thomas DFM, Arthur RJ et al. Multicystic dysplastic kidney: is nephrectomy still appropriate? *J Urol* 1988; 140:1231-1234.
100. Mahony BS, Filly RA, Callen PW. Fetal renal dysplasia: sonographic evaluation. *Radiology* 1984;152:143-146.
101. Estroff JA, Mandell J, Benacerraf BR. Increased renal parenchymal echogenicity in the fetus: Importance and clinical outcome. *Radiology* 1991;181:135-139.
102. Habif DV, Berdon WE, Yeh M-N. Infantile polycystic kidney disease: in utero sonographic diagnosis. *Radiology* 1982; 142:475-477.
103. Romero R, Cullen M, Jeanty P et al. The diagnosis of congenital renal anomalies. II. Infantile polycystic kidney disease. *Am J Obstet Gynecol* 1984;150:259-262.
104. Mahony BS, Callen PW, Filly RA et al. Progression of infantile polycystic kidney disease in early pregnancy. *J Ultrasound Med* 1984;3:277-279.
105. Reuss A, Wladimiroff JW, Stewart PA et al. Prenatal diagnosis by ultrasound in pregnancies at risk for autosomal recessive polycystic kidney disease. *Ultrasound Med Biol* 1990; 16:355-359.
106. Pretorius DH, Lee ME, Manco-Johnson ML. Diagnosis of autosomal dominant polycystic kidney disease in utero and in the young infant. *J Ultrasound Med* 1987;6:249-255.
107. Ceccherini I, Lituania M, Cordone MS et al. Autosomal dominant polycystic kidney disease: prenatal diagnosis by DNA analysis and sonography at 14 weeks. *Prenat Diagn* 1989; 9:751-758.
108. Zerres K, Rudnik-Schoneborn S, Deget F et al. Childhood onst autosomal dominant polycystic kidney disease in sibs: clinical picture and recurrence risk. *J Med Genet* 1993;30: 583-588.
109. Zerres K, Volpel M-C, Wei B. Cystic kidneys. Genetics, pathologic anatomy, clinical picture and prenatal diagnosis. *Hum Genet* 1984;68:104-135.
110. Nyberg DA, Hallesy D, Mahony BS et al. Meckel-Gruber syndrome: Importance of prenatal diagnosis. *J Ultrasound Med* 1990;9:691-696.

Fetal Renal Neoplasm and Adrenal Mass

111. Guilian BB. Prenatal ultrasonographic diagnosis of fetal renal tumors. *Radiology* 1984;152:69-70.
112. Walter JP, McGahan JP. Mesoblastic nephroma: prenatal sonographic detection. *J Clin Ultrasound* 1985;13:686-689.
113. Apuzzio JJ, Unwin W, Adhate A et al. Prenatal diagnosis of fetal renal mesoblastic nephroma. *Am J Obstet Gynecol* 1986; 154:636-637.
114. Rubenstein SC, Benacerraf BR, Retik AB et al. Fetal suprarenal masses: sonographic appearance and differential diagnosis. *Ultrasound Obstet Gynecol* 1995;5:164-167.
115. Ferraro EM, Fakhry J, Aruny JE et al. Prenatal adrenal neuroblastoma: case report with review of the literature. *J Ultrasound Med* 1988;7:275-278.
116. Ho PTC, Estroff JA, Kozakewich H et al. Prenatal detection of neuroblastoma: a ten year experience from the Dana-Farber Cancer Institute and Children's Hospital. *Pediatrics* 1993;92:358-364.
117. Lee W, Comstock CH, Jurcak-Zaleski S. Prenatal diagnosis of adrenal hemorrhage by ultrasonography. *J Ultrasound Med* 1992;11:369-371.
118. Rahman S, Ohlsson A, Fong KW et al. Fetal adrenal hemorrhage in a diamniotic, dichorionic twin. *J Ultrasound Med* 1997;16:297-300.

Fetal Genital Tract

119. Reece EA, Winn HN, Wan M et al. Can ultrasonography replace amniocentesis in fetal gender determination during the early second trimester? *Am J Obstet Gynecol* 1987;156:579-581.

120. Birnholz JC. Determination of fetal sex. *N Engl J Med* 1983; 309:942-944.
121. Elejalde BR, de Elejalde MM, Heitman T. Visualization of the fetal genitalia by ultrasonography: a review of the literature and analysis of its accuracy and ethical implications. *J Ultrasound Med* 1985;4:633-639.
122. Bronshtein M, Rottem S, Yoffe N et al. Early determination of fetal sex using transvaginal sonography: technique and pitfalls. *J Clin Ultrasound* 1990;18:302-306.
123. Meizner I, Levy A, Katz M et al. Prenatal ultrasonographic diagnosis of fetal scrotal inguinal hernia. *Am J Obstet Gynecol* 1992;166:907-909.
124. Cooper C, Mahony BS, Bowie JD et al. Prenatal ultrasound diagnosis of ambiguous genitalia. *J Ultrasound Med* 1985;4: 433-436.
125. Benacerraf BR, Saltzman DH, Mandell J. Sonographic diagnosis of abnormal fetal genitalia. *J Ultrasound Med* 1989;8: 613-617.
126. Bronshtein M, Riechler A, Zimmer E. Prenatal sonographic signs of possible fetal genital anomalies. *Prenat Diagn* 1995; 15:215-219.
127. Hogdall C, Siegel-Bartelet J, Toi A et al. Prenatal diagnosis of Opitz (BBB) syndrome in the second trimester by ultrasound detection of hypospadias and hypertelorism. *Prenat Diagn* 1989;9:783-793.
128. Hill SJ, Hirsch JH. Sonographic detection of hydrometrocolpos. *J Ultrasound Med* 1985;4:323-325.
129. Garel L, Filiatrault D, Brandt M et al. Antenatal diagnosis of ovarian cysts: natural history and therapeutic implications. *Pediatr Radiol* 1991;21:182-184.
130. Meizner I, Levy A, Katz M et al. Fetal ovarian cysts: prenatal ultrasonographic detection and postnatal evaluation and treatment. *Am J Obstet Gynecol* 1991;164:874-878.
131. Rizzo N, Gabrielli S, Perolo A et al. Prenatal diagnosis and management of fetal ovarian cysts. *Prenat Diagn* 1989;9:97-103.
132. Nussbaum AR, Sanders RC, Hartman DS et al. Neonatal ovarian cysts: sonographic-pathologic correlation. *Radiology* 1988;168:817-821.
133. Shozu M, Kazutomo A, Yamashiro G et al. Changing ultrasonographic appearance of a fetal ovarian cyst twisted in utero. *J Ultrasound Med* 1993;12:415-417.
134. Brandt ML, Luks FI, Filiatrault D et al. Surgical indications in antenatally diagnosed ovarian cysts. *J Pediatr Surg* 1991; 26:276-282.

CHAPTER 38

The Fetal Heart

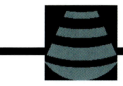

Elizabeth R. Stamm, M.D.
Julia A. Drose, B.A., R.D.M.S., R.D.C.S.

CHAPTER OUTLINE

Sonographic evaluation of the fetal heart can identify fetal cardiac abnormalities that impact obstetric care in a variety of ways, including mode of delivery, place of delivery, opportunity for termination, intrauterine therapy, and parental reassurance. Congenital heart disease (CHD) is a significant problem with an incidence of between 2 to 6.5 cases per 1000 live births. In 85% of cases of congenital heart disease, both environmental and genetic factors are involved (Table 38-1).[1-4] The remaining 15% of cardiac anomalies are associated with a monogenetic or chromosomal abnormality.[2] The risk of congenital heart disease increases to 2% to 3% with an affected sibling and to approximately 10% with two affected siblings or an affected mother.[2,5] The risk to offspring of affected mothers is substantially higher than that to those with affected fathers, suggesting that cytoplasmic inheritance may play a role in the genetics of CHD (Tables 38-2 and 38-3). Only 50% of recurrent heart lesions are of the same type as the previously diagnosed defect.[6]

Extracardiac malformations occur in 25%,[7] and chromosomal anomalies occur in 13% of live-born neonates with CHD.[8-10] Fifty percent of fetuses with nonimmune hydrops and cardiac anomalies have a chromosomal anomaly, and an additional 10% will have extracardiac anomalies.[11] Hydrops in the setting of CHD is predictive of a very poor prognosis.

Indications for fetal echocardiography are detailed in the box on p. 1126. Although the most common indications for formal fetal echocardiography are family history of CHD and fetal arrhythmia, the majority of these fetuses will have normal hearts.

TABLE 38-1
CONGENITAL HEART DISEASE AND ASSOCIATED RISK FACTORS

Factor	Frequency (%)	Most Common Lesions
Maternal Conditions		
Diabetes	3-5	TGA, VSD, coarctation
Lupus erythematosus	30-50	Heartblock
Phenylketonuria	25-50	TOF, VSD, ASD, coarctation
Infection		
Rubella	35	TOF, PS, VSD, ASD, PDA, Cardiomegaly, TA
CMV		
Drugs		
Accutane (retinoic acid)		Truncus, TGA, TOF, DORV, VSD, AO arch interruption, or hypoplasia
Alcohol	25-30	VSD, ASD, PDA, DORV, PA, TOF, dextrocardia
Amantadine		Single vent with PA
Amphetamines	5-10	VSD, TGA, PDA
Azathioprine		PS
Carbamazepine		ASD, PDA
Chlordiazepoxide		Congenital heart malformations
Codeine		Congenital heart malformations
Cortisone		VSD, coarctation
Coumadin		Congenital heart malformations
Cyclophosphamide		TOF
Cytarabine		TOF
Daunorubicin		TOF
Dextroamphetamine		ASD
Diazepam		Congenital heart malformations
Dilantin (hydantoin)		AS, VSD, ASD, coarctation
Lithium	10	Ebstein anomaly, TA, ASD, dextrocardia, MA, PDA
Methotrexate		Dextrocardia
Oral contraceptives		Congenital heart malformations
Paramethadione		TOF
Penicillamine		VSD
Primidone		VSD
Progesterone		TOF, truncus, VSD
Quinine		Congenital heart malformations
Thalidomide	5-10	TOF, VSD, ASD, truncus
Trifluoperazine		TGA
Trimethadione	15-30	ASD, VSD, TGA, TOF, HLHS, AS, PS
Valproic acid		TOF, coarctation, HLHS, AS, ASD, VSD, interrupted AO arch, PA without VSD
Warfarin (coumadin)		Congenital heart malformations
Syndromes		
Apert		VSD, coarctation, TOF
Arthrogryposis multiplex congenita		VSD, coarctation, AS, PDA
Atrial myxoma, familial		Myxoma
Beckwith-Wiedemann		Cardiomegaly
C syndrome (Opitz trigonocephaly)		PDA
Carpenter		VSD, PS, TGA, PDA
Cat-eye (22 partial trisomy)	40	TAPVR, VSD, ASD
CHARGE		Congenital heart malformations
CHILD		VSD, ASD
Conradi-Hünermann (chondrodysplasia punctata)		VSD, PDA
de Lange	29	VSD, TOF, DORV, PDA
DiGeorge		VSD, coarctation, truncus
Ellis-van Creveld (chondroectodermal dysplasia)	50	ASD, single atrium

TABLE 38-1
CONGENITAL HEART DISEASE AND ASSOCIATED RISK FACTORS—CONT'D

Factor	Frequency (%)	Most Common Lesions
Fanconi's pancytopenia		ASD, PDA
Goldenhar		TOF, VSD, ASD
Holt-Oram		ASD, VSD
Kartagener		Dextrocardia
Klippel-Feil		VSD, TGA, TAPVR
Laurence-Moon (Bardet-Biedl)		VSD
Leopard		PS
Meckel-Gruber		VSD, ASD, coarctation, PS, PDA
Noonan		PS, VSD, ASD, PDA
Pallister-Hall		ECD
Pierre Robin		ASD
Poland		TOF, ASD, PDA, VSD
Refsum		AV conduction defects
Seckel		VSD, PDA
Smith-Lemli-Opitz		VSD, PDA
Treacher Collins		VSD, ASD, PDA
Rubinstein-Taybi		ASD, VSD, PDA
Silver		TOF, VSD
Short rib polydactyly (non-Majewski type)		TGA, DOLV, DORV, HRH, AVSD
Thrombocytopenia absent radius (TAR)		ASD, TOF, dextrocardia
VACTERL		Congenital heart malformation
Waardenburg		VSD
Weill-Marchesani		PS, VSD
Williams		Supravalvular AS, PS, VSD, ASD
Zellweger		VSD, ASD, PDA
Chromosomal		
Trisomy 13	90	VSD, ASD, dextroposition, PDA
Trisomy 18	99+	Bicuspid AV, PS, VSD, ASD, PDA
Trisomy 21 (Down's)	50	AV canal, VSD, ASD, PDA
Triploidy		ASD, VSD
$5p^-$ (cri-du-chat)	30	Congenital heart malformations
$9p^-$		VSD, PS, PDA
Partial trisomy 10q	50	Congenital heart malformations
$13q^-$		Congenital heart malformations
T 20p syndromes		VSD, TOF
Turner's (45X)	20+	Bicuspid AV, AS, coarctation, VSD, ASD, AVSD
8 trisomy (mosaic)	50	VSD, ASD, PDA
9 trisomy (mosaic)	50	VSD, coarctation, DORV
$13q^-$	25	VSD
$+14q^-$	50	ASD, TOF, PDA
$18q^-$	50	VSD
XXXXY	14	ASD, ARCA, PDA
Diseases/Conditions		
Crouzon		Coarctation, PDA
Neurofibromatosis		PS, coarctation
Tuberous sclerosis		Rhabdomyoma, angioma
Thalassemia major		Cardiomyopathy

Data from Jones KL. *Smith's Recognizable Patterns of Human Malformation.* 3rd ed. Philadelphia: WB Saunders Co; 1988. Nora J, Fraser FC. *Medical Genetics: Principles and Practice.* Philadelphia: Lea & Febiger; 1989. Nyberg DA, Mahony BS, Pretorius DH. *Diagnostic Ultrasound of Fetal Anomalies: Text and Atlas.* Chicago: Year Book Medical Publishers Inc; 1989. Romero R, Pilu G, Jeanty P et al. *Prenatal Diagnosis of Congenital Anomalies.* Norwalk, Conn. Appleton & Lange; 1988. Taybi H. *Radiology of Syndromes and Metabolic Disorders.* Chicago: Year Book Medical Publishers, Inc; 1983.

ARCA, Anomalous right coronary artery; *AS*, aortic stenosis; *ASD*, atrial septal defect; *AVSD*, atrioventricular septal defect; *DOLV*, double outlet left ventricle; *DORV*, double outlet right ventricle; *HLHS*, hypoplastic left heart syndrome; *MA*, mitral atresia; *PA*, pulmonary atresia; *PDA*, patent ductus arteriosus; *PS*, pulmonary stenosis; *TA*, tricuspid atresia; *TAPVR*, total anomalous pulmonary venous return; *TGA*, transposition of the great arteries; *TOF*, tetralogy of Fallot; *truncus*, truncus arteriosus; *VSD*, ventricular septal defect.

TABLE 38-2

RECURRENCE RISKS IN SIBLINGS FOR ANY CONGENITAL HEART DEFECT: COMBINED DATA PUBLISHED DURING TWO DECADES FROM EUROPEAN AND NORTH AMERICAN POPULATIONS

	Suggested Risk (%)	
Defect	**If 1 Sibling**	**If 2 Siblings**
Fibroelastosis	4	12
Ventricular septal defect	3	10
Patent ductus arteriosus	3	10
Atrioventricular septal defect	3	10
Atrial septal defect	2.5	8
Tetralogy of Fallot	2.5	8
Pulmonary stenosis	2	6
Coarctation of aorta	2	6
Aortic stenosis	2	6
Hypoplastic left heart	2	6
Transposition	1.5	5
Tricuspid atresia	1	3
Ebstein anomaly	1	3
Truncus	1	3
Pulmonary atresia	1	3

From Nora JJ, Fraser FC. *Medical Genetics: Principles and Practice.* Philadelphia: Lea & Febiger; 1989.

TABLE 38-3

SUGGESTED OFFSPRING RECURRENCE RISK FOR CONGENITAL HEART DEFECTS GIVEN ONE AFFECTED PARENT (%)

Defect	Father Affected	Mother Affected
Aortic stenosis	3	13-18
Atrial septal defect	1.5	4-4.5
Atrioventricular canal	1	14
Coarctation of aorta	2	4
Patent ductus arteriosus	2.5	3.5-4
Pulmonary stenosis	2	4-6.5
Tetralogy of Fallot	1.5	2.5
Ventricular septal defect	2	6-10

From Nora JJ, Fraser FC. *Medical Genetics: Principles and Practice.* Philadelphia: Lea & Febiger; 1989.

COMMON INDICATIONS FOR FETAL ECHOCARDIOGRAM

- Abnormal four-chamber view on screening ultrasound
- Fetal hydrops
- Polyhydramnios
- Fetal arrhythmia
- Chromosomal anomalies
- Extracardiac anomalies
- Family history (CHD, syndromes associated with CHD)
- Maternal disease (diabetes, collagen vascular, PKU)
- Teratogen exposure (rubella, alcohol, drugs)
- Monitoring response to intrauterine therapy
- Monitoring fetus at risk for decompensation (persistent tachyarrhythmia, hydrops)

CHD, Congenital heart disease; *PKU*, phenylketonuria.

The highest incidence of CHD occurs in patients referred for an abnormal four-chamber view on screening obstetric ultrasound, fetal hydrops, or polyhydramnios, respectively.[12,13] The fact that most fetuses with congenital heart disease have no known risk factors underscores the importance of a meticulous evaluation of the four-chamber heart view on all routine obstetric ultrasounds. When severe structural cardiac anomalies are identified before viability, termination may be offered. Certainly, one of the most important aspects of fetal echocardiography is the psychologic relief it affords parents whenever normal cardiac anatomy and function are documented in a fetus at risk.

NORMAL FETAL CARDIAC ANATOMY AND SCANNING TECHNIQUES

The fetal heart is similar to that of the adult with several anatomic and physiologic differences. The long axis of the fetal heart is perpendicular to the body such that a transverse section through the fetal thorax demonstrates the four cardiac chambers in a single

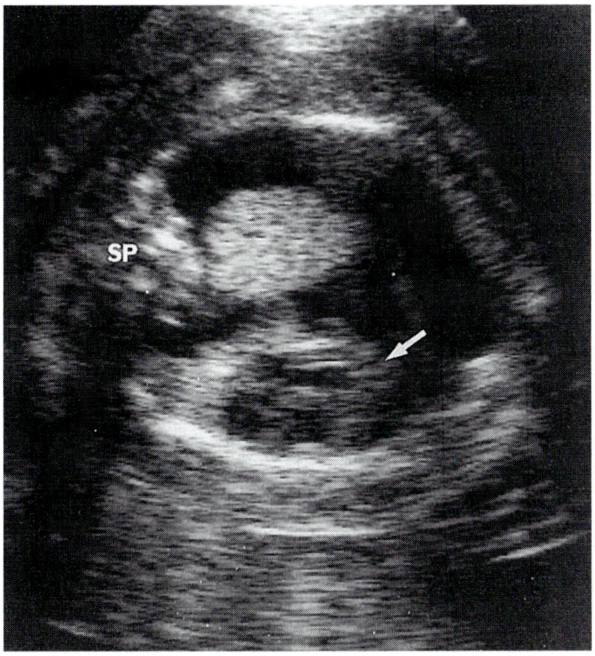

FIG. 38-1. Dextroposition of fetal heart due to a large pleural effusion. Transverse image through the fetal chest showing the heart *(arrow)* being displaced. *SP*, Spine.

view. The adult heart, in contrast, is obliquely oriented with its long axis along a line between the left hip and the right shoulder. The four-chamber view is important because many (43% to 96%) structural anomalies are detectable on this view.[13-16]

Cardiac axis and position is normally such that the apex of the heart points to the left and the bulk of the heart is in the left chest. This is **levocardia**. In **mesocardia,** the heart is central with the apex pointing anteriorly, while in **dextrocardia** the apex is directed rightward and the heart is primarily in the right chest. This abnormality must be distinguished from **dextroposition,** where the heart maintains a normal axis but is displaced to the right by an external process such as a left chest mass or pleural effusion (Fig. 38-1). Abnormal cardiac axis is associated with a 50% mortality and abnormal cardiac position with an 81% mortality.[17]

The fetal cardiovascular system contains several **unique shunts: the ductus venosus, foramen ovale,** and **ductus arteriosus** (Fig. 38-2). Antenatally, the placenta rather than the lungs is the fetus' sole source of oxygen. Oxygenated blood leaves the placenta and travels through the ductus venosus and inferior vena cava to the fetal right atrium. Due to laminar flow, much of this blood is shunted across the foramen ovale to the left atrium and then into the left ventricle, aorta, and the fetal brain. Poorly oxygenated blood from the superior vena cava also enters the right atrium, but preferentially enters the right ventricle and pulmonary artery because of the unique flow pattern. Most of this blood is shunted through the ductus arteriosus into the descending aorta.

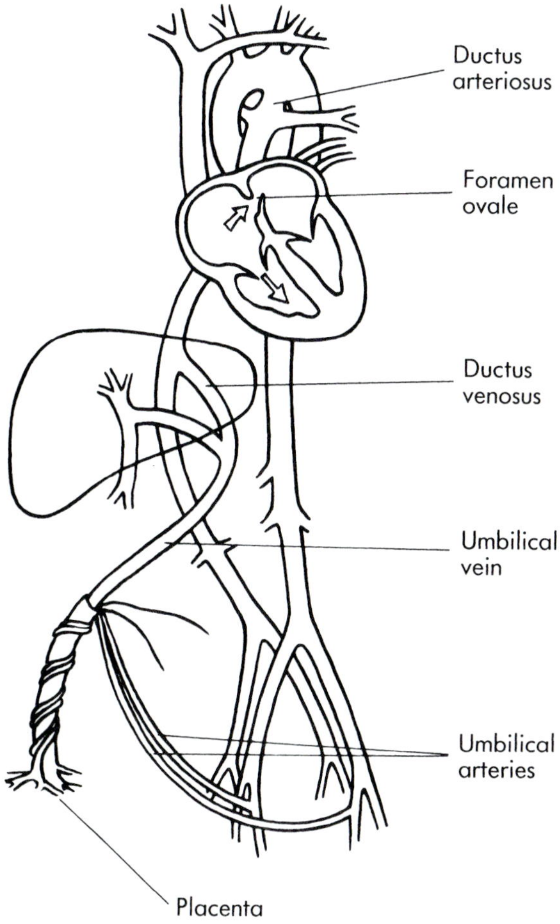

FIG. 38-2. Diagram of fetal circulation. Blood from the umbilical vein is shunted through the ductus venosus to the right atrium and then across the foramen ovale to the left atrium. Most of the fetal cardiac output is shunted to the descending aorta via the ductus arteriosus.

Thus, these shunts function so that the majority of output from both ventricles enters the systemic circulation, rather than a significant portion entering the pulmonary circulation as in the adult (Fig. 38-2). Normal values for measurements of the fetal heart and great vessels are shown in Figs. 38-3 to 38-10.

Fetal echocardiography is best accomplished between 18 and 22 weeks gestation. Before 18 weeks, resolution is frequently limited by the small size of the fetal heart. After 22 weeks the exam may be compromised by a variety of factors, including progressive ossification of the fetal skull, spine, and long bones; the relatively smaller amniotic fluid volume; unaccommodating fetal position; and a larger maternal body habitus. Preliminary data suggest that early screening of the fetal heart may be accomplished with vaginal probe ultrasound as early as 12 to 13 weeks.[18,19]

Scanning the fetal heart requires a systematic approach beginning with determination of the position of the fetus within the uterus and the heart

Text continued on p. 1132.

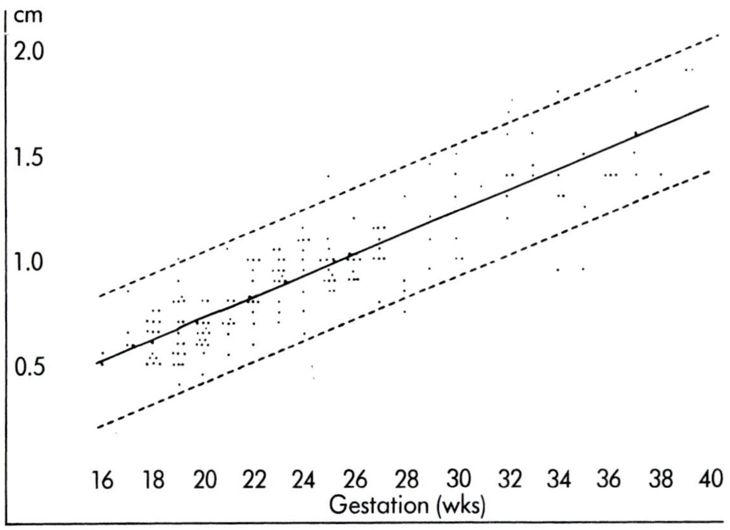

FIG. 38-3. Left ventricular internal dimension versus gestational age (n = 175). The 95% confidence limits represent twice the standard error of the mean. $y = 0.049x - 0.262$; $r = 0.876$; $t = 23.944$; $p < 0.001$; SEM $y \times 2 = 0.3$. (From Allan LD, Joseph MC, Boyd EG et al. M-mode echocardiography in the developing human fetus. *Br Heart J* 1982;47:573-583.)

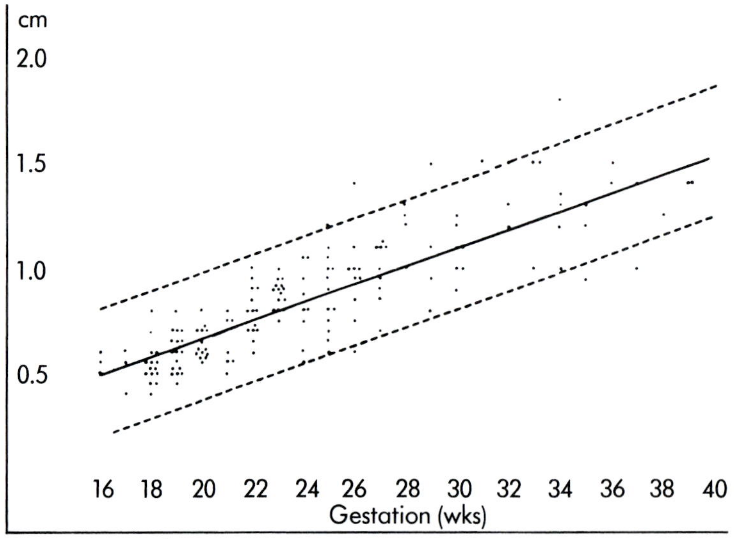

FIG. 38-4. Right ventricular internal dimension versus gestational age (n = 167). The 95% confidence limits represent twice the standard error of the mean. $y = 0.045x - 0.228$; $r = 0.844$; $t = 20.183$; $p < 0.001$; SEM $y \times 2 = 0.306$. (From Allan LD, Joseph MC, Boyd EG et al. M-mode echocardiography in the developing human fetus. *Br Heart J* 1982;47:573-583.)

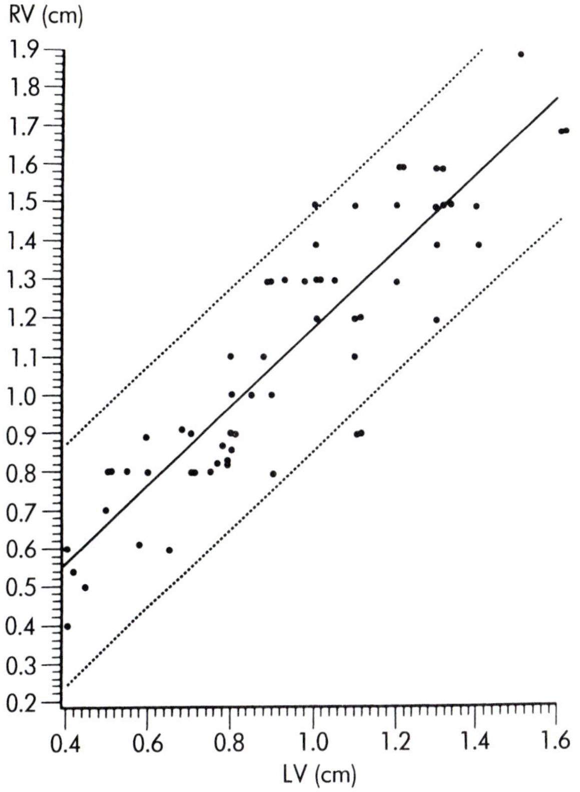

FIG. 38-5. Maximal right ventricular internal dimension (RV) versus maximal left ventricular internal dimension (LV) (n = 62; $y = 1.03x + 0.144$; $r = 0.899$; $p = 0.0001$). (From Shime J, Gresser CD, Rakowski H. Quantitative two-dimensional echocardiographic assessment of fetal cardiac growth. *Am J Obstet Gynecol* 1986;154:294-300.)

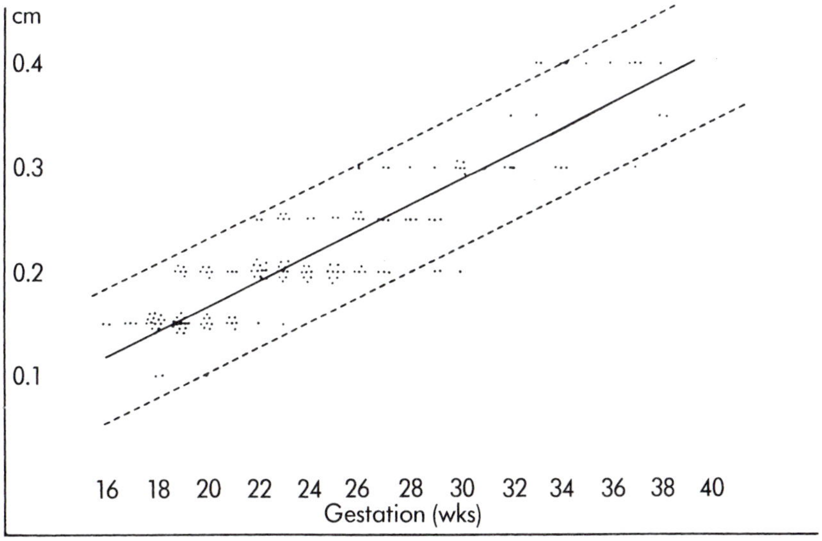

FIG. 38-6. Posterior left ventricular wall thickness versus gestational age (n = 175). The 95% confidence limits represent twice the standard error of the mean. $y = 0.012x - 0.063$; $r = 0.884$; $t = 24.929$; $p < 0.001$; SEM $y \times 2 = 0.66$. (From Allan LD, Joseph MC, Boyd EG et al. M-mode echocardiography in the developing human fetus. *Br Heart J* 1982;47:573-583.)

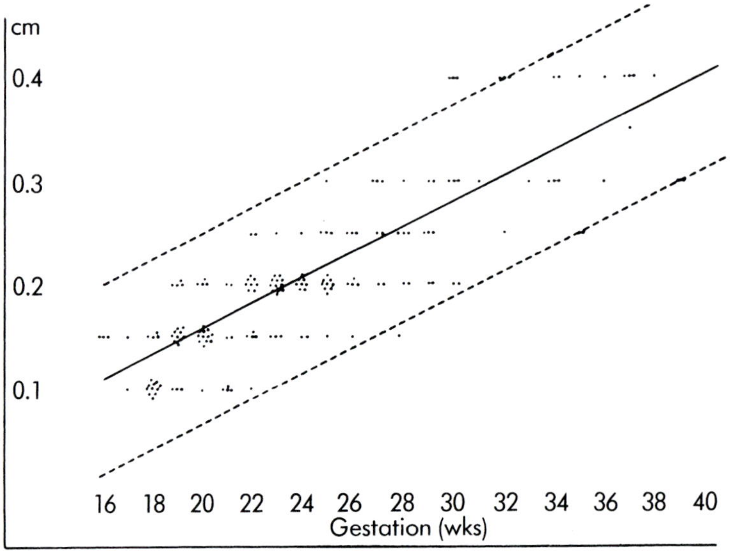

FIG. 38-7. Septal thickness versus gestational age (n = 178). The 95% confidence limits represent twice the standard error of the mean. $y = 0.012x - 0.088$; $r = 0.836$; $t = 20.183$; $p < 0.001$; SEM $y \times = 0.088$. (From Allan LD, Joseph MC, Boyd EG et al. M-mode echocardiography in the developing human fetus. *Br Heart J* 1982;47:573-583.)

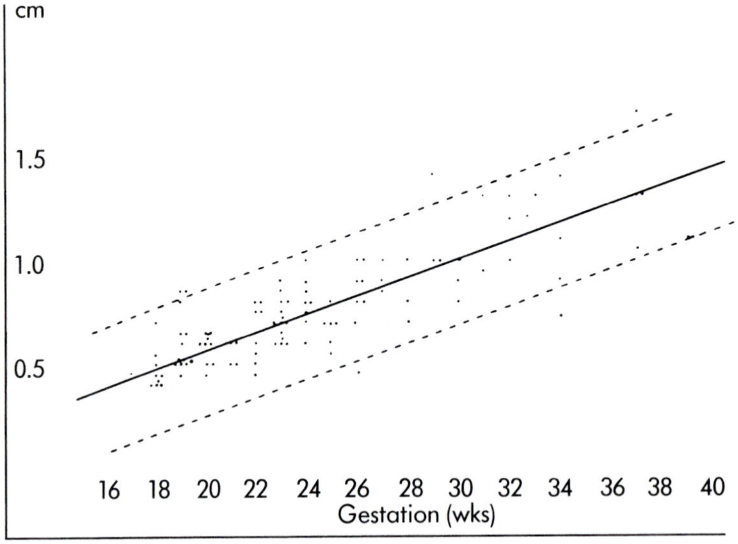

FIG. 38-8. Left atrial internal dimension versus gestational age (n = 107). $y = 0.040x - 0.214$; $r = 0.823$; $t = 14.968$; $p < 0.001$; SEM $y \times 2 = 0.296$. (From Allan LD, Joseph MC, Boyd EG et al. M-mode echocardiography in the developing human fetus. *Br Heart J* 1982;47:573-583.)

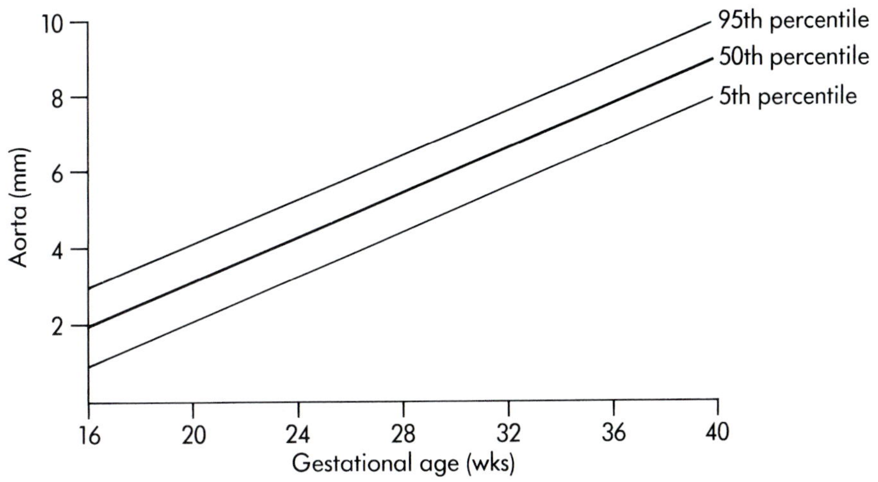

FIG. 38-9. Diameter of aortic root versus gestational age. Norms and confidence limits for echocardiographic measurements. (From Cartier MS, Davidoff A, Warneke LA et al. The normal diameter of the fetal aorta and pulmonary artery: echocardiographic evaluation in utero. *AJR* 1987;149:1003-1007.)

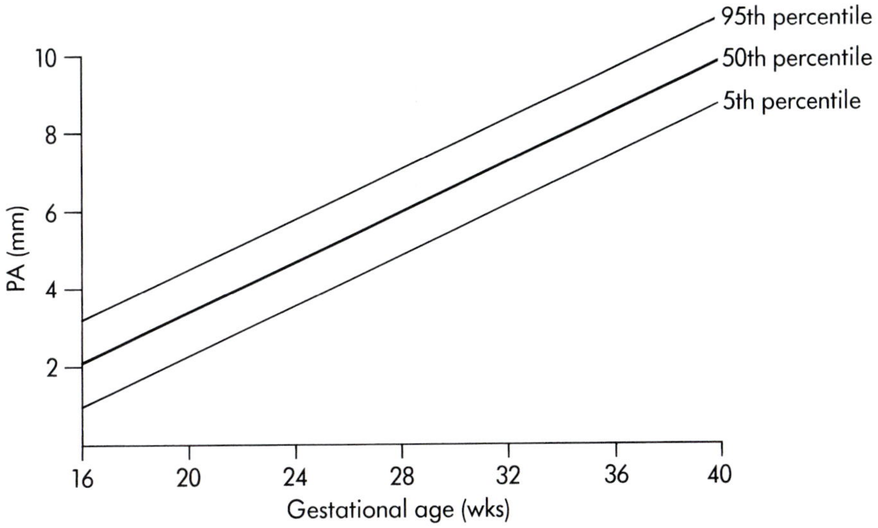

FIG. 38-10. Diameter of pulmonary artery, *PA*, versus gestational age. Norms and confidence limits for echocardiographic measurements. (From Cartier MS, Davidoff A, Warneke LA et al. The normal diameter of the fetal aorta and pulmonary artery: echocardiographic evaluation in utero. *AJR* 1987;149:1003-1007.)

A

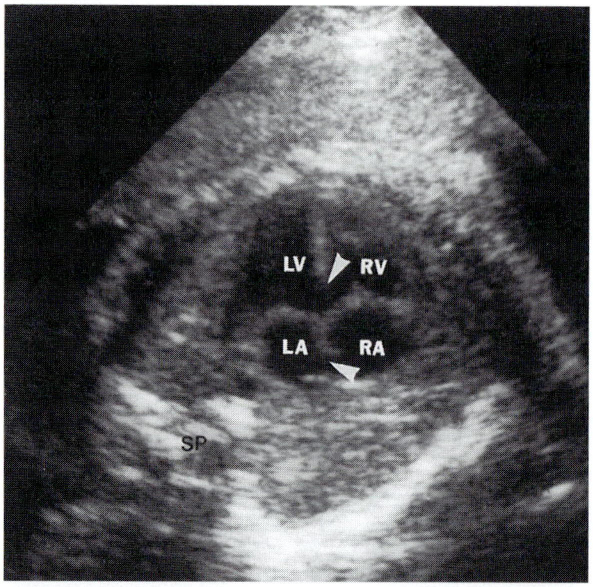

B

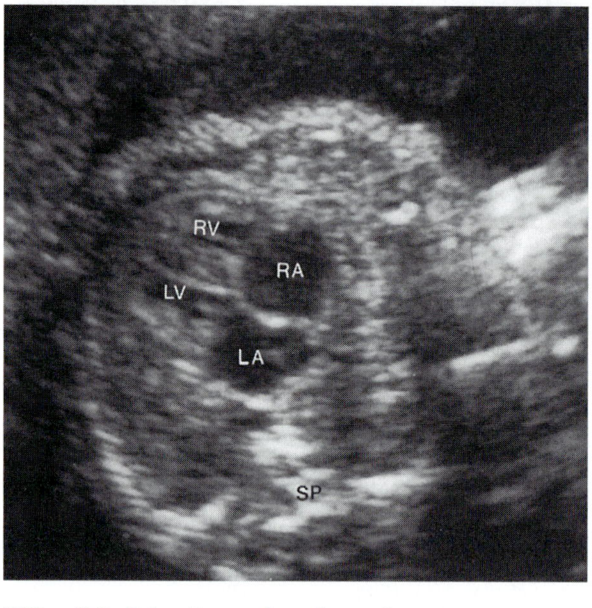

FIG. 38-11. Four-chamber view. **A**, Apical. **B**, Subcostal. The incidence of the sound beam is parallel to the septa in **A** and perpendicular to the septa in **B**. Note the artifactual "dropout" *(arrowheads)* of the ventricular septum and atrial septum in **A**. *LV*, Left ventricle; *RV*, right ventricle; *LA*, left atrium; *RA*, right atrium; *SP*, spine.

within the fetal chest. A transverse view through the fetal thorax above the level of the diaphragm demonstrates four cardiac chambers. **Four-chamber views** can be obtained with the angle of insonation parallel to the interventricular septum (**apical four-chamber view;** Fig. 38-11, *A*) or perpendicular to the septum (**subcostal four-chamber view;** Fig. 38-11, *B*). In this view the echogenic foraminal flap of the foramen ovale can be observed moving into the left atrium at twice the heart rate. With slight angulation, the pulmonary veins may be seen entering the spherical left

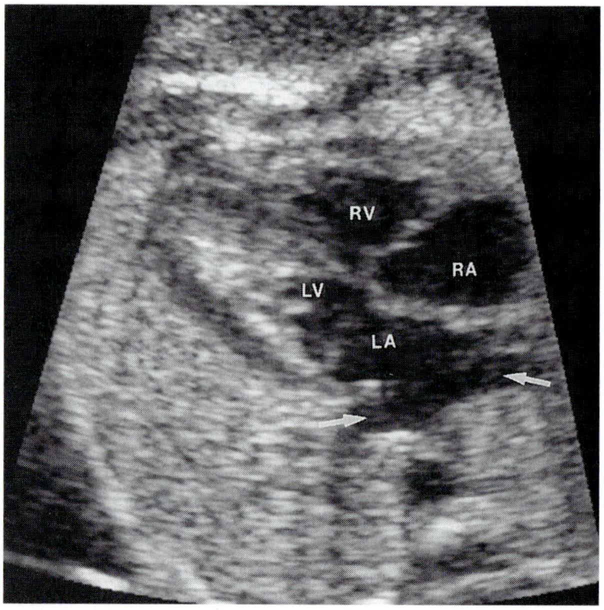

FIG. 38-12. Pulmonary veins (*arrows*) entering the left atrium, *LA*. Subcostal four-chamber view. *LV*, Left ventricle; *RA*, right atrium; *RV*, right ventricle.

atrium (Fig. 38-12) whereas the superior and inferior vena cava may be noted entering the right atrium (Fig. 38-13). The atrioventricular valves are visible in either four-chamber view. The septal leaflet of the tricuspid valve inserts more apically than that of the mitral valve. The left ventricle has a relatively smooth inner wall. The internal surface of the right ventricle is coarse, particularly near the apex, where the moderator band of the trabecula septomarginalis is frequently recognized as a small, bright, echogenic focus. This helps identify the morphologic right ventricle. An additional small, echogenic focus within a ventricle, representing a portion of papillary muscle or chordae tendineae, is seen in 3% to 4% of fetuses. These usually occur in the left ventricle (93%) but may occur in the right ventricle (5%) or both ventricles (2%) and are generally clinically insignificant[20,21] (Fig. 38-14). Recently, these echogenic foci have been associated with chromosomal anomalies such as trisomy 21 and 13. In these cases, the echogenic foci represent calcifications within the papillary muscles.[22-24] Larger echogenic foci within the fetal heart, particularly when associated with other abnormalities such as arrhythmia or hydrops, raise suspicion of a cardiac neoplasm.

From the subcostal four-chamber view, rotating the transducer towards the fetus' right shoulder permits evaluation of the **continuity of the left ventricle with the ascending aorta** (Fig. 38-15). Further rotation in the same direction shows the **right ventricular outflow tract** in continuity with the pulmonary artery (Fig. 38-16). The diameter of the pulmonary artery is approximately 9% larger than that of the aorta between 14 and 42 weeks. The measured differences in

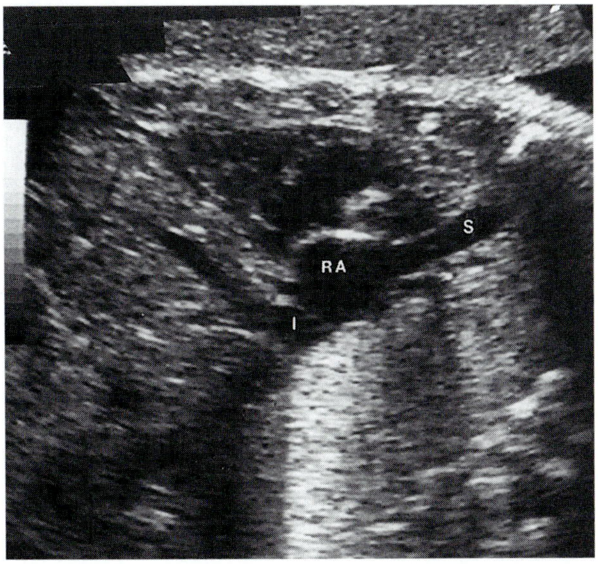

FIG. 38-13. Superior vena cava, *S*, and the inferior vena cava, *I*, entering the right atrium, *RA*. Sagittal view through the fetal chest.

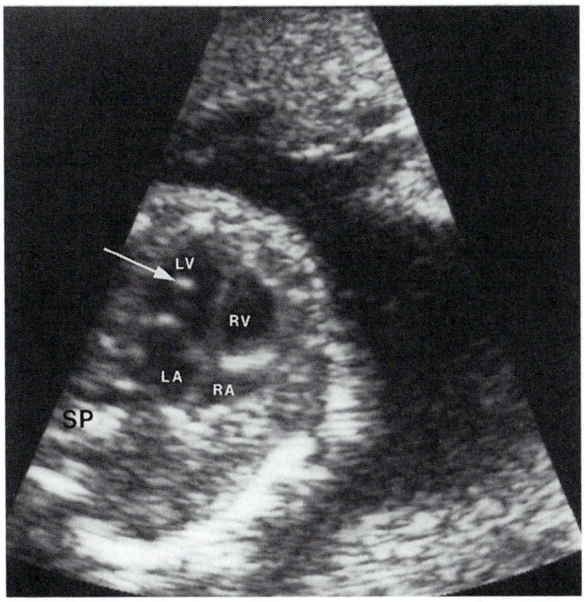

FIG. 38-14. Echogenic focus of the chordae tendineae of the left ventricle (*arrow*). Apical four-chamber view. *LV*, Left ventricle; *RV*, right ventricle; *LA*, left atrium; *RA*, right atrium; *SP*, spine.

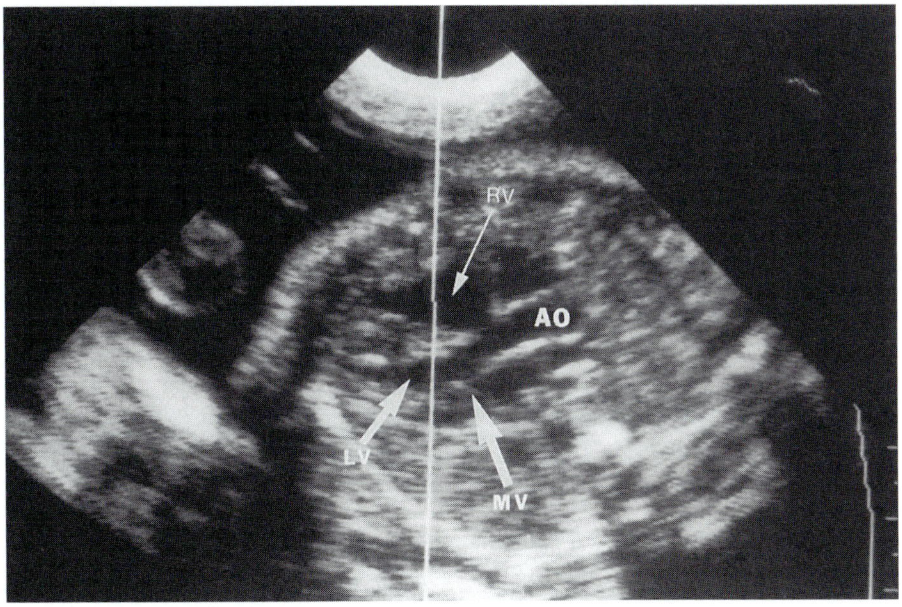

FIG. 38-15. Continuity of aorta with left ventricle, *LV*. The posterior wall of the aorta, *Ao*, is continuous with the anterior leaflet of the mitral valve, *MV*. *RV*, Right ventricle.

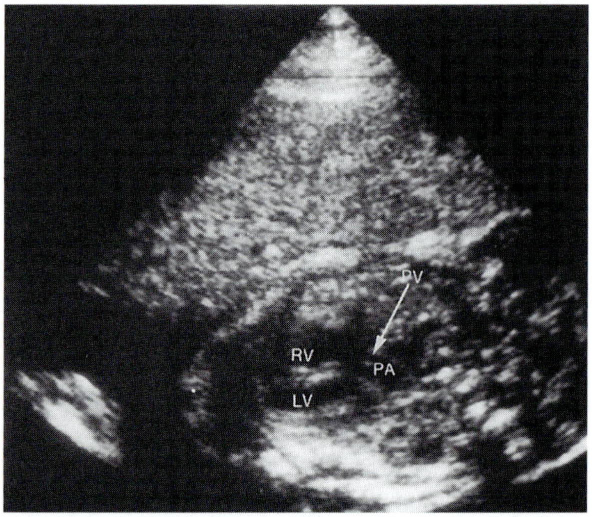

FIG. 38-16. Continuity of pulmonary artery, *PA*, with right ventricle, *RV*. *LV*, Left ventricle; *PV*, pulmonary valve.

these vessels and with M-mode versus two-dimensional (2D) imaging are negligible (2% to 5%) for both the pulmonary artery and the aorta.[25] Further rightward rotation produces a sagittal view of the fetal thorax and a **short-axis view of the ventricles** (Fig. 38-17). Angulation toward the left fetal shoulder from this view shows the aorta as a central circle with the pulmonary artery draping anteriorly and to the left (Fig. 38-18). Directing the transducer from the left shoulder to the right hemithorax demonstrates the distinctive candy-cane shape of the **aortic arch** (Fig. 38-19). The three major vessels to the head and neck and the ductus arteriosus may be seen. The aortic arch should not be confused with the **ductus arch** (Fig. 38-20), which is formed by the right ventricular outflow tract, pulmonary artery, and ductus arteriosus. The ductus arch is broader and flatter than the aortic arch. A four-chamber heart is currently the only cardiac view required for a routine obstetric ultrasound; however, many laboratories consider this single view inadequate and routinely obtain outflow tract views as well. This combination of three images (outflow tracts along with a four-chamber view) allows identification of 80% of detectable structural cardiac anomalies.[16]

M-mode echocardiography (time-motion mode) provides a two-dimensional image of motion over time. It is ideal for hard-copy documentation of fetal heart motion and is useful in evaluating chamber size, wall thickness, and valve and wall motion (Figs. 38-21 and 38-22). Simultaneous M-mode imaging through an atrium and ventricle is helpful in analyzing arrhythmias (Fig. 38-23). Similarly, M-mode imaging through the fetal aorta and atrial wall allows characterization of arrhythmias. Chamber size

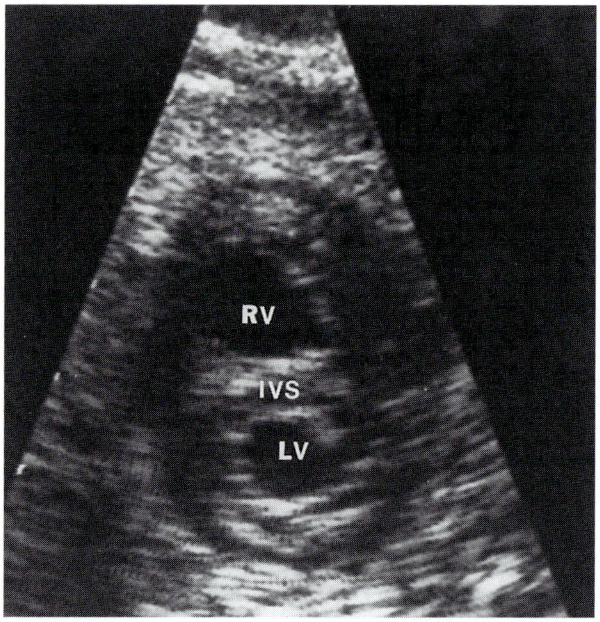

FIG. 38-17. Anterior right ventricle, *RV*, that is normally slightly larger than the left ventricle, *LV*. Short-axis view. *IVS*, Interventricular septum.

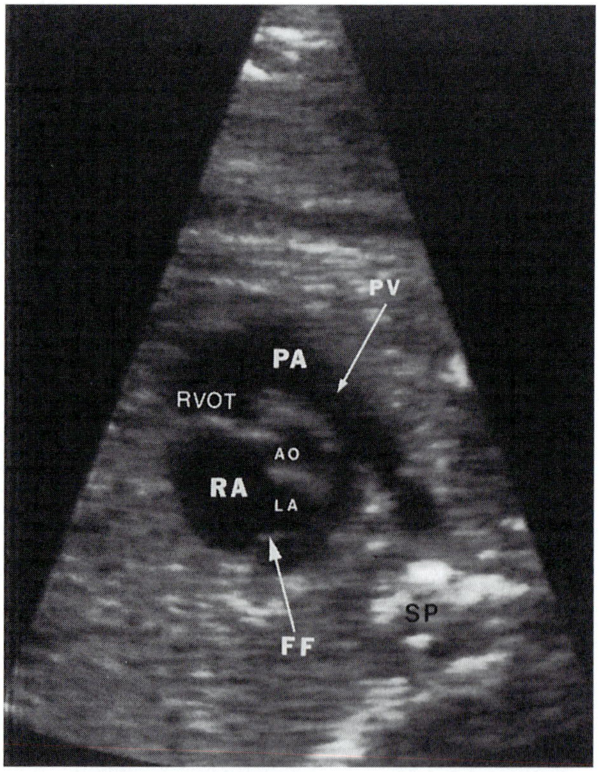

FIG. 38-18. Short-axis view of great vessels. Aorta, *Ao*, in center with pulmonary artery, *PA*, draping anterior. *RVOT*, Right ventricular outflow tract; *LA*, left atrium; *RA*, right atrium; *PV*, pulmonic valve; *FF*, foraminal flap; *SP*, spine.

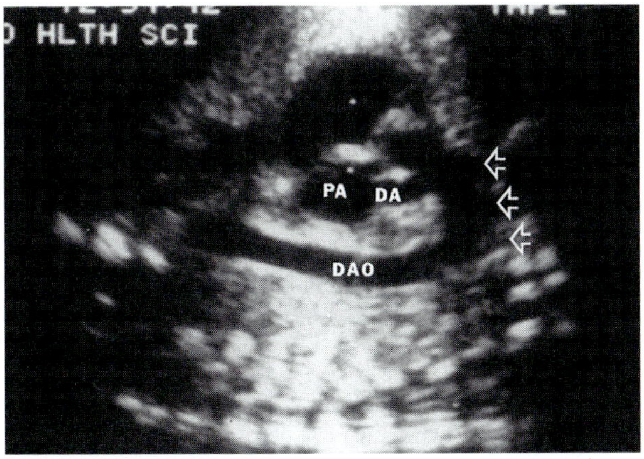

FIG. 38-19. Aortic arch. Sagittal view. Note the three vessels *(open arrows)* arising from top of the arch and the ductus arteriosus, *DA*, inferiorly where it joins pulmonary artery, *PA*. *DAO*, Descending aorta.

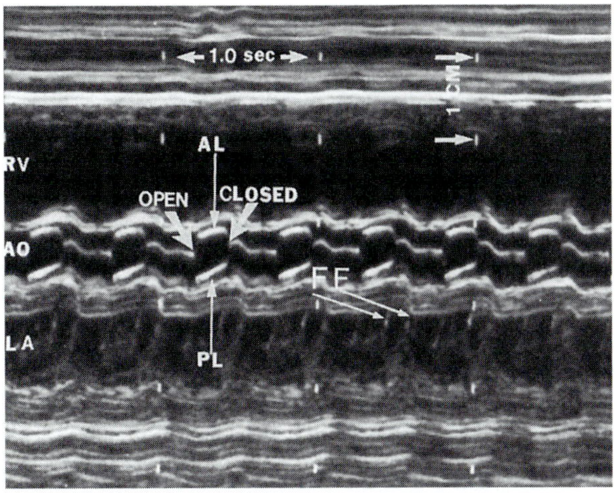

FIG. 38-21. M-mode through level of aortic valve. Heart rate can be calculated by counting the number of beats between markers. The foraminal flap, *FF*, is seen entering the left atrium, *LA*, at twice the heart rate. *AL*, Anterior leaflet; *PL*, posterior leaflet; *RV*, right ventricle; *Ao*, aorta.

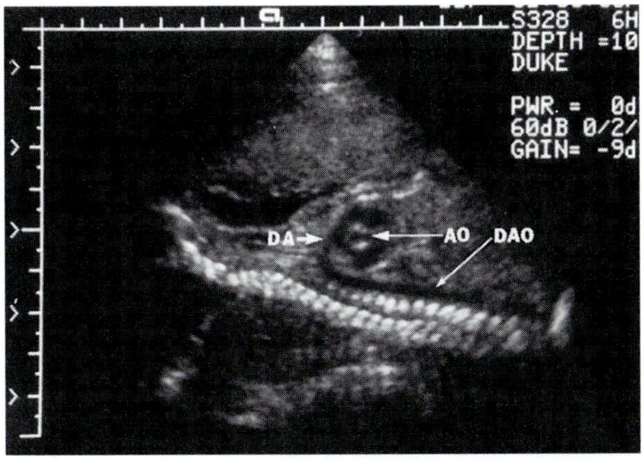

FIG. 38-20. Ductus arch, *DA*, joins the pulmonary artery to the descending aorta, *DAO*. It is broader than the aortic arch and does not give rise to neck vessels. *Ao*, Aorta. (Courtesy Acuson Corp, Mountain View, Calif.)

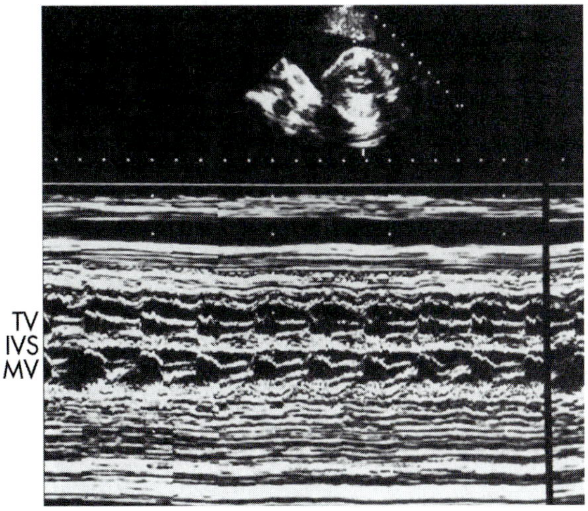

FIG. 38-22. Opening and closing of the atrioventricular valves on M-mode. *TV*, Tricuspid valve; *MV*, mitral valve; *IVS*, interventricular septum.

and function should be evaluated at the level of the atrioventricular (AV) valves. The detailed evaluation of valvular motion afforded by M-mode echocardiography provides additional information.[26]

Spectral Doppler evaluation of the fetal heart can be used to determine the velocity of flow through the vessels or valves (Fig. 38-24) as well as regurgitant flow into the chambers of the heart (Fig. 38-25). Variation in flow velocity may reflect structural or functional cardiac abnormalities. For example, a stenotic AV valve will be associated with an abnormal flow pattern through the affected valve. Doppler is useful in assessing the functional significance of structural abnormalities and arrhythmias.

Color flow Doppler ultrasound permits a rapid interrogation of flow patterns within the heart and

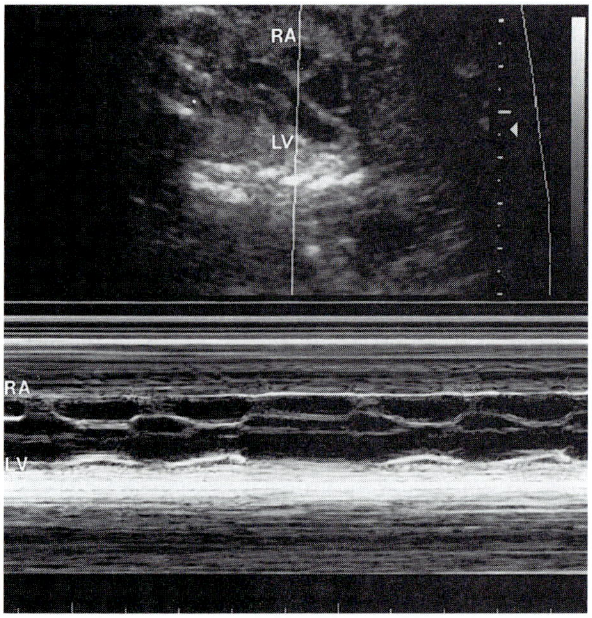

FIG. 38-23. Simultaneous M-mode tracing through the fetal right atrial wall, *RA*, and left ventricular wall, *LV*. *S*, Septum.

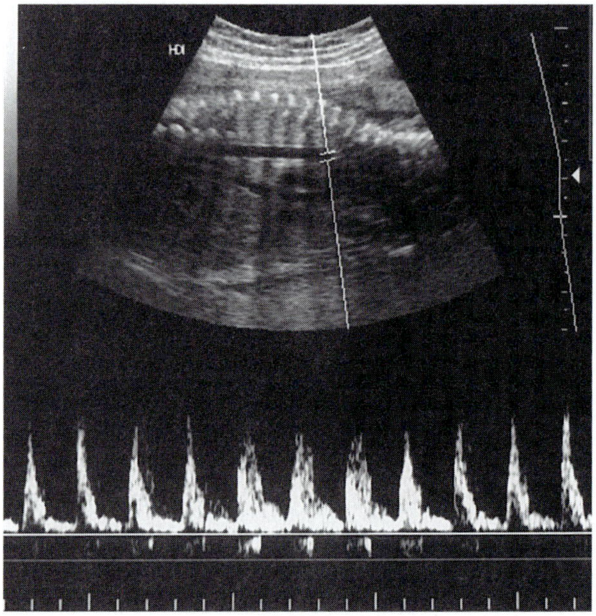

FIG. 38-24. Normal flow through the aortic arch *(arrows)* in a fetal heart pulsed wave Doppler tracing.

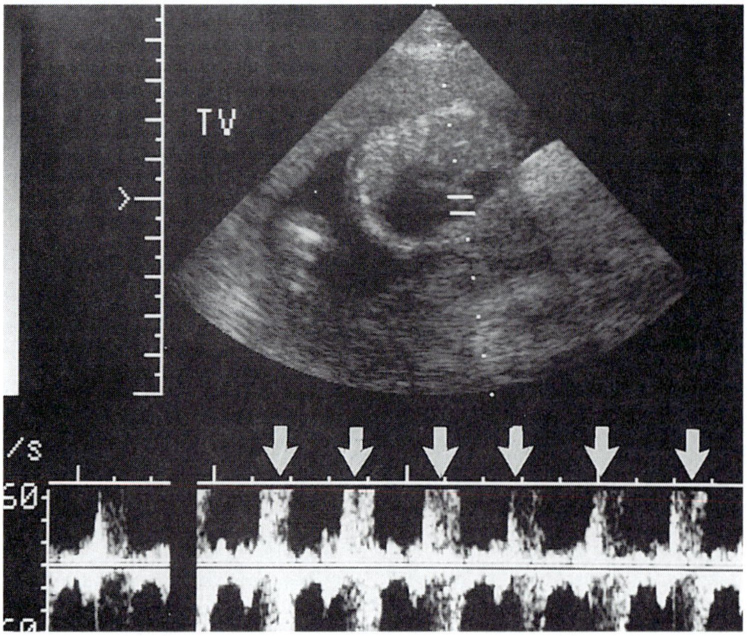

FIG. 38-25. Ebstein's anomaly, demonstrating aliasing of regurgitant flow within the right atrium *(arrows)*. Pulsed wave Doppler tracing in a fetal heart.

great vessels (Figs. 38-26 and 38-27), allowing functional and structural abnormalities to be more rapidly characterized. For example, valvular stenosis is clearly demonstrated with color flow Doppler, as is reversed flow through insufficient valves or in the great vessels. Color flow Doppler mapping significantly reduces the amount of time required for Doppler evaluation of the heart, while improving the accuracy of fetal echocardiography, particularly in the setting of complex cardiac anomalies.[27-30] Subtle lesions such as small ventricular septal defects are more reliably and easily identified with the use of color flow Doppler.

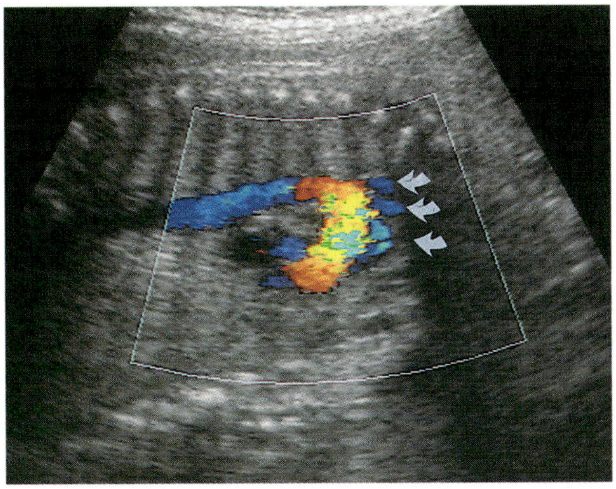

FIG. 38-26. Normal flow throughout the aortic arch and descending aorta. Color flow Doppler imaging. Head and neck vessels arising from the arch *(arrows)* can also be seen with color.

STRUCTURAL ANOMALIES

Atrial Septal Defect

An atrial septal defect (ASD) results from an error in the amount of tissue resorbed or deposited in the interatrial septum. It is the fifth most common form of congenital heart disease and is the most common form in adult patients.[31,32] ASDs occur in 1 per 1500 live births[33,34] and comprise 6.7% of congenital heart disease in live-born infants.[31] ASDs occur twice as commonly in females as males.[35,36] ASDs are associated with a variety of cardiac, extracardiac, and chromosomal abnormalities. ASDs can be classified by embryogenesis, size, or relationship to the fossa ovalis.

Embryologically, between the fourth and sixth weeks of gestation, the primitive atrium is divided into right and left halves. The septum primum, a crescent-shaped membrane, develops along the cephalad portion of the atrium and grows caudally toward the endocardial cushions. The space between these two structures, termed the ostium primum, disappears when the septum primum fuses with the endocardial cushion. Prior to complete fusion, however, multiple small fenestrations develop in the septum primum, coalescing to form the ostium secundum.

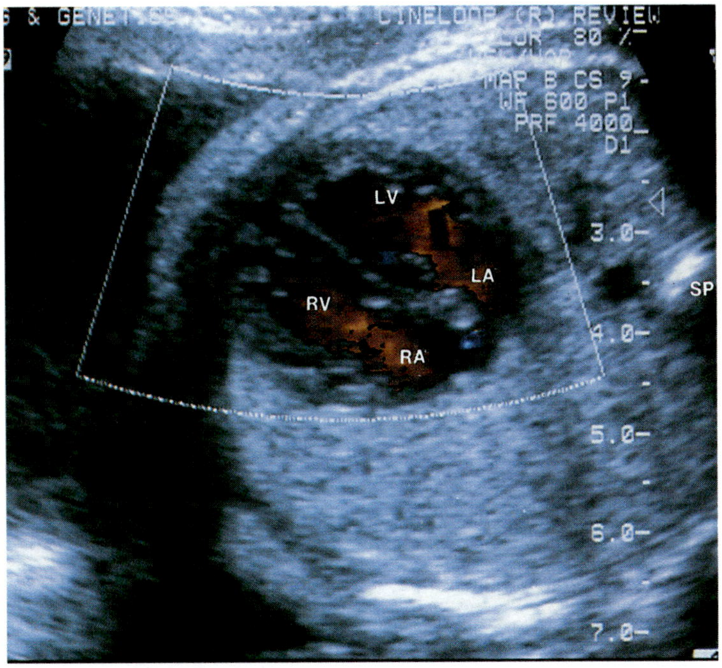

FIG. 38-27. Normal flow from the right atrium, *RA*, and left atrium, *LA*, into the right ventricle, *RV*, and left ventricle, *LV*, respectively. Apical four-chamber view using color flow Doppler imaging. *SP*, Spine.

A second crescent-shaped membrane subsequently develops just to the right of the septum primum. As this membrane grows toward the endocardial cushion, it partially covers the ostium secundum. Its crescent-shaped lower border never entirely fuses with the endocardial cushion, leaving an opening, the foramen ovale (Fig. 38-28).

Ostium secundum ASDs comprise greater than 80% of all ASDs and generally occur in isolation. This defect is caused by excessive resolution of the septum primum (foraminal flap) or by inadequate growth of the septum secundum (Fig. 38-29, *A*).

The **ostium primum ASD** is the second most common type. It is located low in the atrial septum, near the AV valves. Although the ostium primum ASD may occur alone, more commonly, it is associated with a more complex congenital cardiac anomaly, the atrioventricular septal defect (Fig. 38-29, *B*).

The **sinus venosus ASD** is a rare defect that can be divided into two types: (1) sinus venosus ASD of the superior vena cava (with the defect adjacent to the superior vena cava), and (2) sinus venosus ASD of the inferior vena cava (with the defect adjacent to the inferior vena cava). The first type is often associated with anomalous pulmonary venous return (Fig. 38-29, *C*).

The **prenatal sonographic diagnosis of ASD** is difficult because the normal patent foramen ovale, which allows blood to flow from the right to the left atrium *in utero*, itself represents an ASD of sorts. It is difficult to distinguish a small pathologic ASD from the normal patent foramen ovale.

Currently available high-resolution ultrasound equipment allows a detailed evaluation of the atrial septum that was previously impossible. The foraminal flap, or septum primum, is clearly visualized on the four-chamber view. It has a "loose pocket" configuration, appearing either circular or linear in shape as it opens into the left atrium[37,38] (Figs. 38-30 and 38-31). The characteristic appearance of the septum primum is clearly demonstrated on M-mode imaging (Fig. 38-32).

The septum secundum, which is thick and relatively stationary, makes up the majority of the atrial septum. The foramen ovale is an opening in the septum secundum. The septum secundum and foramen ovale are well visualized in the subcostal four-chamber view. The maximal size of the normal foramen ovale differs

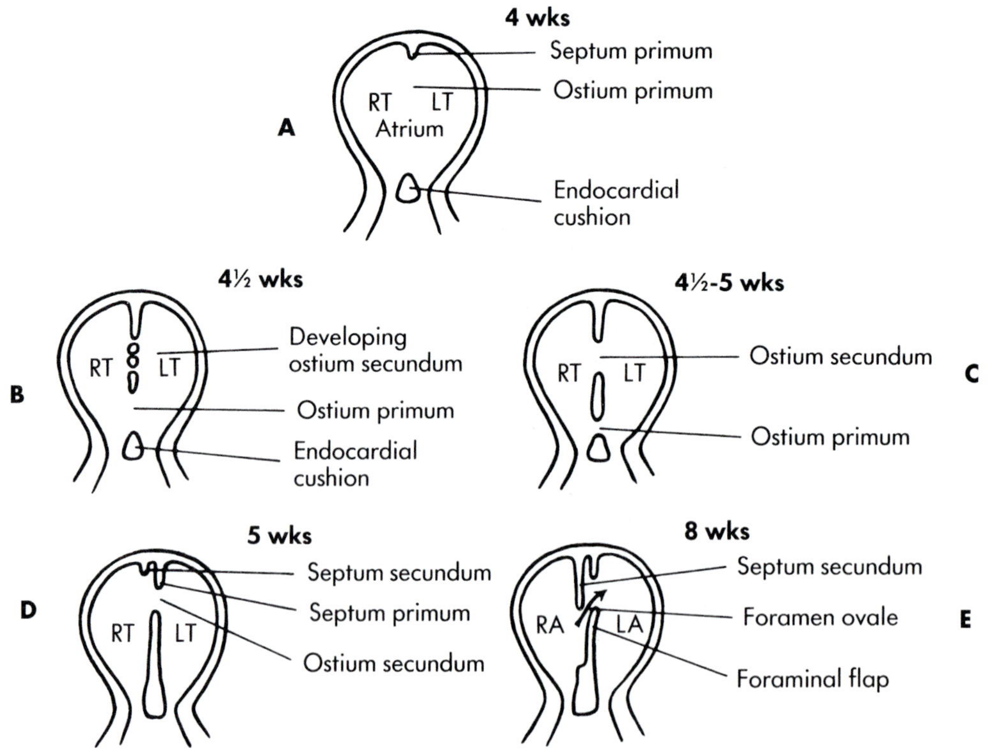

FIG. 38-28. Development of the intratrial septum (viewed facing the patient). **A,** At 4 weeks gestation the septum primum is small. A large ostium primum is present. **B,** At 4 1/2 weeks, enlargement of the septum primum results in reduction in size of the ostium primum. Perforations in the septum primum develop. **C,** Perforations in the septum primum coalesce to form the ostium secundum. **D,** At 5 weeks, the septum primum has fused to the endocardial cushions, and the septum secundum begins to develop to the right of the septum primum. **E,** At 8 weeks, the septum secundum has enlarged, now covering the ostium secundum. Blood flows from the right atrium through the valve mechanism (foraminal flap) of the foramen ovale.

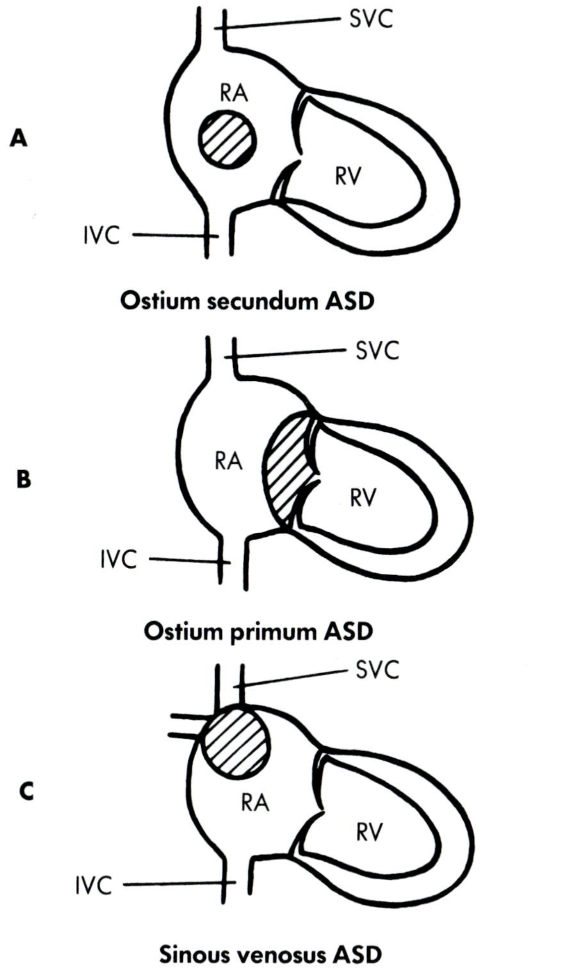

FIG. 38-29. Types of atrial septal defect. Schema of the atrial septum viewed from the right atrium. **A,** Ostium secundum ASD. **B,** Ostium primum ASD. **C,** Sinus venosus ASD.

by 1 mm or less from the aortic root diameter at all gestational ages.[39] An ostium secundum ASD appears as a larger than expected defect in the central portion of the atrial septum near the foramen ovale. Alternatively, it can appear as a deficient foraminal flap.

If the lowest portion of the atrial septum (just adjacent to the AV valves) is deficient, an **ostium primum defect** should be suspected (Fig. 38-33). Color flow Doppler imaging may be helpful in the diagnosis of larger ASDs. However, small ASDs are

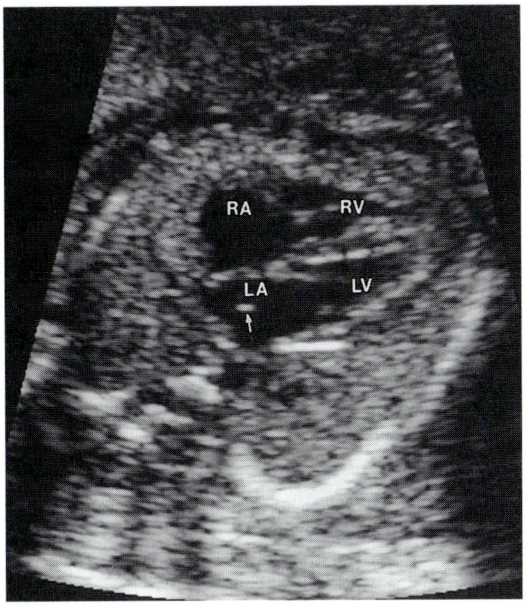

FIG. 38-31. Linear appearance of the foraminal flap *(arrow)* as it enters the left atrium, *LA*. Subcostal four-chamber view. *LV*, Left ventricle; *RA*, right atrium; *RV*, right ventricle.

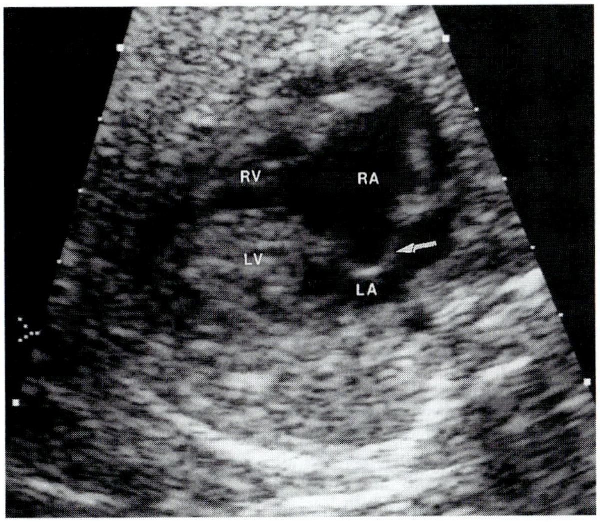

FIG. 38-30. Circular appearance of the foraminal flap *(arrow)* entering the left atrium, *LA*. Subcostal four-chamber view of the fetal heart. *LV*, Left ventricle; *RA*, right atrium; *RV*, right ventricle.

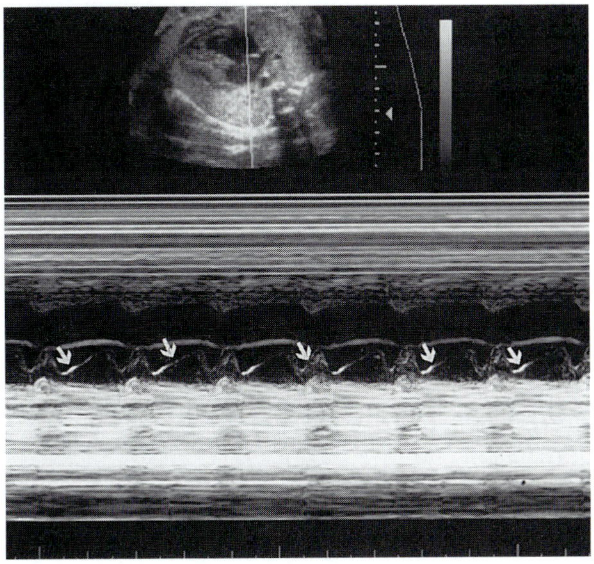

FIG. 38-32. M-mode tracing of the foraminal flap (*arrows*) within the left atrium.

commonly obscured by the normal flow through the patent foramen ovale[40,41] (Fig. 38-34).

A large, right-to-left shunt is physiologic *in utero*, thus an ASD generally does not compromise the fetus hemodynamically. After birth, the shunt may cause right ventricular overload and pulmonary hypertension. **Spontaneous closure** of an ASD will occur in approximately two thirds of cases.[42] It is not uncommon for patients with small ASDs to remain entirely asymptomatic well into their fifties.[43]

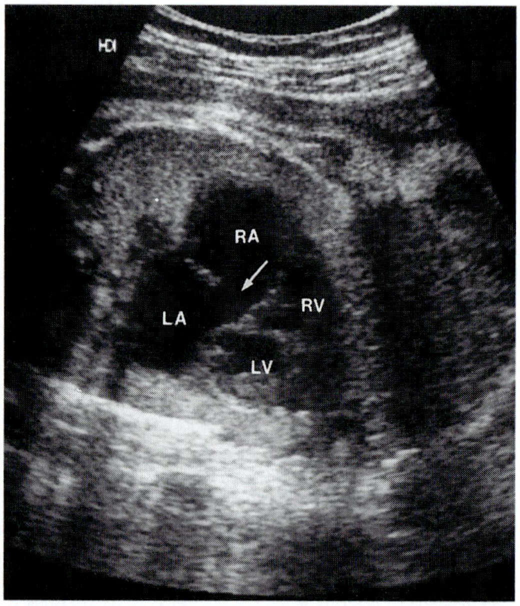

FIG. 38-33. Ostium primum ASD (*arrow*) in a fetus with an endocardial cushion defect. Four-chamber view. *LA*, Left atrium; *LV*, left ventricle; *RA*, right atrium; *RV*, right ventricle.

Ventricular Septal Defect

Ventricular septal defect (VSD) is the most common cardiac anomaly, accounting for 30% of heart defects in live-born infants and 9.7% in fetuses.[31,32,44] It accounts for 50% of all cardiovascular lesions. VSDs are associated with other cardiac anomalies half of the time.[45] Of the structural cardiac defects, VSDs have the **highest recurrence rate** and are the **most teratogen associated defect.** They may be classified according to their position in the interventricular septum (Fig. 38-35):

- Membranous VSD; and
- Muscular VSD (inlet, trabecular, outlet).[45]

Eighty percent of VSDs occur in the membranous portion of the septum.[46]

The subcostal four-chamber view provides optimal evaluation of the interventricular septum. At sonography, a VSD appears as an area of discontinuity in the interventricular septum. When the defect is small, this diagnosis is problematic, and nearly one third of VSDs are missed on the four-chamber view.[14,40,47-51] Color flow Doppler imaging dramatically improves the accuracy of the diagnosis of VSD.[40,51,52] Small VSDs that are not detectable on two-dimensional

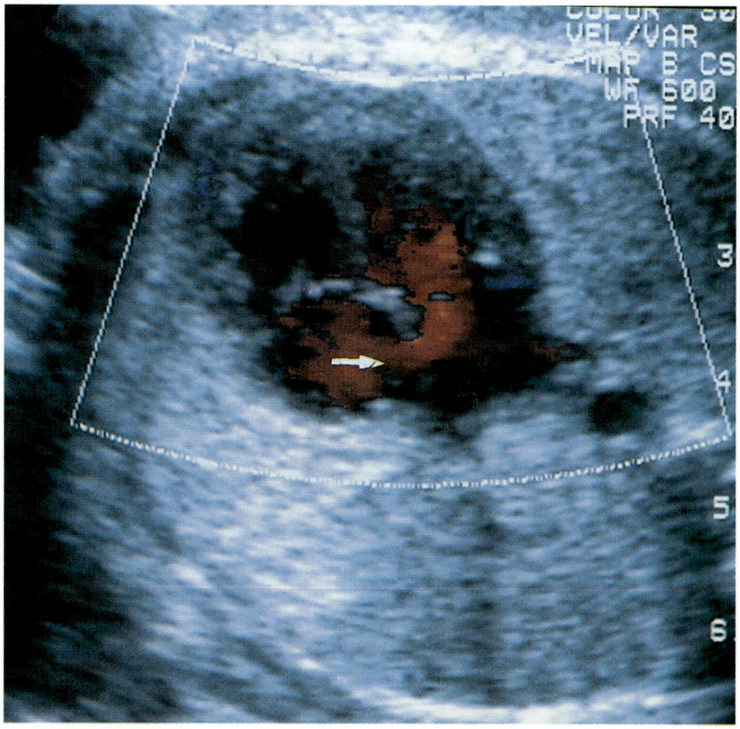

FIG. 38-34. Normal flow through the foramen ovale by color flow Doppler imaging (*arrow*). Apical four-chamber view.

echocardiography may be documented with color flow mapping[28] (Fig. 38-36). In the setting of an **isolated VSD,** color flow Doppler imaging typically shows bidirectional interventricular shunting with a systolic right-to-left shunt and a late diastolic left-to-right shunt. Unidirectional shunting across a VSD suggests additional cardiac anomalies.[27]

The **prognosis** for infants with an isolated VSD is excellent, and many go undetected. Forty percent of VSDs close in the first year of life, and 60% have resolved by 5 years.[53-55] However, large defects detected in the fetus have been associated with an 84% mortality.[56] Concurrent cardiac, extracardiac, and chromosomal anomalies (trisomy 13, 18, 21, and 22) are associated with a worse prognosis.

Atrioventricular Septal Defect

Atrioventricular septal defect (AVSD) refers to a spectrum of cardiac abnormalities involving various degrees of deficiency of the interatrial and interventricular septa

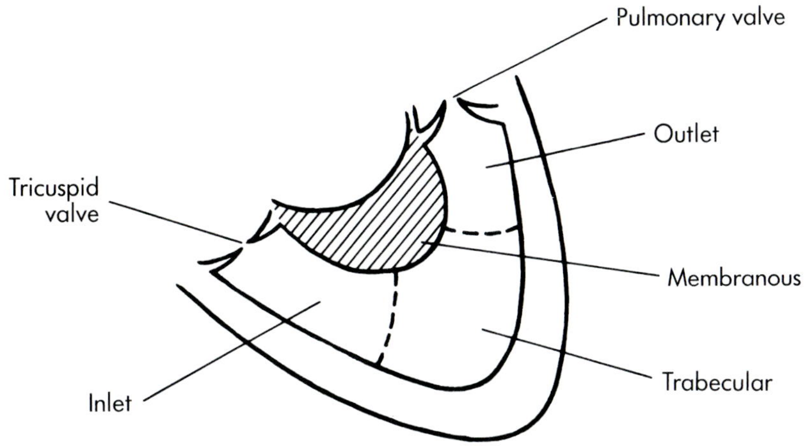

FIG. 38-35. Interventricular septum viewed from the right ventricle. The membranous septum and the three portions of the muscular septum (inlet, outlet, and trabecular) are demonstrated. VSDs may occur in any of these locations.

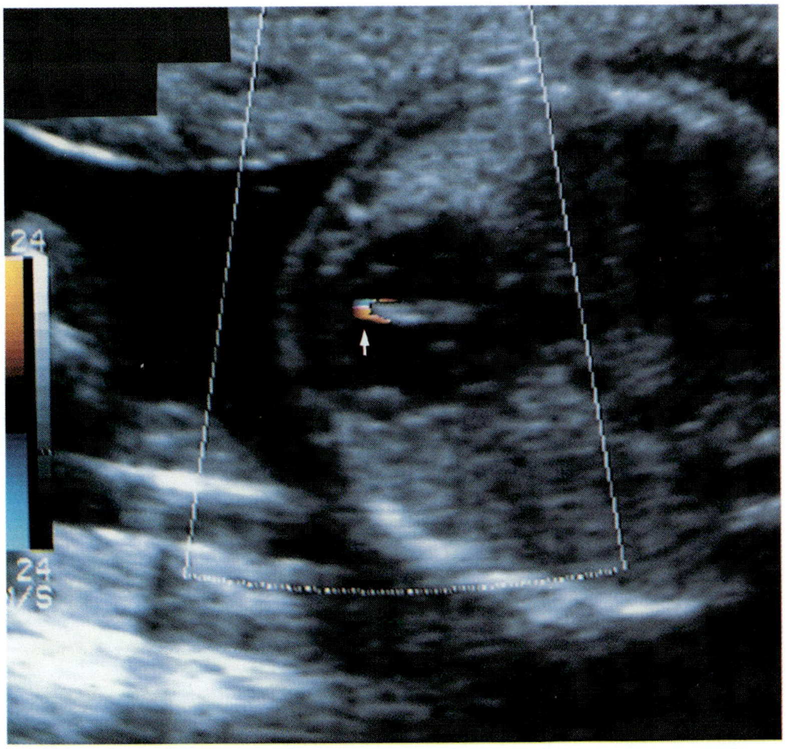

FIG. 38-36. Small VSD in the muscular portion of the interventricular septum. Four-chamber view of the fetal heart using color flow Doppler imaging *(arrow)*.

and of the mitral and tricuspid valves. These defects arise when the endocardial cushions fail to fuse properly and were previously called endocardial cushion defects or AV canal defects. Nearly two thirds of fetuses with AVSD have additional cardiac anomalies.[57-59] Approximately one third are associated with left atrial isomerism (both atria anatomically like the left), and of these the majority have complete heart block.[56,57] Chromosomal (especially **Down syndrome**) or extracardiac anomalies are associated in 78%.[56]

Embryologically, in the primitive heart, the common atrium and ventricle communicate via the AV canal. Development of the endocardial cushion results in division of the single large AV canal into two separate orifices, separating the atria from the ventricles (Fig. 38-37). The interatrial and interventricular septa develop concurrently, eventually dividing the single atrium and ventricle into right and left portions. When the endocardial cushions fail to fuse properly, normal development of the mitral and tricuspid valves cannot occur, and an AVSD results.

AVSDs are divided into complete and incomplete forms[60] (Fig. 38-38). In both, the AV canal has a single large valve with five leaflets. In the **complete type,** the five leaflets are separate whereas in the **incomplete form,** two of the leaflets (bridging leaflets) are connected by a narrow strip of tissue. Complete AVSD has variable amounts of deficient tissue in the atrial and ventricular septa. The incomplete form is associated with an ostium primum ASD and a cleft in the anterior "mitral" leaflet of the single AV valve. At fetal echocardiography, 97% of AVSDs are complete, although after birth only 69% are complete.[57,61] The fetal incidence of AVSD is four times greater than that in the live-born population, indicating a high incidence of *in utero* demise.[31,32]

Sonographically, a defect in the atrial and/or ventricular septum with an associated single abnormal AV valve is seen (Fig. 38-39). Demonstration of the bridging leaflet may allow differentiation between complete and incomplete forms of AVSD.[47]

Color flow Doppler ultrasound demonstrates an open area of flow across the endocardial cushion defect and the abnormal AV valve (Fig. 38-40). Color flow Doppler imaging is particularly useful in the detection of valvular insufficiency.[62] Holosystolic valvular insufficiency is closely associated with fetal hydrops and a worsening prognosis.[63] Frequently a left ventricular to right atrial jet can be identified across the ostium primum defect before the onset of holosystolic valvular insufficiency.[27]

Cardiac malformations associated with AVSD include septum secundum ASD, hypoplastic left heart, valvular pulmonary stenosis, coarctation of the aorta,

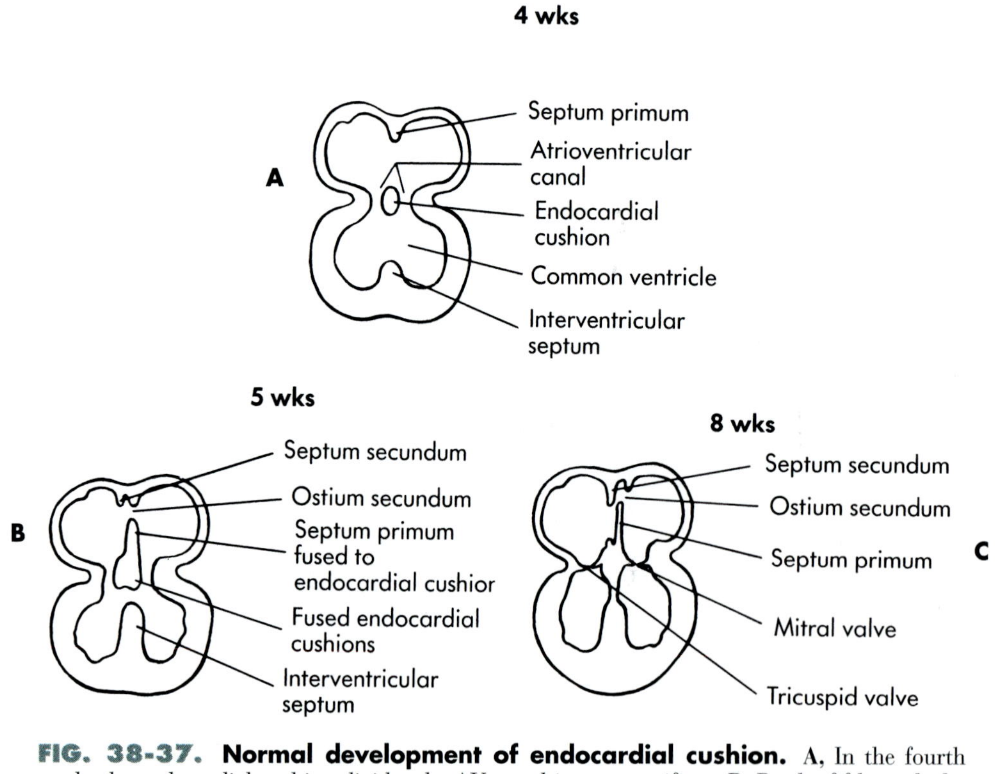

FIG. 38-37. Normal development of endocardial cushion. **A,** In the fourth week, the endocardial cushion divides the AV canal into two orifices. **B,** By the fifth week the communication between the atria, the ostium secundum, is smaller. The ventricular septum has grown, nearly obliterating the communication between the ventricles. **C,** At 8 weeks, complete development of the endocardial cushion and AV valves results in four distinct cardiac chambers.

tetralogy of Fallot, and others. Chromosomal anomalies are common, occurring in 75% of live births with AVSD,[9] and karyotyping is indicated.

The fetus with AVSD and associated defects has a poor prognosis. When hydrops is present, few or none survive the neonatal period.[64] Early operative intervention has increased late survival to 96% at 20 years rather than nearly 50% of untreated patients dying by 6 months.[65,66]

Ebstein Anomaly

Ebstein anomaly is characterized by inferior displacement of the tricuspid valve, frequently with tethered attachments of the leaflets, tricuspid dysplasia, and right ventricular dysplasia[67-71] (Fig. 38-41). Ebstein anomaly makes up approximately 7% of cardiac anomalies in the fetal population and has an incidence of 0.5% to 1% in high-risk populations.[49,72,73] It occurs in approximately 1 per 20,000 live births.[74]

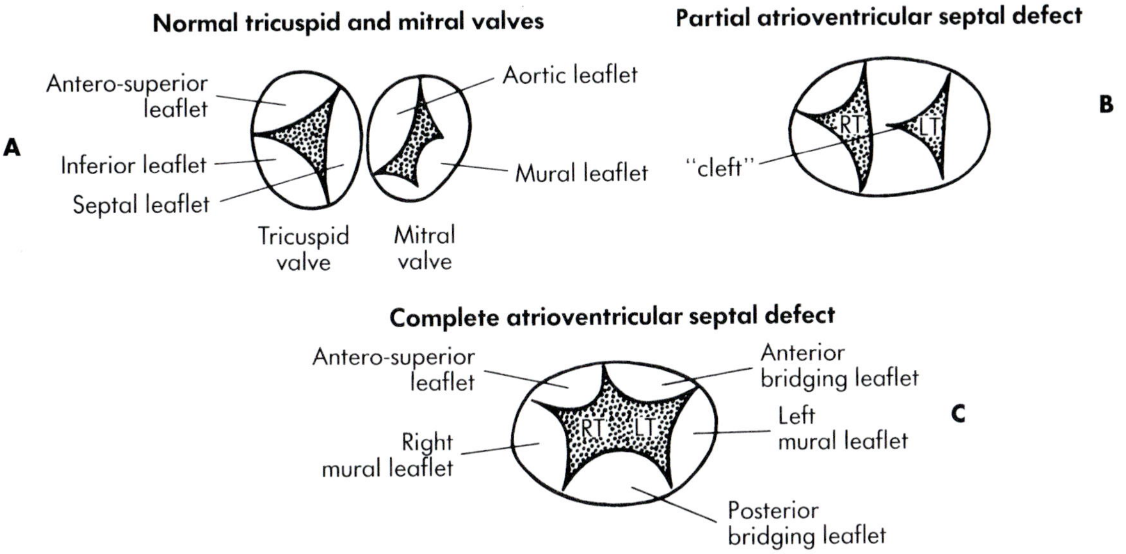

FIG. 38-38. Valve leaflet morphology. A, The normal heart. **B,** Partial AVSD. **C,** Complete AVSD.

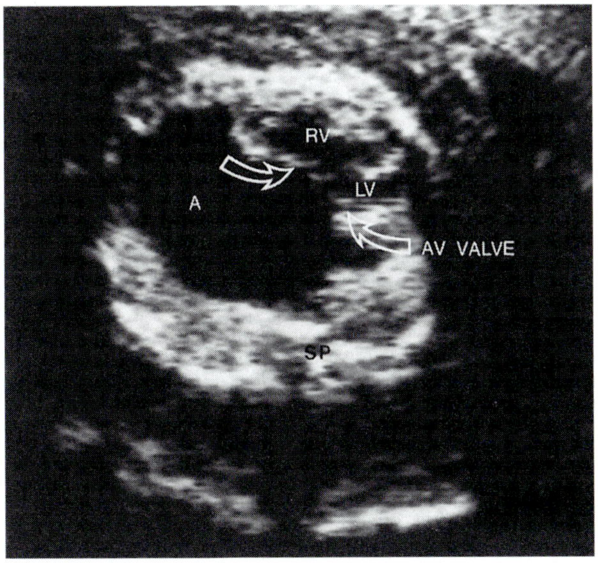

FIG. 38-39. Atrioventricular septal defect. The atrial septum is absent, resulting in a single large atrium, *A*. The VSD is seen between the arrows marking the abnormal AV valve leaflets. *Sp*, Spine; *LV*, left ventricle; *RV*, right ventricle.

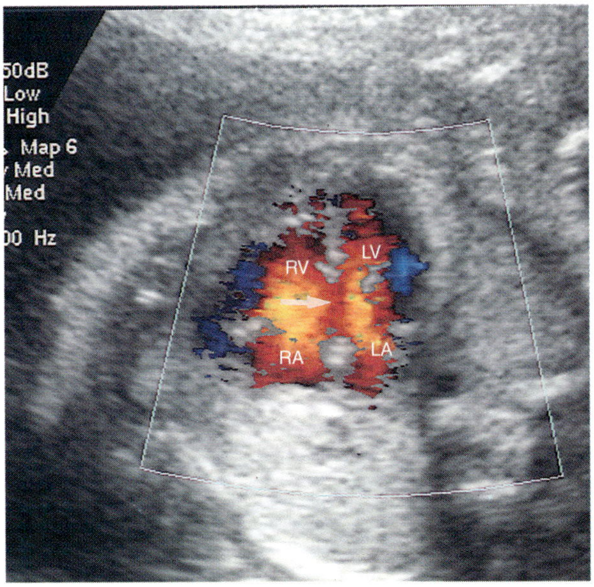

FIG. 38-40. Atrioventricular septal defect. Apical four-chamber view in a fetal heart using color flow Doppler imaging to demonstrate the open endocardial cushion defect *(arrow)*. *LA*, Left atrium; *LV*, left ventricle; *RA*, right atrium; *RV*, right ventricle.

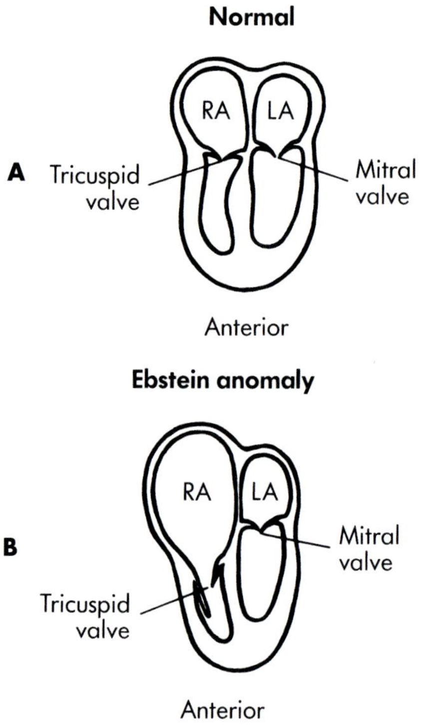

FIG. 38-41. Normal tricuspid valve and right ventricle compared with Ebstein anomaly. **A,** Normal. **B,** The tricuspid valve is apically displaced, resulting in an enlarged atrium and a small functional right ventricle.

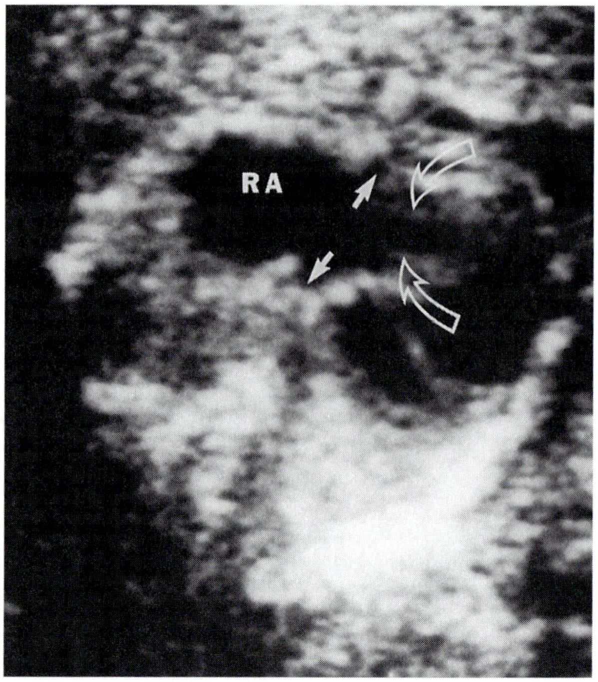

FIG. 38-42. Normal tricuspid valve and right ventricle compared with Ebstein anomaly. **A,** Normal. **B,** The tricuspid valve *(open arrows)* is displaced inferiorly. Note the "atrialized" right ventricle *(solid arrows)* and enlarged right atrium. *RA,* Right atrium.

Ebstein anomaly is most commonly associated with **maternal lithium exposure,** suggesting that lithium is a specific teratogen.[74-79] This view may be biased because most of the data comes from lithium registries in which physicians tend to report abnormal more frequently than normal hearts. The only major study that attempted to avoid this bias reported a cardiac malformation in 7% of lithium-exposed fetuses, but failed to link lithium with Ebstein anomaly.[80] Ebstein anomaly may be associated with a variety of structural cardiovascular defects, particularly pulmonary atresia or stenosis,[81] arrhythmias, and chromosomal anomalies.[69,82-85]

Ebstein anomaly is readily detected *in utero*.[82,86] The **sonographic diagnosis** rests on recognition of apical displacement of the tricuspid valve into the right ventricle, an enlarged right atrium containing a portion of the "atrialized" right ventricle, and a reduction in size of the functional right ventricle (Fig. 38-42). **Differential diagnosis** includes tricuspid valvular dysplasia, Uhl anomaly, and idiopathic right atrial enlargement, but none of these has an inferiorly displaced tricuspid valve, the most reliable sign of Ebstein anomaly. Ebstein anomaly is one of the few structural defects that may cause significant cardiac dysfunction *in utero*, frequently with cardiomegaly, hydrops, and tachyarrhythmias.[69] Doppler examination is helpful in demonstrating tricuspid valve regurgitation, which causes further enlargement of the right atrium and ventricle.[87] Tethered distal attachments of the tricuspid valve, marked right atrial enlargement, and left ventricular compression with narrowing of the pulmonary outflow tract are all associated with a poor prognosis.[69] **Arrhythmias,** particularly supraventricular tachycardias, are common with Ebstein anomaly and can further compromise the fetus. Overall, the 3-month mortality rate of patients diagnosed *in utero* is 80%.[69,86]

Hypoplastic Right Heart Syndrome

Hypoplastic right ventricle generally occurs secondary to pulmonary atresia with an intact interventricular septum. It has an incidence of 1.1% among stillbirths.[31] Tricuspid atresia and other defects may be present, but are uncommon.[88] Pathophysiologically, hypoplasia of the right ventricle develops because of reduction of blood flow secondary to inflow impedance from tricuspid atresia or outflow impedance caused by pulmonary arterial atresia.

Typical **sonographic findings** include a small right ventricle with concentric hypertrophy and a small or absent pulmonary artery[88] (Fig. 38-43). Doppler examination may be helpful in demonstrating decreased flow through the tricuspid valve or

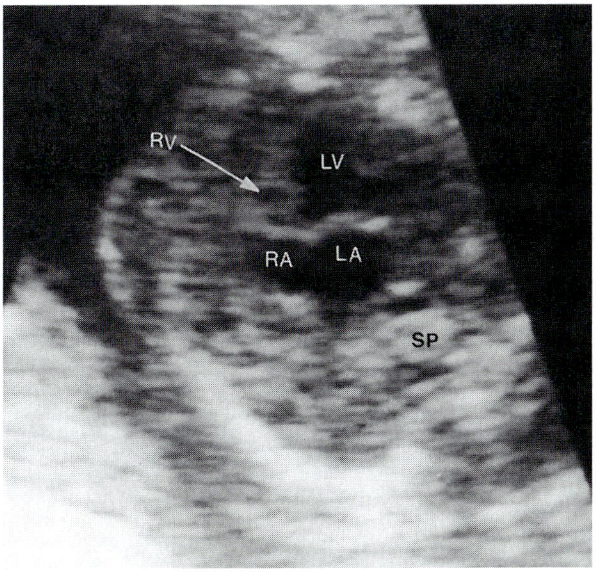

FIG. 38-43. Hypoplastic right ventricle. Apical four-chamber view shows the small right ventricular chamber *(arrow)*. *RV*, Right ventricle; *RA*, right atrium; *LV*, left ventricle; *LA*, left atrium; *Sp*, spine.

pulmonary artery. Congestive heart failure and hydrops may develop from tricuspid regurgitation. Following birth, closure of the ductus arteriosus frequently results in neonatal death. Prognosis has improved with preoperative prostaglandin infusions to maintain the patency of the ductus.[89]

Hypoplastic Left Heart Syndrome

Hypoplastic left heart is a syndrome in which the left ventricular cavity is pathologically reduced in size. It constitutes approximately 7% to 9% of all congenital cardiac lesions.[90] It has a 2:1 male predominance and a recurrence risk of 0.5%.[90,91] The small left ventricle results from decreased blood flow into or out of the left ventricle. The primary abnormalities include **aortic atresia, aortic stenosis,** and **mitral valve atresia.** It is associated with **coarctation of the aorta** in 80% of cases.[92] The primary sonographic feature of hypoplastic left heart syndrome is a small left ventricle (Fig. 38-44). The mitral valve is typically hypoplastic or atretic as is the aorta.[93] Color flow Doppler imaging is extremely helpful in the setting of hypoplastic left heart, commonly demonstrating the characteristic single area of flow at the AV valve level and bidirectional flow in the proximal aorta when associated coarctation of the aorta is present.[28]

This syndrome has an **extremely poor prognosis** with a 25% mortality within the first week of life and untreated infants dying within 6 weeks.[94] A variety of operative procedures have been attempted, but all have a poor prognosis. Heart transplantation has been attempted with limited success.[90,95-97]

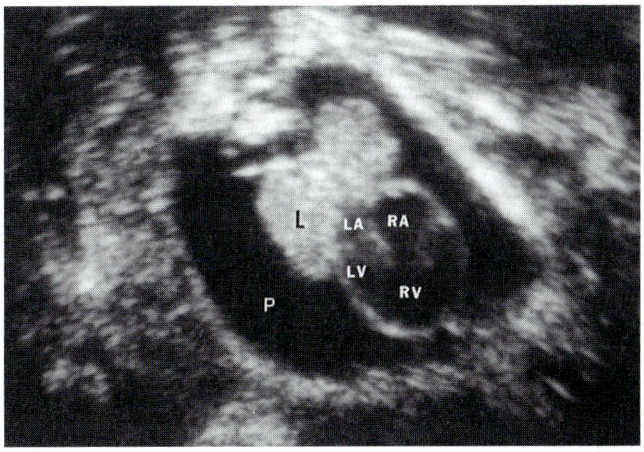

FIG. 38-44. Hypoplastic left ventricle. The left side of the heart is small. The function of the heart is compromised, resulting in hydrops. Anechoic pleural fluid, *P*, surrounds the heart and the compressed echogenic lungs, *L*, posterior to the heart. *LA*, Left atrium; *RA*, right atrium; *LV*, left ventricle; *RV*, right ventricle.

Univentricular Heart

This abnormality consists of a heart in which two AV valves or a common AV valve empty into a single ventricle. The ventricle may (type A) or may not (type B) have an outflow tract.[98] Univentricular heart is rare, accounting for approximately 2% of CHD.[32] It results from a failure of the interventricular septum to develop. The single chamber has a left ventricular morphology in 85% of cases.[99] Cardiac anomalies frequently associated with univentricular heart include pulmonary stenosis (64%), ASD (23%), and common atrium (14%).[100] Asplenia or polysplenia occurs in 13%.[101]

Sonographically, a single ventricle with absence of the interventricular septum is seen. Doppler examination is helpful in determining whether an outflow tract is present. Differential diagnosis includes a large VSD and hypoplastic right or left heart.

Patients with outflow tract stenosis have a poorer prognosis.[98] Death is commonly caused by congestive heart failure or arrhythmia.[102] Pulmonary artery banding and shunts yield a 70% postoperative 5-year survival rate. Ventricular septation has a postoperative survival rate of approximately 56%.[100,103]

Tetralogy of Fallot

Tetralogy of Fallot consists of:

- A VSD;
- An overriding aorta;
- Hypertrophy of the right ventricle; and
- Stenosis of the right ventricular outflow tract.

It accounts for 5% to 10% of CHD[31] and has been associated with a variety of cardiac and extracardiac abnormalities and chromosomal anomalies in 12% to 50%.[56] This abnormality occurs when the conus septum is located too far anteriorly, thus dividing the conus into a smaller anterior right ventricular portion and a larger posterior part. Therefore, closure of the interventricular septum is incomplete, causing the aorta to override both ventricles.[104]

The characteristic structural defects can be demonstrated by **fetal echocardiography** (Fig. 38-45). The VSD typically occurs in the perimembranous portion of the septum. Right ventricular hypertrophy rarely occurs *in utero*, but the dilated aorta is reliably seen.[105,106] Pulmonary atresia or stenosis, or a dilated pulmonary artery secondary to absence of the valve, may be appreciated. The diagnosis of tetralogy of Fallot has been made prior to 15 weeks gestation with the use of vaginal probe ultrasound.[19] Color flow Doppler imaging is helpful in making the diagnosis of tetralogy of Fallot.[107]

Cardiac surgery has improved the survival rate to 85%.[108,109] The presence of congestive heart failure in the fetus or newborn is associated with a 17% to 41% mortality.[110,111]

Truncus Arteriosus

Truncus arteriosus comprises 1.3% of fetal cardiac anomalies and is characterized by a single large vessel arising from the base of the heart. This vessel supplies the coronary arteries and the pulmonary and systemic circulations. Aortic anomalies occur in 20% and noncardiac anomalies in 48% of patients with truncus arteriosus.[112] In nearly all cases, a VSD is present. The truncal valve may have two to six cusps and generally overrides the ventricular septum. **Four types** of truncus arteriosus have been identified by Collett and Edwards[113]:

- **Type I** has a pulmonary artery that bifurcates into right and left branches after it arises from the ascending portion of the truncal vessel;
- **Type II** has right and left pulmonary arteries arising separately from the posterior truncus;
- **Type III** has pulmonary arteries that arise from the sides of the proximal truncus; and
- **Type IV** has systemic collateral vessels from the descending aorta as the source of flow.

The single large truncal artery with overriding of the ventricular septum and an associated VSD has been identified with **fetal echocardiography** (Fig. 38-46). This anomaly has been diagnosed before 15 weeks gestation with transvaginal ultrasound.[19] Color flow Doppler imaging is particularly helpful in the setting of truncus arteriosus because it facilitates accurate localization of the pulmonary arteries and rapidly detects truncal valvular insufficiency. Prognosis is poor with an overall mortality of 70%.[112]

Double Outlet Right Ventricle

Double outlet right ventricle (DORV) comprises less than 1% of all CHD and occurs when more than 50% of both the aorta and pulmonary artery arise from the right ventricle.[114,115] DORV is classified into **three types:**

- Aorta posterior and to the right of the pulmonary artery;
- Aorta and pulmonary artery parallel with the aorta to the right (Taussig-Bing syndrome); and

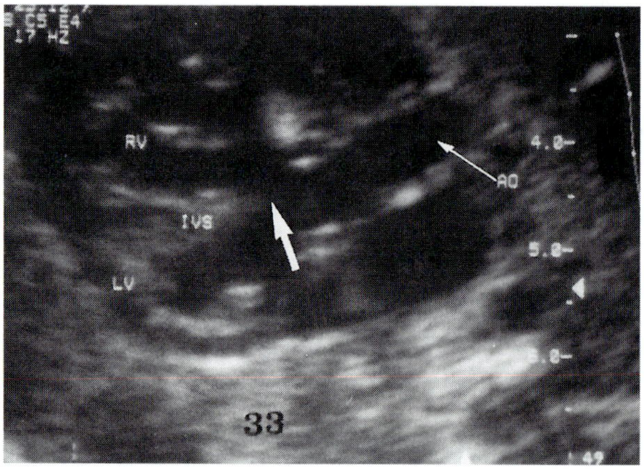

FIG. 38-45. Tetralogy of Fallot. The aorta, *AO*, overrides both ventricular chambers. A high VSD *(arrow)* is seen. *RV*, Right ventricle; *LV*, left ventricle; *IVS*, interventricular septum. (Courtesy Swedish Medical Center, Englewood, Colo.)

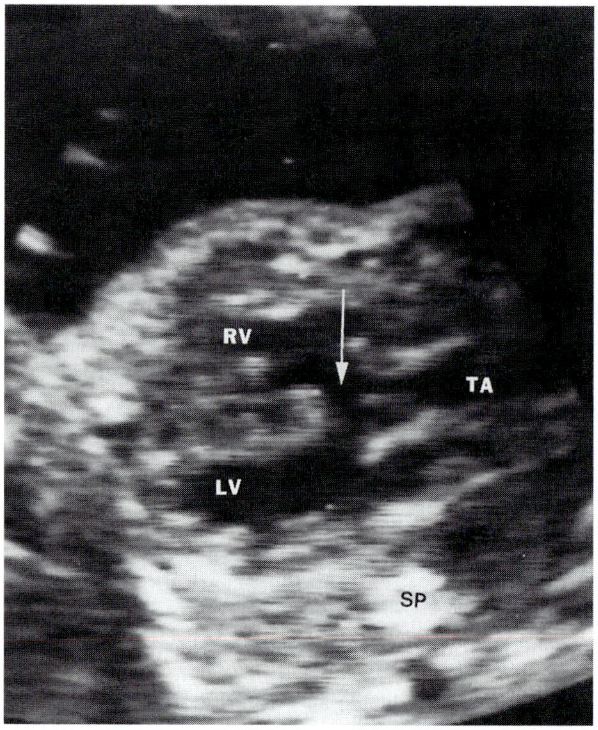

FIG. 38-46. Truncus arteriosus. The single great artery, *TA*, overrides both chambers. A ventricular septal defect *(arrow)* is present. No pulmonary artery was seen, helping to differentiate from tetralogy of Fallot. *RV*, Right ventricle; *LV*, left ventricle; *Sp*, spine.

• Aorta and pulmonary artery parallel with the aorta anterior and to the left.

DORV is associated with other cardiac defects (particularly VSD), maternal diabetes, and maternal alcohol consumption.[2,115] With surgical intervention, a 10-year survival rate of up to 97% has been reported.[114]

Sonographically, the aorta and pulmonary artery arise from the right ventricle (Fig. 38-47). Differential diagnosis includes transposition of the great vessels and tetralogy of Fallot.

Transposition of Great Arteries

Transposition of the great arteries (TGA) can be subdivided into **two types:** (1) complete or dextrotransposition (D-TGA), occurring in 80% of fetuses with transposition; and (2) congenitally corrected or levotransposition (L-TGA), occurring in 20%. In both types, ventriculo-arterial discordance is present. The aorta leaves the right ventricle and the pulmonary artery leaves the left ventricle).

Complete transposition of the great arteries (D-TGA) is defined as atrioventricular concordance (the atria and ventricles are correctly paired) with ventriculo-arterial discordance. It comprises 5.5% of heart disease in the fetal population.[32] It is classified into **two types,** depending on the absence (70%) or presence of a VSD. A variety of cardiac anomalies are associated with D-TGA, including pulmonic stenosis, which rarely occurs in the absence of a VSD. In 8% of cases, other organ systems are involved. Chromosomal anomalies have not been associated with TGA.

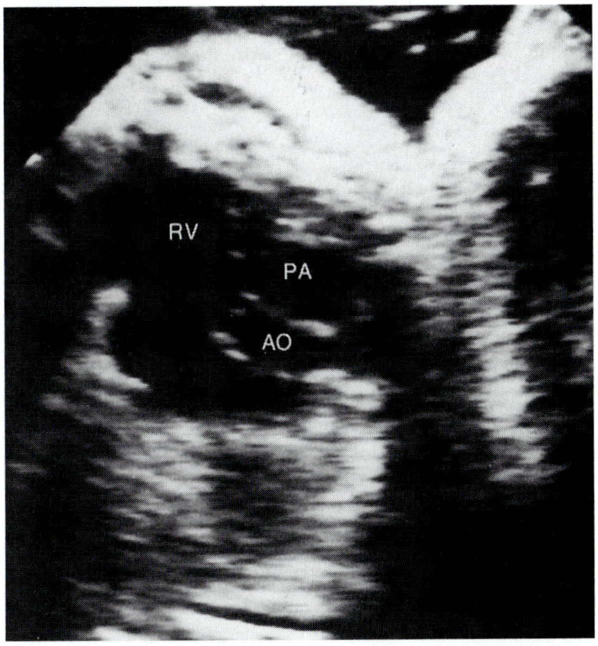

FIG. 38-47. Double outlet right ventricle. The aorta, *Ao*, and pulmonary artery, *PA*, exit the right ventricle, *RV*, parallel to each other with the aorta to the left (type 3). (Courtesy Swedish Medical Center, Englewood, Colo.)

In D-TGA, the aorta arises from the right ventricle, receives systemic blood, and returns it to the systemic circulation. The pulmonary artery arises from the left ventricle, receives pulmonary venous blood, and returns it to the lungs. Generally, the aortic root lies anterior and slightly to the right of the pulmonary outflow tract. With closure of the ductus arteriosus and foramen ovale after birth, this condition is incompatible with life unless there is an associated shunt allowing mixing of the separate right and left circulations.

The antenatal diagnosis of D-TGA is difficult. **Sonographic diagnosis** depends on demonstrating that the great vessels exit the heart in parallel, rather than crossing each other in normal fashion. This is optimally seen in the short-axis view of the great vessels. The diagnosis of TGA is simplified with color flow Doppler imaging because it allows more rapid characterization of the abnormal flow patterns and clearly demonstrates the abnormal parallel configuration of the great vessels.[27,87]

Most neonates with D-TGA require immediate treatment. Initially, a temporizing shunt is created prior to definitive treatment. With operative intervention, a 12-month survival can be expected in 80%.[116]

Corrected transposition of the great arteries (L-TGA) is characterized by AV discordance with ventriculo-arterial discordance. It comprises 1% of CHD and 20% of cases of transposition of the great arteries in the fetal population.[32] The aorta, which arises from the right ventricle, is anterior and to the left of the pulmonary artery. VSD and pulmonic stenosis occur in approximately half the cases.[99,117] Malformation and inferior displacement of the morphologic tricuspid valve may be present. Pathophysiologically, the flow of blood through the heart to the pulmonic and to the systemic circulations is normal, even though the morphologic right ventricle is on the left and the morphologic left ventricle is on the right.

As in D-TGA, the antenatal **sonographic diagnosis** is difficult and hinges on demonstrating a parallel arrangement to the great vessels. Color flow Doppler mapping is extremely helpful in making the diagnosis. Differentiating D-TGA from L-TGA entails identification of the morphologic right and left ventricles. This is problematic.

In the absence of associated cardiac anomalies, patients with corrected TGA may remain asymptomatic throughout their lives.

Anomalous Pulmonary Venous Return

Anomalous pulmonary venous return (APVR) can be divided into two subgroups: **total anomalous pulmonary venous return** (TAPVR), in which none of the pulmonary veins drain into the left atrium, and

partial anomalous pulmonary venous return (PAPVR), in which at least one of the pulmonary veins has an anomalous connection. TAPVR constitutes 2.3% of cases of CHD.[118] There are **four types** of anomalous pathways:

- The pulmonary veins drain into a vertical vein that empties into the innominate vein and then into the superior vena cava;
- The pulmonary veins drain into the coronary sinus and then into the right atrium;
- The pulmonary veins drain directly into the right atrium; and
- The pulmonary vein drains into the portal vein and into the inferior vena cava via the ductus venosus.

TAPVR is associated with AVSDs, polysplenia, and asplenia syndromes.

Embryologically, TAPVR is thought to result from failure of obliteration of the normal connections between the primitive pulmonary vein and the splanchnic, umbilical, vitelline, and cardinal veins.

The antenatal **sonographic diagnosis** of TAPVR is rare because it is difficult to identify the abnormal venous connections in the fetal population since these anomalous vessels are generally extremely small and variable in their course. Only a few reports detail the prenatal diagnosis of TAPVR.[119,120]

Often the first sign of APVR is mild right ventricular and pulmonary artery prominence, and a careful search for the four normal pulmonary veins should be undertaken in this setting. Color flow or pulsed wave Doppler imaging (Figs. 38-48 and 38-49) may be helpful in documenting the normal pulmonary venous anatomy or in detecting and following the anomalous connections.

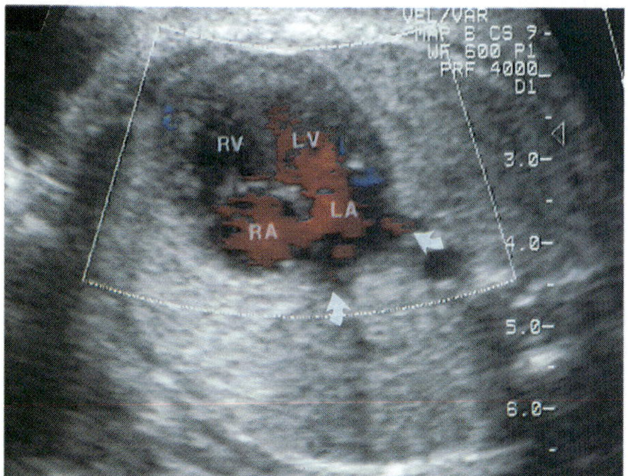

FIG. 38-48. Normal pulmonary veins entering the left atrium (*arrows*). Apical four-chamber view using color flow Doppler imaging. *LA*, Left atrium; *LV*, left ventricle; *RA*, right atrium; *RV*, right ventricle.

Duplex Doppler imaging should be used to evaluate blood flow across the AV valves or aortic and pulmonic valves. A ratio of right-to-left flow greater than 2:1 is highly suspicious for TAPVR.[119]

The diagnosis of TAPVR must be entertained when the four normal pulmonary veins entering the left atrium are not visible. A small left atrium resulting from decreased blood return and from the lack of normal incorporation of the common pulmonary vein into the left atrium is also suggestive of TAPVR. Approximately one third of patients with TAPVR will have associated cardiac anomalies.[121] These are variable.

TAPVR causes little hemodynamic disturbance *in utero*, though hydrops occasionally results. Left untreated, the majority of infants die before 1 year of age.[121]

Coarctation of Aorta

Coarctation is a narrowing of the aortic lumen, usually at the ductus arteriosus. Its severity ranges from a slight narrowing at the distal end of the arch to severe hypoplasia of the entire arch. Coarctation has an incidence of 6% prenatally.[32] Nearly 90% of the cases are associated with other cardiac anomalies, including abnormal (bicuspid or stenotic) aortic valve, VSD, DORV, AVSD, and others. Chromosomal abnormalities occur in 5%, and nearly 5% of coarctations are associated with maternal diabetes.[44,122]

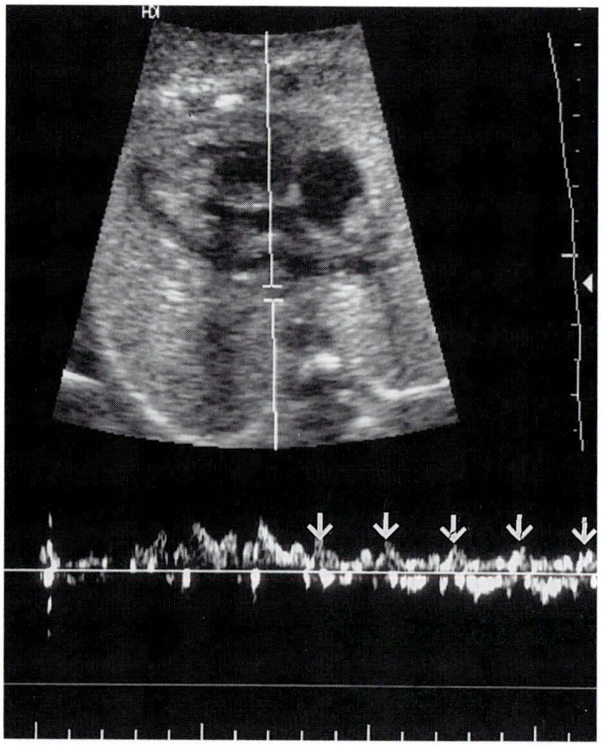

FIG. 38-49. Normal pulmonary vein (*arrows*). Pulsed wave Doppler tracing.

Three **embryologic theories** have been proposed to explain the origin of coarctation of the aorta: (1) a primary developmental defect with failure of connection of the fourth and sixth aortic arches with the descending aorta,[123] (2) aberrant ductal tissue at the level of the aortic arch,[124,125] and (3) decreased blood flow through the aortic isthmus *in utero*.[126]

Sonographic detection of coarctation is difficult. Ventricular size discrepancy with a prominent right ventricle and relatively small left ventricle[40,126] with a right-to-left ventricle diameter ratio greater than 2 standard deviations above the norm[127,128] is suggestive of coarctation of the aorta. Likewise, a discrepancy in pulmonary artery to ascending aorta diameter that falls greater than 2 standard deviations above the normal ratio of 1.18 ± 0.06[128] is suggestive of coarctation.[127] Doppler and color flow Doppler imaging may be useful in identifying the area of narrowing.

The most consistent and useful sign of coarctation, however, appears to be the presence of distal aortic arch hypoplasia[127] when compared with normal values.[129]

Preliminary data suggest that coarctation may progress in utero. For this reason, serial echocardiograms may be useful when there is a strong suspicion of aortic coarctation.[127]

Although isolated coarctation has a good prognosis, a 39% mortality has been reported when other anomalies are associated.[130]

Aortic and Pulmonic Stenosis

Aortic and pulmonic stenosis are strictures or obstructions to the ventricular outflow tract. Aortic stenosis occurs in approximately 5.2% and pulmonic stenosis in 7.4% of newborns.[31] **Aortic stenosis** is divided into supravalvular, valvular, and subvalvular types. Supravalvular stenosis occurs above the sinuses of Valsalva and may be associated with William's syndrome. Valvular aortic stenosis is more frequent in males. It may be associated with a bicuspid aortic valve and chromosomal abnormalities.[131] Subvalvular aortic stenosis may be associated with inherited disorders, asymmetric septal hypertrophy, or hypertrophic obstructive cardiomyopathy. Infants of diabetic mothers may have a transient form of left ventricular outflow tract obstruction secondary to asymmetric septal hypertrophy.

Pulmonic stenosis may occur at the valve level or at the infundibulum. Dysplastic and stenotic pulmonary valves are seen in Noonan syndrome and with maternal rubella. Pulmonic stenosis is associated with total APVR, ASD, supravalvular aortic stenosis, and tetralogy of Fallot.

Sonographically, prenatal detection of **aortic stenosis** is difficult (Fig. 38-50). The supravalvular type has not been reported *in utero*. Thickening of the aortic valve, poststenotic dilatation of the aorta, and ventricular enlargement are clues to valvular aortic stenosis. Thickening of the interventricular septum may be seen in subvalvular aortic stenosis.

Dilatation of the proximal pulmonary artery and hypertrophy of the right ventricle suggest **pulmonic stenosis.** Prenatal identification of pulmonic stenosis is difficult. Color flow Doppler imaging is particularly helpful in distinguishing pulmonary and aortic atresia from valvular stenosis.[27]

A mortality rate of 23% in the first year of life has been reported with aortic stenosis.[132] Prognosis has improved with appropriate surgery with the mortality rate being between 1.9% and 9%.[133,134] Similarly, pulmonic stenosis has a variable outcome and may be effectively managed with closed transventricular valvotomy or percutaneous balloon valvoplasty.[135,136]

Cardiosplenic Syndrome

Cardiosplenic syndromes are syndromes associated with **asplenia** and **polysplenia.** Both are defects of lateralization in which symmetric development of normally asymmetric organs or organ systems occurs. **Asplenia** (Ivemark's syndrome) and **polysplenia** syndromes are usually considered separate clinical entities; however, they have many characteristics in common, including situs inversus or situs ambiguous of various visceral organs and complex congenital heart defects.[137]

Pathologically, in **asplenia or bilateral right-sidedness,** left-sided organs are a mirror image of normally right-sided organs. This results in right atrial isomerism, bilateral trilobed lungs, bilateral right bronchi and pulmonary arteries, ipsilateral location of both the aorta and inferior vena cava (IVC) (either left

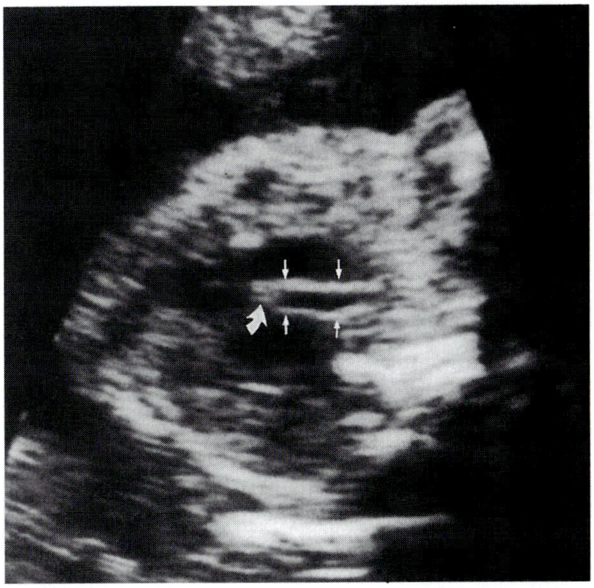

FIG. 38-50. Aortic stenosis. The aortic valve *(curved arrow)* is echogenic and stenotic. The typical poststenotic dilatation is not present in this case, which had fibrotic thickening of the ascending aorta *(small arrows)*.

or right side), absence of the spleen, a midline horizontal liver, and bilateral superior vena cavae.[138] In **polysplenia or bilateral left-sidedness,** the right lung and bronchial tree morphologically mirror those of the left. In many instances, intrahepatic interruption of the IVC with azygous continuation is present as are multiple spleens and left atrial isomerism.[139]

A variety of **associated cardiac anomalies** have been reported with these syndromes. These include TAPVR or PAPVR, ASD, VSD, univentricular heart, transposition, double outlet right ventricle, pulmonary stenosis, pulmonary atresia, aortic atresia, and aortic stenosis. Coarctation, hypoplastic left ventricle, mitral stenosis, cor triatriatum, dextrocardia, right atrial hypoplasia, endocardial cushion defect, and tetralogy of Fallot have also been observed.[139-142] Cardiac anomalies are more complex and severe in asplenia.[140] **Complete AV block** in conjunction with an AV canal has been associated with polysplenia. Polysplenia syndrome is the second most common disease associated with fetal heart block (after L-transposition).[141]

Cardiosplenic syndromes should be considered when congenital heart disease occurs in conjunction with an arrhythmia. If these syndromes are suspected, a careful **sonographic** search for the fetal spleen, which has been visualized at 20 weeks gestation, and of the fetal stomach is indicated.[141,143] Other abnormal relationships, such as ipsilateral aorta and IVC (associated with asplenia) or interruption of the IVC with continuation of the azygous vein (associated with polysplenia), may be documented sonographically.

The mortality rate with cardiosplenic syndromes is extremely high. **Treatment** for polysplenia and asplenia depends largely on the type and number of associated anomalies. Because cardiac malformations associated with polysplenia are often less severe, they are more amenable to surgical correction than are lesions associated with asplenia.[143,144] The association with complete heart block poses a significant threat to survival.

ASPLENIA

Bilateral right sidedness
Right atrial isomerism
Bilateral trilobed lungs
Bilateral right bronchi
Bilateral right pulmonary arteries
Ipsilateral location of both aorta and IVC
Absence of the spleen
Midline horizontal liver
Bilateral superior vena cavae
Severe and complex heart anomalies

POLYSPLENIA

Bilateral left sidedness
Interruption of IVC
Azygous continuation of IVC
Multiple spleens
Left atrial isomerism
Complete AV block

Cardiac Tumors

Cardiac tumors in the infant are rare. Ten percent of tumors are malignant.[145,146] Until the infant is 1 year of age, approximately 75% of all tumors and cysts of the heart and pericardium are rhabdomyomas (58%) and teratomas (19%). Cardiac fibromas account for approximately 12% of the tumors in this age group. Other less frequent tumors include mesothelioma of the AV node and cardiac hemangioma (approximately 2% each). Although myxomas are the most common heart neoplasm (comprising 50% of cardiac tumors over all age groups), they are virtually nonexistent in the neonatal population.[146]

Of patients with cardiac rhabdomyomas, 30% to 78% have **tuberous sclerosis.**[147-149] Other signs of tuberous sclerosis are rarely found in fetal life. Unfortunately, the absence of cardiac neoplasms in a fetus at risk for tuberous sclerosis does not exclude this disease.[150]

Sonographically, fetal cardiac tumors usually appear as solid, echogenic masses. **Rhabdomyomas** (cardiac hamartomas) may be singular or multiple tumors and are located within the heart, typically arising from the interventricular septum[151-153] (Fig. 38-51). Intracardiac clot may closely mimic rhabdomyoma. **Teratomas** may appear as cystic or solid masses. These are intrapericardial in origin.[150,154,155]

Several series report the appearance or enlargement of fetal rhabdomyomas on sequential examinations.[150,156] This finding underscores the importance of **serial fetal echocardiograms** in fetuses at risk for rhabdomyomas.

Infants with cardiac rhabdomyomas have a guarded **prognosis.** Although spontaneous regression of the tumor has been reported, sudden death is not uncommon.[146] Before reaching their second year, 60% to 75% of infants die.[157] Cardiac tumors may become hemodynamically significant by causing obstruction to the outflow tracts or AV valves, resulting in congestive heart failure, hydrops, pericardial effusion, and arrhythmias.[147,158] Prognosis depends on a variety of factors, including size, number, and the exact location of the tumor as well as associated arrhythmias and anomalies.

Cardiomyopathy

Cardiomyopathy encompasses a diverse group of cardiac disorders with variable etiologies and anatomic and functional characteristics. All result in an alteration in cardiac function. Cardiomyopathies represent 1.8% of CHD in live-born infants.[118]

A variety of conditions can cause fetal cardiomyopathy, including viral and bacterial infections, inborn errors of metabolism, endocardial fibroelastosis, and maternal diabetes (Fig. 38-52). Infectious agents act by damaging the myocardium and producing a myocarditis with resultant cardiomyopathy[159] (Fig. 38-53). In the setting of storage diseases, the myocardium becomes hypertrophic secondary to the accumulation of various products within the myocardial cells. Endocardial fibroelastosis (EF) is a poorly understood process in which diffuse endocardial thickening involves one or more cardiac chambers. EF is commonly divided into two broad categories: primary and secondary.

Primary or isolated endocardial fibroelastosis occurs in the absence of other structural cardiac anomalies. In this condition, the affected ventricle may be either dilated, hypertrophic, or "constricted" (which implies profound hypertrophy).[160]

Secondary endocardial fibroelastosis occurs in the setting of a structural cardiac anomaly and may result in dilatation or hypertrophy of the affected chambers. The dilated form may occur with coarctation of the aorta, aortic valvular disease, mitral valvular disease, and other lesions. The constricted form is frequently associated with aortic stenosis or atresia.

In both types, the mural endocardium is largely replaced by collagen and elastic tissue, giving it a glistening white appearance grossly[84] and a striking echogenic appearance at echocardiography (Fig. 38-54). Color flow Doppler imaging may be valuable in the evaluation of cardiomyopathy. Preliminary data suggest that one of the first signs of EF may be tricuspid regurgitation, which is easily identified with color flow mapping.[28]

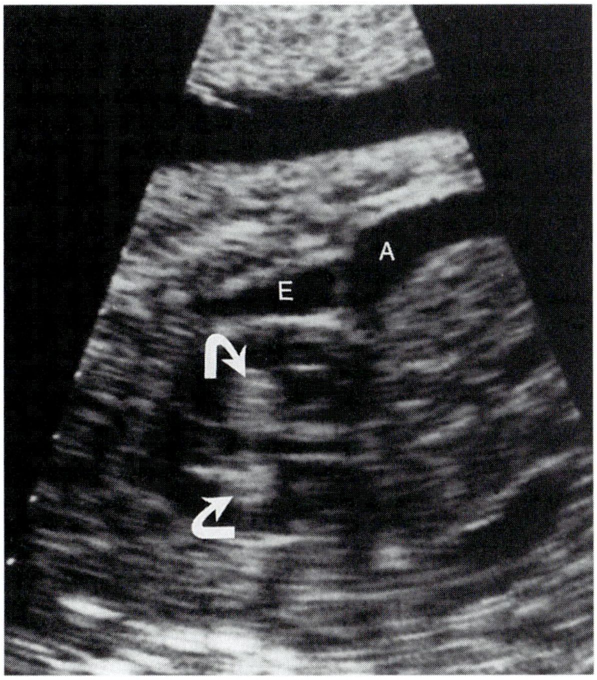

FIG. 38-51. Rhabdomyomas. Biventricular echogenic masses *(arrows)* are seen in a fetus with tuberous sclerosis. Pleural effusions, *E*, and ascites, *A*, are present.

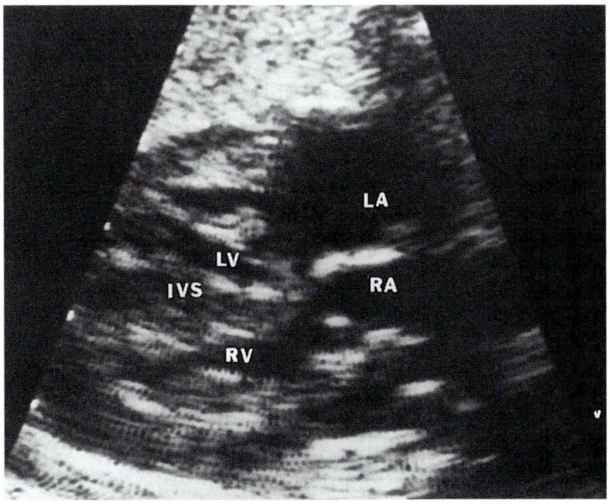

FIG. 38-52. Hypertrophic cardiomyopathy. There is hypertrophic thickening of the interventricular septum, *IVS*, in this fetus of a diabetic mother. Typically, the obstructive hypertrophy is transient and usually not clinically significant. *LA*, Left atrium; *RA*, right atrium; *LV*, left ventricle; *RV*, right ventricle.

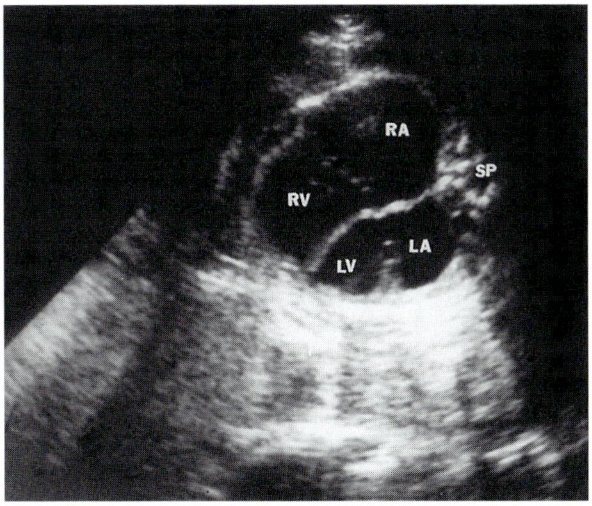

FIG. 38-53. Cardiomyopathy. An enlarged heart with dilated chambers, right greater than left, is seen in fetus with cytomegalovirus. *RA*, Right atrium; *LA*, left atrium; *RV*, right ventricle; *LV*, left ventricle; *Sp*, spine.

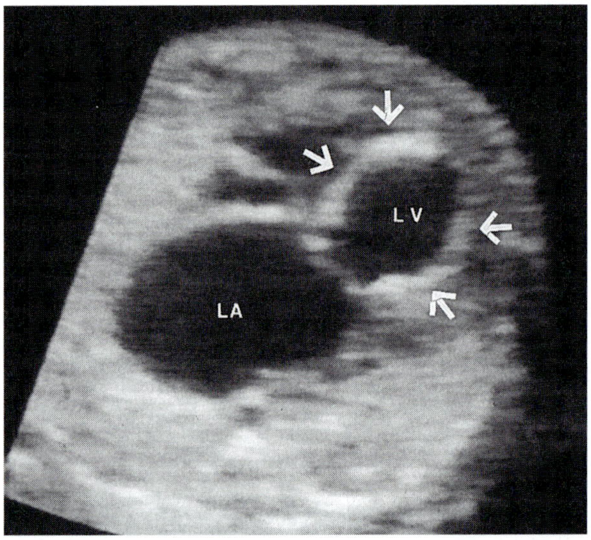

FIG. 38-54. Endocardial fibroelastosis (*arrows*) of the left ventricle, *LV*. Four-chamber view. *LA*, Left atrium; *RA*, right atrium; *RV*, right ventricle.

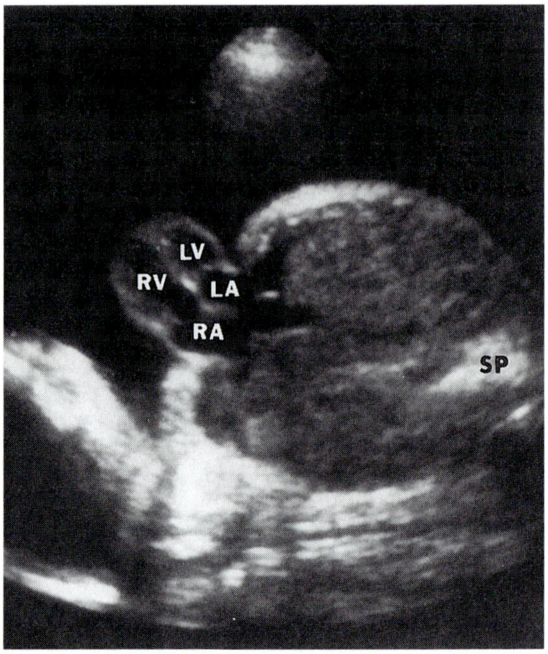

FIG. 38-55. Isolated ectopia cordis. The four-chamber heart is located outside the thorax—type 1. *RA*, Right atrium; *LA*, left atrium; *RV*, right ventricle; *LV*, left ventricle; *Sp*, spine.

A high incidence of **asymmetric septal hypertrophy** (ASH) has long been recognized in **infants of diabetic mothers.**[161] The characteristics of this type of cardiomyopathy have been well documented echocardiographically.[162-164] More recently, it has been clearly demonstrated that not only are the hearts of fetuses of diabetic mothers significantly larger than those of fetuses with unaffected mothers, but that cardiac enlargement is caused by free wall hypertrophy and right ventricle dilatation in addition to septal hypertrophy.[165]

Regardless of the etiology, severe cardiomyopathy results in decreased cardiac function and a tendency to congestive heart failure. This may be secondary to obstruction of ventricular emptying in obstructive forms of cardiomyopathy or to pump failure in nonobstructive forms.

The **sonographic** diagnosis of **obstructive cardiomyopathy** depends on the demonstration of hypertrophy of the ventricular wall or septum. **Nonobstructive cardiomyopathy** can be diagnosed by demonstrating dilatation of one or more cardiac chambers along with poor ventricular contractility.

Thirty seven percent of live-born infants with cardiomyopathy have **associated anomalies.**[118] The **prognosis** for fetal cardiomyopathy is variable, depending on the severity of the cardiac lesion, the underlying etiology, and associated anomalies. When hydrops accompanies cardiomyopathy, the prognosis is poor.

Ectopia Cordis

Ectopia cordis is a rare malformation in which the heart is located outside the thoracic cavity. It results from failure of fusion of the lateral body fold in the thoracic region. There are four types:

- **Thoracic** (60%), in which the heart is displaced from the thoracic cavity through a sternal defect;
- **Abdominal** (30%), in which the heart is displaced into the abdomen through a diaphragm defect;
- **Thoracoabdominal** (7%), in which the heart is displaced from the chest through a defect in the lower sternum with an associated diaphragmatic or ventral abdominal wall defect (pentalogy of Cantrell); and
- **Cervical** (3%), with displacement of the heart into the neck area.[166]

A variety of cardiac and chromosomal anomalies are associated with ectopia cordis. The sonographic diagnosis is generally not difficult, although the abdominal and cervical types have not been reported *in utero* (Fig. 38-55). The prognosis is very poor, with most infants dying within a few days of birth.[167]

ARRHYTHMIAS

Premature Atrial and Ventricular Contractions

Premature atrial contractions (PACs) and premature ventricular contractions (PVCs) are abnormal atrial or ventricular contractions originating from locations other than the sinus node. PACs account for nearly 75% and PVCs for 8% of fetal arrhyth-

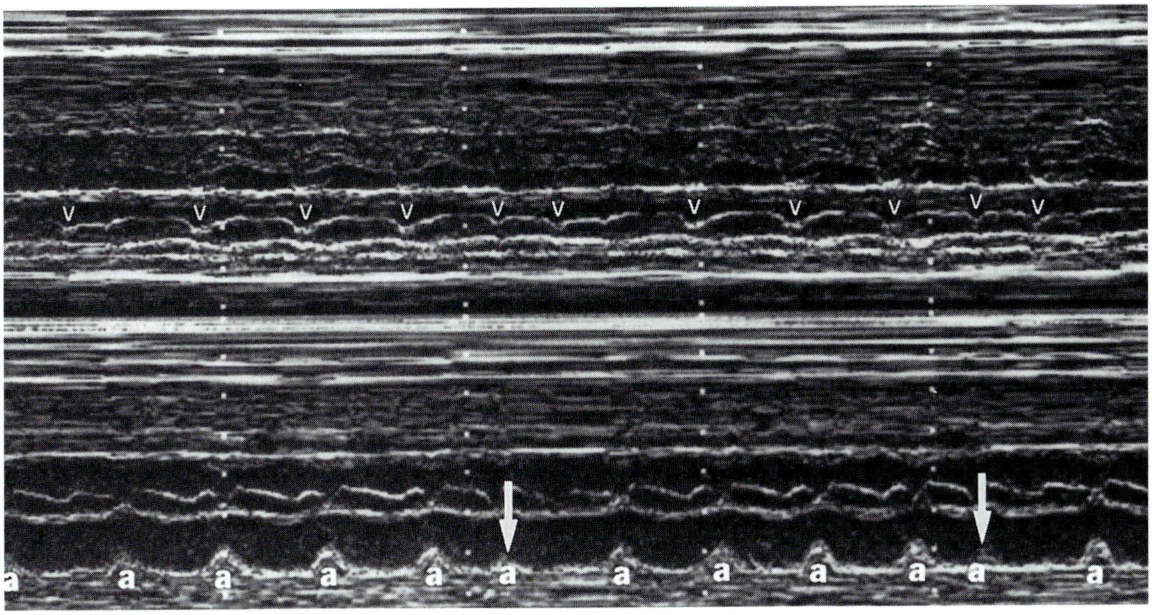

FIG. 38-56. Premature atrial contractions (PACs). M-mode tracing through the walls of the atria, *a*, and ventricles, *v*, shows two premature atrial beats *(arrows)*, which are conducted. Note the pause following the PAC is not fully compensatory.

mias.[29,168] PACs may be associated with redundancy of the foraminal flap (atrial septal aneurysm).[169,170] In 1% to 2% of PACs, a structural cardiac anomaly is present.[26]

PACs may be conducted or nonconducted. In either case, the atrial pacemaker is "reset" so that the next normal atrial beat is also early when compared with normal preextrasystolic beats. PVCs have an early ventricular contraction that is not preceded by an atrial contraction. The atrial pacemaker is not reset, and the next normal beat occurs when expected as if the rhythm were regular. Thus, **PVCs are compensatory,** allowing the preexisting rhythm to continue, whereas **PACs are generally less than compensatory.** PACs and PVCs may be distinguished by M-mode sonography (Fig. 38-56). It is necessary for the M-mode to traverse a structure that responds to atrial contraction and one that responds to ventricular contraction. PACs followed by ventricular contraction are described as "conducted" whereas a PAC that is not followed by a ventricular contraction is "blocked." These must be differentiated from AV block in which a PAC does not occur. Conducted PACs can be distinguished from PVCs by noting that a PAC precedes the early ventricular beat and that, in the majority of cases, PACs are less than compensatory whereas PVCs are generally compensatory.

Premature contractions are entirely benign arrhythmias in the majority of cases. Most disappear *in utero* or in the early neonatal period. One to two percent of PACs may evolve into sustained tachyarrhythmia.[171]

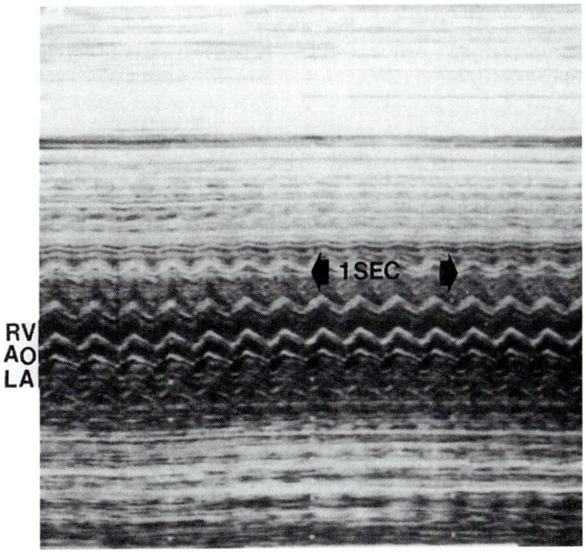

FIG. 38-57. Supraventricular tachycardia. M-mode scan through the ventricle, *RV*, showing a heart rate of 270 beats per minute. *Ao*, Aorta; *LA*, left atrium.

Tachycardia

Fetal tachycardia is a heart rate greater than 180 beats per minute. Supraventricular tachycardias are more common in the fetus than ventricular tachycardias. **Supraventricular tachycardias** are classified as:

- **Paroxysmal supraventricular tachycardia**—an atrial rate of 180 to 300 beats per minute and a conduction rate of 1:1 (Fig. 38-57);

- **Atrial flutter**—atrial rate of 300 to 400 beats per minute frequently associated with heart block and a conduction rate of 2:1 to 4:1, yielding a ventricular rate from 60 to 200 beats per minute; and
- **Atrial fibrillation**—atrial rate of greater than 400 beats per minute and an irregular ventricular response at a rate of 120 to 160 beats per minute.

Ventricular tachycardia is defined as a rapid heart rate associated with three or more consecutive premature ventricular systoles. Of cases of supraventricular tachycardia, 5% to 10% are associated with CHD.[172]

Fetal cardiac rhythm disturbances are usually first suspected on the basis of auscultatory findings. **M-mode and Doppler** echocardiography are useful in identifying and characterizing tachycardias by observing the atrial and ventricular rates. The M-mode tracing is obtained through the heart to allow independent assessment of atrial and ventricular wall motion. Further information can be obtained from simultaneous recordings of the atrial wall or AV and semilunar valve motion. Doppler evaluation has demonstrated a decrease in mean flow velocities and cardiac output during supraventricular tachycardia.[173] Fetal supraventricular tachyarrhythmia is a medical emergency that may lead to fetal cardiovascular compromise, hydrops, and death.

Most fetal tachycardias have a good **prognosis** and can be treated *in utero* with various pharmacologic agents. Careful interrogation of the tricuspid valve with color flow and duplex Doppler imaging is warranted in the setting of fetal tachycardia because tricuspid valvular dysfunction with tricuspid regurgitation can be the first indication of imminent congestive failure and hydrops.[174,175] In the presence of hydrops, immediate and aggressive **therapy** is warranted.[168,171,176-179] Digitalis is the drug most commonly used in the treatment of fetal tachyarrhythmias. Since digoxin rapidly crosses the placenta, fetal tachyarrhythmias can be treated by administering digitalis to the mother. However, the fetus may require higher serum digoxin levels than the adult, necessitating higher maternal serum levels to achieve adequate digitalization of the fetus. Careful monitoring with **serial fetal echocardiograms** and maternal serum digoxin levels is warranted. **Prognosis** in the setting of fetal tachyarrhythmia depends on a number of factors, including type and duration of arrhythmia, presence of structural cardiac anomalies, gestational age, and response to intrauterine therapy.[173]

Bradycardia

Fetal bradycardia is a "prolonged" heart rate of less than or equal to 100 beats per minute. Although the term prolonged is subjective, episodes of bradycardia lasting more than 10 seconds and up to several minutes have been defined as pathologic.[176,180] Approximately 5% of fetal arrhythmias are classified as bradycardia.[26] Transient bradycardia can be related to an increase in intrauterine pressure, occasionally secondary to the pressure of an ultrasound transducer.[181,182] Sinus bradycardia without fetal hypoxia is rare.[183] Below 80 beats per minute, sinus bradycardia may be associated with fetal asphyxia. Heart rates lower than 100 beats per minute during the first trimester have an increased risk of fetal demise.[184] The fetus with sustained bradycardia should have

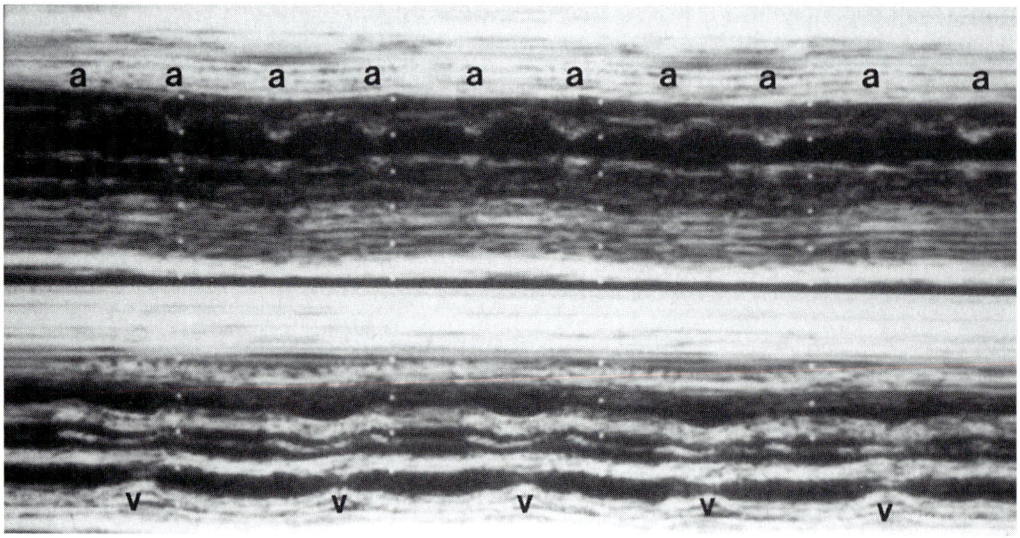

FIG. 38-58. Second-degree heart block. M-mode tracing through the atria, *a*, and ventricles, *v*, shows two atrial contractions for each ventricular beat (2:1 block). There is bradycardia with a heart rate of 60 beats per minute.

careful follow-up and monitoring for signs of cardiac failure. Persistent bradycardia may warrant early delivery. *In utero* treatment has met with limited success.[185]

Congenital Heart Block

Failure of transmission of impulses from the atrium to the ventricles results in atrioventricular block (AVB).

Atrioventricular block is classified into three types:

- **First-degree block**—a prolonged PR interval resulting in a conduction delay, but without markedly abnormal rate or rhythm (this has not been diagnosed *in utero*);
- **Second-degree block** with blockage of a single atrial beat (Mobitz type 1) or intermittent conduction abnormalities such that the ventricular rate is a fraction of the atrial rate (Mobitz type 2; Fig. 38-58); and
- **Third-degree or complete heart block**—the ventricular and atrial rates are entirely dissociated.

In the normal heart, an electrical impulse originates from the sinoatrial (SA) node, travels to the AV node, and through the Purkinje system to the ventricles. AVB can result from immaturity or complete absence of the conducting system or from abnormalities at the level of the AV node. This rare disorder is associated with maternal collagen vascular disease (systemic lupus erythematosus).[186] After one affected child, further pregnancies carry a 30% risk for AVB.[187] Serial fetal **echocardiograms** are useful in the fetus at risk for congenital complete heart block related to maternal lupus. This monitoring may allow early detection and treatment of the immune-mediated fetal myocarditis and congenital complete heart block associated with this disease. Aggressive early treatment with plasmapheresis and corticosteroid therapy may avert permanent fetal cardiac damage and result in a normal healthy baby.[188,189]

In the absence of associated structural abnormalities, the **prognosis** for a fetus with congenital heart block is good; however, at least 40% of fetuses with complete heart block have structural cardiac abnormalities.[26] When associated cardiac anomalies exist, the prognosis is poor. Fetuses with AVB are at risk for heart failure and should be monitored closely.

REFERENCES

1. Jones KL. *Smith's Recognizable Patterns of Human Malformation.* 3rd ed. Philadelphia: WB Saunders Co; 1988.
2. Nora JJ, Fraser FC. *Medical Genetics: Principles and Practice.* Philadelphia: Lea & Febiger; 1989.
3. Nyberg DA, Mahony BS, Pretorius DH. *Diagnostic Ultrasound of Fetal Anomalies: Text and Atlas.* Chicago: Year Book Medical Publishers Inc; 1989.
4. Romero R, Pilu G, Jeanty P et al. *Prenatal Diagnosis of Congenital Anomalies.* Norwalk, Conn: Appleton & Lange; 1988.
5. Nora JJ, Nora AH. Maternal transmission of congenital heart diseases: new recurrence risk figures and the question of cytoplasmic inheritance and vulnerability to teratogens. *Am J Cardiol* 1987;59:459-463.
6. Reed KI. Fetal echocardiography. *Semin US CT MR* 1991; 12:2-10.
7. Greenwood RD, Rosenthal A, Parisi L et al. Extracardiac abnormalities in infants with congenital heart disease. *Pediatrics* 1975;55(4):485-492.
8. Berg KA, Boughman JA, Astemboroski JA et al. Implications for prenatal cytogenetic analysis from Baltimore-Washington study of live born infants with confirmed congenital heart defects (CHD). *Am J Hum Genet* 1986;39:A50.
9. Berg KA, Clark EB, Astemborski JA et al. Prenatal detection of cardiovascular malformations by echocardiography: an indication for cytogenetic evaluation. *Am J Obstet Gynecol* 1988;159:477-481.
10. Wladimiroff JW, Stuart PA, Sachs ES et al. Prenatal diagnosis and management of congenital heart defects: significance of associated fetal anomalies and prenatal chromosome studies. *Am J Med Genet* 1985;21:285-290.
11. Allan LD. Fetal echocardiography. *Clin Obstet Gynecol* 1988;31(1):61-79.
12. Callan NA, Maggio M, Steger S et al. Fetal echocardiography: indications for referral, prenatal diagnosis and outcomes. *Am J Perinatol* 1991;8(6):390-394.
13. Bromley B, Estroff JA, Sanders SP et al. Fetal echocardiography: accuracy and limitations in a population at high and low risk for heart defects. *Am J Obstet Gynecol* 1991; 166:1473-1481.

Normal Fetal Cardiac Anatomy and Scanning Techniques

14. Vergani P, Mariani S, Ghidini A et al. Screening of congenital heart diseases with the four-chamber view of the fetal heart. *Am J Obstet Gynecol* 1992;167:1000-1003.
15. Copel JA, Pilu G, Green J et al. Fetal echocardiographic screening for congenital heart disease: the importance of the four-chamber view. *Am J Obstet Gynecol* 1987;157:648-655.
16. Kirk JS, Riggs TW, Comstock CH et al. The prospective evaluation of fetal cardiac anatomy: a comparison of 4 and 5 chamber views in 5967 patients. *Am J Obstet Gynecol* 1993; 168:291.
17. Comstock CH. Normal fetal heart axis and position. *Obstet Gynecol* 1987;70:255-259.
18. Dolkart LA, Reimers FT. Transvaginal fetal echocardiography in early pregnancy: normative data. *Am J Obstet Gynecol* 1991;165:688-691.
19. Achiron R, Weissman A, Retstein Z et al. Transvaginal echocardiographic examination of the fetal heart between 13 and 15 weeks gestation in a low risk population. *J Ultrasound Med* 1994;13(10):783-789.
20. Levy DW, Mintz MC. Left ventricular echogenic focus: a normal finding. *AJR* 1988;150:85-86.
21. Petrikovsky BM, Challenger M, Wyse LJ et al. Natural history of echogenic foci within ventricles of the fetal heart. *Ultrasound Obstet Gynecol* 1995;5(2):92-94.
22. Roberts DJ, Genest D. Cardiac histologic pathology characteristics of trisomies 13 and 21. *Hum Pathol* 1992;23:1130-40.
23. Lehman CD, Nyberg DA, Winter TC III et al. Trisomy 13 syndrome: prenatal ultrasound findings in a review of 33 cases. *Radiology* 1995;194:217-222.
24. Bromley B, Lieberman E, Laboda LA et al. Echogenic intracardiac focus, a sonographic sign for Down syndrome? *Obstet Gynecol* 1995;86:998-1011.

25. Cartier MS, Davidoff A, Warneke LA et al. The normal diameter of the fetal aorta and pulmonary artery: echocardiographic evaluation *in utero*. *AJR* 1987;149:1003-1007.
26. Reed KL. Fetal arrhythmias: etiology, diagnosis, pathophysiology and treatment. *Semin Perinatol* 1989;13:294-304.
27. Gembruch U, Chatterjee MS, Bald R et al. Color Doppler flow mapping of fetal heart. *J Perinatal Med* 1991;19(1-2):27-32.
28. Chiba Y, Kanzaki T, Kobayashi H et al. Evaluation of fetal structural heart disease using color flow mapping. *Ultrasound Med Cardiol* 1990;16(3):221-229.
29. Benacerraf BR, Sanders SP. Fetal echocardiography. *Radiol Clin North Am* 1990;28(1):131-147.
30. Sharland GK, Chita SK, Allan LD. The use of colour Doppler in fetal echocardiography. *Int J Cardiol* 1990;28(2):229-236.
31. Hoffman JIE, Christianson R. Congenital heart disease in a cohort of 19,502 births with long-term follow-up. *Am J Cardiol* 1978;42:641-647.
32. Allan LD, Crawford DC, Anderson RH et al. The spectrum of congenital heart disease detected echocardiographically in prenatal life. *Br Heart J* 1985;54:523-526.
33. Keith JD. Atrial septal defect: ostium secundum, ostium primum, and atrioventricularis communis (common AV canal). In: Keith JD, Rowe RD, Vlad P, eds. *Heart Disease in Infancy and Childhood.* 3rd ed. New York: Macmillan Publishing Co; 1978:330-404.
34. Samanek M. Children with congenital heart disease: probability of natural survival. *Pediatr Cardiol* 1992;13:152-158.
35. Fyler DC. Atrial septal defect secundum. In Fyler DC, ed. *Nadas' Pediatric Cardiology.* Philadelphia: Hanley and Belfus; 1992:513-524.
36. Feldt RH, Avasthey P, Yoshim ASVF et al. Incidence of congenital heart disease in children born to residents of Olmsted County, Minnesota, 1950-1969. *Mayo Clin Proc* 1971;46: 794-799.
37. Crelin ES, ed. *Anatomy of the Newborn: An Atlas.* Philadelphia: Lea & Febiger; 1969.
38. Kachalia P, Bowie JD, Adams DB et al. *In utero* sonographic appearance of the atrial septum primum and septum secundum. *J Ultrasound Med* 1991;10:423-426.
39. Wilson AD, Rao PS, Aeschlmann S. Normal fetal foramen flap and transatrial Doppler velocity pattern. *J Am Soc Echocardiogr* 1990;3(6):491-494.
40. Benacerraf BR, Pober BR, Sanders SP. Accuracy of fetal echocardiography. *Radiology* 1987;165:847-849.
41. DeVore GR, Horenstein J, Siassi B et al. Fetal echocardiography. VII. Doppler color flow mapping: a new technique for the diagnosis of congenital heart disease. *Am J Obstet Gynecol* 1987;157:1054-1064.
42. Cockerham JT, Martin TC, Guiterrez FR et al. Spontaneous closure of secundum atrial septal defect in infants and young children. *Am J Cardiol* 1983;52:1267-1271.
43. Steele PM, Fuster V, Cohen M et al. Isolated atrial septal defect with pulmonary vascular obstructive disease: long-term follow-up and prediction of outcome after surgical correction. *Circulation* 1987;76(5):1037-1042.
44. Ferencz C, Rubin JD, McCarter RJ et al. Cardiac and non-cardiac malformations: observations in a population-based study. *Teratology* 1987;35:367-378.
45. Goor DA, Lillehei CW. *Congenital Malformations of the Heart.* New York: Grune & Stratton; 1975.
46. Grahm TP, Bender HW, Spach MS. Ventricular septal defects. In: Moss AJ, Adams FH, Emmanouilides GC, eds. *Heart Disease in Infancy, Childhood, and Adolescence.* 2nd ed. Baltimore: Williams & Wilkins; 1977.
47. Allan LD, Crawford DC, Anderson RH et al. Echocardiographic and anatomical correlations in fetal congenital heart disease. *Br Heart J* 1984;52:542-548.
48. Allan LD, Tynan M, Campbell S et al. Identification of congenital cardiac malformations by echocardiography in mid trimester fetus. *Br Heart J* 1981;46:358-362.
49. Parness IA, Yeager SB, Sanders SP et al. Echocardiographic diagnosis of fetal heart defects in mid trimester. *Arch Dis Child* 1988;63:1137-1145.
50. Yagel S, Sherer D, Hurwitz A. The significance of ultrasonic prenatal diagnosis of ventricular septal defect. *J Clin Ultrasound* 1985;13:588-590.
51. Brown DL, Emerson DS, Cartier MS et al. Congenital cardiac anomalies: prenatal sonographic diagnosis. *AJR* 1989;153: 109-114.
52. Sutherland GR, Smyllie JH, Ogilvie BC et al. Color flow imaging in the diagnosis of multiple ventricular septal defects. *Br Heart J* 1989;62:43-49.
53. Hoffman JIE. Natural history of congenital heart disease: problems in its assessment with special reference to ventricular septal defect. *Circulation* 1968;37:97-125.
54. Hoffman JIE, Rudolph AM. The natural history of isolated ventricular septal defect with special reference to selection of patients for surgery. *Adv Pediatr* 1970;17:57-79.
55. Hoffman JIE, Rudolph AM. The natural history of ventricular septal defects in infancy. *Am J Cardiol* 1965;16:634-653.
56. Crawford DC, Chita SK, Allan LD. Prenatal detection of congenital heart disease: factors affecting obstetric management and survival. *Am J Obstet Gynecol* 1988;159:352-356.
57. Machado MVL, Crawford DC, Anderson RH et al. Atrioventricular septal defect in prenatal life. *Br Heart J* 1988;59:352-355.
58. Carvalho JS, Rigby ML, Shinebourne EA et al. Cross-sectional echocardiography for recognition of ventricular topology in atrioventricular septal defects. *Br Heart J* 1989; 61:285-288.
59. Freedom RM, Culham JAG, Moes CAF. *Angiography of Congenital Heart Disease.* New York: Macmillan Publishing Co; 1984:58.
60. Becker AE, Anderson RH. Atrioventricular septal defects: what's in a name? *J Thorac Cardiovasc Surg* 1982;83:461-469.
61. Fontana RS, Edwards JE. *Congenital Cardiac Disease: A Review of 357 Cases Studied Pathologically.* Philadelphia: WB Saunders Co; 1962.
62. Shenker L, Reed KL, Marx GR et al. Fetal cardiac Doppler flow studies in prenatal diagnosis of heart disease. *Am J Obstet Gynecol* 1988;158:1267-1273.
63. Gembruch U, Knopfle G, Chatterjee M et al. Prenatal diagnosis of atrioventricular canal malformations with up-to-date echocardiographic technology: report of 14 cases. *Am Heart J* 1991;121:1489-1497.
64. Allan LD, Crawford DC, Sheridan R et al. Aetiology of non-immune hydrops: the value of echocardiography. *Br J Obstet Gynecol* 1986;93:223-225.
65. Clapp SK, Perry BL, Farooki ZQ et al. Surgical and medical results of complete atrioventricular canal: a 10-year review. *Am J Cardiol* 1987;59:454-458.
66. King RM, Puga FJ, Daniel GK et al. Prognostic factors in surgical treatment of partial atrioventricular canal. *Circulation* 1986;74(suppl):42-46.
67. Genten E, Blount SG Jr. The spectrum of Ebstein's anomaly. *Am Heart J* 1967;73(3):395-425.
68. Lev M, Liberthson RR, Joseph RH et al. The pathologic anatomy of Ebstein's disease. *Arch Pathol* 1970;90:334-343.
69. Roberson DA, Silverman NH. Ebstein's anomaly: echocardiographic and clinical features in the fetus and neonate. *J Am Coll Cardiol* 1989;14:1300-1307.

70. Zuberbuhler JR, Becker AE, Anderson RH et al. Ebstein's malformation and the embryological development of the tricuspid valve. *Pediatr Cardiol* 1984;5:289-296.
71. Anderson KR, Zuberbuhler JR, Anderson RH et al. Morphologic spectrum of Ebstein's anomaly of the heart: a review. *Mayo Clin Proc* 1979;54:174-180.
72. Stewart PA, Wladimiroff JW, Reuss A et al. Fetal echocardiography: a review of 6 years experience. *Fetal Ther* 1987; 2:222-231.
73. Sarland GK, Chita SK, Allan LD. Tricuspid valve dysplasia or displacement in intrauterine life. *J Am Coll Cardiol* 1991; 117(4):944-949.
74. Nora JJ, Nora AH, Toews WH. Lithium, Ebstein's anomaly and other congenital heart defects. *Lancet* 1974;2:594-595.
75. Nora JJ, Nora AH. The evolution of specific genetic and environmental counseling in congenital heart disease. *Circulation* 1978;57(2):205-213.
76. Schou M, Goldfield MD, Weinstein MR et al. Lithium and pregnancy. I. Report from the Register of Lithium Babies. *Br Med J* 1973;2:135-136.
77. Weinstein MR, Goldfield MD. Cardiovascular malformations with lithium use during pregnancy. *Am J Psychol* 1975;132(5):529-531.
78. Park JM, Sridaromont S, Ledbetter EO et al. Ebstein's anomaly of the tricuspid valve associated with prenatal exposure to lithium carbonate. *Am J Dis Child* 1980;134:703-704.
79. Kallen B, Tandberg A. Lithium and pregnancy: a cohort study on manic-depressive women. *Acta Psychiatr Scand* 1983;68:134-139.
80. Brady HR, Horgan JH. Lithium and the heart: unanswered questions. *Chest* 1988;93(1):166-169.
81. Roberson HA, Silverman NH, Zuberbuhler JP. Congenitally enlarged tricuspid orifice: its differentiation from Ebstein's malformation in association with pulmonary atresia with an intact ventricular septum. *Pediatr Cardiol* 1990;11:86-90.
82. Oberhoffer R, Cook AC, Lang D et al. Correlation between echocardiographic and morphological investigations of lesions of the tricuspid valve diagnosed *in utero*. *Br Heart J* 1992;68:580-585.
83. Handler JB, Burger TJ, Miller RH et al. Partial atrioventricular canal in association with Ebstein's anomaly: echocardiographic diagnosis and surgical correction. *Chest* 1981; 80:515-517.
84. Fink BW. *Congenital Heart Disease: A Deductive Approach To Its Diagnosis.* Chicago: Year Book Medical Publishers Inc; 1985:137-146.
85. Copel JA, Cullen M, Green JJ et al. The frequency of aneuploidy in prenatally diagnosed congenital heart disease: an indication for fetal karyotyping. *Am J Obstet Gynecol* 1988; 158:409-413.
86. Hornberger LK, Sahn DJ, Kleinman CS et al. Tricuspid valve disease with significant tricuspid insufficiency in the fetus: diagnosis and outcome. *J Am Coll Cardiol* 1991;17:167-173.
87. Gembruch U, Hansmann M, Redel DA et al. Fetal two-dimensional Doppler echocardiography (color flow mapping) and its place in prenatal diagnosis. *Prenat Diagn* 1989; 9:535-547.
88. Grundy H, Burlbaw J, Gowdamarajan R et al. Antenatal detection of hypoplastic right ventricle with fetal M-mode echocardiography: a report of 2 cases. *J Reprod Med* 1987; 32:301-304.
89. DeLeval M, Bull C, Stark J et al. Pulmonary atresia and intact ventricular septum: surgical management based on a revised classification. *Circulation* 1982;66:272.
90. Schaffer RM, Corio FJ. Sonographic diagnosis of hypoplastic left heart syndrome *in utero*. *J Diagn Med Sonogr* 1988; 6:319-320.
91. Yagel S, Mandelberg A, Hurwitz A et al. Prenatal diagnosis of hypoplastic left ventricle. *Am J Perinatol* 1986;3:6-8.
92. Hawkins JA, Dody DB. Aortic atresia: morphologic characteristics affecting survival and operative palliation. *J Thorac Cardiovasc Surg* 1984;88:620.
93. Saide A, Folger GM. Hypoplastic left heart syndrome: clinical, pathologic and hemodynamic correlation. *Am J Cardiol* 1972; 29:190.
94. Dody DB. Aortic atresia. *J Thorac Cardiovasc Surg* 1980; 79:462.
95. Dody DB, Knott HW. Hypoplastic left heart syndrome: experience with an operation to establish functionally normal circulation. *J Thorac Cardiovasc Surg* 1977;74:624.
96. Levitsky S, van der Horst RL, Hastreiter AR et al. Surgical palliation in aortic atresia. *J Thorac Cardiovasc Surg* 1980; 79:456.
97. Behrendt DM, Rocchini A. An operation for the hypoplastic left heart syndrome: preliminary report. *Ann Thorac Surg* 1981;32:284.
98. Hallerman FJ, Davis GD, Ritter DG et al. Roentgenographic features of common ventricle. *Radiology* 1966; 87:409.
99. Becker AE, Anderson RH. *Pathology of Congenital Heart Disease.* London: Butterworth Publishers; 1981.
100. Moodie DS, Ritter DG, Tajik AH et al. Long-term follow-up after palliative operation for univentricular heart. *Am J Cardiol* 1984;53:1648.
101. Moodie DS, Ritter DG, Tajik AH et al. Long-term follow-up in the unoperated univentricular heart. *Am J Cardiol* 1984; 53:1124.
102. Fontana RS, Edwards JE. *Congenital Cardiac Disease: A Review of 357 Cases Studied Pathologically.* Philadelphia: WB Saunders Co; 1962.
103. McKay R, Pacifico AD, Blackstone EH et al. Septation of the univentricular heart with left anterior subaortic outlet chamber. *J Thorac Cardiovasc Surg* 1982;84:77.
104. Netter F. *The Ciba Collection of Medical Illustrations. V. Heart.* New Jersey: CIBA; 1978.
105. Lev M, Rimoldi HJA, Rowlatt UF. The quantitative anatomy of cyanotic tetralogy of Fallot. *Circulation* 1964;30:531.
106. DeVore GR, Siassi B, Platt LD. Fetal echocardiography. VIII. Aortic root dilatation—a marker for tetralogy of Fallot. *Am J Obstet Gynecol* 1988;159:129-136.
107. Anderson CF, McCurdy CM, McNamara MF et al. Case of the day 8 diagnosis: color Doppler aided diagnosis of tetralogy of Fallot. *J Ultrasound Med* 1994;13(4):341-342.
108. Coirier RA, McGoon DC, Danielson GK et al. Late results after repair of tetralogy of Fallot. *J Thorac Cardiovasc Surg* 1977;73:900.
109. Garson A, Nihill MR, McNamara DG et al. Status of the adult and adolescent after repair of tetralogy of Fallot. *Circulation* 1979;59:1232.
110. Kleinman CS, Donnerstein RL, DeVore GR et al. Fetal echocardiography for evaluation of *in utero* congestive heart failure: a technique for study of nonimmune fetal hydrops. *N Engl J Med* 1982;306:568.
111. Lakier JB, Stanger P, Heymann MA et al. Tetralogy of Fallot with absent pulmonary valve: natural history and hemodynamic considerations. *Circulation* 1974;50:167.
112. Fyler DC. Report of the New England Regional Infant Cardiac Program. *Pediatrics* 1980;375-461.
113. Collett RW, Edwards JE. Persistent truncus arteriosus: a classification according to anatomic types. *Surg Clin North Am* 1949;29:1245-1270.
114. Kirklin JW, Pacifico AD, Blackstone EH, et al. Current risks in protocols for operations for double outlet right ventricle; derivation from an 18-year experience. *J Thorac Cardiovasc Surg* 1986;92:913-930.

115. Stewart PA, Waldimiroff JW, Becker AE. Early prenatal detection of double outlet right ventricle by echocardiography. *Br Heart J* 1985;54:340-342.
116. Trusler GA, Castaneda AR, Rosenthal A et al. Current results of management of transposition of the great arteries with special emphasis on patients with associated ventricular septal defects. *J Am Coll Cardiol* 1987;10:1061-1071.
117. Allwork SP, Bentall HH, Becker AE et al. Congenitally corrected transposition: a morphologic study of 32 cases. *Am J Cardiol* 1976;38:910-922.
118. Ferencz C, Rubin JD, McCarter RJ et al. Congenital heart disease: prevalence at live birth: the Baltimore-Washington infant study. *Am J Epidemiol* 1985;121:31-36.
119. Allan LD. Structural cardiac abnormalities. In: Allan LD, ed. *Manual of Fetal Echocardiography*. Lancaster, England: MTP Press Ltd; 1986:75-79.
120. DiSessa TG, Emerson DS, Felker RE et al. Anomalous systemic and pulmonary venous pathways diagnosed *in utero* by ultrasound. *J Ultrasound Med* 1990;9:311-317.
121. Bonham-Carter RE, Capriles M, Noe Y. Total anomalous pulmonary venous drainage: a clinical and anatomic study of 75 children. *Br Heart J* 1969;31:45.
122. Allan LD, Crawford DC, Tynan M. Evolution of coarctation of the aorta in intrauterine life. *Br Heart J* 1984;52:471-473.
123. Rosenberg H. Coarctation of the aorta: morphology and pathogenesis considerations. In: Rosenberg HS, Bolande RP, eds. *Perspectives in Pediatric Pathology, Vol. I.* Chicago: Year Book Medical Publishers Inc; 1973.
124. Bruins C. Competition between aortic isthmus and ductus arteriosus: reciprocal influence of structure and flow. *Eur J Cardiol* 1978;8:87.
125. Hutchins GM. Coarctation of the aorta explained as a branch point of the ductus arteriosus. *Am J Pathol* 1971;63:203.
126. Benacerraf BR, Saltzman DH, Sanders SP. Sonographic signs suggesting the prenatal diagnosis of coarctation of the aorta. *J Ultrasound Med* 1989;8:65-69.
127. Hornberger LK, Sahn DJ, Kleinman CS et al. Antenatal diagnosis of coarctation of the aorta: a multicenter experience. *J Am Coll Cardiol* 1994;23:417-423.
128. Sahn DJ, Lange LW, Allen HD et al. Quantitative real-time cross-sectional echocardiography in the developing normal human fetus and newborn. *Circulation* 1980;62:588-597.
129. Hornberger LK, Weintraub RG, Pesonen E et al. Echocardiographic study of the morphology and growth of the aortic arch in the human fetus: observations related to the prenatal diagnosis of coarctation. *Circulation* 1992;86:741-747.
130. Hesslein PS, Gutgesell HP, McNamara DG. Prognosis of symptomatic coarctation of the aorta in infancy. *Am J Cardiol* 1983;51:299.
131. Clark CE, Henry WL, Epstein SE. Familial prevalence and genetic transmission of idiopathic hypertrophic subaortic stenosis. *N Engl J Med* 1973;289:709.
132. Campbell M. The natural history of congenital aortic stenosis. *Br Heart J* 1968;30:514.
133. Messina LM, Turley K, Etanger P et al. Successful aortic valvotomy for severe congenital valvular aortic stenosis in the newborn infant. *J Thorac Cardiovasc Surg* 1984;88:92-96.
134. Jones M, Barnhardt GR, Morrow AG. Late results after operations for left ventricular outflow track obstruction. *Am J Cardiol* 1982;50:569.
135. Merrill WH, Shuman TA, Graham TP et al. Surgical intervention in neonates with critical pulmonary stenosis. *Ann Surg* 1987;205:(6)712-718.
136. Marantz PM, Huhta JC, Mullins CE et al. Results of balloon valvuloplasty in typical and dysplastic pulmonary valve stenosis: Doppler echocardiographic follow-up. *J Am Coll Cardiol* 1988;12(2):476-479.
137. Niikawa N, Kohsaka S, Mizumoto M et al. Familial clustering of situs inversus totalis, and asplenia and polysplenia syndromes. *Am J Med Genet* 1983;16:43-47.
138. Rose V, Izukawa T, Moes CAF. Syndromes of asplenia and polysplenia: a review of cardiac and non-cardiac malformations in 60 cases with special reference to diagnosis and prognosis. *Br Heart J* 1975;37:840-852.
139. Peoples WM, Moller JH, Edwards JE. Polysplenia: a review of 146 cases. *Pediatr Cardiol* 1983;4:129-137.
140. Zlotogora J, Elian E. Asplenia and polysplenia syndromes with abnormalities of lateralization in a sibship. *J Med Genet* 1981;18:301-302.
141. Stewart PA, Becker AE, Wladimiroff JW et al. Left atrial isomerism associated with asplenia: prenatal echocardiographic detection of complex congenital cardiac malformations. *J Am Coll Cardiol* 1984;4:1015-1020.
142. Garcia OL, Mehta AV, Pickoff AS et al. Left atrial isomerism and complete atrioventricular block: a report of 6 cases. *Am J Cardiol* 1981;48:1103-1107.
143. Schmidt W, Yarkoni S, Jeanty P et al. Sonographic measurements of the fetal spleen: clinical implications. *J Ultrasound Med* 1985;4:667-672.
144. de Arugo LML, Silverman NH, Filley RA. Prenatal detection of left atrial isomerism by ultrasound. *J Ultrasound Med* 1987;6:667-670.
145. McAllister H Jr. Primary tumors of the heart and pericardium. *Pathol Annu* 1979;14:325-327.
146. Dennis MA, Appareti K, Manco-Johnson ML et al. The echocardiographic diagnosis of multiple fetal cardiac tumors. *J Ultrasound Med* 1985;4:327-329.
147. Smythe JF, Dyek JD, Smallhorn J et al. Natural history of cardiac rhabdomyomas in infancy and childhood. *Am J Cardiol* 1990;66:1247-1249.
148. Simcha A, Wells B, Tynan M et al. Primary cardiac tumors in childhood. *Arch Dis Child* 1971;46:508-514.
149. Crawford DC, Garrett C, Tynan M et al. Cardiac rhabdomyomata as a marker for the antenatal detection of tuberous sclerosis. *J Med Genet* 1983;20:303-312.
150. Groves AM, Fagg NLK, Cook AC et al. Cardiac tumors in intrauterine life. *Arch Dis Child* 1992;67:1189-1192.
151. Bender B, Yunis E. The pathology of tuberous sclerosis. *Pathol Annu* 1982;17:339-341.
152. Journel H, Roussey M, Plais MH et al. Prenatal diagnosis of familial tuberous sclerosis following detection of cardiac rhabdomyoma by ultrasound. *Prenat Diagn* 1986;6:283-289.
153. DeVore GR, Hakim S, Kleinman CS et al. The *in utero* diagnosis of an intraventricular septal cardiac rhabdomyoma by means of real time-directed, M-mode echocardiography. *Am J Obstet Gynecol* 1982;143:967-969.
154. Cyr DR, Guntheroth WG, Neiberg DA et al. Prenatal diagnosis of an intrapericardial teratoma: a cause for non-immune hydrops. *J Ultrasound Med* 1988;7:87-90.
155. Banfield F, Dick M, Behrendt DM et al. Intrapericardial teratoma: a new and treatable cause of hydrops fetalis. *Am J Dis Child* 1980;134:1174-1175.
156. Garva G, Buoso G, Beltrame GL et al. Cardiac rhabdomyomas as a marker for the prenatal detection of tuberous sclerosis: case report. *Br J Obstet Gynecol* 1990;97:1154-1157.
157. Spooner E, Ferrina M. Case report: left ventricular rhabdomyoma causing subaortic stenosis: the two dimensional echocardiographic appearance. *Pediatr Cardiol* 1982;2:67-70.
158. Riggs T, Sholl JS, Ilbawi M et al. *In utero* diagnosis of pericardial tumor with successful surgical repair. *Pediatr Cardiol* 1984;5:23-26.

159. Drose J, Dennis M, Thickman D. Ultrasound diagnosis of *in utero* infection in pregnancy: a review of 19 cases. *Radiology* 1991;178:369-374.
160. Schryer MJP, Karnauchow PN. Endocardial fibroelastosis. Etiologic and pathogenetic considerations in children. *Am Heart J* 1974;88:557-565.
161. Sheehan PQ, Rowland TW, Shah BL et al. Maternal diabetic control and hypertrophic cardiomyopathy in infants of diabetic mother. *Clin Pediatr* 1986;25(5):266-271.
162. Lendrum B, Pildes RS, Serratto M et al. The spectrum of myocardial abnormality in infants of diabetic mothers. *Pediatr Cardiol* 1979;1(2):172.
163. Gutgesell HP, Speer ME, Rosenberg HS. Characterization of the cardiomyopathy in infants of diabetic mothers. *Circulation* 1980;61:441-450.
164. Halliday HL. Hypertrophic cardiomyopathy in infants of poorly controlled diabetic mothers. *Arch Dis Child* 1981;56: 258-263.
165. Veille JC, Hanson R, Sivakoff M et al. Fetal cardiac size in normal, intrauterine growth retarded and diabetic pregnancies. *Am J Perinatol* 1993;10(4):275-279.
166. Kanadasunpheram R, Verzin JA. Ectopia cordis in man. *Thorax* 1962;17:159.
167. Ghidini A, Sirtori M, Romero R et al. Prenatal diagnosis of pentalogy of Cantrell. *J Ultrasound Med* 1988;7:467-472.
168. Lingman G, Lundstrom NR, Marsal K et al. Fetal cardiac arrhythmia: clinical outcome in 113 cases. *Acta Obstet Gynecol Scand* 1986;65:263-267.
169. Steward PA, Wladimiroff JW. Fetal atrial arrhythmias associated with redundancy/aneurysm of the foramen ovale. *J Clin Ultrasound* 1988;16:643-650.
170. Rice MJ, McDonald RW, Reller MD. Fetal atrial septal aneurysm: a cause for fetal arrhythmias. *J Am Coll Cardiol* 1988;12:1292-1297.
171. Kleinman CS. Prenatal diagnosis and management of intrauterine arrhythmias. *Fetal Ther* 1986;1:92-95.
172. Shenker L. Fetal cardiac arrhythmias. *Obstet Gynecol Surg* 1971;34:561.
173. Reed KL, Sahn DJ, Marks GR et al. Cardiac Doppler flows during fetal arrhythmias: physiologic consequences. *Obstet Gynecol* 1987;70:1-6.
174. Chao RC, Ho ES-C, Hsleh K-S. Fetal atrial flutter and fibrillation: prenatal echocardiographic detection and management. *Am Heart J* 1992;124(4):1095-1098.
175. Silverman NH, Kleinman CS, Rudolph AM et al. Fetal atrioventricular valve insufficiency associated with non-immune hydrops: a two-dimensional echocardiographic and pulsed Doppler ultrasound study. *Circulation* 1985;72:825-832.
176. Cameron A, Nicholson S, Nimrod C et al. Evaluation of fetal cardiac dysrhythmias with two-dimensional, M-mode, and pulsed Doppler ultrasonography. *Am J Obstet Gynecol* 1988;158:286-290.
177. Kleinman CS, Copel JA, Weinstein EM et al. Treatment of fetal supraventricular tachyarrhythmias. *J Clin Ultrasound* 1985;13:265-273.
178. Kleinman CS, Donnerstein RL, Jaffe CC et al. Fetal echocardiography: a tool for evaluation of *in utero* cardiac arrhythmias and monitoring of *in utero* therapy: analysis of 71 patients. *Am J Cardiol* 1983;51:237-243.
179. Wiggins JW, Bowes W, Clewell W et al. Echocardiographic diagnosis and intravenous digoxin management of fetal tachyarrhythmias and congestive heart failure. *Am J Dis Child* 1986;140:202-204.
180. Allan LD, Anderson RH, Sullivan ID et al. Evaluation of fetal arrhythmia by echocardiography. *Br Heart J* 1983;50:240-245.
181. Komaromy B, Gall J, Lampe L. Fetal arrhythmia during pregnancy and labor. *Br J Obstet Gynecol* 1977;84:492-496.
182. Mendoza GJ, Orlandino A, Steinfeld L. Intermittent fetal bradycardia induced by midpregnancy fetal ultrasonographic study. *Am J Obstet Gynecol* 1989;160:1038-1040.
183. Minagawa Y, Akaiwa A, Hidaka T et al. Severe fetal supraventricular bradyarrhythmia without fetal hypoxia. *Obstet Gynecol* 1987;70:454-456.
184. Laboda LA, Estroff JA, Benacerraf BR. First trimester bradycardia: a sign of impending fetal loss. *J Ultrasound Med* 1989;8:561-563.
185. Carpenter RJ, Strasburger JF, Garson A et al. Fetal ventricular pacing for hydrops secondary to complete atrioventricular block. *J Am Coll Cardiol* 1986;8:1434-1436.
186. McCue CM, Mantakas ME, Tingelstad JB et al. Congenital heart block in newborns of mothers with connective tissue disease. *Circulation* 1977;56(1):82-90.
187. Crawford D, Chapman M, Allan LD. Assessment of persistent bradycardia in prenatal life. *Br J Obstet Gynecol* 1985;92: 941-944.
188. Friedman D. Fetal echocardiography in the assessment of lupus pregnancies. *Am J Reprod Immunol* 1992;28:164-167.
189. Buyon J, Roubey R, Swersky S et al. Complete congenital heart block: risk of occurrence and therapeutic approach to prevention. *J Rheumatol* 1988;15:1104.

CHAPTER 39

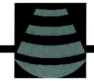

Fetal Abdominal Wall Defects

Jeanne A. Cullinan, M.D.
David A. Nyberg, M.D.

CHAPTER OUTLINE

The development of the anterior abdominal wall represents a complex process involving migration and enfolding of the lateral body folds as well as regression of early embryonic structures. The most common abdominal wall anomalies include gastroschisis and omphalocele. Rarer conditions include pentalogy of Cantrell, limb-body wall complex, bladder exstrophy, and cloacal exstrophy. Key factors for assessment are the site and size of the abdominal wall defect with respect to the umbilical cord as well as associated anomalies.

PRENATAL DIAGNOSIS

With the advent of widespread maternal serum alpha-fetoprotein screening (MSAFP) coupled with prenatal sonography, detection and diagnosis of abdominal wall anomalies have become increasingly common.[1] MSAFP screening may indicate a possible abdominal wall defect.[1] The exposed abdominal contents in the case of gastroschisis often result in an elevated MSAFP value. Screening is more variable in the case of an omphalocele because of the presence of the limiting membrane. A prospective study of 8000 patients combining sonography at 19 weeks with MSAFP correctly diagnosed all cases of gastroschisis and omphalocele.[2] However, despite the recent advances in the sonographic evaluation of these fetuses, large series have reported that up to a third of these defects may go undetected.[3,4] Walkinshaw et al. reported on an unselected population scanned between 1984 and 1988.[5] Examinations between 16 and 22 weeks gestation detected 60% of the defects with a false-positive rate of 5.3%. A recent Swedish report noted that the prenatal diagnosis was correct in 65 of the 70 cases.[6] These discrepancies are the result of a number of factors, including instrumentation, technique, and operator expertise. As these factors improve, the prenatal diagnosis of these disorders may be enhanced. The site, size, and contents of the defect, in combination with other associated anomalies, have an impact on the neonatal management and prognosis of these infants (Table 39-1). Recent neonatal survival has been reported as 96% in 32 infants with either gastroschisis or uncomplicated omphalocele.[6] Prenatal diagnosis allows for a combined clinical team approach in patient counseling and prenatal and neonatal management with a resultant improved neonatal outcome.

TABLE 39-1
TYPICAL PATHOLOGIC AND CLINICAL FEATURES OF ANTERIOR ABDOMINAL WALL DEFECTS

	Gastroschisis	Omphalocele	LBWC	Cloacal Exstrophy
Location	Right paraumbilic	Midline cord insertion site	Lateral	Infraumbilic
Size defect	Small (2-4 cm)	Variable (2-10 cm)	Large	Variable
Membrane	−	+	+ (contiguous with placenta)	"
Liver involvement	−	Common	+	+
Ascites	−	Common	−	"
Bowel thickening	+	− (unless ruptured membrane)	−	"
Bowel complications	Common	−	−	−
Cardiac anomalies	Rare (ASD, PDA)	Common (complex)	Common	10%-15%
Other anomalies	Rare	Common	Always (scoliosis, cranial defects, limb defects)	Always (genitourinary, spinal)
Chromosome abnormalities	−	Common	−	"

LBWC, Limb-body wall complex (body stalk anomaly); *ASD*, atrial septal defect; *PDA*, patent ductus arteriosus.

EMBRYOLOGY

By the sixth menstrual week, the flat embryonic disk begins the complex process of **folding**. This will occur at the cranial, caudal, and lateral ends of the embryo. As the cranial end of the embryo folds, the base of the yolk sac is partially incorporated into the foregut, while the caudal portion becomes part of the hindgut. The enfolding of the lateral components forms the anterior abdominal wall. This process is completed by 8 menstrual weeks except for persistence of the central body stalk (Fig. 39-1, *A*).[7,8] At this time, because of the volume of the solid viscera in the abdomen, the midgut is forced into the extraembryonic coelom in the proximal umbilical cord in a process known as **physiologic herniation**. As the midgut elongates, this ventral U-shaped loop has a cranial loop that will develop into the small intestines and a caudal loop that will develop into the cecum and proximal two thirds of the large bowel. The yolk sac is attached to the apex of this midgut loop. The cranial portion of the loop undergoes rapid development, forming the ileal loops. The end result is that the bowel undergoes a 90-degree counterclockwise rotation along the axis of the superior mesenteric artery (Fig. 39-1, *B*). By approximately the 12th menstrual week, the midgut has returned to the abdominal cavity while undergoing an additional 180-degree counterclockwise rotation, making a total of 270 degrees rotation (Fig. 39-1, *C*).[7] This physiologic midgut herniation can be observed sonographically (Fig. 39-2).[9] Cyr et al. reported the diameter of normal bowel herniation to be 1 cm or less while Bowerman et al. reported a greatest diameter of 7 mm.[10,11] Green and Hobbins have reported a small persistent bulge in the base of the umbilical cord at 12 weeks in 20% of fetuses.[12] For this reason, diagnosis should be delayed until 14 weeks in most cases, since it may be difficult to differentiate pathologic from physiologic herniation. Occasionally, the diagnosis may be made in the first trimester because of the presence of a large defect.[13]

GASTROSCHISIS

Gastroschisis is a **right-sided, relatively small, full-thickness paraumbilical defect of the abdominal wall** (Fig. 39-3).[14] Because of the full-thickness defect, free-floating loops of bowel are seen in the amniotic fluid. Left-sided gastroschises have been reported, but they are rare.[15,16] The defect occurs between 42 and 47 menstrual days.[7] Theories concerning the etiology of this defect include abnormal involution of the right umbilical vein[17] or disruption of the omphalomesenteric artery with ischemia.[18] The theory of vascular disruption is supported by recent work regarding cocaine usage,[19] cigarette smoking,[20] and pseudoepinephrine usage.[21] These substances act as vasoactive agents, potentially resulting in gastroschisis when exposure occurs at critical developmental periods. Gastroschisis is generally sporadic, but a few familial cases have been reported.[22] The reported frequency is 1 per 4000 live births.[23] There has been a report of an increase in the incidence of gastroschisis,[24-26] but comparable studies have failed to confirm this finding.[27,28] In contrast to omphalocele, gastroschisis is usually not associated with an increase in chromosomal abnormal-

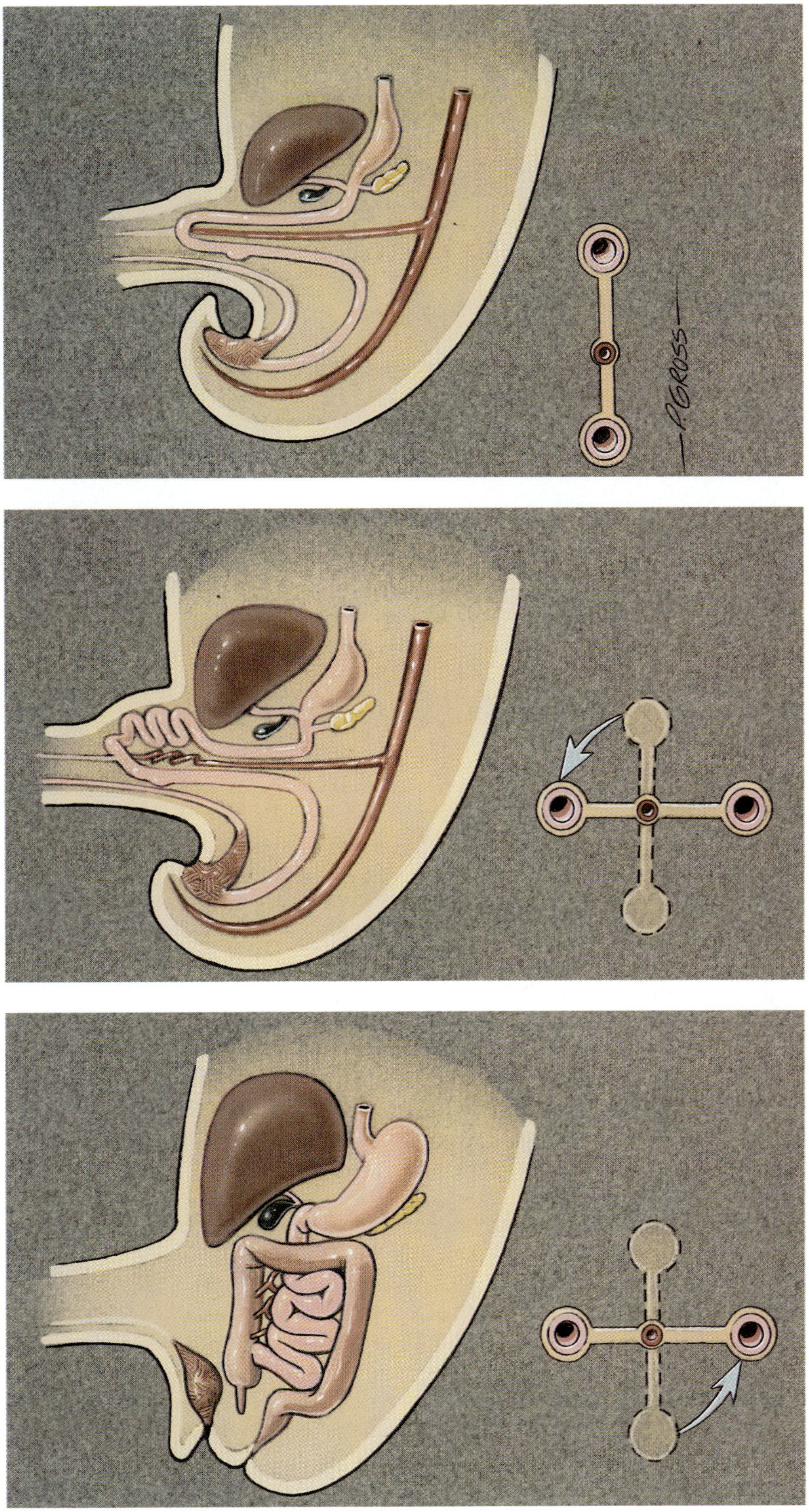

FIG. 39-1. Normal development of the anterior abdominal wall. A, Cross-sectional view of a sagittal representation of the fetal abdomen at approximately 9 weeks demonstrates the small bowel herniation into the base of the proximal umbilical cord. **B,** This bowel undergoes a 90-degree rotation along the axis of the superior mesenteric artery. **C,** At approximately 12 weeks the bowel returns to its normal position in the abdominal cavity, undergoing an additional 180-degree rotation along the axis of the superior mesenteric artery.

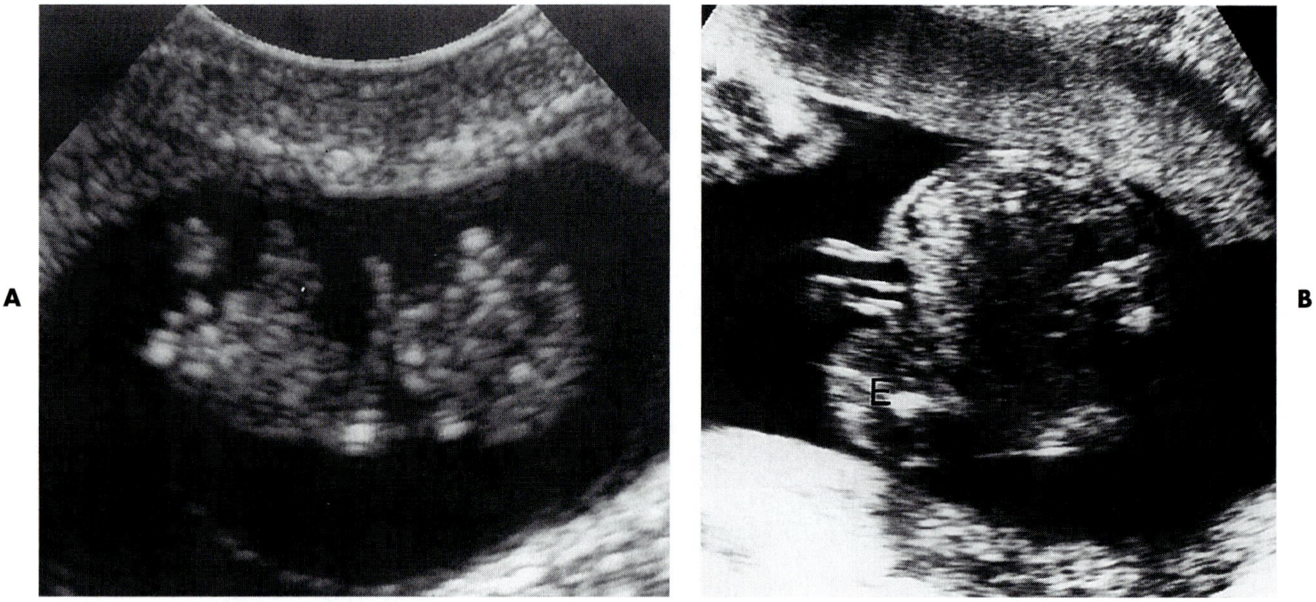

FIG. 39-2. Normal physiologic herniation of the small bowel. A, A small echogenic focus is seen at the base of the umbilical cord in this sagittal image of a 9-week fetus. **B,** In the second trimester, this bowel has returned to the abdominal cavity. An intact anterior abdominal wall with a three-vessel cord is seen inserting at the level of the umbilicus. A fetal extremity, *E,* is seen adjacent to the abdominal wall.

SONOGRAPHIC CRITERIA FOR THE DIAGNOSIS OF GASTROSCHISIS

- Full-thickness abdominal wall defect
- Paraumbilical location of the defect; generally right-sided
- Small (i.e., 2 to 4 cm) defect
- Free-floating loops of bowel in the amniotic fluid
- No enveloping membrane

ities, underscoring the need for accurate distinction between these disorders.[29,30]

Bowel-related abnormalities are the most common and important complications of gastroschisis.[31-37] Small bowel is always eviscerated. This is often accompanied by the large bowel and may be associated with evisceration of the stomach or solid organs. All fetuses with gastroschisis demonstrate either bowel malrotation or nonrotation. Intestinal ischemia or stenosis may be present in 7% to 30% of fetuses. This may be the result of compression of the mesenteric vessels as they exit the small defect or from torsion around the mesenteric axis. This ischemia may lead to bowel gangrene, perforation, or meconium peritonitis. The clinical outcome of the fetus relates to these complications.[33,34] Gastroschisis is usually **not associated with extragastrointestinal anomalies**, although cardiac and genitourinary abnormalities have been reported.[32,36-40] When extragastrointestinal defects are identified, an alternative diagnosis should be considered.

Because the condition of the bowel is the single most important factor in determining neonatal outcomes, this has led to an attempt to determine the optimum time of delivery by following the sonographic appearance of the bowel. With advancing gestation, thickening of the eviscerated bowel may be identified. The etiology of the bowel damage remains controversial. It may be the result of a chemical peritonitis induced by exposure to the amniotic fluid[41] or damage caused by constriction at the site of the abdominal wall defect.[42,43] Although mild dilatation of exposed bowel is commonly seen, development of bowel ischemia or obstruction must be considered when progressive bowel dilatation is noted.[32] Bond et al. reported on 11 cases in which bowel dilatation and mural thickening and not the size of the defect correlated with neonatal outcome.[32] Langer advocated use of a threshold curve of bowel dilatation generated from data of 24 fetuses to predict those infants at risk for neonatal complications.[44] Pryde et al., in a series of 20 pregnancies, reported that an absolute cut-off of more than 17 mm bowel dilatation was associated with increased morbidity and mortality.[45] This is in contrast to Babcock et al., who found 11 mm bowel dilatation to be predictive of adverse fetal outcomes.[46] The lack of agreement in the absolute measurement of the bowel diameter in these series probably relates to the small sample size coupled with variable clinical presentations of these infants.

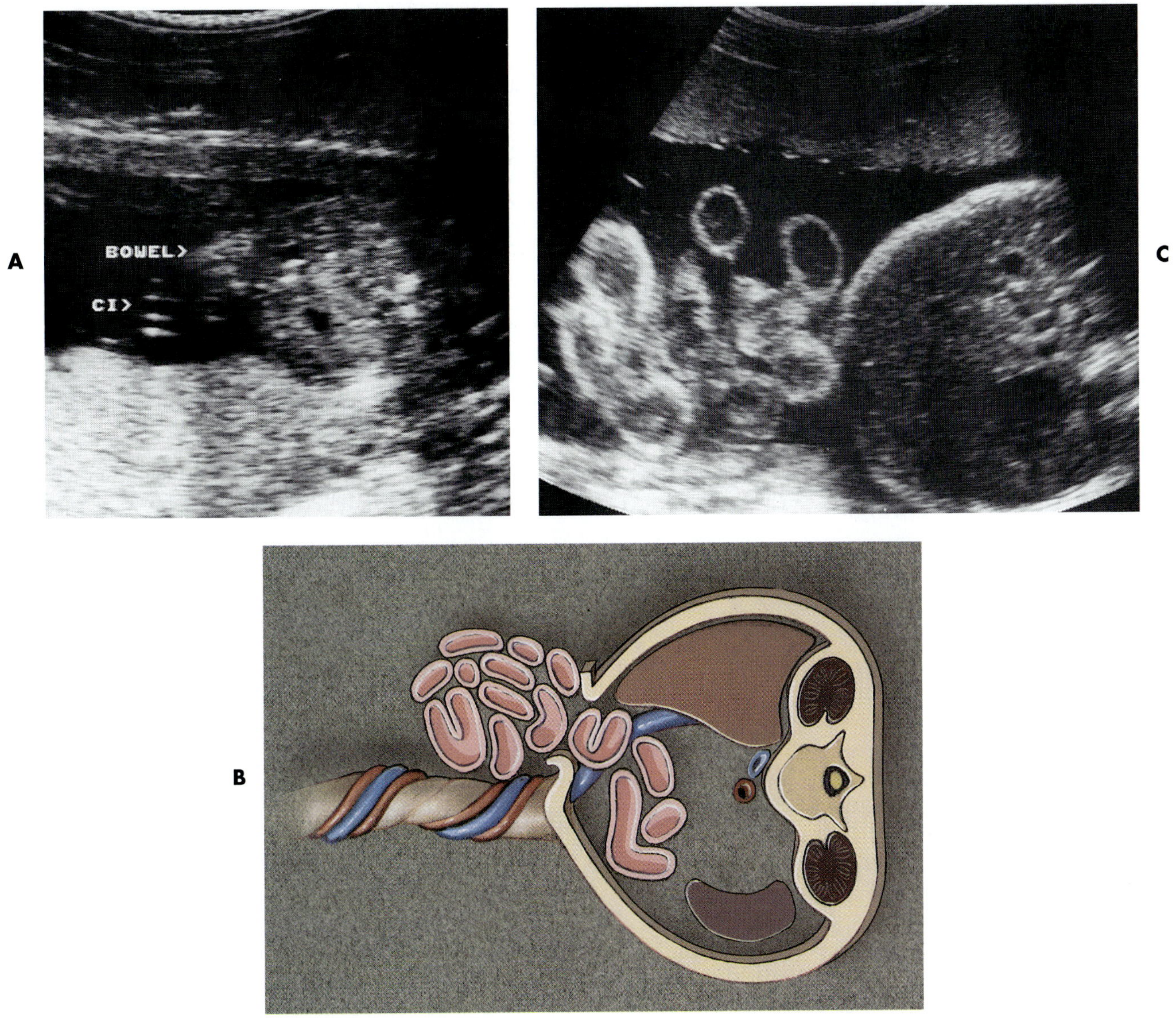

FIG. 39-3. Gastroschisis. **A,** A right paraumbilical defect is identified in the anterior abdominal wall with herniation of free loops of the small bowel into the amniotic cavity in this 16-week fetus. The stomach bubble is seen in the left upper quadrant. **B,** Schema of this finding. **C,** With advancing gestation, it is more difficult to determine the relationship of the abdominal wall defect to the umbilicus. The free-floating bowel loops are consistent with a diagnosis of gastroschisis.

Prematurity and intrauterine growth retardation are often seen in fetuses with gastroschisis.[15,47] The risk of growth retardation approached 50% in a recent series.[48] This, coupled with a risk of fetal distress and a 12.5% incidence of stillbirth, led the authors to suggest serial biophysical assessment of these pregnancies. The prognosis for gastroschisis is better than other abdominal wall defects, since it is usually not associated with other anomalies or with chromosomal defects. The survival rate approaches 90% with aggressive neonatal management,[37] with most deaths related to prematurity, sepsis, or bowel ischemia.[49] Although the mode of delivery remains controversial,[36,50-53] a planned coordinated team approach is to be encouraged.

OMPHALOCELE

An omphalocele is a **midline defect of the anterior abdominal wall at the level of the umbilicus**. This allows for herniation of the intraabdominal contents into the umbilical cord. This anomaly may be the result of failure of the lateral fold to migrate and the body wall to close.[54] An alternative theory is that this defect is due to persistence of the primitive body stalk.[55] The result is a failure of the bowel to return to its normal intraabdominal position. The incidence of this disorder is similar to that of gastroschisis.[56]

The abdominal wall defect is located centrally at the base of the abdominal cord (Fig. 39-4). The omphalo-

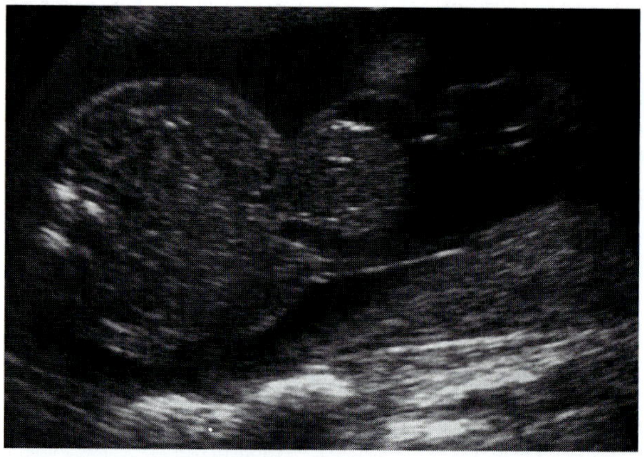

FIG. 39-4. Omphalocele. A central abdominal wall defect is seen at the base of the umbilical cord. Liver is contained within the sac. (Courtesy Ants Toi, M.D., University of Toronto.)

cele may contain bowel and/or solid organs. The contents of the omphalocele are covered by a limiting membrane composed of peritoneum and amnion separated by Wharton's jelly.[7] Bowel dilatation and thickening are not characteristic of this disorder because of the presence of the limiting membrane. Ascites may be demonstrated, implying the presence of the membrane (Fig. 39-5).[57] The size and contents of the defect vary considerably in this disorder.[54,58-60] In most cases, the sac contains liver, with or without bowel (Fig. 39-6). In some cases, only bowel is identified in the sac, which may represent persistence of the primitive body stalk beyond 12 weeks.[54,58] The limiting membrane may be difficult to demonstrate because of technical factors. Its presence may be inferred when the intraabdominal contents appear to be contained rather than free-floating in the amniotic fluid. A false-positive diagnosis of an omphalocele may be made when scanning the fetus in an oblique plane or with compression of the fetal abdomen.[61,62] Rarely, rupture of the membrane may occur, complicating the diagnosis.[31,63]

Sonographic evaluation of omphalocele includes documentation of the size, contents, and location of the defect. An additional diagnostic feature is the presence of the intrahepatic portion of the umbilical vein coursing through the central portion of the defect.[38] An important consideration is the diagnosis of **associated** anomalies, which may be seen in 67% to 88% of fetuses with an omphalocele.[55,64] Because up to 50% of associated anomalies are of cardiac origin,[65-67] a detailed cardiac examination is critical in the evaluation of these fetuses. Gastrointestinal anomalies occur in 40% of fetuses as well as anomalies of the musculoskeletal, genitourinary, and central nervous systems.[14] As expected, given the failure of the bowel to return to the abdominal cavity, malrotation is always present in this condition.

SONOGRAPHIC CRITERIA FOR DIAGNOSIS OF OMPHALOCELE

Central anterior abdominal wall defect containing bowel/solid viscera
Mass encompassed by umbilical cord
Limiting membrane covering the defect

Omphalocele is associated with a number of syndromes. The most notable of these is the **Beckwith-Wiedemann** syndrome, an autosomal dominant disorder characterized by gigantism, macroglossia, and pancreatic hyperplasia.[68,69] Trisomy 11p has been associated with this syndrome.[22] Although an omphalocele is not a prerequisite of this disorder, it is seen in 5% to 10% of infants at delivery.* Additional sonographic criteria include protrusion of the tongue, cardiac anomalies, and visceromegaly of the liver, spleen, or kidney.

There is a correlation with **chromosomal abnormalities and omphalocele.** Trisomies 13 and 18 are the most frequent chromosomal abnormalities associated with an omphalocele, followed by trisomy 21, 45, XO, and triploidy.[54,64,65] The antenatal rate of trisomy 13 and 18 in fetuses with an omphalocele is seven times that of term live-borns.[56] Omphaloceles are associated with chromosomal abnormalities in 30% to 40% of fetuses in prenatal series. One third of fetuses with trisomy 13 and 10% to 50% with trisomy 18 will have an omphalocele.[71,72] Fetuses with sacs containing only bowel carry a significantly higher risk of chromosomal abnormalities than those containing liver.[55,64,73] Additional risk factors for a chromosomal abnormality include abnormal amniotic fluid volume, concurrent anomalies, and advanced maternal age.[54,64,65] For this reason, chromosomal evaluation should be performed on all fetuses diagnosed with an omphalocele.

An accurate determination of associated anomalies is the most important determinant of **fetal survival.** Stillbirth is common,[74] and neonatal death is highly correlated with associated anomalies.[64,75] Hughes et al. noted that survival correlated with major anomalies and abnormal amniotic fluid volume and not the size of the defect or the presence of ascites.[64] As in gastroschisis, the mode of delivery is controversial,[36,51,52,76] but planned delivery at tertiary centers is to be encouraged. Neonatal survival in uncomplicated omphalocele approaches that of gastroschisis, while fetuses with associated major anomalies or chromosomal defects have greater than 80% mortality.[34,36,37,77]

*References 34, 36, 37, 54, 70.

A

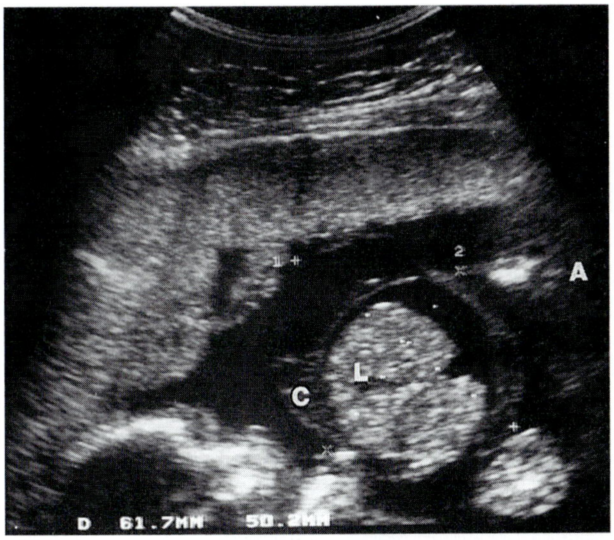

C

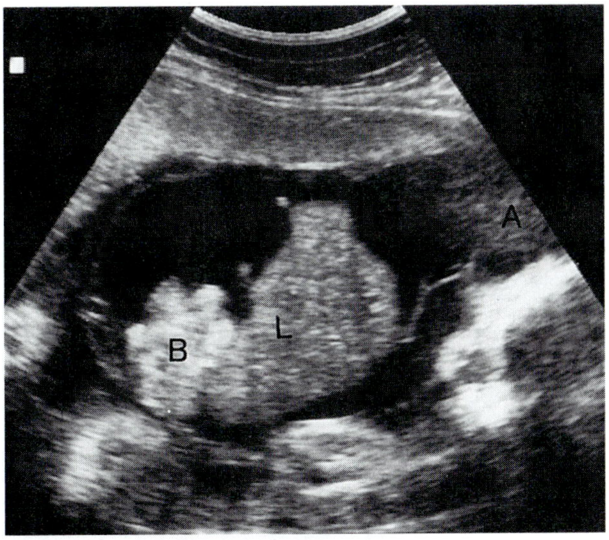

B

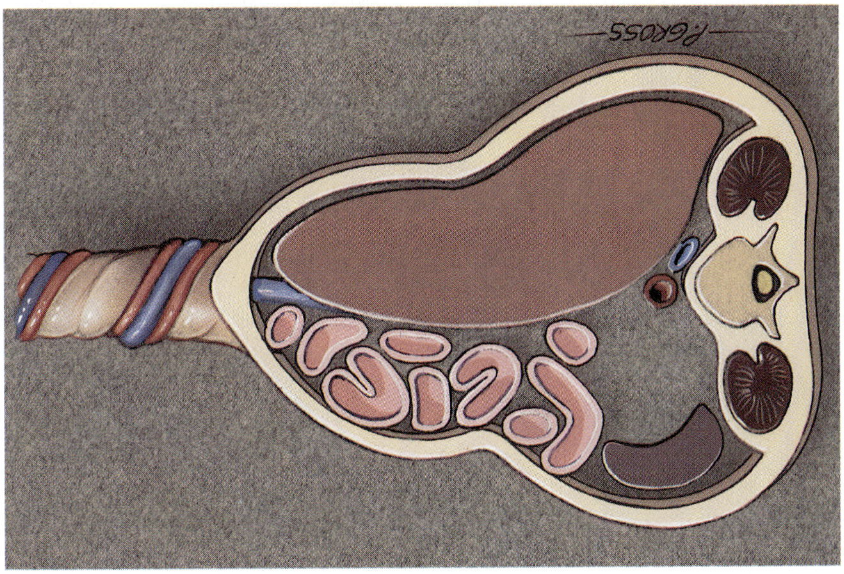

FIG. 39-5. Omphalocele. **A,** Ultrasound scan on an 18-week fetus through the omphalocele in a paraumbilical location shows liver, *L*, cord insertion, *C*, abdomen, *A*. Abdominal ascites is noted as well as a limiting membrane. **B,** Schema of this disorder. **C,** With advancing gestation, the relationship of the umbilical cord is more difficult to assess with respect to the abdominal contents. The limiting membrane suggests the diagnosis of an omphalocele. (Courtesy Joseph Brunner, M.D., Dept. of Obstetrics and Gynecology, Vanderbilt University Medical Center, Nashville, Tenn.)

PENTALOGY OF CANTRELL

The etiology of this condition is uncertain, but it is thought to result from **failure of fusion of the lateral folds in the thoracic region with variable extension inferiorly**.[55] There is failure of development of the transverse septum of the diaphragm.[22] The condition represents an association of an **omphalocele and an ectopic heart** (Fig. 39-7). Other associated findings are secondary to these two major defects. The syndrome consists of the following: anterior diaphragmatic hernia, midline abdominal wall defect, cardiac anoma-

SONOGRAPHIC CRITERIA FOR PENTALOGY OF CANTRELL

- Midline anterior wall defect usually involving the upper abdomen
- Ectopic heart
- Pericardial or pleural effusions
- Craniofacial anomalies
- Ascites
- Two-vessel cord

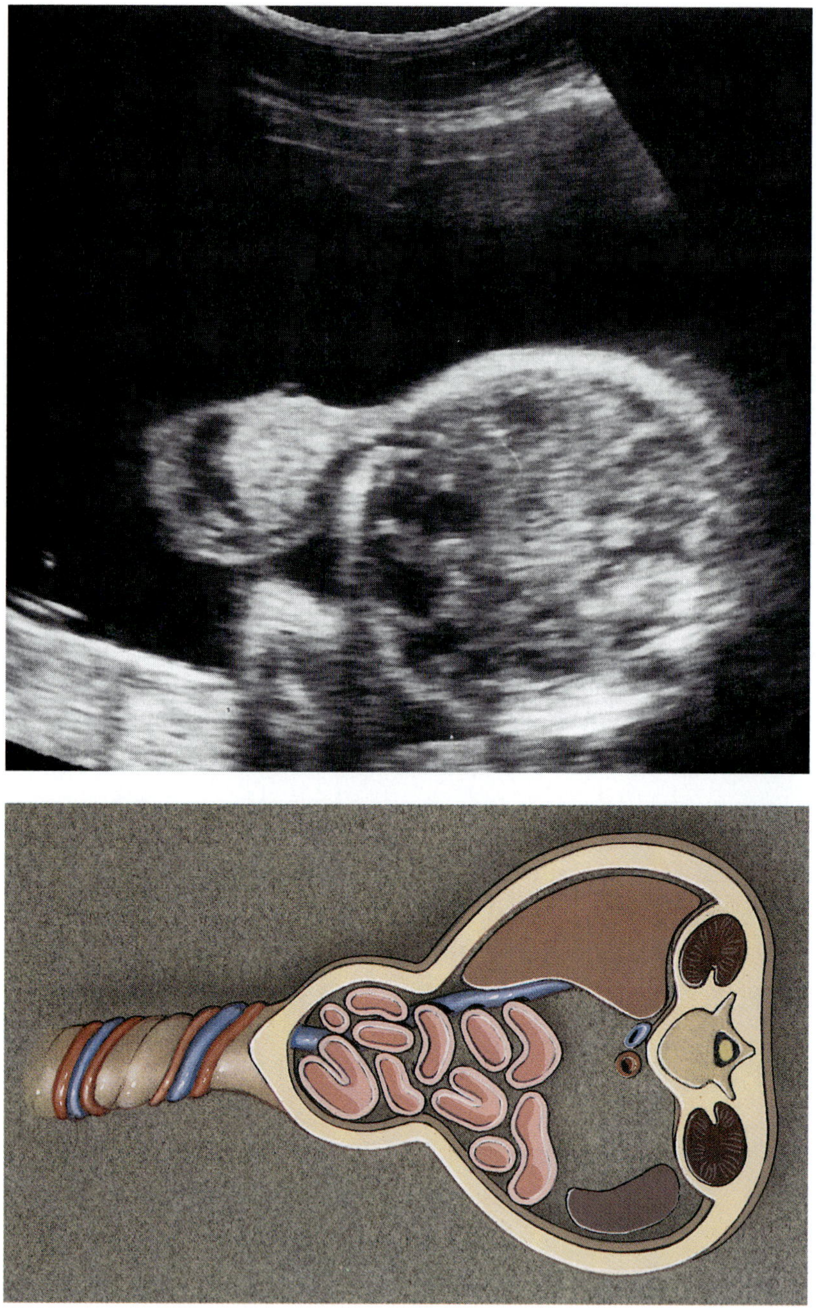

FIG. 39-6. Omphalocele. **A,** In this 17-week fetus, small bowel is identified herniating into the base of the umbilical cord with no other abdominal contents noted. **B,** Schema of this finding.

lies, defect of the diaphragmatic pericardium, and lower sternal defect.[78] An association has been reported with chromosomal abnormalities[79-82] as well as noncardiac anomalies, including craniofacial anomalies, vertebral anomalies, two-vessel cord, and ascites. The condition is rare,[22] with only about 50 reported cases.

The demonstration of both an omphalocele and an ectopic heart should suggest the diagnosis of pentalogy of Cantrell. Siles et al. reported on the association of an omphalocele and a pericardial effusion with no other sonographic findings.[78] When there is consideration of this syndrome, chromosomal determination should be encouraged. **Prognosis** depends on the severity of the anomalies, but most prenatally diagnosed cases have a fatal outcome.[81,83]

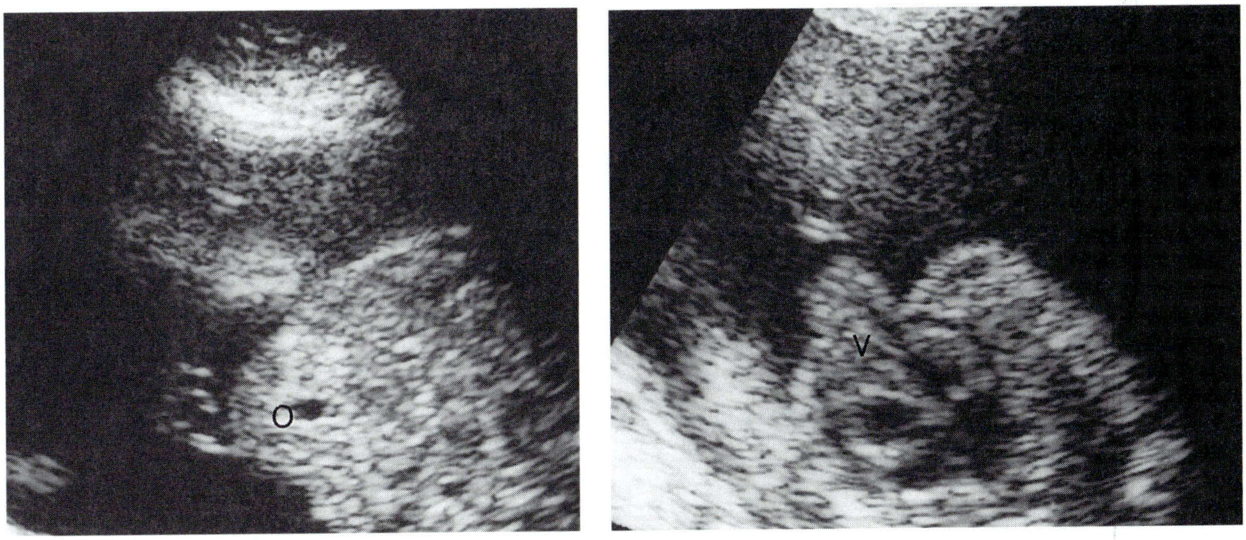

FIG. 39-7. Ectopia cordis with pentalogy of Cantrell. **A,** Transverse scan in the second trimester shows a supraumbilical midline omphalocele, *O*. **B,** Scan at a more cephalic level shows the cardiac ventricles, *V*, eviscerated into the amniotic fluid. A complex cardiac anomaly and cleft lip were also present. (Courtesy Leo Drolshagen, M.D., Fort Smith, Ark.)

LIMB-BODY WALL COMPLEX

The limb-body wall complex, or the body stalk anomaly, is a complex malformation caused by the **failure of the ventral body wall to close.** The cause of this complex remains controversial. Although some investigators view this as an extreme form of the amniotic band syndrome, this would not account for many of the associated anomalies identified in this complex.[84,85] The most plausible theory is that an early vascular accident results in disruptive body wall events and internal malformations.[86-88] The maldevelopment of the cranial, caudal, and lateral body fold results in a short or absent umbilical cord with evisceration of the abdominal organs that are attached to the placenta.[89,90] An eccentric ventral wall defect involving the abdomen and/or thorax, cranial and facial defects, and abnormalities of the placental membranes and umbilical cord are hallmarks of this complex (Fig. 39-8).[84,87,88,91]

The abdominal wall defect is **often left-sided** as opposed to the right-sided defect usually noted with gastroschisis.[85] In a series of 25 infants with limb-body wall complex, **major anomalies** seen included: limb defects (95%), severe scoliosis (77%), internal organ malformations (95%), and craniofacial anomalies (56%).[84] Limb defects included clubfoot, absent limbs or digits, arthrogryposis, polydactyly, and syndactyly. Internal malformations included cardiac defects, absence of the diaphragm, bowel atresia, and renal anomalies. Craniofacial defects included facial clefts, encephalocele, or exencephaly. Amniotic bands are seen in as many as 40% of cases.[92] Some of these malformations may be positional in origin and relate to the fetal attachment to the placenta and hyperextension.[90] The incidence of the disorder is 1 per 14,273 births[89] with no known chromosomal association.

The distorted fetal position and severity of the anomalies may make sonographic evaluation difficult. The fetal trunk is adherent to the placenta with no demonstrable umbilical cord. The limb abnormalities may be difficult to document by sonography, with clubfoot seen in over 30% of cases.[84] Accurate differentiation from other forms of abdominal wall defects is crucial since the limb-body wall complex is universally fatal.

SONOGRAPHIC HALLMARKS OF THE LIMB-BODY WALL COMPLEX

Large ventral wall defect of the abdomen and thorax (often left-sided)
Craniofacial anomalies
Marked scoliosis and/or spinal dysraphism
Limb defects
Short or absent umbilical cord
Amniotic bands

BLADDER AND CLOACAL EXSTROPHY

Bladder and cloacal exstrophy represent **midline defects of the infraumbilical anterior abdominal wall.**[93] Although these disorders share an embry-

A

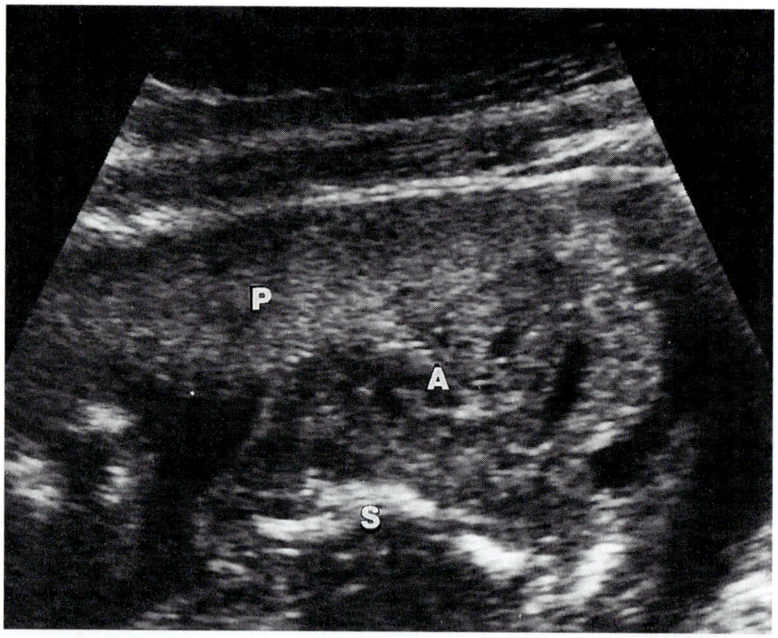

B

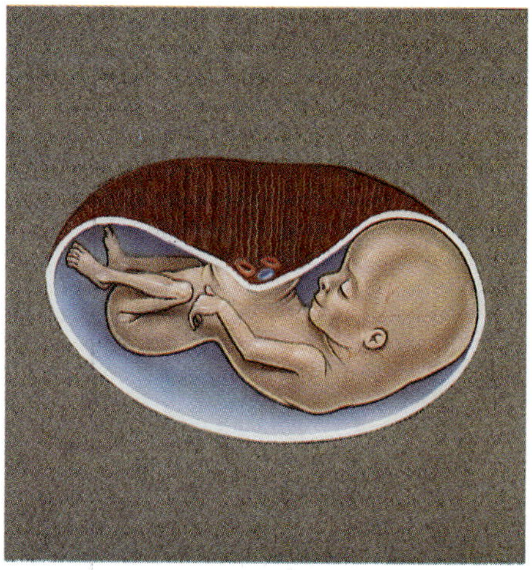

C

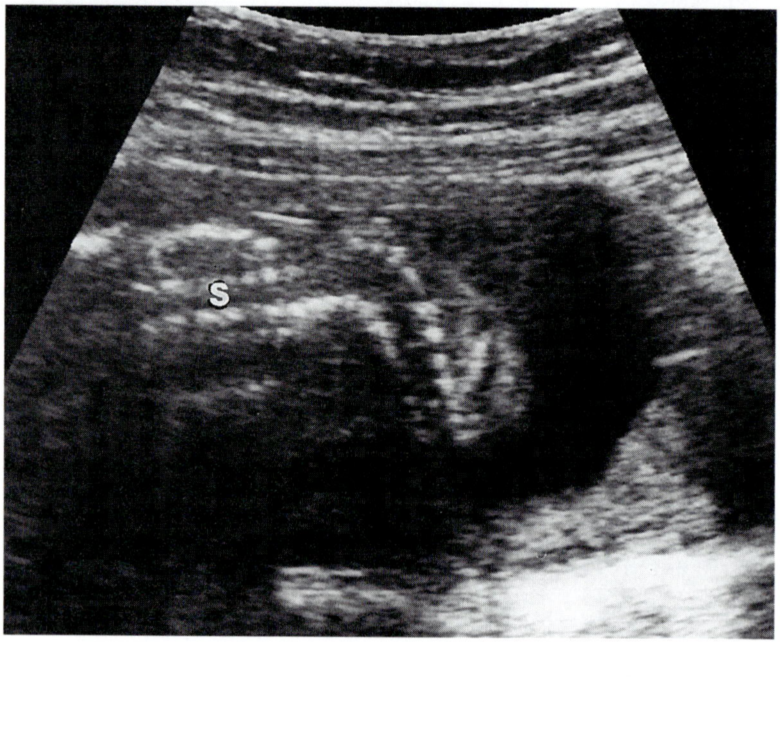

FIG. 39-8. Limb-body wall complex. A, There is difficulty differentiating the anterior abdominal wall from the adherent placenta, *P*, in this 17-week fetus. *A*, Abdominal wall defect; *S*, spine. **B,** Illustration of the relationship of the fetus to the placenta in this condition. **C,** Significant scoliosis is identified.

ologic origin, they differ in the extent and severity of anomalous findings. These are rare defects with an incidence of 1 per 33,000 live births in bladder exstrophy and 1 per 200,000 to 400,000 live births in the case of cloacal exstrophy.[93-96] In fetuses with bladder exstrophy, there is failure of mesenchymal cell to migrate between the ectoderm and cloaca at 6 weeks menstrual age. This produces a failure of muscle development of the anterior abdominal wall with inappropriate eversion of the bladder mucosa (Fig. 39-9).[7] In general, this is usually an isolated defect. The **OEIS complex** has been reported, which is characterized by an omphalocele, bladder exstrophy, imperforate anus, and spinal abnormalities.[97] Cloacal exstrophy is a more complex constellation of findings due to the embryologic maldevelopment of the cloacal membrane. The extent of the defect depends on the timing of the insult.[98] There is nondevelopment of the urorectal septum. This causes a failure in the separation of the urogenital septum from the rectum.[97] As a result, there is persistence of two embryonic rests of bladder mucosa laterally. The two hemibladders are separated by intestinal mucosa, which probably corresponds to the cecum since the

A

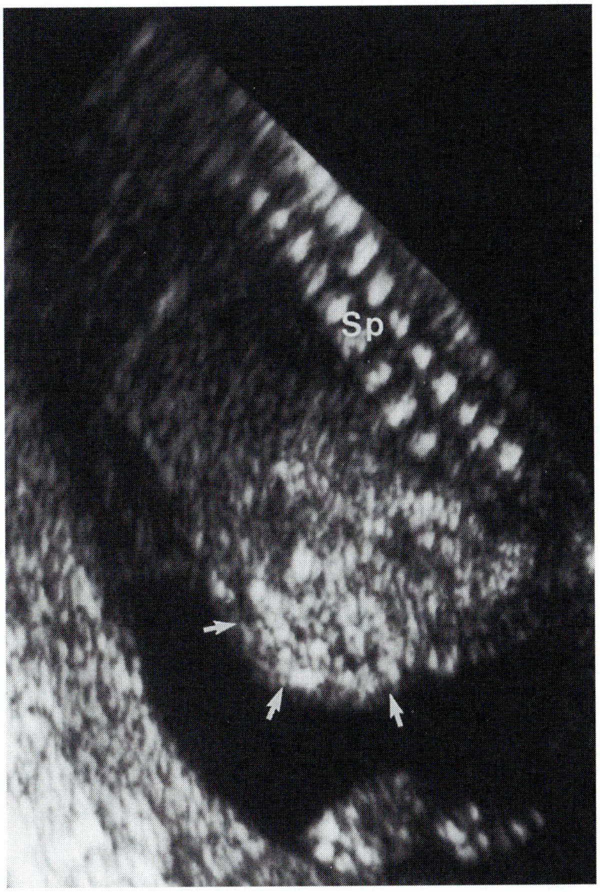

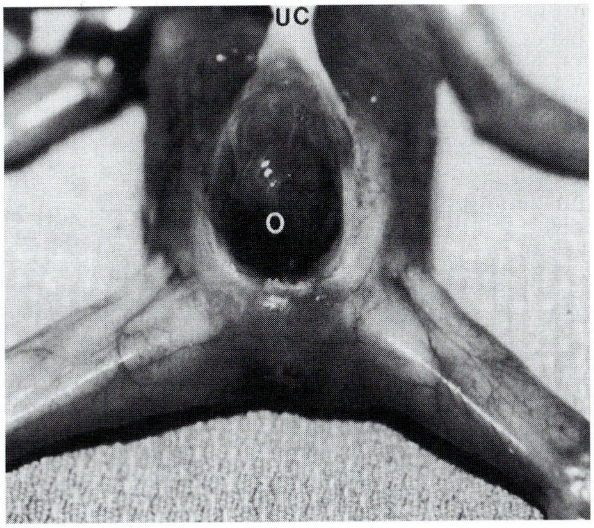

B

FIG. 39-9. Bladder exstrophy. **A,** Transvaginal sonogram at 16 weeks, performed because of suspicion of an abdominal wall defect on transabdominal scans, shows a small soft-tissue mass *(arrows)* protruding from the anterior abdominal wall. The urinary bladder was not visualized, suggesting a differential diagnosis of bladder or cloacal exstrophy. *Sp,* Spine. **B,** Postmortem photograph confirms bladder exstrophy with an associated infraumbilical omphalocele, *O.* Anorectal atresia is also present. *UC,* Umbilical cord.

ileum enters it (Fig. 39-10).* **Associated anomalies** include involvement of the central nervous system, the genitourinary system, anomalous genitalia, limb defects, and a two-vessel cord.[97,98] Because there is infrequent occurrence of these syndromes, the genetics of these disorders is uncertain,[102] and chromosomal evaluation should be considered.

Sonographic findings in bladder exstrophy include inability to identify the bladder. The abdominal wall defect may be obscured by the everted bladder mucosa. The only finding to suggest this anomaly may be a soft-tissue mass protruding from the lower anterior abdominal wall.[103]

Other **associated anomalies** that may be seen include a narrow thorax, kyphoscoliosis, clubfeet, and renal anomalies. Hydrocephalus and ascites have also been reported, but the incidence of these is not uniformly present.[104] It is necessary to differentiate this disorder from other anterior abdominal wall defects. This is accomplished by determining the site of the defect with respect to the umbilicus. Meizner et al. have reported that color flow Doppler imaging may aid in the diagnosis, particularly if overlying structures obstruct visualization of the abdominal wall.[104]

*References 7, 94-96, 99-101.

SONOGRAPHIC FINDINGS IN CLOACAL EXSTROPHY

Large infraumbilical anterior wall defect with irregular anterior wall mass
Absent bladder
Malformation of the genitalia
± Neural tube defect

Prenatal differentiation between these two disorders may be difficult, but small series have described successful prenatal diagnosis of these syndromes.[104,105] These disorders should be considered when there is demonstration of an infraumbilical defect and an absent urinary bladder. An attempt to correctly diagnose these two conditions is important because of the differences in fetal outcome. The **prognosis for bladder exstrophy is favorable,** although multiple procedures may be necessary.[106] Because of the complexity of the anomalies in **cloacal exstrophy, the prognosis is less favorable** and relates to the severity of the defects. Prior reports have noted a mortality of 55%.[100] Recent advances in supportive care and surgical tech-

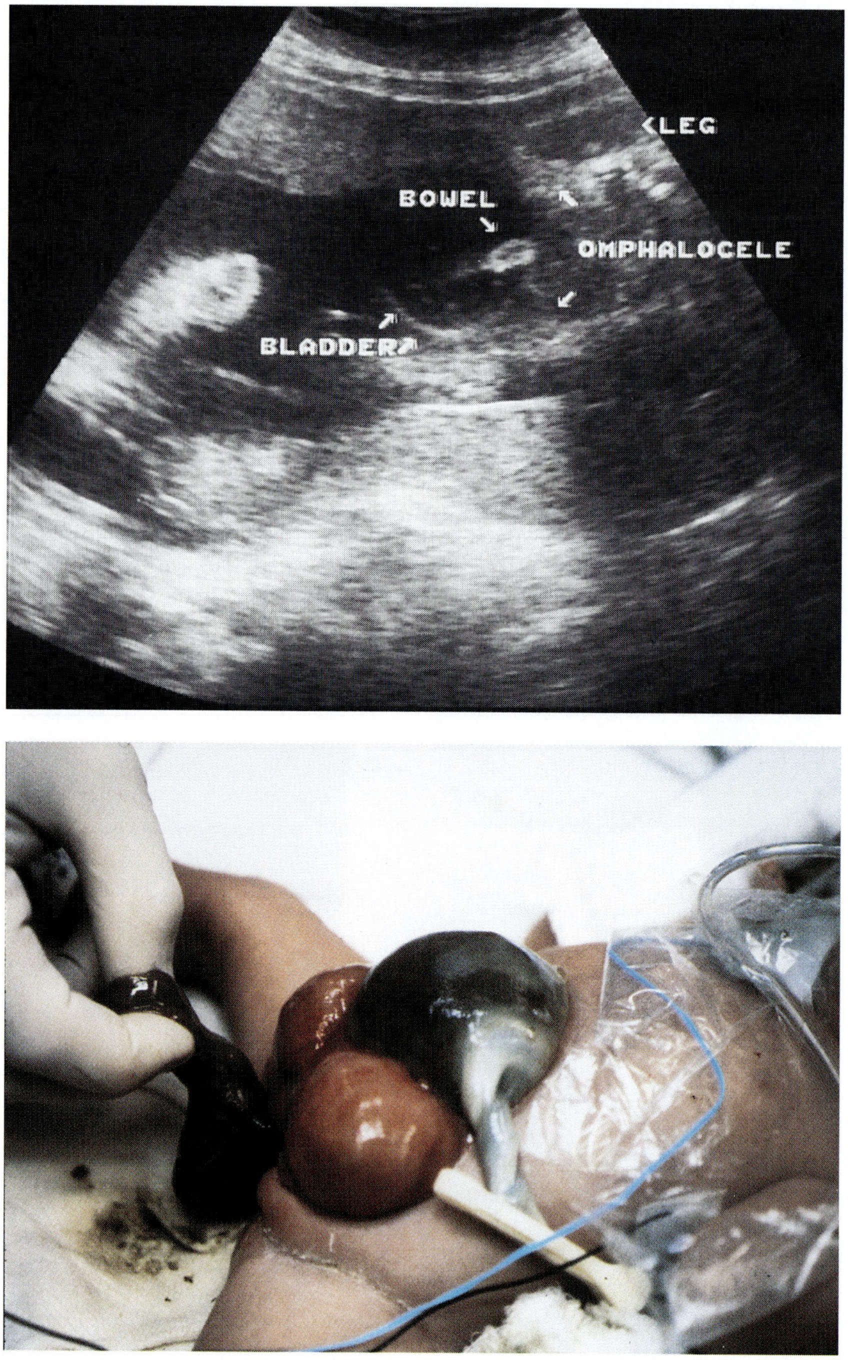

FIG. 39-10. Cloacal exstrophy. **A,** There is a poorly defined soft-tissue mass seen in the infraumbilical abdominal wall as well as lateral hemibladders in this fetus. **B,** Postmortem photograph illustrates the soft-tissue paraumbilical mass inferiorly and the hemibladders, which are separated by extruding bowel. (Courtesy Joseph Brunner, M.D., Dept. of Obstetrics and Gynecology, Vanderbilt University Medical Center, Nashville, Tenn.)

niques have resulted in improved reports of survival, with Hurvitz et al. reporting a 90% postoperative survival rate.[107]

CONCLUSION

Important findings to document in the prenatal assessment of the fetus with an abdominal wall anomaly include the site and size of the defect as well as the presence of a limiting membrane. When coupled with associated anomalies, it is often possible to determine the appropriate clarification of the anomaly. The correct diagnosis has significant clinical implications for predicting the likelihood of chromosomal abnormalities as well as the prognosis, which varies considerably among these disorders. Increased awareness of these uncommon conditions should result in improved diagnosis and management.

ACKNOWLEDGEMENTS

We wish to thank Joylonna Burgoyne for secretarial assistance, Tom Ebers for editorial support, and Paul Gross for the artwork in this chapter.

REFERENCES

Prenatal Diagnosis

1. Palomaki GE, Hill LE, Knight GJ et al. Second-trimester maternal serum alpha-fetoprotein levels in pregnancies associated with gastroschisis and omphalocele. *Obstet Gynecol* 1988;71:906-909.
2. Luck CA. Value of routine ultrasound scanning at 19 weeks: a four year study of 8849 deliveries. *Br Med J* 1992;304: 1474-1478.
3. Morrow RJ, Whittle MJ, McNay MB et al. Prenatal diagnosis and management of anterior abdominal wall defects in the west of Scotland. *Prenat Diagn* 1993;13:111-115.
4. Robert JP, Burge DM. Antenatal diagnosis of abdominal wall defects: a missed opportunity? *Arch Dis Child* 1990;65:687-689.
5. Walkinshaw SA, Renwick M, Hebisch G et al. How good is ultrasound in the detection and evaluation of anterior abdominal wall defects? *Br J Radiol* 1992;67:298-301.
6. Eurenius K, Axelsson O. Outcome for fetuses with abdominal wall defects detected by routine second trimester ultrasound. *Acta Obstet Gynecol Scand* 1994;73:25-29.

Embryology

7. Moore KL. *The Developing Human.* 4th ed. Philadelphia: WB Saunders Co; 1988:217-285.
8. Emanuel PG, Garcia GI, Angtuaco TL. Prenatal detection of anterior abdominal wall defects with ultrasound. *RadioGraphics* 1995;15:517-530.
9. Schmidt W, Yarkoni S, Crelin ES et al. Sonographic visualization of physiologic anterior abdominal wall hernia in the first trimester. *Obstet Gynecol* 1987;69:911.
10. Cyr DR, Mack LA, Schoenecker SA et al. Bowel migration in the normal fetus: US detection. *Radiology* 1986;161:119.
11. Bowerman R, Aulla N, Ginsberg H. High resolution sonographic identification of fetal midgut herniation into the umbilical cord: differentiation from fetal anterior abdominal wall defects. *J Ultrasound Med* 1988;109 (Suppl):7.
12. Green JJ, Hobbins JC. Abdominal ultrasound examination of the first trimester fetus. *Am J Obstet Gynecol* 1988;159:165.
13. Brown DL, Emerson DS, Schulman LP et al. Sonographic diagnosis of omphalocele during 10th week of gestation. *AJR* 1989;153:825-826.

Gastroschisis

14. Hutchin P. Somatic anomalies of the umbilicus and anterior abdominal wall. *Obstet Gynecol Surg* 1965;120:1075-1090.
15. Tibboel D, Raine P, McNee M et al. Developmental aspects of gastroschisis. *J Pediatr Surg* 1986;21:865.
16. Tibboel D, Kluck AWM, van der Kamp AWM et al. The development of the characteristic anomalies found in gastroschisis—experimental and clinical data. *Z Kinderchir* 1986;40:355.
17. Devries PA. The pathogenesis of gastroschisis and omphalocele. *J Pediatr Surg* 1980;15:245-251.
18. Hoyme HE, Higginbottom MC, Jones KL. The vascular pathogenesis of gastroschisis: intrauterine interruption of the omphalomesenteric artery. *Semin Perinatol* 1983;7:294.
19. Hume RF Jr, Gingas JL, Martin LS et al. Ultrasound diagnosis of fetal anomalies associated with in utero cocaine exposure: further support for cocaine-induced vascular disruption teratogenesis. *Fet Diagn Ther* 1994;9:239-245.
20. Goldbaum G, Daling J, Milham S. Risk factors for gastroschisis. *Teratology* 1990;42:397-403.
21. Werler MM, Mitchell AA, Shapiro S. First trimester maternal medication use in relation to gastroschisis. *Teratology* 1992;45:361-367.
22. Goncalves LF, Jeanty P. Ultrasound evaluation of abdominal wall defects. In: Callen PW, ed. *Ultrasonography in Obstetrics and Gynecology*. Philadelphia: WB Saunders Co; 1994:370-388.
23. Goldstein RB. Ultrasound evaluation of the fetal abdomen. In: Callen PW, ed. *Ultrasonography in Obstetrics and Gynecology*. Philadelphia: WB Saunders Co; 1994:347-369.
24. Roeper PJ, Harris J, Lee G et al. Secular rates and correlates for gastroschisis in California (1968-1977). *Teratology* 1987;35:203-210.
25. Lindham S. Omphalocele and gastroschisis in Sweden, 1967-1976. *Acta Paediatr Scand* 1981;70:55-60.
26. Hemmenki K, Salonieme I, Kyronen P et al. Gastroschisis and omphalocele in Finland in the 1970's: prevalence at birth and its correlates. *J Epidemiol Commun Health* 1982;36:289-293.
27. Baird PA, MacDonald EC. An epidemiologic study of congenital malformations of the anterior abdominal wall in more than half a million consecutive live births. *Am J Hum Genet* 1981;33:470-478.
28. Calzolari E, Volpato S, Bianchi F et al. Omphalocele and gastroschisis: a collaborative study of five Italian congenital malformation registries. *Teratology* 1993;47:47-55.
29. Caniano DA, Brokaw B, Ginn-Pease ME. An individualized approach to the management of gastroschisis. *J Pediatr Surg* 1990;25:287-300.
30. Nicolaides KH, Snijders RJM, Cheng HH et al. Fetal gastrointestinal and abdominal wall defects: associated malformations and chromosomal abnormalities. *Fet Diagn Ther* 1992;7:102-115.
31. Hertzberg BA. Sonography of the fetal gastrointestinal tract: anatomic variants, diagnostic pitfalls and abnormalities. *AJR* 1994;162:1175-1182.
32. Bond SJ, Harrison MR, Filly RA. Severity of intestinal damage in gastroschisis: correlation with prenatal sonographic findings. *J Pediatr Surg* 1988;23:520-525.

33. Luck SR, Sherman J, Raffensperger JG et al. Gastroschisis in 106 consecutive newborn infants. *Surgery* 1985;98:677-683.
34. Mabogunje OOA, Mahour GH. Omphalocele and gastroschisis: trends in survival across two decades. *Am J Surg* 1984;148:679-686.
35. Martin LW, Torres AM. Omphalocele and gastroschisis: symposium on pediatric surgery. *Surg Clin North Am* 1985;65:1235-1244.
36. Kirk EP, Wah R. Obstetric management of the fetus with omphalocele or gastroschisis: a review and report of one hundred twelve cases. *Am J Obstet Gynecol* 1983;146:512-518.
37. Mayer T, Black R, Matlak ME et al. Gastroschisis and omphalocele. *Am Surg* 1980;192:783-787.
38. Paidas MJ, Crombleholme TM, Robertson FM. Prenatal diagnosis and management of the fetus with an abdominal wall defect. *Semin Perinatol* 1994;18:196-214.
39. Redford DH, McNay MB, Whittle MJ. Gastroschisis and exomphalos: precise diagnosis by midpregnancy ultrasound. *Br J Obstet Gynaecol* 1985;92:54.
40. Sermer M, Benzie RJ, Pitson L et al. Prenatal diagnosis and management of congenital defects of the anterior abdominal wall. *Am J Obstet Gynecol* 1987;156:308.
41. Kluck P, Tibboel D, Van Der Kamp AWM et al. The effect of fetal urine on the development of bowel in gastroschisis. *J Pediatr Surg* 1983;18:47-50.
42. Langer JC, Longaker MT, Crombleholme TM et al. Etiology of intestinal damage in gastroschisis. I. Effects of amniotic fluid exposure and bowel constriction in a fetal lamb model. *J Pediatr Surg* 1989;24:992-997.
43. Langer JC, Bell JG, Castillo RO et al. Etiology of intestinal damage in gastroschisis. II. Timing and reversibility of histological changes, mucosal function and contractility. *J Pediatr Surg* 1990;25:1122-1126.
44. Langer JC, Khanna J, Caco C et al. Prenatal diagnosis of gastroschisis: development of objective sonographic criteria for predicting outcome. *Obstet Gynecol* 1993;81:53-56.
45. Pryde PG, Bardicef M, Treadwell MC et al. Gastroschisis: can antenatal ultrasound predict infant outcomes? *Obstet Gynecol* 1994;84:505-510.
46. Babcock CJ, Hedrick MH, Goldstein RB et al. Gastroschisis: can sonography of the fetal bowel accurately predict postnatal outcome? *J Ultrasound Med* 1994;13:701-706.
47. Carpenter MW, Curci MR, Dibbins AW et al. Perinatal management of ventral wall defects. *Obstet Gynecol* 1984;64:646.
48. Crawford RA, Ryan G, Wright VM et al. The importance of serial biophysical assessment of fetal well-being in gastroschisis. *Br J Obstet Gynecol* 1992;99:899-902.
49. Higginbottom MC, Jones KL, Hall BD et al. The amniotic band disruption complex: timing of amniotic rupture and variable spectra of consequent defects. *J Pediatr* 1979;95:544–549.
50. Lenke RR, Hatch EI. Fetal gastroschisis: a preliminary report advocating the use of cesarean section. *Obstet Gynecol* 1986;67:395.
51. Moretti M, Khoury A, Rodriquez J et al. The effect of mode of delivery on the perinatal outcome in fetuses with abdominal wall defects. *Am J Obstet Gynecol* 1990;163:833-838.
52. Sipes SL, Weiner CP, Sipes DR et al. Gastroschisis and omphalocele: does either antenatal diagnosis or route of delivery make a difference in perinatal outcome? *Obstet Gynecol* 1990;76:195-199.
53. Bethel CAE, Seashore JH, Touloukian RJ. Cesarean section does not improve outcome in gastroschisis. *J Pediatr Surg* 1989;24:1-4.

Omphalocele

54. Nyberg DA, Fitzsimmons J, Mack LA et al. Chromosomal abnormalities in fetuses with omphalocele: significance of omphalocele contents. *J Ultrasound Med* 1989;8:299-308.
55. Nyberg DA, Mack LA. Abdominal wall defects. In: Nyberg DA, Mahony BS, Pretorius DH, eds. *Diagnostic Ultrasound of Fetal Anomalies: Text and Atlas.* St Louis: Mosby–Year Book; 1990:395-432.
56. Snijders JM, Brizot ML, Faria M et al. Fetal exomphalos at eleven to fourteen weeks of gestation. *J Ultrasound Med* 1995;14:469-574.
57. Bair JH, Russ PD, Pretorius DH et al. Fetal omphalocele and gastroschisis: a review of 24 cases. *AJR* 1986;147:1047-1051.
58. Seashore JH. Congenital abdominal wall defects. *Clin Perinatol* 1978;5:62-77.
59. Schaffer RM, Barone C, Friedman AP. The ultrasonographic spectrum of fetal omphalocele. *J Ultrasound Med* 1983;2:219-222.
60. Brown BSJ. The prenatal ultrasonographic features of omphalocele: a study of 10 patients. *J Can Assoc Radiol* 1985;36:312-316.
61. Lindfors KK, McGahan JP, Walter JP. Fetal omphalocele and gastroschisis: pitfalls in sonographic diagnosis. *AJR* 1986;147:797-800.
62. Salzman L, Kuligowska E, Semine A. Pseudoomphalocele: pitfall in fetal sonography. *AJR* 1986;146:1283-1285.
63. Hansen KH, Pedersen SA, Kristoffersen K. Prenatal rupture of omphalocele. *J Clin Ultrasound* 1987;15:191.
64. Hughes MD, Nyberg DA, Mack LA et al. Fetal omphalocele: prenatal detection of concurrent anomalies and other predictors of outcome. *Radiology* 1989;173:371-376.
65. Crawford DC, Chapman MG, Allan LD. Echocardiography in the investigation of anterior abdominal wall defects in the fetus. *Br J Obstet Gynecol* 1985;92:1034.
66. Greenwood RD, Rosenthal A, Nadas AS. Cardiovascular malformations associated with omphalocele. *J Pediatr* 1974;85:818.
67. Calisti A. The fetus with an abdominal wall defect: management and outcome. *J Perinat Med* 1987;15:105.
68. Winter SC, Curry CJR, Smith JC et al. Prenatal diagnosis of the Beckwith-Wiedemann syndrome. *Am J Med Genet* 1986;24:137-141.
69. Weinstein L, Anderson C. In utero diagnosis of Beckwith-Wiedemann syndrome by ultrasound. *Radiology* 1980;134:474.
70. Schwaitzberg SD, Pokorny WJ, McGill CW et al. Gastroschisis and omphalocele. *Am J Surg* 1982;144:650-654.
71. Smith DW. *Recognizable Patterns of Human Malformations.* Philadelphia: WB Saunders Co; 1982:10-19.
72. Smith DW, Patau K, Therman E et al. The no. 18 trisomy syndrome. *J Pediatr* 1962;57:338-345.
73. De Veciana M, Major CA, Porto M. Prediction of an abnormal karyotype in fetuses with omphalocele. *Prenat Diagn* 1994;14:487-492.
74. Gilbert WM, Nicolaides KH. Fetal omphalocele: associated malformations and chromosomal defects. *Obstet Gynecol* 1987;70:633.
75. van de Geijn EJ, van Vugt JM, Sollie JE et al. Ultrasonographic diagnosis and perinatal management of fetal abdominal wall defects. *Fet Diagn Ther* 1991;6:2-10.
76. Sermer M, Benzie RJ, Pitson L et al. Prenatal diagnosis and management of congenital defects of the anterior abdominal wall. *Am J Obstet Gynecol* 1987;156:308-312.
77. Knight PJ, Sommer A, Clatworthy HW. Omphalocele: a prognostic classification. *J Pediatr Surg* 1981;16:599-604.

Pentalogy of Cantrell

78. Siles C, Boyd PA, Manning N et al. Omphalocele and pericardial effusion: possible sonographic markers for the pentalogy of Cantrell or its variants. *Obstet Gynecol* 1996;87:840-842.

79. Abu-Yousel MM, Wray AB, Williamson RA et al. Antenatal ultrasound diagnosis of variant of pentalogy of Cantrell. *J Ultrasound Med* 1987;6:535-538.
80. Klingensmith WC III, Cioffi-Ragan DT, Harvey DE. Diagnosis of ectopia cordis in the second trimester. *J Clin Ultrasound* 1988;16:204-206.
81. Ghidini A, Sirtori M, Romero R et al. Prenatal diagnosis of pentalogy of Cantrell. *J Ultrasound Med* 1988;7:467-472.
82. Fox JE, Gloster ES, Mirchandani R. Trisomy 18 with Cantrell pentalogy in a stillborn infant. *Am J Med Genet* 1988;31:391.
83. Craigo S, Gillieson MS, Cetrulo CL. Pentalogy of Cantrell. *Fetus* 1992;3:7548.

Limb-Body Wall Complex

84. Van Allen MI, Curry C, Gallagher L. Limb-body wall complex. I. Pathogenesis. *Am J Med Genet* 1987;28:529-548.
85. Moerman P, Fryns JP, Vandenberghe K et al. Constrictive amniotic bands, amniotic adhesions and limb-body wall complex: discrete disruption sequences with pathologic overlap. *Am J Med Genet* 1992:42:470-479.
86. Hartwig NG, Vermeij-Keers C, De Vries HE et al. Limb-body wall malformation: an embryologic etiology? *Hum Pathol* 1989;20:1071-1077.
87. Van Allen MI, Myhre S. Ectopia cordis thoracalis with craniofacial defects resulting from early amnion rupture. *Teratology* 1985;32:19-24.
88. Smith DW. *Recognizable Patterns of Human Malformations.* Philadelphia: WB Saunders Co; 1982:488-496.
89. Shalev E, Eliyahu S, Battino S et al. First trimester transvaginal sonographic diagnosis of body stalk anatomy. *J Ultrasound Med* 1995;14:641-642.
90. Giacoia GP. Body stalk anomaly: congenital absence of the umbilical cord. *Obstet Gynecol* 1992;80:527-529.
91. Van Allen MI, Curry C, Walden L et al. Limb-body wall complex. II. Limb and spine defects. *Am J Med Genet* 1987;28:549-565.
92. Soper RT, Kilger K. Vesico-intestinal fissures. *J Urol* 1986;92:390.

Bladder and Cloacal Exstrophy

93. Mueke EC. Exstrophy of the bladder, epispadias and other bladder anomalies. In: Walsh PC, Retik AB, Stamey TA et al, eds. *Campbell's Urology.* 5th ed. Philadelphia: WB Saunders Co; 1992;1772-1821.
94. Engel RME. Exstrophy of the bladder and associated anomalies. *Birth Defects* 1974;10:146-149.
95. Bartholomew TH, Gonzales ET Jr. Urologic management in cloacal dysgenesis. *Urology* 1978;11:549-557.
96. Tank ES, Lindenaner SM. Principles of management of exstrophy of the cloaca. *Am J Surg* 1970;119:95-100.
97. Kutzner DK, Wilson WG, Hogge WA. OEIS complex (cloacal exstrophy): prenatal diagnosis in the second trimester. *Prenat Diagn* 1988;8:247-253.
98. Fujiyoshi Y, Nakamura Y, Takanori C et al. Exstrophy of the cloacal membrane. *Arch Pathol Lab Med* 1987;111:157.
99. Patten RM, Van Allen MI, Mack LA et al. Limb-body wall complex: in utero sonographic diagnosis of a complicated fetal malformation. *AJR* 1986;146:1019-1024.
100. Howel C, Caldamone A, Snyder H et al. Optimal management of cloacal exstrophy. *J Pediatr Surg* 1983;18:365-369.
101. Kay R, Tank ES. Principles of management of the persistent cloaca in the female newborn. *J Urol* 1977;117:102-114.
102. Jeffs RD. Exstrophy, epispadias, and cloacal and urogenital sinus abnormalities. *Pediatr Clin North Am* 1987;34:1233.
103. Mirk P, Callisti A, Fieni A. Prenatal sonographic diagnosis of bladder exstrophy. *J Ultrasound Med* 1986;5:291-293.
104. Meizner I, Levy A, Barnhard Y. Cloacal exstrophy sequence: an exceptional ultrasound diagnosis. *Obstet Gynecol* 1995;86:446-450.
105. Pinette MG, Pan Y-Q, Pinette SG et al. Prenatal diagnosis of fetal bladder and cloacal exstrophy by ultrasound: a report of three cases. *J Reprod Med* 1996;41:132-134.
106. Canning DA, Gearhart JP. Exstrophy of the bladder. In: Ashkroft KW, Holder TM, eds. *Pediatric Surgery.* 2nd ed. Philadelphia: WB Saunders Co; 1993:678-693.
107. Hurvitz RS, Manzoni GA, Ransley PG et al. Cloacal exstrophy: a report of 34 cases. *J Urol* 1987;138:1060-1064.

CHAPTER 40

Chromosome Abnormalities

Jo-Ann M. Johnson, M.D., F.R.C.S.C.
David A. Nyberg, M.D.

CHAPTER OUTLINE

PHENOTYPIC EXPRESSION OF CHROMOSOMAL DEFECTS

Approximately 1 in 160 liveborn infants has a demonstrable chromosome abnormality; at least half of them will lead to conditions requiring medical intervention. The most common liveborn chromosome abnormality and the most common genetic cause of mental retardation is **trisomy 21, or Down syndrome,** which occurs in approximately 1 in 700 livebirths.[1] The incidence of trisomy 21 as well as of other chromosome abnormalities increases with maternal age.[2] Other abnormalities include the autosomal trisomies (47, + 13; 47, + 18) as well as abnormalities of the sex chromosomes (47,XXX; 47,XYY). The phenotypes of both trisomy 13 and 18 are more severe than that of trisomy 21, and the majority of those infants die in utero or in early infancy, with major malformations. The sex-chromosome abnormalities, on the other hand, are rarely associated with phenotypic abnormalities and often go undetected.[3] Other autosomal trisomies are very rarely seen, most likely because they are lethal and result in very early pregnancy loss.

Turner's syndrome is the most common chromosome complement among abortuses, an intriguing observation because liveborn 45,XO females manifest relatively few life-threatening anomalies and are not mentally retarded.[3] **Triploidy** represents a complete extra set of chromosomes and is estimated to occur in approximately 1% of conceptuses.[4] Most of these end in miscarriage, however, with triploidy accounting for approximately 20% of chromosome abnormalities identified in spontaneous abortions. Unlike other chromosome abnormalities, Turner's syndrome (45,XO) and triploidy are not associated with maternal age.

The recognition of the association between chromosome abnormalities and maternal age has prompted the recommendation that all women who will be 35 years of age or over at the time of delivery (late maternal age, or LMA) be offered invasive prenatal testing with either amniocentesis or chorionic villus sampling (CVS). However, at least 80% of children with chromosome abnormalities are born to women under 35 years of age because they represent 95% of the pregnant population.[5] Since the inherent risks and costs of prenatal chromosome analysis preclude unselected chromosome testing of all pregnant women, noninvasive screening for these disorders has become a primary focus of prenatal diagnostic efforts.

In recent years, the improved resolution of real-time ultrasonography has allowed for detailed delineation of normal and abnormal fetal anatomy.

Since most fetuses with major chromosomal defects have either external or internal abnormalities that can be detected by a detailed ultrasound examination, ultrasound is emerging as a powerful, noninvasive screening tool for the prenatal detection of cytogenetic abnormalities.

After the first trimester, each chromosomal defect is associated with its own syndromic pattern of abnormalities. The most common pathologic and sonographic features of the five main chromosomal syndromes (trisomies 21, 18, and 13, triploidy, and Turner's syndrome) are described in the boxes on pages 1178 and 1179.

The phenotypic expression of chromosome abnormalities *in utero* and at birth differs, with certain abnormalities' being detected more frequently prenatally. In a series of 461 fetuses with chromosomal abnormalities undergoing second trimester ultrasound examina-

COMMON PATHOLOGIC AND SONOGRAPHIC FEATURES OF TRISOMY 21

*Cystic hygroma
*Nuchal thickening
*Nonimmune hydrops
*Hydrothorax

CRANIOFACIAL MALFORMATIONS
- Brachycephaly
- Epicanthic folds
- Short nose
- *Round, low ears
- Broad neck
- *Protruding tongue

CENTRAL NERVOUS SYSTEM ABNORMALITIES
- *Mild ventriculomegaly

CARDIOVASCULAR MALFORMATIONS
- ASVD, VSD, ASD, and PDA†

GASTROINTESTINAL TRACT MALFORMATIONS
- *Duodenal atresia
- *Esophageal atresia
- *Anorectal atresia
- *Omphalocele
- *Echogenic bowel

GENITOURINARY TRACT MALFORMATIONS
- *Undescended testis
- *Mild hydronephrosis

SKELETAL MALFORMATIONS
- Flattening of acetabular angles
- *Widening of iliac wings
- Short, broad hands
- *Clinodactyly
- *Short upper and lower extremities
- *Increased space between first and second toes

*Features detectable by prenatal ultrasound
†ASVD-Atrioventricular septal defect; VSD-Ventricular septal defect; ASD-Atrial septal defect; PDA-Patent ductus arteriosus.

COMMON PATHOLOGIC AND SONOGRAPHIC FEATURES OF TRISOMY 18

*Intrauterine growth retardation
*Polyhydramnios or oligohydramnios
*Single umbilical artery (>80%)
*Cystic hygroma
*Nuchal edema
*Nonimmune hydrops

CRANIOFACIAL ABNORMALITIES
- *Dolichocephaly (strawberry-shaped head)
- *Microcephaly
- *Low-set ears or "pixie" ears
- *Micrognathia
- *Cleft lip or palate (10% to 20%)

CENTRAL NERVOUS SYSTEM ABNORMALITIES
- *Choroid plexus cysts
- *Absent corpus callosum
- *Enlarged cisterna magna
- *Hydrocephalus
- *Myelomeningocele (10% to 20%)

CARDIOVASCULAR MALFORMATIONS
- VSD, ASD, PDA,† double-outlet right ventricle, bicuspid aortic and pulmonic valves

GASTROINTESTINAL TRACT ANOMALIES
- *Esophageal atresia/tracheoesophageal fistula
- *Omphalocele
- *Diaphragmatic hernia
- *Anorectal atresia

GENITOURINARY TRACT ANOMALIES
- *Urethrovesical obstruction
- *Renal dysplasia
- *Horseshoe kidney
- *Ambiguous genitalia

SKELETAL MALFORMATIONS
- *Short extremities
- *Radial aplasia
- *Overlapping fingers, flexed hands (>80%)
- *Rockerbottom feet
- *Shortened first toes

*Features detectable by prenatal ultrasound
†VSD-Ventricular septal defect; ASD-Atrial septal defect; PDA-Patent ductus arteriosus

COMMON PATHOLOGIC AND SONOGRAPHIC FEATURES OF TRISOMY 13

*Single umbilical artery

CRANIOFACIAL ABNORMALITIES
- *Microcephaly
- *Cyclopia
- *Anopthalmia
- *Microphthalmia
- *Cleft lip and palate
- *Low-set, deformed ears
- *Capillary hemangiomas

CENTRAL NERVOUS SYSTEM ANOMALIES
- *Holoprosencephaly
- *Agenesis of the corpus callosum

CARDIOVASCULAR MALFORMATIONS
- VSD, ASD, PDA†

GASTROINTESTINAL TRACT MALFORMATIONS
- *Omphalocele, umbilical hernia

UROGENITAL MALFORMATIONS
- *Cystic renal dysplasia
- *Hydronephrosis
- *Duplicated kidney
- Ambiguous genitalia

SKELETAL MALFORMATIONS
- *Polydactyly (70%)
- *Rockerbottom feet
- *Scalp defects

*Features detectable by prenatal ultrasound
†VSD-Ventricular septal defect; ASD-Atrial septal defect; PDA-Patent ductus arteriosus

COMMON PATHOLOGIC AND SONOGRAPHIC FEATURES OF TRIPLOIDY

*Severe early-onset (second trimester) intrauterine growth restriction (43%)
*Third-trimester hydramnios
***CONGENITAL HEART DISEASE (>80%)**
- Ventricular septal defect, atrial septal defect
- Dextrocardia

CENTRAL NERVOUS SYSTEM MALFORMATIONS (>70%)
- *Holoprosencephaly
- *Agenesis of corpus callosum
- *Mild ventriculomegaly
- *Meningomyelocele

CRANIOFACIAL MALFORMATIONS
- *Micrognathia
- *Sloping forehead
- *Cleft lip and/or palate
- Microphthalmia

EXTREMITY ABNORMALITIES
- *Postaxial polydactyly
- Camptodactyly
- *Overlapping digits
- *Syndactyly

RENAL MALFORMATIONS
- *Renal cortical cysts
- *Hydronephrosis
- *Horseshoe kidney

ABDOMINAL WALL ABNORMALITIES
- *Omphalocele
- *Molar placenta

*Features detectable by prenatal ultrasound

COMMON PATHOLOGIC AND SONOGRAPHIC FEATURES OF TURNER'S SYNDROME (45,XO)

*Cystic hygroma
*Nonimmune hydrops
CRANIOFACIAL MALFORMATIONS
- *Brachycephaly
- *Abnormal ears
- *Small mandible

CARDIOVASCULAR MALFORMATIONS
- *Coarctation of the aorta

GENITOURINARY TRACT MALFORMATIONS
- *Horseshoe kidneys
- *Double renal pelvis

SKELETAL MALFORMATIONS
- *Cubitus valgus
- *Short stature

*Features detectable by prenatal ultrasound

tion at the Harris Birthright Research Centre for Fetal Medicine,[4] the most commonly reported abnormalities in **trisomy 21** (n = 155) were nuchal thickening (38%), mild hydronephrosis (30%), relative shortening of the femur (28%), and cardiac abnormalities (26%). In **trisomy 18** (n = 137), 74% of the fetuses had intrauterine growth restriction (IUGR), 72% had abnormal hands or feet, and 54% had a strawberry-shaped head; other common abnormalities were cardiac problems (52%) and choroid plexus cysts (47%). Intrauterine growth restriction was the most common feature of **trisomy 13** (n = 154) (61%), followed by abnormal hands and feet (52%), cardiac abnormalities (43%), holoprosencephaly (39%), and facial clefting (39%). In **triploidy** (n = 50), there were two different phenotypic expressions, depending on the origin of the extra set of chromosomes. When the extra set was paternally derived, it was associated with a molar placenta, and the pregnancy rarely persisted beyond 20 weeks. When the extra set was maternally derived, the pregnancy more often persisted into the third trimester. The placenta was of normal consistency but the fetuses demonstrated severe asymmetrical IUGR (100%). There were commonly other abnormalities as well, including abnormal hands and feet (75%) and short femur (60%) (see box at top of this page). In **Turner's syndrome** (n = 65), the most common abnormalities were cystic hygromata (88%) and nonimmune hydrops (80%). In addition, 59% of cases were associated with relative shortening of the femur, 55% with IUGR, and 48% with cardiac abnormalities.

CHROMOSOMAL DEFECTS IN FETAL ABNORMALITIES

An underlying chromosome abnormality should be considered when fetal abnormalities are detected by sonography. The risk depends upon a number of factors, including the type of abnormality and the incidence of associated defects. In addition, the risk of a chromosome abnormality increases with maternal age and decreases with gestational age. The lower prevalence of chromosome abnormalities at livebirth reflects the natural attrition rate of chromosomally abnormal fetuses during pregnancy.

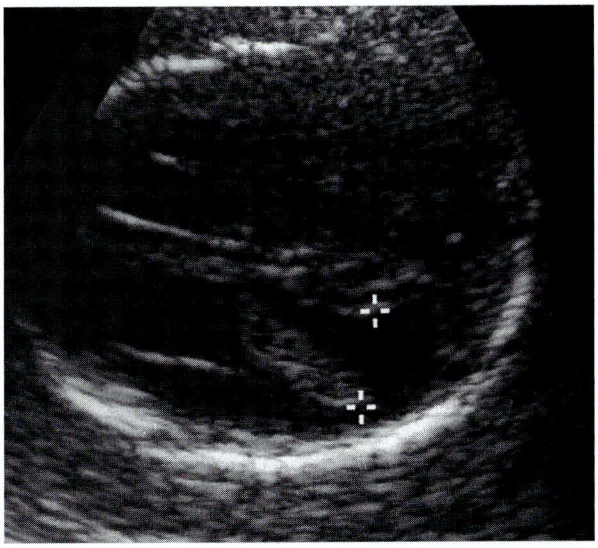

FIG. 40-1. Mild cerebral ventricular dilatation with trisomy 21. Transverse view of the cranium, through the lateral ventricles, demonstrates mild dilatation of the lateral ventricles (LV) at 18 weeks' gestation.

Central Nervous System Abnormalities

Ventriculomegaly. Ventriculomegaly represents a common endpoint for a variety of pathologic processes that can generally be divided into three categories: increased intraventricular pressure, primary neuronal loss, and abnormalities in brain development.[6-8] Increased intraventricular pressure is most commonly due to obstruction of normal cerebrospinal fluid flow. This can be the result of a number of processes, including Dandy-Walker malformation, Chiari II malformation, X-linked aqueductal stenosis, infection, and chromosomal abnormalities. Neuronal loss may be due to infection or vascular insufficiency. Abnormalities of brain development include agenesis of the corpus callosum and holoprosencephaly.[8]

Regardless of the cause, it is clear that severe fetal ventriculomegaly is associated with a poor prognosis, especially when associated with additional malformations (70% to 85% of cases).[6,9,10]

Mild or Borderline Ventriculomegaly. The detection of mild ventricular dilatation may be an important clue to the presence of fetal abnormalities, including chromosome abnormalities (Fig. 40-1). The ventricles are measured in the axial plane of the fetal head along the posterior portion of the lateral ventricle. Measurements obtained in the distal body, atrium, or proximal horn of a normal-sized ventricle appear to be reasonably constant, provided the cursors are placed at the edge of the ventricular lumen and are perpendicular to the ventricular axis and not to the cerebral midline. A potential source of error in measurement is the failure to be certain that the plane of section is truly axial.

The size of the lateral ventricles remains relatively constant throughout gestation, showing a mean diameter 6.1 ± 1.3 mm,[11] with slightly larger ventricles in males than in females (6.4 mm versus 5.8 mm).[12] **Ventriculomegaly is suspected when the lateral atrial ventricular diameter reaches 10 mm.** Early ventricular dilatation may also appear as visibly enlarged ventricles with separation of the choroid from the ventricular wall, yet the ventricle measures less than 10 mm in diameter. In this case, the choroid appears to "dangle" in the ventricle; this is a good visual clue to enlargement.[13] An abnormal relationship is defined as a separation of 3 mm or more between the choroid and the medial ventricular wall.[14]

> **FETAL VENTRICULOMEGALY**
>
> Definitions
> Ventricular atrial diameter ≥ 10 mm
> "Borderline" or mild 10-12 mm
> Frank ventriculomegaly ≥ 13 mm
> Choroid clearly separated from ventricular wall (≥ 3 mm)

Fetuses with mild ventricular dilatation are at risk for chromosome abnormalities, particularly in the presence of other malformations. In a series by Bromley et al., 5 of 43 fetuses (12%) with mild ventriculomegaly (ventricular diameter 10 to 12 mm) had abnormal karyotypes (3, trisomy 21; 2, trisomy 18), and all of these fetuses had other findings.[15] However, even in the absence of additional abnormalities (e.g., isolated ventriculomegaly), the risk of a chromosome abnormality has been shown to be approximately 2% to 3%.[12,15] In addition, while the outcome of mild, isolated ventriculomegaly with a normal karyotype is generally favorable, such children are at increased risk of mild to moderate developmental or motor handicaps in childhood.[11,15,16] Thus, while more information is needed, particularly long-term follow-up, the following recommendations can be made regarding the lateral ventricles:

- Measurement of the lateral atrial ventricular width should be a standard part of the obstetric ultrasound examination.
- A ventricular atrial diameter of >10 mm is considered abnormal.
- Occasionally, the ventricle appears visibly dilated and the choroid is clearly separated from the ventricular wall, yet the ventricle measures less than 10 mm; a small percentage of these may also be abnormal.
- Borderline or mild ventriculomegaly is defined as a lateral atrial ventricular measurement of 10 to 12 mm. Male fetuses are more likely to have borderline ventricular dilatation as a normal variant than are female fetuses.

- A measurement of >13 mm is considered frank ventriculomegaly.
- A detailed sonogram should be undertaken when ventriculomegaly is detected. If additional abnormalities are detected, karyotype analysis should be offered. The risk of aneuploidy for isolated ventriculomegaly may be as high as 2% to 3%. Additional investigations should include a screen for congenital infection and for platelet alloantibodies, as these may be associated with ventriculomegaly.

In cases of isolated mild ventriculomegaly with a normal karyotype, a favorable outcome can be expected in the majority of cases; however, long-term follow-up studies are not yet available. Serial ultrasound examinations during pregnancy and postnatally should be considered.

Holoprosencephaly. Holoprosencephaly is characterized by failure of proper cleavage of the prosencephalon which also causes abnormal midfacial development. Sonographic diagnosis can be made by identifying a single ventricle with absence of midline structures and fused thalami (Fig. 40-2). In published studies describing fetal holoprosencephaly, the mean prevalence of chromosomal defects was 33%; the prevalence was 4% for fetuses with apparently isolated holoprosencephaly and 39% for those with additional abnormalities.[4] The most common chromosomal defects associated with holoprosencephaly were trisomies 13 and 18.

Microcephaly. Microcephaly occurs with an incidence with about 1 per 1000 births. It is associated with chromosomal defects, genetic syndromes, hemorrhage, infection, teratogens, and radiation.

Microcephaly is defined by a biparietal diameter (BPD) below the first percentile or by a head-circumference-to-femur-length ratio below the 2.5 percentile of the normal range for gestation. In milder cases, diagnosis requires a progressive decrease in head circumference until it falls below the fifth percentile in the presence of normal growth of the abdomen and femur. This may not become apparent before 26 weeks of gestation. In a series by Nicolaides et al.[17] microcephaly was found in 2.5% of 2086 fetuses karyotyped because of fetal malformations or IUGR. Eight (15%) of these had chromosomal abnormalities. Eydoux et al.[18] reported chromosomal defects in 5 of 20 cases (25%). Of the 13 chromosomally abnormal fetuses in these two studies, 12 had additional abnormalities, and the most common chromosomal defect was **trisomy 13**. It is important to note, however, that the majority of fetuses with trisomy 13 do not have microcephaly and those that do usually have **holoprosencephaly.**

Choroid Plexus Cysts. Choroid plexus cysts (CPCs) are fluid-filled structures of varying sizes surrounded by normal tissue in the choroid plexus of the lateral cerebral ventricles. These cysts are found in approximately 1% to 3% of fetuses at 16 to 24 weeks of gestation.[19,20] A higher frequency of CPCs has been observed in fetuses with chromosomal abnormalities, particularly trisomy 18. Among three studies reporting the ultrasound features of trisomy 18, the mean prevalence of CPCs was about 50%.[17,21,24] The risk for trisomy 18 and unusually large cysts increases with additional anomalies (Fig. 40-3). Among 38 fetuses with trisomy 18 and CPCs reported by Snijders et al.[24] 97%

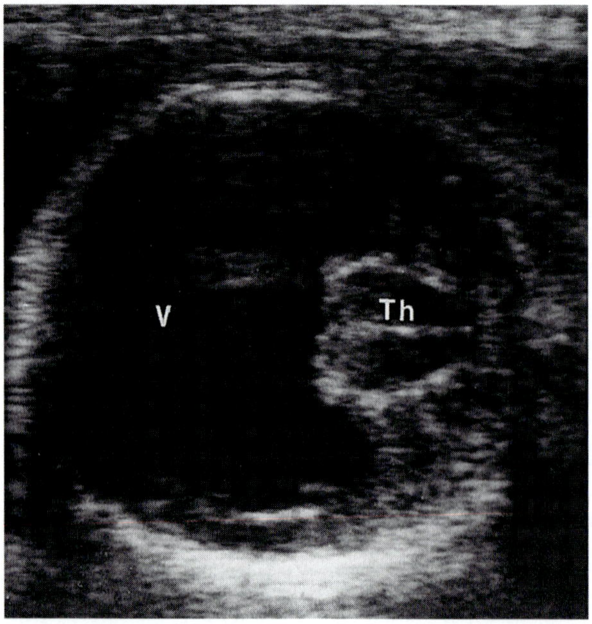

FIG. 40-2. Holoprosencephaly and trisomy 13. Transverse view of the head at 25 weeks shows a single ventricle (V), absence of midline structures, and fused thalami (Th).

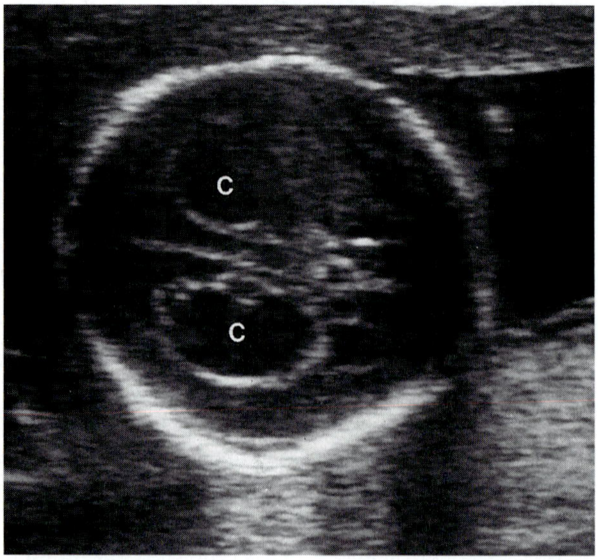

FIG. 40-3. Choroid plexus cysts and trisomy 18. Transverse view at the level of the lateral ventricle shows large bilateral choroid plexus cysts (C).

had other detectable anomalies, including 5.2% with one additional abnormality and 92.1% with two or more abnormalities.[4,24] On the other hand, in a meta-analysis by Gross et al.[25] only 2 cases of trisomy 18 were identified among 748 fetuses with apparently isolated CPCs (1 in 374). These data do not support offering karyotyping in fetuses with isolated CPCs.

The prevalence of trisomy 18 increases with increasing maternal age and with younger gestational age. Snijders et al. have published charts estimating the risk for trisomy 18 according to maternal age in midtrimester fetuses with isolated CPCs and in those with one and two or more additional anomalies.[4] These tables are useful for providing more accurate risk assessments for individual patients. From a general perspective, however, we **recommend** the following regarding the **identification of CPCs** in the **midgestation fetus**:

- The detection of fetal CPCs should stimulate the sonographer to search for additional features of trisomy 18 (Table 40-2 on page 1197). If the cysts are apparently isolated, the risk of trisomy 18 is only **marginally increased**, and **maternal age should be the main factor in deciding whether or not fetal karyotyping should be performed.**
- If one additional abnormality is found, the maternal-age-related risk is increased about **twenty fold.**
- If two or more additional abnormalities are found, the risk is increased by almost one thousand times and karyotyping should be offered irrespective of maternal age.
- Amniocentesis might be considered for unusually large choroid cysts, even if they are isolated.

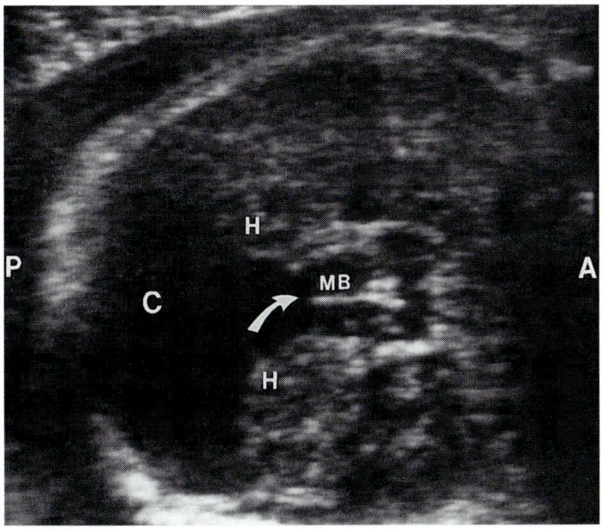

FIG. 40-4. Dandy-Walker variant with mosaic trisomy 13. Transverse view of the head shows posterior fossa cyst (C) and absence of the cerebellar vermis *(curved arrows)*. A, anterior. P, posterior. MB, midbrain. H, cerebellar hemisphere.

Absent Corpus Callosum. Agenesis of the corpus callosum may be an isolated finding with no pathologic significance, but it is also found in association with chromosomal defects and genetic syndromes.[26] Snijders et al. diagnosed the absence of the corpus callosum in 7% of 137 fetuses with trisomy 18, but never as an isolated abnormality.[4] In three additional studies on a total of 17 fetuses with an absent corpus callosum, trisomy 13 was reported in one fetus who also had additional abnormalities.[26-28]

Posterior Fossa Abnormalities. The posterior fossa consists of the cerebellum and cisterna magna and normally measures <10 mm in the anteroposterior dimension. Abnormalities of the posterior fossa with enlargement of the cisterna magna or a posterior fossa cyst may been seen with a spectrum of abnormalities, including the **Dandy-Walker malformation, the Dandy-Walker variant**, and **cerebellar hypoplasia** (Fig. 40-4, 40-5). In combined data from a total of five series evaluating 101 fetuses with an enlarged cisterna magna, the mean frequency of associated chromosome defects was 44%.[17,29-32] The risk of a chromosomal abnormality was much higher with the Dandy-Walker variant in the absence of hydrocephalus as compared with the Dandy-Walker malformation with hydrocephalus. The most common chromosome abnormality was **trisomy 18**.

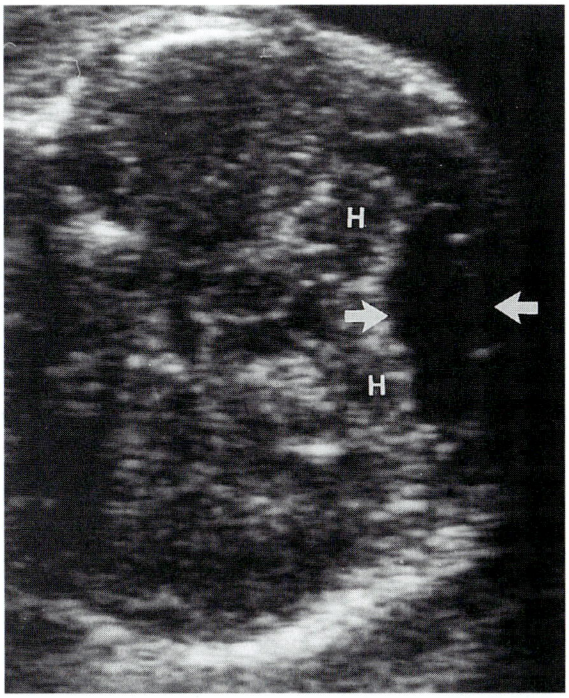

FIG. 40-5. Large cisterna magna with trisomy 18. Scan at 30 weeks shows large cisterna magna *(arrows)* measuring 1.3 cm in AP dimension. Growth restriction and polyhydramnios were also identified. H, cerebellar hemisphere.

Abnormal Shape of Head

Strawberry-shaped Skull. Some fetuses with trisomy 18 may show flattening of the occipit and narrowing of the frontal part of the head, giving rise to a strawberry-shaped skull (Fig. 40-6). A narrow frontal region is most likely due to hypoplasia of the face and frontal cerebral lobes. In a series of 54 fetuses with strawberry-shaped heads, all had additional malformations, and 44 (81%) had chromosomal defects (most commonly, trisomy 18).[33]

Brachycephaly. Brachycephaly is characterized by shortening of the occipitofrontal diameter. It is found in association with chromosomal defects and genetic syndromes such as Robert's syndrome.[4] Although it is well recognized in postnatal life that children with trisomy 21 have brachycephalic heads, no difference in the mean cephalic index has been found in a group of second-trimester fetuses with trisomy 21 as compared to normal controls.[34,35]

Facial Abnormalities

Fetal facial defects are commonly found in association with many chromosome abnormalities and genetic syndromes.

Facial Clefts. Cleft lip and/or palate is found in approximately 1 in 700 livebirths (Fig. 40-7).

Chromosomal defects are found in less than 1% of newborns with cleft lip/palate but are much more common when the cleft has been detected prenatally. In seven prenatal series reporting a total of 118 cases, 40% had chromosome defects, most commonly **trisomy 13 and 18.**[31,36-41] In all cases, additional abnormalities were present. The high prevalence of chromosomal defects in prenatal studies reflects both the insensitivity of ultrasound for detection of isolated cleft lip/palate and the higher rate of anomalies in prenatal series. More severe types of cleft lip/palate are also associated with a higher risk of chromosomal abnormalities, and prenatal ultrasound is more likely to detect these types. Among a series of 65 fetuses with cleft lip with or without cleft palate, Nyberg et al.[42] found the highest frequency of chromosome abnormalities with bilateral cleft lip and palate (30%) and gaping midline cleft lip and palate (52%); unilateral cleft lip or unilateral cleft lip/palate had a low frequency of chromosome abnormalities.

Micrognathia. Micrognathia is a nonspecific finding in a wide range of genetic syndromes and chromosomal defects (Fig. 40-8). In two studies reporting on 65 cases of micrognathia diagnosed antenatally, 40 (62%) were chromosomally abnormal, most commonly with trisomy 18.[37,40] In all chromosomally abnormal fetuses, there were additional abnormalities and/or IUGR.

Ocular and Nasal Abnormalities. Hypotelorism, cyclops, nasal aplasia/hypoplasia, or proboscis are abnormalities often seen in the presence of

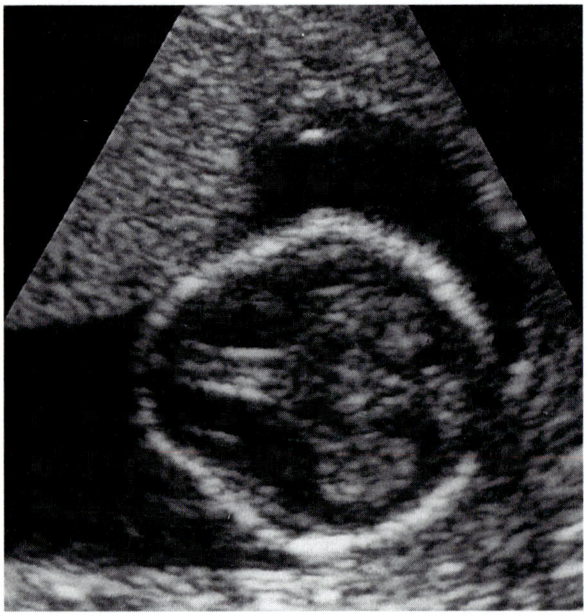

FIG. 40-6. Strawberry-shaped head with trisomy 18. No neural tube defect was present.

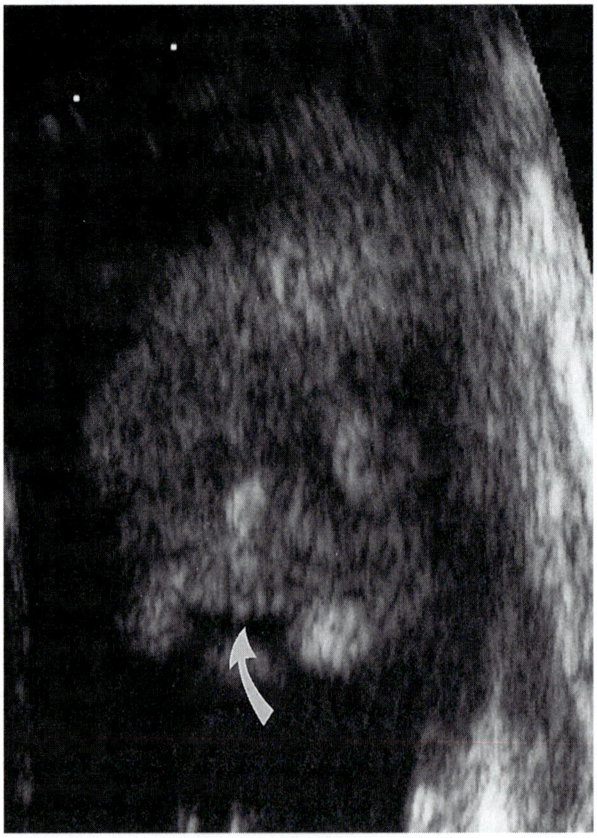

FIG. 40-7. Midline cleft lip and palate with trisomy 13. Coronal view of the face shows the gaping midline cleft lip and palate *(curved arrow)*. Also note absence of discrete nose, indicating hypoplastic midface.

holoprosencephaly and are usually associated with **trisomy 13**, and less commonly with trisomy 18.[37] In fact, the presence of facial defects increases the risk for chromosomal abnormalities in fetuses with holoprosencephaly.[43]

Macroglossia. Macroglossia and a flat facial profile are common postnatal features of trisomy 21. These abnormalities are rarely diagnosed antenatally unless other features of trisomy 21 are also found. In a series of 69 fetuses with trisomy 21, Nicolaides et al.[37] found macroglossia in 10% of those examined before 28 weeks and in 20% of those diagnosed after 20 weeks.

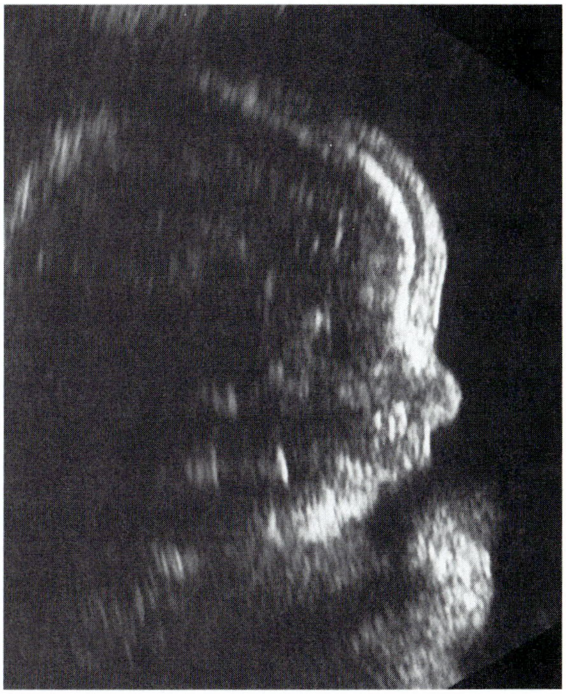

FIG. 40-8. Micrognathia and trisomy 18. Sagittal view of face at 19 weeks showing an abnormally small mandible. Abnormal hands and large VSD were also present.

Neck Abnormalities

Abnormal fluid collections or thickening in the posterior fetal neck carries a high risk for aneuploidy even in the absence of other sonographic markers. These findings may be categorized as a spectrum of abnormalities termed **cystic hygroma** (Fig. 40-9), **nuchal thickening or increased nuchal fold** (Fig. 40-10), and **nuchal sonolucency or translucency** (also known as nuchal edema or nuchal membrane) (Fig. 40-11).

Nuchal Cystic Hygroma. Nuchal cystic hygroma carries a high risk of chromosomal abnormality and is one of the earliest abnormalities that can be detected by ultrasound. It is usually seen as sonolucent, fluid-filled spaces separated into compartments by septations coursing in an anterior-posterior plane. Fetuses with large cystic hygromas associated with generalized lymphedema and nonimmune hydrops have a very poor prognosis (Fig. 40-12).

In a study by Azar et al. that examined only fetuses with septated, cervical, dorsal hygromas, 75% had chromosomal defects, 94% of which were **Turner's syndrome.**[44] Trisomies 21 and 18 made up the majority of the other abnormal karyotypes. The risk for Turner's syndrome was found to be increased if the mother was young, if there was an associated fetal cardiac defect, and if the head-circumference-to-femur-length ratio was large.

Cystic hygroma can be associated with normal chromosomes, in which case **Noonan's syndrome** should be considered, particularly if the fetus is male.[45,46] Noonan's syndrome is associated with short stature, cubitus valgus, and congenital heart disease

A

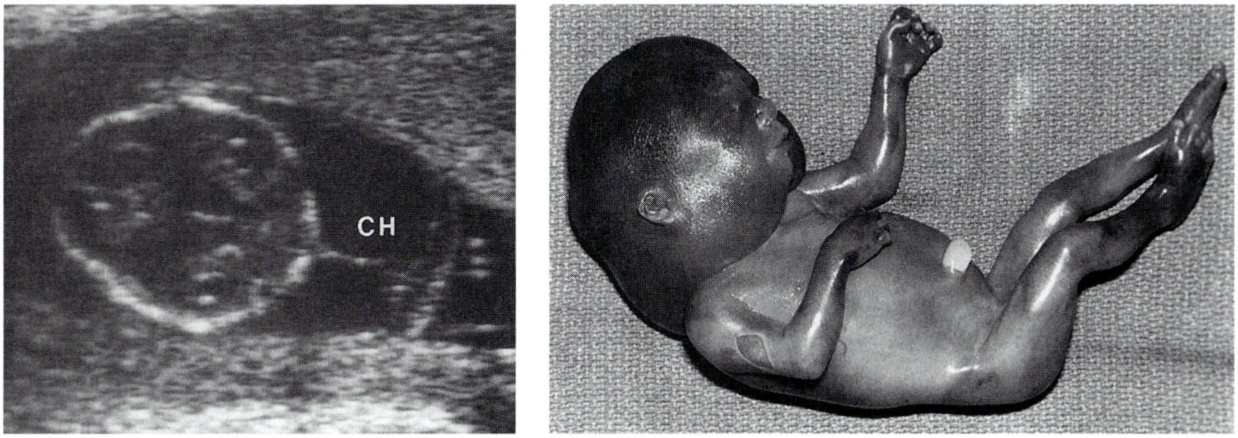

B

FIG. 40-9. Cystic hygroma. A, Cystic hygroma with trisomy 18. Axial view through the head at 14 weeks shows large nuchal cystic hygroma (CH) with midline septation. **B,** Fetus with cystic hygroma.

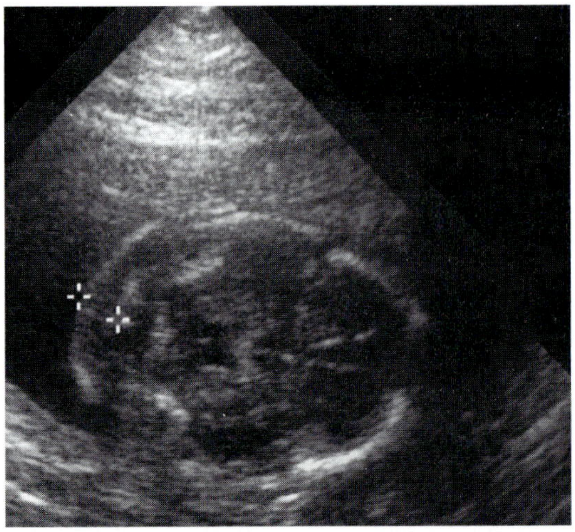

FIG. 40-10. Nuchal thickening and trisomy 21. Axial view at 17 weeks shows nuchal thickening of 8 mm.

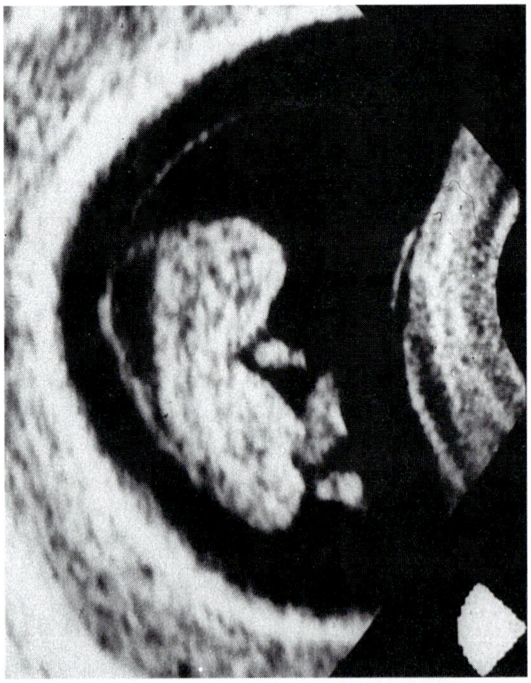

FIG. 40-11. Nuchal translucency and trisomy 21. Transvaginal scan at 9.5 weeks' gestation showing distinct nuchal sonolucency. The karyotype showed trisomy 21. (Courtesy of Ants Toi, M.D., University of Toronto.)

and is thought to be the male counterpart of Turner's syndrome but with a normal karyotype.[47] Patients with Noonan's syndrome have mental retardation, which is not usually a factor in Turner's syndrome.

Nuchal Fold. As many as 80% of infants with trisomy 21 have redundant skin in the posterior part of the neck.[45,48] Benacerraf et al., in 1985,[49] was the first to suggest the usefulness of measuring this fea-

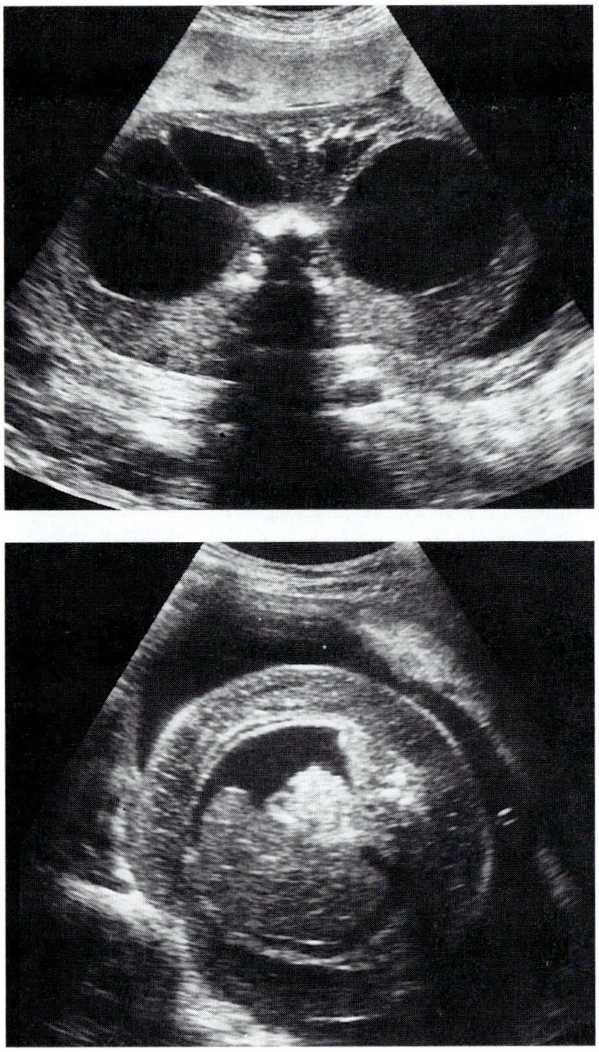

A

B

FIG. 40-12. Cystic hygroma with nonimmune hydrops in a fetus with Turner's syndrome (45XO). **A**, Large nuchal cystic hygroma with septations. **B**, There is also generalized lymphedema and nonimmune hydrops. (Courtesy of Ants Toi, M.D., University of Toronto.)

ture to detect fetuses with trisomy 21. In a series of 1704 patients undergoing amniocentesis between 15 and 20 weeks of gestation for late maternal age, 11 fetuses had trisomy 21; 45% of these had nuchal thickness of 6 mm or more, compared with only 0.6% of normal fetuses. Subsequent prospective studies (Table 40-1) have reported variable results, with sensitivities ranging from 16% to 75%, and false-positive rates from 0 to 8%.[50-58] Differences in measurement techniques may have contributed to these variable results. The **nuchal fold measurement should be made from the outer skull table to the skin surface,** with the transducer in an axial plane through the thalami, cerebellum, and occipital bone (Fig. 40-11). Improper angling can produce an incorrectly wide value and

TABLE 40-1
PROSPECTIVE SERIES OF PREDICTION FOR DOWN SYNDROME BY MEANS OF NUCHAL THICKNESS

Series	Sensitivity (%)	False Positives (%)	PPV (%)
Benacerraf et al., 1987[50]	43 (12/28)	0.1 (4/3816)	75 (12/16)
Nyberg et al., 1990[51]	16 (4/25)	0.3 (1/350)	8*
Ginsberg et al., 1990[52]	41 (5/12)	0.0 (0/212)	100 (8/8)†
Crane and Gray, 1991[53]	75 (12/16)	1.4 (47/338)	8*
Devore and Alfi, 1993[54]	20 (7/35)	0.5 (14/2742)	39
Watson et al., 1994[55]	50 (7/14)	2.0 (27/1382)	21 (7/34)
Donnenfeld et al., 1994[56]	18 (1/13)	1.2 (16/1382)	6 (1/17)
Grandjean et al., 1995[57]	39 (17/44)	8.5 (273/3205)	2*
Borrell et al., 1996 ($\geq$ 6mm)[58]	33 (6/18)	0.1 (2/1424)	33*
Borrell et al., 1996 ($\geq$ 5mm)[58]	78 (14/18)	2.1 (30/1424)	5*

PPV, positive predictive value
*Adjusted to prevalence of Down syndrome in the general population.
†Positive predictive value for aneupoloidy
From Borell A, Costa D, Martinez JM et al. Early midtrimester fetal nuchal thickness: effectiveness as a marker of Down syndrome. *Am J Obstet Gynecol* 1996;175:45-49.

false-positive results.[59] Because nuchal thickness increases with gestational age, a threshold of 5 mm has been suggested for between 14 and 18 weeks.[58,60]

Nuchal Translucency. Nuchal translucency (NT) is a term used to describe a sonolucent area in the nuchal region of the neck that is typically observed in the first trimester between 10 and 14 weeks.[61,62] Unlike cystic hygroma, it does not show discrete fluid collections or internal septations. The mechanism of the nuchal translucency is uncertain. Some have proposed that it is simply a variation of the normal development of the lymphatic system, with transient fluid accumulation in the fetal cervical spine region that in many cases resolves by 18 to 20 weeks' gestation, whether aneuploidy is present or not (Fig. 40-13). Persistence of nuchal fluid into the middle to late second trimester and/or the presence of septations probably represent truly abnormal development of the lymphatic system (e.g., cystic hygroma) with a higher risk of aneuploidy.[63] Among karyotypically abnormal fetuses, it is likely that NT is a precursor to nuchal thickening.

Measurement of nuchal translucency should be performed with the fetus in the sagittal plane. Care must be taken to distinguish between the fetal skin and amnion because at this stage both structures appear as thin membranes (Fig. 40-12). As defined by Nicolaides, the maximal area of translucency is measured between the occipital bone and the subcutaneous interface.[61] Nuchal translucency normally increases with gestational age, and thresholds for abnormal NT have been described in relation to crown-rump length. In general, a measurement of 3 **mm or more is considered abnormal,** although at

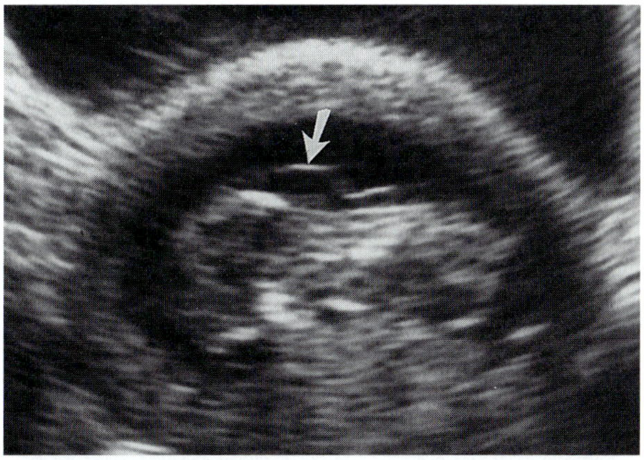

A

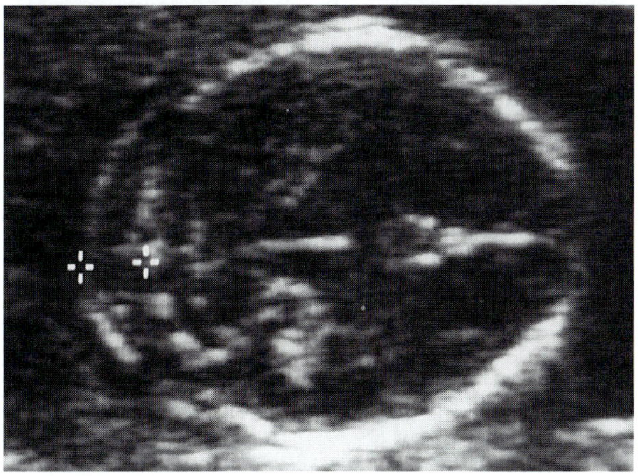

B

FIG. 40-13. Resolution of nuchal translucency with trisomy 21. A, Scan at 12 weeks shows nuchal translucency (*arrow*) over dorsum of fetus. **B,** Follow-up scan at 17 weeks shows borderline nuchal measurement. No other abnormalities were demonstrated.

younger gestational ages, even 2 mm may be abnormal.

Increased NT has been associated with a variety of chromosome abnormalities, including trisomies 21, 18, and 13. In a study by Pandya et al.[64] involving 1763 fetuses between 10 and 13 weeks' gestation, NT measurement of greater than 3 mm detected 75% of fetuses with trisomy 21, with a false-positive rate of 3.6%.[64] The incidence of chromosomal defects (19% overall) increased with both maternal age and translucency thickness. The observed number of trisomies 21, 18, and 13 in fetuses with translucencies of 3, 4, 5, and greater than 6 mm was approximately 3 times, 18 times, 28 times, and 36 times higher than the respective number expected on the basis of maternal age.[64] The incidence of sex-chromosome aneuploidies was similar to that expected.

Natural History of Nuchal Translucency. Two questions arise when considering the natural history of nuchal translucency. **First, do chromosomally abnormal fetuses with abnormal NT in the first trimester have a higher risk of intrauterine death?** If so, the effectiveness of NT as a screening method would be exaggerated. One study by Pandya et al. suggests that an increased NT does not identify those trisomic fetuses destined to die *in utero*.[65] He followed six fetuses with trisomy 21 diagnosed in the first trimester because of an increased NT whose mothers had elected to continue their pregnancies. At the second trimester scan, the nuchal translucency had resolved in five of six cases. One fetus had persistent nuchal thickness, three had cardiac septal defects, two had echogenic bowel, and one had mild hydronephrosis. All were subsequently liveborn.

The second question is: **What is the significance of an abnormal nuchal translucency in fetuses with normal chromosomes?** The answer is important for appropriate patient management. Many studies have now shown that such fetuses are normal although they are more likely to have other major congenital anomalies.[66] In a study by Pandya et al. of 565 chromosomally normal fetuses with NT measurements between 3 and 9 mm, survival decreased with increasing nuchal translucency from 97% for 3 mm to 53% for greater than 5 mm.[67,68] In all babies that survived, the translucency had resolved by 20 weeks' gestation. One of the survivors has Stickler syndrome, but the others are apparently healthy. The incidence of structural defects, primarily cardiac, diaphragmatic, renal, and abdominal wall, was approximately 4%, which is higher than expected in the general population. Three patients tested positive for infectious disorders (one case each of parvovirus, cocksackie B virus, and toxoplasmosis). In addition, a relationship between cardiac septal defects and increased NT has been shown for both karyotypically abnormal and normal fetuses. Among fetuses with trisomy 21 examined at 10 to 14 weeks, Hyett et al.[69] reported the frequency of cardiac defects was 10% in fetuses with an NT thickness of greater than 3 mm and over 75% when the NT thickness was greater than 4 mm. Hyett suggested that the increased nuchal translucency in these cases may have been the result of abnormal cardiac development, with fluid collection representing an early sign of cardiac failure.

Nuchal Translucency and Screening. Whether NT screening should be performed is currently the subject of extensive investigation. Certainly, first trimester scanning including measurement of NT thickness has the advantage of offering early invasive testing (early amniocentesis or chorionic villus sampling) if NT thickness raises the possibility of chromosome abnormality. Also, screening with NT thickness is potentially useful in multiple pregnancies because alternative methods of screening (e.g., maternal biochemistry) are not applicable in such cases. Selective termination of an affected fetus carries a lower risk of miscarriage of the normal fetus if performed before 16 weeks' gestation compared to after 16 weeks' gestation (5.4% versus 14.4%, respectively).[70] Of interest is that NT thickness appears to be independent of biochemical markers (PAPP-A and human chorionic gonadotropin) during the first trimester.[71,72]

On the other hand, the accuracy of NT as a screening test in low-risk populations remains uncertain.[73,74] Kornman et al. found that NT thickening identified only 2 of 10 aneuploid fetuses before 13 weeks, and they concluded that NT "as a screening technique in general ultrasound practice at this stage is imprudent."[73] Further studies will be required to determine the exact role of first trimester NT screening. Until then, the following **conclusions regarding NT can be reached:**

- Increased NT may be a useful marker for abnormalities or other anomalies during the first trimester (10 to 14 weeks).
- The risk of anomalies and the mortality rate increase with the degree of NT.
- NT commonly resolves during the second trimester, whether or not the chromosomes are abnormal.
- Patients should be offered chromosome analysis if NT thickening greater than or equal to 3 mm is shown. If chromosome analysis is normal, patients should be followed with a targeted obstetric sonogram including detailed cardiac evaluation at 18 to 22 weeks. If this examination is normal and the NT has resolved, the prognosis is good and the vast majority of such fetuses will be found to be normal at birth.

Nonimmune Hydrops (NIH). Nonimmune hydrops (NIH) is defined as an **excess of total body water** evident as an extracellular accumulation of fluid in tissues and serous cavities without any identifiable circulating antibody against red blood cell antigens. With the decreasing frequency of rhesus immunization, NIH has become a relatively more frequent cause of hydrops.

The sonographic diagnosis of hydrops is straightforward. The excess body fluid accumulation is seen as subcutaneous edema, pleural and pericardial effusions, ascites, polyhydramnios, and/or placental thickening (Fig. 40-14).

Fluid accumulation must involve more than one site for the term hydrops to be used. If the fluid accumulation is limited to only one body cavity, the situation should be described in terms of the involved site (e.g., ascites or pleural effusions), as this may help in narrowing the differential diagnosis. In general, when NIH is fully developed, the prognosis is very poor, with a greater than 80% mortality rate.[75]

In a review of over 600 cases, NIH was found to be associated with a large variety of causes, including hematologic, cardiovascular, pulmonary, renal, gastrointestinal, hepatic, neoplastic, chromosomal, hereditary, infectious, and placental disorders.[75] The diagnosis of NIH is an indication to offer invasive prenatal diagnostic testing, including percutaneous umbilical blood sampling (PUBS). This permits the direct evaluation of fetal blood, including hematologic parameters, immunoglobulin titers, viral cultures, and rapid chromosome analysis. **Turner's syndrome and trisomy 21 are the most common causes of NIH among the chromosomal abnormalities associated with hydrops.**[17,75] Rare cases of other chromosomal rearrangements including mosaicisms, translocations, and deletion of the short arm of chromosome 13, and pericentric inversions also have been reported in fetuses with hydrops.

Thoracic Abnormalities

Diaphragmatic Hernia. Diaphragmatic hernia occurs in approximately 1 in 3000 live births (Fig. 40-15). It can be diagnosed sonographically by demonstrating the stomach, intestines, or liver within the fetal thorax, usually associated with a mediastinal shift to the opposite side. In addition, polyhydramnios and ascites may be present. In 7 prenatal series totaling 173 fetuses with diaphragmatic hernia, the incidence of chromosomal defects was 18%, most commonly **trisomy** 18.[17,31,76,80] The prevalence was higher for those with multiple additional abnormalities (34%) than for those with apparently isolated lesions (2%).

Cardiovascular Abnormalities

The risk of a chromosome abnormality varies with the specific type of cardiac anomaly, with the **highest risk** being present for **atrioventricular septal defect (endocardial cushion defect), double-outlet-right-ventricle**, and **hypoplastic left-heart syndrome** (Fig. 40-16). In a population-based, case-controlled study, chromosome disorders were

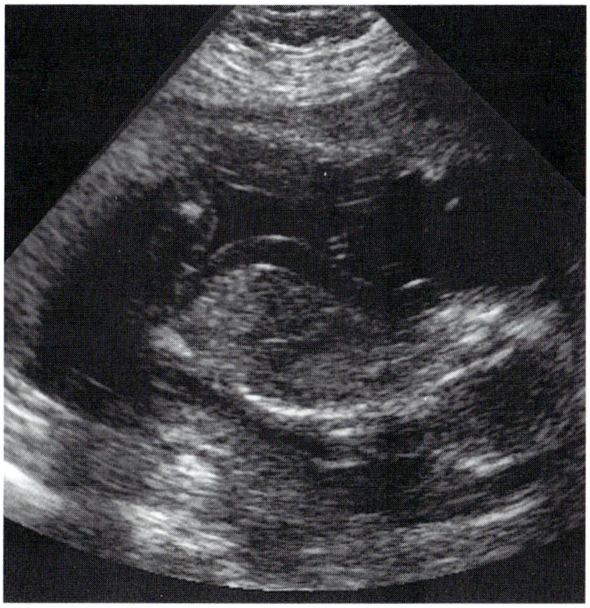

FIG. 40-14. Nonimmune hydrops and trisomy 18. Scan at 13 weeks shows diffuse edema with hydrops.

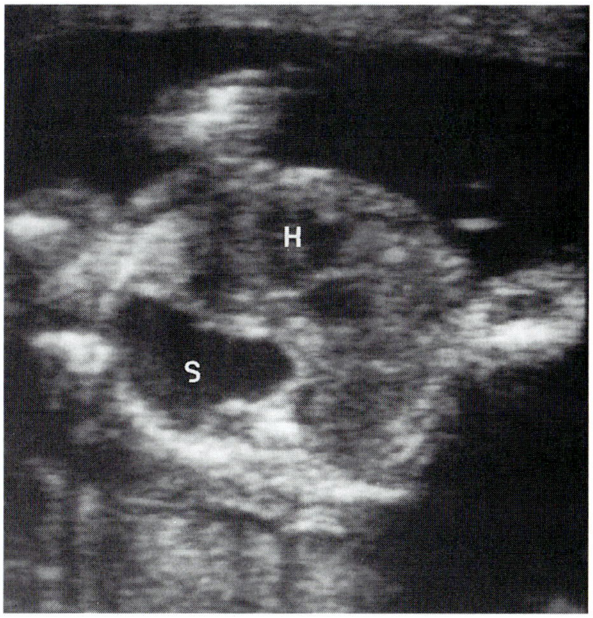

FIG. 40-15. Diaphragmatic hernia and trisomy 18. Transverse view of the thorax at 22 weeks shows fluid-filled stomach (S) in the left hemithorax. H, heart.

reported in 13% of livebirths with a cardiovascular malformation, compared with only 0.1% of infants without a cardiovascular malformation.[81] In contrast, 22% to 32% of fetuses with a sonographically detectable cardiac defect proved to have a chromosome abnormality. The most common defects were trisomies 21, 18, and 13, and Turner's syndrome. The incidence of chromosomal defects was significantly higher in fetuses with additional abnormalities (65%) compared with apparent isolated cardiac abnormalities (16%).[82,83]

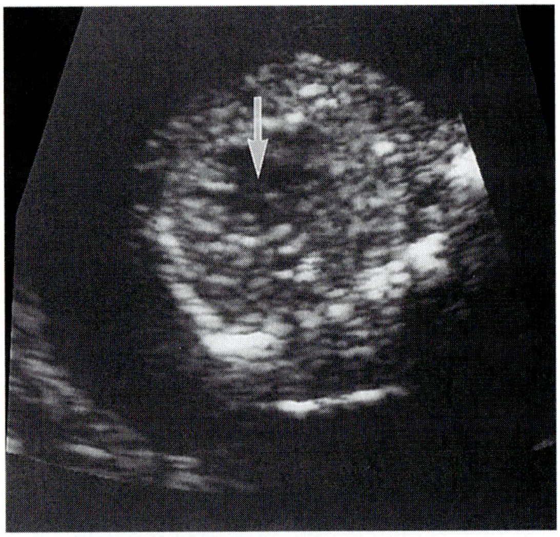

FIG. 40-16. Cardiac defect with trisomy 18. Transverse view of the heart at 17 weeks shows large septal defect *(arrow)*.

Echogenic Cardiac Foci. Echogenic intracardiac foci (EIF), also referred to as **echogenic chordae tendineae**, may be found in either or both ventricles of the fetal heart and may be single or multiple. The most common finding is a single focus in the left ventricle. The prevalence of these foci in routine second trimester scans is approximately 1% to 3%, and their size varies from 1 to 6 mm.[84,85] Histologic studies suggest these foci are due to mineralization within a papillary muscle.[86] Follow-up studies of fetuses with echogenic foci have demonstrated normal cardiac function.[85] Most studies describe the echogenic foci as benign variants with no clinical significance.[85,86] However, an association with chromosome abnormalities has been shown. In a series of fetuses with **trisomy 13,** 40% of affected fetuses examined during the second trimester showed EIF[87] (Fig. 40-17) and in a separate series of fetuses with **trisomy 21**, 18% showed this finding[88] (Fig. 40-18). These figures are remarkably similar to an autopsy study that showed microcalcification of the papillary muscle in 39% of fetuses with trisomy 13 and in 18% of fetuses with trisomy 21.[89] As an isolated finding, it is estimated that EIF increases the risk of trisomy 21 by twofold.

Gastrointestinal Abnormalities

Congenital abnormalities of the abdominal wall and gastrointestinal tract are often amenable to surgical

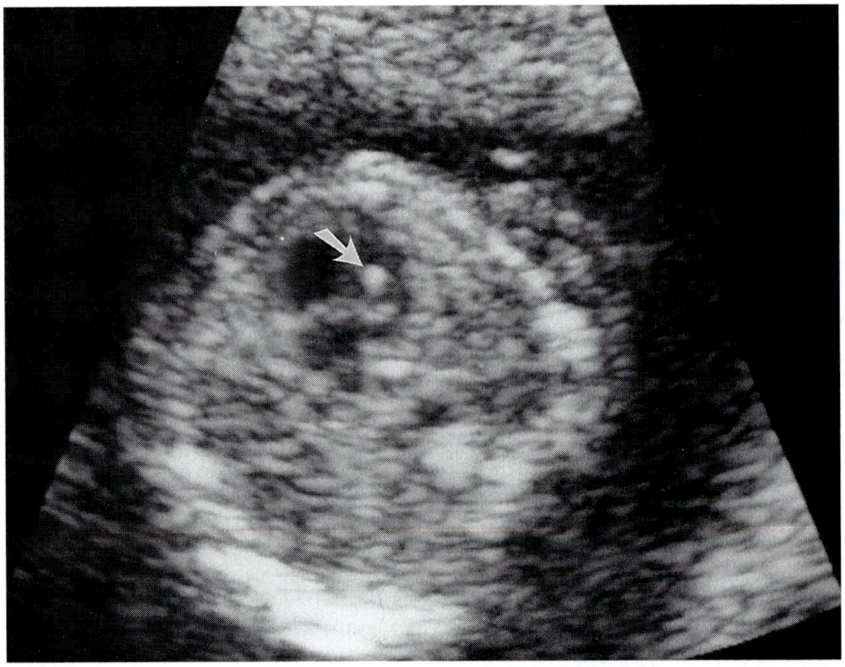

FIG. 40-17. Echogenic chordae tendineae (intracardiac echogenic focus) and trisomy 13). Transverse view of the heart shows echogenic focus *(arrow)* in the left ventricle of the heart. The left ventricle and left atrium also appear disproportionately small.

correction, and postnatal studies have established that their prognosis is dependent primarily upon the presence or absence of other major organ system malformations and chromosome abnormalities. Since these conditions can now be diagnosed antenatally, accurate prenatal evaluation of the primary defect and associated abnormalities, if present, is essential for effective pregnancy management.

Duodenal Atresia. **Chromosomal abnormalities are found in about 30% of fetuses with duodenal atresia detected prenatally, most commonly trisomy 21.**[81] Unfortunately, the characteristic sonographic findings of duodenal atresia ("double bubble" and polyhydramnios) are not usually apparent until after 24 weeks (Fig. 40-19). Nonetheless, knowledge of the fetal karyotype is useful for patient counseling and optimal obstetrical management of affected pregnancies. Therefore, chromosome analysis should be offered whenever duodenal atresia is identified prenatally.

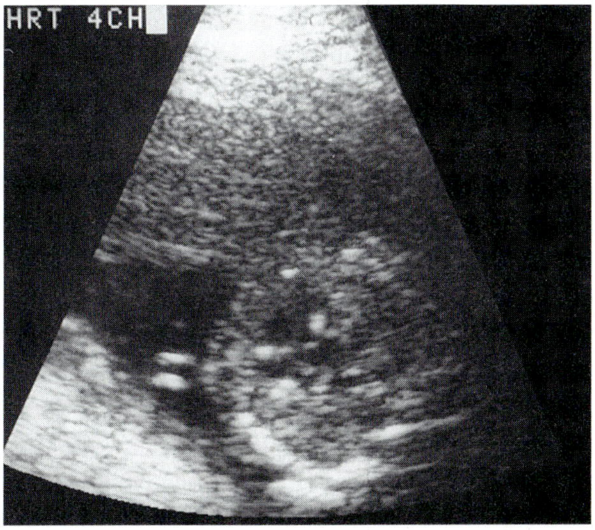

FIG. 40-18. Echogenic chordae tendinae and trisomy 21. Transverse view of the heart shows echogenic focus in the left ventricle of the heart without other abnormalities.

Absent Stomach Bubbles. Nicolaides et al. reported the antenatal findings and outcomes in 24 cases of absent fetal stomach bubbles with polyhydramnios.[90] In 20 fetuses with the presumptive diagnosis of esophageal atresia, there were 17 (80%) with trisomy 18, 5 of which were also associated with an omphalocele. Only 1 of these 20 fetuses survived. In 2 of the 24 cases, the lack of a visible stomach bubble was found to be due to absent fetal swallowing because of athrogryposis. Both of these fetuses were chromosomally normal but they died in the neonatal period because of pulmonary hypoplasia. In 2 additional cases, the lack of a visible stomach was the result of esophageal compression due to a cystic adenomatoid malformation of the lung in one case and the result of bilateral pleural effusions in the second case; the former had normal female karyotype and the latter had trisomy 21. Thus, in all cases in which the fetal stomach cannot be visualized, detailed evaluation of the remaining fetal anatomy should be carried out, and consideration should be given to fetal karyotyping.

Bowel Obstruction. Jejunal and ileal obstructions are visualized as multiple, fluid-filled loops of bowel in the abdomen. In contrast to duodenal atresia, they are rarely associated with additional abnormalities. In a combined series of 589 infants with jejunal and ileal atresia there were 5 cases of Down syndrome.[91] In an additional series of 24 fetuses with di-

A

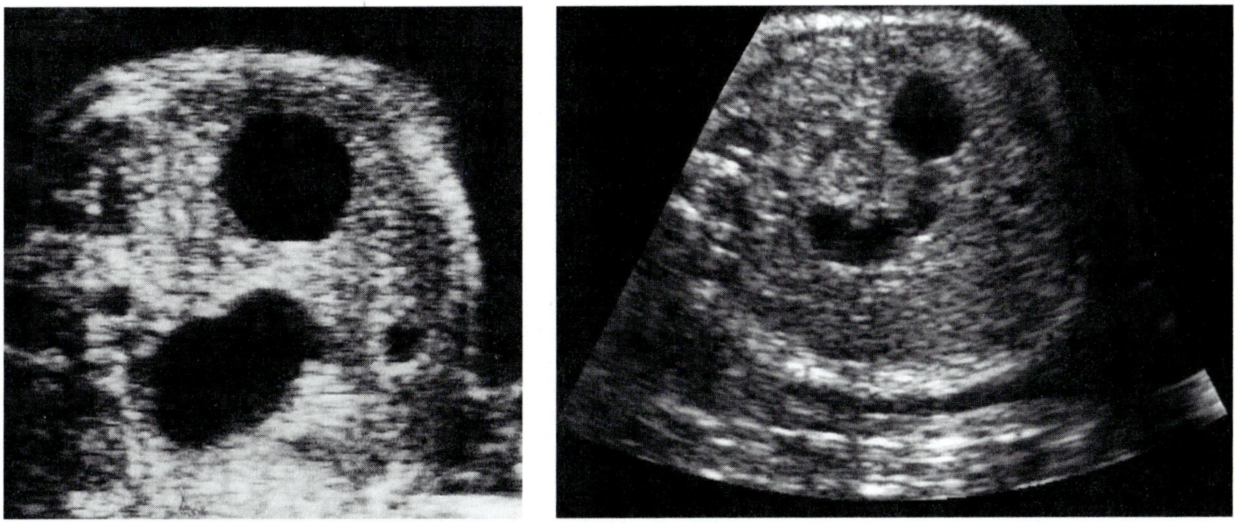

B

FIG. 40-19. Duodenal atresia and trisomy 21. A, Transverse view of the abdomen at 30 weeks shows "double-bubble" duodenal atresia. Karyotype analysis yielded trisomy 21. *B*, Ultrasound appearance of duodenal atresia at 20 weeks' gestation.

lated bowel, the karyotype was normal in all but 1 case in which the fetus also had additional abnormalities.[88]

Echogenic Bowel. The association between echogenic bowel and trisomy 21 was first established by Nyberg et al. who noted echogenic bowel in 7 of 68 (10%) trisomy 21 fetuses scanned between 14 and 24 weeks' gestation.[92] This group and other investigators have confirmed this association. In addition, echogenic bowel is a nonspecific finding seen in some fetuses with bowel atresia, volvulus, congenital infection, and meconium ileus secondary to cystic fibrosis.[93] An increased risk of IUGR and fetal demise has also been described with echogenic abdominal masses.

Recommendations regarding echogenic bowel:

- Recognition of echogenic bowel is subjective, though it is generally considered echogenic if its **echogenicity on ultrasound is similar to that of surrounding bone** (Fig. 40-20).
- Echogenic bowel found in the midtrimester should prompt a search for additional abnormalities. Even if isolated, however, the risk for chromosome abnormality is estimated to be 5.5 times the baseline risk.
- If amniocentesis is offered for chromosomal analysis, testing for congenital infection and cystic fibrosis should be considered.
- If these tests are normal, serial ultrasonographic evaluation of fetal growth and antenatal biophysical profile testing should be considered.

Abdominal Cysts. These include ovarian, mesenteric, adrenal, and hepatic cysts. In one series of 27 fetuses with abdominal cysts, 26 had normal karyotypes, suggesting these findings are **not** usually associated with chromosome defects.[88]

Abdominal Wall Defects

Omphalocele. The incidence of omphalocele is about 1 per 3000 livebirths. When it is an isolated, surgically correctable abnormality, the postnatal survival approaches 90%. It may, however, be associated with chromosomal defects, X-linked, autosomal dominant, and autosomal recessive disorders.

CAUSES OF ABSENT STOMACH BUBBLE

Esophageal atresia
Absent fetal swallowing
  e.g. -Arthrogryposis
Esophageal compression
  e.g. -Cystic adenomatoid malformation of lung
    -Pleural effusions

ECHOGENIC BOWEL MAY BE ASSOCIATED WITH:

Trisomy 21
Bowel atresia
Volvulus
Meconium ileus
Congenital infection

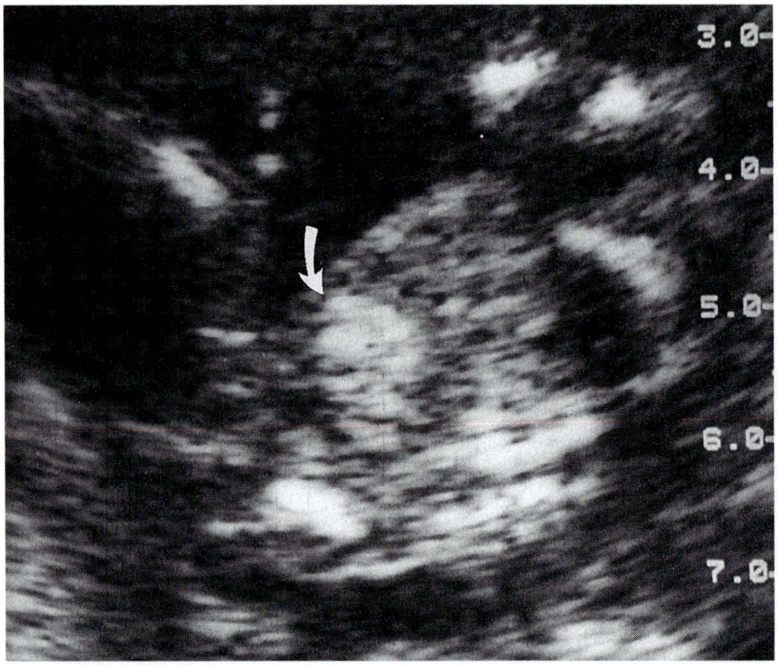

FIG. 40-20. Echogenic bowel and trisomy 21. Echogenic bowel in the lower fetal abdomen (*curved arrow*) is identified.

The **ultrasound diagnosis** is based on demonstrating the following;

- A midline anterior abdominal wall defect;
- A herniated sac with visceral contents (bowel and/or liver); and
- The umbilical cord inserting at the apex of the sac.

The prevalence of chromosomal defects in liveborn infants with omphalocele is approximately 10%, mainly trisomies 18 and 13. In antenatal series, the reported prevalence is about 36%, with trisomy 18 being the most common defect. **Chromosome abnormalities are more likely when the omphalocele sac contains only bowel (67%) compared to cases where the liver is included (16%)**[94] (Fig. 40-21). In addition, the karyotype is more likely to be abnormal when omphalocele is associated with additional abnormalities (46% versus 13% for isolated omphalocele).[94]

Gastroschisis. Gastroschisis occurs in approximately 1 in 10,000 livebirths. It consists of an isolated evisceration of the intestine, usually through a **right-sided,** paraumbilical abdominal wall defect. **Prenatal diagnosis** is based on demonstrating:

- A normally situated umbilicus; and
- Herniated loops of intestine that are free-floating in the amniotic fluid.

The vast majority of cases are **sporadic,** and associated chromosomal defects are rare. In 4 reports on a total of 63 fetuses with gastroschisis, there were no chromosomal defects.[88]

Genitourinary Abnormalities

The risk for fetal chromosome abnormalities when fetal renal defects are identified by ultrasound is significantly increased compared with the maternal-age-related risk; it is threefold when the renal defect is isolated and up to thirtyfold when there are multiple defects.[95] In a study by Nicolaides et al.[95] of 682 fetuses with renal defects, the overall incidence of chromosome abnormalities was 85 in 682, or 12% (trisomies, n = 63; deletions, n = 9; triploidies, n = 5; and sex chromosome aneuploidies, n = 8). The risk of chromosome

SONOGRAPHIC DIAGNOSIS OF ABDOMINAL WALL DEFECTS

Omphalocele
Midline anterior location
Visceral contents (bowel and/or liver) contained within herniated sac
Umbilical cord inserts at apex of sac

Gastroschisis
Right-sided paraumbilical
Herniated loops of bowel free-floating in amniotic fluid
Umbilicus normally situated

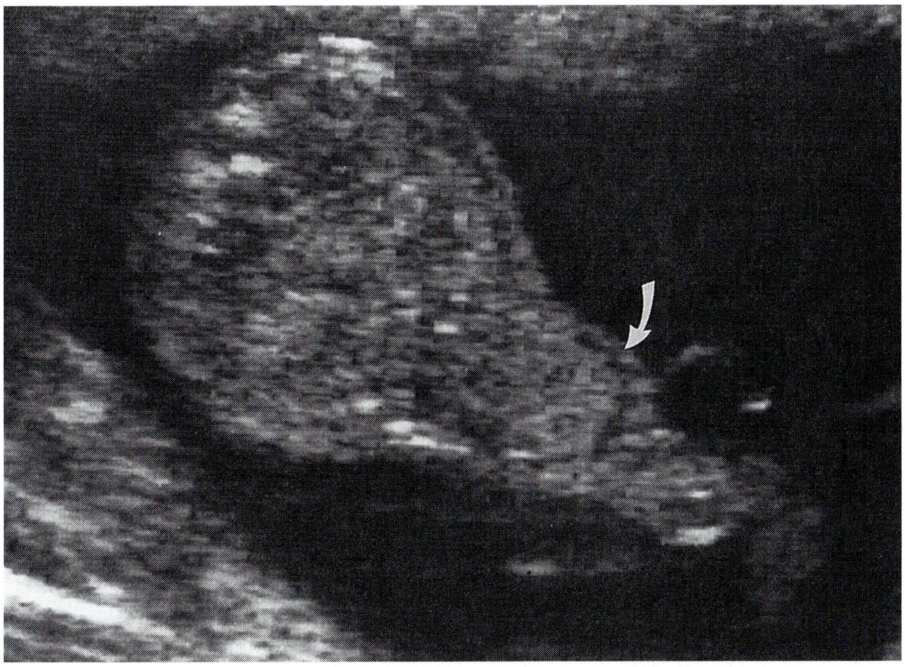

FIG. 40-21. Bowel-containing omphalocele and trisomy 18. Transverse view of the abdomen shows bowel-containing omphalocele (*curved arrow*).

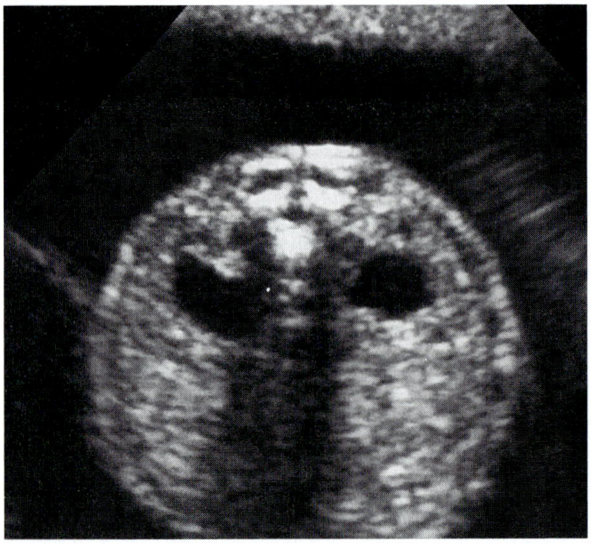

FIG. 40-22. Renal pyelectasis and trisomy 21. Transverse view of the kidney shows mild bilateral renal pyelectasis with the renal pelvis measuring 7 mm in AP dimension.

abnormalities was similar whether the fetuses had unilateral or bilateral involvement, urethral or ureteric obstruction, oligohydramnios or normal amniotic fluid volume, or different types of renal defects. The patterns of chromosome abnormalities and consequently those of the associated malformations were, however, related to the different types of renal defects. For example, in **mild hydronephrosis,** the most common chromosome abnormality was trisomy 21 (approximately a 1% risk), whereas in moderate/severe hydronephrosis, multicystic kidneys, or renal agenesis, the most common abnormalities were trisomy 18 and 13, each with its own associated syndromal defects.

Based on this evidence, **chromosomal analysis is recommended** for fetuses with renal abnormalities, particularly in the presence of other associated malformations.

Isolated Mild Hydronephrosis and Trisomy 21. Mild hydronephrosis, or pyelectasis, is a common finding during routine obstetric ultrasound evaluation. If defined as an anteroposterior renal pelvic diameter of greater than or equal to 3.5 mm, mild pyelectasis has been found in 2.0% to 2.8% of the normal population, and in as many as 25% of fetuses with trisomy 21 (Fig. 40-22).[96] The prevalence of chromosome abnormalities has been estimated at 1.1% when isolated as compared to 5.4%, 22.9%, and 63.3% in the presence of 1, 2, or 3 additional abnormalities, respectively.[97] One study of 5944 consecutive midtrimester fetuses found that pyelectasis had a sensitivity of 17% for trisomy 21; the rate fell to 4% when it was isolated.[96] Snijders and Nicolaides estimate that isolated, mild pyelectasis increases the risk of trisomy 21 1.6 times over the baseline risk.

Skeletal Abnormalities

A well-known characteristic of children with trisomy 21 is short stature associated with disproportionately short proximal long bones (femur and humerus). This characteristic has been suggested as a potentially useful method for screening fetuses for trisomy 21 in the second trimester. However, there is a large overlap in bone measurement between the group with trisomy 21 and the group without it. In addition, the sensitivities and specificities for detecting trisomy 21 using femur length vary considerably among studies.[50,98-100] Sensitivities as high as 69% with false-positive rates as low as 2% to 7% have been reported,[50,100] but others have reported sensitivities of less than 20% in the detection of trisomy 21 using femur length alone.[50,98-101] The humerus length appears to be a slightly more specific indicator, but the differences among races and populations make the use of this marker impractical in general population screening for trisomy 21.[100]

Extremity Malformations. Extremity malformations are commonly found in a wide range of chromosome defects. The detection of abnormal hands or feet at the time of routine ultrasound examination should stimulate a search for other markers of chromosomal abnormalities.

Clubfoot (Talipes Equinovarus). Clubfoot has been associated with multiple chromosomal abnormalities, including **trisomies 18** and **13.** Other associations include **neural tube** or **brain abnormalities, oligohydramnios, skeletal dysplasias,** and **arthrogryposis.**[4]

In 3 series comprising 127 cases of prenatally diagnosed clubfoot, 32% had chromosomal defects, **mainly trisomy 18.**[17,102,103] All the fetuses with chromosomal defects had multiple abnormalities. These data suggest that isolated clubfoot is commonly missed by prenatal sonography.

Identification of clubfoot is an indication for chromosome analysis when additional malformations are detected. Because associated abnormalities may be subtle or undetectable, chromosome analysis should also be considered when clubfoot is seen as an apparently isolated finding.

Limb Reduction Abnormalities (Micromelia). Limb reduction abnormalities have been reported to be associated with chromosome abnormalities, particularly trisomy 18.[104-106] Among fetuses with trisomy 18, up to 16% may demonstrate a limb reduction abnormality (8% in the upper limb and 8% in the lower limb).[106] Limb reduction abnormalities of the upper extremities may also be associated with radial aplasia.

Other Limb Abnormalities. Fetuses with trisomy 18 frequently demonstrate **flexion deformities** of the hands and **overlapping fingers,** most commonly seen as the second finger overlapping the third finger (Fig. 40-23, 40-24). **Polydactyly** is found in approximately 80% of fetuses with trisomy 13.

A 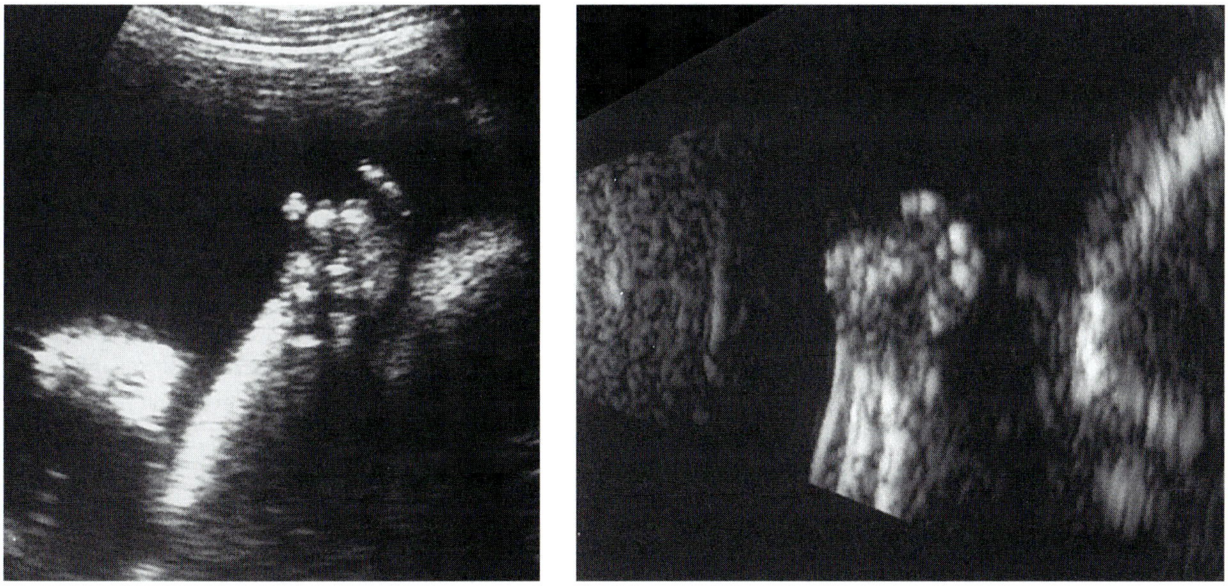 B

FIG. 40-23. Clenched hands and trisomy 18 in two different fetuses. A and B, In both cases, the hands remained clenched, with the fingers overlapping, throughout the examination.

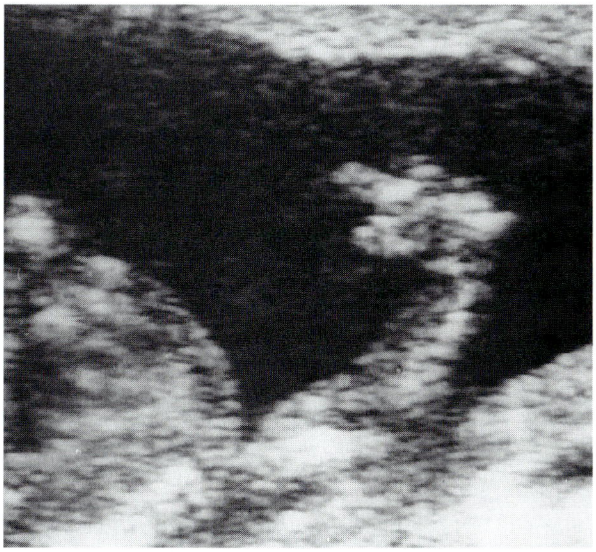

FIG. 40-24. Flexion deformity and trisomy 18. View of the arm shows flexion deformity at the wrist, with clenched hand.

Triploidy is often characterized by syndactyly, although this finding is extremely difficult to demonstrate sonographically. Trisomy 21 is frequently accompanied by hypoplasia of the middle phalanx of the fifth digit, resulting in clinodactyly.[107] It is also associated with a widened space between the first and second toes (sandal toes).[108]

The Iliac Angle. Dysmorphic pelvic features are a well-known pediatric sign of trisomy 21. In these children, the iliac crest is flattened and opened, producing a widened iliac crest. A recent study by Kliewer et al.[109] has reported that this wide iliac flare is a useful ultrasound marker for identifying, in the second trimester, fetuses at risk for trisomy 21. The **iliac angle is measured in the axial view of the fetal pelvis.** It is defined as the angle formed by the convergence of lines drawn along the posterolateral aspect of the right and left iliac wings of the ilium, measured with a hand-held goniometer.

In Kliewer's study, the iliac angle was measured in 19 fetuses with trisomy 21 and in 87 fetuses with normal karyotypes between 15 and 20 weeks of gestation. The mean iliac angle was 60° in the normal fetuses and 75° in the fetuses with trisomy 21, which was a highly significant difference. They determined that, based on a prevalence rate of trisomy 21 of 1 in 800 in the general population, the likelihood a fetus would have trisomy 21 is 1 in 270 for an iliac angle of 70° and 1 in 50 for an angle of 80°.[109] Such odds ratios approach a risk of 1 in 250, which is generally considered a reasonable cut-off point for amniocentesis. Because of the overlap between measurements in fetuses with and without trisomy 21, an angle of 80°, which is associated with high specificity, is likely to be the most appropriate angle to use for the general population. While these results need to be verified in larger studies, this measurement may be a promising adjunct in screening for trisomy 21.

Single Umbilical Artery

A single umbilical artery is a common abnormality, occurring in up to 1% of all deliveries. Infants with this abnormality are at increased risk for congenital abnormalities, chromosome abnormalities, IUGR, prematurity, and perinatal mortality.[110-112] A single umbilical artery is also more common in autopsy series and in stillbirths.

The incidence of congenital malformations associated with a single umbilical artery has been reported to range from 18.4% to 68.0%, with a 21.0% incidence in one prospective series.[113-115] Detection of a single umbilical artery should prompt a detailed ultrasound examination including fetal echocardiography to rule out concurrent abnormalities. In the absence of associated abnormalities, an isolated single umbilical artery does not increase the risk of chromosome aberrations.[116] Thus, most authorities agree that **identification of a single umbilical artery should initiate a careful search for additional anomalies, but it is not in itself an indication for chromosome analysis.**

Abnormal Amniotic Fluid Volume

Polyhydramnios is often the initial or primary manifestation of an underlying fetal disorder.[117,118] The greater the degree of polyhydramnios, the greater the likelihood of finding a major malformation and an accompanying chromosome disorder. **The presence of both polyhydramnios and IUGR has been stated to be characteristic of trisomy 18, although oligohydramnios may also be seen with trisomy 18.**[119]

In a series of 156 cases of hydramnios associated with congenital malformations, 55.0% of cases had more than one malformation, 13.4% had a chromosome abnormality (most commonly trisomies 18 and 21), and 32.0% had multiple malformations.[120] The most common abnormalities detected were congenital heart disease, musculoskeletal malformations, and anomalies of the gastrointestinal tract. These abnormalities are consistent with what is known of the pathophysiology of polyhydramnios.

Intrauterine Growth Restriction

Oligohydramnios may reflect an underlying chromosome abnormality when seen in association with intrauterine growth restriction or renal malformations. In a series by Snijders et al. of 458 fetuses referred between 17 and 39 weeks' gestation with IUGR (abdominal circumference measuring less than the fifth percentile) the **incidence of chromosome abnormality was** 19%.[121] The most common chromosome defect in the group referred **prior to 26 weeks'** gestation was **triploidy**, whereas in those referred **later than 26 weeks'** gestation, the most common defect was **trisomy 18**. Compared with those IUGR fetuses with a normal karyotype, the **chromosomally abnormal group** had the following:

- A higher incidence of associated fetal abnormalities (96% had multisystem defects characteristic of the chromosome syndrome);
- A higher mean head circumference/abdominal circumference ratio;
- A higher incidence of **normal** or increased amniotic fluid volume; and
- A higher incidence of **normal** waveforms from the uterine or umbilical arteries or both.

It has been previously suggested that assessment of body proportionality provides information concerning the underlying pathophysiology of IUGR. For example, **IUGR-associated chromosome abnormalities** were thought to be associated with **early-onset, symmetric impairment** in growth of all parts of the body. In contrast, **placental insufficiency** was thought to be associated with **late-onset, asymmetric impairment** in growth affecting primarily the abdomen and sparing the head and femur. This is not always the case, however. Fetuses with triploidy have been shown to demonstrate severe early-onset asymmetric growth restriction whereas fetuses with chromosome abnormalities other than triploidy tend to be symmetrically growth-restricted prior to 30 weeks and asymmetrically growth-restricted when diagnosed after 30 weeks.

In summary, IUGR should prompt careful search for associated malformations. If they are detected, **fetal karyotyping** should be offered, as there is a high risk of chromosome abnormality, **particularly if the IUGR is associated with normal amniotic fluid volume and a normal umbilical artery waveform.** In the absence of associated malformations, karyotyping should still be considered, as the risk of a chromosome abnormality is close to 2% to 4%.

APPROACH TO THE PATIENT WITH ULTRASOUND FETAL ANOMALIES

Risk Assessment

The detection of a fetal abnormality by ultrasound, regardless of whether it appears major or "minor," should prompt the sonographer to embark on a detailed search for associated malformations. In fetuses with multiple abnormalities, the frequency of chromosomal defects is high and fetal karyotyping should be offered irrespective of maternal age.

When apparently isolated or "subtle" abnormalities (e.g., mild hydronephrosis) are present, there are large differences in the reported prevalence of associated chromosome defects, and it is less clear whether karyotyping should be offered. This is especially true when the prevalence of the abnormality is high in the general population and the prognosis, in the absence of a chromosomal defect, is good.

Factors that will influence the patient's risk include:

- **The type of defect**;
- **The number of abnormalities present**;

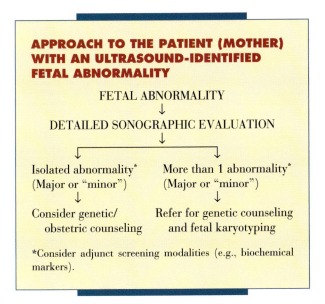

APPROACH TO THE PATIENT (MOTHER) WITH AN ULTRASOUND-IDENTIFIED FETAL ABNORMALITY

FETAL ABNORMALITY
↓
DETAILED SONOGRAPHIC EVALUATION
↓

Isolated abnormality* (Major or "minor")	More than 1 abnormality* (Major or "minor")
↓	↓
Consider genetic/ obstetric counseling	Refer for genetic counseling and fetal karyotyping

*Consider adjunct screening modalities (e.g., biochemical markers).

ABNORMALITIES ASSOCIATED WITH INCREASED PROBABILITY OF FETAL CHROMOSOME ABNORMALITY, EVEN IF ISOLATED

Borderline ventriculomegaly
Posterior fossa abnormalities
Cystic hygroma
Nuchal fold
Nuchal translucency
Atrioventricular septal defect
Double outlet right ventricle
Omphalocele
Duodenal atresia
Echogenic bowel
Genitourinary abnormalities
Nonimmune hydrops

RISK OF KARYOTYPIC ABNORMALITY DEPENDS ON:

Type of abnormality present
Number of abnormalities present
Maternal age (MA)
  Risk increases with increasing MA
Gestational age (GA)
  Risk decreases with increasing GA

TABLE 40-2
SONOGRAPHIC SCORING SYSTEM FOR TRISOMIES BASED ON THE PRESENCE OR ABSENCE OF SPECIFIC ABNORMALITIES[123]

Ultrasound Feature	Score
Structural abnormality	2
Thickened nuchal fold	2
Short femur	1
Short humerus	1
Pyelectasia	1
Choroid plexus cysts	1
Echogenic bowel	1

- **The gestational age of the fetus**; and
- **The maternal age.**

It is well documented that the risk of trisomies increases with maternal age (trisomy 21, 18, and 13). Turner's syndrome is usually due to loss of the paternal X chromosome and consequently the frequency of conception of 45,XO embryos, unlike that of trisomies, is unrelated to maternal age. In addition, the prevalence of triploidy is not related to maternal age but is strongly related to gestational age because of the very high rate of intrauterine lethality. In fact, the incidence of all of the chromosome defects (except for the sex-chromosomal abnormalities) decreases with gestational age. For trisomies 21, 18, and 13, the rate of intrauterine lethality between 16 weeks and birth is 28%, 71%, and 43%, respectively.[122] For Turner's syndrome, 75% are lost between 16 weeks and birth and for triploidy, 100% are lost.

The overall risk for chromosome defects increases with the total number of abnormalities identified. It is thus recommended that whenever an abnormality or marker is detected at routine ultrasound examination, a thorough check be made for other features of the chromosomal defect known to be associated with that marker; should additional abnormalities be identified, the risk of a chromosome defect is dramatically increased.

The Sonographic Scoring System

Benacerraf et al., in 1994,[123] proposed a scoring system for the risk of trisomies according to the presence or absence of specific abnormalities (Table 40-2). In her system, two points are arbitrarily given to thickened nuchal fold and to any other major structural malformation. The other markers, which include short femur, short humerus, pyelectasis, and echogenic bowel, each receive 1 point. According to Benacerraf, when a cutoff limit of 2 is used to indicate an increased risk of trisomy 21, approximately 80% of fetuses with trisomy 21 are identified sonographically at a false-positive rate of 4.4%. The higher the score, the higher the risk that a woman is carrying a fetus with trisomy 21. Furthermore, Benacerraf has reported that a sonographic score of zero can dramatically reduce the age-related risk of an older woman for carrying a fetus with trisomy 21. Nyberg et al., expanding on this concept, have recently proposed a method of assessing the risk of fetal trisomy 21 based on sonographic findings and maternal age.[123] They have devised a computer program that assesses an individual patient's risk for carrying a fetus with trisomy 21 based on the presence or absence of various sonographic findings (nuchal thickening, echogenic bowel, pyelectasis, shortened femur, shortened humerus, and echogenic cardiac foci). A likelihood ratio is assigned for each finding based on published data, and an overall postultrasound risk assessment is calculated as an odds ratio from the combination of ultrasound findings and the patient's a priori risk based on maternal age. This allows the individual at-risk patient to make a more informed choice about whether to proceed with invasive diagnostic testing.

REFERENCES

1. Hook EB, Cross PK, Schreinemachers DM. Chromosomal abnormality rates at amniocentesis and in live-born infants. *JAMA* 1983;249:2034-2038.
2. Hook EB. Rates of chromosome abnormalities at different maternal ages. *Obstet Gynecol* 1981;58:282-285.
3. Norton ME. Biochemical and ultrasound screening for chromosomal abnormalities. *Seminars in Perinat* 1994;18:256-265.
4. Snijders RJM, Nicolaides KH. *Ultrasound markers for fetal chromosome defects*. London, New York: Parthenon Publishing Group; 1996.
5. Adams M, Erikson J, Layde P et al. Down's syndrome: recent trends in the United States. *JAMA* 1981;246:758-760.
6. Cardoza JD, Goldstein RB, Filly RA. Exclusion of fetal ventriculomegaly with a single measurement: the width of the lateral ventricular atrium. *Radiology* 1988;169:711-714.
7. Abramowicz J, Jaffe R. Diagnosis and intrauterine management of enlargement of the cerebral ventricles. *J Perinat Med* 1988;16:165-173.
8. Bertino RE, Nyberg DA, Cyr DR, Mack LA. Prenatal diagnosis of agenesis of the corpus callosum. *J Ultrasound Med* 1988;7:251-260.
9. Chervenak FA, Duncan C, Ment LR, Hobbins JC. Outcome of fetal ventriculomegaly. *Lancet* 1984;2:179-181.
10. Nyberg DA, Mack LA, Hirsch J et al. Fetal hydrocephalus: sonographic detection and clinical significance of associated anomalies. *Radiology* 1987;163:187-191.
11. Patel MD, Filly AL, Hersh DR, Goldstein RB. Mild fetal lateral cerebral ventriuclomegaly: clinical course and outcome. *Radiology* 1994;192:759-764.
12. Filly RA, Goldstein RB. The fetal ventricular atrium; fourth down and 10 mm to go. *Radiology* 1994;193:315-317.
13. Cardoza JD, Filly RA, Podrasky AE. The dangling choroid plexus: a sonographic observation of value in excluding ventriculomegaly. *AJR* 1989;151:767-770.
14. Hertzberg BS, Lile R, Foosaner DE et al. Choroid plexus-ventricular wall separation in fetuses with normal-sized cerebral ventricles at sonography: postnatal outcome. *Am J Roentgenol* 1994;163:405-410.
15. Bromley B, Frigoletto FD, Benacerraf BR. Mild fetal lateral cerebral ventriculomegaly: clinical course and outcome. *Am J Obstet Gynecol* 1991;164:863-867.
16. Goldstein RB, LaPidus AS, Filly RA et al. Mild lateral cerebral ventricular dilatation *in utero*: clinical significance and prognosis. *Radiology* 1990;176:237-242.
17. Nicolaides KH, Snijders RJM, Gosden CM et al. Ultrasonographically detectable markers of fetal chromosomal abnormalities. *Lancet* 1992;340:704-707.
18. Eydoux P, Choiset A, LePorrier N et al. Chromosomal prenatal diagnosis: study of 936 cases of intrauterine abnormalities after ultrasound assessment. *Prenat Diagn* 1989;9:255-268.
19. Walkinshaw S, Pilling D, Spriggs A. Isolated choroid plexus cysts: the need for routine offer of karyotyping. *Prenat Diagn* 1994;14:663-667.
20. Chinn DH, Miller E, Worthy LM et al. Sonographically detected fetal choroid plexus cysts; frequency and association with aneuploidy. *J Ultrasound Med* 1991;10:255-258.
21. Chitkara U, Cogswell C, Norton K et al. Choroid plexus cysts in the fetus: a benign anatomic variant or pathologic entity? Report of 41 cases and review of the literature. *Obstet Gynecol* 1988;72:185-189.
22. Hertzberg BS, Kay HH, Bowie JD. Fetal choroid plexus lesions: relationship of antenatal sonographic appearance to clinical outcome. *J Ultrasound Med* 1989;8:77-82.
23. Achiron R, Barkai G, Kaznelson MBM et al. Fetal lateral ventricle choroid plexus cysts: the dilemma of amniocentesis. *Obstet Gynecol* 1991;78:815-818.
24. Snijders RJM, Shawwa L, Nicolaides KH. Fetal choroid plexus cysts and trisomy 18: assessment of risk based on ultrasound findings and maternal age. *Prenat Diagn* 1994; 14:1119-1127.
25. Gross SJ, Shulman LP, Tolley EA et al. Isolated fetal choroid plexus cysts and trisomy 18: a review and meta-analysis. *Am J Obstet Gynecol* 1995;172:83-87.
26. Fergani P, Ghidini A, Strobelt N et al. Prognostic indicators in the prenatal diagnosis of agenesis of corpus callosum. *Am J Obstet Gynecol* 1994;170:753-758.
27. Comstock C, Culp D, Gonzalez J et al. Agensis of the corpus callosum in the fetus: its evolution and significance. *J Ultrasound Med* 1985;4:613-616.
28. Lockwood CJ, Ghidini A, Aggarwal R et al. Antenatal diagnosis of partial agenesis of the corpus callosum: a benign cause of ventriculomegaly. *Am J Obstet Gynecol* 1988;159: 184-186.
29. Estroff JA, Scott MR, Benacerraf BR. Dandy-Walker variant: prenatal sonographic features and clinical outcome. *Radiology* 1992;185:755-758.
30. Nyberg DA, FitzSimmons J, Mack LH et al. Chromosomal abnormalities in fetuses with omphalocele: significance of omphalocele contents. *J Ultrasound Med* 1989;8:299-308.
31. Wilson RD, Chitayat D, McGillivray BC. Fetal ultrasound abnormalities: correlation with fetal karyotype, autopsy findings, and postnatal outcome—five-year prospective study. *Am J Med Genet* 1992;44:586-590.
32. Watson WJ, Katz VL, Chescheir NC et al. The cisterna magna in second trimester fetus with abnormal karyotypes. *Obstet Gynecol* 1992;79:723-725.
33. Nicolaides KH, Salvesen D, Snijders RJM et al. Strawberry-shaped skull: associated malformations and chromosomal defects. *Fetal Diagn Ther* 1992c;7:137-137.
34. Perry TB, Benzie RJ, Cassar N. Fetal cephalometry by ultrasound as a screening procedure for the prenatal detection of Down syndrome. *Br J Obstet Gynaecol* 1984;91:138-143.
35. Shah YG, Eckl CJ, Stinson SK et al. Biparietal diameter/femur length ratio, cephalic index, and femur length measurements: not reliable screening techniques for Down syndrome. *Obstet Gynecol* 1990b;75:186-188.
36. Nicolaides KH, Salvesen DR, Snijders RJM et al. Fetal facial defects: associated malformations and chromosomal abnormalities. *Fetal Diagn Ther* 1993;8:1-9.
37. Hsieh FJ, Lee CH, Wu CC et al. Antenatal ultrasonic findings of craniofacial malformations. *J Formosan Med Assoc* 1991; 90:550-554.

38. Benacerraf BR, Mulliken JB. Fetal cleft lip and palate: sonographic diagnosis and postnatal outcome. *Plast Reconstr Surg* 1993;184:239-242.
39. Saltzman DH, Benacerraf BR, Frigoletto FD. Diagnosis and management of fetal facial clefts. *Am J Obstet Gynecol* 1986;155:377-379.
40. Turner GM, Twining P. The facial profile in the diagnosis of fetal abnormalities. *Clin Radiol* 1993;47:389-395.
41. Bronshtein M, Blumenfeld I, Kohn J et al. Detection of cleft lip by early second-trimester transvaginal sonography. *Obstet Gynecol* 1994;84:73-76.
42. Nyberg DA, Sickler GK, Hegge FN et al. Fetal cleft lip with and without cleft palate: ultrasound classification and correlation with outcome. *Radiology* 1995;195:677-684.
43. Berry SM, Gosden CM, Snijders RJM et al. Fetal holoprosencephaly: associated malformations and chromosomal defects. *Fetal Diagn Ther* 1990;5:92-99.
44. Azar G, Snijders RJM, Gosden CM et al. Fetal nuchal cystic hygromata: associated malformations and chromosomal defects. *Fetal Diagn Ther* 1991;6:46-57.
45. Zarabi M, Mieckowski CG, Mazer J. Cystic hygroma associated with Noonan's syndrome. *J Clin Ultrasound* 1983;11:398.
46. Rahmani MR, Fong KW, Connor TP. The varied sonographic appearance of cystic hygromas *in utero*. *J Ultrasound Med* 1986;5:165.
47. Smith DW. Recognizable patterns of human malformation. In: *Major Problems in Clinical Pediatrics*. Philadelphia: WB Saunders Co; 1978:11-23, 30-31, 72-75.
48. Hall B. Mongolism in newborn infants. *Clin Pediatrics* 1966;5:4.
49. Benacerraf BR, Barss VA, Laboda LA. A sonographic sign for the detection in the second trimester of the fetus with Down's syndrome. *Am J Obstet Gynecol* 1985;151:1078.
50. Benacerraf BR, Gelman R, Frigoletto FD. Sonographic identification of second-trimester fetuses with Down syndrome. *N Engl J Med* 1987;317:1371-1376.
51. Nyberg DA, Resta RG, Luthy DA et al. Prenatal sonographic findings of Down syndrome: review of 94 cases. *Obstet Gynecol* 1980;76:370-377.
52. Ginsberg N, Cadkin A, Pergament E et al. Ultrasonographic detection of second-trimester fetus with trisomy 18 and trisomy 21. *Am J Obstet Gynecol* 1990;163:1186-1190.
53. Crane JP, Gray DL. Sonographically measured nuchal skinfold thickness as a screening tool for Down syndrome: results of a prospective clinical trial. *Obstet Gynecol* 1991;77:533-536.
54. DeVore GR, Alfi O. The association between an abnormal nuchal skin fold, trisomy 21, and ultrasound abnormalities identified during the second trimester of pregnancy. *Ultrasound Obstet Gynecol* 1993;3:387-394.
55. Watson WJ, Miller RC, Mendard MK et al. Ultrasonographic measurement of fetal nuchal skin to screen for chromosomal abnormalities. *Am J Obstet Gynecol* 1994;170:583-586.
56. Donnenfeld AE, Carlson DE, Palomaki GE et al. Prospective multicenter study of second-trimester nuchal skinfold thickness in unaffected and Down syndrome pregnancies. *Obstet Gynecol* 1994;84:844-847.
57. Grandjean H, Sarramon MF, Association Française pour le Dépistage et la Prévention des Handicaps de l'Enfant Study Group. Sonographic measurement of nuchal skinfold thickness for detection of Down syndrome in the second-trimester fetus: a multicenter prospective study. *Obstet Gynecol* 1995; 85:103-106.
58. Borrell A, Costa D, Martinez JM et al. Early midtrimester fetal nuchal thickness: effectiveness as a marker of Down syndrome. *Am J Obstet Gynecol* 1996;175:45-49.
59. Toi A, Simpson GF, Filly RA. Ultrasonically evident fetal nuchal skin thickening: is it specific for Down syndrome? *Am J Obstet Gynecol* 1987;156:150-153.
60. Gray DL, Crane JP. Optimal nuchal skin-fold thresholds based on gestational age for prenatal detection of Down syndrome. *Am J Obstet Gynecol* 1994;171:1282-1286.
61. Nicolaides KH, Brizot ML, Snijders RJM. Fetal nuchal translucency: ultrasound screening for fetal trisomy in the first trimester of pregnancy. *Br J Obstet Gynecol* 1994; 101:782-786.
62. Nicolaides KH, Azar G, Byrne D et al. Fetal nuchal translucency: ultrasound screening for chromosomal defects in first trimester of pregnancy. *Br Med J* 1992;304:867-869.
63. Landwehr JB, Johnson MP, Hume RF et al. Abnormal nuchal findings on screening ultrasonography: aneuploidy stratification on the basis of ultrasonographic anomaly and gestational age at detection. *Am J Obstet Gynecol* 1996;175:995-999.
64. Pandya PP, Altman D, Brizot ML et al. Repeatability of measurement of fetal nuchal translucency thickness. *Ultrasound Obstet Gynecol* 1995a;5:337-340.
65. Pandya PP, Snijders RJM, Johnson S et al. Natural history of trisomy 21 fetuses with fetal nuchal translucency. *Ultrasound Obstet Gynecol* 1995;5:381-383.
66. Johnson MP, Johnson A, Holzgreve W et al. First-trimester simple hygroma: cause and outcome. *Am J Obstet Gynecol* 1993;168:156-161.
67. Pandya PP, Kondylios A, Hilbert L et al. Chromosomal defects and outcome in 1,105 fetuses with increased nuchal translucency. *Ultrasound Obstet Gynecol* 1995;5:15-19.
68. Pandya PP, Brizot ML, Kuhn P. et al. First trimester fetal nuchal translucency thickness and risk for trisomies. *Obstet Gynecol* 1994;84:420-423.
69. Hyett JA, Moscoso G, Kypros H et al. First-trimester nuchal translucency and cardiac septal defects in fetuses with trisomy 21. *Am J Obstet Gynecol* 1995;172:1411-1413.
70. Evans MI, Goldberg JD, Dommergues M et al. Efficacy of second-trimester selective termination for fetal abnormalities: international collaborative experience among the world's largest centers. *Am J Obstet Gynecol* 1994;171:90-94.
71. Brizot ML, Snijders RJM, Bersinger NA et al. Maternal serum pregnancy-associated placental protein A and fetal nuchal translucency thickness for the prediction of fetal trisomies in early pregnancy. *Obstet Gynecol* 1994;84:918-922.
72. Brizot ML, Snijders RJM, Butler J et al. Maternal serum hCG and fetal nuchal translucency thickness for the prediction of fetal trisomies in the first trimester of pregnancy. *Br J Obstet Gynaecol* 1995;102:127-132.
73. Kornman LH, Morssink LP, Beekhuis JR et al. Nuchal translucency cannot be used as a screening test for chromosomal abnormalities in the first trimester of pregnancy in a routine ultrasound practice. *Prenat Diagn* 1996;16:797-805.
74. Bewley S, Roberts LJ, Mackinson AM et al. First trimester fetal nuchal translucency: problems with screening the general population. *Br J Obstet Gynaecol* 1995;102:386-388.
75. Jauniaux E, Maldergem LV, Munter CG et al. Nonimmune hydrops fetalis associated with genetic abnormalities. *Obstet Gynecol* 1990;75:568-572.
76. Benacerraf BR, Adzick NS. Fetal diaphragmatic hernia: ultrasound diagnosis and clinical outcome in 19 cases. *Am J Obstet Gynecol* 1987a;156:573-576.
77. Gagnon S, Fraser W, Fouquette B et al. Nature and frequency of chromosomal abnormalities in pregnancies with abnormal ultrasound findings: an analysis of 117 cases with review of the literature. *Prenat Diagn* 1992;12:9-18.
78. Thorpe-Beeston JG, Gosden CM, Nicolaides KH. Choroid plexus cysts and chromosomal defects. *Br J Radiol* 1990; 63:783-786.
79. Fogel M, Copel JA, Cullen MT et al. Congenital heart disease and fetal thoracoabdominal anomalies: association *in utero* and the importance of cytogenetic analysis. *Am J Perinatol* 1991;8:411-416.

80. Sharland GK, Lockhart SM, Heward AJ et al. Prognosis in fetal diaphragmatic hernia. *Am J Obstet Gynecol* 1992;166:9-13.
81. Paladini D, Calabro R, Palmieri S et al. Prenatal diagnosis of congenital heart disease and fetal karyotyping. *Obstet Gynecol* 1992;81:679-682.
82. Copel JA, Pilu G, Kleinman CS. Congenital heart disease and extracardiac anomalies: associations and indications for fetal echocardiography. *Am J Obstet Gynecol* 1986;154:1121-1132.
83. Copel JA, Cuyllen M, Green JJ et al. The frequency of aneuploidy in prenatally diagnosed congenital heart disease: an indication for fetal karyotyping. *Am J Obstet Gynecol* 1988;158:409-413.
84. Twining P. Echogenic foci in the fetal heart: incidence and association with chromosomal disease abstract. *Ultrasound Obstet Gynecol* 1992;3(suppl 2):190.
85. How HY, Villafane J, Parihus RR et al. Small hyperechoic foci of the fetal cardiac ventricle: a benign sonographic finding? *Ultrasound Obstet Gynecol* 1994;4:205-207.
86. Brown DL, Roberts DJ, Miller WA. Left ventricular echogenic focus in the fetal heart: pathologic correlation. *J Ultrasound Med* 1994;13:613-616.
87. Lehman C, Nyberg DA, Winter T et al. Trisomy 13 syndrome: prenatal US findings in review of 36 cases. *Radiology* 1995;194:217-2.
88. Bromley B. Lieberman E, Laboda LA et al. Echogenic intracardiac focus: a sonographic sign for Down syndrome? *Obstet Gynecol* 1995;86:998-1001.
89. Roberts DJ, Genest D. Cardiac histologic pathology characteristic of trisomies 13 and 21. *Hum Pathol* 1992;23:1130-1140.
90. Nicolaides KH, Snijders RJM, Cheng H et al. Fetal gastrointestinal and abdominal wall defects: associated malformations and chromosomal defects. *Fetal Diagn Ther* 1992; 7:102-115.
91. Nyberg DA, Dubinsky T, Resta RG et al. Echogenic fetal bowel during the second trimester: clinical importance. *Radiology* 1993;188:527-533.
92. MacGregor SN, Tamura R, Sabbagha R et al. Isolated hyperechoic fetal bowel: significance and implications for management. *Am J Obstet Gynecol* 1995;173:1254-1258.
93. Nyberg DA, FitzSimmons J, Mack LH et al. Chromosomal abnormalities in fetuses with omphalocele: significance of omphalocele contents. *J Ultrasound Med* 1989;8:299-308.
94. Nicolaides KH, Cheng H, Abbas A et al. Fetal renal defects: associated malformations and chromosomal defects. *Fetal Diagn Ther* 1992;7:1-11.
95. Benacerraf BR, Mandell J, Estroff JA et al. Fetal pyelectasis: a possible association with Down syndrome. *Obstet Gynecol* 1990;76:58-60.
96. Snijders RJM, Sebire NJ, Faria M et al. Fetal mild hydronephrosis and chromosomal defects: relation to maternal age and gestation. *Fetal Diagn Ther* 1995;10:349-355.
97. Johnson MP, Barr M Jr, Treadwell MC et al. Fetal leg and femur/foot length ratio: a marker for trisomy 21. *Am J Obstet Gynecol* 1993;169:557-563.
98. Lockwood CJ, Lynch L, Berkowitz RL. Ultrasonographic screening for the Down syndrome fetus. *Am J Obstet Gynecol* 1991;165:124-128.
99. Nyberg DA, Resta RG, Luthy DA et al. Humerus and femur length shortening in the detection of Down's syndrome. *Am J Obstet Gynecol* 1993;168:534-538.
100. Hill LM, Guzick D, Belfar HL et al. The current role of sonography in the detection of Down syndrome. *Obstet Gynecol* 1989;74:620-623.
101. Benacerraf BR. Antenatal sonographic diagnosis of congenital clubfoot: a possible indication for amniocentesis. *J Clin Ultrasound* 1986b;14:703-706.
102. Jeanty P, Romero R, D'Alton M et al. *In utero* sonographic detection of hand and foot deformities. *J Ultrasound Med* 1985;4:595-601.
103. Kajii T. Phocomelia in trisomy 18 syndrome. *Lancet* 1967;1:385-386.
104. Bofinger MK, Dignan PSJ, Schmidt RE et al. Reduction malformations and chromosome anomalies. *Am J Dis Child* 1973;125:135-143.
105. Pfeiffer RA, Santelmann R. Limb anomalies in chromosomal aberrations. *Birth Defects* 1977;13:319-337.
106. Benacerraf BR, Osathanondh R, Frigoletto FD Jr. Sonographic demonstration of hypoplasia of the middle phalanx of the fifth digit: a finding associated with Down syndrome. *Am J Obstet Gynecol* 1988;159:181-183.
107. Jeanty P. Prenatal detection of simian crease. *J Ultrasound Med* 1990;9:131-136.
108. Kliewer MA, Hertzberg BS, Freed KS et al. Dysmorphologic features of the fetal pelvis in Down syndrome: prenatal sonographic depiction and diagnostic implications of the iliac angle. *Radiology* 1996;201:681-684.
109. Bryan EM, Kohler HG. The missing umbilical artery: prospective study based on a maternity unit. *Arch Dis Child* 1974;49:844-846.
110. Byrne J, Blane WA. Malformations and chromosome anomalies in spontaneously aborted fetuses with single umbilical artery. *Am J Obstet Gynecol* 1985;151:340-343.
111. Lenoski EF, Medovy H. Single umbilical artery: incidence, clinical significance and relation to autosomal trisomy. *Can Med Assoc J* 1962;87:1229-1232.
112. Hermann U, Sidiropoulos D. Single umbilical artery: prenatal findings. *Prenat Diagn* 1988;8:275-279.
113. Leung A, Robson W. Single umbilical artery: a report of 159 cases. *Am J Dis Child* 1989;1453:108-112.
114. Romero R, Pilu G, Jeanty P et al. *Prenatal diagnosis of congenital anomalies.* East Norwalk, Conn.: Appleton & Lange; 1988.
115. Nyberg DA, Mahony BS, Lath D et al. Single umbilical artery: prenatal detection of concurrent anomalies. *J Ultrasound Med* 1991;10:247-253.
116. Barkin SZ, Pretorius DH, Beckett MK et al. Severe polyhydramnios: incidence of anomalies. *AJR* 1987;148:155-159.
117. Landy HJ, Isada NB, Larsen JW Jr. Genetic implications of idiopathic hydramnios. *Am J Obstet Gynecol* 1987;157:114-117.
118. Liang ST, Yam AWC, Tang MHY et al. Trisomy 18: the value of late prenatal diagnosis. *Eur J Obstet Gynecol Reprod Biol* 1986;22:95-97.
119. Stoll CG, Alembik Y, Dott B. Study of 156 cases of polyhydramnios and congenital malformations in a series of 118,265 consecutive births. *Am J Obstet Gynecol* 1991; 165:586-590.
120. Snijders RJM, Shrrod C, Gosden CM et al. Fetal growth retardation: associated malformations and chromosomal abnormalities. *Am J Obstet Gynecol* 1993;168:547-555.
121. Hook EB. Chromosome abnormalities and spontaneous fetal death following amniocentesis: further data and associations with maternal age. *Am J Hum Genet* 1983;35:110-116.
122. Benacerraf BR, Nadel A, Bromley B. Identification of second-trimester fetuses with autosomal trisomy by use of a sonographic scoring index. *Radiology* 1994;193:135-140.
123. Nyberg DA, Luthy DA, Winter TC. The "genetic sonogram": computerized calculation of patient specific risk for fetal Down syndrome abstract. *Ultrasound Obstet Gynecol* 1996; 8:202.

CHAPTER 41

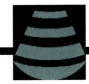

The Fetal Musculoskeletal System

Phyllis Glanc, M.D., F.R.C.P.C.
David Chitayat, M.D., F.C.C.M.G., F.A.B.M.G., F.R.C.P.C.
E. Michel Azouz, M.D., F.R.C.P.C.

CHAPTER OUTLINE

The skeletal dysplasias are a heterogeneous group of disorders affecting the growth and development of the musculoskeletal system. The **prevalence of skeletal dysplasias** diagnosed prenatally or during the neonatal period is **2.4 to 4.5 per 10,000**, and over 200 subtypes have been reported (Table 41-1).[1,2] The majority of cases have no family history. Many fetal skeletal dysplasias can be accurately identified by ultrasound, but that remains a challenging task because of the low incidence and wide range of appearances of these anomalies. Fortunately, the **majority of lethal anomalies**, including thanatophoric dysplasia, achondrogenesis, and osteogenesis imperfecta type IIA, can be **diagnosed**

solely on the basis of **antenatal ultrasound.**[3] Often a combination of ultrasound, radiologic and pathologic investigations, and DNA analysis is necessary to classify a given musculoskeletal dysplasia. A prenatal diagnosis of a musculoskeletal anomaly will provide an opportunity for genetic counseling, pregnancy termination, or tertiary level care where appropriate. A **multidisciplinary team approach** involving the sonographer, obstetrician, perinatologist, and medical geneticist will optimize the accuracy of prognosis and recurrence risk. This information is crucial to the family and to medical personnel involved in planning clinical management for the current as well as for future pregnancies. A **"key features" approach to the sonographic diagnosis** of the common skeletal dysplasias will simplify the differential diagnosis.

NORMAL FETAL SKELETON

Development

The high level of intrinsic contrast the fetal extremities provide place them among the earliest structures that can be evaluated on ultrasound. By the end of the embryonic period, the differentiation of bones, joints, and musculature is similar to that of an adult, and muscular activity has begun.[4] Transvaginal ultrasound can demonstrate the limb buds by 7 weeks' gestation; the foot and hand plates are visible by 8 weeks' gestation.[5] Osteogenesis begins in the clavicle and mandible by 8 weeks' gestation. By 11 to 12 weeks, the primary ossification centers of the long bones, scapulae, and ilia as well as the limb articulations and phalanges can be identified. The ischium, metacarpals, and metatarsals ossify during the fourth month of gestation. The pubis, calcaneus, and talus ossify during the fifth and sixth months. Ossification of the other tarsal and carpal bones occurs postnatally.[6] The direction of growth in the long bones is from proximal to distal, and the lower extremities lag slightly behind the upper extremities.[4]

Of the secondary ossification centers, only the **distal femoral epiphysis** (**DFE**), the **proximal tibial epiphysis** (**PTE**), and occasionally the **proximal** humeral epiphysis **ossify prenatally**. The unossified epiphysis appears hypoechoic, with a variably, mildly echogenic center. Ossification begins centrally. The **DFE** can ossify as early as 29 weeks' menstrual age and as late as 34 weeks. When it measures >7mm, the menstrual age is generally greater than 37 weeks.[7,8] The **PTE** begins to ossify by 35 menstrual weeks.[8] In the normal fetus the combination of a DFE greater than or equal to 3 mm and the presence of a PTE is a reliable **predictor** of **pulmonic maturity**.[9] Intrauterine growth retardation may delay ossification of the DFE and PTE.

The **fascial planes** are echogenic compared to the relatively hypoechoic cartilage. The **fetal musculature** is slightly more echogenic than cartilage. The **fetal joint spaces,** in particular the knee, appear echogenic because of the combination of synovium, fat, and microvasculature.[4]

The normal development and ultimate **function** of the fetal musculoskeletal system **depend on fetal movements** that occur by the second half of the first trimester. In the absence of normal fetal motion, the bones will be underdeveloped. Joint contractures and postural deformities may also occur.

TABLE 41-1
APPROXIMATE BIRTH PREVALENCE OF SKELETAL DYSPLASIAS

Skeletal Dysplasia	Approximate Birth Prevalence per 100,000
LETHAL DYSPLASIAS	
Thanatophoric dysplasia	2.4 to 6.9
Achondrogenesis	0.9 to 2.3
Osteogenesis imperfecta type IIA	1.8
Hypophosphatasia congenita	1.0
VARIABLE-PROGNOSIS DYSPLASIAS	
Rhizomelic CDP	0.5 to 0.9
Campomelic dysplasia	1.0 to 1.5
Asphyxiating thoracic dystrophy	0.8 to 1.4
Chondroectodermal dysplasia	0.7
Osteogenesis imperfecta (other types)	1.8
NONLETHAL DYSPLASIAS	
Heterozygous Achondroplasia	3.3 to 3.8
OVERALL	**24.4 to 75.0**

Extremity Measurements

It is standard practice to assess **femur length** as part of the routine evaluation of fetal size and morphology. Although measurement of the other long bones is not required in a routine obstetric ultrasound, an overall evaluation of the fetal skeleton should be performed to ensure the **presence** and **bilateral symmetry of the tubular bones.** Available charts provide guidance for correlating the length of the extremities with the gestational age (Table 41-2).

The **longest femur measurement, excluding** both the **proximal and distal epiphyses**, is usually chosen. The inclusion of the "distal femur point," or the specular reflection of the lateral aspect of the DFE cartilage, is the most common reason for **overestimating femur length** (Fig. 41-1, *A*).[10] An oblique femur length measurement will result in **undermeasurement.** The lateral border of the femur in the near field of the transducer appears straight, whereas the medial border of the femur in the far field has a curved appearance (Fig. 41-1, *B*).[11]

In the **lower extremity,** the lateral bone is the fibula and the medial bone is the tibia. The tibia and fibula end at the same level distally. In the **upper extremity,** pronation may cause the radius and ulna to "cross" so it will be difficult to distinguish the ulna from the radius by utilizing lateral and medial positions. The ulna is distinguished from the radius by its longer proximal extent and its relationship to the fifth digit distally (Fig. 41-2). The radius and ulna end at the same level distally.

TABLE 41-2

NORMAL EXTREMITY LONG-BONE LENGTHS AND BIPARIETAL DIAMETERS AT DIFFERENT MENSTRUAL AGES*

Menstrual Age	Biparietal Diameter	Bone					
		Femur	Tibia	Fibula	Humerus	Radius	Ulna
13	2.3 (0.3)	1.1 (0.2)	0.9 (0.2)	0.8 (0.2)	1.0 (0.2)	0.6 (0.2)	0.8 (0.3)
14	2.7 (0.3)	1.3 (0.2)	1.0 (0.2)	0.9 (0.3)	1.2 (0.2)	0.8 (0.2)	1.0 (0.2)
15	3.0 (0.1)	1.5 (0.2)	1.3 (0.2)	1.2 (0.2)	1.4 (0.2)	1.1 (0.1)	1.2 (0.1)
16	3.3 (0.2)	1.9 (0.3)	1.6 (0.3)	1.5 (0.3)	1.7 (0.2)	1.4 (0.3)	1.6 (0.3)
17	3.7 (0.3)	2.2 (0.3)	1.8 (0.3)	1.7 (0.2)	2.0 (0.4)	1.5 (0.3)	1.7 (0.3)
18	4.2 (0.5)	2.5 (0.3)	2.2 (0.3)	2.1 (0.3)	2.3 (0.3)	1.9 (0.2)	2.2 (0.3)
19	4.4 (0.4)	2.8 (0.3)	2.5 (0.3)	2.3 (0.3)	2.6 (0.3)	2.1 (0.3)	2.4 (0.3)
20	4.7 (0.4)	3.1 (0.3)	2.7 (0.2)	2.6 (0.2)	2.9 (0.3)	2.4 (0.2)	2.7 (0.4)
21	5.0 (0.5)	3.5 (0.4)	3.0 (0.4)	2.9 (0.4)	3.2 (0.4)	2.7 (0.4)	3.0 (0.4)
22	5.5 (0.5)	3.6 (0.3)	3.2 (0.3)	3.1 (0.3)	3.3 (0.3)	2.8 (0.5)	3.1 (0.4)
23	5.8 (0.5)	4.0 (0.4)	3.6 (0.2)	3.4 (0.2)	3.7 (0.3)	3.1 (0.4)	3.5 (0.2)
24	6.1 (0.5)	4.2 (0.3)	3.7 (0.3)	3.6 (0.3)	3.8 (0.4)	3.3 (0.4)	3.6 (0.4)
25	6.4 (0.5)	4.6 (0.3)	4.0 (0.3)	3.9 (0.4)	4.2 (0.4)	3.5 (0.3)	3.9 (0.4)
26	6.8 (0.5)	4.8 (0.4)	4.2 (0.3)	4.0 (0.3)	4.3 (0.3)	3.6 (0.4)	4.0 (0.3)
27	7.0 (0.3)	4.9 (0.3)	4.4 (0.3)	4.2 (0.3)	4.5 (0.2)	3.7 (0.3)	4.1 (0.2)
28	7.3 (0.5)	5.3 (0.5)	4.5 (0.4)	4.4 (0.3)	4.7 (0.4)	3.9 (0.4)	4.4 (0.5)
29	7.6 (0.5)	5.3 (0.5)	4.6 (0.3)	4.5 (0.3)	4.8 (0.4)	4.0 (0.5)	4.5 (0.4)
30	7.7 (0.6)	5.6 (0.3)	4.8 (0.5)	4.7 (0.3)	5.0 (0.5)	4.1 (0.6)	4.7 (0.3)
31	8.2 (0.7)	6.0 (0.6)	5.1 (0.3)	4.9 (0.5)	5.3 (0.4)	4.2 (0.3)	4.9 (0.4)
32	8.5 (0.6)	6.1 (0.6)	5.2 (0.4)	5.1 (0.4)	5.4 (0.4)	4.4 (0.6)	5.0 (0.6)
33	8.6 (0.4)	6.4 (0.5)	5.4 (0.5)	5.3 (0.3)	5.6 (0.5)	4.5 (0.5)	5.2 (0.3)
34	8.9 (0.5)	6.6 (0.6)	5.7 (0.5)	5.5 (0.4)	5.8 (0.5)	4.7 (0.5)	5.4 (0.5)
35	8.9 (0.7)	6.7 (0.6)	5.8 (0.4)	5.6 (0.4)	5.9 (0.6)	4.8 (0.6)	5.4 (0.4)
36	9.1 (0.7)	7.0 (0.7)	6.0 (0.6)	5.6 (0.5)	6.0 (0.6)	4.9 (0.5)	5.5 (0.3)
37	9.3 (0.9)	7.2 (0.4)	6.1 (0.4)	6.0 (0.4)	6.1 (0.4)	5.1 (0.3)	5.6 (0.4)
38	9.5 (0.6)	7.4 (0.6)	6.2 (0.3)	6.0 (0.4)	6.4 (0.3)	5.1 (0.5)	5.8 (0.6)
39	9.5 (0.6)	7.6 (0.8)	6.4 (0.7)	6.1 (0.6)	6.5 (0.6)	5.3 (0.5)	6.0 (0.6)
40	9.9 (0.8)	7.7 (0.4)	6.5 (0.3)	6.2 (0.1)	6.6 (0.4)	5.3 (0.3)	6.0 (0.5)
41	9.7 (0.6)	7.7 (0.4)	6.6 (0.4)	6.3 (0.5)	6.6 (0.4)	5.6 (0.4)	6.3 (0.5)
42	10.0 (0.5)	7.8 (0.7)	6.8 (0.5)	6.7 (0.7)	6.8 (0.7)	5.7 (0.5)	6.5 (0.5)

*Mean values (cm); value of 2 SD in parentheses

From Merz E, Mi-Sook KK, Pehl S. Ultrasonic mensuration of fetal limb bones in the second and third trimesters. *J Clin Ultrasound* 1987;5:175.

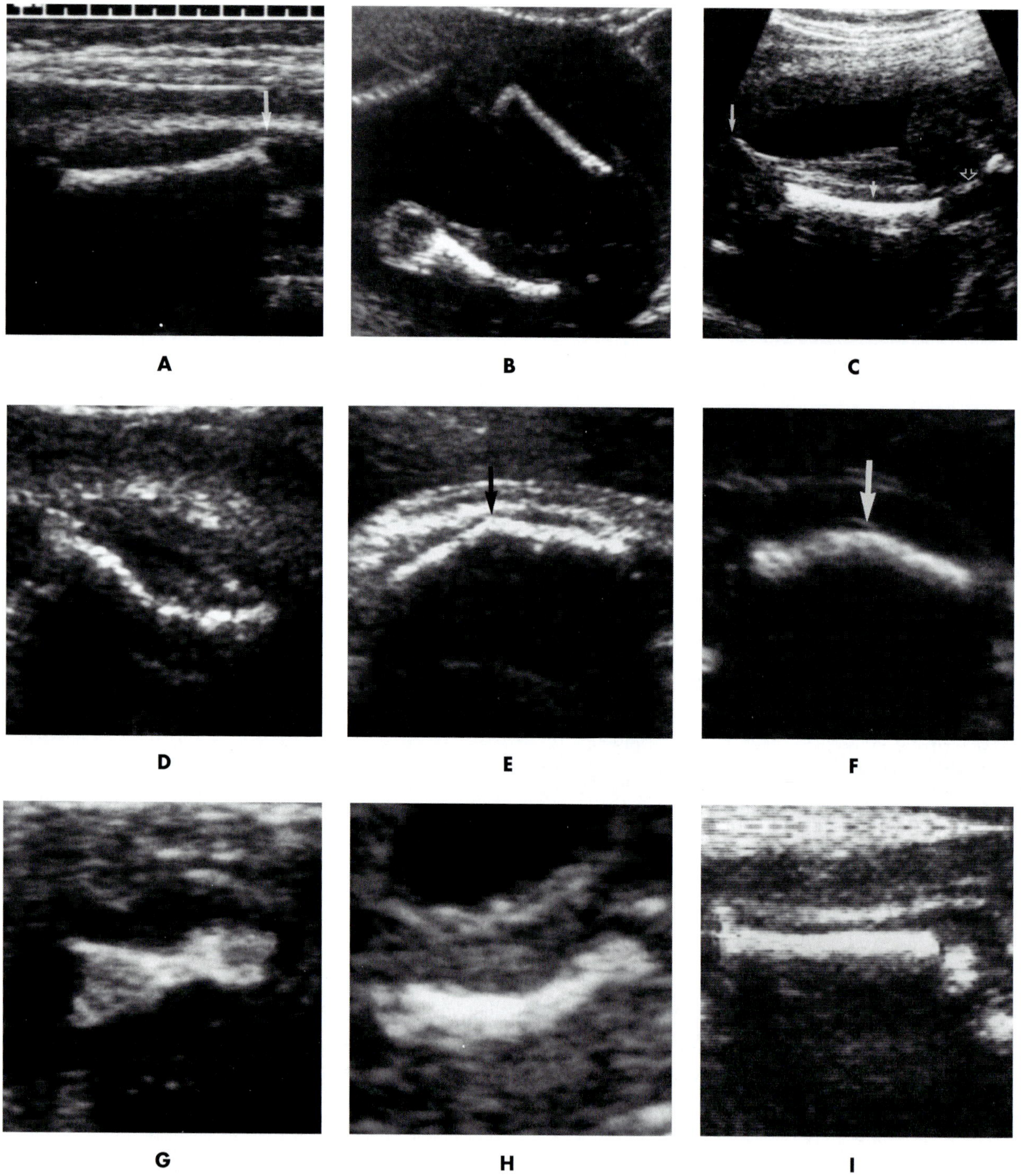

FIG. 41-1. Femurs: normal and abnormal appearance. A, **Normal femur:** measure the longest length, excluding the proximal and distal epiphysis and the specular reflection of the lateral aspect of the distal femoral epiphysis (*arrow*). **B, Normal femur** in the near field, straight lateral border versus the curved medial border in the far field of the transducer. **C, Isolated hypoplastic left** femur (*open arrow*), normal tibia (*small arrow*) and foot (*arrow*). **D, Osteogenesis imperfecta type IIA**: Innumerable fractures with exuberant callus formation result in a "wrinkled" bone contour. **E, Osteogenesis imperfecta type I**: isolated femoral fracture with acute angulation (*arrow*). **F, Campomelic dysplasia**: mild shortening and a gentle curved ventral femoral bowing (*arrow*). **G, Hypophosphatasia congenita**: severe micromelia (relatively broad metaphysis, short diaphysis). **H, Thanatophoric dysplasia:** curved, "telephone receiver" femur. **I, Chondrodysplasia punctata:** third trimester appearance of a stippled epiphysis. (C only, courtesy of Ants Toi, M.D., University of Toronto; D and E only, courtesy of Shia Salem, M.D., University of Toronto.)

The **clavicles** grow in a linear fashion, approximately **1 mm per week.** The gestational age in weeks is approximately the length of the clavicle in millimeters from 14 weeks to term. By 40 weeks' gestation they measure approximately 40 mm.[12]

Foot length is a useful parameter to use when estimating gestational age.[13,14] The foot is measured from the skin edge overlying the calcaneus to the distal end of the longest toe (the first or second toe) on either the plantar or the sagittal view (Fig. 41-3). The ossified femur length is almost equivalent to the foot length, so the **femur length to foot length ratio equals 1.0.** If the fetus is constitutionally small or there is symmetric intrauterine growth retardation, the ratio is generally greater than or equal to 0.9. In most skeletal dysplasias characterized by limb shortening, the ratio is generally less than 0.9 because of the relative sparing of the hands and feet.

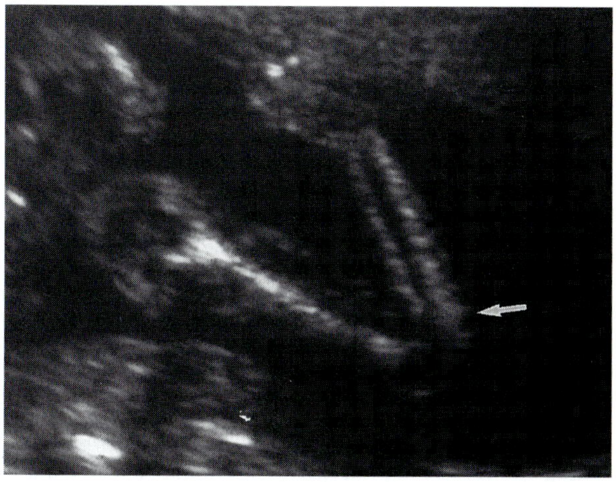

FIG. 41-2. Upper extremity. The radius and ulna end at the same level distally; the ulna is distinguished by its longer proximal extent (*arrow*) at the elbow.

Approach to the Sonographic Evaluation of a Fetus with Skeletal Dysplasia

A prenatal evaluation of a skeletal dysplasia is indicated if there is a positive family history or an abnormal length or appearance of the bones on sonography.[15,16]

Positive Family History. A positive family history of a sibling or parents having skeletal dysplasia or consanguineous parents should prompt an intensive ultrasound investigation with a focus on targeted abnormalities and serial measurements. A his-

KEY FEATURES IN THE ASSESSMENT OF SKELETAL DYSPLASIAS

Family history
Serial measurements
Degree of limb shortening
Pattern of limb shortening
Presence of bowing, fractures, angulations
Spine
Thoracic measurements
Hands and feet
Calvarium and facial features

A

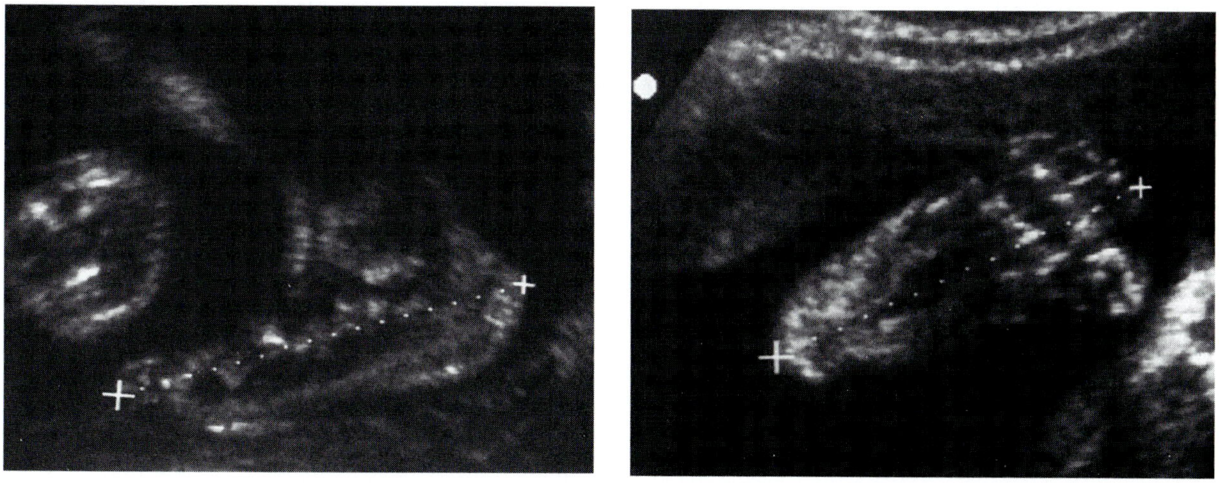

B

FIG. 41-3. Foot length measurement. From the skin edge overlying the calcaneus to the distal end of the longest toe. **A,** Sagittal measurement; note the normal squared appearance of the heel. **B,** Plantar measurement.

tory of consanguinity is important, as many of the skeletal dysplasias have an autosomal recessive mode of inheritance. Heterozygous achondroplasia, the most common of the nonlethal skeletal dysplasias, has an autosomal dominant pattern of inheritance. Unfortunately, 80% of cases are due to a new dominant mutation.

Abnormal Length or Appearance of the Bones. An **abnormal femur length** is traditionally defined as below −2 standard deviations (SD) for gestational age.[16,17] Using this cut-off, 2.5% of all fetuses would be classified as having short limbs, which exceeds the expected frequency of skeletal dysplasias, so further investigations will be needed to distinguish the fetus with a skeletal dysplasia. When there is a positive family history or the ultrasound findings suggest shortened long bones, a detailed assessment of fetal morphology and determination of the degree of limb shortening[16] is performed.

When one or all of the long bones measure below −2SD for gestational age, a follow-up ultrasound should be done in 3 to 4 weeks to evaluate interval growth. **If interval femur growth is normal, there is a high likelihood that the fetus does not have skeletal dysplasia.** However, if further deviation from the mean by at least 1 SD is detected, it should suggest the presence of a skeletal dysplasia or intrauterine growth retardation (IUGR). When the femur length measures below −4 SD for gestational age there is a high likelihood of a skeletal dysplasia. Kurtz et al.[16] have shown that the number of millimeters below the 2SD line is a simple screening tool to evaluate **femoral shortening** with the following guidelines:

- If the **femur length is 1 to 4 mm below the −2SD line, further serial measurements are required** to determine if a skeletal dysplasia is present.
- If the **femur length is >5 mm below −2SD, there is a high likelihood of a skeletal dysplasia.**

Occasionally, severe IUGR may manifest predominantly as shortened extremities. Associated findings of normal or decreased skin-fold measurements, oligohydramnios, and abnormal umbilical artery waveforms are suggestive of the diagnosis of IUGR,[18] whereas redundant, thickened skin folds and polyhydramnios are a common accompaniment of short-limb dysplasias. **As a rule, the earlier the detection of limb shortening, the worse the prognosis.**

Patterns of limb shortening[3,19] should be assessed to determine which long-bone segments are most severely affected (Fig. 41-4). Rather than millimeters, we find it useful to standardize measurements to weeks of size to determine disproportion. There are four main patterns: **rhizomelia**, shortening of the proximal segment (femur and humerus); **mesomelia**, shortening of the middle segment (radius, ulna and tibia, fibula); **acromelia**, shortening of the distal segment (hands and feet); and **micromelia**, shortening of the entire limb (mild, mild and bowed, or severe).

PATTERNS OF LIMB SHORTENING

Rhizomelia: Shortening of the proximal segment
Femur and humerus
Mesomelia: Shortening of the middle segment
Radius, ulna and tibia, fibula
Acromelia: Shortening of the distal segment
Hands and feet
Micromelia: Shortening of the entire limb
Mild, mild and bowed, severe

The **shape, contour, and density** of the bones should be assessed for the presence of bowing, angulations, fractures, or thickening. Anterior bowing of the tibia and also of the femur and humerus may suggest the diagnosis of campomelic dysplasia. Bone **fractures** may appear as angulations or interruptions in the bone contour or as thick, "wrinkled" contours corresponding to callus formation (Fig. 41-1, *D*). Decreased or absent acoustic shadowing is a marker for **decreased mineralization** of the long bones. When evident, this is helpful, but in its absence the bone mineralization may still be abnormal. The most reliable sign of demineralization is abnormal compressibility of the calvarium. Osteogenesis imperfecta type IIA typically presents with signs of abnormal mineralization and bone fractures.

The **spine** is assessed for segmentation anomalies, kyphoscoliosis, platyspondyly, demineralization, myelodysplasia, and caudal regression syndromes. Although platyspondyly is the most common spine abnormality, it is a difficult prenatal diagnosis.[20] Demineralization of the spine can result in the appearance of "ghost vertebrae" or in the nonvisualization of the three ossification centers of the spine. A progressively narrowed lumbar interpedicular distance is associated with achondroplasia; a widened interpedicular distance is associated with myelodysplasia.

The **thoracic circumference** is measured at the level of the four-chamber heart and compared to nomograms (Table 41-3 on p. 1208). The **thoracic length** (from the neck to the diaphragm) is also measured, and the ribs are assessed to determine if they are short (Table 41-4 on p. 1209). A short, narrow thorax usually implies pulmonary hypoplasia, the single most important factor in determining whether or not a given anomaly is lethal or nonlethal. A thoracic to abdominal circumference ratio of < 0.8 may be abnormal.

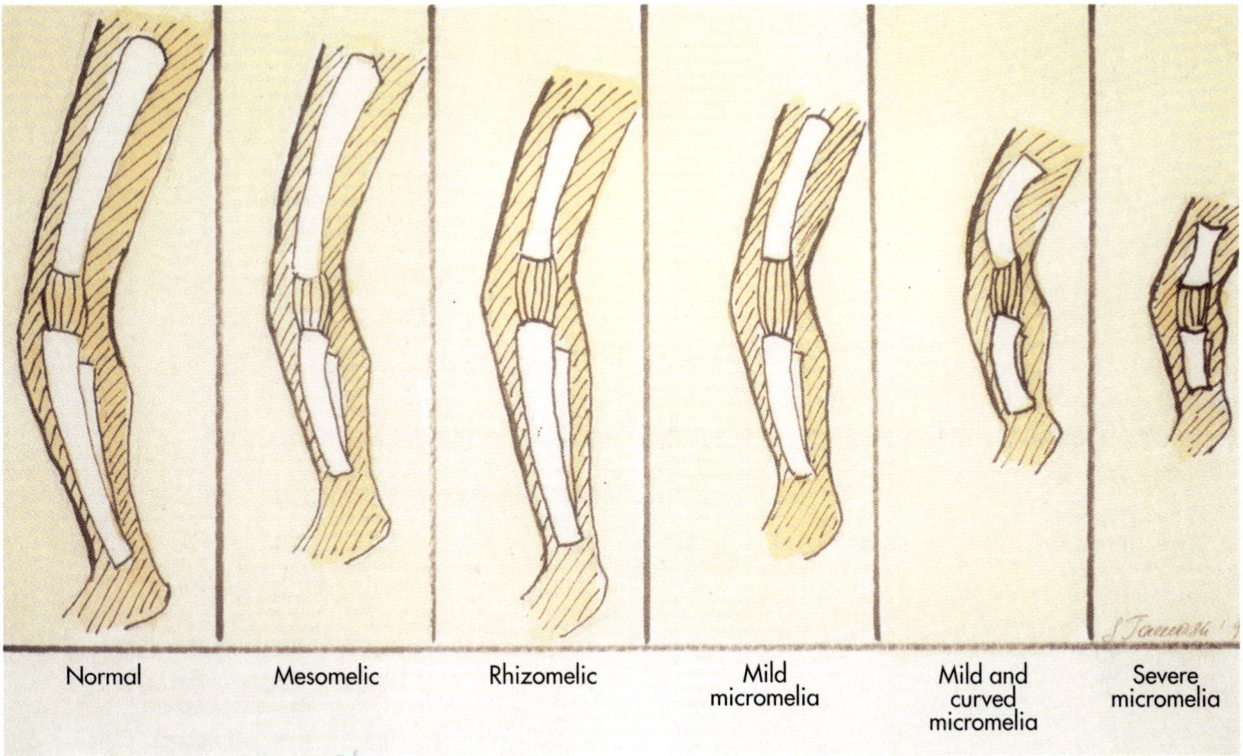

FIG. 41-4. Patterns of limb shortening. Normal, mesomelia, rhizomelia, mild micromelia, mild and curved micromelia, and severe micromelia. (Drawing courtesy of J. Tomash, M.D., University of Toronto.)

The **hands and feet** are examined for typical deformities such as clubfoot or clubhand. A hitchhiker thumb or abducted thumb is associated with diastrophic dwarfism. Fixed postural deformities may suggest the diagnosis of arthrogryphosis. **Polydactyly** is associated with short-rib polydactyly dysplasias, chondroectodermal dysplasia, and asphyxiating thoracic dystrophy, as well as with chromosomal abnormalities.

The fetal **cranium** is assessed for the presence of macrocranium, frontal bossing, cloverleaf skull deformity, underlying brain abnormalities, and facial abnormalities such as saddle nose, hypertelorism, and cleft lip and palate. Abnormal calvarial mineralization, as in osteogenesis imperfecta or hypophosphatasia congenita, may result in skull compressibility and an abnormally bright or echogenic falx compared to the demineralized calvarium.

Role of Radiographs. The role of **prenatal radiography** is **limited**. Typically, two films might be performed: an AP view, placing the fetus over the hollow of the pelvis, and an angulated view with the fetus projected down, away from the sacrum. The appearance of short limbs of normal shape and the presence of growth recovery lines can be useful in distinguishing severe intrauterine growth retardation from a skeletal dysplasia.[18] **Postnatal radiography,** in contrast, plays an extremely **important** role in completing the diagnosis of skeletal dysplasias by evaluating the characteristic radiologic features found in many skeletal anomalies.

In many cases, the diagnosis remains unknown, and consultation with registries such as the International Skeletal Registry in Los Angeles, California, may be helpful.

LETHAL SKELETAL DYSPLASIAS

The lethal skeletal dysplasias are characterized by **severe micromelia** and **decreased thoracic circumference** with **pulmonary hypoplasia**. Death is caused by **pulmonary hypoplasia** as a result of a hypoplastic thorax. Associated findings include polyhydramnios and thick, redundant skin folds. Polyhydramnios may be related to esophageal compression by the small chest, gastrointestinal abnormalities, and hypotonia. In many of the short-limb skeletal dysplasias, the skin and subcutaneous layers continue to grow at a rate proportionately greater than the long bones, resulting

TABLE 41-3
NORMAL THORACIC CIRCUMFERENCE (CM) CORRELATED WITH MENSTRUAL AGE

Gestational Age (Weeks)	No.	Predictive Percentiles								
		2.5	5	10	25	50	75	90	95	97.5
16	6	5.9	6.4	7.0	8.0	9.1	10.3	11.3	11.9	12.4
17	22	6.8	7.3	7.9	8.9	10.1	11.2	12.2	12.8	13.3
18	31	7.7	8.2	8.8	9.8	11.0	12.1	13.1	13.7	14.2
19	21	8.6	9.1	9.7	10.7	11.9	13.0	14.0	14.6	15.1
20	20	9.5	10.0	10.6	11.7	12.9	13.9	15.0	15.5	16.0
21	30	10.4	11.0	11.6	12.6	13.7	14.8	15.8	16.4	16.9
22	18	11.3	11.9	12.5	13.5	14.6	15.7	16.7	17.3	17.8
23	21	12.2	12.8	13.4	14.4	15.5	16.6	17.6	18.2	18.8
24	27	13.2	13.7	14.3	15.3	16.4	17.5	18.5	19.1	19.7
25	20	14.1	14.6	15.2	16.2	17.3	18.4	19.4	20.0	20.6
26	25	15.0	15.5	16.1	17.1	18.2	19.3	20.3	21.0	21.5
27	24	15.9	16.4	17.0	18.0	19.1	20.2	21.3	21.9	22.4
28	24	16.8	17.3	17.9	18.9	20.0	21.2	22.2	22.8	23.3
29	24	17.7	18.2	18.8	19.8	21.0	22.1	23.1	23.7	24.2
30	27	18.6	19.1	19.7	20.7	21.9	23.0	24.0	24.6	25.1
31	24	19.5	20.0	20.6	21.6	22.8	23.9	24.9	25.5	26.0
32	28	20.4	20.9	21.5	22.6	23.7	24.8	25.8	26.4	26.9
33	27	21.3	21.8	22.5	23.5	24.6	25.7	26.7	27.3	27.8
34	25	22.2	22.8	23.4	24.4	25.5	26.6	27.6	28.2	28.7
35	20	23.1	23.7	24.3	25.3	26.4	27.5	28.5	29.1	29.6
36	23	24.0	24.6	25.2	26.2	27.3	28.4	29.4	30.0	30.6
37	22	24.9	25.5	26.1	27.1	28.2	29.3	30.3	30.9	31.5
38	21	25.9	26.4	27.0	28.0	29.1	30.2	31.2	31.9	32.4
39	7	26.8	27.3	27.9	28.9	30.0	31.1	32.2	32.8	33.3
40	6	27.7	28.2	28.8	29.8	30.9	32.1	33.1	33.7	34.2

From Chitgara U, Rosenberg J, Chevenak FA et al. Prenatal sonographic assessment of thorax: normal values. *Am J Obstet Gynecol* 1987;156:1069.

TABLE 41-4

NORMAL THORACIC LENGTH (CM) CORRELATED WITH MENSTRUAL AGE

Gestational Age (Weeks)	No.	Predictive Percentiles								
		2.5	5	10	25	50	75	90	95	97.5
16	6	0.9	1.1	1.3	1.6	2.0	2.4	2.8	3.0	3.2
17	22	1.1	1.3	1.5	1.8	2.2	2.6	3.0	3.2	3.4
18	31	1.3	1.4	1.7	2.0	2.4	2.8	3.2	3.4	3.6
19	21	1.4	1.6	1.8	2.2	2.7	3.0	3.4	3.6	3.8
20	20	1.6	1.8	2.0	2.4	2.8	3.2	3.6	3.8	4.0
21	30	1.8	2.0	2.2	2.6	3.0	3.4	3.7	4.0	4.1
22	18	2.0	2.2	2.4	2.8	3.2	3.6	3.9	4.1	4.3
23	21	2.2	2.4	2.6	3.0	3.4	3.8	4.1	4.3	4.5
24	27	2.4	2.6	2.8	3.1	3.5	3.9	4.3	4.5	4.7
25	20	2.6	2.8	3.0	3.3	3.7	4.1	4.5	4.7	4.9
26	25	2.8	2.9	3.2	3.5	3.9	4.3	4.7	4.9	5.1
27	24	2.9	3.1	3.3	3.7	4.1	4.5	4.9	5.1	5.3
28	24	3.1	3.3	3.5	3.9	4.3	4.7	5.0	5.4	5.4
29	24	3.3	3.5	3.7	4.1	4.5	4.9	5.2	5.5	5.6
30	27	3.5	3.7	3.9	4.3	4.7	5.1	5.4	5.6	5.8
31	24	3.7	3.9	4.1	4.5	4.9	5.3	5.6	5.8	6.0
32	28	3.9	4.1	4.3	4.6	5.0	5.4	5.8	6.0	6.2
33	27	4.1	4.3	4.5	4.8	5.2	5.6	6.0	6.2	6.4
34	25	4.2	4.4	4.7	5.0	5.4	5.8	6.2	6.4	6.6
35	20	4.4	4.6	4.8	5.2	5.6	6.0	6.4	6.6	6.8
36	23	4.6	4.8	5.0	5.4	5.8	6.2	6.5	6.8	7.0
37	22	4.8	5.0	5.2	5.6	6.0	6.4	6.7	7.0	7.1
38	21	5.0	5.2	5.4	5.8	6.2	6.6	6.9	7.1	7.3
39	7	5.2	5.4	5.6	6.0	6.4	6.8	7.1	7.3	7.5
40	6	5.4	5.6	5.8	6.1	6.5	6.9	7.3	7.5	7.7

From Chitgara U, Rosenberg J, Chevenak FA et al. Prenatal sonographic assessment of thorax: normal values. *Am J Obstet Gynecol* 1987;156:1072.

TABLE 41-5
SEVERE MICROMELIA WITH DECREASED THORACIC CIRCUMFERENCE

	Bone Mineralization	Fractures	Macrocrania	Short Trunk Length
Thanatophoric dysplasia*†	Normal	No	Yes	No
Achondrogenesis	Patchy demineralization	Occasional	Yes	Yes
Osteogenesis imperfecta type II	Generalized demineralization	Innumerable	No	Yes
Hypophosphatasia	Patchy or generalized demineralization	Occasional	No	No

*Homozygous achondroplasia is similar to thanatophoric dysplasia but distinguishable as both parents are affected with the heterozygous form of achondroplasia.
†Short-rib polydactyly dysplasias are similar to thanatophoric dysplasia, but there is no macrocrania and polydactyly is present.

SONOGRAPHIC ASSESSMENT OF BONES

Long bones:
- Degree of limb shortening
- Pattern of limb shortening
- Degree of mineralization
- Presence of fractures, bowing or angulation
- Abnormal shape or contour
- Limb reduction anomalies
- Hyoplastic or aplastic bones

Spine:
- Degree and pattern of demineralization
- Platyspondyly
- Segmentation or curvature anomalies
- Caudal regression syndrome
- Myelodysplasia

Thorax:
- Thoracic length and circumference
- Hypoplastic ribs
- "Bell-shaped" thorax of pulmonary hypoplasia
- Convex contour in cross-section

Hands and feet:
- Postural deformities
- Abnormal number of digits
- Syndactyly

Calvarium:
- Macrocranium
- Frontal bossing
- Craniosynostosis
- Compressibility/abnormal degree of mineralization

Facial features:
- Cleft lip and palate
- Hypertelorism and hypotelorism
- Flat nasal bridge/"saddle nose"

IS THERE A LETHAL SKELETAL DYSPLASIA?

Characteristic features
- Severe micromelia
- Pulmonary hypoplasia

Distinguishing features
- Abnormal mineralization
- Fractures
- Presence or absence of macrocranium
- Thoracic length

in relatively thickened skin folds which can be mistaken for hydrops fetalis.

Approximately 60% of all the lethal skeletal dysplasias are either thanatophoric dysplasia or achondrogenesis. With osteogenesis imperfecta type II, these three skeletal dysplasias will account for two thirds of lethal skeletal dysplasias.[1] Pretorius et al.[3] suggest that it is possible to make the correct diagnosis of a lethal short-limbed dwarf in 85% of cases, with a correct specific diagnosis in approximately 54% of cases. The "**key features**" that are assessed include **degree of micromelia,** mineralization, macrocranium, and thoracic length and circumference (Table 41-5).

Thanatophoric Dysplasia

Thanatophoric dysplasia is the most common of the lethal skeletal dysplasias. The birth prevalence is 0.24 to 0.69 per 10,000, with a high mutation rate. The key features are **severe micromelia** with a **rhizomelic** predominance, **macrocrania,** and decreased thoracic circumference and a normal trunk length.

The extremities are so foreshortened that they tend to protrude at right angles to the body; the skin

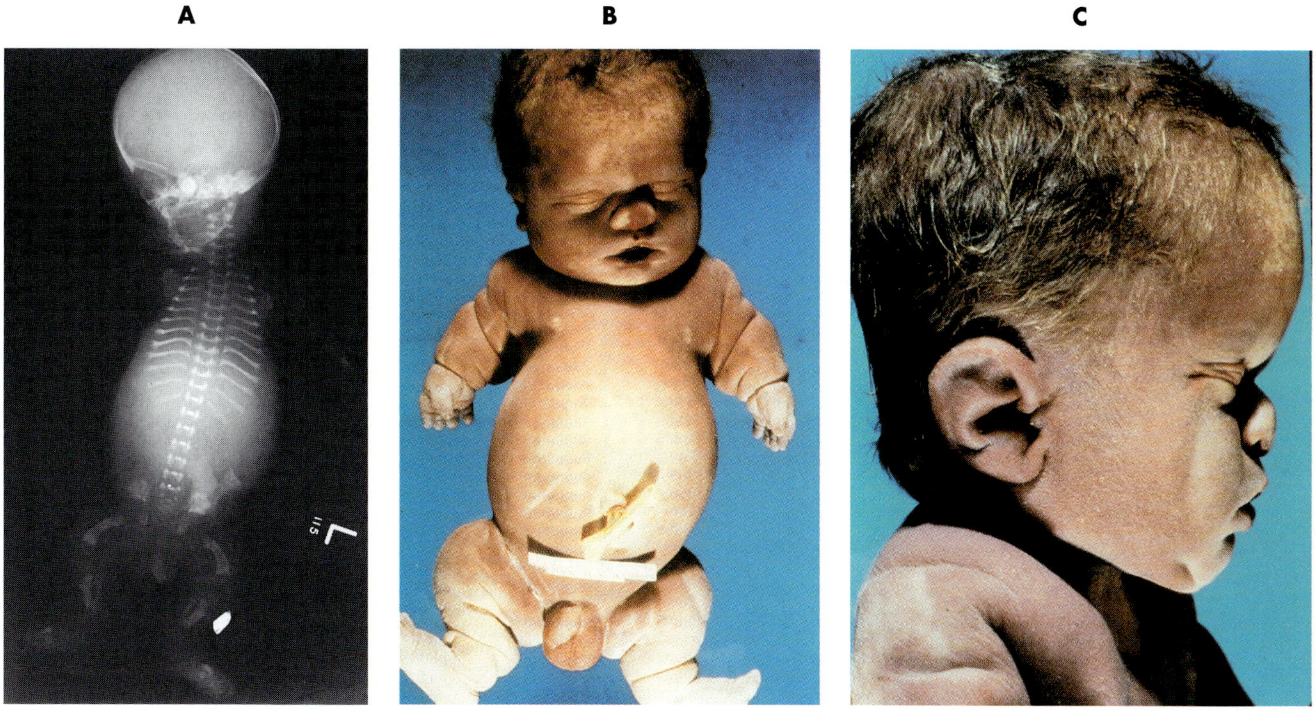

FIG. 41-5. Thanatophoric dysplasia at 33 weeks. **A,** AP radiograph shows normal mineralization, short, curved extremity bones, severe platyspondyly with U-shaped vertebral bodies, narrow thorax with shortened ribs. **B,** AP specimen photograph shows severe micromelia with relative sparing of the hands and feet, telescoping of the redundant skin folds, small, bell-shaped thorax. **C,** Profile specimen photograph shows macrocranium, frontal bossing, flattened nasal bridge.

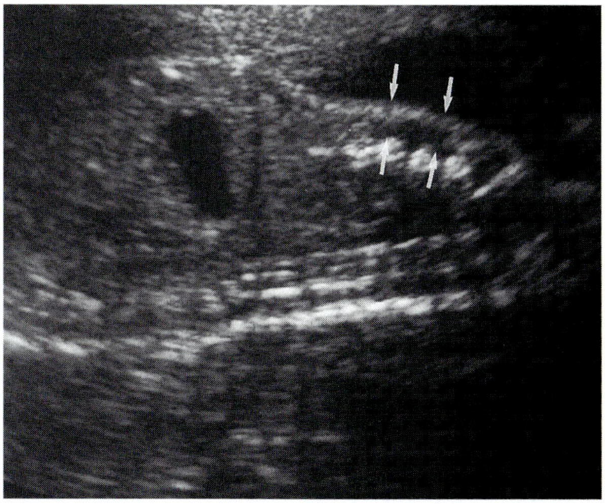

FIG. 41-6. Thanatophoric dysplasia at 33 weeks. Sagittal sonogram shows disproportionately small thorax on right and relatively protuberant abdomen on left, signifying a lethal condition on the basis of pulmonary hypoplasia; thickened redundant anterior chest wall tissues (*arrows*).

folds are thickened and redundant. Clinical presentation is commonly due to large-for-dates measurements secondary to polyhydramnios (Fig. 41-5 and Fig. 41-6).

Langer et al.[21] distinguished two types of thanatophoric dysplasia. **Type 1 (TD1),** the common form, displays the typical "**telephone receiver**" shape of the extremities (Fig. 41-1, *H*), a bowed appearance, with marked curves present at the ends of the severely shortened tubular bones. This type can occur with or without a very mild variant of cloverleaf skull deformity, frontal bossing, and a flattened nasal bridge. Platyspondyly (flattened vertebral bodies) is present.

In **type 2** (**TD2**) the **femora are typically straight**, with flared metaphyses. The most characteristic feature is the "**cloverleaf**" deformity of the skull. This is a trilobed appearance of the skull on the coronal plane that results from premature craniosynostosis of the lambdoid and coronal sutures (Fig. 41-7). Other conditions that may be associated with this unusual skull deformity are homozygous achondroplasia, campomelic dysplasia, and trisomy 13. The vertebral bodies are not as flattened as in TD1. Both types are autosomal dominant conditions caused by a new dominant mutation. They

A B

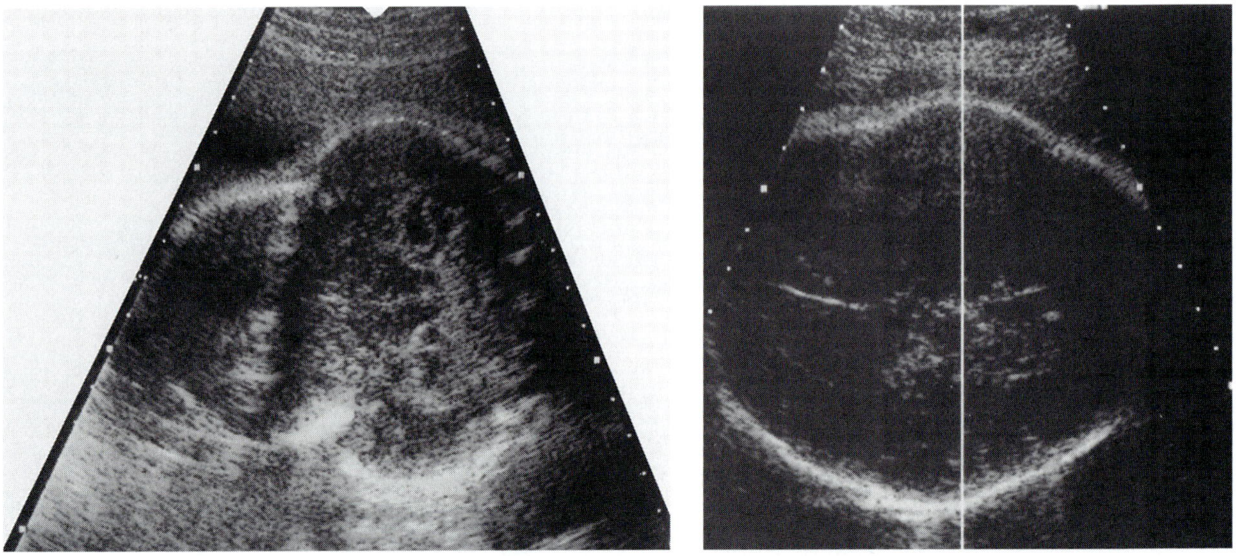

FIG. 41-7. Cloverleaf deformity of thanatophoric dysplasia. **A,** Severe variant. **B,** Mild variant. (Courtesy of Greg Ryan, M.D., University of Toronto.)

A B

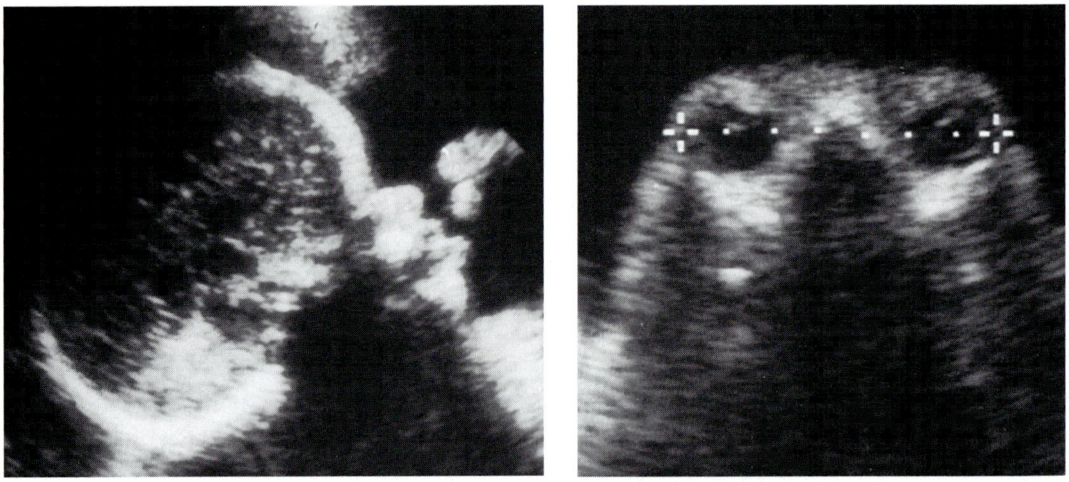

FIG. 41-8. Homozygous achondroplasia at 34 weeks. **A,** Lateral profile is similar to thanatophoric dysplasia with macrocranium, frontal bossing, and flat nasal bridge. **B,** Axial image through the orbits and nasal bones confirms a flat nasal bridge.

are associated with advanced paternal age and have a negligible recurrence risk.[22]

Thanatophoric dysplasia has many phenotypic similarities to **homozygous achondroplasia.** Both conditions may appear identical from ultrasound and radiographic perspectives. They can be distinguished by the positive family history of homozygous achondroplasia, in which both parents are affected with the heterozygous form of achondroplasia (Fig. 41-8). Mutation analysis of the gene affected in achondroplasia, the fibroblast growth factor receptor-3 (FGFR-3) reveals sporadic heterozygous mutation in both TD1 and TD2.[23] Another condition indicated by bowed tubular bones is **campomelic** dwarfism, which is distinguished from TD by a moderate and bowed form of micromelia, typically affecting the tibias and having characteristic associated anomalies.

Platyspondyly, or flattened vertebral bodies, is one of the most characteristic features on AP radiographs of a thanatophoric dwarf. There is a U or H configuration of the vertebral bodies and a relatively increased height of the disc spaces. This feature can be extremely difficult to assess on a prenatal ultrasound. Platyspondyly appears on ultrasound as a wafer-thin vertebral body with a relatively larger, hypoechoic intervertebral disc space on either side of the vertebral body (Fig. 41-9). The ratio of vertebral

A

B

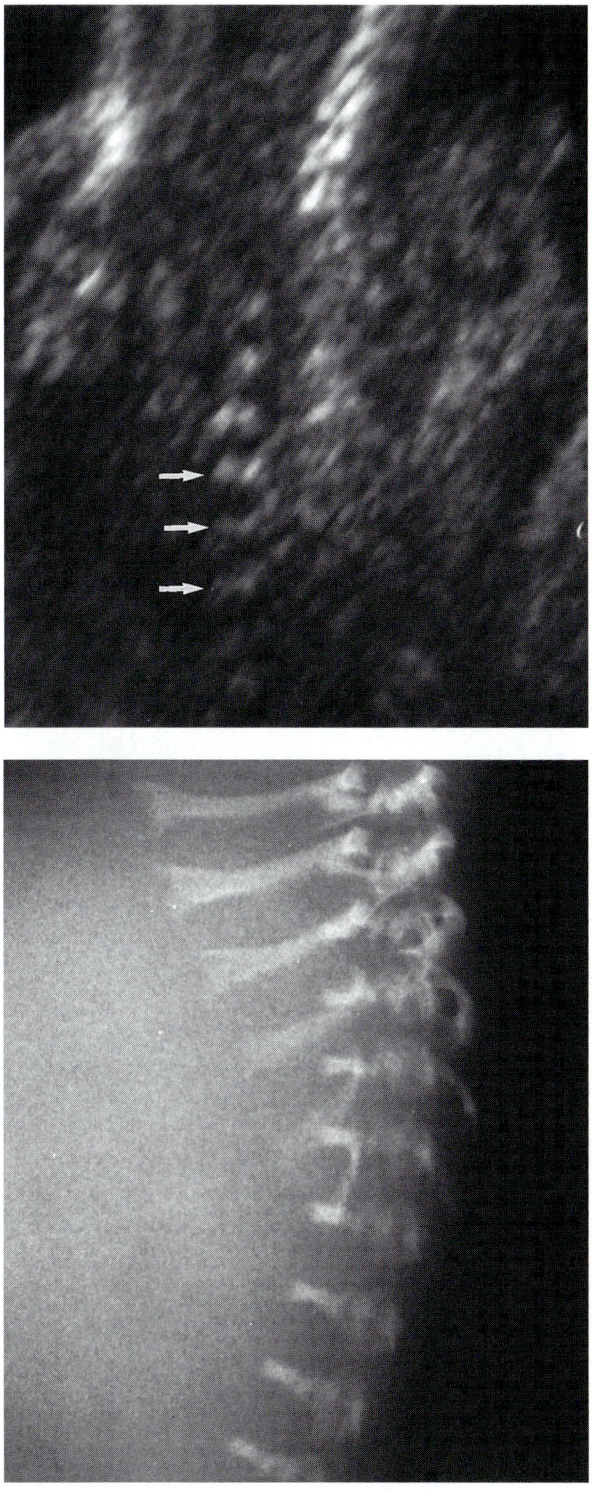

FIG. 41-9. Thanatophoric dysplasia at 33 weeks. **A,** Platyspondyly appears on ultrasound as a wafer-thin vertebral body (*arrows*) with relatively larger hypoechoic intervertebral disc space on either side of the vertebral body. **B,** Correlative lateral spine radiograph.

TABLE 41-6
ACHONDROGENESIS: KEY FEATURES (ALL HAVE DECREASED THORACIC CIRCUMFERENCE)

Prototype	Percentage	Micromelia	Fractures	Calvarial Mineralization	Vertebral Mineralization
I	20%	Severe	Occasional	Decreased	Decreased
II	20%	Severe	No	Normal	Decreased
III	40%	Moderate	No	Normal	Decreased
IV	20%	Moderate	No	Normal	Normal

body height to vertebral interspace (disc and body) in thanatophoric dysplasia is lower than in normal cases. Platyspondyly also occurs in many cases of achondrogenesis and osteogenesis imperfecta type II.[20]

Associated anomalies include **holoprosencephaly**, **agenesis of the corpus callosum**, and **ventriculomegaly**. These generally occur in association with the cloverleaf deformity. Other anomalies may include **horseshoe kidneys, hydronephrosis, congenital heart disease** (atrial septal defect and tricuspid insufficiency), **radioulnar synostosis,** and **imperforate anus.**[24]

Achondrogenesis

Achondrogenesis is the second most commonly occurring lethal skeletal dysplasia. The birth prevalence is 0.09 to 0.23 per 10,000 births. It is a phenotypically diverse group of chondrodysplasias characterized by **severe micromelia, macrocranium, decreased thoracic circumference and trunk length,** and **decreased mineralization** (Table 41-6).

The **pattern of demineralization** is most marked in the vertebral bodies, ischium, and pubic bones, leading to a markedly shortened trunk length, decreased thoracic circumference, and occasional fractures.[24-26] Classically, due to predominant demineralization of the vertebral body, only two echogenic posterior elements appear in a transverse image of the spine—the neural arches. This is in contrast to hypophosphatasia congenita where the predominant spine deossification involves the posterior elements, with only patchy involvement of the vertebral bodies. Polyhydramnios and thick, redundant skin folds are a common accompaniment.

Type 1, or the Parenti-Fraccaro form, is the most severe. Approximately 20% of cases of achondrogenesis are of this type. It is autosomal recessive and is characterized by a severe form of micromelia evidenced by short, cuboid bones and metaphyseal scalloping. There is partial or complete lack of ossification of the calvarium, vertebral bodies, and sacral and pubic bones. The ribs are thin and have occasional fractures. Due to the extremely limited skeletal frame, the subcutaneous tissues can appear grotesquely redundant and show multiple telescoped skin folds.

Type 2, or the Langer-Saldino form, accounts for 80% of cases of achondrogenesis. It is also autosomal recessive and is characterized by normal calvarial ossification and by absent ossification in the vertebral column and sacral and pubic bones (Fig. 41-10). The Langer-Saldino form demonstrates relatively longer tubular bones and body length in association with an increased survival time.

Whitley and Gorlin[25] proposed subdividing achondrogenesis into four prototypes based on roentgenographic criteria and measurements. Their prototype 1 is identical to the Parenti-Fraccaro form; prototypes 2, 3, and 4 form a spectrum of decreasing severity. The degree of micromelia is less severe and there are no rib fractures. There is normal calvarial ossification. All prototypes but prototype 4 (20%) present with severely retarded or absent skeletal ossification of the vertebral bodies and pelvic bones, leading to a markedly shortened trunk length.

These two key features of **achondrogenesis**—abnormal mineralization and shortened trunk length—distinguish it from **thanatophoric dysplasia** which has normal mineralization and a normal trunk length. Both display macrocrania and severe micromelia.

Osteogenesis Imperfecta

Osteogenesis imperfecta (OI) is a clinically and genetically heterogeneous group of collagen disorders characterized by mutations in collagen genes that result in brittle bones and multiple fractures (Table 41-7). The incidence is 1 out of 60,000; all types are autosomal dominant, apart from a subcategory of OI type III that follows an autosomal recessive mode of inheritance. **Prenatal diagnosis** is possible based on DNA extracted from chorionic villi or on collagen extracted from cultured fibroblasts obtained from chorionic villus sampling as early as 10 weeks[27] when the mutation or collagen abnormality on the proband or index case is known. A modification of the Silence classification is most commonly used to distinguish the subtypes of osteogenesis imperfecta.[28,29]

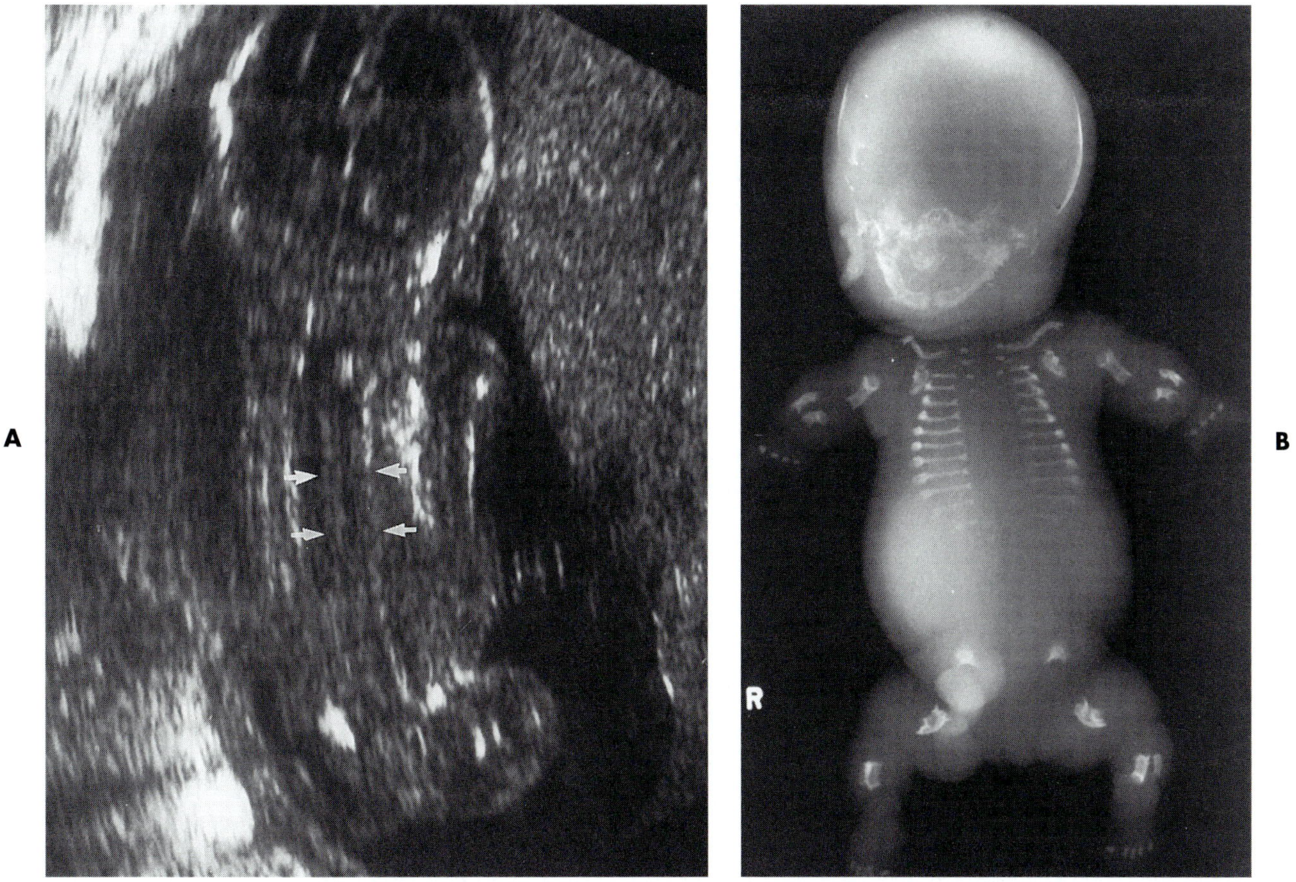

FIG. 41-10. Achondrogenesis at 18 weeks. **A,** Coronal sonogram shows small thorax, redundant subcutaneous tissues, absent spine ossification (*arrowheads*), normal calvarial ossification. **B,** Postmortem radiograph shows macrocranium, normal calvarial ossification, absent spine ossification, and severe micromelia. (Courtesy of Shia Salem, M.D., University of Toronto.)

TABLE 41-7
CLASSIFICATION OF OSTEOGENESIS IMPERFECTA: KEY FEATURES

Type	Genetics	Pattern-shortening	Beading of Ribs	Fracture	Ultrasound Mineralization	Prognosis
I	AD	None	Normal	Isolated	Normal	Good
IIA	AD	Severe micromelia	Thick and beaded	Innumerable	Decreased	Lethal
IIB	AD	Moderate 1° femur Broad bones	Minimal	Numerous	Normal	Lethal
IIC	AD	Moderate micromelia Thin bones	Thin and beaded	Numerous	Normal	Lethal
III	AD or AR	Lower than upper extremity	Thin and beaded	Many	Variable	Deforming
IV	AD	None	Normal	Isolated	Normal	Good

AD, autosomal dominant; AR, autosomal recessive

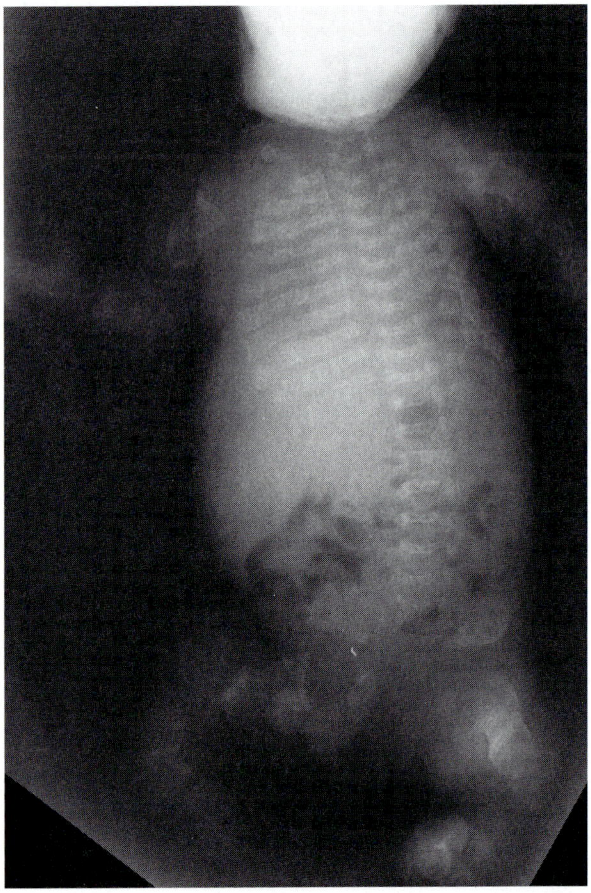

FIG. 41-11. Osteogenesis imperfecta type IIA at 32 weeks. Postmortem radiograph shows severe micromelia, thickened bone with wavy contours due to innumerable fractures and exuberant callus formation, shortened ribs with multiple fractures and platyspondylisis.

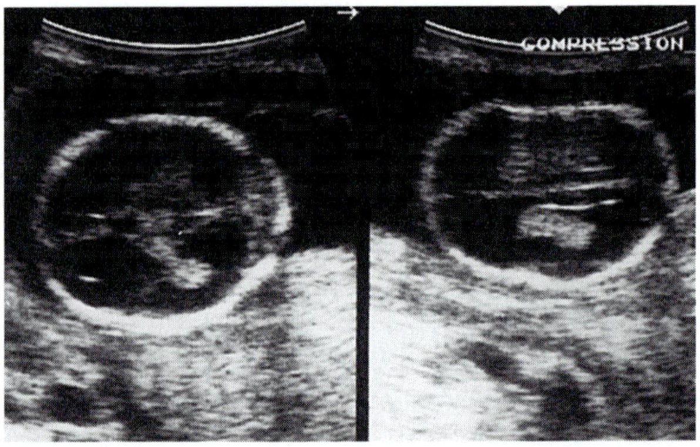

FIG. 41-12. Osteogenesis imperfecta type IIA at 17 weeks. Left image: rounded head contour. Right image: gentle transducer compression on the demineralized calvarium results in flattening of the cranial contour. (Courtesy of Ants Toi, M.D., University of Toronto.)

Osteogenesis imperfecta type II is the neonatal, lethal form. In most cases, it is the result of a new, dominant mutation in the COL1A1 gene.[29] However, the recurrence risk of only 6% to 7% is due to parental or germ-line mosaicism. Multiple repetitive *in utero* fractures occur secondary to defective collagen formation, resulting in fragile bones.

Osteogenesis imperfecta type IIA makes up 80% of the cases of OI type II and is uniformly lethal. The birth prevalence is approximately 0.18 per 10,000 births. Most cases are sporadic and can be detected on prenatal ultrasound (Fig. 41-11). The key features are **severe micromelia, decreased thoracic circumference and trunk length,** and **decreased mineralization and multiple bone fractures.**

The tubular bones exhibit a classical "accordion" or "wrinkled" contour. The bones are **angulated,** bowed, and **thickened** because of repetitive *in utero* fractures with exuberant callus formation (Fig. 41-1, *D*). The bones are **demineralized,** so there is diminished or absent acoustic shadowing. On ultrasound, the bones may appear thickened, as a demineralized bone reflects sound waves to a lesser degree than does a normally ossified bone. Multiple rib fractures cause the lateral **chest contour** to be characteristically **concave** rather than convex. The **ribs** are **hypoplastic** and have a continuous beaded or wavy appearance secondary to repetitive fractures and callus formation. **Platyspondyly** caused by compression fractures of many vertebral bodies may be present. **Demineralization of the cranial vault** can be observed by looking for a localized deformation of the cranial vault under transducer pressure (Fig. 41-12), the "bright falx sign" in which the falx appears brighter or more echogenic than the demineralized cranial vault and there is unusual clarity of detail in the near field. The cranial vault is of normal size, but the thoracic circumference is decreased and the trunk length is shortened.

In a retrospective analysis, Munoz et al.[29] concluded that if the following three criteria are fulfilled one can correctly make the specific **diagnosis of osteogenesis imperfecta type IIA: femur length is >3SD below the mean,** there is **demineralization of the calvarium,** and there are **multiple fractures within a single bone.** A normal sonogram after 17 weeks would exclude this diagnosis.

Osteogenesis imperfecta type IIB is a variably lethal autosomal dominant form with moderate shortening of the femurs. The ribs are relatively normal with incomplete beading and isolated fractures.

Osteogenesis imperfecta type IIC is a lethal autosomal dominant form with mild shortening of all the long bones. The bones remain thin, and there is mild

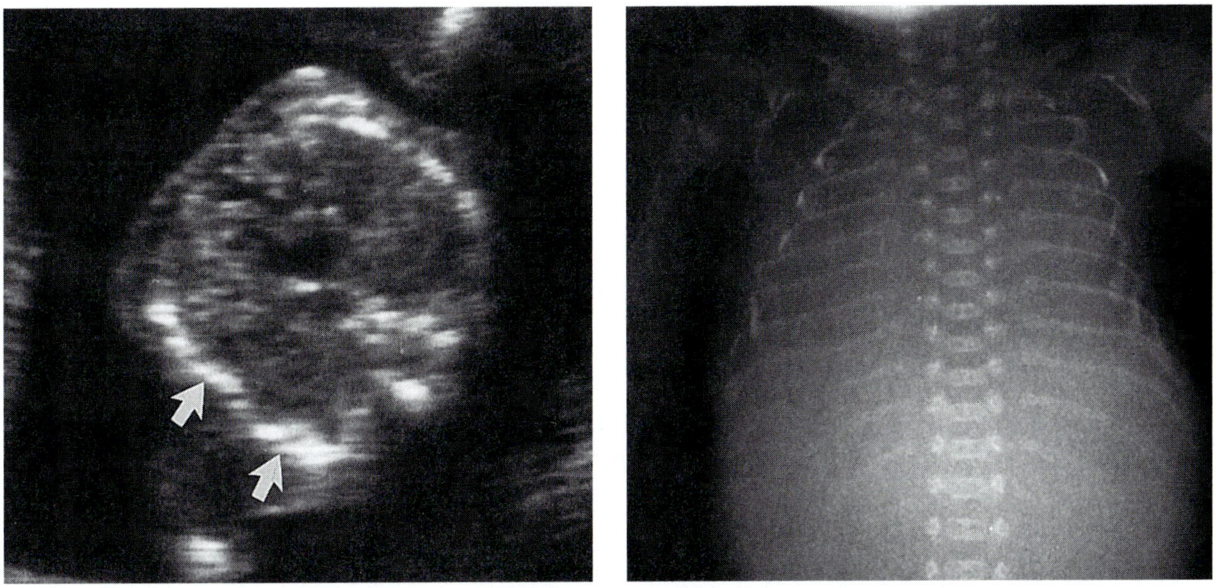

A

B

FIG. 41-13. Osteogenesis imperfecta type IIC at 20 weeks. **A,** Cross-sectional image of the thorax shows normal-length ribs with multiple fractures (*arrows*) resulting in a wavy contour. **B,** Postmortem radiograph shows the ribs are thin and have multiple fractures.

beading of the ribs (Fig. 41-13). The sclerae are normal. Osteogenesis type I, III, and IV are described in the section on nonlethal skeletal dysplasias.

Hypophosphatasia Congenita

Hypophosphatasia congenita, the lethal neonatal form of hypophosphatasia, is an autosomal recessive skeletal dysplasia caused by a **deficiency of alkaline phosphatase,** a tissue-specific isoenzyme.[30] The birth frequency of hypophosphatasia congenita is approximately 1 out of 100,000. Second trimester, detailed fetal ultrasound in combination with monoclonal antibody testing of a chorionic villus sampling and measurement of alkaline phosphatase activity in cultured amniocytes can be used for prenatal diagnosis of this disorder (Fig. 41-14).

The key features are **severe micromelia, decreased thoracic circumference with normal trunk length,** and **decreased mineralization with occasional fractures.**

The demineralized long bones may be bowed and may have occasional angulations due to **fractures.** The **cranial vault fails to mineralize** and may be compressible under locally applied transducer pressure. The **bones** are thin and **delicate** in appearance, even **entirely absent** at times. Because of the **variable expressivity** of this disorder, the demineralization can vary from a diffuse form to a patchy distribution with severe involvement of the spine and calvarium. The ribs are short, resulting in a **decreased thoracic circumference,** but the **trunk length is normal.** There is **no macrocrania**; polyhydramnios is a common finding.

The main **differential diagnosis** is osteogenesis imperfecta type IIA. Both display a severe form of micromelia, demineralization, decreased thoracic circumference, and a normal-sized cranial vault that is compressible due to demineralization. In osteogenesis imperfecta type IIA, the greater degree of bone fragility results in innumerable fractures and a thickened, wavy appearance of the bones in contrast to the thin, almost delicate appearance of the bones in hypophosphatasia congenita. The normal trunk length and cranial vault size can aid in distinguishing hypophosphatasia from achondrogenesis. Typically, in hypophosphatasia congenita, the posterior elements are poorly ossified, whereas the vertebral bodies are maximally affected in achondrogenesis.[31,32]

Campomelic Dysplasia

Campomelic dysplasia, or "bent limb" dysplasia, is a rare autosomal dominant condition resulting, in most cases, from a new dominant mutation. The reported incidence is 0.5 to 1.0 per 100,000 births. Most cases are lethal because of respiratory insufficiency on the basis of **laryngotracheomalacia** in combination with a mildly **narrowed thorax.**

The characteristic skeletal features of campomelic dysplasia are a **short and ventrally bowed tibia and femur,** a **hypoplastic or absent fibula,** and **talipes equinovarus** (clubfoot), and **hypoplastic scapulae** (Fig. 41-15).

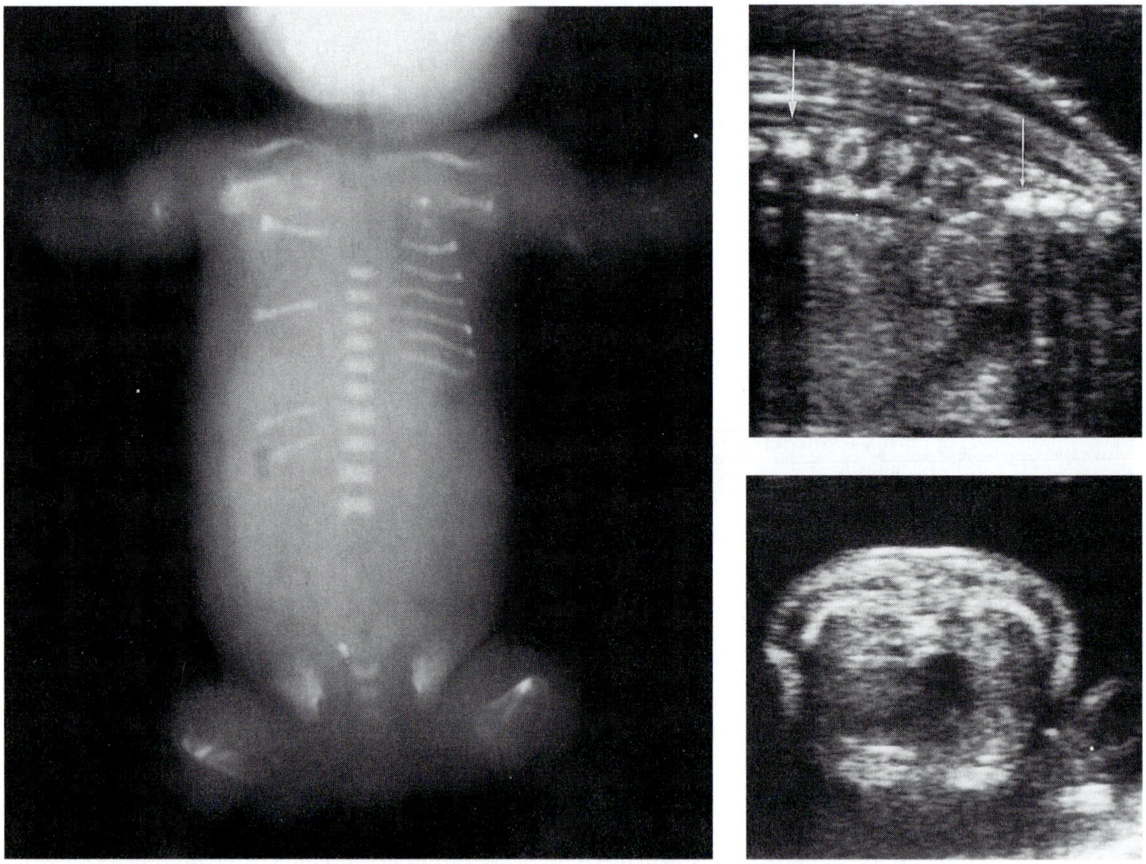

A

B

C

FIG. 41-14. Hypophosphatasia congenita at 27 weeks. **A,** Postmortem radiograph shows thin, delicate bones, "absent bones," and hypoplastic ribs in association with severe micromelia. **B,** Sagittal view of the lumbosacral spine shows normal acoustic shadowing of vertebral bodies cephalad and caudad (*arrows*) to a demineralized segment where the vertebral bodies have a "ghost" outline and no acoustic shadowing. **C,** Cross-sectional view of thorax shows hypoplastic thin ribs and absent spine ossification. Typically, the ribs encircle approximately 70% to 80% of the thorax.

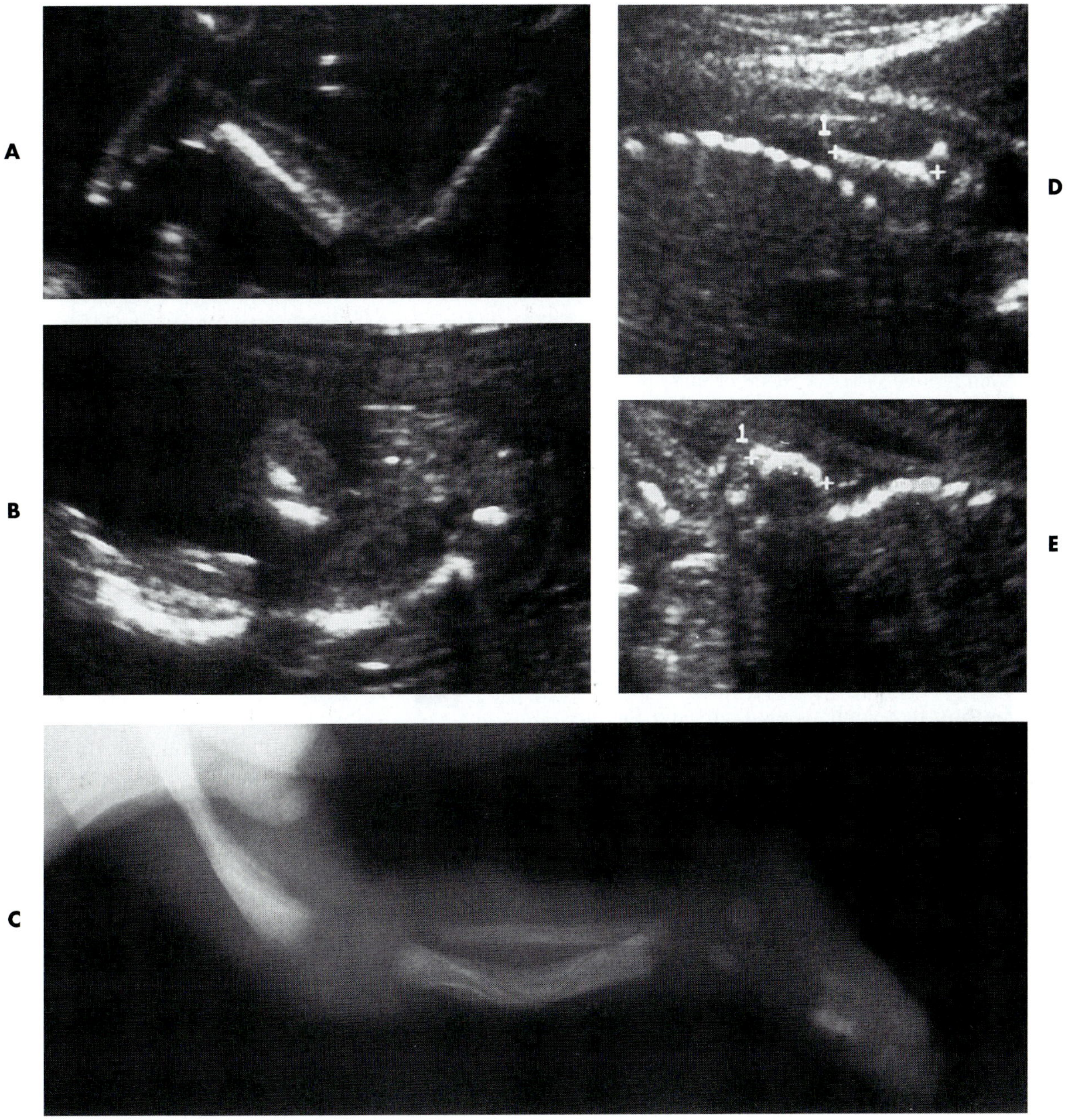

FIG. 41-15. Campomelic dysplasia of triplet B at 27 weeks. **A,** Triplet A shows the normal length and curvatures in the lower extremity. **B,** Triplet B's lower extremity shows the shortened femur and tibia with ventral bowing. **C,** Triplet B's radiograph shows ventral bowing of the tibia and femur. **D,** Triplet A: normal Y-shaped appearance of the scapula (graticules). **E,** Triplet B: short and curved dysplastic scapula (graticules). Note bell-shaped deformity of thorax, suggesting a lethal anomaly.

Bowing may also occur in the upper extremities. Other characteristic skeletal features include scoliosis, dislocated hips, and facial abnormalities. Approximately 33% of cases have congenital heart disease, brain abnormalities such as ventriculomegaly, and renal abnormalities, including pyelectasis.

Sex reversal is found in about 75% of the affected 46 XY cases, with a gradation of defects ranging from ambiguous genitalia to normal female genitalia. The gene responsible for campomelic dysplasia is sex-determining protein homeobox 9 or SOX9, which is expressed in the fetal brain, the testes, and the perichondrium and chondrocytes of the long bones and ribs.[33]

Short-Rib Polydactyly Dysplasias

Short-rib polydactyly dysplasias (SRPDs) are a heterogeneous group of **rare** and **lethal** skeletal dysplasias with an autosomal recessive mode of inheritance. All forms are characterized by **severe micromelia** and **decreased thoracic circumference.**

The cranial vault measurements and bone mineralization are normal. **Polydactyly and cardiac** and **genitourinary abnormalities** are found in most cases.

Thanatophoric dysplasia is distinguished by the absence of polydactyly and the presence of the typical facial features, macrocrania, and platyspondyly. Chondroectodermal dysplasia (CED) and asphyxiating thoracic dystrophy (ATD) have similar features, but the shortening of the limbs and the narrowing of the thorax are less severe.

The SRPDs are subdivided into four groups[30,34]: type I Saldino-Noonan; type II Majewski; type III Verma-Naumoff; and type IV Beemer-Langer (which can present without polydactyly). They can be distinguished by radiographic and clinical features.

Chondrodysplasia Punctata

Chondrodysplasia punctata (CDP), or "**stippled epiphyses,**" is a heterogeneous group of disorders that result in many small calcifications (ossification centers) in the cartilage in the ends of bones and around the spine. Among the known conditions associated with CDP are single gene disorders, such as Conradi-Hunerman CDP (X-linked dominant), rhizomelic CDP (AR), and Zellweger syndrome (cerebro-hepato-renal syndrome); chromosome abnormalities such as trisomy 21 and 18; and teratogen exposure through, e.g., warfarin or alcohol.

Rhizomelic CDP is an autosomal recessive condition caused by a peroxisomal disorder that evidences severe symmetric, predominantly rhizomelic (proximal or root) forms of limb shortening.[30,35] The incidence is approximately 1 in 110,000 births, and it is generally lethal prior to the second year of life. The humeri tend to be relatively shorter than the femora and have metaphyseal cupping. The enlarged epiphyses with the characteristic stippling may occasionally be identified on ultrasound in the third trimester (Figs. 41-1, 41-16). Other abnormalities include dysmorphic facial features, joint contractures, coronal clefting of the vertebral bodies, brain abnormalities, and severe mental retardation.

Conradi-Hunerman CDP, or the **nonrhizomelic form of CDP,** is an X-linked dominant condition with intermediate severity and good prognosis.[36] The disorder occurs exclusively in females. It is lethal in hemizygous males. The characteristic skeletal abnormalities are asymmetric dysplastic skeletal changes with bone stippling. The punctate calcifications occur predominantly in the axial skeleton, although stippling may also be identified in the long bones. Stature is usually reduced and kyphoscoliosis with shortening of the long bones, particularly the femur and humerus, and dysmorphic facial features are common.[37]

Other lethal skeletal dysplasias include atelosteogenesis, fibrochondrogenesis, boomerang dysplasia, de la Chapelle dysplasia, and Schneckenbecken dysplasia. These are rare and difficult to diagnose specifically on ultrasound.

NONLETHAL OR VARIABLE-PROGNOSIS SKELETAL DYSPLASIAS

The nonlethal skeletal dysplasias form a larger group with milder and later onset of skeletal abnormalities. The majority of the cases present with mesomelic (middle) and acromelic (distal) dysplasias and are autosomal recessive. Their diagnoses are based on clinical and radiologic findings. The nonlethal skeletal dysplasias that have characteristic ultrasound findings are described in Tables 41-8, 41-9, and 41-10.

Heterozygous Achondroplasia

This is the **most common nonlethal skeletal dysplasia.**[1] Eighty percent of cases are the result of a spontaneous dominant mutation associated with advanced paternal age, and the remainder are inherited from parental heterozygous achondroplasia. The incidence is approximately 1 out of 26,000. Previously considered a diagnosis of the third trimester, **recent studies have shown that a second trimester diagnosis is possible.**[38-40]

The key features are **mild to moderate forms of rhizomelic limb shortening** more prominent in the upper limbs; **macrocranium, frontal bossing, depressed nasal bridge, midface hypoplasia;** and **brachydactyly,** with a **trident configuration**

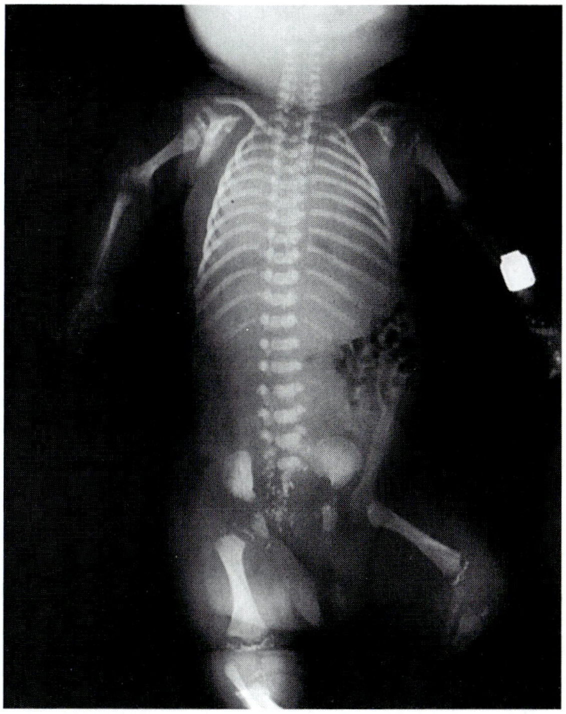

FIG. 41-16. Chondrodysplasia punctata, rhizomelic form. Stippled calcification within the epiphyseal cartilages.

TABLE 41-8
RHIZOMELIC DYSPLASIA: KEY FEATURES

Dysplasia	Prognosis	Degree of Limb Shortening	Key Sonographic Features
Heterozygous achondroplasia	Nonlethal	Mild	Progressive discrepancy FL and BPD
Chondrodysplasia punctata—rhizomelic form	Lethal	Moderate–severe	Stippled epiphysis in third trimester
Diastrophic dysplasia	Variably lethal	Mild–moderate	Hitchhiker thumb, postural deformities, dislocations, joint contractures, clubfoot

TABLE 41-9
MICROMELIC DYSPLASIA, MILD: KEY FEATURES

Dysplasia	Prognosis	Key Sonographic Features
Asphyxiating thoracic dystrophy	May be lethal	Long narrow thorax, renal anomalies (cystic dysplasia), polydactyly (14%)
Chondroectodermal dysplasia	May be lethal	Long narrow thorax, congenital heart disease, 50% (ASD), polydactyly (100%)

TABLE 41-10
MICROMELIC DYSPLASIA, MILD AND BOWED: KEY FEATURES

Dysplasia	Prognosis	Key Sonographic Features
Osteogenesis imperfecta type III	Nonlethal Progressively deforming	Lower extremities demonstrate greater degree of shortening and fractures/bowing
Campomelic dysplasia	Generally lethal	Ventral-bowing femur and tibia, hypoplastic or absent fibula, hypoplastic scapulae

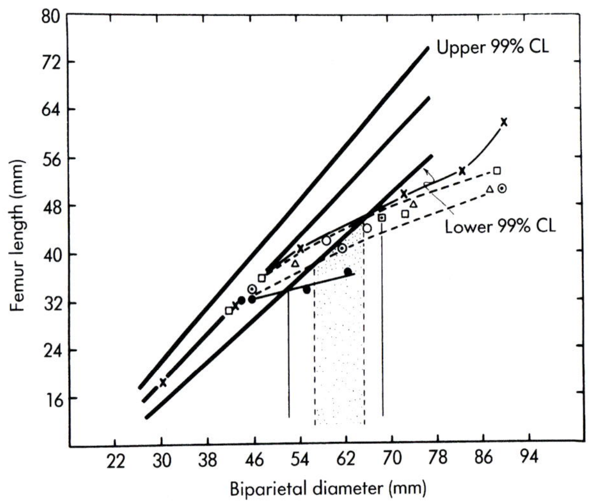

FIG. 41-17. Femur length versus BPD in 7 cases of recurrent heterozygous achondroplasia. The femur length falls below the 99% confidence limit (CL) by the time the BPD corresponds to 27 weeks' gestational age (approximately 69 mm). (From Kurtz AB, Filly RA, Wapner RJ et al. In utero analysis of heterozygous achondroplasia: variable time of onset as detected by femur length measurements. *J Ultrasound Med* 1986;5:137–140.)

of the hand. The BPD typically is above the 97th percentile at term. The interpedicular distances progressively narrow from the upper to the lower lumbar spine.

There is a progressive discrepancy between femur length and biparietal diameter during the third trimester of pregnancy, with the **femur length falling below the first percentile** when **compared to biparietal diameter** (Fig. 41-17).[39] This may occur as early as 21 weeks' or as late as 27 weeks' gestational age.

Patel et al.[38] suggested that fetuses with heterozygous achondroplasia have a femoral length that exceeds 34 mm at 26 weeks' BPD age, whereas fetuses with homozygous achondroplasia do not. In cases where both parents are heterozygous achondroplastic, fetal ultrasound can help to differentiate between normal, heterozygous, and homozygous achondroplasia. Fetuses with femoral lengths below the third percentile compared with the BPD at 17 weeks' BPD age, and with progressive shortening over the following 6 weeks, have homozygous achondroplasia, whereas those in whom a femoral length decrease occurs between 17 and 23 weeks' BPD age have heterozygous achondroplasia.[38]

The identification of the gene responsible for achondroplasia, fibroblast growth factor receptor type 3 (FGFR3), mapped to the short arm of chromosome 4, has allowed the early prenatal diagnosis by DNA analysis on CVS material at 10 to 12 weeks' gestation in cases where the parents are heterozygous for achondroplasia.[23]

Diastrophic Dysplasia

Diastrophic dysplasia (DTD) is an autosomal recessive disorder with a variable degree of expression and a predominantly **rhizomelic** form of micromelia. The term *diastrophic* implies **"twisted"** which reflects the **multiple postural deformities, dislocations, joint contractures,** and **kyphoscoliosis** present.[40]

The **most characteristic feature is the "hitchhiker thumb"** which is due to a lateral positioning of the thumb in association with a hypoplastic first metacarpal. The first toe may have a similar positioning. There is a severe talipes equinovarus which may be refractory to surgical treatment. Other features include micrognathia, cleft palate, and laryngotracheomalacia. The lifespan may be normal if the progressive kyphoscoliosis does not compromise cardiopulmonary function. The DTD gene was mapped to the long arm of chromosome 5 and found to encode a novel sulfate transporter.[42] Mutations in the same gene were reported in achondrogenesis type IB and atelosteogenesis type II.[42]

Asphyxiating Thoracic Dysplasia

Asphyxiating thoracic dysplasia (ATD), or Jeune's syndrome, is an autosomal recessive disorder with variable expressivity. The incidence is 1 out of 70,000 to 130,000 births. The perinatal mortality rate is high as a result of pulmonary hypoplasia, and those who survive may develop renal and hepatic fibrosis at a later stage[9,24,30,41] (Table 41-9). Key features are:

- **Mild to moderate form of micromelia** with rhizomelic predominance in 60%;
- Long **narrow thorax** with short, horizontal ribs, inverted "handlebar" appearance of the **clavicles**;
- **Renal dysplasia** and cysts; and
- Postaxial **polydactyly in 14%**.

Chondroectodermal Dysplasia

Chondroectodermal dysplasia (CED), or **Ellis-van Creveld** syndrome, is an autosomal recessive disorder with an incidence of approximately 1 out of 150,000 births. The condition has a high prevalence among inbred populations, such as the Amish and the Arabs of the Gaza strip.[30] Key features in affected fetuses are a **mild to moderate form of micromelia** with a mesomelic predominance; **ribs that are short and horizontal in orientation;** postaxial or ulnar **polydactyly**[40] (Fig. 41-18) that is almost **100% in the hands and 25% in the feet;**[24] and **congenital**

A B

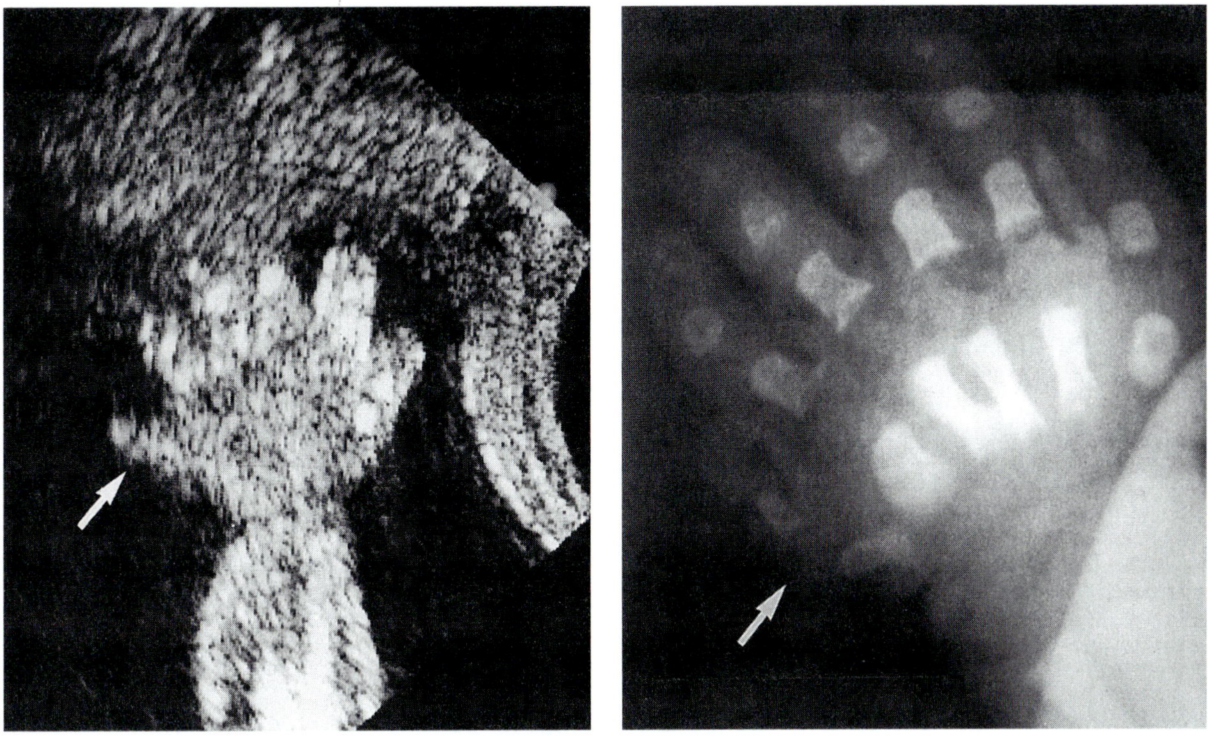

FIG. 41-18. Chondroectodermal dysplasia. Postaxial or ulnar polydactyly (*arrow*). **A,** Sonogram. **B,** Radiograph of another fetus with postaxial polydactyly. Note hypoplastic distal phalanges and fusion of the third and fourth metacarpals. (Courtesy of Greg Ryan, M.D., University of Toronto.)

heart disease, most commonly **atrial septal defect,** in approximately 50%.

The presence of polydactyly and congenital heart disease and the absence of renal cysts help to distinguish this condition from asphyxiating thoracic dystrophy. It is generally a nonlethal disorder, but death due to pulmonary hypoplasia can occur.[19,30]

Osteogenesis Imperfecta Types I, III, IV

Osteogenesis imperfecta type I is a mild, "tarda" variant inherited in an autosomal dominant manner as a result of mutation in the COL1A1 (on chromosome 17) or COL1A2 (on chromosome 7) and possibly in other collagen genes. OI type I is a generalized connective tissue disorder characterized by bone fragility and blue sclerae. The bones are of normal length, and only 5% present at birth with fractures. Most fractures occur from childhood to puberty. There is progressive hearing loss in approximately 50%.

Osteogenesis imperfecta type III has a heterogeneous mode of inheritance. This is a nonlethal, progressively deforming variety of OI that often spares the humeri, vertebrae, and pelvis. Rib involvement is variable. The blue sclerae will normalize, and there is no associated hearing impairment.

Osteogenesis imperfecta type IV is an autosomal dominant form of OI. It is the mildest form, involving isolated fractures. The sclerae are blue at birth but normalize over time. There is no associated hearing impairment.

LIMB REDUCTION DEFECTS AND ASSOCIATED CONDITIONS

This is a heterogeneous group of inherited and noninherited disorders associated with a spectrum of limb defects. The defect can consist of the absence of an entire limb (**amelia**), of part of a limb (**phocomelia**), or of digits (**oligodactyly**), or can involve an increased number of digits (**polydactyly**). It can also affect only the radial or ulnar ray, with or without involvement of the corresponding fingers (Table 41-11). The overall incidence of congenital limb reduction deformities is estimated at 0.40 per 10,000 births. An isolated am-

TABLE 41-11
NOMENCLATURE OF LIMB ANOMALIES

Limb Reduction Anomalies	
Amelia	Absent limb
Adactyly	Absent digits
Acheiria	Absent hand
Apodia	Absent foot
Hemimelia	Absent extremity distal to knee or elbow
Phocomelia	Absent middle segment of limb
Ectrodactyly	Split hand
Ulnar or radial paraxial hemimelia	Absent ulnar and ulnar digits or radius and thumb
Hand and Foot Anomalies	
Clinodactyly	Incurvature of a digit
Camptodactyly	Flexion of a digit
Syndactyly	Fusion of digits
Polydactyly	Extra digits
Oligodactyly	Decreased number of digits

putation may be due to amniotic band syndrome, teratogen exposure, or a vascular accident.

Proximal Focal Femoral Deficiency

Proximal focal femoral deficiency (PFFD) is a rare, sporadic condition, and 35% of those affected are infants of diabetic mothers.[24] There is an **asymmetric** degree of absence of the **subtrochanteric femur,** which may extend to the femoral head and acetabulum.[30] The femoral hypoplasia is often associated with ipsilateral fibular hemimelia which may result in a bowed appearance of the tibia similar to that of campomelic dysplasia; however, PFFD is generally **unilateral**. There can be hypoplasia or aplasia of other long bones, vertebral anomalies, microcephaly, and facial dysmorphism. When associated with the "unusual facies syndrome" the femoral hypoplasia is usually bilateral and there is an autosomal recessive inheritance pattern.

Caudal Regression Syndrome

Caudal regression syndrome consists of partial to total **sacral agenesis** and abnormalities of the lumbar,

A

B

C

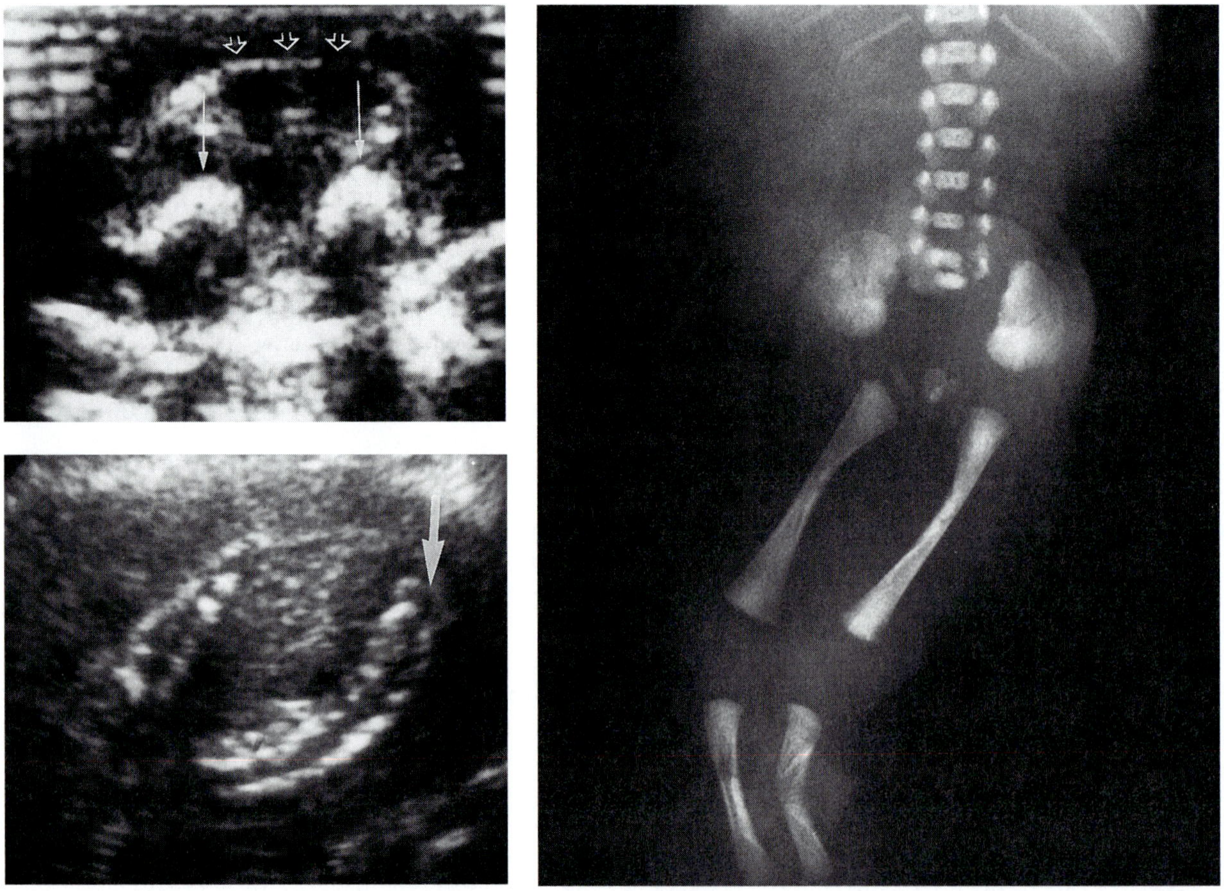

FIG. 41-19. Sirenomelia. **A,** Cross-section, lower extremities: femurs (*arrows*) are closer than expected due to fusion of the soft tissues (*open arrows*). **B,** Sacral agenesis with abrupt termination of the lower spine (*arrow*). **C,** Single fused lower extremity and sacral agenesis.

pelvis, and lower limbs.[43-45] The majority of cases are associated with maternal diabetes but familial cases have been reported. **Sirenomelia** is believed to be the most severe form of this disorder; it is characterized by an absent sacrum, fusion of the lower extremities, anorectal atresia, and renal dysgenesis or agenesis (Fig. 41-19). Severe oligohydramnios and single umbilical artery are commonly present. The birth frequency is approximately 1 out of 60,000.

Amniotic Band Sequence and Limb-Body-Wall Complex

Amniotic band sequence is most probably the result of first trimester rupture of the amnion, resulting in amniotic bands that extend from the chorionic surface of the amnion to the fetal tissue.[46,47] The incidence is approximately 1 out of 1200 livebirths, but is much higher in spontaneous abortions. Depending on the timing and orientation of the bands, the resultant disruption of fetal organs includes **amputations of limbs or digits** (Fig. 41-20), **bizarre facial or cranial clefting,** and **thoracoabdominal schisis**. The distribution is **asymmetric. Constriction ring defects** are the most common finding. Identification of a fibrous band of tissue within a **constricting ring** with distal elephantiasis or protrusion of uncovered bone distally are **pathognomonic** signs. Antenally, an aberrant band attached to the fetus in which characteristic deformities and restriction of motion permit the diagnosis. An amniotic sheet is distinguished from anamniotic band by a thickened base and a free edge.[48]

The **limb-body-wall complex** is a sporadic disorder that occurs in approximately 1 out of 4000

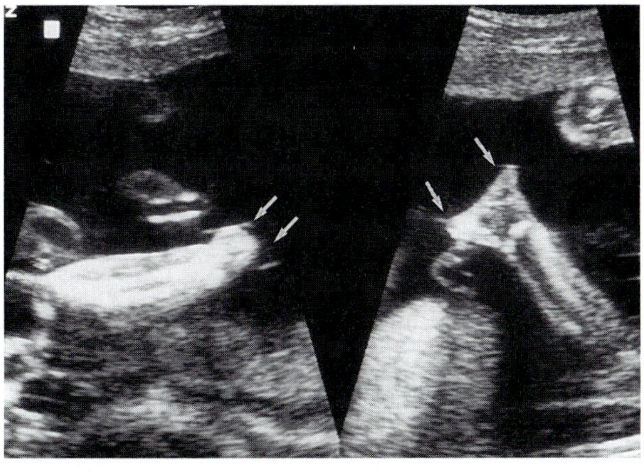

FIG. 41-20. Isolated amputation of the hand. The upper extremity ends abruptly distal to the wrist, in the midcarpal region (*arrows*). (Courtesy of Ants Toi, M.D., University of Toronto.)

livebirths with a similar but invariably more severe and **lethal** complex of fetal malformations.[49] Additional findings include evisceration of internal organs, myelomeningocele, marked scoliosis, and a very **short, straight umbilical cord.** Amniotic bands cannot be identified in all cases. The etiology is hypothesized to be related to early amnion rupture, vascular disruption, or an error in embryological development.

Radial Ray Defects

Radial ray defects are associated with a wide variety of syndromes. Their diagnosis is confirmed by the absence of a visualized distal radius at the same level as the ulna, in association with a radial deviation or clubhand. There may be bowing or hypoplasia of the ulna and a hypoplastic or absent thumb.

Fanconi's panycytopenia syndrome is an autosomal recessive blood dyscrasia in which 80% of cases have an associated unilateral or bilateral **aplastic or hypoplastic thumb and radius**. Prenatal diagnosis is based on increased chromosome breakage and sister chromatid exchange in cultured amniotic fluid cells both before and after exposure to diepoxybutane.[40,50] **Aase syndrome** is an autosomal recessive blood dyscrasia characterized by hypoplastic anemia, a **hypoplastic distal radius**, and a **triphalangeal thumb.** Cardiac defects (VSD) may be associated.

Thrombocytopenia–absent radius syndrome, or TAR, is an autosomal recessive blood dyscrasia characterized by hypomegakaryocytic thrombocytopenia and **bilateral absence of the radii.**[51] The **thumb is always present.** The humerus and lower extremities may be variably involved. One third of such patients have the congenital heart disease tetralogy of Fallot and septal defects. Fetuses are at risk of intracranial hemorrhage, so delivery by cesarean section is recommended.[40]

Holt-Oram syndrome is an autosomal dominant disorder consisting of a **congenital heart defect** (ASD, VSD) in combination with a large variety of **upper limb** anomalies. The limbs are **asymmetrically affected,** the left limb usually showing more effects than the right. The lower extremities are not involved. (Fig. 41-21, *A*).

Robert's syndrome, or pseudothalidomide syndrome, is an autosomal recessive disorder characterized by tetraphocomelia and bilateral cleft lip-palate. The limb reductions are most prominent in the upper extremities.

Other conditions associated with radial ray abnormalities include **trisomy 18 and 13,** the **VACTERL** association, **acrorenal syndrome, Cornelia de Lange's syndrome, Goldenhar's** syndrome, **Nager's acrofacial dysostosis,** and **Klippel-Feil** syndrome.

A

B

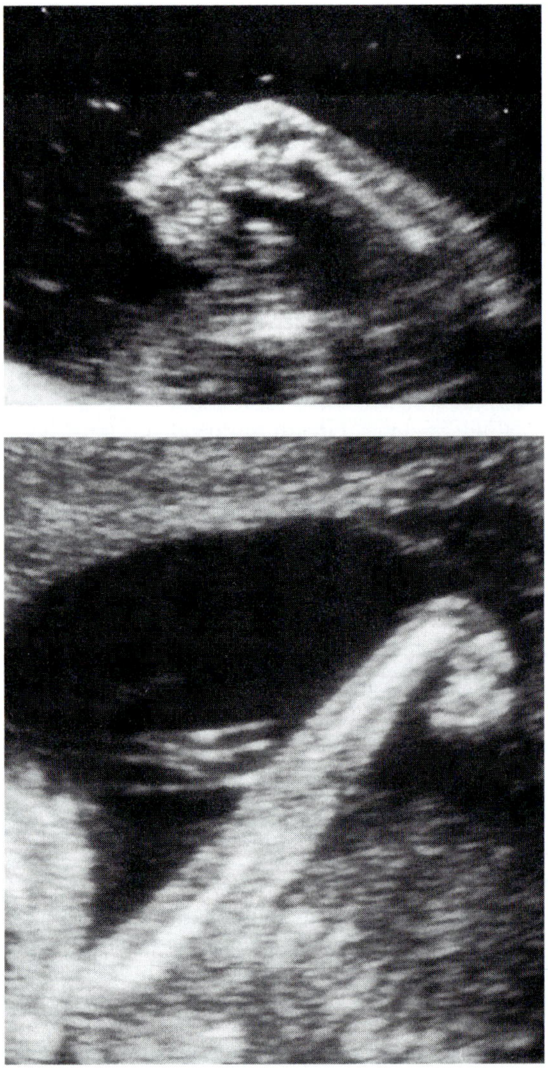

FIG. 41-21. Holt-Oram syndrome. **A,** Radial deviation hand, or clubhand, secondary to radial ray aplasia and ulnar hypoplasia. **Arthrogryphosis multiplex congenita. B,** Fixed elbow extension and wrist flexion with talipomanus or clubhand. (Courtesy of Ants Toi, M.D., University of Toronto.)

Arthrogryphosis Multiplex Congenita

Arthrogryphosis multiplex congenita (AMC) is a heterogeneous group of disorders with **multiple joint contractures of prenatal onset**[52-54] (Fig. 41-21, *B*). Some cases are due to **extrinsic causes** such as oligohydramnios, twinning, or uterine masses. Most of these cases have good prognoses. Among the **intrinsic causes** resulting in AMC are neuromuscular disorders (the majority of cases) and skeletal and connective tissue disorders. The **fetal akinesia sequence** refers to the combination of multiple joint contractures in association with intrauterine growth retardation, underdevelopment of the bones, pulmonary hypoplasia, typical craniofacial abnormalities, and a short umbilical cord.

Limb pterygium, or webbing of the skin across a joint, can involve a single or several joints[55] and etiologically is a heterogeneous disorder.

Asymmetric limb enlargement may be due to hemihypertrophy, cutaneous hemangioma or lymphangioma, elephantiasis secondary to a constricting band, A-V malformations, neurofibromatosis, or the Beckwith-Wiedemann syndrome, among other conditions. **Extremity enlargement** may also be related to thickened subcutaneous tissues as in hydrops fetalis or large-for-gestational-age infants.

Kyphoscoliosis may be a manifestation of an isolated vertebral defect or may be associated with complex syndromes such as VACTERL, limb-body-wall complex, neurofibromatosis, arthrogryphosis, diastrophic dysplasia, or other skeletal dysplasias.

HAND AND FOOT DEFORMITIES

The optimal time for evaluation of the hands and feet is during the second trimester.[56-65] Bromley et al.[5] estimate that in approximately 85% of cases, both hands and feet can be identified on an ultrasound scan within a 5-minute period. **Aneuploidy** is associated with an increased risk of hand and foot anomalies. These include persistent clenched hand, overlapping digits, clinodactyly, polydactyly, syndactyly, simian creases, talipes equinovarus, rockerbottom foot, and sandal toes (Fig. 41-22).

Persistent clenched hand with **overlapping of digits** occur in more than 50% of trisomy 18 fetuses and is generally bilateral (Fig. 41-22, *H*). This characteristic hand appearance is highly suggestive of trisomy 18 but can also occur in other conditions such as fetal akinesia syndrome, among others.

Clinodactyly is the permanent incurvature of a finger. Clinodactyly, due to hypoplasia of the middle phalanx, most commonly involves the fifth finger and is associated with trisomy 13, 15, 18, and 21 (Fig. 41-22, *G*). Clinodactyly occurs in 60% of fetuses with trisomy 21; up to 18% of normal fetuses may have evidence of it to a mild degree.[59] **Camptodactyly** is the permanent flexion of a finger.

Polydactyly is the presence of extra digits on the foot or hand. The majority are isolated findings, but they can be associated with syndromes and chromosome abnormalities. The extra digit may consist of a small soft tissue projection or a complete digit (Fig. 41-18). **Postaxial polydactyly** (ulnar or fibular) is more common and is found in conditions such as chondroectodermal dysplasia, asphyxiating thoracic dystrophy, short-rib polydactyly dysplasia, and

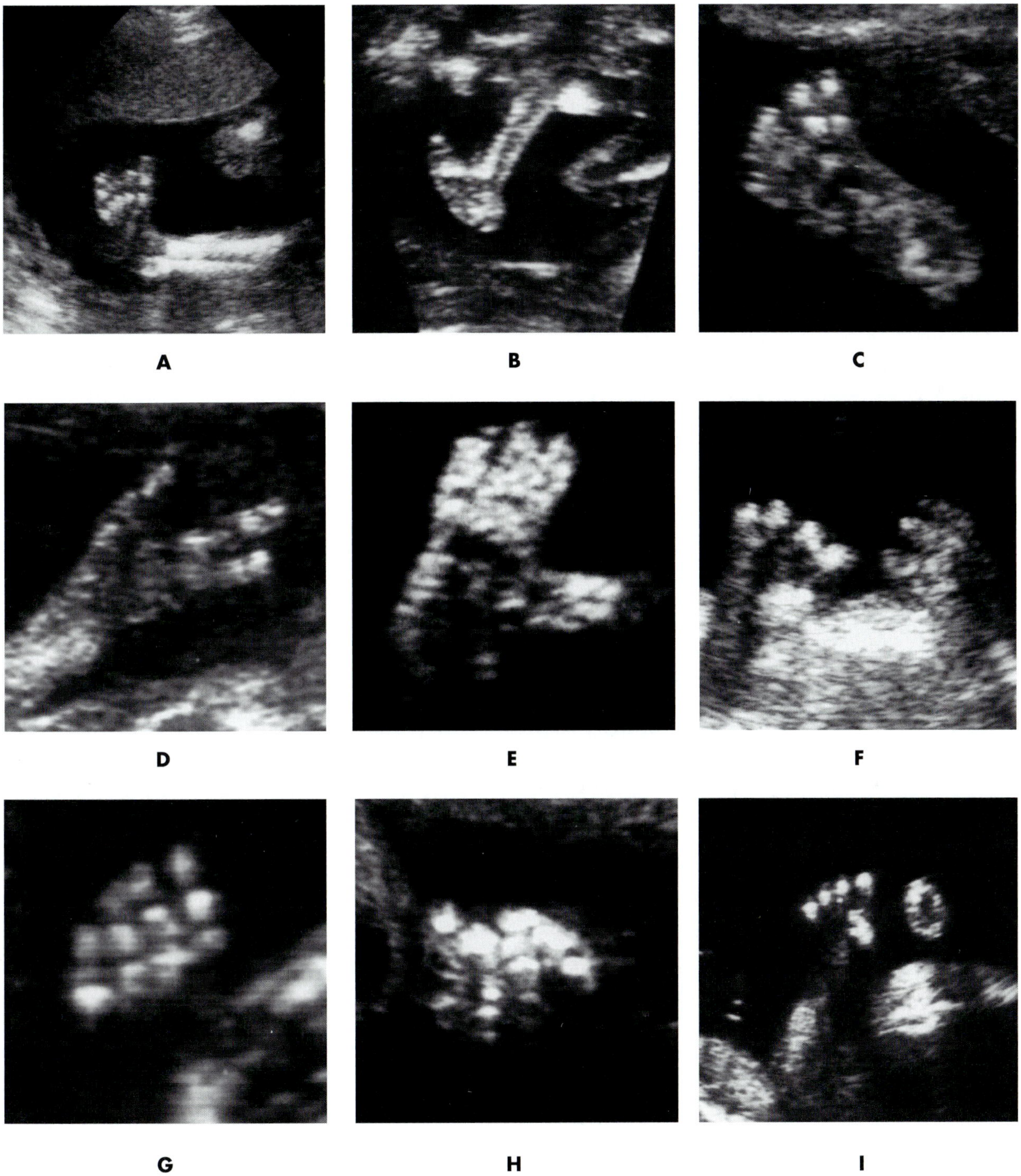

FIG. 41-22. Hand and foot anomalies. A, **Talipes equinovarus:** Inverted plantar flexion with medial deviation of the foot results in visualization of the long axis of the foot (metatarsals) and lower leg in the same plane. Rounded angle between the foot and lower leg. B, **Rockerbottom foot:** Convex sole contour and rounded soft-tissue protrusion posterior to the calf soft tissues. C, **Toe polydactyly:** Six digits. D, **Oligodactyly:** Three digits. E, **Syndactyly:** Soft tissue fusion of the first and second digits. F, **Brachydactyly:** Marked shortening of the hand digits with trident configuration in a homozygous achondroplastic fetus. G, **Clinodactyly:** Hypoplastic middle phalanx fifth digit. H, **Clenched hand with overlapping second digit** in a trisomy 18 fetus. I, **Adduction of the thumb** across the palmar surface may be associated with aqueduct stenosis. (C, E, and H, courtesy of Ants Toi, MD, University of Toronto; D courtesy of Shia Salem, MD, University of Toronto.)

trisomy 13. **Preaxial (radial or tibial) polydactyly** is found in familial conditions such as Fanconi's syndrome, Holt-Oram syndrome, acrocephalosyndactyly, and conditions associated with triphalangeal thumb.[30] **Central polydactyly** can also occur.

Syndactyly refers to cutaneous and/or osseous fusion of digits (Fig. 41-22, *E*). Syndactyly of the third and fourth fingers in association with intrauterine growth retardation in the second trimester suggests the diagnosis of triploidy. An **abducted,** lowset **thumb**, or hitchhiker thumb, is associated with diastrophic dwarfism. **Adducted thumb** may be associated with aqueductal stenosis (Fig. 41-22, *I*).

Ectrodactyly, or the split hand/foot **"lobster claw"** deformity, can occur as an isolated abnormality or in association with other findings such as cleft lip-palate as in ectrodactyly-ectodermal dysplasia clefting syndrome, Cornelia de Lange's syndrome, and Nievergelt syndrome.[40] Many isolated cases are the result of a new dominant mutation or are inherited from parents with minimal manifestations. Thus, a careful examination of the parents is needed before counseling low-recurrence risk.

Talipomanus, or **clubhand,** can be radial or ulnar. **Radial** clubhand is more common and is generally associated with the syndromes or karyotype abnormalities described in the preceding section on radial ray variants (Fig. 41-21). Another abnormality includes a sporadic group of syndromes associated with craniofacial abnormalities, most commonly cleft lip and palate. **Ulnar clubhand** is associated with ulnar ray defects; it is uncommon and may be an isolated finding.

Talipes equinovarus occurs in 0.1 to 0.2% of the population. The recurrence risk after the birth of one affected child is 2% to 3%, and if one of the parents is affected, it is 3% to 4%. The diagnosis is based on the recognition of an inverted and plantar flexed foot in which the metatarsal long axis is in the same plane as the tibia and fibula, in association with a rounded angle of junction between the foot and the lower leg (Figs. 41-22, *A*, 41-23). The majority are isolated malformations; however, fetal karyotyping should be considered if talipes is found in association with other structural abnormalities. Hindfoot equinus (plantar flexion), hindfoot varus (inward rotation), forefoot adduction, and variable forefoot cavus (plantar flexion) can also occur.

Rockerbottom foot is the result of a vertical position of the talus and equinus or vertical position of the calcaneus because of a short Achilles tendon (Fig. 41-22, *B*). The tarsal bones are dislocated dorsally so there is a convex plantar surface with posterior bulging of the calcaneus. It carries a high risk for fetal chromosome abnormalities such as trisomy 18 and 13 when associated with other abnormalities as well as for other syndromes such as fetal akinesia sequence.

Sandal toes, or an exaggerated gap between the first and second digits, is often visualized in the normal fetus but has a higher prevalence in trisomy 21 fetuses[57] (Fig. 41-24).

SKELETAL FINDINGS ASSOCIATED WITH ANEUPLOIDY

When an abnormality in the musculoskeletal system is detected during routine ultrasound examination, a systematic search is performed to detect other defects that may lead to the diagnosis of a specific genetic or chromosomal defect.[24,30,66] During the **second trimester,** an expected femur to measured-femur-length ratio below 0.9, based on biparietal diameter, should prompt a detailed examination to assess for other possible features of aneuploidy. However, in the **third trimester,** a mildly shortened femur is generally associated with asymmetric IUGR, rather than with aneuploidy. A femur to foot ratio > 0.9 is suggestive of IUGR rather than of a bone dysplasia, whereas a femur to foot ratio < 0.9 is suggestive of a skeletal dysplasia.[56-65] In general, chromosomal anomalies are associated with a symmetrical form of IUGR, although triploidy syndrome is an exception.

Trisomy 21, or Down syndrome, is the most common chromosome abnormality in newborns, having an incidence of 1 out of 600 to 800. About 95% of such cases are the result of an additional chromosome 21; 3% are the result of translocation, and 2% are mosaic. Most cases are sporadic; about 33% are born to mothers over 35 years of age. **Characteristic skeletal findings** may include **mild shortening of the femur and humerus, clinodactyly** of the fifth finger, **sandal toes, flat nasal bridge,** frontal bossing, and brachycephaly. The most common **nonskeletal fetal ultrasound findings** include thickened nuchal fold, or cystic hygroma, during the first or second trimester of pregnancy, cardiac abnormality (50%), isolated pleural or pericardial effusions, duodenal atresia (10%), echogenic bowel, pelviectasis, bladder outlet obstruction, simian creases (45%), mild cerebral ventriculomegaly, and nonimmune hydrops fetalis.

Trisomy 18, or **Edwards' syndrome,** is sporadically inherited, with an incidence of 1 out of 5000 livebirths. The **classic hand appearance** is that of a **persistently clenched hand** with the **overlapping** of the second and third **digits** and of the fourth and fifth digits, often in association with clinodactyly of the fifth digit. The findings are usually

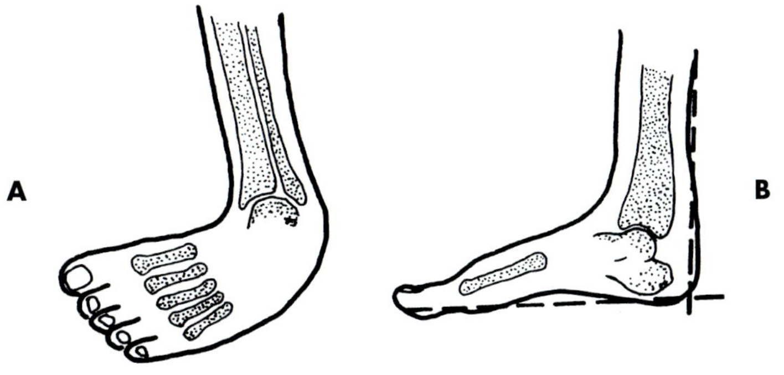

FIG. 41-23. Sonographic in utero diagnosis of clubfoot. A, Clubfoot, left side of the figure, demonstrates inverted plantar flexed and medially deviated foot resulting in visualization of the long axis of the foot and tibia/fibula in the same plane. Note the rounded angle of junction between the lower leg and foot. **B**, Normal right side of the figure demonstrates the normal relationship of tibia and fibula to the metatarsals and the normal squared angle of the lower leg to the foot. (From Jeanty P, Romero R, d'Alton M et al. *In utero* sonographic detection of hand and foot deformities. *J Ultrasound Med* 1985;4:595-601.)

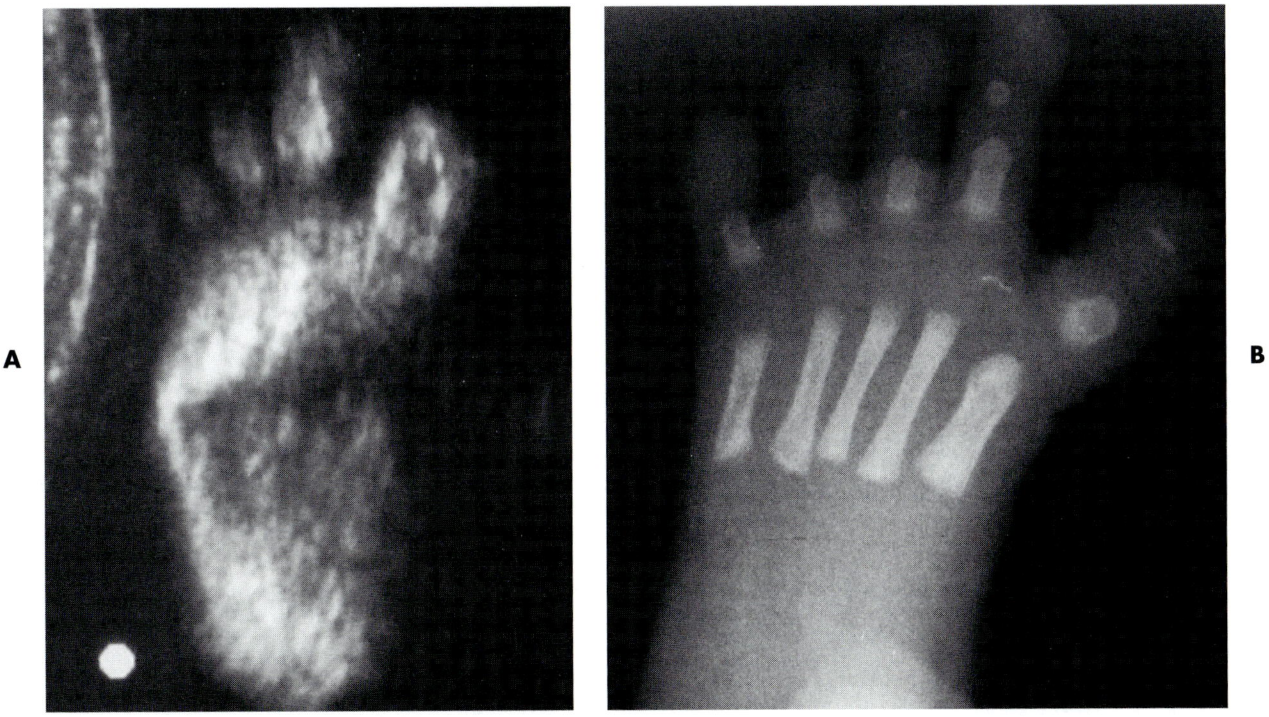

FIG. 41-24. Sandal toes in a 37-week fetus with Nager syndrome. A, Plantar view of the foot shows an exaggerated gap between the first and second toes and a plantar skin furrow. **B,** Correlative x-ray.

MUSCULOSKELETAL FEATURES OF TRISOMY 21

Mild shortening of the femur and humerus
Clinodactyly of the fifth finger
Sandal toes
Flat nasal bridge
Frontal bossing
Brachycephaly

MUSCULOSKELETAL FEATURES OF TRISOMY 18

Persistent clenched hand with overlapping digits
Radial ray aplasia variants
Syndactyly
Talipes equinovarus
Rockerbottom foot
Vertebral and rib anomalies

MUSCULOSKELETAL FEATURES OF TRISOMY 13

Polydactyly
Persistent clenched hand with or without overlapping digits
Clinodactyly
Hypoplastic ribs and pelvic bones
Microcephaly
Hypotelorism
Facial clefts

bilateral and occur in **more than 50% of trisomy 18** cases. **Other musculoskeletal findings** associated with trisomy 18 include **radial ray aplasia** variants in 10% to 50%, **syndactyly** of the second and third toes, simian creases, talipes equinovarus or rockerbottom foot, incomplete clavicle ossification, and vertebral and rib anomalies. **Other features** are early symmetrical IUGR, single umbilical artery (80%), cystic hygroma, cranial abnormalities including "strawberry-shaped" head, choroid plexus cysts, ventriculomegaly, agenesis of the corpus callosum, congenital heart disease, omphalocele, congenital diaphragmatic hernia, and renal anomalies. The prognosis is poor; 90% succumb within the first year of life, and all survivors have profound mental retardation.

Trisomy 13, or Patau's syndrome, is sporadically inherited with an incidence of 1 out of 10,000 livebirths. The **musculoskeletal anomalies** include postaxial **polydactyly** of hands and feet, possible **clenched hand, with or without overlapping digits,** clinodactyly, and possible associated hypoplastic ribs and pelvic bones. Classic **associated findings** include microcephaly, with sloping forehead and hypotelorism, and variants of **holoprosencephaly,** with **facial clefting.** Other findings include cardiac, renal, and gastrointestinal anomalies. Trisomy 13 is not always associated with IUGR.

Triploidy (69,XXX, 69,XXY, or 69,XXY) occurs in 18% of all early miscarriages but the incidence is only 1 out of 2500 births. In 60% it is the result of dispermy and in 40%, the result of diploid sperm or diploid egg. The combination of early severe asymmetrical IUGR, oligohydramnios, and an enlarged hydropic placenta is suggestive of this diagnosis. A partial molar pregnancy may be present. Associated **musculoskeletal findings** include syndactyly of the third and fourth fingers, simian crease, talipes equinovarus, and hitchhiker toe deformity. Other findings may include micrognathia, ventriculomegaly, myelomeningocele, and cardiac abnormalities.

REFERENCES

1. Camera G, Mastroiacovo P. Birth prevalence of skeletal dysplasias in the Italian multicentric monitoring system for birth defects. In: Papadatos CJ, Bartsocas CS, eds. *Skeletal Dysplasias*. New York: Alan R. Liss; 1982:441-449.
2. Lachman RS, Rappaport V. Fetal imaging in the skeletal dysplasias. *Clin Perinatol* 1990;17:703-722.
3. Pretorius DH, Rumack CM, Manco-Johnson ML et al. Specific skeletal dysplasias *in utero*: sonographic diagnosis. *Radiology* 1986;159:237-242.

Normal Fetal Skeleton

4. Mahoney BS, Filly RA. High-resolution sonographic assessment of the fetal extremities. *J Ultrasound Med* 1984; 3:489-498.
5. Bromley B, Benacerraf B. Abnormalities of the hands and feet in the fetus: sonographic findings. *AJR* 1995;165:1239-1243.
6. Greulich WW, Pyles SI, eds. *Radiologic Atlas of Skeletal Development of the Hand and Wrist*, 2nd ed. Stanford, Calif: Stanford University Press; 1959.
7. Mahoney BS, Callen PW, Filly RA. The distal femoral epiphyseal ossification center in the assessment of third-trimester menstrual age: sonographic identification and measurement. *Radiology* 1985;155:201-204.
8. Chin DH, Bolding DB, Callen PW et al. Ultrasonographic identification of fetal lower extremity epiphyseal ossification centers. *Radiology* 1983;147:815-818.
9. Goldstein I, Lockwood CJ, Reece EA et al. Sonographic assessment of the distal femoral and proximal tibial ossification cen-

ters in the prediction of pulmonic maturity in normal women and women with diabetes 1988;159:72-76.
10. Goldstein RB, Filly Ra, Simpson G. Pitfalls in femur length measurements. *J Ultrasound Med* 1987;6:203-207.
11. Abrams SL, Filly RA. Curvature of the fetal femur: a normal sonographic finding. *Radiology* 1985;156:490.
12. Yarkoni S, Schmidt W, Jeanty P et al. Clavicular measurement: a new biometric parameter for fetal evaluation. *J Ultrasound Med* 1985;4:467-470.
13. Campbell J, Henderson A, Campbell SS. The fetal femur/foot length ratio: a new parameter to assess dysplastic limb reduction. *Obstet Gynecol* 1988;72:181-184.
14. Platt LD, Medearis AL, Gregory DR et al. Fetal foot length: relationship to menstrual age and fetal measurements in the second trimester. *Obstet Gynecol* 1988;71:526-531.
15. Lachman RS, Rappaport V. Fetal imaging in the skeletal dysplasias. *Clin Perinatol* 1990;17:703-722.
16. Kurtz AB, Needleman L, Wapner RJ et al. Usefulness of a short femur in the *in utero* detection of skeletal dysplasias. *Radiology* 1990;177:197-200.
17. Goncalves L, Jeanty P. Fetal biometry of skeletal dysplasias: a multicentric study. *J Ultrasound Med* 1994;13:977-985.
18. Pattarelli P, Pretorius D, Edwards D. Intrauterine growth retardation mimicking skeletal dysplasia on antenatal sonography. *J Ultrasound Med* 1990;9:737-739.
19. Spirt BA, Oliphant M, Gottlieb RA et al. Prenatal sonographic evaluation of short-limbed dwarfism: an algorithmic approach. *Radiographics* 1990;10:217-236.
20. Rouse GA, Filly RA, Toomey F et al. Short-limb skeletal dysplasias: evaluation of the fetal spine with sonography and radiography. *Radiology* 1990;174:177-180.

Lethal Skeletal Dysplasias

21. Langer LO et al. Thanatophoric dysplasia and cloverleaf skull. *Am J Genet* 1987;3:167-179.
22. Martinez-Frias ML, Ramos-Arroyo MA, Salvador J. Thanatophoric dysplasia: an autosomal dominant condition? *Am J Med Genet* 1988;31:815-820.
23. Tavormina PL, Shiang R, Thompson LM et al. Thanatophoric dysplasia (types I and II) caused by distinct mutations in fibroblast growth factor receptor 3. *Nat Genet* 1995;9:321-328.
24. Taybi H, Lachman RS. *Radiology of Syndromes, Metabolic Disorders, and Skeletal Dysplasias*, 3rd ed. Chicago: Year Book Medical Publishers Inc; 1990.
25. Whitley CB, Gorlin RJ. Achondrogenesis: New onsology with evidence of genetic heterogeneity. *Radiology* 1983;148: 693-698.
26. DiMaio MS, Barth R, Koprivnikar KE et al. First-trimester prenatal diagnosis of osteogenesis imperfecta type II by DNA analysis and sonography. *Prenat Diag* 1993;13:589-596.
27. Sillence DO, Senn A, Danks DM. Genetic heterogeneity in osteogenesis imperfecta. *J Med Genetics* 1979;16:101-116.
28. Sillence DO, Barlow KK, Garber AP et al. Osteogenesis imperfecta type II delineation of the phenotype with reference to genetic heterogeneity. *Am J Med Genet* 1984;17:407-423.
29. Munoz C, Filly RA, Golbus MS. Osteogenesis imperfecta type II: prenatal sonographic diagnosis. *Radiology* 1990;174:181-185.
30. Meizner I, Bar-Ziv J. *In utero diagnosis of skeletal disorders: an atlas of prenatal sonographic and postnatal radiologic correlation.*: CRC Press; 1993.
31. Bowerman RA. Anomalies of the fetal skeleton: sonographic findings. *AJR* 1995;164:973-979.
32. Spranger JW, Langer LO, Weidemann HR. *Bone Dysplasias: An Atlas of Constitutional Disorders of Skeletal Development.* Philadelphia: WB Saunders Co; 1974:28-23.
33. Kwok C, Weller PA, Guioli S et al. Mutations in SOX9, the gene responsible for campomelic dysplasia and autosomal sex reversal. *Am J Hum Genet* 1995;57:1028-1036.
34. Wu Meng-Hsing, Kuo P-L, Lin S-J. Prenatal diagnosis of recurrence of short-rib polydactyly syndrome. *Am J Med Genet* 1995;55:279-284.
35. Duff P, Harlass FE, Milligan DA. Prenatal diagnosis of chondrodysplasia punctata by sonography. *Obstet Gynecol* 1990;76:497-500.
36. Pryde PG, Bawle E, Brandt F et al. Prenatal diagnosis of nonrhizomelic chondrodysplasia punctata (Conradi-Hünermann syndrome). *Am J Med Genet* 1993;47:426-431.
37. Manzke H, Christophers E, Wiedemann HR. Dominant sex-linked inherited chondrodysplasia punctata: a distinct type of chondrodysplasia punctata. *Clin Genet* 1980;17:97-107.

Nonlethal or Variable-Prognosis Skeletal Dysplasias

38. Patel MD, Filly RA. Homozygous achondroplasia: US distinction between homozygous, heterozygous, and unaffected fetuses in the second trimester. *Radiology* 1995;196:541-545.
39. Kurtz AB, Filly RA, Wapner RJ et al. *In utero* analysis of heterozygous achondroplasia: variable time of onset as detected by femur length measurements. *J Ultrasound Med* 1986; 5:137-140.
40. Romero R, Athanassiadis AP, Jeanty P. *Radiol Clin North Am* 1989; 28:75-98.
41. Kaitila I, Ammala P, Karjalainen O et al. Early prenatal detection of diastrophic dysplasia. *Prenat Diag* 1983;3:237-244.
42. Hastaback J, Superti-Furga A, Wilcox WR et al. Atelosteogenesis type II is caused by mutations in the diastrophic dysplasia sulphate-transporter gene (DTDST): evidence for a phenotypic series involving three chondrodysplasias. *Am J Hum Genet* 1996;58:255-262.

Limb Defects and Associated Conditions

43. Sonek JD, Gabbe SG, Landon MB et al. Antenatal diagnosis of sacral agenesis syndrome in a pregnancy complicated by diabetes mellitus. *Am J Obstet Gynecol* 1990;162:806-808.
44. Sirtori M, Ghidini A, Romero R et al. Prenatal diagnosis of sirenomelia. *J Ultra Med* 1989;8:83-88.
45. Duhamel B. From the mermaid to anal imperforation: the syndrome of caudal regression. *Arch Dis Childhood* 1961;36:152-155.
46. Mahoney BS, Filly RA, Callen PW et al. The amniotic band syndrome: antenatal sonographic diagnosis and potential pitfalls. *Am J Obstet Gynecol* 1985;152:63-69.
47. Patten RM, Van Allen M, Mack LA et al. Limb-body-wall complex: *in utero* sonographic diagnosis of a complicated fetal malformation. *AJR* 1986;146:1019-1024.
48. Randel SB, Filly RA, Callen PW et al. Amniotic sheets. *Radiology* 1988;166:633-636.
49. Van Allen MI, Curry I, Gallagher L. Limb-body-wall complex: pathogenesis. *Am J Med Genet* 1987;28:529-548.
50. Auerbach AD. Fanconi anemia. *Dermatol Clin* 1995;13:41-49.
51. Hall G. Thrombocytopenic and absent radius (TAR) syndrome. *J Med Gen* 1987;24:79-83.
52. Ohlsson A, Fong KW, Rose TH et al. Prenatal sonographic diagnosis of Pena-Shokeir syndrome type 1, or fetal akinesia syndrome. *Am J Med Gen* 1988;29:59-56.
53. Bay BJ, Cubberley D, Morris C et al. Prenatal diagnosis of distal arthrogryphosis. *Am J Med Gen* 1988;29:501-510.
54. Goldberg JD, Chervenak FA, Lipman RA et al. Antenatal sonographic diagnosis of arthrogryphosis multiplex congenita. *Prenat Diag* 1986;6:45-49.
55. Hall JG, Reed S, Gershanik J et al. Limb pterygium syndromes: a review and report of eleven patients. *Am J Med Gen* 1982;12:377-409.

Hand and Foot Deformities

56. Jeanty P, Romero R, d'Altoan M et al. *In utero* sonographic detection of hand and foot deformities. *J Ultrasound Med* 1985;4:595-601.
57. Bromley B, Benacerraf B. Abnormalities of the hands and feet in the fetus: sonographic findings. *AJR* 1995;165:1239-1242.
58. Reiss RE, Foy PM, Mendiratta V et al. Ease and accuracy of evaluation of fetal hands during obstetrical ultrasonography: a prospective study. *J Ultrasound Med* 1995;14:813-820.
59. Benacerraf BR, Osathanondh R, Frigoletto FD. Sonographic demonstration of hypoplasia of the middle phalanx of the fifth digit: a finding associated with Down syndrome. *Am J Obstet Gynecol* 1988;159:181-183.
60. Hegge FN, Presscott GH, Watson PT. Utility of a screening examination of the fetal extremities during obstetrical sonography. *J Ultrasound Med* 1986;5:639-645.
61. Benacerraf BR, Gelman R, Frigoletto FD. Sonographic identification of second trimester fetuses with Down's syndrome. *N Engl J Med* 1987;317:1371-1376.
62. Benacerraf BR, Frigoletto FD. Prenatal ultrasound diagnosis of clubfoot. *Radiology* 1985;155:211-213.
63. Hashimoto BE, Filly RA, Callen PW. Sonographic diagnosis of clubfoot *in utero*. *J Ultrasound Med* 1986;5:81-83.
64. Benacerraf BR, Frigoletto FD, Greene MF. Abnormal facial features and extremities in human trisomy syndromes: prenatal US appearance. *Radiology* 1986;159:243-246.

Skeletal Findings Associated with Aneuploidy

65. Avni EF, Rypens F, Zappa M et al. Antenatal diagnosis of short-limb dwarfism: sonographic approach. *Pediatr Radiol* 1996;26:171-178.
66. Ultrasound markers for fetal chromosomal defects. In: *Frontiers in Fetal Medicine Series*. Snijders RJM, Nicolaides KH, eds. New York: Parthenon Publishing Grp; 1996.

CHAPTER 42

The Fetal Face and Neck

Ants Toi, M.D., F.R.C.P.C.

CHAPTER OUTLINE

Facial and associated cranial malformations have significant implications for a person's physiologic and social well-being. Facial alterations are common in many syndromes and may suggest specific diagnoses when found in association with other anomalies (Table 42-1). As a result, the face should be evaluated whenever anomalies are suspected. Some labs[2-4] now examine the face during routine scanning even though it is not included as a requirement of a routine sonographic obstetric examination in the current guidelines such as those of the American College of Radiology (ACR) or the American Institute of Ultrasound in Medicine (AIUM).[5,6]

EMBRYOLOGY

Facial development starts by about 5 menstrual weeks and is essentially complete by 10 weeks.[7,8] It is closely associated with the development of the brain.[9,10]

Facial structures develop from **five main facial processes** that move together and fuse (Fig. 42-1). The **nasofrontal process** starts superiorly and moves inferiorly to form the midforehead, nose and central upper lip, central maxilla including teeth, and anterior palate. From the sides, the two **maxillary prominences** move medially to form the cheeks, lateral upper lips, maxilla, and hard palate. Inferiorly, the two **mandibular prominences** move medially and fuse to form the mandible.[7,8] Subsequent migration of mesoderm supports these primary structures, and mesodermal abnormalities may account for some of the unusual cleftings that can occur.[11]

The nose, eyes, and ears undergo major shifts in position with facial development. The **nose** starts above the orbits as two widely spread nasal placodes that move medially and inferiorly. The **eyes** start laterally and move medially. The **ears** start below the mandible and move laterally and upward. By 11 to 12 menstrual weeks the facial structures are essentially in their final positions and the face appears normal.

TABLE 42-1
FACIAL ANOMALIES AND ASSOCIATED MALFORMATIONS

Term	Meaning	Associated With*
Anophthalmia	Congenital absence or severe hypoplasia of eye(s)	
Cyclopia	Fusion of orbits and eyes into one, typically with nose as supraorbital proboscis	Holoprosencephaly
Hypotelorism	Eyes too closely positioned; at ultrasound, measured as excessively small space between globes; in infants, measured as decreased interpupillary distance or on x-ray as decreased interorbital distance	Holoprosencephaly Maternal PKU Trisomy 13
Hypertelorism	Eyes too widely positioned; measured as hypotelorism (above)	Frontal encephalocele; multiple syndromes (Apert, Crouzon, Carpenter); hydantoin, frontonasal dysplasia
Ethmocephaly	Two separate, closely positioned eyes and supraorbital proboscis	Holoprosencephaly
Cebocephaly	Two separate, closely positioned eyes and a centrally placed nose with a single, blindly ending nostril	Holoprosencephaly
Facies	Facial appearance	Many syndromes have a characteristic appearance
Micrognathia Retrognathia	Abnormally small jaw, especially with lower jaw recession (small chin) measured from mandibular condyle to point of mandible	Pierre Robin syndrome Treacher Collins syndrome
Prognathism	Large, forward-jutting jaw	Beckwith-Wiedemann syndrome
Macroglossia	Abnormally large or hypertrophic tongue	Beckwith-Wiedemann syndrome Hypothyroidism

*For expanded lists of associations see Jones KL. *Smith's Recognizable Patterns of Human Malformation.* 4th ed. Philadelphia: WB Saunders Co; 1988.

The **eye** develops as a stalk from the neuroectoderm of the forebrain which forms the retina. This induces changes in the overlying ectoderm and mesoderm which form the remaining structures of globe, eyelids, and bony orbit.

The **ear** develops from otic placodes at the side of the hindbrain, which form the inner ear. An outpouching of the pharynx forms the middle ear. The external ear develops from surface swellings low in the neck near the first and second branchial grooves, the auricular hillocks, which fuse to form the auricle.[7,8] Subsequently, the ear migrates upward and rotates to a more vertical position. Failures in development, movement, and fusion result in various abnormal appearances. Low-set, rotated ears are a common feature of many syndromes in which the normal cephalad migration of the pinna is impeded.[7,9]

OVERVIEW OF ANOMALIES

Craniofacial anomalies are common and may occur as often as 1 in 600 births.[12] At ultrasound, facial anomalies were found in 13 of 7100 (0.2%) fetuses in a mixed high- and low-risk population[13] and in 18 of 223 (8.1%) fetuses in a high-risk population.[12] Abnormality **detection rates** were in excess of 78% and no false-positive diagnoses occurred. Detected abnormalities included anophthalmia, single nostril, proboscis, absent nose, flat nose, hypertelorism, hypotelorism, clefting of nose, lip, and palate, and micrognathia. Lesions that were missed included cleft palate, flattened nose, and cleft lip, but typically these were only components of more complex lesions that were detected at sonography. More recently, in screening situations under 24 weeks in which facial views were routinely performed, the detection of abnormalities ranged from 7% to 33%.[3,4] Polyhydramnios occurred in about 60% of cases, and

FACIAL ANOMALIES

High association with
- Other abnormalities
- Chromosomal aberrations
- Polyhydramnios
- Syndromes

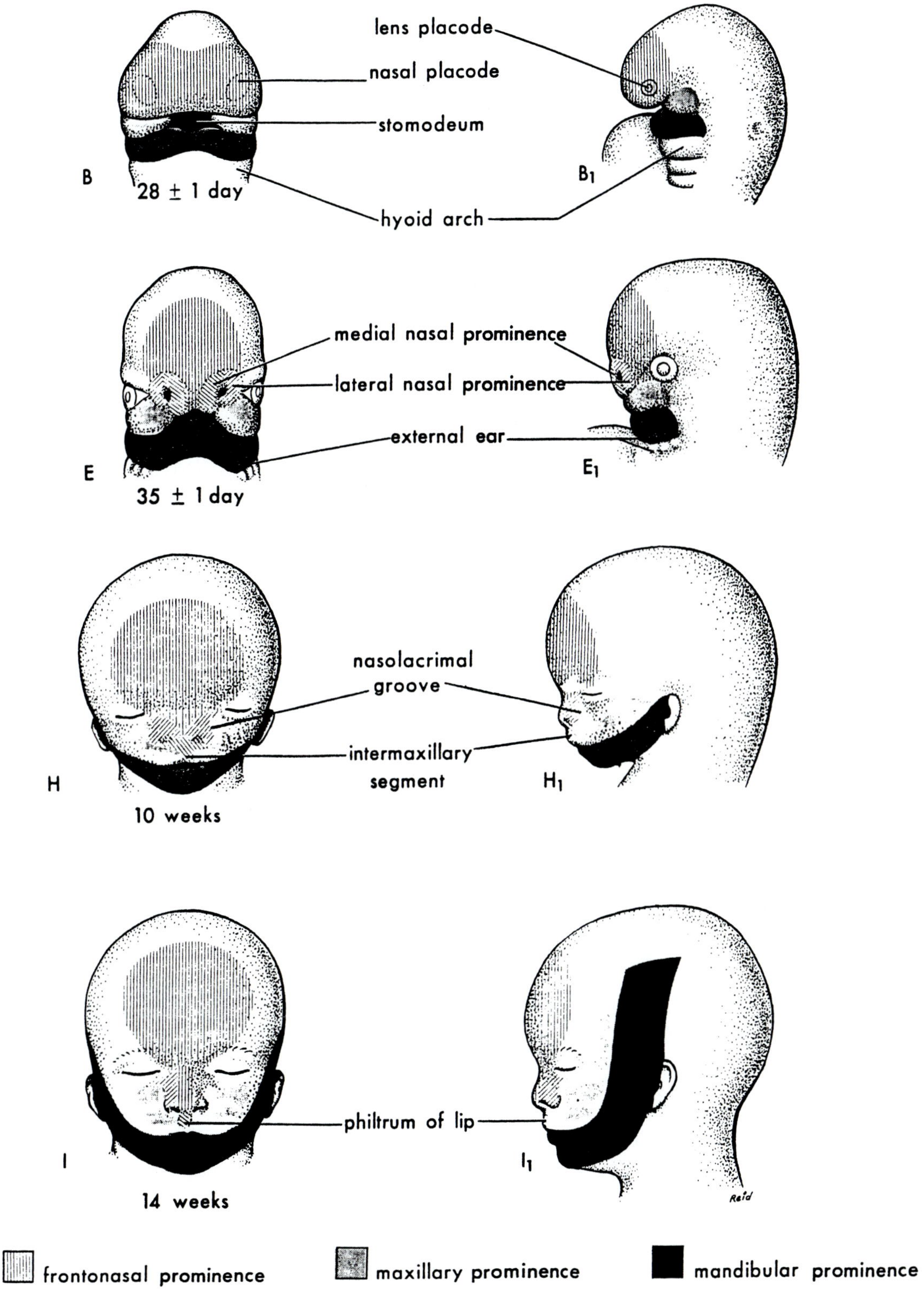

FIG. 42-1. Stages in development of the fetal face. Note the initial wide separation of the eyes, high wide separation of the nostrils (nasal placodes), and low position of the ears. (Modified from Moore KL. *Essentials of Human Embryology*. Toronto: BC Decker; 1988.)

other nonfacial anomalies were found in more than 50%. Risk factors included family history, other anomalies detected by ultrasound, chromosome aberrations, and teratogen exposure.[12,13]

Chromosomal abnormalities are common with facial malformations. Nicolaides found chromosomal abnormality as follows: micrognathia, 66%; macroglossia, 77%; cleft lip/palate, 48%; severe hypotelorism, 45%; nasal hypoplasia, proboscis, single nostril, 32%. Macroglossia was associated mainly with trisomy 21; micrognathia with trisomy 18 and triploidy; facial clefting with trisomy 13 and 18; ocular and nasal defects with trisomy 13. All the fetuses with facial abnormalities and abnormal chromosomes also had additional ultrasound abnormalities.[14]

Numerous **drugs** can affect facial development. These include alcohol, codeine, diazepam (Valium), retinoic acid (Retin A), antiepileptic drugs, and others.[15]

A B C D

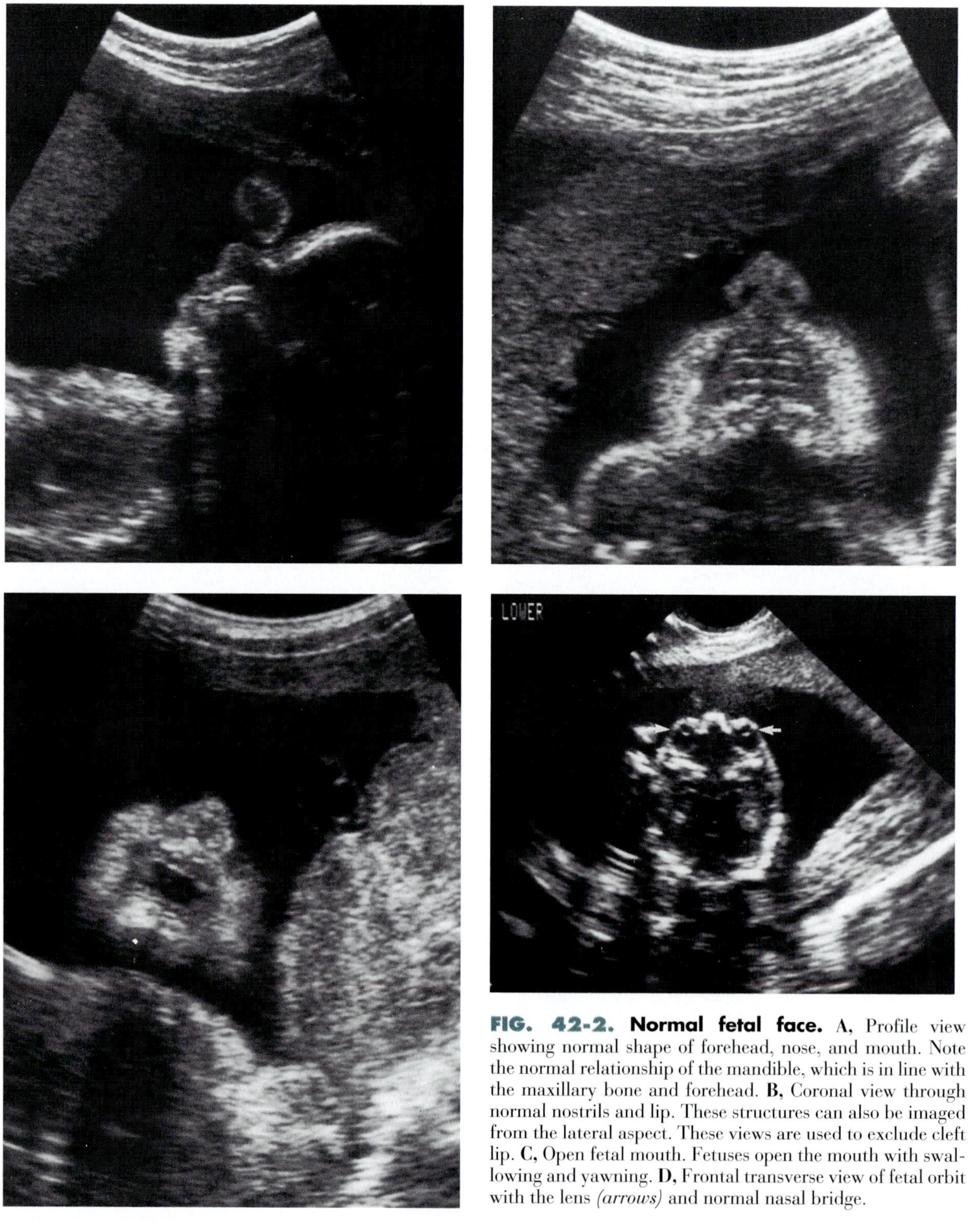

FIG. 42-2. Normal fetal face. **A,** Profile view showing normal shape of forehead, nose, and mouth. Note the normal relationship of the mandible, which is in line with the maxillary bone and forehead. **B,** Coronal view through normal nostrils and lip. These structures can also be imaged from the lateral aspect. These views are used to exclude cleft lip. **C,** Open fetal mouth. Fetuses open the mouth with swallowing and yawning. **D,** Frontal transverse view of fetal orbit with the lens *(arrows)* and normal nasal bridge.

NORMAL SONOGRAPHIC EXAMINATION

The main features of the eyes and orbital contents, nose, lips, cheeks, ears, tongue, pharynx, and neck vessels are accessible to ultrasound delineation.[16,17] Fetal eye movements,[18,19] mouth movements, swallowing, and regurgitation have been observed.[20,21] Normality of the features is determined mainly by simple appearance,[22] but measurement nomograms are available for the orbits[23,24] and are becoming available for general morphometrics.[25]

A complete **facial survey** is possible in most patients. It includes axial views of the orbits; coronal and axial views of the nose, lips, and anterior palate; profile; and views of the ears and neck (Fig. 42-2). The structures should be adequately visible in about 90% of patients, but visibility can be restricted by fetal position, oligohydramnios, and maternal obesity.[12] In patients who have an identified risk for a specific syndrome that has a characteristic facial appearance, we have found it useful to review the images in texts such as that by Jones[1] or to ask the parents to provide photos of the affected individuals so that the examination can be targeted to these specific changes.

Recently, new computer assisted technology has allowed three-dimensional scanning of fetal structures with surface rendition that can give strikingly clear depiction of the "facies"[26,27] (Fig. 42-3, *A*, *B*, and *C*).

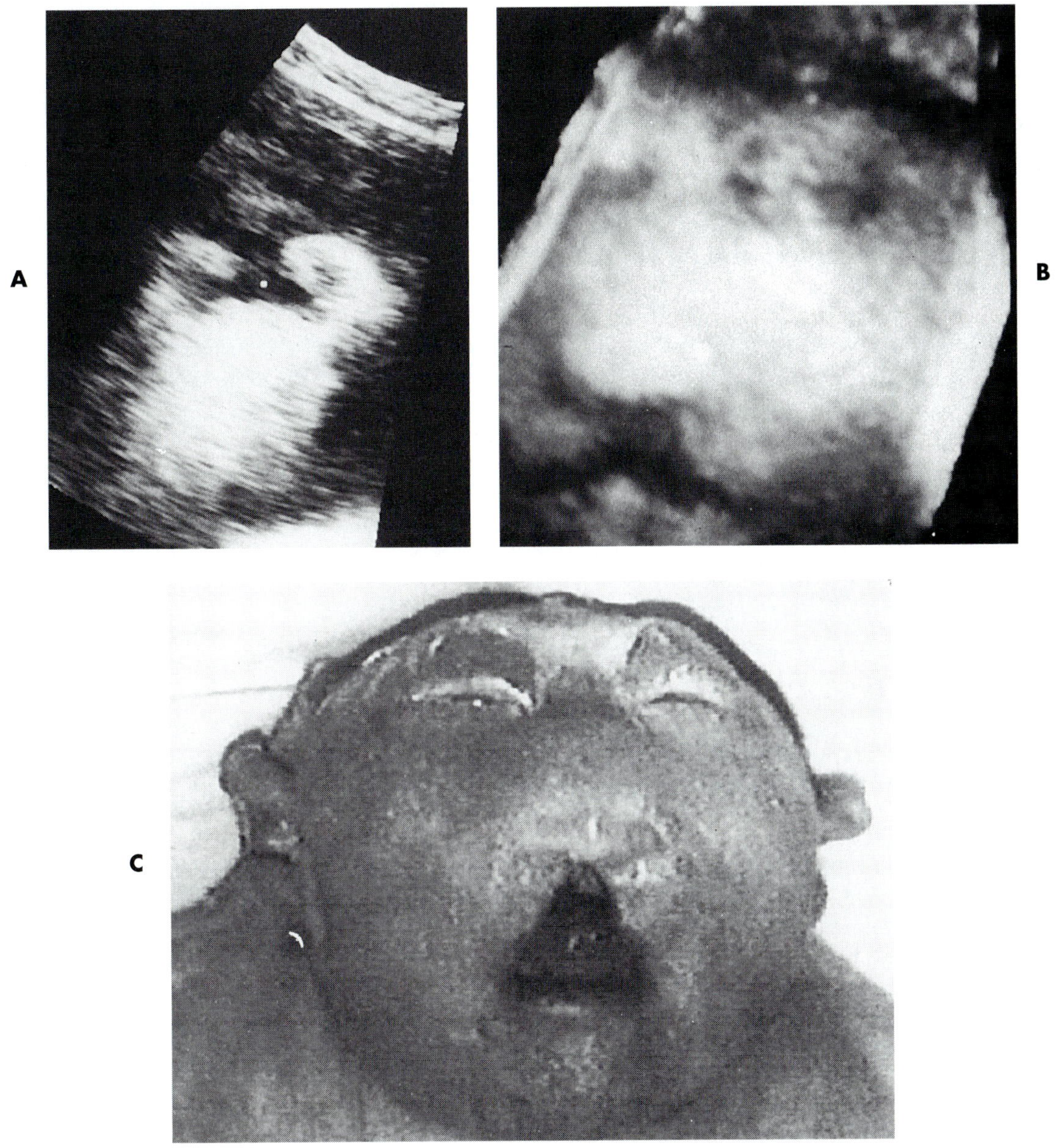

FIG. 42-3. Median cleft lip with hypotelorism and flat nose. **A,** Standard axial 2D view through the upper lip shows cleft. **B,** Comparison 3D surface, rendered view. **C,** Photo of fetus correlates well with the 3D representation. (Courtesy of Dolores Pretorius, M.D.)

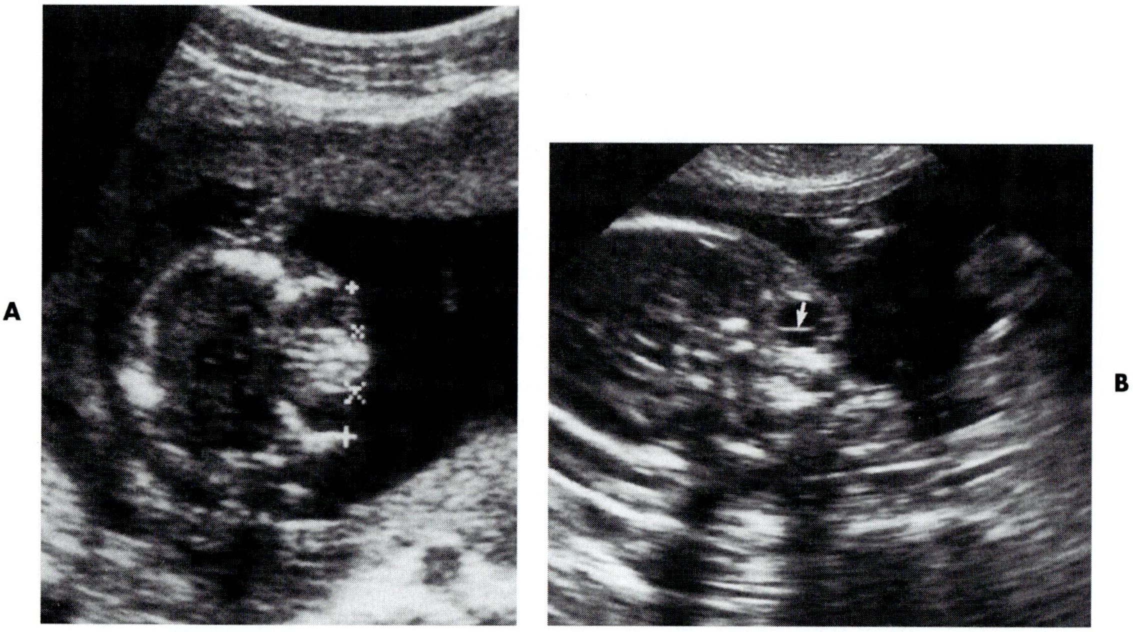

FIG. 42-4. Fetal eyes and orbits. **A,** Lateral view of orbits with measurements of outer orbital dimension (+...+) and interorbital dimension (×...×). **B,** Normal hyaloid artery *(arrow)* in globe coursing from the posterior part of the orbit to the lens at 21 menstrual weeks.

ORBITAL DISORDERS

The **eyes** can be identified by 10 weeks. By 24 weeks the globe, lens, vitreous body, anterior chamber, eye muscles, optic nerve, and ophthalmic artery may be seen.[16] Nomograms are available for inner and outer orbital diameters to diagnose hypotelorism and hypertelorism. A rule of thumb for judging eye separation is that the globes should be separated by about the diameter of a globe. If the space between the orbits appears larger or smaller than the width of one eye, then measurements can be employed to document and confirm this impression. The outer orbital diameters can be used to date the pregnancy when biparietal diameter cannot be measured[23,24] (Fig. 42-4, *A*).

The hyaloid artery, which nourishes the lens, can be seen between 16 and 30 weeks' gestation (Fig. 42-4, *B*). It appears as an echogenic line coursing from the posterior globe through the vitreous to the back of the lens. It regresses during normal pregnancy and should not be mistaken for an abnormality.[7,28,29]

Abnormalities of eye spacing (hypotelorism and hypertelorism) are the most commonly detected orbital disorders. Usually, abnormalities of eye spacing are associated with other anomalies (Table 42-2). Other orbital and periorbital lesions are also being recognized with increasing frequency, including anophthalmia (unilateral or bilateral) (Fig. 42-5), microphthalmia, cataracts (Fig. 42-6, *A* and *B*),[12,13,30] lacrimal duct cysts,[31] facial hemangiomas, dermoid cysts, exophthalmos,[32] and retinal nonattachment.[33,34]

TABLE 42-2
COMMON ABNORMALITIES ASSOCIATED WITH ABNORMAL EYE SPACING[1]

Hypotelorism	Hypertelorism
Holoprosencephaly	Cleft lip sequences
Maternal phenylketonuria	Anterior encephalocele
Trisomy 13	Craniosynostosis
	Apert syndrome
	Pena-Shokir syndrome
	Noonan's syndrome
	Frontonasal dysplasia
	Fetal hydantoin (Dilantin)
	Crouzon syndrome

Hypotelorism

Hypotelorism, or reduced interorbital distance, is commonly associated with holoprosencephaly (Fig. 42-7, *A-D*). Fetuses with both findings commonly have abnormal chromosomes, especially trisomy 13 (Table 42-2). **Holoprosencephaly** is the result of simultaneous failure of induction of facial and forebrain structures. The most severe alobar form has a single cerebral monoventricle and is most likely to be associated with characteristic facial anomalies. There is a typical range of facial changes associated with holoprosencephaly[10,11,35,36] (Fig. 42-8). These include normal faces, cyclopia, ethmocephaly, cebocephaly, midline facial cleft, and bilateral facial cleft.

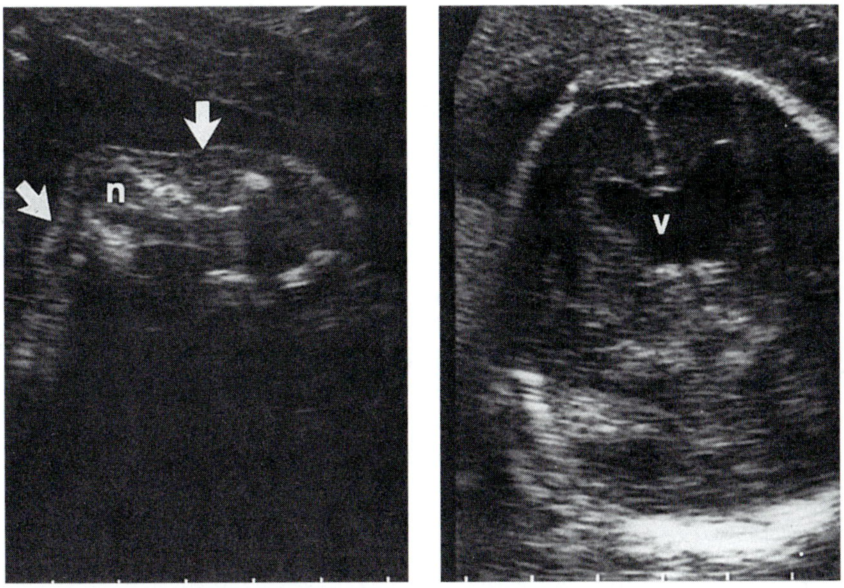

FIG. 42-5. Anophthalmia at 22 weeks. The left image is taken transversely through the fetal face at orbit level. Note that there is no globe in either orbit *(arrows)* beside the nose (n). This fetus also had **lobar holoprosencephaly** as seen on the right image where there is a single ventricle (V) but the interhemispheric sulcus is visible separating the left and right hemispheres.

A

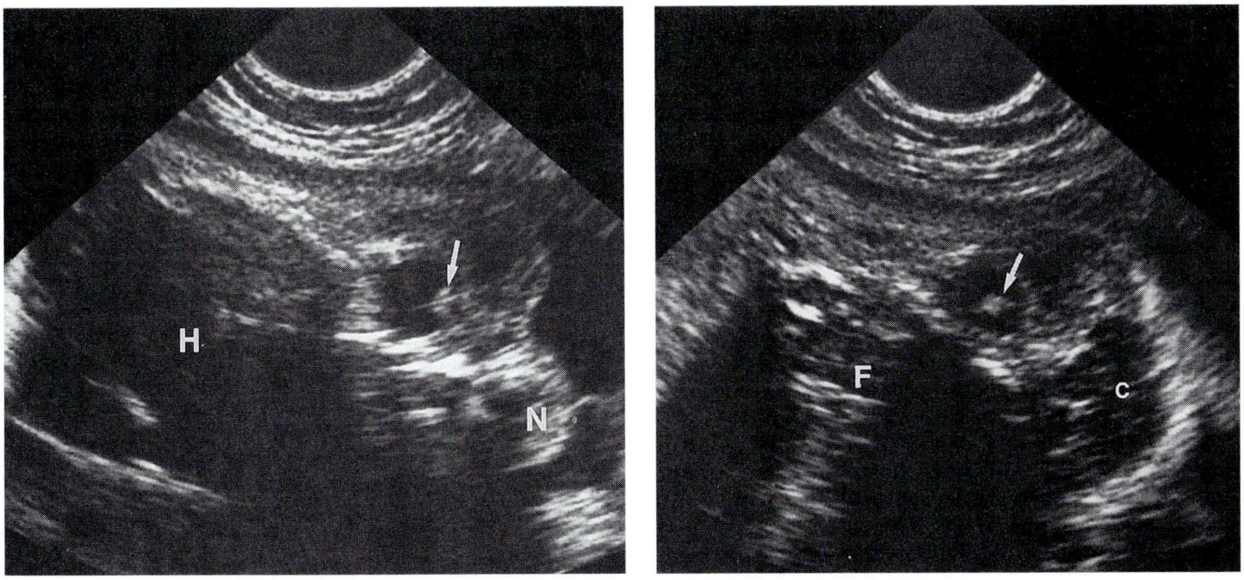

B

FIG. 42-6. Cataract visible as an abnormally echogenic lens (*arrow*) at 30 weeks' gestation. **A,** Axial view through fetal head (H) at orbit level shows echogenic lens *(arrow)* with hyaloid artery visible between the lens and the back of the globe. Nose (N). **B,** Coronal view through fetal face at level of orbit. F, forehead. C, chin. Only the upper globe is visible and the lower globe is obscured by fetal nasal structures. The echogenic lens with cataract *(arrow)* is visible. This fetus also had hydrops and generalized facial swelling.

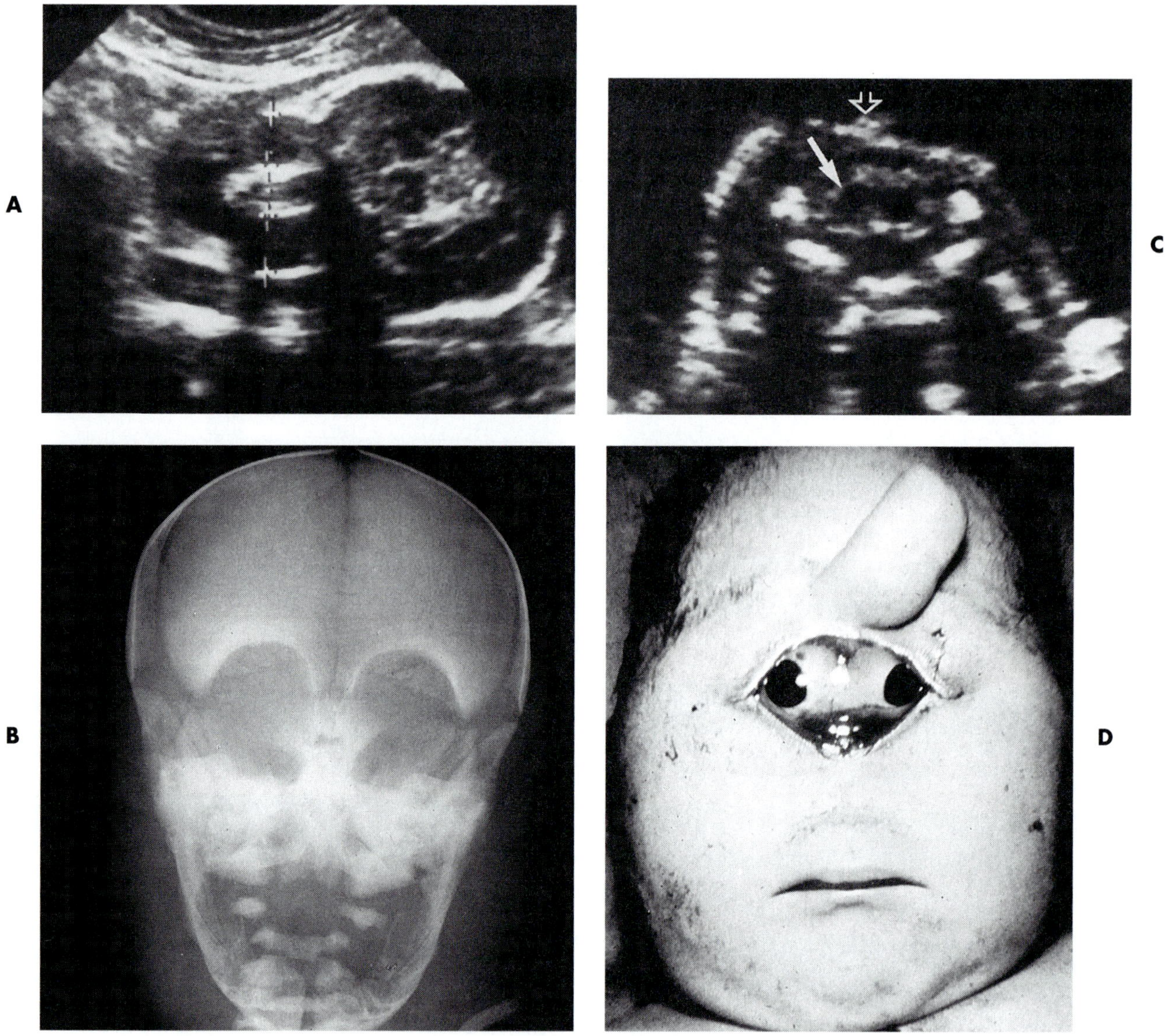

FIG. 42-7. Hypotelorism. **A,** Transverse view through orbits at 34 menstrual weeks shows the narrow interorbital distance also visible on **B,** postnatal x-ray. Normally the orbits are separated by about the width of one orbit. **C,** Postnatal transverse frontal scan of fetal face through the "orbit" of a fetus with cyclopia and proboscis at 18 menstrual weeks. Note the fused, dumbbell-shaped globes *(solid arrow)* and small supraorbital nubbin of nasal structure, the proboscis (*open arrow*). Only the outer orbital bony margin is present, and the medial bony walls are absent in this malformation. **D,** Cyclops with fused globes, supraorbital proboscis, and absent nose. (Courtesy of Margot Van Allan, M.D., The Hospital for Sick Children, Toronto.)

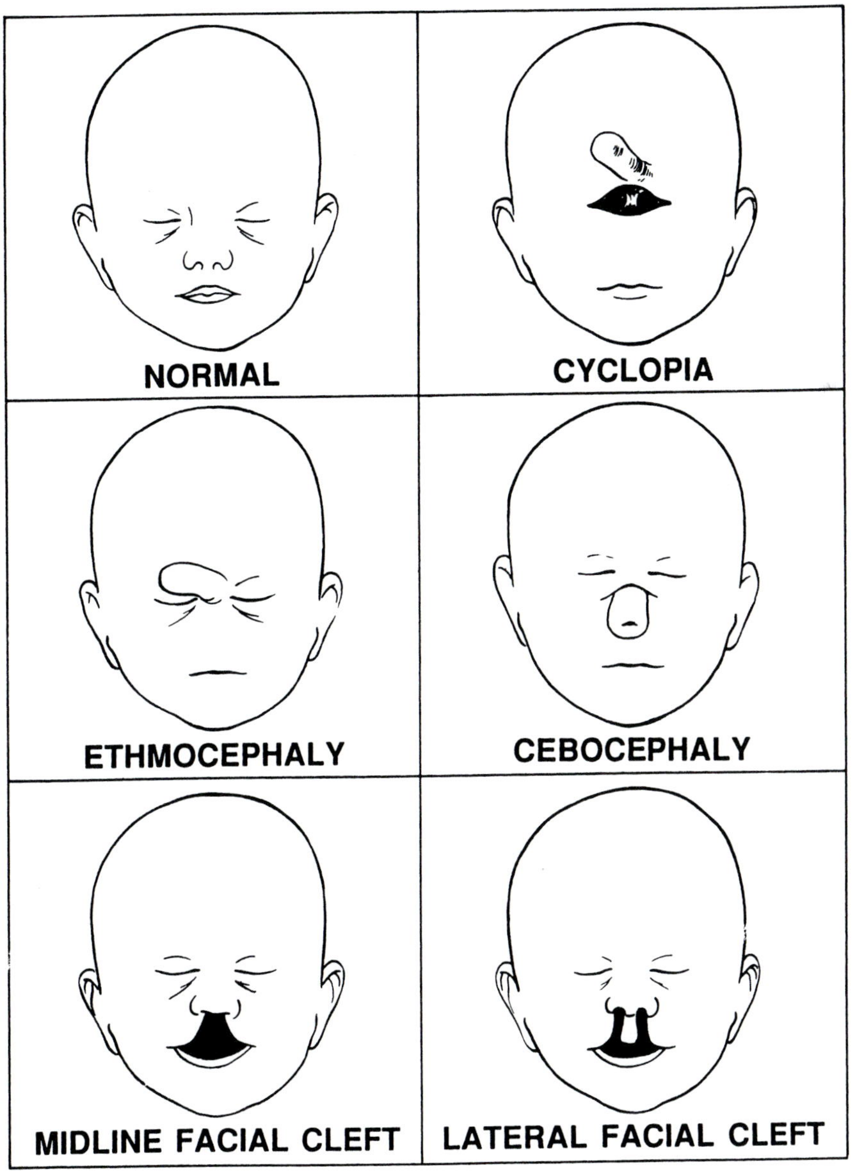

FIG. 42-8. Different facial malformations seen with holoprosencephaly. (From Nyberg D, Mahony B, Pretorius D. *Diagnostic Ultrasound of Fetal Anomalies: Text and Atlas:* Year Book Medical Pub; 1990.)

RANGE OF FACIAL FINDINGS SEEN WITH HOLOPROSENCEPHALY

Normal	
Cyclopia	Single orbit with a single partly fused eye and supraorbital, trunk-like nose (proboscis)
Ethmocephaly	Extreme hypotelorism with proboscis or absent nose
Cebocephaly	Hypotelorism with flattened rudimentary nose with single nostril
Midline facial cleft	Midline gap in upper lip with flattened nose
Bilateral facial cleft	Bilateral lip clefting

Hypertelorism

Hypertelorism implies increased orbital separation as measured by interpupillary distance or on posteroanterior orbital x-rays taken postnatally. Simple separation of the inner canthi of the eyelids (telecanthus) should not be mistaken for true orbital separation. For example, in Down syndrome, the inner canthi are widely separated due to the mongoloid fold (telecanthus), but the globes are actually too close together (hypotelorism). Hypertelorism may be isolated or may occur as part of multiple syndromes (especially with myelomeningocele and the Chiari II malformation or with frontal encephalocele)[37] (Fig. 42-9) or may be associated with chromosome abnormalities or result from teratogen exposure.[1]

Median Cleft-Face Syndrome

The median cleft-face syndrome (frontonasal dysplasia malformation complex) (Fig. 42-10) is characterized by hypertelorism, median clefting of the nose, cranium bifidum occulta, various degrees of lip, maxilla, and palate clefting, and a V-shaped anterior hairline. It is thought to result from arrest of development, migration, and fusion of the nasal and maxillary structures, resulting in persisting embryonic appearances that allow brain structures to be displaced inferiorly as an anterior encephalocele.[11,37] *In utero*, the associated cranial abnormalities frequently lead to the discovery of the facial changes.[38]

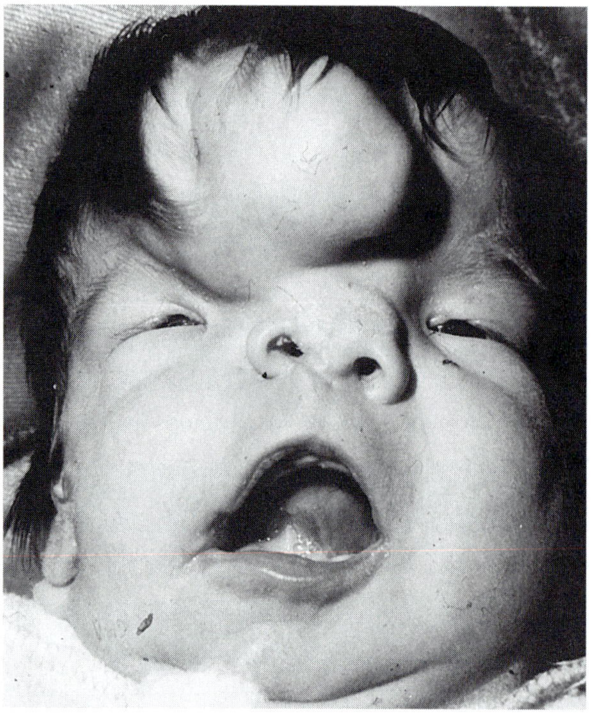

FIG. 42-9. Hypertelorism associated with bulging frontal encephalocele.

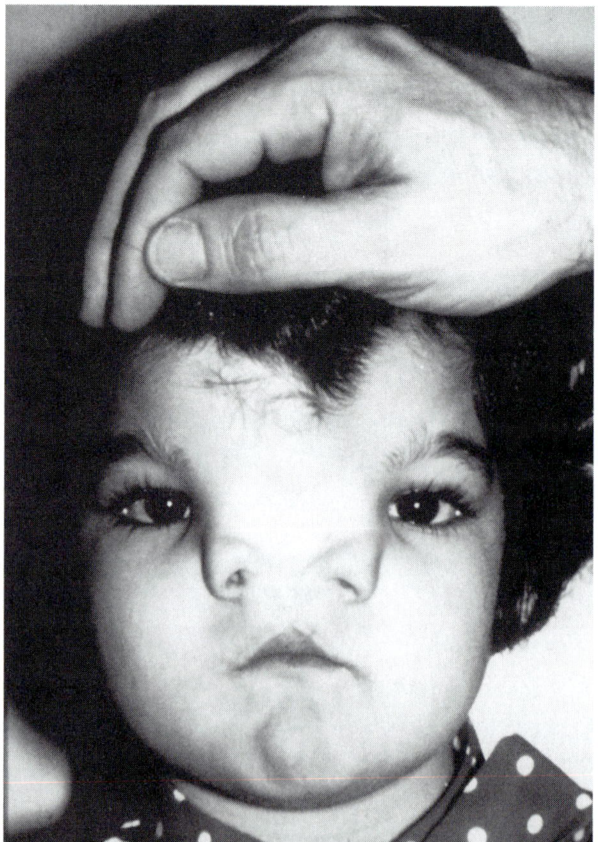

FIG. 42-10. Hypertelorism in girl with median cleft face after surgical repair of the midline lip clefting. Note marked separation of the eyes and right and left nasal structures. (Courtesy of Margot Van Allan, M.D., The Hospital for Sick Children, Toronto.)

MOUTH

Cleft Lip and Palate

Clefting is the major abnormality of the mouth. Clefts usually follow lines of fusion of the maxilla, primary palate, and secondary palate (Fig. 42-11). However, bizarre clefting of mouth and face can be caused by bands related to amniotic band syndrome. These do not follow embryologic developmental patterns. Nyberg has classified clefting about the mouth into **five patterns**:[39]

- Cleft lip alone;
- Unilateral cleft lip and palate;
- Bilateral cleft lip and palate;
- Midline cleft lip and palate; and
- Facial defects associated with amniotic bands.

Cleft lip with or without cleft palate is a common anomaly that occurs at a rate of about 0.4 to 1.7 per 1000 deliveries.[9,40,41] It results from abnormalities of fusion of the nasofrontal and maxillary processes and primary and secondary palatal processes and is modified by failure of migration of supporting mesenchymal tissue into facial regions.[9] The fused nasal prominences form the central intermaxillary segment which has a labial component forming the central part of the lip and a triangular palatal bony component including the four upper incisor teeth, alveolar ridge, and primary palate which extends to the incisive foramen just behind the teeth.[42]

Nomenclature is somewhat confusing. The term **"cleft lip and palate"** generally implies anterior clefting involving the lip and primary palate. The term **"cleft palate"** implies clefting of the secondary palate in the roof of the mouth. However, if there is major clefting of the lip and primary palate, then it is common for the defect also to involve at least parts of the secondary palate in continuity (Fig. 42-11).

Cleft lip may involve only the upper lip (**incomplete**) (Fig. 42-12), or may extend to involve the nose (**complete**) (Fig. 42-13), or may extend to involve the primary palate and secondary hard and soft palates to varying degrees. Isolated **cleft palate** implies clefting of the secondary palate and can involve the soft palate and/or the hard palate. The minimal lesion is a cleft uvula. Also, there may be a deficiency of the bony secondary palate, with the mucosa of the roof of the mouth remaining intact.

Cleft lip/palate is the most common variant (45%), followed by isolated cleft palate (30%) and cleft lip (25%).[9,41,42] Bilateral clefting is common. In this case, the central premaxilla drifts anteriorly as a mass visible below the nose (Fig. 42-14).

Associated abnormalities, which may be lethal, occur in 2% to 50% of instances[39,41,43] and are commonly seen in combination with chromosomal aberrations. Clefting occurs in 40% of fetuses with trisomy 18 and in 60% of fetuses with trisomy 13.[43]

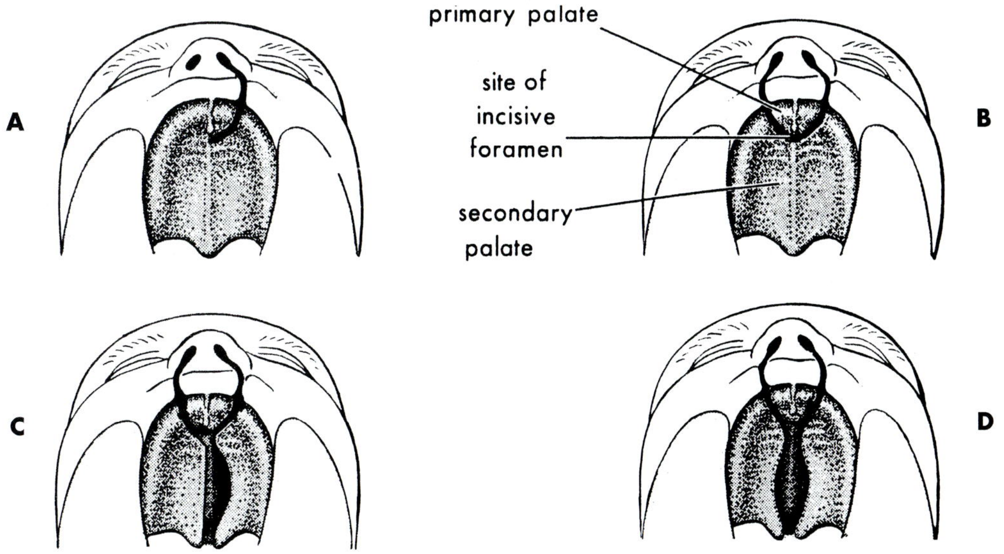

FIG. 42-11. Patterns of clefting of lip and palate. **A,** Isolated complete cleft lip/palate. This involves the lip and nose and the primary palate. **B,** Bilateral cleft lip/palate. In this instance the medial part of the lip and alveolar ridge, the premaxilla, which usually protrudes anteriorly, can be recognized as a mass below the nose (see Fig. 42-14). **C & D,** Bilateral cleft lip/palate. In this instance the lip clefting extends to involve one or both sides of the secondary hard palate in continuity, a common variant. (Modified from Moore KL, Persaud TVN. *The Developing Human.* 5th ed. Philadelphia: WB Saunders Co; 1993.)

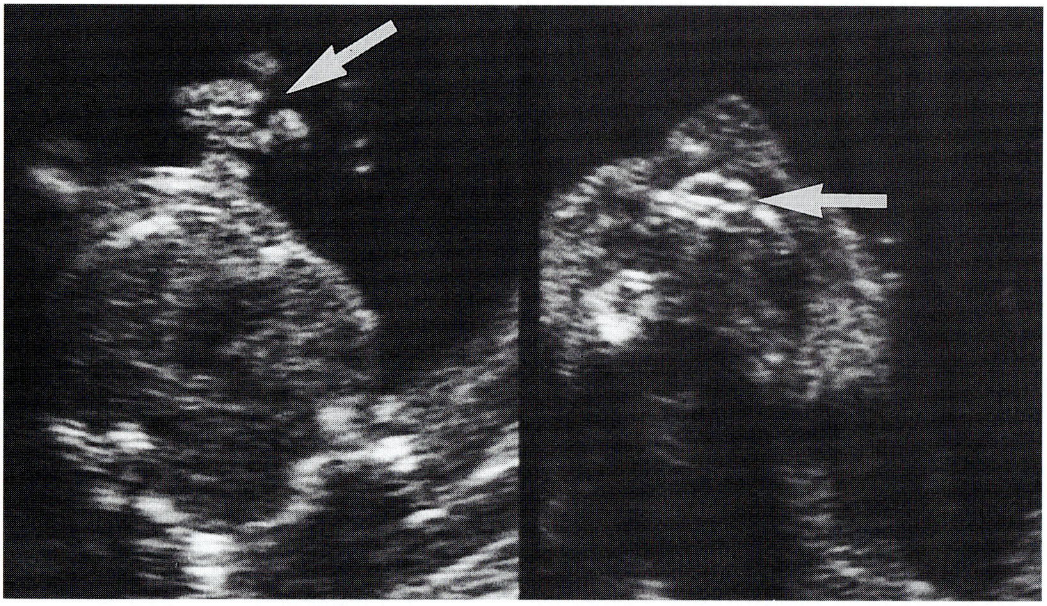

FIG. 42-12. Incomplete cleft lip at 23 weeks seen at coronal views illustrating a possible diagnostic pitfall. The left image is taken to just include the lip and shows the cleft *(arrow)*. The image on the right is deeper into the face and includes the bony alveolar ridge which is intact *(arrow)*. This is an incomplete cleft lip since the nose is not involved. It is important to examine the lips superficially as in the left image to see the cleft. Images made too deeply and posteriorly through the alveolar ridge, such as the right image, will miss clefting.

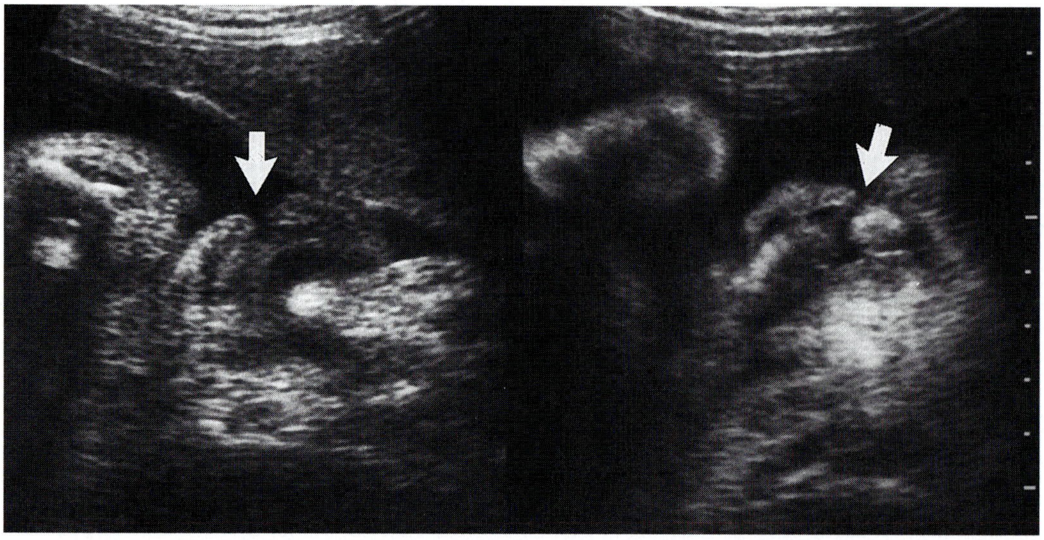

FIG. 42-13. Cleft lip and palate at 38 weeks showing the two common ultrasound orientations to detect clefting. Left image is axial through the lip and shows a cleft *(arrow)*. Right image is coronal through the tip of the nose, lips, and chin. Note the cleft *(arrow)* which extends into and deforms the nostril (complete cleft lip).

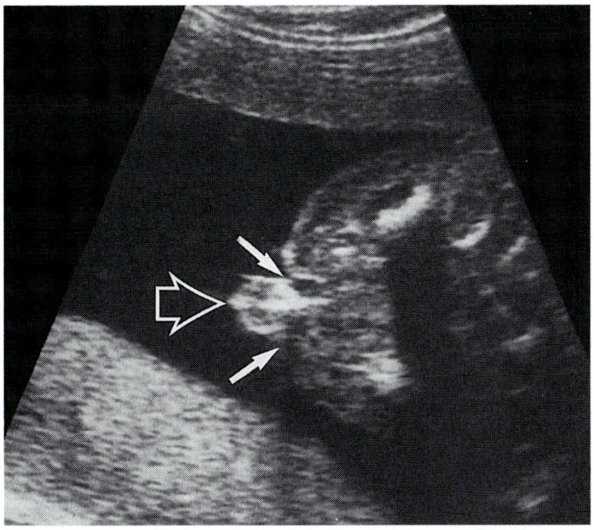

FIG. 42-14. Bilateral complete cleft lip/palate *(small arrows)* with the premaxilla protruding anteriorly as a mass *(open arrow)*. Axial view through fetal lip at 25 weeks.

Isolated cleft palate is more likely to be associated with additional anomalies (13% to 50%) than is isolated cleft lip (7% to 13%) or cleft lip/palate (2% to 11%).[44] The fetuses with associated chromosomal abnormalities usually have additional sonographic abnormalities.[14,39] Median cleft face (Fig. 42-15, *A* and *B*) is more likely to be associated with mental retardation than is isolated lateral clefting.[41]

Recurrence risk for cleft lip/palate and cleft palate, if there is no other affected first- or second-degree relative, is 3% to 5%. However, the rate increases to 10% to 20% and even higher if there are other affected relatives.[41]

Sonographically, clefting is diagnosed by viewing the nose, upper lip, and alveolar margin in the coronal direction, either from the forehead or the side,[22,45] or transaxially from the front (Fig. 42-13). Lip clefting is more readily detected than is palatal clefting and has been reported as early as 16 weeks' gestation.[43] The combination of polyhydramnios and a small stomach should lead to a detailed examination of the face, since clefting can disturb swallowing.[40] When clefting is discovered, the fetus should be examined for other anomalies and karyotyping should be performed.

There are many other patterns of clefting that are less common.[46] The most common of them is seen in

A

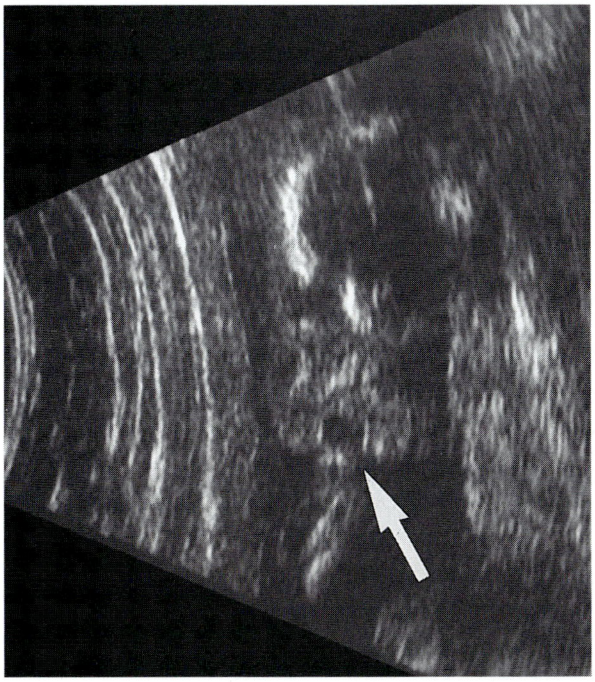

B

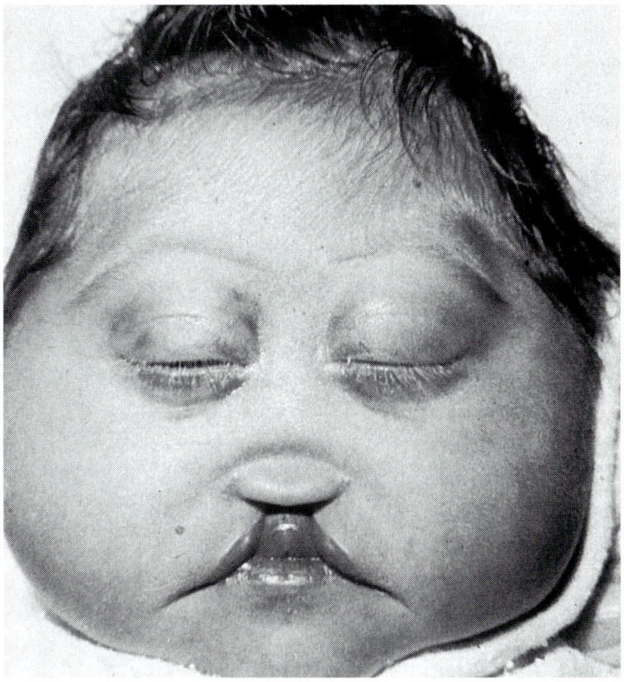

FIG. 42-15. Midline cleft lip/palate. A, Coronal view through the median cleft lip and palate *(arrow)* shows fetal face at 17 weeks. **B,** Fetal face shows midline cleft, flat nose, hypotelorism, and microcephaly. Fetuses with this anomaly generally have additional anomalies, particularly in the brain. This fetus had trisomy 18, hypotelorism, holoprosencephaly, microencephaly, dysplastic kidneys, and congenital heart disease.

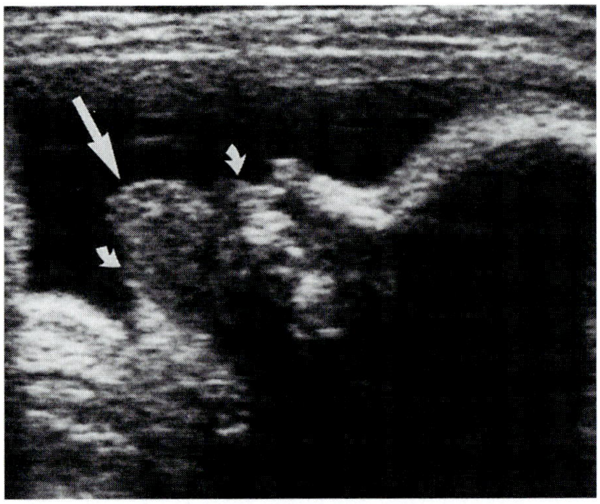

FIG. 42-16. Macroglossia in Beckwith-Wiedemann syndrome at 33 weeks. Note the massive tongue *(straight arrow)* protruding from the fetal mouth (lips, *curved arrows*). At no time could the fetus draw its tongue entirely into its mouth. This fetus also had macrosomia and large but otherwise normal-appearing kidneys.

amniotic band syndrome which can cause bizarre clefts in nonanatomic orientations. Some of these are thought to result from the fetus's swallowing part of the membrane which then causes the defect through the effects of pressure. Not unusually, the cleft courses through and disrupts the orbit, maxilla, and lip. Most of these fetuses have additional, major lethal anomalies.

Other Facial Disorders

The **tongue** can normally be seen moving in the mouth; it is an uncommon site for problems. Macroglossia is rare but can be seen in several disorders. In the Beckwith-Wiedemann syndrome, the tongue is grossly enlarged and protrudes beyond the lips (Fig. 42-16). Associated anomalies include macrosomia, omphalocele, renal hyperplasia and dysplasia, and an increased incidence of Wilms' tumor and hepatoblastoma.[1] The large tongue can cause neonatal breathing and feeding difficulties. Lesser degrees of macroglossia are common with trisomy 21.[14]

The **mandible** is readily demonstrated in transverse and profile views. Shortening of the mandible (micrognathia or retrognathia) can be detected prenatally and is present in numerous syndromes[1,12-14,42,47] (Fig. 42-17, *A* and *B*). Prenatally identified micrognathia is commonly associated with polyhydramnios and karyotypic abnormalities and has a poor prognosis.[48] Though the mandible forms through fusion of two lateral processes, clefts of the lower lip and mandible are rare.[42]

The normal **hypopharynx** contains fluid and changes with swallowing. The esophagus is not normally

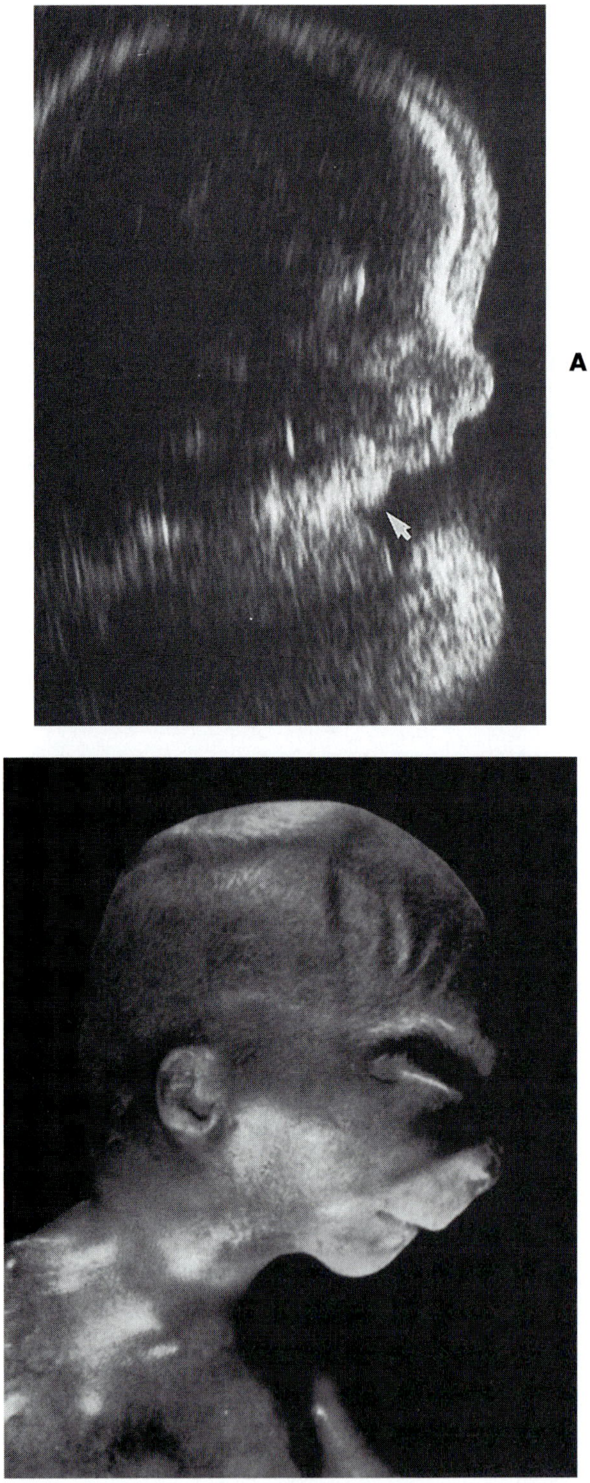

A

B

FIG. 42-17. Micrognathia. A, Profile at 31 weeks shows mandible *(arrow)* posteriorly positioned relative to nose and upper lip and **B,** confirmed postnatally.

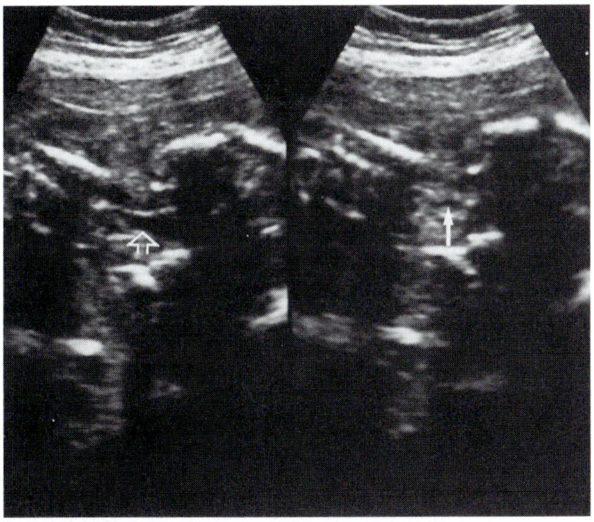

FIG. 42-18. Fetal swallowing. Lateral coronal views of the hypopharynx at 21 weeks' menstrual age. The left image shows the normal appearance of the fluid-filled hypopharynx *(open arrow)*. The right image taken during swallowing shows the hypopharynx closed as a thin line *(solid arrow)*. A few seconds later, the appearance again was that of the normal fluid-filled pharynx.

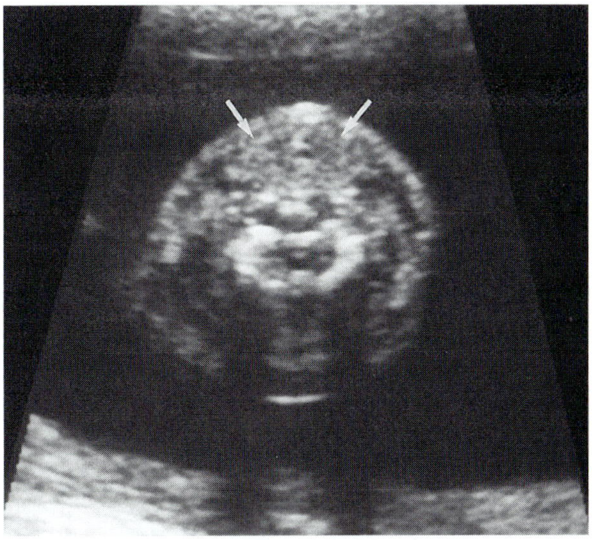

FIG. 42-19. Normal fetal thyroid *(arrows)*. Axial view through fetal neck at 21 weeks. The trachea is visible between the thyroid lobes. The carotid arteries/jugular veins are just behind the lobes.

visible, but with gastrointestinal obstruction, it can be recognized as transiently fluid-filled tube coursing between the aorta and heart (Fig. 42-18).

A rare **teratoma (epignathus)** occurs in the oropharynx and may cause polyhydramnios by obstructing swallowing. In most cases it causes fatal respiratory obstruction after delivery.[49]

EARS

The **ears** are readily visible. They participate in numerous syndromes.[50] They may be abnormally low, rotated, prominent, or of abnormal shape or size.[13,16,50,51] Normal ear length has been measured by Birnholz who also found that in trisomies, especially 13 and 18, the ears tend to be short—less than 1.5 standard deviations below the mean.[50]

NECK

Normal Anatomy

The soft tissues of the fetal neck are normally not assessed in detail on routine scanning but should be evaluated with polyhydramnios to look for obstructive lesions and fluid collections.[52,53] The pulsatile carotid arteries, trachea, and fluid-filled hypopharynx are normally visible. Nomograms of neck diameter are available.[54]

Fetal Thyroid

The fetal thyroid functions by 12 weeks. Normal measurements have been described from 20 weeks onward (Fig. 42-19). The 95th percentile for width at 20 weeks is 22 mm and by 40 weeks it increases to 35 mm.[55] Thyroid enlargement, or goiter, can be detected prenatally and may be seen with fetal hyper- or hypothyroidism. Maternal Graves' disease and the drugs used to treat hyperthyroidism can affect the fetus and cause fetal hyper- or hypothyroidism.[56] About 1% to 12% of mothers with Graves' disease will have hyperthyroid fetuses. Fetal manifestations of thyroid dysfunction include IUGR, oligohydramnios, tachycardia, polyhydramnios, and hyperextension of the neck. Mothers with known thyroid disease should be monitored for development of fetal goiter, as it can be treated *in utero* to avoid fetal thyroid dysfunction and other malfunctions related to thyroid enlargement, which include problems at delivery due to persistent neck hyperextension and respiratory embarrassment.[57]

Cystic Hygroma (Nuchal Cysts Syndrome)

A large, septated nuchal fluid collection is called a **cystic hygroma**; this is a specific pathologic term used to describe a multilocular lymphatic malformation lined by lymphatic endothelium. While most nuchal collections are lymphatic in origin, this is not true in every case.[58] Hygromas are thought to arise from failure of the lymphatic system to develop a communication to the venous system in the neck, and they may be associated with cutaneous edema and collections of fluid in serous cavities (hydrops). Most fetuses with large hygromas, especially if associated with hydrops, will die *in utero*.[59] Chromosomal anomalies are common, especially Turner's and Down syndrome, but hygromas may occur in fetuses with normal chromosomes as well as in association with fetal alcohol syndrome, multiple pterygium syndrome, and as a postmortem effect.[58]

At **sonography,** they are large nuchal fluid collections with random septations and, characteristically, a thicker midline septum (Fig. 42-20). They

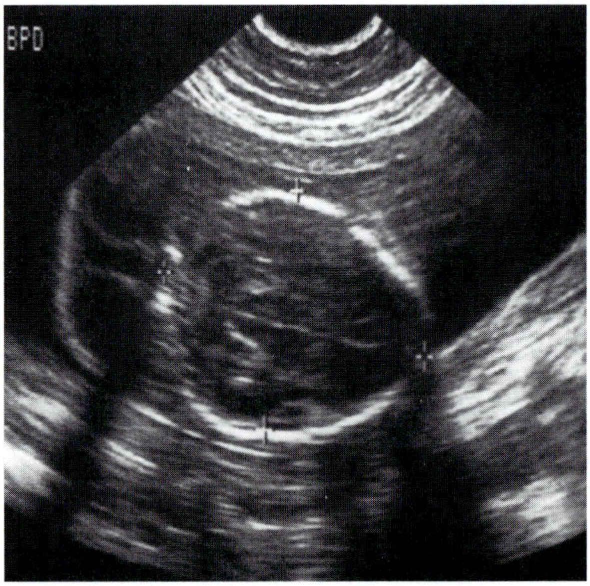

FIG. 42-20. Cystic hygroma (nuchal cysts syndrome). Axial view at 18 weeks' menstrual age shows the hygroma discovered on a routine scan in a male fetus who also had many other anomalies. Note the typical midline septation and normal intracranial structures (cerebellum), which help differentiate this nuchal hygroma from encephalocele.

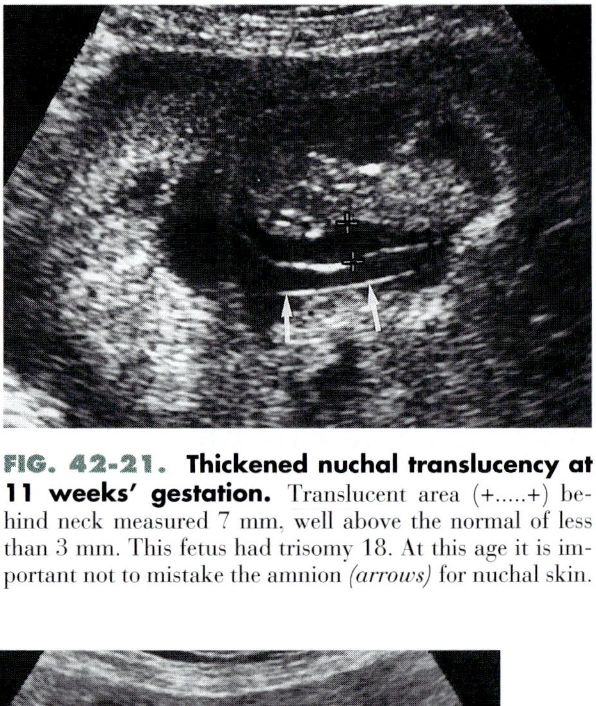

FIG. 42-21. Thickened nuchal translucency at 11 weeks' gestation. Translucent area (+.....+) behind neck measured 7 mm, well above the normal of less than 3 mm. This fetus had trisomy 18. At this age it is important not to mistake the amnion *(arrows)* for nuchal skin.

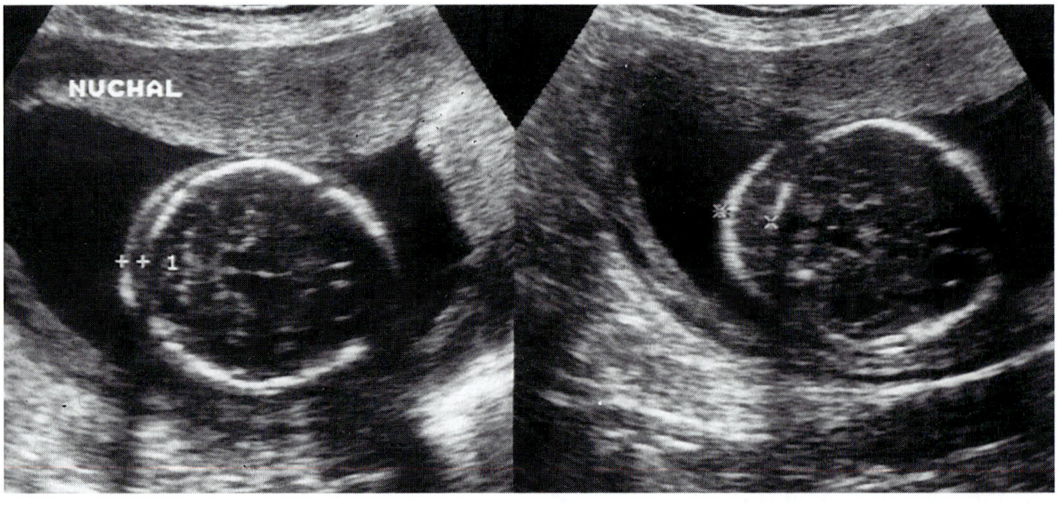

FIG. 42-22. Down syndrome fetus with nuchal thickening. Note the excess soft tissues between the caliper marks on the right image. The measurement is taken as shown from the outer surface of the occipital bone to the skin surface. The normal measurement should be less than 6 mm in fetuses under 20 weeks. The left image shows the pitfall of measuring too high on the occiput where the measurement is normal. The thickening is typically more prominent lower toward the neck and should be measured as low on the occipital bone as possible, as in the right image.

differ from encephaloceles in that the skull, brain, and spine are normal. Additional fluid collections in the soft tissues at the sides of the neck often occur with cystic hygromas.

Hygromas have been detected as nuchal bulges as early as 10 weeks. It is important to avoid mistaking for a hygroma the normal sonolucent space (fetal nuchal translucency) between fetal nuchal skin and the denser spinal tissues that can be seen between 10 to 14 weeks' gestation.[60]

Measurements of **fetal nuchal translucency** have been suggested as a screen for chromosomal disorders. The normal measurement, taken between 10 and 13 weeks, is under 2.5 mm. It is measured as the maximal thickness between the skin and the soft tissue overlying the cervical spine, taking care to distinguish between fetal skin and amnion.[61] Increased thickness is associated with trisomies 21, 18, and 13, triploidy, and Turner's syndrome (Fig. 42-21). Chromosomally normal fetuses with thickening showed a slight increase in structural defects involving mainly cardiac, diaphragmatic, renal, and abdominal wall structures.[62] (See also Chapter 40 on chromosomal abnormalities.)

Nuchal Thickening and Down Syndrome

Benacerraf has reported skin thickening of 6 mm or more in the occipital region between 15 and 19 weeks as suspicious for Down syndrome.[63] The thickening is due to subcutaneous edema, and usually no distinct fluid collection is present. This is probably a mild manifestation of the same process that causes cystic hygromas and, in fact, some fetuses with Down syndrome have massive hygromas. Demonstration of increased nuchal thickness under 20 weeks' gestation has detected 42% of Down syndrome fetuses, with a false-positive rate of 0.1%.

The **nuchal measurement** is taken on a transaxial view of the fetal head, measuring from the outer surface of the occipital bone to the outer surface of the overlying skin (Fig. 42-22).[63] Care must be taken to avoid overrotating the transducer to minimize false-positive results.[64]

Neck Masses

Masses constitute the main prenatally diagnosed abnormality involving the neck. Such masses commonly include cystic hygroma, hemangioma, teratoma, and goiter.[52,53,65] During pregnancy these masses can obstruct swallowing and cause polyhydramnios and absence of fluid in the fetal stomach. If they are large, dystocia may result from the effects of the masses or from neck extension. After delivery, respiration and swallowing can be obstructed.

REFERENCES

1. Jones KL. *Smith's Recognizable Patterns of Human Malformation.* 4th ed. Philadelphia: WB Saunders Co; 1988.
2. Campbell S, Pearch JM. The prenatal diagnosis of fetal structural anomalies by ultrasound. *Clinics in Obstet Gynecol* 1983; 10:475-506.
3. Levy S, Schaaps JP, De Havay P et al. End result of routine ultrasound screening for congenital anomalies: the Belgian multicentric study 1984-1992. *Ultrasound Obstet Gynecol* 1995; 5:366-371.
4. Crane JP, LeFevre ML, Winborn RC et al. A randomized trial of prenatal ultrasonographic screening: impact on detection, management and outcome of anomalous fetuses (RADIUS study). *Am J Obstet Gynecol* 1994;171:392-399.
5. Guidelines for performance of antepartum obstetrical ultrasound examination. *American Institute of Ultrasound in Medicine;* 1991.
6. ACR standard for antepartum obstetrical ultrasound. American College of Radiology Standards; 1995.

Embryology

7. Moore KL, Persaud TVN. *The Developing Human.* 5th ed. WB Saunders Co; 1993.
8. Maniglia AJ. Embryology, teratology, and arrested developmental disorders in otolaryngology. *Otolaryng Clin North Am* 1981;14:25-38.
9. Stewart RE. Craniofacial malformations: clinical and genetic considerations. *Pediatr Clin North Am* 1978;25:485-515.
10. DeMyer W, Zeman W, Palmer CG. The face predicts the brain: diagnostic significance of median facial anomalies for holoprosencephaly (arrhinencephaly). *Pediatrics* 1964;34:256-263.
11. Pashley NRT, Krause CJ. Cleft lip, cleft palate and other fusion disorders. *Otolaryngol Clin North Am* 1981;14:125-143.

Overview of Anomalies

12. Pilu G, Reece A, Romero R et al. Prenatal diagnosis of craniofacial malformations with ultrasonography. *Am J Obstet Gynecol* 1986;155:45-50.
13. Hegge FN, Prescott GH, Watson PT. Fetal facial abnormalities identified during obstetric sonography. *J Ultrasound Med* 1986; 5:679-684.
14. Nicolaides KH, Salvesen DR, Snijders RJ et al. Fetal facial defects: associated malformations and chromosomal abnormalities. *Fetal Diagn Ther* 1993;8:1-9.
15. Koren G, Edwards MB, Miskin M. Antenatal sonography of fetal malformations associated with drugs and chemicals. *Am J Obstet Gynecol* 1987;176:79.

Normal Sonographic Examination

16. Jeanty P, Romero R, Staudach A et al. Facial anatomy of the fetus. *J Ultrasound Med* 1986;5:607-616.
17. De Elejalde MM, Elejalde BR. Visualization of the fetal face by ultrasound. *J Craniofac Gen Dev Biol* 1984;4:251-257.
18. Birnholz JC. The development of human fetal eye movement patterns. *Science* 1981;213:679-681.
19. De Elejalde MM, Elejalde BR. Ultrasonic visualization of the fetal eye. *J Craniofac Gen Dev Biol* 1985;5:319-326.
20. Cooper C, Mahoney BS, Bowie JD et al. Ultrasound evaluation of the normal fetal upper airway and esophagus. *J Ultrasound Med* 1985;4:343-346.
21. Bowie JD, Clair MR. Fetal swallowing and regurgitation: observation of normal and abnormal activity. *Radiology* 1982; 144:877-878.
22. Benacerraf BR, Frigoletto FD, Bieber FR. The fetal face: ultrasound examination. *Radiology* 1984;153:495-497.

23. Jeanty P, Cantraine F, Cousaert E et al. The binocular distance: a new way to estimate fetal age. *J Ultrasound Med* 1984; 3:241-243.
24. Mayden KL, Tortora M, Berkowitz RL et al. Orbital diameters: a new parameter for prenatal diagnosis and dating. *Am J Obstet Gynecol* 1982;144:289-297.
25. Escobar LF, Bixler D, Padilla LM et al. Fetal craniofacial morphometrics: *in utero* evaluation at 16 weeks' gestation. *Obstet Gynecol* 1988;72:674-679.
26. Pretorius DH, Nelson TR. Fetal face visualization using three-dimensional ultrasonography. *J Ultrasound Med* 1995;14:349-356.
27. Pretorius DH, House M, Nelson TR et al. Evaluation of normal and abnormal lips in fetuses: Comparison between three- and two-dimensional sonography. *AJR* 1995;165:1233-1237.

Orbital Disorders

28. Birnholz JC, Farrell EE. Fetal hyaloid artery: timing of regression with ultrasound. *Radiology* 1988;166:781-783.
29. Berrocal T, de Orbe A, Prieto C et al. Ultrasound and color Doppler imaging of ocular and orbital disease in the paediatric age group. *RadioGraphics* 1996;16:251-272.
30. Garry EA, Rawnsley E, Marin-Padilla JM et al. *In utero* detection of fetal cataracts. *J Ultrasound Med* 1993;4:234-236.
31. Davis KW, Mahony BS, Carroll BA et al. Antenatal sonographic detection of benign dacrocystoceles (lacrimal duct cysts). *J Ultrasound Med* 1987;6:461-465.
32. Menashe Y, Baruch GB, Rabinovitch O et al. Exophthalmus (sic)—prenatal ultrasonic features for diagnosis of Crouzon syndrome. *Prenat Diag* 1989;9:805-808.
33. Farrell SA, Toi A, Leadman ML et al. Prenatal diagnosis of retinal detachment in Walker-Warburg syndrome. *Am J Med Genetics* 1987;28:619-624.
34. Chitayat D, Toi A, Babul R et al. Prenatal diagnosis of retinal nonattachment in the Walker-Warburg syndrome. *Am J Med Genet* 1995;56:351-358.
35. McGahan JP, Nyberg DA, Mack LA. Sonography of facial features of alobar and semilobar holoprosencephaly. *AJR* 1990; 154:143-148.
36. Nyberg DA, Mahony BS, Pretorius DH. *Diagnostic Ultrasound of Fetal Anomalies: Text and Atlas:* Year Book Medical Pub; 1990:212.
37. DeMyer W. The median cleft face syndrome. *Neurology* 1967; 17:961-971.

Mouth

38. Chervenak FA, Tortora M, Mayden K et al. Antenatal diagnosis of median cleft face syndrome: sonographic demonstration of cleft lip and hypertelorism. *Am J Obstet Gynecol* 1984;149: 94-97.
39. Nyberg DA, Sickler GK, Hegge FN et al. Fetal cleft lip with and without cleft palate: US classification and correlation with outcome. *Radiology* 1995;195:677-684.
40. Bundy AL, Saltzman DH, Emerson D et al. Sonographic features associated with cleft palate. *J Clin Ultrasound* 1986; 14:486-489.
41. CP, Wong D. Management of children with cleft lip and palate. *Can Med Assoc J* 1980;12:19-24.
42. Gorlin RJ, Cohen MM, Levin LS. Syndromes of the head and neck. In: *Orofacial Clefting Syndromes: General Aspects.* Oxford University Press; 1990.
43. Saltzman DH, Benacerraf BR, Frigoletto FD. Diagnosis and management of fetal facial clefts. *Am J Obstet Gynecol* 1986; 155:377-379.
44. Fraser FC. The genetics of cleft lip and cleft palate. *Am J Hum Genet* 1970;22:336-352.
45. Seeds JW, Cefalo RC. Technique of early sonographic diagnosis of bilateral cleft lip and palate. *Obstet Gynecol* 1983; 62(suppl):2S-7S.
46. Tessier P. Anatomical classification of facial, cranio-facial and latero-facial clefts. *J Max-fac Surg* 1976;4:69-92.
47. Benacerraf BR, Frigoletto FD, Greene MF. Abnormal facial features and extremities in human trisomy syndromes: prenatal US appearance. *Radiology* 1986;159:243-246.
48. Bromley B, Benacerraf BR. Fetal micrognathia: associated anomalies and outcome. *J Ultrasound Med* 1994;13:529-533.
49. Chervenak FA, Tortora M, Moya FR et al. Antenatal sonographic diagnosis of epignathus. *J Ultrasound Med* 1984;3: 235-237.

Ears

50. Birhnolz JC, Farrell EE. Fetal ear length. *Pediatrics* 1988; 81:555-558.
51. Hill LM, Thomas ML, Peterson CS. The ultrasonic detection of Apert syndrome. *J Ultrasound Med* 1987;6:601-604.

Neck

52. Grundy H, Glasmann A, Burlbaw J et al. Hemangioma presenting as a cystic mass in the fetal neck. *J Ultrasound Med* 1985;4:147-150.
53. Barone CM, Van Natta FC, Kourides IA et al. Sonographic detection of fetal goiter, an unusual cause of hydramnios. *J Ultrasound Med* 1985;4:625-627.
54. Hata K, Hata T, Takamiya O et al. Ultrasonographic measurements of the fetal neck correlated with gestational age. *J Ultrasound Med* 1988;7:333-337.
55. Bromely B, Frigoletto FD, Cramer D et al. The fetal thyroid: normal and abnormal sonographic measurements. *J Ultrasound Med* 1992;11:25-28.
56. Davidson KM, Richards DS, Schatz DA et al. Successful *in utero* treatment of fetal goiter and hypothyroidism. *N Engl J Med* 1991;324:543-546.
57. Abuhamad AZ, Fisher DA, Warsof SL et al. Antenatal diagnosis and treatment of goitrous hypothyroidism: case report and review of the literature. *Ultrasound Obstet Gynecol* 1995; 6:368-371.
58. Elejalde BR, de Elejalde MM, Leno. Nuchal cysts syndromes: etiology, pathogenesis, and prenatal diagnosis. *Am J Med Genet* 1985;21:417-432.
59. Chervenak FA, Isaacson G, Blakemore KJ et al. Fetal cystic hygroma, cause and natural history. *N Engl J Med* 1983;309:822-825.
60. Hertzberg BS, Bowie JD, Carroll BS et al. Normal sonographic appearance of the fetal neck late in the first trimester: the pseudomembrane. *Radiology* 1989;171:427-429.
61. Pandya PP, Goldberg H, Walton B et al. The implementation of first-trimester scanning at 10-13 weeks' gestation and the measurement of fetal nuchal translucency thickness in two maternity units. *Ultrasound Obstet Gynecol* 1995;5:20-25.
62. Pandya PP, Kondylios A, Hilbert L et al. Chromosomal defects and outcome in 1015 fetuses with increased nuchal translucency. *Ultrasound Obstet Gynecol* 1995;5:15-19.
63. Benacerraf BR, Frigoletto FD. Soft-tissue nuchal fold in the second-trimester fetus: standards for normal measurements compared with those in Down's syndrome. *Am J Obstet Gynecol* 1987;157:1146-1149.
64. Toi A, Simpson GF, Filly RA. Sonographically evident fetal nuchal skin thickening: is it specific for Down's syndrome? *Am J Obstet Gynecol* 1987;156:150.
65. Shipp TD, Bromley B, Benacerraf B. The ultrasonographic appearance and outcome for fetuses with masses distorting the fetal face. *J Ultrasound Med* 1995;14:673-678.

CHAPTER 43

The Fetal Brain

Ants Toi, M.D., F.R.C.P.C.
Eric E. Sauerbrei, B.Sc., M.Sc., M.D., F.R.C.P.C.

CHAPTER OUTLINE

Anomalies of the central nervous system (CNS) are the most common cause of referral for prenatal diagnosis and they cause the greatest anxiety for parents.[1-3] CNS anomalies occur with a frequency of about 1.4 to 1.6 per 1000 livebirths but are seen in about 3% to 6% of stillbirths. The increased use of maternal serum alpha-fetoprotein (MS-AFP) screening has resulted in increased numbers of pregnancies being referred for evaluation of the CNS and suspected anomalies.[4] Fortunately, ultrasound carefully performed by a knowledgeable examiner following established guidelines is proving very sensitive in evaluating the CNS.[1]

DEVELOPMENTAL ANATOMY

Embryology

Central nervous system development starts at about the fifth menstrual week (the third week after conception) as the growth of cells destined to form the notochord infiltrates into the embryonal disc. This induces overlying embryonal tissue to thicken and, ultimately, to fold over and fuse as the neural tube. The fusion starts in the middle of the embryo and subsequently extends to the cranial and caudal ends. The anterior end, the rostral neuropore, closes by about 5½ menstrual weeks and the caudal end closes about half a week later. By the sixth week, the cephalic end enlarges to become the brain and expands and flexes to form the final brain structures (Table 43-1).[1,5] By 12 to 15 menstrual weeks, almost all structures are in their final form. Exceptions are the corpus callosum, cerebellar vermis, neuronal migration from the periventricular germinal matrix, development of the sulci and gyri, and myelinization.

The **corpus callosum** starts developing at about this time and is complete at about 18 to 20 weeks. During its development, the corpus callosum induces the formation of the two septi pellucidi and the **cavum septi pellucidi et vergae.** The cerebellar **vermis** starts development superiorly and grows from above down; it is complete at about 18 weeks. At about this time also, the brain cells start to migrate from their original site, the germinal layer that lines the ventricles, to their final position at the surface of the cortex where they form the gray matter. After this migration in the third trimester, the cerebral cortex starts becoming convoluted to form the gyri and sulci.

TABLE 43-1
DIFFERENTIATION OF BRAIN REGIONS FROM PRIMARY VESICLES

Primary Vesicles	Secondary Vesicles	Mature Structures
Forebrain	Telencephalon	Cerebral hemispheres
		Basal ganglia
		Olfactory system
	Diencephalon	Thalamus
		Hypothalamus
Midbrain	Mesencephalon	Midbrain
Hindbrain	Metencephalon	Pons
		Cerebellum
Myelencephalon		Medulla

From Moore KL. *Essentials of Human Embryology*. Toronto: B.C. Decker Inc; 1988.

Sonographic Anatomy

First Trimester: Conception to 13 Weeks.

The early embryo is best examined transvaginally. The cephalic end is identifiable by about 8 weeks (Fig. 43-1, *A*). By 10 to 11 weeks, bones of the vault show mineralization (Fig. 43-1, *B*). At this age, the brain

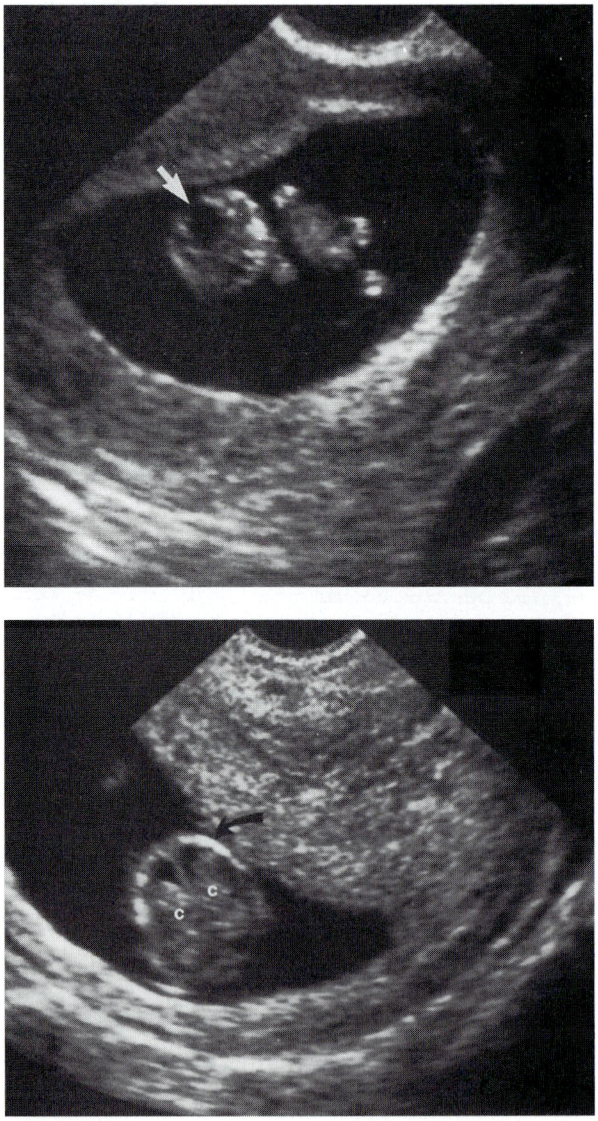

A

B

FIG. 43-1. Early fetal head images with the transvaginal probe. **A,** At 9 menstrual weeks, the cranium can be clearly differentiated from the trunk, which has limb buds. The intracranial cystic structure is the fetal rhombencephalic cavity, a normal space that subsequently becomes the fourth ventricle (*arrow*). **B,** Scan at 11½ menstrual weeks. The cortex is exceedingly thin at this age and the cerebral area consists mainly of ventricles filled with choroid (c). The echogenic ossification of the frontal bones (*arrow*) helps to rule out anencephaly.

mantle is very thin. The ventricles are large and filled with choroid, which is believed to provide nourishment for the developing brain.[6] A large echo-free space behind the hindbrain represents the **rhombencephalic cavity,** which decreases in size as the cerebellum begins to form (Fig. 43-1, *A*).[7] This normally echo-free space appears quite prominent in first trimester scanning and should not be mistaken for abnormality.

Second and Third Trimesters: 14 Weeks to Term. From this time on, most of the cerebral structures can be identified ultrasonically. **Three standard views** that show the major structures have been suggested. Consistent adherence to these three views may lead to the detection of over 95% of sonographically detectable cerebral anomalies.[8,9] These standard views, which are all transaxial from the side of the head, are:

- the thalamic view;
- the ventricular view; and
- the cerebellar view.

The **thalamic** plane is the view used to measure the biparietal and occipitofrontal diameters (BPD and OFD)[10] (Fig. 43-2, *A*). It displays the thalamus, third ventricle, fornices, basal ganglia, insula, and ambient cistern. The **ventricular** view is slightly higher than the thalamic and shows the bodies and, more importantly, the atria of the lateral ventricles as well as the interhemispheric fissure (Fig. 43-2, *B*). The **atrium** of the lateral ventricle is at the base of the occipital horn where it joins with the temporal horn and the body of the ventricle. The atrium is an important landmark at which ventricular size is measured. The **cerebellar** view is obtained by rotating the transducer into a suboccipito-bregmatic plane centered on the thalamus to show the cerebellar hemispheres (Fig. 43-2, *C*). This view shows the cerebellum, the cisterna magna, the cavum septi pellucidi, and, frequently, the anterior horns of the lateral ventricles. McLeary has described the normal appearances and measurements of the cerebellum. He finds that cerebellar measurements may be used to determine gestational age if the head has undergone molding.[11] The **cisterna magna** is the CSF space between the cerebellum and the occipital bone (Fig. 43-2, *C*). This should be noted at every study. Its obliteration suggests Arnold-Chiari II malformation, which is a common finding in spina bifida.

Head shape should be noted at all of these views. The normal shape is ovoid (Fig. 43-2). Bifrontal indentation, or **lemon** shape (Fig. 43-13, *A*), occurs with spina bifida, some dwarfs, and about 1% of normal fetuses. A **strawberry** shape is seen with chromosomal abnormality, especially trisomy 18. It consists of shortened occipitofrontal length **(brachycephaly)** (Fig. 43-4) and a somewhat triangular shape with pointing anteriorly and flattening at the occiput. A **cloverleaf** shape is seen with some dwarfs, especially thanatophoric dwarfs, and in some fetuses with cranial synostosis. This deformity is best seen coronally. In it, the top of the head is small and there is bulging bilaterally in the low temporal and squamosal region. Bizarre shapes can be seen with **craniosynostoses**, depending on which sutures fuse. Craniosynostoses may be idiopathic and sporadic or may occur as part of other syndromes.[12] **Dolichocephaly** describes a head that is elongated from front to back and narrow from side to side. This is generally due to head-molding in breech presentation but it can be a fixed deformity.

Cranial bone mineralization should be noted, especially if the view of the brain is unexpectedly clear. Conditions with poor mineralization, such as **osteogenesis imperfecta** (Fig. 43-5) and **hypophosphatasia**, should be considered in these instances.

These three views form a useful starting point but the examination should not be limited to them alone. The entire brain should be examined, using whatever projections are needed to show all the structures (Fig. 43-2, *D*). On occasion, the transvaginal probe may have to be employed; when the head is deep in the pelvis, it allows a better view of the brain.[13]

CRANIAL MEASUREMENTS OBTAINED AT 2ND AND 3RD TRIMESTER SCAN

Definite:
- Biparietal diameter (BPD)
- Occipitofrontal diameter (OFD)
- Occipital horn
- Nuchal fold (second trimester)

If concerned:
- Cerebellum transverse diameter
- Cisterna magna

CRANIAL STRUCTURES TO NOTE AT EACH SCAN

Head shape
Bone density
Ventricle
Cavum septi pellucidi
Thalamus
Cerebellum and vermis
Cisterna magna
Nuchal fold

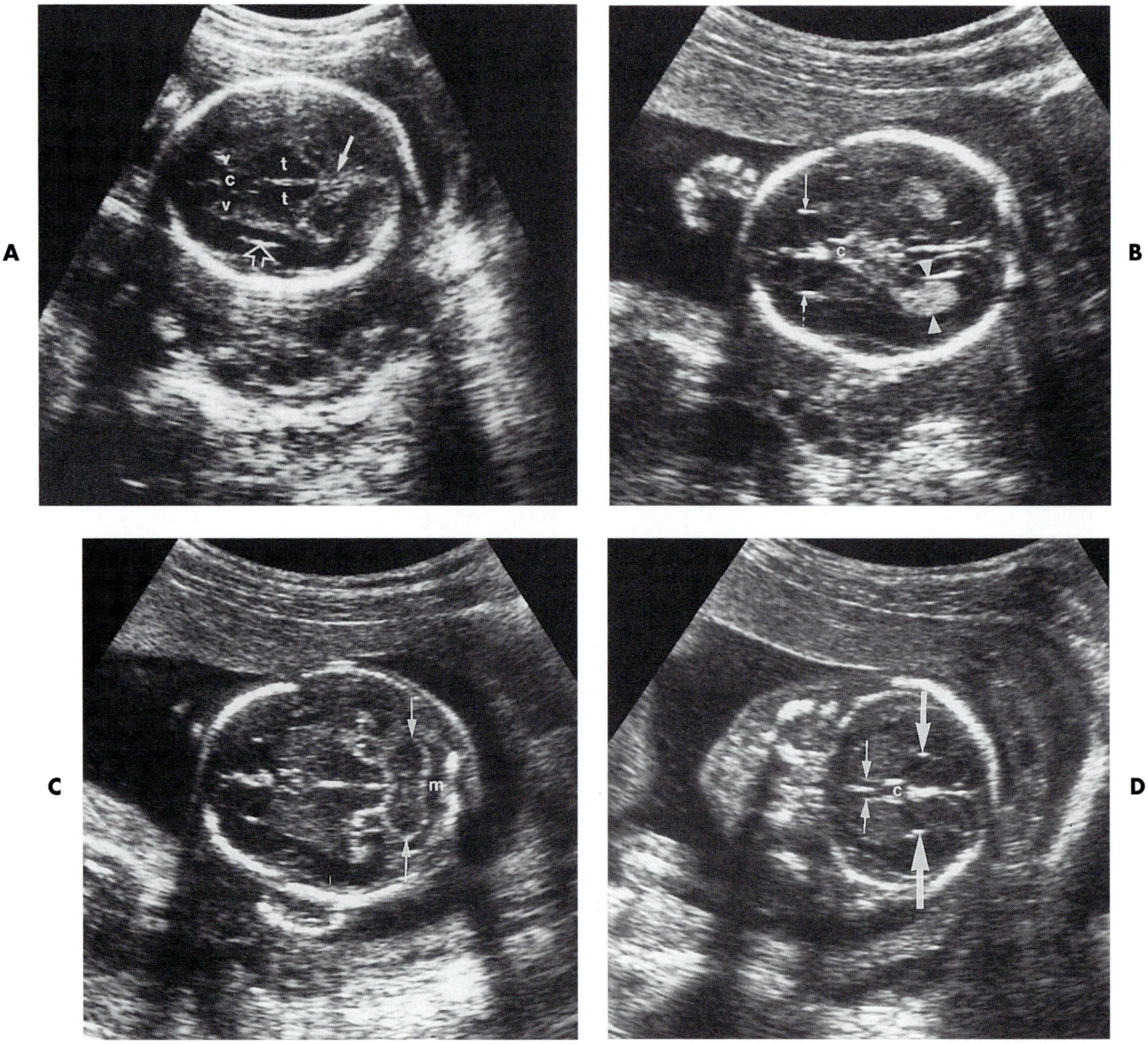

FIG. 43-2. Standard planes for viewing cerebral structures. **A**, Thalamic view at 20 menstrual weeks. This transverse view through the diamond-shaped thalamus-hypothalamus complex (t) contains the slitlike midline third ventricle. The echogenic triangular area behind the thalamus and between the occipital lobes is the ambient cistern (*arrow*), which contains CSF but is rendered echogenic because of strands of meninges supporting the brain structures. The insula is a short, brightly echogenic line (*open arrow*) containing the pulsating middle cerebral artery branches. It is surrounded by normal white matter that is very hypoechoic and should not be mistaken for fluid. The echogenic band between thalamus and insula is the basal ganglia. Anteriorly are the tips of the anterior horns of the lateral ventricles (v) and between them is the boxlike cavum septi pellucidi (c). **B**, Ventricular view at 18 weeks. The atrium of the occipital horn is filled with echogenic choroid and the point of measurement indicated (*arrowheads*). The normal measurement is < 10 mm. Note that the choroid fills over 60% of the atrium, and the measurement between the medial ventricle wall and the choroid is under 3 mm. Compare this to Fig. 43-8, *B*. The tips of the anterior horns are visible (*arrows*). Cavum septi pellucidi (c). **C**, Cerebellar view at 18 menstrual weeks is obtained by rotating the transducer from the thalamic view so that the cerebellar hemispheres (*arrows*) come into view connected in the midline by the slightly more echogenic vermis. The cisterna magna (m) is visible between the cerebellum and the occipital bone. Also visible in this view are the thalamus, third ventricle, anterior horns, and cavum septi pellucidi. **D**, Coronal view at 19 weeks through the coronal suture shows anterior horns. This demonstrates how various projections can display distinct parts of the anatomy clearly. Anterior horns of lateral ventricles (*large arrows*) and large nerve runks, the fornices (*small arrows*), are clearly visible. Orbits and chin are to the left. Contrast the normal V-shaped configuration of the anterior horns to the U shape seen in agenesis of the corpus callosum (Fig. 43-26, *B*). Cavum septi pellucidi (c).

A

B

C

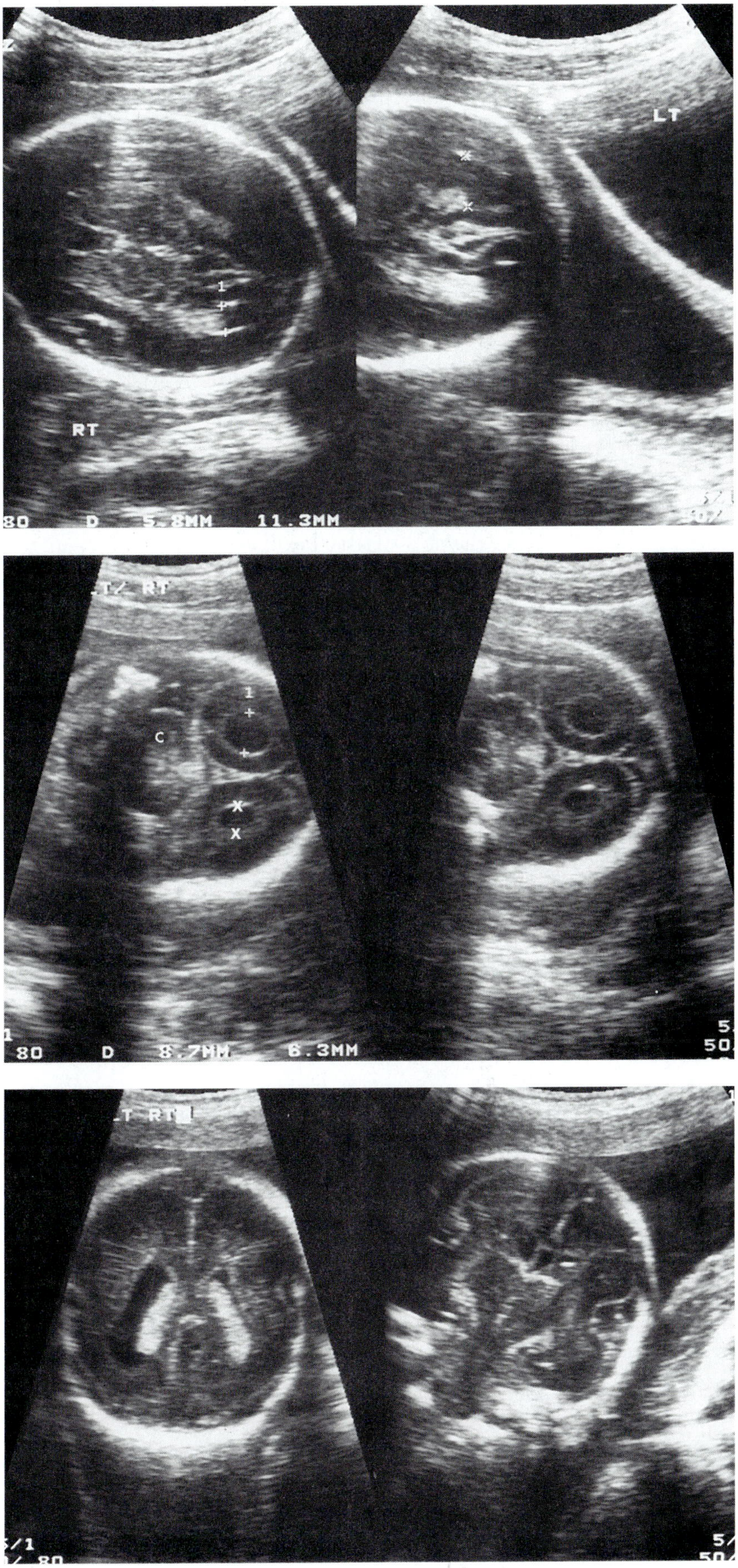

FIG. 43-3. Assessment of the proximal (upper) ventricle at 23 weeks. **A,** Axial view left shows the usually measured lower ventricle. On the right, by viewing through the posterior squamosal suture, we can see and measure (×...×) the upper ventricle in the axial plane as well. **B,** Coronal view through the lambdoid suture shows asymmetry of the occipital horns (+...+) and (×...×) in the occipital lobes above the cerebellum. Neck is to the left, vertex to right. Cerebellum (c). **C,** Views taken through the anterior fontanelle analogous to neonatal head ultrasound. The left image shows the occipital horns and the right image shows the anterior horns and confirms slight ventricular asymmetry.

VENTRICULOMEGALY AND HYDROCEPHALUS

Definition

The term **ventriculomegaly** (VM) describes large ventricles. The head itself may be normal, large, or even smaller than expected for menstrual age. **Hydrocephalus** (HC) refers to enlarged ventricles associated with increased intracranial pressure and/or head enlargement. Ventriculomegaly is the most common cranial abnormality.

Enlargement of the lateral cerebral ventricles is not the primary problem but, rather, part of the manifestation of diverse cerebral disorders. Although ventriculomegaly is an obvious manifestation of many cerebral disorders, one must remember that it is not the size and appearance of the ventricles that is clinically important but the underlying changes in the brain. Cerebral functional alterations are predicted only variably by ventricular size or cortical thinning or appearance.[14-17]

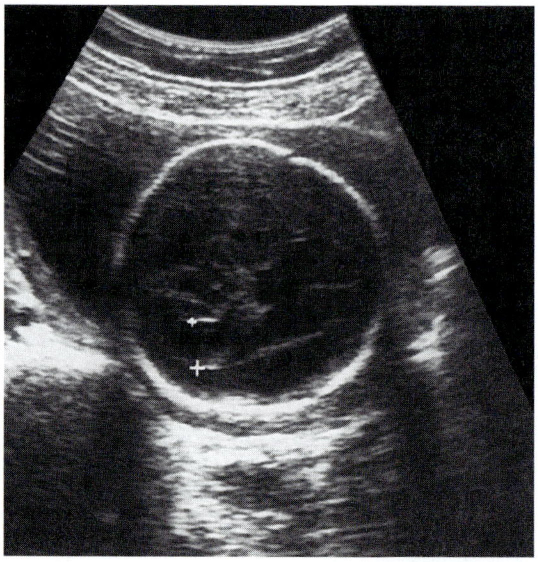

FIG. 43-4. Brachycephaly and slight strawberry shape at 24 weeks in fetus with trisomy 18. Cephalic index is 96% (normal is 80%). There is also borderline ventriculomegaly of 11 mm.

Pathogenesis

Cerebrospinal fluid (CSF) is secreted by the choroid plexus of the lateral, third, and fourth ventricles as well as by the cerebral capillaries.[18] It flows from the lateral ventricles through the foramina of Monro, third ventricle, aqueduct of Sylvius, and fourth ventricle and out the foramina of Magendie and Luschka into the subarachnoid space of the posterior fossa. Then it courses over the surface of the brain to the Pacchionian granulations, which are distributed at the top of the head adjacent to the superior sagittal sinus. Ventricular enlargement generally results from obstruction of CSF flow **in** the brain (**intraventricular obstructive hydrocephalus**). Alternatively, the site of blockage may be **outside** the ventricular system or there may be failure of absorption (**extraventricular obstructive hydrocephalus**, or **communicating hydrocephalus**). Less commonly, ventriculomegaly results from excess CSF secretion with choroid plexus papillomas or follows cerebral destruction as a result of diverse insults (hydrocephalus ex vacuo) (Fig. 43-6). In liveborn infants with ventriculomegaly, 43% are associated with aqueductal stenosis, 38% have extraventricular, or communicating, hydrocephalus, 13% have a Dandy-Walker malformation, and 6% have other lesions.[18]

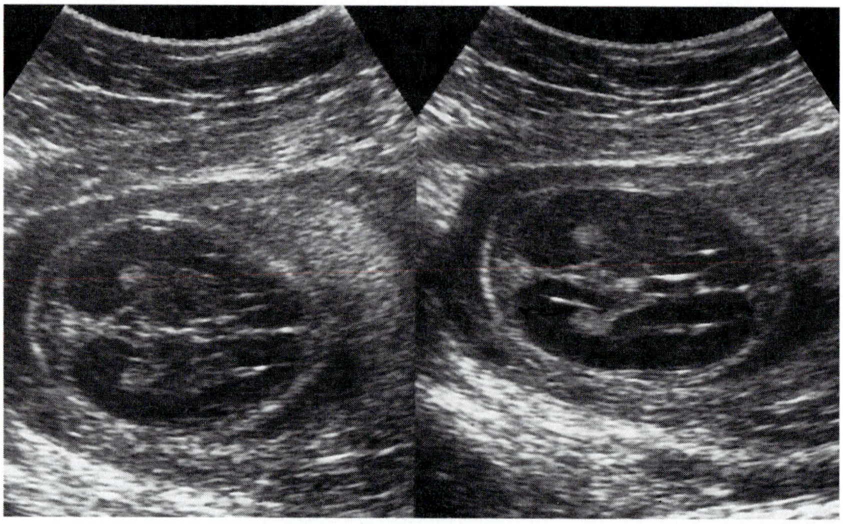

FIG. 43-5. Almost absent cranial mineralization at 19 weeks due to osteogenesis imperfecta, type 2. The entire brain is seen too clearly because there is no bone to absorb sound. The right image is taken with slight pressure on the transducer to show how readily the soft skull deforms and assumes a dolichocephalic shape.

Ultrasound Examination of the Ventricles

The detection of ventricular enlargement is the clue to the detection of most cerebral anomalies.[8] Several techniques have been described to evaluate ventricular size: occipital horn (atrial) measurement, ventricle-to-hemisphere ratio, anterior horn measurement, and anatomic appearances.

The size of the head is **not** helpful in detecting ventriculomegaly, and frequently the BPD remains normal even with severe ventricular enlargement.[19]

Atrial Size. This is the **most useful** measurement of the ventricles. The **atrium** of the lateral ventricles is the site of confluence of the bodies, occipital horns, and temporal horns. Although authors say they measure the atrium, they are probably really measuring the transverse diameter of the occipital horn just behind the atrium where the walls of the ventricle become parallel. Cardoza reports that between 14 and 38 menstrual weeks the **transverse atrial measurement** is constant at 7.6 mm (standard deviation 0.6 mm). Measurements above 10 mm suggest ventriculomegaly with a low false-positive rate[20] (Figs. 43-2, *B*, 43-8, *B*, and 43-9). This measurement is easily obtained during routine obstetric scanning; it assesses the part of the ventricle that undergoes the earliest and most marked enlargement. The walls of the occipital horn are reasonably parallel throughout their length and thus the measurement is relatively insensitive to errors in cursor placement along the axis of the ventricle. However, if the plane of view is tilted and not axial or if there is an improper choice of ventricle boundary, then a falsely large measurement will be obtained.[21]

There is a slight difference in atrial size between the sexes, with female ventricles being slightly smaller than male ventricles. The female mean atrial diameter is 5.8 ± 1.3 mm, and the male diameter is 6.4 ± 1.3 mm.[22]

Mahoney reports that the **distance between the medial atrial wall and the choroid** is 1 to 2 mm in normal fetuses over 15 weeks' gestation. Measurements of 3 mm and greater were associated with abnormal outcomes when combined with other fetal abnormalities[23] (Fig. 43-8).

Even if the ventricle measurement is normal, i.e., 10 mm, separations of choroid over 3 mm from the ventricle wall can be significant. Hertzberg found that 20% of such fetuses had abnormal outcomes.[24]

Usually, only the distal ventricular atrium is measured, as the near ventricle is hidden in artifact created by the skull bone. It is assumed that the ventricles are symmetrical. It is also possible to directly measure the proximal occipital ventricle by exploiting access provided by the squamosal and lambdoid sutures and the posterior and posterolateral fontanelle (Fig. 43-3, *A*, *B*, *C*). We have found that the **atria are generally symmetrical.** They differed by less than 1,

MEASUREMENTS OF VENTRICLE SIZE

Occipital horn	<10 mm
Ventricle to choroid	<3 mm
Anterior horns	<20 mm under 24 weeks
Ventricle/hemisphere ratio	Depends on gestation age

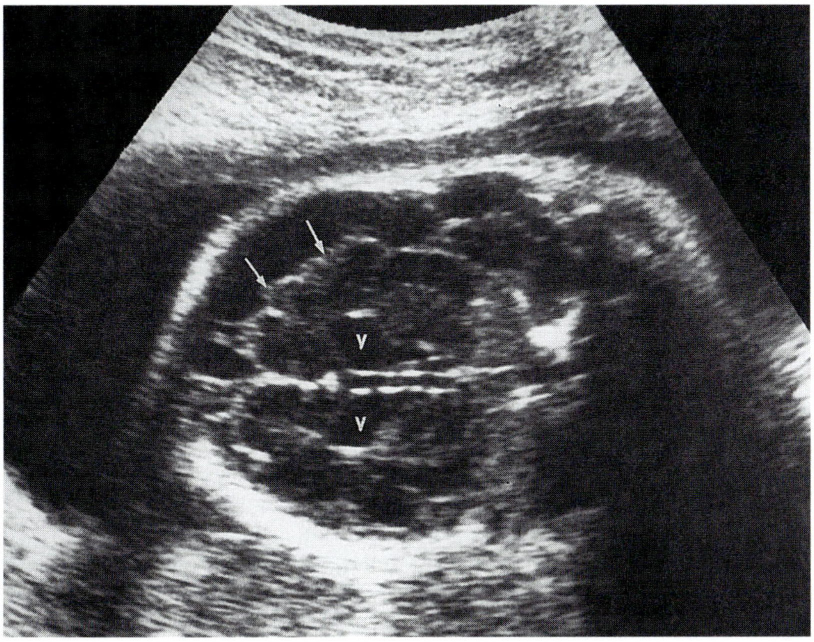

FIG. 43-6. Hydrocephalus ex vacuo at 28 weeks. The ventricles (v) are large. The brain has shrunk and its surface (*arrows*) has fallen away from the skull, leaving a wide CSF-filled subarachnoid space. This fetus had multiple other anomalies, including caudal regression and neurenteric cyst.

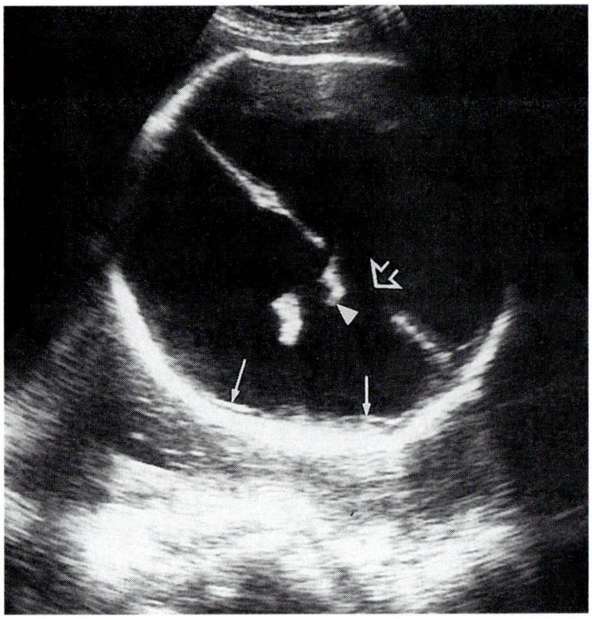

FIG. 43-7. Massive ventriculomegaly at 35 weeks due to aqueduct stenosis. The septum pellucidum has fenestrated (*open arrow*), allowing the upper choroid (*arrowhead*) to fall across the midline. The cortex is markedly thinned (*small arrows*) but present, allowing differentiation from hydranencephaly.

mm in 86% of fetuses, by less than 2 mm in 98% of fetuses, and by less than 3 mm in all the normal fetuses we studied. Differences of more than 3 mm should be viewed with caution.[25] Further assessment of symmetry is possible by evaluating the anterior horns through the anterior fontanelle as in neonatal scanning, either transabdominally or transvaginally, if the head is low in the pelvis (Fig. 43-3, *C*).

Although 10 mm has been considered the upper limit of normal, there are recent reports of normal fetuses with ventricles over 10 mm who have normal outcomes[26] and some have suggested raising the upper limit of normal to 11 to 12 mm. We agree with those who feel that 10 mm should remain the criterion above which further investigation should occur.[27]

Ventricle-to-Hemisphere Ratio. This ratio was one of the earliest techniques used to determine ventricle size, but it has now been largely supplanted by other techniques. The measurements are taken at the widest part of the head on the axial view; the distance from the falx to the ventricular wall is then compared to the width of the hemisphere. This ratio varies throughout pregnancy. Existing nomograms define the normal ranges starting at 15 menstrual weeks[28-30] (Fig. 43-9). At 16 weeks this ratio can be as high as 74% but it should decrease to less than 35% by 25 weeks. Care must be taken to identify the ventricular walls by noting the contained choroid so that the supraventricular venous lines are not mistaken for ventricles[29,31] (Fig. 43-8).

Combined Anterior Horn Measurement. We have found that the total distance between the left and right anterior ventricles never exceeds 20 mm as long as the BPD is under 6.5 cm (Fig. 43-2, *B*). This measurement is less sensitive than the individual occipital measurement, but it becomes especially useful when ventricular separation is suspected as with agenesis of the corpus callosum.

Anatomic Appearances. Qualitative appearances suggesting **ventricular enlargement** include a convex wall at the anterior horn of the lateral ventricle and asymmetry of the choroids, which fall with gravity ("droopy" or "dangling" choroids) (Fig. 43-10) when unsupported by ventricular walls.[32] With massive enlargement, the interhemispheric structures, particularly the septum pellucidum, undulate and can fenestrate; the upper choroid can fall across the midline through this hole and into the lower ventricle (Fig. 43-7).

The insula, the extreme capsule of the basal ganglia, the supraventricular veins, and reverberation echoes of the proximal skull should not be mistaken for ventricular walls (Fig. 43-2, *A*). In the second trimester the normal white matter is so homogeneous that it has been mistaken for abnormal intracranial fluid (Fig. 43-2).

Prognosis

Once enlarged ventricles are discovered, it is important to search for the etiology and any associated abnormalities because they determine the prognosis.[23,27,33-39]

Additional anomalies occur in 70% to 83% of cases but even experienced observers can miss 20% to 39% of them. About 40% of the additional anomalies are intracranial and 60% are extracranial; infants with these additional problems have mild to severe mental or physical handicaps, or they die.[39] Spina bifida is the most common association. Findings that suggest **associated spina bifida** are ventriculomegaly, effacement of the cisterna magna, and deformation of the cerebellum **(the banana sign)**[33-35] as well as scalloping of the frontal bones **(the lemon sign).**[33-36] When ventriculomegaly is present, an umbilical cord with only a single artery (i.e., two-vessel cord) strongly suggests associated extracranial anomalies and a high risk of chromosomal disorders.[37]

Parents of many fetuses with **isolated ventriculomegaly** select termination of pregnancy. Of the 28% to 46% of fetuses with true isolated ventriculomegaly who survive, 50% to 80% may have normal mental and functional outcomes.[27] Because of the high risk for poor outcomes, parents are offered pregnancy termination if ventricular enlargement is discovered early. If pregnancy is continued and the ventricles pro-

A

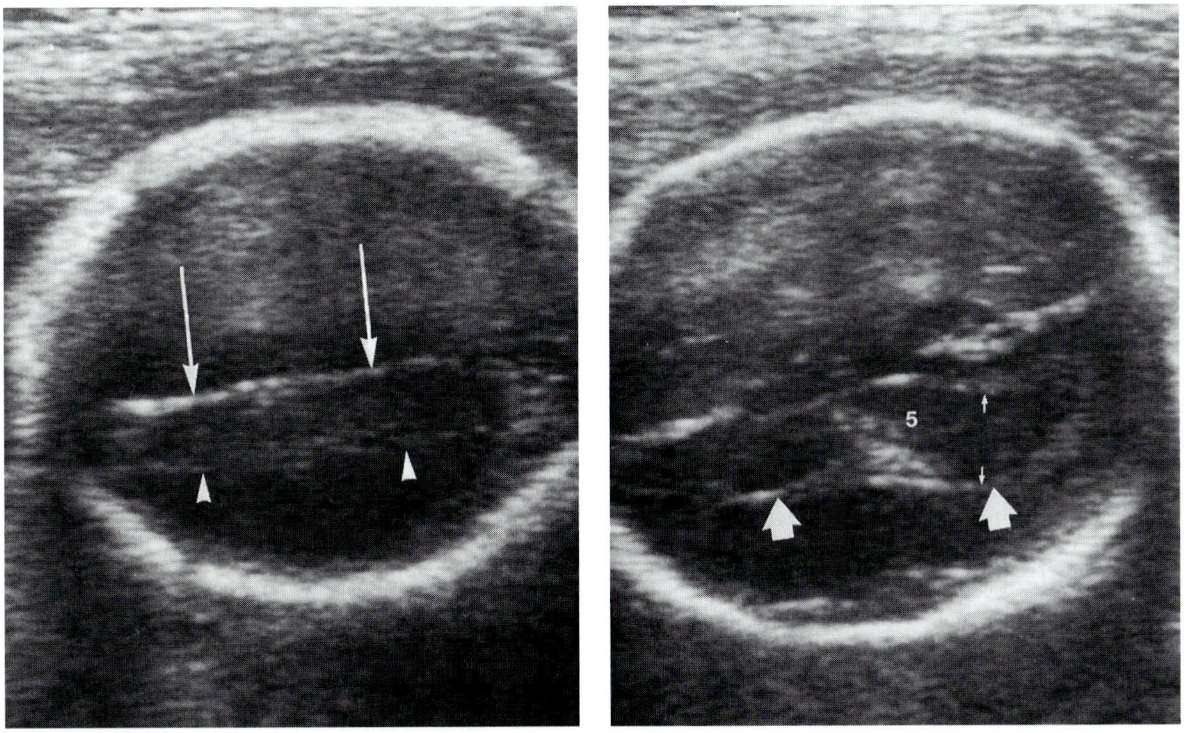

B

C

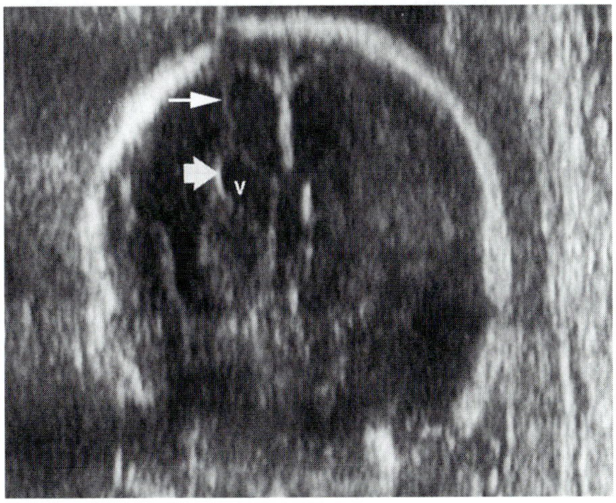

FIG. 43-8. Supraventricular marginal venous echoes at 26 menstrual weeks versus ventricular walls. **A,** Transverse view above the level of the ventricles shows echoes from the marginal veins (*arrowheads*) parallel to the interhemispheric fissure (*long arrows*). **B,** Transverse view at the ventricular plane shows mild ventricular enlargement with the occipital horn measuring over 10 mm *(small arrows)* and the choroid separated from the medial wall of the occipital horn by 5 mm (5). The ventricular margin (*broad arrows*) is curved and diverges from the midline unlike the venous "line" which is straight and parallels the midline. **C,** Coronal view through the region of the thalamus. The lateral ventricle wall echo (*short arrow*) is lateral to the supraventricular venous echo (*longer arrow*), which goes from the top of the ventricle (v) to the surface of the hemisphere.

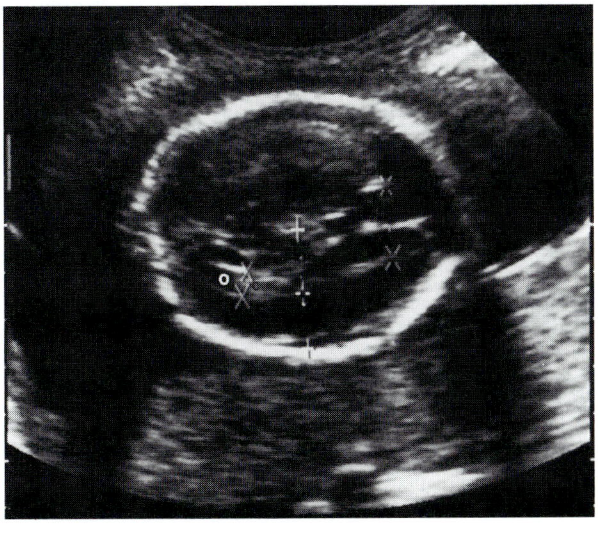

FIG. 43-9. Techniques of ventricle measurement. Ventricular view at 22 menstrual weeks. Transverse view, slightly higher than the thalamic view, shows the slightly diverging outer wall of the lateral ventricles from anterior (right) to occiput (left). The echogenic choroid fills the atrial region of the ventricle (small black c). The medial and lateral walls of the occipital horn (o) are visible. The normally hypoechoic white matter surrounding the ventricles should not be mistaken for fluid. The common ventricular measurements are shown. The **occipital horn** (×...×) is the most important measurement and is less than 10 mm at all gestational ages. **Ventricle-to-hemisphere ratio:** ventricle is measured from the midline to the lateral ventricle wall [+...+]; hemisphere is measured from the midline to the inner table of the skull [+...+]; combined **anterior horns** (×...×), which always are less than 20 mm for BPDs under 6.5 cm.

A

B

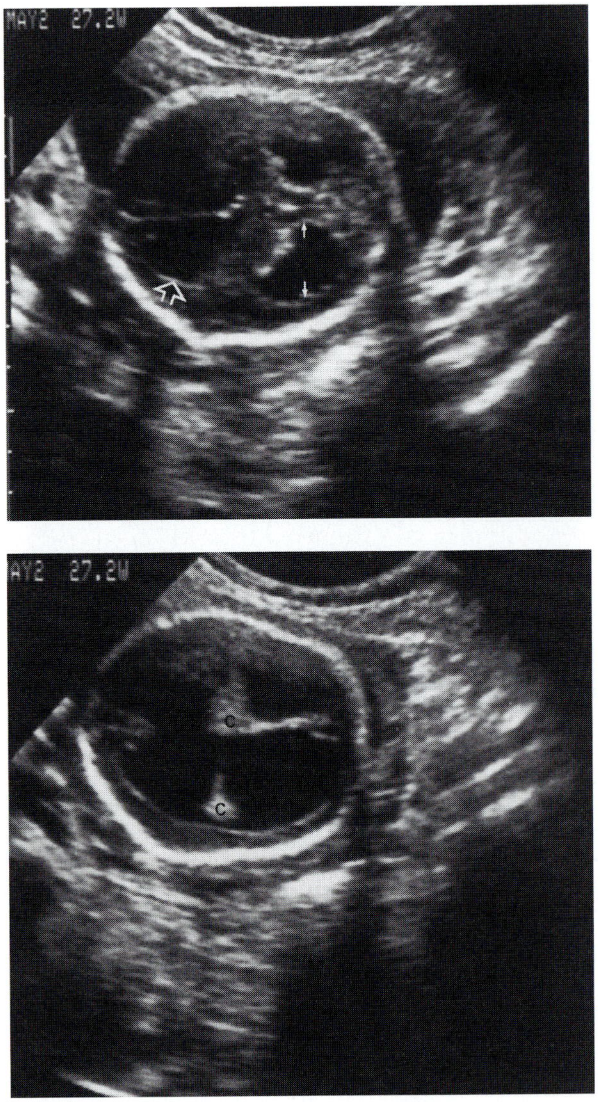

FIG. 43-10. Ventriculomegaly at 27 menstrual weeks. **A,** Thalamic view shows large occipital horns measuring over 10 mm (*arrows*) and a convex wall to the anterior horn (*open arrow*). **B,** Ventricular view shows obvious ventricular enlargement with convex surface of the lateral ventricle wall that parallels the bony calvarium. Note the drooping, or dangling, choroids (c).

gressively enlarge, then delivery is performed at pulmonary maturity.[39] Currently there is a moratorium on *in utero* intervention and ventriculo-amniotic shunting.[40,41]

SPECIFIC ABNORMALITIES

Congenital CNS abnormalities can be classified according to **time of insult** in prenatal life, as abnormalities reflect the time of noxious influence rather than the cause. Etiologic classification is not as useful as are specific malformation patterns[42,43] (Table 43-2).

TABLE 43-2
CLASSIFICATION OF CONGENITAL CNS MALFORMATIONS[36]

Disorder	Time of Onset
Dorsal induction	
Anencephaly	4th week
Encephalocele/iniencephaly	4th week
Spina bifida/Chiari II malformation	4th week
Caudal regression	4th to 7th week
Ventral induction	
Holoprosencephaly	5th to 6th week
Dandy-Walker malformation	7th to 10th week
Neuronal proliferation, differentiation	
Microcephaly	2nd to 4th month
Macrocephaly	2nd to 4th month
Vascular malformations, tumors	2nd to 3rd month
Migration	
Agenesis of corpus callosum	3rd to 5th month
Acquired injury	
Porencephaly	3rd to 4th month
Aqueductal stenosis	
Unclassified	

From van der Knaap MS, Valk J. Classification of congenital abnormalities of the CNS. *AJNR* 1988;9:315-316.

Errors of Dorsal Induction

Errors of induction and development of the neural plate and canal (neurulation) result in defects of closure, including anencephaly, encephaloceles, spinal dysraphism, and Chiari malformations.

Acrania, Anencephaly, Exencephaly. **Acrania,** or absence of the cranial vault, or calvaria ("calvarium" is improper English, although it is commonly used to describe the bones and structures that form the covering of the brain), is common to all these lesions. **Anencephaly** occurs in about 1 in 1000 births and is characterized by the absence of the cranial vault, cerebral hemispheres, and diencephalic structures and their replacement by a flattened, amorphous vascular-neural mass (area cerebrovasculosa) (Fig. 43-11, *A*). The amorphous mass may resemble brain structures uncovered by bone (**exencephaly**) (Fig. 43-11, *B*), but in all cases there is absence of normally formed calvaria and brain superior to the orbits.[44,45] Facial structures and orbits are present. Spinal and non-CNS abnormalities and polyhydramnios are common.[46,47] On occasion, the dysraphic abnormality involves the head and entire spine (craniorachischisis). The outcome of anencephaly is invariably

A

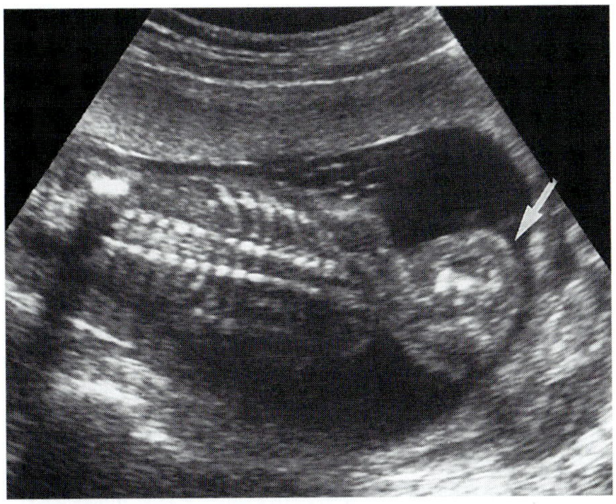

B

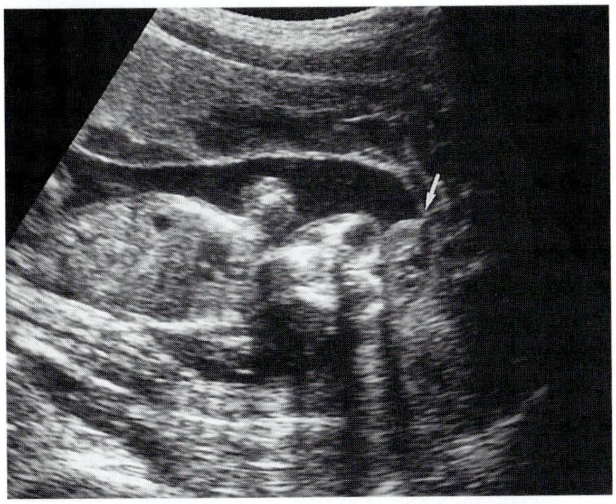

C

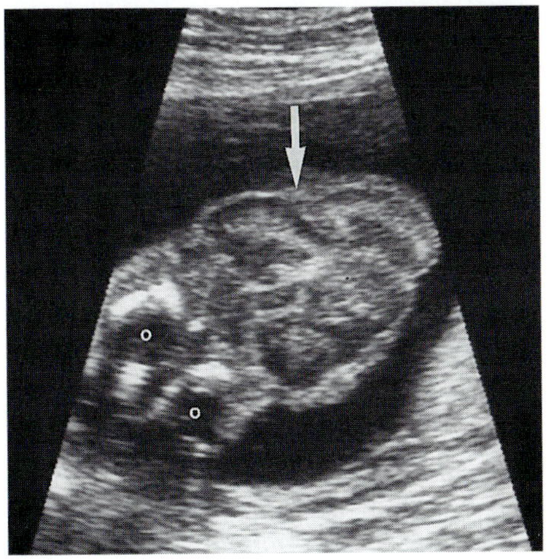

FIG. 43-11. Anencephaly. A, Sagittal view of fetus at 14 menstrual weeks shows the spine ending in a clump of basal skull bones without a formed cranial vault (*arrow*). Disorganized neural tissue, the vasculosa, may mimic the brain but skull bones are always absent. **Amniotic band syndrome at 15 weeks mimics anencephaly, B,** but this fetal head and brain were stuck to the uterine wall by obvious bands (*arrow*). Unlike anencephaly, this condition is sporadic and not likely to recur. **Exencephaly at 19 weeks. C,** Substantial brain-like tissue (*arrow*) above the base of the skull. Orbits (o). Some feel that exencephaly is an early phase of anencephaly and that continuing trauma to this unprotected tissue will result in its destruction, ultimately leaving the typical appearance of anencephaly.

fatal, and pregnancy termination is offered at any gestational age.[48]

Although the diagnosis has been suggested as early as 10½ weeks, detection prior to 14 menstrual weeks can be difficult since the malformed mass can mimic the normally developing brain (exencephaly), especially at transabdominal scanning, but the cranial bones are not ossified.[46,49] Using transvaginal probes, ultrasonically visible ossification of frontal bones is not apparent until 11½ weeks (Fig. 43-1B), and anencephaly should not be diagnosed before this age. It has been suggested that **exencephaly** may be an early phase of anencephaly. In early pregnancy, area cerebrovasculosa can be prominent and resemble brain structures (exencephaly), and it is postulated that they become destroyed during continuing pregnancy and assume the characteristic flattened appearance of anencephaly.[45,49,50]

There are subclassifications of anencephaly related to the location of the opening, the amount of cerebral tissue remaining, and the associated spinal involvement, but they are of academic interest only, as all are lethal. All have a similar recurrence rate.[51]

Differential diagnosis includes amniotic band syndrome and large encephaloceles. Absence or disruption of the cranial vault may also occur with early amnion rupture syndrome (**amniotic band syndrome**) (Fig. 43-11, *C*). These fetuses generally have an asymmetric defect, abnormality, or amputation of other body parts and occasional oligohydramnios. Membranes may be visible in amniotic fluid or the fetus may be stuck to the side of the uterus or placenta. Although anencephaly increases the likelihood of normal tube defects in subsequent pregnancies, early amnion rupture is sporadic and without increased recurrence risk.[47] Large encephaloceles generally have more calvarial development than does anencephaly, but on occasion they can look very similar. In either case, the prognosis remains hopeless.

Encephaloceles. Encephaloceles are herniations of intracranial structures through a defect in the cranium. They may contain only meninges and CSF (cranial meningocele) or brain tissue (encephalocele). Most occur in the midline in the occipital (75%) or frontal regions (13%) but some are parietal (12%)[52] (Fig. 43-12, *A-D*). They can extend into the nasal and sphenoid areas where their identification can be difficult.[48,53-55] They can occur as isolated lesions or be associated with other anomalies or syndromes commonly involving the head, spine, face, skeleton, or kidneys.[48]

Ultrasonically, an encephalocele manifests as a cystic mass at the surface of the skull, commonly in the midline. Contained brain tissue or a visible bony defect confirms the diagnosis but these may be difficult to detect. The **differential diagnosis** includes cystic hygroma, hemangioma, teratoma, branchial cleft cyst, and scalp edema.[48,54]

The **Meckel-Gruber syndrome** is an autosomal recessive lethal condition having encephalocele, cystic renal dysplasia, and polydactyly as its dominant features.[56] The detection of either cystic kidneys or an encephalocele should lead to a search for the other components of this surprisingly common syndrome.

The **prognosis** depends on the location of the mass, the amount of brain herniation, and associated anomalies. Mortality can be up to 44%, and 40% to 91% can be intellectually impaired.[55] If discovered before viability, pregnancy termination is offered. Later in pregnancy, management depends on the size and location of the encephalocele and associated anomalies.[48]

> **SIGNS OF OPEN SPINA BIFIDA**
>
> Lemon sign
> Ventriculomegaly
> Banana sign
> Shape of cerebellum around brainstem
> Effacement of cisterna magna
> Slightly small fetal measurements
> Spinal defects
> Family history
> Elevated MS-AFP
>
> NB: Closed spina bifida has normal-appearing head!

Spina Bifida. Spina bifida is classified as **open** or **closed**, depending on whether the spinal lesion is skin-covered (closed) or not (open). The open lesions are more commonly diagnosed prenatally and are said to account for about 80% of spina bifida. In the case of open lesions, 80% show elevation of maternal serum alpha-fetoprotein (MS-AFP) and commonly show intracranial changes. In contrast, most closed lesions, even if large, have no intracranial changes, and the MS-AFP levels are normal. Thus it is important to examine the spine even if the head appears normal so as to avoid missing an obvious deformity of closed spina bifida.

Most cases of open spina bifida are first suspected following detection of characteristic associated changes in the head and, in fact, we find it rare for open spina bifida to occur without some cerebral distortion. The characteristic **head changes** of **open spina bifida** (Fig. 43-13) include[9] ventriculomegaly,[57] the lemon sign (bifrontal scalloping or indentation),[58,59] the banana sign (Chiari II malformation),[59-61] cisterna magna effacement,[62] and BPD and body measurements that are **small** for gestational age.

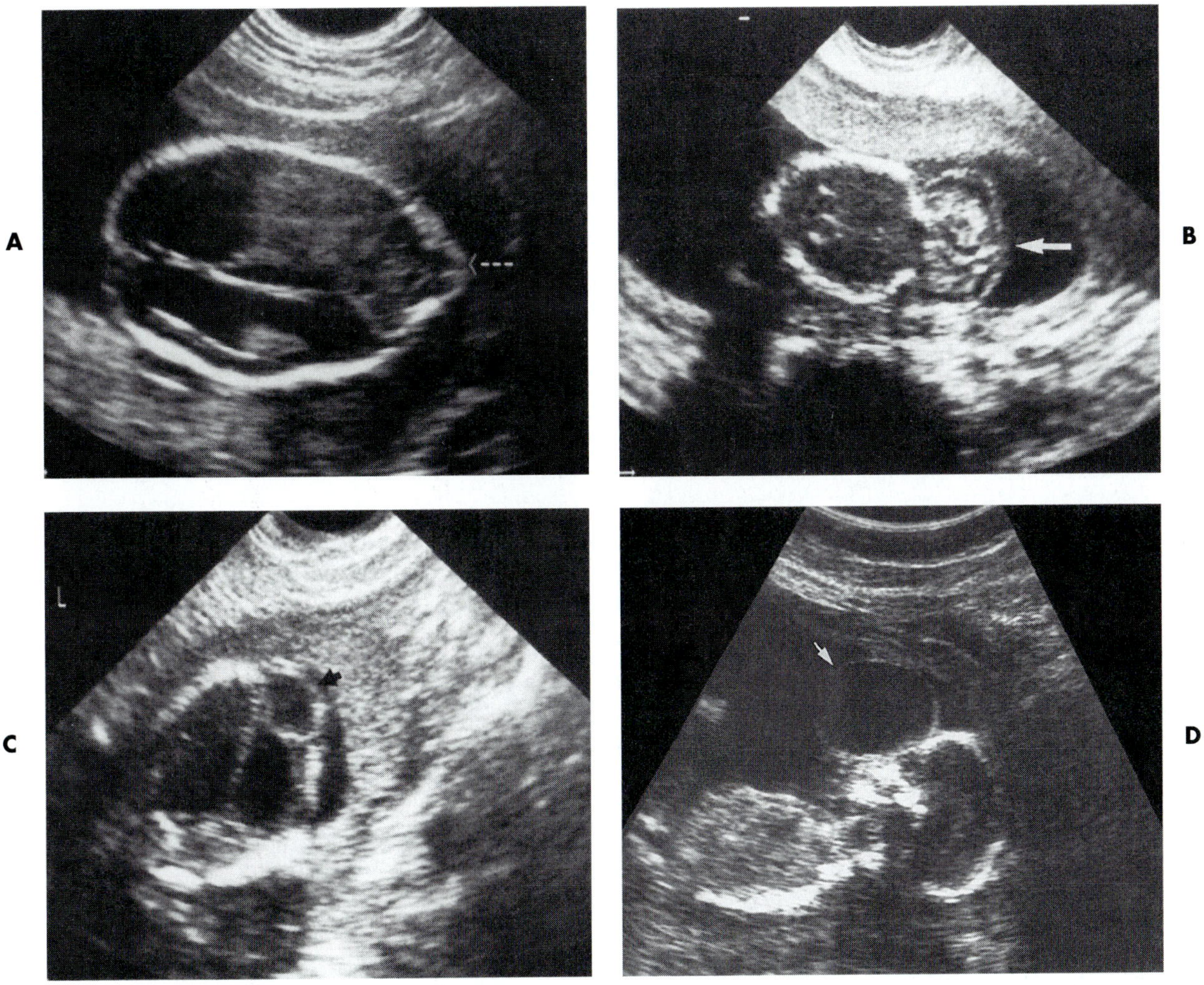

FIG. 43-12. Encephaloceles. **A,** Transverse cerebellar view at 18 menstrual weeks shows ventriculomegaly and a small occipital encephalocele (*arrow*), which contains part of the cerebellum. **B,** Transverse view at 22 menstrual weeks shows a large midline encephalocele with considerable brain tissue (*arrow*) herniating through the occipital bony skull defect. The head is microcephalic. **C,** Coronal view at 21 menstrual weeks shows asymmetrical parietal encephalocele (*arrow*). Nonmidline locations for these lesions are uncommon. **D,** Anterior encephalocele (*arrow*) at 18 weeks. This herniated through a defect between the orbits.

Ventriculomegaly with spina bifida that has occipital horns over 10 mm is common but usually occurs in later pregnancy (Fig. 43-13, *A*). Babcook found it in 44% of fetuses under 24 weeks' gestation and in 94% after 24 weeks. It was commonly associated with severe posterior fossa deformities.[57] We find that though the absolute atrial measurement in such fetuses may be under 10 mm, it is common to see that the choroid appears too small and is a droopy, or dangling, choroid (Fig. 43-9, *B*) even early in the second trimester. After delivery and after repair of the skin lesion, virtually all infants develop progressive enlargement of ventricles and head (hydrocephalus) and require shunting.

The **lemon sign** is commonly associated with spina bifida (Fig. 43-13, *A*). It is seen in 89% to 98% of spina bifida fetuses under 24 weeks' gestation but becomes less obvious later.[58,59] It can also occur in normal fetuses and others with diverse abnormalities including encephalocele, Dandy-Walker malformation, thanatophoric dysplasia, and others.[63]

The **banana sign** and **effacement of the posterior fossa** are the result of hypoplasia of the posterior fossa with spina bifida (Fig. 43-13, *B-D*). The result is compression of the cerebellum which, in turn, conforms to the remaining available space. The fluid in the cisterna magna is displaced (**cisterna magna effacement**) by the cerebellum. Also, the cerebellar ton-

A
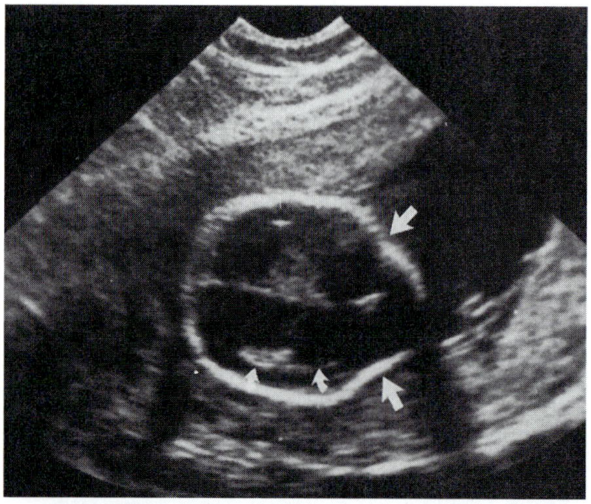

B
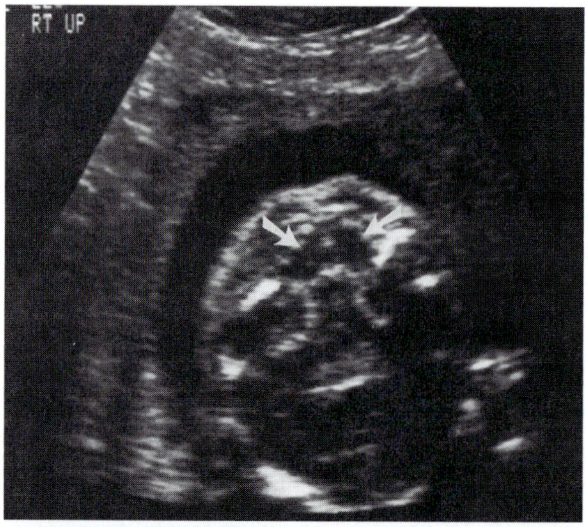

C
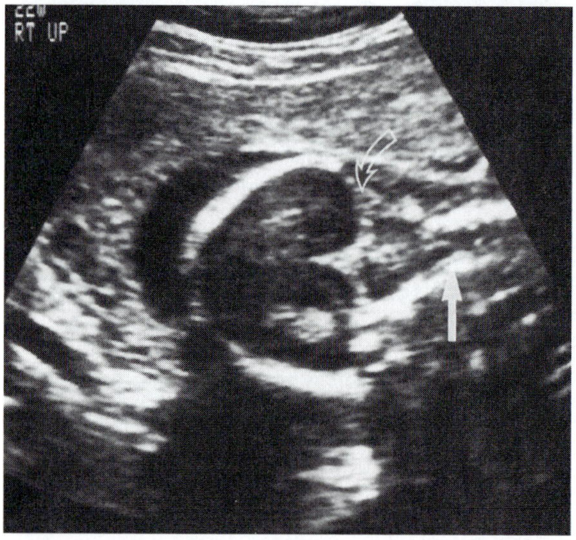

D
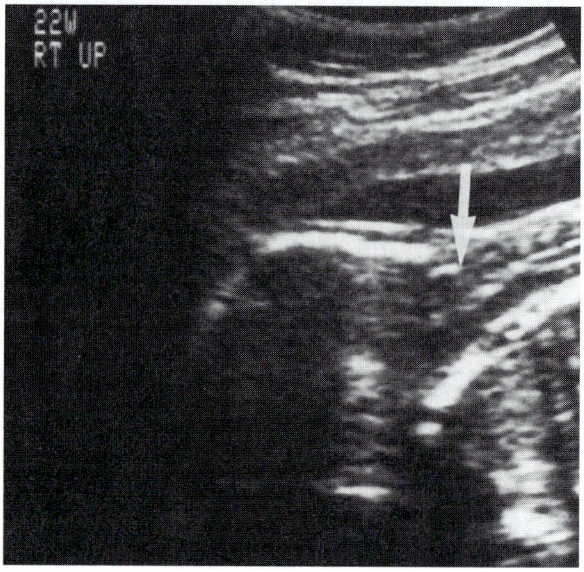

E
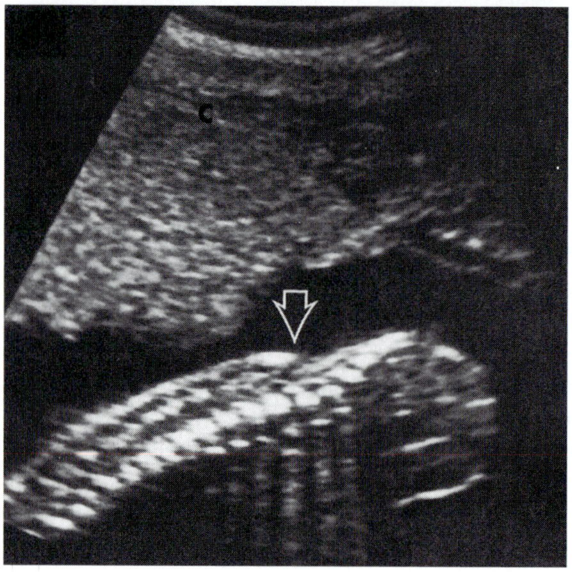

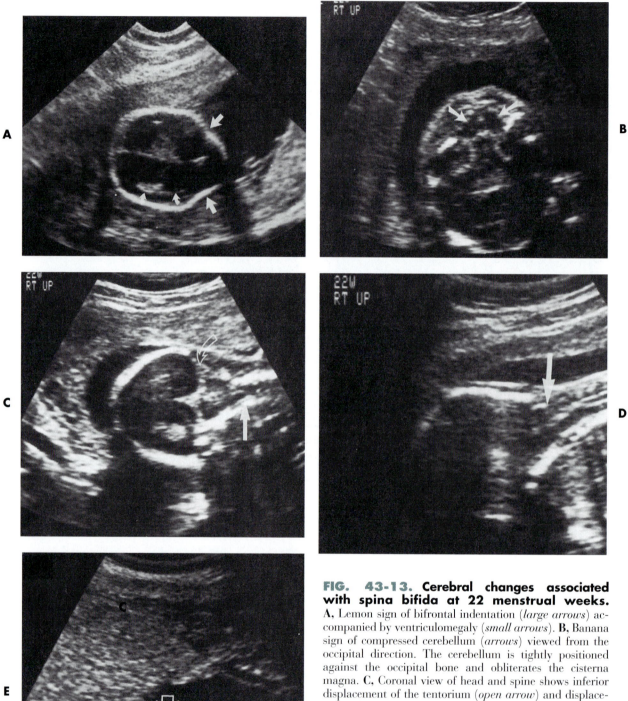

FIG. 43-13. Cerebral changes associated with spina bifida at 22 menstrual weeks. **A,** Lemon sign of bifrontal indentation (*large arrows*) accompanied by ventriculomegaly (*small arrows*). **B,** Banana sign of compressed cerebellum (*arrows*) viewed from the occipital direction. The cerebellum is tightly positioned against the occipital bone and obliterates the cisterna magna. **C,** Coronal view of head and spine shows inferior displacement of the tentorium (*open arrow*) and displacement of the cerebellar tonsils and vermis low into the cervical spinal canal (*solid arrow*) due to Chiari II malformation. **D,** Dorsal midsagittal view shows the cerebellar vermis (*arrow*) well below the occipital bone. This is an alternative view used to evaluate for Chiari II malformation and cisterna magna obliteration. **E,** Dorsal midsagittal lumbosacral spine view shows the open spinal defect and skin defect starting at about the fifth lumbar vertebra (*arrow*) and extending to the sacral tip. This spinal lesion was not appreciated at several examinations of this pregnancy although all observers detected the head abnormalities.

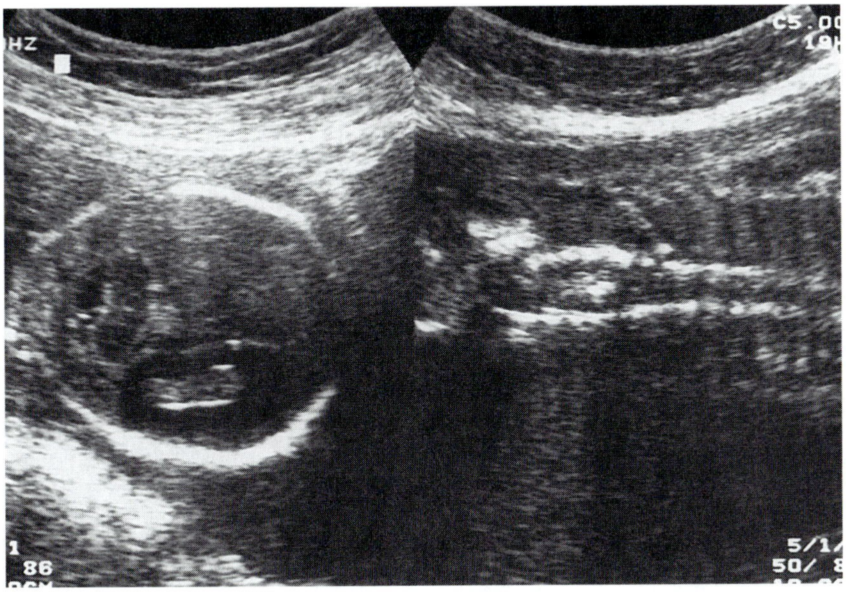

FIG. 43-14. Closed skin covered spina bifida at 19 weeks. The right image shows massive dysraphism from about T10 to S5. On the left image, note the normal ventricles, cerebellum, and cisterna magna. Cranial signs are generally absent with closed spina bifida and the MS-AFP is normal since the lesion is skin-covered.

sils and vermis herniate inferiorly through the foramen magnum. Its lateral parts wrap around the brainstem laterally and the cerebellum assumes a C-curved shape, the **banana sign**. These findings constitute the ultrasonographic Chiari II malformation. In fact, the Chiari II malformation has many more subtle components as described by neuroradiologists.[64] On occasion, the cerebellum may be displaced so far inferiorly into the bony base of the skull that it cannot be imaged with ultrasound. Some describe this as an absent cerebellum with spina bifida. This absence is generally artifactual due to shadowing by bone. It is rare for the cerebellar compression in Chiari II to actually result in cerebellar atrophy.

Remember that even large, closed, skin-covered spina bifidas typically have no cranial findings, so a normal cranial examination does not justify a hurried and incomplete spinal assessment (Fig. 43-14). The MS-AFP will also be normal in such patients.

Fetuses with isolated NTD have an increased incidence of chromosomal abnormality ranging from 6.7% to 16%, and antenatal genetic evaluation should be offered.[65,66]

The intracranial changes are similar for all levels of spinal abnormality, so the functional **prognosis** depends primarily on the level of the spinal lesion.[67]

The **iniencephaly** sequence is a rare and special case of dysraphism involving the back of the cranium and the contiguous upper spine ("inion" refers to the nape of the neck) and is associated with segmentation errors of the upper spine. The resulting deformity markedly shortens the neck, and the head is dorsiflexed (which is known as the star-gazing position). Associated anomalies are common. Outcome is fatal. There may be an association with anencephaly or Kippel-Feil syndrome. In Kippel-Feil syndrome, there is segmentation error and shortening in the cervical vertebrae, but no dysraphism.[56]

Errors of Ventral Induction

Errors of ventral induction occur in the rostral end of the embryo and result in brain abnormalities. Usually, they also affect facial development.

Holoprosencephaly. Holoprosencephaly is a continuum of cerebral malformations resulting from incomplete cleavage or diverticulation of the primitive forebrain into two cerebral hemispheres. Holoprosencephaly is commonly associated with midline facial anomalies.[68,69] It occurs in about 1 in 5000 to 1 in 16,000 livebirths. As many affected fetuses abort, the overall incidence may be as high as 1 in 250.[68,69]

Even though the deformity has a continuous spectrum, it is divided into **three groups**: alobar (lacking two hemispheric lobes), semilobar (partial formation of lobes), and lobar (two hemispheres present). The **alobar variety** is the most severe: there is no cerebral separation into two hemispheres but a single mantle of neural tissue with a single ventricle; there is no falx or interhemispheric fissure; there is thalamic fusion and absent corpus callosum (Fig. 43-15, 43-16, and 43-17). The **semilobar** and **lobar varieties** show greater degrees of differentiation, with the semilobar having partial cleavage into hemispheres and the lobar having complete cleavage. **Midline facial abnormalities** occur in about 80% of cases, including hypotelorism, midline maxillary cleft, cyclopia (single eye with supraorbital proboscis), ethmocephaly (hypotelorism with proboscis) (Fig. 43-17, *B*), and cebocephaly (hypotelorism and single-nostril nose). Extracranial

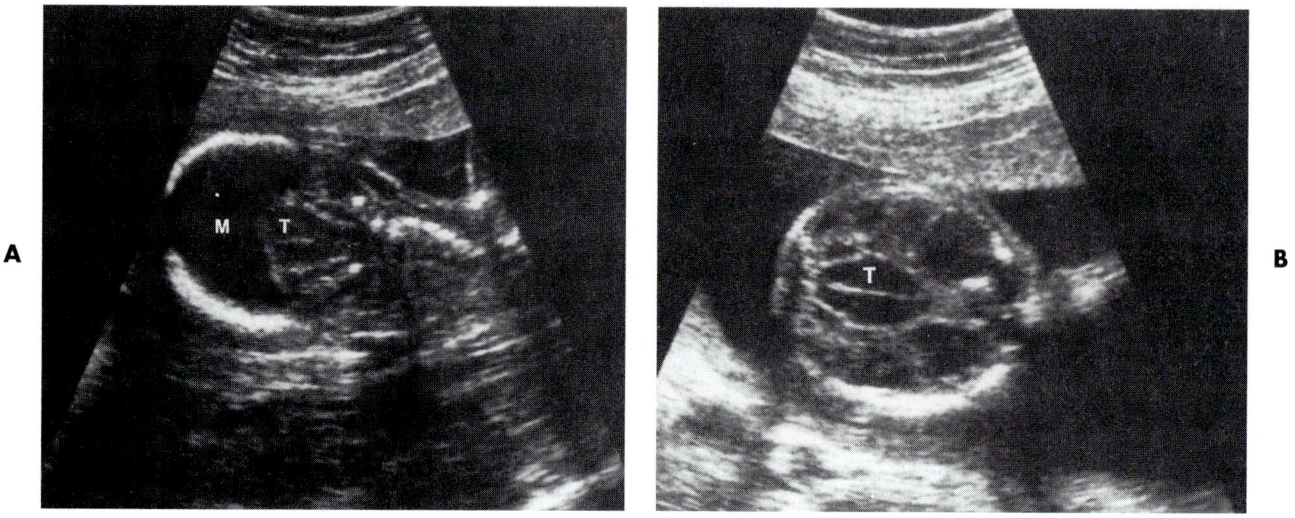

FIG. 43-15. Alobar holoprosencephaly. **A,** Coronal view at 19 menstrual weeks shows fused nubbin of thalamus (T) and large monoventricle (M) with virtually no cerebral tissue and absence of interhemispheric fissure and falx. **B,** Transverse view of same fetus lower in the head showing the rounded, elongated thalamus (T), which frequently is the initial clue to thalamic fusion associated with holoprosencephaly. This fetus also had facial anomalies which are common with the most severe lobar form of holoprosencephaly.

FIG. 43-16. "Cup" type of alobar holoprosencephaly. **A,** Coronal view shows mantle (m) of cerebrum without interhemispheric fissure, the monoventricle, and fused thalami (t). *Continued.*

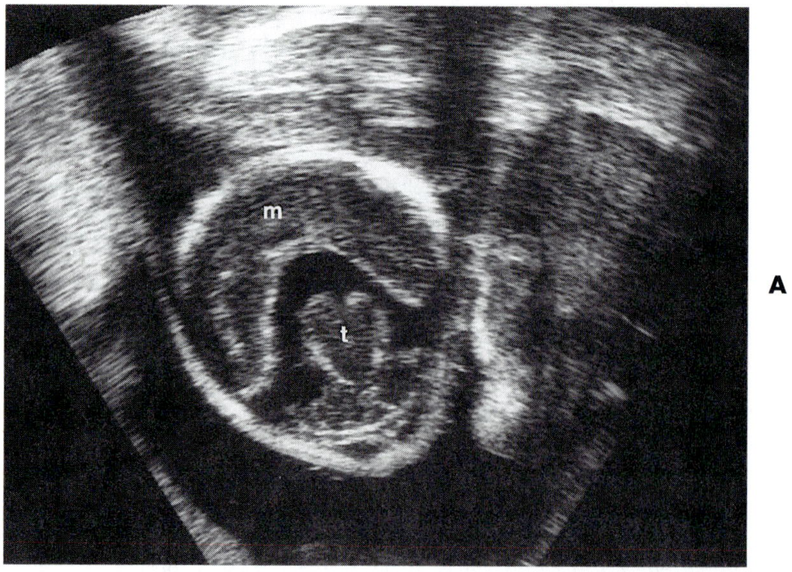

B

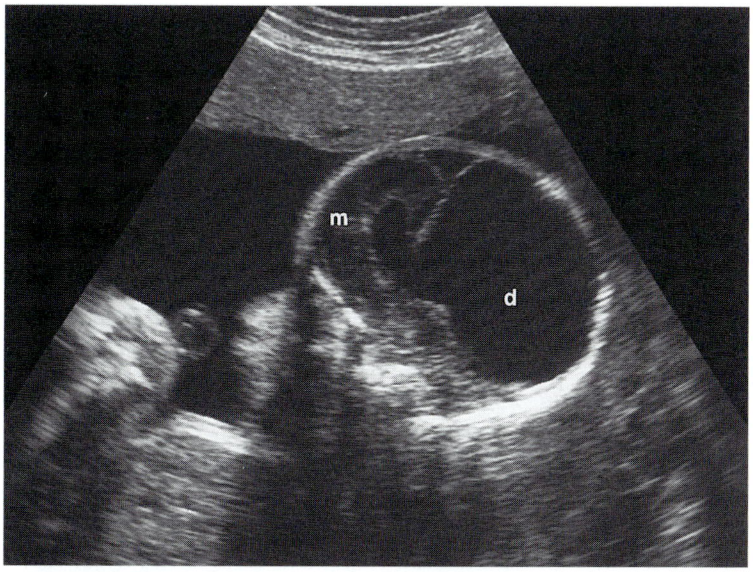

FIG. 43-16, cont'd. "Cup" type of alobar holoprosencephaly. **B,** Midsagittal view shows the anterior "cup" of mantle (m) and a large dorsal cyst (d).

A

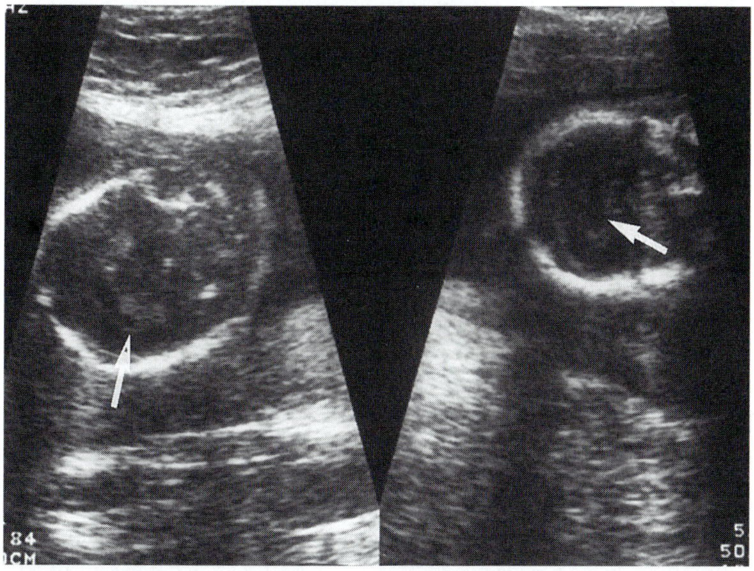

B

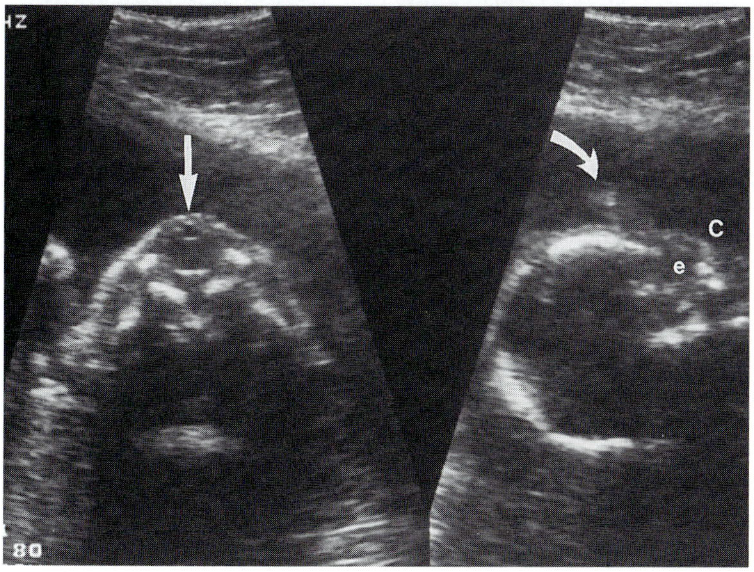

FIG. 43-17. "Ball" type of alobar holoprosencephaly at 20 weeks. **A,** Single, small, central monoventricle (*straight arrow*) surrounded by thick cerebral mantle in axial (left) and coronal (right) views. **B,** Facial anomaly of cyclops with proboscis associated with holoprosencephaly. Left image transversely across face at orbit level has only a single midline eye (*straight arrow*). Right profile view shows supraorbital soft-tissue proboscis (*curved arrow*) above the single eye (e). Chin (c).

anomalies are also common, especially if the face is abnormal.[68-70]

Many cases are sporadic but 50% have chromosomal abnormalities, especially trisomy 13.[68] The prognosis is poor, and those with the more severe alobar and semilobar types are profoundly retarded and often die shortly after birth.

At **sonography**, the diagnostic features of the alobar and semilobar types are absence of the falx and fusion of the thalami. The **alobar type** has **three variants:** the "pancake," the "cup" (Fig. 43-16), and the "ball" (Fig. 43-17).[71] The pancake type has a small, flattened plate of cerebrum anteriorly with a large dorsal cyst posteriorly. The cup type has more anterior cerebrum forming an anterior cup-like mantle and a dorsal cyst. The ball type has a single, featureless monoventricle surrounded by a mantle of ventricle of varying thickness. A dorsal cyst continuous with the single ventricle may be present in the occiput.[68] Many authors emphasize detection of associated facial abnormalities in making the diagnosis.[72,73] With the **semilobar type**, rudimentary occipital horns may be seen (Fig. 43-18). The lobar form, since it forms lobes, may be difficult if not impossible to diagnose prenatally. Features that suggest **lobar holoprosencephaly** include absence of the cavum septi pellucidi, with fusion and squaring of the frontal horns and an abnormal appearance of two large nerve trunks, the fornices, which are rudimentary and appear fused into a single tract in the third ventricle.[74,75]

Alobar holoprosencephaly has been diagnosed as early as 10.5 weeks through demonstration of a single ventricle, single orbit, and proboscis.[76] In such early cases, it is important to not mistake the normal rhombencephalic cavity, which represents the developing fourth ventricle, for holoprosencephaly (Fig. 43-1, *A*). The presence of facial changes is important in this regard.

Differential diagnosis includes severe hydrocephalus and hydranencephaly. With early diagnosis, we offer termination of pregnancy. With late diagnosis, we provide conservative therapy and karyotyping because of the high incidence of aneuploidy.

Dandy-Walker Malformation. The Dandy-Walker malformation (DWM) is characterized by a cyst in the posterior fossa and a defect in the cerebellar vermis through which the cyst communicates with the fourth ventricle (Fig. 43-19, *A*). The lateral ventricles are variably enlarged *in utero* but may be normal only to enlarge after birth.[77] The Dandy-Walker **variant** (DWV) is more common than the full syndrome. It has less vermian agenesis, a smaller cyst, and minimal, if any, lateral ventricular enlargement (Fig. 43-19, *B*).[78-80]

Care must be taken to **avoid overdiagnosis of the Dandy-Walker variant.** There are two major pitfalls: too early a diagnosis and an incorrect scan plane. Vermian development is not complete until about 18 weeks. Scans made earlier than 18 weeks may demonstrate an incompletely formed vermis which can be mistaken for DWV by the unwary. The diagnosis of DWV should not be made until after 18 weeks.[81] The scan plane must be correct when assessing the posterior fossa. We find that a plane that includes the cavum septi pellucidi anteriorly and the cerebellum posteriorly works well (Fig. 43-2, *C*). Choice of too steep a plane will result in a false-positive diagnosis of DWM and megacisterna magna.[82]

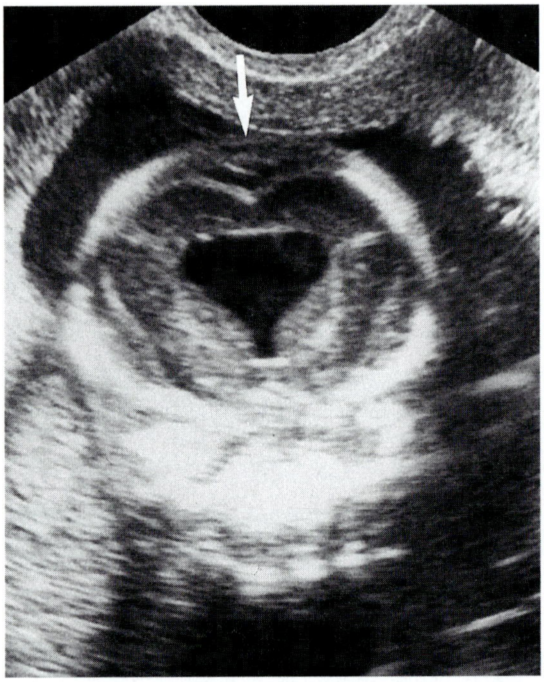

FIG. 43-18. Semilobar holoprosencephaly at 20 weeks. There is a single monoventricle but there is also rudimentary development of falx and interhemispheric fissure (*arrow*).

Associated anomalies of the CNS and other structures are common, including agenesis of the corpus callosum, neuronal migration disorders, cerebral lipomas, congenital heart disease, genitourinary abnormalities, and polydactyly.[83]

It was initially believed that the Dandy-Walker malformation resulted from failure of fenestration of the foramina of Magendie and Luschka, but now the condition is believed to represent a more generalized developmental abnormality of the roof of the fourth ventricle. It has a multifactorial etiology, and most cases are seen in association with many genetic and nongenetic syndromes.[84,85] Intellectual impairment and fetal death are common; the latter is frequently dependent on associated non-CNS anomalies.[85,86] If the malformation is discovered before viability, termi-

A 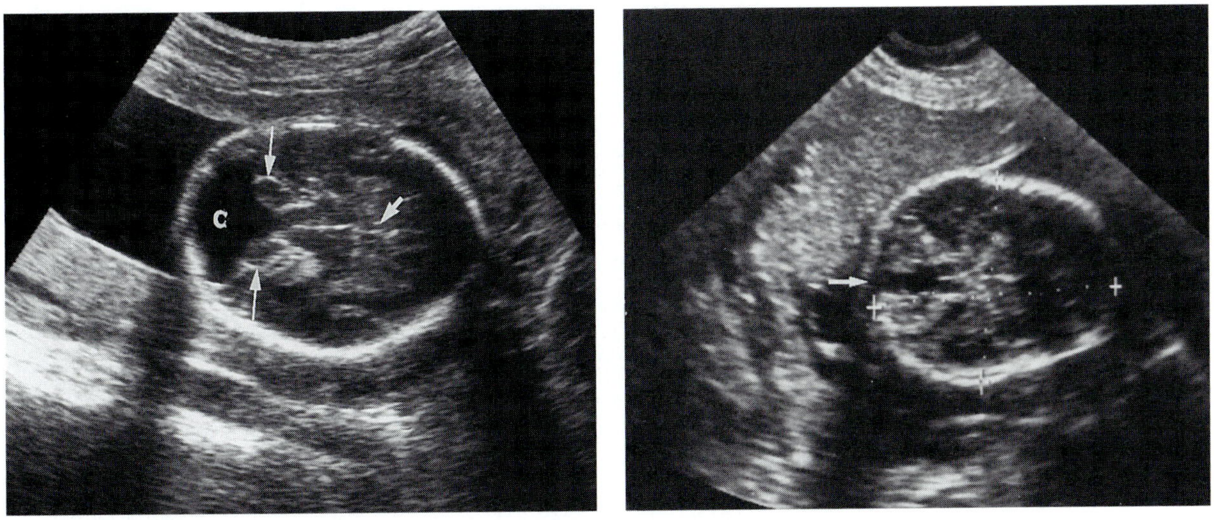 B

FIG. 43-19. Dandy-Walker malformation at 21 weeks. **A,** The large posterior fossa cyst (c) communicates with the fourth ventricle and splays the cerebellum (*arrows*). The vermis is absent. The cavum septi pellucidi is also absent (*thick arrow*), a clue to the associated agenesis of the corpus callosum in this case. **Dandy-Walker variant. B,** Transverse cerebellar view at 31 menstrual weeks with a cleft between the cerebellar hemispheres (*arrow*) where the vermis is absent. The ventricles are not dilated. This lesion is easily missed if the cerebellar vermis is not routinely imaged.

nation of pregnancy is offered because of the poor prognosis, including high mortality, likelihood of intellectual impairment, and association with other anomalies.

Ultrasound diagnosis depends on demonstration of the major components of the DWM (Fig. 43-19, *A*):

- vermian agenesis or hypoplasia;
- posterior fossa cyst communicating with the fourth ventricle;
- identification of characteristic associated anomalies that can help confirm the diagnosis, including elevated tentorium, ventriculomegaly, agenesis of the corpus callosum, and systemic anomalies.[85]

The **differential diagnosis** between DWM and DWV includes a posterior fossa arachnoid cyst that may be midline and associated with ventriculomegaly. Unlike a fetus with DWM, a fetus with DMV has an intact vermis separating the cyst from the fourth ventricle, and the cyst may be asymmetric, but on occasion the two conditions look very similar.[87]

The **posterior fossa arachnoid cyst**[80] is a unilocular collection of CSF within the layers of the arachnoid membrane, which does not communicate with the ventricles or subarachnoid spaces. There is no association with congenital abnormalities. It occurs sporadically. The cerebellum and brain stem are compressed but normal; compression can cause obstructive hydrocephalus. Differentiation from other Dandy-Walker cysts can be difficult, even postpartum. Treatment involves unroofing the cyst or inserting a shunt. Even though they are benign, these cysts can result in secondary injury to the brain through hydrocephalus or hemorrhage.

Arachnoid Cysts. These cysts can occur anywhere in the cranium. They represent fluid collections in the layers of the arachnoid membrane. Symptoms arise if they compress the brain or cause hydrocephalus (Fig. 43-20).

Megacisterna magna refers to an enlargement of the cisterna magna beyond 10 mm (Fig. 43-21). The vermis is intact. This can be a normal finding, but some affected children have hydrocephalus or developmental delay related to associated supratentorial abnormalities. Chromosomal abnormalities, especially trisomy 18, are also common and have been seen in 55% of these infants. They should be suspected, especially if the ventricles are of normal size.[79,88]

Neuronal Proliferation, Differentiation, and Destruction

Hydranencephaly. This rare congenital disorder shows an almost total absence of the cerebrum but an intact cranial vault and meninges. It is the most severe degree of porencephaly, or brain destruction.[89,90] Occlusion of the supraclinoid carotid arteries is said to be the most common cause, but hydranen-

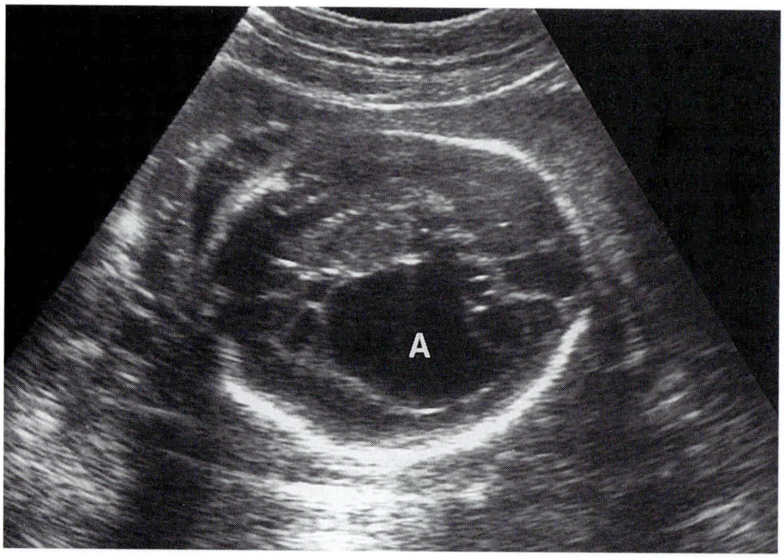

FIG. 43-20. Arachnoid cyst (A) in the supratentorial, interhemispheric position at 25 weeks. Occasionally tumors with cystic degeneration can look like this.

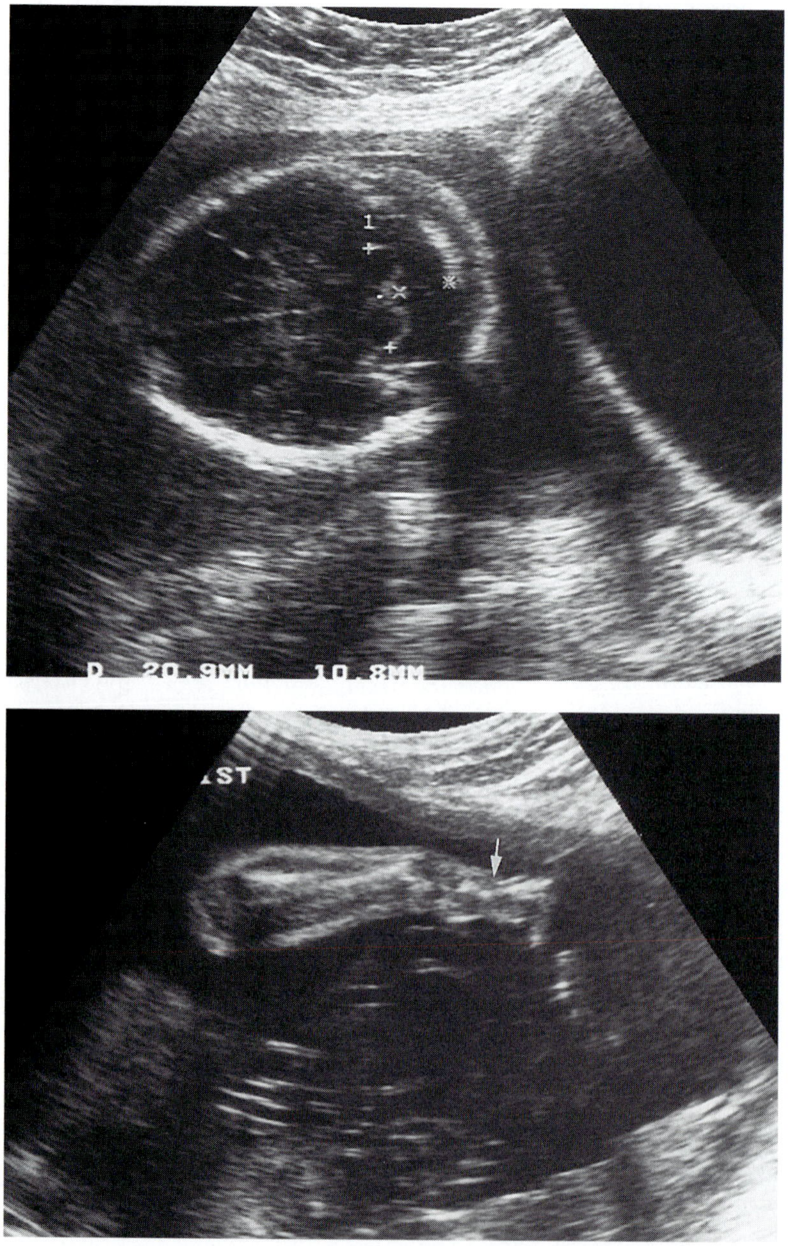

A

B

FIG. 43-21. Megacisterna magna at 25 weeks. A, The CM (x. . .x) is over 10 mm. The crebellum (+...+) is small and under the tenth centile. This fetus has cerebellar hypoplasia due to olivo-ponto-cerebellar dysplasia. **Abnormal hand position due to neurologic deficit with olivo-ponto-cerebellar dysplasia. B,** The metacarpophalangeal joints were in fixed hyperextension *(arrow)* and fingers in fixed flexion. All fetal limb movements were abnormal.

cephaly may result from other conditions, including infection.[89-91] Prognosis is hopeless, and death commonly follows delivery.[90]

Pathologically, hydranencephaly is characterized by fluid surrounding the basal ganglia and brain stem, variable absence of the cerebral hemispheres, intact meninges, and a variably incomplete falx. It may not develop until later pregnancy. One case has been detected by 24 weeks of gestation and another has been shown in evolution starting at about 27 weeks of gestation.[90-92]

Ultrasonically, the cerebrum is variably destroyed and replaced by fluid. It lacks the thinned cortical mantle that is present in severe hydrocephalus. The thalamus, basal ganglia, and lower brain stem are intact. The falx is present to a variable degree but may be displaced or hypoplastic (Fig. 43-22). The head size is commonly normal but may be small or large. Hydranencephaly is not associated with other anomalies.[90-91] Differentiation from marked hydrocephalus is important, since isolated hydrocephalus can be successfully shunted after delivery and may have a good outcome. With hydrocephalus, ventricle shape is preserved even if the cortex is markedly thinned (Fig. 43-7), whereas with hydranencephaly, there generally are irregular tissue masses visible in the frontal and occipital regions where there is some brain sparing due to blood supply from the anterior and posterior cerebral circulation.

The **differential diagnosis** includes severe hydrocephalus, alobar holoprosencephaly, massive congenital subdural hydroma, and postanoxic and infective encephalopathy.[89]

Schizencephaly. Schizencephaly is a rare condition characterized by roughly symmetrical clefts or defects in the parietal or temporal brain that extend from the ventricles to the cortical surface.[92] The appearance is that of the brain being split (*schiz*-encephaly) into an anterior and a posterior part by these bilateral, roughly symmetrical, porencephaly-like lesions. The etiology is unknown. Some consider it a destructive process due to vascular injury similar to hydranencephaly and porencephaly. Others feel that there is a more fundamental error in neuronal migration. Developmental delay is common.[93,94]

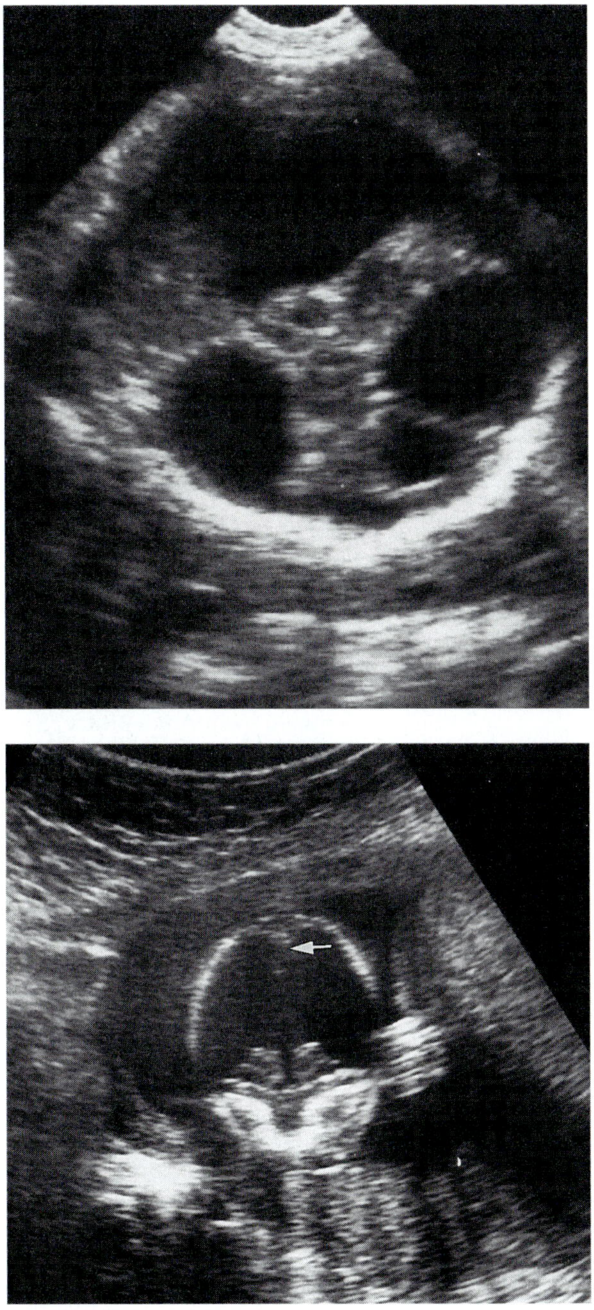

A

B

FIG. 43-22. Hydranencephaly. A, Transverse thalamic view at 38 weeks shows asymmetrical cerebral destruction with preserved interhemispheric fissure. **B,** Hydranencephaly at 17 weeks shows cranium filled with fluid. At first, the appearance suggests alobar holoprosencephaly, but the presence of the falx (*arrow*) and lack of thalamic fusion as seen by the large third ventricle help confirm hydranencephaly.

Lissencephaly. This term describes a brain surface that is smooth and lacks the normal sulci and gyri. Normally, as the neurons migrate from the periventricular germinal matrix to the cortical surface, they enlarge the cortex which then undergoes folding to accommodate the increased tissue, thus forming sulci and gyri. Abnormal migration of neurons from the germinal matrix to the surface results in abnormal development of sulci and gyri. The brain surface remains flat and smooth (lissencephaly or agyria) or develops broad, flat gyri (pachygyria). Children with this malformation have severe functional disturbance. Diagnosis is not possible until the third trimester, as it depends on the demonstration of abnormal sulci, but these only start developing at about 28 weeks. Typically, there is mild ventriculomegaly, poor development of sulci, a large open Sylvian fissure, and possibly an abnormal, poorly developed corpus callosum. With severe lissencephaly, the brain, in essence, retains its appearance from the early second trimester.[94] Ultrasound diagnosis is possible only in severe cases and requires attention to the appearance and presence of the normal development of sulci. MRI has been used to confirm the diagnosis *in utero*.[95]

Microcephaly. Microcephaly implies a disproportionately small head for age and body size. Precise diagnostic definition is difficult but clinically, a head circumference less than 2 to 3 standard deviations (SD) below the mean for age and sex is associated with subnormal mental ability; the smaller the head circumference, the lower the performance level.[96,97] After delivery, the diagnosis is usually made when the head circumference is less than 3 SD below the mean for gestational age. Note that some individuals with such a small head size still have normal intelligence. Incidence at birth ranges from 1 in 6250 to 1 in 8500.[97]

Smallness of the head resulting from calvarial abnormalities (e.g., craniosynostosis) is not generally included under this diagnosis because in these cases, intelligence is spared. Rather, the diagnosis implies failure of brain development (**micrencephaly**) following multiple **prenatal causes**, including genetics, environment, asphyxia, infectious (cytomegalovirus) maternal phenylketonuria, drugs (e.g., alcohol), and irradiation. At pathologic examination the brain may be small but normal or may have diverse findings, including porencephaly, abnormal gyri, absent corpus callosum, and ventriculomegaly.[98] Associated CNS and non-CNS abnormalities are common.

Ultrasonically, the diagnosis of microcephaly is difficult but must be suspected if the BPD is more than 3 SD below the mean for gestational age. Other criteria include small head circumference, abnormal head/abdomen circumference ratio, small femur/head circumference ratio, and small frontal lobe size[97-100] (Figs. 43-12, *B* and 43-23, *A-C*). Measurements are poor for diagnosis and in one study, only 4 of 24 fetuses with small measurements confirmed the diagnosis at delivery.[99]

The diagnosis has been made as early as 15.5 weeks in pregnancies known to be at risk, but microcephaly may not be evident until late in pregnancy when the BPD fails to grow normally.[101,102]

Macrocephaly (Megaloencephaly). True **megaloencephaly** with true cerebral gigantism, or enlarged brain, is rare. More commonly, other conditions such as ventricular enlargement, cerebral infiltrations, or storage diseases and tumors cause the enlargement. In true megaloencephaly, intelligence may be normal or subnormal. Cesarean delivery may be necessary.[103,104]

Migration

Agenesis of Corpus Callosum (ACC). The corpus callosum (CC) is the largest neural commissure connecting the cerebral hemispheres. Absence may be complete or partial, developmental or acquired.[105] It may be an isolated abnormality with very little, if any, functional disturbance, but it commonly occurs with CNS (85%) or other (62%) abnormalities.[106-108]

At about 12 weeks, the corpus callosum starts to develop from the lamina terminalis near the anterior end of the third ventricle. At first, it is a bundle of fibers connecting the left to the right hemisphere. This bundle develops in an anteroposterior fashion, beginning anteriorly with the rostrum and then forming the genu, body, and the splenium posteriorly. It forms the septi pellucidi and the cavum septi pellucidi et vergae as it grows.

Two septi pellucidi form initially; the space between them is the cavum septi pellucidi. Specifically, the part of this space anterior to the foramina of Monro is called the cavum septi pellucidi, and the posterior part of the same space is called the cavum vergae. In common usage, "cavum septi pellucidi" refers to both of these spaces. In early childhood, the cavum closes and the two septi fuse, after which they are called the "septum pellucidum," in the singular.

Callosal development is complete by 20 weeks. Developmental disturbances interrupt the formation of the more posterior parts but still later insults can cause secondary atrophy of previously developed central parts.[104] **Associated anomalies** of nearly every CNS structure may be present, most commonly gyral dysplasias, heterotopias (cortical gray matter cells in abnormal positions), and hypoplasias, including the cerebellar vermis (the Dandy-Walker malformation). Common non-CNS anomalies involve the face, limbs, and genitourinary tract. This high incidence of associated malformations suggests that ACC is part of a widespread developmental disturbance.[104,106] Prognosis relates to the associated anomalies.[109,110] Because callosal development is not complete until 20 weeks, early diagnosis of ACC may be difficult.[111] At ultrasound, the cavum septi pellucidi is generally seen by 17 weeks. Because its formation is associated with the development of the corpus callosum, when the cavum is not present at 17 to 20 weeks, there should be suspicion of ACC. We offer termination of pregnancy if absence of the corpus callosum is detected early, but early diagnosis has been difficult, with up to 50% of cases missed in the second trimester, even by experienced observers.

Ultrasonic appearances are subtle on the usual axial scans performed *in utero* (Figs. 43-24, *A*, *B* and 43-25, *A*). They include:

- disproportionate enlargement of occipital horns (colpocephaly);
- lateral displacement of both medial and lateral ventricular walls;
- angular configuration of ventricles with pointing of anterior ends;

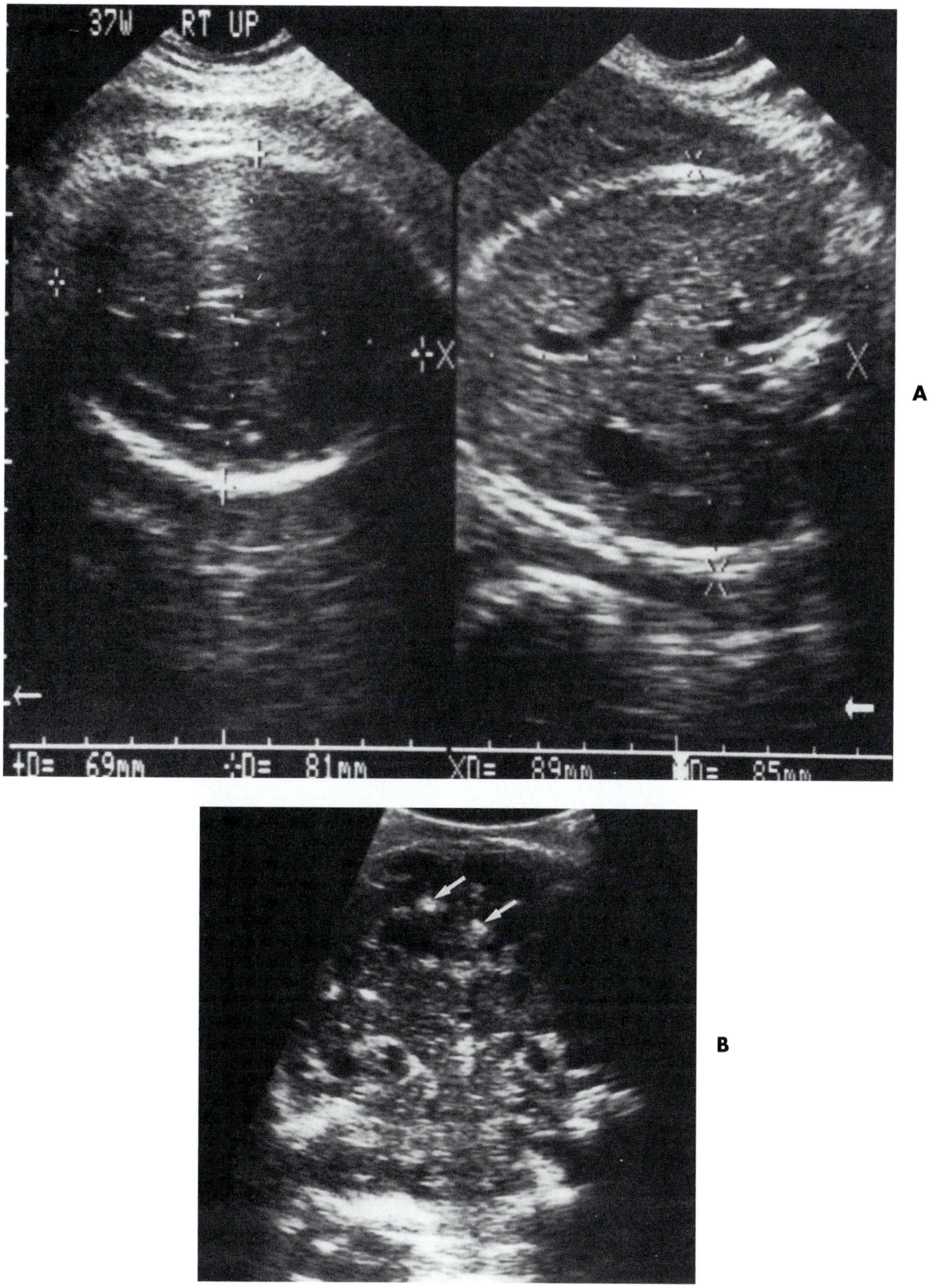

FIG. 43-23. Microcephaly. **A,** Comparative head (left) and abdominal circumference (right) views at 37 menstrual weeks show the abnormally small, symmetrical head. Brain structures are abnormal but poorly visible due to obscuration by overlying bone. **B,** Coronal scan shows intracerebral calcifications (*arrows*). Screen for infection was negative. Autopsy diagnosis was a rare autosomal recessive lissencephaly.

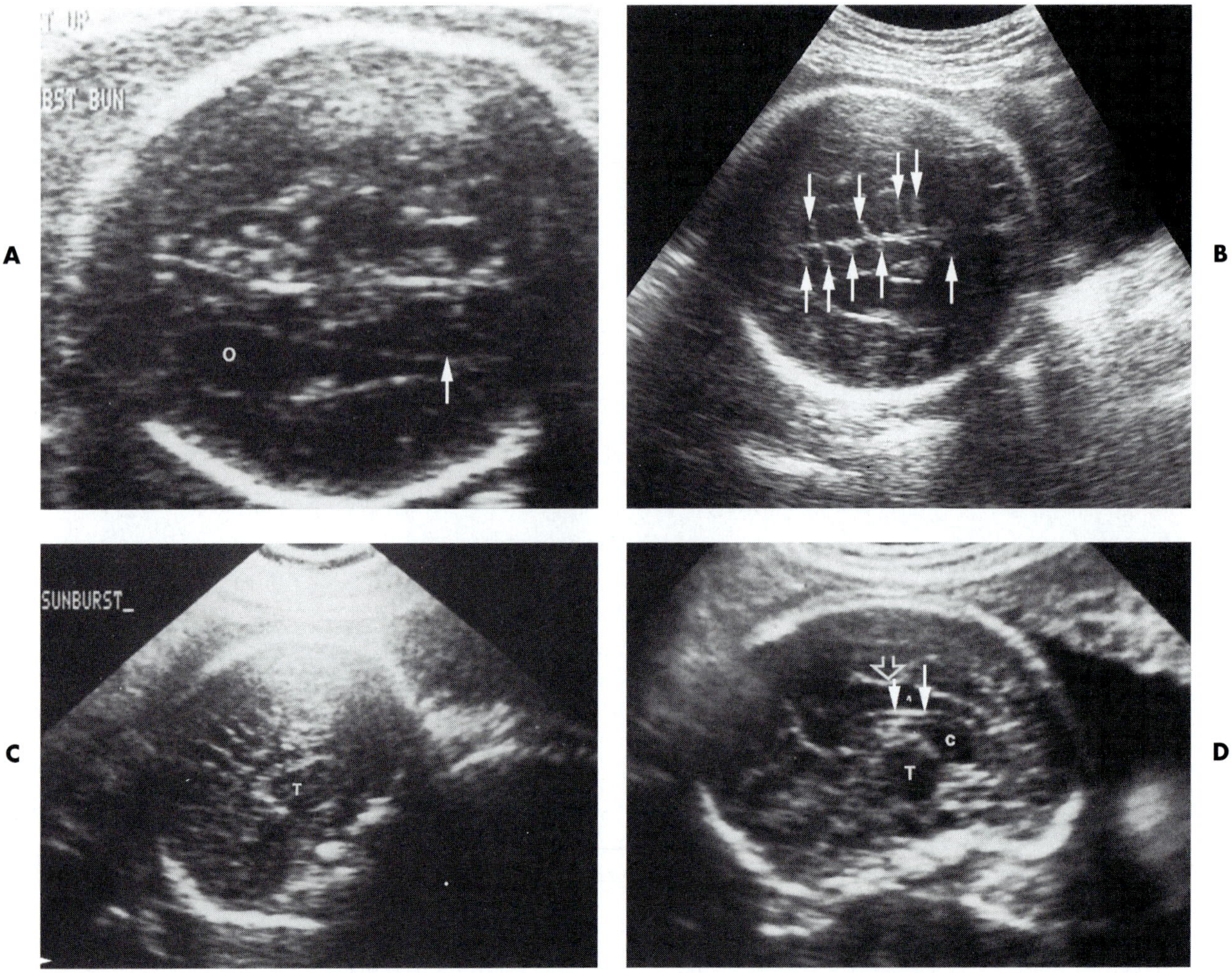

FIG. 43-24. Agenesis of corpus callosum. A, Transverse ventricular view at 35 menstrual weeks shows characteristic borderline dilation of occipital horns (o) and pointed, slightly spread anterior horns (*arrow*). This ventricle configuration is called colpocephaly. **B,** Axial ventricular view at 33 weeks demonstrates too many sulci perpendicular to the interhemispheric fissure (*arrows*), the axial correlate of the "sunburst" sign. The ventricle is also enlarged. **C,** Midsagittal view shows typical sunburst radiation of interhemispheric sulci from the thalamus (T) and absent corpus callosum and cavum septi pellucidi. **D,** Normal fetal head for comparison shows the normal sweeping pattern of the cingulate sulcus (*open arrow*), corpus callosum (*small arrows*), and cavum septi pellucidi (C); thalamus (T).

- absent cavum septi pellucidi; and
- in third trimester, too many sulci perpendicular to the interhemispheric fissure (Fig. 43-24, *B*).

Once the diagnosis is suspected, the less commonly used coronal and parasagittal views help to confirm the diagnosis. On the coronal views, the third ventricle is elevated, the medial walls of the anterior horns are indented from their medial aspect by the bundles of Probst (Fig. 43-25, *B*), and an interhemispheric cyst may be present. On parasagittal views, the CC is not present and the sulci on the interhemispheric brain surface show a "sun-burst" orientation radiating from the third ventricle[112] (Fig. 43-24, *C*). Under about 24 weeks, the metopic suture of the frontal bone and anterior fontanelle offer a clear window for seeing the CC in a midsagittal view (Figs. 43-24, *D* and 43-25, *D*). If the head is deep in the pelvis, transvaginal scans can provide especially clear views. Color Doppler scans can be used to demonstrate an abnormal course of the cingulate and pericallosal arteries.

Occasionally, fetuses with callosal abnormalities develop a lipoma close to the midline near the expected anterior end of the corpus callosum.[113]

Acquired Lesions

Aqueductal Stenosis. This form of ventricle enlargement follows mechanical or functional obstruction at the **aqueduct of Sylvius** (Fig. 43-26). Aqueduct narrowing is present in about 20% to 30% of patients with ventriculomegaly and results from di-

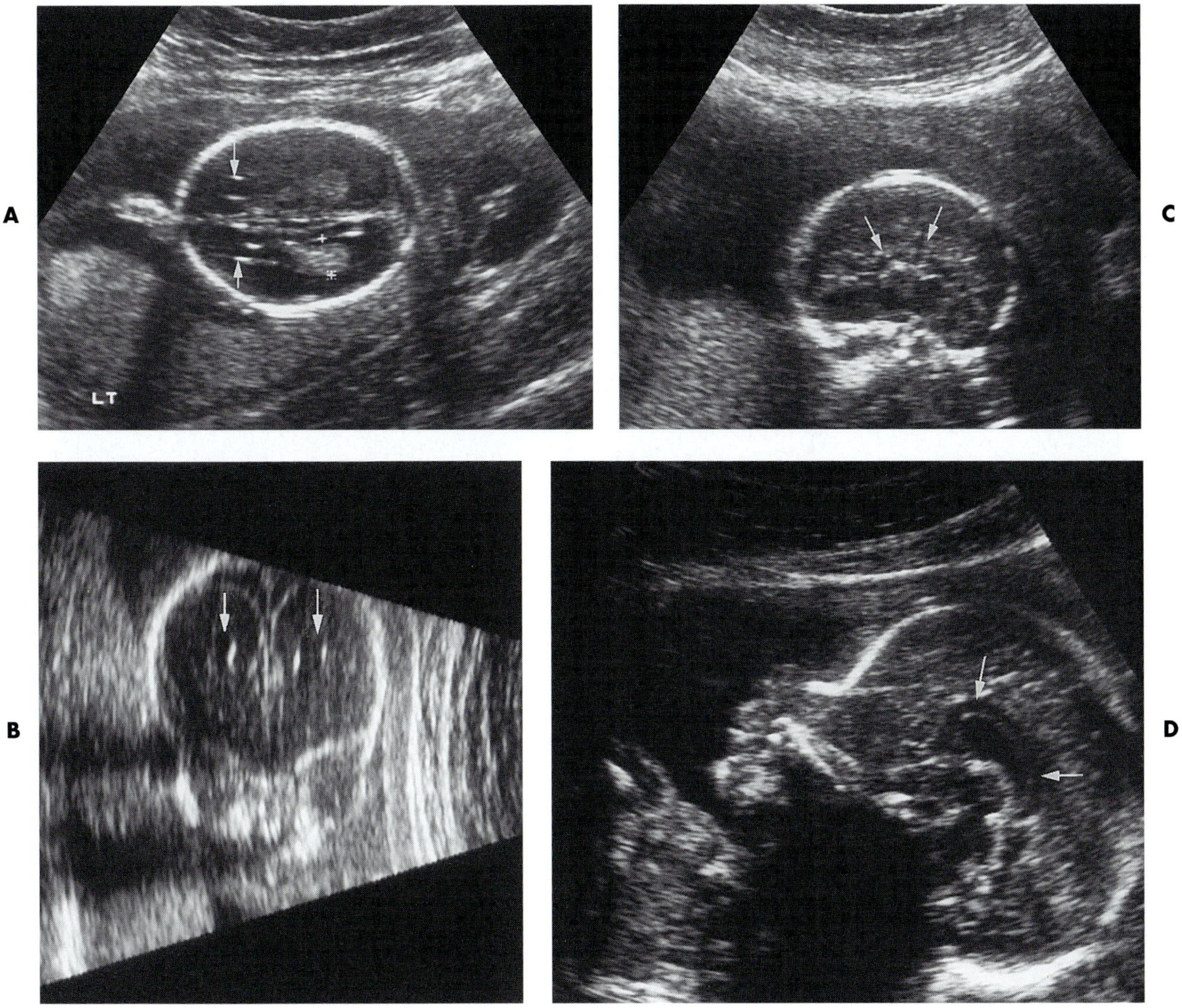

FIG. 43-25. Agenesis of corpus callosum at 19 weeks. **A,** Ventricular view shows laterally displaced anterior horns (*arrows*) and there is no cavum septi pellucidi. Rather, the hemispheres appear abnormally separated. **B,** Coronal view shows abnormal vertical or U-shaped orientation of the anterior horns with medial walls displaced laterally by bundles of Probst, and there is no cavum septi pellucidi between the ventricles. (Compare to Fig. 43-2, *D.*) **C,** Midsagittal view confirms absence of the corpus callosum and CSP in their expected location (*arrows*). This fetus is too young to have developed sulci and the sunburst pattern has not yet developed. **D,** Normal 22-week corpus callosum and CSP (*arrows*) imaged through the metopic suture.

verse causes.[39] If present as an isolated, nonprogressive abnormality, a functionally and mentally normal outcome can be seen in 50% to 80% of instances, even if severe cortical thinning is present, though postpartum ventricular shunting may be required.[15,114] Although the hydrocephalus of aqueductal stenosis is readily diagnosed, associated anomalies occur in 70% to 83% of cases and escape detection in 20% to 39% of cases. Those with associated anomalies do poorly.[39] If discovered before viability, termination is offered. Cesarean section is indicated for macrocephaly, fetal distress, and obstetric complications, but it is avoided if other serious, associated anomalies are present. In such patients, vaginal delivery may require drainage of fluid from the ventricles to allow head passage (cephalocentesis). If there is progressive ventricular enlargement, delivery is recommended as soon as pulmonary maturity is established.[41] Prenatal, *in utero* ventriculo amniotic shunting has been attempted in the past but without clear improvement in outcome and the procedure is not currently practiced.[40,48]

Causes may be genetic, congenital, or infectious, or there may be other, less common etiologies such as an X-linked recessive gene.[114,115]

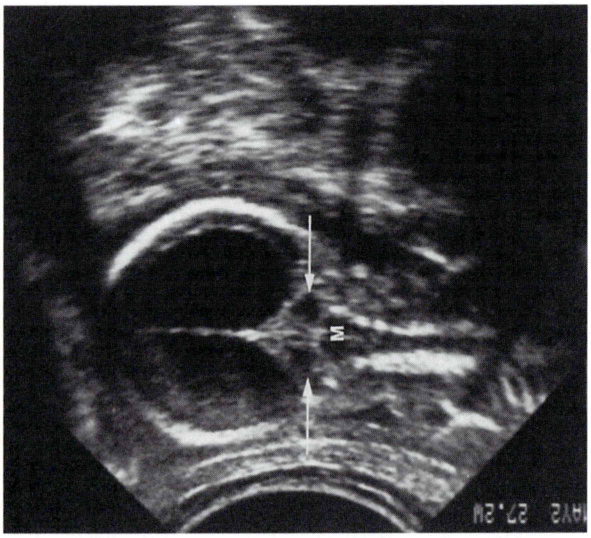

FIG. 43-26. Aqueduct stenosis. Coronal view at 27 menstrual weeks shows massively dilated lateral ventricles. Note preservation of cerebellar lobar configuration (*arrows*) and position of the cisterna magna (M) unlike that in the Chiari malformation.

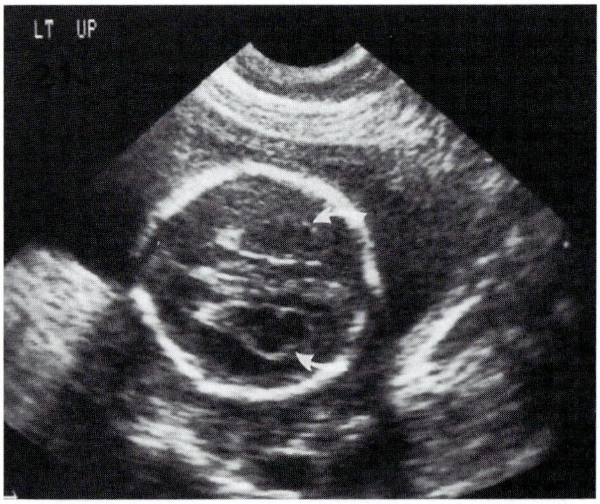

FIG. 43-27. Choroid plexus cysts. Transverse ventricular view at 21 menstrual weeks shows entire choroid plexus replaced with cysts bilaterally (*arrows*). Although most fetuses with small cysts are normal, those with extensive cysts or other anomalies may have chromosomal abnormalities, especially trisomy 18, as was present in this fetus.

At **ultrasound,** the lateral and third ventricles are enlarged, occasionally asymmetrically, but there is no enlargement of the fourth ventricle. The cerebellum, posterior fossa, and cisterna magna may appear normal (Fig. 43-26).

Intracranial Calcifications. Calcifications are rare. They occur late in gestation (Fig. 43-23, *C*), are commonly associated with fetal infections, and suggest a poor prognosis. Anatomically, they occur in areas of cell necrosis and may line ventricles or occur in the parenchyma and be associated with severe CNS changes, including microcephaly, ventriculomegaly, and porencephalic cysts.

Differential diagnosis of fetal intracranial calcifications includes intrauterine infections (especially cytomegalovirus and toxoplasmosis; see below), teratomas, tuberous sclerosis, Sturge-Weber syndrome, and venous sinus thrombosis.[116]

Choroid Plexus Cysts (CPCs). Cystic spaces occur in the choroid in about 3% of fetuses between 13 and 24 weeks of gestation. Most are small and incidental and disappear without consequence. Occasionally, they may be associated with chromosomal abnormalities, especially trisomy 18 or infection.[117] In these cases, the cysts tend to be large and to involve most of the substance of the choroid. They are most commonly associated with other findings of trisomy 18[117] (Fig. 43-27).

The relationship of CPCs to chromosomal problems, especially trisomy 18, remains controversial. Literature reviews now suggest that the association of isolated CPCs and chromosomal abnormality is about 1 in 150 to 1 in 390.[118,119] This is about the same risk as an amniocentesis. In contrast, if any other anomalies are present, then the risk for abnormal chromosomes rises to about 1 in 3.[119] It is advisable to use CPCs as an indication to perform detailed scanning rather than invasive testing.[119]

Infections. The **TORCH** group of organisms (**To**xoplasma, **R**ubella, **C**ytomegalovirus (CMV), and **H**erpes simplex virus) can cross the placenta and cause encephalitis followed by microcephaly, ventriculomegaly, and calcifications. Diagnosis is made by demonstrating maternal seroconversion or specific fetal immunoglobulin M in fetal blood obtained by cordocentesis.[120]

The severity of brain injury generally relates to the age of infection rather than to the agent. CMV is the most common infection; it may infect about 1% of newborns, followed by toxoplasmosis and congenital rubella. CMV is a common virus usually acquired through association with groups of people, especially children, because there is normally a high incidence of infection in the population. Toxoplasmosis is acquired through contact with uncooked meat and contact with animals, particularly cats, and kitty litter. Herpes simplex encephalitis can be transplacentally acquired, but is more commonly acquired during fetal passage through an infected birth canal.[121]

Both CMV and toxoplasmosis can cause similar cerebral changes that range from mild to very severe. They include microcephaly, ventriculomegaly, calcifications, and abnormal cortex formation such as lissencephaly and polymicrogyria. In CMV, calcifications tend to be in the periventricular area (Fig. 43-28, *A*, *B*) in contrast to toxoplasmosis calcifications which are more likely to affect the cortex and

A

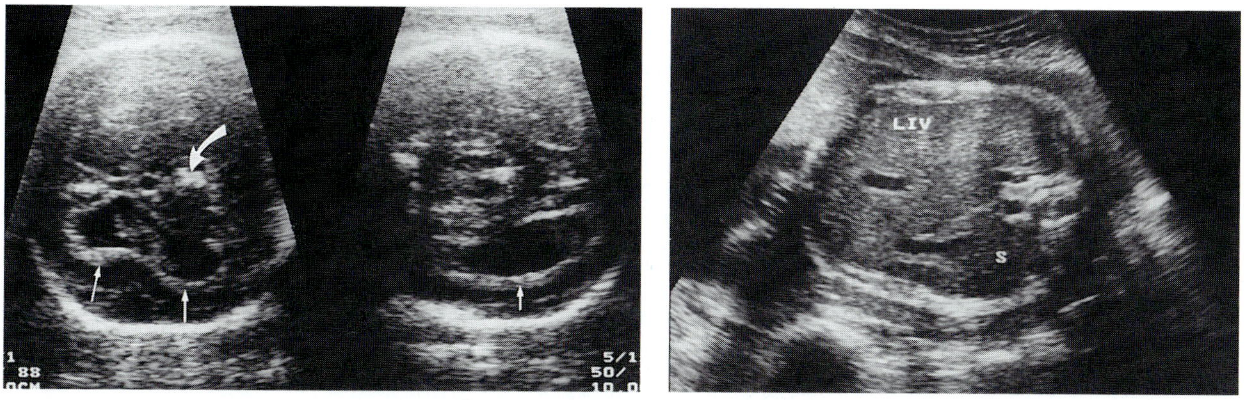

B

FIG. 43-28. Fetal cytomegalovirus (CMV) infection at 28 weeks. **A,** Cranial changes with CMV infection including enlarged ventricles with thick, calcified walls (*straight arrows*). There is also calcification in the brainstem (*curved arrow*). **B,** Hepatosplenomegaly compressing the fetal stomach helps confirm fetal infection. Liver (LIV). Spleen (S).

A

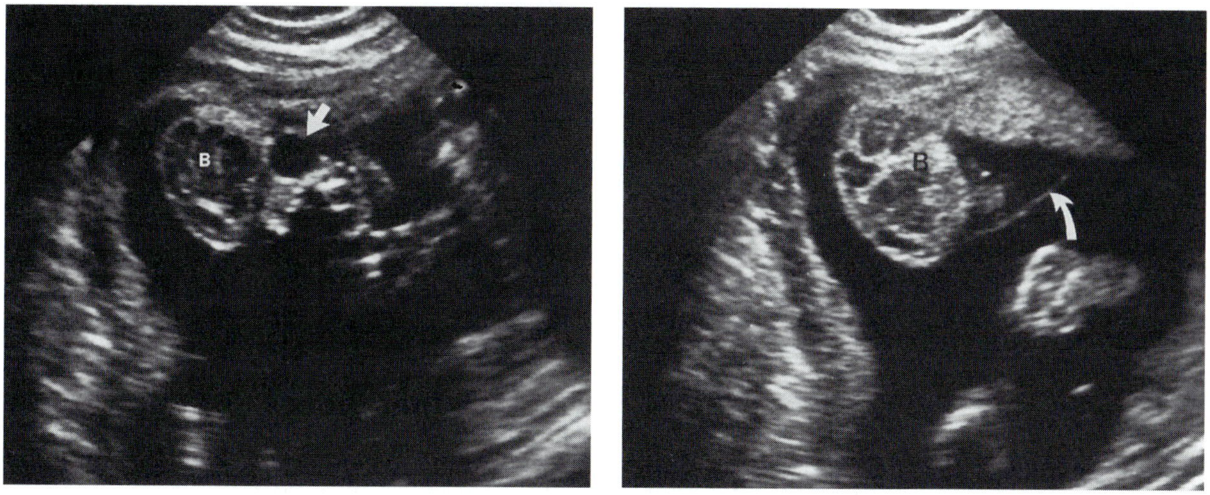

B

FIG. 43-29. Early amnion rupture sequence (amniotic band syndrome). **A,** Coronal view through face shows disorganized brain tissue (B) not covered by skull. This is similar to anencephaly, but unlike anencephaly, only one orbit is present (*arrow*). **B,** View through disorganized brain (B) shows lack of skull bones and the presence of a membrane or band (*curved arrow*) attaching the head to the uterine wall, characteristic of early amnion rupture sequence. (See also Fig. 43-11, *C*.)

basal ganglia.[121] Other generalized changes also occur, including heart failure, pleural effusion, hepatosplenomegaly, echogenic bowel, hepatic calcification, and ascites.

Early Amnion Rupture Sequence (amniotic band syndrome, amniotic band disruption complex, and limb-body-wall complex). This sporadic malformation occurs in about 1 in 1200 livebirths but is about five times more common in stillbirths. Its etiology is not clear, but there is a common theme of early rupture of the amnion, attachment of the strands to the fetus, and secondary fetal disruptions, deformations, and malformations, some of which relate to vascular injuries.[122] Fetuses with this disorder can have bizarre changes that may mimic other malformations.[123] The type and severity of the abnormality relate to the timing of the rupture. Early lesions at about 5 menstrual weeks result in craniofacial abnormalities such as anencephaly, unusual and asymmetric encephaloceles, unusual facial clefting, and placental attachment to fetal head and abdomen. Occurrence at 7 weeks results in limb reductions and abnormalities as well as thoraco abdominal defects, frequently with scoliosis. Occurrence after 9 weeks results in limb abnormalities, such as hypoplasias, amputations, and deformities.[56,122] Although the extremities are most commonly involved, about one third of affected children have craniofacial anomalies, including facial clefting, asymmetric encephaloceles, anencephaly, holoprosencephaly, and hydrocephalus.[122] Prognosis varies with the specific lesions. Fortunately, there is negligible risk of recurrence.

Sonographically (Figs. 43-11, *C* and 43-29, *A, B*) the diagnosis should be suspected if clefts, malforma-

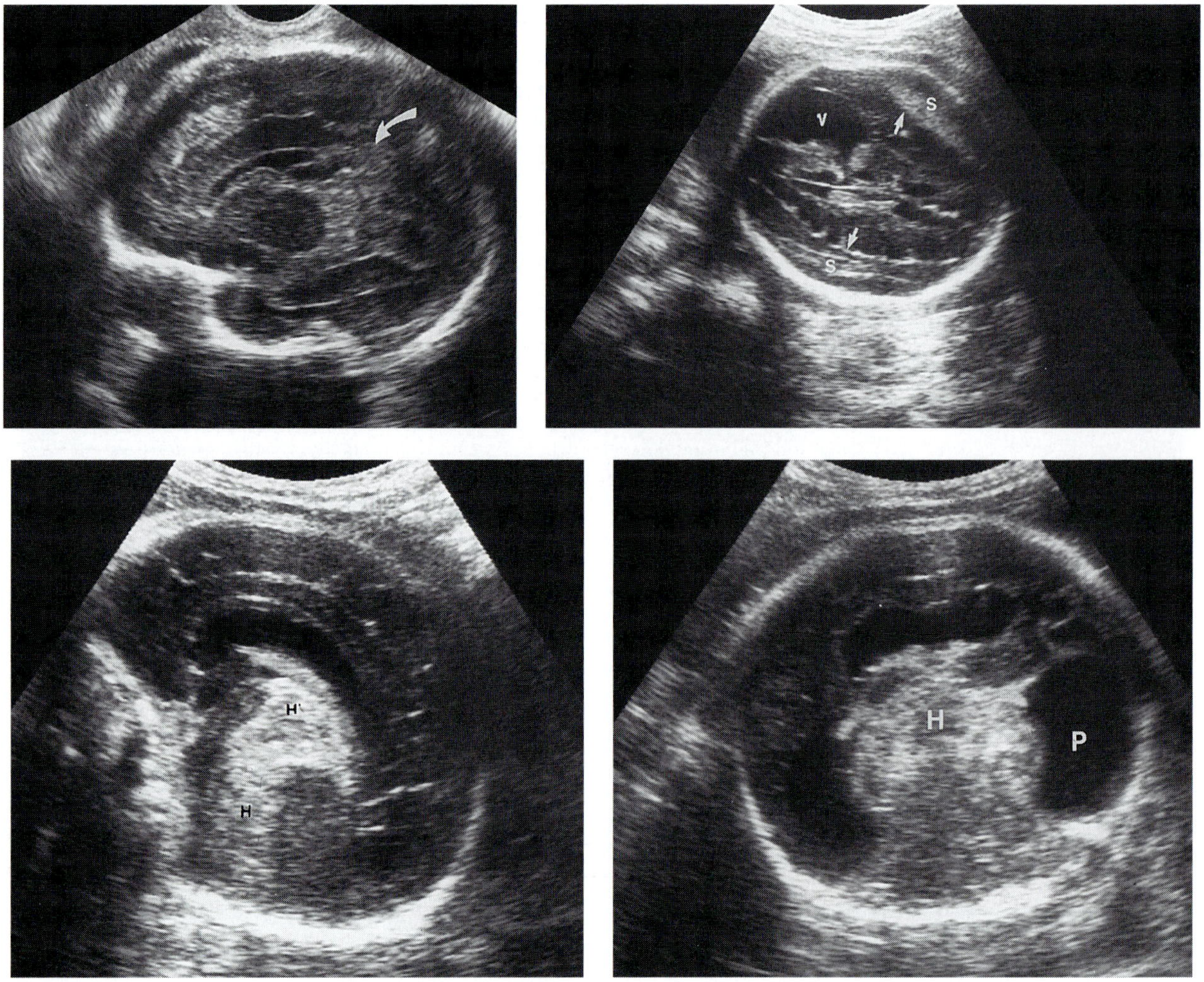

FIG. 43-30. Intracranial hemorrhage. **A,** Parasagittal view of grade 4 intracerebral hemorrhage with clot (*arrow*) excavating into the occipital cortex. **B,** Bilateral subdural hemorrhages (s) compressing the brain (*arrows*) and associated with slight asymmetric ventricular enlargement (V). These hemorrhages resolved spontaneously and the child is well after delivery. No cause was found. Most children with this finding do poorly. **C,** Parasagittal and **D,** coronal views of midcerebral hemorrhage (H) at 38 weeks. The post hemorrhagic porencephalic cyst (P) helps to differentiate this from tumor such as teratoma. Hypoxia was the likely etiology. This fetus died shortly after the examination.

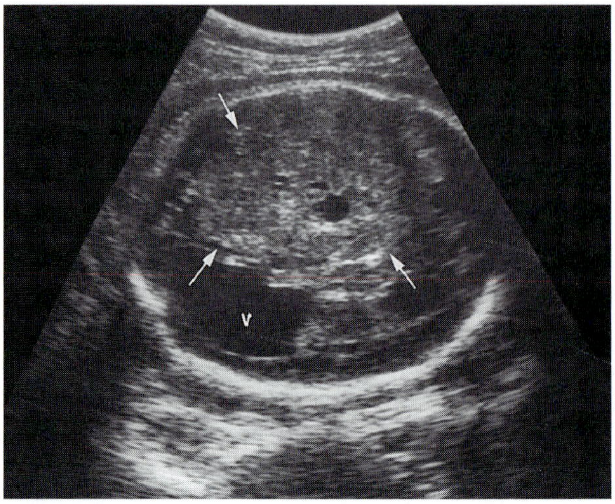

FIG. 43-31. Intracranial teratoma at 34 weeks forming an echogenic mass with small cystic spaces (*arrows*) displacing the midline to one side. The visible lateral ventricle (V) is dilated.

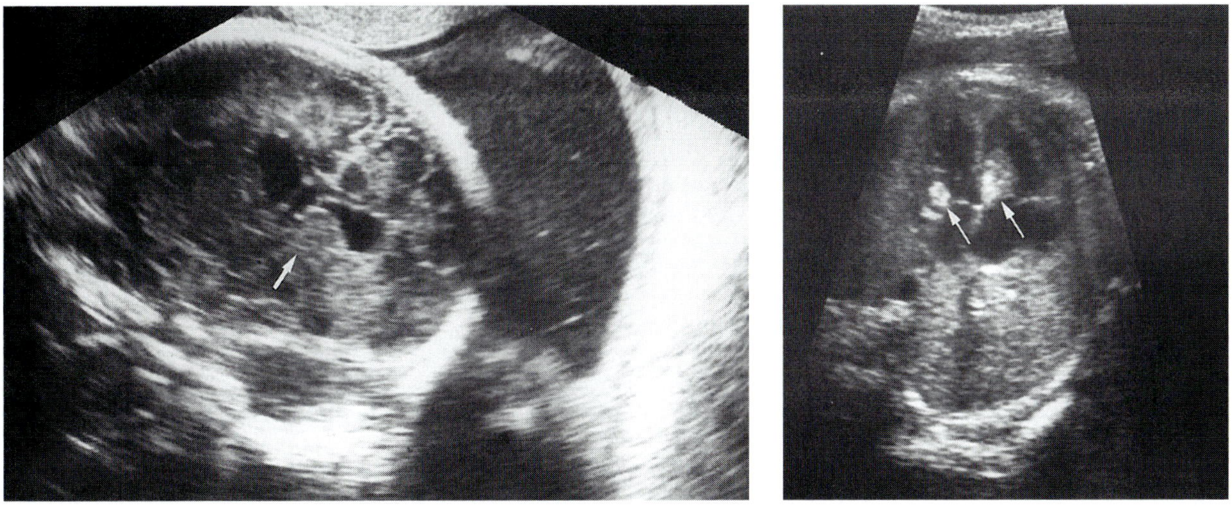

FIG. 43-32. Tuberous sclerosis at 30 weeks. **A,** A typical hamartoma, or giant-cell tumor, is visible at the foramen of Monro indenting the anterior horn of the lateral ventricle (*arrow*). Both ventricles are dilated. **B, Rhabdomyomas** involving the heart are clearly visible as echogenic masses in left and right ventricle (*arrows*).

tions, and amputations in nonembryologic distributions, asymmetric encephaloceles, and thoracoabdominal disruptions exist, even if the bands that relate to these malformations are not apparent.[123] In such cases, the fetus can appear to be "stuck" to a part of the uterus or placenta.

Vein of Galen Aneurysm. A variety of arteriovenous malformations drain into the vein of Galen and result in its distention as a single, dilated, midline fluid collection. The dilation usually does not occur until the third trimester. The shunting may be severe enough to result in fetal or neonatal heart failure.[124,125] Once suspected, the diagnosis is readily confirmed with Doppler ultrasound. (See Chapter 52.) Also, neck vessels will appear prominent, and signs of heart failure can be present. The prognosis is poor, with many cases dying in the neonatal period from heart failure which becomes increasingly severe after delivery despite attempts at embolization therapy.

Sonographically, the dilated vein is visible as a fluid space close to the midline behind the thalamus and midbrain. Most are not diagnosed until the third trimester.[125] **Differential diagnosis** includes other midline fluid collections, such as arachnoid cysts, cysts associated with agenesis of the corpus callosum, and porencephaly.

Hemorrhagic Lesions. These are uncommon. Fetal hypoxia due to abruption or amnionitis is the most common etiology. The changes are similar to those seen with neonatal asphyxia. (See Chapter 52 on neonatal scanning.) In addition, trauma or maternal platelet antibodies can result in bleeding into any part of the brain. Several of our cases have been spontaneous and no etiology has been discovered. Prognosis is variable, depending on the site and the extent of bleeding (Fig. 43-30, *A-D*).

Tumors. Congenital brain tumors are rare. Most are identified in the third trimester, the head having appeared normal at earlier scans. However, a teratoma has been detected at 22 weeks. **Teratomas** are the most common lesion and they account for 50% of brain tumors detected *in utero*.[126] Typically, they form large, central, echogenic masses with cystic spaces and occasional calcifications (Fig. 43-31). Other tumors that have been identified include glioblastoma, neuroblastoma, craniopharyngioma,[127,128] tuberous sclerosis-associated masses, subependymal hamartomas, and giant-cell tumors[129] (Fig. 43-32, *A*). The **prognosis** is dismal and most infants die or are severely disabled.[126-128] With tuberous sclerosis, echogenic cardiac rhabdomyomas may be more obvious than the cerebral masses (Fig. 43-32, *B*).

ACKNOWLEDGMENTS

The authors thank Dr. Margot van Allan for her kind assistance with portions of this chapter and Rose Baldwin for assistance with the manuscript.

REFERENCES

1. Campbell S, Pearce JM. The prenatal diagnosis of fetal structural anomalies by ultrasound. *Clin Obstet Gynecol* 1983;10:475-506.
2. Manchester DK, Pretorius DH, Avery C et al. Accuracy of ultrasound diagnoses in pregnancies complicated by suspected fetal anomalies. *Prenat Diagn* 1988;8:109-117.
3. Porter KB, Wagner PC, Cabaniss ML. Fetal board: a multidisciplinary approach to management of the abnormal fetus. *Obstet Gynecol* 1988;72:275-278.
4. Main DM, Mennuti MT. Neural tube defects: issues in prenatal diagnosis and counselling. *Obstet Gynecol* 1986;67:1-16.

Developmental Anatomy

5. Moore KL. *Essentials of Human Embryology*. Toronto: Decker Inc; 1988.
6. Crade M, Patel J, McQuown D. Sonographic imaging of the glycogen stage of the fetal choroid plexus. *AJR* 1981;137:489-491.
7. Cyr DR, Mack LA, Nyberg DA et al. Fetal rhombencephalon: normal ultrasound findings. *Radiology* 1988;166:691-692.
8. Filly RA, Cardoza JD, Goldstein RB et al. Detection of central nervous system anomalies: a practical level of effort for a routine sonogram. *Radiology* 1989;172:403-408.
9. Nyberg DA. Recommendations for obstetric sonography in the evaluation of the fetal cranium. *Radiology* 1989;172:309-311.
10. Shepard M, Filly RA. A standardized plane for biparietal diameter measurement. *J Ultrasound Med* 1982;1:145-150.
11. McLeary RD, Kuhns LR, Barr M. Ultrasonography of the fetal cerebellum. *Radiology* 1984;151:439-442.
12. Romero R, Pilu G, Jeanty P et al. Craniostenoses. In: Prenatal Diagnosis of Congenital Anomalies. East Norwalk, Conn.: Appleton & Lange; 1988:369-373.
13. Benacerraf BR, Estroff JA. Transvaginal sonographic imaging of the low fetal head in the second trimester. *J Ultrasound Med* 1989;8:325-328.

Ventriculomegaly and Hydrocephalus

14. Young HF, Nulsen FE, Weiss MH et al. The relationship of intelligence and cerebral mantle in treated infantile hydrocephalus. *Pediatrics* 1973;52:38-44.
15. Shurtleff DB, Foltz EL, Loeser JD. Hydrocephalus: a definition of its progression and relationship to intellectual function, diagnosis and complications. *Am J Dis Child* 1973;125:688-693.
16. Lorber J. The results of early treatment of extreme hydrocephalus. *Develop Med Child Neurol* 1968;16(suppl):21-29.
17. Stein SC, Schut L, Ames MD. Selection for early treatment of meningomyelocele: a retrospective analysis of selection procedures. *Dev Med Child Neurol* 1975;17:311-319.
18. Vintzileos AM, Ingardia CJ, Nochimson DJ. Congenital hydrocephalus: a review and protocol for perinatal management. *Obstet Gynecol* 1983;62:539-549.
19. Callen PW, Chooljian D. The effect of ventricular dilation upon the biometry of the head. *J Ultrasound Med* 1986;5:17-19.
20. Cardoza JD, Goldstein RB, Filly RA. Exclusion of fetal ventriculomegaly with a single measurement: the width of the lateral ventricular atrium. *Radiology* 1988;169:711-714.
21. Heiserman J, Filly RA, Goldstein RB. Effect of measurement errors on sonographic evaluation of ventriculomegaly. *J Ultrasound Med* 1991;10:121-124.
22. Patel MD, Goldstein RB, Tung S, Filly RA. Fetal cerebral ventricular atrium: difference in size according to sex. *Radiology* 1995;194:713-715.
23. Mahony BS, Nyberg DA, Hirsch JH et al. Mild idiopathic lateral ventricular dilatation *in utero*: sonographic evaluation. *Radiology* 1988;169:715-721.
24. Hertzberg BS, Lile R, Foosaner DE et al. Choroid plexus-ventricular wall separation in fetuses with normal-sized cerebral ventricles at sonography: postnatal outcome. *AJR* 1994;163:405-410.
25. Toi A, Brown A. Measurement of the upper (proximal) fetal cerebral ventricle. *Ultrasound Obstet Gynecol* 1996;8(suppl 1):75.
26. Farrell TA, Herzberg BS, Kliewer MA et al. Fetal lateral ventricles: reassessment of normal values for atrial diameter at ultrasound. *Radiology* 1994;193:409-411.
27. Filly RA, Goldstein RB, Callen PW. Fetal ventricle: importance in routine obstetric sonography. *Radiology* 1991;181:1-7.
28. Jeanty P, Dramaix-Wilmet M, Delbeke D et al. Ultrasonic evaluation of fetal ventricular growth. *Neuroradiology* 1981;21:127-131.
29. Pretorius D, Drose J, Manco-Johnson M. Fetal lateral ventricular ratio determination during the second trimester. *J Ultrasound Med* 1986;5:121-244.
30. Johnson ML, Dunne MC, Mack LA et al. Evaluation of fetal intracranial anatomy by static and real-time ultrasound. *J Clin Ultrasound* 1980;8:311-318.
31. Herzberg BS, Bowie JD, Burger PC et al. The three lines: origin of sonographic landmarks in the fetal head. *AJR* 1987;149:1009-1012.
32. Benacerraf BR, Birnholz JC. The diagnosis of fetal hydrocephalus prior to 22 weeks. *J Clin Ultrasound* 1987;15:531-536.
33. Campbell J, Gilbert WM, Nicolaides KH et al. Ultrasound screening for spina bifida: cranial and cerebellar signs in a high-risk population. *Obstet Gynecol* 1987;70:247-250.
34. Goldstein RB, Podarsky AE, Filly RA et al. Effacement of the fetal cisterna magna in association with myelomeningocele. *Radiology* 1989;172:409-413.
35. Benacerraf BR, Stryker J, Frigoletto FD. Abnormal ultrasound appearance of the cerebellum (banana sign): indirect sign of spina bifida. *Radiology* 1989;171:151-153.
36. Filly RA. The "lemon" sign: a clinical perspective. *Radiology* 1988;167:573-575.
37. Nyberg DA, Shepard T, Mack LA et al. Significance of a single umbilical artery in fetuses with central nervous system malformations. *J Ultrasound Med* 1988;7:265-273.
38. Nyberg DA, Mack LA, Hirsch J et al. Fetal hydrocephalus: sonographic detection and clinical significance of associated anomalies. *Radiology* 1987;163:187-191.
39. Drugen A, Krause B, Canady A et al. The natural history of prenatally diagnosed cerebral ventriculomegaly. *JAMA* 1989;261:1785-1788.
40. Chervenak FA, Berkowitz RL, Tortora M et al. The management of fetal hydrocephalus. *Am J Obstet Gynecol* 1985;151:933-942.
41. Vintzileos AM, Campbell WA, Weinbaum PJ et al. Perinatal management and outcome of fetal ventriculomegaly. *Obstet Gynecol* 1987;69:5-11.

Specific Abnormalities

42. Van der Knaap MS, Valk J. Classification of congenital abnormalities of the CNS. *AJNR* 1988;9:315-326.
43. Poe LB, Coleman LL, Mahmud F. Congenital central nervous system anomalies. *RadioGraphics* 1989;9:801-826.
44. Hendricks SK, Cyr DR, Nyberg DA et al. Exencephaly—clinical and ultrasonic correlation to anencephaly. *Obstet Gynecol* 1988;72:898-901.
45. Cox GC, Rosenthal SJ, Hosapple JW. Exencephaly: sonographic findings and radiologic-pathologic correlation. *Radiology* 1985;155:755-756.

46. Goldstein RB, Filly RA, Callen PW. Sonography of anencephaly: pitfalls in early diagnosis. *J Clin Ultrasound* 1989;17:397-402.
47. Goldstein RA, Filly RA. Prenatal diagnosis of anencephaly: spectrum of sonographic appearances and distinction from the amniotic band syndrome. *AJR* 1988;151:547-550.
48. Vintzileos AM, Campbell WA, Nochimson DJ et al. Antenatal evaluation and management of ultrasonically detected fetal anomalies. *Obstet Gynecol* 1987;69:640-660.
49. Wilkins-Haug L, Freedman W. Progression of exencephaly to anencephaly in the human fetus: an ultrasound perspective. *Prenatal Diag* 1991;11:227-233.
50. Achiron R, Achiron A. Transvaginal fetal neurosonography: the first trimester of pregnancy. In: Chervenak FA, Kurjak A, Comstock CH eds. Progress in Obstetric and Gynecological Sonography Series: Ultrasound and the Fetal Brain. Parthenon Pub; 1995:90-108.
51. Salmanca A, Gonzalez-Gomez R, Padilla MC et al. Prenatal ultrasound seminography of anencephaly: sonographic-pathological correlations. *Ultrasound Obstet Gynecol* 1992; 2:95-100.
52. Goldstein RB, LaPidus AS, Filly RA. Fetal cephaloceles: diagnosis with ultrasound. *Radiology* 1991;180:803.
53. Fitz CR. Midline anomalies of the brain and spine. *Radiol Clin North Am* 1982;20:95-104.
54. Cullen MT, Athanassiadis AP, Romero R. Prenatal diagnosis of anterior parietal encephalocele with transvaginal sonography. *Obstet Gynecol* 1990;75:489-491.
55. Carlan SJ, Angel JL, Leo J et al. Cephalocele involving the oral cavity. *Obstet Gynecol* 1990;75:494-496.
56. Jones KL. *Smith's Recognizable Patterns of Human Malformation*. 4th ed. Philadelphia: WB Saunders Co; 1988.
57. Babcook CJ, Goldstein RB, Barth RA, et al. Prevalence of ventriculomegaly in association with meningomyelocele: correlation with gestation age and severity of posterior fossa deformity. *Radiology* 1994;190:703-707.
58. Nyberg DA, Mack LA, Hirsch J, Mahoney BS. Abnormalities of fetal cranial contour in . . . *Radiology* 1988;167:387-392.
59. Van den Hof MC, Nicolaides KH, Campbell J et al. Evaluation of the lemon and banana signs in one hundred thirty fetuses with open spina bifida. *Am J Obstet Gynecol* 1990;162:322-327.
60. Benacerraf BR, Stryker J, Frigoletto FD. Abnormal US appearance of the cerebellum (banana sign): indirect sign of spina bifida. *Radiology* 1989;171:151-153.
61. Campbell J, Gilbert WM, Nicolaides KH et al. Ultrasound screening for spina bifida: cranial and cerebellar signs in a high-risk population. *Obstet Gynecol* 1987;70:247-250.
62. Goldstein RB, Podarsky AE, Filly RA. Effacement of the fetal cisterna magna in association with myelomeningocele. *Radiology* 1989;172:409-413.
63. Ball RH, Rilly RA, Goldstein RB, Callen PW. The lemon sign: not a specific indicator of myelomeningocele. *J Ultrasound Med* 1993;12:131-134.
64. Barkovich AJ. Congenital malformations of the brain. In: Pediatric Neuroimaging. 2nd ed., New York: Raven Press; 1995:238-246.
65. Harmon JP, Hiett AK, Palmer CG et al. Prenatal ultrasound detection of isolated neural tube defects: is cytogenetic evaluation warranted? *Obstet Gynecol* 1995;86:595-599.
66. Kennedy D, Chitayat D, Toi A et al. Chromosome abnormalities in antenatally diagnosed neural tube defects. *Am J Human Genetics* 1996;59(suppl):A323.
67. Cochrane DD, Wilson DR, Steinbock P, Farquharson DF et al. Prenatal spinal evaluation and functional outcome of patients born with myelomeningocele: information for improved prenatal counselling and outcome prediction. *Fetal Diagn Ther* 1996;11:159-168.
68. Nyberg DA, Mack LA, Bronstein A et al. Holoprosencephaly: prenatal sonographic diagnosis. *AJR* 1987;149:1051-1058.
69. Cohen MM Jr, Sulik KK. Perspectives on holoprosencephaly: part II. *J Craniofac Genet Dev Biol* 1992;12:196-244.
70. Byrd SE, Naidich TP. Common congenital brain anomalies. *Radiol Clin North Am* 1988;26:755-772.
71. McGahan JP, Ellis W, Lindfors KK et al. Congenital cerebrospinal fluid-containing intracranial abnormalities: sonographic classification. *J Clin Ultrasound* 1988;16:531-544.
72. Greene MF, Benacerraf BR, Frigoletto FD. Reliable criteria for the prenatal sonographic diagnosis of alobar holoprosencephaly. *Am J Obstet Gynecol* 1987;156:687-689.
73. McGahan JP, Nyberg DA, Mack LA. Sonography of facial features of alobar and semilobar holoprosencephaly. *AJR* 1990; 154:143-148.
74. Pilu G, Sandri F, Perolo A et al. Prenatal diagnosis of lobar holoprosencephaly. *Ultrasound Obstet Gynecol* 1992;2:88-94.
75. Pilu G, Ambrosetto P, Sandri F et al. Intraventricular fused fornices: a specific sign of fetal lobar holoprosencephaly. *Ultrasound Obstet Gynecol* 1994;4:65-67.
76. Nelson LH, King M. Early diagnosis of holoprosencephaly. *J Ultrasound Med* 1992;11:57-59.
77. Hirsch JF, Pierre-Kahn A, Reiner D et al. The Dandy-Walker malformation: a review of 40 cases. *J Neurosurg* 1984; 61:515-522.
78. Fitz CR. Disorders of ventricles and CSF spaces. *Semin Ultrasound CR, MR* 1988;9:216-230.
79. Altman NR, Naidich TP, Braffman BH. Posterior fossa malformations. *AJNR* 1992;13:691-724.
80. Kollias SS, Ball WS, Prenger EC. Cystic malformations of the posterior fossa: differential diagnosis clarified through embryonic analysis. *RadioGraphics* 1993;13:1211-1231.
81. Bromley B, Nadel AS, Pauker S et al. Closure of the cerebellar vermis: evaluation with second trimester US. *Radiology* 1994;193:761-763.
82. Laing F, Frates MC, Brown DL et al. Sonography of the fetal posterior fossa: false appearance of mega-cisterna magna and Dandy-Walker variant. *Radiology* 1994;192:247-251.
83. Hart MN, Malamud N, Ellis WG. The Dandy-Walker syndrome: a clinicopathological study based on 28 cases. *Neurology* 1972;22:771-780.
84. Murray JC, Johnson JA, Bird TD. Dandy-Walker malformation: etiologic heterogenicity and empiric recurrence risks. *Clin Genet* 1985;28:272-283.
85. Gardner E, O'Rahilly R, Prolo D. The Dandy-Walker and Arnold-Chiari malformations: clinical, developmental, and teratological considerations. *Arch Neurol* 1975;32:393-407.
86. Nyberg DA, Cyr DR, Mack LA et al. The Dandy-Walker malformation: prenatal sonographic diagnosis and its clinical significance. *J Ultrasound Med* 1988;7:65-71.
87. Roach ES, Laster DW, Sumner TE et al. Posterior fossa arachnoid cyst demonstrated by ultrasound. *J Clin Ultrasound* 1982;10:88-90.
88. Nyberg DA, Mahony BS, Hegge FN et al. Enlarged cisterna magna and the Dandy-Walker malformation: factors associated with chromosomal abnormalities. *Obstet Gynecol* 1977;77:436-42.
89. Dublin AB, French BN. Diagnostic image evaluation of hydranencephaly and pictorially similar entities, with emphasis on computed tomography. *Radiology* 1980;137:81-91.
90. Greene MF, Benacerraf B, Crawford JM. Hydranencephaly: ultrasound appearance during *in utero* evolution. *Radiology* 1985;156:779-780.
91. Hadi HA, Mashini IS, Devoe LD et al. Ultrasonographic prenatal diagnosis of hydranencephaly. *J Reprod Med* 1986; 31:254-256.

92. Edmondson SR, Hallak M, Carpenter RJ Jr et al. Evolution of hydranencephaly following intracerebral hemorrhage. *Obstet Gynecol* 1992;79:870.
93. Suchet IB. Schizencephaly: antenatal and postnatal assessment with colour-flow Doppler imaging. *Can Assoc Radiol J* 1994;45:193-200.
94. Barkovich JA, Gressens P, Evrard P. Formation, maturation and disorders of the brain neocortex. *AJNR* 1992;13:423-446.
95. Okamura K, Murotsuki J, Sakai T et al. Prenatal diagnosis of lissencephaly by magnetic resonance image. *Fetal Diagn Ther* 1993;8:56-59.
96. O'Connell EJ, Feldt RH, Stickler GB. Head circumference, mental retardation and growth failure. *Pediatrics* 1965; 36:62-66.
97. Chervenak FA, Jeanty P, Cantraine F et al. The diagnosis of fetal microcephaly. *Am J Obstet Gynecol* 1984;149:512-517.
98. Kurtz AB, Wapner RJ, Rubin CS et al. Ultrasound criteria for *in utero* diagnosis of microcephaly. *J Clin Ultrasound* 1980;8:11-16.
99. Goldstein I, Reece A, Pilu G et al. Sonographic assessment of the fetal frontal lobe: a potential tool for prenatal diagnosis of microcephaly. *Am J Obstet Gynecol* 1988;158:1057-1062.
100. Chervenak FA, Rosenberg J, Brightman RC et al. A prospective study of the accuracy of ultrasound in predicting fetal microcephaly. *Obstet Gynecol* 1987;69:908-910.
101. Nguyen The H, Pescia G, Deonna TH et al. Early prenatal diagnosis of genetic microcephaly. *Prenat Diagn* 1985;5:345-347.
102. Bromley B, Benacerraf BR. Difficulties in the prenatal diagnosis of microcephaly. *J Ultrasound Med* 1995;14:303-305.
103. DeMyer W. Megaloencephaly in children. *Neurology* 1972; 22:4-642.
104. Pilu G, Bovicelli L. Sonography of the fetal cranium. *Clin Diagn Ultrasound* 1989;25:221-259.
105. Barkovich JA, Norman D. Anomalies of the corpus callosum: correlation with further anomalies of the brain. *AJR* 1988;151:171-179.
106. Parrish ML, Roessmann U, Levinsohn MW. Agenesis of the corpus callosum: a study of the frequency of associated malformations. *Ann Neurol* 1979;6:349-354.
107. Byrd SE, Harwood-Nash DC, Fitz CR. Absence of the corpus callosum: computed tomographic evaluation in infants and children. *J Can Assoc Radiol* 1978;29:108-112.
108. Blum A, Andre M, Droulle P et al. Prenatal echographic diagnosis of corpus callosum agenesis: the Nancy experience 1982-1989. *Genet Counsel* 1990;38:115-126.
109. Vergani P, Ghidini A, Mariani S et al. Antenatal sonographic findings of agenesis of corpus callosum. *Am J Perinatol* 1988;5:105-108.
110. Vergani P, Ghidini A, Stobelt N et al. Prognostic indicators in the prenatal diagnosis of agenesis of corpus callosum. *Am J Obstet Gynecol* 1994;170:753-758.
111. Bennett GL, Bromley B, Benacerraf BR. Agenesis of the corpus callosum: prenatal detection usually is not possible before 22 weeks of gestation. *Radiology* 1996;199:447-450.
112. Bertino RE, Nyberg DA, Cyr DR. Prenatal diagnosis of agenesis of the corpus callosum. *J Ultrasound Med* 1988;7:251-260.
113. Georgy BA, Hesselink JR, Jernigan TL. MR imaging of the corpus callosum. *AJR* 1993;160:949-55.
114. Lorber J. Medical and surgical aspects in the treatment of congenital hydrocephalus. *Neuropediatric* 1971;2:239-246.
115. Burton BK. Recurrence risks in congenital hydrocephalus. *Clin Genet* 1979;16:47-53.
116. Ghidini A, Sirtori M, Vergani P et al. Fetal intracranial calcifications. *Am J Obstet Gynecol* 1989;160:86-87.
117. Hertzberg BS, Kay HH, Bowie JD. Fetal choroid plexus lesions: relationship of antenatal sonographic appearance to clinical outcome. *J Ultrasound Med* 1989;8:77-82.
118. Gross SJ, Shulman LP, Tolley EA et al. Isolated fetal choroid plexus cysts and trisomy 18: a review and meta-analysis. *Am J Obstet Gynecol* 1995;172:83-7.
119. Gupta JK, Cave M, Lilford RJ et al. Clinical significance of fetal choroid plexus cysts. *Lancet* 1995;346:724-729.
120. Spirit BA, Oliphant M, Gordon LP. Fetal central nervous system abnormalities. *Radiol Clin North Am* 1990;28:59-73.
121. Barkovitch JA. Infections of the nervous system. In: Pediatric Neuroimaging. 2nd ed., New York: Raven Press; 1995: 569-618.
122. Hudgins RJ, Edwards MSB, Ousterhour DK et al. Pediatric neurosurgical implications of amniotic band disruption complex. *Pediatr Neurosci* 1985-1986;12:232-239.
123. Mahony BS, Filly RA, Callen PW et al. The amniotic band syndrome: antenatal and diagnosis and potential pitfalls. *Am J Obstet Gynecol* 1985;152:63-68.
124. Sepulveda W, Platt CC, Fisk NM. Prenatal diagnosis of cerebral arteriovenous malformation using color Doppler ultrasonography: case report and review of the literature. *Ultrasound Obstet Gynecol* 1995;6:282-286.
125. Doren M, Tercanli S, Holzgreve W. Prenatal sonographic diagnosis of a vein of Galen aneurysm: relevance of associated malformation for timing and mode of delivery. *Ultrasound Obstet Gynecol* 1995;287-289.
126. Lipman SP, Pretorius DH, Rumack CM et al. Fetal intracranial teratoma: US diagnosis of three cases and a review of the literature. *Radiology* 1985;157:491-494.
127. Comstock CH, Chervenak FA. Transabdominal sonography of the fetal forebrain. In: Progress in Obstetric and Gynecological Sonography Series: Ultrasound and the Fetal Brain. Chervenak FA, Kurjak A, Comstock CH., eds. Parthenon Pub; 1995:43-82.
128. Guibaud L, Champion F, Buenerd A et al. Fetal intraventricular glioblastoma: ultrasonographic, magnetic resonance imaging and pathologic findings. *J Ultrasound Med* 1997; 16:285-288.
129. Barkovich AJ. The phakomatoses. In: Pediatric Neuroimaging. 2nd ed. New York: Raven Press; 1995:296-304.

CHAPTER 44

The Fetal Spine

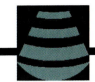

Eric E. Sauerbrei, B.Sc., M.Sc., M.D., F.R.C.P.C.
Ants Toi, M.D., F.R.C.P.C.

CHAPTER OUTLINE

DEVELOPMENTAL ANATOMY

Embryology of the Neural Tube

The brain, spinal cord, and spinal canal develop from the neural tube, which forms very early in pregnancy from embryonic ectoderm. The entire process of formation and closure of the embryonic neural tube occurs in approximately 12 days (i.e., from conceptual age 16 to 28 days, or menstrual age 30 to 42 days, or crown-rump length of 1.2 to 5.0 mm). Initially the neural plate (16 days after conception) is a small plane of tissue that invaginates into a groove (18 days after conception). This neural groove begins to fuse along the middorsal aspect of the embryo (21 days after conception) and fusion progresses cranially and caudally until only a small cranial opening (anterior neuropore) and small caudal opening (caudal neuropore) remain.

The anterior neuropore closes at about 24 days after conception and the caudal neuropore at 26 to 28 days after conception (CRL = 5 mm). The newly formed lumen of the neural tube becomes the small central canal of the spinal cord and the walls develop into the spinal cord and the components of the spinal canal.[1]

Ossification of the Fetal Spine

Sonograms clearly portray ossified structures in the fetal spine but the unossified components are difficult to delineate. It is thus important for sonographers and sonologists to understand the temporal and spatial ossification patterns during fetal development to optimize spinal evaluation.

Each vertebra will develop **three ossification centers:** the **centrum,** the **right neural process,** and the **left neural process.**[2] The centrum will form the central portion of the vertebral body and the neural processes will form the posterolateral portions of the vertebral body and the pedicles, transverse processes, laminae, and articular processes.

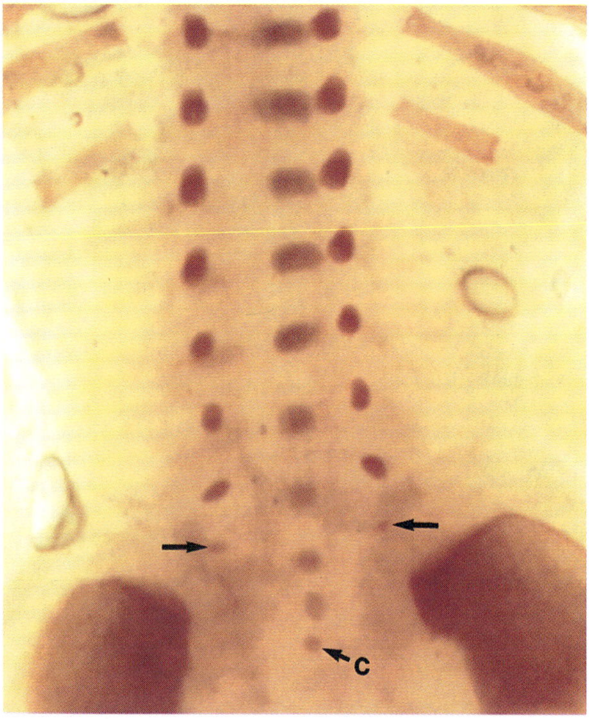

FIG. 44-1. Spine ossification specimen at 13 weeks' gestation. Ossification in the neural processes has progressed down to level S1. Within the neural process, ossification begins at the junction of the pedicle and lamina seen in the lumbar spine as a small localized focus. *Arrows*, ossification in S1 neural processes; *C*, centrum of S3.

Ossification begins in the fetal spine at approximately 10 weeks' gestation.[3] By 13 weeks' gestation, early ossification has appeared in the neural processes from C1 down to L5 or S1 (Fig. 44-1).[4] Between 13 and 20 weeks' gestation, ossification in the neural processes gradually extends into the laminae and pedicles; the ossification is always more complete in the thoracic vertebrae than in the lumbar and sacral vertebrae (Fig. 44-2).

Evaluation for spina bifida usually occurs before 20 weeks' gestation (often at 16 to 18 weeks' gestation, at the time of genetic amniocentesis). Although there is individual variability in spinal ossification, by 18 weeks' gestation there is usually enough ossification in the neural processes from C1 to S1 to scan effectively for spina bifida. By 18 to 20 weeks, ossification in the thoracic vertebrae is well advanced (Fig. 44-3) and in the lumbar spine less advanced (Fig. 44-4). However, there is enough ossification to diagnose or rule out spina bifida with ultrasound.

SCANNING TECHNIQUES

Optimal Scan Planes

To completely characterize an ultrasound scan plane, one must specify the ultrasound probe position and the orientation of the scan plane within the fetus. Two terms are therefore required to describe any scan plane used to examine the fetal spine. The first term describes the **probe position** with respect to the fetal body (e.g., posterior, lateral, anterior, posterolateral, etc.) and the second term describes the **orientation of the tomographic scan plane with respect to the long axis of the fetal spine** (e.g., transaxial, or perpendicular to long axis of fetal spine; longitudinal, or parallel to long axis of fetal spine).

SCAN PLANES FOR SPINA BIFIDA DETECTION

Posterior transaxial
Lateral transaxial
Lateral longitudinal
Posterior longitudinal
Posterior angled transaxial scan

In clinical practice, the most useful **scan planes** to assess the fetal neural processes are posterior transaxial (Fig. 44-5), lateral transaxial (Fig. 44-6), lateral longitudinal (coronal; Fig. 44-7), posterior longitudinal (sagittal; Fig. 44-8), and posterior angled transaxial scan (Fig. 44-9).

The fifth scan plane, the posterior angled transaxial, can occasionally be useful to visualize the pedicles and laminae simultaneously. Because the laminae course caudal to the transaxial plane, which contains the centrum and pedicles, only the angled scan plane can depict the pedicles and laminae simultaneously in their entirety (Fig. 44-9).

Level 1 Sonograms (Screening Sonograms)

With no clinical suspicion of spina bifida, it is impractical to examine every vertebra in four or five scan planes. The first step in assessing for spina bifida is scanning the head, because most fetuses with spina bifida have signs of a Chiari II malformation in the brain at 16 to 20 weeks' gestation: obliterated cisterna magna (**banana sign**) and/or concave frontal bones (**lemon sign**) and/or dilated lateral ventricles.[5] Even in experienced hands, the actual spina bifida defect is detected in only 80% to 90% of cases.[6] Then the position of the fetal spine should be determined. The scan plane is then placed perpendicular to the long axis of the fetal spine (**posterior transaxial or lateral transaxial;** Figs. 44-5 and 44-6). The sonographer should scan from one end of the spine to the other while maintaining the scan plane perpendicular to the spine, no matter how the spine is curved. This is repeated several times fairly quickly. In the process one builds up an impression of the three-dimensional

A

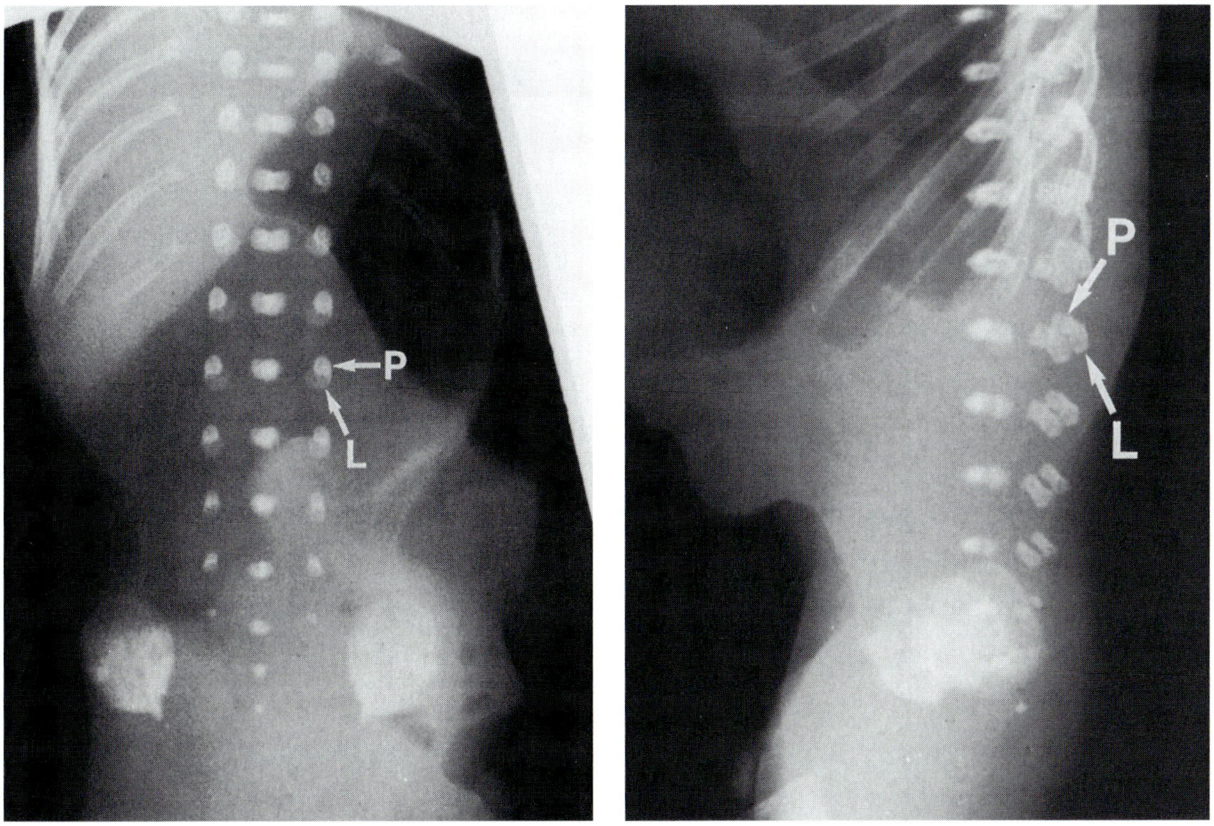

B

FIG. 44-2. Spine ossification on radiographs at 14 weeks' gestation. **A**, AP and **B**, lateral radiographs. Well-developed ossification in the centra now extends down to level S3. Ossification in the lumbar neural processes extends into the lamina (*L*) and pedicles (*P*). The neural process ossification starts to resemble the shape of the cartilaginous neural process rather than the focal dot-like ossification at 13 weeks' gestation.

A

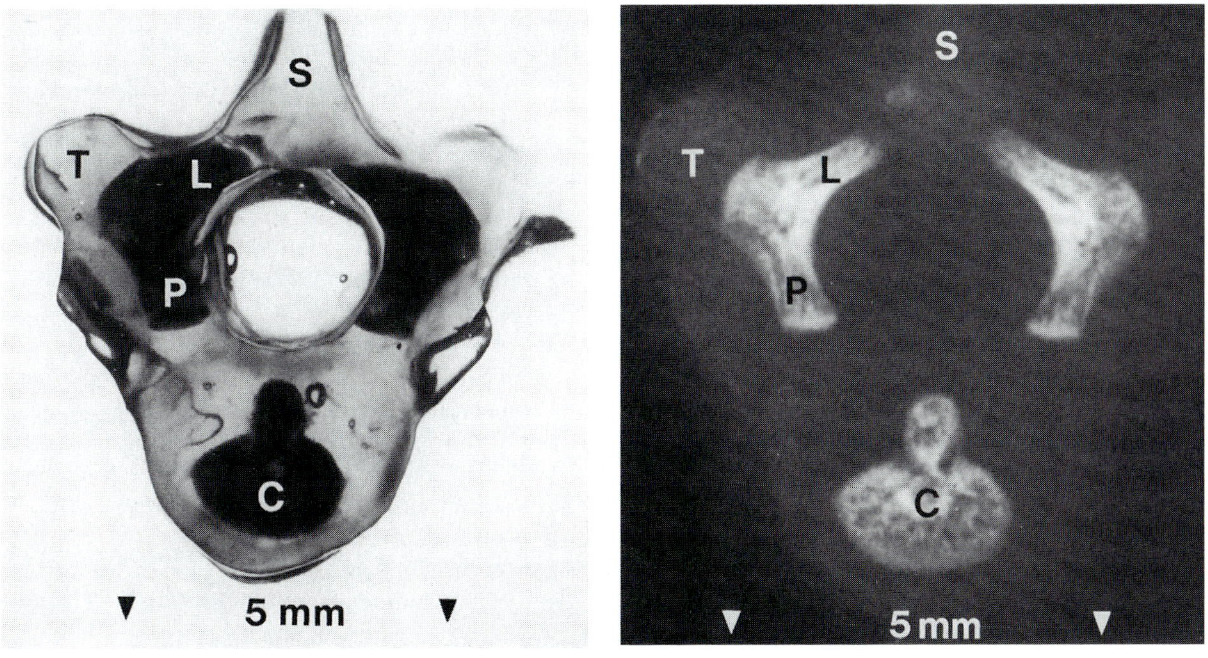

B

FIG. 44-3. Vertebral ossification of T9 at 16 weeks' gestation. **A**, specimen and **B**, radiograph. Ossification already extends quite far into the pedicles (*P*) and laminae (*L*). Note the early ossification in the base of the transverse processes (*T*). The width of the vertebra is about 5 mm. *C*, ossification within the centrum; *T*, transverse process (cartilage); *S*, spinous process (cartilage).

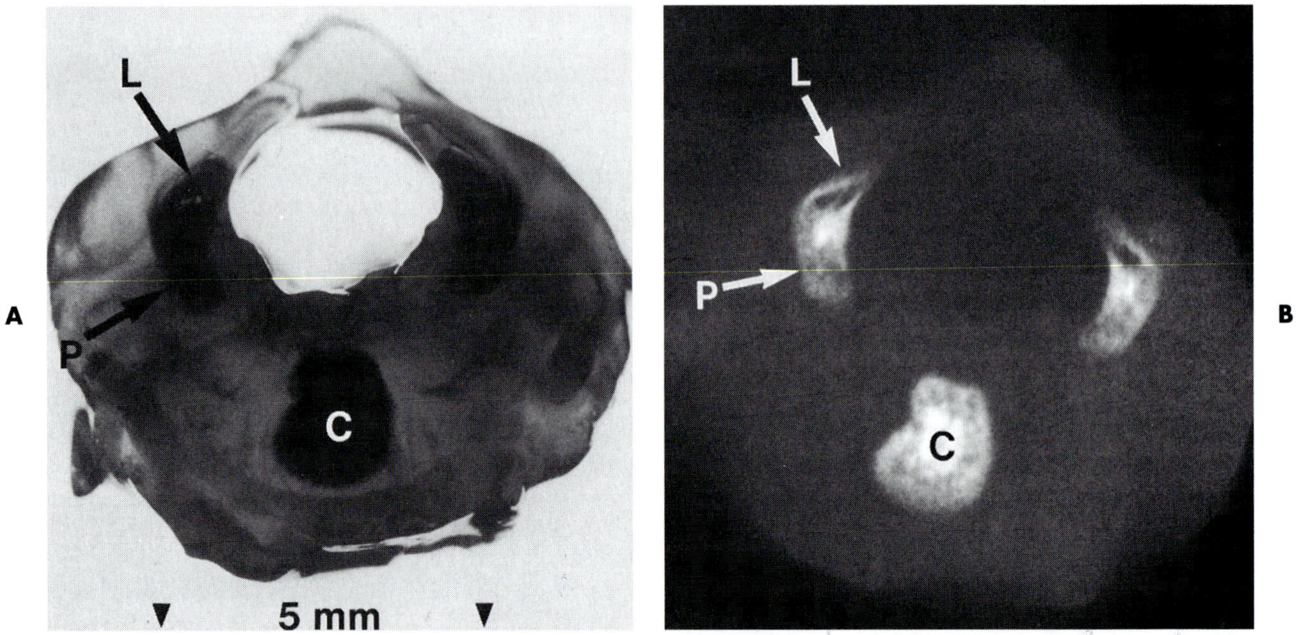

FIG. 44-4. Vertebral ossification of L5 at 17 weeks' gestation. A, specimen and **B,** radiograph. There is usually enough ossification at this gestation in the pedicles (*P*) and laminae (*L*) to determine the true course of these structures in radiographs and ultrasound scans. The width of the vertebra is about 5 mm. (*C*) ossification within the centrum.

structures of the spine. Then the scan plane should be repositioned parallel to the long axis of the fetal spine to obtain **posterior longitudinal** or **lateral longitudinal** scans.

The screening scans of the fetal head and spine in low-risk patients are performed with a conventional ultrasound probe (3.5 MHz or 5.0 MHz). An experienced sonographer or sonologist can obtain a reasonably thorough study of the fetal spine at 18 to 20 weeks' gestation in 2 to 3 minutes.

Level 2 Sonograms (Detailed Sonograms)

A detailed sonogram of the fetal spine is requested for several reasons: previous suspicious ultrasound, family history of neural tube defect, and raised serum and/or amniotic fluid alpha-fetoprotein. The study may require the use of different probes (sector, linear, different frequencies) and possibly different machines. In thinner patients in the first half of pregnancy it may be possible to use a higher frequency probe (e.g., 7.5 MHz) and in some cases an endovaginal probe may be useful (Fig. 44-9, B). Ideally, the sonographer will examine all levels of the spine in posterior transaxial, lateral transaxial, lateral longitudinal, and posterior longitudinal scan planes. This may not be possible within a short time interval because of fetal position, but fetal position usually changes enough in 30 to 45 minutes at 18 to 20 weeks to obtain all scan planes. If the spine cannot be visualized optimally, then a repeat scan can be performed in 1 or 2 days.

SPINA BIFIDA

Definition, Incidence, and Prevalence

Spina bifida implies a physical defect in the structure of the spinal canal that may result in a communication of its contents (meninges, cerebrospinal fluid, and neural tissue) to the exterior space. These defects usually occur along the dorsal midline (most often in the lumbosacral area) but rarely may occur anteriorly. Neural tube defects (NTDs) include spina bifida and equivalent lesions of the head (e.g., encephalocele, anencephaly).

Spina bifida occurs at **different rates** in different parts of the globe. In addition, there are differing rates among races and there is an east-west gradient ranging from a high in Great Britain to a low on the west coast of Canada (Table 44-1).[7,8] Although most recent studies have documented a worldwide decline in the incidence of neural tube defects, the responsible factors have not been elucidated. There is no correla-

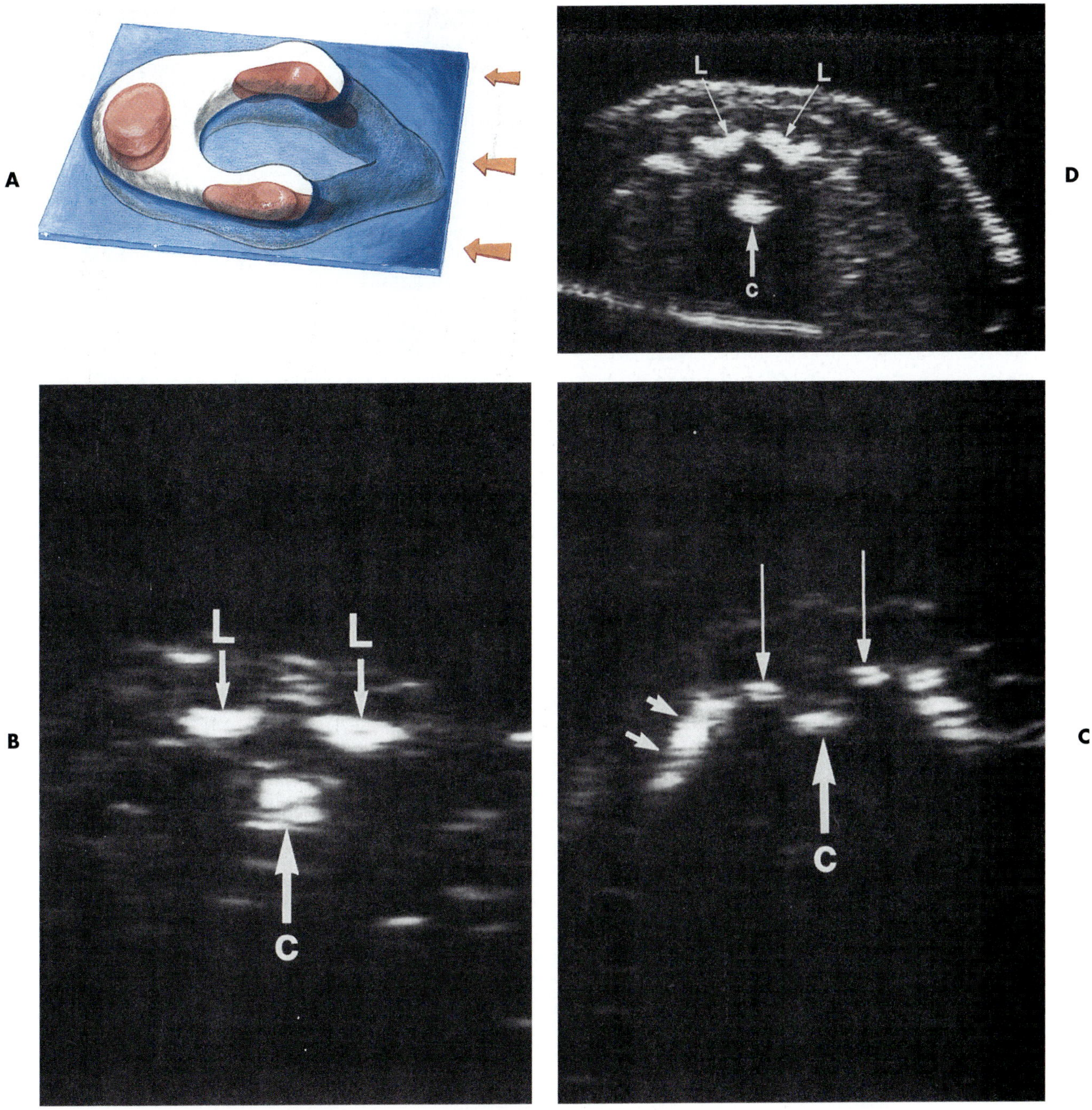

FIG. 44-5. Posterior transaxial scan planes. **A,** diagram. The incident sound beam *(arrows)* reflects off the posterior surfaces of the laminae and centrum. Therefore, this scan plane demonstrates clearly the laminae and centrum but not the pedicles. The shaded structures represent the ossified portions of the vertebra. **B,** the L3 vertebra at 17 weeks' gestation demonstrates the ossified laminae (*L*) and the ossified centrum (*C*)**.** The pedicles are not visualized. **C,** scan of S1 vertebra at 17 weeks' gestation shows early ossification at the junction of the lamina and pedicle on each side *(longest arrows)*. With this amount of ossification, it is not possible to determine the course of the laminae and thus it is difficult to rule out spina bifida of this vertebra. (*C*) ossified centrum; *short arrows,* iliac wing. **D,** scan of the lower thoracic vertebra T10 at 24 weeks' gestation shows advanced ossification in the laminae *(longer arrows)*. The ossification almost reaches midline. Despite advanced ossification in the pedicles, the pedicles are not visualized in this scan plane. (*C*) Ossified centrum.

A

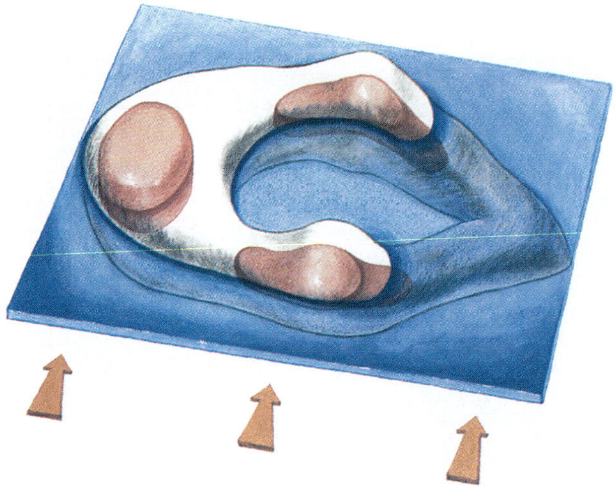

B

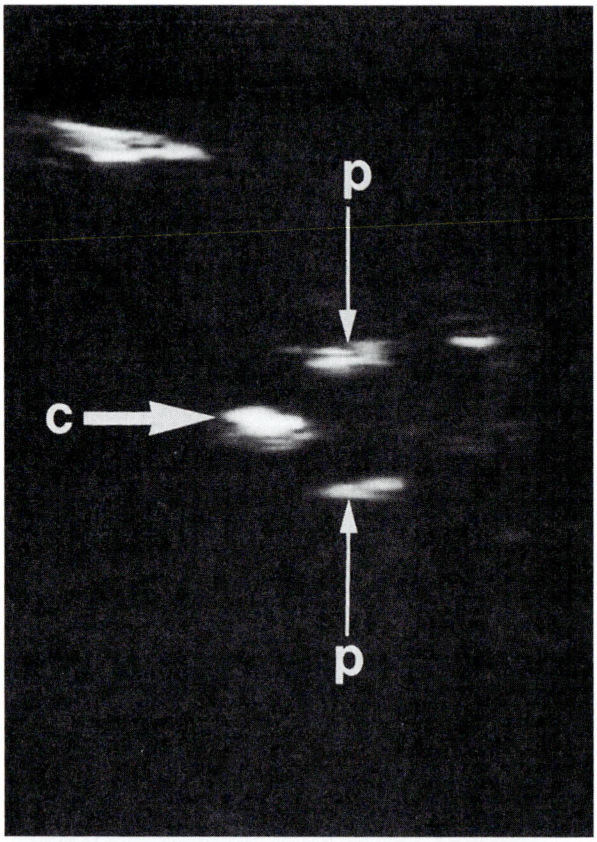

FIG. 44-6. Lateral transaxial scan planes. A (diagram). The incident sound beam *(arrows)* reflects off the lateral surfaces of the centrum and the near pedicle and off the medial surface of the far pedicle. Therefore, this scan plane clearly shows the centrum and pedicles but not the laminae. The laminae course toward midline (hence the sound beam is not perpendicular to the lamina surface) and caudally (hence it is out of the plane of the sound beam). The shaded structures are ossified portions of the vertebra. **B,** scan of vertebra L3 at 17 weeks' gestation shows the ossified pedicles (*P*) and the ossified centrum (*C*). The laminae are not visualized.

A

B

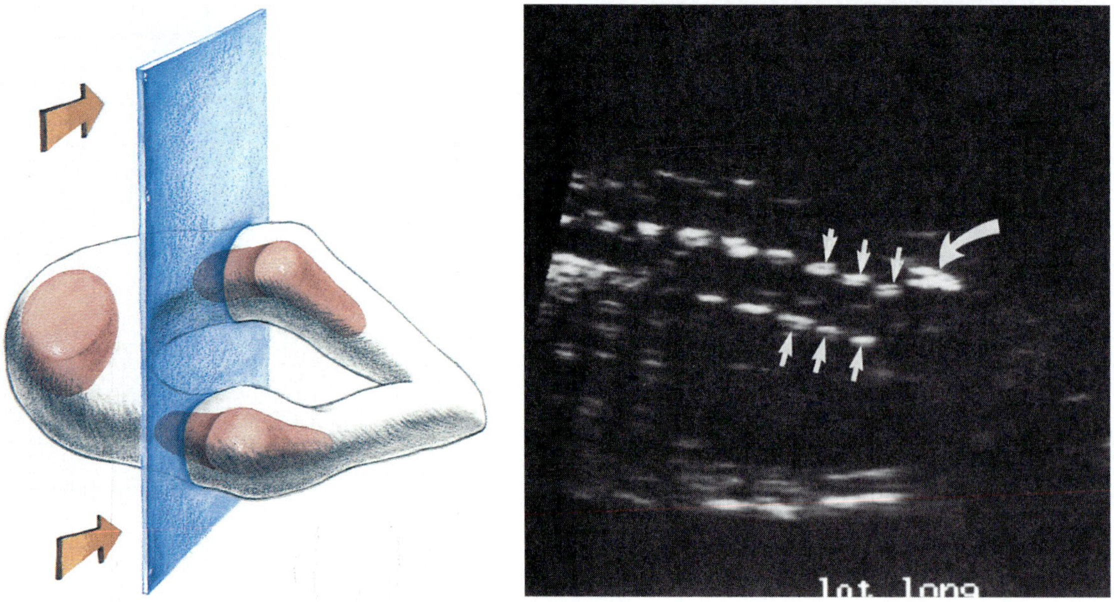

FIG. 44-7. Lateral longitudinal scan plane. A (diagram). The incident sound beam *(arrows)* reflects off the lateral surface of the near pedicle and the medial surface of the far pedicle. Therefore this scan plane will show the cross-section of the pedicles of each vertebra. The centrum and laminae will not be visualized in this scan plane. The shaded structures are ossified portions of the vertebra. When the tomographic scan plane is thick or placed closer to the centrum, the pedicles and centrum may be visualized. The centra will then appear as an extra set of echogenic dots between the series of pedicles in the lateral longitudinal scan plane. **B,** the lateral longitudinal scan of the lumbar spine at 16 weeks' gestation shows the ossified pedicles *(straight arrows)*. The lumbar pedicles usually form a series of parallel echogenic foci, although they may normally diverge by 1 to 2 mm. Note the faint echogenic structures between the pedicles; these represent echoes from the centra that intercept the edge of the insonating beam. *Curved arrow,* iliac wing.

A

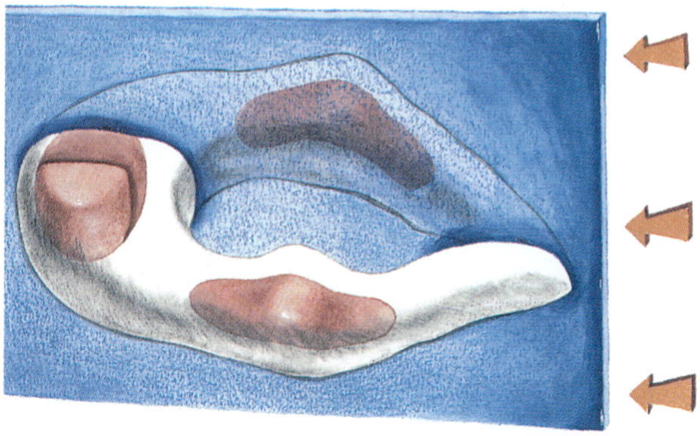

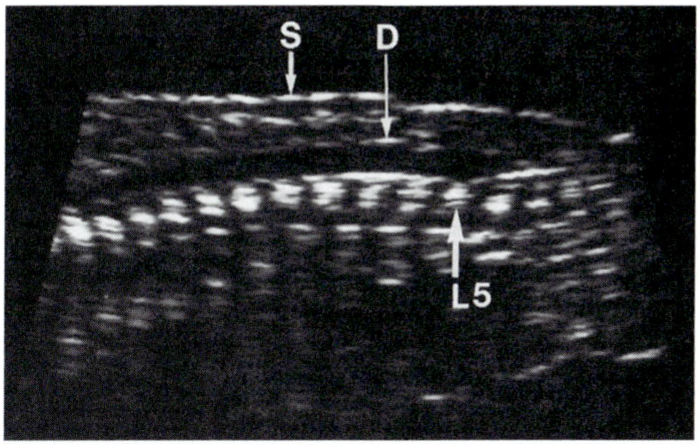

B

FIG. 44-8. Posterior longitudinal scan plane. A (diagram). The incident sound beam *(arrows)* reflects off the posterior surface of the centrum. If there is no ossification in the laminae near the midline, the laminae will not be visible on the scan; only the centra will be seen in the scan. If the laminar ossification is present near the midline, then the centra and laminae will be seen as echogenic foci. The shaded structures are ossified portions of the vertebra. **B,** the posterior longitudinal scan of the lumbosacral spine at 15 weeks' gestation shows ossification in the centra of the lower thoracic, lumbar, and sacral spine (*L5*, centrum of vertebra L5). In this midline scan, no ossification is present posterior to the posterior surface of the dural sac (*D*). *S*, skin surface.

A

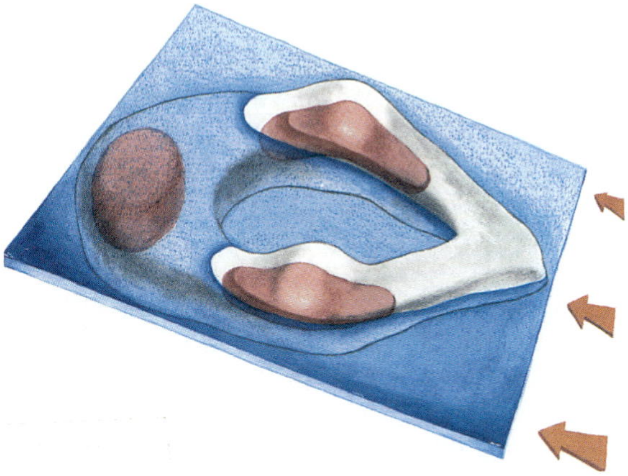

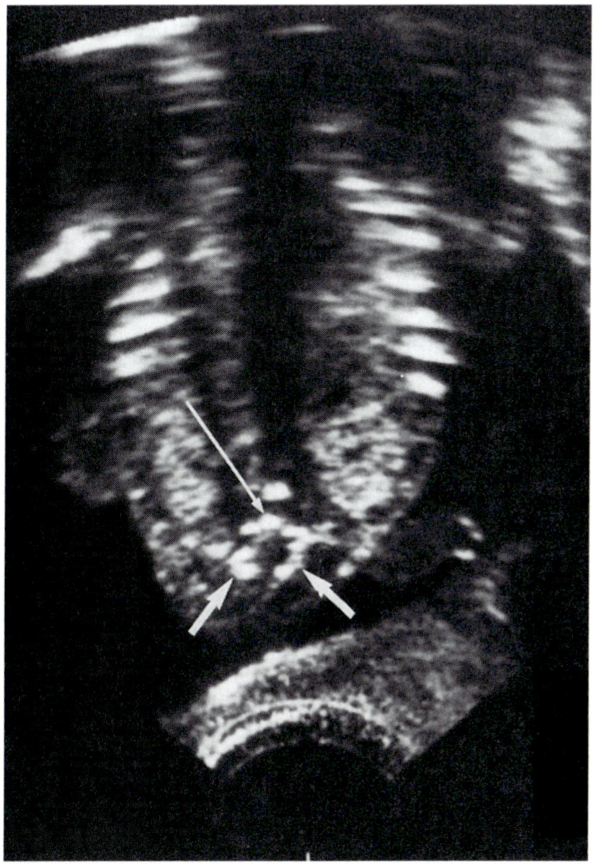

B

FIG. 44-9. Posterior angled transaxial scan plane. A (diagram). The incident sound beam *(arrows)* reflects off the posterior aspects of the laminae and portions of the pedicles. The beam may also reflect off the ossified centrum. This scan plane can depict the entire "ring" of ossification of the spinal canal, whereas the posterior transaxial and lateral transaxial cannot. The shaded structures are ossified portions of the vertebra. **B,** the endovaginal scan (at 18 weeks) clearly outlines the curvilinear structure of each neural arch (lamina plus pedicle; *short arrows)* and the ossified centrum *(long arrows)*. Together these structures form the ossified ring of the spinal canal, in this case, in the midlumbar spine.

TABLE 44-1
PREVALENCE OF NEURAL TUBE DEFECTS (NTDS)

Geographic Area	Prevalence per 1000 Births
Great Britain 1	6.1
Newfoundland	3.2
New Brunswick	2.5
Nova Scotia	2.0
Eastern Ontario	1.7
British Columbia	1.5
United States, overall	1.1

tion between the incidence of NTDs and such factors as maternal age, parity, season of birth, birth weight, or gestational age. The risk of NTDs rises to 20 to 30 per 1000 births given a previous infant with NTDs. This constitutes about a tenfold increase in risk over the general population.[9] Other risk factors that increase the chance of neural tube defects include ingestion of valproic acid (taken for seizure disorders) (10 to 20 per 1000 live births), maternal diabetes (20 per 1000 live births), parent of fetus with spina bifida (11 per 1000 live births), and sibling of fetus with multiple vertebral defects and scoliosis (15 to 30 per 1000 live births).[10]

Between 1970 and 1989 in the United States, the new-born incidence of neural tube defects had decreased from 1.3 per 1000 live births to 0.6 per 1000 live births.[11] At least part of this decline is due to improved prenatal detection and subsequent induced abortion. Note that the rate of pregnancy termination varies considerably within the United States, e.g., 9% in Arkansas to 42% in Hawaii and Atlanta.[12] In the United Kingdom, approximately 80% of pregnancies diagnosed with neural tube defects end in elective termination or stillbirth.[13]

Pathogenesis and Pathology

Most cases of spina bifida probably result from failure of closure of the embryologic neural tube, although some cases may be caused by rupture of the neural tube after primary closure. Although most examples of NTDs occur as isolated malformations in chromosomally normal individuals, they can also occur as part of syndromes inherited as single Mendelian traits (e.g., Meckel syndrome) or as part of syndromes caused by chromosome imbalance (e.g., trisomy 18 or triploidy). A number of studies[14] have found the **incidence** of NTDs to be about 10 times higher in spontaneously aborted pregnancies than in term births, indicating that *in utero* selection against embryos with such defects is quite effective.

Folic acid deficiency appears to play a role in the development of neural tube defects. In women at high risk for carrying a fetus with a neural tube defect, routine folic acid supplementation around the time of conception confers a 72% decrease in probability of neural tube defect.[15] For women at increased risk for pregnancies with neural tube defect, a minimum daily supplement of 0.8 mg of folic acid is recommended.[16] For women who are not at increased risk, the U.S. Public Health Service recommends that all women who are capable of becoming pregnant consume 0.4 mg of folic acid per day in order to reduce the risk of a pregnancy affected with spina bifida or other neural tube defects.[17]

The **pathology** of spina bifida involves a physical defect that may involve all layers from the dura to the skin surface (80% to 85% of cases; spina bifida aperta) or only deeper layers (15% to 20% of cases; spina bifida occulta). The latter cases are usually associated with an overlying skin dimple, a patch of hair on the skin, or a subcutaneous lipoma.[18] In adults, spina bifida occulta may be seen radiographically in 3% of the population, but these radiographic incidental findings are not clinically significant.[19]

In **spina bifida aperta,** the defect may be open to the extradermal space or it may be covered by a thin meningeal membrane. In the latter, a cystic mass is associated with the defect (**spina bifida cystica**) and this usually contains cerebrospinal fluid (CSF) and neural tissue (**myelomeningocele**); less commonly (less than 10% of spina bifida cystica), the sac contains only CSF (**meningocele**).[19]

Screening Tests for Spina Bifida

Because most cases of NTD occur in families with no history of such abnormalities, measurement of **maternal serum alpha-fetoprotein (MS-AFP)** is becoming more popular. In the province of Ontario, Canada (population 9,000,000), all pregnant women are currently offered a maternal serum screen test which consists of measuring alpha-fetoprotein (AFP), β subunit human chorionic gonadotropin (hCG), and unconjugated estriol (uE3). If all women were to have this **triple screen** serum test at 16 weeks' gestation, then 90% to 95% of open neural tube defects would be detected, in addition to approximately 66% of fetuses with trisomy 21 (Down syndrome) and trisomy 18 (Edwards' syndrome).

AFP is a glycoprotein (molecular weight 70,000) produced by fetal liver. Some of it enters the amniotic fluid via fetal urine and a small amount crosses the placenta to maternal serum. Normal AFP levels in amniotic fluid and maternal serum vary with gestational age. MS-AFP and amniotic fluid AFP are elevated in **neural tube defects** that are not covered by skin. If the upper limit of normal MS-AFP is taken to be 2.5 **multiples of the median** (MOM) for a given gestational age, then MS-AFP will be elevated in approximately 90% of open NTDs. Note, however, that about 2% of **normal pregnancies** will have an elevated MS-AFP; that is, of all the elevated test results for MS-AFP, most fetuses will be normal. At this stage, a detailed ultrasound exam is required to determine which fetuses actually have a neural tube defect.

MS-AFP is also elevated in multifetal pregnancy, fetal death, fetomaternal transfusion, and in other fetal anomalies such as omphalocele and gastroschisis (50% to 60% of cases), congenital nephrosis (Finnish type, 100% of cases), and infrequently in esophageal or duodenal atresia, polycystic kidney disease, renal agenesis, urinary obstruction, epidermolysis bullosa, sacrococcygeal teratoma, cystic hygroma, osteogenesis imperfecta, cloacal exstrophy, and cyclopia. Detailed fetal sonography will also detect most of these causes of elevated MS-AFP.

If the maternal serum AFP is elevated and there is no sonographic explanation for the abnormal test result (e.g., wrong dates, multiple fetuses, dead fetus, anencephaly, spina bifida, abdominal wall defect, or any other of the above fetal abnormalities that can cause elevated AFP), then amniocentesis should be offered. If the amniotic fluid AFP is normal and there is no **acetyl cholinesterase** (**ACHE**) present, then the likelihood of a neural tube defects is very low. If the amniotic fluid AFP is elevated and ACHE is present, then a neural tube defect or abdominal wall defect may well be present but undetected by sonography.

Between 1989 and 1990, 1.1 million women in California had maternal serum AFP tests in early pregnancy.[20] From these tests, 1390 fetal abnormalities were found (1.3 fetal anomalies per 1000 pregnancies), consisting of 710 neural tube defects (417 anencephalies, 247 spina bifidas, and 46 encephaloceles) and 680 nonneural abnormalities (286 anterior abdominal wall defects, 163 Down syndrome, and 231 other chromosomal abnormalities).

CAUSES OF ELEVATED MS-AFP

Multifetal pregnancy
Fetal death
Fetomaternal transfusion
Omphalocele and gastroschisis
Congenital nephrosis
Esophageal or duodenal atresia
Polycystic kidney disease
Renal agenesis
Urinary obstruction
Epidermolysis bullosa
Sacrococcygeal teratoma
Cystic hygroma
Osteogenesis imperfecta
Cloacal exstrophy
Cyclopia

Sonographic Findings in the Spine

Spina bifida may occur anywhere in the fetal spine but it is most common in the lumbosacral area.[21] Ultrasound findings in the spine consist of abnormalities of the ossified posterior elements and related soft tissues.

In spina bifida (Fig. 44-10), the laminae fail to converge toward midline, and this is best visualized with the posterior transaxial scan plane (Fig. 44-10, *A*, *B*). If the pedicles are normally positioned and if there is no myelomeningocele, the posterior transaxial scana plane is the only one that will depict the abnormality with reliability. When the pedicles are displaced more laterally than usual, then the lateral transaxial (Fig. 44-10, *C*) and lateral longitudinal (Fig. 44-10, *D*) scan planes will also demonstrate the bony abnormalities of spina bifida. All of these scan planes will usually demonstrate the meningocele or myelomeningocele if it is present (Fig. 44-11). The posterior longitudinal scan gives the best demonstration of a myelomeningocele (Fig. 44-11, *B*) and of the soft-tissue defect when no cystic mass is present (Fig. 44-10, *E*).

In most cases of spina bifida, there is abnormal divergence or splaying of the pedicles over several vertebral levels. This is best appreciated in the lateral longitudinal views where multiple interpedicular distances can be evaluate simultaneously (Fig. 44-10, *D* and F). However, it must be noted that there is normally divergence of the pedicles in the cervical spine compared to the thoracic spine (Fig. 44-11, *C*), and there may be mild divergence (by 1 to 2 mm) in the lumbar spine compared with the thoracic spine in normal fetuses (Fig. 44-1).

Sonography can also be used to determine the level and extent of the spinal abnormality by using the following landmarks:

- T12 corresponds to the medial ends of the most caudal ribs;
- L5 lies at the superior margin of the iliac wing;
- S4 is the most caudal ossification center in the second trimester.

Associated Cranial Abnormalities

Chiari II malformation is highly associated with spina bifida. This cranial lesion may be easier to identify between 16 and 24 weeks' gestation than the spinal lesions. Thus, cranial malformations may "tip off" the sonographer that a detailed study of the spine is required to search for spina bifida. Alternately, the cranial abnormalities are useful confirmatory signs when the ultrasound demonstrates evidence of spina bifida in the fetal spine.

The biparietal diameter may be lower than expected, compared to all other predictors of gestational age (even when the lateral ventricles are enlarged),[22,23] but three qualitative findings are more useful in clinical practice. These are nonvisualization of the cisterna magna and deformation of the cerebellar shape (**banana sign,** Fig. 44-12); concave frontal bones (**lemon sign,** Fig. 44-12); and dilatation of the lateral ventricles.

Most infants (>97%) with spina bifida have an associated Chiari II malformation affecting the posterior fossa structures. This often leads to enlargement of the lateral ventricles, which is usually mild in the second trimester. **Ventriculomegaly** is seen in 44% to 86% of fetuses with spina bifida.[5,24-26] The most common single cause of ventriculomegaly is spina bifida, although only 30% to 40% of fetuses with enlarged ventricles actually have spina bifida. The Chiari II malformation also gives rise to obliteration of the cisterna magna (Fig. 44-12),[27,28] whereas the cisterna magna should be fluid-filled in normal fetuses of 16 to 28 weeks' gestation. The compression of the cerebellum may change its shape in the transaxial scan plane, giving the **banana sign** (Fig. 44-12).[25,29] In two different series, obliteration of the cisterna magna was noted in 22 of 23 cases with spina bifida at 16 to 27 weeks' gestation[29] and in 18 of 20 cases at 24 weeks' gestation and less.[28]

For unknown reasons, there is usually a concave deformity of the fetal frontal bones in the second trimester (Fig. 44-12), the **lemon sign.**[30] Various authors have shown that 85% of fetuses with spina bifida before 24 weeks' gestation have the lemon sign.[25,26,31,32] Therefore, absence of the lemon sign is a useful indirect indicator that spina bifida is not present. In practice, however, the lemon sign can be difficult to portray unequivocally; ultimately, one must examine the spine itself to assess for the presence and extent of spina bifida.

The lemon sign spontaneously resolves in the third trimester.[31] In addition, it can be seen in fetuses without spina bifida.[26,31] In fact, this may be the case in up to 1% of normal infants, so the lemon sign must not be taken as proof that spina bifida is present. It

FETAL BRAIN FINDINGS IN SPINA BIFIDA

Nonvisualization of the cisterna magna
Deformation of the cerebellar shape
Banana sign
Concave frontal bones
Lemon sign
Dilatation of the lateral ventricles
Ventriculomegaly

A
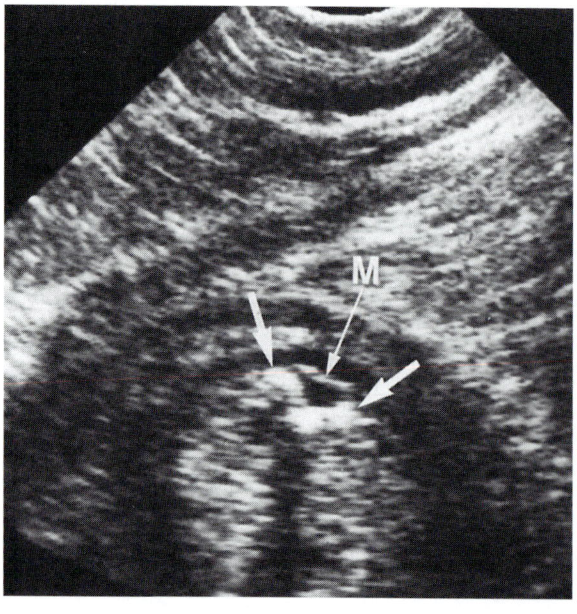

B
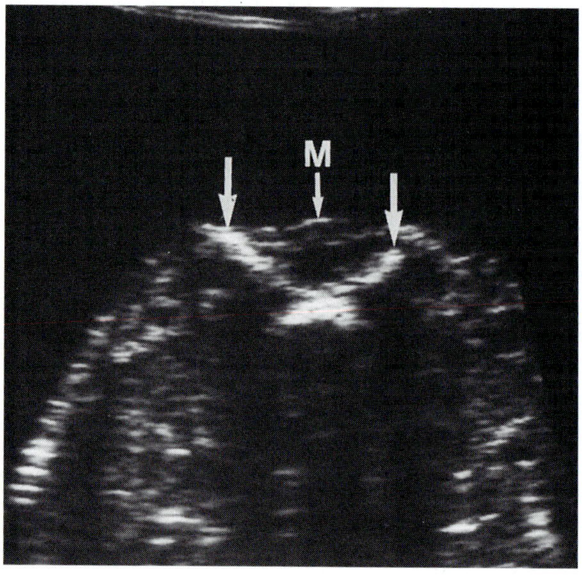

FIG. 44-10. Spina bifida aperta. **A,** *in utero* posterior transaxial scan shows splaying of the lumbar laminae *(arrows)* away from midline. Only a thin membrane (*M*) overlies the spinal defect posteriorly. **B,** posterior transaxial scan of the specimen after delivery shows in more detail the splaying of the laminae *(arrows)* away from midline and the membrane (*M*) covering the defect.

Continued.

C

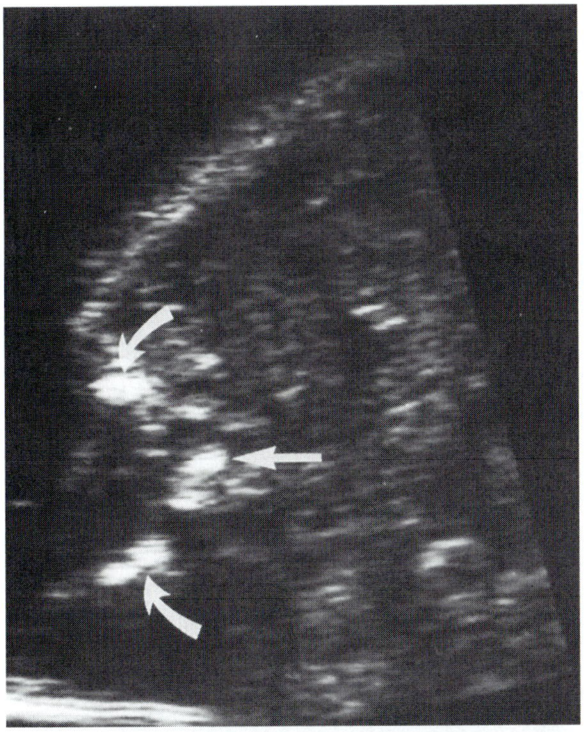

D

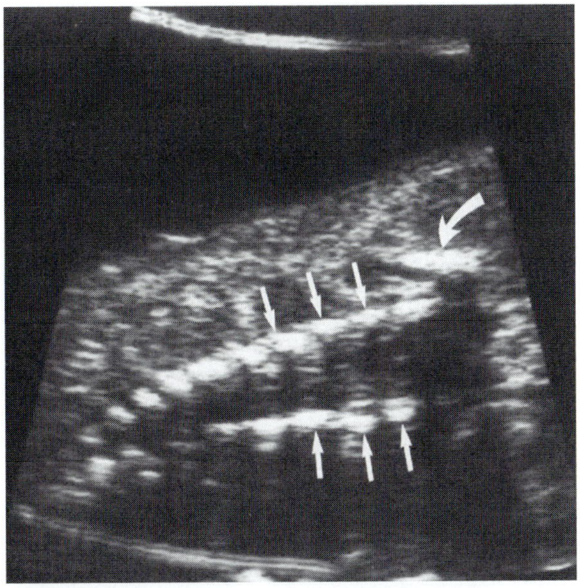

E

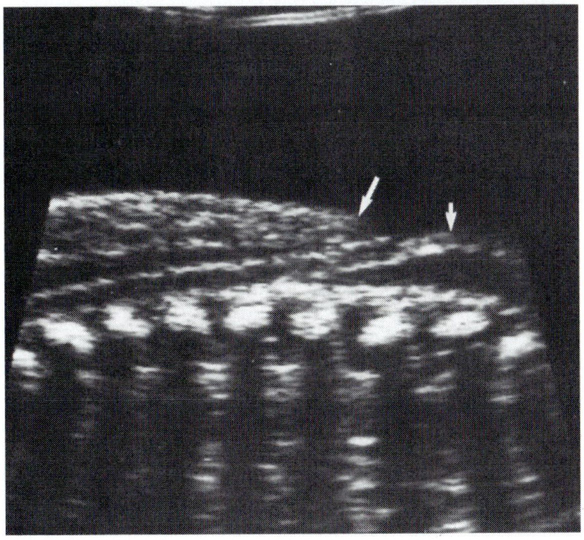

F

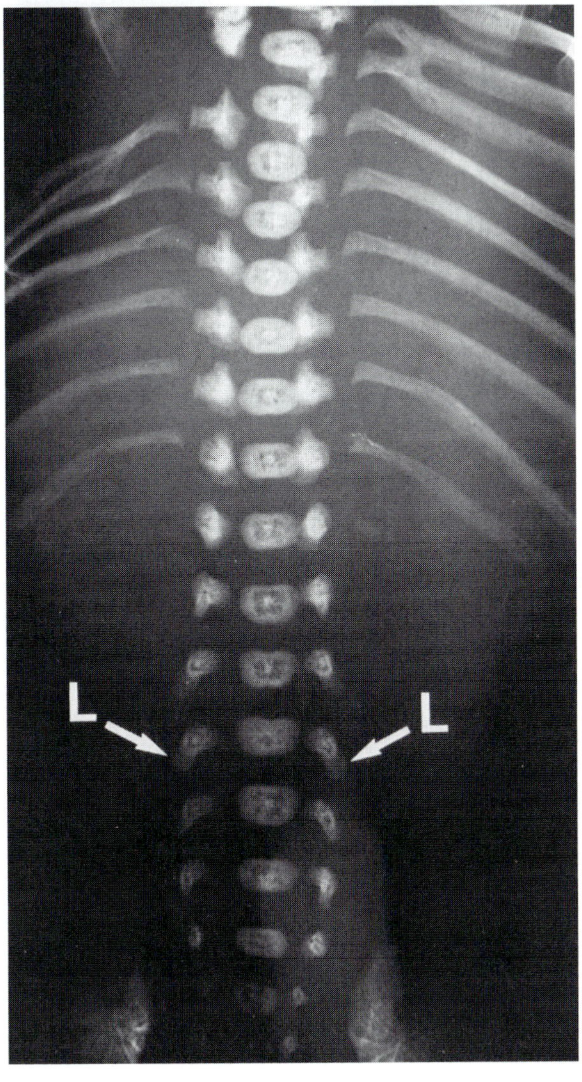

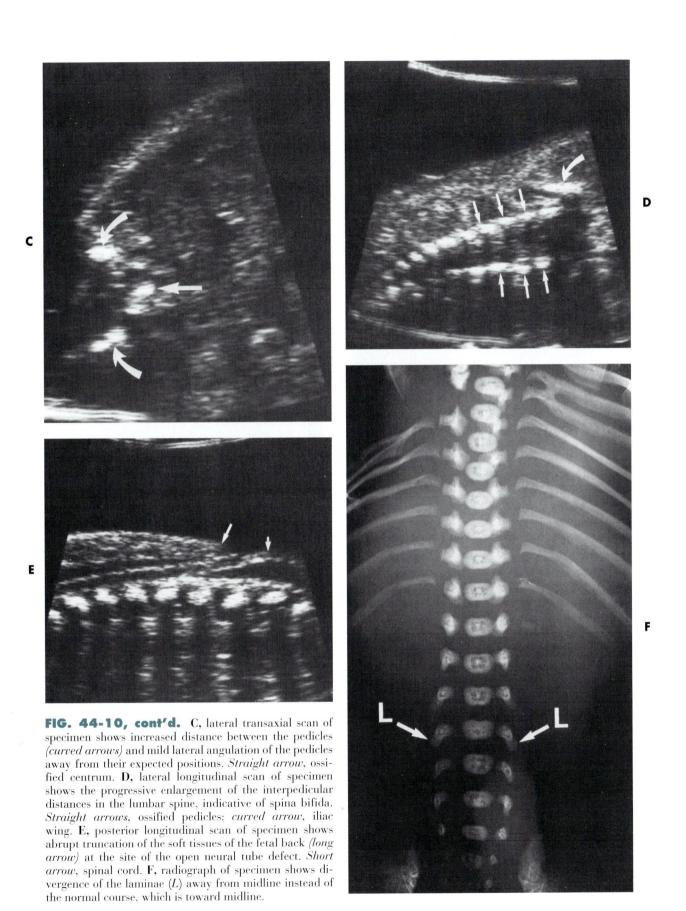

FIG. 44-10, cont'd. **C,** lateral transaxial scan of specimen shows increased distance between the pedicles *(curved arrows)* and mild lateral angulation of the pedicles away from their expected positions. *Straight arrow,* ossified centrum. **D,** lateral longitudinal scan of specimen shows the progressive enlargement of the interpedicular distances in the lumbar spine, indicative of spina bifida. *Straight arrows,* ossified pedicles; *curved arrow,* iliac wing. **E,** posterior longitudinal scan of specimen shows abrupt truncation of the soft tissues of the fetal back *(long arrow)* at the site of the open neural tube defect. *Short arrow,* spinal cord. **F,** radiograph of specimen shows divergence of the laminae (*L*) away from midline instead of the normal course, which is toward midline.

A

B

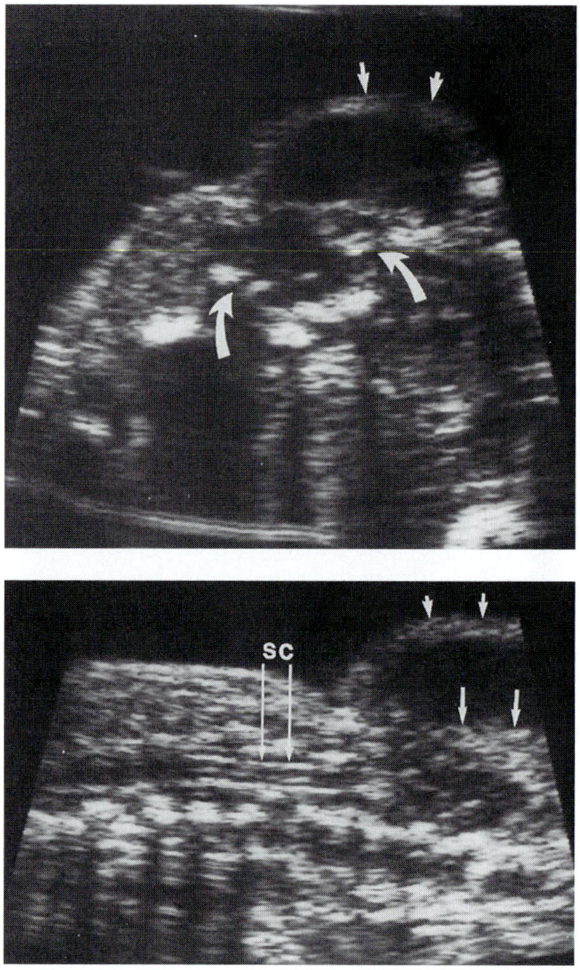

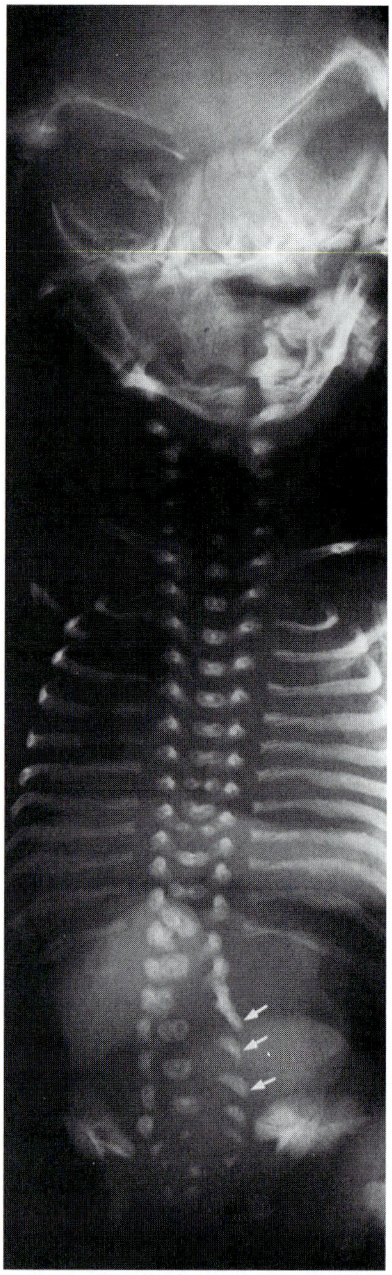

C

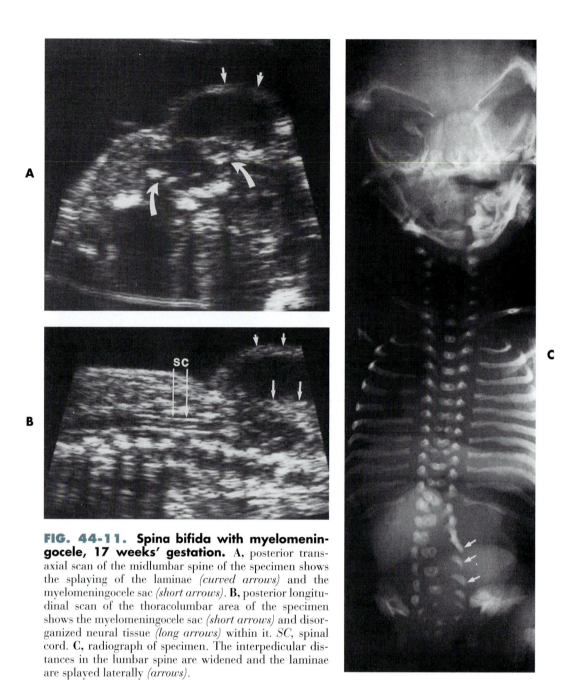

FIG. 44-11. Spina bifida with myelomeningocele, 17 weeks' gestation. **A,** posterior transaxial scan of the midlumbar spine of the specimen shows the splaying of the laminae *(curved arrows)* and the myelomeningocele sac *(short arrows)*. **B,** posterior longitudinal scan of the thoracolumbar area of the specimen shows the myelomeningocele sac *(short arrows)* and disorganized neural tissue *(long arrows)* within it. *SC,* spinal cord. **C,** radiograph of specimen. The interpedicular distances in the lumbar spine are widened and the laminae are splayed laterally *(arrows)*.

should prompt detailed examination of the posterior fossa (to search for obliteration of the cisterna magna and the banana sign) and examination of the fetal spine for direct evidence of spina bifida.

Associated Noncranial Abnormalities

Foot deformities (primarily club foot) and dislocation of the hips are frequently associated with spina bifida.[33] These arise because of imbalanced muscular action resulting from peripheral nerve involvement with the neural tube defect. In fetuses with open spida bifida (i.e., not skin-covered), 24% demonstrate additional morphological abnormalities in second trimester sonography: renal abnormalities, choroid plexus cysts, VSD, omphalocele, and IUGR.[34]

Associated Chromosomal Abnormalities

Babcock et al.[34] found that 9 of 52 fetuses with spina bifida (17%) had chromosomal abnormalities, including 5 with trisomy 18, 2 with trisomy 13, 1 with triploidy, and 1 with translocation. Of the 9 fetuses with spina bifida and chromosomal abnormalities, 2 of 9 (22%) had no other morphological abnormality demonstrable by sonography. The authors suggest that cytogenetic analysis is justified if spina bifida is detected prenatally.

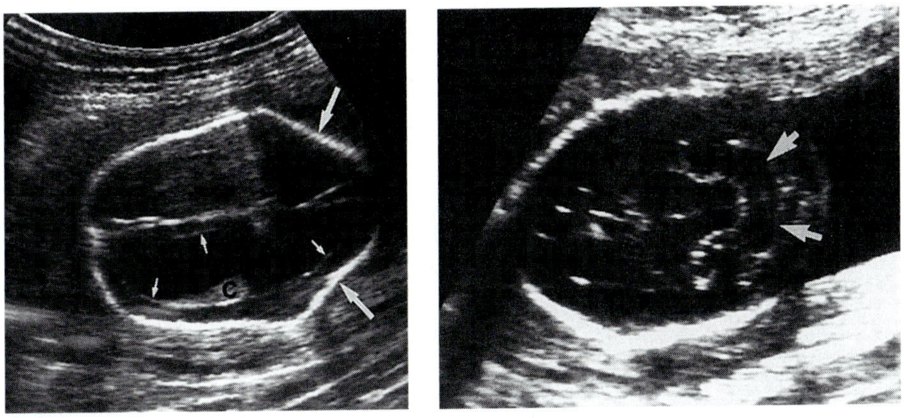

FIG. 44-12. Lemon sign and ventriculomegaly. **A,** the transaxial sonogram of the fetal head demonstrates concave deformity of the frontal bone *(long arrows)*, as well as dilatation of the lateral ventricles *(small arrows)* at 19 weeks' gestation. The choroid plexus (*C*) rests along the dependent portion of the deep lateral ventricle. The near ventricle is obscured due to reverberation artifact from the proximal cranial vault. **Banana sign. B,** the transaxial sonogram of the fetal head at 18 weeks' gestation demonstrates compression and deformity of the cerebellum *(arrows)*. This abnormal cerebellar shape creates the banana sign.

Prognosis

It is difficult to predict the long-term prognosis in a fetus with an identified myelomeningocele. However, the outcome tends to be better for smaller lesions (i.e., few number of levels involved), low lesions (lower lumbar, sacral), closed defects, and those with little or no hydrocephalus and no compression of the hindbrain due to the Chiari II malformation.[9,29,35,36] In a large study of more than 880 patients published in 1988,[37] the survival and prognosis, given the surgical and medical treatment modalities currently available, were documented. Of live deliveries with spina bifida, about 85% survive past age 10; 2% die in the neonatal period. Of the survivors, about 50% suffer some sort of learning disability. About 25% of survivors have an IQ above 100 and about 75% have an IQ above 80. About 33% of survivors develop symptoms and signs related to pressure on the hindbrain and brainstem (e.g., pain, weakness, and spasticity in the arms), and some may require cervical laminectomy to relieve the pressure. The mortality from respiratory failure in such affected children is about 33%.

MYELOCYSTOCELE

Myelocystocele is an uncommon form of spinal dysraphism; there is dilatation of the spinal cord's central canal which herniates posteriorly through the spinal canal to form an exterior sac. There may be no associated spina bifida lesion. The sac is composed of three layers (from inner to outer): the **hydromyelia sac** lined by ependyma (a syrinx), the **meningeal layer** which is contiguous with the meninges around the spinal cord, and the **skin.**

The fluid within the inner sac is continuous with the fluid of the central canal of the spinal cord; the fluid between the hydromyelia sac and the meningeal layer is continuous with the subarachnoid fluid.

Myelocystocele may occur at any level of the spine but spina bifida cystica in the cervical and upper thoracic area is more frequently of this type. Myelocystocele is commonly associated with Chiari II malformation.[38-40]

Prenatal and postnatal **sonography** demonstrates a "cyst within a cyst" appearance in a myelocystocele (Fig. 44-13). Splaying of the laminae and pedicles may or may not be present. More detail is visible postnatally with sonography and MRI when hydromyelia, cord deformity, and a thin communication channel between the spinal cord canal and the cyst may be evident.

The **prognosis** for a myelocystocele is worse than for a simple meningocele; infants with a simple meningocele often remain normal neurologically after surgical repair. The prognosis with myelocystocele is worse because there is usually some degree of associated myelodysplasia (i.e., dysplasia of the spinal cord). Although neurological function is normal in the immediate postoperative period, neurologic deficits often become apparent later in life.

DIASTEMATOMYELIA

Diastematomyelia implies a partial or complete sagittal cleft in the spinal cord, the distal conus of the

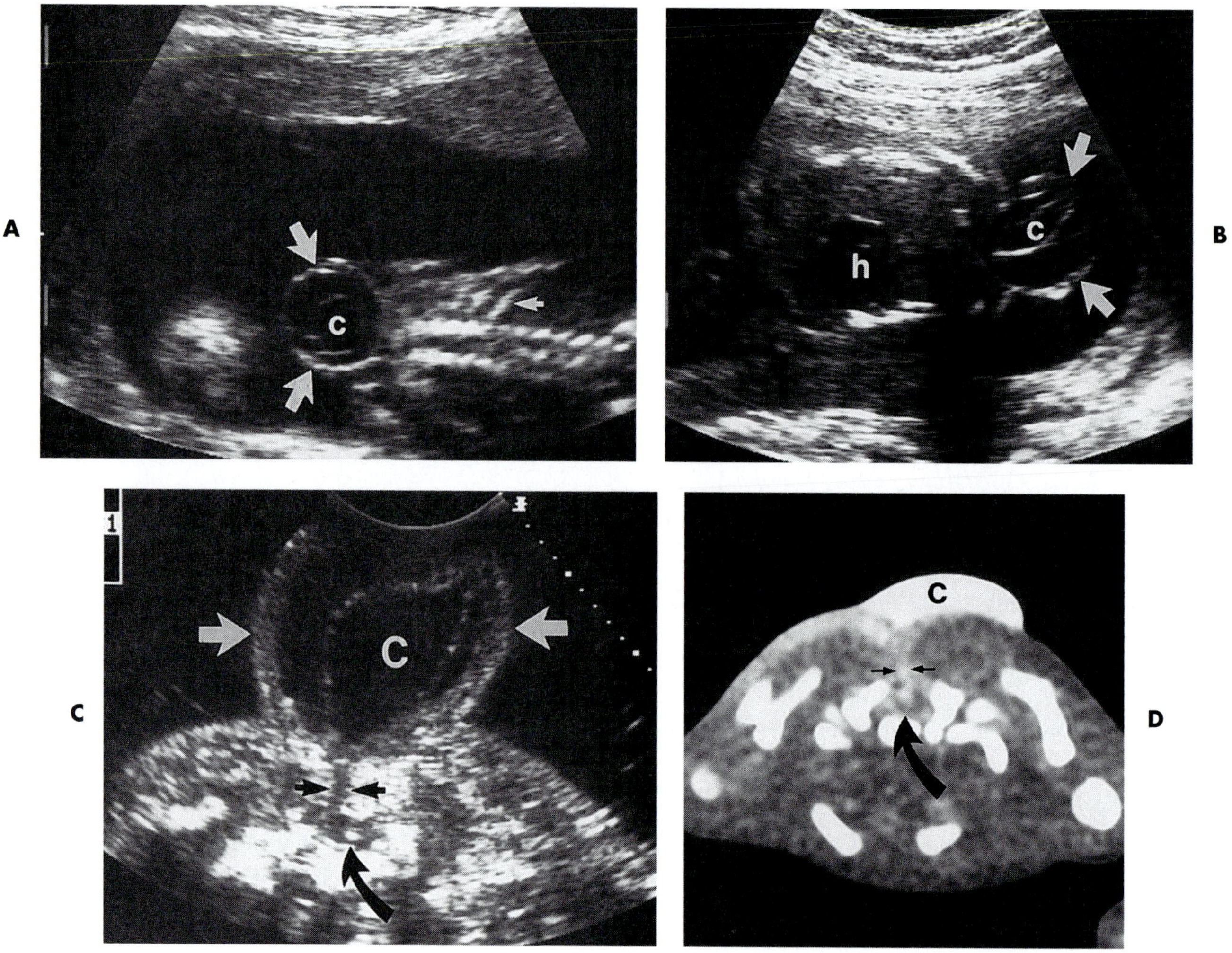

FIG. 44-13. Myelocystocele. **A,** coronal sonogram of fetal thoracic spine at 18 weeks' gestation demonstrates a double-walled cystic mass *(big arrows)* with inner cystic component (*c*) arising from the upper thoracic area *(small arrow* = rib arising from thoracic spine area). **B,** transaxial sonogram of the fetal chest 1 week later in the same patient demonstrates a double-walled cystic mass *(arrows)* arising along the posterior aspect of the fetal chest. *c* = inner cystic component. *h* = fetal heart. Note that the inner cystic component is slightly smaller and flattened compared to the scan 1 week earlier. No abnormality was noted in the ossified neural arch. **C,** sonogram of the specimen demonstrates the double-walled cystic mass *(big arrows)* arising from the posterior thorax. Note the hypoechoic tract *(small arrows)* extending from the posterior aspect of the spinal cord *(curved arrow)* toward the central cystic component (*C*) of the posterior mass. **D,** CT scan of the specimen in the same scan plane. Note the hyperdense tract *(small arrows)* between the spinal cord *(curved arrow)* and the posterior cystic mass (*C*). The cystic mass has been injected with dense water-soluble contrast material that extended into the tract. No abnormality is present in the ossified neural arch (i.e., the laminae and pedicles).

Continued.

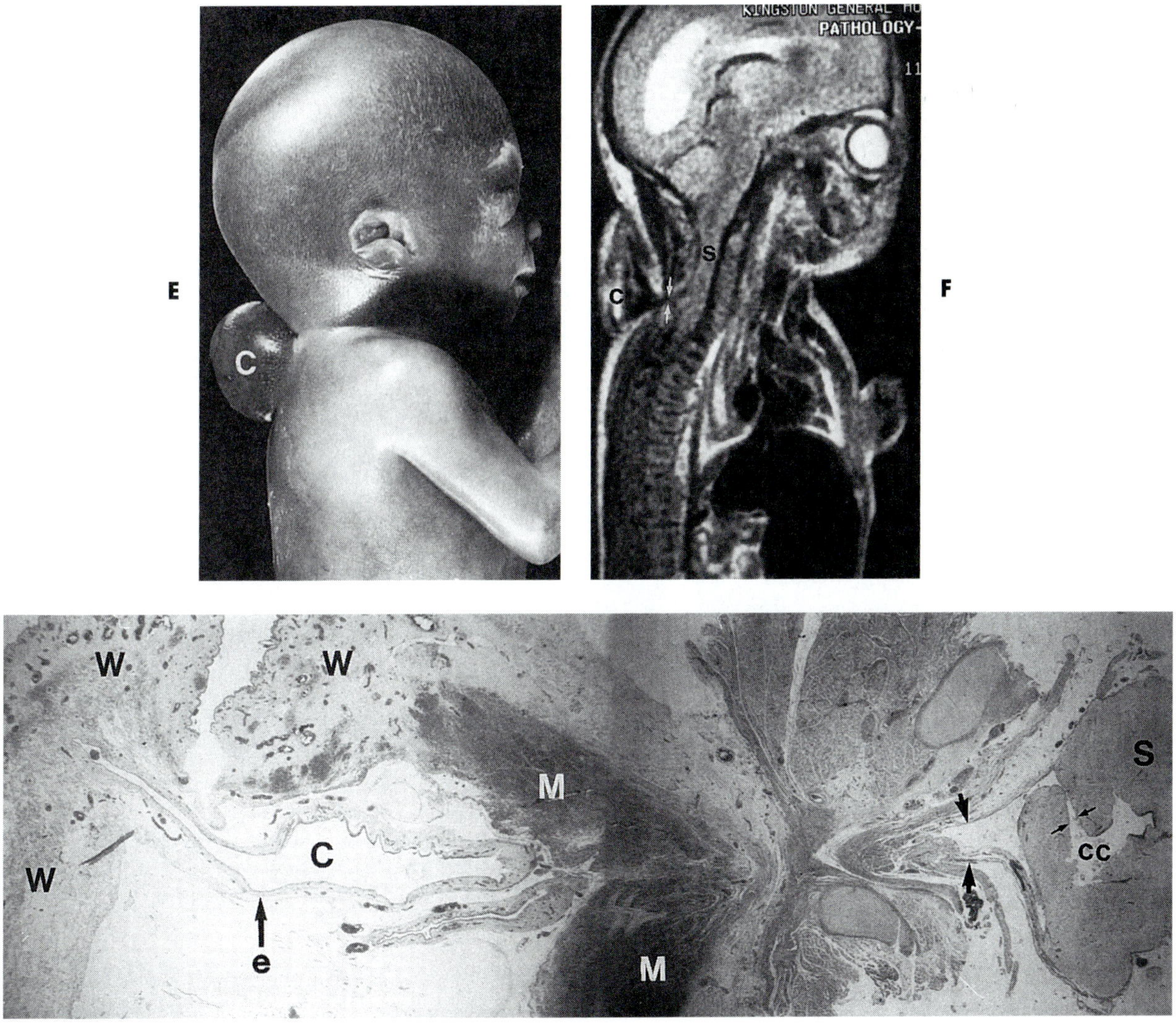

FIG. 44-13, cont'd. **E,** lateral picture of the specimen demonstrates the posterior cystic mass (*C*) arising from the upper thorax. **F,** sagittal MR scan of the fetal specimen demonstrates the cystic mass along the upper thoracic area. Note the small tract *(arrows)* extending from the posterior aspect of the spinal cord (*S*) toward the cystic mass (*C*). **G,** histologic section through the cystic mass and spinal cord. Note the abnormal channel *(larger arrows)* communicating with the posterior aspect of the spinal cord (*S*). Note also the defect in the posterior spinal cord *(small arrows)* communicating with the central canal (*cc*) of the spinal cord. C = the central cystic component of the posterior mass. *e* = the ependymal lining of the central cyst which communicated with the central canal of the spinal cord. *W* = outer wall of the cystic mass.

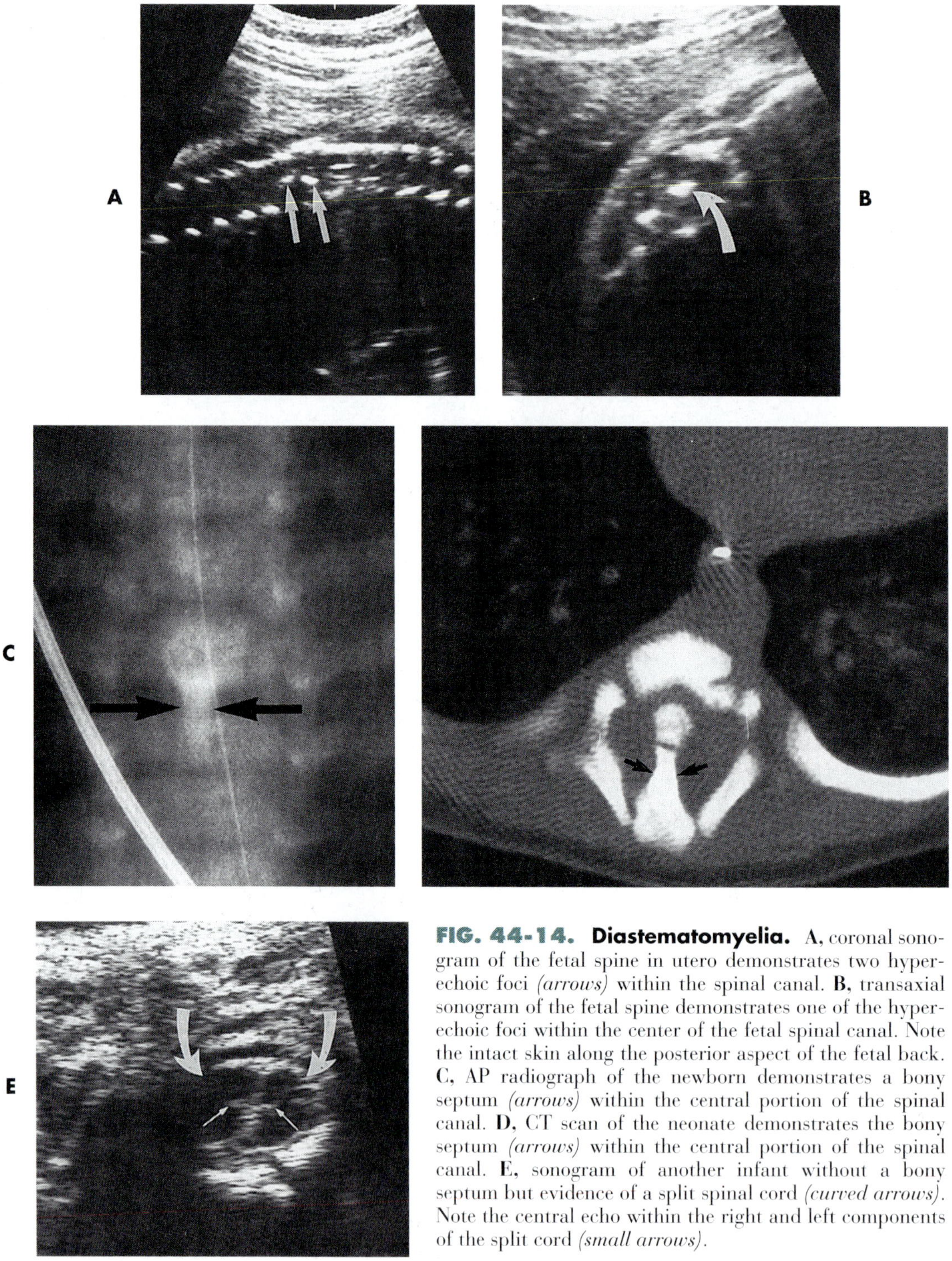

FIG. 44-14. Diastematomyelia. **A**, coronal sonogram of the fetal spine in utero demonstrates two hyperechoic foci *(arrows)* within the spinal canal. **B**, transaxial sonogram of the fetal spine demonstrates one of the hyperechoic foci within the center of the fetal spinal canal. Note the intact skin along the posterior aspect of the fetal back. **C**, AP radiograph of the newborn demonstrates a bony septum *(arrows)* within the central portion of the spinal canal. **D**, CT scan of the neonate demonstrates the bony septum *(arrows)* within the central portion of the spinal canal. **E**, sonogram of another infant without a bony septum but evidence of a split spinal cord *(curved arrows)*. Note the central echo within the right and left components of the split cord *(small arrows)*.

cord, or filum terminale. This may be associated with a spina bifida defect and/or hydromyelia, which is dilatation of the cord's central canal.

If the defect involves the spinal cord only, and there is no associated fibrous or bony septum, prenatal sonography will not detect the abnormality. Postnatal sonography, CT, and MRI can demonstrate the lesion (Fig. 44-14). If the hemicords are split by a bony septum, the septum will appear as an abnormal hyperechoic focus which is best demonstrated in the posterior transaxial and lateral longitudinal scan planes (Fig. 44-14).[41-43] An associated spina bifida lesion may also be evident in these scan planes.

A

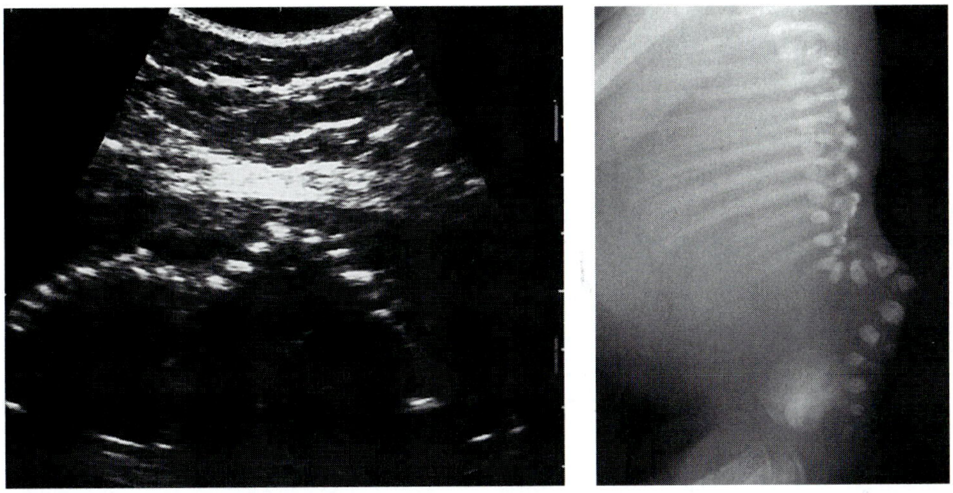

B

FIG. 44-15. Fetal kyphosis. **A,** sagittal scan of the fetus demonstrates an S-shaped curvature to the thoracolumbar spine. **B,** the lateral radiograph of the neonate demonstrates the S-shaped curvature of the thoracolumbar spine.

SCOLIOSIS AND KYPHOSIS

Kyphosis is exaggerated curvature of the spine in the sagittal plane. **Scoliosis** is lateral curvature of the spine. Kyphosis and scoliosis may be positional and nonpathological or permanent and pathological. Pathological kyphosis and scoliosis are usually associated with spina bifida or ventral abdominal wall defects.[44] Less common associations include limb-body wall complex, amniotic band syndrome, arthrogryposis, skeletal dysplasias, VACTERL association,[45,46] and caudal regression syndrome. Mild scoliosis may be due to a hemivertebra anomaly.[44,47]

The posterior longitudinal scan plane is the best to assess for kyphosis; the lateral longitudinal scan plane is the best to assess for scoliosis (Fig. 44-15). Since oligohydramnios can cause positional curvature in the fetal spine, a confident diagnosis of pathological kyphosis or scoliosis should be made only if the curvature is severe. Possible associated anomalies must then be sought because prognosis is dependent on the coexistent anomalies.

A **hemivertebra** represents underdevelopment or nondevelopment of one half of a vertebral body, i.e., one of the two early chondrification centers is deficient. The remaining ossification center is displaced laterally with respect to the vertebrae above and below it, leading to a short-segment mild scoliosis. The abnormalities are best seen in the lateral longitudinal scan plane. Fetuses with an isolated hemivertebra have an excellent prognosis, whereas those with other fetal anomalies (e.g., Potter's syndrome; cardiac, intestinal, intracranial, and limb anomalies) have a poor prognosis.[48] The presence of associated anomalies reduces survival to approximately 50%. If oligohydramnios is also present, the mortality approaches 100%.[48]

CAUDAL REGRESSION

Caudal regression implies a spectrum of abnormalities ranging from absence of part of the sacrum to absence of the lumbar spine.[49,50] The severest form is **sirenomelia (mermaid syndrome),** which includes absence of the sacrum, fusion of the legs, anorectal atresia, renal dysgenesis or agenesis, and possibly cardiac defects.[51] **Sacral agenesis** is a form of caudal regression. It may be associated with kyphoscoliosis, pelvic bone deformity, and club foot.

In caudal regression, prenatal **sonography** demonstrates the absence of sacral and possibly lumbar vertebrae (Fig. 44-16). The legs may be hypoplastic in caudal regression syndrome. In sirenomelia the legs are fused. If there is renal dysgenesis or agenesis, the main ultrasound finding is oligohydramnios and the spine and limb deformities may be difficult to identify. If gastrointestinal, cardiac, or brain lesions are present, these may be more obvious than the spinal and leg abnormalities.

The incidence of caudal regression is much higher in infants of diabetic mothers (250 times higher)[52,53] although the majority (85%) of cases occur in pregnancies uncomplicated by diabetes mellitus.

Caudal regression is often associated with anomalies seen in the **VACTERL** sequence which implies anomalies in the following systems: **V**ertebral, **A**nal, **C**ardiovascular, **T**racheo-**E**sophageal, **R**enal, and **L**imb.[54] There is considerable overlap between

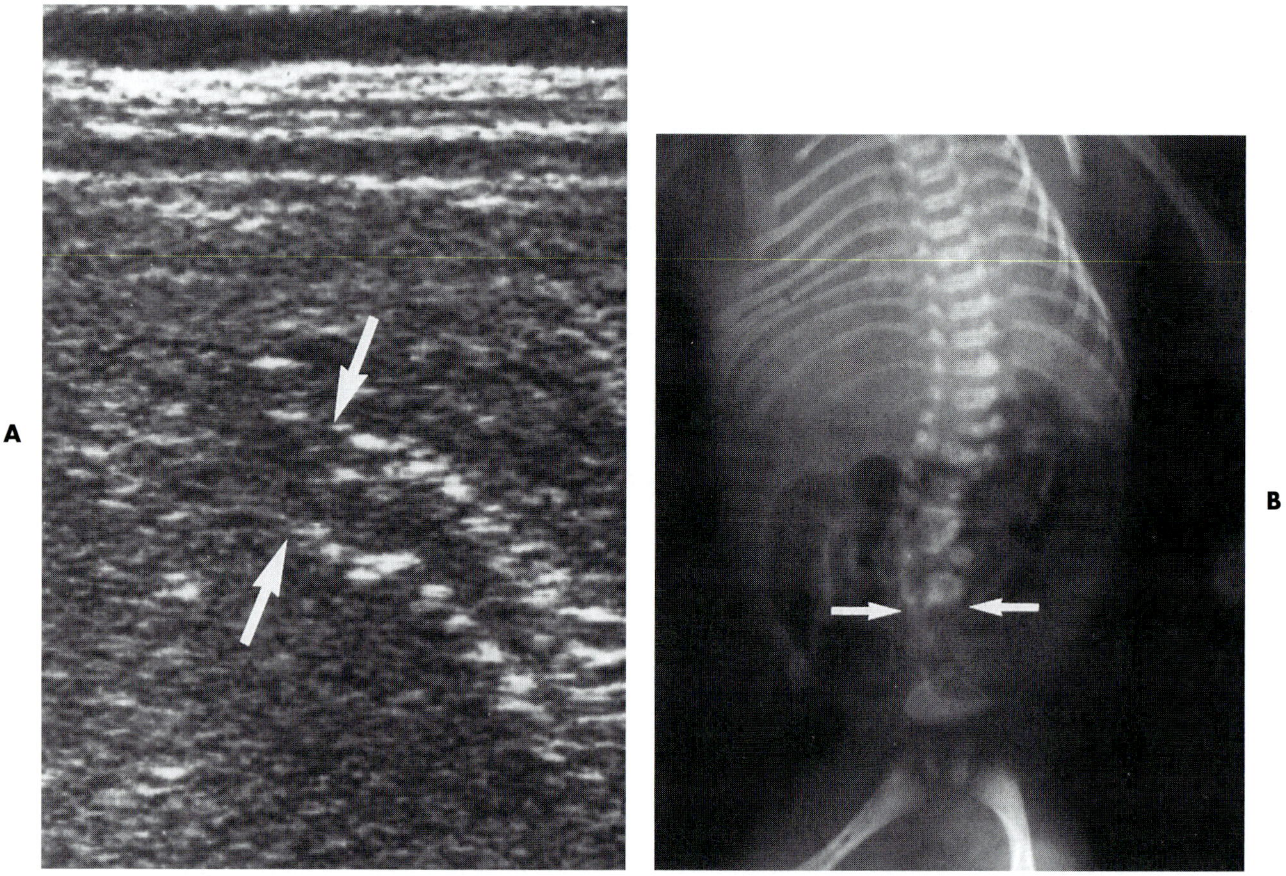

FIG. 44-16. Caudal regression syndrome (sacral agenesis). **A**, lateral longitudinal scan of lumbar spine shows an abrupt termination *(arrows)* of ossified structures in lower lumbar spine. **B**, radiograph of specimen. There is abrupt termination *(arrows)* of the lumbar spine and absence of the sacrum. The pelvic bones are small and deformed.

the caudal regression syndrome and the VACTERL sequence.

The **prognosis** of affected infants depends on the severity and extent of involvement. All infants with sirenomelia die in infancy. In sacral agenesis, with no internal organ involvement, there are usually deficits in the legs and altered control of the urinary bladder. In others with internal organ involvement, the prognosis is related to these defects.

SACROCOCCYGEAL TERATOMA

Fetal teratomas may arise from the sacrum or coccyx, from other midline structures from the brain to the coccyx, or from the gonads.[55] Because teratomas arise from totipotential cells, the neoplasms may contain elements of many tissues, including neural, respiratory, and gastrointestinal. Sacrococcygeal tumor is rare (1 in 35,000 births).[56]

Sacrococcygeal teratomas may be classified into **four types:**[55]

Type I (47%):	External mass predominant
Type II (34%):	External mass with significant internal component
Type III (9%):	Internal mass predominant, with smaller external component
Type IV (10%):	Presacral mass only

Sonography commonly demonstrates a mass in the rump or buttocks area adjacent to the spine.[57] Most teratomas (85%) are either solid or mixed (solid plus cystic); 15% are mostly cystic, which is a benign sign. Calcifications are frequently present. Large masses may displace and distort neighboring structures such as the rectum and urinary bladder (Fig. 44-17). Compression of the distal ureters may cause hydronephrosis. Larger solid tumors may develop significant arteriovenous shunting causing fetal cardiac failure and hydrops.[57] The development of fetal hydrops in the presence of a sacrococcygeal teratoma

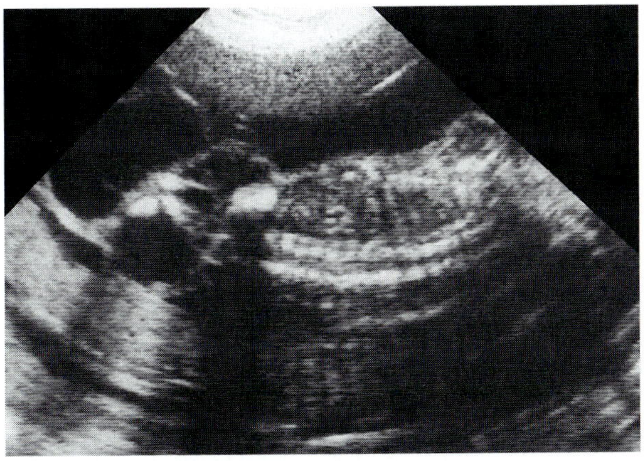

FIG. 44-17. Sacrococcygeal teratoma. Coronal scan at 23 weeks' gestation shows a complex septated cystic mass protruding from the buttock region exterior to the pelvis at the caudal end of the fetal spine. (Courtesy of Stephanie R. Wilson, M. D., University of Toronto.)

DIFFERENTIAL DIAGNOSIS OF A PRESACRAL FETAL MASS

Sacrococcygeal teratoma
Chordoma
Anterior myelomeningocele
Neurenteric cyst
Neuroblastoma
Sarcoma
Lipoma
Bone tumor
Lymphoma
Rectal duplication

carries a poor prognosis, and these findings should precipitate a cesarean section for fetal salvage.[58-62]

The **differential diagnosis** of a presacral fetal mass also includes chordoma, anterior myelomeningocele, neurenteric cyst, neuroblastoma, sarcoma, lipoma, bone tumor, lymphoma, and rectal duplication. Amniotic fluid alpha-fetoprotein is often elevated in sacrococcygeal tumor and acetylcholinesterase is often present in the amniotic fluid. These results rule out most other etiologies except a myelomeningocele.

If a fetal sacrococcygeal teratoma is suspected from prenatal sonograms, serial sonograms (e.g., every 1 to 4 weeks) should be arranged to monitor the pregnancy to assess for complications, especially signs of fetal cardiac failure. Complete fetal assessment should also include the internal characteristics of the tumor, the size of the tumor, and associated fetal anomalies.

For masses less than 4.5 cm diameter, without associated abnormalities, elective vaginal delivery is recommended. For masses greater than 4.5 cm diameter, elective cesarean section may be advisable because of the risk of dystocia and hemorrhage during vaginal delivery. *In utero* surgery for anteriovenous shunting has been described for treatment of fetal hydrops from congestive heart failure in early pregnancy (less than 30 weeks' gestation) but this should be considered only in experienced hands.[59]

REFERENCES

Developmental Anatomy

1. Moore KL. *The Developing Human: Clinically Oriented Embryology*. 4th ed. Philadelphia: WB Saunders Co; 1988.
2. O'Rahilly R, Muller F, Meyer DB. The human vertebral column at the end of the embryonic period proper: the column as a whole. *J Anat* 1980;131:565-575.
3. Bagnall KM, Harris PF, Jones PRM. A radiographic study of the human fetal spine: the sequence of development of the ossification centers in the vertebral column. *J Anat* 1977;24:791-802.
4. Ford DM, McFadden KD, Bagnall KM. Sequence of ossification in human vertebral neural arch centers. *Anat Rec* 1982; 203:175-178.

Scanning Techniques

5. Babook CJ, Goldstein RB, Barth RA et al. Prevalence of ventriculomegaly in association with myelomeningocele: correlation with gestational age and severity of posterior fossa deformity. *Radiology* 1994;190:703-707.
6. Thiagarajah S, Henke J, Hogge WA et al. Early diagnosis of spina bifida: the value of cranial ultrasound markers. *Obstet Gynecol* 1994;76:54-57.

Spina Bifida

7. Sadovnick AD, Baird PA. Incidence of neural tube defects in liveborn and stillborn infants in British Columbia over a 10-year period. *Can Med Assoc J* 1983;129:1109-1110.
8. Hunter AGW. Neural tube defects in eastern Ontario and western Quebec: demography and family data. *Am J Med Genet* 1984;19:45-63.
9. Main DM, Mennuti MT. Neural tube defects: issues in prenatal diagnosis and counseling. *Obstet Gynecol* 1986;67:1-16.
10. Lescale KB, Eddleman KA, Chervenak FA. The fetal neck and spine. In: McGahan JP, Porto M, eds. *Diagnostic Obstetrical Ultrasound*. Philadelphia: JB Lippincott Company; 1994:195.
11. Yen IH, Khoury MJ, Erickson JD et al. The changing epidemiology of neural tube defects, United States, 1968-1989. *Am J Dis Child* 1992;146:857-861.
12. Cragan JD, Roberts HE, Edmonds LD et al. Surveillance for anencephaly and spina bifida and the impact of prenatal diagnosis, United States, 1985-1994. *MMWR DCD Surveillance Summaries* 1994;44:1-13.
13. Anonymous. Folic acid to prevent neural tube defects. *Drug Therap Bull* 1994;32:31-32.
14. Byrne J, Warburton D. Neural tube defects in spontaneous abortions. *Am J Med Genet* 1986;23:327-333.
15. MRC Vitamin Study, 1991;338:131-137.
16. VanAllen MI, Fraser FC, Dallairel et al. Recommendations on the use of folic acid supplementation to prevent the recurrence of neural tube defects. Clinical Teratology Committee, Canadian College of Medical Geneticists [comment]. *Can Med Assoc J* 1993;149:1239-1243.
17. Anonymous. Recommendations for the use of folic acid to reduce the number of cases of spina bifida and other neural tube defects [review]. *MMWR* 1991;41:1-7.
18. Emery JL, Lendon RG. Lipomas of the cauda equina and other fatty tumors related to neurospinal dysraphism. *Dev Med Child Neurol* 1969;20(suppl):62-70.

19. Warkany J. *Congenital malformations.* Chicago: Year Book Medical Publishers Inc; 1971.
20. Filly RA, Callen PW, Goldstein RB. Fetoprotetin screening programs: what every obstetric sonologist should know. In: Callen PW, ed. *Ultrasonograph Obstet Gynecol.* Philadelphia: WB Saunders Co; 1994:24-34.
21. Ames MD, Schut L. Results and treatment of 171 consecutive myelomeningoceles: 1963 to 1968. *Pediatrics* 1972;50:466-470.
22. Roberts AB, Campbell H, Boreham J et al. Fetal head measurements in spina bifida. *Br J Obstet Gynecol* 1980;87:927-928.
23. Wald N, Cuckle H, Boreham J et al. Small biparietal diameter of fetuses with spina bifida: implications for antenatal screening. *Br J Obstet Gynecol* 1980;87:219-221.
24. Nyberg DA, Mack LA, Hirsch J et al. Fetal hydrocephalus: sonographic detection and clinical significance of associated anomalies. *Radiology* 1987;163:187-191.
25. Nicolaides KH, Campbell S, Gabbe SG. Ultrasound screening for spina bifida: cranial and cerebellar signs. *Lancet* 1986; 2:72-74.
26. Campbell J, Gilbert WM, Nicolaides KH et al. Ultrasound screening for spina bifida: cranial and cerebellar signs in a high-risk population. *Obstet Gynecol* 1987;70:247-250.
27. Pilu G, Romero R, Reece A et al. Subnormal cerebellum in fetuses with spina bifida. *Am J Obstet Gynecol* 1988;158:1052-1056.
28. Goldstein RB, Podrasky AE, Filly RA et al. Effacement of the fetal cisterna magna in association with myelomeningocele. *Radiology* 1989;172:409-413.
29. Benacerraf BR, Stryher J, Frigoletto JD Jr et al. Abnormal appearance of the cerebellum (banana sign): indirect sign of spina bifida. *Radiology* 1989;171:151-153.
30. Furness ME, Barbary JE, Verco PW. A pointer to spina bifida: fetal head shape in the second trimester. In: Gill RW, Dadd MJ, eds. *WFUMB (World Federation of Ultrasound in Medicine and Biology).* Sidney: Pergamon Press Inc; 1985:296.
31. Nyberg DA, Mack LA, Hirsch J et al. Abnormalities of the fetal cranial contour in sonographic detection of spina bifida: evaluation of the "lemon" sign. *Radiology* 1988;167:387-392.
32. Penso C, Redline RW, Benacerraf BR. A sonographic sign which predicts which fetuses with hydrocephalus have an associated neural tube defect. *J Ultrasound Med* 1987;6:307-311.
33. Sharrard WJW. The mechanism of paralytic deformity in spina bifida. *Dev Med Child Neurol* 1962;4:310-313.
34. Babcook CJ, Goldstein RB, Filly RA. Prenatally detected fetal myelomeningocele: is karyotype analysis warranted? *Radiology* 1995;194:491-494.
35. Lorber J. Results of treatment of myelomeningocele: an analysis of 524 unselected cases with special reference to possible selection for treatment. *Dev Med Child Neurol* 1971;13:279-303.
36. Kollias SS, Goldstein RB, Cogen PH, Filly RA. Prenatally detected myelomeningoceles: sonographic accuracy in estimation of the spinal level. *Radiology* 1992;185:109-112.

Myelocystocele

37. Nelson MD Jr, Bracchi M, Naidish TP et al. The natural history of repaired myelomeningocele. *RadioGraphics* 1988;8:695-706.
38. Steinbok P, Cochrane DD. The nature of congenital posterior cervical or cervicothoracic midline cutaneous mass lesions. Report of eight cases. *J Neurosurg.* 1991;75:206-212.
39. Bhargava R, Hammond DI, Benzie RJ et al. Prenatal demonstration of a cervical myelocystocele. *Prenat Diag* 1992;653-659.
40. Steinbok P. Dysraphyic lesions of the cervical spinal cord (review). *Neurosurg Clin N Am* 1995;6:367-376.

Diastematomyelia

41. Raghavendra BN, Epstein FJ, Pinto RS et al. Sonographic diagnosis of diastematomyelia. *J Ultrasound Med* 1988;7:111-113.
42. Anderson NG, Joran S, MacFarlane MR, Lovell-Smith M. Diastematomyelia: diagnosis by prenatal sonography. *AJR* 1994;163:911-914.
43. Korsvik HE, Keller MS. Sonography of occult dysraphism in neonates and infants with MR imaging correlation. *Radiographics* 1992;12:297-306.

Scoliosis and Kyphosis

44. Harrison LA, Pretorius DH, Budorick NE. Abnormal spinal curvature in the fetus. *J Ultrasound Med* 1992;11:473-479.
45. Patten RM, Van Allen MI, Mack LA et al. Limb-body wall complex: *in utero* sonographic diagnosis of a complicated fetal malformation. *Am J Roentgenol* 1986;146:1019-1024.
46. VanAllen MI, Curry C, Walden CE et al. Limb-body wall complex: II: Limb and spine defects. *Am J Med Gen* 1987;28:549-565.
47. Benacerraf BR, Greene MF, Barss VA. Prenatal sonographic diagnosis of congenital hemivertebra. *J Ultrasound Med* 1986; 5:257-259.
48. Zelop CM, Pretorius DH, Benacerraf BR. Fetal hemivertebrae: associated anomalies, significance, and outcome. *Obstet Gynecol* 1993;81:412-416.

Caudal Regression

49. Mariani AJ, Stern J, Khan AU et al. Sacral agenesis: an analysis of 11 cases and review of the literature. *J Urol* 1979;122:684-686.
50. Renshaw TS. Sacral agenesis: a classification and review of twenty-three cases. *J Bone Joint Surg* 1978;60A:373-383.
51. Kallen B, Winberg J. Caudal mesoderm pattern of anomalies: from renal agenesis to sirenomelia. *Teratology* 1973;9:99-12.
52. Mills JL. Malformations in infants of diabetic mothers. *Teratology* 1982;25:385-394.
53. Sonek JD, Gabbe SG, Landon MB et al. Antenatal diagnosis of sacral agenesis syndrome in a pregnancy complicated by diabetes mellitus. *Am J Obstet Gynecol* 1990;162:806-808.
54. Khoury MJ, Cordero JF, Greenberg F. A population study of the VACTERL association: evidence for its etiologic heterogeneity. *Pediatrics* 1983;71:815-820.

Sacrococcygeal Teratoma

55. Bloechle M, Ballman R, Zienert A et al. Fetal teratoma: diagnosis and management. *Zentralblatt fur Gynakologie* 1992; 114:175-180.
56. Altman RP, Randolph JG, Lilly JR. Sacrococcygeal teratoma: American Academy of Pediatrics surgical section survey. *J Pediatr Surg* 1974;9:389-398.
57. Sheth S, Nussbaum AR, Sanders RC et al. Prenatal diagnosis of sacrococcygeal teratoma: sonographic-pathologic correlation. *Radiology* 1988;169:131-136.
58. Bond SJ, Harrison MR, Schmimdt KG et al. Death due to high output cardiac failure in fetal sacrococcygeal teratoma: rationale for fetal surgery. *J Pediatr Surg* 1991;25:1287-1291.
59. Langer JC, Harrison MR, Schmidt KG et al. Fetal hydrops and death from sacrococcygeal teratoma: rationale for fetal surgery. *Am J Obstet Gynecol* 1989;160:1145-1150.
60. Gross SJ, Benzie RJ, Sermer M et al. Sacrococcygeal teratoma: prenatal diagnosis and management. *Am J Obstet Gynecol* 1987;156:393-396.
61. Teal LN, Angtuaco TL, Jiminez JF, Quirk JG Jr. Fetal teratomas, antenatal diagnosis and clinical management. *J Clin Ultrasound* 1988;16:329-336.
62. Robertson FM, Crombleholme TM, Frantz ID 3rd et al. Devascularization and staged resection of giant sacrococcygeal teratomas in the premature infant. *J Pediatr Surg* 1995;30: 309-311.

CHAPTER 45

Fetal Hydrops

Daniel E. Challis, M.B., B.S., F.R.A.C.O.G., D.D.U.
Greg Ryan, M.B., M.R.C.O.G., F.R.C.S.C.
Ann Jefferies, M.D., F.R.C.P.C.

CHAPTER OUTLINE

CHAPTER OUTLINE, cont'd.

Hydrops is defined as an abnormal accumulation of serous fluid in at least two body cavities or tissues. The **major classification of hydrops** is based on two groups of etiologies—**immune** and **nonimmune.** Non-immune hydrops (NIH) is defined by the absence of a detectable circulating antibody against red blood cells (RBC) in the mother. Prior to the widespread introduction of Rhesus (Rh) immunoglobulin[1,2] in the 1970s, most cases of hydrops were immune,[3] whereas today most are nonimmune.

NIH was initially described in 1892 amongst a series of hydropic cases[4] and was first differentiated from immune hydrops in 1943 in a "fetus unassociated with erythroblastosis."[5] Recent reviews document the changing pattern of hydrops.[6-9] Although "hydrops" is a relatively common indication for tertiary level fetal evaluation, each specific etiology is relatively rare.

Hydrops represents a terminal stage for many conditions, the majority of which are fetal in origin. The onset of hydrops usually signifies fetal decompensation. Immune causes can be successfully treated *in utero*, as can many nonimmune causes. Whereas in the past NIH carried a 100% mortality, this is no longer the case. A team approach utilizing sonographers, obstetrical perinatologists, neonatologists, and geneticists will provide optimal care and help to decide which cases are suitable for therapeutic intervention. Parents can be counseled that a steadily growing number of carefully selected cases may be amenable to some form of prenatal therapy, with the possibility of a good outcome. A comprehensive approach must be taken to the investigation of hydrops, both for the management of the index case and for future counseling. The cornerstones of this investigation are detailed ultrasound and fetal blood sampling. Early referral to a tertiary perinatal care center is encouraged for the optimal evaluation of each case.

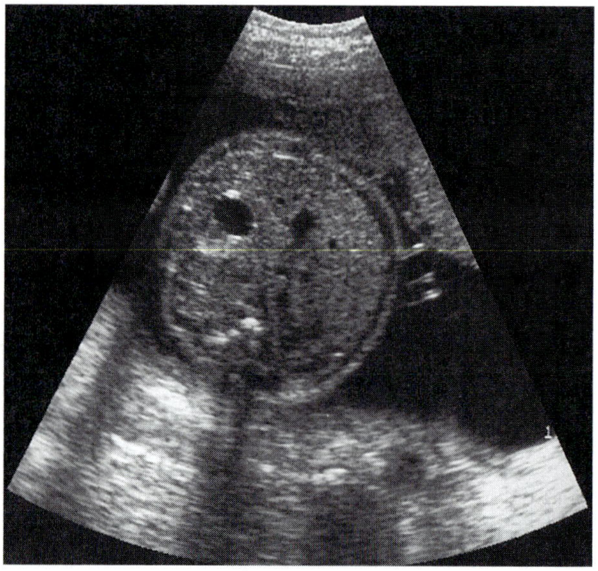

FIG. 45-1. Pseudoascites at 27 weeks' gestation. Transverse abdominal image shows a thin hypoechoic rim surrounding the fetal organs, raising the possibility of ascites. This rim is produced by the normal abdominal wall musculature. (Courtesy of Stephanie R. Wilson, M.D., University of Toronto.)

SONOGRAPHIC FEATURES OF HYDROPS

SONOGRAPHIC FEATURES OF HYDROPS

- Ascites
- Pleural effusions
- Pericardial effusions
- Subcutaneous edema
- Placental edema
- Arterial or venous Doppler abnormalities
- Alteration of fetal "well being"

The initial **sonographic diagnosis** of hydrops is straightforward (see box). The fetus may show unexpected **ascites, pleural** or **pericardial effusions**, or **subcutaneous edema** at a routine sonographic assessment or the patient may be referred because of a clinical suspicion of **polyhydramnios.** Fluid collections in the fetal chest or abdomen are easily seen at any gestation. A small ring of **"pseudoascites"** (less than 2 mm in thickness) is a normal finding and usually represents the hypoechoic muscular layer of either the diaphragm or the abdominal wall.[10] This pseudoascites usually disappears when the transducer angle is changed (Fig. 45-1). Similarly, small, angle-dependent pericardial effusions may be normal. A tiny amount of free peritoneal fluid is physiologic and is a feature one commonly employs to visualize structures such as the diaphragm.

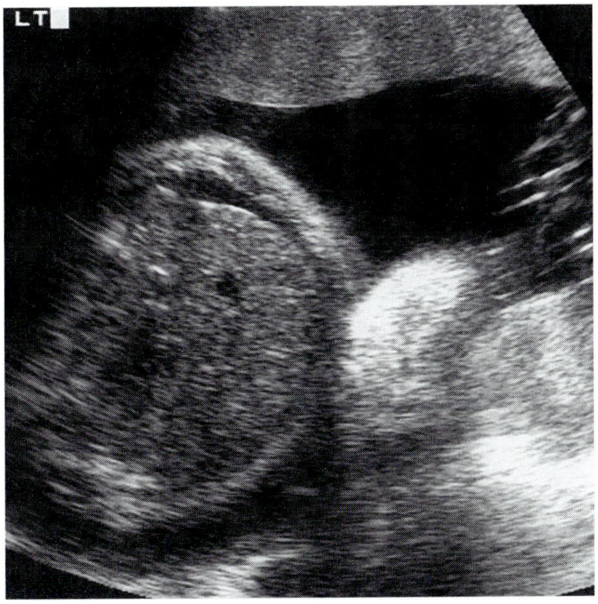

FIG. 45-2. Small rim of ascites. Transverse view through fetal abdomen at 26 weeks shows a rim of black fluid between the abdominal wall and the liver.

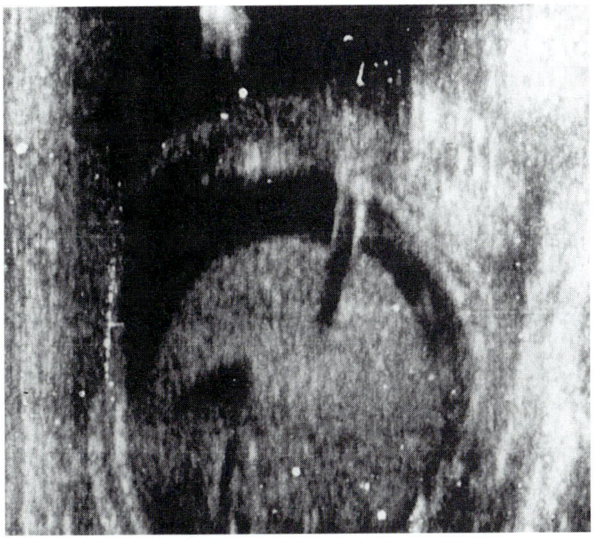

FIG. 45-3. Moderate-large ascites at 34 weeks. Transverse view through fetal abdomen shows a large rim of fluid around the visceral organs.

Ascites

Small collections of **ascitic fluid** may be seen to outline abdominal viscera, including bowel loops or bladder, and may cause an apparent increase in their echogenicity due to the fluid/tissue interface (Fig. 45-2). Larger accumulations, particularly in the anterior peritoneal cavity, will outline other visceral organs, and the umbilical vein can be seen prominently, traversing the fluid space (Fig. 45-3). **Bowel loops** may appear to be either free-floating (e.g., illumine hydrops) or a matted echogenic posterior mass (e.g., meconium peritonitis). Ascitic fluid may track through the patent processus vaginalis into the scrotum, causing a **hydrocoele.** Rarely, chronic chest compression from massive ascites may result in lethal pulmonary hypoplasia.

Pleural Effusions

Pleural effusions may initially be unilateral or bilateral. Small effusions are seen as a thin echolucent rim surrounding lung tissue, and they may also outline mediastinal structures. Large unilateral effusions suggest a local cause or etiology such as **chylothorax** (Fig. 45-4). Large bilateral effusions cause the lungs to appear as free-floating "bat wings" beside the heart. As effusions enlarge, compression or kinking of mediastinal vascular structures causes upper-body edema, and functional esophageal obstruction leads to secondary polyhydramnios.

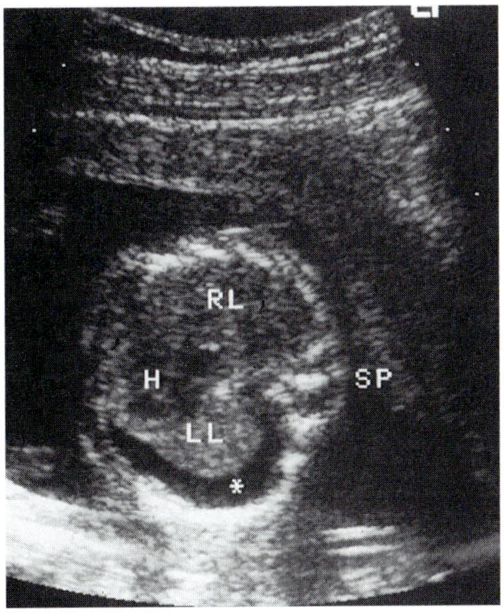

FIG. 45-4. Unilateral small pleural effusion. Transverse sonogram shows a rim of fluid *(asterisk)* around the convexity of the left lung (LL), heart (H), right lung (RL), spine (Sp). This case resolved without pleuroamniotic shunting.

Edema

Subcutaneous edema may be generalized, localized, or limited to the upper or lower body, depending on the etiology. Edema is often most easily seen over the fetal scalp (Fig. 45-5) or face, where a thickening and layering of skin overlies bone. Subcutaneous edema may also be seen over the limbs and abdominal wall.

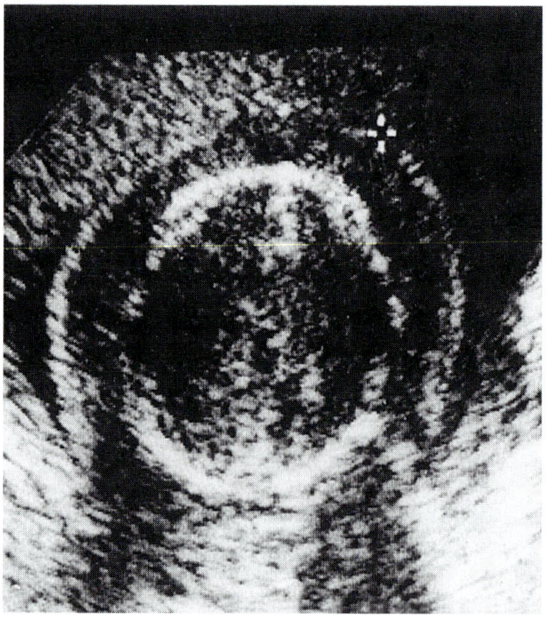

FIG. 45-5. Severe skull edema. Nonimmune hydrops associated with trisomy 21. Sonogram shows a rim of echo-poor fluid surrounding the skull.

Placental Edema

Placental edema is a variable and usually late sign in hydrops. The placental **echotexture** is altered and may be described as **thickened, echogenic, spongy,** or having the classic **ground glass** appearance. Placental **dimensions,** especially thickness, are increased over the normal (4 to 5 cm in the third trimester).[11-13] When placental edema is secondary to the hydropic process in the fetus, the entire placenta is usually affected. This finding may be used to exclude primary placental causes of hydrops (e.g., vascular malformations).

Pattern of Hydrops

The **distribution** and size of fluid collections and edema should be noted, for they may provide a clue to etiology. In immune hydrops, ascites appears first, whereas subcutaneous edema appears with more advanced anemia. Intrathoracic collections are generally a very late sign.

In some cases, it may not be possible to differentiate sonographically between hydrops resulting from a systemic insult and hydrops resulting from a local cause of fluid collection (with secondary NIH). For example, isolated pleural effusions resulting from primary hydrothoraces may appear no different from pleural effusions resulting from systemic causes early in the development of generalized NIH. Although the signs are not reliable, it seems that pleural and pericardial effusions appear earlier and more prominently with thoracic pathologies, while ascites appears earlier and predominates with anemia and primary abdominal pathologies. For example, massive ascites with associated bowel echogenicity is typical of either **parvovirus** infection (where it is very tense) or **meconium peritonitis** (where it is usually more fluctuant).

Localized fluid collections may progress to hydrops because of pressure or metabolic effects, and thus the pattern of hydrops may change over time.

IMMUNE HYDROPS

Pathogenesis

Immune hydrops occurs in a pregnancy when a sensitized mother has **antibodies** to fetal red blood cells (RBC). Hemolysis occurs when circulating maternal immunoglobulin G (IgG)-class antibodies cross the placenta and attack antigen-positive fetal red cells. The majority of cases (80%) still occur in the presence of **Rh (D)** antibodies but several atypical blood group antibodies, such as **Kell,** still frequently cause hydrops. The result is anemia, extramedullary erythropoiesis, hepatosplenomegaly, hypoalbuminemia, and an outpouring of immature nucleated red blood cells **(erythroblastosis fetalis).** Ultimately, tissue hypoxia, fetal hydrops, cardiac failure, and death occur. Hydrops develops only when the fetal hemoglobin (Hb) deficit is <7 g/dL,[14] probably because of reduced oncotic pressure secondary to hypoalbuminemia, possibly combined with high-output cardiac failure[15] (Fig. 45-6). Eventually there is fetal decompensation, with metabolic and lactic acidosis[16,17] which exacerbate the high-output cardiac failure. Once decompensation commences, progression of hydrops may be rapid and demise may occur in 24 to 48 hours.

Treatment

A complete discussion of alloimmune disease is beyond the scope of this chapter, and we will restrict ourselves to the hydropic fetus. Immune hydrops is an absolute indication for **fetal blood sampling** (FBS) and transfusion while *in utero*. This was initially performed fetoscopically,[18] a technique since superseded by ultrasound-guided needling procedures.[19] **Fetal intravascular transfusion** (IVT) has proved lifesaving in the hydropic fetus in whom **intraperitoneal transfusion** (IPT) is often unsuccessful because of poor absorption of blood from the peritoneal cavity, possibly due to reduced fetal breathing movements.[20] With IVT, 70% to 85% of hydropic and 85% to 95% of nonhydropic fetuses can survive.[21,22]

Noninvasive Assessment of Severity of Alloimmunization

The development of immune hydrops is a fetal emergency and requires invasive testing. When hydrops is

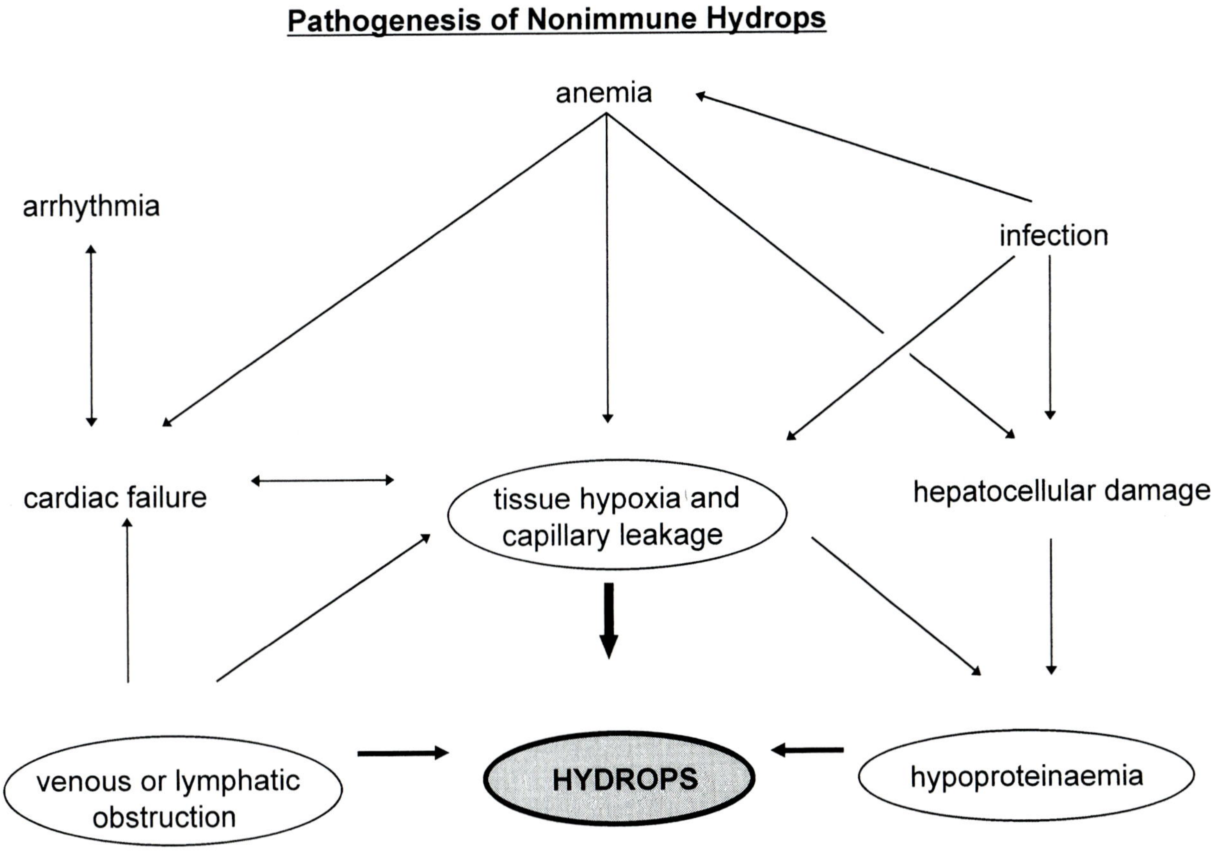

FIG. 45-6. Pathogenesis of hydrops: schematic diagram.

present, the fetal prognosis is guarded. The tried and tested approach to the management of alloimmune disease involves a **progression of investigations**:

- assessment of antibody titers;
- amniotic fluid spectrophotometry;
- fetal blood sampling.[15,22]

As each invasive procedure carries its own inherent risk, there is a need for better noninvasive methods of assessing alloimmune anemia. A number of the structural and functional responses to severe alloimmunization can be assessed sonographically.[23] **Liver** and **spleen size** have been correlated with **severity of fetal anemia** as their volume increases due to extramedullary hematopoiesis. These measurements are associated with a high number of false-negative results, possibly in rapidly progressive disease where there has not been time for organomegaly to develop.[24,25]

The **compensatory response** to severe anemia is a **hyperdynamic fetal circulation** leading to increased blood flow velocities in the umbilical vein, intrahepatic vein, ductus venosus, thoracic aorta, and carotid and middle cerebral arteries. Pulsed Doppler studies of numerous vessels have been reported in alloimmune hydrops, both before and after fetal transfusion.[24,26-31] It appears that a combination of sonographic approaches can play an increasingly important role in the noninvasive assessment of the fetus with alloimmune anemia[24] (see also Chapter 49).

NONIMMUNE HYDROPS

Nonimmune hydrops (NIH) occurs in 1 out of 1500 to 1 out of 4000 pregnancies. It can occur at any gestation and is a common pathological finding in first and second trimester spontaneous abortions. When generalized subcutaneous edema is present, the appearances may be referred to as **anasarca** (Fig. 45-7). The etiology varies geographically. In North America and Europe, the **most common causes** are cardiovascular, infective, and chromosomal.[7] In Southeast Asia, the most common etiology is homozygous thalassaemia.[6]

Pathogenesis

NIH represents the terminal stage for many conditions (see box on pages 1308–1309), and several different pathogenic mechanisms may act simultaneously. These include heart failure, hypoxia, anemia, hypopro-

CAUSES OF HYDROPS FETALIS

IMMUNE: *Anemia	*Rhesus alloimmunization
	*Other red cell antigen alloimmunization
NONIMMUNE:	
Fetal	
Cardiovascular	
Malformation	Left or right heart hypoplasia
	A-V canal
	Single ventricle
	Closure of foramen ovale or ductus arteriosus
	Severe AV valve regurgitation
	Endocardial fibroelastosis
	Ebstein's anomaly
	Biventricular outflow tract obstruction
	Cardiac tumors
	Myocarditis/cardiomyopathy
Arrhythmia	
*Tachyarrhythmia	*Supraventricular tachycardia (SVT)
	*Paroxysmal atrial tachycardia (PAT)
	*Atrial flutter
	*Wolff-Parkinson-White syndrome
*Bradyarrhythmia	*Complete heart block
	*Unspecified bradycardia
High-output failure	Placental chorioangioma
	Other large fetal angiomas
	Sacrococcygeal teratoma
	Vein of Galen aneurysm
	*Twin/twin transfusion (recipient, usually)
	*Acardiac twin (donor)
Neck/Thoracic anomalies	Cystic hygroma
	*Chylothorax/Hydrothorax
	*Congenital cystic adenomatoid malformation
	*Diaphragmatic hernia
	Pulmonary sequestration
	Thoracic tumors
Gastrointestinal anomalies	
Hepatic	Cirrhosis
	Hepatitis
	Tumor
Bowel	Atresias
	Volvulus
	Meconium peritonitis
Urinary tract anomalies	Congenital nephrotic syndrome
	*Lower urinary tract obstruction
	*Upper urinary tract obstruction
	Prune belly syndrome
	Polycystic kidneys
Chromosomal	45,X
	Trisomy 21
	Trisomy 18
	Trisomy 13
	Triploidy
Anemia	α thalassaemia (homozygous)
	*Human parvovirus (HPV) B19 infection

*Conditions in which prenatal therapy has been successful.

CAUSES OF HYDROPS FETALIS, cont'd.

Anemia, cont'd.	G6PD deficiency
	*Feto-maternal hemorrhage
	*Twin/twin transfusion (donor)
Infection	Cytomegalovirus (CMV)
	*Parvovirus (HPVB19)
	*Toxoplasmosis
	Syphilis
	Coxsackie
	Rubella
	Listeriosis
Genetic disorders	
Metabolic disorders	Gaucher's disease
	GM1 gangliosidosis
	Sialidosis
	Mucopolysaccharidosis
	Hurler's syndrome
Skeletal dysplasias	Achondroplasia
	Achondrogenesis
	Osteogenesis
	Thanatophoric dysplasia
	Asphyxiating thoracic dystrophy
	Short rib polydactyly syndromes
Fetal hypokinesis	Arthrogryposis
	Neu-Laxova syndrome
	Pena-Shokeir syndrome
	Multiple pterygia
	Congenital myotonic dystrophy
Idiopathic (approx. 15% to 20%)	
Maternal	Severe diabetes mellitus
	Severe anemia
	Severe hypoproteinemia
Placental	Chorioangioma
	Venous thrombosis
	Cord torsion, knot or tumor

teinemia, hepatitis, arrhythmia, infection, and vascular or lymphatic obstruction (Fig. 45-6). Fluid collections are the end result of a redistribution of body fluids among the intravascular, intracellular, and interstitial compartments, secondary to an imbalance in capillary ultrafiltration and interstitial fluid return.[32] Hypoxia and/or circulatory failure may result in capillary damage which then leads to plasma protein and fluid loss from the intravascular compartment.[33] Animal models of hydrops utilizing induced tachycardia or fetal anemia suggest that elevations in venous pressures and venomotor tone lead to increased pressures in the microcirculation, causing fluid loss.[34]

Classification

Causes of NIH are most commonly **fetal** but may also be may be **maternal** or **placental** (see box above). **Maternal** causes (such as poorly controlled diabetes mellitus) are rare and should be differentiated from maternal complications that are secondary to fetal hydrops (such as preeclampsia). **Placental** causes (such as **chorioangiomata** and other vascular shunts) are relatively rare and are usually associated with high output failure states (see also Chapter 49).

Fetal Causes

A classification scheme for **fetal causes** is suggested in the box above. There is some overlap in the groupings, which may represent only associations and not causations. Many reports are from specialized units,[35] so certain rarer conditions tend to be overrepresented. Machin[7] has extensively reviewed cases from the past decade and has taken into account both general and specialized series.

Cardiovascular Anomalies. The most common causes in most series are **cardiovascular,** which

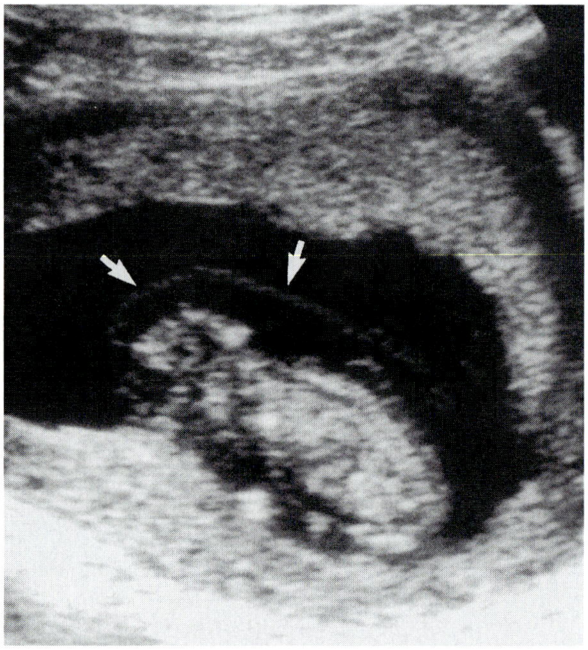

FIG. 45-7. Anasarca in an 11-week fetus with cystic hygroma. Sonogram shows the skin as a faint line *(arrows)* separated from the body by a rim of hypoechoic fluid.

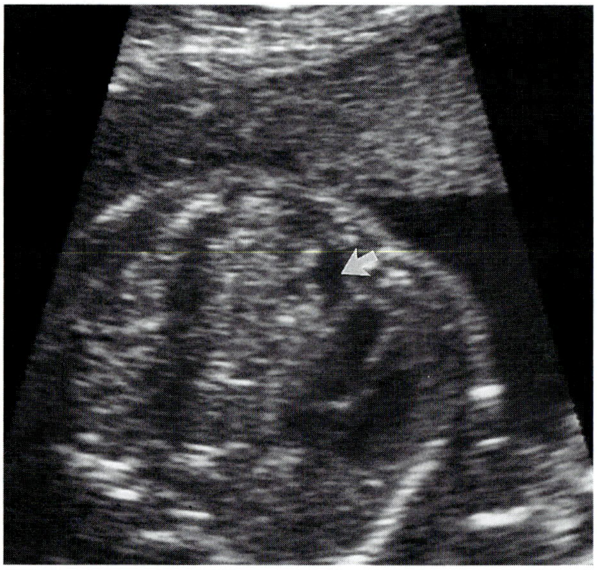

FIG. 45-8. Small pleural effusions seen in association with diaphragmatic hernia. Transverse view of the fetal thorax at 26 weeks shows the fluid as a small hypoechoic collection adjacent to the herniated bowel *(arrow)*. (Courtesy of Ants Toi, M.D., University of Toronto)

represent about 25% of cases.[8,36-40] These can be subdivided into structural malformations, arrhythmias, valvular disorders, tumors, premature closure of communicating structures, and high-output failure states. Of 50 fetuses from three series of hydrops in cardiac disease, 18 had **structural** disorders (36%), 17 had **tachyarrhythmias** (34%), 10 had **complete heart block** (CHB) (20%), and 5 had primary **myocardial** diseases (10%).[35,41,42] Structural and rhythm disorders of the fetal heart are discussed in more detail in Chapter 38.[39]

Structural cardiac anomalies. Numerous structural cardiac anomalies are associated with the development of hydrops. Most result in **congestive cardiac failure** *in utero* with associated right-sided outflow obstruction.[43] The presence of hydrops with congenital structural heart disease carries a dismal prognosis, with some series reporting no survivors.[44] Some fetuses with structural cardiac anomalies also have associated rhythm disturbances.

Arrhythmias. Arrhythmias associated with hydrops include both brady- and tachyarrhythmias. Tachyarrhythmias include **supraventricular tachycardia** (SVT) and **atrial fibrillation/flutter** which may be amenable to treatment. In one series of fetuses with tachycardia, 22 of 51 (43%) had signs of hydrops.[45] Of these 22 fetuses, 16 had SVT and 6 had atrial flutter. The mean ventricular rate in hydropic fetuses (249 beats per minute) was significantly higher than in nonhydropic cases (231 beats per minute).

CHB in particular is associated with a high incidence of structural cardiac malformations. A detailed fetal echocardiographic assessment is always warranted in cases of CHB.[35] Hydrops is seen more commonly with ventricular rates <60 beats per minute and where heart block accompanies structural abnormalities. The coexistence of structural heart disease with CHB has a very poor prognosis.[46] In fetal complete heart block (CHB) 30% to 50% of cases are associated with maternal anti-Ro (ssA) or anti-La (ssB) antibodies. **Umbilical vein pulsations** have been reported as a poor prognostic sign in the presence of cardiac failure.[47]

Neck/Thoracic Anomalies. Hydrops results from obstruction of venous or lymphatic return due to maldevelopment, compression, or kinking, or from cardiac tamponade. **Mediastinal masses, pleural effusions,** and **diaphragmatic hernias** may also cause NIH by similar mechanisms[48] (Fig. 45-8) (see also Chapter 16).

Gastrointestinal Anomalies. These relatively rare causes of NIH may be related to other primary pathology (e.g., infection).[49] Abdominal masses presumably act by compression of venous return, although hypoproteinemia or AV shunting may also play a role. **Meconium peritonitis** may be idiopathic or associated with fetal **cystic fibrosis** (CF) in 30% to 70% of cases.[50] Bowel rupture and leakage of contents results in an intense sterile chemical peritonitis, often

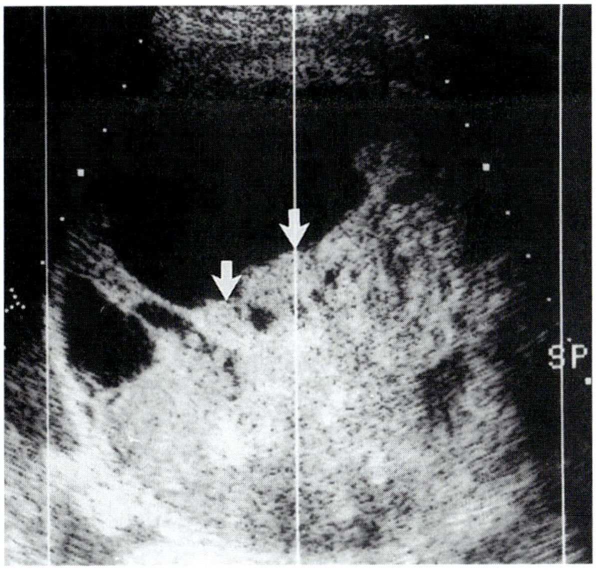

FIG. 45-9. Meconium peritonitis secondary to cystic fibrosis. Transverse view of fetal abdomen show ascites with matted, posteriorly positioned gut *(arrows)*; spine (SP).

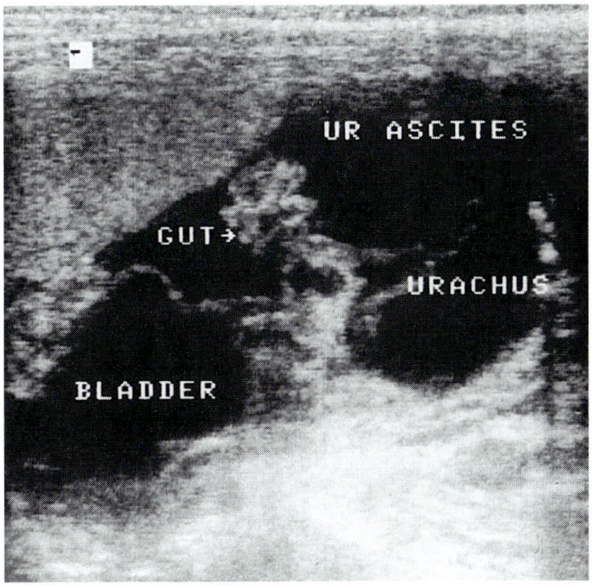

FIG. 45-10. Urinary ascites in obstructive uropathy with bladder rupture. Sonogram shows a large amount of ascites and a partially collapsed bladder in the presence of oligohydramnios.

with very marked ascites[51] (Fig. 45-9). Fluid collections may appear clear or particulate on ultrasound. The bowel will usually have a "bunched up" or "matted" appearance, and often flecks or areas of calcification will be visible. Where this diagnosis is suspected, the parents should be offered carrier testing for the common CF mutations.

Urinary Tract Anomalies. These are uncommon causes of NIH. It is unclear why hydrops may occur in lower urinary tract obstruction, although isolated ascites is usually urinary in origin following bladder rupture (Fig. 45-10). It is also common for urine to leak transiently into the peritoneal cavity following aspiration or shunting procedures for lower urinary tract obstruction (see also Chapter 37).

Chromosomal Anomalies. These comprise the second most common group, overall.[52] **Turner's syndrome** is classically associated with **cystic hygroma** in the first and early second trimester (see Chapters 40 and 42). Many of these disorders result in early spontaneous abortion. **Trisomies 21, 18, 13,** and **triploidy** have all been associated with NIH, although it is often unclear exactly why hydrops develops. The finding of multiple structural anomalies, a prominent cystic hygroma, or nuchal translucency may be suggestive of this etiology in the hydropic fetus. The physiological basis for thickened nuchal fold is not understood; however, it may be secondary to cardiovascular malformations in aneuploidy.[53]

Anemia. Anemia is due to decreased RBC production, increased hemolysis, or hemorrhage. If the process is gradual, the fetus mounts a compensatory erythropoietic response and NIH develops only when the anemia exceeds the fetal ability to keep pace.[14-16] Hydrops seems to result from a combination of high-output cardiac failure and hypoxic capillary damage causing protein leakage.

Decreased production. Affected homozygotes with **α-thalassaemia** cannot manufacture globin chains required to form HbF *in utero*, and HbA after birth.[54] Instead, Hb Bart is formed *in utero* that has such a high oxygen affinity that tissue hypoxia results, leading in turn to capillary damage, protein leakage, cardiac failure, and hydrops. Other causes of decreased production include a generalized marrow aplasia, as found in parvovirus infection,[55] or fetal leukemia.[37]

Hemolysis. G6PD deficiency has been reported as a rare cause of NIH resulting from increased hemolysis. Hemolysis may also play a part in the anemia that is secondary to *in utero* infection.

Hemorrhage. Blood loss may occur either into another fetus in **twin/twin transfusion syndrome** (TTTS),[56] into the fetus itself (e.g., intracranial), into a tumor (e.g., sacrococcygeal), or transplacentally.[7]

In TTTS, the donor is usually growth-restricted and anemic and may have severe **oligohydramnios** ("stuck twin"), whereas the recipient is usually larger

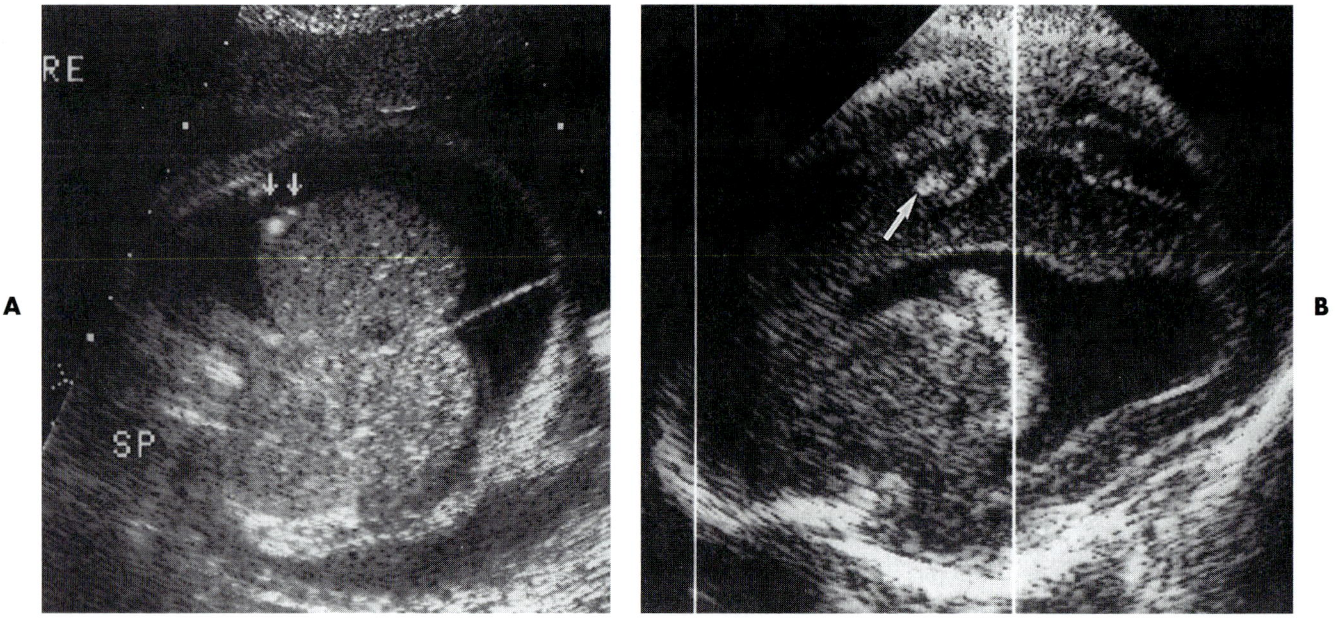

FIG. 45-11. A hydropic fetus with congenital toxoplasmosis at 33 weeks showing **A,** ascites with hepatic calcifications *(arrows);* spine (Sp). **B,** Ventriculomegaly with intracranial calcifications *(arrow).* This patient was commenced on high-dose antibiotic therapy, and the calcifications had resolved by the time of delivery.

and polycythemic with a persistently large bladder and associated hydramnios, giving the clinical picture of a **polyhydramnios/oligohydramnios sequence.**[56] It is thought that the recipient becomes hydropic because of volume overload, although this can also occur in the donor because of anemia and tissue hypoxia.[3] TTTS occurs only in **monochorionic** placentas, because of their vascular communications[57] (see Chapter 35).

Infection. Intrauterine infections may cause NIH as a result of multiple organ damage, hepatitis causing decreased protein production, or hypoxic capillary damage causing protein leakage[58] (Fig. 45-7). **Parvovirus, toxoplasmosis,** and **cytomegalovirus** (CMV) have a predilection for erythroid precursors and cause a generalized marrow aplasia.[38,55] The marrow may be particularly sensitive to infection between 17 and 22 weeks of gestation. In contrast to most other congenital infections, parvovirus is rarely associated with any adverse long-term sequelae. Spontaneous recovery from congenital parvovirus infections with hydrops has been reported.[59]

Toxoplasmosis may also cause anemia, intracerebral and intrahepatic calcifications, ventriculomegaly, and chorioretinitis, and can present with NIH, particularly ascites (Fig. 45-11 and Fig. 45-12). The prenatal diagnosis of toxoplasmosis can pose a difficult diagnostic challenge; it relies on the demonstration of maternal seroconversion and/or demonstration of the parasite in amniotic fluid by various PCR or isolation techniques.[60,61] **Rubella** and **syphilis** are still encountered as causes of NIH, predominantly in developing countries.

Genetic Conditions. A host of nonchromosomal genetic conditions may cause NIH,[52] and some are listed in the box on p. 1308. The mechanisms are poorly understood and are probably multifactorial. In storage diseases the most likely mechanism is hepatic infiltration resulting in hypoproteinemia or vascular obstruction.

Idiopathic Cases. The number of idiopathic cases of NIH (for which we still cannot identify an obvious cause) has decreased in recent series[6-8] and will continue to do so as our investigative abilities improve.

INVESTIGATION OF NONIMMUNE HYDROPS

A thorough, systematic prenatal evaluation can establish a cause for NIH in 80% to 85% of cases. This is important for the management of the current pregnancy and essential for future **genetic counseling.** The box on p. 1314 outlines a suggested protocol for the investigation of NIH, in which some investigations are recommended universally (unless a cause is immediately obvious), whereas others may be performed selectively.

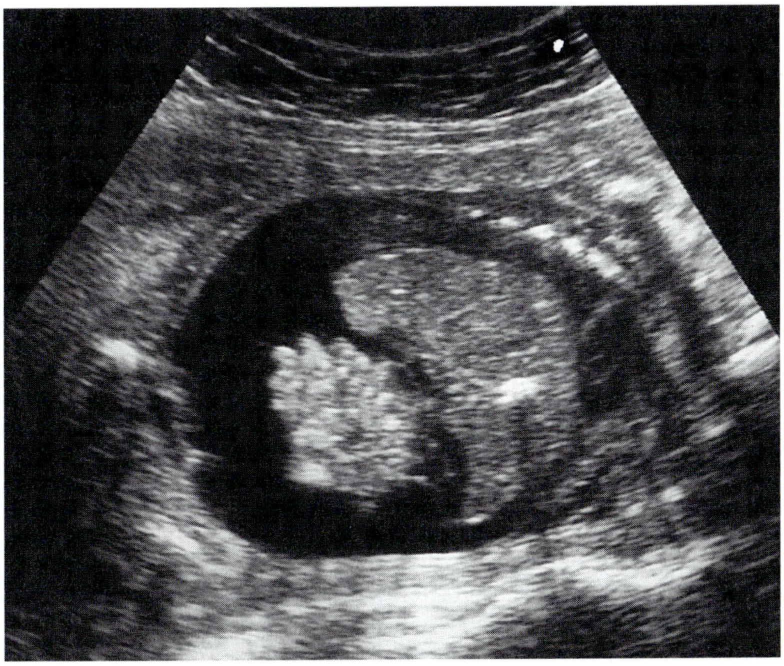

FIG. 45-12. NIH, intrauterine infection. View of fetal body shows massive ascites with fluid surrounding the liver and gut. There is a bright shadowing focus from a liver calcification.(Courtesy of Stephanie R. Wilson, M.D., University of Toronto).

History

A detailed history may provide the first clues to etiology and may help to prioritize the subsequent investigations. For example, homozygous α-thalassaemia is particularly prevalent in patients of Southeast Asian origin; a maternal history of SLE or diabetes may be relevant; previous pregnancy losses may be related to one of the inborn errors of metabolism or chromosomal rearrangements; the family history or the presence of consanguinity may suggest other genetic conditions; parvovirus infection is more likely to occur in teachers or daycare workers.[62]

Detailed Ultrasound

A comprehensive sonographic evaluation should be the initial step (see the top box on p. 1315). Polyhydramnios is a common association; indeed, a uterine fundus that is large for dates on clinical examination often prompts the initial ultrasound that identifies the hydrops. Collections of fluid in the body cavities and tissues are unmistakable (Fig. 45-1), and their relative distribution and timing of development may give a clue to the etiology.[40] A thorough **anatomical scan** may identify the responsible structural anomaly. Ultrasound "markers" may suggest a chromosomal cause[63] (see Chapter 40). The degree of polyhydramnios should be assessed, as it may pose an imminent threat of premature rupture of the membranes or preterm labor. The fetal bladder should be visualized to exclude urinary ascites due to bladder rupture. A systematic head-to-toe survey of fetal anatomy should be performed, searching for other clues to the etiology of the hydrops. Bone lengths and density should be evaluated to exclude skeletal dysplasias which may be associated with NIH. Stigmata of congenital infection such as microcephaly and calcification within the fetal brain or liver should be excluded. A dedicated fetal **echocardiographic** assessment is warranted in most cases.[35] Each finding should be evaluated in detail to determine if there are other structural abnormalities that may mimic hydrops (see the bottom box on p. 1315).

Maternal Investigations

The initial blood work should **exclude immune** hydrops by identifying maternal blood type and any RBC antibodies. Other baseline tests include a complete blood count (CBC) and indices, Kleihauer-Betke test, infection screen (TORCH and parvovirus IgG and IgM), and glucose. Further selective investigations are suggested in the box on p. 1314.

Fetal Investigations

Karyotype. Fetal karyotype may be determined from fetal blood, chorionic villi (CVS), amniotic fluid, or fluid from one of the fetal body cavities, as appropriate. This depends on gestation, accessibility, and urgency of the need for results. A rapid karyotype can be successfully obtained from fluid collections in most anatomical sites.[64]

Fluorescent *in situ* Hybridization (FISH) techniques can be used to count chromosomes for common aneuploidies (trisomies 13, 18, and 21 and monosomy X) as well as for identifying other specific

INVESTIGATION OF NONIMMUNE HYDROPS

History Age, racial background	
Occupation	Schoolteacher/daycare worker
Medical history	DM, SLE, hemoglobinopathy
Obstetrical history	Stillbirth, neonatal deaths
Family history	Stillbirths/recurrent miscarriages
	Congenital anomalies
	Inherited conditions
	Consanguinity
Complications during pregnancy	Vaginal bleeding
	Viral illness
Investigations **IN ALL CASES**	**IN SELECTED CASES ONLY**
Mother	
Indirect Coombs' test	Karyotype
Blood group	MSAFP
CBC and indices	Hb electrophoresis
Kleihauer-Betke	SS-A, SS-B antibodies
Glucose screen	Glucose tolerance test
TORCH/HPVB19 IgM, IgG	G6PD pyruvate kinase
VDRL	Uric acid, LFTs
	HLA typing
Father	Hb electrophoresis
	Karyotype
Fetus	
Ultrasound	Fetal echocardiogram
Detailed anatomy	Structure (2-D)
Amniotic fluid volume	M-mode
Doppler (venous and arterial)	Doppler
Biophysical profile	Color flow mapping
Nonstress test	
Fetal blood	
CBC, platelets	Hb electrophoresis
Direct Coombs' test	Blood gas
Blood group	
Karyotype	Liver function tests
WBC differential	Specific enzyme assays
TORCH/HPVB19 (IgM)	TORCH/HPVB19 (DNA)
Protein/albumin	Electron microscopy
Placenta Karyotype (CVS)	Specific metabolic tests
Amniotic fluid	
Karyotype/FISH	Viral DNA
CMV culture	L/S ratio
Other viral C&S	Restriction endonucleases
Bacterial C&S	Amniotic fluid AFP
	Organic acids
Fetal effusions	
Lymphocyte count (pleural)	Karyotype
Protein/albumin	Viral culture and/or DNA
Post mortem Placental pathology	Establish cell line
Full autopsy	Liver and muscle enzymes
Skeletal survey	
Neonate	Work-up similar to above, as appropriate

EVALUATION OF HYDROPS SHOULD INCLUDE A METHODICAL SONOGRAPHIC STUDY TO ASSESS THE FOLLOWING:

Fetus	Biometry
	Full anatomical study
	Careful search for associated structural anomalies
	Sonographic "markers" of aneuploidy
	Distribution and size of fluid collections
	Ascites
	Pleural effusions
	Pericardial effusions
	Distribution and thickness of skin edema
	Fetal echocardiography
	Normal bladder (usually excludes urinary ascites)
Placenta	Thickness
	Texture
	Exclusion of arteriovenous malformations
Amniotic fluid	Semiquantitative assessment
Functional assessment	Biophysical studies
	Doppler blood flow studies (arterial and venous)
	Functional cardiac assessment

STRUCTURES THAT MAY MIMIC HYDROPS ON ULTRASOUND

Abnormality in Hydrops	*May be falsely suggested by:*
Pleural effusions	Type I CCAML
	Diaphragmatic hernia
	Bronchogenic cyst
Ascites	Pseudoascites
	Obstructed or mature bowel
	Obstructive uropathy
	Hydrocoeles
Pericardial effusions	Cardiac aneurysms
	Pseudo/physiological effusions
Subcutaneous edema	Loop of umbilical cord
	Cystic hygroma
	Prominent fat layer in well-nourished fetus

deletions and chromosome rearrangements. This technique can provide a result from amniotic fluid specimens in 24 to 48 hours.[65,66] In practice, the confirmation or exclusion of the most common aneuplodies is usually sufficient to direct the management of the pregnancy.

Amniotic fluid is preferable for viral culture or PCR for toxoplasmosis and CMV,[61] and can also give an indication of fetal lung maturity in later gestations. CVS is an alternative at any gestation for obtaining a rapid karyotype or for DNA testing in specific circumstances. Although fetal karyotyping is an important part of the investigation of nonimmune hydrops, amniotic fluid or CVS specimens alone may not reveal the cause; thus, fetal blood sampling remains the diagnostic mainstay.

Fetal Blood Sampling (FBS). This is a key investigation in most cases. Basic fetal blood work should include a direct Coombs' test, CBC and indices, karyotype, protein, albumin, and viral-specific IgM. Other tests are done selectively (see top box in left column)[67] and some samples can be kept in storage for subsequent evaluation. With this approach, one can find an answer within 48 hours in the majority of cases. The risks of fetal loss due to this procedure is approximately 1.4%,[19,68] although in the sick fetus with NIH, loss rates of up to 7% to 25% may be more realistic.[69-71] Blood is usually sampled from the fixed cord root or the intrahepatic vein,[72] although less ideal alternatives are a free loop of cord or the heart.[73,74] If it is anticipated that the fetus may require transfusion (e.g., parvovirus infection), it is prudent to have some crossmatched blood ready, to avoid the risks of a second procedure. In the investigation of NIH, platelets should also be immediately available for any FBS in case the fetus is severely thrombocytopenic.

Cavity Aspiration. It is usually a simple matter to advance the needle simultaneously into the fetal chest, abdomen, or amniotic fluid at the time of FBS. This can be diagnostic (e.g., to diagnose chylothorax or for rapid karyotype[64]) and occasionally therapeutic, and it does not increase the overall procedure risk.

Other Investigations

After birth, the placenta should be sent for pathology and a **skeletal survey** may be helpful. If the baby is dead, permission for an **autopsy** should be obtained. If a metabolic condition is suspected to be the cause of the hydrops, then a fetal cell line should be established for future investigations. Further investigations may be prompted by additional physical findings. A genetics or fetal medicine opinion may help in identifying appropriate investigations and with particular counseling issues.[75] A comprehensive evaluation of each case greatly aids future genetic counseling.

FETAL WELFARE ASSESSMENT IN NONIMMUNE HYDROPS

If appropriate, fetal well-being should be assessed simultaneously.[76] It should be remembered that many of the tests for fetal well-being need careful interpretation in preterm pregnancies[77] (see also Chapter 34).

Ultrasound

Over recent years there has been increasing interest in the use of noninvasive ultrasound techniques for fetal welfare assessment in pregnancies complicated by NIH. All of the commonly used modalities have been studied, including biophysical assessment, pulsed Doppler velocitometry of the umbilical and intrafetal vessels, and functional cardiac assessment.

Fetal Doppler evaluation may give some indication of anemia,[28,29] well-being,[78-80] and cardiac failure.[81,82] Umbilical vein pulsations probably represent severe tricuspid valvular regurgitation and have been correlated with poor perinatal outcomes[47,81] (see also Chapter 49).

Functional Cardiac Assessment in Nonimmune Hydrops

Although not yet in routine clinical use, functional cardiac assessment may potentially offer a more accurate method for fetal welfare assessment in NIH and related conditions by indicating the degree of cardiac and circulatory failure.

It has been suggested that there are five measurements of **cardiac function** that may be useful in assessing the degree of cardiac decompensation. These include:

- Cardiothoracic ratio measurement to assess **cardiomegaly;**
- Assessment of **venous flow velocity waveforms** in the inferior vena cava, intrahepatic or umbilical veins, which will indicate the degree of tricuspid regurgitation;[47,82-84]
- **Tricuspid regurgitation,** which can be assessed directly using color flow;
- Measurement of **peak systolic velocities** in the descending aorta; and
- A measurement of cardiac contractility such as **ventricular shortening fractions,** which may be taken using an M-mode line, including both ventricles in the four-chamber view placed just below the A-V valves.

Invasive Testing

Fetal blood can be analyzed for gases and pH. Attempts have been made to correlate hypercarbia, hypoxia, and acidosis with outcomes and to compare these with other fetal welfare tests in IUGR pregnancies; however, their clinical utility seems limited, and there are few data on their significance in NIH.[85-88]

PRENATAL THERAPY

Cases in which some form of prenatal therapy has been successful, as determined by the birth of a healthy child, are identified in the box on p. 1317 (see also Chapter 50).

It is important to complete a full maternal and fetal work-up prior to consideration of prenatal therapy, as many fetuses will be excluded on the basis of nontreatable or lethal disorders.

Arrhythmias

Many of the tachyarrhythmias are amenable to **antiarrhythmic therapy,** almost always transplacentally; however, rarely direct fetal administration may be required[45,89] (see also Chapter 38). **Digoxin** has been the mainstay of treatment for many years, and maternal administration may require the use of high doses, sometimes to the extent of mild toxicity. Numerous other antiarrhythmics, including **flecainide, adenosine, verapamil,** and **amiodarone** at standard pediatric dosages (mg/kg), have been used. Digoxin has also been given when intrauterine congestive failure due to other causes is suspected, and it has even been empirically combined with lasix, albumin, and blood,[8] but without data to support its efficacy.

Twin Gestation

Untreated twin/twin transfusion syndrome (**TTTS**) has a very high mortality (90%),[56] and various interventions have been attempted (see also Chapter 35). Aggressive **serial amniocentesis** has become widely used to improve outcome.[90] Success with **fetoscopic laser ablation** of communicating vessels has also been reported.[91] It is currently not clear whether therapeutic amniocentesis or endoscopic techniques are associated with better outcomes, as current series show similar survival rates for both procedures (60% to 70%). **Selective fetocide** is contraindicated because of the risks to the other monochorionic twin. **Cord occlusion** and cord embolization have been attempted in acardiac twins to prevent cardiac failure in the donor.[8,92]

Pleural Drainage

Thoracic causes of NIH such as **chylothorax,** and congenital cystic adenomatoid malformation of the lung (**CCAML**) type 1 have been successfully treated by chest shunt insertion *in utero*.[93-96] The main rationale for invasive therapy in these cases is to prevent **pulmonary hypoplasia** and to prevent or reverse hydrops and hydramnios. Cases must be carefully selected, as some effusions may resolve spontaneously, whereas others proceed to develop NIH, hydramnios, and premature labor and/or intrauterine death.[97,98] **Aneuploidy** must be excluded in cases of chylothorax, as it is present in about 6% of these fetuses.[99]

THERAPY IN NONIMMUNE HYDROPS

Cause	Pathological Process	Therapy
Primary hydrothorax	Interrupted thoracic duct/mediastinal shift	Pleuroamniotic shunt placement
Parvovirus B19 infection	Anemia due to bone marrow suppression	Fetal red cell transfusion
Feto-maternal hemorrhage	Anemia	Fetal red cell transfusion
Twin/twin transfusion	?Hyper/hypovolemia	Therapeutic amniocentesis/ laser ablation
Cardiac tachyarrhythmia	Decreased cardiac output	Antiarrhythmic drugs
Cardiac bradyarrhythmia	Decreased cardiac output	Cardiac pacing Positive chronotropes
Obstructive uropathy	Probably back pressure effects	Shunt placement
Diaphragmatic hernia	Lung compression	Shunt placement or aspiration Open fetal surgery
Chest masses	Probably pressure effects and SVC kinking	Shunt placement or aspiration Open fetal surgery
Toxoplasmosis	Infection	Antibiotics

We drain all isolated large effusions initially, using a fine needle. The analysis of this fluid may suggest a diagnosis (e.g., high lymphocyte count),[100] allows rapid karyotyping,[64] evaluates the ability of the lung to reexpand, and may occasionally be therapeutic. Effusions that recollect rapidly may benefit from ongoing drainage, and shunt placement should be considered. Therapeutic drainage immediately prior to delivery may facilitate neonatal resuscitation.[101]

Obstructive Uropathy

Urinary tract obstructions are rarely associated with NIH, although they may present as urinary ascites. Vesicoamniotic drainage may have a role in carefully selected cases. No prenatal drainage procedures have yet been subjected to scientific scrutiny by randomized trials.

Diaphragmatic Hernia

NIH related to a diaphragmatic hernia has been successfully treated by thoracentesis.[102] Several cases of diaphragmatic hernias, CCAML,[103] and sacrococcygeal teratoma[104] causing progressive hydrops have been definitively repaired antenatally, although open fetal surgery has been associated with high loss rates, mainly due to preterm labor.

Anemia

The most significant application of fetal therapy is in fetal anemia. Initially, fetal transfusion was confined to Rh disease[15] but the same principles and expertise have been applied to nonimmune causes of anemia such as **parvovirus** infection[105] and severe **fetomaternal hemorrhage.**[106] It is very controversial as to whether fetal transfusion should be offered for otherwise lethal conditions such as homozygous α-thalassaemia. Theoretically, there might be a role in G6PD deficiency. **Stem cell transfusion** is an exciting potential future option for some genetic causes of NIH.[107]

Infections

Maternal or fetal **antibiotic** therapy is possible in various fetal infections leading to NIH.[60] However, in most infections, apart from parvovirus and toxoplasmosis, there may be major adverse long-term sequelae which may be a contraindication for such treatment. By the time hydrops occurs, irreversible damage may have been done. Some adverse sequelae may be prevented by early diagnosis and antenatal antibiotic therapy. This is particularly true for infections due to toxoplasmosis and it underlines the need for accurate antenatal diagnosis.[60,61] Aggressive prenatal antibiotic therapy instituted at diagnosis can result in resolution of the intracerebral calcifications by the time of delivery.

Idiopathic Cases

In cases where all known causes of hydrops have been excluded, survival rates of up to 70% have been reported with the appropriate use of antenatal treatment.[6,108]

PROGNOSIS

The overall **mortality** in NIH as a whole is still high.[6,8] Some of the improvement over earlier reports[3,36] is attributable to the growing number of cases that are amenable to ***in utero* therapy.** Unfortunately, the majority of cases still represent a terminal process that may be irreversible; that explains the grim outlook for many fetuses. Although the prognosis overall has improved somewhat in recent years, most series are small and represent variable mixtures of causes, so they are difficult to compare.[109] Attempts have been made to identify predictors of outcome in NIH with limited success.[47,110] The key to further improvement in prognosis lies in early comprehensive evaluation and accurate diagnosis, with the institution of appropriate **prenatal therapy.** Pregnancies should no longer be "written off" as prenatal treatment may be beneficial in carefully selected cases.

OBSTETRICAL MANAGEMENT

Counseling

Counseling a couple with the recent diagnosis of hydrops is a challenge. It is impossible to be specific about prognosis without a diagnosis, emphasizing the need for a diagnostic workup as described above. In the first and early second trimesters, many couples will opt for pregnancy termination with or without investigation because of the poor outlook of these gestations. Nonetheless, it is important to complete the diagnostic workup because of the implications for future pregnancies. A discussion regarding invasive procedures should include the realistic appraisal of risks and benefits. A **team approach,** with consultation involving neonatology, obstetrics, pediatric surgery, and genetics will usually assist patients in making informed choices.[111]

Maternal Complications

Maternal complications may occur in association with NIH. Hypoproteinemia, edema, hypertension, and laboratory findings consistent with a diagnosis of **preeclampsia** may develop.[112] This association was noted previously with severe Rh disease and was often called the **"mirror syndrome,"** where edema develops in the mother of a hydropic fetus. We have seen dramatic amelioration of this condition once the fetal problem has resolved. The maternal condition may occasionally be severe enough to warrant delivery.

Fetal Monitoring

Ongoing viable pregnancies should be closely monitored for **fetal well-being** until delivery by biophysical profile scoring, including nonstress test (NST) and Doppler analysis of fetal hemodynamics as described above (see also Chapter 49).

Delivery

Mode of delivery should be decided on usual obstetrical grounds, taking into account the underlying prognosis.[113] Uterine overdistention secondary to hydramnios carries the dangers of **abruptio placenta** or **cord prolapse** when the membranes rupture. There is an increased risk of postpartum hemorrhage due to uterine atony. Prematurity secondary to hydramnios is a major contributing factor to the poor outcome of some neonates, and both **therapeutic amniocentesis** and **indomethacin** have been used to decrease the amniotic fluid volume,[114] although the latter therapy should be used with caution after 32 weeks because of the potential for premature ductus arteriosus closure *in utero*.

Predelivery Aspiration Procedures

Fluid collections may be drained under ultrasound guidance prior to delivery to assist with neonatal **resuscitation.**[100] This is particularly applicable to pleural effusions. Massive ascites may also be drained to prevent dystocia, particularly when vaginal birth is planned. Therapeutic amniocentesis prior to induction of labor may be considered in cases with massive hydramnios to decrease the chance of malpresentation and cord prolapse.

Recurrence Risk Evaluation

An assessment of recurrence risk for future pregnancies depends on making an accurate diagnosis. For this reason, autopsy examination is to be recommended to parents in cases of fetal loss, especially for cases where a definitive diagnosis has not been made during the pregnancy. Where consent for autopsy is denied, useful diagnostic information may sometimes be obtained from radiographs, clinical photography (Fig. 45-13), and studies of cord blood. Rarely have recurrences been reported for apparently idiopathic cases.[115]

NEONATAL MANAGEMENT

The diagnosis of NIH presents a challenge to the neonatologist in terms of both management and diagnosis. Antenatal diagnosis permits delivery in an appropriate setting with neonatal personnel in attendance. At our institution, 76% of cases of NIH were diagnosed more than 24 hours before delivery. Only 9% of cases were undiagnosed before delivery.

Delivery Room Stabilization

All viable pregnancies complicated by hydrops should be delivered at a tertiary care center with facilities for neonatal resuscitation and subsequent diagnosis and management. Ultrasound examination shortly prior to delivery is helpful to delineate the presence and extent of pleural/pericardial effusions and ascites. It is important to have this information to ascertain what equipment may be necessary and what procedures may be required for stabilization following delivery. At our center, approximately 48% of infants with NIH required full cardiopulmonary resuscitation (CPR) at the time of delivery, and 60% required drainage of one or more body cavities.

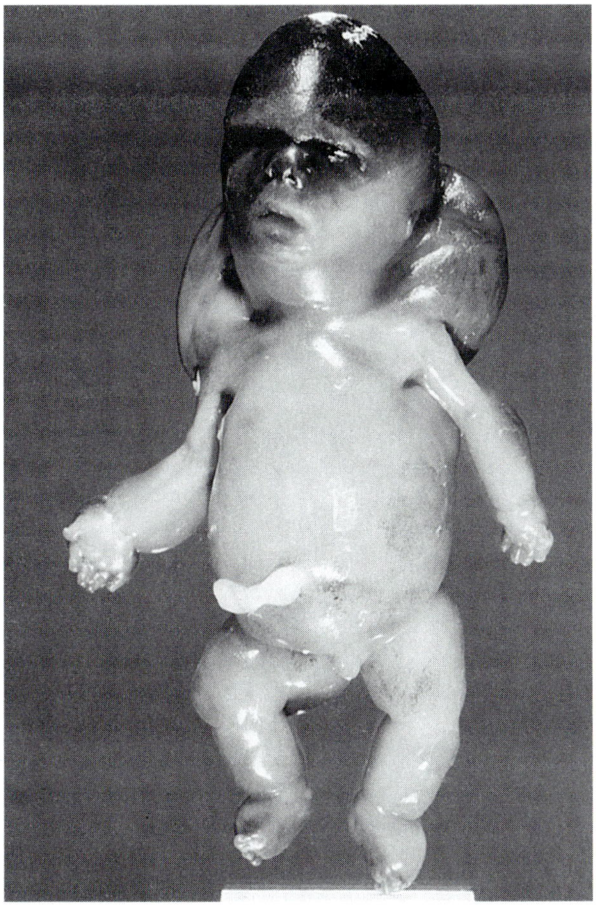

FIG. 45-13. Fetus with hydrops. A postmortem photograph shows prominent bilateral cystic hygromas in addition to diffuse subcutaneous edema.

Resuscitation of infants with NIH always follows the standard ABCs of resuscitation:

Airway. Intubation may be difficult, as edema may impair visualization of the cords.

Breathing. Many infants require some form of assisted ventilation, often with high pressures (>25 cm H_2O). The presence of pulmonary hypoplasia or pleural effusions and ascites that inhibit chest expansion may make ventilation difficult. Endotracheal surfactant administration may improve ventilation. Using information from antenatal ultrasound, needle thoracentesis, chest tube insertion, or paracentesis may greatly facilitate ventilation. Ultrasound guidance may be helpful in these procedures. Pericardiocentesis is required only in extreme situations.

Circulation. Despite the presence of edema, these infants often have a decreased intravascular volume and require the use of an appropriate volume expander (saline, albumin, blood). Lines should be placed in the umbilical artery and vein for ongoing monitoring and intravenous access. Administration of inotropes may be required.

Investigations

Neonatal investigations should represent a continuation of antenatal investigations and be geared toward the suspected etiology. Ultrasound of the chest/abdomen may need to be obtained. Ultrasound may be used to follow the extent of pleural effusions postnatally, thus minimizing radiation exposure. An **echocardiogram** may be necessary to obtain an anatomic diagnosis and assess ventricular function. **Cranial ultrasound** examination should be performed to document the presence of intraventricular hemorrhage and/or periventricular leukomalacia.

Outcome

A review of 46 cases of NIH who delivered at our institution beyond 24 weeks gestation showed an overall **mortality** of 44%.[116] Six infants were stillborn, 12 cases were resolved *in utero* before delivery, and 14 infants were liveborn but died after birth. Predictors of mortality were the presence of congenital anomalies and/or chromosomal abnormalities. There are few data regarding long-term outcome in survivors.

CONCLUSION

Hydrops usually represents a state of fetal decompensation, in response to a variety of insults. Immune causes have been successfully treated *in utero* for over a decade, whereas nonimmune causes, until recently, have carried a 100% mortality. An increasing number of these are now also becoming amenable to prenatal therapy, with the potential for a good outcome. Care should be provided by a coordinated team of perinatologists, sonographers, neonatologists, and geneticists to optimize selection of those cases that may be most appropriate for antenatal therapeutic intervention. A comprehensive approach should be taken to the investigation of hydrops, both for the management of the index case and for future counseling; the cornerstones of which are detailed ultrasound and invasive fetal testing. Early referral to a tertiary perinatal center is essential for optimal management of this condition.

REFERENCES

1. Freda V, Gorman J, Pollack W. Rh factor: prevention of immunization and clinical trial on mothers. *Science* 1966; 151:828-830.
2. Bowman J. The management of Rh-isoimmunization. *Obstet Gynecol* 1978:52:385.
3. Macafee C, Fortune D, Beischer N. Non-immunological hydrops fetalis. *Br J Obstet Gynaecol* 1970:77:226-237.
4. Ballantyne J. *The Diseases and Deformities of the Fetus.* Edinburgh: Oliver & Boyd; 1892.
5. Potter E. Universal edema of the fetus unassociated with erythroblastosis. *Am J Obstet Gynecol* 1943;43:130-134.

6. Anandakumar C, Biswas A, Wong YC et al. Management of non-immune hydrops: 8 years' experience. *Ultrasound Obstet Gynecol* 1996;8:196-200.
7. Machin GA. Hydrops revisited: literature review of 1,414 cases published in the 1980s. *Am J Med Genet* 1989;34:366-390.
8. Hansmann M, Gembruch U, Bald R. New therapeutic aspects in nonimmune hydrops fetalis based on four hundred and two prenatally diagnosed cases. *Fetal Diagn Ther* 1989;4:29-36.
9. Andersen H, Hutchinson A, Fortune D. Non-immune hydrops fetalis: changing contribution to perinatal mortality. *Br J Obstet Gynaecol* 1983;90:636-639.

Sonographic Features of Hydrops

10. Hashimoto BE, Filly RA, Callen PW. Fetal pseudoascites: further anatomic observations. *J Ultrasound Med* 1986;5:151-152.
11. Hoddick WK, Mahony BS, Callen PW et al. Placental thickness. *J Ultrasound Med* 1985;4:479-482.
12. Chitkara U, Wilkins I, Lynch L et al. The role of sonography in assessing severity of fetal anemia in Rh- and Kell-isoimmunized pregnancies. *Obstet Gynecol* 1988;71:393-398.
13. Nicolaides KH, Fontanarosa M, Gabbe SG et al. Failure of ultrasonographic parameters to predict the severity of fetal anemia in rhesus isoimmunization. *Am J Obstet Gynecol* 1988;158:920-926.

Immune Hydrops

14. Nicolaides K, Warenski J, Rodeck C. The relationship of fetal plasma protein concentration and hemoglobin level to the development of hydrops in rhesus isoimmunization. *Am J Obstet Gynecol* 1985;152:341-344.
15. Ryan G, Morrow RJ. Fetal blood transfusion. *Clin Perinatol* 1994;21:573-589.
16. Nicolaides K. Studies on fetal physiology and pathophysiology in rhesus disease. *Semin Perinatol* 1989;13:328-337.
17. Soothill PW, Nicolaides KH, Rodeck CH. Effect of anemia on fetal acid-base status. *Br J Obstet Gynecol* 1987;94:880-883.
18. Rodeck C, Kemp J, Holman C et al. Direct intravascular fetal blood transfusion in severe rhesus isoimmunization. *Lancet* 1981;625-627.
19. Daffos F, Capella-Povolsky M, Forestier F. Fetal blood sampling during pregnancy with use of a needle guided by ultrasound: a study of 606 consecutive cases. *Am J Obstet Gynecol* 1985;153:655-660.
20. Menticoglou SM, Harman CR, Manning FA et al. Intraperitoneal fetal transfusion: paralysis inhibits red cell absorption. *Fetal Ther* 1987;2:154-159.
21. Harman C, Bowman J, Manning F et al. Intrauterine transfusion—intraperitoneal versus intravascular approach: a case-control comparison. *Am J Obstet Gynecol* 1990;162:1053-1059.
22. Tannirandorn Y, Rodeck CH. New approaches in the treatment of hemolytic disease of the fetus. *Baillieres Clin Haematol* 1990;3:289-320.
23. Oepkes D. Ultrasonography and Doppler in the management of red cell alloimmunized pregnancies. *Rijksuniversiteit of Leiden* 1995.
24. Oepkes D, Brand R, Vandenbussche FP et al. The use of ultrasonography and Doppler in the prediction of fetal hemolytic anemia: a multivariate analysis. *Br J Obstet Gynaecol* 1994;101:680-684.
25. Oepkes D, Meerman RH, Vandenbussche FP et al. Ultrasonographic fetal spleen measurements in red blood cell-alloimmunized pregnancies. *Am J Obstet Gynecol* 1993;169:121-128.
26. Copel JA, Grannum PA, Belanger K et al. Pulsed Doppler flow-velocity waveforms before and after intrauterine intravascular transfusion for severe erythroblastosis fetalis. *Am J Obstet Gynecol* 1988;158:768-774.
27. Warren PS, Gill RW, Fisher CC. Doppler flow studies in rhesus isoimmunization. *Semin Perinatol* 1987;11:375-378.
28. Mari G, Moise KJJ, Deter RL et al. Flow velocity waveforms of the vascular system in the anemic fetus before and after intravascular transfusion for severe red blood cell alloimmunization. *Am J Obstet Gynecol* 1990;162:1060-1064.
29. Mari G, Adrignolo A, Abuhamad AZ. Diagnosis of fetal anemia with Doppler ultrasound in the pregnancy complicated by maternal blood group immunization. *Ultrasound Obstet Gynecol* 1995;5:400-405.
30. Moise KJJ, Mari G, Fisher DJ et al. Acute fetal hemodynamic alterations after intrauterine transfusion for treatment of severe red blood cell alloimmunization. *Am J Obstet Gynecol* 1990;163:776-784.
31. Oepkes D, Vandenbussche FP, Van Bel F et al. Fetal ductus venosus blood flow velocities before and after transfusion in red-cell alloimmunized pregnancies. *Obstet Gynecol* 1993;82:237-241.

Nonimmune Hydrops (NIH)

32. Apkon M. Pathophysiology of hydrops fetalis. *Semin Perinatol* 1995;19:437-446.
33. Blair DK, Vander Straten MC, Gest AL. Hydrops in fetal sheep from rapid induction of anemia. *Pediatr* 1994;35:560-564.
34. Stevens DC, Hilliard JK, Schreiner RL et al. Supraventricular tachycardia with edema, ascites, and hydrops in fetal sheep. *Am J Obstet Gynecol* 1982;142:316-322.
35. Allan L, Crawford D, Sheridan R. Etiology of nonimmune hydrops: the value of echocardiography. *Br J Obstet Gynaecol* 1986;93:223-228.
36. Machin GA. Differential diagnosis of hydrops fetalis. *Am J Med Genet* 1981;9:341-350.
37. Watson J, Campbell S. Antenatal evaluation and management in nonimmune hydrops fetalis. *Obstet Gynecol* 1986;67:589-593.
38. Holzgreve W, Curry C, Golbus M et al. Investigation of nonimmune hydrops fetalis. *Am J Obstet Gynecol* 1984;150:805-812.
39. Poeschmann RP, Verheijen RH, Van Dongen PW. Differential diagnosis and causes of nonimmunological hydrops fetalis: a review. *Obstet Gynecol* 1991;46:223-231.
40. Saltzman DH, Frigoletto FD, Harlow BL et al. Sonographic evaluation of hydrops fetalis. *Obstet Gynecol* 1989;74:106-111.
41. Hornberger L. Hydrops and congenital heart disease. Ontario-Quebec *Perinatal Investigators Meeting*. Kingston, Canada, 1996.
42. Kleinman CS, Donnerstein RL, DeVore GR et al. Fetal echocardiography for evaluation of *in utero* congestive heart failure. *N Engl J Med* 1982;306:568-575.
43. Groves AM, Fagg NL, Cook AC et al. Cardiac tumors in intrauterine life. *Arch Dis Child* 1992;67:1189-1192.
44. Hornberger LK, Sahn DJ, Kleinman CS et al. Tricuspid valve disease with significant tricuspid insufficiency in the fetus: diagnosis and outcome. *JACC* 1991;17:167-173.
45. Van Engelen AD, Weijtens O, Brenner JI et al. Management outcome and follow-up of fetal tachycardia. *JACC* 1994;24:1371-1375.
46. Schmidt KG, Ulmer HE, Silverman NH et al. Perinatal outcome of fetal complete atrioventricular block: a multicenter experience. *JACC* 1991;17:1360-1366.
47. Gudmundsson S, Huhta JC, Wood DC et al. Venous Doppler ultrasonography in the fetus with nonimmune hydrops. *Am J Obstet Gynecol* 1991;164:33-37.
48. Giacoia GP Right-sided diaphragmatic hernia associated with superior vena cava syndrome. *Am J Perinatol* 1994;11:129-131.
49. Pletcher BA, Williams MK, Mulivor RA et al. Intrauterine cytomegalovirus infection presenting as fetal meconium peritonitis. *Obstet Gynecol* 1991;78:903-905.

50. Irish MS, Gollin Y, Borowitz DS et al. Meconium ileus: antenatal diagnosis and perinatal care. *Fetal Maternal Med Rev* 1996;8:79-93.
51. Mayock DE, Hickok DE, Guthrie RD. Cystic meconium peritonitis associated with hydrops fetalis. *Am J Obstet Gynecol* 1982;142:704-705.
52. Jauniaux E, Van Maldergem L, De Munter C et al. Nonimmune hydrops fetalis associated with genetic abnormalities. *Obstet Gynecol* 1990;75:568-572.
53. Morosco G. Fetal nuchal translucency: a need to understand the physiological basis. *Ultrasound Obstet Gynecol.* 1995; 5:6-8.
54. Tan SL, Tseng AM, Thong PW. Bart's hydrops fetalis—clinical presentation and management—an analysis of 25 cases. *Aust N Z J Obstet Gynaecol* 1989;29:233-237.
55. Anand A, Gray ES, Brown T et al. Human parvovirus infection in pregnancy and hydrops fetalis. *N Engl J Med* 1987;316:183-186.
56. Blickstein I. The twin-twin transfusion syndrome. *Obstet Gynecol* 1990;76:714-722.
57. Bajoria R, Wigglesworth J, Fisk NM. Angioarchitecture of monochorionic placentas in relation to the twin-twin transfusion syndrome. *Am J Obstet Gynecol* 1995;172:856-863.
58. Barron S, Pass R. Infectious causes of hydrops fetalis. *Semin Perinatol* 1995;19:493-501.
59. Humphrey W, Magoon M, O'Shaughnessy R. Severe nonimmune hydrops secondary to parvovirus B-19 infection: spontaneous reversal *in utero* and survival of a term infant. *Obstet Gynecol* 1991;78:900-902.
60. Daffos F, Forestier F, Capella-Povolsky M. Prenatal management of 746 pregnancies at risk for congenital toxoplasmosis. *N Engl J Med* 1988;318:271-275.
61. Boyer KM, McAuley JB. Congenital toxoplasmosis. *Semin Pediatric Infectios Dis* 1994;5:42-51.

Investigation of Nonimmune Hydrops

62. Adler SP, Manganello AM, Koch WC et al. Risk of human parvovirus B19 infections among school and hospital employees during endemic periods. *J Infect Dis* 1993;168:361-368.
63. Benacerraf B. Prenatal sonography of autosomal trisomies. *Ultrasound Obstet Gynecol* 1991;1:66-75.
64. Teoh TG, Ryan G, Johnson JM et al. The role of fetal karyotyping from unconventional sources. *Am J Obstet Gynecol* 1996;175:873-877.
65. Divane A, Carter NP, Spathas DH et al. Rapid prenatal diagnosis of aneuploidy from uncultured amniotic fluid cells using five-color fluorescence *in situ* hybridization. *Prenat Diagn* 1994;14:1061-1069.
66. Ward BE, Gersen SL, Carelli MP et al. Rapid prenatal diagnosis of chromosomal aneuploidies by fluorescence *in situ* hybridization: clinical experience with 4,500 specimens. *Am J Hum Genet* 1993;52:854-865.
67. Galjaard H. Fetal diagnosis of inborn errors of metabolism. *Baillieres Clin Obstet Gynecol* 1987;1:547-567.
68. Ghidini A, Sepulveda W, Lockwood CJ et al. Complications of fetal blood sampling. *Am J Obstet Gynecol* 1993;168:1339-1344.
69. Bernaschek G, Yildiz A, Kolankaya A et al. Complications of cordocentesis in high-risk pregnancies: effects on fetal loss or preterm delivery. *Prenat Diagn* 1995;15:995-1000.
70. Maxwell DJ, Johnson P, Hurley P et al. Fetal blood sampling and pregnancy loss in relation to indication. See comments. *Br J Obstet Gynaecol* 1991;98:892-897.
71. Weiner C, Wenstrom K, Sipes S et al. Risk factors for cordocentesis and fetal intravascular transfusion. *Am J Obstet Gynecol* 1991;165:1020-1025.
72. Nicolini U, Nicolaidis P, Fisk N. Fetal blood sampling from the intrahepatic vein: analysis of safety and clinical experience with 214 procedures. *Obstet Gynecol* 1990;76:47-53.
73. Westgren M, Selbing A, Stangenberg M. Fetal intracardiac transfusions in patients with severe rhesus isoimmunisation. *Br Med J* 1988;296:885-886.
74. Ryan G, Rodeck CH. Fetal blood sampling. In: Simpson JL, Elias S, eds. *Essentials of Prenatal Diagnosis.* New York: Churchill Livingstone, 1993.
75. Evans MI, Hume RF, Jr., Johnson MP et al. Integration of genetics and ultrasonography in prenatal diagnosis: just looking is not enough. *Am J Obstet Gynecol* 1996;174:1925-1931.

Fetal Welfare Assessment in Nonimmune Hydrops

76. Manning F. Assessment of fetal condition and risk: analysis of single and combined biophysical variable monitoring. *Semin Perinatol* 1985;9:168.
77. Challis DE, Trudinger BJ. Assessment of well-being in the preterm fetus. *Fetal Maternal Med Rev* 1995;7:13-29.
78. Rizzo G, Capponi A, Arduini D et al. The value of fetal arterial, cardiac and venous flows in predicting pH and blood gases measured in umbilical blood at cordocentesis in growth-retarded fetuses. *Br J Obstet Gynaecol* 1995;102:963-969.
79. Gembruch U, Krapp M, Baumann P. Changes of venous blood flow velocity waveforms in fetuses with supraventricular tachycardia. *Ultrasound Obstet Gynecol* 1995;5:394-399.
80. Respondek ML, Kammermeier M, Ludomirsky A et al. The prevalence and clinical significance of fetal tricuspid valve regurgitation with normal heart anatomy. *Am J Obstet Gynecol* 1994;171:1265-1270.
81. Tulzer G, Gudmundsson S, Wood DC et al. Doppler in nonimmune hydrops fetalis. *Ultrasound Obstet Gynecol* 1994; 4:279-283.
82. Chiba Y, Kanzaki T. Fetal cardiac function in non-immune hydrops. In: Arduini D, Rizzo G, Romanini C, eds. *Fetal Cardiac Function.* New York: Parthenon Publishing, 1995.
83. Chiba Y, Kobayashi H, Kanzaki T. Quantitative analysis of cardiac function in non-immunological hydrops fetalis. *Fetal Diagn Ther*, 1990;5:175-188.
84. Tulzer G, Gudmundsson S, Huhta JC et al. The value of Doppler in evaluation and prognosis of fetuses with nonimmunologic hydrops fetalis. *Gynakol Rundsch* 1991;2:152-153.
85. Sonek J, Nicolaides KH. The role of cordocentesis in the diagnosis of fetal well-being. *Clin Perinatol* 1994;21:743-764.
86. Yoon BH, Romero R, Roh CR. Relationship between the fetal biophysical profile score, umbilical artery Doppler velocimetry, and fetal blood acid-base status determined by cordocentesis. *Am J Obstet Gynecol* 1993;169:1586-1594.
87. Soothill PW, Ajayi RA, Campbell S et al. Fetal oxygenation at cordocentesis, maternal smoking and childhood neuro-development. *Eur J Obstet Gynecol Reprod Biol* 1995;59:21-24.
88. Nicolini U, Nicolaidis P, Fisk NM. Limited role of fetal blood sampling in prediction of outcome in intrauterine growth retardation. *Lancet* 1990;336:768.

Prenatal Therapy

89. Hansmann M, Gembruch U, Bald R et al. Fetal tachyarrhythmias: transplacental and direct treatment of the fetus: a report of 60 cases. *Ultrasound Obstet Gynecol* 1991;1:162-170.
90. Elliott JP, Urig MA, Clewell WH. Aggressive therapeutic amniocentesis for treatment of twin-twin transfusion syndrome. *Obstet Gynecol* 1991;77:537-540.
91. Ville Y, Hecher K, Ogg D et al. Successful outcome after Nd: YAG laser separation of chorioangiopagus twins under sonoendoscopic control. *Ultrasound Obstet Gynecol* 1992; 2:429-431.
92. Quintero RA, Romero R, Reich H et al. *In utero* percutaneous umbilical cord ligation in the management of complicated monochorionic multiple gestations. *Ultrasound Obstet Gynecol* 1996;8:16-22.

93. Morrow RJ, Macphail S, Johnson J et al. Mid-trimester thoraco-amniotic shunting for the treatment of fetal hydrops. *Fetal Diagn Ther* 1995;10:92-94.
94. Weiner C, Varner M, Pringle K et al. Antenatal diagnosis and palliative treatment of nonimmune hydrops fetalis secondary to pulmonary extralobar sequestration. *Obstet Gynecol* 1986;68:275-280.
95. Rodeck C, Fisk N, Fraser D et al. Long-term in utero drainage of fetal hydrothorax. *N Engl J Med* 1988;319:1135-1138.
96. Nicolaides KH, Azar GB. Thoraco-amniotic shunting. *Fetal Diagn Ther* 1990;5:153-164.
97. Weber AM, Philipson EH. Fetal pleural effusion: a review and meta-analysis for prognostic indicators. *Obstet Gynecol* 1992;79:281-286.
98. Hagay Z, Reece A, Roberts A et al. Isolated fetal pleural effusion: a prenatal management dilemma. *Obstet Gynecol* 1993; 81:147-152.
99. Achiron R, Weissman A, Lipitz S et al. Fetal pleural effusion: the risk of fetal trisomy. *Gynecol Obstet Invest* 1995;39:153-156.
100. Eddleman KA, Levine AB, Chitkara U et al. Reliability of pleural fluid lymphocyte counts in the antenatal diagnosis of congenital chylothorax. *Obstet Gynecol* 1991;78:530-532.
101. Cardwell MS. Aspiration of fetal pleural effusions or ascites may improve neonatal resuscitation. *South Med J* 1996;89: 177-178.
102. Benacerraf BR, Frigoletto FD Jr. *In utero* treatment of a fetus with diaphragmatic hernia complicated by hydrops. *Am J Obstet Gynecol* 1986;155:817-818.
103. Harrison MR, Adzick NS, Jennings RW et al. Antenatal intervention for congenital cystic adenomatoid malformation. *Lancet* 1990;336:965-967.
104. Bullard K. Before the horse is out of the barn: fetal surgery for hydrops. *Semin Perinatol* 1995;19:462-473.
105. Sahakian V, Weiner CP, Naides SJ et al. Intrauterine transfusion treatment of nonimmune hydrops fetalis secondary to human parvovirus B19 infection. *Am J Obstet Gynecol* 1991; 164:1090-1091.
106. Cardwell M. Successful treatment of hydrops fetalis caused by fetomaternal hemorrhage: a case report. *Am J Obstet Gynecol* 1988;158:131.
107. Johnson J, Elias S. Prenatal treatment: medical and gene therapy in the fetus. *Clin Obstet Gynecol* 1988;31:390-406.
108. Ayida GA, Soothill PW, Rodeck CH. Survival in non-immune hydrops fetalis without malformation or chromosomal abnormalities after invasive treatment. *Fetal Diagn Ther* 1995; 10:101-105.

Prognosis

109. Wilson DC, Halliday HL, McClure G et al. The changing pattern of fetal hydrops. *Ulster Med J* 1990;59:119-121.
110. Carlson DE, Platt LD, Medearis AL et al. Prognostic indicators of the resolution of nonimmune hydrops fetalis and survival of the fetus. *Am J Obstet Gynecol* 1990;163:1785-1787.

Obstetrical Management

111. Steiner R. Hydrops fetalis: role of the geneticist. *Semin Perinatol* 1995;19:516-524.
112. Van Selm M, Kanhai H, Gravenhorst J. Maternal hydrops syndrome: a review. *Obstet Gynecol Surv* 1991;46:785-788.
113. Kuller JA, Katz VL, Wells Sr et al. Cesarean delivery for fetal malformations. *Obstet Gynecol Surv* 1996;51:371-375.
114. Kirshon B, Mari G, Moise K. Indomethacin therapy in the treatment of symptomatic polyhydramnios. *Obstet Gynecol* 1990;75:202-205.
115. Harper A, Kenny B, O'Hara MD et al. Recurrent idiopathic non-immunologic hydrops fetalis: a report of two families, with three and two affected siblings [letter; comment]. *Br J Obstet Gynaecol* 1993;100:796.

Neonatal Management

116. Jefferies AL, Ryan G. Improved outcome for fetal and neonatal non-immune hydrops. *Pediatr Res* 1995;37:215A.

CHAPTER 46

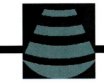

Cervical Incompetence and Preterm Labor

Katherine W. Fong, M.B., B.S., F.R.C.P.(C)
Dan Farine, M.D., F.R.C.S.C.

CHAPTER OUTLINE

Evaluation of the maternal cervix is an integral part of the obstetric ultrasound examination. Sonographic depiction of the cervix and appropriate measurements may facilitate the diagnosis and management of incompetent cervix and preterm labor.

Changes in the length, funneling of the cervix, and dilatation of the cervical canal are important sonographic findings. However, they have very different implications at different gestational ages. For example, a dilated cervix prior to 12 weeks gestation indicates an inevitable abortion. During the second trimester, the same finding in the absence of uterine contractions and ruptured membranes is diagnostic of incompetent cervix. In the third trimester, a dilated cervix may imply impending premature labor. The obstetrician is confronted with the following clinical dilemmas: Do I have to perform elective cerclage to prevent pregnancy loss due to cervical incompetence?

Do I have to perform an emergency cerclage for a cervix that has dilated? Do I have to modify the patient's behavior for impending preterm labor?

There are different techniques for sonographic assessment of the cervix. Interpretation of the scan requires knowledge of the normal anatomy of the cervix and abnormal cervical changes, as well as familiarity with the clinical entities of incompetent cervix and preterm labor and their management.

SONOGRAPHIC TECHNIQUE

There are **three approaches** to scanning the cervix: transabdominal, transperineal, and transvaginal. Knowing the **advantages** and **limitations** of each scanning technique enables the clinician to combine or change approaches according to the clinical situation.

Transabdominal Approach

The technique as originally described by Sarti et al. used static scanners and emphasized the necessity of a **full urinary bladder.**[1] With present day real-time equipment, using a 3.5-MHz sector or convex transducer, the examination can be performed with ease. Scanning should be initiated in the midline of the lower abdomen just above the symphysis pubis. It is important that longitudinal scans are obtained parallel to the long axis of the cervix. When the endocervical canal comes into view, slight adjustment or angulation of the transducer may be necessary to visualize the entire canal from the internal os to the external os (Fig. 46-1). Following this, the transducer is rotated 90 degrees to obtain transverse views of the cervix. Using digital calipers, the cervical length, cervical width, and the width of the cervical canal at the level of the internal os can be measured.

Overdistention of the bladder should be avoided. Increased bladder pressure can compress the lower uterine segment, leading to false cervical elongation and/or masking of cervical dilatation. This problem can be overcome by rescanning the cervix after partial emptying. One can subjectively assess bladder distention relative to pelvic size or use a bladder diameter of 45 to 60 mm.[2]

When the urinary bladder is empty, amniotic fluid can be used as the acoustic window to scan the cervix with some success in the second trimester.[3] Sagittal views are obtained with the transducer angled downward from just below the umbilicus. The cervix assumes a more vertical orientation and appears bulkier (Fig. 46-2).

With the transabdominal approach, demonstration of the cervix becomes more difficult with increasing gestation. In the third trimester, despite a full urinary bladder and maneuvers such as **Trendelenburg positioning of the mother or external manipulation of the fetus,** the cervix is not adequately visualized in approximately 30% of patients.[4] This is due to overlying fetal parts, particularly acoustic shadowing from the fetal head, and/or maternal obesity. These limitations can be overcome by either transperineal or transvaginal sonography.

Transperineal (Translabial) Approach

Description of the current technique is credited to Jeanty et al.[5] Any commercially available 3.5-MHz sector transducer can be used. Higher-frequency (5-MHz) transducers do not usually provide adequate penetration necessary for visualization of the cervix. To minimize the risk of infection, the transducer is covered with plastic wrap over which is placed clean gel. Scanning is performed with an **empty bladder.** With the patient supine and hips abducted, the transducer is placed between the labia minora at the vaginal introitus. The ultrasonic beam is oriented in a sagittal plane along the direction of the vagina. Images are displayed in the conventional manner with the head toward the left of the screen (Fig. 46-3). The vagina is seen in a vertical plane between the bladder and the rectum. The cervix is oriented horizontally, at a right angle with the vagina (Fig. 46-4).

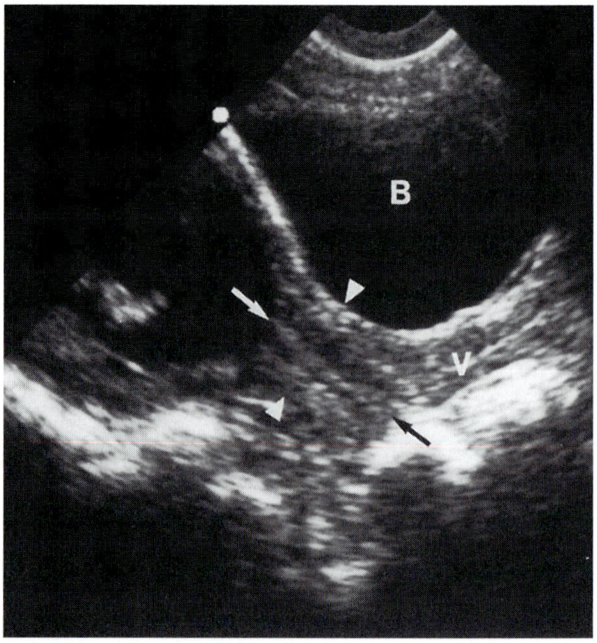

FIG. 46-1. Normal cervix, transabdominal full bladder technique. Longitudinal midline scan of the lower uterine segment. The cervix is defined in length *(arrows)* from the external os to the internal os. The hyperechoic cervical canal is seen between the two arrows. The cervical width is denoted by arrowheads. *V*, Vagina; *B*, Bladder.

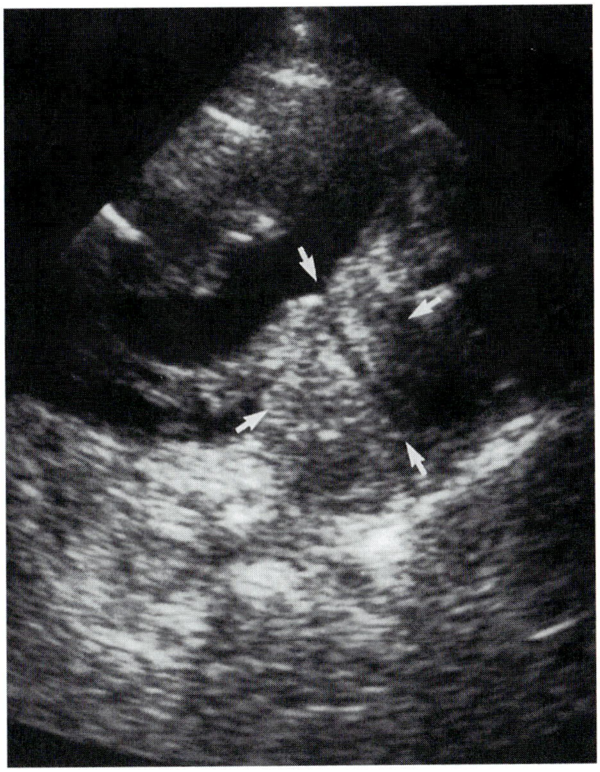

FIG. 46-2. Normal cervix, transabdominal empty bladder technique. Longitudinal midline scan of the lower uterine segment obtained by scanning through the amniotic fluid. The cervix *(arrows)* has a near vertical orientation. The cervical canal is hypoechoic in this patient.

Transperineal sonography is an effective technique for imaging the cervix during the **third trimester** of pregnancy, and patient acceptance is good. In two recent studies, the entire cervix was successfully visualized in 86% and 96% of patients.[6,7] If the region of the external os is obscured by rectal gas, elevating the patient's buttocks on a thick cushion may improve visualization of the cervix.[8] Transperineal sonography may be **especially valuable in patients with ruptured membranes** when digital examination and **transvaginal sonography** are **contraindicated** because of potential risk of uterine infection. It is also helpful if **vaginismus** prevents the transvaginal approach.

Transvaginal Approach

Dedicated endovaginal transducers (5 MHz or higher frequency) are necessary. The examination is performed with an **empty urinary bladder.** With the patient supine and hips abducted, the transducer, covered with a condom, is placed in the vagina and oriented in a sagittal plane along the length of the cervical canal (Fig. 46-5). Higher-frequency transducers and closer proximity to the structures studied allow for **better resolution,** although there is the disadvantage of a limited field of view. Vaginal probes with a wide scanning angle (> 90 degrees) allow visualization of the cervix in its entirety regardless of cervical length. The transducer is inserted only 3 to 4

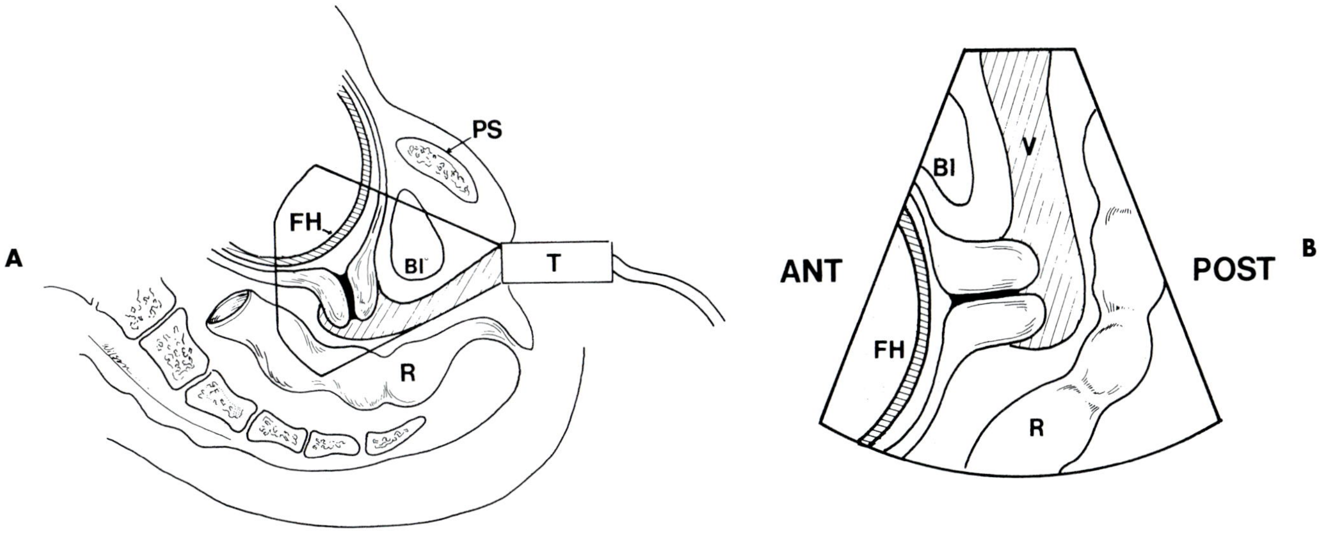

FIG. 46-3. Anatomic landmarks—transperineal approach. **A,** Sagittal illustration of the female pelvis with transducer, *T*, positioned at the vaginal introitus shows typical scanning plane during transperineal sonography. **B,** Scanning plane depicted in **A** is rotated 90 degrees counterclockwise before display on the ultrasound monitor. As a result, the cervix is oriented horizontally at approximately 90 degrees to the vagina, *V*. *PS*, Pubic symphysis; *Bl*, bladder; *FH*, fetal head; *R*, rectum. (From Mahony BS, Nyberg DA, Luthy DA et al. Translabial ultrasound of the third-trimester uterine cervix: correlation with digital examinations. *J Ultrasound Med* 1990;9:717-723.)

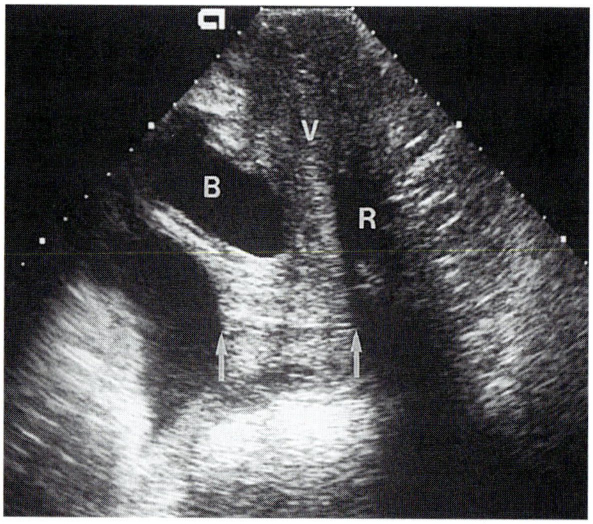

FIG. 46-4. Transperineal scan of normal third-trimester cervix. The cervix *(arrows)* is oriented horizontally, approximately perpendicular to the ultrasound beam. The vagina, *V*, is oriented in a nearly vertical plane. *B*, Bladder; *R*, rectum.

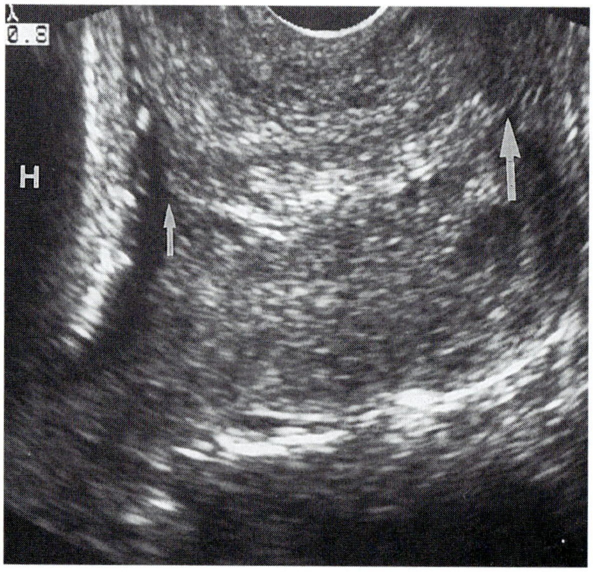

FIG. 46-5. Transvaginal scan of normal cervix. The echogenic cervical canal is imaged from the external os *(large arrow)* to the internal os *(small arrow)*. *H*, Fetal head.

cm into the vagina to avoid contact with the cervix and to image the cervix in the effective focal range of the transducer.

Several reports suggest that the transvaginal technique is superior to both the transabdominal technique and digital examination in obtaining an adequate evaluation of the cervix.[9,10] Also, it is a reproducible method.[11] A study comparing patient acceptance for transvaginal scanning and transabdominal scanning reported that patients found transvaginal scanning less painful and less annoying.[12]

Potential complications include increased risk of amnionitis following rupture of membranes, stimulation of contractions in cases with preterm labor, and induction of vaginal bleeding in cases with placenta previa, although the latter is not likely to occur in experienced hands.[4]

Technical Limitations and Pitfalls

Technical limitations and pitfalls of these three scanning approaches are summarized in Table 46-1.

NORMAL CERVIX

Sonographically, the cervix appears as a distinct soft-tissue structure containing mid-range echoes. The endocervical canal often appears as an echogenic line (representing the mucous plug) surrounded by a hypoechoic zone attributed to endocervical glands. Occasionally, the endocervical canal may appear hypoechoic. The lower uterine segment and cervix normally have a Y-shaped configuration.

Cervical Length

Cervical length is obtained by measuring the length of the endocervical canal from the internal cervical os to the external cervical os. There have been numerous ultrasound studies that evaluated cervical length in normal pregnancy.* With the **transabdominal technique,** there is a **wide variation** in the cervical length measurements because of lack of standardization of bladder volumes. **Transvaginal sonography** avoids the problem of cervical distortion and is a **more accurate** method. The largest study to date was reported by Iams et al.[11] In this prospective, multicenter study, vaginal sonography was performed at 24 and 28 weeks gestation in women with singleton pregnancies at low risk for preterm delivery. The cervical length was normally distributed at both examinations, mean ± SD was 35.2 ± 8.3 mm at 24 weeks and 33.7 ± 8.5 mm at 28 weeks.

Table 46-2 lists the results from several prospective studies of cervical length. Measurements of cervical length obtained transabdominally are generally longer when compared with those obtained transvaginally. No transperineal study of cervical length in normal pregnancy has been reported. In the **normal population, the mean cervical length is greater than 30 mm.** Gradual cervical effacement and shortening begin at about 30 weeks gestation. The difference in the cervical length of primigravid and multigravid women is not clinically significant.[2,11,17]

Comparison of ultrasound measurement to clinical examination. Since digital examination measures only the length from the external cervical os

*References 2, 3, 10, 11, 13-17.

TABLE 46-1
CERVICAL ASSESSMENT: TECHNICAL LIMITATIONS AND PITFALLS

	TAS	TPS	TVS
Technical Factors			
Presenting fetal part	++	–	–
Large maternal body habitus	++	+	–
Limited field of view	–	+	++
Poor depth penetration (due to high-frequency transducer)	–	–	+
Bowel gas	–	+	–
Gas in vagina	–	++	+
Pitfalls			
Overdistended bladder	+	–	–
Uterine contractions	++	++	++
Fluid in vaginal vault (mistaken for cervical dilatation)	++	+	–
Cervical fibroid	++	++	++
Visualization of Internal Os and Cervix in Third Trimester	70%	86%-96%	99.5%

TAS, Transabdominal; *TPS*, transperineal; *TVS*, transvaginal sonography.
++ indicates major/significant limitation or pitfall.
+ indicates possible limitation or pitfall.
– indicates not a limitation or pitfall.

TABLE 46-2
CERVICAL LENGTH IN NORMAL PREGNANCY

Studies	No. of Patients	Gestation	Mean Length (mm)	1 SD (mm)
Transvaginal Approach				
Iams[11]	2915	24 wks	35.2	8.3
	2531	28 wks	33.7	8.5
Tongsong[13]	639	28-30 wks	37.0	5.0
Andersen[10]	38	1st trimester	39.8	8.5
	77	2nd trimester	41.6	10.2
	62	3rd trimester	32.3	11.6
Transabdominal Approach (with Bladder Distention)				
Ayers[2]	142	8-33 wks	52.0	6.0
Podobnik[14]	80	1st trimester	49.7	3.1
	80	2nd trimester	47.8	3.2
	80	3rd trimester	44.3	3.9
Andersen[10]	32	1st trimester	53.2	16.9
	67	2nd trimester	43.7	13.8
	36	3rd trimester	39.5	9.8

to the cervical-vaginal junction, there is only a fair degree of association between transvaginal measurements of cervical length and measurements obtained by digital examination (correlation coefficient of 0.49).[18,19] Digital examination underestimates cervical length by a mean difference of 12 mm in more than 80% of women in the second and third trimesters.[18]

Cervical Width

The cervical width is obtained by measuring the anteroposterior diameter of the cervix at the midpoint between the internal and external cervical os. This dimension increases with gestational age. Nomograms have been published for cervical width from 10 to 37 weeks gestation.[16,20] In practice, this measurement is not widely used for diagnosis.

Cervical Canal and Internal Os

Normally, the internal os is closed, with its "knuckles" apposed. The membranes are frequently closely applied to the internal os. Studies with transabdominal ultrasound have shown that in **normal pregnancy the mean width of the cervical canal is 5 mm** (SD 1 mm), and there is no significant change from 10 to 36 weeks of gestation.[14,16]

ABNORMAL CERVICAL APPEARANCES

Shortening of the Cervix

For **transabdominal** sonography, **30 mm** has been suggested as the **lower limit of normal** for cervical length.[16,21] With **transvaginal** sonography, **25 mm corresponds to the 10th percentile for cervical length** in the study by Iams et al., and it has been suggested as the cut-off point.[11] A cervical length of 15 mm corresponds with approximately 50% effacement on digital examination, and a cervical length of 10 mm corresponds with approximately 75% effacement (Fig. 46-6).[7] Progressive shortening of the cervix is more significant than a single abnormal cervical length measurement.[22] The clinician should also be aware that shortening of the cervix in the absence of any other changes may not alter the prognosis of the pregnancy.[23]

Funneling of Internal Os/Early Herniation of the Fetal Membranes

Sonography can reveal funneling or early herniation of the membranes into the internal cervical os when there is still an intact external cervical os (Fig. 46-7). This occurs before physical changes in the cervix can be detected by digital and speculum examination.[24] **Funneling** of the internal os has been reported as **an early sign of incompetent cervix.**[10,22] Funneling is defined by Iams et al. as a protrusion of the amniotic membranes 3 mm or more into the internal os.[11] It was seen in 3% to 7% of the low-risk population at both 24 and 28 weeks gestation, and it correlated with an increased risk of premature delivery.[11] However, some patients with funneling of the internal os carry to term without intervention.[11,19] There is no agreement as to what constitutes significant funneling. Michaels et al. considered protrusion of the membranes for a distance of > 6 mm as significant.[22] Also, there is no standard method to measure funneling of the cervix. Measurement of the length and the width of the funnel and the length of the closed cervical canal are suggested (Fig. 46-8).[25]

Dilated Cervical Canal

Studies with **transabdominal** ultrasound have suggested using a cervical canal width of **8 mm or more as abnormal.**[14,24] On **transvaginal** sonography, an anteroposterior diameter of the internal os of **> 5 mm** before 30 weeks gestation is regarded as significant dilatation (Fig. 46-9).[26]

The amount of dilatation of the internal os on ultrasonography did not correlate well with cervical dilatation by digital examination.[7,26] This may reflect the inaccuracy of digital examination as well as the inability of the examining finger to reach beyond the external os.

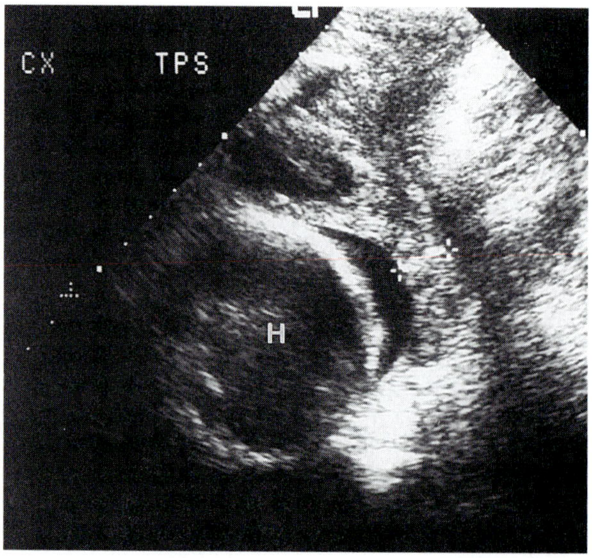

FIG. 46-6. Moderate cervical effacement, transperineal scan. The cervix measures 15 mm long and is 50% effaced. *Cursors*, Cervix; *H*, fetal head.

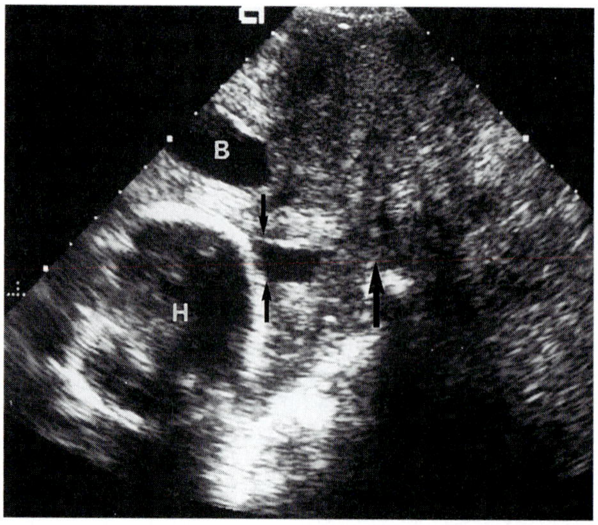

FIG. 46-7. Early herniation of membranes. Transperineal longitudinal scan demonstrates protrusion of the membranes into the proximal cervical canal. The external os *(large arrow)* remains closed. The width of cervical funneling *(small arrows)* is 7 mm. *B*, Bladder; *H*, fetal head.

Bulging Amnion

With advanced herniation of the membranes, a spectrum of sonographic findings has been described (Figs. 46-10 and 46-11).[27,28] In the most severe cases, the amniotic sac may prolapse into the vagina with the products of conception, and delivery most likely will ensue.

Pitfalls in Sonographic Diagnosis

Changes in the configuration of the lower uterine segment and internal cervical os can occur with varying degrees of bladder distention. True cervical dilatation can be masked by a **distended bladder** that compresses the cervix and obliterates the fluid within the endocervical canal.

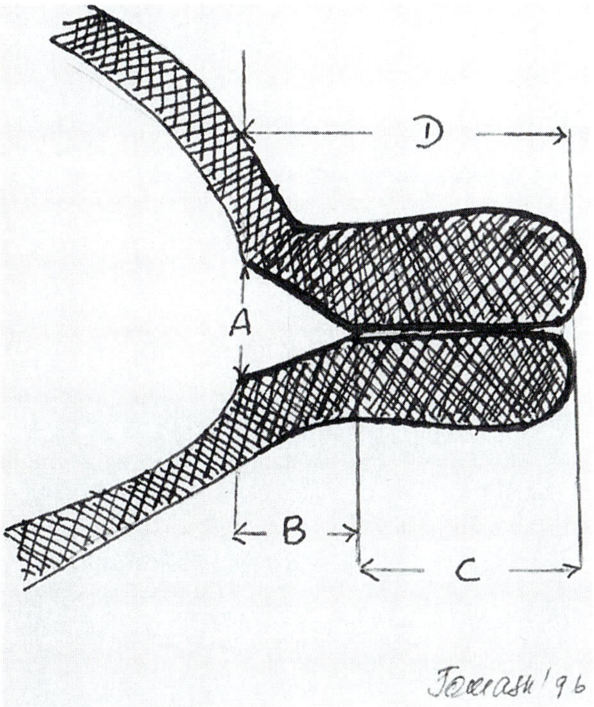

FIG. 46-8. Measurements of cervix. *A*, Funnel width (width of internal os). *B*, Funnel length. *C*, Length of the closed cervical canal. *D*, Length of the cervix from internal os to external os.

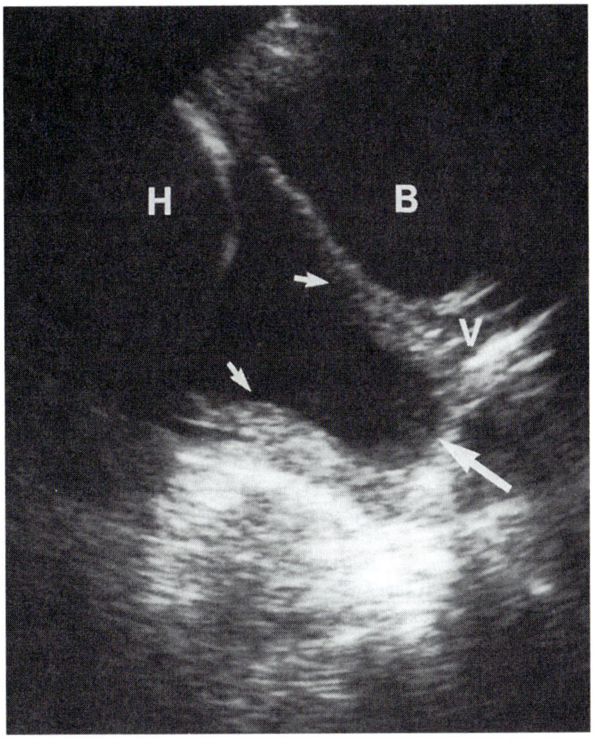

FIG. 46-10. Advanced herniation of membranes. Transabdominal longitudinal scan shows an open cervical canal from the internal os *(small arrows)* to the external os *(large arrow)*. *V*, Vagina; *B*, bladder; *H*, fetal head.

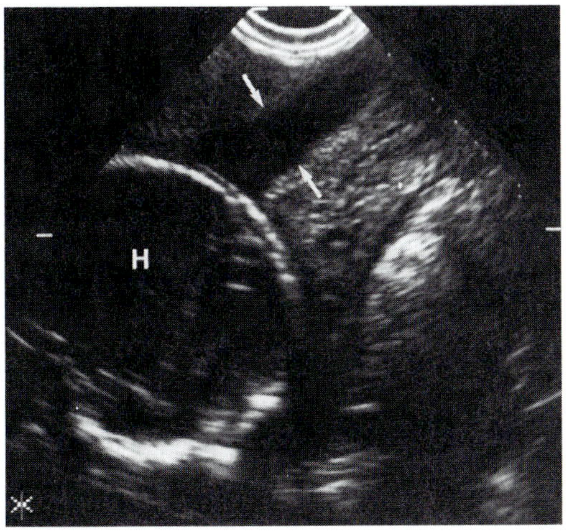

FIG. 46-9. Dilated cervical canal. Transvaginal longitudinal scan demonstrates fluid in the cervical canal *(arrows)*, which measures 1.2 cm in width. *H*, Fetal head.

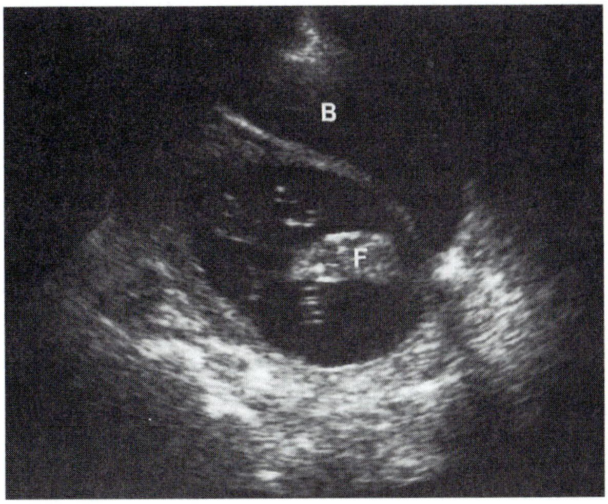

FIG. 46-11. True hourglassing. Transabdominal longitudinal scan shows bulging amnion containing a foot, *F*, and loops of umbilical cord. *B*, Bladder.

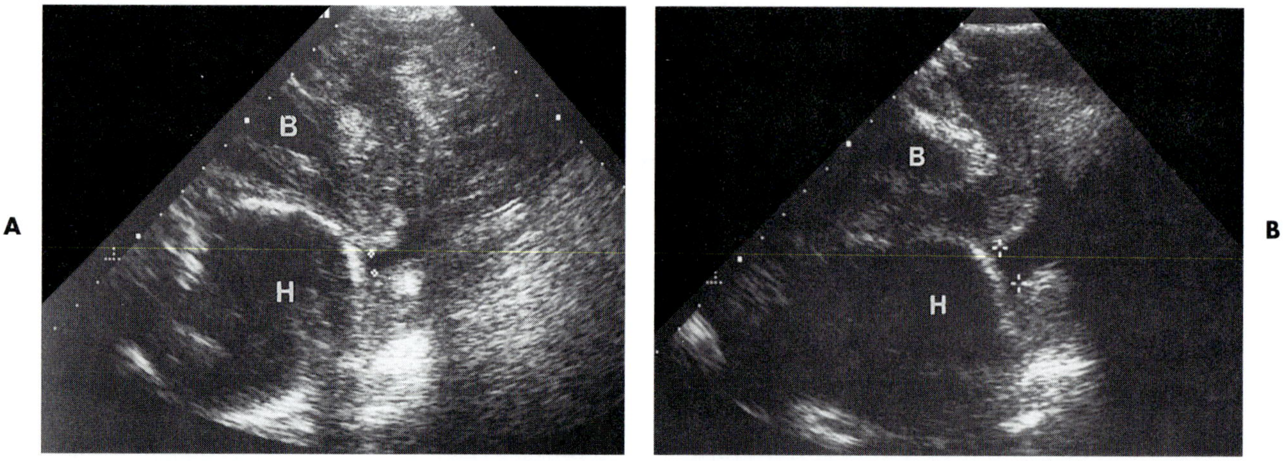

FIG. 46-12. Dynamic dilatation of the cervix, transperineal ultrasound. **A,** Initially, the internal os measures 6 mm *(cursors)*. **B,** Image obtained 5 minutes later shows the internal os dilated to 12 mm. The cervix is short, measuring 15 mm. *B*, Bladder; *H*, fetal head.

Development of cervical incompetence is not a static but rather a **dynamic** process.[29,30] The cervix can change spontaneously, sometimes dramatically, over the course of a sonographic examination. It may appear completely normal at one point in the examination and grossly abnormal at another (Fig. 46-12). Therefore, in patients at risk for cervical incompetence or in whom initial ultrasound images demonstrate a questionable cervical abnormality, **the cervix should be imaged more than once** and **observed continuously** over a period of several minutes. As well, if suspicious but nondiagnostic changes are noted on the sonogram, the study must be repeated in 24 to 48 hours.

Functional evaluation of the cervix, such as the application of mild fundal pressure, has been shown to induce funneling and dilatation that were not otherwise present.[31] This maneuver, also called "cervical stress test," may lead to earlier diagnosis of cervical incompetence.

Although the sonographic appearance of prolapse of the amniotic sac is almost pathognomonic, confusion might occur if a **contraction of the lower uterine segment** occurs.[28,32] The resulting **false "hourglass membranes"** should be distinguishable from true bulging amniotic membranes because the internal cervical os is still closed in the former situation (Fig. 46-13). Furthermore, with delayed scanning after the contraction relaxes, the appearance will return to normal. A **low-lying leiomyoma,** especially if hypoechoic, or a **large amount of fluid in the vagina** may also produce a similar picture, but these can be excluded by recognition of a closed internal cervical os.

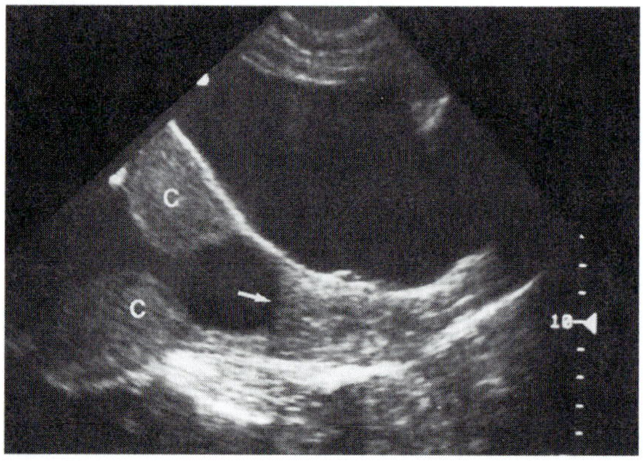

FIG. 46-13. Contraction—false "hourglass membranes." Transabdominal longitudinal scan shows a contraction of the lower uterine segment, *C*, simulating the appearance of prolapse of the amniotic sac. Note the closed internal cervical os *(arrow)*.

INCOMPETENT CERVIX

Clinical Aspects

An incompetent cervix is unable to retain an intrauterine pregnancy until term because of some deficiency in cervical structure or function. The reported incidence varies from 0.05% to 1% of all pregnancies,[33] but it may account for as many as 16% of second-trimester losses.[34]

Cervical incompetence can be acquired or congenital. In the majority of patients, it is the result of **traumatic injury to the cervix,** including cervical laceration, amputation, conization, and excessive cervical dilatation before diagnostic curettage or therapeutic abortion.[35] Congenital cervical incompetence is uncommon. It is diagnosed when a woman's first pregnancy course is consistent with cervical incompetence and there is no past history of cervical trauma. Congenital cervical incompetence has been reported in women exposed to diethylstilbestrol (DES) in utero.[36] It may also be associated with uterine malformations.

The **classic obstetric history** is characterized by **painless cervical dilatation and recurrent second-trimester loss.** Cervical incompetence is generally not associated with labor, bleeding, or ruptured membranes and usually occurs earlier than other causes of preterm labor, typically at 18 to 26 weeks.[37] However, a significant number of multigravid patients with an incompetent cervix do not have the classic obstetric history. In these patients and in the primigravid patients, clinical symptoms are useless in identifying this condition. When they present with cervical dilatation and/or prolapse of the fetal membranes into the vagina, it is an obstetric emergency, with a high pregnancy loss rate.

In the woman who is not pregnant, investigations such as hysterosalpingography, Hegar dilator test, and hysteroscopy are not widely used clinically for diagnosis,[37-40] because extrapolation of the findings to the cervix in pregnancy may be inappropriate.

Cervical Cerclage

Therapy for cervical incompetence consists of conservative management and cervical cerclage, a surgical procedure in which a purse string suture is applied to the cervix, using one of two techniques (Shirodkar or McDonald). In patients with a documented history of incompetent cervix, the suture is usually inserted **electively at 13 to 16 weeks gestation** (when the chance of miscarriage is minimal, yet prior to the silent dilatation that typically occurs after 16 weeks gestation). However, there is a lack of satisfactory evidence concerning the efficacy of cervical cerclage. The recent multicenter, randomized, controlled trial of cervical cerclage was conducted in women deemed to be at increased risk of cervical incompetence, but obstetricians were not sure if a cerclage should be inserted.[41] This study showed a reduction in deliveries before 33 weeks following cerclage, from 17% to 13%. This result was only marginally significant, probably because of inclusion of less classic cases of cervical incompetence. The use of cervical cerclage was associated with a doubling of the risk of puerperal fever.[41] Another study reports a 2% procedure-related pregnancy loss, usually due to premature rupture of membranes or preterm labor.[42] The actual selection of women for whom the apparent benefits of cerclage outweigh its risks remains difficult. When the membranes are bulging into the vagina, an emergency cerclage seems to be indicated in view of the high pregnancy loss without cerclage. Even with emergency cerclage, there is still a pregnancy loss rate of about 30%.[43]

Ultrasound Prediction of Incompetent Cervix

Since the outcome of early or prophylactic cervical cerclage is much better than cerclage placed after the cervix has dilated and membranes are bulging, it is important to diagnose incompetent cervix early.

Several studies described differences in cervical measurements between patients with clinical diagnosis of cervical incompetence and normal controls.[14,44,45] The cervix is shorter, and the overall width of the cervix is increased.[14,44,45] As early as 12 weeks gestation, funneling of the internal cervical os or dilated endocervical canal can be identified in some cases.[14,22,24]

However, there are **no clear criteria** for the diagnosis of cervical incompetence concerning the early signs: **cervical shortening, funneling of internal os,** and **dilated endocervical canal.** Different investigators have used different cervical lengths as indications for cervical cerclage and different criteria for diagnosis of cervical incompetence. There has been no prospective study that randomizes patient management according to ultrasound findings. Therefore the exact predictive value of ultrasound for therapeutic maneuvers and pregnancy outcome is not known at present. So far, none of the studies allows us to quantify the risk of a short or dilated cervix or funneling of the internal os for cervical incompetence. When these signs are present in a specific patient, it is advisable to describe the sonographic findings, to mention that these are associated with incompetent cervix, and to suggest close follow-up.

Scanning Patients with Suspected Cervical Incompetence

In a patient suspected to have painless dilatation (possible previous cervical incompetence, vaginal discharge, pelvic pressure), an ultrasound examination can confirm dilatation of the cervix and herniation of the amniotic sac into the vagina. Ultrasound examination is preferable to digital or speculum examination as it can provide more information (e.g., is the fetus in the uterus or vagina and to what extent is the cervix dilated behind the bulging membranes).[28] This information may be crucial for management. Furthermore, there is less risk of rupturing the membranes or introducing an infection.

Insertion and Follow-Up of Cervical Cerclage

It has been reported that the cerclage suture is often not optimally inserted (i.e., placed too far below the internal cervical os).[46] Sonography has been used in the operating room to guide the placement of cerclage sutures, especially when the cervix is short.[47,48]

More frequently, it is used to evaluate the efficacy of surgical treatment. On sonographic examination of the cervix, the sutures appear as hyperechoic linear structures, usually with acoustic shadowing. The anterior and posterior components of the sutures can be demonstrated in both the longitudinal and transverse views (Fig. 46-14). The shadowing is most prominent in the region of the surgical knot, which is usually placed anteriorly. It is important to **determine the location of the sutures** in relation to both the internal and the external cervical os and to **measure the length of the closed cervical canal.**[49] Periodic follow-up sonograms may detect complications such as a "slipping suture," funneling of the internal os, or protrusion of the membranes beyond the sutures before they are clinically apparent (Fig. 46-15). These findings can be valuable in patient management and in determining the necessity for a second cerclage procedure.[50] In a recent study using transvaginal ultrasound to predict cerclage outcome, funneling of the internal os and shortening of the closed cervical canal above the cerclage were associated with a higher risk of preterm delivery.[51]

PRETERM LABOR

Clinical Aspects

Preterm labor (prior to 37 weeks gestation) is diagnosed when regular uterine contractions accompany anatomic changes in the cervix or rupture of the amniotic membranes. Preterm birth occurs in 5% to 10% of all pregnancies and is the second most important contributor to perinatal mortality after congenital anomalies.[52-54]

In spite of intensive research efforts and many new techniques and technologies, the frequency of preterm labor and preterm birth has not changed in the last 30 years. There are many reasons for the lack of success:

- **Indeterminate etiology.** The etiology and mechanism of preterm labor are still poorly understood. There are possibly several different etiologies such as infection and uterine distention.[55,56]
- **Poor identification of at-risk population.** Several scoring systems have been developed to identify women at higher risk for preterm births, based mainly on previous history and cervical changes on digital examination. However, the majority of preterm births still occur in women that

A

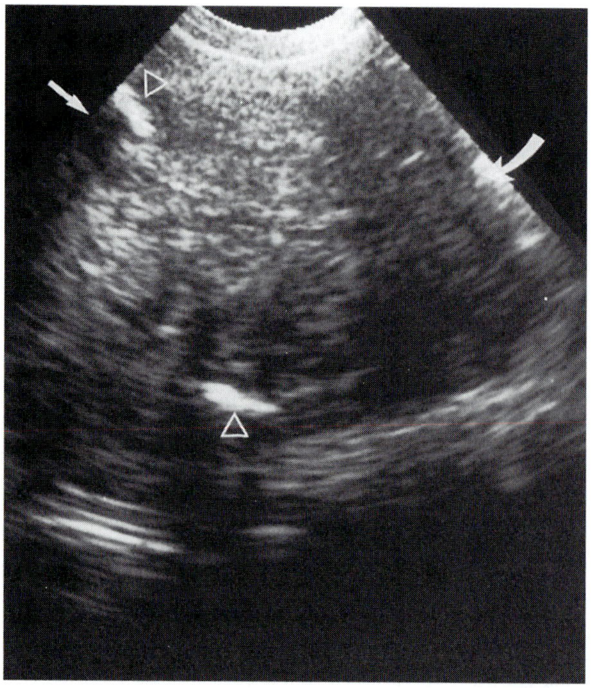

B

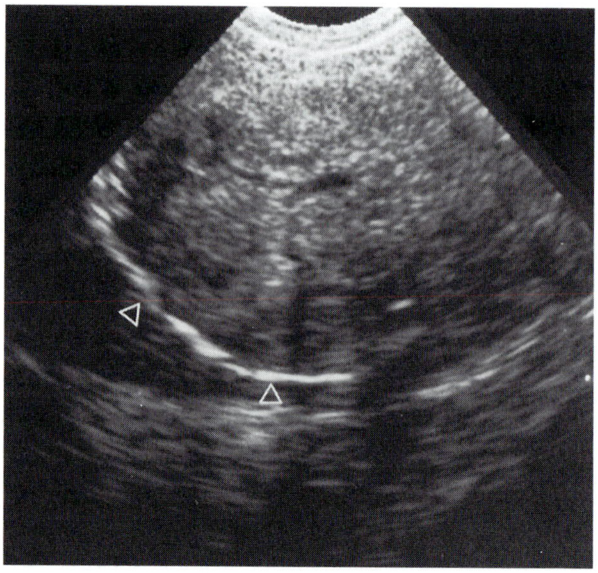

FIG. 46-14. Shirodkar cerclage. A, Transvaginal longitudinal scan demonstrates the cervical canal from the external os *(large arrow)* to the internal os *(small arrow)*. The echogenic sutures *(arrowheads)* are placed close to the internal os. **B,** Transverse scan shows circular configuration of suture material *(arrowheads)* within the cervix.

were not identified as high risk. In addition, most women identified to be at risk for preterm birth have term deliveries.

Two new approaches, ultrasound assessment of the cervix and the fibronectin level in vaginal secretion,[57] may better define women at high risk for preterm labor. However, no data are available on the value of combining these two tests.

- **Late diagnosis.** The criteria for diagnosis of preterm labor include painful contractions and cervical changes. This clinical approach is used because half of the women that present with painful contractions are not in labor. However, using the present criteria, the diagnosis may be made long after the process has begun, certainly long enough for alterations in the dimensions of the cervix to occur.
- **Ineffective therapy.** The current medical therapy (betamimetic drugs, MgSO4) does not prolong pregnancy by more than 72 hours and does not improve neonatal outcome. The limited effect of these medications is further reduced if therapy is started after advanced cervical changes have occurred.[58,59] Nonmedical interventions that include behavior modifications such as bed rest, restricted activity, and care from health care providers may improve outcome.

Ultrasound Prediction of Preterm Labor/Risk for Preterm Delivery

It seems that there is a continuum between incompetent cervix and preterm labor, since incompetent cervix is sometimes not clinically silent, and preterm labor is often preceded by shortening and funneling of the cervix. Thus differentiating these conditions based on symptomatology and gestational age may be difficult. Furthermore, it is not clear at what point in pregnancy a cerclage should not be done.[43]

There have been several studies that identified women with either short cervices or dilatation/funneling of the internal os to be at higher risk for preterm delivery (Table 46-3).

Shortening of the Cervix. Several studies have demonstrated an inverse relationship between the length of the cervix, as measured by ultrasonography during pregnancy, and the frequency of spontaneous preterm delivery.[11,13,26,60] The shorter the cervix, the greater the likelihood of preterm delivery, as shown in Fig. 46-16. However, different cut-off points of cervical length and different definitions of preterm birth (< 35 weeks versus < 37 weeks) were used by different investigators, and the study populations were different (low risk versus

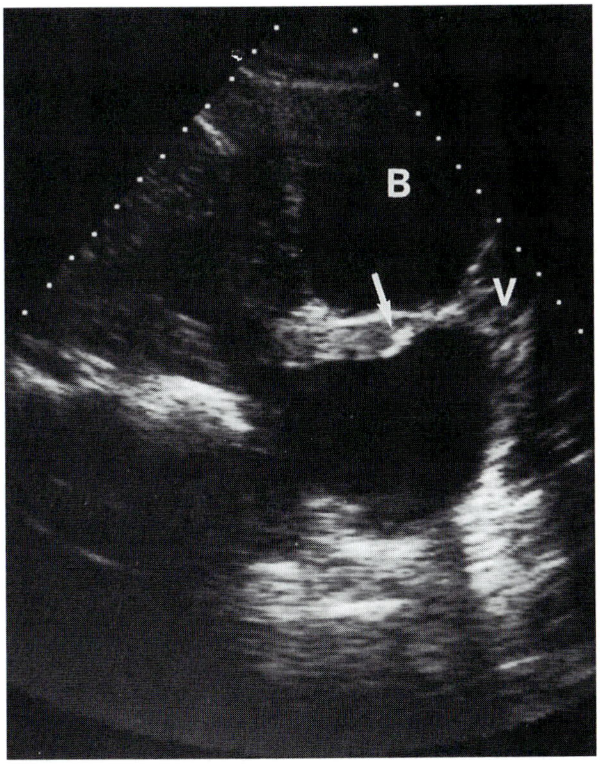

FIG. 46-15. Failed cervical cerclage. Transabdominal longitudinal scan demonstrates protrusion of the membranes beyond the McDonald suture *(arrow)* into the vagina, *V*. *B*, Bladder.

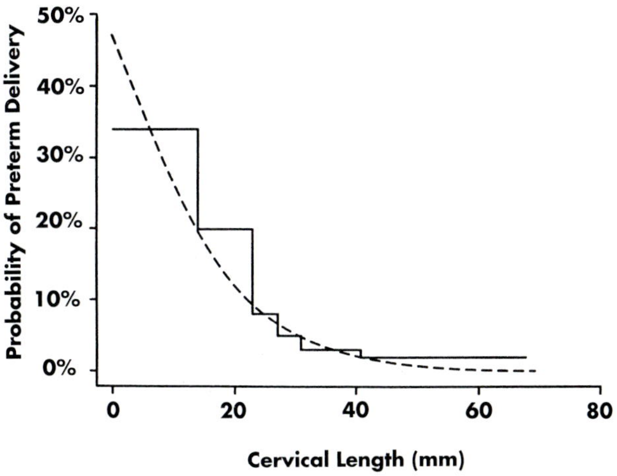

FIG. 46-16. Probability of spontaneous preterm delivery before 35 weeks gestation. Observed frequency of spontaneous preterm delivery *(solid line)* and estimated probability from logistic-regression analysis *(dashed line)*, according to cervical length measured by transvaginal ultrasonography at 24 weeks gestation.(From Iams JD, Goldenberg RL, Meis PJ, et al. The length of the cervix and the risk of spontaneous premature delivery. *N Engl J Med* 1996;334:567-572. © Massachusetts Medical Society.)

TABLE 46-3
CERVICAL CHANGES ON TRANSVAGINAL SONOGRAPHY AND RISK OF PRETERM DELIVERY

Author	Gestation (wk)	Cut-off (mm)	Preterm Delivery Relative Risks
Short Cervix			
Iams[11]*	24	26	6.19
	28	26	9.57
Tongsong[13]**	28-30	35	2.77
Andersen[60]**	10-30	39	3.75
Okitsu[26]**	6-40	< 1.5 SD	3.94
Funneling			
Iams[11]*	24	3	5.02
	28	3	4.78
Dilated Internal Os			
Okitsu[26]**	< 30	5	9.5

Relative Risks + 95% CI

0.2 1 5 20 200

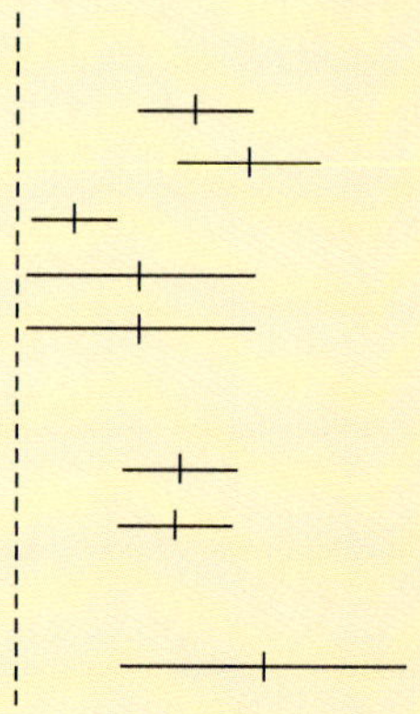

Outcome Better — Outcome Worse

* < 35 wk; ** < 37 wk

high risk). Therefore it is difficult to be sure what is the optimal cervical length that is clinically useful for predicting preterm delivery risk. We recommend using the cut-off point reported by Iams et al. and to consider **cervical length < 25 mm as short.**[11] The actual length should be reported because **very short cervices have a very high association with preterm labor.**

Dilatation/Funneling of Internal Os. A dilated internal os of **more than 5 mm before 30 weeks gestation** was associated with preterm delivery more often than an undilated internal os (33% versus 3.5%).[26] It is the most significant predictor of preterm delivery. Funneling or herniation of membranes into the internal os is also correlated with an increased risk of preterm delivery.[11]

Clinical Implications of Ultrasound Findings Associated with Preterm Labor. There is a definite correlation between cervical changes and the risk of preterm delivery. However, **the majority of women with short cervices or funneling will not have a preterm delivery** because these findings have low positive predictive values. The mechanism linking cervical changes and preterm labor is still unexplained. So far, there are no studies in which women with abnormal ultrasound findings were randomized into different management regimes. Therefore sonographic information cannot be used to alter clinical management at this time, but a repeat examination is recommended to detect any progression of the cervical changes.

CONCLUSION

Sonography provides an objective and noninvasive method for evaluation of the cervix. Sonographic changes may be the earliest indicators of incipient cervical failure, often before they can be detected by digital and speculum examination, and before the presence of clinical symptoms associated with preterm labor or incompetent cervix. However, future research should try to standardize the definitions of abnormal cervical shortening, funneling and dilatation of the internal os, and the obstetric management of these ultrasound findings, so that the clinical significance of early sonographic changes in the cervix can be established.

REFERENCES

Sonographic Technique

1. Sarti DA, Semple WF, Hobel CJ et al. Ultrasonic visualization of a dilated cervix during pregnancy. *Radiology* 1979;130:417-420.
2. Ayers JW, DeGrood RM, Compton AA et al. Sonographic evaluation of cervical length in pregnancy: diagnosis and management of preterm cervical effacement in patients at risk for premature delivery. *Obstet Gynecol* 1988;71:939-944.
3. Bowie JD, Andreotti RF, Rosenberg ER. Sonographic appearance of the uterine cervix in pregnancy: the vertical cervix. *AJR* 1983;140:737-740.
4. Farine D, Fox HE, Jacobson S et al. Is it really placenta previa? *Eur J Obstet Gynecol* 1989;31(2):103-108.
5. Jeanty P, d'Alton M, Romero R et al. Perineal scanning. *Am J Perinatol* 1986;3:289-295.
6. Hertzberg BS, Bowie JD, Weber TM et al. Sonography of the cervix during the third trimester of pregnancy: value of the transperineal approach. *AJR* 1991;157:73-76.

7. Mahony BS, Nyberg DA, Luthy DA et al. Translabial ultrasound of the third-trimester uterine cervix: correlation with digital examinations. *J Ultrasound Med* 1990;9:717-723.
8. Hertzberg BS, Kliewer MA, Baumeister LA et al. Optimizing transperineal sonographic imaging of the cervix: the hip elevation technique. *J Ultrasound Med* 1994;13:933-936.
9. Brown JE, Thieme GA, Shah DM et al. Transabdominal and transvaginal endosonography: evaluation of the cervix and lower uterine segment in pregnancy. *Am J Obstet Gynecol* 1986;155:721-726.
10. Andersen HF. Transvaginal and transabdominal ultrasonography of the uterine cervix during pregnancy. *J Clin Ultrasound* 1991;19:77-83.
11. Iams JD, Goldenberg RL, Meis PJ et al. The length of the cervix and the risk of spontaneous premature delivery. *N Engl J Med* 1996;334:567-572.
12. Slavik T. Transvaginal sonography: the technician's view. *J Ultrasound Med* 1988;7:214.

Normal Cervix

13. Tongsong T, Kamprapanth P, Srisomboon J et al. Single transvaginal sonographic measurement of cervical length early in the third trimester as a predictor of preterm delivery. *Obstet Gynecol* 1995;86:184-187.
14. Podobnik M, Bulic M, Smiljanic N et al. Ultrasonography in the detection of cervical incompetency. *J Clin Ultrasound* 1988; 16:383-391.
15. Zemlyn S. The length of the uterine cervix and its significance. *J Clin Ultrasound* 1981;9:267-269.
16. Varma TR, Patel RH, Pillai U. Ultrasonic assessment of cervix in normal pregnancy. *Acta Obstet Gynecol Scand* 1986;65: 229-233.
17. Kushnir O, Vigil DA, Izquierdo L et al. Vaginal ultrasonographic assessment of cervical length changes during normal pregnancy. *Am J Obstet Gynecol* 1990;162:991-993.
18. Sonek JD, Iams JD, Blumenfeld M et al. Measurement of cervical length in pregnancy: comparison between vaginal ultrasonography and digital examination. *Obstet Gynecol* 1990; 76:172-175.
19. Andersen HF, Ansbacher R. Ultrasound: a new approach to the evaluation of cervical ripening. *Semin Perinatol* 1991;15:140-148.
20. Smith CV, Anderson JC, Matamoros A et al. Transvaginal sonography of cervical width and length during pregnancy. *J Ultrasound Med* 1992;11:465-467.

Abnormal Cervical Appearances

21. Riley L, Frigoletto FD, Benacerraf BR. The implications of sonographically identified cervical changes in patients not necessarily at risk for preterm birth. *J Ultrasound Med* 1992;11:75-79.
22. Michaels WH, Montgomery C, Karo J et al. Ultrasound differentiation of the competent from the incompetent cervix: prevention of preterm delivery. *Am J Obstet Gynecol* 1986; 154:537-546.
23. Vaalamo P, Kivikoski A. The incompetent cervix during pregnancy diagnosed by ultrasound. *Acta Obstet Gynecol Scand* 1983;62:19-21.
24. Varma TR, Patel RH, Pillai U. Ultrasonic assessment of cervix in at risk patients. *Acta Obstet Gynecol Scand* 1986;65:147-152.
25. Gomez R, Galasso M, Romero R et al. Ultrasonographic examination of the uterine cervix is better than cervical digital examination as a predictor of the likelihood of premature delivery in patients with preterm labor and intact membranes. *Am J Obstet Gynecol* 1994;171:956-964.
26. Okitsu O, Mimura T, Nakayama T et al. Early prediction of preterm delivery by transvaginal ultrasonography. *Ultrasound Obstet Gynecol* 1992;2:402-409.
27. Fried AM. Bulging amnion in premature labor: spectrum of sonographic findings. *AJR* 1981;136:181-185.
28. McGahan JP, Phillips HE, Bowen MS. Prolapse of the amniotic sac "hourglass membranes." *Radiology* 1981;140:463-466.
29. Parulekar SG, Kiwi R. Dynamic incompetent cervix uteri: sonographic observations. *J Ultrasound Med* 1988;7:481-485.
30. Hertzberg BS, Kliewer MA, Farrell TA et al. Spontaneously changing gravid cervix: clinical implications and prognostic features. *Radiology* 1995;196:721-724.
31. Guzman ER, Rosenberg JC, Houlihan C et al. A new method using vaginal ultrasound and transfundal pressure to evaluate the asymptomatic incompetent cervix. *Obstet Gynecol* 1994; 83:248-252.
32. Karis JP, Hertzberg BS, Bowie JD. Sonographic diagnosis of premature cervical dilatation: potential pitfall due to lower uterine segment contractions. *J Ultrasound Med* 1991;10:83-87.

Incompetent Cervix

33. Cousins L. Cervical incompetence: a time for reappraisal. *Clin Obstet Gynecol* 1980;23:467-479.
34. Stromme WB, Haywa EW. Intrauterine fetal death in the second trimester. *Am J Obstet Gynecol* 1963;85:223-233.
35. Lash AF, Lash SR. Habitual abortion: the incompetent internal os of the cervix. *Am J Obstet Gynecol* 1950;59:68-76.
36. Singer MS, Hockman M. Incompetent cervix in a hormone-exposed offspring. *Obstet Gynecol* 1978;51:625-626.
37. Ansari AH, Reynolds RA. Cervical incompetence: a review. *J Reprod Med* 1987;32:161-171.
38. Lash AF. Incompetent internal os of the cervix: diagnosis and treatment. *Am J Obstet Gynecol* 1960;79:552-556.
39. Jeffcoate TNA, Wilson JK. Uterine causes of abortion and premature labor. *NY State J Med* 1956;56:680-690.
40. Hall D, Hann LE. Gynecologic radiology: benign disorders. In: Taveras JM, Ferrucci JT, eds. *Radiology: Diagnosis, Imaging, Intervention.* Philadelphia: JB Lippincott Co; 1988:15.
41. MacNaughton MC, Chalmers IG, Dubowitz V et al. Final report of the Medical Research Council/Royal College of Obstetricians and Gynecologists multicentre randomized trial of cervical cerclage. *Br J Obstet Gynecol* 1993;100:516-523.
42. Harger JH. Cervical cerclage: patient selection, morbidity and success rates. *Clin Perinatol* 1983;10:321-341.
43. Aarts JM, Brons TJ, Bruinse HW. Emergency cerclage: a review. *Obstet Gynecol Surv* 1995;50:459-69.
44. Brook I, Feingold M, Schwartz A. Ultrasonography in the diagnosis of cervical incompetency in pregnancy: a new diagnostic approach. *Br J Obstet Gynaecol* 1981;88:640-643.
45. Feingold M, Brook I, Zakut H. Detection of cervical incompetence by ultrasound. *Acta Obstet Gynecol Scand* 1984:63:407-440.
46. Lysikiewicz A, Canterino J, Robinson RP et al. Ultrasonic follow-up of cervical cerclage placement. *Am J Obstet Gynecol* 1996;174:414.
47. Wheelock JB, Johnson TR, Graham D et al. Ultrasound-assisted cervical cerclage. *J Clin Ultrasound* 1984;12:307-308.
48. Fleischer AC, Lombardi S, Kepple DM. Guidance for cerclage using transrectal sonography. *J Ultrasound Med* 1989;8:589-590.
49. Parulekar SG, Kiwi R. Ultrasound evaluation of sutures following cervical cerclage for incompetent cervix uteri. *J Ultrasound Med* 1982;1:223-228.
50. Rana J, Davis SE, Harrigan JT. Improving the outcome of cervical cerclage by sonographic follow-up. *J Ultrasound Med* 1990;9:275-278.
51. Andersen HF. Prediction of cervical cerclage outcome by endovaginal ultrasonography. *Am J Obstet Gynecol* 1994;171: 1102-1106.

Preterm Labor

52. Lye, SJ. The initiation and inhibition of labor—toward a molecular understanding. *Semin Reprod Endocrinol* 1994; 12(4):284-294.
53. Kierse MJCN. New perspectives for the effective treatment of preterm labor. *Am J Obstet Gynecol* 1995;173:618-628.
54. Moutquin JM, Milot-Roy V, Irion O. Preterm birth prevention: effectiveness of current strategies. *JSOGC* 1996;18:571-588.
55. Challis JRG, Lye SJ. Parturition. In: Knobil E, Neill JD, eds. *The Physiology of Reproduction.* New York: Raven Press; 1994:985-1031.
56. Lockwood CJ. Recent advances in elucidating the pathogenesis of preterm delivery, the detection of patients at risk and preventive therapy. *Curr Opinion Obstet Gynecol* 1994;6:7-18.
57. Iams JD, Casal D, McGregor JA et al. Fetal fibronectin improves the accuracy of diagnosis of preterm labor. *Am J Obstet Gynecol* 1995;173:141-145.
58. Hannah ME. The Canadian consensus on the use of tocolytics for preterm labour. *J SOGC* 1995;17:1089-1115.
59. Creasy RK. Preterm labor and delivery. In: Creasy RK, Resnik R, eds. *Maternal Fetal Medicine: Principles and Practice.* 3rd ed. Philadelphia: WB Saunders; 1994:497-498.
60. Andersen HF, Nugent CE, Wanty SD et al. Prediction of risk for preterm delivery by ultrasonographic measurement of cervical length. *Am J Obstet Gynecol* 1990;163:859-867.

CHAPTER 47

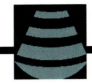

Sonographic Evaluation of the Placenta

Beverly A. Spirt, M.D., F.A.C.R.
Lawrence P. Gordon, M.D.

CHAPTER OUTLINE

Evaluation of the location, size, shape, and echotexture of the placenta as well as the retroplacental area should be part of every antenatal ultrasound examination. A thorough understanding of the normal placental anatomy as well as pathologic conditions is necessary to interpret the sonographic appearance. Many clinical problems are ascribed to the placenta, even though an anatomic or pathologic explanation is not apparent. Thus, recognition of the many normal variations is crucial in order to avoid overinterpretation of sonographic findings.

NORMAL GROWTH AND DEVELOPMENT

Embryology

After fertilization and subsequent cell division the **morula,** consisting of an inner and an outer cell layer, is formed. The morula enters the uterus and, upon the accumulation of fluid, becomes a **blastocyst.** The inner cell layer of the blastocyst will become the embryo, and the outer cell layer will form the placenta.

The blastocyst attaches to the endometrium on day 5–6, at which point rapid proliferation of the

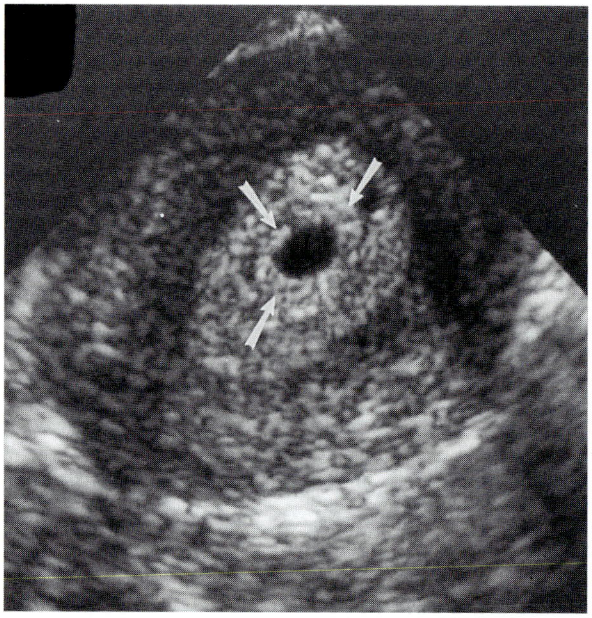

FIG. 47-1. Early gestational sac. Transvaginal scan at 4 weeks' menstrual age shows gestational sac surrounded by hyperechoic rim of villi *(arrows)*.

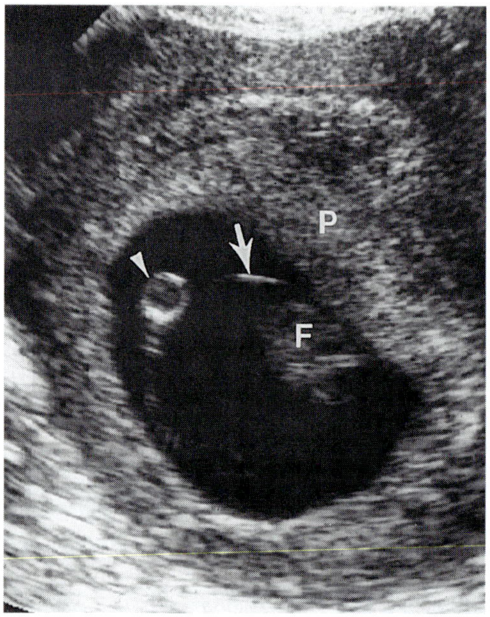

FIG. 47-2. Chorioamniotic separation. Transvaginal scan at 8.5 weeks demonstrates amniotic membrane *(arrow)*. P, placenta. *Open arrow*, fetus. *Arrowhead*, yolk sac.

trophoblast, the outer cell layer, begins. The trophoblast differentiates into two layers: an outer layer of multinucleated syncytiotrophoblast and an inner layer of mitotically active cytotrophoblast. During implantation, the syncytiotrophoblast erodes into the endometrial vessels and glands. A lacunar network develops around the syncytiotrophoblast and fills with maternal blood and endometrial glandular secretion, forming the primitive uteroplacental circulation. The lacunar network is the precursor of the intervillous space.

Between 13 and 21 days after conception (4 to 5 weeks' menstrual age) the primary stem villi, which form from columns of cytotrophoblast, surround the periphery of the gestational sac. At sonography, the early gestational sac is distinguished by its hyperechoic rim representing the surrounding villi (Fig. 47-1).

At approximately 8 weeks' menstrual age those villi on the side of the endometrial cavity begin to regress, leaving a smooth surface known as the ***chorion laeve.*** The remaining villi, which are oriented toward the endometrium, continue to branch and proliferate. This portion of the sac is known as the ***chorion frondosum*** and it forms the bulk of the placenta (Fig. 47-2).

When the amniotic sac reaches the size of the chorionic sac, the amnion and chorion fuse; this occurs at approximately 12 weeks' menstrual age. Chorioamniotic separation (nonfusion) can, however, persist to term (Fig. 47-3).[1]

During the third month, folds of the basal plate are pulled up between the proliferating branches of the villous tree. These folds, which contain decidua, are known as placental septa (Fig. 47-4, *A* and *B*). They divide the maternal surface into 15 or 20 lobules that have no physiologic significance.[2]

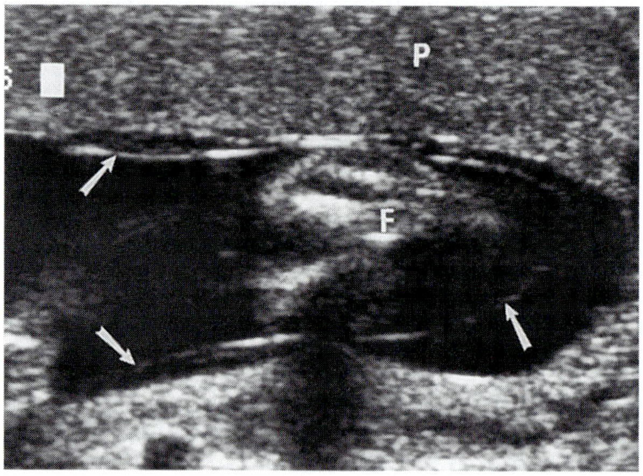

FIG. 47-3. Persistent chorioamniotic separation, confirmed at delivery. At 21 weeks, circumferential membranes *(arrows)* are seen surrounding the entire amniotic sac. P, placenta. F, fetus. (From Spirt BA, Gordon LP. The placenta and cervix. In: McGahan JP, Porto M, eds. *Diagnostic Obstetrical Ultrasound.* Philadelphia: JB Lippincott Co; 1994.)

At sonography, the diffuse granular echo pattern of the placenta is produced by echoes from the villi, which are bathed in maternal blood. Draining veins are visible along the entire basal plate and in the septa[3-6] (Fig. 47-4, *A*, *C*, and *D*), and they are especially

A B C D

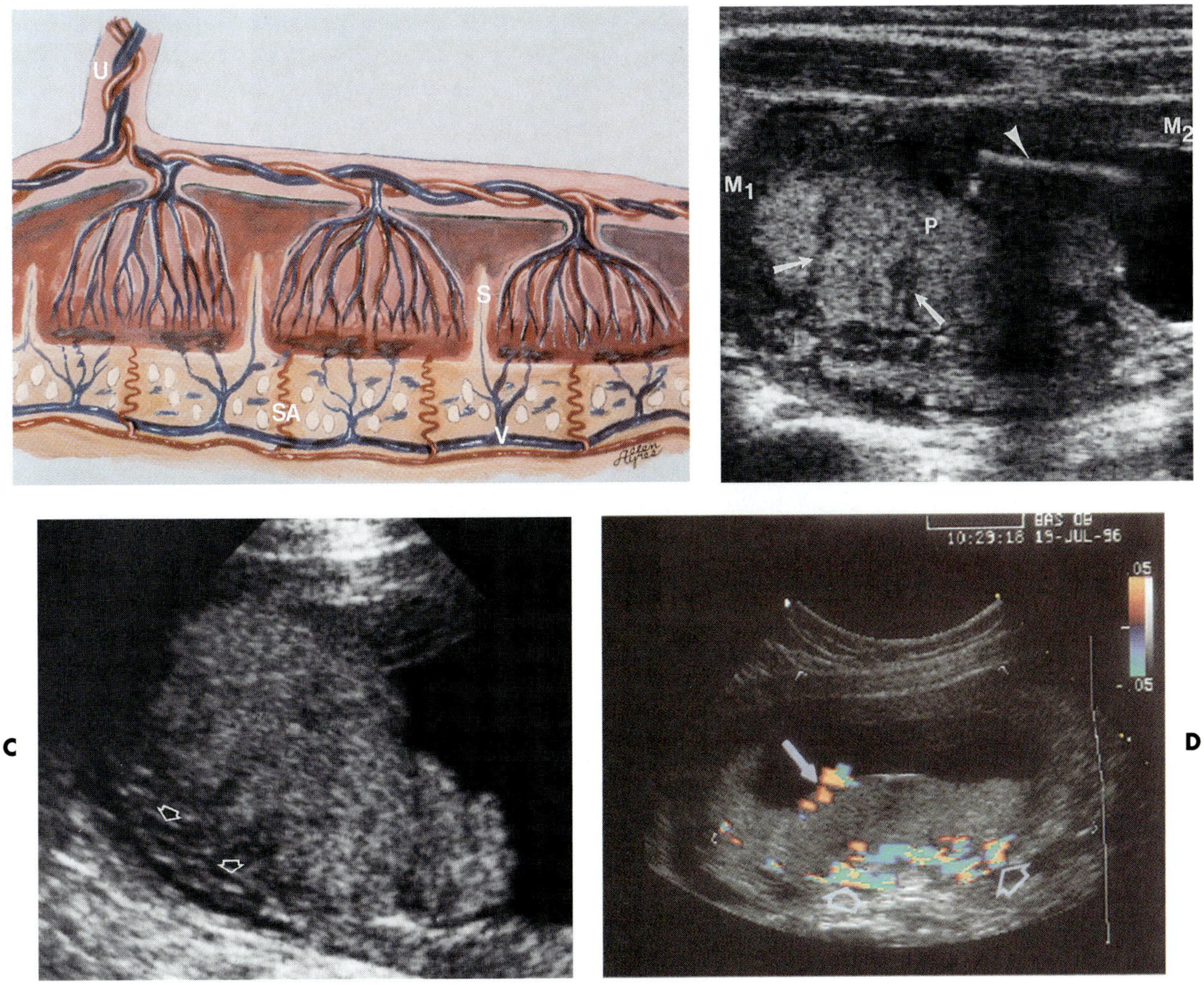

FIG. 47-4. Placental circulation. **A,** U, umbilical cord. SA, spiral arteriole. V, draining vein. S, septum. (From Spirt BA, Kagan EH. Sonography of the placenta. *Semin Ultrasound* 1980;1:293-310.) **B,** Posterior placenta (P) with septa *(arrows)* at 18 weeks. *Arrowhead*, fetal femur. The retroplacental myometrium (M_1) appears relatively hypoechoic. Myometrium (M_2) elsewhere appears hyperechoic compared with amniotic fluid. **C,** Sagittal scan at 16 weeks shows venous drainage *(open arrows)* of posterior placenta. **D,** Color flow Doppler image at 15 weeks demonstrates venous drainage *(open arrows)* of posterior placenta. *Arrow*, umbilical cord vessels.

prominent if the placenta is located posteriorly because of the effect of gravity.[7,8] The spiral arterioles that supply maternal blood to the intervillous space are too small to be consistently visible at sonography.

Calcification

The sonographic texture of the placenta remains unchanged throughout pregnancy except for the deposition of calcium (Fig. 47-5, *A*), which is a physiologic phenomenon that occurs throughout pregnancy.[2] The calcium is microscopic during the first two trimesters but may be macroscopic thereafter, most commonly after 33 weeks.[9,10] Calcium deposits are found primarily in the basal plate and septa but may also be seen in the subchorionic and perivillous spaces. Placental calcification has no proven clinical or pathologic significance.[2,11,12]

Histologic,[13,14] chemical,[15] radiographic[9] as well as sonographic[10] techniques have been used to study this phenomenon. The incidence of placental calcification increases exponentially with increasing gestational age from about 29 weeks.[9,10,13,15] Some degree of calcification is seen in over 50% of placentas after 33 weeks (Fig. 47-5, *B*).[9,10] Postmature placentas do not show increased calcification.[2,9,13,15] Placental calcification occurs more commonly in women of lower parity.[9,10,13] It appears to be related to maternal serum calcium levels; placental calcification is more common in placentas from late summer and early fall births, when maternal serum calcium levels are high.[9,14,15]

A

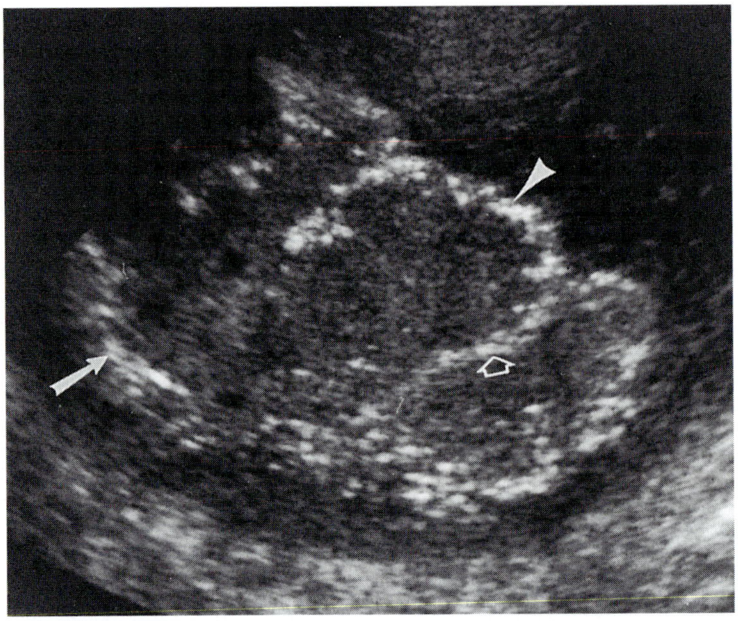

B

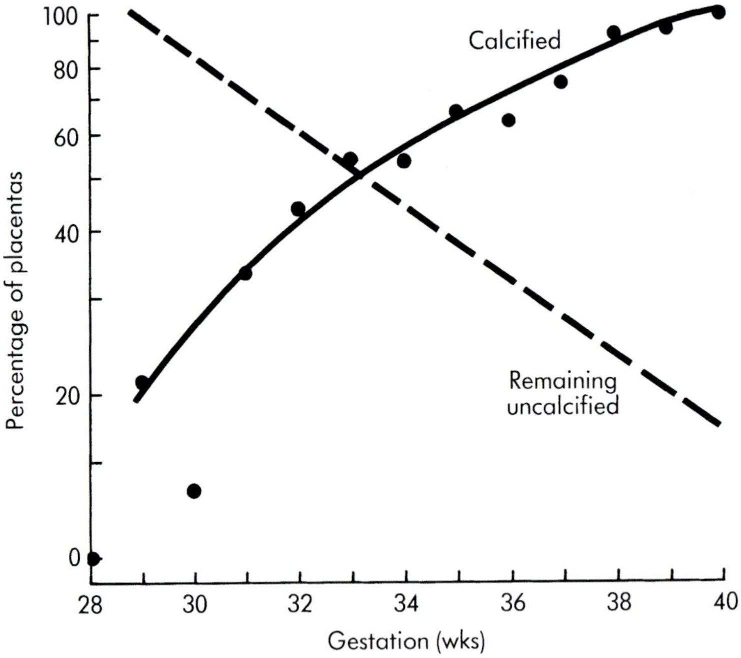

FIG. 47-5. Placental calcification. **A,** At 38 weeks, calcification is seen in basal plate *(arrow)*, septa *(open arrows)*, and subchorionic region *(arrowhead)* of posterior placenta. **B,** Placental calcification vs. gestational age. (**Fig. 5B** from Spirt BA, Cohen WN, Weinstein HM. The incidence of placental calcification in normal pregnancies. *Radiology* 1982;142:707-711.)

Since there is no proof that placental calcification has any significance, grading the degree of calcification seen at sonography is not worthwhile.

Umbilical Cord

The normal umbilical cord has **three blood vessels:** two arteries and one vein, surrounded by Wharton's jelly (Fig. 47-6, *A* and *B*). Documentation of the number of vessels in the umbilical cord should be included in every obstetrical sonogram. While the incidence of a single umbilical artery is 1% or less,[2,16] approximately 10% to 20% of these cases will have one or more additional malformations,[16,17] including trisomy 18, trisomy 13, urinary tract anomalies, CNS abnormalities, cardiac anomalies, omphalocele, sirenomelia, and the VATER association (Fig. 47-6, *C*).

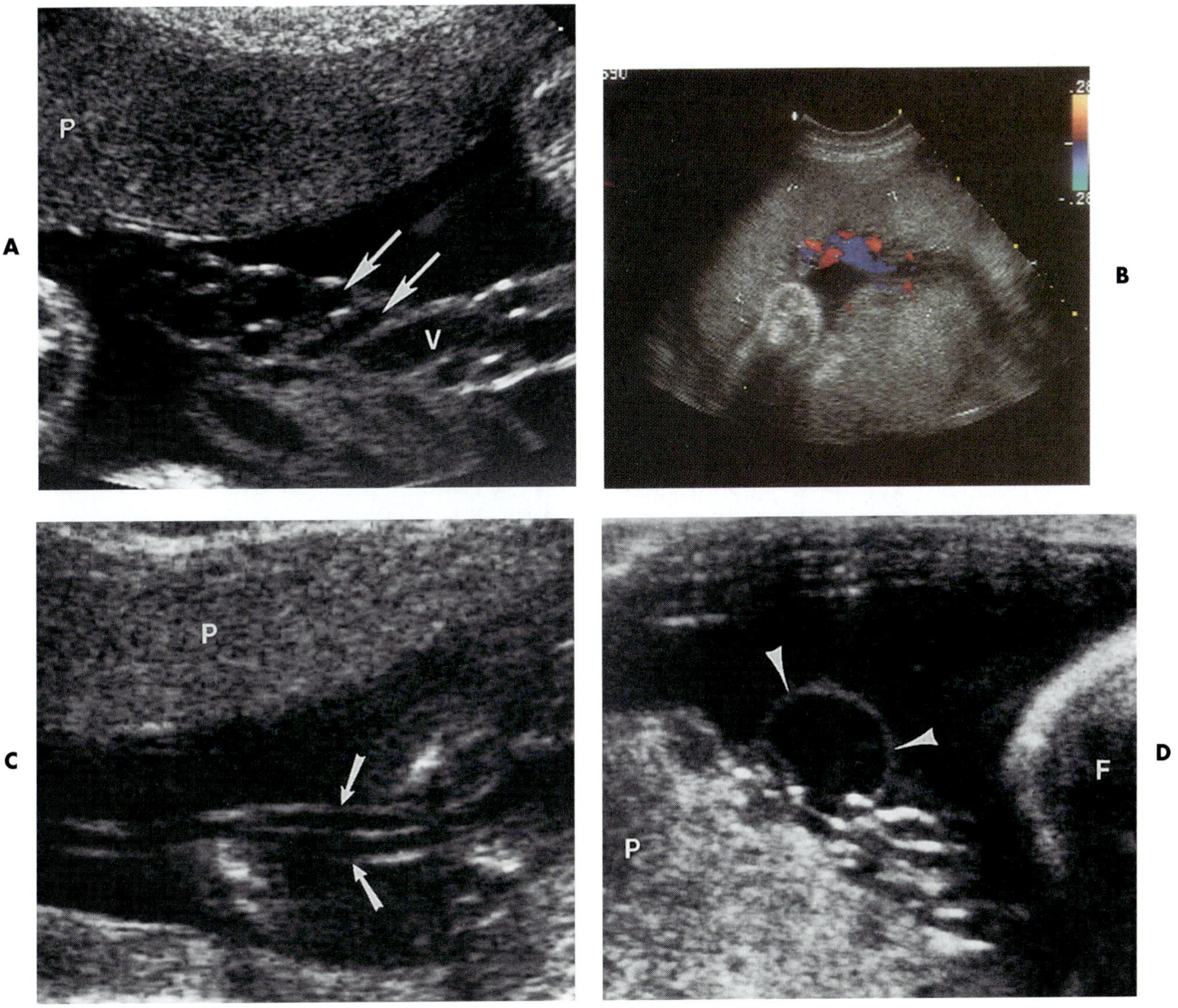

FIG. 47-6. Umbilical cord. **A, Normal three-vessel cord** is seen at 28 weeks and **B,** at 33 weeks. Note equal-sized umbilical arteries *(arrows)* and larger caliber umbilical vein (V). P, placenta. **C, Two-vessel cord** *(arrows)* is seen in case of trisomy 13. Note that the single umbilical artery and the umbilical vein are of equal size. P, placenta. **D, Umbilical cord cyst** *(arrowheads)* at 33.5 weeks. P, placenta. F, fetus.

The umbilical cord normally measures 1 to 2 cm in diameter.[2] Enlargement may be caused by hematoma[18] or edema,[2] or it may be a normal variant.[19]

Tumors of the umbilical cord are rare.[2] **Hemangioma** of the cord has been diagnosed antenatally by ultrasound, appearing as an echogenic mass that is usually closer to the placental end of the cord.[20,21] The differential diagnosis includes umbilical cord **hematoma,** which may vary in echo texture depending on the age of the lesion, and **teratoma.**

Cysts may occur. They are usually derived from either the omphalomesenteric duct or the allantois (Fig. 47-6, *D*).[2,22] Mucoid degeneration of Wharton's jelly may also produce the appearance of a cyst.

Umbilical cords usually insert on the fetal surface of the placenta, most commonly in an eccentric location.[2] Marginal insertion (**battledore placenta**) occurs in less than 6% of placentas and is likely to be of no clinical significance.[2] In up to 1.6% of deliveries, the cord inserts on the membranes at a variable distance from the placenta (**velamentous insertion**) (Fig. 47-7).[2] In this situation, the unprotected intramembranous umbilical vessels may bleed in the antepartum period and are susceptible to damage during labor and delivery. Vessels traversing the internal os of the cervix (**vasa previa**) (Fig. 47-8)[23] may also rupture during delivery. Color flow Doppler is useful in the antenatal detection of vasa previa.

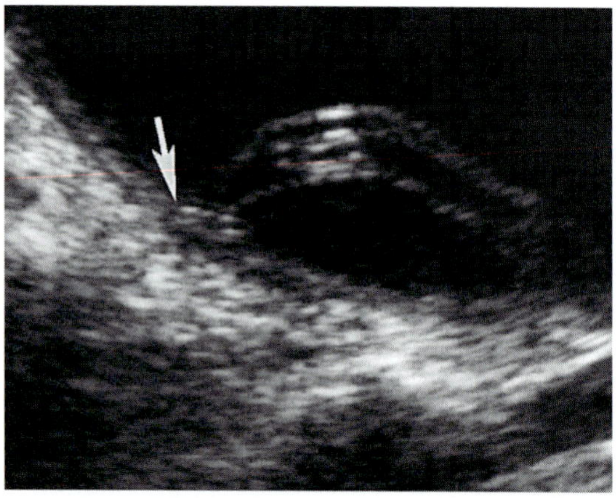

FIG. 47-7. Velamentous insertion. Sector scan at 25 weeks shows membranous insertion of the umbilical cord *(arrow)*. (From Spirt BA, Gordon LP. Sonography of the placenta. In: Fleischer AC, Manning FA, Jeanty P, Romero R, eds. *Sonography in Obstetrics and Gynecology: Principles and Practice*. Stamford: Appleton & Lange; 1996.)

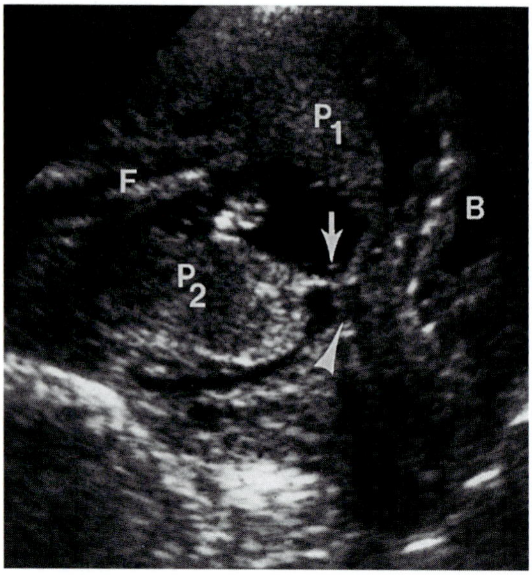

FIG. 47-8. Vasa previa. Midline sagittal sector scan at 25 weeks shows vessel *(arrow)* overlying internal cervical os *(arrowhead)*. Placenta was on the left, with anterior (P_1) and posterior (P_2) extensions. Vasa previa was confirmed at cesarian section. B, maternal bladder. F, fetus.

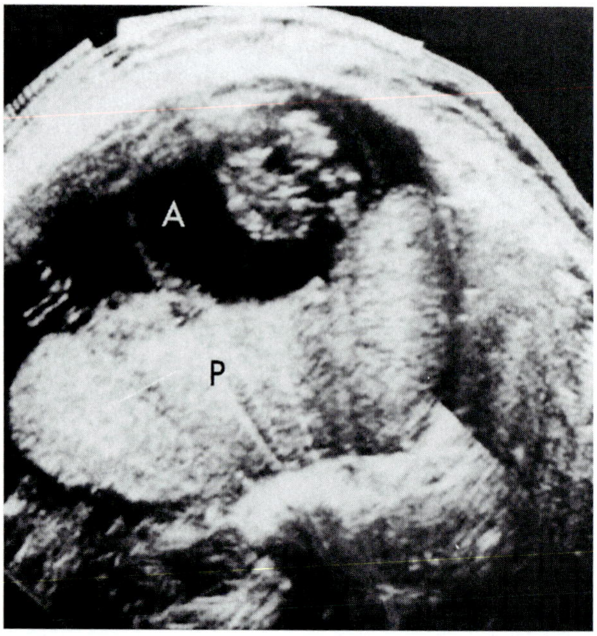

FIG. 47-9. Maternal-fetal Rh incompatibility. Transverse scan at 28 weeks shows grossly enlarged placenta (P). Note marked fetal ascites (A). (Courtesy of Edward Bell, M.D., Syracuse, New York. From Spirt BA, Kagan EH, Rozanski RM. Sonography of the placenta. In: Sanders RC, James AE, eds. *The Principles and Practice of Ultrasonography in Obstetrics and Gynecology*. 2nd ed. New York: Appleton-Century-Crofts; 1980.)

SIZE

The placenta is a fetal organ and, as such, is proportionate to the size of the fetus. A small placenta is expected with a small baby; this does not imply that the placenta is abnormal or that a small placenta results in a small baby.[2,11] Placental size does not in itself predict placental function.

Although methods to measure the size of the placenta have been described,[24-27] visual assessment is usually sufficient to decide whether a placenta is abnormally large or small. **Large placentas** (Fig. 47-9) are associated with various conditions, including blood group incompatibilities, maternal diabetes, severe maternal anemia, fetal anemia, fetal hydrops, and homozygous alpha-thalassemia. Large placentas with hydatidiform change are found in cases of triploidy (see below).

Small placentas are seen in disorders characterized by underperfusion, such as maternal hypertension, toxemia, and severe diabetes, as well as in some cases of multiple congenital anomalies and chromosomal abnormalities.[28]

MACROSCOPOIC APPEARANCE: NORMAL

Variations in Shape

Succenturiate Lobes. Focal areas of noninvolution of the chorion laeve result in accessory (**succenturiate**) lobes of the placenta (Fig. 47-10). These may be single or multiple and of varying size. They occur in 3% to 8% of placentas.[2,28] Fetal blood vessels coursing through the membranes connect these lobes to the main placenta. Succenturiate lobes are visible at sonography.[29,30] It is important to identify them be-

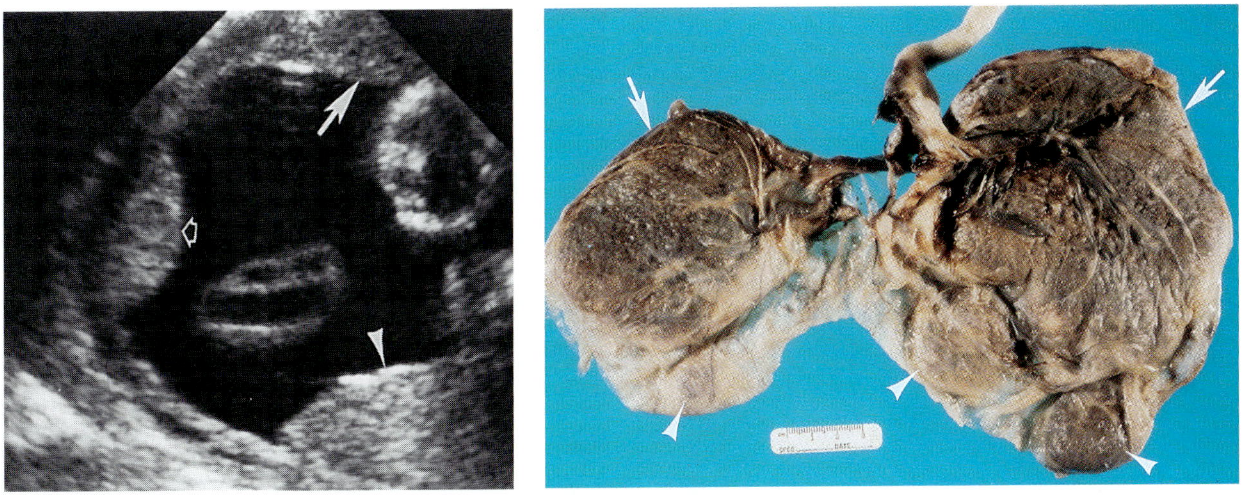

FIG. 47-10. Succenturiate lobes. **A,** Sagittal scan at 31 weeks shows three separate placental lobes. *Arrow*, main placenta. *Arrowhead*, next largest lobe. *Open arrow*, small lobe. **B,** Fetal surface of term placenta. Note two large lobes *(arrows)* and three small lobes *(arrowheads)*. (From Spirt BA, Gordon LP. Sonography of the placenta. In: Fleischer AC, Manning FA, Jeanty P, Romero R, eds. *Sonography in Obstetrics and Gynecology: Principles and Practice*. Stamford: Appleton & Lange; 1996.)

cause of the complications that can result, including retention of the accessory lobe following delivery, implantation of the accessory lobe over the cervical os, and bleeding from the vessels connecting the succenturiate lobe to the main placental mass.

Extrachorial Placenta. The fetal membranes do not extend to the edge of the placenta in 18% to 30% of placentas.[2] Two types of extrachorial placentas occur: **circummarginate,** in which the membranes form a flat ring at the site of attachment to the chorionic plate, and **circumvallate,** in which there is a fold in the membranes at the site of attachment (Fig. 47-11). The thick membranous folds of a circumvallate placenta may be identified at sonography (Fig. 47-12). In our experience, they are best visualized prior to 20 weeks. Either form of extrachorial placenta may be partial or complete. Circummarginate placentas have no clinical significance.[2] Complete circumvallate placentas have been associated with an increased incidence of antepartum bleeding, marginal hemorrhage, threatened abortion, and premature labor.[2,31-33]

Other. **Annular** (ring-shaped) placentas and **placenta membranacea** have been associated with antepartum and postpartum hemorrhage. Placenta membranacea is a rare condition in which the entire surface of the amniotic sac is covered with villi due to failure of regression during early pregnancy. The annular placenta, also rare, is probably a variant of placenta membranacea.[2]

Intraplacental Lesions

Several common macroscopic intraplacental lesions are visible at sonography but are devoid of clinical sig-

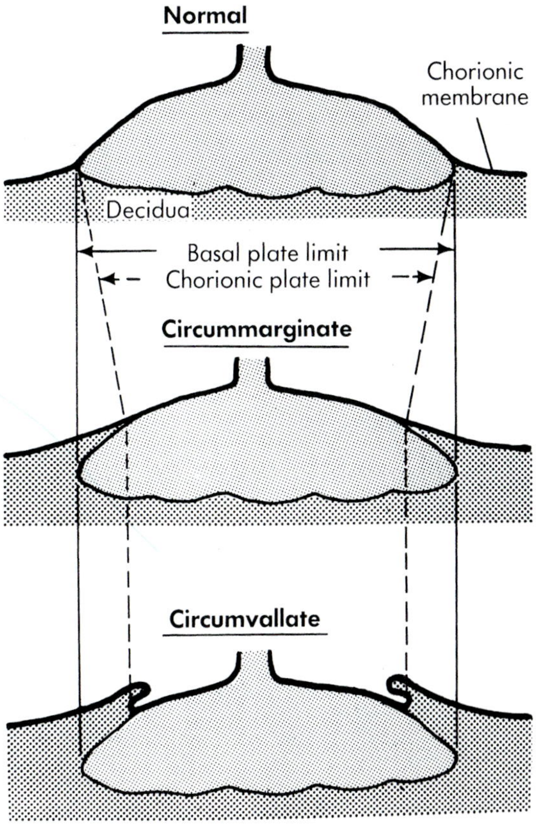

FIG. 47-11. Diagram in cross-section comparing extrachorial to normal placenta. Normally, the membranes extend to the edge of the placenta. With a circummarginate placenta, the transition from villous to membranous chorion occurs at a distance from the edge of the placenta. A circumvallate placenta is similar but has a fold in the membranes at the site of transition. (From Spirt BA, Kagan EH. Sonography of the placenta. *Semin Ultrasound* 1980;1:293-310.)

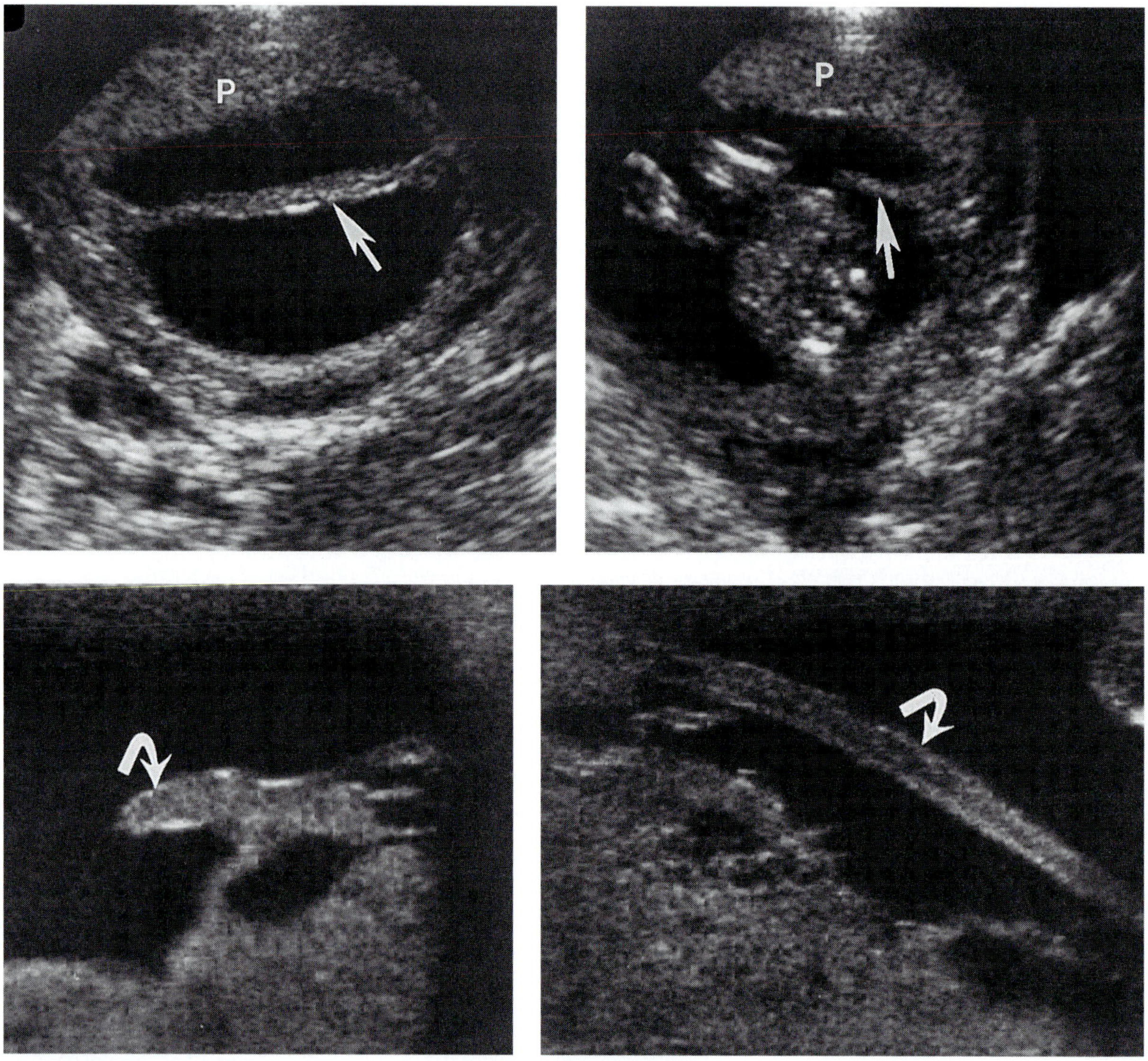

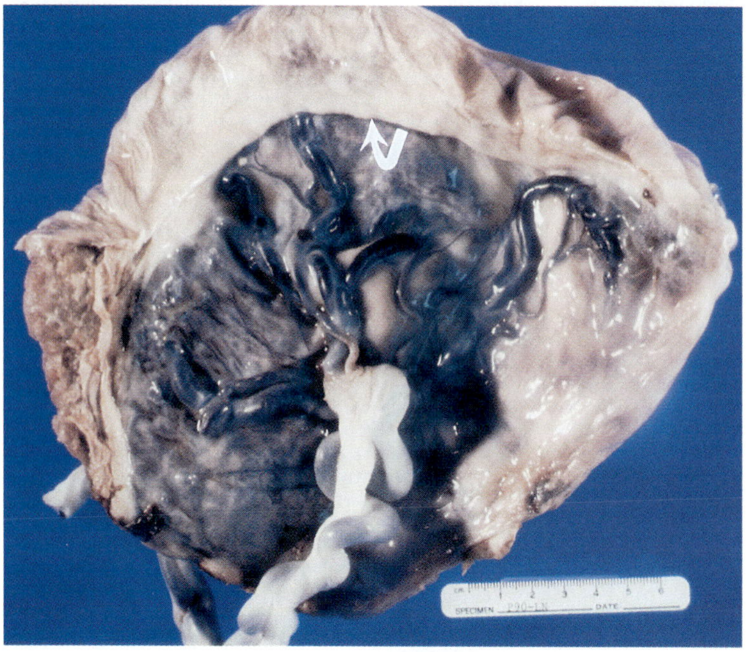

FIG. 47-12. Circumvallate placenta. **A,** Transverse and **B,** sagittal scans at 14 weeks show thick membranous fold *(arrows)* involving one portion of placenta. At delivery, a partial circumvallate placenta was found. **C,** Transverse and **D,** oblique images at 26.5 weeks show thick membrane fold *(arrows)* involving a portion of the placenta. **E,** A partial circumvallate placenta was confirmed at delivery. *Curved arrow,* membrane fold. (**C, D, E** from Spirt BA, Gordon LP. Imaging of the placenta. In: Taveras JM, Ferrucci JT, eds. *Radiology: Diagnosis-Imaging-Intervention.* Philadelphia: JB Lippincott Co; 1992.)

nificance. These include subchorionic fibrin deposition, perivillous fibrin deposition, intervillous thrombosis, and septal cysts.

Subchorionic Fibrin Deposition. Plaques of subchorionic fibrin are found in 20% of placentas from uncomplicated pregnancies at delivery.[2] They are a result of pooling and stasis of blood in the subchorionic space, leading to thrombosis and the deposition of fibrin. They contain laminated fibrin without villi.

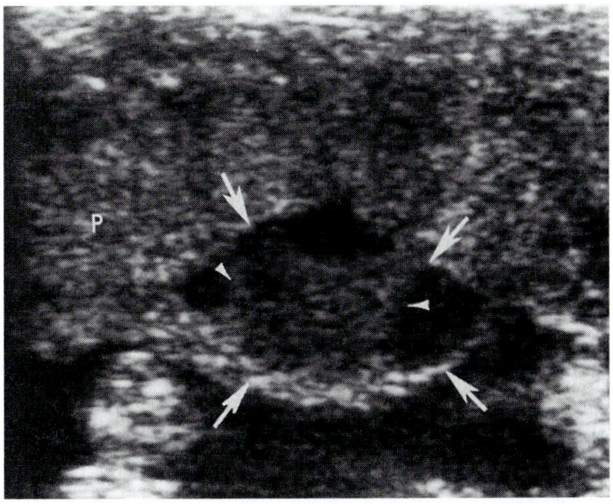

FIG. 47-13. Subchorionic fibrin deposition. Transverse linear array scan at 26 weeks shows subchorionic anechoic/hypoechoic lesion *(arrows)*. Solid echoes correspond to flow observed at real-time examination *(arrowheads)*. P, placenta.

Subchorionic anechoic/hypoechoic lesions that correlate with subchorionic fibrin deposition at delivery may be identified at sonography as early as 12 weeks (Fig. 47-13).[34] They may be quite prominent (Fig. 47-14), but they usually decrease in size as term approaches and fibrin is laid down. Slow flow may be demonstrated in these lesions at real-time sonography. However, color Doppler often fails to demonstrate the flow (Fig. 47-15).

Perivillous Fibrin Deposition. Perivillous fibrin deposition occurs to some degree in almost every placenta[35] and is visible macroscopically in about 25%.[11] It is caused by turbulence and stasis of maternal blood in the intervillous space, with secondary fibrin deposition. At sonography, it appears as intraplacental anechoic/hypoechoic lesions[36] in which flow is sometimes visible. The lesions may contain echogenic foci that represent areas of villi trapped in fibrin (Fig. 47-16). Microscopically, nonlaminated fibrin is seen surrounding villi that have become fibrotic and avascular.

Intervillous Thrombosis. Approximately 36% of term placentas contain intervillous thromboses,[2] lesions caused by fetal bleeding into the intervillous space.[37] These contain laminated fibrin and are visible sonographically as intraplacental anechoic/hypoechoic lesions[38] (Fig. 47-17). At sonography, flow may be seen in those lesions that are at an earlier stage.

Intervillous thromboses are not considered to be clinically significant.[2] However, there is an increased incidence of intervillous thrombosis in cases of Rh

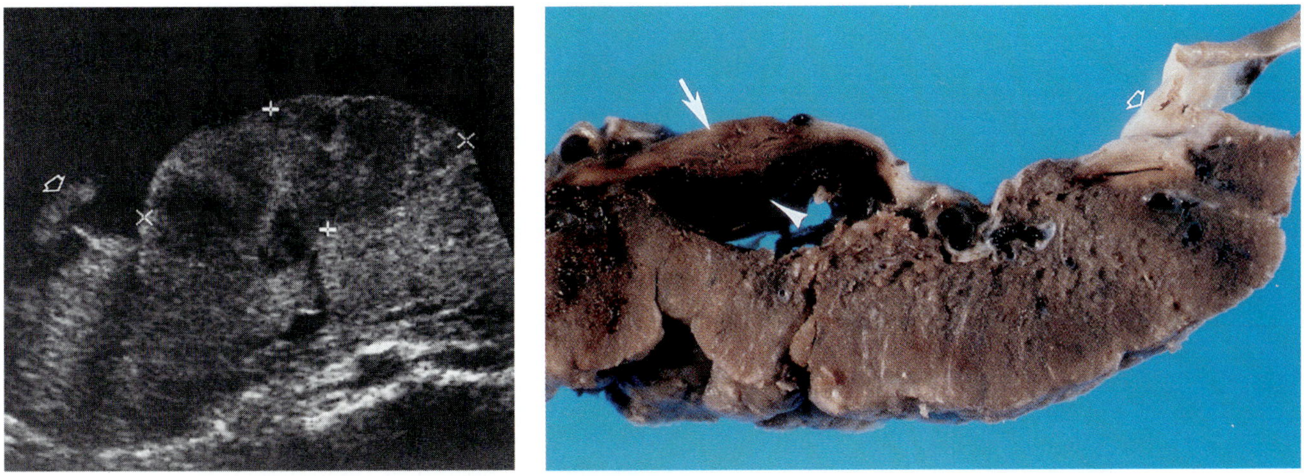

B

FIG. 47-14. Subchorionic fibrin deposition. **A**, Sagittal scan at 26.5 weeks shows prominent hypoechoic subchorionic lesion *(cursors)* that contained slow flow. Note membrane fold *(open arrow)*. **B**, At term, corresponding lesion contained laminated fibrin *(arrow)* along with blood *(arrowhead)*. Fresh blood fell out upon sectioning. *Open arrow*, membrane fold of partial circumvallate placenta. (Same patient as in 47-12 **C, D, E.**) (From Spirt BA, Gordon LP. Imaging of the placenta. In: Taveras JM, Ferrucci JT, eds. *Radiology: Diagnosis-Imaging-Intervention.* Philadelphia: JB Lippincott Co; 1992.)

isoimmunization,[39-41] suggesting that these lesions may lead to sensitization.

Some investigators have postulated a relationship between elevated maternal serum alpha-fetoprotein levels and lesions in the placenta.[42-44] However, if such a relationship is valid it should be true only in lesions that contain fetal blood such as intervillous thromboses.

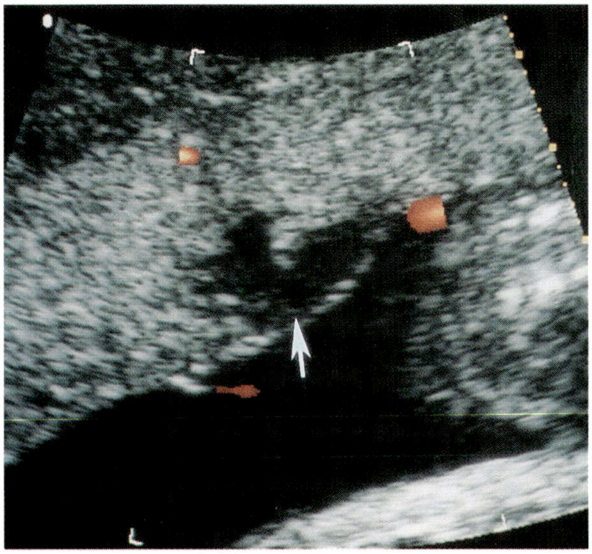

FIG. 47-15. Subchorionic fibrin deposition. Slow flow was visualized in subchorionic hypoechoic lesion *(arrow)* at real-time sonography, but color flow was not present. P, placenta.

"Maternal Lakes." "Maternal lakes" are not described in the pathology literature. The term appears in the ultrasound literature as a description of anechoic lesions in the placenta that correspond to blood-filled spaces at delivery. Many of these lesions represent an early stage in the evolution of intervillous thromboses or perivillous fibrin deposition (Figs. 47-18 and Fig. 47-19).

The common denominator of the lesions described above is the combination of blood and fibrin that produces the anechoic and/or hypoechoic appearance seen at sonography. Flow may be visualized within these lesions.

Septal Cysts. Up to 19% of term placentas contain septal cysts.[2] They are located at the apex of the septa and are probably a result of obstructed venous drainage.[2] Septal cysts have been documented sonographically as anechoic/hypoechoic intraplacental lesions.[45]

Septal cysts, perivillous fibrin deposition, and intervillous thromboses are indistinguishable at sonography.

A

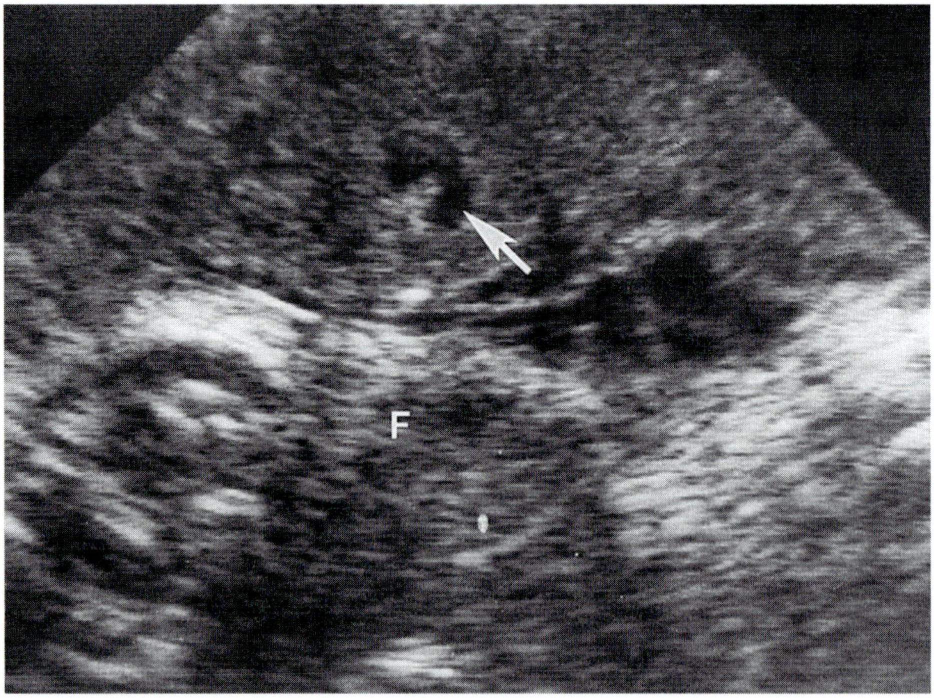

FIG. 47-16. Perivillous fibrin deposition. **A,** Sector scan at 35 weeks shows intraplacental anechoic lesion with echogenic area within *(arrow)*. F, fetus.

Continued.

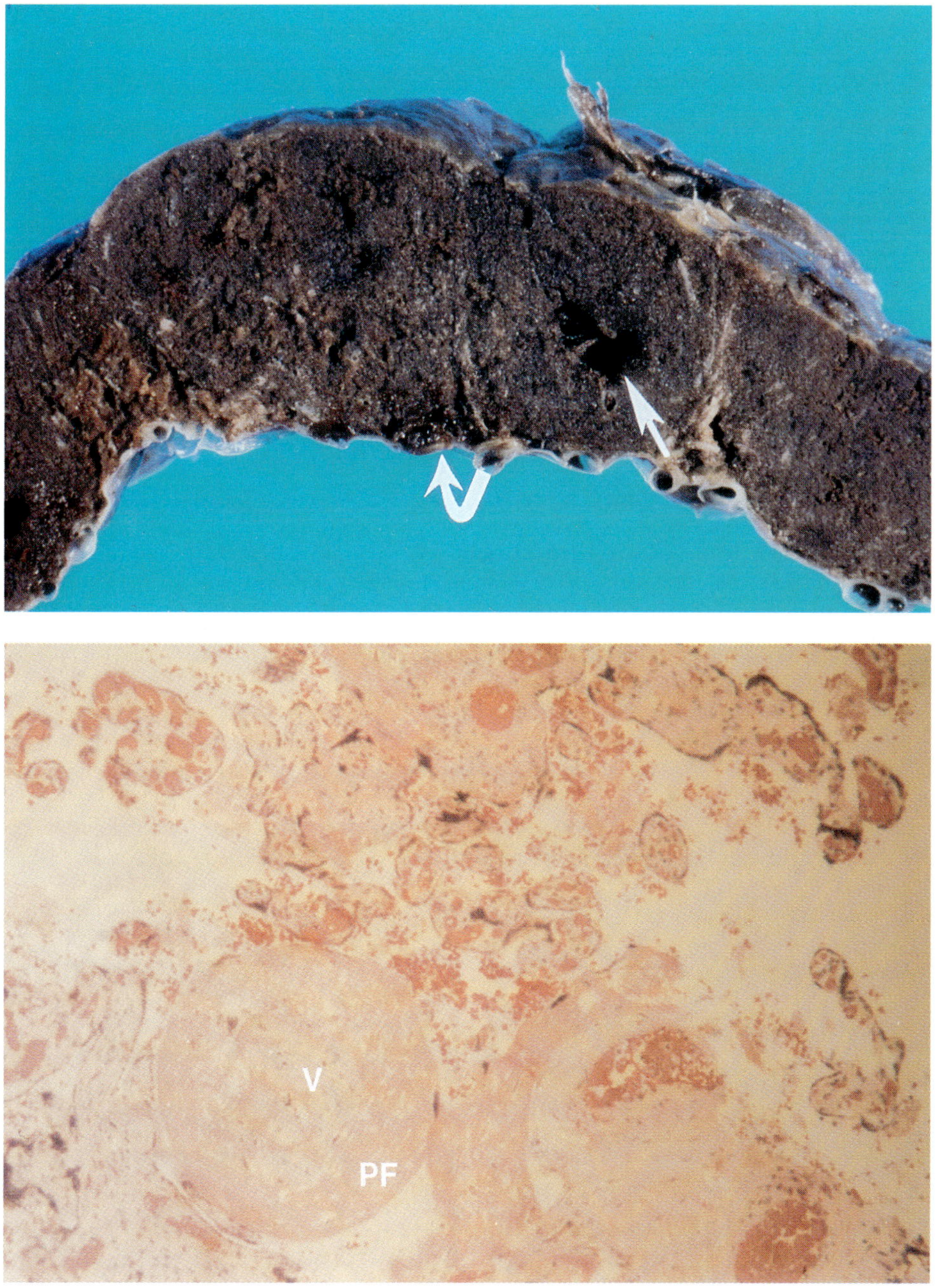

B

C

FIG. 47-16, cont'd. **B,** Cross-section of placenta following delivery shows corresponding lesion *(arrow)*, with solid component corresponding to echogenic region in **A**. Empty space contained blood, which fell out upon sectioning. *Curved arrow,* fetal surface. **C,** Photomicrograph of solid portion of lesion shows perivillous fibrin (PF) surrounding villi (V). (**C** from Spirt BA, Gordon LP. Sonography of the placenta. In: Fleischer AC, Romero R, Manning FA et al., eds. *The Principles and Practice of Ultrasonography in Obstetrics and Gynecology*. 4th ed. Norwalk: Appleton & Lange; 1991.)

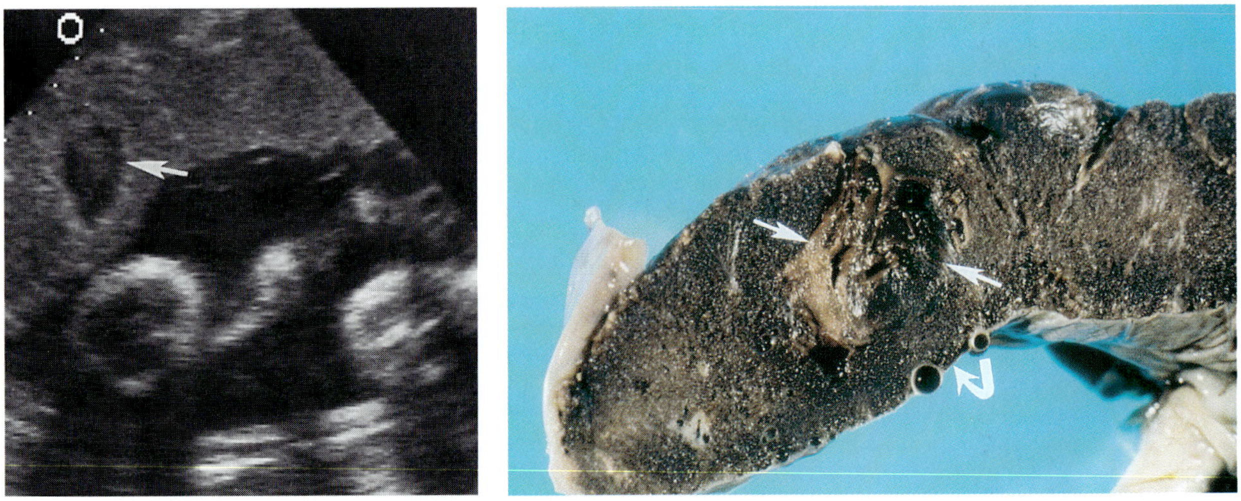

FIG. 47-17. Intervillous thrombosis. **A,** Sagittal scan at 37 weeks shows hypoechoic intraplacental lesion with visible flow *(arrows)* in anterior placenta. (Courtesy of John McKennan, M.D., Mohawk Valley General Hospital, Ilion, New York.) **B,** At term, corresponding lesion *(arrows)* contained blood and laminated fibrin. *Curved arrow,* fetal surface. (From Spirt BA, Gordon LP. Imaging of the placenta. In: Taveras JM, Ferrucci JT, eds. *Radiology: Diagnosis-Imaging-Intervention.* Philadelphia: JB Lippincott Co; 1992.)

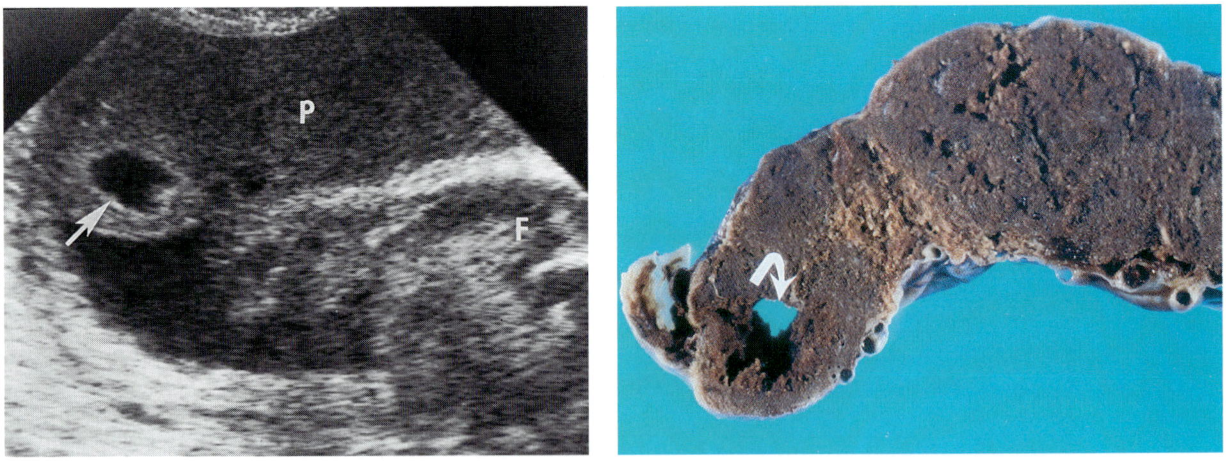

FIG. 47-18. Maternal lake (same patient as in Fig. 47-16.). **A,** Sector scan at 35 weeks shows anechoic intraplacental lesion *(arrow)*. F, fetus. **B,** At delivery, the lesion *(curved arrow)* contained blood that fell out at sectioning. As this placenta contained several areas of perivillous fibrin deposition, it is likely that this lesion represents a stage in the evolution of that entity. (**B** from Spirt BA, Gordon LP. Sonography of the placenta. In: Fleischer AC, Romero R, Manning FA et al., eds. *The Principles and Practice of Ultrasonography in Obstetrics and Gynecology,* 4th ed. Norwalk: Appleton & Lange; 1991.)

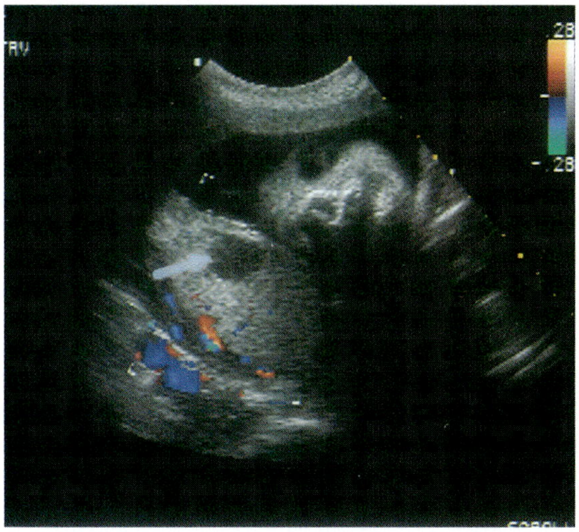

FIG. 47-19. Maternal lake. Slow flow in hypoechoic intraplacental lesion *(arrow)* was visualized at real-time sonography but not with color Doppler imaging.

MACROSCOPIC APPEARANCE: ABNORMAL

Infarcts

Infarcts appear macroscopically as triangular-shaped lesions based on the maternal surface of the placenta. Microscopically, they contain villi that have undergone coagulation necrosis due to disruption of the maternal blood supply. Small areas of infarction occur in 25% of term placentas and are of no clinical significance.[2,11] However, infarction that involves more than 10% of the placenta is considered to be extensive and is associated with IUGR, fetal hypoxia, and fetal demise.[11] The placenta is known to have a large reserve capacity; it can lose up to 30% of its villi and still maintain its function.[2,11] In cases of extensive infarction, it is the underlying disorder that is the cause of the fetal complications and not the loss of placental villi.[11]

Because infarcts are the most likely of the common macroscopic lesions to have clinical significance in the sense that they are a manifestation of an underlying disorder, it would be useful to identify them antenatally. Infarcts cannot, however, be visualized at sonography unless they are complicated by hemorrhage.[45] This is probably because infarcts contain ghost villi, while those lesions that are demonstrable at sonography contain fluid, blood, or fibrin.

Nontrophoblastic Tumors

Primary Placental Tumors. There are two known nontrophoblastic primary placental tumors: the rare **teratoma**[46] and the **chorioangioma.**[47] Small chorioangiomas can be found in up to 1% of carefully sectioned placentas.[2,35] They are usually solitary, but multiple lesions may occur. Most chorioangiomas are located within the substance of the placenta. Lesions measuring greater than 5 cm in diameter are rare and may protrude from the fetal surface (Fig. 47-20).

Chorioangiomas are usually separated from the surrounding placental tissue by a pseudocapsule. Histologically, they consist of small, capillary-sized vessels. Large vessels of varying sizes may be present;

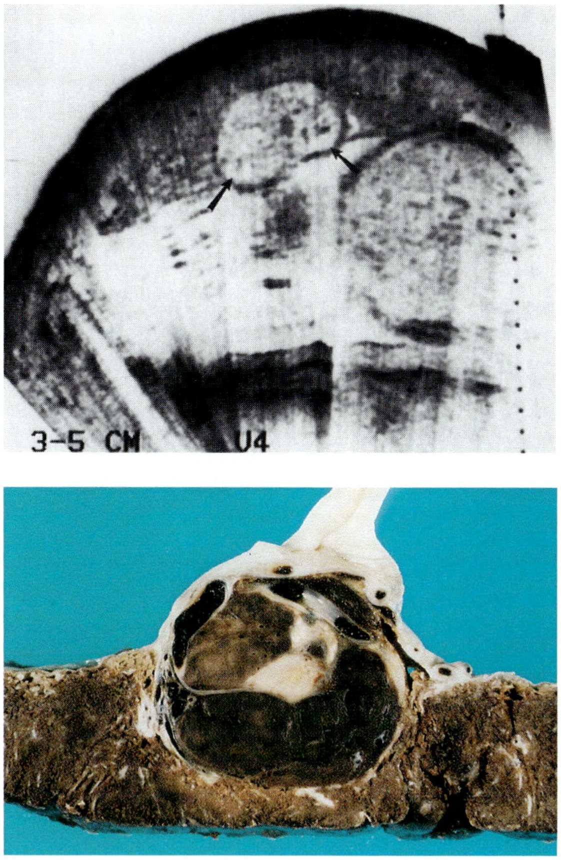

A

B

FIG. 47-20. Chorioangioma. A, Transverse static image at 24 weeks demonstrates solid subchorionic mass *(arrows)*. (From Spirt BA, Gordon LP, Oliphant M. Prenatal Ultrasound: A Color Atlas with Anatomic and Pathologic Correlation. New York: Churchill Livingstone; 1987.) **B,** Cross-section of placenta shows mass protruding from fetal surface. Note multiple vessels of varying size. I, area of infarct. (From Spirt BA, Gordon LP, Cohen WN et al. Antenatal diagnosis of chorioangioma of the placenta. *AJR* 1980;135:1273-1275.)

> **THREE CATEGORIES OF NONTROPHOBLASTIC TUMORS THAT OCCUR IN THE PLACENTA**
>
> Primary placental tumors
> Metastasis from maternal neoplasms
> Metastasis from fetal neoplasms

they are similar to hemangiomas elsewhere in the body. The sonographic appearance is that of a well-demarcated, complex mass within the placenta. If it is sufficiently large, it distorts the fetal surface. Larger vessels may be identified within the lesion.[48]

Most chorioangiomas have no clinical significance. However, large tumors may cause fetal as well as maternal complications, including polyhydromnios, fetal hydrops, fetal cardiomegaly and congestive heart failure, and neonatal thrombocytopenia.[47]

Metastatic Lesions. Reported cases of maternal neoplasms that have metastasized to the placenta include melanoma, carcinoma of the breast, and carcinoma of the lung. Fetal neuroblastoma and leukemia have been detected in the placenta as well.[47]

Hydatidiform Change

Multiple diffuse anechoic intraplacental lesions of varying sizes are abnormal and correlate with hydatidiform change. The differential includes true mole, partial mole, and triploidy.

True Hydatidiform Mole. A hydatidiform mole represents total replacement of the normal placenta by grossly dilated, hydropic villi. It is thought to arise as a result of abnormal fertilization. An empty ovum fertilized by a single sperm with duplication of the paternal haploid set of chromosomes will result in a 46,XX karyotype. 46,YY is nonviable. An empty ovum fertilized through dispermy will yield either 46,XX or 46,XY karyotypes. From 3% to 13% of classical hydatidiform moles are 46,XY; the remainder are 46,XX.[49-51]

At **sonography,** a hydatidiform mole presents a classic pattern of a solid collection of echoes with anechoic spaces too numerous to count (Fig. 47-21). These represent vesicles that result from edema and distention of the villi, producing the typical gross appearance of a "bunch of grapes." It is usually accompanied by absence of the fetal stromal blood vessels. The vesicles vary in size from 1 to 30 mm[49] and seem to increase in size with gestational age. With the relatively smaller villi seen in earlier gestation, the uterus may have a more homogeneous appearance. In this situation, transvaginal sonography is useful to confirm the diagnosis of hydatidiform mole (Fig. 47-22).

Massive bilateral ovarian enlargement with multiple theca lutein cysts may occur in the presence of a mole. This is thought to be a reaction to the high levels of human chorionic gonadotropin (hCG).

A true mole in association with a fetus is most likely to occur in the case of multiple ovulation in which one ovum was empty. Thus, if a hydatidiform mole is seen in association with a fetus, another placenta should be present as well (Fig. 47-23). Rarely, a fetus may occur in a complete mole.[50]

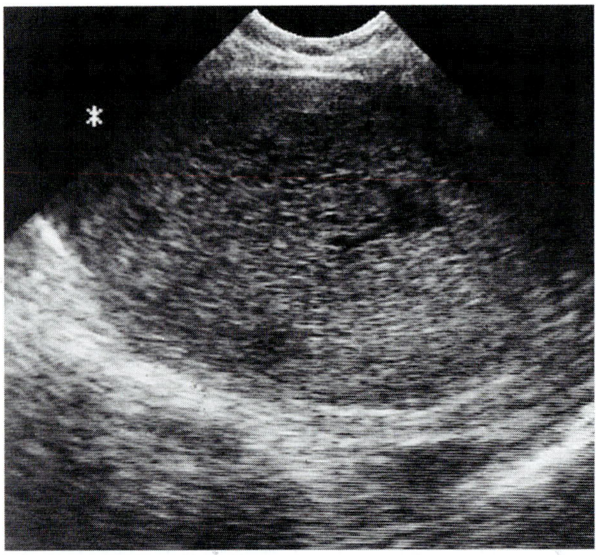

FIG. 47-21. Hydatidiform mole. Sagittal sector scan shows typical vesicular echo pattern of hydatidiform mole filling the entire uterus. (From Spirt BA, Gordon LP. Practical aspects of placental evaluation. *Semin Roentgenol* 1991;26:32-49.)

While not in itself a neoplastic condition, hydatidiform mole is often considered to be premalignant because of its close association with choriocarcinoma. Approximately 10% of patients with hydatidiform mole go on to develop persistent trophoblastic disease, including invasive mole and choriocarcinoma.[49]

Choriocarcinoma is characterized by sheets of malignant trophoblast and the absence of identifiable villi. In approximately 50% of cases in the western hemisphere, choriocarcinoma was preceded by a hydatidiform mole; the incidence is higher in the Far East.[49]

Persistent trophoblastic disease should be suspected clinically on the basis of continued hCG elevation following evacuation of a hydatidiform mole.

Partial Mole. A placenta in which there are villi interspersed with enlarged, edematous (hydropic) villi in association with a fetus is known as a partial mole. Most partial moles have a triploid karyotype (69 chromosomes).[49-52] The fetus is usually abnormal. At sonography, the placenta is enlarged and contains areas of multiple, diffuse anechoic lesions (Fig. 47-24).

There is evidence that patients with partial mole may develop persistent disease requiring chemotherapy.[49,53-56] Thus, follow-up hCG levels are necessary in patients with partial moles as well as in those with complete moles.

THE RETROPLACENTAL AREA

The retroplacental myometrium and decidua can be visualized throughout pregnancy. It is important to

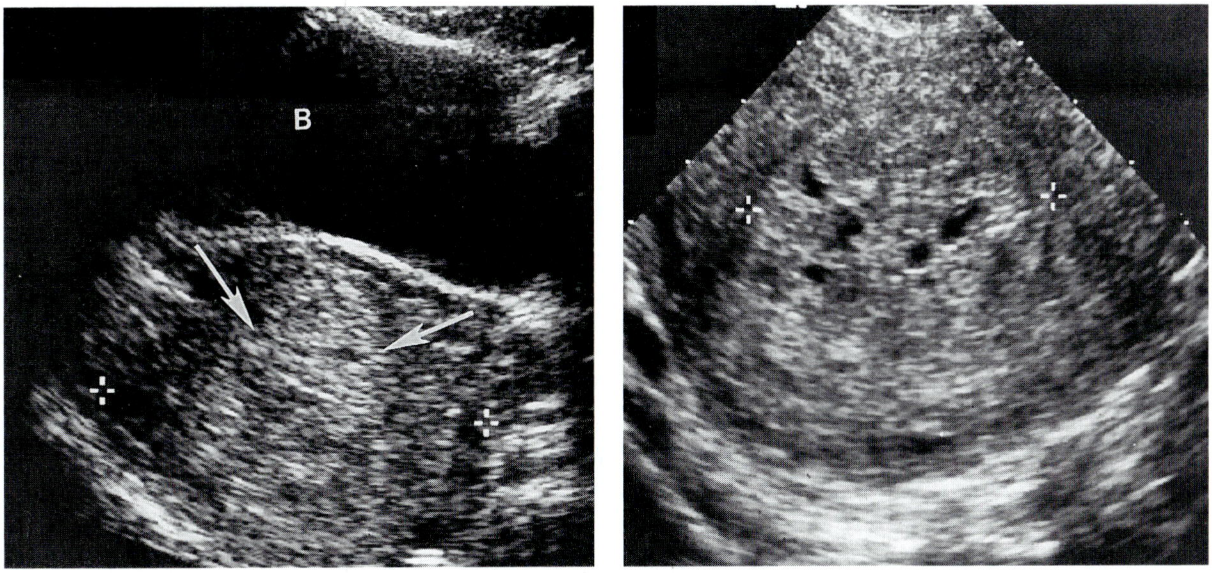

FIG. 47-22. Early hydatidiform mole. **A,** Transabdominal scan of the uterus at 12 weeks' amenorrhea shows inhomogeneous echogenic uterine contents *(arrows)*. B, bladder. **B,** Transvaginal scan clearly shows the typical vesicular pattern of hydatidiform mole *(cursors)*.

document the presence of the hypoechoic retroplacental myometrium and decidua; absence of the normal retroplacental structures may be seen in placenta creta.[57,58]

Placenta Creta

In this condition the placenta adheres to (***placenta accreta vera***), invades (***placenta increta***), or completely penetrates (***placenta percreta***) the myometrium (Fig. 47-25) because of partial or complete absence of the decidua basalis. At sonography, multiple intraplacental "lakes" have been documented in cases of placenta creta.[59-61] These are likely a result of the aberrant blood flow that occurs in the absence of normal decidua. There is an increased risk of placenta creta in patients with a history of prior cesarian section or uterine scars of other etiology.[2] Antepartum rupture of the uterus may occur. A hysterectomy must usually be performed due to failure of the placenta to separate from the uterus. In over 30% of cases, placenta creta is associated with placenta previa. Thus, placenta creta should be suspected when placenta previa is documented. If the decidual defect is small, and in the absence of myometrial invasion, placenta creta may not be detected at sonography.

Contractions

Myometrial and placental thickening occurs as a transient event due to normal uterine contractions (Figs. 47-26 and 47-27) which are imperceptible to the mother. These are most commonly seen toward the end of the first trimester and in the second trimester, and

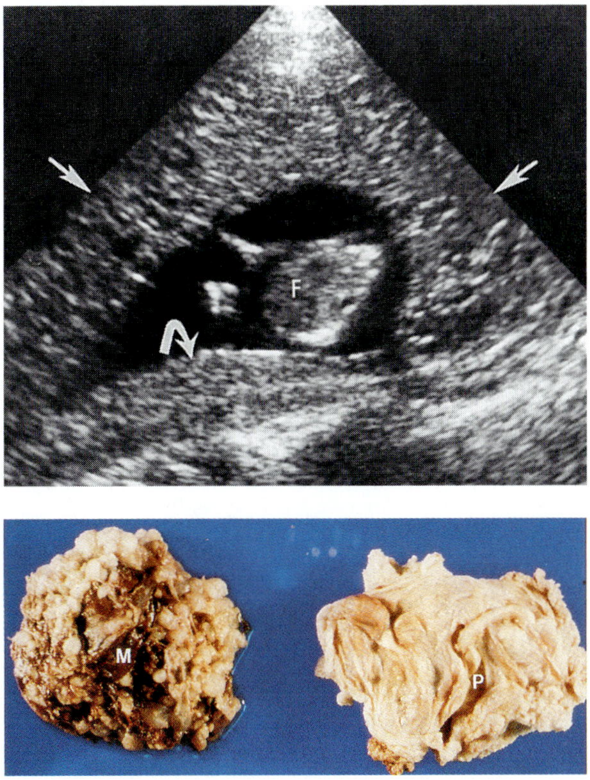

FIG. 47-23. Hydatidiform mole and coexistent fetus. **A,** Sagittal sector scan at 13 weeks shows large anterior hydatidiform mole *(arrows)* and separate posterior placenta *(curved arrow)*. F, fetus. (From Spirt BA, Gordon LP. Imaging of the placenta. In: Taveras JM, Ferrucci JT, eds. Radiology: Diagnosis-Imaging-Intervention. Philadelphia: JB Lippincott Co; 1992.) **B,** A hydatidiform mole (M) was delivered along with a normal placenta (P). (From Spirt BA, Gordon LP. Practical aspects of placental evaluation. *Semin Roentgenol* 1991;26:32-49.)

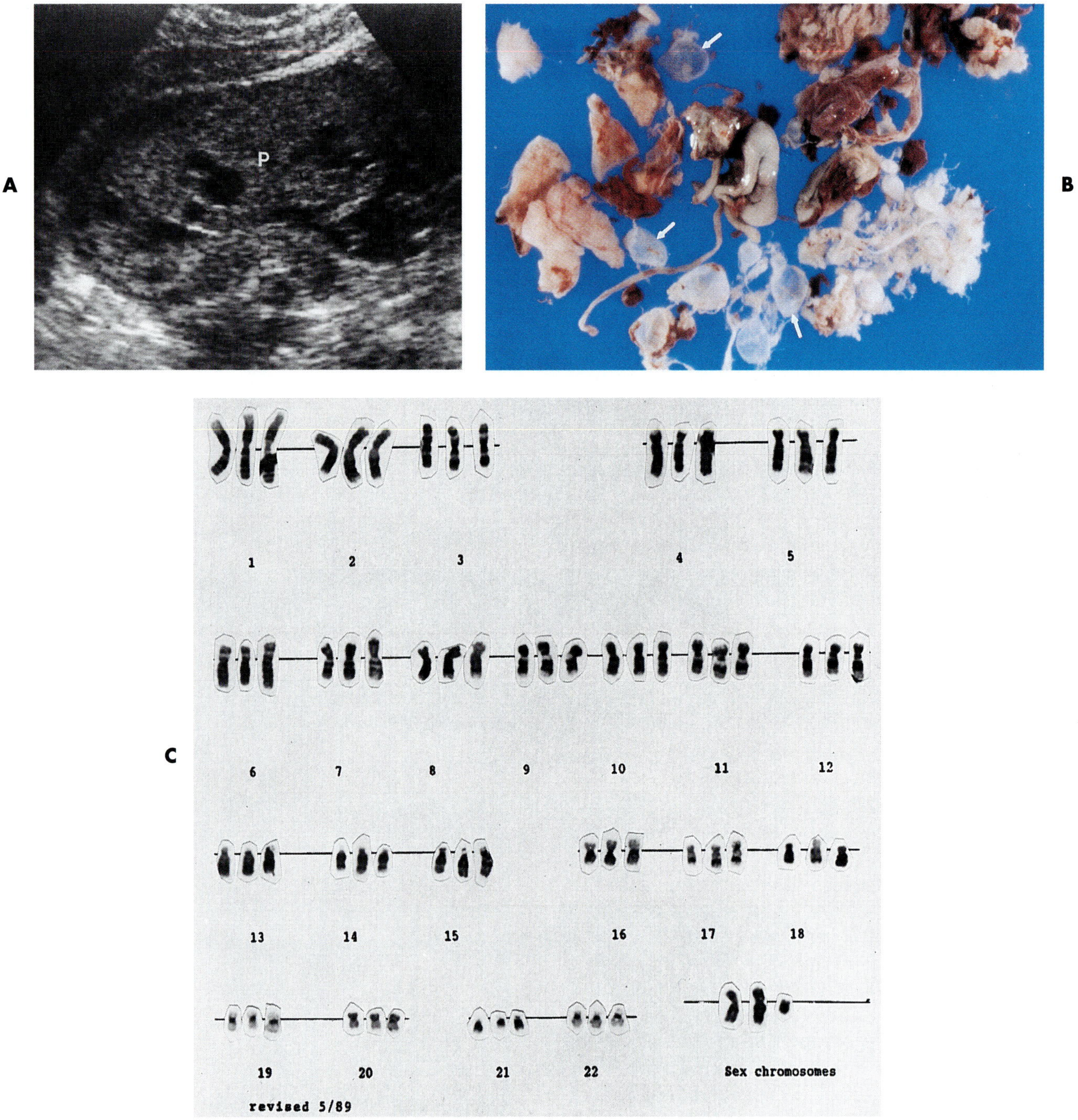

FIG. 47-24. Partial mole (triploidy). **A,** Sagittal scan at 16 weeks shows large placenta (P) with multiple anechoic lesions of varying sizes. Fetal demise had occurred. (From Spirt BA. The placenta, umbilical cord and membranes. In: Wilson SR, ed. *Ultrasound: Categorical Course Syllabus.* Reston, Va: American Roentgen Ray Society; 1993.) **B,** Note areas of normal villi interspersed with hydropic vesicles *(arrows)*. **C,** Chromosomal analysis confirmed triploidy. (**B, C** from Spirt BA, Gordon LP. Sonography of the placenta. In: Fleischer AC, Manning FA, Jeanty P, Romero R. *Sonography in Obstetrics and Gynecology: Principles and Practice.* 5th ed. Stamford: Appleton & Lange; 1996.)

often result in confusion at sonography because they can mimic a retroplacental mass such as a leiomyoma or hematoma, as well as placenta previa (see below). Contractions will change over a short period of time (usually 20 to 30 minutes), while a leiomyoma or a hematoma would not change significantly during such a time span. The presence of multiple leiomyomas in the uterus also helps to distinguish this entity from a contraction.

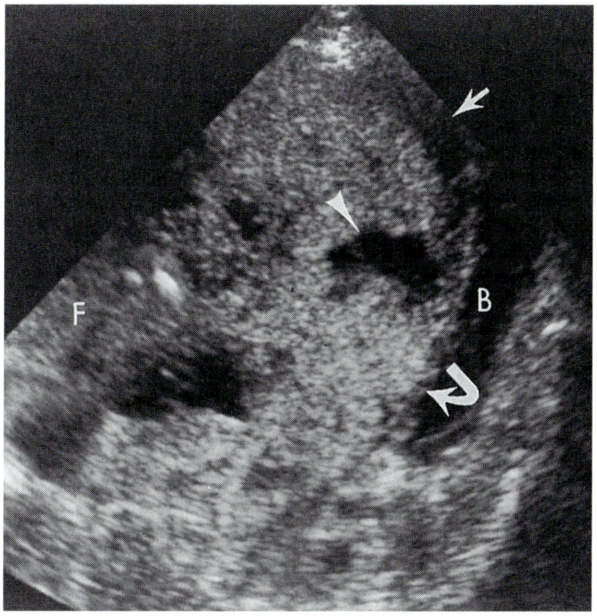

FIG. 47-25. Placenta creta. Sagittal scan at 20.5 weeks. The retroplacental myometrium/decidua *(arrows)* disappears inferiorly where the placenta invades the myometrium *(curved arrow)*. Note the prominent placental lake *(arrowhead)*. B, maternal bladder. F, fetus. P, placenta. (From Spirt BA, Gordon LP. Practical aspects of placental evaluation. *Semin Roentgenol* 1991;26:32-49.)

ANTEPARTUM HEMORRHAGE

Bleeding from placenta previa and abruption usually occurs at or near term, while submembranous and small retroplacental hematomas may be seen throughout pregnancy.[62-65]

Placenta Previa

Placenta previa refers to a placenta that covers part or all of the internal os of the cervix (Fig. 47-28). It occurs in approximately 0.7% of births, with increased frequency in older mothers and in women who smoke.[66]

Two situations mimic placenta previa at sonography: an overdistended bladder and myometrial contractions. The overly full bladder presses against the lower uterine segment, bringing the anterior wall against the posterior wall and causing an artificially elongated cervix. A normally implanted placenta may thus appear to cover the internal os[7,57-59] (Fig. 47-29). Rescanning after emptying of the bladder will resolve this problem.

ANTEPARTUM HEMORRHAGE MAY BE DIVIDED INTO THREE CATEGORIES

Placenta previa
Abruption
Retroplacental or submembranous hematomas

A 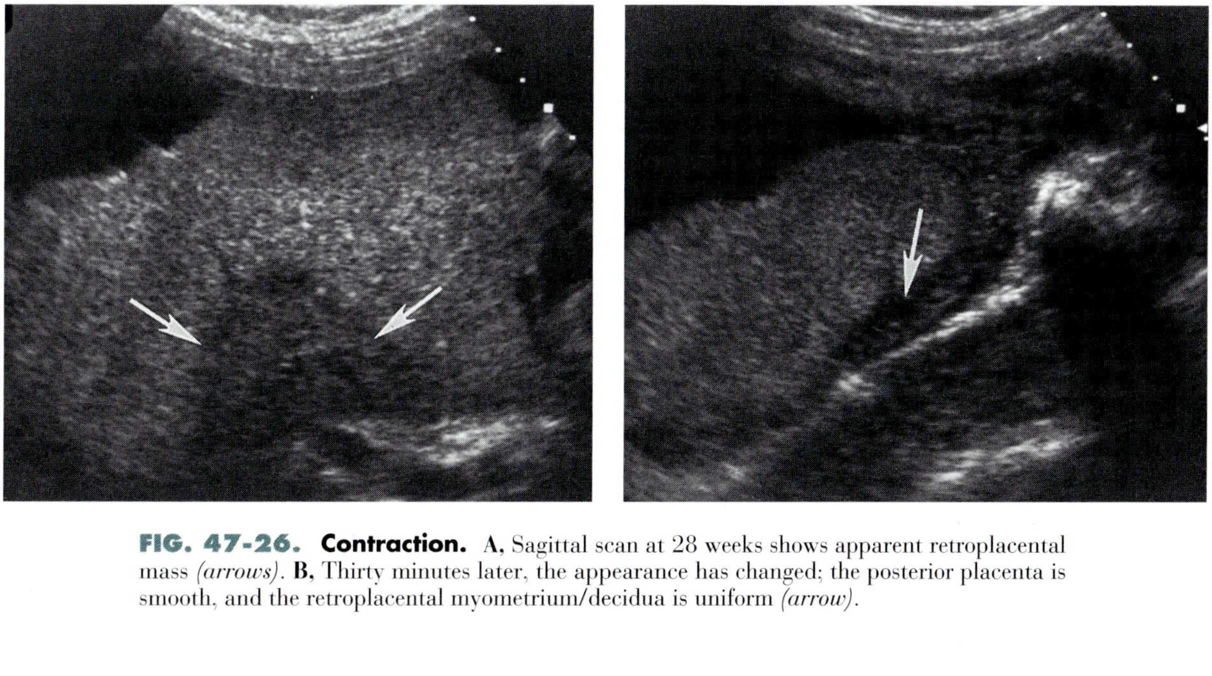 B

FIG. 47-26. Contraction. A, Sagittal scan at 28 weeks shows apparent retroplacental mass *(arrows)*. **B,** Thirty minutes later, the appearance has changed; the posterior placenta is smooth, and the retroplacental myometrium/decidua is uniform *(arrow)*.

A

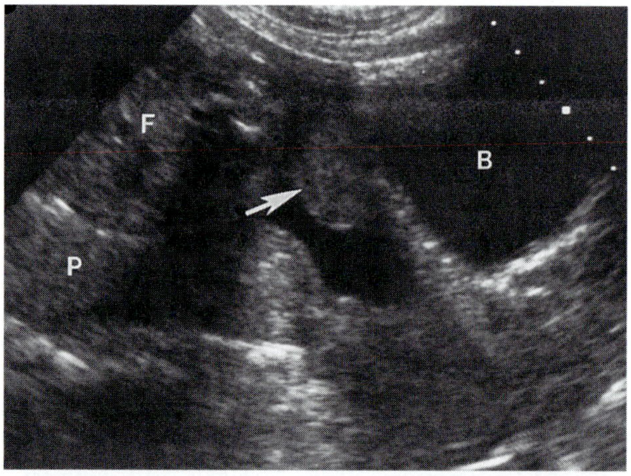

B

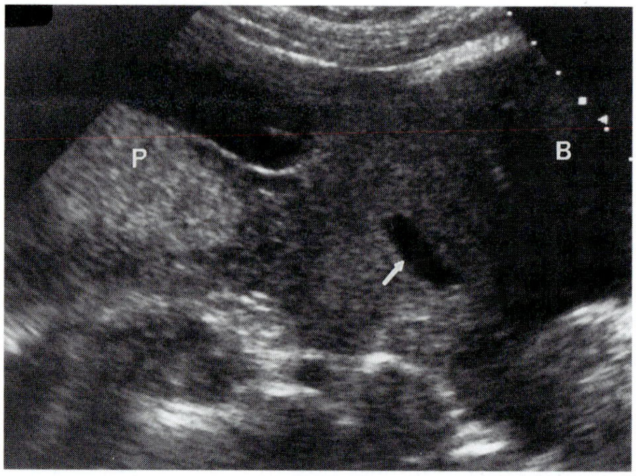

C

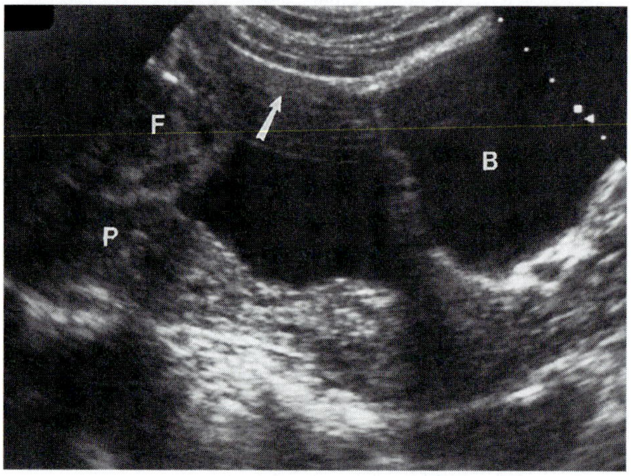

FIG. 47-27. Contraction. **A**, Sagittal scan at 28 weeks shows posterior placenta and apparent anteroinferior succenturiate lobe *(arrow)*. **B**, A few minutes later, the inferior myometrium has markedly thickened, with a small area of amniotic fluid in the center *(arrow)*. **C**, Eighteen minutes later, the contraction has disappeared and the anterior myometrium *(arrow)* has thinned. P, placenta. B, maternal bladder. F, fetus.

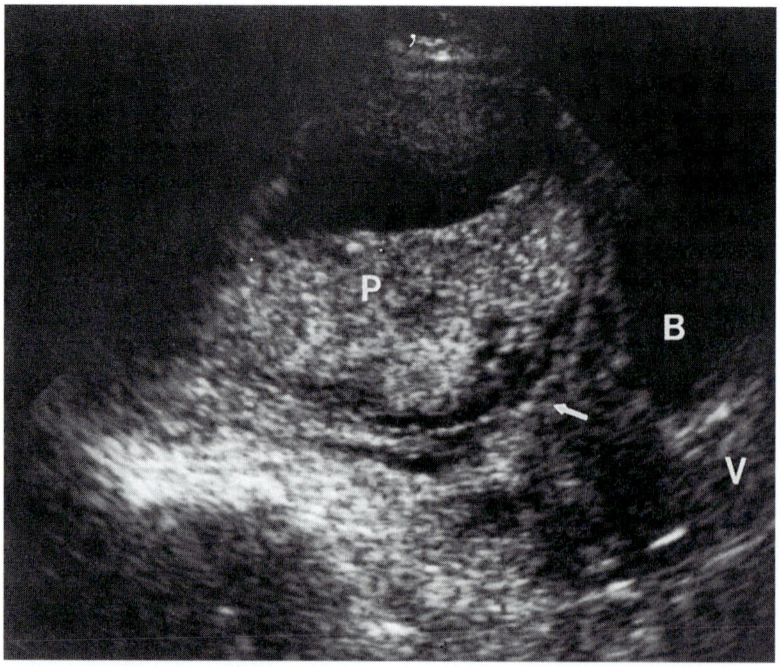

FIG. 47-28. Placenta previa. Sagittal scan at 28 weeks shows posteroinferior placenta (P) completely covering the internal cervical os *(arrow)*. Placenta previa was confirmed at cesarian section. B, maternal bladder. V, vagina. (From Spirt BA, Gordon LP. Practical aspects of placental evaluation. *Semin Roentgenol* 1991;26:32-49.)

A

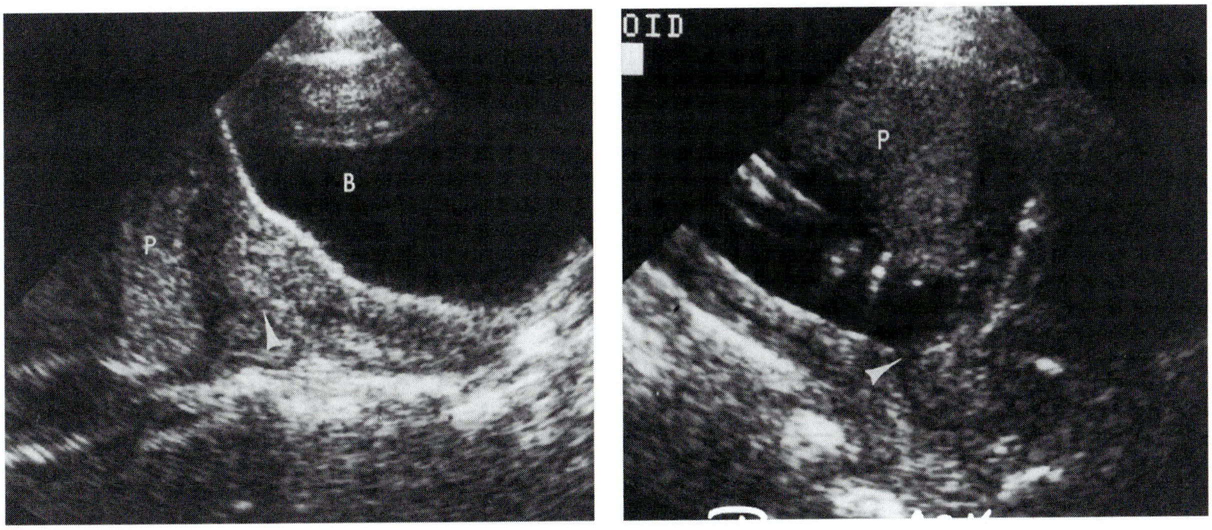

B

FIG. 47-29. Bladder effect. **A,** Midline sagittal sector scan at 19 weeks shows overdistended bladder (B). Placenta (P) overlies apparent cervical os *(arrowhead)*. B, Following voiding, anterior placenta (P) is well away from internal cervical os *(arrowhead)*. (From Spirt BA, Gordon LP. Practical aspects of placental evaluation. *Semin Roentgenol* 1991;26:32-49.)

A

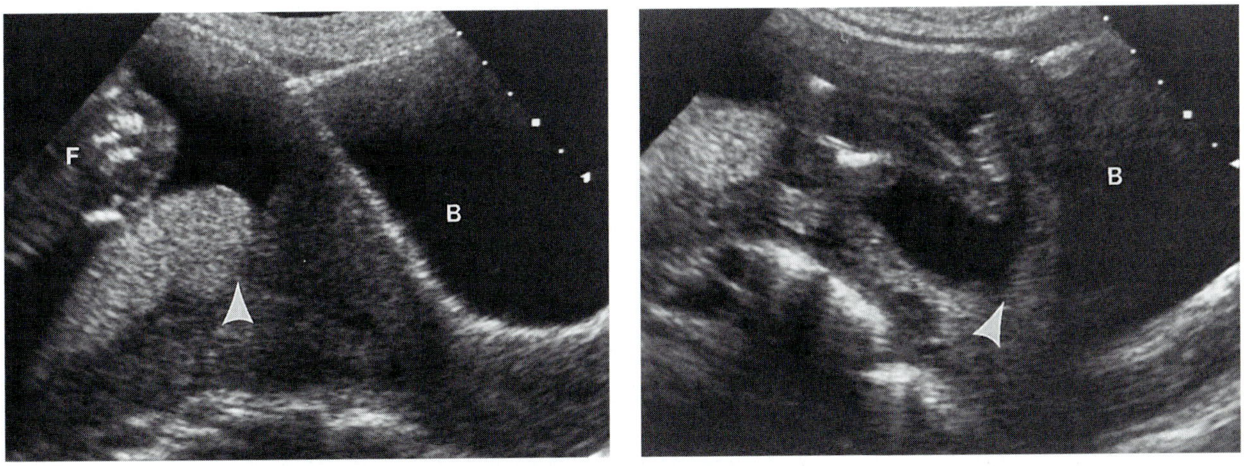

B

FIG. 47-30. Contraction mimicking placenta previa. **A,** Sagittal midline sector scan at 19 weeks shows posterior placenta covering area of internal cervical os *(arrowhead)*. B, maternal bladder. F, fetus. **B,** Repeat scan 45 minutes later shows that the posterior placenta is well away from the internal cervical os *(arrowhead)*.

Contractions in the first and second trimesters commonly mimic placenta previa (Fig. 47-30). Most false-positive ultrasound diagnoses of early placenta previa are, in fact, due to contractions.[69,70] Therefore, in any case of suspected placenta previa, the patient should be reimaged after a 20- to 30-minute interval and, if necessary, again after an hour to assess the true relationship of the placenta to the internal cervical os.

After about 20 weeks, the cervix is often obscured by the fetal head at transabdominal sonography. In that situation, transperineal sonography is useful to establish the position of the placenta with respect to the cervix.[71]

Abruptio Placenta

Abruptio placenta is an acute clinical syndrome manifested by pain, vaginal bleeding, and hypovolemic shock, necessitating rapid delivery. Often there is no time for sonography to be performed. In patients who are sufficiently stable to have an ultrasound examination, an ill-defined echogenic collection, either hyperechoic or isoechoic with respect to the placenta, is seen in the retroplacental area (Fig. 47-31). Abruptio placenta has been associated with maternal hypertension[28] and with cocaine abuse.[72]

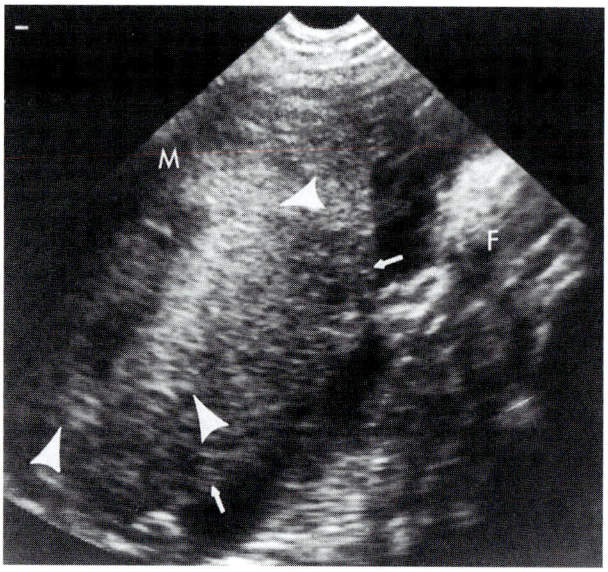

FIG. 47-31. Abruptio placenta. Sagittal sector scan at 35 weeks shows inhomogeneous echogenic collection *(arrowheads)* between placenta *(arrows)* and myometrium (M). Interface between placenta and hematoma is not clearly delineated. F, fetus. At cesarian section, a 75% abruption was found. (Courtesy of Medical Imaging Department, Crouse-Irving Memorial Hospital, Syracuse, New York.)

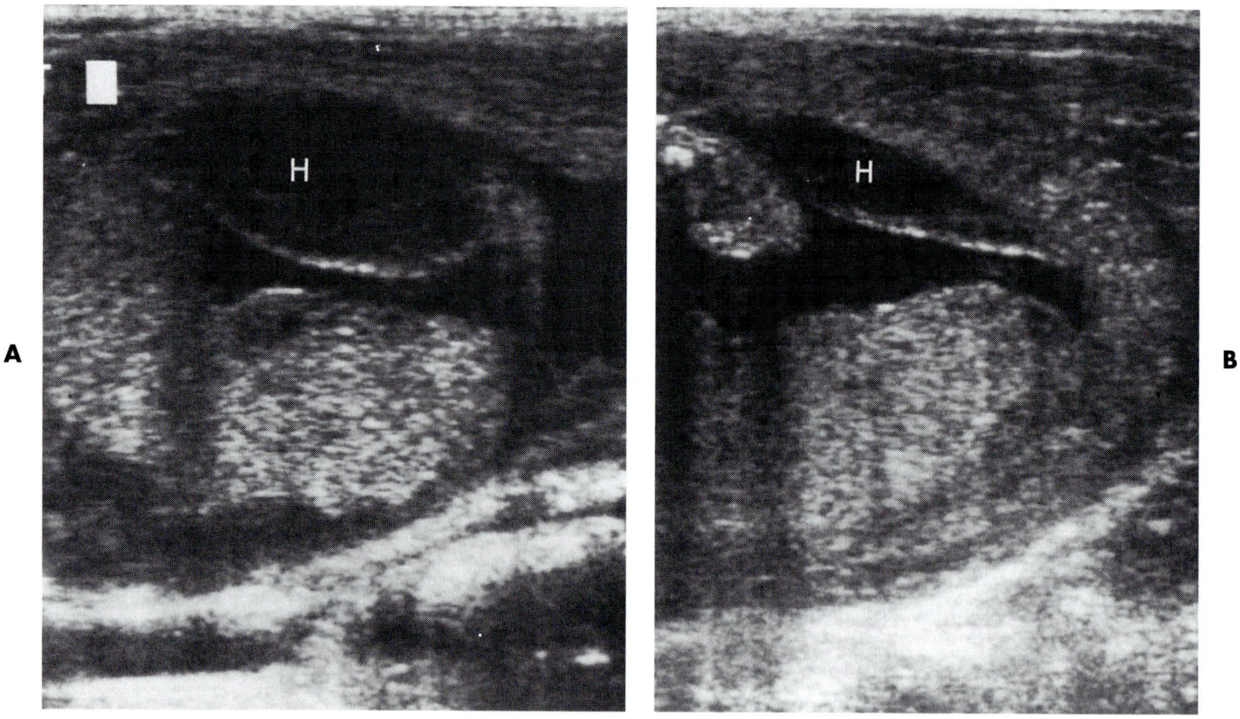

FIG. 47-32. Subchorionic hematoma. **A,** Sagittal linear array scan at 27 weeks shows anterior hypoechoic subchorionic collection (H) adjacent to posterior fundal placenta. The patient had been bleeding. **B,** Follow-up scan at 30 weeks shows that the hematoma (H) has decreased in size.

"Chronic" Retroplacental/ Submembranous Hematoma

Submembranous hematomas may be seen at sonography as early as 9 weeks' menstrual age.[65,73] They range in appearance from hypoechoic or hyperechoic to anechoic, depending on the age of the hematoma (Fig. 47-32). They are usually seen to decrease in size at follow-up examination. At delivery careful examination of the placenta and membranes will show a layer of organized hematoma or fibrin.[62]

Small submembranous hematomas (less than 60 ml) are not associated with an increased risk of spontaneous abortion.[65] Submembranous and retroplacental hematomas should be followed sonographically to insure that they decrease in size.

REFERENCES

Normal Growth and Development

1. Kaufman AJ, Fleischer AC, Thieme GA et al. Separated chorioamnion and elevated chorion: sonographic features and clinical significance. *J Ultrasound Med* 1985;4:119-125.
2. Fox H. *Pathology of the Placenta*. Philadelphia: WB Saunders Co; 1978.
3. Crawford JM. Vascular anatomy of the human placenta. *Am J Obstet Gynecol* 1962;84:1543-1567.
4. Ramsey EM, Corner GW, Donner MW. Serial and cineradiographic visualization of maternal circulation in the primate (hemochorial) placenta. *Am J Obstet Gynecol* 1963;86:213-225.
5. Wigglesworth JF. Vascular anatomy of the human placenta and its significance for placental pathology. *J Obstet Gynecol Br Commonw* 1969;76:979-989.
6. Ramsey EM. Circulation in the maternal placenta of the Rhesus monkey and man with observations on the marginal lakes. *Am J Anat* 1956;98:159-190.
7. Spirt BA, Kagan EH, Rozanski R. Sonographic anatomy of the normal placenta. *J Clin Ultrasound* 1979;7:204-207.
8. Smith DF, Foley DW. Real-time ultrasound and pulsed Doppler evaluation of the retroplacental clear area. *J Clin Ultrasound* 1982;10:215-219.
9. Tindall VR, Scott JS. Placental calcification. A study of 3,025 singleton and multiple pregnancies. *J Obstet Gynecol Br Commonw* 1965;72:356-373.
10. Spirt BA, Cohen WN, Weinstein HM. The incidence of placental calcification in normal pregnancies. *Radiology* 1982; 142:707-711.
11. Fox H. General pathology of the placenta. In: Fox H., ed. Haines and Taylor *Obstetrical and Gynaecological Pathology, 3rd ed.* Edinburgh: Churchill Livingstone; 1987:972-1000.
12. Spirt BA, Gordon LP. The placenta as an indicator of fetal maturity: fact and fancy. *Semin Ultrasound* 1984;5:290-297.
13. Wentworth P. Macroscopic placental calcification and its clinical significance. *J Obstet Gynecol Br Commonw* 1965;72:215-222.
14. Fujikura D. Placental calcification and seasonal difference. *Am J Obstet Gynecol* 1963;87:46-47.
15. Jeacock MK. Calcium content of the human placenta. *Am J Obstet Gynecol* 1963;87:34-40.
16. Heifetz SA. Single umbilical artery: a statistical analysis of 237 autopsy cases and review of the literature. *Perspec Pediatr Pathol* 1984;8:345-378.
17. Froehlich LA, Fujikura T. Follow-up of infants with single umbilical artery. *Pediatrics* 1973;52:6-13.
18. Sutro WH, Tuck SM, Loesevitz A et al. Prenatal observation of umbilical cord hematoma. *AJR* 1984;142:801-802.
19. Casola G, Scheible W, Leopold GR. Large umbilical cord: a normal finding in some fetuses. *Radiology* 1985;156:181-182.
20. Ghidini A, Romero R, Eisen RN et al. Umbilical cord hematoma: prenatal identification and review of the literature. *J Ultrasound Med* 1990;9:297-300.
21. Juniaux E, Moscoso G, Chitty L et al. An angiomyxoma involving the whole length of the umbilical cord: prenatal diagnosis by ultrasonography. *J Ultrasound Med* 1990;9:419-422.
22. Rosenberg JC, Chervenak FA, Walker BA et al. Antenatal sonographic appearance of omphalomesenteric duct cyst. *J Ultrasound Med* 1986;5:719-720.
23. Reuter KL, Davidoff A, Hunter T. Vasa previa. *J Clin Ultrasound* 1988;16:346-348.

Size

24. Hellman LM, Kobayashi M, Tolles WE et al. Ultrasonic studies of the volumetric growth of the human placenta. *Am J Obstet Gynecol* 1970;108:740-750.
25. Hoddick WK, Mahony BS, Callen PW et al. Placental thickness. *J Ultrasound Med* 1985;4:479-482.
26. Ghosh A, Tang MHY, Lam YH et al. Ultrasound measurement of placental thickness to detect pregnancies affected by homozygous alpha-thalassaemia-1. *Lancet* 1994;344;988-989.
27. Ko TM, Tseng LK, Hsu PM et al. Ultrasonographic scanning of placental thickness and the prenatal diagnosis of homozygous alpha-thalassemia 1 in the second trimester. *Prenat Diag* 1995;15:7-10.
28. Perrin EVKD, Sander CH. Introduction: how to examine the placenta and why. In: Perrin EVKD, ed. *Pathology of the Placenta*. New York: Churchill Livingstone; 1984:11-12.

Macroscopic Appearance: Normal

29. Spirt BA, Kagan EH, Gordon LP et al. Antepartum diagnosis of a succenturiate lobe: sonographic and pathologic correlation. *J Clin Ultrasound* 1981;9:139-140.
30. Jeanty P, Kirkpatrick C, Verhoogen C et al. The succenturiate placenta. *J Ultrasound Med* 1983;2:9-12.
31. Scott JS. Placenta extrachorialis (placenta marginata and placenta circumvallate): a factor in antepartum hemorrhage. *J Obstet Gynaecol Br Commonw* 1960;67:904-918.
32. Naftolin F, Khudr G, Benirschke K, et al. The syndrome of chronic abruptio placentae, hydrorrhea, and circumvallate placentae. *Am J Obstet Gynecol* 1973;116:347-350.
33. Cutillo DP, Swayne LC, Schwartz JR. Intra-amniotic hemorrhage secondary to placenta circumvallate. *J Ultrasound Med* 1989;8:399-401.
34. Spirt BA, Kagan EH, Rozanski RM. Sonolucent areas in the placenta: sonographic and pathologic correlation. *AJR* 1978; 131:961-965.
35. Benirschke K, Kaufman P. *Pathology of the Human Placenta*. New York: Springer-Verlag; 1995.
36. Spirt BA, Gordon LP, Kagan EH. Sonography of the placenta. In: Sanders RC, James AE, eds. *The Principles and Practice of Ultrasonography in Obstetrics and Gynecology. 2nd ed.* New York: Appleton-Century-Crofts; 1980.
37. Kaplan C, Blanc WA, Elias J. Identification of erythrocytes in intervillous thrombi: a study using immunoperoxidase identification of hemoglobins. *Hum Pathol* 1982;113:554-557.
38. Spirt BA, Gordon LP, Kagan EH. Intervillous thrombosis: sonographic and pathologic correlation. *Radiology* 1983; 147:197-200.
39. Hoogland HJ, de Haan J, Vooys GP. Ultrasonographic diagnosis of intervillous thrombosis related to Rh isoimmunization. *Gynecol Obstet Inves* 1979;10:237-245.
40. Javert CT, Reiss C. The origin and significance of macroscopic intervillous coagulation hematomas (red infarcts) of the human placenta. *Surg Gynecol Obstet* 1952;94:257-269.
41. Devi B, Jennison RF, Langley FA. Significance of placental pathology in transplacental hemorrhage. *J Clin Path* 1968;21: 322-331.
42. Perkes EA, Baim RS, Goodman KJ et al. Second-trimester placental changes associated with elevated maternal serum fetoprotein. *Am J Obstet Gynecol* 1982;144:935-938.
43. Fleischer AC, Kurtz AB, Wapner RJ et al. Elevated alpha-fetoprotein and a normal fetal sonogram: association with placental abnormalities. *AJR* 1988;150:881-883.
44. Kelly RB, Nyberg DA, Mack LA et al. Sonography of placental abnormalities and oligohydramnios in women with elevated alpha-fetoprotein levels: comparison with control subjects. *AJR* 1989;153:815-819.
45. Harris RD, Simpson WA, Pet LR et al. Placental hypoechoic/anechoic areas and infarction: sonographic-pathologic correlation. *Radiology* 1990;176:75-80.

Macroscopic Appearance: Abnormal

46. Williams VL, Williams RA. Placental teratoma: prenatal ultrasonographic diagnosis. *J Ultrasound Med* 1994;13:587-589.

47. Fox H. Non-trophoblastic tumours of the placenta. In: Fox H, ed. Haines and Taylor *Obstetrical and Gynaecological Pathology*. 3rd ed. Edinburgh: Churchill Livingstone; 1987: 1030-1044.
48. Spirt BA, Gordon L, Cohen WN et al. Antenatal diagnosis of chorioangioma of the placenta. *AJR* 1980;135:1273-1275.
49. Elston CW. Gestational trophoblastic disease. In: Fox H, ed. Haines and Taylor *Obstetrical and Gynaecological Pathology 3rd ed.* Edinburgh: Churchill Livingstone; 1987:1045-1078.
50. Mazur MT, Kurman RJ. Gestational trophoblastic disease. In: Kurman RJ; ed. *Blaustein's Pathology of the Female Genital Tract.* 3rd ed. New York: Springer-Verlag; 1987:835-875.
51. Szulman A. Trophoblastic disease: complete and partial hydatidiform mole. In: Perrin EVDK, ed. *Pathology of the Placenta.* New York: Churchill Livingstone; 1984:183-197.
52. Szulman AE, Surti U. The syndromes of hydatidiform mole, I: cytogenetic and morphologic correlations. *Am J Obstet Gynecol* 1978;131:665-671.
53. Szulman AE, Wong LC, Hsu C. Residual trophoblastic disease in association with partial hydatidiform mole. *Obstet Gynecol* 1981;57:392-394.
54. Szulman AE, Surti U. The clinicopathologic profile of the partial hydatidiform mole. *Obstet Gynecol* 1982;59:597-602.
55. Teng NH, Ballon SC. Partial hydatidiform mole with diploid karyotype: report of three cases. *Am J Obstet Gynecol* 1984; 150:961-964.
56. Berkowitz RS, Goldstein DP, Bernstein MR. Natural history of partial molar pregnancy. *Obstet Gynecol* 1985;66:677-681.

The Retroplacental Area

57. Pasto ME, Kurtz AB, Rifkin MD et al. Ultrasonographic findings in placenta increta. *J Ultrasound Med* 1983;2:155-159 and *Ultrasound Med* 1992;11:333-343.
58. DeMendonca LK. Sonographic diagnosis of placenta accreta: presentation of six cases. *J Ultrasound Med* 1988;7:211-215.
59. Hoffman-Tretin JC, Koenigsberg M, Rabin A et al. Placenta accreta: additional sonographic observations. *J Ultrasound Med* 1992;11:20-34.
60. Finberg HJ, Williams JW. Placenta accreta: prospective sonographic diagnosis in patients with placenta previa and prior cesarean section. *J Ultrasound Med* 1992;11:333-343.
61. Lerner JP, Deane S, Timor-Tritsch IE. Characterization of placenta accreta using transvaginal sonography and color Doppler imaging. *Ultrasound Obstet Gynecol* 1995;5:198-201.
62. Spirt BA, Kagan EH, Rozanski RM. Abruptio placenta: sonographic and pathologic correlation. *AJR* 1979;133:877-881.
63. Nyberg DA, Cyr DR, Mack LA. Sonographic spectrum of placental abruption. *AJR* 1987;141:161-164.
64. Nyberg DA, Mack LA, Benedetti TJ. Placental abruption and placental hemorrhage: correlation of sonographic findings with fetal outcome. *Radiology* 1987;164:357-336.
65. Pedersen JF, Mantoni M. Prevalence and significance of subchorionic hemorrhage in threatened abortion: a sonographic study. *AJR* 1990;154:535-537.
66. Naeye RL. Functionally important disorders of the placenta, umbilical cord, and fetal membranes. *Human Pathology* 1987;18:680-691.
67. Zemlyn S. The effect of the urinary bladder in obstetrical sonography. *Radiology* 1978;128:169-175.
68. Bowie JD, Andreotti RF, Rosenberg ER. Ultrasound appearance of the uterine cervix in pregnancy: the vertical cervix. *AJR* 1983;140:737-740.
69. Artis AA, Bowie JD, Rosenberg ER, et al. The fallacy of placental migration: effect of sonographic techniques. *AJR* 1985;144:79-81.
70. Spirt BA. Unpublished data.
71. Hertzberg BS, Bowie JD, Carroll BA et al. Diagnosis of placenta previa during the third trimester: role of transperineal sonography. *AJR* 1992;159:83-87.
72. Townsend RR, Laing FC, Jeffrey RB. Placental abruption associated with cocaine abuse. *AJR* 1988;150:1339-1340.
73. Stabile I, Campbell S, Grudzinskas JG. Threatened miscarriage and intrauterine hematomas: sonographic and biochemical studies. *J Ultrasound Med* 1989;8:289-292.

CHAPTER 48

Gestational Trophoblastic Neoplasia

•

Margaret A. Fraser-Hill, M.D., F.R.C.P.C.
Stephanie R. Wilson, M.D., F.R.C.P.C.

CHAPTER OUTLINE

Gestational trophoblastic neoplasia (GTN) is a spectrum of disorders characterized by abnormal proliferation of pregnancy-related trophoblasts with progressive malignant potential.[1] GTN includes molar pregnancy, invasive mole, choriocarcinoma, and placental-site trophoblastic tumor (PSTT). Collectively, the last three conditions are referred to as **persistent trophoblastic neoplasia,** or PTN.

In a normal pregnancy, one of the primary functions of placental trophoblast is to gain access to the maternal circulation. Normal trophoblast infiltrates maternal tissues, invades vessels, and can even be transported to the lungs.[2] This capacity for invasion is shared by all trophoblastic tumors and is responsible for many of the distinctive pathologic, clinical, and imaging features of this fascinating group of lesions. GTN has been known since ancient times. Hippocrates described molar pregnancy as "dropsy of the uterus" and attributed it to unhealthy water. The term hydatidiform mole has been recognized for over three centuries and refers to cystic degeneration of chorionic villi in molar pregnancy. Prior to the middle of this century, malignant GTN was uniformly fatal. Remarkably, it is now the **most curable gynecologic malignancy** as the result of several important advances, including the availability of a sensitive and reliable tumor marker (human chorionic gonadotropin, or hCG), the exquisite sensitivity of most lesions to antifolic chemotherapy, and the use of aggressive multimodality regimens combining chemotherapy, radiation therapy, and surgery in selected patients unresponsive to conventional protocols.[1,3] In general, once the diagnosis of GTN has been established, therapeutic decisions rest mainly on clinical criteria. Diagnostic imaging has an important role to play in diagnosis and management.

MOLAR PREGNANCY

Molar pregnancy is the most common and benign form of GTN, with an incidence of 1 in 1000 pregnancies in North America.[1,3-5] Advancing maternal age, prior history of molar pregnancy, and Asian ancestry are established risk factors.[4,5] Molar pregnancy has the distinctive histologic characteristics of cystic or grape-like (hydatidiform) degeneration of chorionic villi, absent or inadequate vascularization of chorionic villi, and abnormal proliferation of placental trophoblast.[1,3,5-12] Hydatidiform mole is classified as either complete molar pregnancy or partial molar pregnancy on the basis of cytogenetic, morphologic, and clinical features.

Complete Molar Pregnancy

Complete molar pregnancy is characterized by a diploid karyotype of 46,XX in approximately 70% to 85% of cases. In complete molar pregnancy, chromosomal DNA is exclusively paternal in origin. This occurs when an ovum with absent or inactive maternal chromosomes is fertilized by a normal haploid sperm. Endoreduplication of paternal chromosomes produces a **diploid karyotype** of 46,XX (46,YY is lethal). Occasionally, fertilization of an empty ovum by two haploid sperm results in the 46,XY pattern.[10-12] At pathology, there is **no fetal development** in complete molar pregnancy. The placenta is entirely replaced by abnormal, hydropic chorionic villi with excessive trophoblastic proliferation.[1-3,8,9] Although the degree of trophoblastic proliferation ranges from mild to severe, up to 50% of cases are severe.[8,9] Excessive trophoblastic proliferation results in **classic symptoms and signs** that frequently suggest the diagnosis. These include excessive uterine size for dates, markedly elevated serum hCG (greater than 100,000 mIU/ml), hyperemesis gravidarum, toxemia, hyperthyroidism, and respiratory failure. Theca lutein cysts of the ovaries occur in approximately 15% to 30% of cases and reflect excessive hCG levels. Vaginal bleeding, present in over 90% of cases, is the most frequent presenting symptom.[7-9] Passage of vesicles (hydropic villi) occurs in up to 80% of cases and is considered specific for the condition.[7]

Partial Molar Pregnancy

In contrast, **partial molar pregnancy** has a **triploid karyotype** of 69,XXX, 69,XXY, or 69,XYY. Most partial moles have one set of maternal chromosomes and two sets of paternal chromosomes resulting from fertilization of a normal ovum by two haploid sperm. This condition, in which the extra set of chromosomes is paternally derived, is known as diandric triploidy. Triploidy of maternal origin is not associated with GTN.[10-12] At pathology, partial molar pregnancy has well-developed but generally **anomalous (triploid) fetal tissues.** Hydropic degeneration of placental villi is focal, interspersed with normal placental villi. Trophoblastic proliferation is mild.[1-3,7] The clinical diagnosis of partial molar pregnancy is rarely made prospectively. Symptoms and signs are less frequent and less severe because trophoblastic proliferation is mild. Missed or incomplete abortion is the most common clinical diagnosis.[8,9]

Diagnosis and Management

The diagnosis of molar pregnancy should be considered in patients presenting with first trimester vaginal bleeding, rapid uterine enlargement, excessive uterine size for dates, hyperemesis gravidarum, and preeclampsia before 24 weeks. Serum hCG levels in molar pregnancy are abnormally elevated, commonly over 100,000 mIU/ml, in contrast to normal pregnancy levels of less than 60,000 mIU/ml.[7]

Sonographic Features. The classic **sonographic features of complete molar pregnancy** are well-known and include an enlarged uterus containing echogenic tissue that expands the endometrial canal (Fig. 48-1, *A*). Hydropic villi within molar tissue appear as innumerable, diffusely and uniformly distributed cystic spaces ranging in size from a few millimeters to 2 to 3 cm.[13-16] In the second trimester, transabdominal sonographic diagnosis is highly accurate. Transvaginal scans may not add significant diagnostic information or improve outcome.[17] However, early molar gestations may possess atypical features that make transabdominal diagnosis more difficult. In first trimester molar gestations, molar tissue appears as a predominantly solid and echogenic mass because very tiny hydropic villi are not adequately resolved by transabdominal sonography. This appearance is nonspecific, simulated by incomplete abortion or blood clot.[18] Transvaginal US is more sensitive than transabdominal sonography and may depict hydropic villi earlier and to better advantage than transabdominal US (Fig. 48-1, *B*).[19,20] Transvaginal sonography of early molar pregnancy may also depict a solid, echogenic mass within a gestational sac.[21] In complete moles, a fetus is absent except in the rare event of a coexistent twin pregnancy (Fig. 48-2). In such cases, sonography is accurate in establishing the diagnosis. Differentiation from partial molar pregnancy rests on identifying a separate, normal placenta[22] (Fig. 48-2). The ovaries may be greatly enlarged in complete molar pregnancy by multiple, bilateral theca lutein cysts. These may be clear or hemorrhagic and can be a source of pelvic pain.[7,20] The sonographic appearance is similar to that seen in ovarian hyperstimulation from ovulation induction therapy. Theca lutein cysts represent an in vivo bioassay for endogenous hCG and are most marked when trophoblastic proliferation is severe.

The **sonographic features of partial molar pregnancy** are less frequently described and they overlap with other conditions. Partial molar pregnancy is commonly mistaken for missed or incomplete abortion.[18] In partial molar pregnancy, the placenta is excessive in

A

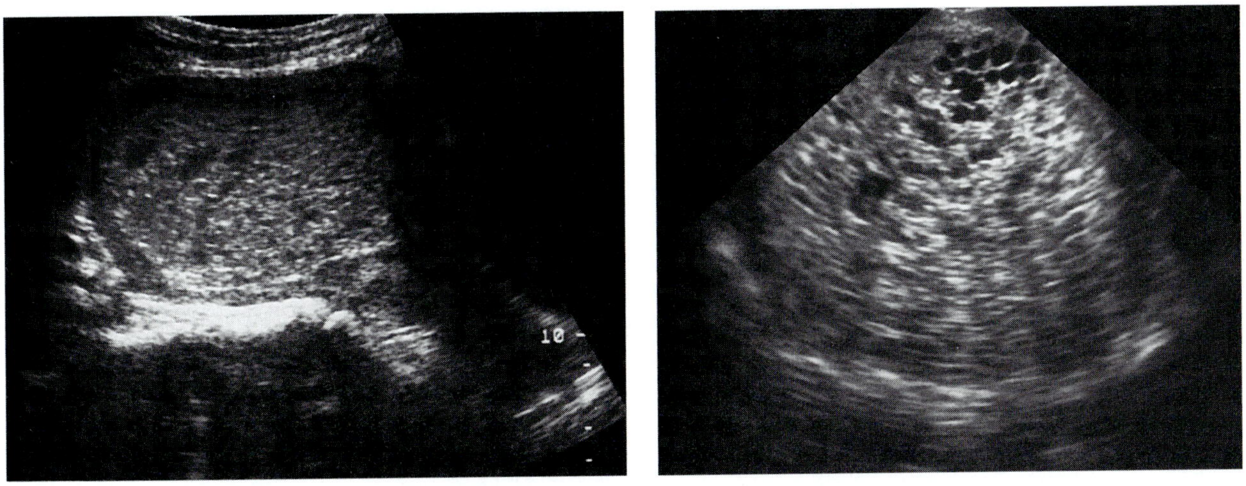

B

FIG. 48-1. Complete molar pregnancy, classic appearance. **A,** Transabdominal scan shows a vesicular echogenic mass filling the endometrial canal. **B,** Transvaginal high-resolution sonogram shows innumerable uniformly distributed cystic spaces that correspond to hydropic chorionic villi at pathology.

A

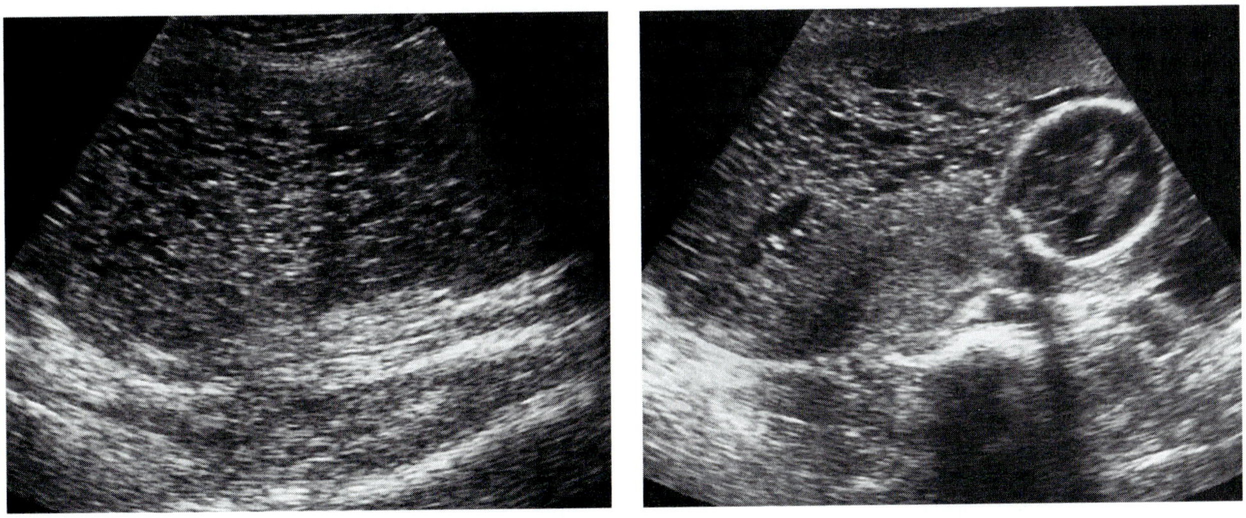

B

FIG. 48-2. Complete mole with a coexistent fetus in an 18-week gestation. **A,** Sagittal scan of right side of uterus shows a large echogenic mass with innumerable tiny cystic spaces, the classic morphology for a complete mole. **B,** Transverse image shows the mole on the left side of the image. There is a normal fetus, head shown here, and a normal anterior placenta. This condition has a poor prognosis.

size and contains numerous cystic spaces distributed in a nonuniform manner. A gestational sac is present and is frequently deformed in shape.[13,14] A growth-retarded fetus is present and may show anomalies of triploidy including syndactyly and hydrocephalus (Fig. 48-3).[1,7,13] Placental hydropic degeneration (unrelated to trophoblastic neoplasia) can also possess similar sonographic features.[13,15] Hydropic degeneration is a common occurrence in first trimester abortion of any cause. The associated cystic spaces may be difficult or impossible to differentiate from an early mole. Therefore, careful evaluation of the products of conception should be recommended to avoid the possibility of missing a diagnosis of mole in cases with equivocal ultrasound features.

Therapy and Prognosis. Therapy of molar pregnancy is uterine evacuation, and the majority are adequately treated in this fashion. Approximately 80% of complete moles and 95% of partial moles will subsequently follow a benign course.[7-9] However, accurate diagnosis and classification of molar pregnancy are important because of the risk of persistent trophoblastic neoplasia (PTN). For this reason, all patients with molar pregnancy are monitored with weekly serum hCG determinations and are counseled to avoid pregnancy for at least one year.

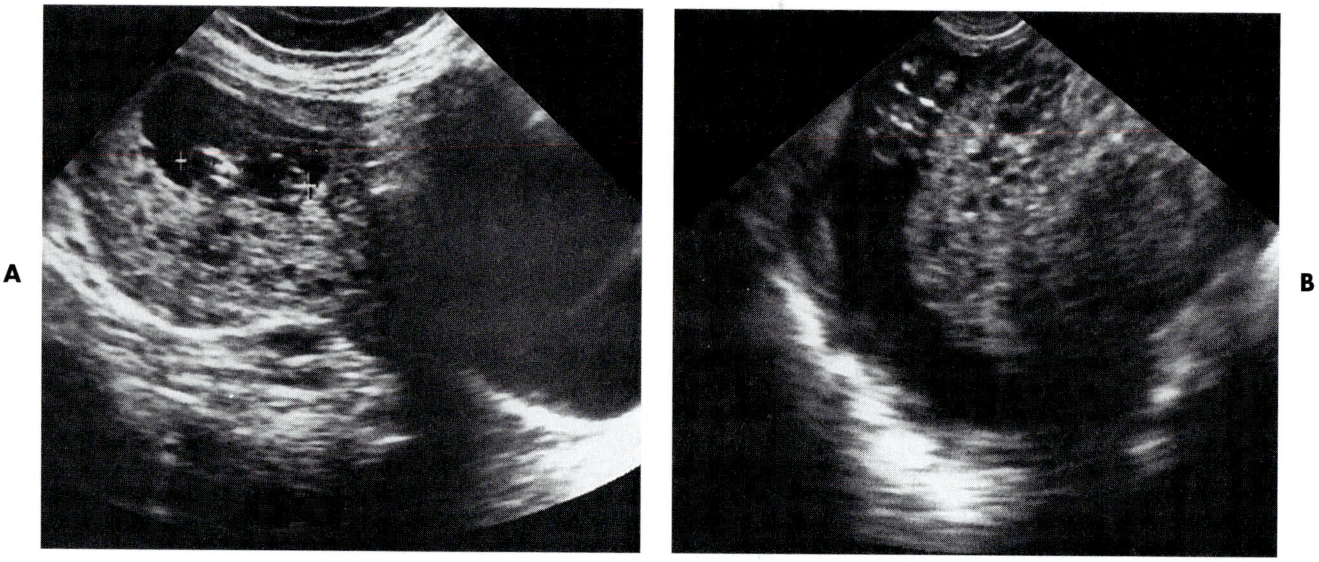

FIG. 48-3. Partial mole at 16 weeks. **A,** Suprapubic scan shows a gravid uterus. There is a small, dead, growth-retarded fetus of approximately 12-week size. The placental tissue is large and has multiple vesicular spaces consistent with hydropic villi. There is no normal placenta. **B,** Transvaginal scan shows the small fetus relative to the large, abnormal posterior placenta.

PERSISTENT TROPHOBLASTIC NEOPLASIA

Persistent trophoblastic neoplasia (PTN) is a life-threatening complication of pregnancy that encompasses invasive mole, choriocarcinoma, and the extremely rare placental-site trophoblastic tumor (PSTT). PTN occurs most commonly in the setting of molar pregnancy; up to 20% of complete moles develop persistent disease requiring additional therapy.[4,7-9,23-25] Complete moles with severe degrees of trophoblastic proliferation are at the highest risk. Persistent disease develops in 50% or more of these cases.[4,7,8,23,24] The risk is similarly high for complete molar pregnancy with a coexisting fetus, probably because of delayed diagnosis.[22] The risk of persistent disease after partial molar pregnancy is much lower, occurring in approximately 5% of cases.[9,11,14,23,25] Uncommonly, PTN develops in the setting of a normal term delivery, spontaneous abortion, or, very rarely, ectopic pregnancy.[4,6,7,11]

Invasive Mole

Invasive mole (chorioadenoma destruens) is the most common form of PTN, accounting for 80% to 95% of cases.[23] It is defined histologically by the presence of formed chorionic villi and proliferating trophoblast deep in the myometrium.[1,2,7] It is considered biologically benign and is usually confined to the uterus; however, uterine penetration or perforation can occur, with the potential for death from severe hemorrhage.[1,2,7,25] Lesions can invade beyond the uterus to parametrial tissues, adjacent organs, and blood vessels.[1,2,7] Invasive molar villi may embolize to distant sites including lung and brain.

Choriocarcinoma

Choriocarcinoma is a very rare malignancy with an incidence of 1 in 30,000 pregnancies.[1,7] As with other forms of PTN, the most important risk factor for choriocarcinoma is molar pregnancy. Molar gestations precede 50% to 80% of cases, and 1 in 40 molar pregnancies gives rise to choriocarcinoma. Choriocarcinoma is a purely cellular lesion defined histologically by the absence of formed villi and the invasion of the myometrium by abnormal, proliferating trophoblast.[1,6] Vascular invasion, hemorrhage, and necrosis are prominent features.[6] Distant metastases are common and most frequently affect the lungs, followed by the liver and brain, gastrointestinal tract, and kidney. Respiratory compromise may be the initial presentation.[7,26] Venous invasion and retrograde metastases to the vagina and pelvic structures are also common.[5,26]

Placental-Site Trophoblastic Tumor

Placental-site trophoblastic tumor (PSTT) is the rarest and most fatal form of GTN.[2,3,27] Like choriocarcinoma and invasive mole, PSTT can follow any type of gestation but most commonly follows term delivery.[6] PSTT may be confined to the uterus, may be locally invasive in the pelvis or distantly metastatic to the lungs, lymph nodes, peritoneum, liver, pancreas, or brain. Vaginal bleeding is the most common presenting symptom.[6] Surgical therapy is recommended because these lesions tend to be resistant to chemotherapy, and the risk of metastases is high. Unlike choriocarcinoma, PSTT does not prominently feature necrosis, vascular invasion, and hemorrhage.[2,3,6] Histologically, PSTT is distinct from other forms of trophoblastic neoplasia. It arises from nonvillus, "intermediate" trophoblast that infiltrates the decidua, spiral arteries, and myometrium at the placental bed.[2,6] PSTT presents a diagnostic challenge because it is frequently difficult to distinguish from the normal intermediate trophoblastic infiltration at the placental site. Furthermore, unlike other forms of PTN, serum hCG is not a reliable marker for PSTT. Histochemical staining of intermediate trophoblast for hCG is weak or absent, while staining for human placental lactogen (hPL) is strongly positive. Unfortunately, serum hPL is not a reliable predictor of tumor behavior.[5,27]

Diagnosis and Management

Because PTN arises most commonly in the setting of molar pregnancy, the diagnosis is usually based on abnormal regression of hCG after uterine evacuation. A histologic diagnosis is not considered mandatory. Curettage risks uterine perforation and does not significantly alter management or outcome.[25] Patients are treated on the basis of clinical staging that includes computed tomography of the brain, chest, abdomen, and pelvis.[25,26] While the diagnosis of PTN is straightforward in most cases, there are instances when PTN may go unrecognized. This most commonly occurs when inadequate pathologic examination fails to detect hydatidiform mole in a first trimester abortion. PTN developing in such cases or after nonmolar gestations will be mistaken for incomplete abortion or retained products of conception. Recognition of PSTT is further complicated by negative or low hCG levels. In addition, patients with PTN may present with a confusing variety of nongynecologic problems, including respiratory compromise and cerebral, gastrointestinal, or urologic hemorrhage.[23,26] In difficult cases, imaging may be the first to suggest the diagnosis. In all cases, sonography has an important role to play in staging disease and monitoring response to therapy.

Human Chorionic Gonadotropin. With the exception of PSTT, hCG is a sensitive and specific marker for detecting and monitoring PTN. Elaborated by placental trophoblast, hCG is composed of alpha and beta subunits that must combine to form the biologically active parent hormone. While the alpha subunit of hCG is similar to that of pituitary glycoprotein hormones, luteinizing hormone (LH), follicle stimulating hormone (FSH), and thyroid stimulating hormone (TSH), the beta subunit is unique and confers the specific biological activity on hCG.[28-30]

Quantitative measurements of hCG employ **radioimmunoassay** (RIA), an exquisitely sensitive technique that quantifies the amount of hormone present in small samples of serum or other body fluids. Care must be exercised when choosing an assay to diagnose PTN and monitor response to therapy. Assays that measure total hCG or beta-hCG are recommended for these patients.[29,31]

Normal mean disappearance time of hCG in benign moles ranges from 7 to 14 weeks, with a median of 11 weeks. The maximum disappearance time can be as long as 60 weeks. Clinical criteria for abnormal hCG regression have not been uniformly defined. Some clinicians institute therapy when hCG levels plateau or increase for 2 to 4 weeks or have not returned to normal by 8 weeks. Others treat when hCG has not regressed completely by 6 months. These empirical criteria account for the variation in the reported frequency of PTN following molar pregnancy. **Standardized regression curves** constructed from large numbers of patients provide a more objective means of diagnosing persistent disease and monitoring response to therapy[31] (Fig. 48-4, *A*, *B*). By 6 weeks, hCG levels deviate beyond the 95th percentile of the standard curve in 50% of cases of PTN. By 14 weeks, over 90% of cases are detected in this fashion. Standardized curves avoid the misdiagnosis of PTN in benign moles with minor, transitory plateaus or increases in hCG that remain in the normal range. When hCG continues to be positive after 6 months, expectant management is recommended as long as levels continue to fall. In general, PTN should be diagnosed and treated when hCG levels plateau or increase for 3 consecutive weeks with at least one measurement outside the normal regression corridor. Once hCG levels have normalized, the risk of PTN is low (less than 1% of cases); however, it is recommended that all patients with molar pregnancy be followed for at least one year.[31]

Sonography and Duplex Color Doppler. Sonography is currently the best imaging modality for assessing uterine and pelvic disease in PTN. It is well tolerated, accessible, inexpensive, and reproducible—ideal for serial examinations. **Sonographic features of PTN** are less familiar than those of primary molar pregnancy. While transvaginal sonography is frequently unnecessary for the diagnosis of primary molar pregnancy,[21] it is an essential diagnostic tool in PTN. The small, myometrial lesions typical of this condition may not be apparent through transabdominal scanning.[13,32-35]

Invasive mole, choriocarcinoma, and PSTT may appear similar sonographically.[13,15,36-39] Morphologic features reflect tissue invasion, necrosis, and hemorrhage. The most frequently described sonographic abnormality in PTN is a **focal, echogenic myometrial**

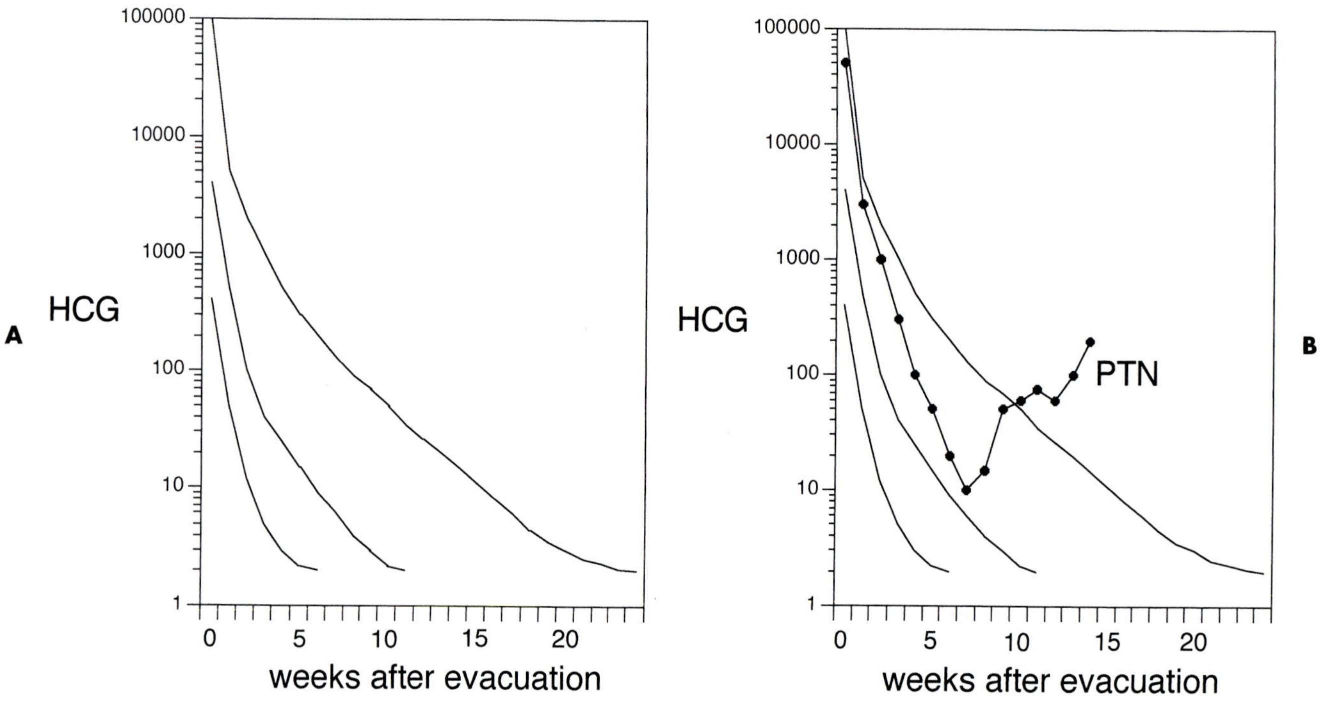

FIG. 48-4. Human chorionic gonadotropin (hCG) regression curve. **A,** Normal regression curve for serum hCG following molar pregnancy. Lines from top to bottom represent the 95th, 50th, and 5th percentiles of spontaneous hCG regression in patients with benign moles. Median disappearance time is 11 weeks. **B,** In 90% of cases, PTN shows abnormal hCG regression by 14 weeks. The dotted line represents abnormal serum hCG regression in a patient with postmolar PTN. Standardized regression curves are a more objective means of identifying persistent disease than are empirical clinical criteria. (Modified from Yedema KA, Verheijen RH, Kenemans P et al. Identification of patients with persistent trophoblastic disease by means of a normal human chorionic gonadotropin regression curve. *Am J Obstet Gynecol* 1993;168:787-792.)

nodule[13,14,16,26,33-39] (Fig. 48-5). The lesion usually lies close to the endometrial canal but it may be found deep in the myometrium. Lesions may appear solid and uniformly echogenic, hypoechoic, or complex and multicystic, like molar tissue. Anechoic regions resulting from tissue necrosis and hemorrhage appear as thick-walled, irregular cavities within solid tumors[33,37,38] (Fig. 48-6). In other cases, echo-free areas within lesions represent vascular spaces[40] (Fig. 48-7, *A, B*). PTN may also present as **bulky uterine enlargement** when tumor replaces the entire myometrium. In these cases, the myometrium assumes a heterogeneous, lobulated appearance (Fig. 48-8). There may be extension beyond the uterus to the parametrium, pelvic side wall, and adjacent organs. In extreme cases, PTN appears as a **large, undifferentiated pelvic mass** (Fig. 48-9). In the correct setting (e.g., recent molar pregnancy, rising serum hCG, and a previously documented normal sonogram), sonography can be diagnostic; however, sonography is not completely specific. Common, benign conditions, including adenomyosis and fibroids, may appear similar to PTN.[16,40,41] Accurate diagnosis depends on correlation with clinical findings and serum hCG levels.

After effective therapy, sonographic abnormalities usually resolve and uterine morphology returns to normal. Lesions become progressively more hypoechoic and smaller in size (Fig. 48-8, *C*). Eventually, no residual abnormality is apparent in many cases.[33,35] However up to 50% of patients will have persistent abnormalities after therapy that may be difficult to distinguish from active lesions sonographically.[36]

Normal uterine bloodflow. In the normal uterus, myometrial vascularity is always visible on color Doppler. Color flow is generally limited to discrete, regularly arranged vessels in the peripheral one half to one third of the myometrium. Smaller vessels radiate at intervals toward the endometrium. Duplex Doppler shows signals of low velocity and high impedance. Myometrial color flow can appear increased in normal subjects with prominent parametrial vascular complexes and in conditions such as fibroids and adenomyosis. In pregnancy, myometrial color vascularity may be focally increased in the re-

A 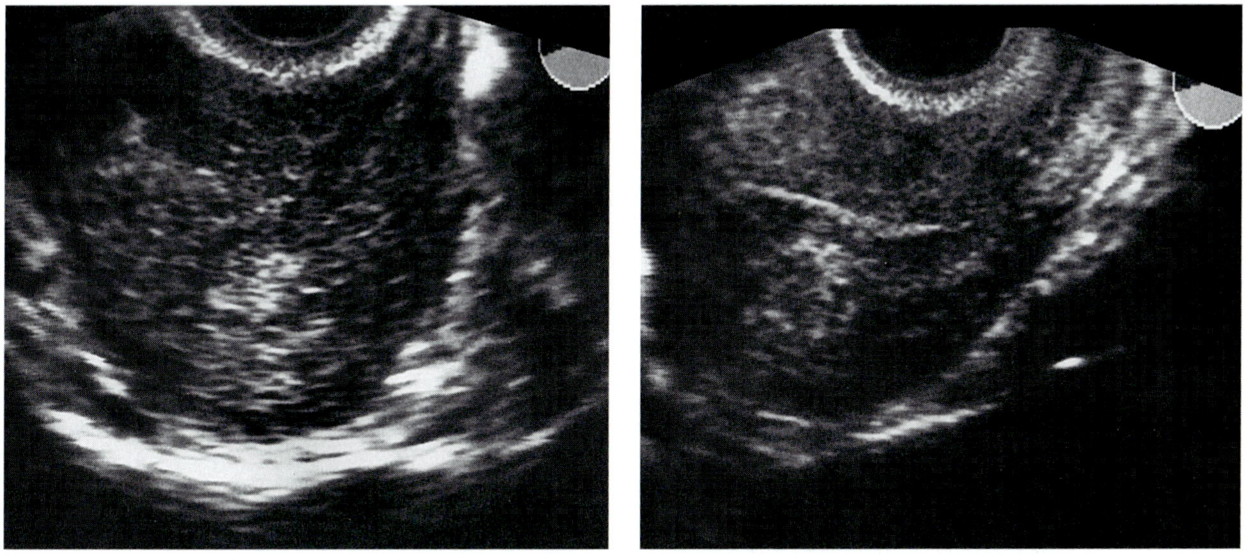 B

FIG. 48-5. Focal echogenic myometrial nodule of persistent trophoblastic neoplasia (PTN). **A,** Transverse transvaginal sonogram shows central focal uterine echogenicity which could be mistaken for a thick endometrium. **B,** Sagittal image shows that the echogenic area lies within the myometrium posterior to a normal endometrial canal. (From Fraser-Hill MA, Burns PN, Wilson SR. Transvaginal ultrasound and duplex color Doppler of persistent trophoblastic neoplasia. *Radiology* 1993; 189(P):374-375.)

A 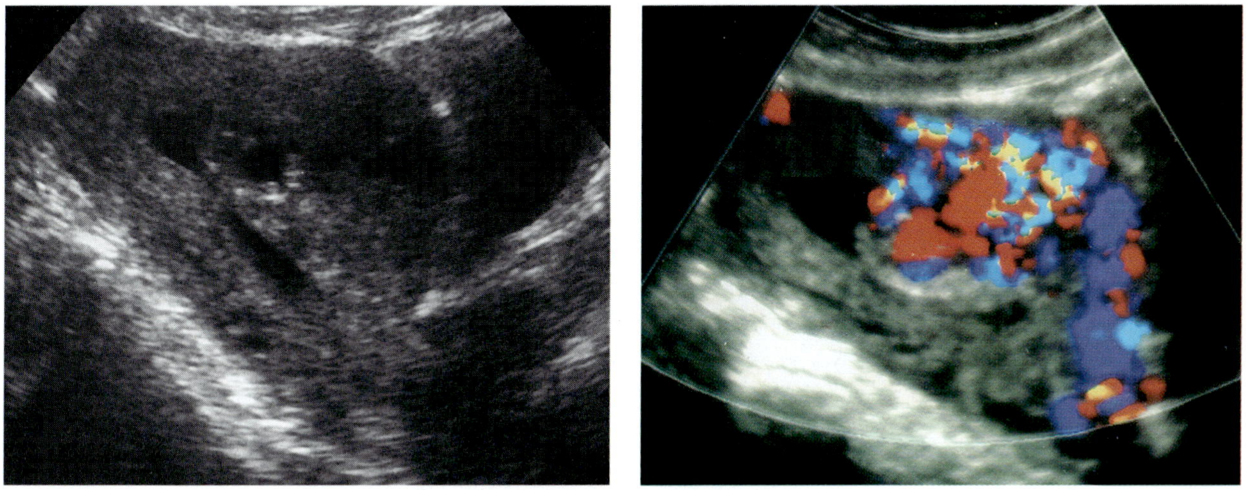 B

FIG. 48-6. Cystic spaces representing vessels and hemorrhage in persistent trophoblastic neoplasia (PTN). **A,** Sagittal sonogram shows a bulky uterus with a complex anterior myometrial mass and blood (cystic spaces could be filled with fluid, here blood, or blood vessels) in the endometrial cavity. **B,** Color Doppler shows a florid color mosaic pattern in the very anterior myometrial tumor and blood (dot filled by color) in the endometrial cavity. (From Fraser-Hill MA, Burns PN, Wilson SR. Transvaginal ultrasound and duplex color Doppler of persistent trophoblastic neoplasia. *Radiology* 1993; 189(P):374-375.)

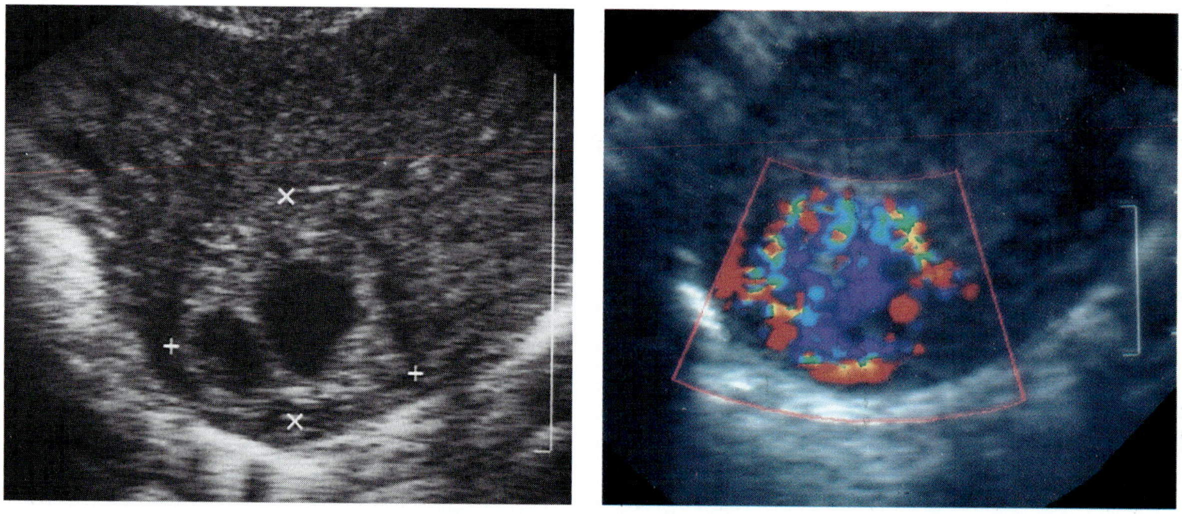

FIG. 48-7. Cystic myometrial mass with vascular spaces in persistent trophoblastic neoplasia (PTN). **A,** Sagittal transvaginal sonogram shows a focal echogenic nodule with well-defined cystic spaces. **B,** Color Doppler shows a florid color mosaic pattern with aliasing. The cystic spaces fill in with color, confirming their vascular nature. (From Fraser-Hill MA, Burns PN, Wilson SR. Transvaginal ultrasound and duplex color Doppler of persistent trophoblastic neoplasia. *Radiology* 1993; 189(P):374-375.)

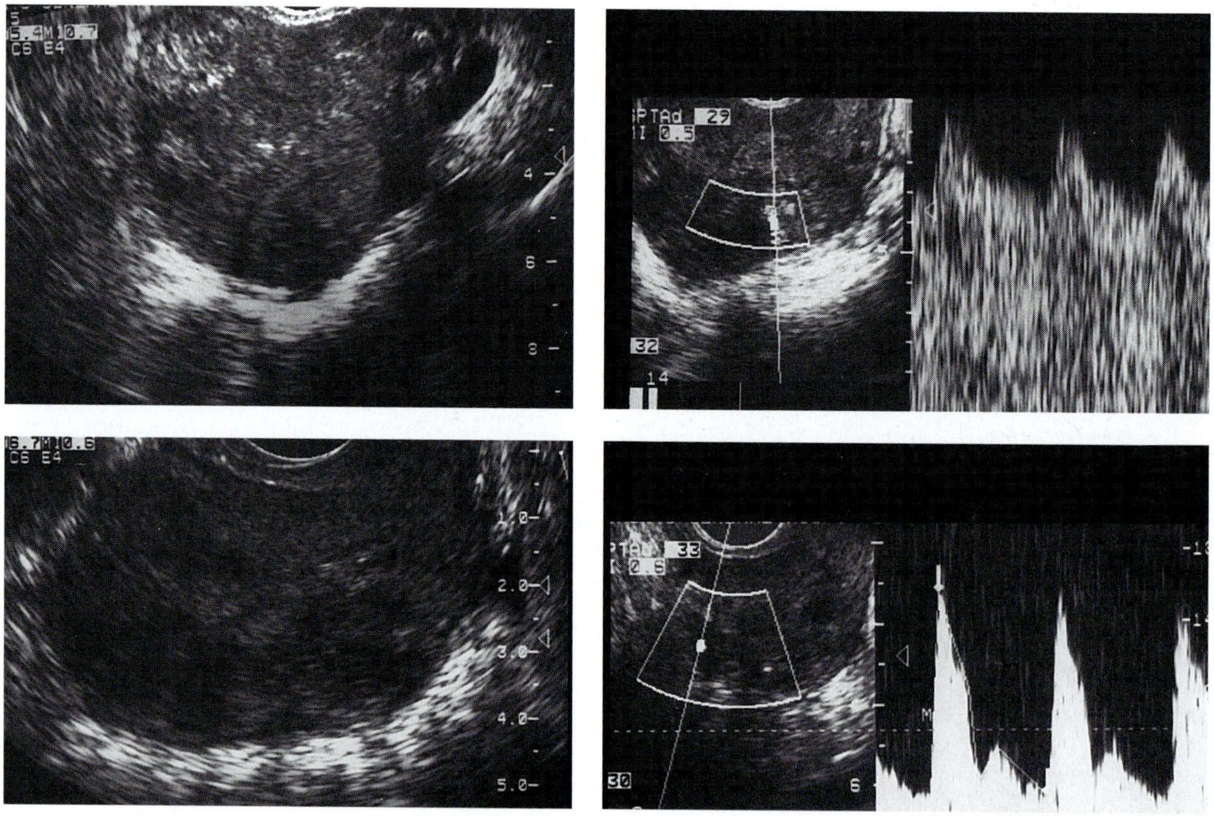

FIG. 48-8. Bulky, lobulated uterus mimicking fibroids in persistent trophoblastic neoplasia (PTN); Doppler improves specificity. **A,** Transvaginal sonogram shows a bulky nonhomogeneous uterus with several areas suggesting fibroids. Color Doppler showed florid diffuse color with aliasing. **B,** Spectral waveforms show high-velocity, low-resistance flow PSV 70 cm/sec, PI 0.35, RI 0.29. C and **D, Postchemotherapy, beta hCG is negative. PTN is gone.** **C,** Transvaginal sonogram has improved, but uterus maintains a somewhat bulky and lobulated contour. Focal nodules are not as evident. Color Doppler showed minimal blood flow. **D,** Spectral waveform shows normal low-velocity, high-impedance flows. PSV 15 cm/sec, PI 1.43, RI 0.74. (From Fraser-Hill MA, Burns PN, Wilson SR. Transvaginal ultrasound and duplex color Doppler of persistent trophoblastic neoplasia. *Radiology* 1993; 189(P):374-375.)

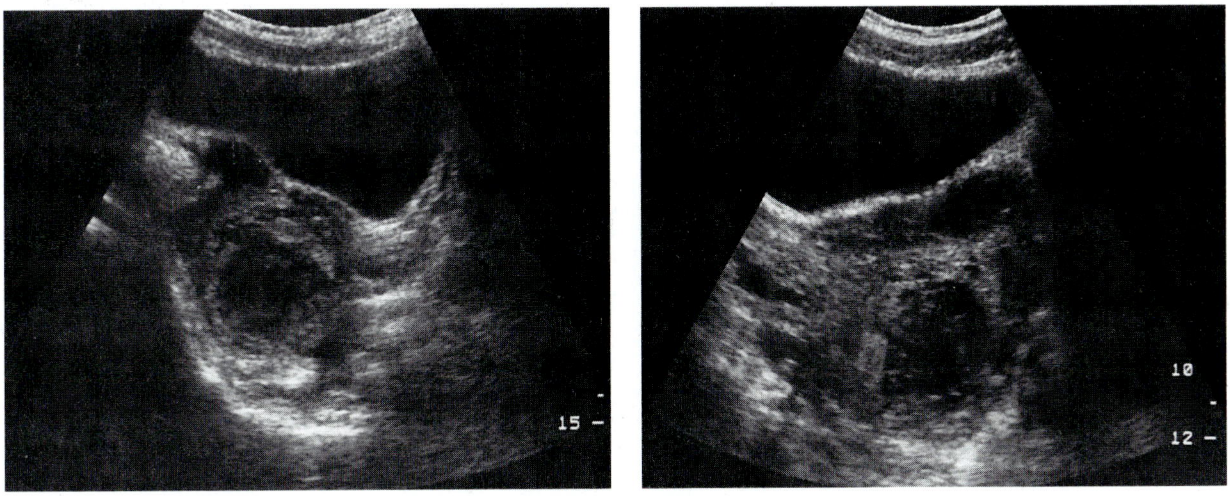

FIG. 48-9. Choriocarcinoma after a normal term pregnancy, producing a large, ill-defined pelvic mass in persistent trophoblastic neoplasia (PTN). **A,** Sagittal and **B,** transverse sonograms show a large, poorly defined, complex pelvic mass with both cystic and solid components. The uterus could not be identified. Doppler showed trophoblastic signals everywhere within this mass. PTN was not suspected clinically or on sonography until Doppler was performed. (From Fraser-Hill MA, Burns PN, Wilson SR. Transvaginal ultrasound and duplex color Doppler of persistent trophoblastic neoplasia. *Radiology* 1993; 189(P):374-375.)

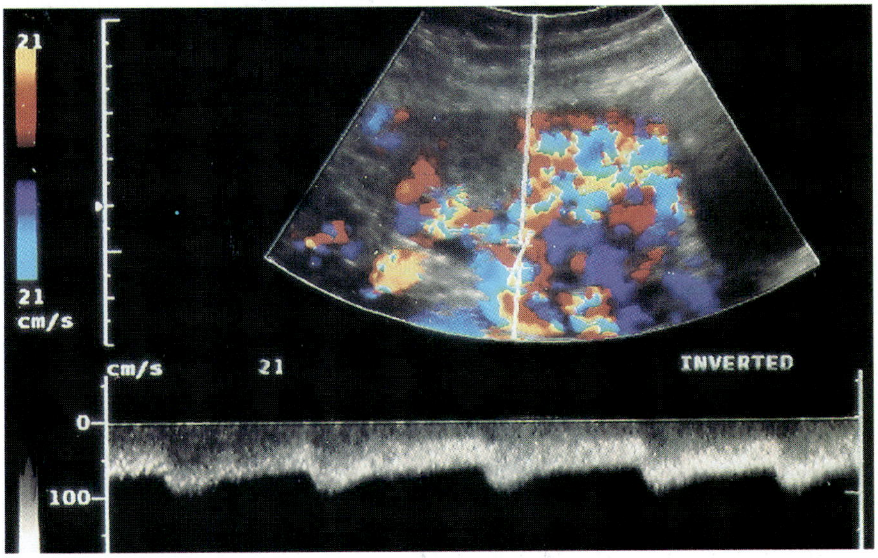

FIG. 48-10. Classic florid color mosaic pattern seen in PTN. Color Doppler transvaginal image shows consistent extensive aliasing. Spectral waveform shows high-velocity, low-impedance flow. (From Fraser-Hill MA, Burns PN, Wilson SR. Transvaginal ultrasound and duplex color Doppler of persistent trophoblastic neoplasia. *Radiology* 1993; 189(P):374-375.)

gion of placental implantation. Endometrial color flow, usually absent in the nongravid uterus, is nonspecific and is seen in normal pregnancy, incomplete abortion, retained products of conception, endometrial polyps, cancer, and PTN.

Duplex and color Doppler features of PTN reflect the marked hypervascularity of invasive trophoblast.[32,41-46] The extreme vascularity of trophoblastic neoplasia has long been known from angiography.[46] Uterine spiral arteries feed directly into prominent vascular spaces that then communicate with draining veins.[3,46] These **functional arteriovenous shunts** produce abnormal uterine hypervascularity and high-velocity, low-impedance blood flow on duplex interrogation.[41,42,44] **Color Doppler features** typical of PTN include extensive color aliasing, admixture of color signals, loss of discreteness of vessels, and chaotic vascular arrangement. Regions of abnormal color Doppler frequently appear larger than corresponding sonographic abnormalities[32] (Fig. 48-10).

Duplex Doppler features of PTN relate to the arteriovenous shunting. "Trophoblastic" blood flow has

A
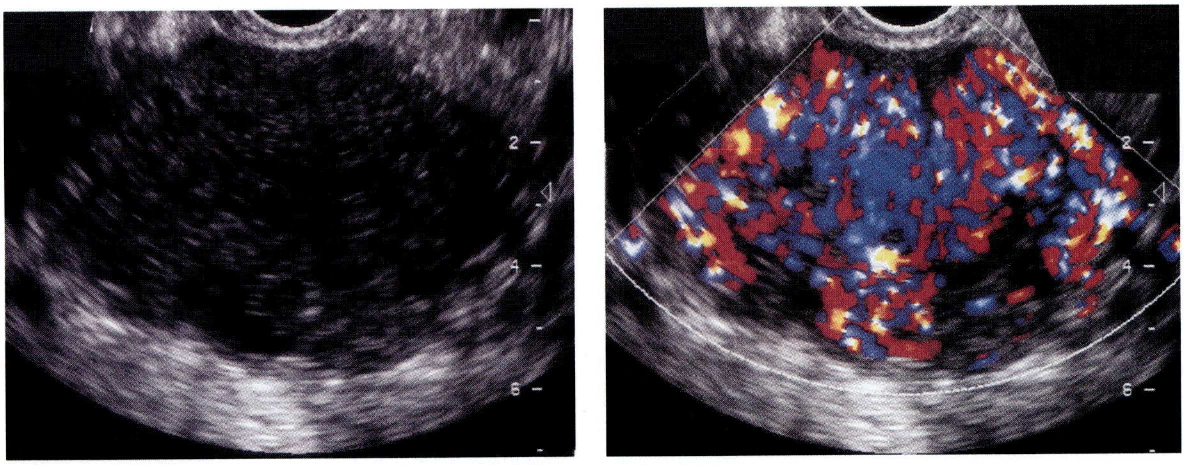

B

FIG. 48-11. Arteriovenous malformation of the uterus in a young woman with severe menorrhagia following spontaneous abortion with dilatation and curettage. Beta hCG was negative. AVM was treated successfully with embolotherapy. **A,** Transvaginal transverse sonogram shows a vague, subtle abnormality of the entire myometrium. **B,** Color Doppler image shows a florid mosaic pattern with color aliasing and prominent parametrial vessels. The sonographic and Doppler features are indistinguishable from PTN. Only beta hCG is discriminatory. (From Huang M, Muradali D,Thurston W, Burns PN, Wilson SR. Uterine arteriovenous malformations (AVM): ultrasound features with MRI correlation. *Radiology;* in press.)

A
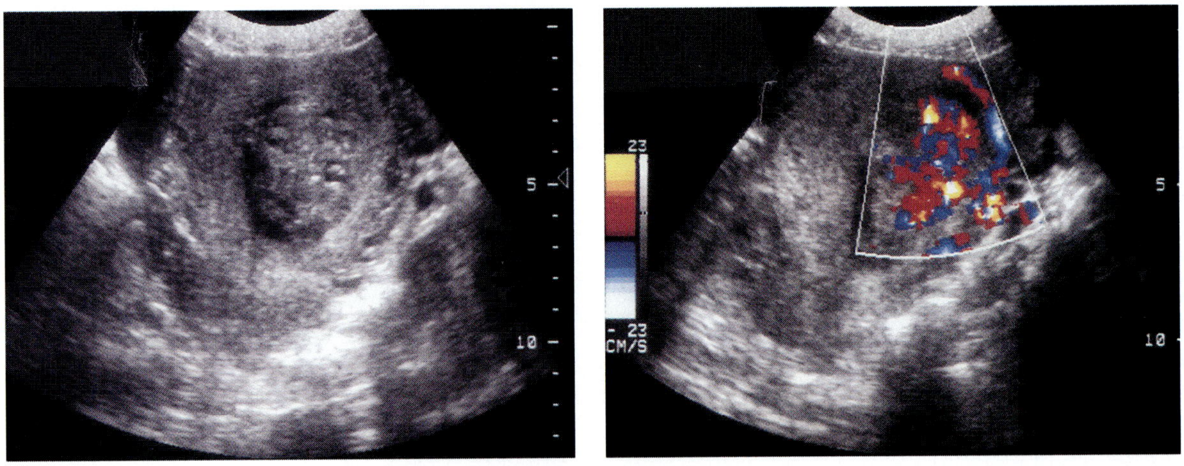

B

FIG. 48-12. Placental-site trophoblastic tumor (PSTT). 28-year-old woman, gravida 10, para 2, with heavy bleeding requiring transfusion. Beta hCG negative. **A,** Transverse transvaginal sonogram shows a central, complex, 3 cm-diameter uterine mass involving both the endometrial canal and the myometrium. **B,** Color Doppler shows extensive color, more extensive than the gray scale abnormality. (From Fraser-Hill MA, Burns PN, Wilson SR. Transvaginal ultrasound and duplex color Doppler of persistent trophoblastic neoplasia. *Radiology* 1993; 189(P):374-375.)

characteristic high peak systolic velocity (PSV) and low resistance index (RI).[32,41-46] PSV is usually greater than 50 cm/s and is often over 100 cm/s. RI is usually less than 0.50 and is often well below 0.40[32,41,46] (Fig. 48-10). In contrast, normal myometrial blood flow usually has a PSV of less than 50 cm/s and an RI in the range of 0.70. Endometrial blood flow normally has a low resistance pattern but is distinguished from trophoblastic flow by low peak velocity in the range of 10 to 15 cm/s.[32] The sensitivity and specificity of Doppler in PTN are yet to be determined by a large prospective series.

Duplex and color Doppler are noninvasive and reliable alternatives to conventional angiography for detecting and staging pelvic PTN.[44] In our experience, the contribution of Doppler is greater in patients with PTN than in patients with primary molar gestation. Abnormal vascularity may be difficult or impossible to detect in primary molar pregnancy but it is a major feature of PTN. Qualitative assessments of vascularity on color Doppler are not diagnostic of PTN. However, the extreme degree of myometrial vascularity in PTN is matched by few other conditions. We have not seen similar color Doppler hypervascularity except in extremely rare uterine arteriovenous malformations (Fig. 48-11), a potential pitfall.[47]

Trophoblastic signals on spectral Doppler are not unique to PTN. They are found in all conditions with functioning trophoblast, including missed abortion, incomplete abortion, retained products of conception, and ectopic pregnancy.[48-50] These potential pitfalls are distinguished from PTN by clinical findings, sonographic morphology, and pathology. However, PSTT should remain a consideration even with a normal hCG (Fig. 48-12). High-velocity, low-impedance flow similar to that of PTN occurs in many other conditions, including pelvic inflammatory disease, pelvic abscess from appendicitis or diverticulitis, and benign and malignant ovarian neoplasms. These are distinguished from PTN by clinical findings, sonographic morphology, and serum hCG. Uncommon uterine fibroids and very rare uterine arteriovenous malformations may have similar high-velocity, low-impedance blood flow (Fig. 48-11, *A, B*). If present in a patient at risk for PTN, these lesions could cause false-positive Doppler diagnoses. In most cases, the diagnosis of PTN is fairly straightforward, and additional information provided by Doppler is supportive but not critical. However, when PTN is clinically unsuspected, duplex color Doppler may provide the first indication of trophoblastic disease by showing marked hypervascularity and typical trophoblastic blood flow within lesions. Doppler also improves diagnostic specificity by showing normal uterine waveforms when PTN is absent and sonography is abnormal (for instance, when adenomyosis mimics the appearance of PTN or when persistent, nonspecific abnormalities remain after effective therapy)[32,45] (Fig. 48-8, *A, B, C, D*).

Therapy and Prognosis. Therapy of PTN is initiated when abnormal hCG regression occurs after molar pregnancy, when metastases appear, or when there is a histologic diagnosis of choriocarcinoma or PSTT. PTN is broadly classified as non-metastatic or metastatic on the basis of staging computed tomography of the brain, chest, abdomen, and pelvis.[25,26] Nonmetastatic PTN has an excellent prognosis. Single-agent therapy with methotrexate achieves sustained remission in virtually 100% of cases.[25,51] Metastatic PTN is subdivided into low-risk and high-risk groups. Virtually all patients with low-risk metastatic disease are cured with simple chemotherapy.[26,51] In contrast, patients with high-risk disease have a significantly worse prognosis and a high likelihood of failure with single-agent therapy. High-risk, poor-prognosis disease is indicated by duration of disease for more than 4 months, pretreatment hCG levels greater than 40,000 mIU/ml, presence of brain or liver metastases, antecedent term pregnancy, and prior history of failed chemotherapy. These patients are treated aggressively with appropriate combinations of intense multiagent chemotherapy, adjuvant radiotherapy, and surgery. By tailoring therapy in this way, even high-risk patients have cure rates of 80% to 90%.[26,52]

REFERENCES

1. Crum CP. Female genital tract. In: *Robbins Pathologic Basis of Disease*. 5th ed. Philadelphia: WB Saunders Co; 1994:1081-1086.
2. Paradinas FJ. Pathology and classification of trophoblastic tumors. *Gynecologic Oncology*. 2nd ed. New York: Churchill Livingstone; 1992:1013-1026.
3. DiSaia PJ, Creaseman WT. Gestational trophoblastic neoplasia. In: *Clinical Gynecologic Oncology*. 4th ed. St. Louis: Mosby–Year Book; 1993:210-237.

Molar Pregnancy

4. Semer DA, Macfee MS. Gestational trophoblastic disease: epidemiology. *Sem Oncology* 1995;22(2):109-113.
5. Palmer JR.: Advances in the epidemiology of gestational trophoblastic disease. *J Reprod Med* 1994;39(3):155-162.
6. Redline RW, Abdul-Karim FW. Pathology of gestational trophoblastic disease. *Sem Oncology* 1995; 22(2): 96-109
7. O'Quinn AG, Barnard DE. Gestational trophoblastic diseases. In: *Current Obstetric and Gynecologic Diagnosis and Treatment*. 8th ed. East Norwalk: Appleton & Lange; 1994:967-976.
8. Goldstein DP, Berkowitz RS. Current management of complete and partial molar pregnancy. *J Reprod Med* 1994;39(3):139-146.
9. Rose PG. Hydatidiform mole: diagnosis and management. *Sem Oncology* 1995;22(2):149-156.
10. Roberts DJ, Mutter GL. Advances in the molecular biology of gestational trophoblastic disease. *J Reprod Med* 1994;39(3): 201-208.
11. Wolf NG, Lage JM. Genetic analysis of gestational trophoblastic disease: A review. *Sem Oncology* 1995;22(2):113-120.
12. Kajii T, Ohama K. Androgenic origin of hydatidiform mole. *Nature* 1977;268:633-634.
13. DeBaz BP, Lewis TJ. Imaging of gestational trophoblastic disease. *Sem Oncology* 1995;22(2):130-141.
14. Berkowitz RS, Goldstein DP, Bernstein MR. Evolving concepts of molar pregnancy. *J Reprod Med* 1991;36(1):40-44.
15. Reid MH, McGahan JP, Oi R. Sonographic evaluation of hydatidiform mole and its look-alikes. *AJR* 1983;140:307-311.
16. Fleischer AC, James AE, Krause DA et al. Sonographic patterns in trophoblastic diseases. *Radiology* 1978;126:215-220.
17. Teng FY, Magarelli PC, Montz FJ. Transvaginal probe ultrasonography: diagnostic or outcome advantages in women with molar pregnancies. *J Reprod Med* 1995;40(6):427-430.
18. Woodward RM, Filly RA, Callen PW. First trimester molar pregnancy: nonspecific ultrasonic appearance. *Obstet Gynecol* 1980;55:315-335.
19. Crade M, Weber P. Appearance of molar pregnancy 9.5 weeks after conception: use of transvaginal US for early diagnosis. *J Ultrasound Med* 1991;10:473-474.
20. Sherer DM, Allen T, Woods J. Transvaginal sonographic diagnosis of a hydatidiform mole occurring 2 weeks after curettage for an incomplete abortion. *J Clin Ultrasound*;1991:224-226.

21. Bronson RA, Van de Vegte GL. An unusual first trimester sonographic finding associated with the development of hydatidiform mole: the hyperechoic ovoid mass. *AJR* 1993;160: 137-138.
22. Steller MA, Genest DR, Bernstein MR et al. Natural history of twin pregnancy with complete hydatidiform mole and coexisting fetus. *Obstet Gynecol* 1994;83:35-42.

Persistent Trophoblastic Neoplasia

23. Greenfield AW. Gestational trophoblastic disease: prognostic variables and staging. *Sem Oncology* 1995;22(2):142-148.
24. Rice LW, Genest DR, Berkowitz RS et al. Pathologic features of sharp curettings in complete hydatidiform mole: predictors of persistent gestational trophoblastic disease. *J Reprod Med* 1991; 36(1):17-20.
25. Kennedy AW. Persistent nonmetastatic gestational trophoblastic disease. *Sem Oncology* 1995;22(2):161-165.
26. Soper JT. Identification and management of high-risk gestational trophoblastic disease. *Sem Oncology* 1995;22(2):172-184.
27. Finkler NJ. Placental-site trophoblastic tumor: diagnosis, clinical behavior and treatment. *J Reprod Med* 1991;39(1):27-30.
28. Tyrey L. Human chorionic gonadotropin: properties and assay methods. *Sem Oncology* 1995;22(2):121-129.
29. Cole LA, Kohorn EI, Kim GS. Detecting and monitoring trophoblastic disease: new perspectives on measuring human chorionic gonadotropin levels. *J Reprod Med* 1994;39(3):193-200.
30. Ozturk M. Human chorionic gonadotropin, its free subunits and gestational trophoblastic disease. *J Reprod Med* 1991; 36(1):21-26.
31. Yedema KA, Verheijen RH, Kenemans PK et al. Identification of patients with persistent trophoblastic disease by means of a normal human chorionic gonadotropin regression curve. *Am J Obstet Gynecol* 1993;168(3):787-792.
32. Fraser-Hill MA, Burns PN, Wilson SR. Transvaginal ultrasound and duplex color Doppler of persistent trophoblastic neoplasia. *Radiology* 1993; 189(P):374-375.
33. Magii G, Spagnolo D, Valsecchi L et al. Transvaginal ultrasonography in persistent trophoblastic tumor. *Am J Obstet Gynecol* 1993;169(5):1218-1223.
34. Ansbacher R, Hopkins MP, Roberts JA et al. Localization of trophoblastic disease with vaginal ultrasonography: a report of 2 cases. *J Reprod Med* 1990;35(8):835-838.
35. Schneider DF, Bukovsky I, Weinraub Z et al. Case report: transvaginal ultrasound diagnosis and treatment follow-up of invasive gestational trophoblastic disease. *J Clin Ultrasound* 1990;18:110-113.
36. Long MG, Boultbee JE, Begent RHJ et al. Ultrasonic morphology of the uterus and ovaries after treatment of invasive mole and gestational choriocarcinoma. *Br J Radiology* 1990; 63:942-945.
37. Caspi B, Elchalal U, Dgani R et al. Invasive mole and placental-site trophoblastic tumor: two entities of gestational trophoblastic disease with a common ultrasonographic appearance. *J Ultrasound Med* 1991;10:517-519.
38. Sakamoto C, Oikawa K, Kashimura M et al. Sonographic appearance of placental-site trophoblastic tumor. *J Ultrasound Med* 1990;9:533-535.
39. Goshen R, Lavy Y, Hochner-Celnikier D et al. More on the importance of transvaginal ultrasonography follow-up in the treatment of persistent hydatidiform mole. *Am J Obstet Gynecol* 1994;171(6):1675-1676.
40. Abulafia O, Sherer DM, Fultz PJ et al. Unusual endovaginal ultrasonography and magnetic resonance imaging of placental-site trophoblastic tumor. *Am J Obstet Gynecol* 1994;170(3): 750-752.
41. Taylor KJW, Schwartz PE, Kohorn EI. Gestational trophoblastic neoplasia: diagnosis with US. *Radiology* 1987; 165:445-448.
42. Desai RK, Desberg AL. Diagnosis of gestational trophoblastic disease: value of endovaginal color flow Doppler sonography. *AJR* 1991;157:787-788.
43. Kazuhiro S, Sadayuki S, Ishigaki T et al. Intratumoral blood flow: evaluation with color flow echography. *Radiology* 1987; 165:683-685.
44. Dobkin GR, Berkowitz RS, Goldstein DP et al. Duplex ultrasonography for persistent gestational trophoblastic tumor. *J Reprod Med* 1991;36(1):14-16.
45. Chan FY, Chau MT, Pun TC et al. A comparison of colour Doppler sonography and the pelvic arteriogram in assessment of patients with gestational trophoblastic disease. *Br J Obstet Gynaecol* 1995;102(9):720-7255.
46. Hendrickse JPV, Cockshott WP, Evans KTL et al. Pelvic angiography in the diagnosis of malignant trophoblastic disease. *N Engl J Med* 1964;271:859-865.
47. Huang M, Muradali D,Thurston W et al. Uterine arteriovenous malformations (AVM): ultrasound features with MRI correlation. *Radiology*; in press.
48. Kurjak A, Zalud I, Schulman H. Ectopic pregnancy: transvaginal color Doppler of trophoblastic flow in questionable adnexa. *J Ultrasound Med* 1991;10:685-689.
49. Taylor KJW, Ramos IM, Feyock AL et al. Ectopic pregnancy: duplex Doppler evaluation. *Radiology* 1989;173:93-97.
50. Pellerito JS, Taylor KJW, Quedens-Case C et al. Ectopic pregnancy: evaluation with color flow imaging. *Radiology* 1992;183:407-411.
51. Feldman S, Goldstein DP, Berkowitz RS. Low-risk metastatic gestational trophoblastic tumors. *Sem Oncology* 1995;22(2): 166-171.
52. Lurain JR. High-risk metastatic gestational trophoblastic tumors: current management. *J Reprod Med* 1994;39(3):217-222.

CHAPTER 49

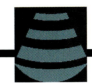

Doppler Assessment of Pregnancy

Carl A. Nimrod, M.B., F.R.C.S.C.
Stuart F. Nicholson, M.D., F.R.C.P.C.

CHAPTER OUTLINE

Doppler ultrasound provides a safe, noninvasive, and rapid method to assess the physiology and pathophysiology of the fetal and maternal circulations. It is used largely to assess fetal well-being, and excellent correlations exist with the fetal acid/base status.

Although Doppler does not appear to be sensitive enough to be used as a screening test for intrauterine growth retardation (IUGR), it does correlate well with fetal compromise, often giving earlier warning of fetal distress than other tests.[1-3] The indication for its use is confined to high-risk pregnancies.

There is a variable time interval between the appearance of abnormal Doppler results and the onset of severe fetal distress necessitating delivery. With IUGR, depending on the degree of abnormality, this can range from a few days in a fetus with reversal of end-diastolic flow, to several weeks in a fetus with elevated Doppler indices.

An abnormal Doppler result is more worrisome in the presence of severe pregnancy-induced hypertension and oligohydramnios.[4] Furthermore, combined arterial and venous Doppler abnormalities, with or without evidence of fetal cardiac dysfunction, are ominous signs.

OMINOUS SIGNS IN ASSOCIATION WITH ABNORMAL DOPPLER FINDINGS

Severe pregnancy-induced hypertension
Oligohydramnios
Combined arterial and venous Doppler abnormalities

INSTRUMENTATION

Continuous wave (CW), pulsed wave (PW), and color flow Doppler instrumentation have all been used for fetal blood flow assessments. The major advantage of **continuous wave Doppler** is its ability to measure high velocities. This is offset, however, by the disadvantage of interference by Doppler signals from blood flow along the line of the ultrasound beam but at depths different from the region of interest.

Pulsed wave Doppler is limited to measuring velocities that produce frequency shifts less than one half the pulse repetition frequency (PRF).[5] Use of pulsed Doppler does not present a problem in most obstetrical cases, as the maximum velocities seen in normal fetal vessels are less than 1 m/sec. However, Doppler of very deep vessels may be problematic, as the PRF must be reduced. In addition, in assessing stenotic cardiac anomalies, higher velocities may be present. Pulsed Doppler has the advantage of being used with an imaging probe that has a selectable sample volume to insure that the desired vessel is being studied. This is of particular value in the fetus because of the small vessel size and variable position resulting from fetal movement.

Color flow Doppler allows the routine assessment of vessels that cannot be imaged and are seen only by virtue of the color flow signal. This reduces examination time and also reduces interobserver and intraobserver variation.[6] **Power Doppler** allows visualization of small vessels with low flow and, although there is no directional flow information, quantitative information can be obtained. Many machines now combine all of these features on the same probe, allowing greater selectivity and efficiency.

The fetal sonographer has the responsibility to know the **acoustic output** of the actual Doppler machine being used, as there is a theoretical danger of higher exposure because of the longer pulse lengths, the higher pulse repetition rates, and the higher output necessitated for Doppler studies. It is generally possible to keep the acoustic exposure in an acceptable range by turning the output to the minimum and using higher gains. Some machines allow an attenuator to be added to the Doppler transducer. As for all ultrasound examinations, the lowest power setting that produces diagnostic results should be used, especially in the first trimester.

A **filter** is present on all Doppler machines to remove low-frequency noise from vessel wall echoes. For many studies, such as adult echocardiograms, an 800 Hz filter is used. If this high a filter were used for fetal studies, slow venous flow could not be assessed, and absent or mild reversal of diastolic flow would be masked (flows up to 43 cm/sec would be masked by an 800 Hz filter at a carrier frequency of 2.5 MHz and a Doppler angle of 55°). Filter setting should be 50 to 100 Hz, or the lowest possible setting for the machine.

DOPPLER ANALYSIS

An ultrasound beam striking a moving target, such as a red blood cell, will be reflected with a change in frequency proportional to the speed of the target. As flowing blood always contains cells with a range of velocities, the reflected ultrasound beam will contain a range of frequency shifts. The **flow velocity waveform** (FVW) is a graph of the frequency shifts present in the sample volume and the changes over time. If the angle between the vessel and the ultrasound beam is known, the target velocities can be calculated from the Doppler shift equation $V = Fd \times c/F \times 2\cos Q$, where V = velocity of blood, Fd = Doppler shift, c = speed of sound in tissue, F = Doppler frequency, and Q is the angle between the vessel and the Doppler beam. The maximum Doppler shift is obtained when the smallest angle of incidence is used; this is readily apparent as an audible, high-pitched signal.

Quantitative Analysis

Assessment of **blood flow volume** requires measurement of the vessel's cross-sectional area and the beam/vessel angle. This can be done reliably only in large straight vessels, such as the aorta and the umbilical vein. The error in measuring vessel diameter is squared, so that, for example, a 1-mm error in measuring the diameter of a 4-mm vessel will produce a 44% error in area. Volume flow does, however, provide information about the circulation that is not obtainable by other means. Volume of flow may be calculated with the following formula: $Q = V \times A$, where V is the mean velocity averaged over the cardiac cycle

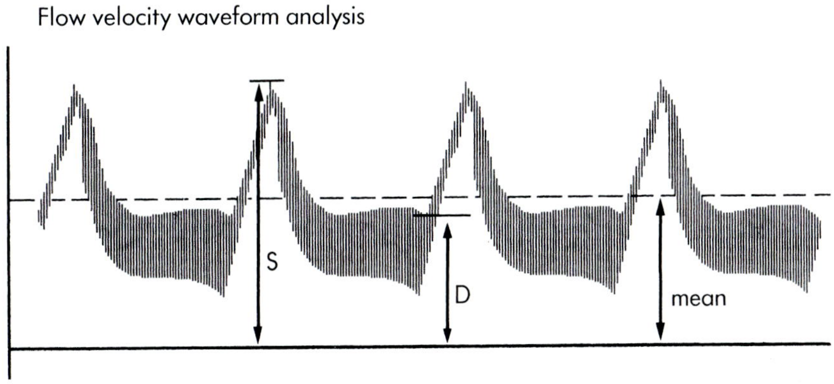

$$\text{S/D ratio} = \frac{S}{D}$$

$$\text{Pulsatility index} = \frac{S\text{-}D}{\text{mean}}$$

$$\text{Resistance index} = \frac{S\text{-}D}{S}$$

FIG. 49-1. Semiquantitative indices used to characterize the Doppler flow velocity waveform.

and A is the cross-sectional area of the vessel. V is calculated from the Doppler shift equation, but must be the average of the velocities across the vessel; hence, the sample volume must include the entire vessel.

Semiquantitative Analysis

The use of continuous wave Doppler without imaging and the interrogation of tortuous vessels such as the umbilical artery preclude measurement of absolute velocity, as the Doppler angle is unknown. Therefore, a variety of **arterial indices** have been developed that use a ratio of systolic (S) and diastolic (D) velocities so that the results are **angle-independent** (Fig. 49-1).

Pulsatility index [PI = (S − D)/mean velocity],[7] **resistance index** [RI = (S − D)/S],[8] **S/D ratio,**[9] and **D/S ratio**[10] are all thought to reflect downstream impedance. As impedance increases, the pulsatility of the flow velocity waveform (FVW) increases. Adamson et al.[11] embolized the placental microcirculation to produce an increase in resistance that was reflected by linear changes in the D/S ratio, PI, and RI, with absent diastolic flow being reached after a sixfold increase in resistance. The S/D ratio had a hyperbolic correlation. Constriction of the umbilical arteries with angiotensin II did not produce changes in the shape of the FVW despite large decreases in umbilical blood flow. However, all indices seem to show a similar sensitivity (80%) for the **prediction of fetal compromise.**[12] It is worth noting that the S/D ratio will become infinity once diastolic velocities reach zero, while RI approaches one. PI will continue to show change even with no diastolic flow, causing it to be favored by some investigators. Others prefer the S/D or D/S ratios because of their simplicity. Interobserver and intraobserver errors are less than 10%, but three or more waveforms should be measured and the results averaged. The flow velocity waveform also depends on **upstream factors,** such as cardiac contractility, stroke volume, and proximal stenosis. Computer analysis of the waveform allows measurement of acceleration and deceleration times and percentage flow in systole and diastole.[13] A correction can be made for fetal heart rate, as an increased rate does not allow as much time for diastolic runoff, reducing pulsatility.[14] Care must also be taken to avoid the effects of fetal breathing and motion by measuring during periods of fetal apnea (Fig. 49-2).

Recently, **venous flow velocity ratios** have been described to semiqualitatively assess flow in the IVC and ductus venosus (Fig. 49-3).

Qualitative Analysis

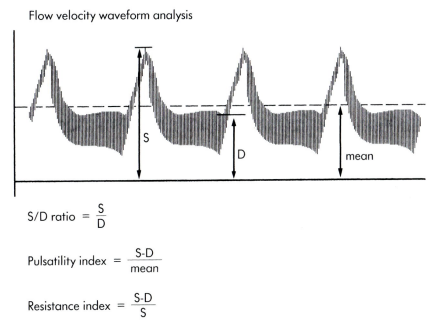

A variety of changes can be seen, including **loss of diastolic flow, reversal of flow,** and **notching** of the fetal flow velocity waveform. It is almost universal in the normal fetal-maternal circulation that diastolic velocities increase as term approaches, because of decreasing placental or other vascular resistance (Fig. 49-4). Specific changes will be discussed in reference to individual vessels and diseases. Color flow Doppler provides a qualitative measure of flow to various organs such as the placenta and allows the assessment of

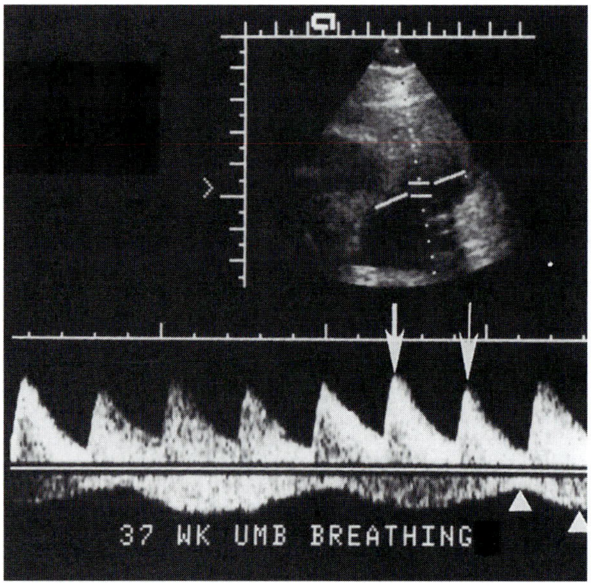

FIG. 49-2. Umbilical artery and vein in the umbilical cord. Flow velocity waveform shows that flow in both the artery and vein is affected by fetal breathing movements. Note the varying heights of the systolic peaks in the arterial flow (*arrows*) and the sinusoidal variation of the venous flow (*arrowheads*).

the distribution of vessels too small to be imaged in those organs.

NORMAL DOPPLER FINDINGS

Most studies of Doppler blood flow in the fetomaternal circulation have focused on the umbilical arteries, the fetal aorta, and the maternal uterine arteries, but smaller vessels, including the cerebral arteries, have become major areas of interest. Potential areas for examination include:

- The **maternal** uterine, ophthalmic, and middle cerebral arteries;
- The **fetal** umbilical artery, umbilical vein, aorta, inferior vena cava, and cerebral vessels;
- The **fetal** ductus venosus;
- The **fetal** heart for intracardiac flow;
- The **placenta**; and
- Other areas such as the renal arteries.

Maternal Arteries

Uterine Arteries. A more easily reproducible waveform pattern for maternal Doppler is obtained when the endovaginal approach is used in conjunction with color flow mapping. This also facilitates the identification of the myometrial arcuate, radial, and spiral arteries from which specific Doppler signals can be

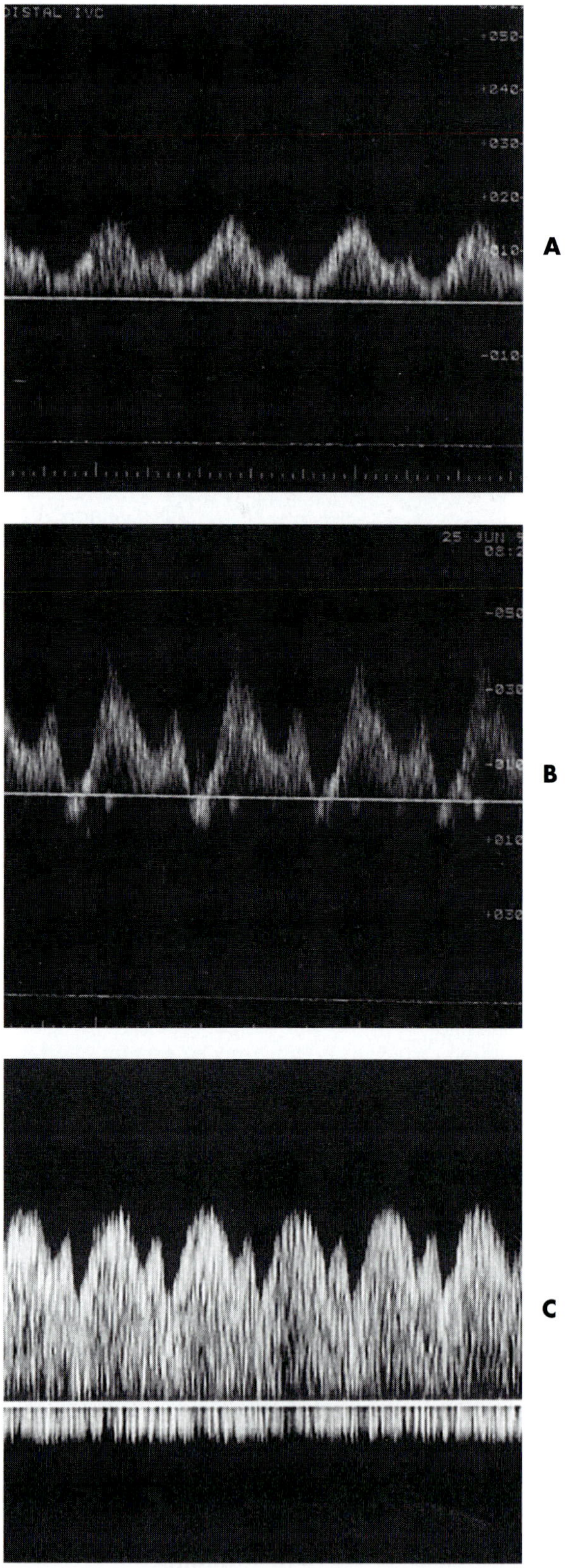

FIG. 49-3. Venous waveforms inferior vena cava. A, **Distal inferior vena cava** shows a biphasic waveform. B, **IVC close to the fetal heart** shows the triphasic waveform. C, **Ductus venosus** shows the typical pattern.

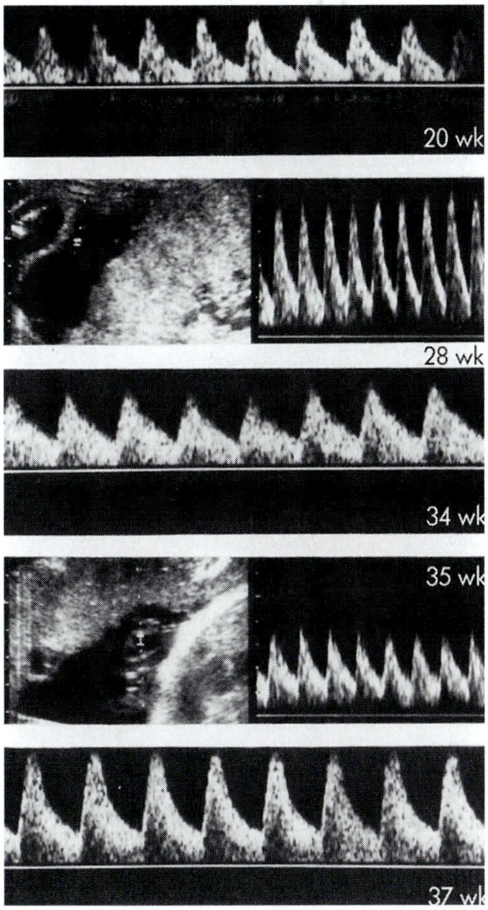

FIG. 49-4. Umbilical artery. Flow velocity waveform at different gestational ages. Diastolic flow increases, but there is some variability in the appearance of the waveform depending on the patient and the machine used.

obtained, primarily because of their anatomic location (Fig. 49-5).

In general terms, there is a small but significant decline in the Doppler indices in these vessels as **gestation advances.** Increasingly low resistance of the bed of the placenta results from placental angiogenesis and endovascular trophoblastic migration of the spiral arteries converts them into larger, tortuous channels. The latter process is complete by 18 weeks' gestation.[15] After 20 weeks' gestation, the pulsatility in these vessels is very similar to the pulsatility at term.

In recent years, **maternal cerebral vasculature** has become the subject of Doppler investigation, particularly as it relates to **preeclampsia.**[16] Williams et al.[17] have demonstrated that peak systolic velocities increase from 47 cm/sec to 65 cm/sec in the intrapartum period of hypertensive patients and continue to rise to 80 cm/sec at 48 hours postpartum before returning to normal. These velocities appear to be the highest in cases of eclampsia (137 cm/sec), secondary

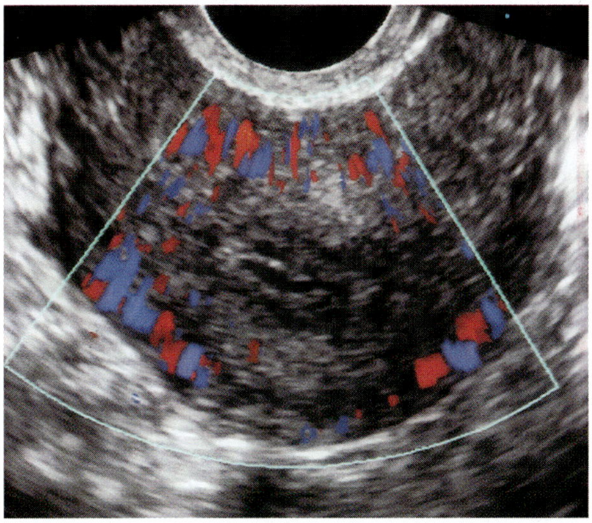

FIG. 49-5. Normal myometrial blood flow in a nonpregnant uterus shown with color flow Doppler.

to the increased arteriolar vasospasm and vascular resistance that are the hallmarks of this condition.

Maternal **ophthalmic** and central **retinal** arteries also hold a promise for the future (Fig. 49-6 and Table 49-1), as the nomograms created by McKenzie[18] provide an accessible window for easy monitoring of maternal cardiovascular changes.

Fetal Vessels

A high resistance pattern[19,20] is present in the embryonic period with absent end-diastolic flow (Fig. 49-7). Toward the end of the first trimester, end-diastolic flow appears and increases in velocity as normal gestation advances.

Umbilical Artery. Doppler waveforms can be obtained easily from the umbilical arteries with continuous or pulsed Doppler[21-23] (see box on p. 1376). A **decline in the S/D ratio** and **PI** occurs **with gestational age** irrespective of the technique or equipment used[24] (Fig. 49-8).

Fetal breathing affects the ratios,[25] and fetal heart-rate increases cause a decrease in pulsatility.[14] Ratios are higher, too, if measured at the fetal end of the cord rather than at the placental end,[26] perhaps because of damping of the pressure pulse as it travels down the cord. If considerable variation occurs on repeated measurements, it may be that the two arteries are dissimilar.[27] Recent observations also show that the measurements can be made reliably during labor.[28] A single umbilical artery is easily identified on color Doppler flow mapping (Fig. 49-9) by a cross-section through the cord or by scanning in the region of the fetal bladder.

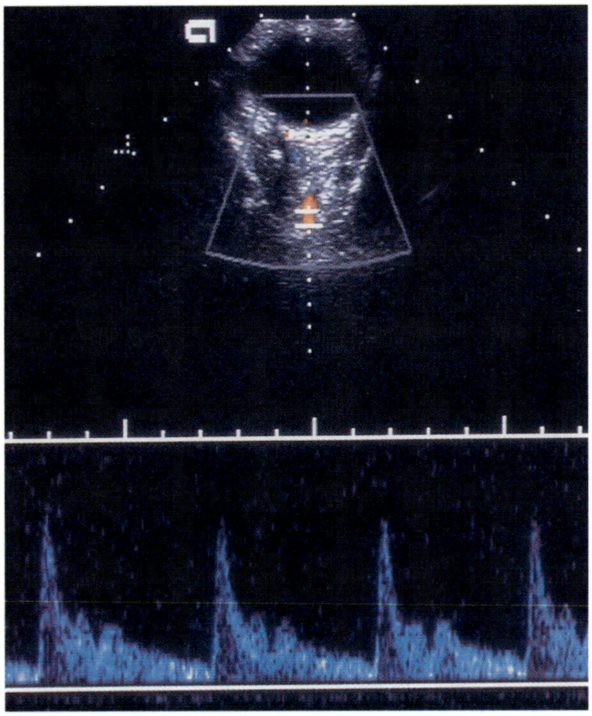

FIG. 49-6. Ophthalmic artery. Color and pulsed Doppler in a pregnant woman.

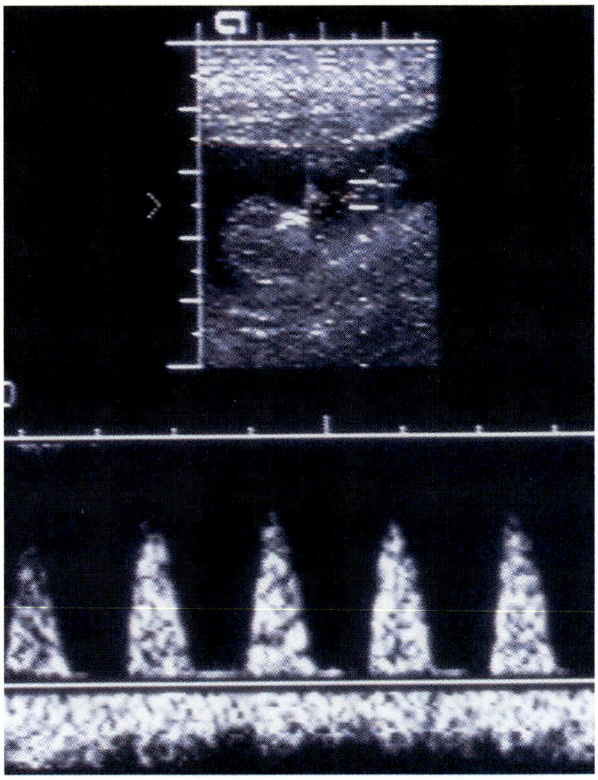

FIG. 49-7. Embryonic umbilical artery and vein from the nonhuman primate.

TABLE 49-1
DOPPLER INDICES: MEAN (STANDARD DEVIATION) FOR OA AND CRA AT DIFFERENT GESTATIONAL AGES

	20-<24	24-<28	28-<32	32-<36	36-41
Central Retinal Artery					
S/D	2.82(0.51)	2.78(0.67)	2.64(0.46)	2.76(0.57)	2.48(0.5)
RI	0.63(0.06)	0.62(0.07)	0.61(0.06)	0.62(0.07)	0.58(0.07)
PI	1.29(0.3)	1.37(0.46)	1.26(0.27)	1.33(0.36)	1.15(0.33)
Ophthalmic Artery					
S/D	4.47(0.9)	4.41(0.83)	4.18(1.19)	3.85(0.98)	3.82(0.89)
RI	0.76(0.06)	0.77(0.04)	0.74(0.07)	0.72(0.06)	0.72(0.06)
PI	1.92(0.35)	1.98(0.36)	1.9(0.53)	1.75(0.4)	1.81(0.46)

From Mackenzie F, De Vermette R, Nimrod C et al. Doppler sonographic studies on the ophthalmic and central retinal arteries in the gravid woman. *J Ultrasound Med* 1995;14:643-647.

NORMAL UMBILICAL ARTERY WAVEFORM

Embryo	No end-diastolic flow
Fetus	Increasing diastolic flow
S/D ratio	Declines with increasing gestational age
PI	Declines with increasing gestational age

Umbilical Vein. During the **embryonic period, venous flow is pulsatile,** constant, and of low velocity, with variation noted during fetal breathing movements (Fig. 49-10) (see box on p. 1378). The pulsatile component is not a feature of the second trimester; its presence at that time is of grave clinical significance. The size of the vein allows volume flow to be calculated. This increases throughout pregnancy, although it remains almost constant when corrected for fetal weight [29,30] (100 to 120 ml/kg/min).

FIG. 49-8. Normal systolic/diastolic (S/D) ratios in **A,** the maternal arcuate arteries, **B,** umbilical arteries, and **C,** fetal aorta in the last half of pregnancy. Lines are mean, and 95% confidence limits are derived by linear regression. (From Cameron A, Nicholson S, Nimrod CA et al. Duplex ultrasonography of the fetal aorta, umbilical artery, and placental arcuate artery throughout normal human pregnancy. *J Can Assoc Radiol* 1989;40:145-149.)

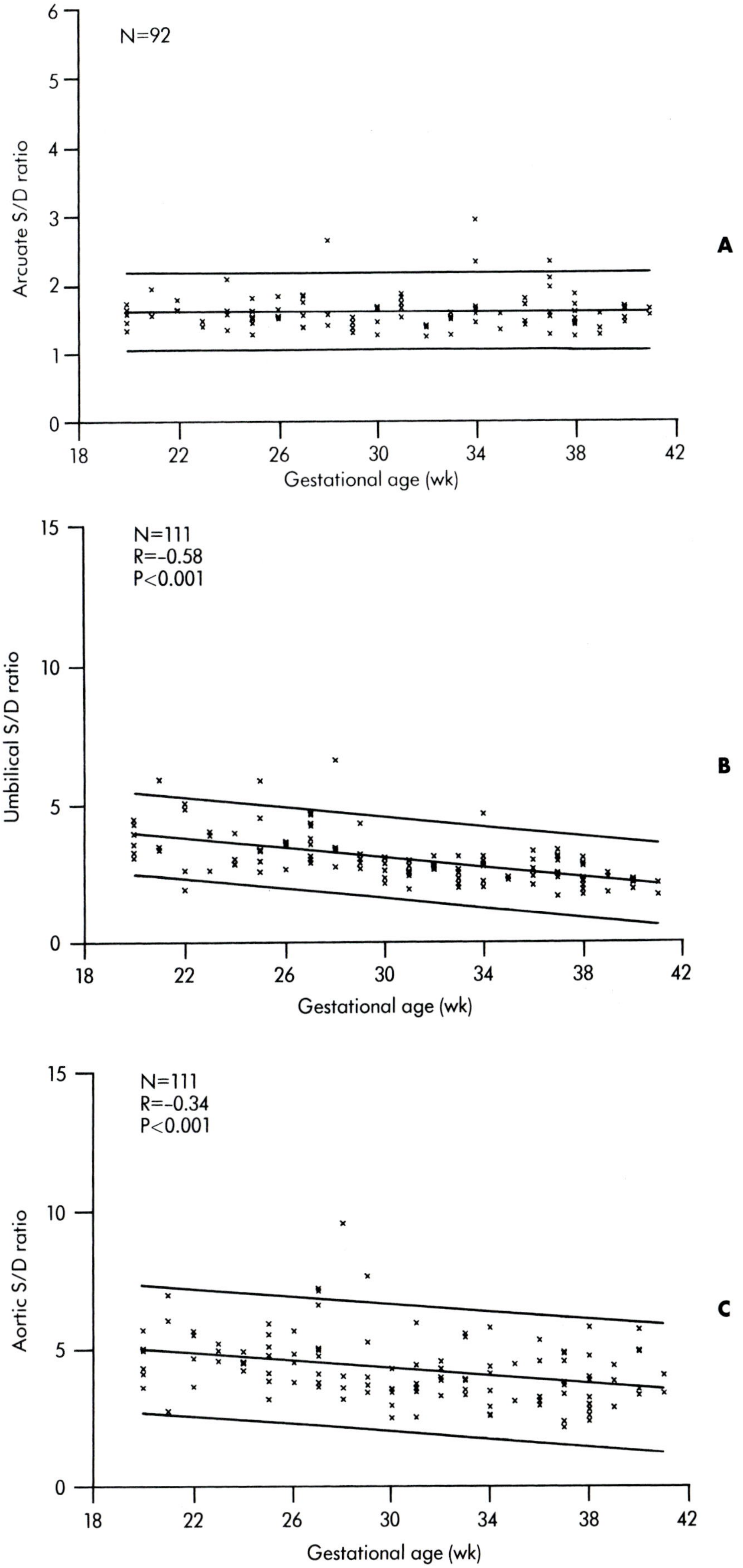

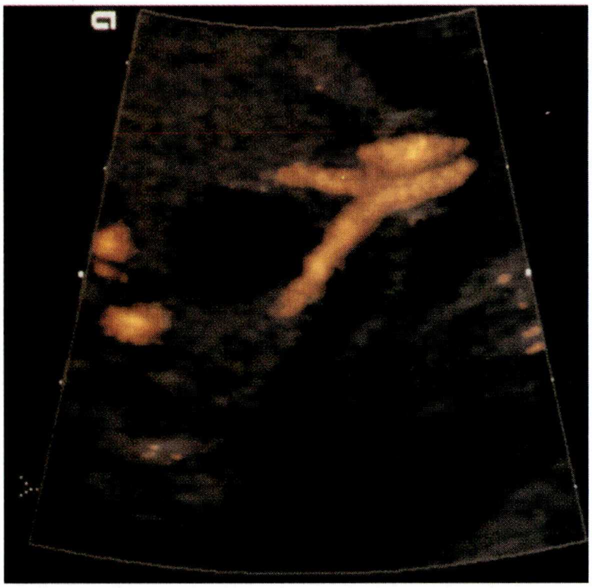

FIG. 49-9. Imaging three-vessel cord. Color Doppler imaging of umbilical arteries seen adjacent to the fetal urinary bladder.

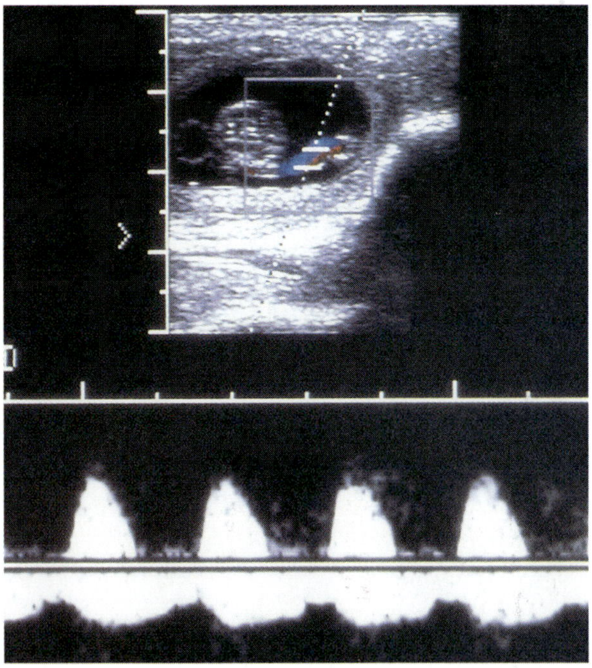

FIG. 49-10. Pulsatile embryonic umbilical vein.

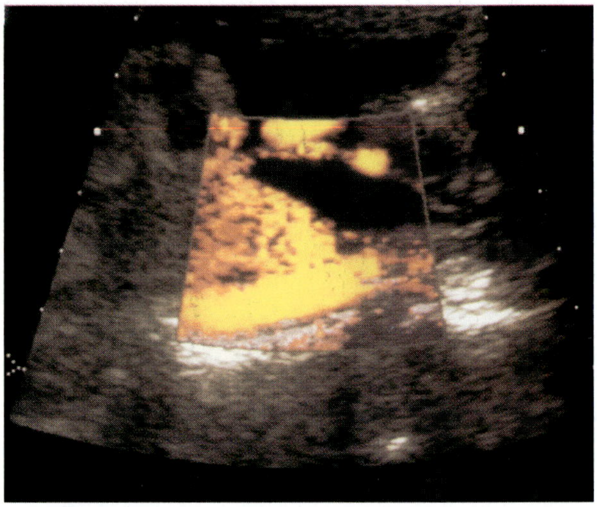

FIG. 49-11. Hypoechoic placental cyst on power Doppler sonogram.

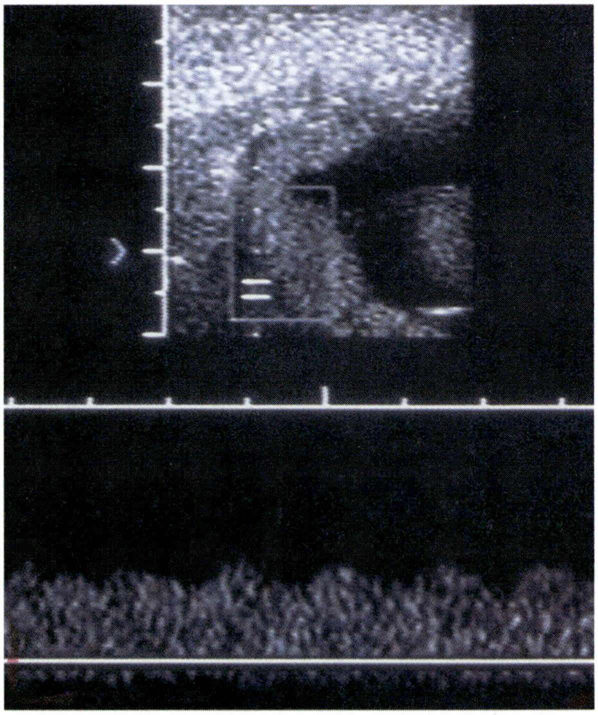

FIG. 49-12. Pulsatile, unidirectional, low-impedance intervillous flow in a hemichorial placenta.

NORMAL UMBILICAL VEIN WAVEFORM

Embryo	Pulsatile, low velocity
Fetus	Nonpulsatile

Placenta. Color Doppler and power Doppler have provided excellent mapping of vascular and nonvascular parenchymal structures in the placenta. Placental cysts, chorioangiomas, and areas of abruption are more easily characterized with the use of Doppler (Fig. 49-11).

A

B

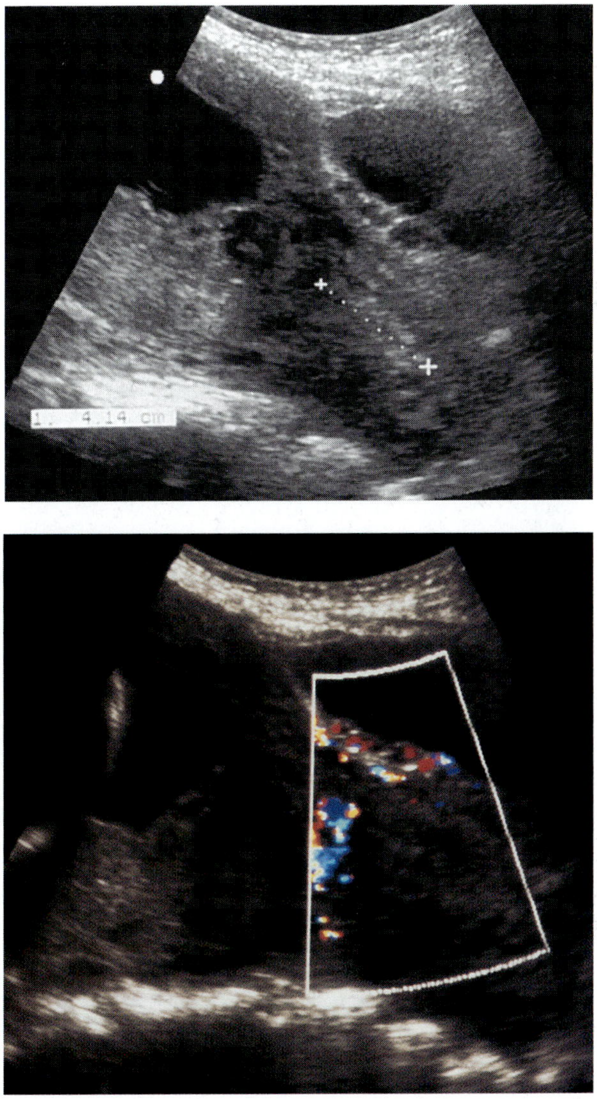

FIG. 49-13. Placenta percreta. A, Real-time image of placenta percreta demonstrating vascular lacunae. **B,** Color Doppler demonstrates vascular invasion into the urinary bladder mucosa.

The future holds promise for the study of intervillous blood flow (Fig. 49-12) because of the increasing sensitivity of Doppler instrumentation.

The diagnosis of placenta accreta has been enhanced by the demonstration of vascular penetration of placental vessels into the myometrium (Fig. 49-13).

Descending Aorta. Flow in the fetal aorta is measured just above or near the diaphragm to avoid the effects of major branches. Waveform indices can be measured and quantitative measurements can also be made (Fig. 49-14).

Flow volume and systolic, diastolic, and mean velocity increase as **pregnancy progresses,** with a plateau in velocities near term.[21] **S/D ratios decrease** with **gestational age** because of increasing diastolic velocities. Presumably this results from the decreasing placental resistance, as 60% to 70% of flow in the descending aorta is to the placenta.[31] As in the umbilical vein, volume flow corrected for fetal weight is fairly constant to term (200 to 250 ml/kg/min).[29,30]

Inferior Vena Cava (IVC). Interest has increased in the venous circulation and its role in the assessment of the fetal cardiovascular integrity.[32-34] The **normal waveform pattern** is triphasic when measured close to the fetal heart. A biphasic pattern emerges as the sampling site moves caudally in the IVC, with the highest peak occurring during ventricular systole when the atrium refills, and a second, smaller peak occurring during the rapid ventricular-filling phase of early diastole. The IVC is measured just below the diaphragm. Measurement too close to the right atrium can show reverse flow of the *a* wave of atrial contraction at the end of normal diastole. IVC flow is sensitive to intrathoracic pressure and changes during fetal breathing movements. The waveform is also influenced by heart rate, with a bradycardia allowing a prolonged diastolic surge, while the diastolic and systolic peaks tend to merge during a tachycardia (Fig. 49-15).

Hypoxia has been shown to increase the amplitude of vena caval pulsations,[35] and an enlarged *a* wave may be indicative of increased atrial pressure/tricuspid regurgitation.

Middle Cerebral Artery. Studies of the **middle cerebral artery** are useful, as they provide an opportunity to assess the brain-sparing effect in IUGR fetuses.[36,37] The preferential flow to the brain results in an increased diastolic flow during fetal asphyxia. Color Doppler flow mapping easily aids in the identification of the anterior, middle, and posterior cerebral arteries (Fig. 49-16). The ratio of MCA to umbilical artery PI, the cerebral/placental ratio, allows for the assessment of brain-sparing. The presence of **continuous flow** in the brain is a **normal feature** and is seen even in embryonic life. It is suggestive of a protective effect for the brain from the highly pulsatile arterial flow.

Ductus Arteriosus. Right ventricular output in the fetus is 1.1 to 1.3 times left ventricular output, with most of the blood bypassing the high-resistance pulmonary circulation to supply the lower body and placenta via the ductus arteriosus.[38] Huhta et al. have demonstrated that ductal flow can be routinely assessed at 20 weeks' gestation, with **ductal systolic velocities** ranging from **50 to 140 cm/sec.**[39] These are the highest velocities found in the normal fetal cardiovascular system. Diastolic velocities range from 6 to 30 cm/sec. This information can be used to detect early ductal constriction with pulmonary hyperten-

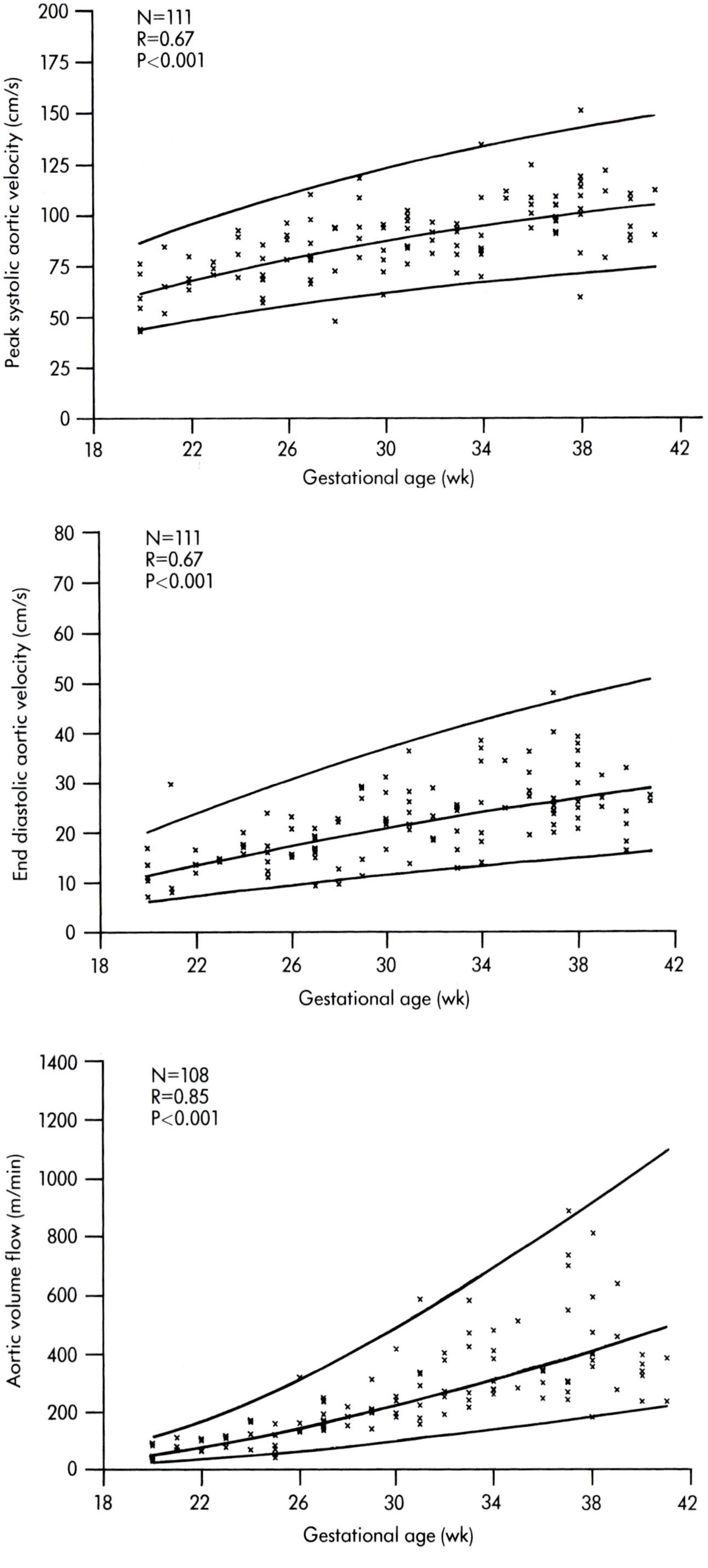

FIG. 49-14. Normal fetal aorta values for quantitative measurements in the last half of pregnancy. Lines are mean, and 95% confidence limits are derived by curvilinear regression. (From Cameron A, Nicholson S, Nimrod CA et al. Duplex ultrasonography of the fetal aorta, umbilical artery, and placental arcuate artery throughout normal human pregnancy. *J Can Assoc Radiol* 1989;40:145-149.)

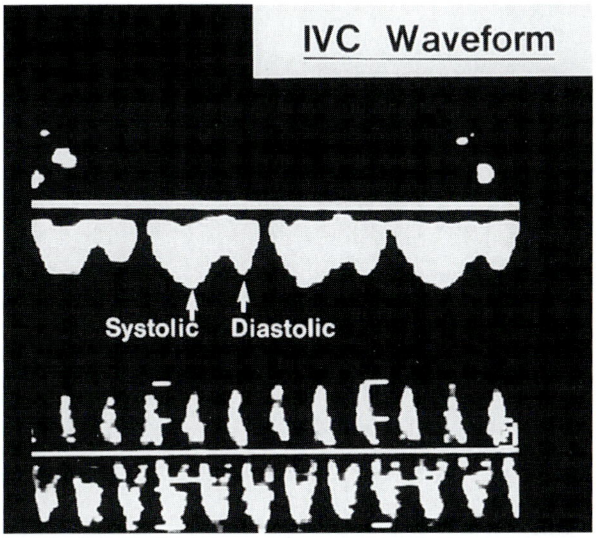

FIG. 49-15. Supraventricular tachycardia causes a biphasic IVC waveform.

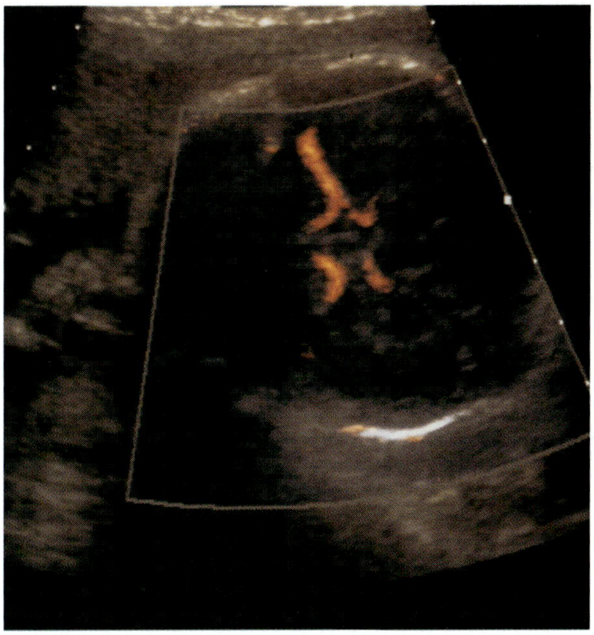

FIG. 49-16. Fetal circle of Willis. Color Doppler sonogram.

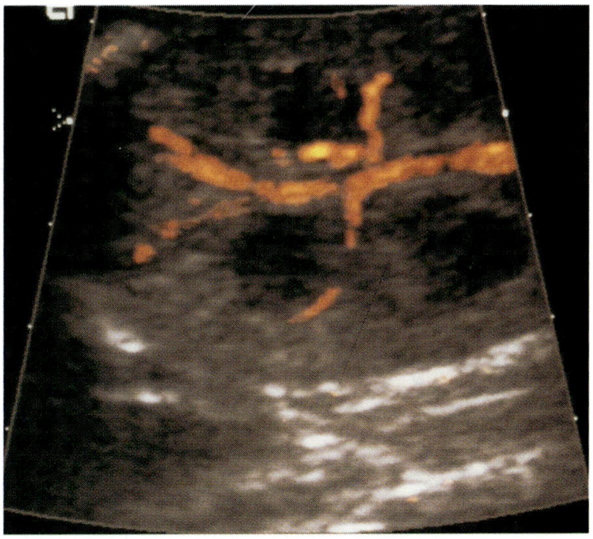

FIG. 49-17. Fetal renal arteries. Color Doppler sonogram shows renal vessels on both sides of the aorta.

sion in fetuses of mothers receiving indomethacin for premature labor.[39]

Other Arteries. Color flow and power Doppler allow the assessment of blood flow in vessels that cannot be reliably found using only duplex scanners. In oligohydramnios, possibly due to renal agenesis, the demonstration of renal artery (Fig. 49-17) and parenchymal flow clearly establishes the presence of kidneys. The PI in the fetal renal arteries decreases linearly from 18 to 42 weeks, with increasing diastolic flow.[40]

PATHOLOGIC DOPPLER FINDINGS

Pulsed Doppler ultrasound has been used in a variety of obstetrical diseases to elucidate pathophysiology,[41] to aid in earlier diagnosis, and to assess fetal well-being and fetal response to various therapies or interventions. Contributions to pathophysiology are limited to the circulatory systems of the mother and fetus and may have implications for therapy. There is currently no role for the use of Doppler as a screening test in low-risk pregnancies. However, the application of pulsed Doppler as a second-level test in complex pregnancies offers considerable advantages over other methods of fetal health surveillance in the prediction of perinatal death.[42]

Intrauterine Growth Retardation (IUGR)

Small-for-gestational-age (SGA) babies make up 10% of all pregnancies but include an assortment of diagnoses, such as chromosomal and other fetal anomalies, placental insufficiency, congenital infections, and even structurally normal small babies. A number of these diseases appear to act through the common pathway of placental insufficiency, but as expected, the Doppler FVW varies widely in this diverse group. Factors related to reduced blood flow in the intervillous space include smoking, maternal hypertension, cocaine use, and poor nutrition.

Abnormal Doppler indices and **waveform shape** have been shown in the **uterine artery** as early as 20 weeks gestation,[43] suggesting that reduction in maternal blood flow may be one of the earliest changes in some forms of IUGR. **Reduced diastolic velocities** in the umbilical arteries indicate that placental resistance is rising and correlate with the loss of small vessels seen pathologically.[44] This change can be created in the animal model by injection of microspheres to block the placental vascular bed.[11] **Volume flow** in the **umbilical vein** is **reduced,** confirming the loss of perfusion.[45] Changes can be seen in the fetal aorta and cerebral and venous circulations that correspond to the compensatory changes seen with hypoxia[46] as the fetus attempts to protect its vital organs in the face of reduced placental function. Cardiac changes may then occur secondary to changes in factors affecting preload and afterload as well as myocardial oxygenation.

What Are the Doppler Changes and How Commonly Do They Occur?

When pulsed Doppler is used to monitor fetal health status in the IUGR patient, **elevation of the Doppler indices** in the **umbilical artery** or **aorta** is usually the **first sign** of compromised placental function. The increase in placental vascular resistance manifests itself in the altered ratio, and if this is followed serially, a worsening ratio is good evidence of further compromise. The fetus compensates by shunting blood from its limbs, gut, and muscle to the cerebral and coronary circulations. As a consequence, pulsed Doppler of the **middle cerebral artery** illustrates a **reduction in its pulsatility**. This can be seen as a change in the normal cerebral-placental ratio from greater than 1 to less than 1 (sensitivity = 75% to 85%, specificity = 93% to 100%).[47,48] **Progressive worsening** is manifested by **absent** diastolic flow followed by a **reversal of diastolic flow** in both the **aorta** and **umbilical artery**[49-51] and may occur first in the aortic isthmus.[52] By that time, the **venous circulation** also demonstrates modifications in the flow velocity waveforms:

- An increased *a* wave coupled with a decreased diastolic forward peak in the IVC waveform[41] (Fig. 49-18);
- Lack of continuous forward flow in the ductus venosus;[41] and
- A pulsatile umbilical vein.[53,54]

These venous flow changes may indirectly reflect changes in the cardiac status, particularly tricuspid regurgitation and increased right atrial pressure.

The maternal uterine artery may show reduced end-diastolic flow in IUGR cases.[55] A difference in S/D ratios between right and left uterine arteries correlates well with poorer outcome.[56]

Overall, excellent placental histopathologic correlation with umbilical Doppler has been demonstrated, primarily illustrating a reduction in the tertiary stem villi in compromised cases.

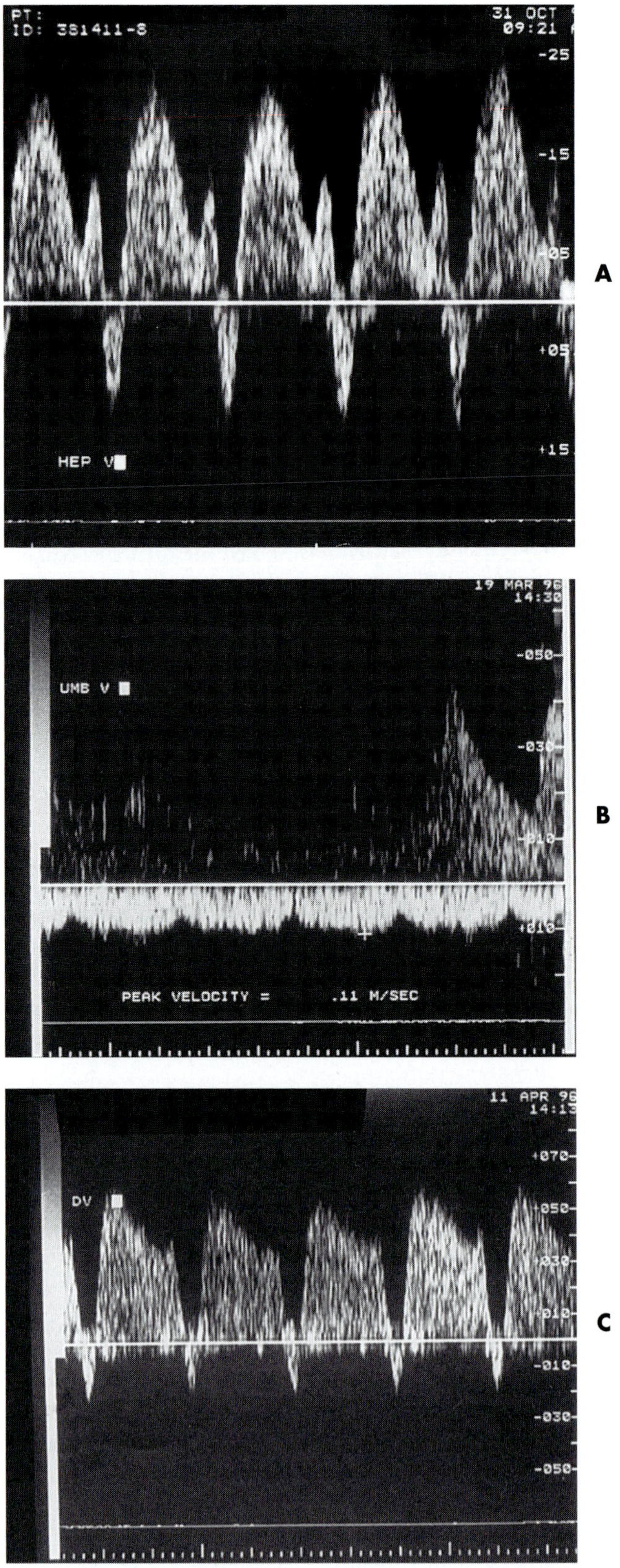

FIG. 49-18. Abnormal fetal venous waveforms. **A,** Abnormal IVC waveform. **B,** Pulsatile umbilical vein. **C,** Abnormal ductus venosus.

What Does an Abnormal Doppler Parameter Mean?

Each of the parameters seems to measure something different. The umbilical artery waveforms and total venous flow reflect changes in the placental vascular bed, whereas the cerebral waveforms reflect the compensatory response of the fetal brain to the reduced placental function. As aortic flow is the product of cardiac contractility and stroke volume acting against the resistance of the cerebral, peripheral, and placental circulations, the relative impedance of these parts of the fetal circulation determines in which direction blood will flow in diastole. The aortic pattern, therefore, reflects cardiac performance as well as the redistribution in the peripheral circulation, as the fetus attempts to compensate for the inadequate placental flow. IVC and other venous patterns may be the best measure of deteriorating cardiac function as cardiac chamber size and filling pressure increase. The number of abnormal Doppler parameters, as well as the extent of abnormality, correlate well with the degree of fetal compromise, particularly if cardiac performance is affected. Doppler parameters may begin to become abnormal in IUGR 4 or more weeks before the fetus appears to deteriorate as judged by cardiotopography.[51,57] **It is therefore of the utmost importance to use the test results in light of other findings.** A single abnormal result does not necessarily mean that delivery should be undertaken. However, the persistent presence of reversed end-diastolic flow in either the aorta (Fig. 49-19), the umbilical artery and ductus venosus, or a pulsatile umbilical vein all represent ominous signs.[58]

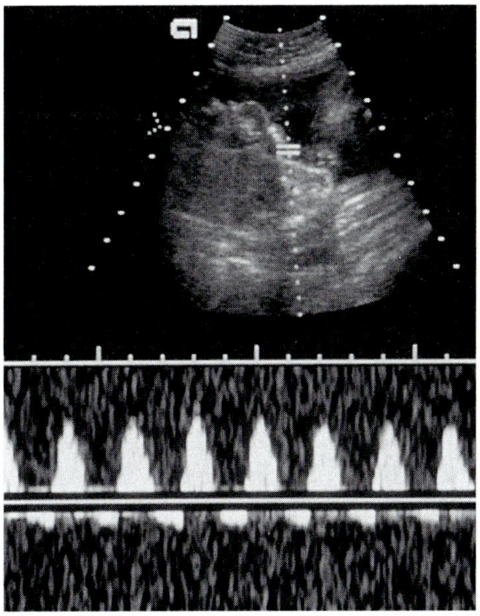

FIG. 49-19. Reverse flow in the umbilical artery.

> **OMINOUS DOPPLER FEATURES**
>
> Reversed end-diastolic flow
> - Fetal aorta
> - Umbilical artery
> - Ductus venosus
>
> Pulsatile umbilical vein

What Correlations Exist among Doppler, Other Biophysical Tests, and the Acid/Base Status in Growth-restricted Fetuses?

Several recent meta-analyses have explored the value of pulsed Doppler in randomized clinical trials.[59] Thornton and Lilford assessed the relative risk for death in the absence of end-diastolic flow in the umbilical artery to be 80.[60] The work of Alfirevic and Neilson in high-risk pregnancies also indicates that the provision of Doppler information to physicians confers significant benefit to obstetrical outcomes.[61] Specifically, a 44% reduction in antenatal admissions (Fig. 49-20), a 20% reduction in induction of labor, a 52% decline in cesarean section for fetal distress, and a 38% reduction in perinatal mortality (Fig. 49-21) are some of the benefits.

In addition, a 7-year follow-up Swedish study of 159 children indicated that fetuses with flow disturbances in utero had a higher association with neurodevelopmental impairment than did control children.[62]

A comparison between umbilical artery Doppler and biophysical profile in predicting the acid/base status of fetuses showed that umbilical Doppler was the better predictor of acidemia and hypercarbia (Table 49-2).[63]

In a separate study by Rizzo et al. assessing umbilical artery, aorta, renal artery, middle cerebral artery, cardiac outflow tract, IVC, and ductus venosus just prior to cordocentesis, logistic regression demonstrated that the IVC percentage reverse flow most closely reflected acidemia and hyperapnea, while hypoxemia was best predicted by the middle cerebral artery (Table 49-3).[64]

PREGNANCY-INDUCED HYPERTENSION (PIH)

PIH occurs in approximately 7% of all primigravidas,[65] varying in time of onset and severity and having high perinatal morbidity and mortality. If impaired perfusion of the intervillous space is present, the same Doppler changes seen in IUGR can be seen in PIH.[66] Patients

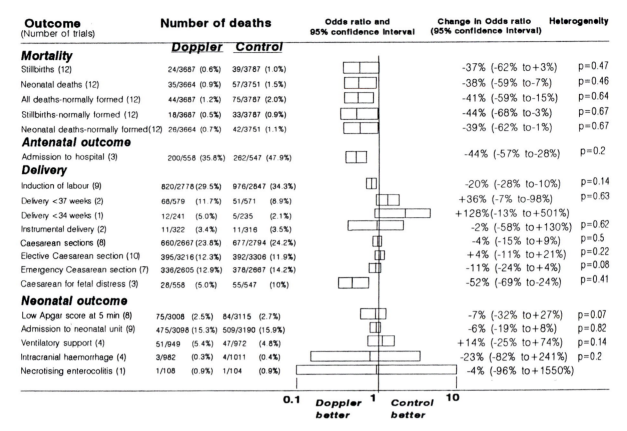

Outcome (Number of trials)	Number of deaths: Doppler	Number of deaths: Control	Change in Odds ratio (95% confidence interval)	Heterogeneity
Mortality				
Stillbirths (12)	24/3687 (0.6%)	39/3787 (1.0%)	-37% (-62% to+3%)	p=0.47
Neonatal deaths (12)	35/3664 (0.9%)	57/3751 (1.5%)	-38% (-59% to-7%)	p=0.46
All deaths-normally formed (12)	44/3687 (1.2%)	75/3787 (2.0%)	-41% (-59% to-15%)	p=0.64
Stillbirths-normally formed (12)	18/3687 (0.5%)	33/3787 (0.9%)	-44% (-68% to-3%)	p=0.67
Neonatal deaths-normally formed(12)	26/3664 (0.7%)	42/3751 (1.1%)	-39% (-62% to-1%)	p=0.67
Antenatal outcome				
Admission to hospital (3)	200/558 (35.8%)	262/547 (47.9%)	-44% (-57% to-28%)	p=0.2
Delivery				
Induction of labour (9)	820/2778 (29.5%)	976/2847 (34.3%)	-20% (-28% to-10%)	p=0.14
Delivery <37 weeks (2)	68/579 (11.7%)	51/571 (8.9%)	+36% (-7% to-98%)	p=0.63
Delivery <34 weeks (1)	12/241 (5.0%)	5/235 (2.1%)	+128%(-13% to+501%)	
Instrumental delivery (2)	11/322 (3.4%)	11/316 (3.5%)	-2% (-58% to+130%)	p=0.62
Caesarean sections (8)	660/2667 (23.8%)	677/2794 (24.2%)	-4% (-15% to+9%)	p=0.5
Elective Caesarean section (10)	395/3216 (12.3%)	392/3306 (11.9%)	+4% (-11% to+21%)	p=0.22
Emergency Ceasarean section (7)	336/2605 (12.9%)	378/2667 (14.2%)	-11% (-24% to+4%)	p=0.08
Caesarean for fetal distress (3)	28/558 (5.0%)	55/547 (10%)	-52% (-69% to-24%)	p=0.41
Neonatal outcome				
Low Apgar score at 5 min (8)	75/3008 (2.5%)	84/3115 (2.7%)	-7% (-32% to+27%)	p=0.07
Admission to neonatal unit (9)	475/3098 (15.3%)	509/3190 (15.9%)	-6% (-19% to+8%)	p=0.82
Ventilatory support (4)	51/949 (5.4%)	47/972 (4.8%)	+14% (-25% to+74%)	p=0.14
Intracranial haemorrhage (4)	3/982 (0.3%)	4/1011 (0.4%)	-23% (-82% to+241%)	p=0.2
Necrotising enterocolitis (1)	1/108 (0.9%)	1/104 (0.9%)	-4% (-96% to+1550%)	

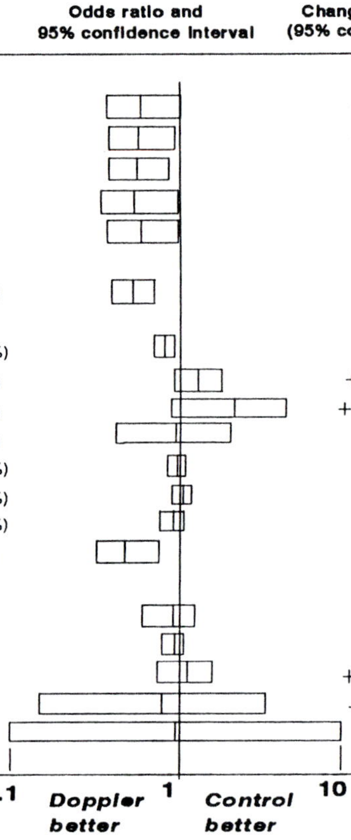

FIG. 49-20. Proportional effect of Doppler ultrasonography on prespecified perinatal outcomes. (From Alfiveric Z, Neilson JP. Doppler ultrasonography in high-risk pregnancies: systematic review with meta-analysis. *Am J Obstet Gynecol* 1995;172:1379-1387.)

Trial	Number of deaths: Doppler	Number of deaths: Control	Change in Odds ratio (95% confidence interval)
Trudinger et al 1987	1/127 (0.8%)	5/162 (3.1%)	-68% (-94% to+65%)
McParland&Pearce 1988	6/254 (2.4%)	20/255 (7.8%)	-68% (-85% to-29%)
Tyrell et al 1990	3/250 (1.2%)	3/250 (1.2%)	0% (-80% to+399%)
Hofmeyr et al 1991	4/438 (0.9%)	8/459 (1.7%)	-47% (-83% to+67%)
Newnham et al 1991	9/275 (3.3%)	9/270 (3.3%)	-2% (-62% to+151%)
Burke et al 1992	4/241 (1.7%)	3/235 (1.3%)	+30% (-71% to+478%)
Almstrom et al 1992	0/214 (0%)	3/212 (1.4%)	-87% (-99% to+28%)
Biljan et al 1992	1/338 (0.3%)	4/336 (1.2%)	-70% (-95% to+72%)
Johnstone et al 1993	12/1132(1.1%)	16/1197(1.3%)	-21% (-62% to+67%)
Pattison et al 1994	6/108 (5.6%)	8/104 (7.7%)	-29% (-76% to+109%)
Neales et al	11/236 (4.7%)	14/231 (6.1%)	-24% (-66% to+70%)
Nienhuis&Hoogland	2/74 (2.7%)	3/76 (3.9%)	-32% (-88% to+403%)
ALL TRIALS	**59/3687 (1.6%)**	**96/3787 (2.5%)**	**-38% (-55% to-15%)**

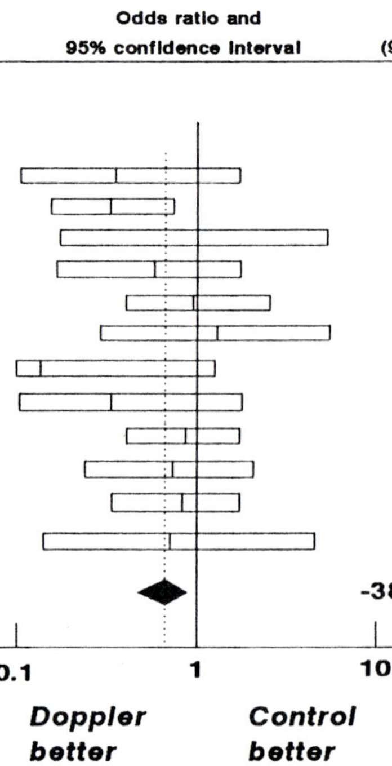

Heterogeneity: x^2=8.67; p=0.56

FIG. 49-21. Proportional effect of Doppler ultrasonography on number of dead babies (stillbirths and neonates) **when used in high-risk pregnancies.** (From Alfiveric Z, Neilson JP. Doppler ultrasonography in high-risk pregnancies: systematic review with meta-analysis. *Am J Obstet Gynecol* 1995;172:1379-1387.)

TABLE 49-2

RELATIONSHIP OF VARIOUS ANTEPARTUM TESTS WITH FETAL ACIDEMIA, HYPERCAPNIA, AND HYPOXIA ANALYZED BY LOGISTIC REGRESSION

Antepartum Tests	Acidemia		Hypercapnia		Hypoxia	
	χ^2	Significance	χ^2	Significance	χ^2	Significance
Umbilical artery Doppler velocimetry (Δ PI)	26.6	$p < 0.000001$	22.9	$p < 0.000005$	1.0	NS
Biophysical profile score	11.1	$p < 0.001$	9.0	$p < 0.005$	2.3	NS
Nonstress test	4.8	$p < 0.03$	2.8	NS	1.3	NS
Fetal breathing movement	11.1	$p < 0.001$	8.5	$p < 0.005$	1.8	NS
Fetal movement	13.5	$p < 0.0005$	11.8	$p < 0.001$	2.9	$p = 0.09$
Fetal tone	5.8	$p < 0.02$	5.1	$p < 0.03$	0.3	NS
Amniotic fluid volume	3.7	NS	3.3	NS	0.2	NS

NS, Not significant.
From Yoon BH, Romero R, Roh CR et al. Relationship between the fetal biophysical profile, umbilical artery, Doppler velocimetry, and fetal blood acid/base status determined by cordocentesis. *Am J Obstet Gynecol* 1993;169:1586-1594.

TABLE 49-3

RELATION OF DOPPLER INDICES WITH FETAL ACIDEMIA, HYPOXEMIA, AND HYPERCAPNIA ANALYZED BY LOGISTIC REGRESSION

	Acidaemia			Hypercapnia			Hypoxaemia		
	R^2	χ^2	P≤	R^2	χ^2	P≤	R^2	χ^2	P≤
IVC% reverse flow	0.46	29.69	0.0001	0.20	12.86	0.0003	0.20	11.11	0.001
AO PV	0.39	24.86	0.0001	0.20	12.91	0.0003	0.19	10.03	0.001
DV S:A	0.28	17.11	0.0001	0.11	7.50	0.006	0.24	14.24	0.0004
PA PV	0.25	13.78	0.0001	0.12	7.62	0.005	0.14	8.28	0.004
DA PI	0.10	6.22	0.005	0.08	3.43	0.05	0.01	0.515	NS
RA PI	0.09	5.79	0.01	0.08	3.98	0.04	0.02	3.03	NS
MCA PI	0.02	2.99	NS	0.15	9.79	0.001	0.26	15.13	0.0001
UA PI	0.02	2.90	NS	0.01	0.94	NS	0.01	1.42	NS

NS, Not significant.
Hypoxemia and hypercapnia were diagnosed when individual values were below 2 SD for pO_2 and pH and above 2 SD for pCO_2 from the expected mean for gestation. The prevalence of fetal hypoxemia, acidemia, and hypercapnia was, respectively, 79.2% (38/48), 41.7% (20/48), 58.3% (28/4).
From Rizzo G, Capponi A, Ardioni D et al. The value of fetal arterial, cardiac and venous flows in predicting pH and blood gases measured in the umbilical blood at cordocentesis in growth retarded fetuses. *Br J Obstet Gynecol* 1995;102:963-969.

with mild PIH did not show any flow abnormalities unless there was IUGR.[67,68] In severe PIH, Doppler studies were often abnormal, and they correlated with poor outcomes and signs of fetal distress. The Doppler changes often preceded the finding of an abnormal nonstress test by 24 hours. The greater the number of abnormal Doppler parameters found in the uterine artery, aorta, and umbilical arteries, the worse was the prognosis. Hypertension generally worsened the fetal prognosis if IUGR was already present. Maternal status has been followed by Doppler of the middle cerebral artery, and promise exists for ascertainment of her response to antihypertensive agents by following maternal ophthalmic artery blood-flow patterns.[69]

MULTIPLE-GESTATION PREGNANCY

Pulsed Doppler remains a useful adjunct in establishing fetal well-being when poor growth in multiple gestation is due to placental insufficiency.

In monochorionic placentation, there may be intraplacental shunts that may cause twin-to-twin transfusion. The unpredictable nature of these shunts has limited the value of pulsed Doppler.[70-73] In the future, power Doppler analysis of these placentas may result in the delineation of the shunts. Until such time, ultrasound monitoring of fetal growth in various organs may be the best evaluative tool available.

HYDROPS

Fetal hydrops is the end result of a number of disease processes. In immune hydrops, an increase in fetal cardiac output as a result of the anemia can be shown by Doppler techniques[74] (879 ± 86 ml/kg/min versus 644 ± 35.3 ml/kg/min in normal controls). Similar findings of a hyperdynamic circulatory state have been found in hydrops caused by alpha-thalassemia.[75] Doppler indices, however, were not useful in predicting fetal hematocrit.[76] In patients with cardiac causes of hydrops, such as supraventricular tachycardia, fetal echocardiography combined with intracardiac Doppler has been helpful in assessing the degrees of cardiac compromise. Animal studies[77] have shown that this hydrops is due to elevation of venous pressure secondary to increased right atrial pressure from right ventricular failure and tricuspid regurgitation. Liver congestion and decreased albumin levels lead to worsening edema, and atrial natriuretic factor[78] also seems to play a role. Again, the percentage of reverse flow in the IVC may hold prognostic value in the evaluation of some forms of nonimmune hydrops.

POSTTERM PREGNANCY

Conservative noninterventional management of the postterm or postdates pregnancies may be complicated by placental insufficiency and fetal compromise. Conversely, an increased cesarean section rate is associated with active induction of labor in the presence of an unfavorable cervix. Biophysical profile and amniotic fluid volume are usually used to guide management but have limitations. In 243 postterm patients randomized into two groups, with one group having the Doppler results available for management and the other group blinded to the Doppler results, we found the cesarean section rate higher in the blinded group (23.6 versus 17.2%).[79] In addition, a greater proportion of patients in the group using the Doppler results were allowed to deliver past 42 weeks ($p < 0.04$), and their hospital stays were shorter. Fetal aortic Doppler was more useful than umbilical S/D ratios and appeared to offer advantages over amniotic fluid volume. Cerebral S/D ratios were significantly lower in patients with abnormal antepartum fetal surveillance tests. Several studies[80,81] now support the thesis that **umbilical artery Doppler is not a particularly sensitive tool in the evaluation of the postdates pregnancy**. Its value may increase if serial studies are performed and the Doppler indices rise rather than fall.

DOPPLER NORMAL AND BIOPHYSICAL PROFILE ABNORMAL

True knot in the cord
A short cord
Fetal neurologic impairment
Fetal maternal transfusion
Fetal viremia

CARDIAC ANOMALIES

The differentiation of congenital heart defects is a problem that requires a specific expertise. A deterioration in cardiac function appears to be the final pathway in fetal compromise leading to fetal death. Therefore, it is important to assess cardiac function in the compromised fetus with a structurally normal heart. In addition to the ultrasound assessment of heart rate and heart size, Doppler helps gauge systolic function by measuring aortic volume flow, systolic velocities, and acceleration time. Diastolic function may be mirrored by changes in the IVC flow velocity waveform. As chamber sizes increase, the development of atrioventricular valve incompetence can be shown by pulsed or color flow Doppler. This continues to be an important tool in the assessment of fetal well-being. Fetal arrhythmias can be difficult to assess with M-mode ultrasound, and we find it easier to determine the timing of atrial and ventricular contraction using simultaneous pulsed Doppler of the IVC and aorta.

CAUTION

At times a significant lack of congruence exists between Doppler findings and those of other biophysical tests, and this may be a signal for further clarification (see box). Several examples of circumstances in which the Doppler is normal but the biophysical profile is abnormal include the existence of a true knot in the cord, a short cord, fetal neurological impairment, fetal maternal transfusion, and fetal viremia.

Appropriate detailed evaluation should include ultrasound for fetal examination, Kleihaeur-Bethe testing, fetal stimulation with anticipation of heart-rate accelerations, or cordocentesis for acid/base status and hematocrit.

THE FUTURE

The recent studies examining the relationship between the nonstress test, the biophysical profile, and various arterial and venous Doppler waveforms and the fetal acid/base status have shed considerable light on the relative value of these tests and perhaps on the sequence in which they deteriorate. Further advances are anticipated as the fetal echo-Doppler relationship is examined more closely.[82] To date, it seems that from a practical standpoint, the umbilical artery and middle cerebral artery will offer most of the arterial information necessary, and the IVC and ductus venous will provide the venous information. Much wider clinical application is anticipated with power Doppler, particularly in the area of assessment of intervillous blood flow. On the maternal side, the full potential offered by cerebral and ophthalmic Doppler is still to be realized.

REFERENCES

1. Schulman H, Winter D, Farmakides G, et al. Pregnancy surveillance with Doppler velocimetry of uterine and umbilical arteries. *Am J Obstet Gynecol* 1989;160:192-196.
2. Jouppila P, Kirkinen P. Increased vascular resistance in the descending aorta of the human fetus in hypoxia. *Br J Obstet Gynaecol* 1984;91:853-856.
3. Trudinger BJ, Cook CM, Jones L, et al. A comparison of fetal heart rate monitoring and umbilical artery waveforms in the recognition of fetal compromise. *Br J Obstet Gynaecol* 1986; 3:171-175.
4. Lombardi SJ, Rosemond R, Ball R et al. Umbilical artery velocimetry as a predictor of adverse outcome in pregnancies complicated by oligohydramnios. *Obstet Gynecol* 1989;74: 338-341.

Instrumentation

5. McDicken WN. *Diagnostic Ultrasonics: Principles and Use of Instruments.* 2nd ed. New York: John Wiley & Sons; 1981:259.

Doppler Analysis

6. Arduini D, Rizzo G, Boccolini MR, et al. Functional assessment of uteroplacental and fetal circulations by means of color Doppler ultrasonography. *J Ultrasound Med* 1990;9:249-253.
7. Gosling RG, King DH. Ultrasonic angiography. In: Marcus AW, Adamson L, eds. *Arteries and Veins.* Edinburgh: Churchill Livingstone; 1975:61-98.
8. Pourcelot L. Diagnostic ultrasound for cerebral vascular diseases. In: Donald J, Levi S, eds. *Present and Future Diagnostic Ultrasound.* Toronto: John Wiley & Sons; 1976:141-147.
9. Gosling RG. Extraction of physiological information from spectrum-analyzed Doppler-shifted continuous ultrasound signals obtained noninvasively from the arterial tree. In: Hull DW, Watson BW, eds. *IEE Medical Electronics Monographs 13-22.* London: Peter Peregrinns; 1976:73-125.
10. Trudinger BJ, Giles WB, Cook CM. Uteroplacental blood flow velocity-time waveforms in normal and complicated pregnancy. *Br J Obstet Gynaecol* 1985;92:39-45.
11. Adamson SL, Morrow RJ, Langille BL, et al. Site-dependent effects of increases in placental vascular resistance on the umbilical arterial velocity waveform in fetal sheep. *Ultrasound Med Biol* 1990;16:19-27.
12. Hoskins PR, Haddad NG, Johnstone FD, et al. The choice of index for umbilical artery Doppler waveforms. *Ultrasound Med Biol* 1989;15:107-111.
13. Thompson RS, Trudinger BJ, Cook CM. A comparison of Doppler ultrasound waveform indices in the umbilical artery I: indices derived from the maximum velocity waveform. *Ultrasound Med Biol* 1986;12:835-844.
14. Yarlagadda P, Willoughby L, Maulik D. Effect of fetal heart rate on umbilical arterial Doppler indices. *J Ultrasound Med* 1989;8:215-218.

Normal Doppler Flows

15. Pijnenborg R, Bland JM, Robertson WB, et al. Uteroplacental arterial changes related to interstitial trophoblast migration in early human pregnancy. *Placenta* 1983;4:387-414.
16. Zunker P, Ley-Pozo J, Louwen F, et al. Cerebral hemodynamics in preeclampsia/eclampsia syndrome. *Ultrasound Obstet Gynecol* 1995;6:411-415.
17. Williams K, Wilson S. Maternal cerebral changes with preeclampsia assessed by transcranial Doppler: a review. *J Soc Obstet Gynecol* 1995;17:759-765.
18. Mackenzie F, De Vermette R, Nimrod C, et al. Doppler sonographic studies on the ophthalmic and central retinal arteries in the gravid woman. *J Ultrasound Med* 1995:14;643-647.
19. Wladimiroff J, Huisman T, Stewart P, et al. Normal fetal Doppler inferior vena cava, transtricuspid, and umbilical artery flow velocity waveforms between 11 and 16 weeks' gestation. *Am J Obstet Gynecol* 1992;166:921-924.
20. Nimrod C, Simpson N, Hafner T, et al. Assessment of early placental development in the cynomolgus monkey (Macaca fascicularis) using color and pulsed wave Doppler sonography. *J Med Primatol* (in press).
21. Cameron A, Nicholson S, Nimrod CA, et al. Duplex ultrasonography of the fetal aorta, umbilical artery, and placental arcuate artery throughout normal human pregnancy. *J Can Assoc Radiol* 1989;40:145-149.
22. Kurjak A, Alfirevic Z, Miljan M. Conventional and color Doppler in the assessment of the fetal and maternal circulation. *Ultrasound Med Biol* 1988;4:337-354.
23. Hendricks SK, Sorensen TK, Wang KY, et al. Doppler umbilical artery waveform indices—normal values from fourteen to forty-two weeks. *Am J Obstet Gynecol* 1989;161:761-765.
24. Abramowicz JS, Arrington J, Levy D, et al. Doppler study of umbilical artery blood flow waveform: should we use an instrument-adapted nomogram? *J Ultrasound Med* 1989;8:183-185.
25. Mulders LG, Muijsers GJ, Jongsma HW, et al. The umbilical artery blood flow velocity waveform in relation to fetal breathing movements, fetal heart rate, and fetal behavioral states in normal pregnancy at 37 to 39 weeks. *Early Hum Dev* 1986;14:283-293.
26. Kay HH, Carroll BA, Bowie JD, et al. Nonuniformity of fetal umbilical systolic/diastolic ratios as determined with duplex Doppler sonography. *J Ultrasound Med* 1989;8:417-420.
27. Short B, Nicholson S, Cameron A, et al. Assessment of the variability between fetal Doppler assessment of the umbilical artery and descending aorta. *Proceedings of the Canadian Association of Radiologists Annual Meeting.* Edmonton; 1988.
28. Brar HS, Platt LD, DeVore GR, et al. Qualitative assessment of maternal uterine and fetal umbilical artery blood flow and resistance in laboring patients by Doppler velocimetry. *Am J Obstet Gynecol* 1988;158:952-956.
29. Lingman G, Marsal K. Fetal central blood circulation in the third trimester of normal pregnancy: a longitudinal study. I. Aortic and umbilical blood flow. *Early Hum Dev* 1986;13:137-150.
30. Eik-Nes SH, Marsal K, Brubakk AO, et al. Ultrasonic measurement of human fetal blood flow. *J Biomed Eng* 1982;4:28-36.
31. Chen HY, Chang FM, Huang HC, et al. Antenatal fetal blood flow in the descending aorta and in the umbilical vein and their ratio in normal pregnancy. *Ultrasound Med Biol* 1988;14:263-268.
32. Harder J, Nimrod C, Davies D, et al. Pulsed Doppler assessment of fetal blood flow in the inferior vena cava in normal and

altered physiological states. In: Lipshitz J, et al., eds. *Perinatal Development of the Heart and Lung.* Ithaca, N.Y.: Perinatology Press; 1987:161-174.
33. Huisman T, Stewart P, Wladimiroff J. Flow velocity waveforms in the fetal inferior vena cava during the second half of normal pregnancy. *Ultrasound in Med Biol* 1991;17:679-682.
34. Reed K, Appleton C, Anderson C, et al. Doppler studies of vena cava flows in human fetuses. *Circulation* 1990;81:498-505.
35. Reuss LM, Rudoph AH, Dae MW. Phasic blood flow patterns in the superior and inferior venae cavae and umbilical vein of fetal sheep. *Am J Obstet Gynecol* 1983;145:70-78.
36. Arbielle P, Body G, Fignon A, et al. Doppler assessment of the intracerebral circulation of the fetus. *Clin Phys Physiol Meas* 1989;10(suppl A):51-57.
37. Mari G, Moise KJ, Deter RL, et al. Doppler assessment of the pulsatility index in the cerebral circulation of the human fetus. *Am J Obstet Gynecol* 1989;160:698-703.
38. De Smedt MC, Visser GH, Meijboom EJ. Fetal cardiac output estimated by Doppler echocardiography during mid- and late gestation. *Am J Cardiol* 1987;60:338-342.
39. Huhta JC, Moise KJ, Fisher DJ, et al. Detection and quantitation of constriction of the fetal ductus arteriosus by Doppler echocardiography. *Circulation* 1987;75:406-412.
40. Viyas S, Nicolaides KH, Campbell S. Renal artery flow-velocity waveforms in normal and hypoxemic fetuses. *Am J Obstet Gynecol* 1989;161:168-172.
41. Hercher K, Campbell S, Doyle P, et al. Assessment of fetal compromise by Doppler ultrasound investigation of the fetal circulation, atrial, intracardiac and venous blood flow velocity studies. *Circulation* 1995;91:129-138.

Pathologic Doppler Findings

42. Divon M. Umbilical artery Doppler velocimetry: clinical utility in high-risk pregnancies. *Am J Obstet Gynecol* 1996;174:10-14.
43. Steel SA, Pearce JM, Chamberlain G. Doppler ultrasound of the uteroplacental circulation as a screening test for severe preeclampsia with intra-uterine growth retardation. *Eur J Obstet Gynecol Reprod Biol* 1988;28:279-287.
44. Giles WB, Trudinger BJ, Baird, PJ. Fetal umbilical artery flow velocity waveforms and placental resistance: pathological correlation. *Br J Obstet Gynaecol* 1985;92:31-38.
45. Giles WB, Lingman G, Marsal K, et al. Fetal volume blood flow and umbilical artery flow velocity waveform analysis: a comparison. *Br J Obstet Gynaecol* 1986;93:466-470.
46. Bilardo CM, Nicolaides KH. Cordocentesis in the assessment of the small-for-gestational-age fetus. *Fetal Ther* 1988;3:24-30.
47. Arbeille P, Body G, Saliba E, et al. Fetal cerebral circulation assessment by Doppler ultrasound in normal and pathological pregnancies. *Eur J Obstet Gynecol Reprod Biol* 1988;29:261-273.
48. Rizzo G, Arduini D, Luciano R, et al. Prenatal cerebral Doppler ultrasonography and neonatal neurologic outcome. *J Ultrasound Med* 1989;8:237-240.
49. Fleischer A, Schulman H, Farmakides G, et al. Umbilical artery velocity waveforms and intrauterine growth retardation. *Am J Obstet Gynecol* 1985;151:502-505.
50. Gudmundsson S, Marsal K. Umbilical and uteroplacental blood flow velocity waveforms in pregnancies with fetal growth retardation. *Eur J Obstet Gynecol Reprd Biol* 1988;27:187-196.
51. Haddad NG, Johnstone FD, Hoskins PR, et al. Umbilical artery Doppler waveform in pregnancies with uncomplicated intrauterine growth retardation. *Gynecol Obstet Invest* 1988;26: 206-210.
52. Fouron JC, Teyssier G, Shalaby L, et al. Fetal central blood flow alterations in human fetuses with umbilical artery reverse diastolic flow. *Am J Perinatol* 1993;10:197-207.
53. Jouppila P, Kirkinen P. Umbilical vein blood flow as an indicator of fetal hypoxia. *Br J Obstet Gynaecol* 1984;91:107-110.
54. Rizzo G, Capponi A, Soragaroli M, et al. Umbilical vein pulsations and acid base status at cordocentesis in growth-retarded fetuses with absent end diastolic velocity in the umbilical artery. *Biol Neonate* 1995;68:163-168.
55. McCowan LM, Ritchie K, Mo LY, et al. Uterine artery flow velocity waveforms in normal and growth-retarded pregnancies. *Am J Obstet Gynecol* 1988;158:499-504.
56. Schulman H, Ducey J, Farmakides G, et al. Uterine artery Doppler velocimetry: the significance of divergent systolic/diastolic ratios. *Am J Obstet Gynecol* 1987;157:1539-1542.
57. Reuwer PJ, Sijmons EA, Rietman GW, et al. Intrauterine growth retardation: prediction of perinatal distress by Doppler ultrasound. *Lancet* 1987;11:415-418.
58. Eronen M, Kari A, Pesonen E, et al. Value of absent or retrograde end-diastolic flow in the fetal aorta and umbilical artery as a predictor of perinatal outcome in pregnancy-induced hypertension. *Acta Paed* 1993;82:919-924.
59. Divon M. Umbilical artery Doppler velocemetry: clinical utility in high-risk pregnancies. *Am J Obstet Gynecol* 1996;174:10-14.
60. Thornton JC, Lilford RJ. Do we need randomised trials of antenatal tests of fetal well being? *Br J Obstet Gynecol* 1993; 100:197-200.
61. Alfirevic Z, Neilson JP. Doppler ultrasonography in high-risk pregnancies: systematic review with meta-analysis. *Am J Obstet Gynecol* 1995;172:1379-1387.
62. Marsal K, Ley D. Intrauterine blood flow and post natal neurological development in growth-retarded fetuses. *Biol Neonate* 1992;62:258-264.
63. Yoon BH, Romero R, Roh CR, et al. Relationship between the fetal biophysical profile, umbilical artery, Doppler velocimetry, and fetal blood acid base status determined by cordocentesis. *Am J Obstet Gynecol* 1993;169:1586-1594.
64. Rizzo G, Capponi A, Ardioni D, et al. The value of fetal arterial, cardiac and venous flows in predicting pH and blood gases measured in the umbilical blood at cordocentesis in growth-retarded fetuses. *Br J Obstet Gynecol* 1995;102:963-969.

Pregnancy-Induced Hypertension

65. MacGillivray I. Some observations on the incidence of preeclampsia. *J Obstet Gynecol Br Comm* 1958;65:536.
66. Fleischer A, Schulman H, Farmakides G, et al. Umbilical artery velocity waveforms and intrauterine growth retardation. *Am J Obstet Gynecol* 1985;151:502.
67. Fleischer A, Schulman H, Farmakides G, et al. Uterine artery Doppler velocimetry in pregnant women with hypertension. *Am J Obstet Gynecol* 1986;154:806-813.
68. Cameron AD, Nicholson SF, Nimrod CA, et al. Doppler waveforms in the fetal aorta and umbilical artery in patients with hypertension in pregnancy. *Am J Obstet Gynecol* 1988;158: 339-345.
69. Guidetti R, Luzi G, Chiodi A. Blood flow measurement in pregnancies complicated by hypertension. *Proceedings of the Sixth Congress of the European Federation of Societies for Ultrasound in Medicine and Biology.* Helsinki; 1987:171.

Multiple Gestation

70. Divon MY, Girz BA, Sklar A, et al. Discordant twins: a prospective study of the diagnostic value of real-time ultrasonography combined with umbilical artery velocimetry. *Am J Obstet Gynecol* 1989;161:757-760.
71. Degani S, Paltiely J, Lewinsky R, et al. Fetal internal carotid artery flow velocity time waveforms in twin pregnancies. *J Perinat Med* 1988;16:405-409.
72. Pretorius DH, Manchester D, Barkin S, et al. Doppler ultrasound of twin transfusion syndrome. *J Ultrasound Med* 1988; 7:117-124.

73. Giles WB, Trudinger BJ, Cook CM. Fetal umbilical artery flow velocity-time waveforms in twin pregnancies. *Br J Obstet Gynaecol* 1985;92:490-497.

Hydrops

74. Copel JA, Grannum PA, Green JJ, et al. Fetal cardiac output in the isoimmunized pregnancy: a pulsed Doppler-echocardiographic study of patients undergoing intravascular intrauterine transfusion. *Am J Obstet Gynecol* 1989;161:361-365.
75. Copel JA, Grannum PA, Green JJ, et al. Pulsed Doppler flow velocity waveforms in the prediction of fetal hematocrit of the severely isoimmunized pregnancy. *Am J Obstet Gynecol* 1989; 161:341-344.
76. Woo JS, Liang ST, Lo RL, et al. Doppler blood flow velocity waveforms in alpha-thalassemia hydrops fetalis. *J Ultrasound Med* 1987;6:679-684.
77. Nimrod CA, Davies D, Harder JA, et al. Ultrasound evaluation of tachycardia-induced hydrops in fetal lambs. *Am J Obstet Gynecol* 1987;157:655-659.
78. Nimrod CA, Keane P, Harder JA, et al. Atrial natriuretic peptide production in association with nonimmune fetal hydrops. *Am J Obstet Gynecol* 1988;159:625-628.

Postterm Pregnancy

79. Nimrod C, Yee J, Hopkins C, et al. The utility of pulsed Doppler studies in the evaluation of the postdate pregnancies. *J Mat Fet Invest* 1991;1:127.
80. Brar H, Hozenstein J, Medaris A, et al. Cerebral, umbilical and uterine resistance using Doppler velocimetry in post term pregnancy. *J Ultrasound Med* 1989;8:187-191.
81. Farmakides G, Schulman H, Doucey J, et al. Uterine and umbilical artery Doppler velocimetry in postterm pregnancy. *J Reprod Med* 1988;33:259-261.

Cardiac Anomalies

82. Hecher K, Snijders R, Campbell S, et al. Fetal venous, intracardiac, and arterial blood flow measurements in intrauterine growth retardation: relationship with fetal blood gases. *Am J Obstet Gynecol* 1995;173:10-15.

CHAPTER 50

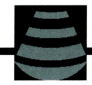

Intervention in Obstetrics

Jo-Ann M. Johnson, M.D., F.R.C.S.C.

CHAPTER OUTLINE

Our generation is the first ever to have a reasonably complete understanding of the development of a baby from conception. Paralleling this has been a virtual explosion in technology permitting highly sophisticated ways to visualize, measure, monitor, and sample the fetus. Of these advances, ultrasonography has been among the most important by permitting a variety of diagnostic interventions to be accomplished with a high degree of accuracy and low fetal and maternal risks. These include the *in utero* sampling of amniotic fluid; placental tissue; fetal blood, skin, liver, and lung; and intrafetal solid and cystic masses. The information obtained from these fetal tissues can then be used to inform the parents whether they carry a fetus affected with a particular genetic, developmental, or acquired disorder for which the fetus is at risk.

As diagnostic skills have improved, so has our understanding of the natural history of fetal disorders, and fetal therapy increasingly is being attempted as a logical sequel to fetal diagnosis. Intrauterine transfusions, therapeutic thoracentesis, and amniotic shunting are just some of the therapeutic interventions now available. We may anticipate that as our knowledge and understanding of fetal disease continue to expand, our ability to diagnose and treat fetal conditions *in utero* will continue to increase.

CHORIONIC VILLUS SAMPLING

Chorionic villus sampling (CVS) is a method of prenatal evaluation that permits the diagnosis of many genetic disorders in the first trimester. The basis for prenatal diagnosis using CVS is that the chorionic villi are mitotic derivatives of the early embryo and therefore reflect the genetic constitution of the fetus. In early embryonic development, the chorionic villi completely surround the gestational sac as a delicate fringe (Fig. 50-1, *A*). The villi along the site of implantation proliferate rapidly, creating an area of increased echogenicity that can be visualized on ultrasound (Fig. 50-1, *B*). This is known as the **chorion frondosum,** which eventually becomes the placenta. The chorionic villi opposite the site of implantation degenerate and are known as the chorion levae. The chorion frondosum is the optimal site for obtaining a chorionic villus sample.

CVS had its beginnings in the late 1960s when it was performed using endoscopic techniques,[1,2] although enthusiasm waned because of the high complication and failure rates compared with amniocentesis. In the mid-1970s, a report from China described successful CVS using a blind catheter-aspiration technique.[3] However, CVS did not receive significant attention until 1982, when a report by Kazy et al. described its benefits for genetic diagnosis[4] and emphasized the role of ultrasound guidance in successful sampling. Since then the technique has developed rapidly, and enough experience has been gained to delineate its safety, accuracy, and reliability.

There are **two basic approaches** for performing CVS: the transcervical (TC-CVS) method and the transabdominal (TA-CVS) method.

Transcervical Chorionic Villus Sampling

Transcervical CVS is usually performed **between 10 and 12.6 weeks** gestation. Prior to the procedure, a real-time ultrasound examination determines the viability and gestational age of the fetus and the location

A

B

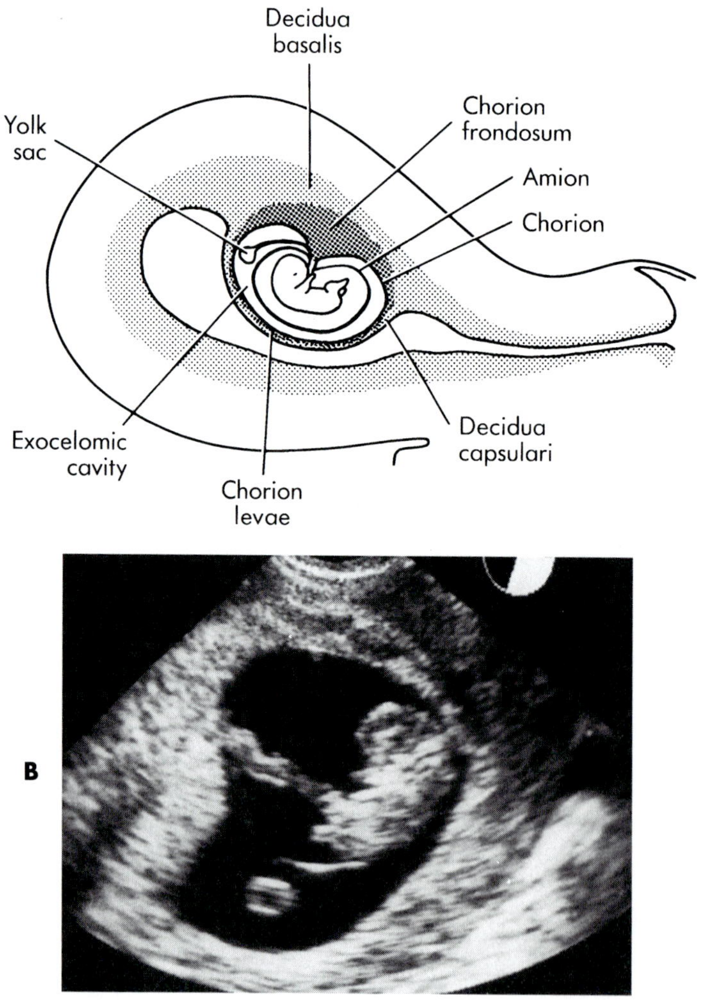

FIG. 50-1. Chorion frondosum, the site for chorionic villus sampling. **A,** Diagram of a normal fetus. Intrauterine anatomy at approximately 10 weeks gestation. **B,** Transvaginal ultrasound of an embryo at 9.6 weeks gestation. The umbilical cord can be seen inserting into the chorion frondosum, which appears thick and echogenic. (Courtesy Ants Toi, M.D., Toronto Hospital, Toronto, Ontario.)

of the chorion frondosum. The patient is then placed in the lithotomy position, a speculum inserted, and the cervix and vagina cleansed with an antiseptic solution. A number of different **transcervical biopsy catheters** are available, all of which contain a malleable metal obturator that may be preformed to negotiate the cervicouterine angle and the pathway to the intended biopsy site (Fig. 50-2, *A*). Under ultrasound guidance, the catheter is passed through the cervix and placed within the villi of the chorion frondosum (Fig. 50-3). The metal obturator is removed and a 20 cc syringe containing media is attached to the catheter. Negative suction is applied to the syringe with simultaneous "to-and-fro" movements of the catheter. The catheter is then withdrawn and the sample examined immediately under a dissection microscope. An estimated wet weight of 10 to 20 mg is sufficient for most diagnoses. If the amount of chorionic villi is determined to be inadequate, the procedure is repeated. A fresh, sterile catheter is used for each pass to minimize the risk of intrauterine infection, and, in general, no more than three passes are attempted. The fetal heart rate, sac configuration, and appearance of the chorion frondosum are visualized carefully after each pass. The only discomfort reported by most patients is the pressure of the ultrasound transducer on the full bladder and the placement of the tenaculum on the cervix, if one is used. Vaginal spotting is common after the procedure but usually subsides within 3 days.

TC-CVS may also be performed using a thin-gauged, rigid, **transcervical biopsy forceps** (see Fig. 50-2, *B*). At our institution, the rounded-tip, curved, steel forceps (1.9 mm in diameter and 25 cm in length) (R.M. Surgical Developments, Surrey, UK) that was first introduced at Queen Charlotte's Maternity Hospital by Rodeck et al., is used.[5]

The procedure is performed in a manner similar to that of the catheter aspiration technique with the forceps being introduced under continuous ultrasound monitoring. Once the forceps tip is visualized within the chorion, the jaws are opened, advanced, and then closed and slowly withdrawn. The sample is removed from the tip of the forceps directly into the transport medium and the tissue inspected for adequacy.

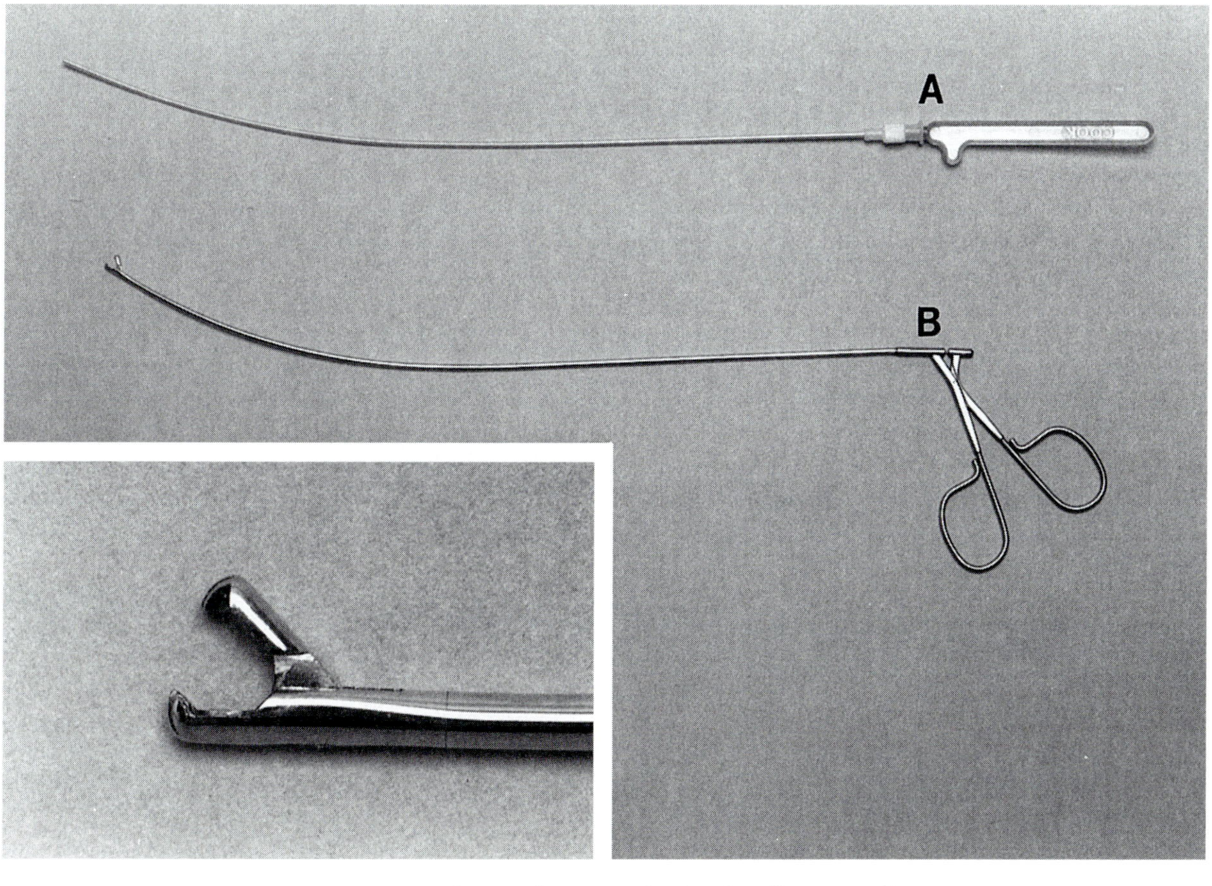

FIG. 50-2. Instruments for performing chorionic villus sampling. **A,** The flexible transcervical biopsy catheter (Portex). When the catheter is in position within the chorion frondosum, the malleable metal obturator is removed, and a syringe is attached to the catheter. **B,** The rigid transcervical biopsy forceps described by Rodeck et al.[5] (R.M. Surgical Developments, Surrey, UK). The insert shows the rounded tip of the rigid forceps magnified.

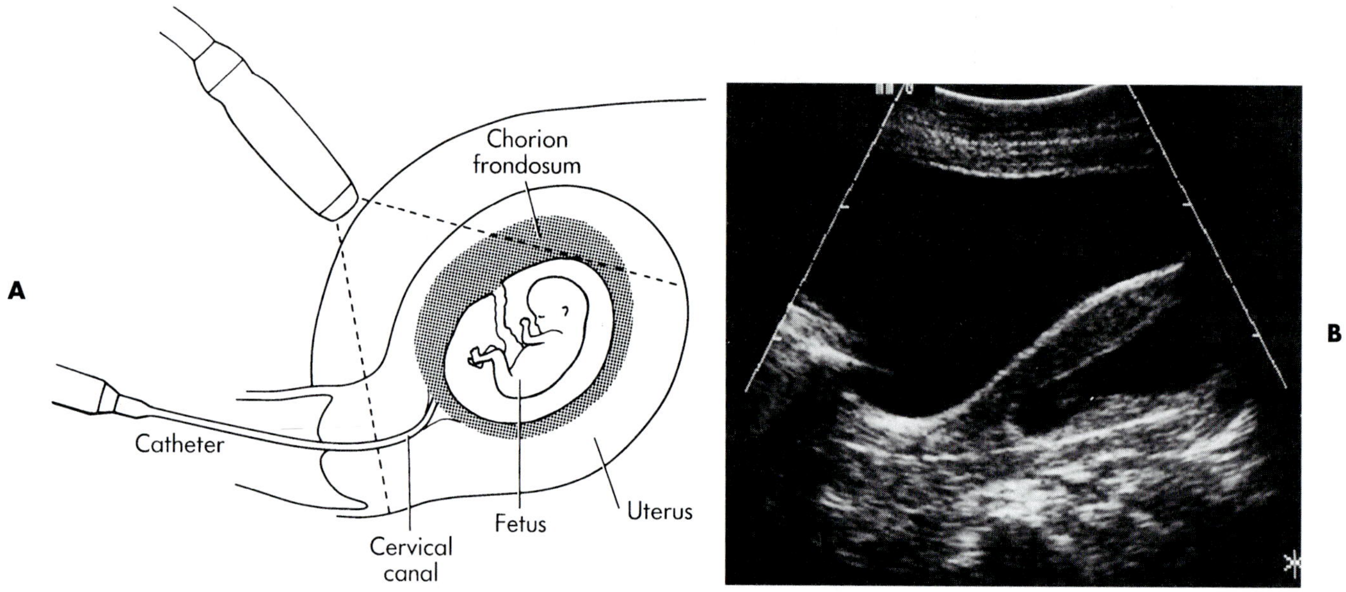

FIG. 50-3. Transvaginal chorionic villus sampling. **A,** Schema of technique showing a transcervical catheter entering the chorion frondosum. **B,** Ultrasound of transcervical CVS. The catheter is visible within the chorion frondosum. (Courtesy Ants Toi, M.D., Toronto Hospital, Toronto, Ontario.)

The **fetal loss rate** associated with TC-CVS has been evaluated in several large series, and a figure of 1% to 2% above the background risk is quoted.[6,7] In two large series comparing CVS with amniocentesis, the risk of fetal loss with CVS was slightly higher than with amniocentesis; however, the difference (0.6% to 0.8%) was not statistically significant.[6,7]

Transabdominal Chorionic Villus Sampling

In transabdominal chorionic villus sampling (TA-CVS), an ultrasound examination is first performed to determine fetal viability, gestational age, and location of the chorion frondosum. An **18 to 20 gauge needle** is then introduced through the maternal abdomen and uterine wall under aseptic conditions, and inserted into the chorion frondosum with ultrasound guidance. A 20 cc syringe is then attached to the needle and negative suction is applied to the syringe while the needle tip is simultaneously moved back and forth to sample several sites. Unlike TC-CVS, TA-CVS can be performed **beyond 12.6 weeks gestation** (10 weeks to term). Because a fine-gauge needle is used, there is less trauma to the placenta compared with that from the transcervical catheter, which is associated with an unacceptably high fetal loss rate beyond 13 weeks gestation.

TA-CVS may also be performed using **rigid, straight biopsy forceps** such as those developed by Nicolini and Rodeck.[5] The forceps are a modified version of fetal skin biopsy forceps (1.35 mm in diameter and 25 cm in length) and are guided by a 17.5 gauge needle (R.M. Surgical Development, Surrey, UK). The procedure is similar to that previously described for TA-CVS. Once the sampling site is reached, the forceps are introduced until they are seen to emerge beyond the tip of the trocar, and the jaws are opened, advanced, and closed again. The forceps is gently rotated as it is withdrawn back into the trocar to facilitate dislodging of the tissue. The advantage of this technique is that multiple samplings can be performed with a single introduction of the trocar. However, the method is associated with more maternal discomfort compared with the single-needle aspiration technique, probably due to the needle size.

The **fetal loss rate** associated with TA-CVS is not significantly different than TC-CVS.[8] TA-CVS appears to be associated with fewer postprocedural complications than TC-CVS, especially spotting and bleeding.

At our institution, the **selection of the route of CVS** is at the discretion of the operator and depends on the location of the chorion, the position of the uterus and bladder, and the presence of uterine or cervical abnormalities. For example, in patients with posterior low-lying chorions, we favor the transcervical route whereas for patients with anterior or posterior fundal placentas we favor the transabdominal approach. The most important criteria for successful CVS are clear visualization of the chorion and the selection of a route of entry that will lead most directly to the thickest part of the chorion without disturbing the membranes or the amniotic cavity.

INDICATIONS FOR INVASIVE PRENATAL TESTING

Late maternal age (≥35 years)
Previous trisomic offspring
Parental chromosome rearrangement
X-linked recessive disorders
Mendelian disorders (other genetic disorders)

Indications for Chorionic Villus Sampling

By far the most common **indication** for offering CVS is late maternal age (≥80%), which is defined as 35 years of age or older at the time of delivery (see box above). Other indications are previous trisomic offspring, parental chromosome rearrangement, X-linked recessive disorders, and Mendelian disorders. Because a large volume of DNA can be extracted from CVS tissue compared with amniocentesis cell cultures, CVS has become the preferred procedure for diagnoses requiring DNA analysis.[9] Gene probes are now available for the prenatal diagnosis of an increasing number of disorders, including the hemoglobinopathies, most families with hemophilia (A and B), Duchenne's muscular dystrophy, cystic fibrosis, and a number of metabolic disorders. It is important to note that CVS is not a substitute for amniocentesis in the prenatal detection of neural tube defects. Maternal serum alpha-fetoprotein (AFP) screening is generally advocated at 15 to 18 weeks of pregnancy after CVS for this purpose. Note also that since anatomy cannot be visualized with certainty in the first trimester, a detailed ultrasound is recommended at 18 weeks to provide reassurance of fetal structural normality in all patients who undergo CVS.

Chorionic Villus Sampling and Limb Reduction Defects

In 1991 Firth et al. reported a cluster of babies with severe limb abnormalities born to women who had undergone TA-CVS between 55 and 66 days of gestation.[10] Subsequent to this publication, additional clusters of cases with transverse **limb reduction defects** (LRDs) born to women who had undergone both TA-CVS and TC-CVS were published.[11,12] In evaluating these reports, a trend of increasingly severe defects with progressively earlier CVS was discernible (e.g., a 20- to 30-fold increase in LRDs when the CVS was performed **before** 9 weeks compared with sampling **after** 9.5 weeks). These reports prompted extensive reevaluation of the safety of CVS by a number of organizations, including the National Institutes of Health (NIH) in the United States and the World Health Organization (WHO). Both have recently concluded that while early gestation and excessive placental trauma may be important in the causation of LRDs associated with CVS, there is **no evidence of an increased risk of limb reduction defects following CVS at 10 weeks gestation or later.**[13] They recommend that while each center must define its own policy concerning the association of CVS with LRDs, the following recommendations should be considered:

- CVS should not be done before 9.5 weeks gestation and should be done with as little damage to the placenta as possible;
- Patients who have had CVS should be offered a detailed follow-up scan at 18 to 20 weeks gestation;
- Patients should be given information about the potential association of CVS with LRDs so they can make an informed decision about whether to proceed with CVS; and
- All affected cases should be reported to the WHO-sponsored registry being kept by Dr. Laird Jackson, Division of Medical Genetics, Thomas Jefferson University, Philadelphia, Pennsylvania, USA.

AMNIOCENTESIS

Amniocentesis is the most common invasive technique used in prenatal diagnosis. Described as early as 1952, it was first used clinically in the early 1960s for the management of Rhesus disease (Rh incompatibility).[14] The procedure then was performed without ultrasound, but since the target (i.e., the pool of amniotic fluid in later gestation) was large, it was usually successful. In 1966, it was reported that fetal cells obtained from amniotic fluid could be cultured and karyotyped.[15] This finding stimulated investigations toward offering second-trimester amniocentesis to women at increased risk for fetal chromosomal abnormalities. Since that time, advances in ultrasound and laboratory technology have resulted in amniocentesis becoming a safe and reliable technique with widespread acceptance.

Amniocentesis is exclusively performed by the **transabdominal route,** although a transvaginal approach has been attempted in the past.[16] An ultrasound is first performed to assess the gestational age and viability of the fetus and the location of the placenta. The abdomen is then cleansed with an antiseptic solution, and a **fine-gauge spinal needle (20 or 22 gauge)** is inserted through the maternal abdomen and uterine wall into the amniotic sac. The ultrasound transducer is usually held away from the puncture site such that the ultrasound beam strikes the needle at right angles, giving a clear echo on the screen. A syringe is attached to the needle and the fluid is aspirated. The first few cubic centimeters are discarded to avoid maternal cell or blood contamination of the culture. A new syringe is then attached and 15 to 20 ml of fluid is aspirated. A postprocedural scan is performed to confirm fetal heart activity and to check the integrity of the sac. The fluid, which contains fetal cells (primarily skin fibroblasts), is then cultured and used for cytogenetic, biochemical, and DNA analysis as indicated.

The **indications** for offering genetic amniocentesis are similar to those of CVS (see box on p. 1395). Because of the slightly higher incidence of interpretive difficulties with CVS, amniocentesis may be preferred for patients at risk of chromosomal rearrangements or mosaicism. Amniocentesis is also used as an **adjunct to obstetric management.** Examples include the measurement of bilirubin levels in Rhesus-sensitized pregnancies and, more recently, for determination of D-antigen status using the polymerase chain reaction (PCR).[17] Amniocentesis is also used for the measurement of the lecithin/sphingomyelin (L/S) ratio and phosphatidoglycerol levels in the determination of fetal lung maturity and for culture and/or PCR analysis in the diagnosis of fetal intrauterine infection. **Therapeutic amniocentesis** (amnioreduction) may be used selectively in cases of hydramnios and twin-to-twin transfusion syndrome (TTS).[18]

Midtrimester Amniocentesis

Amniocentesis can be performed throughout gestation. It is most commonly performed **between 15 and 17 weeks gestation** (midtrimester amniocentesis or MA) for the **purpose of prenatal diagnosis.**

MA combines the **advantages** of low risk to the fetus (≤0.5% fetal loss rate) with high diagnostic accuracy (≥99%).[19-22] It is also performed late enough in gestation to allow for evaluation of fetal anatomy as well as the measurement of amniotic fluid AFP for the detection of neural tube defects.[23] Despite these many positive aspects, MA has several **disadvantages.** These include the fact that because culture is required for most diagnoses, the results are not available until the eighteenth to twentieth week of pregnancy. This can create a tremendous psychologic burden, particularly for those couples for whom selective abortion may be indicated. In addition, there is an increased risk of morbidity and mortality associated with second-trimester termination. Many patients, therefore, find the procedure unacceptable. Although CVS is an alternative in many cases, it is limited in its availability to tertiary level centers with experienced medical and laboratory personnel. For these reasons, a third alternative to MA and CVS has been developed; namely, early amniocentesis.

Early Amniocentesis

Early amniocentesis (EA) is defined as an amniocentesis performed **between 11 and 14 weeks gestation.** It has become feasible in recent years because of advances in ultrasound technology and improved laboratory methodologies. EA may be considered an alternative to midtrimester amniocentesis for patients who want earlier testing but do not wish to bear the additional risks associated with CVS or to whom CVS is not available. It is also a useful alternative to MA for earlier clarification of equivocal CVS results.

The technique of early amniocentesis is similar to midtrimester amniocentesis except that a sharper "thrusting" motion is required to penetrate the membranes to enter the amniotic cavity. It is also recommended that the fluid be aspirated slowly, and 1 ml of fluid per week of gestation be aspirated, although the latter is an arbitrary determination.[24] Although there are fewer cells in the amniotic fluid in early gestation, there are a higher percentage of viable cells, and obtaining a cytogenetic result has not been a problem.[24,25]

Safety and Accuracy of Early Amniocentesis

Preliminary data suggest that the **safety** and **accuracy** of EA are similar to MA, but none of the studies performed to date have had the power to adequately assess the risk of fetal loss, particularly between 11 and 12 weeks of gestation.[26-28] Nonetheless, EA is gradually gaining increased clinical acceptance in many centers in both North America and Europe. To ensure that EA does not become routine in Canada before being adequately assessed, a randomized, controlled, multicentered trial designed to compare the safety and accuracy of EA versus MA has been funded by the Medical Research Council (MRC) of Canada and has recently completed recruitment (over 4,000 patients).

The trial is comparing amniocentesis performed in the gestational period between 11 and 12.6 weeks with amniocentesis performed at the usual time (15 to 16.6 weeks). Analysis of the pilot component of this study has shown no significant difference in safety and accuracy between EA and MA and no difference in the incidence of congenital abnormalities.[29] However, complete analysis of the data from the multicentered trial is required before EA becomes an established technique for first-trimester prenatal diagnosis.

PERCUTANEOUS UMBILICAL BLOOD SAMPLING

Fetal blood sampling, also known as percutaneous umbilical blood sampling (PUBS) or **cordocentesis,** is a technique that permits direct vascular access to the fetus for both diagnostic and therapeutic purposes. First described by Daffos et al. in 1983,[30] the technique has been made possible through advances in high-resolution ultrasound, which allow clear visualization of the umbilical cord and its vessels without the need for endoscopic techniques (e.g., fetoscopy).

PUBS can be performed from as early as the seventeenth week of gestation to term. An ultrasound examination is first performed to determine fetal viability, position, gestational age, presence of associated anomalies, and location of placenta. Clear identification of the insertion site of the umbilical cord in the placenta is a critical step. It is important not to confuse a loop of cord adjacent to the placental mass with the actual insertion site. Cordocentesis is easiest when the placenta is anterior, as access to the posterior placenta may be hampered by the fetus. However, fetal activity can interfere with cord visualization irrespective of the placental location. The procedure is usually performed as an outpatient procedure with facilities to monitor viable pregnancies ($\geq$ 26 weeks) after the procedure. Maternal sedation before the procedure is recommended, and prophylactic antibiotics are used selectively.

The **technique** involves the insertion of a fine-gauge (20 or 22 gauge) spinal needle through the maternal abdomen and uterine wall into the umbilical cord, approximately 2 to 3 cm from its insertion site into the placenta (Fig. 50-4). Although several different approaches can be used for the procedure, the general principle is to insert the needle under sonographic monitoring, manipulating the transducer to maintain the tip of the needle under visualization at all times. Many experienced operators use a "freehand" technique because of the flexibility and ability to adjust the needle pathway. It is also acceptable to employ a needle-guiding device attached to the transducer. Most real-time machines are equipped with an on-screen template of the needle track that can be used to target the sampling site.

After the needle enters the umbilical cord, the trocar is removed and fetal blood is withdrawn into a syringe attached to the hub of the needle. The syringe contains a small amount of anticoagulant such as heparin. The sample is analyzed immediately to determine its origin and purity. Confirmatory tests include a complete blood count, which is compared with the maternal blood count drawn before the procedure; the most useful value is the mean corpuscular volume (MCV), which is higher in fetal red blood cells (RBCs) than in maternal RBCs. A small amount of saline is then injected into the cord with a "flush" on ultrasound documenting correct placement of the needle (Fig. 50-5). A Kleihauer-Betke test is also performed on all the samples.[31]

The **volume** of blood removed varies with gestational age. Generally, we remove an amount corresponding to 6% to 7% of the fetoplacental volume for that gestational age. In most cases, blood is obtained from the umbilical vein. Puncturing the artery is associated with a greater incidence of bradycardia (possibly vasospastic reflex) and longer postprocedural bleeding. When access to the insertion site near the umbilical cord is not possible, fetal blood sampling can also be carried out at the insertion of the cord into the umbilicus,[32] at the intrahepatic portion of the cord,[33] at a free loop of umbilical cord, or by an intracardiac puncture.[32] Of these, sampling the intrahepatic portion of the umbilical vein has become a fa-

A

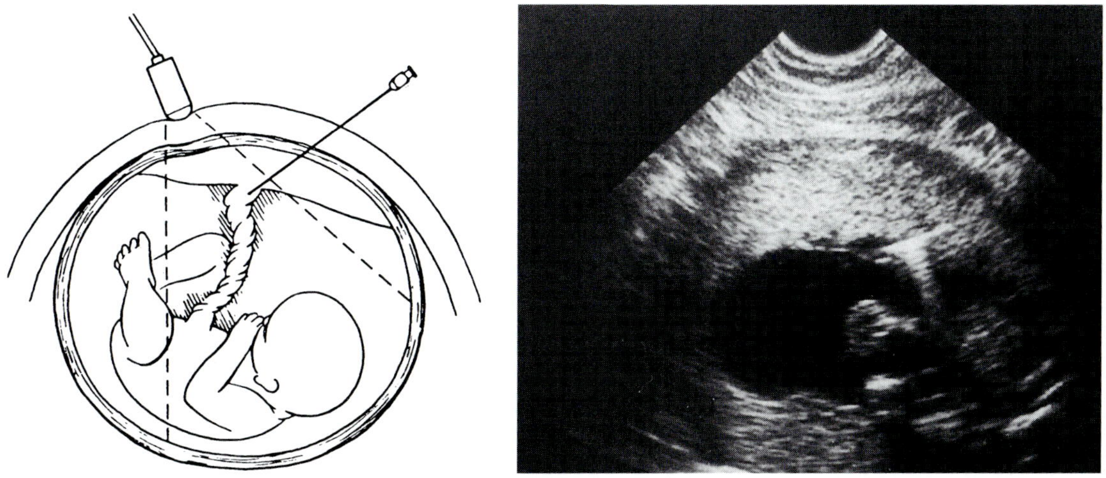

B

FIG. 50-4. Percutaneous umbilical blood sampling (PUBS) needle placement into umbilical cord. **A,** Schema of the technique showing needle placement into the cord insertion site with an anterior placenta. **B,** Ultrasound of PUBS showing needle placement at the cord insertion site of an anterior placenta. (Courtesy Ants Toi, M.D., Toronto Hospital, Toronto, Ontario.)

A

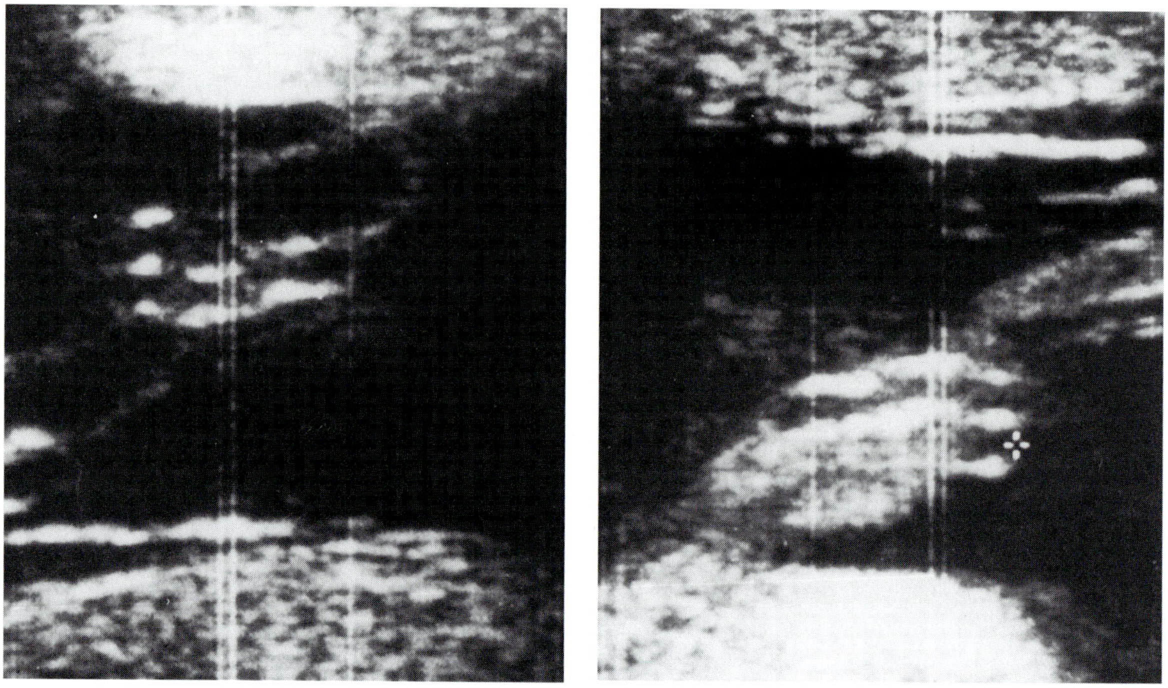

B

FIG. 50-5. Percutaneous umbilical blood sampling (PUBS) saline injection. **A,** Ultrasound of an intrauterine gestation at 30 weeks. Loops of umbilical cord can be seen in the amniotic fluid. **B,** Ultrasound of the same patient as in **A** after injection of saline showing a "flush" in the umbilical cord, documenting correct placement of the needle. (Courtesy Christopher R. Harman, M.D., Women's Hospital, University of Manitoba, Winnipeg, Manitoba.)

vored site at our institution, particularly when access to the cord insertion site is hampered by a posterior placenta or fetal position (Fig. 50-6). The advantages of this approach are a relatively large target, virtually no risk of vasospasm of the cord or maternal contamination, and minimal risk of postprocedure bleeding. This site is particularly favored in the older fetus (greater than 28 weeks) undergoing intravascular transfusion for Rhesus or platelet incompatibility.

The **risks** of PUBS include bleeding from the needle puncture site, infection, and rupture of the membranes. Fortunately, these risks appear to be rare, with data from the International Fetal Blood Sampling Registry in Philadelphia reporting a 1.1% fetal loss rate with PUBS.[34] This is significantly less than that associated with fetoscopy, which is approximately 4% to 6%.[35] In our own experience with more than 500 PUBS over a 7-year period, the direct procedure-related fetal loss rate was approximately 1.6%, with a low incidence of associated complications.

Indications for Percutaneous Umbilical Blood Sampling

The rapidly dividing fetal lymphocytes obtained through PUBS enable reliable chromosomal analysis within 48 to 72 hours. This may be helpful when either a structural abnormality is detected on ultra-

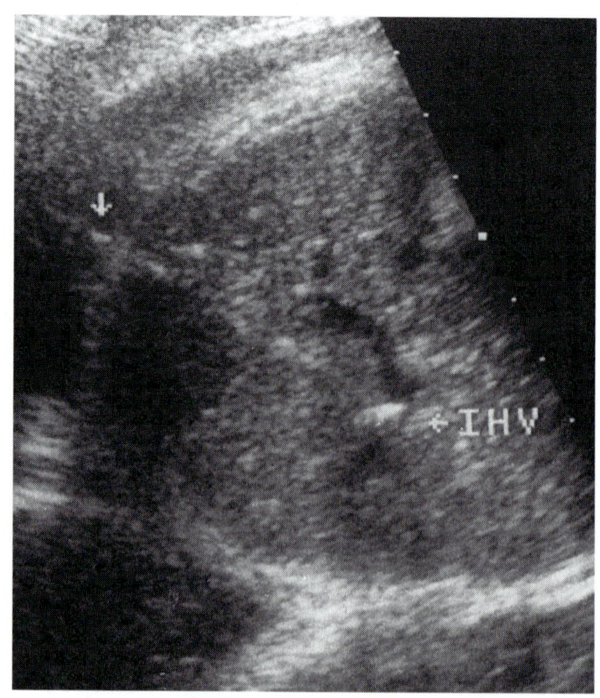

FIG. 50-6. Percutaneous umbilical blood sampling (PUBS) needle in umbilical vein. Transverse view of the fetal abdomen at the level of the intrahepatic portion of the umbilical vein, *IHV*. The arrows show the needle penetrating the fetal abdominal wall. The echogenic tip of the needle is visualized within the IHV.

TABLE 50-1
PERCUTANEOUS UMBILICAL BLOOD SAMPLING (PUBS)

Indications	n	%
Rapid karyotype	1110	37
Isoimmunization	1020	34
Nonimmune hydrops	195	6.5
Intrauterine infection	165	5.5
Idiopathic thrombocytopenic purpura	162	5.3
Twin-to-twin transfusion	63	2.1
Alloimmune thrombocytopenia	63	2.1
Fetal acid-base imbalance	60	2
Hemoglobinopathy	60	2
Coagulation disorders	54	1.8
Immunologic deficiency	30	1
Other (including confirmation of chromosome abnormalities in one of a twin pair found to be discordant for a chromosome abnormality at the time of amniocentesis)	20	

National PUBS Registry (n = 3002), Philadelphia (unpublished data).

sound or severe intrauterine growth retardation (IUGR) suggests aneuploidy (Table 50-1). **Rapid karyotyping** of these fetuses may assist parental counseling and allow for appropriate intervention, optimal planning of delivery, and neonatal management.[36] The use of PUBS for **antepartum fetal blood gas analysis** in the assessment of IUGR has been reported; however, its significance is controversial, and it does not have an established clinical role at present.[37] **Fetal infections** such as toxoplasmosis, cytomegalovirus, or parvovirus can be confirmed either by detection of viral DNA or a fetal IGM response in fetal blood. Although most **genetic conditions** can now be diagnosed by DNA analysis of CVS or amniotic fluid specimens, PUBS is still necessary in certain circumstances. For example, nonimmune hydrops fetalis (NIHF) is a nonspecific end point for many fetal abnormalities and diseases, and PUBS makes the diagnosis of some of its diverse chromosomal, hematologic, infectious, and metabolic etiologies possible. Fetal blood grouping is useful in **blood group incompatibility.** In erythroblastosis fetalis, assessment of the **severity of anemia** and **fetal blood transfusion** by PUBS has become an established practice.[38]

In alloimmune platelet disorders, severe fetal thrombocytopenia may result in spontaneous intracranial hemorrhage. **Fetal platelet** levels may be monitored so that if they are very low, immune globulin (IVIG) and/or prednisone can be given to the mother,[39] or when this fails, platelets can be transfused directly into the fetus.[40]

Fetal arrhythmias may be treated by the direct administration of **antiarrhythmic medication,** although initial treatment should always be the transplacental administration of maternal drugs.[41] In addition, research is being conducted in the administration of **stem cell transplants** to fetuses known to be affected with hematopoietic disorders.

PERCUTANEOUS FETAL TISSUE SAMPLING

Although many inborn errors of metabolism can be diagnosed from chorionic villus samples, cultured fibroblasts, or fetal blood, there are a few diseases that require **direct tissue biopsy** for diagnosis because the affected protein is expressed exclusively in these tissues. There are **two approaches** to obtain fetal tissue; the first and older method uses the fetoscope; the second, more recent method uses ultrasound to guide needles or forceps into the target organ.[42] Ultrasound-guided fetal biopsies cause less maternal trauma because the needles are much finer than the fetoscope, resulting in a lower risk of miscarriage.

Fetal Liver Biopsy

In a few rare disorders of the urea cycle, the biochemical assay has to be done on the liver. **Ornithine transcarbamylase (OTC) deficiency** is an X-linked condition causing failure to convert ammonia into urea.[43] Affected males develop ammonia intoxication after birth and usually die within the first week. Diagnosis *in utero* is not possible from fetal blood or amniotic fluid because the placenta rapidly clears the metabolites.[44] OTC is expressed only in the mitochondria of hepatocytes and intestinal tissue, and thus a liver biopsy is needed to confirm the absence of this enzyme. Since carrier females have minimal or no clinical manifestations, prenatal diagnosis is offered to male fetuses selected by ultrasound.[45] It is best to perform the test at approximately 18 weeks gestation because at earlier gestations the enzyme level in the liver tends to be low.[44] A gene probe is now available, and first-trimester diagnosis is theoretically possible in informed families. Other enzyme deficiencies that are tissue-specific to liver and in which prenatal diagnosis can be accomplished include **phenylalanine hydroxylase** (PAH), glucose-6 phosphatase (G6P-ASE), and **carbamylphosphate synthetase 1** (CPS1).[42]

Fetal liver biopsy should be restricted to specialized centers with operators skilled in invasive procedures. The exact enzyme defect should be known from a previously affected pregnancy, and the carrier state should be identified before embarking on such invasive procedures. The gestation at which the enzyme is first expressed should also be known. Laboratories should have established their own control ranges for enzyme activities for midtrimester fetuses, as these may be lower than neonatal values.

Fetal Skin Biopsy

Histologic and ultrasound studies of fetal skin biopsies are needed to diagnose several of the **skin conditions** that are **genetically transmitted.**[46] Diagnosis is made following electron microscopy of the skin structure and immunohistochemical studies. The disorders prenatally diagnosed include **congenital bullous icthyosiform erythroderma, dystrophic epidermolysis bullosa, harlequin icthyosis, and oculocutaneous albinism.**[46] Although such biopsies were initially performed by fetoscopy between 17 and 20 weeks gestation, ultrasound-guided techniques have been described.[47] Small biopsies are taken by passing biopsy forceps down a 16 to 18 gauge transabdominal needle. The preferential site for biopsy depends on the skin condition in question, and the risk appears to be similar to that of other diagnostic interventions (1% to 2%). It is hoped that in the future many of these disorders will be diagnosed by DNA analysis.

Fetal Muscle Biopsy

Fetal muscle biopsy allows specimens to be obtained from the fetal thigh or calf with apparent safety, although injury to the peroneal nerve is possible. The purpose is to exclude or confirm the diagnosis of **Duchenne's muscular dystrophy** in at-risk male fetuses for whom deletion mutations are not identifiable on DNA analysis. Of the reported cases, no obvious problems occurred, and the scars were not significant in the survivors.[48]

Other Fetal Biopsies

Given the fluctuating indications and replacement with molecular and cellular techniques for liver, skin, and muscle biopsies, it is not surprising that the total number of biopsies of all other fetal organs is less than 100 reported cases.

Fetal Lung Biopsies

Ultrasound recognition of abnormal lung morphology is reliable as early as 18 weeks gestation. Fetal lung biopsies have been successfully performed following ultrasound recognition of **pulmonary masses** by percutaneous ultrasound-directed means. In two reported cases, cystic adenomatoid malformation type 3 (CCAM) was diagnosed and pregnancy termination elected.[49] However, biopsy abnormality of one lung does not necessarily mean the lesion is lethal to the fetus; apparent normality of the other lung does not guarantee viability. In addition, as experience with lung abnormalities, in particular CCAMs, expands, it is apparent that such disorders are not invariably progressive and lethal, but in fact may regress spontaneously or respond to drainage of associated hydrothorax. For these reasons, fetal lung biopsy has not seen an expanding role. It may, however, have value in the future when no lung pathology is seen *in situ*ations where it may be likely. For example, in prolonged rupture of the membranes, chest size is an imperfect means of assessing the likelihood of lethal pulmonary hypoplasia. If pathologic criteria for this disorder were a reliable means to evaluate the adequacy of fetal lung development, this would be important clinical information to guide pregnancy management.

Fetal Tumor Biopsy

Cystic or solid masses identified within the fetus by ultrasound have been biopsied to guide obstetric management. In one report, six cystic hygromas, three sacrococcygeal teratomas, and two ovarian cysts were biopsied.[50] Most of these procedures were done for diagnostic purposes; the rationale would no longer exist at present with high-resolution ultrasonography.

OTHER INTERVENTIONS

Aspiration of Urine or Fluid

Useful information can be obtained by analysis of fetal urine and fluid from the pleural or peritoneal cavities or from cysts.

Vesicoamniotic Shunting

Urinary obstruction in the male fetus caused by posterior valves is not an uncommon problem (Fig. 50-7). The poor perinatal outcome in these fetuses is associated with renal dysplasia caused by the obstruction and

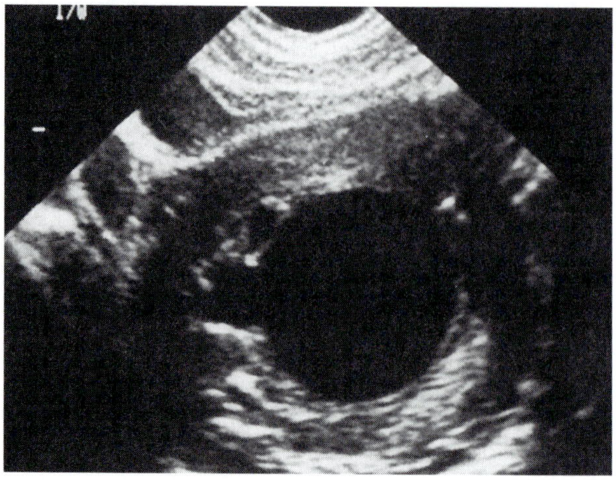

FIG. 50-7. Fetal urinary obstruction. Ultrasound of a fetus at 17 weeks showing bladder and urethral distention resulting from posterior urethral valves. (Courtesy Ants Toi, M.D., Toronto Hospital, Toronto, Ontario.)

back pressure and pulmonary hypoplasia caused by severe oligohydramnios.[51,52] Bypassing the obstruction using a double pigtail vesicoamniotic catheter *in utero* may prevent these complications and has been shown to be effective (Fig. 50-8).[52] Careful case selection, however, is essential, and bypass procedures are restricted to fetuses with normal karyotypes who do not have irreversible renal damage. Vesicoamniotic shunting of a fetus with severe renal dysplasia would not only fail to prevent eventual death from renal failure, but would also not prevent pulmonary hypoplasia if the kidneys were incapable of restoring amniotic fluid volume. Although hyperechogenicity of the renal parenchyma may accurately predict renal dysplasia (sensitivity 73%, specificity 80%),[53] the prognostic accuracy can be increased by evaluating the biochemistry of fetal urine aspirated from the bladder and renal pelvis.[54] The fluid can also be used for karyotype analysis.[55]

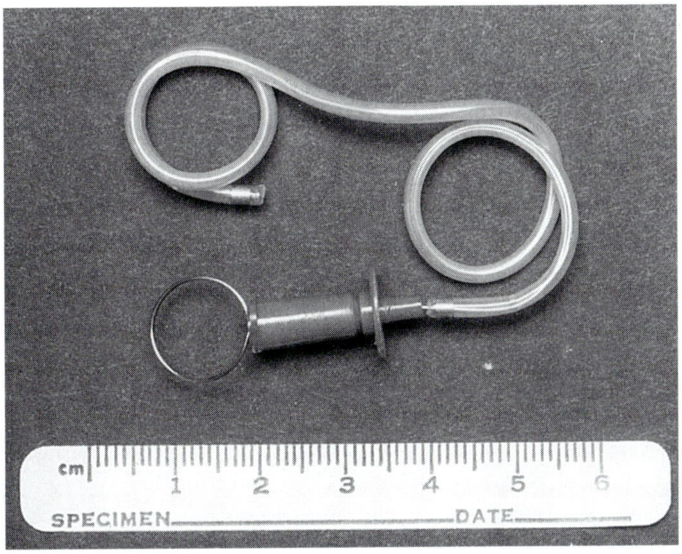

A

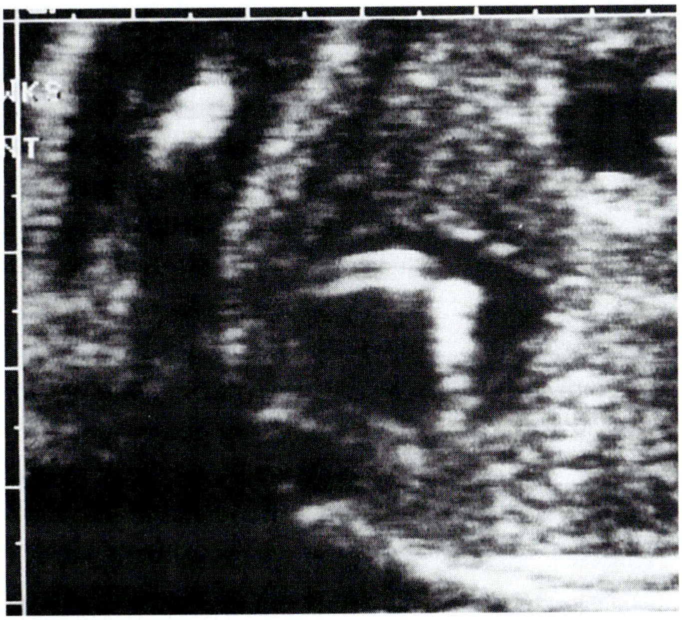

B

FIG. 50-8. Vesicoamniotic shunting. **A,** Double-pigtail catheter used for vesicoamniotic shunting (Rocket-Kings Catheters). The catheter has an external and internal diameter of 0.21 mm and 0.15 mm, respectively, and has radiopaque stainless steel inserts at each end and lateral holes around the coil. The malleable metal obturator allows the catheter to be straightened and threaded into a rigid metal cannula with a trocar (external diameter is 3 mm, length is 15 cm, R.M. Surgical Developments, Surrey, UK). At the time of insertion percutaneously through the maternal abdomen into the fetal bladder, the metal obturator is removed and the catheter resumes its double-pigtail configuration. **B,** Transverse view of the fetal pelvis showing the double-pigtail catheter in correct position (echogenic double lines) in the fetal bladder.

Pleuroamniotic Shunting

Fetal **thoracentesis** for diagnostic and therapeutic purposes has also been reported.[56,57] Fetal hydrothorax may be related to structural or karyotypic abnormalities, fetal infection, or may be part of a more generalized picture of nonimmune fetal hydrops (NIFH). Detailed ultrasound, PUBS, and thoracentesis are important investigations, especially in the presence of hydrops. When the underlying pathology has been excluded, there are a group of fetuses where the primary pathology is related to a delay in the development of lymphatic channels draining the pleural cavity. In such cases, there is a high white cell count in the aspirated fluid. Long-standing pleural effusions may cause pulmonary hypoplasia, and pressure on the heart and great vessels together with increased thoracic pressure can reduce cardiac output and lead to cardiac failure and hydrops. Since the fluid reaccumulates, pleuroamniotic shunts similar to double-pigtail vesicoamniotic catheters have been used and shown to be of benefit, particularly in reversing hydrops.

Aspiration of Other Cysts or Cavities

Aspiration of **ovarian cysts, cystic small bowel, mesenteric cysts, loculated or overt ascites, cystic hygromas,** and **other lymphatic collections** has been done, but most of these procedures do not stand up to critical appraisal in terms of defined benefits. For example, in the case of large fetal ovarian cysts, dystocia is not a problem and neonatal surgery is seldom needed as the cyst itself almost always regresses spontaneously in the newborn period. Massive ascites with prune-belly distention and pulmonary compression is usually a lethal developmental disorder, and drainage is usually not helpful. Inflammatory ascites associated with meconium peritonitis is rarely ever associated with pulmonary compromise, and no drainage is indicated. There may be, however, useful diagnostic information obtained by sampling the ascitic fluid for determining etiology, prognosis, and newborn management.

It is unclear whether drainage of **large fetal bronchopulmonary cysts** is beneficial in terms of allowing reexpansion of the normal but compressed lung. In at least one case, serial drainage in fetal life allowed reexpansion of the lung, and evidence of ongoing repair was confirmed histologically after neonatal lung resection.[58]

In general, fetal tumors and cysts rarely need to be aspirated because the diagnosis can be made by ultrasound examination in most cases. However, if the cyst is very large, the origin is uncertain, or malignant elements may be present, analysis of the tissue or fluid may be diagnostic.

Fetal Intracardiac Procedures

A number of percutaneous ultrasound-guided intracardiac procedures have been reported. **Fetal cardiocentesis** has been performed in cases where a fetal blood sample has been required early in gestation (less than 17 weeks) and as a lifesaving route for transfusion when umbilical or other fetal vessels are not accessible.[59,60] Some groups have used the heart as a routine secondary source for fetal blood typing and transfusion; however, the overall loss rate (2% to 17%) among the various reports is unsatisfactory within the context of routine testing.

Fetal pericardiocentesis has been performed for significant pericardial effusions thought to be potentially life threatening. Fetal viral infection causing pericarditis with pericardial effusion may result in deficient myocardial action, markedly reduced cardiac output, and decreased peripheral perfusion reflected by absent fetal behavior. In this situation, pericardiocentesis has been successful, although reported cases do not provide a level of information as to whether the procedure was necessary or beneficial. In most cases, successful management of pericardial effusions does not involve direct treatment or drainage. Treatment of the underlying condition (e.g., blood transfusion for Rhesus isoimmunization) will result in resolution of the effusion.

We recently reported a case of isolated pericardial effusion associated with a ventricular diverticulum.[61] In this case, there was no evidence of cardiac failure; however, because of the large size of the effusion, the fetus was believed to be at considerable risk of pulmonary hypoplasia from fetal lung compression (Fig. 50-9). Successful drainage of the effusion was carried out under continuous ultrasound guidance. The pericardial effusion did not reaccumulate, and the pregnancy progressed uneventfully. The ventricular diverticulum was confirmed at birth, and the child has remained asymptomatic.

Other intracardiac procedures that have been reported include the placement of percutaneous fetal transthoracic wire leads for complete heart block in the fetus. In addition, ultrasound-guided percutaneous balloon dilatation of deficient aortic valve orifices in the case of critical aortic stenosis has also been reported.[62] These are investigational procedures at present.

Fluid Instillation into the Amniotic Cavity

Ultrasound visualization of fetal anatomy is difficult in patients with severe oligohydramnios. Fluid instillation into the amniotic or peritoneal cavities creates an acoustic window for clear imaging with ultrasound.[63] Such procedures should be carried out under strict aseptic conditions, and prophylactic antibiotics are recommended. The fluid instilled (normal saline) should be at body temperature and the needle guided into the intraamniotic space with ultrasound. Hypoechoic areas suggesting a small pocket of amniotic fluid may be umbilical cord and should be excluded through use of a

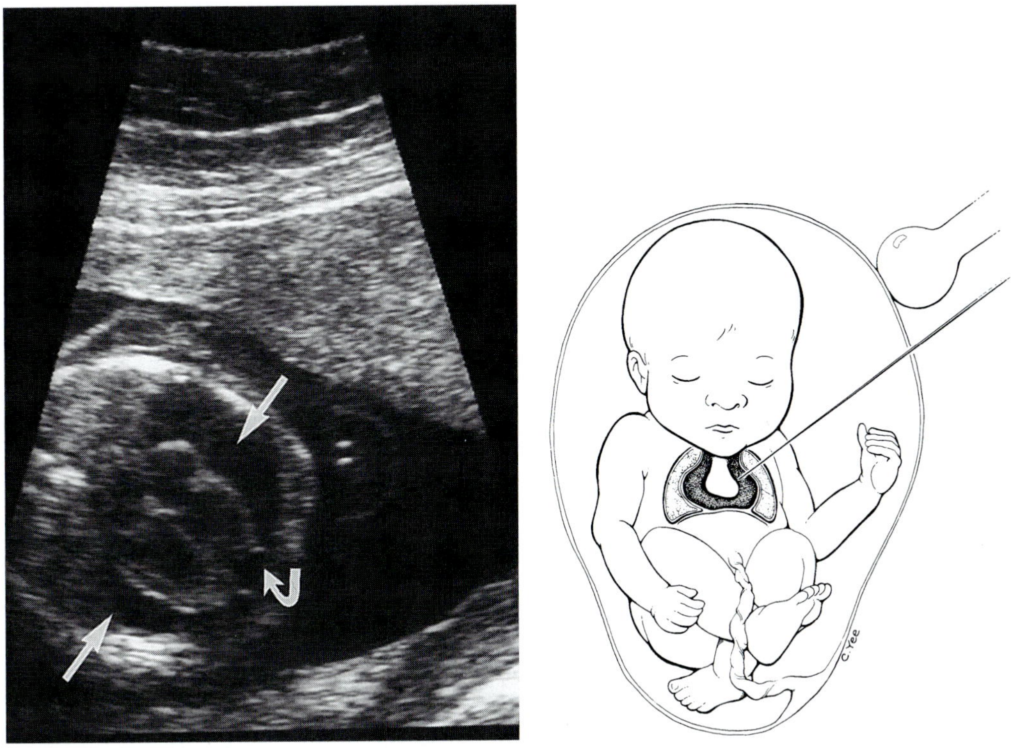

A

B

FIG. 50-9. Pericardial effusion. **A,** Transverse scan through the fetal chest at 20 weeks gestation showing a large pericardial effusion *(arrows)* filling about half of the chest area. A diverticulum *(curved arrow)* is visible at the apex of the right ventricle. **B,** Schema showing a fetal pericardiocentesis using a 22 gauge needle under continuous ultrasound guidance.

Doppler ultrasound. Before any fluid is instilled, a syringe should be attached to the needle for aspiration to see whether amniotic fluid or blood is obtained. Once the needle is in the intraamniotic cavity, if no fluid is aspirated, a small volume of warm saline is injected and the fluid dispersion is observed. Occasionally, there is no dispersion, and if the needle tip is under the fetal skin, a salinoma may become visible on ultrasound.

Amnioinfusion will improve sonographic visualization, especially of the kidneys, and allow the fetus to make body and limb movements, permitting examination of external and internal features. This may be useful, for example, in the evaluation of fetuses with an obstructive uropathy, where it is essential to rule out associated abnormalities before considering vesicoamniotic shunting. As the fetus swallows, the stomach may become visible, and with increased fluid absorption, excretion by the kidneys and bladder may occur. Leakage of fluid from the maternal cervix and vagina will indicate premature rupture of the membranes, and if further verification is needed, a nontoxic dye (indigo carmine) can be used for confirmation.

Intrapartum Amnioinfusion

Repetitive decelerations are caused by compression of the umbilical cord, placenta, and fetal head during labor and are increased with oligohydramnios. The decelerations, if persistent, can lead to fetal acidosis and increased operative delivery for fetal distress. The purpose of amnioinfusion is to prevent this sequence, especially when the usual maneuvers of changing maternal position and giving maternal oxygen fail. This technique may result in fewer cesarean sections performed for fetal distress in cases of premature rupture of the membranes associated with oligohydramnios, but less so with oligohydramnios associated with IUGR in term or postterm pregnancies.[63] The procedure is performed by inserting an intrauterine pressure catheter through the cervix into the amniotic cavity. Up to 1 L of 0.9% saline is infused at 20 to 25 ml per minute through the catheter under ultrasound guidance. The procedure appears to have potential value; however, further evaluation is required.

Therapeutic Amnioreduction

In cases of polyhydramnios, therapeutic drainage of amniotic fluid has been described. Polyhydramnios without any major pathology is not uncommon, especially in multiple pregnancies. It may be associated with severe maternal discomfort, breathlessness, insomnia, and preterm labor. Medical treatment with prostaglandin synthesis antagonists has been tried with some success but is associated with fetal complications, including premature closure of the ductus arteriosus and renal shutdown.[64–66] This may be a major threat, particularly in twins if one has growth retardation and oligohydramnios. Therapeutic drainage of amniotic fluid from the sac with the polyhydramnios is an option.[48] Known as a reduction amniocentesis, this approach is gaining increased acceptance in the management of twin-to-twin transfusion syndrome. Depending on the pathophysiology of the placental bed vascular communications, reduction amniocentesis may allow stabilization of the twin transfusion process enough to enable both twins to gain maturity in a less compromised intrauterine environment. The advantage is improvement over the 60% to 100% perinatal mortality of expectant management alone.[18] The risks include precipitating premature rupture of the membranes, separation of the placenta caused by too rapid decompression, and infection.

CONCLUSION

Improvements in ultrasound technology and other diagnostic interventions have allowed earlier and more accurate evaluation of a vast array of fetal conditions. Invasive obstetric procedures now have a definitive role in the investigation and management of select fetal conditions and have opened up an exciting new range of options for fetal therapy. It should be kept in mind that these procedures should be confined to tertiary level centers with appropriate expertise in identification of the anomalous fetus, obstetric management, and perinatal care. A regionalized, integrated multidisciplinary team approach is fundamental to the optimal management of these cases.

REFERENCES

Chorionic Villus Sampling (CVS)

1. Hanemann N, Mohr J. Antenatal fetal diagnosis in the embryo by means of biopsy with extra embryonic membranes. *Bull Eur Soc Hum Genet* 1968;2:23.
2. Kullander S, Sandahl V. Fetal chromosome analysis after transcervical placental biopsy during early pregnancy. *Acta Obstet Gynecol Scand* 1973;52:355.
3. Tiatung Hospital of Anshan Steel Works. Department of Obstetrics and Gynaecology. Fetal sex prediction by sex chromatin of chorionic villi cells during early pregnancy. *Chin Med J* 1975;1:117-126.
4. Kazy Z, Rozovsky IS, Bakharev VA. Chorion biopsy in early pregnancy: a method of early prenatal diagnosis for inherited disorders. *Prenat Diagn* 1982;2:39.
5. Rodeck CH, Sheldrake A, Beattie B et al. Maternal serum alpha-fetoprotein after placental damage in chorionic villus sampling. *Lancet* 1993;341:500.
6. Canadian Collaborative CVS-Amniocentesis Clinical Trial Group. Multicentered randomized clinical trial of chorionic villus sampling and amniocentesis. First Report. *Lancet* 1989;**i**:2-6.
7. National Institute of Child Health and Human Development. The safety and efficacy of chorionic villus sampling for early prenatal diagnosis of cytogenetic abnormalities. *N Engl J Med* 1989;320:609-617.
8. Brambati B, Lanzani A, Tului L. Transabdominal and transcervical chorionic villus sampling: efficacy and risk evaluation of 2,411 cases. *Am J Med Genet* 1990;35:160-164.
9. Williamson R, Eskdale J, Coleman DV et al. Direct gene analysis of chorionic villi: a possible technique for the first trimester diagnosis of haemoglobinopathies. *Lancet* 1981;**ii**:1125-1127.
10. Firth HV, Boyd PA, Chamberlain P et al. Severe limb abnormalities after chorion villus sampling at 55-66 days' gestation. *Lancet* 1991;337:762-763.
11. Burton BK, Schulz CJ, Burd LI. Limb anomalies associated with chorionic villus sampling. *Obstet Gynecol* 1992;79:726-730.
12. Kuliev AM, Modell B, Jackson L et al. Risk evaluation of CVS. *Prenat Diagn* 13:197-209.
13. Report of National Institute of Child Health and Human Development Workshop on chorionic villus sampling and limb and other defects. *Am J Obstet Gynecol* 1993;169:1-6.

Amniocentesis

14. Bevus DCA. The antenatal prediction of hemolytic disease of the newborn. *Lancet* 1952;**i**:395-398.
15. Steel NW, Bragg WR. Chromosome analysis of human amniotic fluid cells. *Lancet* 1966;**i**:383.
16. Scrimgeour JB. Amniocentesis: technique and complications. In: Emery ACH, ed. *Antenatal Diagnosis of Genetic Diseases.* Edinburgh: Churchill Livingstone; 1973:11-39.
17. Bennett PR, Mervankim LE, Van Kim C et al. Prenatal determination of fetal RhD type by DNA amplification. *N Engl J Med* 1993;329:607-610.
18. Elliot JP, Urig MA, Clewell WH. Aggressive therapeutic amniocentesis for treatment of twin-twin transfusion syndrome. *Obstet Gynecol* 1991;77:537-540.
19. Simpson E, Daillaire L, Miller JR et al. Prenatal diagnosis of genetic disease in Canada: report of a collaborative study. *Can Med Assoc J* 1976:115-739.
20. National Institutes of Health and Development Amniocentesis Registry. *The Safety and Accuracy of Mid-Trimester Amniocentesis.* Rockville, Md: US Dept of Health, Education, and Welfare; 1978:78-190.
21. Medical Research Council 1978. An assessment of the hazards of amniocentesis. *Br J Obstet Gynaecol* 1978:85(suppl 2).
22. Tabor A, Philip J, Marson M et al. Randomized control trial genetic amniocentesis in 4606 low-risk women. *Lancet* 1986:**i**:1278-1293.
23. Brock DJD, Scrimgeor JB, Nelson MM. Amniotic fluid AFP measurements in the early prenatal diagnosis of central nervous system disorders. *Clin Genet* 1975;7:163.
24. Elejalde B, de Elejalde M, Acuna J et al. Prospective study of amniocentesis performed between weeks 9 and 16 of gestation; its feasibility, risks, complications and use in early genetic prenatal diagnosis. *Am J Med Genet* 1990;35:188-196.
25. Hanson FW, Florn EM, Tennant FR et al. Amniocentesis before 15 weeks gestation; outcome, risks and technical problems. *Am J Obstet Gynecol* 1987;156:1524.
26. Golbus MS, Loughman WD, Epstein CJ. Prenatal genetic diagnosis in 3,000 amniocenteses. *N Engl J Med* 1979;300:157–163.
27. Benacerraf B, Greene M, Saltzman B et al. Early amniocentesis for prenatal cytogenetic evaluation. *Radiology* 1988;169:709-710.
28. Godmillow L, Weiner S, Done L. Genetic amniocentesis performed between 12 and 14 weeks gestation. *Am J Hum Genet* 1987;41:818.
29. Johnson JM, Wilson RD, Winsor EJT et al. The early amniocentesis study: a randomized clinical trial of early amniocentesis versus mid-trimester amniocentesis. *Fet Diagn Ther* 1996;11:85-93.

Percutaneous Umbilical Blood Sampling (PUBS)

30. Daffos F, Capella-Pavovisky M, Forestier F. Fetal blood sampling via the umbilical cord using a needle guided by ultrasound. *Prenat Diagn* 1982;3:271-274.
31. Forestier F, Cox WL, Daffos F et al. The assessment of fetal blood samples. *Am J Obstet Gynecol* 1988;158:1184.
32. Romero R, Athanassiadis AP, Inati M. Fetal blood sampling. In: Fleischer AC, Romero R, Manning FA, eds. *The Principles and Practice of Ultrasonography in Obstetrics and Gynecology*. Norwalk, Conn: Appleton & Lange; 1991:455-473.
33. Nicolini U, Santolaya J, Ojo OE et al. The fetal intrahepatic umbilical vein as an alternative to cord needling for prenatal diagnosis and therapy. *Prenat Diagn* 1988;8:665.
34. National PUBS Registry. Philadelphia Proceedings of the 4th Annual Meeting; 1989.
35. Rodeck CH, Campbell S. Sampling pure fetal blood by fetoscopy in the second trimester of pregnancy. *Br Med J* 1978;2:728.
36. Nicolaides KH, Rodeck CH, Gosden CM. Rapid karyotyping in nonlethal fetal malformations. *Lancet* 1986;**i**:283-287.
37. Nicolaides KH, Suto PW, Rodeck CH et al. Ultrasound-guided sampling of umbilical cord and placental blood to assess fetal well-being. *Lancet* 1986;**i**:1065-1067.
38. Harman CR, Bowman JM, Manning FA et al. Use of intravascular transfusion to treat hydrops fetalis in a moribund fetus. *Can Med Assoc J* 1988;138:827-830.
39. Bussell JP, Berkowitz RL, McFarland JG et al. Antenatal treatment of neonatal alloimmune thrombocytopenia. *N Engl J Med* 1988;319:1374-1378.
40. Nicolini U, Rodeck CH, Kochenour NK et al. In utero platelet transfusion for alloimmune for cytopenia. *Lancet* 1988;2:506.
41. Ito S, Magee L, Smallhorn J. Drug therapy for fetal arrythmias. In: Corn G, Ito S, eds. Clinics in perinatology. *Fet Drug Ther* 1994;21(3):543-590.

Percutaneous Fetal Tissue Sampling

42. Golbus MS, McGonigle KF, Goldberg J et al. Fetal tissue sampling. The San Francisco experience with 190 pregnancies. *Western J Med* 1989;150(4):423.
43. Scott CR, Tang CC, Goodman SI et al. X-linked transmission of ornithine transcarbamylase deficiency. *Lancet* 1972; **ii**:1148.
44. Rodeck CH, Patrick AD, Penbrey ME et al. Fetal liver biopsy for prenatal diagnosis of ornithine transcarbamylase deficiencies. *Lancet* 1982;**ii**:297-299.
45. Natuyama E. Sonographic determination of fetal sex from 12 weeks gestation. *Am J Obstet Gynecol* 1984;149:748-757.
46. Brady RAJ, Rodeck CH. Prenatal diagnosis of disorders of the skin. In: Rodeck CH, Nicolaides KH, eds. *Prenatal Diagnosis. Proceedings of the 11th Study Group of the Royal College of Obstetrics and Gynaecologists.* Chichester, England: Wiley; 1984:147-158.
47. Bang J. Intrauterine needle diagnosis. In: Holm, K. *Interventional Ultrasound.* Copenhagen: Munksgaard; 1985: 122-128.
48. Arulkumaran S, Rodeck CH. Invasive prenatal diagnostic techniques. *Fet Med Rev* 1990;2:171-185.
49. Rodeck CH, Nicolaides KH. Fetal tissue biopsy; techniques and indications. *Fet Ther* 1986;46-58.
50. Kurjaka, Alfirevicz, Jurkovic D. Ultrasonically-guided fetal tissue biopsy. *Acta Obstet Gynecol Scand* 1987;66:523-527.

Other Interventions

51. Harrison MR, Golbus MS, Filly RA et al. Management of the fetus with congenital hydronephrosis. *J Pediatr Surg* 1982; 17:728-742.
52. Harrison MR, Filly RA, Parer JT et al. Management of the fetus with a urinary tract malformation. *JAMA* 1981;246:635-639.
53. Mahoney BS, Filly RA, Cowan PW et al. Fetal renal dysplasia: sonographic evaluation. *Radiology* 1984;152:143-146.
54. Nicolini U, Rodeck CH, Fish NN. Shunt treatment for fetal obstructive uropathy. *Lancet* 1987;**ii**:1338-1339.
55. Teoh TG, Ryan G, Johnson JM et al. The role of fetal karyotyping from unconventional sources. *Am J Obstet Gynecol* 1996;175:873-877.
56. Schmidt W, Harms E, Wolfe D. Successful prenatal treatment of non-immune hydrops fetalis due to congenital chylothorax. *Br J Obstet Gynaecol* 1985;92:685-687.
57. Rodeck CH, Fish NN, Fraser DI et al. Long-term in-utero drainage of fetal hydrothorax. *N Engl J Med* 1988;319:1135-1138.
58. Kyle P, Lauge IR, Menticoglou SM et al. Intrauterine thoracentesis of fetal cystic lung malformations. *Fet Diagn Ther* 1994;9:84-87.
59. Westgren M, Selbing A, Stangenbergm. Fetal intracardiac transfusions in patients with severe rhesus-isoimmunization. *Br Med J* 1988;296:885-886.
60. Harman CR, Manning FA, Menticoglous S et al. Fetal exsanguination at intravascular transfusion. *Proc Soc Obstet Gynecol Can* 1990: (Abstract).
61. Johnson JM, Ryan G, Toi A et al. Prenatal diagnosis of a fetal ventricular diverticulum associated with pericardial effusion: successful outcome following pericardiocentesis. *Prenat Diagn* (In press 1996).
62. Maxwell D, Adan L, Tynan MJ. Balloon dilatation of the aortic valve in the fetus: a report of two cases. *Br Heart J* 1991;65:256-258.
63. Genbruch U, Hansmann M. Artificial instillation of amniotic fluid as a new technique for the diagnostic evaluation of cases of oligohydramnios. *Prenat Diagn* 1988;8:33-45.
64. Nageotte MP, Bertucci L, Towers CV et al. Prophylactic amnioinfusion in pregnancies complicated by oligohydramnios; a prospective study. *Obstet Gynecol* 1991;77:677–680.
65. Cabrol D, Landesman R, Muller J et al. Treatment of polyhydramnios with prostaglandin synthetase inhibitor (indomethacin). *Am J Obstet Gynecol* 1987;157:422-426.
66. Moise KJ, Huhta JC, Sharif DS et al. Indomethacin in the treatment of preterm labour; effects on ductus arteriosus. *N Engl J Med* 1988;319:327-331.

CHAPTER 51

Infertility

David A. Wiseman, M.D., F.R.C.P.(C)
Calvin A. Greene, M.D., F.R.S.C.(C)
Roger A. Pierson, M.S., Ph.D.

CHAPTER OUTLINE

ROLE OF ULTRASOUND IN DIAGNOSIS OF INFERTILITY

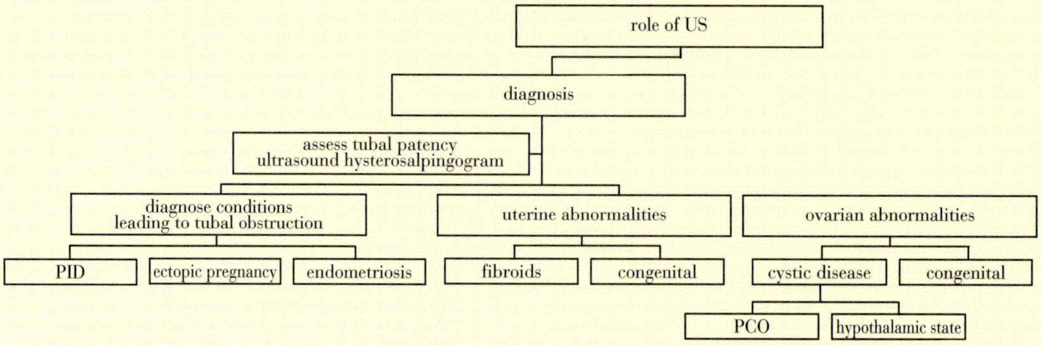

ROLE OF ULTRASOUND IN TREATMENT OF INFERTILITY

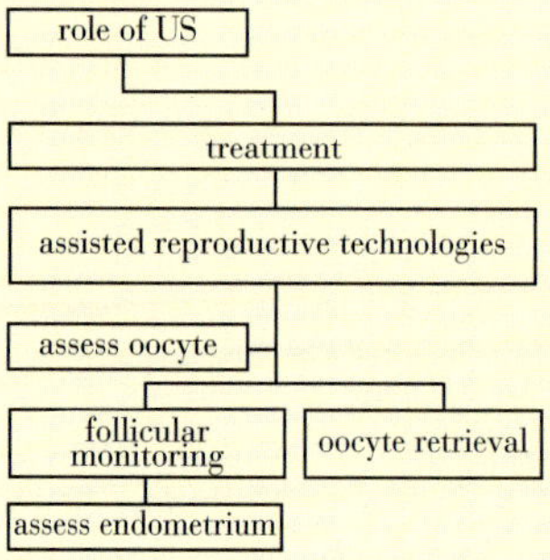

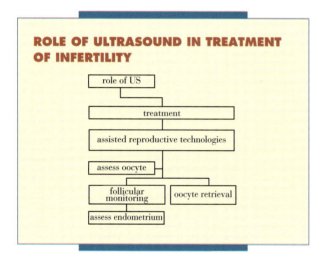

Infertility is defined as the inability to conceive a wanted child after 12 months of unprotected intercourse. In normal day-to-day practice, an individual patient is afflicted with an illness. In contrast, infertility involves a couple. The investigation and management of the infertile couple have become the domain of a multidisciplinary team in which diagnostic and therapeutic ultrasound imaging and interventional techniques play an integral and indispensable role. The cause of a couple's infertility may often be traced to one or other of the couple, but the burden of "infertility" is shared by both. Awareness of this fact should temper the manner in which these patients are seen in ultrasound departments, ensuring whenever possible that both partners participate in procedures and imaging relating to their infertility.

Sensitivity is required in the management of all patients, but the infertile couple is particularly vulnerable. It is therefore critical that practitioners involved in diagnostic imaging be sensitive to the emotional needs of their patients and be able to respond to these needs, as well as provide a quality imaging service. It should not be forgotten that infertile couples hang on every word uttered by their attendants. This clearly means that ultrasonographers and infertility practitioners must work in close harmony, ensuring dissemination to the patients of precise and consistent information.

EPIDEMIOLOGY

The number of patients presenting for the diagnosis and treatment of infertility disorders has increased in recent years. In general, the infertile couple is older and have had no previous children. It is believed that 10% to 15% of reproductive age couples encounter this situation.[1] In the United States in the early 1800s, birth rates were eight births per woman, a number which presently has fallen to two.[2] The cause for this reduced birth rate is multifactorial including medical, environmental, and social factors.

Postponement of pregnancy in lieu of career development or convenience is believed to contribute significantly to the increase in the number of couples presenting with infertility. Several studies have documented a decrease in fecundity with advancing age. In one donor insemination program, the conception rate was 74% in patients under the age of 31, 62% in patients between the ages of 31 and 35, and 54% in women older than 35 years of age.[3] The cause of decreased fertility with age is multifactorial including reduced coital frequency, an accelerated loss of endocrinologically competent oocytes, increased ovulation defects, decreased endometrial receptivity and an increased incidence of other diseases. By far the greatest contributing factor is the decline in endocrinologically competent oocytes. Uterine abnormalities, such as fibroids and endometriosis, are two conditions that increase with age and have a negative impact on fertility. Early spontaneous abortion is a cause of decreased term pregnancy and increases from

10% for women under 30 years of age to 35% in patients in their early forties, with the majority of these being caused by chromosomal abnormalities, especially aneuploidy.[4] Aging also negatively affects male fertility because of decreasing androgen levels; this results in reduced libido, sperm density, and motility.

INVESTIGATION OF THE INFERTILE COUPLE—CLINICAL ISSUES

The box summarizes the objectives in investigating the infertile couple. To achieve these goals, one must understand the basic reproductive process and the conditions that may interfere with reproduction.

GOALS IN THE INVESTIGATION OF THE INFERTILE COUPLE

- To identify the cause of the infertility
- To formulate a treatment program aimed at achieving a successful pregnancy
- To respond to the emotional needs of the infertile couple whether or not treatment is successful
- To monitor the early development of pregnancy, when established

ULTRASOUND AND THE NORMAL REPRODUCTIVE PROCESS

For successful initiation and establishment of human pregnancy, ovulation must occur. **Ovulation,** by definition, is the rupture of a mature ovarian follicle and the expulsion of the follicular fluid and cumulus complex. Ovulation depends upon the precisely regulated growth and development of a preovulatory follicle and is the culmination of a complex series of physiologic events set in motion by a surge of luteinizing hormone (LH). Recruitment of a cohort of follicles into the pool of developing follicles, physiologic selection of the follicle destined to ovulate, preferential growth of the preovulatory follicle and its timely acquisition of LH receptors are of paramount importance for successful ovulation. It is now apparent that optimal follicle growth is necessary for normal ovulation and luteal function. It is important to recall that development of the preovulatory follicle and the oocyte occurs in concert so that the oocyte is in the correct stage of maturation for fertilization to occur.

Ovulation occurs on approximately Day 14 following menstruation in a "textbook" 28-day menstrual cycle.[5-9] However, it is possible for ovulation to occur at almost any time during a cycle, and few cycles seem to reflect the theoretical norm, especially in women experiencing difficulty in conception. Transabdominal ultrasound scanning has been used for many years to detect ovulation in women.[10] However, images of rupture of the follicle and evacuation of the follicular fluid and cumulus/oocyte complex have only recently been demonstrated by ultrasonography. On the average, ovulation appeared to take approximately 10 minutes from initiation to complete follicular evacuation. However, the time required for ovulation varied from less than 1 minute to more than 20 minutes. The site of follicular evacuation was immediately detectable. A sequence of images showing **stages of folliculllar evacuation** is shown (Fig. 51-1). The point of follicular rupture from the surface of the ovary may be recognized for up to 1 week and the luteal gland typically remains identifiable by ultrasonography until the subsequent ovulatory cycle.[11] An example of an **early site of ovulation** is shown (Fig. 51-2). Detailed evaluation of ovulation and early luteogenesis in clinically normal women and patients referred for idiopathic infertility is revealing previously undescribed flaws in the ovulatory process.[12]

There is considerable variation in the duration of ovulation and the morphologic aspects of follicular rupture and emptying. Additional studies are ongoing to elucidate various physiologic and biomechanical aspects of ovulation and to develop quantitative methods of evaluating the ovulatory process. Clinical applications resulting from these investigations include assessment of the potential for ovulation of individual follicles of preovulatory diameter in infertile women.

The use of ultrasonography to monitor follicular growth and confirm the occurrence of ovulation is becoming an integral part of clinical research and practice. Research is beginning to assess the efficacy of computer-assisted image analysis and enhancement for examining the echotextural characteristics and vascular patterns of individual preovulatory follicles to evaluate the probability of ovulation. We anticipate that such image display algorithms will become a standard modality.[13] A highly processed surface map originating from an ultrasound image of a **normal preovulatory follicle** immediately prior to ovulation is shown (Fig. 51-3). Similarly, a role for color-flow Doppler ultrasonography in assessing follicular development and ovulation remains to be elucidated. The technique is easily applied to the study of follicles, ovulation, and early luteogenesis, however, the clinical relevance has not yet been determined.

The oocyte released by the process of ovulation must be captured by the tubal fimbria and transported to the ampulla of the fallopian tube where fertilization occurs. Spermatogenesis occurs within the testes, and the spermatozoa must be deposited into the lower genital tract of the woman around the time of ovulation.

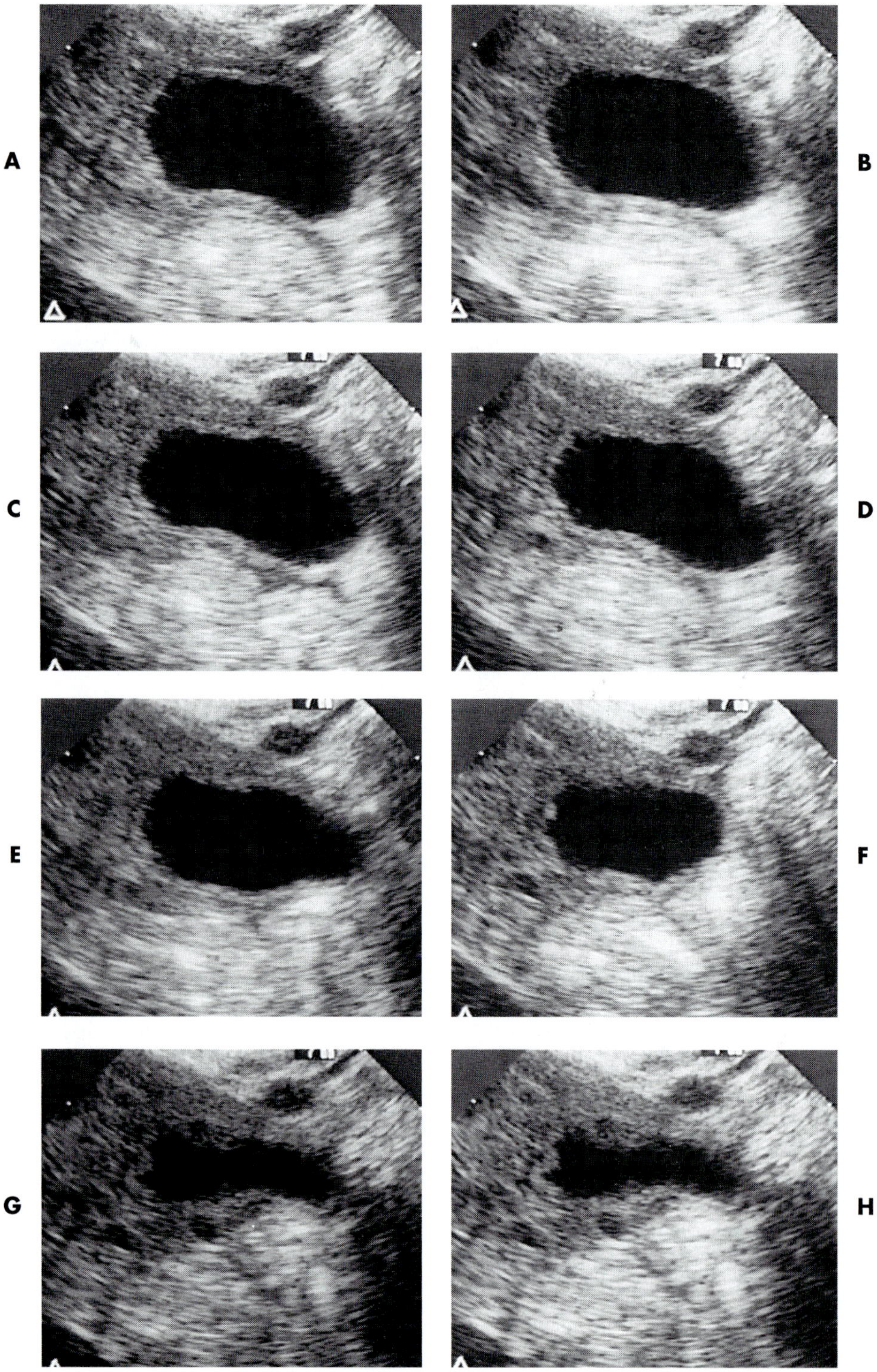

FIG. 51-1. Sequential ultrasonographic images taken during ovulation. Images (**A** through **H**) were captured at approximately 0.5 second intervals. The ovulation, from onset to complete follicular ovulation, took approximately 6.5 seconds.

The spermatozoa then must penetrate the cervical mucus, traverse the uterine cavity, and then enter and travel down the fallopian tube. **Fertilization** occurs if the fallopian tube is patent and normal. Following fertilization, the embryo is transported along the fallopian tube to the uterus. **Implantation** occurs if a satisfactory endometrium has developed that is capable of nourishing a pregnancy. Uterine tissues are the target tissues for the reproductively active hormones in the peripheral circulation (primarily estradiol 17b and progesterone). Several other endocrine and paracrine secretory products also are involved in achieving the

A

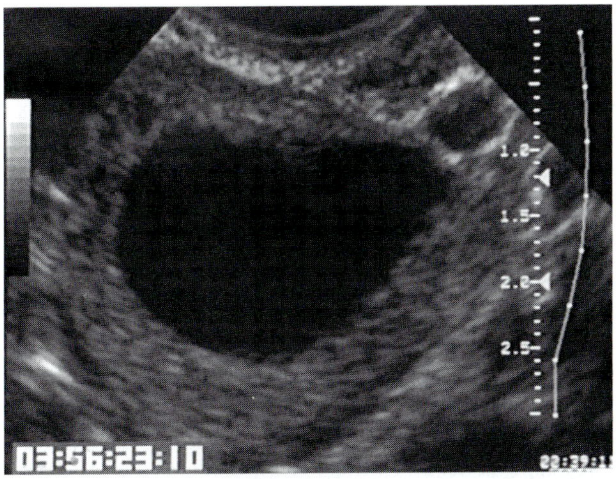

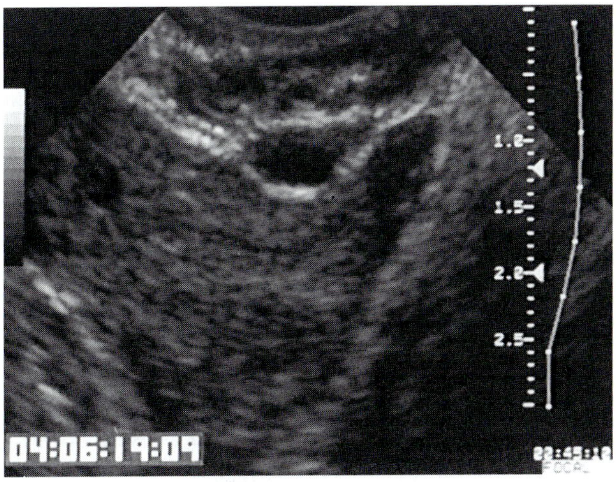

B

C

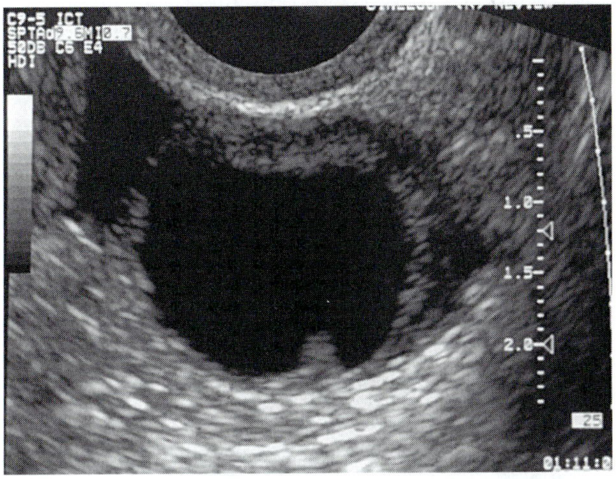

FIG. 51-2. Ovulation. **A,** Ultrasonographic image of a imminently preovulatory follicle. Image recorded 1 second before onset of ovulation. **B,** Site of ovulation of the follicle in A at complete follicular evacuation. The ovulation event took approximately 10 minutes from onset to complete follicular evacuation (timescale, bottom left corner). **C,** In a different patient, an image of an imminently preovulatory follicle with the cumulus-oocyte complex observed protruding from the interior inferior aspect of the follicle wall.

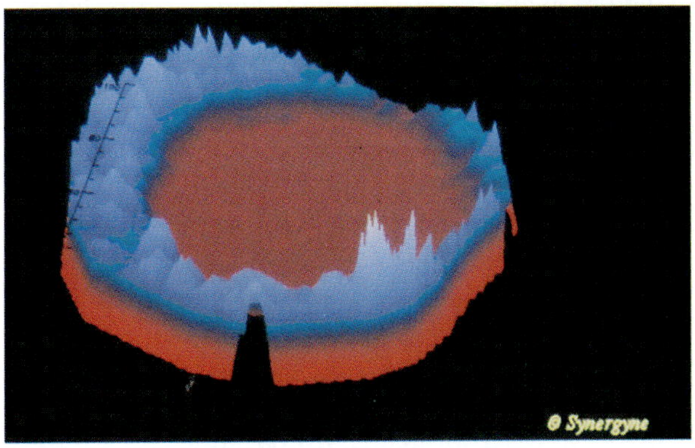

FIG. 51-3. Highly processed ultrasound image of a normal preovulatory follicle rendered and shaded for height-biased image analysis. Note the thick, well-developed follicular walls (*light blue*), the transition zone from follicular fluid to follicle wall (*dark blue*) and the deep red tones representing follicular fluid.

ultimate goal of turning the uterus into a receptive environment for implantation of the blastocyst.[14] Because of the intimate relationship of ovarian and uterine function, detailed examinations of the endometrium provide a great deal more information on uterine receptivity than peripheral hormone assays. The changes in the endometrium during the follicular and luteal phases of the menstrual cycle are directly related to the circulating concentrations of estrogen and progesterone and provide a conceptual bioassay for the reproductively active hormones.

The endometrium undergoes dramatic morphologic changes which mirror those of the ovaries during a normal menstrual cycle. These alterations in functional anatomy may be rapidly assessed with ultrasonographic imaging technology.[15-18] The endometrial detail that may be appreciated with high-resolution transvaginal ultrasound is striking. The inner and outer strata of the endometrium may be identified and the changes in echotexture of the stratum functionalis during the follicular and luteal phases of the menstrual cycle assessed.[18]

The **immediately postmenstrual endometrium** exhibits a single hyperechoic line representing the uterine lumen surrounded by a thin layer (2 to 3 mm) of hyperechoic tissue. During the periods of follicular selection, development and growth, the **proliferative endometrium** is under estrogen stimulation and is characterized by the appearance of a triple line pattern. The central echogenic line is produced by the lumen of the uterine endometrial cavity and the outer lines represent the basal layer of the endometrium or interface between the endometrium and myometrium. The hypoechoic areas between the echogenic central line and the outer lines of the proliferative endometrium represent the functional layer of the endometrium. The functional layer (the hypoechoic area) gradually increases in thickness during the follicular phase of the ovarian cycle (proliferative phase of the menstrual cycle) exactly as observed in the histologic examination of tissues collected at endometrial biopsy. Occasionally, a hypoechoic "halo" surrounding the basal layer is observed. This probably represents the vascular network within the myometrium which intimately surrounds the endometrium.[19] Immediately before ovulation when the dominant ovarian follicle is at its peak of estrogen activity, the **endometrial stratum functionale** triple-line configuration becomes pronounced and quite thick (e.g., 10 to 14 mm). The hyperechoic endometrium typically constitutes less than approximately half of the endometrial thickness with a hyperechoic stratum basalis and a hypoechoic functionalis.[19-21]

After ovulation, the endometrium progresses from the proliferative phase to the **secretory phase.** The functional layer during early luteogenesis, typically 6 days following ovulation, undergoes a transition from hypoechoic to hyperechoic textures. The endometrium also becomes progressively thicker.[15-17,19,22,23] During the early secretory phase, the stratum basalis appears hyperechoic and the stratum functionalis comprises more than 50% of the endometrial thickness, although it does not typically encompass the entire endometrial cavity. It has been suggested that stromal edema is necessary for the increased echotextural values observed when the uterus is under the influence of progesterone during the luteal phase. The increased echotextural values probably arise from interfaces of intracellular stromal fluid and adjacent glands and vessels. In the mid- to late secretory phase, the functionalis appears homogeneous, hyperechoic and extends from the stratum basalis to the uterine lumen.

The **degree of synchronicity between the ovaries and uterus** may be serially evaluated and may be indicative of subtle defects in reproductive hormone production or action. For example, the presence of ovarian follicles of ostensibly preovulatory diameter combined with a thin, hyperechoic uterus would indicate a potentially low estradiol milieu. Similarly, endometrial hypertrophy in the absence of appropriate ovarian structures may be indicative of other clinical problems. The accuracy of ultrasonographic staging of the endometrium is 76% to 93% when compared with classic histologic dating of the same uterine tissues, although the accuracy will undoubtedly increase with the new generation of ultrasound instruments.[14] The importance of integrating the results of ultrasonographic examinations of the ovaries and uterus is amplified in this regard; satisfactory luteal function is expected when the endometrium is at least 11 mm in thickness during the midluteal phase.

The **thickness of the endometrium** is typically measured in the sagittal plane at the thickest point in the uterine body. The measurement extends from the junction of the stratum basalis and myometrium on superior aspect to the same location on the inferior aspect, encompassing the entire width of the endometrium.[14,24] It has been demonstrated in several studies that measurement of endometrial thickness is a highly efficient attribute for distinguishing potential conception cycles from cycles which will not produce a pregnancy even if a fertilized embryo is present.[24,25] Ultrasonographic evaluation of the endometrium also may have predictive value for the outcome of treatments to ameliorate infertility. Several studies have been performed where the probability of implantation was correlated with the thickness of the endometrium when fertilized ova were transferred into the uterus following *in vitro* fertilization. During *in vitro* fertilization cycles, patients who exhibited an endometrial thickness of less than 7 mm on the day of hCG administration did not conceive. In preliminary studies, it was also demonstrated that an early luteal transformation on the day of oocyte aspiration did not favor conception.[24]

The **myometrium** has an even level of echogenicity and does not appear to exhibit easily identifiable changes during the menstrual cycle. It serves as the reference for changes in the echoicity of the endometrium during the menstrual cycle. Myometrial echotexture appears homogenous throughout the body of the uterus. The vasculature of the uterus is distinct, especially at the interface with the broad ligament. Uterine blood vessels in women who have previously been pregnant are demonstrably larger than those of nulligravida women and should be noted in women experiencing secondary infertility.

Disruption of one or more of these fundamental mechanisms may lead to infertility or pregnancy loss. Finally, as Hilgers et al.[26] have shown, timing of coitus is critical. In **"fertility focused intercourse,"** pregnancy was achieved in 76%, 90%, and 98% of cases by the first, third, and sixth cycles, respectively. Normal fertility has been considered to be between 20% and 22% per cycle, and approximately 50% after three cycles.[26]

INVESTIGATION OF INFERTILITY

Specific abnormalities can be identified that may interfere at each step of the reproductive process. Some of these lesions can be stated categorically to cause infertility. Others interfere with natural reproduction but may not be absolute causes of infertility. Rarely, unusual or unexpected causes of infertility are encountered (Fig. 51-4).

Etiologies of infertility include **male factor** (23%), **ovulatory dysfunction** (18%), **tubal damage** (14%), **endometriosis** (6%), **coital dysfunction** (5%), **abnormal cervical mucus** (3%), and **unexplained infertility** (28%). It is important to note that the most common causes of infertility include conditions not amenable to investigation with ultrasound.

The infertility investigation begins after a detailed history and physical examination of both members of the couple is completed.

The **man** is assessed early in the investigative process. Semen analysis is performed and sperm are studied for motility, sperm density, morphology, signs of infection and presence of antisperm antibodies. If the screening semen analysis is entirely normal, attention is then directed toward the **woman**. The assessment of the woman includes tests to confirm ovulation, ensure normal pelvic anatomy and tubal patency, and prove that the cervix and uterine cavity are normal.

Disorders of ovulation account for 18% of all infertility problems. On history alone, it is possible to triage couples into those in which the woman is probably ovulatory and those who are not.

The anovulatory woman will require a full endocrinologic work-up to detect the pathophysiologic basis for the ovulatory dysfunction.[2] In couples in which the woman is apparently ovulatory, the occurrence of ovulation should be confirmed by basal body charts or luteal phase serum progesterone determination. Serial ultrasound may also be used to confirm normal follicular development and the occurrence of ovulation.

Anovulation may be caused by **hypothalamic or pituitary factors, premature ovarian failure or polycystic ovarian syndrome.** All causes of anovulation that are treatable may be approached using ovarian stimulation to induce follicular development and ovulation; however, the manner in which the ovarian stimulation varies dramatically with the condition underlying ovulatory failure. Women with hypothalamic defects do not usually respond to clomiphene citrate therapy. Hypogonadotropic anovulation secondary to Kallmann's syndrome may be successfully treated with pulsatile gonadotropin-releasing agonist (GnRHa) administered with a subcutaneous or intravenous (IV) infusion pump. Women who use the infusion pump for ovulation induction usually require only intermittent ultrasound examinations during the early phase of stimulation. Only one or two dominant

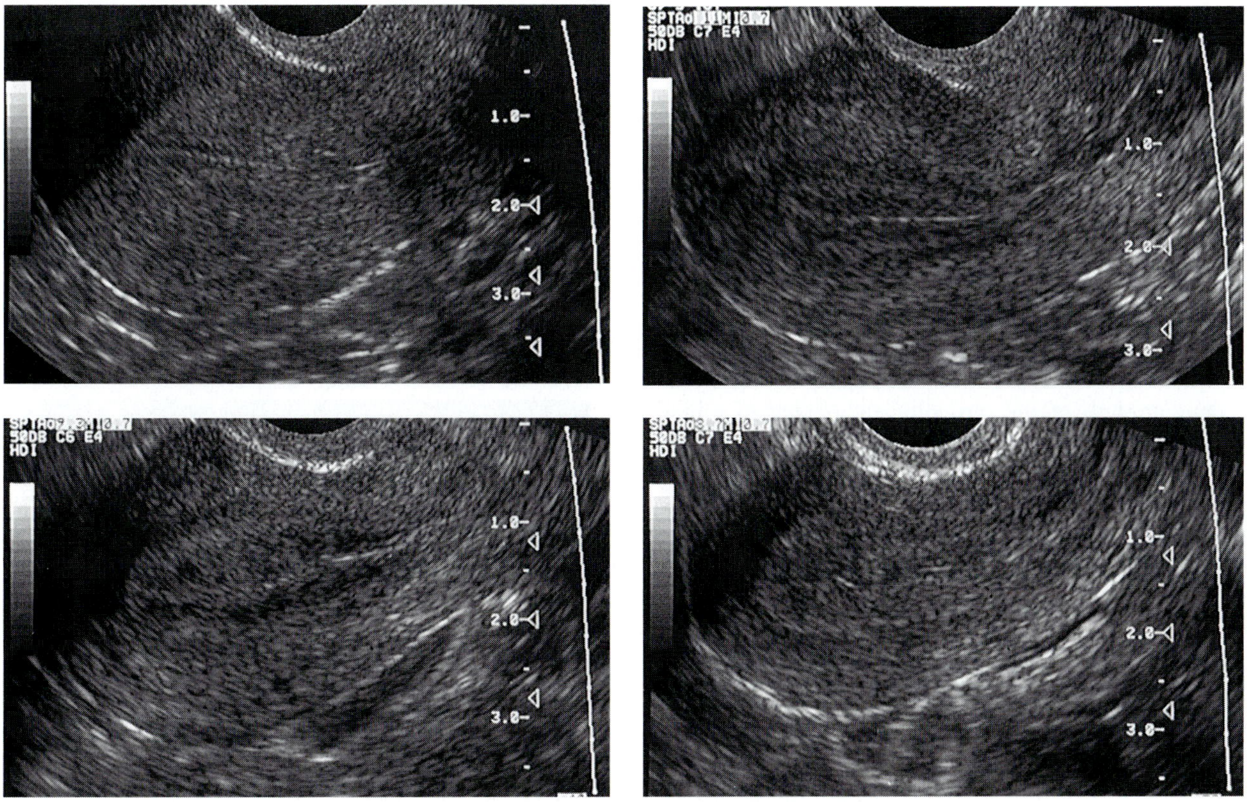

FIG. 51-4. Profound changes in the endometrial echoes. Transverse, midsagittal images of the uterus during the **A,** immediately postmenstrual phase, **B,** midfollicular phase, **C,** preovulatory phase, and **D,** midluteal phase of the cycle. See text for full description.

follicles tend to develop in response to GnRH infusion in contrast to superstimulation observed with human menopausal gonadotropins (hMG) ovulation induction. Human chorionic gonadotropin (hCG) is administered when preovulatory dominant follicles attain 18 mm to 20 mm by ultrasonographic examination. If GnRH therapy is not successful, hMG stimulation may be considered. Anovulatory women with hypothalamic menorrhea who are treated with hMG and ovulatory women stimulated with hMG typically respond to ovarian stimulation similarly; they are equally susceptible to multiple ovulation and ovarian hyperstimulation syndrome.

Assessment of the cause of ovulatory failure is an important aspect of infertility investigations. If follicular rupture and release of a properly matured oocyte do not occur, conception is not possible. Therefore, ultrasonographic confirmation of ovulation, or its failure, is important for many patients undergoing clinical evaluation for ovulatory dysfunction.

Failure of ovulation probably occurs by one of two mechanisms. Although transvaginal US has been used for detailed descriptions of **luteinized, unruptured follicle syndrome** (LUF), its existence remains a subject of debate (Fig. 51-5).[27,28] The physiologically selected follicle attains preovulatory diameter and fails to rupture and release the oocyte/cumulus complex. The oocyte/cumulus complex apparently remains trapped within the lumen of the follicular structure, whereas the walls of the follicle thicken and acquire echotexture characteristics similar to those displayed by luteinized tissue following normal ovulations. The follicular fluid/follicle interface acquires hazy, indistinct borders. The LUF remains identifiable for the duration of the menstrual cycle and apparently regresses following a time course similar to that of clinically normal corpora lutea. Basal body temperature charts and midcycle progesterone concentrations remain within clinically normal limits. Menstrual periods may be reported to be normal or somewhat lighter than normal for individual patients.

A second mechanism for failure of ovulation involves growth of the physiologically selected follicle beyond normal preovulatory diameter without rupture of the follicle wall and release of the oocyte (Fig. 51-6).[28] The now **dysfunctional dominant follicle** appears to remain static in diameter and echotexture for one to several days and then regresses. The rate of follicular regression appears to be highly variable, although in several instances in our laboratory, the rate of regression has been the same as the rate of follicular growth. There does not appear to be luteinization of the follicular wall as would occur in normally ovulated follicles or LUF syndrome. The walls of the follicle appear thin and are comprised of high-amplitude echoes. The follicular fluid/follicle interface typically appears sharp and distinct. Menstrual periods following this type of ovulatory failure typically occur within a normal cycle length, although the amount of flow appears quite variable. Unilocular ovarian cysts filled with clear fluid also represent a form of ovulatory failure, although it is not known whether the determinants of cyst formation reside with the developing follicle or with the mechanism of ovulation (Fig. 51-7).

Polycystic ovarian syndrome (PCOS) is a common cause of infertility and is represented by a broad spectrum of endocrine, morphologic, and causative characteristics.[29] The diagnosis of PCOS has been traditionally made on clinical history and endocrine assessment; however, the ultrasonographic appearance of the ovaries in PCOS patients may be used to strongly support the clinical diagnosis. The ultrasonographic morphology of PCOS has been well described.[30] An image representative of one of the ultrasonographic morphologies characteristic of PCOS is shown. Routine ultrasound examinations performed at the time of first consultation for infertility may be used to identify ovarian morphologic features suggestive of PCOS and the course of subsequent investigations directed.

The patterns of follicular turnover, initiation of follicular growth and physiological selection of a dominant follicle are poorly understood in PCOS patients; however, most women with PCOS will respond to ovarian stimulation. Some PCOS patients are refractory to exogenous stimulation and a satisfactory method of ovulation has not yet been determined. Therapies instituted with some GnRHa ovulation induction protocols have recently shown promise in safer, more effective stimulation of the ovaries of these women.[31] We anticipate that new research will elucidate specific defects in the processes of follicular growth and development and allow the application of more effective, safer ovulation induction schemes.

It is difficult to induce ovulation in patients with PCOS. It is extremely difficult to control the course of ovarian stimulation because all follicles visualized

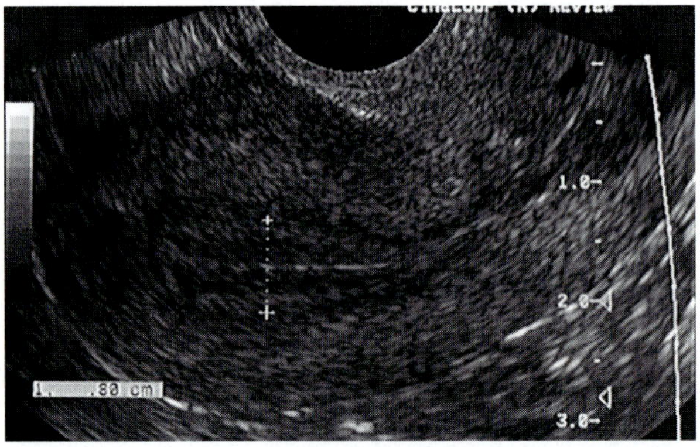

FIG. 51-5. Measuring endometrial thickness. Midsagittal image of the uterus during the follicular phase of the menstrual cycle (B pattern from Fig. 51-4) showing the proper placement of the calipers.

within the ovaries tend to respond to the exogenous follicle stimulating hormone (FSH). In women with severe PCOS, physiologic selection of a few dominant follicles does not occur and ovarian hyperstimulation often results. Multiple ovulations leading to higher-order multiple conceptions represent only one of the risks associated with even the least aggressive stimulation. **Ovarian hyperstimulation syndrome** occurs more commonly in PCOS patients when greater numbers of follicles respond to hCG in an aberrant fashion. In PCOS patients, serial transvaginal ultrasonography is crucial in the assessment of ovarian responses to stimulation of the ovaries throughout the ovulation induction protocol. When the ovaries hyperrespond, it is important to abort the stimulation cycle or to have the facilities required to convert the patients to an assisted

A B

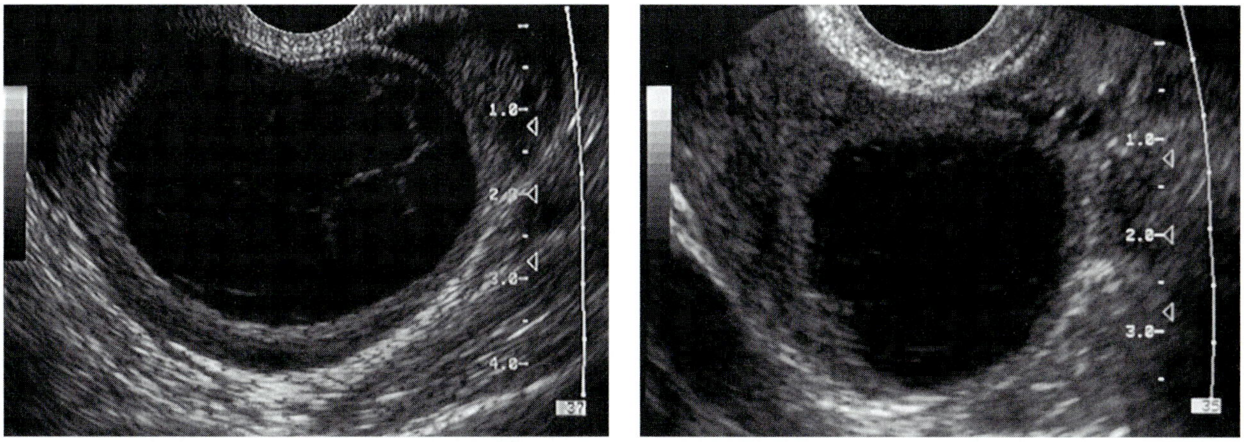

FIG. 51-6. Ovulatory failures classified as **A,** hemorrhage anovulatory follicle and **B,** luteinized unruptured follicle (LUF). **A,** Note the fibrin network interspersed within the fluid of the lumen of the hemorrhagic follicle. The walls of the structure are thin and no luteinized tissue is observed. **B,** Echoes consistent with cellular debris and hemorrhage are observed within the lumen of the LUF. Note the thick, luteinized walls of the LUF. Serum progesterone levels in women with LUF are frequently in the low, clinically normal range, although failure of ovulation can be documented.

A B

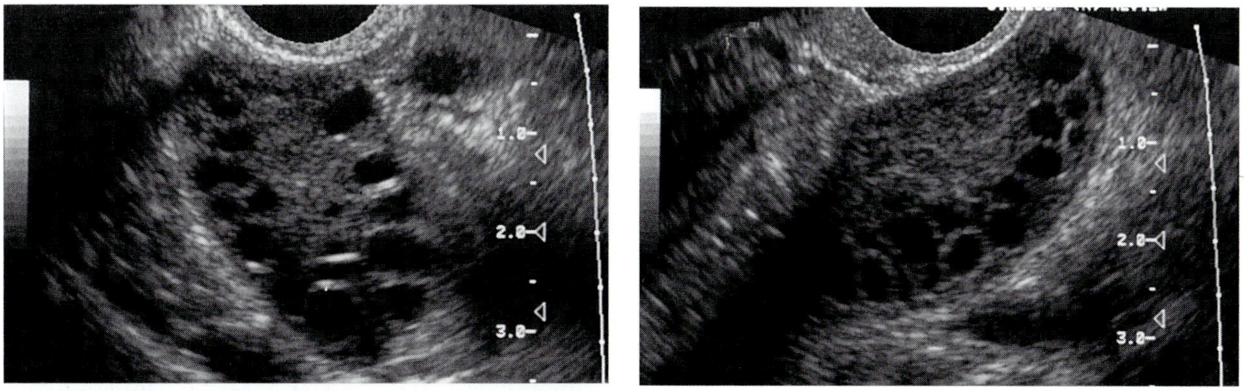

C

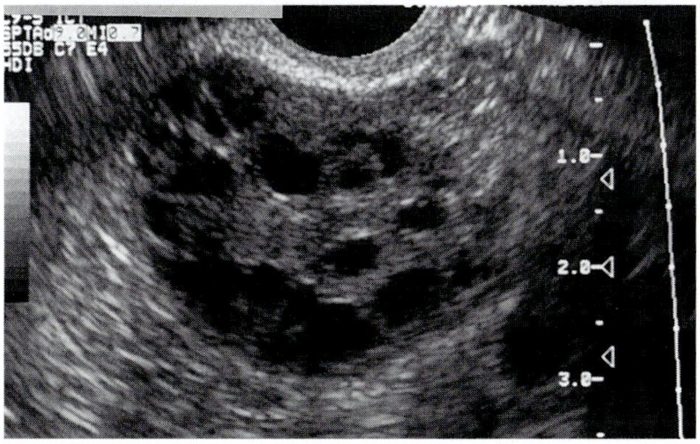

FIG. 51-7. Characteristic sonographic appearance of polycystic ovary syndrome. A through C, The string-of-pearls appearance of small follicles around the periphery of the ovary is characteristic of the syndrome. Note the multiple, small (3 to 6 mm) follicles and lack of a dominant, or preovulatory, follicle.

reproductive technology protocol where the follicles are aspirated and thus at least partially avoid the complications of severe ovarian hyperstimulation.

Pelvic and uterine anatomy are assessed by hysterosalpingography (now accomplished both radiographically and under ultrasound surveillance (discussed in Chapter 15)) initially, and laparoscopy and hysteroscopy if the couple's infertility persists. This is particularly important in women with a history of **appendicitis, pelvic inflammatory disease (PID), septic abortion, intrauterine device (IUD) usage, tubal surgery or ectopic pregnancy,** and those with signs and symptoms of **endometriosis.**

Hysterosalpingography is best performed 2 to 5 days following cessation of the menstrual flow. If both tubes are patent, a pregnancy rate of 58% may be anticipated, whereas with unilateral patency, a pregnancy rate of 50% can be expected.[2] There is evidence that the hysterosalpingogram can have a therapeutic effect. Patients with patent tubes have an increased pregnancy rate following hysterosalpingography. This effect is more profound with oil contrast than water-soluble preparations.

In some clinics, the **postcoital test** is used to **assess the movement of sperm** through the cervical mucus. Mucus of poor quality may act as a barrier to sperm transport. In the postcoital test, cervical mucus is removed after intercourse just before ovulation and the sperm number and quality are assessed. A normal result is greater than five sperm per high-power field (20 is ideal). The postcoital test result is also evaluated on five observations of the cervical mucus sample that may affect sperm transport including Spinnbarkheit (stretchability >9 cm), volume (>0.2 ml), presence of ferning, viscosity, and cellularity (11 cells per high-power field). If the sperm are not moving or twitching in the cervical mucus the possibility of antisperm antibodies on the sperm or in the cervical mucus should be considered.

ULTRASOUND DIAGNOSIS OF CONDITIONS LEADING TO INFERTILITY

The oviducts are paired structures, approximately 10 cm in length, attached to the superolateral aspects of the uterine cornua terminating with fingerlike fimbriae adjacent to the ovaries. The free border of each ovary is typically covered by the fimbriae and ampullae.[32] The oviducts are the site of fertilization and serve not only to transport the ovum between the ovary and uterus, but fulfill several important roles in the final stages of sperm and oocyte maturation as well.

Sonographic Hysterosalpingography

Confirmation of oviductal patency is of paramount importance to anyone working with infertility patients. The traditional method of assessing patency of the oviducts is with hysterographic studies (HSG) of the uterine cavity and oviducts using fluoroscopy and radiopaque contrast which is injected into the uterus in the radiology department. The desire to limit patient exposure to ionizing radiation, reduce costs, and simplify routine work-ups for infertile couples has led to the development of sonographic techniques to assess the uterine tubal patency which may be performed in the office or clinical setting.

Early studies used transabdominal sonography and saline injection into the uterine cavity to visualize the contours of the uterine cavity and predict tubal patency, primarily by observation of fluid collections within the cul-de-sac.[33-35] The technique was enhanced by the addition of ultrasound contrast media which resulted in improved demarcation of the uterine walls. This technique has largely been replaced with **transvaginal sonography** and **transcervical injection** of either **saline** or **ultrasonographic contrast media.**[36] The technique and instruments are essentially the same as for radiographic hysterosalpingography. The ultrasound probe and hysterosalpingographic instruments are placed in the vagina and intermittent injections of saline or contrast media are performed. The uterine walls are examined for smoothness and irregularities of the contours of the uterine lumen. The probe is then directed toward the adnexae and more medium is injected to observe spillage into the peritoneal cavity.

More recently, **color-flow Doppler sonography** has been used to improve **visualization of spillage from the oviducts.**[36,37] The technique is the same as previously described except that the color-flow Doppler detection window is located over the area of interest prior to the injection of small amounts of media. The first window is located over the lower uterine segment to ascertain the location and sealing of the HSG catheter; a small burst of fluid is injected to verify placement of the catheter and settings of the Doppler window. The second and third windows are located in the transverse plane at the uterotubal junction, allowing visualization of the proximal oviduct and are then moved to visualize the distal oviduct and cul-de-sac. The same anatomic locations are subsequently visualized on the contralateral side. Confirmation of tubal patency is based on the appearance of color flow through the fallopian tube and ipsilateral cul-de-sac. Failure to visualize flow in any part of the tube or cul-de-sac is interpreted as evidence of an obstruction. Tubal patency documented by color-flow Doppler hysterosalpingography compares favorably with radiographic hysterosalpingography.[36] The most recent studies report sensitivity and specificity of 87%. False-positive results were reported to be 9% and false-negative results were 20%.

After conclusion of the fluid injection, a full ultrasound scan of the uterus and adnexae is performed to identify any change from the baseline or preprocedural scan. The second scan is useful to identify **pelvic adhesions** and **hydrosalpinges**. Fluid collections not identified in the preliminary scan may suggest **pelvic adhesions. Hydrosalpinges** are typically easily identified. Scans of free fluid in the cul-de-sac without evidence of loculations or septae are suggestive of absence of significant pelvic adhesions. The uterine cavity may be distended by injection of 2 to 5 ml of saline or contrast media following assessment of tubal patency. This addition to the examination yields detailed visualization of the cavity in both the transverse and longitudinal planes and the identification of **polyps, submucous fibroids, adhesions, or foreign bodies.**

Examination of the uterus and fallopian tubes using high-resolution sonography and color-flow mapping techniques is a safe, easy, and effective method to evaluate women experiencing reproductive disorders. The techniques may be easily incorporated into office or clinic procedures which allows the physician to interpret the results immediately. The advantages include decreased risks of allergic reactions and lower costs. Color-flow mapping makes visualization of flow easier and lowers the risk of misinterpretation, facilitating a rapid and accurate method of assessing tubal patency and the evaluation of the uterine cavity.

Uterine Abnormalities

Uterine Fibroids (Leiomyoma). The study of uterine lesions has been greatly enhanced with the use of transvaginal sonography.[38,39] Uterine leiomyomata are frequently diagnosed in the myometrium. The location and size of individual leiomyomata may be mapped. Changes in the diameter and echotexture of leiomyomata in consecutive examinations may be assessed. Correlation of the presence of leiomyomata with infertility or reproductive failure is not clear; however, serial transvaginal assessment may help in elucidating mechanisms of infertility or reproductive failure in the presence of leiomyomata.[38] Although the relationships between sonographic and surgical findings are under investigation, it appears useful to establish a uterine map for localization of leiomyomata prior to surgical excision. In addition, it may be appropriate to use sonography in the decision-making process when medical treatment for size reduction of leiomyomata is contemplated. For example, administration of gonadotropin releasing hormone analogues (GnRHa) prior to surgery may reduce organ damage and blood loss during surgical excision (Fig. 51-8).

Congenital Anomalies. Congenital abnormalities in the uterine cavity may also be diagnosed using high-resolution transvesical and/or transvaginal ultrasonography (Fig. 51-9).[40-42] Congenital abnormalities may contribute to infertility by repeated early pregnancy loss. Although hysterosalpingography is the usual infertility investigation dedicated to the diagnosis of uterine cavity abnormalities, it is possible to screen for anomalies such as an **arcuate, unicornuate and bicornuate or septate uterus** using transvaginal ultrasonography at the time of initial re-

A

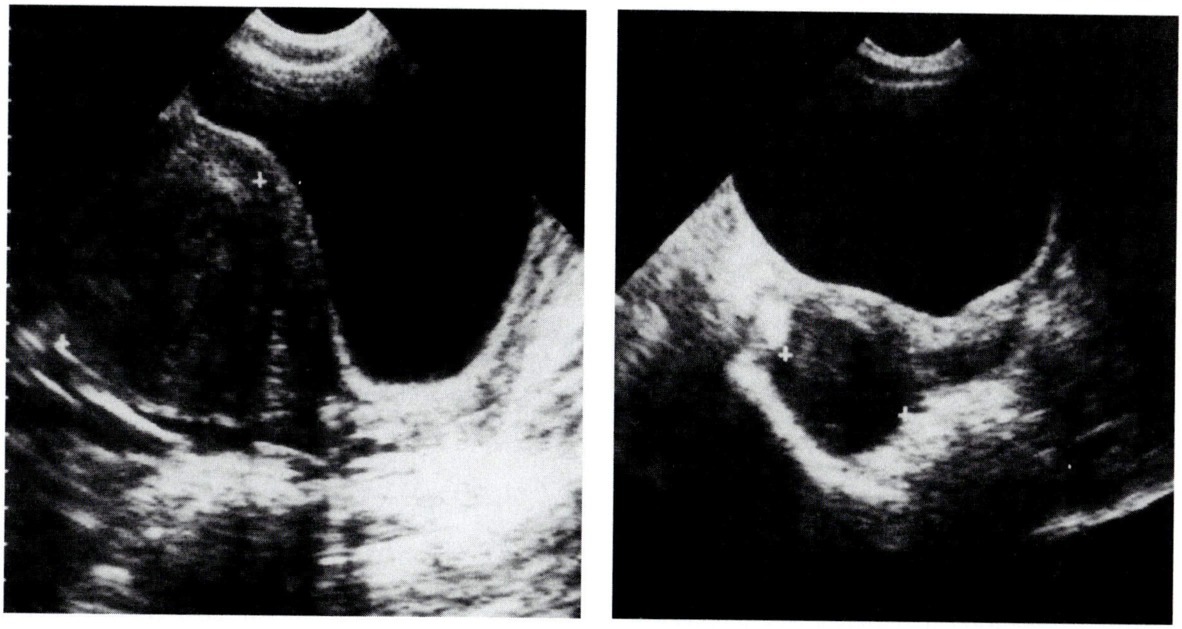

B

FIG. 51-8. Fibroid (+ marks lesion). Sagittal scans before, **A,** and after, **B,** treatment with GnRH agonist show diminution in size.

A

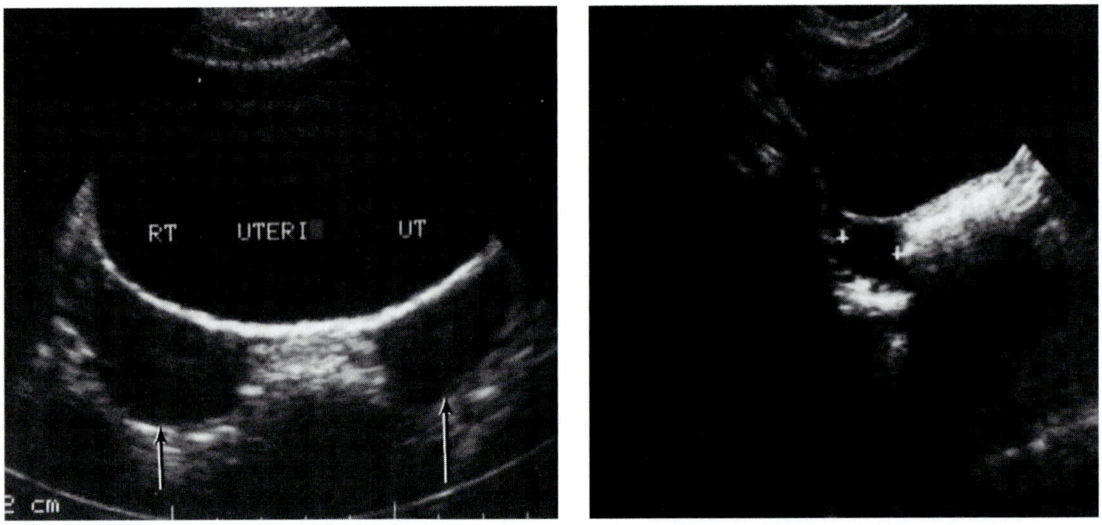

B

FIG. 51-9. Uterus didelphys. **A,** Transverse (transabdominal) sonogram shows two uterine bodies *(arrows)*. There was also a double cervix and double vagina. **B,** Ovarian ultrasound performed to determine side of ovulation shows a dominant follicle in the right ovary.

ferral. **Uterus didelphys** may also be visualized as complete separation of the female reproductive tract.[40,42] If an anomaly is suspected following sonographic examination, definitive hysterosalpingography may be used to establish the exact contour of the uterine cavity. The advantages of this approach are that the ultrasonographic examination is noninvasive, is performed without contrast and reduces the potential chance of infection. Saline-enhanced sonography may provide additional information regarding intrauterine morphology. In addition, a color-flow Doppler investigation may be used to identify the vascular supply to various portions of the uterus and may be valuable prior to reconstructive surgery.

Diagnosis of **adenomyosis** with sonography has been attempted, although definitive diagnosis with ultrasound technology has proven difficult. A combined approach of hysterosalpingography and transabdominal ultrasonography has not been successful; however, adenomyosis has been successfully evaluated using transvaginal ultrasonography.[38,43] Additionally, it has been suggested that color-flow mapping with transvaginal sonography may be useful in the assessment of adenomyosis although this condition remains out of the realm of routine evaluation.[39]

Nabothian cysts of various diameters are frequently noted at the external cervical os. The presence of these cysts is probably not noteworthy; however, small cysts may also be seen at the junction of the internal cervix and the lower uterine segment and at various intrauterine locations. The correlation of these small cystic structures with infertility is not known although it is probably inconsequential. Survey studies are ongoing.

Gartner's cysts result from the remnants of the embryonic Wolffian duct system and are frequently observed along the lateral aspects of the cervix and lower uterine segment. Single, fluid-filled cystic structures, multilocular complexes and long, sometimes tortuous cylindrical morphologies are among the many iterations of Gartner's cystic complexes; a role for these structures is not known in the investigation of infertility.

Ovarian Factors

Cystic Ovarian Disease.

The **Stein-Leventhal syndrome (polycystic ovary syndrome or PCO)** probably represents the best-known endocrine abnormality associated with infertility, but there are several other ovulatory disorders with which the ultrasonographer should be familiar. These conditions can occasionally be suspected on the basis of ultrasound examination and the physician thereby alerted. In most cases, however, ultrasound does not offer a definitive diagnosis.

Polycystic ovary disease (PCO) is a complex endocrine disturbance resulting from chronic anovulation. Symptoms, signs, ultrasound findings, and hormonal values are quite variable, making the diagnosis anything but certain in many cases. The most common symptoms are amenorrhea, hirsutism, obesity, and infertility. The pathophysiology of this condition is quite complex. The inciting cause of PCO is still debated, but FSH and LH are in a "steady state." This results in the recruitment and early development of multiple follicles. The steady-state production of LH causes an increased concentration of androgen in the ovarian microenvironment. The androgen is converted peripherally to estrogen, but its local concentration in the ovary im-

A

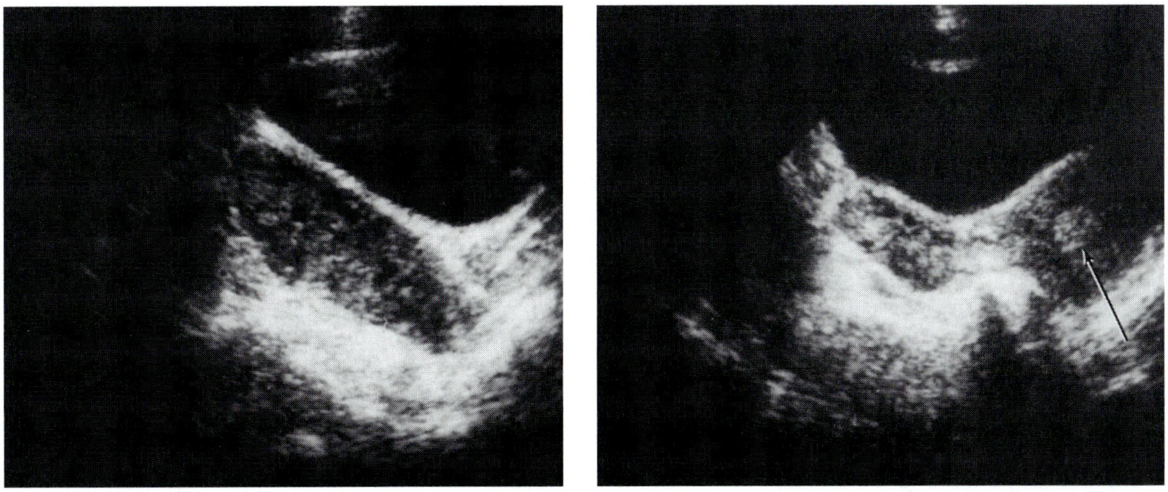

B

FIG. 51-10. Polycystic ovary disease. **A**, Sagittal scan of right ovary and, **B**, transverse scan of pelvis show multiple tiny ovarian cysts, ovarian enlargement, and thickened endometrium *(arrow)*.

TABLE 51-1
FINDINGS IN POLYCYSTIC OVARY DISEASE

	Parisi	Tabbakh	Hann
Total number of patients diagnosed PCO	25	20	28
Number of patients with enlarged ovaries	25 (100%)	15 (75%)	20 (71%)
Average ovarian surface area (N=4.8 cm^2)	12.9	9.8	Not measured
Average ovarian volume (N=5.7 cm^3)	Not measured	15.5%	14.3
Cases with multiple cysts	75%	55%	39%
Cases with hypoechoic ovaries	25%	25%	25%
Cases with "normal" ovarian echotexture	0%	20%	29%

Data from Parisi L, Tramonti M, Derchi L, et al: Polycystic ovarian disease: ultrasonic evaluation and correlations with clinical and hormonal data. *J Clin Ultrasound* 1984;12:21-26; el Tabbakh GH, Lotfy I, Azab I, et al: Correlation of the ultrasonic appearance of the ovaries in polycystic ovarian disease and the clinical, hormonal and laparoscopic findings. *Am J Obstet Gynecol* 1986;154:(4)892-895; and Hann LE, Hall DA, McArdle C, et al: Polycystic ovarian disease: sonographic spectrum. *Radiology* 1984;150:(2)531-534.

pedes follicular maturation, resulting in atresia. The peripheral high estrogen has a positive-feedback effect on the pituitary/hypothalamus, stimulating increased LH production, thereby completing this "vicious circle." The correct diagnosis of PCO is important not only from the perspective of diagnosing a cause of infertility, but it may also be life saving, as patients with elevated estrogen have a significantly **increased risk of endometrial carcinoma** and possibly **ovarian malignancy**.[44]

The **ultrasound examination** (Table 51-1) may have variable results. In the majority of cases, ovarian size is increased (70% to 100%) as is the surface area. Multiple cysts are present in 40% to 80% of cases (Fig. 51-10). Several authors describe a hypoechoic ovary and comment on thickened "irregular contour." There is very little correlation between ultrasound findings and symptoms or their duration. The presence of a **very prominent thick endometrial echo** is suggestive of PCO,[45] especially if other ultrasound, clinical, and endocrinologic findings point to this diagnosis. **Treatment** of PCO may be initiated with a trial of clomiphene citrate (CC). Ultrasound is often performed near the expected midcycle (after a progesterone-induced withdrawal bleed) in an attempt to document ovulation in patients so treated. If ovulation fails to occur, then hCG may be added midcycle to induce ovulation, which may not have occurred because of a failed midcycle surge of LH. As many as 75% of patients with PCO treated with clomiphene will ovulate, but many less than this will conceive. Wedge resection is

A

B

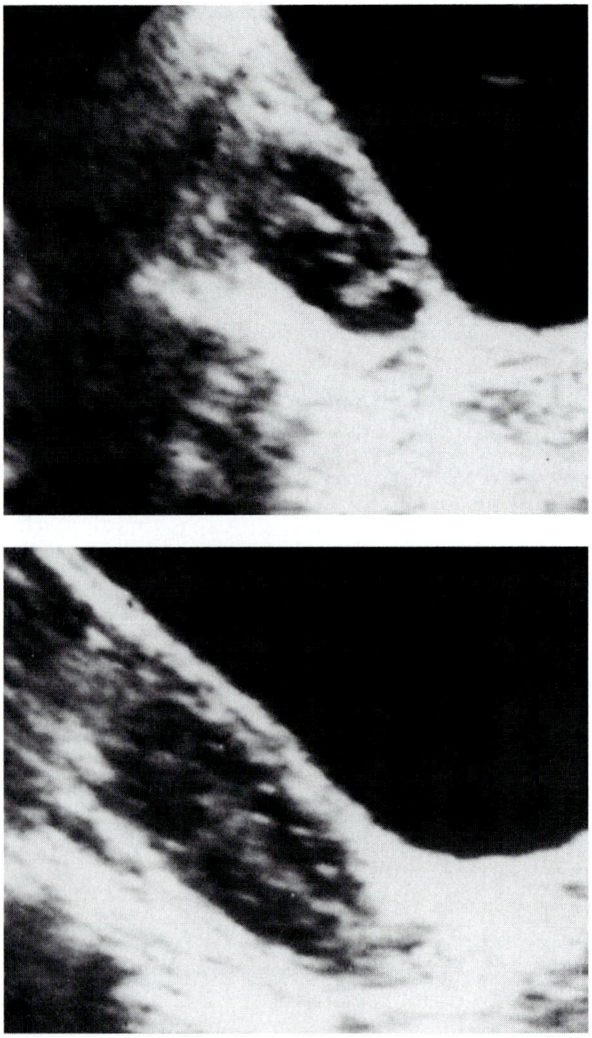

FIG. 51-11. The ovary in hypothalamic amenorrhea. **A,** Patient on birth control pill. **B,** Patient with hypothalamic amenorrhea after cessation of the BCP. Note the cohort of atretic follicles. An identical appearance may also be seen: at menarche, in women doing extreme forms of physical training, in lactating women, and in the normal follicular phase of the menstrual cycle.

still used by some as a means of treatment, but its mechanism of action is uncertain.[45]

Cystic ovarian disease with "hypothalamic amenorrhea." There is another group of cystic ovarian disease entities that are encountered not infrequently.[46,47] This group of patients includes a wide variety of normal and pathologic conditions, including patients who have developed amenorrhea secondary to weight loss,[46] extensive exercise, or lactation, or after cessation of taking the birth control pill (Fig. 51-11). In our experience, these cysts are most often circumferentially oriented in the ovary. Patients with these types of cysts almost invariably have low estrogen states, and therefore, the endometrial echo is very often attenuated (the opposite of patients with PCO). The distinction between this so-called "hypothalamic amenorrhea" and PCO oligomenorrhea is not one that can be invariably established by ovarian morphologic assessment. The ultrasound examination can, however, offer some direction. After the appropriate hormonal/clinical assessment a precise diagnosis may be made.

Endometriosis

Endometriosis is one of the most common benign gynecologic conditions, estimated to be present in 10% to 25% of women with gynecologic disorders, having a prevalence of 1% in reproductive age women. The symptoms of endometriosis include the triad of infertility, dyspareunia, and dysmenorrhea. The incidence of endometriosis in infertile women is 40%. Endometriosis is defined as the presence of functional endometrial tissue outside the uterine cavity. There are several types of deposits, including plaques, implants, nodules, and endometriomas. An endometrioma is a cystic structure lined with endometrial epithelium.

Among patients with endometriosis the prevalence of infertility is estimated to be approximately 30% to 40%. Although the pathophysiology in severe endometriosis is almost certainly related to mechanical factors, such as tubal obstruction, other factors have been implicated to explain infertility in mild cases.

Ultrasound has a limited role in the diagnosis of endometriosis largely confined to identifying endometriomas. **Endometriomas** are typically hypoechoic, multiple or single, cystic-appearing lesions. Endometriomas vary in size and have a low-amplitude uniform echotexture in the cavity of the cyst often best appreciated with endovaginal imaging.

Often, diffuse forms of endometriosis escape detection with ultrasound.[48] Friedman et al.[48] were only able to detect endometriosis with ultrasound in 4 of 37 patients. In another study, the authors were able to correctly detect endometriosis in 13 of 13 patients.[49]

Ectopic Pregnancy

With the development of endovaginal scanning techniques, the reliability and the role of ultrasound in diagnosis of this entity have been clearly established. The triad of an empty uterus, free fluid, and an adnexal mass coupled with a positive pregnancy test should always alert the sonographer and clinician to the possibility of ectopic pregnancy. Some experts suggest that this combination of findings is accurate in 95% of cases. In 10% of cases, a definitive diagnosis can be made by the demonstration of a live ectopic pregnancy. Of current interest is the recent demonstration of conservative and "semi-invasive" management strategies,[50-52] including nonsurgical treatment of selected patients,[51,52] by injection of the fetus with potassium chloride[51] or methotrexate.

Pelvic Inflammatory Disease

More than 3 million cases of gonorrhea and 3 to 5 million cases of chlamydia occur annually in the United States.[53] Of women with salpingitis, 25% will experience long-term complications, the most notable being infertility, which occurs in 20%. Predisposing factors for pelvic inflammatory disease (PID) include:

- Prior episode of gonococcal salpingitis
- Multiple sexual partners
- Use of IUD

At least two infectious agents have been implicated in acute salpingitis, with gonorrhea accounting for 33% to 80% of cases. Clinically, the diagnosis of PID should be suspected in patients with lower abdominal pain, purulent discharge, and fever. The ultrasound findings are often nonspecific. Initially the uterus may be enlarged with indistinct margins. In the early phase of the illness there may be mild adnexal enlargement with loss of tissue plane definition. As the process becomes more severe, ill-defined areas of decreased echogenicity may be seen. These may be purely cystic or solid in appearance and may be associated with fluid in the cul-de-sac. The fluid accumulations often extend posterior to the uterus. Ultimately frank abscess may develop. The differential diagnosis from hematoma, ectopic pregnancy, and endometriosis may be extremely difficult.

Follicular Development In Natural Ovarian Cycles

The ability of ultrasound to document morphologic changes in the ovary and uterus during normal and induced cycles has had great significance to reproductive medicine.[54-57] Hackeloer et al.,[58] in 1979, was the first to demonstrate with ultrasound sequential **follicular development of the normal menstrual cycle** (Fig. 51-12).[58] Since then, ultrasound has had an expanded role in the diagnosis and treatment of reproductive disorders particularly as it has been applied to follicular monitoring and endometrial development in natural and induced cycles.

The ovary is usually visualized during ultrasound scanning of the pelvis either abdominally or transvaginally. It is most often located above the iliac vessels but may be found in the cul-de-sac or adherent to the uterus. It is hypoechoic compared with the surrounding structures often with translucent follicles which may vary in size from a few millimeters to 2.5 centimeters. **Follicular development** begins in embryonic life and the primordial follicles are suspended in their development in the diplotene stage of the first meiotic prophase. At all times, including pregnancy, there is a continuous process of follicular growth and atresia. Although born with approximately 2,000,000 follicles only about 400 to 600 will actually mature and ovulate. When the supply is exhausted menopause is reached. During **each menstrual cycle,** under the influence of endocrine, autocrine, and paracrine hormones and peptides, a cohort of follicles are recruited. They become ultrasonically visible as fluid accumulates in the follicular antrum by day 5 to 7. By this same time, usually one dominant follicle has developed which will continue to grow and ovulate. The remainder of the recruited follicles undergo a process of atresia, called apoptosis. By day 8 to 10 the dominant follicle can be detected ultrasonographically as the largest follicle and is observed to grow in a linear fashion approximately 2 mm/day.[59] The maximum mean diameter reaches approximately 20 mm before ovulation occurs (range, 16 to 28 mm).[54,58,60] In natural cycles there is a remarkable correlation between the mean follicular diameter of the dominant follicle and estradiol (E_2) levels.[58] This supports the belief that 90% to 95% of measurable E_2 in a normal cycle is elaborated by the dominant follicle.[54] The E_2 level usually peaks 24 to 36 hours before ovulation. This rise in E_2 triggers the LH surge that usually results in resumption of meiosis and luteinization of the granulosa cells with subsequent production of progesterone. The LH surge usually begins 34 to 36 hours before follicular rupture.[61] It is also responsible for prostaglandin and other eicosanoid production that are required for the digestion of the follicular wall and release of the oocyte. In natural cycles the dominant follicle will be apparent by days 8 to 10. In 5% to 10% of cycles, more than one ovulatory follicle will develop.

Before ovulation the granulosa cell layer separates from the hypervascular and edematous thecal layer. This may be seen sonographically approximately 24 hours before ovulation as a line of decreased echogenicity surrounding the follicle. Folding and separation of the granulosa cell layer result in a crenated appearance and often precede ovulation by 6 to 10 hours. The expanded cumulus oophorus may be seen projecting from the wall into the follicle. Follicular rupture has been observed and may last between 1 and 20 minutes.[62] After ovulation the **corpus hemorrhagicum** is found and may be identified sonographically as early as one hour later. (Fig. 51-13). The follicle at this time may have one of a number of appearances, including increased echogenicity secondary to intrafollicular hemorrhage, or if no bleeding has occurred, the cyst may be sonolucent. It is also usually of diminished size when compared with its preovulatory dimensions. Over the next 4 to 5 days, it may increase in size to 2 to 3 cm as the resulting **corpus luteum** (CL) produces progesterone. However, if pregnancy fails to occur, the CL regresses in size and function.

Ovulation can be assessed by real-time ultrasonography[63] and evidence of ovulation can be seen

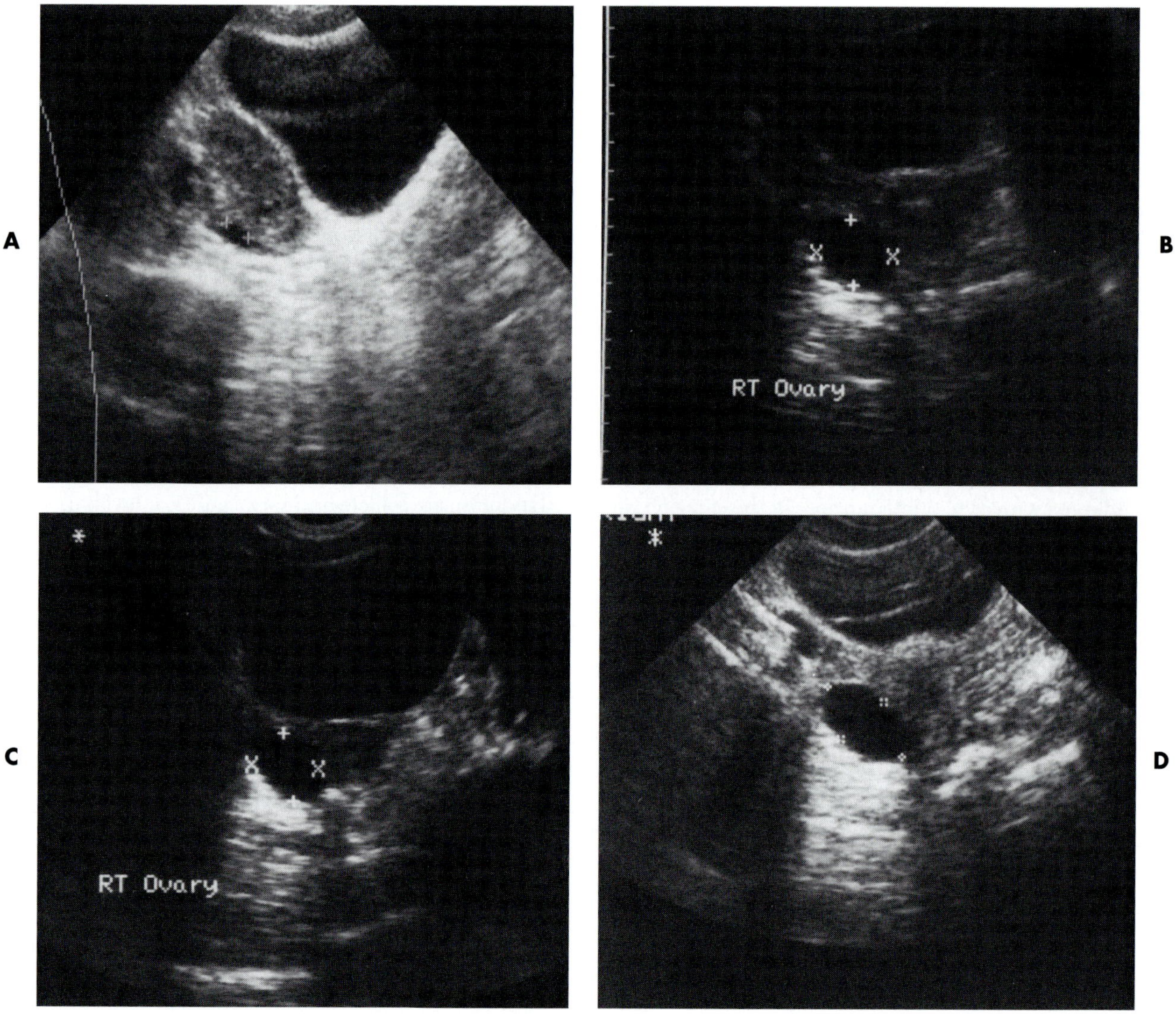

FIG. 51-12. Normal nonstimulated cycle. **A,** Day 4, follicle measured 0.74 cm in diameter. **B,** Day 7, follicle diameter measured 2.5 cm. **C,** Day 10, follicle measured 2.6 cm in mean diameter. **D,** Day 13, follicle measured 2.85 cm. Ovulation could be expected within 24 hours of day 13.

in approximately 80% of cycles. It may be signaled by a sudden reduction in size of a previously observed large follicle, development of a corpus hemorrhagicum or corpus luteum, or the appearance of fluid in the posterior cul-de-sac that was not seen previously. The volume of the fluid in the posterior cul-de-sac has been determined to be greater than that attributable to the release of fluid from the follicle itself.[64] Mittelschmerz is not associated with follicular rupture as once believed, but rather this discomfort occurs with the rapid growth of the dominant follicle immediately prior to ovulation.[65] Mittelschmerz is usually experienced by women on the same day as the LH peak (77% of cases) and therefore precedes follicular rupture as can be documented by ultrasound.[54] When present, the rise in basal body temperature occurs approximately two days after the LH peak and is coincident with the production of progesterone.

Follicular monitoring with ultrasound can be accomplished either transvaginally or transabdominally at any time during the menstrual cycle.[66,67] Certain pathologic conditions including uterine, tubal, and ovarian abnormalities may be better assessed if visualized by transabdominal scanning. However, in most cases, the transvaginal approach will provide the best information. This is attributed to the superior resolution and high-quality images that can be obtained by this method. As well, transvaginal scanning precludes the need for a full bladder and is therefore a more comfortable and easy-to-schedule procedure.

The periods of greatest interest in assessing follicular development are the late follicular phase and the time of ovulation. Serial ultrasound examinations

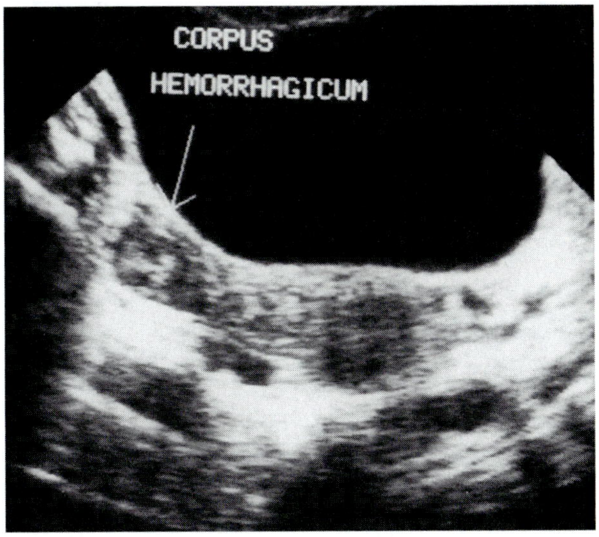

FIG. 51-13. Corpus hemorrhagicum. The follicle is smaller and more echogenic after rupture.

when coupled with endocrine tests at these times may reveal subtle abnormalities of follicular selection, growth, function, and ovulation.[68] Subtle abnormalities in follicular growth, when detected, may be corrected by a variety of therapies which usually involve induction of ovulation. Studies of this nature appear to be most useful in the elucidation of problems associated with idiopathic infertility. Although serial ultrasound examinations during several ovarian cycles may appear to be a daunting task, aberrations in follicular development or ovulation may usually be identified within a few cycles.

Identification of Follicular Phase Defects. Serum estradiol concentrations and ultrasonographically determined growth profiles of preovulatory follicles normally run parallel courses.[6,7] Therefore, serial ultrasonography and evaluation of systemic estrogen levels are extremely useful in the isolation and identification of follicular phase defects. Patients may present with estradiol concentrations that appear to be within clinically normal limits for the preovulatory phase of the menstrual cycle; however, sonography may reveal several follicles of 5 to 10 mm in diameter and the absence of a dominant preovulatory follicle. Alternatively, ultrasound examination during the late follicular phase may reveal a follicle of ostensibly preovulatory diameter (e.g., 22 mm) and the patient may exhibit clinically low levels of estradiol. The follicle subsequently regresses over what would normally be the luteal phase of the cycle.

Subtle defects in follicular recruitment, development, physiologic selection of the ovulatory follicle, follicular maturation and ovulation probably play a greater role in unexplained infertility than is generally appreciated. Seemingly minor disturbances in the continuum of folliculogenesis, ovulation, and luteogenesis may be responsible for failure of conception. Synchronous development and maturation of the oocyte and follicle in addition to the acquisition of cell surface receptors which enable the follicle to respond to FSH or LH currently are under intense scrutiny. Assessment of follicular dynamics and mapping the fates of individual follicles in normative and infertile patients also are under active investigation.

Follicular tracking has a number of other clinical applications (see box on p. 1424). As previously described the precise time of spontaneous ovulation can be predicted with follicular measurements in conjunction with LH testing in natural and induced cycles. The timing for artificially triggered ovulation with LH or HCG can also be determined by follicular monitoring. This information facilitates timed intercourse and may improve pregnancy rates when insemination of sperm is so timed. When treating infertility patients with Müllerian anomalies or absent, damaged, or blocked fallopian tubes, it may be necessary to determine the side of ovulation in a treatment cycle. With this knowledge, intrauterine insemination (IUI) of sperm would not be undertaken when a dominant follicle is not on the functional side and therefore, treatments that cannot possibly be successful are avoided.

INDICATIONS FOR FOLLICULAR TRACKING

Use of Ultrasound in Assisted Reproduction

Ultrasonographic imaging and controlled ovarian superstimulation have become intrinsic parts of therapies involved in the assisted reproductive technologies (ART). Careful monitoring of the results of ovarian stimulation regimens is an especially important aspect of any ART therapy. The protocols for the use of ovarian stimulatory agents vary tremendously; however, ultrasonography remains the common denominator for monitoring the progress of stimulation. Ovarian stimulation with clomiphene citrate, human menopausal gonadotropins (hMG), GnRHa, or other pharmaceutical agents designed to enhance follicular development may be used to induce ovulation in anovulatory women, mimic a normal menstrual cycle with the intent of synchronizing maturation of the oocyte and follicle, or to superstimulate the ovaries to collect oocytes for use in the ART.

In any of the assisted reproductive technologies, regardless of technical complexity, accurate timing is critical for administration of human chorionic gonadotropin (hCG) and oocyte retrieval or insemination. The role of ultrasonography is the evaluation of

INDICATIONS FOR FOLLICULAR TRACKING

Natural cycles

Assessment of follicular growth and ovulation (luteinized unruptured follicle)
Prediction of ovulation
- Timed intercourse
- Intrauterine insemination of sperm

Determination of side of ovulation
- Blocked or absent fallopian tube when performing intrauterine insemination of sperm
- When Müllerian abnormalities may alter intrauterine insemination technique

Induced cycles

Human menopausal gonadotropin ovarian hyperstimulation
- *In vitro* fertilization
- Intrauterine insemination of sperm

Clomiphene citrate ovulation induction
- Timed intercourse
- Intrauterine insemination of sperm

Gonadotropin releasing hormone ovulation induction
- Ovulation triggering with human chorionic gonadotropin hormone or luteinizing hormone

the development of a cohort of follicles recruited and stimulated with the exogenous hormones on a daily basis in a rapid, noninvasive manner. In addition, the application of new computer-assisted ultrasound image analysis algorithms is beginning to make possible the interpretation of physiologic status of individual follicles during the stimulation protocol.

INDUCTION OF OVULATION

Induction of ovulation refers to the use of exogenous agents to stimulate the growth and development of follicles within the ovary and/or enhancement of the process of follicular rupture and release of an oocyte. Ovulation induction therapy may be performed for many reasons varying from simply providing adequate stimulation to achieve a single ovulation to the production of a cohort of oocytes for *in vitro* fertilization (IVF) or other ART.

The primary goal of ovarian superstimulation is to bypass atresia in a follicle or cohort of follicles, sustain development to a preovulatory state and obtain properly matured oocytes for fertilization. In women who have clinically normal ovarian cycles, induction of ovulation may be also be described as *controlled ovarian hyperstimulation*.

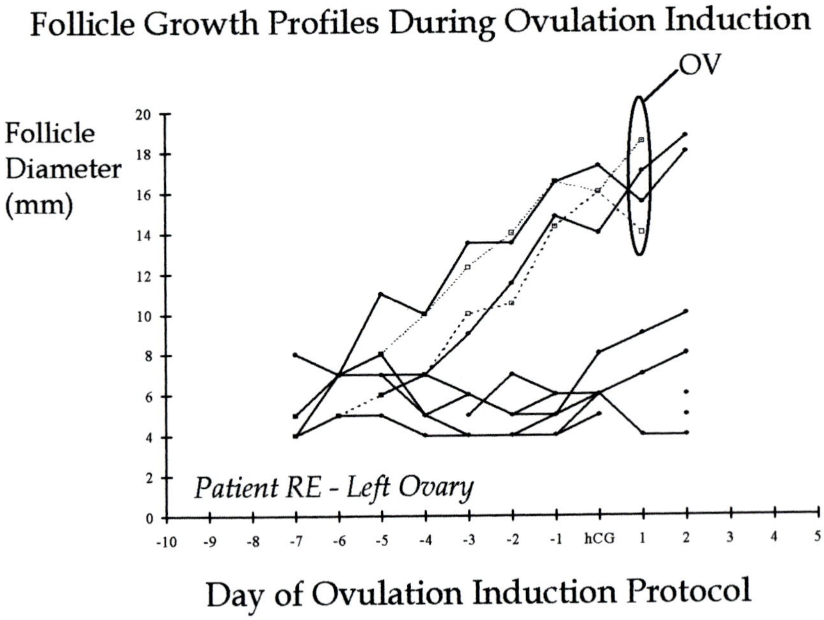

FIG. 51-14. Follicle growth profiles of each individually identified follicle in one ovary during an ovulation induction protocol. Dashed lines represent the profiles of follicles which ovulated in response to an ovulation-inducing dose of human chorionic gonadotropin (hCG). Solid lines represent the profiles of follicles that did not ovulate.

Ultrasonography is essential in determining the numbers and fates of individual follicles stimulated by exogenous gonadotropins. **The follicular kinetics of an ovarian superstimulation protocol** are shown (Fig. 51-14). It is also important to note that the expected linear relationship between circulating estradiol 17 concentrations and follicular diameter may not exist during ovulation induction.[69] Ultrasonography is thus a crucial element of ovulation induction protocols (Fig. 51-15). Similarly, new time-series and surface image analyses of the ultrasound images of follicles during ovulation protocols are showing profound differences between follicles which are healthy and eventually ovulate, and those who are atretic (Figs. 51-16 and 51-17). Using these exciting new types of imaging, the dosage of gonadotropins may be altered to achieve optimal follicular development.

Timing of hCG administration is critical in all ovulation induction protocols. In monitoring the course of an ovulation induction, the responses of individual follicles to the ovulatory dose of hCG may be as important as monitoring the number and rates of growth of the follicles. The number of ovulatory follicles should be determined and unruptured follicles remaining in the ovaries assessed (Fig. 51-18).[70] If conception does not occur, the induction protocol may be altered to achieve a better response.

A

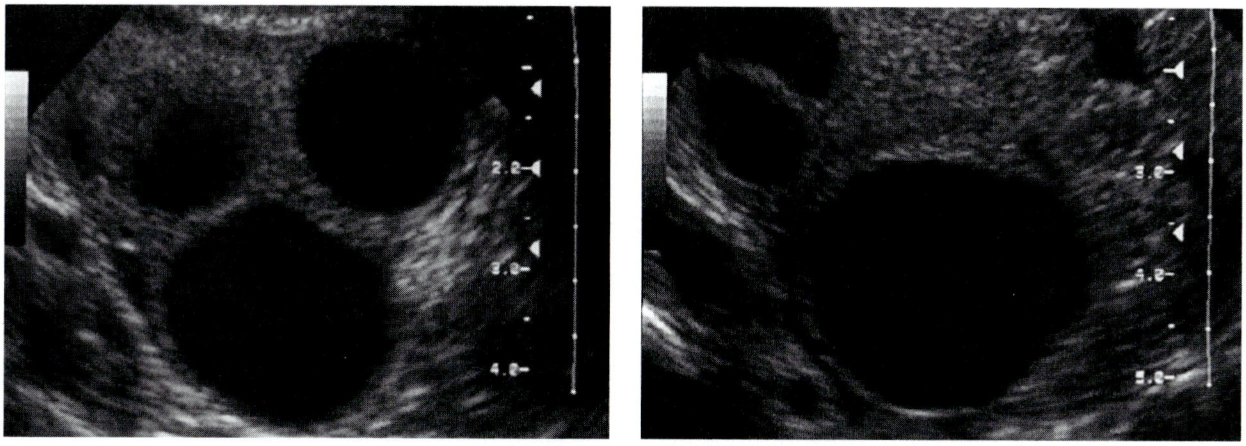

B

FIG. 51-15. Follicle changes after ovarian superstimulation. **A,** Two preovulatory diameter (20-mm) follicles recorded during an ovarian superstimulation protocol 24 hours following an ovulation-inducing injection of hCG. **B,** Same follicles 48 hours following hCG. Note that the superior follicle has ovulated, whereas the follicle in the inferior aspect of the image has not.

A

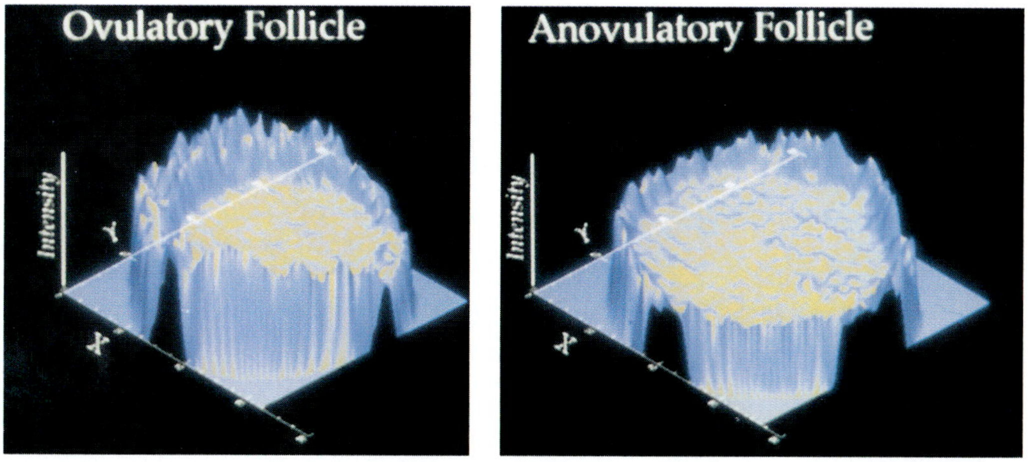

B

FIG. 51-16. Profound graphic differences in the image representing the follicle which ovulated versus the one which did not. Images of the follicles in Fig. 51-15 processed for surface image analysis. The X and Y coordinates represent distance in two dimensions on the image (i.e., length and width) and Z represents pixel intensity. This technique allows discriminatory examination of the surfaces and rapid visual assessment of ultrasonographic attributes associated with follicle health (state of viability or atresia).

Clomiphene Citrate

The primary indication for clomiphene citrate therapy is anovulation. Women exhibiting the oligo-ovulation associated with mild polycystic ovarian syndrome also are good candidates for clomiphene citrate therapy. Amenorrhea or oligomenorrhea is secondary to both of these conditions. The standardized dosage regimen is intended to mimic the increased circulating FSH levels seen in the early follicular phase of the menstrual cycle. Increased FSH levels during this period should initiate development of a follicle which attains an appropriate diameter and state of maturity. This follicle will induce an LH surge allowing ovulation at the appropriate time of the menstrual cycle.

Clomiphene citrate is a weak estrogen agonist with a long half-life that exerts its effect by binding to hypothalamic estrogen receptors and facilitates increased gonadotropin secretion. The FSH elaborated by clomiphene citrate binding recruits follicles and sustains their continued development. The normal physiological mechanism for selection and dominance of preovulatory follicles may be overridden and more than one preovulatory follicle may develop, as with any therapy which is based upon supraphysiologic FSH doses. **Multiple follicular development ranges** from 20% to 60% per cycle. Follicles induced with clomiphene citrate appear to follow a normal course of preovulatory development. Estrogen levels are consistent with those observed in spontaneous cycles and the diameter of preovulatory follicles is reportedly 22 mm to 23 mm.[71-73] Intensive ultrasonographic monitoring, although desirable, is not mandatory with clomiphene citrate inductions of ovulation, because ovarian hyperstimulation is rare and the multiple pregnancy rate is approximately 5%. However, not all follicles induced with clomiphene citrate ovulate (Fig. 51-19), and analysis of the follicle wall echotexture reveals thin, high-amplitude echoes and follicular fluid echoes which are dramatically different from those of unstimulated preovulatory follicles or follicles stimulated with the menopausal gonadotropins (Fig. 51-20).[74]

Clomiphene citrate is administered as an oral medication and therapy is typically initiated on day 5 of the menstrual cycle. Standard starting doses are 50 or 100 mg daily from day 5 to day 9. Most women will exhibit a spontaneous LH surge and ovulate approximately 5 to 7 days following completion of the clomiphene citrate regimen. If a pregnancy is not established within three to four cycles of clomiphene citrate use, then serial ultrasound examinations during the follicular phase are well justified. If the standard starting doses do not initiate the development of follicles at the appropriate time, the dose of clomiphene citrate may be increased and/or administered for a longer period (e.g., 10 days). In many instances, the follicles may not ovulate until they attain a diameter of 30 to 35 mm, or alternatively, do not ovulate and regress.[66]

The administration of hCG to initiate the changes associated with ovulation may then be required. It is important to appreciate that hCG should not be administered as an empiric therapy or according to a specific menstrual cycle date. The timing for administration of the hCG injection is best performed following serial ultrasonographic examination to ascertain progressive growth of the dominant follicles. The hCG injection should be administered when the follicles are 18 to 20 mm in diameter; ovulation would be expected to occur within 34 to 48 hours.[70,71] Clinically, it has been assumed that menstrual bleeding 30 to 40 days following clomiphene citrate administration in amenorrheic women indicates that ovulation has occurred. New research on normal and aberrant ovulation may be interpreted to mean that ovulation with the release of an oocyte is not a foregone conclusion if menses result and even if circulating progesterone levels are in the low, clinically normal range.[70] Luteinized unruptured follicles or hemorrhage anovulatory follicles are subtle defects in ovulation which appear to be more common than previously believed. Therefore, it is increasingly important to verify ovulation with follow-up ultrasonographic examinations and assessment of midluteal phase progesterone concentrations.

CLOMIPHENE CITRATE

Clomid (clomiphene citrate)

Indication

Absent/infrequent ovulation/unexplained infertility

Mechanism

Binds to estrogen receptors and "fools" the hypothalamus/pituitary into thinking estrogen is low causing an increase in follicle-stimulating and luteinizing hormone secretion

Administered

50-200 mg orally days 5 to 9

Ultrasound

May show multiple follicles/one dominant

May be used to time human chorionic gonadotropin administration

Results

75% of pregnancies occur in the first three cycles

75% ovulate

Pregnancy rate 15%-40%

5%-7% multiple pregnancy (usually twins)

Severe hyperstimulation syndrome rare

HUMAN MENOPAUSAL GONADOTROPIN

Indication
- Absent/infrequent ovulation
- Failed Clomid induction/unexplained infertility

Mechanism
- Contains follicle-stimulating hormone ± luteinizing hormone and causes follicular development

Administered
- Intramuscular or subcutaneous injection

Ultrasound
- Multiple follicles
- Used for timing human chorionic gonadotropin administration
- Used for diagnosis of hyperstimulation syndrome

Results
- 90% ovulate
- Pregnancy rate 15% to 20%/cycle
- 15% to 20% multiple pregnancy rate

Human Menopausal Gonadotrophins

Ovulation induction with the hMG typically follows a complex regimen which involves the daily injection of supraphysiologic doses of FSH and LH. The relative purity of the FSH component varies with the drug chosen for the stimulation. Some of the gonadotropin preparations contain approximately equal quantities of FSH and LH whereas others contain an FSH to LH ratio of approximately nine to one. New advances in the purification of hMG have seen the development of ultrapure products with less than 1% LH components. It is also expected that pure FSH derived from recombinant sources will soon become available for clinical use.

Ovulation induction with hMG may be carried out in many variations in women with normal ovarian cyclicity or anovulation. Anovulatory women may be started on an induction protocol at any time, whereas protocols in cyclic women are initiated on specific days. In some centers, initial follicle recruitment is stimulated with clomiphene citrate or GnRH analogues and then completed with hMG, other protocols use hMG exclusively. Menstrual cycles for groups of women with normal ovulatory cycles may be synchronized using GnRH analogues or oral contraceptives to suppress ovarian activity. Women in our program whose cycles are synchronized in this manner typically begin taking oral contraceptives to suppress the ovaries no later than day 5 of their natural menstrual cycle and continue taking them for at least 2 weeks prior to beginning ovulation induction. On a specified date, all women stop ovarian suppression and we begin ovulation induction. Typically, we begin hMG stimulation on cycle day 3. Intensive ultrasonographic surveillance is then initiated after 5 days of hMG injections. Alternatively, hMG injections may be initiated on day 3 to day 5 of a natural menstrual cycle. Depending on the follicular response of each woman, the daily dose of gonadotropins may be increased or decreased to either stimulate more follicles or to prevent ovarian hyperstimulation, respectively.

Ovarian response to induction with hMG should be assessed by daily measurement of serum estradiol and ultrasonography. Both methods of surveillance play complementary roles in controlled ovarian hyperstimulation; however, the importance of intensive ultrasonographic monitoring during the stimulation cycle cannot be overemphasized. When the largest follicle first attains a predetermined diameter (e.g., 18 to 20 mm), hCG 5000 or 10,000 IU is administered to trigger the final phases of follicular maturation leading to ovulation. An image of preovulatory follicles on the day after hCG administration is shown (Fig. 51-18). Oocyte retrieval for the assisted reproductive technologies is scheduled for 30 to 34 hours following hCG. Ovulation is expected to occur 34 to 48 hours following hCG administration in women undergoing IUI using prewashed husband's sperm. Ultrasonographic examinations should be continued until all follicles have either ovulated or shown ultrasonographically detectable signs of atresia. Images of an ovary following **multiple ovulation** show multiple collapsed follicles with crenated walls.

The relationship between follicular size and oocyte maturity has not yet been determined. However, hCG is usually administered when the leading preovulatory follicle attains 18 to 20 mm. Oocyte maturity has been postulated to occur at a mean follicular diameter of 15 to 16 mm in hMG stimulated cycles; however, it is possible that follicle diameter does not correlate well with the stage of maturity and quality of the oocyte.[74,75] No differences in the fertilization rate of oocytes aspirated from follicles in various size categories were observed in a recent study although the lack of differences may also have been caused by *in vitro* maturation of the oocytes.[27] The characteristics and appropriate sizes of follicles that produce mature oocytes ready for fertilization remain the subject of much controversy and research. These observations underscore the importance of monitoring the development of individual follicles; any follicle that attains 14 mm in diameter has the potential to ovulate fertilizable oocytes. Some reports have suggested that reduced oocyte quality and fertilization rates result from ova of smaller follicles; however, the prospects for *in vitro* maturation of immature oocytes were not considered at that time.[76]

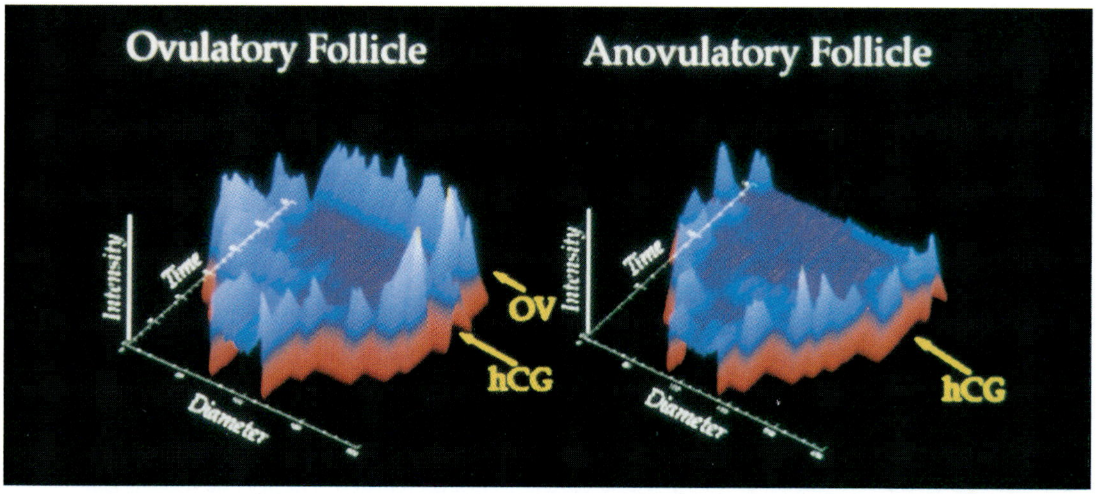

FIG. 51-17. Three dimensions in graphic display are follicle diameter, pixel intensity, and time. Time-series analysis of the follicles in Fig. 51-15. Visual assessment of the surface features representing various portions of the follicles provides important clues regarding the physiologic status at different time points during follicle development or regression. Visual clues enable the identification of time-related structural changes which may be quantitatively characterized. Physiologically important time periods may be identified with this technique and specific images selected for more detailed analysis.

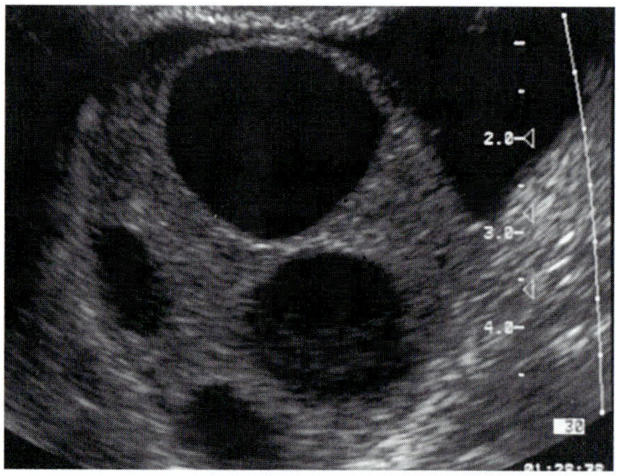

FIG. 51-18. An unovulated follicle remaining in the ovary of a woman in an ovarian superstimulation, ovulation induction protocol. Three ovulation sites are observed in the inferior aspect of the ovary, and the unovulated follicle is observed in the superior aspect. The most important ultrasound scan performed in the ovulation-induction protocol is the one 48 to 72 hours after the ovulation-inducing dose of human chorionic gonadotropin (hCG) to evaluate the efficacy of the treatment regimen.

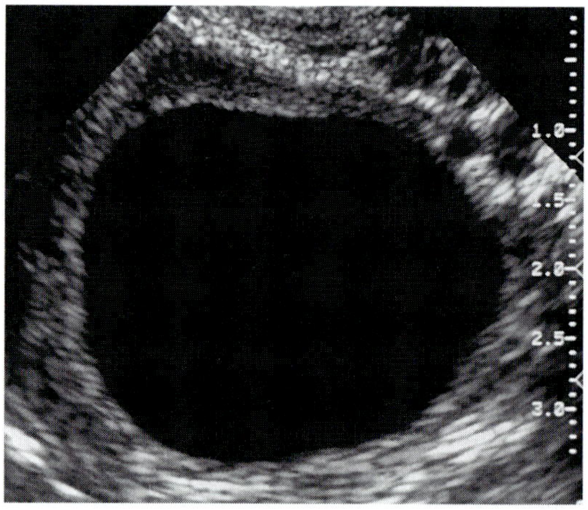

FIG. 51-19. Preovulatory follicle (23 mm) stimulated by administration of clomiphene citrate.

Gonadotropin-Releasing Hormone Agonists

Gonadotropin-releasing hormone agonists initiated before ovarian stimulation with hMG have had a positive effect on the induction of ovulation. Natural GnRH is a 10-amino acid peptide elaborated in the hypothalamus. Substitutions in the amino acid sequence either enhance or diminish the biological response to the synthetic peptide. Some GnRH analogues have as much as 5 to 20 times the potency of the native molecule. The half-life of many of the agonists is short, thus necessitating frequent administration. The number of follicles available for use in the assisted reproductive technologies is usually higher in

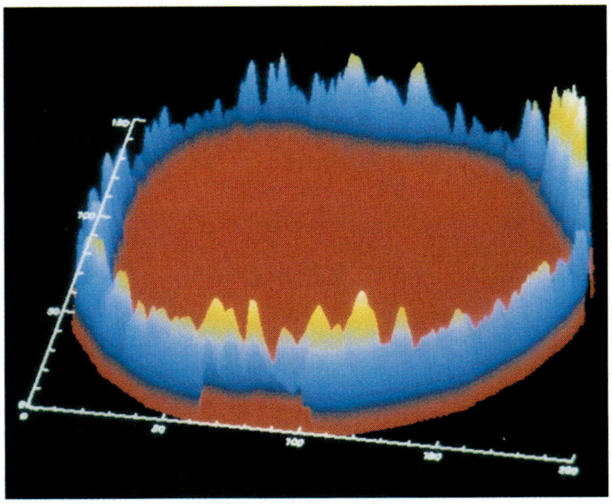

FIG. 51-20. Ultrasound image of follicle in Fig. 51-19 processed for quantitative image analysis. Note the deep red coloration of the area representing the follicular fluid, sharp transition zone at the fluid-follicle interface and relatively thin, high-amplitude follicle walls.

THE ASSISTED REPRODUCTIVE TECHNOLOGIES

IVF	*In vitro* fertilization Retrieval of oocytes, fertilization in the laboratory and cervical transfer of embryos into the endometrial cavity.
GIFT	Gamete intrafallopian transfer The placement of retrieved oocytes and sperm into the fallopian tube by laparoscopy.
ZIFT	Zygote intrafallopian transfer The placement of zygotes into the fallopian tube, usually by laparoscopy.
TET	Tubal embryo transfer The placement of embryos directly into the fallopian tube transcervically or at the time of laparoscopy.
ICSI	Intercytoplasmic sperm insertion The injection of a single spermatozoon into an oocyte under microscopic control.

women who respond poorly to traditional ovulation induction as a result of the synergistic combination of GnRHa and exogenous gonadotropins.[77,78] GnRHa help to decrease ovarian androgen production and high late-follicular phase LH levels in situations where oocyte retrieval is contemplated. The addition of GnRHa to the stimulation protocol typically results in fewer cycle cancellations. In addition, more oocytes of higher quality are usually retrieved from stimulation protocols which include GnRHa.[79]

Human Chorionic Gonadotropin

Human chorionic gonadotropin has LH-like activity and is administered to induce the final preovulatory changes in the oocyte/follicle complex and ovulation. Optimal timing for hCG administration is usually determined from the diameter of preovulatory follicles, their ultrasonographic appearance and circulating estradiol-17 levels during spontaneous or induced cycles. hCG and controlled ovarian superstimulation are used in combination with timed artificial insemination, oocyte retrieval for *in vitro* fertilization, gamete, or zygote intrafallopian transfer.

Irrespective of the ART procedure to be used, hCG is consistently used to induce the final phases of follicular and oocyte maturation. It is therefore imperative that the **timing of the hCG administration be perfect to ensure ovulation,** or retrieval of oocytes in the optimal condition for fertilization. If hCG is administered too early in follicular development, the follicles are not capable of responding and most probably will regress without ovulating. If the hCG is administered too late, many follicles will respond by failing to ovulate; ovarian hyperstimulation syndrome then becomes an issue. Similarly, if hCG is administered too early, or too late, in oocyte retrieval cycles, immature or postmature oocytes may be retrieved.

ULTRASOUND IN THE ASSISTED REPRODUCTIVE TECHNOLOGIES

The ART include those procedures that retrieve oocytes from the ovary in an attempt to initiate a pregnancy. There is an ever-increasing list of variations of these technologies (see box above). However, the first and most common ART at present is IVF. On November 10, 1977, Dr. P. Steptoe performed laparoscopic oocyte retrieval at midcycle on a 30-year-old woman who was suffering from irreversible bilateral tubal occlusion. A single oocyte was retrieved and fertilized *in vitro*. The resulting eight-cell embryo was transferred to the woman's uterus 2.5 days later. On July 25, 1978, the first IVF mother delivered by cesarean section a 2700-g infant girl. This birth heralded the beginning of a new era in the medical management of infertility.[80] With the exception of the laboratory management of gametes and embryos, ultrasonography plays an important role in each step of the IVF process.

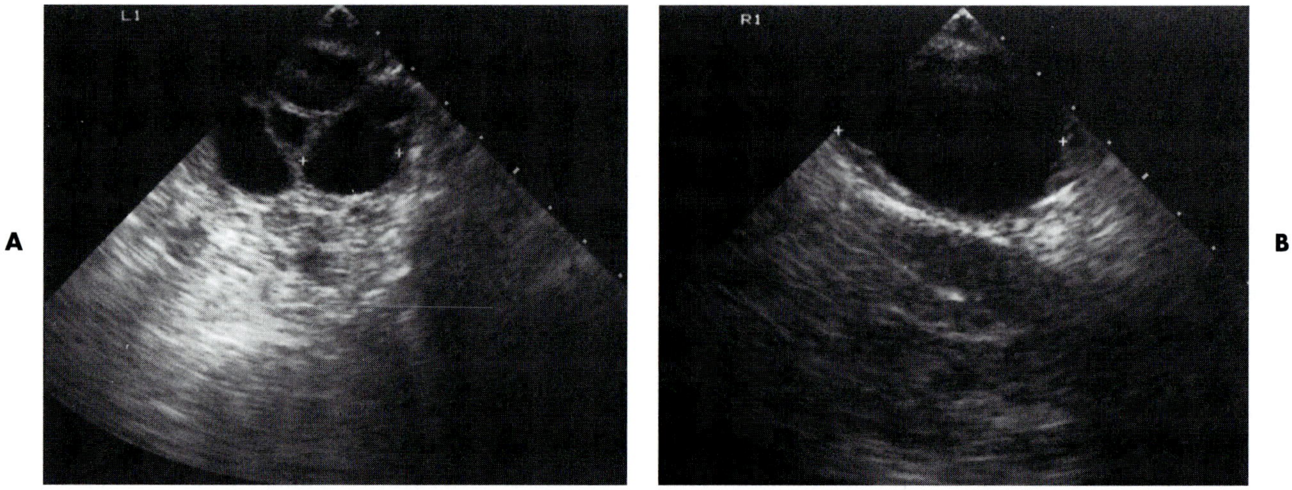

FIG. 51-21. Large right ovarian cyst, in a patient on clomid citrate–hMG-hCG protocol, shows, **A,** multiple left follicles and **B,** a right functional cyst proven to be benign by aspiration at time of retrieval.

Patient Selection and Precycle Treatment for IVF

The original requirement for a patient to enter an IVF program was **irreversible tubal occlusion,** a final common pathway of many disease processes. These disease processes include bilateral ectopic pregnancy, PID, and endometriosis. More recently, the indications for IVF have been expanded to include patients with a wide variety of infertility disorders, including **unexplained infertility, endometriosis, fertilization defects, and male factor infertility.** With the first report of a successful pregnancy initiated by intracytoplasmic sperm insertion (ICSI) in 1992 the treatment of male factor infertility was revolutionized.[81] Men previously believed to be either infertile or sterile can now become biologic parents through this new method of sperm microinjection into oocytes retrieved by IVF. The minimal requirements for participating in IVF include a normal uterine cavity and a source of oocytes and sperm. Age, general health, and mental health must also be considered in the final decision to admit a couple to IVF treatment.

In preparation for an IVF cycle, a basic work-up is indicated including general blood work, an endocrine survey, evaluation of the endometrial cavity through hysterosalpingography or hysteroscopy, and a baseline ultrasound. Anomalies of the uterus, including congenital abnormalities, fibroids and polyps, are identified and the uterine position noted. The adnexa are best evaluated both by transabdominal and transvaginal studies. The accessibility of the ovaries to transvaginal oocyte retrieval is documented and normal ovaries and fallopian tubes confirmed prior to initiating treatment. **Ovarian cysts** (Fig. 51-21) and **hydrosalpinges** are not infrequently discovered in baseline studies and may interfere with ovarian hyperstimulation, hamper oocyte retrieval or interfere with successful blastocyst implantation. Abnormalities detected by baseline studies are dealt with prior to initiating treatment.

Ovarian Stimulation and Monitoring of IVF Cycles

Although the initial success by Steptoe[80] was achieved in a spontaneous menstrual cycle it soon became apparent that IVF pregnancy rates could be dramatically improved if more oocytes could be retrieved and fertilized. The resulting greater number of embryos that are available provide patients with an increased opportunity for implantation and successful pregnancy. Although there has been an increased interest recently in natural cycle IVF,[82] most treatment protocols involve **ovarian hyperstimulation** in an attempt to produce multifollicular recruitment and development. Clomiphene citrate was shown initially to improve pregnancy rates but is now seldom used in IVF stimulation protocols.[83] At present, most IVF centers routinely use hMG (either recombinant or extracted from postmenopausal urine) in combination with a GnRha preparation to maximize oocyte recovery and pregnancy rates. **Ovarian response to the treatment protocol** is followed by serial endovaginal ultrasounds and estradiol (E_2) determinations. The timing of administration of hCG to reinitiate meiosis and produce oocyte maturity

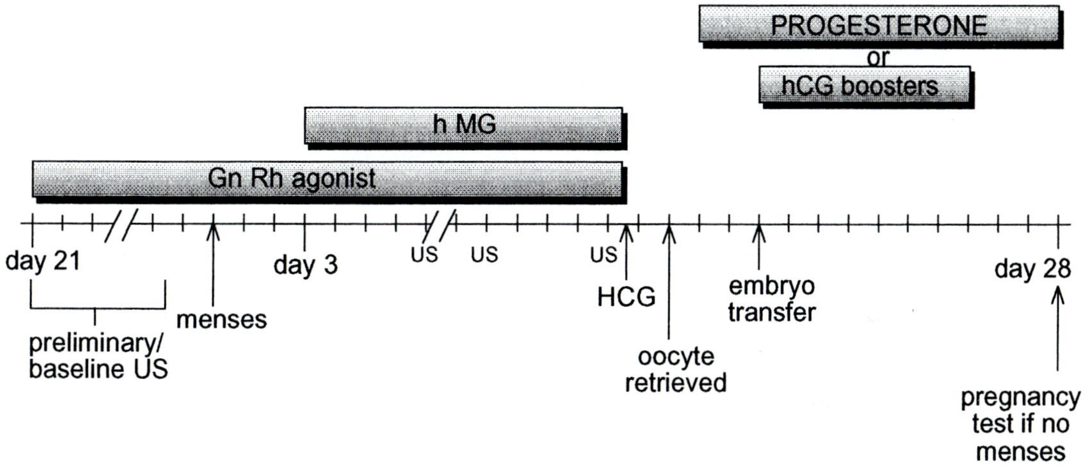

FIG. 51-22. Typical ovarian hyperstimulation protocol. The ultrasound studies include a preliminary examination prior to the treatment cycle. During the treatment cycle, ultrasound examinations are performed every second day until the leading follicle achieves a mean diameter of 18 mm.

is dependent upon E levels and ultrasound measurements of the lead follicles. In general, hCG is given when the three lead follicles reach a mean diameter of 1.6 to 1.8 cm and the E_2 level is in a satisfactory range. In programs where pituitary suppression with a GnRha is being used, the day and time of retrieval are determined by the timing of hCG administration (Fig. 51-22). If GnRha suppression is not used, then oocyte retrieval must occur after a timed interval following the LH surge. In either case, transvaginal ultrasound–guided oocyte retrieval follows 34 to 36 hours later.

Oocyte Retrieval

The first oocyte retrieval was accomplished via a laparotomy. In 1977, Steptoe[80] successfully retrieved oocytes laparoscopically. For some time, laparoscopy became the standard way of retrieving eggs and although it was a invasive technique with operative risks, oocytes were recovered from 60% to 95% of all follicles punctured.[84-87] In 1982, Lenz[88] and later Wikland[89] reported a method of ultrasonically guided transvesical retrieval that produced oocyte recovery rates comparable to laparoscopy. Over the 4 to 5 years during which time transvesical oocyte retrieval was popular,[90] it became apparent that this method, too, suffered from certain disadvantages. Most notable of these disadvantages was the often relatively poor quality of follicular imaging. A search for an alternate oocyte retrieval method yielded two alternatives: transurethral and transvaginal.[87,88,91] The transurethral approach quickly fell out of favor. The **transvaginal approach** for oocyte retrieval is now the most commonly employed. The number of oocytes retrieved by this method is increased compared with other techniques and therefore, the chance of achieving a pregnancy is greater (Fig. 51-23).[92] Using high-frequency endovaginal probes (5 to 7.5 MHz), imaging is usually excellent and the procedure can be performed safely and comfortably with IV sedation using a benzodiazepine (such as Valium) and analgesia (a narcotic such as Fentanyl).[93] General anesthesia may occasionally be required because of patient anxiety or extreme patient discomfort. A needle guide attached to the ultrasound probe shaft allows for precise follicular puncture and aspiration. Rarely, the ovary is fixed beyond the visual field of the endovaginal probe. In these cases, an ultrasound-guided transabdominal approach or laparoscopic retrieval may be necessary.

Transvaginal oocyte retrieval is performed in a surgical suite adjacent to the IVF laboratory. The patient is placed in the dorsal lithotomy position and the vagina is cleansed with sterile saline. A vaginal probe sheathed with a sterile cover is advanced to the vaginal vault and the pelvis scanned. It is important to scan each ovary in two planes, because occasionally, a vessel may be intimately applied to the margins of the ovary and may simulate a follicle. The long aspiration needle, with a scored tip to enhance its echogenicity, is advanced slowly into the center of the follicle. Negative pressure of 100 mm Hg is created by a small vacuum pump immediately upon entering the follicle and the follicular fluid collected in a warmed test tube (Fig. 51-24). Collapse of the follicle is immediate and is observed on the ultrasound

A

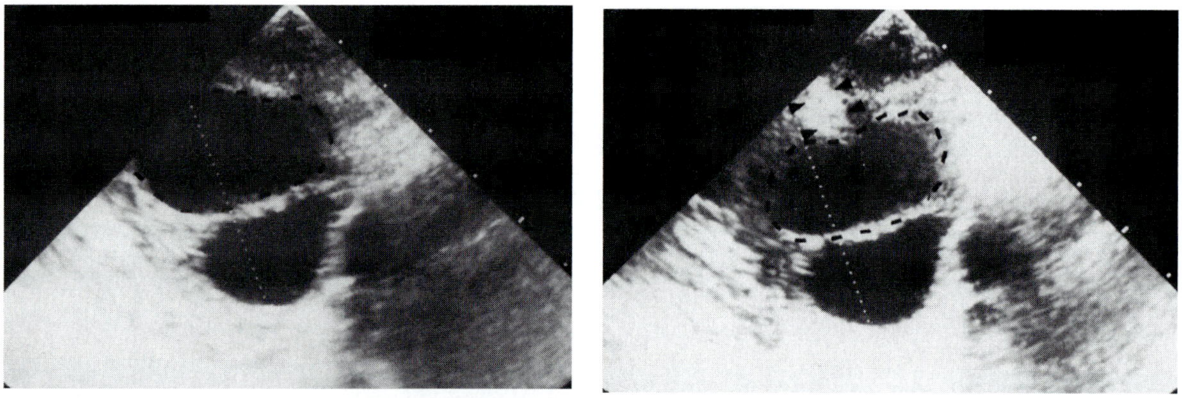

B

C

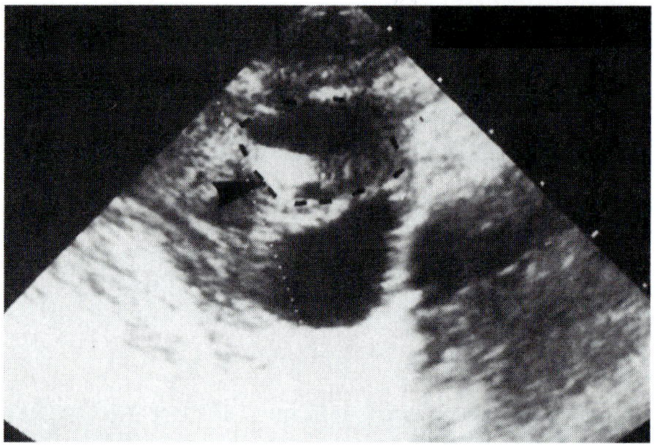

FIG. 51-23. Transvaginal oocyte retrieval needle tip. **A,** Follicle before puncture. **B,** Needle tip (*arrowheads*) indenting leading edge of follicle. **C,** Needle in collapsing follicle.

screen. An attempt to curette the follicles to improve oocyte recovery is made by manipulation of the needle. All follicles in excess of 1.0 cm are punctured and aspirated. In some IVF programs follicles are repeatedly irrigated and aspirated although this has not proven to significantly improve oocyte retrieval rates. The follicular fluid is immediately examined by the embryologist and the oocytes recovered. After all follicles are aspirated the pelvis is scanned to ensure no significant bleeding is present. A small amount of fluid (blood and peritoneal fluid) is invariably seen. This should not cause alarm unless it is excessive or increasing. Minimal vaginal bleeding results from the vaginal vault needle punctures. Vaginal packing is rarely required for excessive or relentless vaginal bleeding. **Complications of transvaginal oocyte retrieval** are uncommon, but may include peritonitis, pelvic abscess, bleeding and inadvertent damage to adjacent organs by the retrieval needle. Literature has reported at least one death as a result of transvaginal retrieval; this death occurred because of puncture to a pelvic wall vessel. Obviously, care must be taken during the procedure to avoid puncturing blood vessels or loops of bowel. If the latter should occur then the needle should be changed to reduce the possibility of introducing infection prior to completing the retrieval.

Embryo Transfer

The number of oocytes retrieved, depending on the patient's response to ovarian hyperstimulation, may vary from 2 to 55. Once collected, they are classified according to the appearance of the oocyte-corona-cumulus complex. Mature oocytes are incubated for approximately 4 hours and inseminated with prepared sperm. Immature oocytes are matured *in vitro* and inseminated when appropriate. A fertilization check is performed the following morning. Approximately 75% to 80% of mature oocytes will fertilize and approximately 85% of these will subsequently cleave. Embryos are cultured for 1 to 3 days and therefore transferred in the pronuclear to 12-cell stage.

Embryo transfer is usually performed in the dorsal lithotomy position with a sterile speculum to expose the cervix. The embryos are placed between the "two warm blankets" of the endometrial layers approximately 1 cm from the top of the uterine fundus. In some programs, endometrial cavity length is measured by ultrasound but the distance is better determined by sounding the uterus prior to the treatment cycle. Ultrasound can be used to observe the embryo transfer catheter entering the cavity and releasing the transfer medium with the embryo.[94] However, there is no clear advantage to

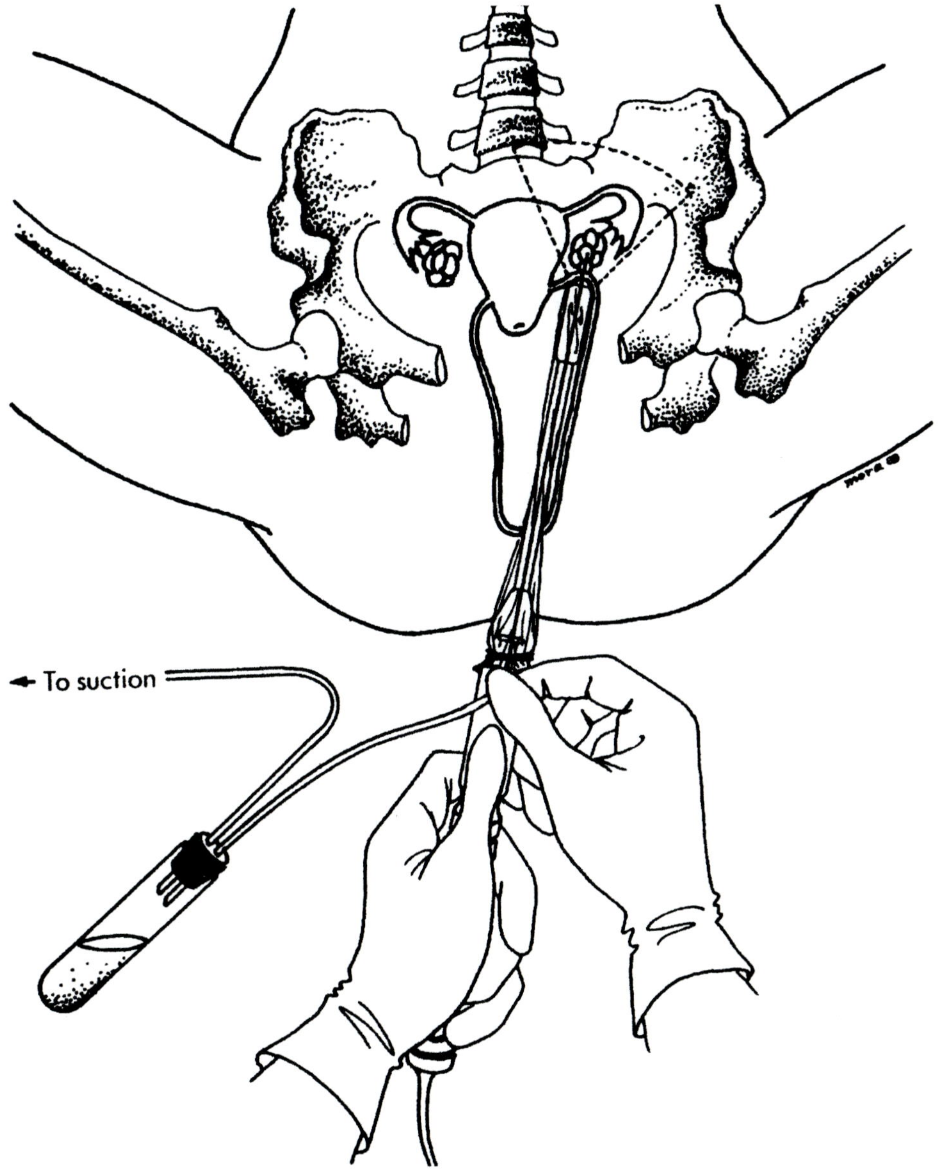

FIG. 51-24. Schematic depiction of transvaginal oocyte retrieval. (From Wiseman DA, Short WB, Pattinson HA, et al. Oocyte retrieval in an *in vitro* fertilization program: comparison of four methods. *Radiology* 1989; 173:99-102.)

this technique. Following embryo transfer hCG injections or progesterone are administered in an attempt to better support the endometrial lining and improve the chances for implantation. If pregnancy occurs, serum and urine βhCG tests will be positive after approximately 12 days following embryo transfer. When pregnancy occurs an ultrasound is performed 4 to 6 weeks after oocyte retrieval to confirm the pregnancy location and to determine the number of viable embryos.

CRYOPRESERVATION OF EXCESS EMBRYOS

Under usual circumstances, 2 to 4 embryos are transferred in the stimulated cycle. If there are excess good-quality embryos, they can be cryopreserved in liquid nitrogen for further attempts at pregnancy. These thaw cycle embryo replacements can be performed in either a natural cycle or one prepared with estradiol/progesterone (E/P). Both methods appear to be equally successful.[95] In the case of a natural thaw the embryo transfer is timed to coincide with the period of maximum endometrial receptivity. This occurs 3 days after the LH surge. Confidence intervals are calculated to identify the earliest likely day of the LH surge and an ultrasound is performed that day to identify and measure the dominant follicle. Based on that mean follicular size, it is determined when the follicle will reach a size of 1.6 cm (assuming a growth of 2 mm a day). Upon reaching that diameter, daily LH levels are measured to identify the surge. Embryo transfer is accomplished 3 days later. For patients traveling long distances and for those with irregular menstrual cycles, E/P replacement cycles are often more convenient. This method of ensuring endometrial preparedness involves administering sequential estrogen and progesterone and replacing the embryos 3 days after progesterone is initiated. With both methods, it is useful to undertake an ultrasound for endometrial thickness at the time of the LH surge or before starting progesterone. This is to ensure an **endometrial thickness of at least 6 mm**—the minimum thickness believed to support a pregnancy.[96]

IVF OUTCOMES

When reporting IVF pregnancy rates, clinical pregnancies are often cited and are those where products of conception are seen on the 4- to 6-week ultrasound. However, the most significant statistic is **live births per oocyte retrieval.** Many clinics report to a registry, which is available to the public, and is run by the Society for Assisted Reproductive Technology (SART) of the American Society of Reproductive Medicine. In 1993, 267 clinics reported 33,543 cycles of IVF with an 18.3% delivery rate for oocyte retrieval.[97] However, many clinics now achieve success rates in the range of 30% to 40%. The pregnancy rate per embryo transfer for cryopreserved embryos in the same year was 13.3%.[97] The greater the number of IVF cycles the patient enters into the greater the possibility she will ultimately be successful. The most profound impact on success rates is maternal age due to decreased fecundity and increased miscarriage with advancing reproductive age. Miscarriage rates in IVF pregnancies are slightly higher than natural conception at 20%. The risk of congenital anomalies in live born infants from IVF is the same as in the background population.[98] Obstetrical outcome is related to **maternal age** and the **number of fetuses.**

OTHER ASSISTED REPRODUCTIVE TECHNOLOGIES

Gamete intrafallopian transfer (**GIFT**) has a greater chance for successful pregnancy in some infertility clinics compared with their IVF programs. GIFT involves ovarian hyperstimulation and monitoring much like IVF. Oocyte retrieval may be undertaken transvaginally by ultrasound or performed under direct vision at the time of laparoscopy. The oocytes are loaded into a catheter with capacitated sperm and the contents of the catheter injected into the ampulla of the fallopian tube. This is usually accomplished by laparoscopic injection but has also been successfully performed using transvaginal ultrasound guidance.[99] GIFT is usually used for treatment of patients with unexplained infertility but may also be indicated for the treatment of endometriosis related infertility. It is believed by some to be a more "natural" form of ART as **fertilization occurs *in vivo*** in the milieu of the fallopian tube. This technique is acceptable to some religious groups that object to *in vitro* fertilization. The major disadvantage of GIFT is the need for a laparoscopy. Obviously, at least one fallopian tube must be patent and normal. The SART Registry in 1993 reported a delivery rate of 28.6% per gamete transfer.[97]

Zygote intrafallopian transfer (**ZIFT**) is a modification of IVF where oocytes are retrieved transvaginally and fertilized *in vitro*. However, rather than culturing the embryos to day 2 or 3, as with IVF, 1-day-old zygotes are placed into the fallopian tube by a laparoscopic or transcervical tubal technique. The theoretical advantage to ZIFT is that it allows the embryo to develop in the fallopian tube. However, the validity of this assumption is in question.[100] The SART Registry in 1993 reported a

28.6% delivery rate per zygote transfer.[97] The Foothills Hospital regional fertility program experience from January 1, 1996 through December 31, 1996 is summarized in Table 51-2.

BIOLOGIC EFFECTS OF ULTRASOUND

Patients undergoing ART procedures are frequent visitors to the ultrasound suite. For example, in an IVF cycle patients undergo approximately four ultrasounds scans for follicular tracking and an additional scan at the time of oocyte retrieval. Considering the degree of ultrasound exposure, it is easy to understand the concern that exists about the biologic effects of ultrasound waves. No clinical study to date has shown a significant adverse effect. In one animal study, ultrasound was applied to superovulated mouse embryos in a fashion similar to that encountered in normal clinical situations.[101] Fertilization and speed of embryo development and implantation were then evaluated. No difference between the two groups in fertilization or early development was identified. The authors did note a slight increase in the number of failed implantations. The etiology of this effect remains unexplained. The final conclusion of the 1988[102] and 1989[92] US IVF Embryo Transfer Registry Report, as well as a 1984 collaborative world report on IVF,[103]

TABLE 51-2
1996 PREGNANCY RATES/ET (%) ACCORDING TO AGE AND DIAGNOSIS

	Cause of Infertility					
	Tubal Occlusion N = 120	Male Factor N = 87	Non Tubal Female Factor N = 35	Unexplained Infertility N = 43	Combined Female & Male Factor N = 36	Total 351
Age < 34						
*2.9 embryo						
N = 187						
**PR/ET	55.7	59.3	57.9	54.8	63.6	57.8
***IR/ET	28.9	34.7	36.8	28.6	45.2	33
						Take home rate 55.4%****
Age 35-38						
*3.5 embryo						
N = 105						
**PR/ET	53.7	64.0	25.0	47.6	60.0	53.3
***IR/ET	24.6	30	7.1	18.8	20.0	22.7
						Take home rate 47.1%****
Age > 39						
*3.9 embryo						
N = 59						
**PR/ET	27.8	25.0	50.0	33.3	50.0	33.9
***IR/ET	10.4	5.9	13.8	9.5	12.5	10.0
						Take home rate 21.7%****
Total N = 351						
**PR/ET	50.8	57.5	48.6	46.6	61.1	
***IR/ET	24.2	29.5	23.0	19.5	32.7	

*The average # of embryos transferred in each group per IVF treatment cycle.

**PR/ET—Pregnancy Rate/Embryo Transfer = Presence of Gest Sac Seen on U/S per IVF Cycle

***IR/ET—Implantation/Embryo Transferred = # of Gest Sacs seen on U/S per Embryo Transferred

****Take home rate—Describes the probability of taking home a live baby following a cycle of IVF.

Foothills Hospital Regional Fertility Program pregnancy rates for varying age groups and diagnoses, January 1, 1996 to December 31, 1996.

emphatically states that there is no increased risk of fetal anomalies in that experience (6500 live births).

COMPLICATIONS OF OVARIAN HYPERSTIMULATION

Ovarian hyperstimulation syndrome (OHS) is a frequent iatrogenic complication of ovulation induction. It is most commonly seen after ovulation with hMG and ovulation triggering with hCG but has also been rarely seen after administration of clomiphene citrate and gonadotropin releasing hormone. This syndrome is characterized by **weight gain, cystic ovarian enlargement, ascites, and pleural effusions.** The manifestations of the OHS are related to third-space losses secondary to increased vascular permeability. Several vasoactive mediators have been implicated but at the present time, it appears that the most likely mediator is angiotensin II, produced by the ovarian renin-angiotensin cascade. Depletion of intravascular fluids, proteins, and electrolytes in the most severe form may result in **hypotension, oliguria, electrolyte abnormalities, hemoconcentration, and thromboembolic complications.** As well, **ovarian torsion** may result because of the large size of the ovaries secondary to multifollicular development.[103] Classification systems that categorize OHS into mild, moderate, and severe forms have been proposed and revised based on clinical signs and symptoms.[104-106] Included in these criteria is ovarian size (mild, <5 cm; moderate, 5-12 cm; and severe, >12 cm). The likelihood of developing OHS is greater in oligo-ovulatory women and in those patients with a history of previous OHS. OHS does not occur in the absence of hCG and therefore, if the ovulatory dose of hCG is not given, this condition will not occur. Approximately two thirds of OHS cases occur in conception cycles, particularly multifetal pregnancies. This is due to the rapidly rising levels of hCG. In patients at risk for OHS because of high E_2 levels and multiple follicles (>25),[107] it may be prudent to abandon that treatment cycle and restart later with a reduced dosage of hMG. Alternately, in IVF cycles, it may be decided to proceed to oocyte retrieval but to cryopreserve all satisfactory embryos for delayed transfer. Patients at risk for OHS receive progesterone, and not hCG, for luteal phase support. Mild and moderate forms of OHS are expected and a common occurrence of ovulation induction (23% to 33%)[108,109] and are usually treated symptomatically at home. However, for the 1% to 3% of patients that develop severe OHS which may be life threatening, hospitalization is mandatory. Ultrasound-guided paracentesis, either abdominally or vaginally, may be required. Resolution of the syndrome will occur within 2 to 3 weeks.

Another frequent complication arising from ovarian induction is **multiple pregnancy** (Fig. 51-25). Of the deliveries resulting from IVF as reported by SART, 69.5% were singletons, 27.5% twins, 5.4% triplets, and .4% were of higher order.[97] In clomiphene citrate cycles, the twin frequency is 5% to 7%, and there is very little probability of more than twins. HMG cycles have a multiple pregnancy rate of approximately 20% to 30%, most of which are twins, but certainly higher order pregnancies are not uncommon. Infertility specialists usually regard twins as a bonus. However, triplet- and higher-order pregnancies are at high risk for preterm birth and other obstetrical complications with the attendant risks to the mother and infants. For this reason, **ultrasound-guided fetal reduction** is often considered for multiple pregnancies, particularly those above triplets.[110]

It is surprising to some experts that the incidence of **ectopic pregnancy** (EP) in IVF is 4.4% per established pregnancy.[97] It is most likely to occur in patients with preexisting tubal disease. Perhaps even more surprising is that the incidence of **heterotrophic pregnancy** is 1 in 100 in IVF, whereas this incidence occurs with the frequency of 1 in 25,000 after natural conception.[111] These facts mandate careful early ultrasound studies to establish the intrauterine location of the pregnancy and to try to ensure that the patient does not have an ectopic or heterotrophic pregnancy.

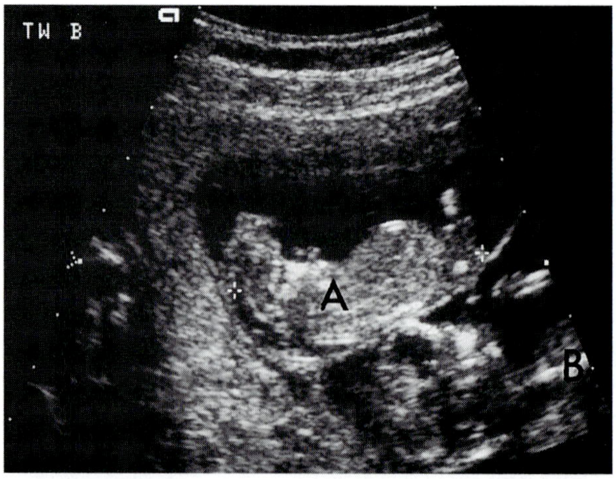

FIG. 51-25. *In vitro* fertilization—twin pregnancy. Twin A (*upper left*) anencephalic; twin B (*lower right*) normal. Twin A underwent ultrasound-guided fetacide.

REFERENCES

Epidemiology

1. Mosher WD, Pratt WF. Fecundity and infertility in the United States: Incidence and trends. *Fertil Steril* 1991;56:192.
2. Speroff L, Glass LH, Kase NG. Clinical investigations of the infertile couple. In: *Gynecologic Endocrinology and Infertility, ed 5.* Williams and Wilkins; 1994;809-840.
3. Federation CECOS, Schwartz D, Mayaux JM. Female fecundity as a function of age: results of artificial insemination in 2193 multiparous women with azoospermic husbands. *N Engl J Med* 1982;306:404.
4. Warburton D, Kline J, Stein Z et al. *Perinatal Genetics: Diagnosis and Treatment.* New York: Academic Press; 1986.

Ultrasound and the Normal Reproductive Process

5. Timor-Tritsch IE, Ruttem S. Transvaginal ultrasonography in the management of infertility. In: Kurjak A (ed): *Ultrasound and Infertility.* Boca Raton, CRC Press 1989;125.
6. Bomsel-Helmreich O. Ultrasound and the preovulatory human follicle. *Oxford Rev Reprod Biol* 1985;7:1.
7. Hackeloer BJ, Fleming R, Robinson HP et al. Correlation of ultrasonic and endocrinologic parameters of human follicular development. *Am J Obstet Gynecol* 1979;135:122-128.
8. Hall DA, Hann LE, Ferrucci Jr. JT et al. Sonographic morphology of the normal menstrual cycle. *Radiology* 1979; 133:185.
9. Lenz S. Ultrasonic study of follicular maturation, ovulation and development of corpus luteum during normal menstrual cycles. *Acta Obstet Gynecol Scand* 1985;64:15-19.
10. Queenan JT, O'Brien GD, Bains LM et al. Ultrasound scanning of ovaries to detect ovulation in women. *Fertil Steril* 1980;34(2):99.
11. Nakata M, Selstam G, Olofsson J, B'ckstr'm T. Investigation of the human corpus luteum by ultrasonography: a proposed scheme for clinical investigation. *Ultrasound Obstet Gynecol* 1992:190.
12. Pierson RA, Chizen DR. Transvaginal ultrasonographic assessment of normal and aberrant ovulation. In: Jaffe R, Pierson RA, Abramowicz JS, editors: *Imaging in Infertility and Reproductive Endocrinology.* Philadelphia: Lippincott; 1994:129-142.
13. Pierson, RA, Adams GP. Computer-assisted image analysis, diagnostic ultrasonography, and ovulation induction: strange bedfellows. *Theriogenology* 1995;43:105-112.
14. Lindenberg S. Ultrasonographic assessment of the endometrium during the normal menstrual cycle. In: Jaffe R, Pierson RA, Abramowicz JS, editors: *Imaging in Infertility and Reproductive Endocrinology.* Philadelphia: Lippincott; 1994:47-51.
15. Brandt TD, Levy EB, Grant TH, et al. The endometrial echo and its significance in female infertility. *Radiology* 1985; 157:225.
16. Fleischer AL, Kalemeris GC, Entman SS. Sonographic depiction of the endometrium during normal cycles. *Ultrasound Med Biol* 1986;12:271.
17. Fleischer AC, Kalemeris GC, Machin JE et al. Sonographic depiction of normal and abnormal endometrium with histopathologic correlation. *J Ultrasound Med* 1986;5:445.
18. Lenz S, Lindenberg S. Ultrasonic evaluation of endometrial growth in women with normal cycles during spontaneous and stimulated cycles. *Human Reprod* 1990;5:377.
19. Fleischer AC, Gordon AN, Entman SS, et al. Transvaginal scanning of the endometrium. *J Clin Ultrasound* 1990; 18:337.
20. Fleischer AC, Gordon AN, Entman SS, Kepple DM. Transvaginal scanning of the endometrium. *J Clin Ultrasound* 1990;18:337.
21. Grunfeld L, Walker B, Bergh PA, et al. High-resolution endovaginal ultrasonography of the endometrium: a noninvasive test for endometrial adequacy. *Obstet Gynecol* 1991; 78:200.
22. Grunfeld L, Walker B, Bergh PA et al. High-resolution endovaginal ultrasonography of the endometrium: a noninvasive test for endometrial adequacy. *Obstet Gynecol* 1991;78:200.
23. Ritchie WG. Sonographic evaluation of normal and induced ovulation. *Radiology* 1986;161:1.
24. Gonen Y, Casper RF. Prediction of implantation by the sonographic appearance of the endometrium during controlled ovarian stimulation for in vitro fertilization (IVF). *J In Vitro Fert Embryo Transfer* 1990;7:146.
25. Shoham Z, Di Carlo C, Patel A et al. Is it possible to run a successful ovulation induction program based solely on ultrasound monitoring? The importance of endometrial measurements. *Fertil Steril* 1991;56:836.
26. Hilgers TW, Daly KD Prebil AM et al: *J Rep Med* 1992; 37:864-866.

Investigation of Infertility

27. Haines CJ, Emes AL: The relationship between follicle diameter, fertilization rate and microscopic embryo quality. *Fertil Steril* 1991;55:205-207.
28. Pierson RA, Chizen DR, Olatunbosun AO. The role of ultrasonography in ovulation induction. In: Jaffe R, Pierson RA, Abramiwicz JS, editors: *Imaging in Infertility and Reproductive Endocrinology.* Philadelphia: Lippincott, 1994:155-166.
29. Falcone T, Bourque J, Granger L et al. Polycystic ovary syndrome. *Curr Prob Obstet Gynecol Fert* 1993;16:65-95.
30. Hann LE, Hall DA, McArdle CR et al. Polycystic ovarian disease: sonographic spectrum. *Radiol* 1984:150:531-534.
31. Filicori M, Flamigni C, Meriggiola MC et al. Endocrine response determines the clinical outcome of pulsatile gonadotropin releasing hormone ovulation induction in different ovulatory disorders. *J Clin Endocrinol Metab* 1991; 72:965-972.

Ultrasound Diagnosis of Conditions Leading to Infertility

32. Crouch JE. *Functional Human Anatomy.* Philadelphia: Lea & Febiger, 1978:561-596.
33. Richman TS, Viscomi GN, De Cherney et al: Fallopian tubal patency assessed by ultrasound following fluid injection. *Radiology* 1984;152:507-510.
34. Randolph JR, Yu KY, Schmidt CL et al: Comparison of real-time ultrasonography, hysterosalpingography and laparoscopy in the evaluation of uterine abnormalities and tubal patency. *Fertil Steril* 1986;46:828-832.
35. Timor-Tritsch I, Shraga R: Transvaginal ultrasonographic study of the fallopian tube. *Obstet Gynecol* 1987;70:424-428.
36. Stern J, Coulam CB. Color Doppler hysterosalpingography. In: Jaffe R, Pierson RA, Abramowicz JS, eds: *Imaging in Infertility and Reproductive Endocrinology*, Philadelphia: Lippincott, 1994:335-343.
37. Peters AJ, Coulam CB. Hysterosalpingography with color Doppler ultrasonography. *Am J Obstet Gynecol* 1991;164: 1530-1534.
38. Bree RL. Transvaginal ultrasound in infertility. In: *Syllabus of the Endovaginal Ultrasound Course.* American Institute of Ultrasound in Medicine 1989:45.
39. Hata T, Hata H, Daisaku S et al. Transvaginal Doppler color flow mapping. *Gynecol Obstet Invest* 1989;27:217.
40. Daya S. Ultrasonographic Evaluation of Uterine Anomalies. In: Jaffe R, Pierson RA, and Abramowicz JS, eds: *Imaging in*

Infertility and Reproductive Endocrinology. Philadelphia: Lippincott, pp 63-91.
41. Malini S, Valdes C, Malinak R. Sonographic diagnosis and classification of anomalies of the female genital tract. *J Ultrasound Med* 1984;3:397.
42. Reuter KL, Daly DC, Cohen SM. Septate versus bicornuate uteri: errors in imaging diagnosis. *Radiology* 1989;172:749.
43. Siedler D, Laing FC, Jeffrey RB, Wing VW. Uterine adenomyosis, a difficult sonographic diagnosis. *J Ultrasound Med* 1987;6:345.
44. Coulam CB, Annegers JF, Kranz JS. Chronic anovulation syndrome and associated neoplasia. *Obstet Gynecol* 1983;61: 403-407.
45. Franks S, Adams J, Mason H et al. Ovulatory disorders in women with polycystic ovary syndrome. *Clin Obstet Gynecol* 1985;12:605-632.
46. Treasure JL, Gordon PA, King EA et al. Cystic ovaries: a phase of anorexia nervosa. *Lancet* 1985;1379-1381.
47. Seang LT, Jacobs HS. Recent advances in the management of patients with amemorrhea. *Clin Obstet Gynecol* 1985;12: 725-747.
48. Friedman H, Vogelzang RL, Mendelson E et al. Endometriosis detection by U/S with laparoscopic correlation. *Radiology* 1985;157:217-220.
49. Coleman BG, Arger PH, Mulhern CB. Endometriosis: clinical and ultrasonic correlation. *AJR* 1979;132:747-749.
50. Pouly JL, Hubert M, Gerard M. Conservative laparoscopy treatment of three hundred and twenty one ectopic pregnancies. *Fertil Steril* 1986;46(6):1093-1097.
51. Timor-Tritsch IE, Baxi L, Peisner DB. Transvaginal salpingocentesis: a new technique for treating ectopic pregnancy. *Am J Obstet Gynecol* 1989;160:459-461.
52. Feichtinger W, Kemefer P. Conservative treatment of ectopic pregnancy by transvaginal aspiration under sonographic control and methotrexate injection. *Lancet* 1987;1:381-382.
53. Behrman SJ, Kistner W, Patton GW. *Progress in infertility*. Boston: Little Brown; 1988.
54. Richie GM. Ultrasound in the evaluation of normal and induced ovulation. *Fertil Steril* 1980;43(2):167-181.
55. McArdle CR, Seibel M, Weinstein F et al. Induction of ovulation monitored by ultrasound. *Radiology* 1983;148(3):809-812.
56. Vargyas JM, Marrs R, Kletzky OA et al. Correlation of ultrasonic measurement of ovarian follicle size and serum estradiol levels in ovulatory patients following clomiphene citrate for *in vitro* fertilization. *Am J Obstet Gynecol* 1982;144(5):569-573.
57. Gonzalez CJ, Curson R, Parsons J. Transabdominal versus transvaginal ultrasound scanning of ovarian follicles: are they comparable? *Fertil Steril* 1988;50(4):657-659.
58. Hackeloer BJ, Fleming R. Robinson HP et al. Correlation of ultrasonic and endocrinologic parameters of human follicular development. *Am J Obstet Gynecol* 1979;135:122-128.
59. Picker RH, Smith DH, Tucker MH et al. Ultrasonic signs of imminent ovulation. *J Clin Ultrasound* 1983;11(1):1-3.
60. Hackeloer BJ: The role of ultrasound in female infertility management. *Ultrasound Med Biol* 1984;10:35-50.
61. Hoff JD, Quigley ME, Yen SSC. Hormonal dynamics at midcycle: a reevaluation. *J Clin Endocrinol Metab* 1983;57:792.
62. Pierson RA, Chizen DR. Transvaginal diagnostic ultrasonography in evaluation and management of infertility. *J Sogc* 1991;37:37-48.
63. Pierson RA, Martinuk SD, Chizen DR et al. Ultrasonographic visualization of human ovulation. In: *Proc Reinier de Graaf Symposium-From Ovulation to Implantation*. Maastricht, The Netherlands. 1990: In press.
64. O'Herlitty C, De Crespigny L, Lopata A et al. Preovulatory follicular size; a comparison of ultrasound and laparascopic measurements. *Fertil Steril* 1980;3(1):24-26.
65. Fleischer AC, Herbert CM, Sacks GA et al. Sonography of the endometrium during conception and nonconception cycles of in vitro fertilization and embryo transfer. *Fertil Steril* 1986; 46(30):442-447.
66. Itskovitz J, Boldes R, Levron J et al. Transvaginal ultrasonography in the diagnosis and treatment of infertility. *J Clin Ultrasound* 1990;18(4):248-257.
67. Hackeloer BJ, Sallam HN. Ultrasound scanning of ovarian follicles. *Clin Obstet Gynecol* 1983;10(3):603-619.
68. Renaud RL, Macler J, Dervain I et al. Echographic study of follicular maturation and ovulation during the normal menstrual cycle. *Fertil Steril* 1980;33(3):272.

Induction of Ovulation

69. Marrs R, Vargyas D, March C. Correlation of ultrasonic and endocrinologic measurements in human menopausal gonadotropin therapy. *Am J Obstet Gynecol* 1983;145:417-421.
70. Pierson RA, Chizen DR. Normal and aberrant ovulation. In Jaffe R, Pierson RA, Abramowicz JS, eds: *Imaging in Infertility and Reproductive Endocrinology*. Philadelphia: Lippincott 1994:129-142.
71. O'Herlihy C, Pepperell RJ, Robinson H. Ultrasound timing of human chorionic gonadotrophin administration in clomiphene citrate stimulated cycles. *Obstet Gynecol* 1982;59: 40-45.
72. Vargyas J, Marrs R, Kletsky O et al. Correlation of ultrasonic measurement of ovarian follicular size and serum estradiol levels in ovulatory patients following clomiphene citrate for in vitro fertilization. *Am J Obstet Gynecol* 1982;144:569-573.
73. Leerentveld R, VanGent I, DerStoep M, Wladimiroff JW. Ultrasonographic assessment of Graafian follicle growth under monofollicular and multifollicular conditions in clomiphene citrate stimulated cycles. *Fertil Steril* 1985;40: 461-465.
74. Pierson RA, Adams GP. Computer-assisted image analysis, diagnostic ultrasonography, and ovulation induction: strange bedfellows. *Theriogenology*. 43:105-112.
75. Silverberg KM, Olive DL, Burns WN et al: Follicular size at the time of human chorionic gonadotropin administration predicts ovulation outcome in human menopausal gonadotropin stimulated cycles. *Fertil Steril* 1991;56:296-300.
76. Veek LL, Wortham JWE, Witmyer J et al. Maturation and fertilization of morphologically immature human oocytes in a program of in vitro fertilization. *Fertil Steril* 1983;39:594-602.
77. Dor J, Ben-Shlomo I, Levran D et al. The relative success of gonadotropin releasing hormone analogue, clomiphene citrate and gonadotrophin in 1,099 cycles of in vitro fertilization. *Fertil Steril* 1992;58:986-990.
78. Hugues JN, Torresani T, Herve F et al. Interest of growth hormone releasing hormone administration for improvement of ovarian responsiveness to gonadotropins in poor responder women. *Fertil Steril* 1991;55:945-951.
79. Rutherford AJ, Subak-Sharpe RJ, Dawson KJ et al. Improvement of an in vitro fertilization after treatment with buserelin, an agonist of luteinizing hormone releasing hormone. *Br Med J Clin Res Ed* 1988;296:1765-1768.

Ultrasound in the Assisted Reproductive Technologies

80. Steptoe PC, Edwards RG. Birth after re-implantation of a human embryo. *Lancet* 1978;2:366.

Patient Selection and Precycle Treatment for IVF

81. Palermo G, Joris H, Devroey P et al. Pregnancies after intracytoplasmic injection of a single spermatozoon into an oocyte. *Lancet* 1992;340:17-18.

Ovarian Stimulation and Monitoring of IVF Cycles

82. Paulson RJ, Sauer MV, Francis MM et al. In vitro fertilization in unstimulated cycles: the University of Southern California experience. *Fertil Steril* 1992;57:290.

Oocyte Retrieval

83. Wood C, Trounson AO, Leeton JF et al. Clinical features of eight pregnancies resulting from in vitro infertilization and embryo transfer. *Fertil Steril* 1982;38:22-29.
84. Wiseman DA, Short WB, Pattinson HA et al. Oocyte retrieval in an *in vitro* fertilization program: comparison of four methods. *Radiology* 1989;173:99-102.
85. Robertson RD, Picker RH, O'Neil C et al. An experience of laparoscopic and transvesical oocyte retrieval in an in vitro fertilization program. *Fertil Steril* 1986;45(1):88-92.
86. Lewin A, Margalioth EJ, Rabinowitz R et al. Comparative study of ultrasonically guided percutaneous aspiration with local anesthesia and laparoscopic aspiration of follicles in an in vitro fertilization program. *Am J Obstet Gynecol* 1985; 151(5):621-625.
87. Marrs RP. Does the method of oocyte collection have a major influence on in vitro fertilization? *Fertil Steril* 1986;46(2): 193-195.
88. Lenz S, Lauritsen JG. Ultrasonically guided percutaneous aspiration of human follicles under local anesthesia: a new method of collecting oocytes for in vitro fertilization. *Fertil Steril* 1982;38(6):673-677.
89. Wikland M, Nilsson L, Hansson R et al. Collection of human oocytes by the use of sonography. *Fertil Steril* 1983;39(5): 603-608.
90. Taylor PJ, Wiseman DA, Mahadevan M et al. "Ultrasound rescue": with a successful alternative form of oocyte recovery in patients with periovarian adhesions. *Am J Obstet Gynecol* 1986;54:240-244.
91. Parson J, Pampiglione JS, Sadler AP et al. Ultrasound directed follicle aspiration for oocyte collection using perurethral technique. *Fertil Steril* 1990;53(1):97-102.
92. Hartz SC. In vitro fertilization-embryo transfer (IVF-ET) in the United States: 1989 results from the IVF-ET registry. *Fertil Steril* 1991;55(1):14-21.
93. Miller DL, Wall RT. Fentanyl and diazepam for analgesia and sedation during radiologic special procedures. *Radiology* 1987;162:195-198.

Embryo Transfer

94. Strickler R, Christianson C, Crane JP et al. Ultrasound guidance for human embryo transfer. *Fertil Steril* 1985;43(1):54-61.

Cryopreservation of Excess Embryos

95. Pattinson HA, Greene CA, Fleetham J et al. Exogenous control of the cycle simplifies thawed embryo transfer and results in a pregnancy rate similar to that for natural cycles. *Fertil Steril* 1992;58(3):627-629.
96. Gonen Y, Casper RF. Prediction of implantation by the sonographic appearance of the endometrium during controlled ovarian stimulation for IVF. *J In Vitro Fert Embryo Transfer* 1990;7:146-152.

IVF Outcomes

97. Society for Assisted Reproductive Technology, The American Fertility Society, Assisted Reproductive Technology in the United States and Canada. 1991 results from the Society for Assisted Reproductive Technology generated from the American Fertility Society Registry. *Fertil Steril* 1993;59:956.
98. Shoham Z, Zosmer A, Insler V. Early miscarriage and fetal malformations after induction of ovulation (by clomiphene citrate and/or human menotropins), in vitro fertilization, and gamete intrafallopian transfer. *Fertil Steril* 1991;55:1.

Other Assisted Reproductive Technologies

99. Lucena E, Ruiz JA, Medoza JC et al. Vaginal intratubal insemination (VITI) and vaginal GIFT, endosonographic technique: early experience. *Hum Reprod* 1989;4(6):658-662.
100. Balmaceda JP, Alam V, Roszjtein D et al. Embryo implantation rates in oocyte donation: a prospective comparison of tubal versus uterine transfers. *Fertil Steril* 1992;57:362.

Biologic Effects of Ultrasound

101. Puissant F, Lejeune LF. Effects on mature mouse oocytes of ultrasound treatment applied before in vitro fertilization. *Obstet Gynecol* 1984;12:421-422.
102. Hartz SC. In vitro fertilization-embryo transfer in the United States: 1988 results from the IVF-ET registry. *Fertil Steril* 1990;53(1):13-20.
103. Mashiach S, Bider D, Moran O et al. Adnexal torsion of hyperstimulated ovaries in pregnancies after gonodotropin therapy. *Fertil Steril* 1990;53:76.

Complications of Ovarian Hyperstimulation

104. Rabau E, Serr DM, David A et al. Human menopausal gonadotropins for anovulation and sterility. *Am J Obstet Gynecol* 1967;98:92-98.
105. Schenker JG, Weinstein D. Ovarian hyperstimulation syndrome; a current survey. *Fertil Steril* 1978;30:255-268.
106. Golan A, Ron-El R, Herman A et al. Ovarian hyperstimulation syndrome: an update review. *Obstet Gynecol* 1989;6: 430-440.
107. Blankstein J, Shalev J, Saadon T et al. Ovarian hyperstimulation syndrome: prediction by number and size of preovulatory ovarian follicles. *Fertil Steril* 1987;47(4):597-601.
108. Polishuk WA, Schenker JG. Ovarian overstimulation syndrome. *Fertil Steril* 1969;20:443.
109. Tulandi T, Mcinnes RA, Arronet GH. Ovarian hyperstimulation syndrome following ovulation induction with HMG. *Int J Fertil* 1984;29:113.
110. Evans MI, Dommergues M, Wapner RJ et al. Efficacy of transabdominal multifetal pregnancy reduction: collaborative experience among the world's largest centers. *Obstet Gynecol* 1993;82:61.
111. Savare J, Norup P, Thomsen SG et al. Heterotropic pregnancies after in vitro fertilization and embryo transfer: a Danish survey. *Hum Reprod* 1993;8:116.

PART VI

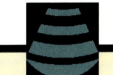

Pediatric Sonography

CHAPTER 52

Neonatal and Infant Brain Imaging

•

Terese I. Kaske, M.D.
Carol M. Rumack, M.D., F.A.C.R.
Curtis L. Harlow, M.D.

CHAPTER OUTLINE

CHAPTER OUTLINE, cont'd.

Sonography of the brain is an integral part of care in the neonate, particularly among high-risk premature infants. Current ultrasound technology allows for rapid evaluation of infants in the intensive care nursery with virtually no risk.[1] The advantages of sonography over computed tomography (CT) or magnetic resonance imaging (MRI) include portability, lower cost, speed, lack of ionizing radiation, and no need for sedation. Screening of premature infants for intracranial hemorrhage has proven highly sensitive and specific. Ultrasound can also be valuable in the evaluation and follow-up of hydrocephalus and periventricular leukomalacia (PVL). Prenatal diagnosis of central nervous system (CNS) malformations, infection, or masses is now often followed up in the neonatal period by MRI or CT. Ultrasound can be useful for the follow-up of therapy or for follow-up of complications. Pulsed, color, and power Doppler imaging of cranial blood flow may prove valuable if the differential diagnosis includes a vascular lesion and is useful in infants receiving extracorporeal membrane oxygenation.[2-5] A new use for sonography has been described in evaluation of normal cranial sutures which may allow diagnosis of craniosynostosis and other abnormal sutures.[6]

EQUIPMENT

In the premature infant, a 7.5-MHz transducer is recommended to obtain the highest resolution possible. A 5-MHz transducer is necessary to allow for adequate sound penetration of a larger infant's head.[7] Electronic phased array transducers with a 120-degree sector angle and multifocal zone capability are generally used for imaging through the anterior fontanelle. Some manufacturers have transducers with very small footplates that are well suited to premature infants or smaller fontanelles. These transducers are also useful when scanning from the posterior mastoid area or foramen magnum (posterior fontanelle views).[8] Small linear array transducers can provide quality images for scanning in the axial plane through the squamous portion of the temporal bone. This thin bone window usually requires a 3.5-MHz transducer. The multifocal zone capability provides excellent resolution throughout the field of view, but requires a cooperative patient as the scanning speed is slowed significantly. Cineloop features that allow review and retrieval of images, before the frozen image, are invaluable in an uncooperative infant.[4]

A high-quality, multi-image, multiformat camera is important to record permanent digital or hard copies of the examination. Digital storage allowing post-processing of images can improve quality and save film. It may be useful to videotape an examination for later review. This can prevent the repetition of an examination if there is a questionable finding on the individual images. Areas of increased or decreased echogenicity can be extremely subtle on hard-copy film, but they become much more apparent when integrated with multiple images of a moving picture in realtime.

SONOGRAPHIC TECHNIQUE

Currently, most brain sonographic examinations are performed through the anterior fontanelle in both the coronal and sagittal planes. Good skin-to-transducer coupling can be achieved by an acoustic coupling gel. Occasionally, a standoff pad can be useful to evaluate superficial abnormalities such as subdural hemorrhage, but a higher resolution transducer may be best to evaluate the nearfield in detail. Most recently, color Doppler has been used to evaluate fluid collections.[9] If extracerebral fluid collections are expected, they may be better evaluated with CT or MRI. Axial scanning has been used extensively in the past, particularly for accurate measurements of ventricular dimensions. Presently, axial scanning is used in Doppler imaging to evaluate the circle of Willis.[7,10,11] Additional innovative methods of cranial scanning using the posterior and posterolateral fontanelles and foramen magnum, as well as transcranial Doppler imaging have been described.[4,8,12-13] The posterior scanning techniques are useful when evaluating the posterior fossa and the occipital horns; the foramen magnum approach may be useful when evaluating the spinal canal—for instance in patients with Chiari malformation. The anterior fontanelle remains open until approximately 2 years of age, but is suitable for scanning only until about 12 to 14 months, and this scanning is rarely performed in patients over 6 months of age.[12] The smaller the fontanelle, the smaller the acoustic window and the more difficult the examination will be.[7,10,11]

Every effort should be made to maintain normal body temperature in premature infants. Their small size results in a high surface-to-volume ratio and rapid heat loss when they are exposed. Use of overhead warming lamps, blankets, and warmed coupling gel should be routinely used. If the infant is in an isolette, heat loss may be minimized by using access side holes as an entry site for the transducer.

Hand washing and cleansing of the transducer between patients are of paramount importance to avoid the spread of infection in the intensive care nursery. Simply cleansing the transducer head with alcohol should be adequate. A transducer should never be autoclaved because this will destroy it. When absolute sterility is required, such as during operative sonography, the transducer can be placed inside of a sterile surgical glove or sterile transducer cover with coupling gel. Sterile aqueous gel or saline solution can be used as a coupler outside of the glove.

Standard brain scanning includes sagittal and coronal planes. Nonstandard planes can and should be used if they are helpful to outline pathologic states. Whenever possible, the transducer should be held firmly between the thumb and index finger, and the lateral aspect of the hand should rest on the infant's head for stability.

Coronal Brain Scans

Coronal images are obtained by placing the scan head transversely across the anterior fontanelle (Fig. 52-1). The plane of the ultrasound beam is then made to sweep in an anterior to posterior direction, completely through the brain.[14] Care must be taken to maintain symmetric imaging of each half of the brain and skull. At least six standard, frozen images should be made during this anterior to posterior scan.[11,12,14,15] The box on p. 1448 lists the structures to be seen on the normal images.

The most anterior section (Fig. 52-2, *A*) should be just anterior to the frontal horns of the lateral ventricles. Visualization of the anterior cranial fossa, frontal lobes of the cerebral cortex with the orbits deep to the floor of the skull base is obtained.

Moving posterior (Fig. 52-2, *B*) the frontal horns of the lateral ventricles appear as symmetric anechoic, comma-shaped areas with the hypoechoic caudate

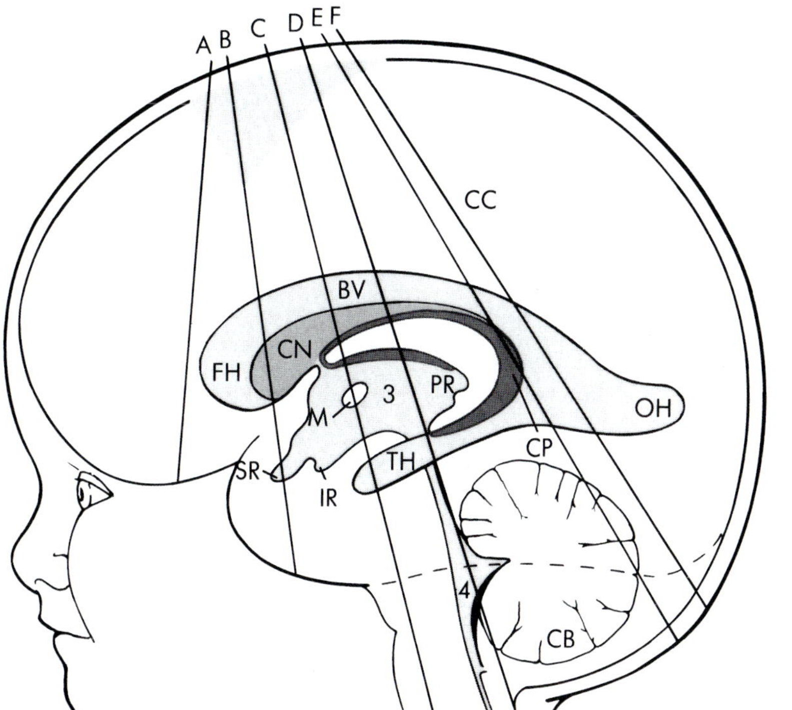

FIG. 52-1. Schematic representation of coronal planes used in brain scanning through anterior fontanelle (**A** to **F** correspond front to back). CC—Cerebral cortex; BV—body of lateral ventricle; FH—frontal horn; OH—occipital horn; CN—caudate nucleus; M—massa intermedia; PR—pineal recess; 3—third ventricle; TH—temporal horn; SR—supraoptic recess; IR—infundibular recess; CP—choroid plexus; 4—fourth ventricle; CB—cerebellum. (From Rumack CM, Johnson ML: *Perinatal and Infant Brain Imaging*, St. Louis, 1984, Mosby–Year Book.)

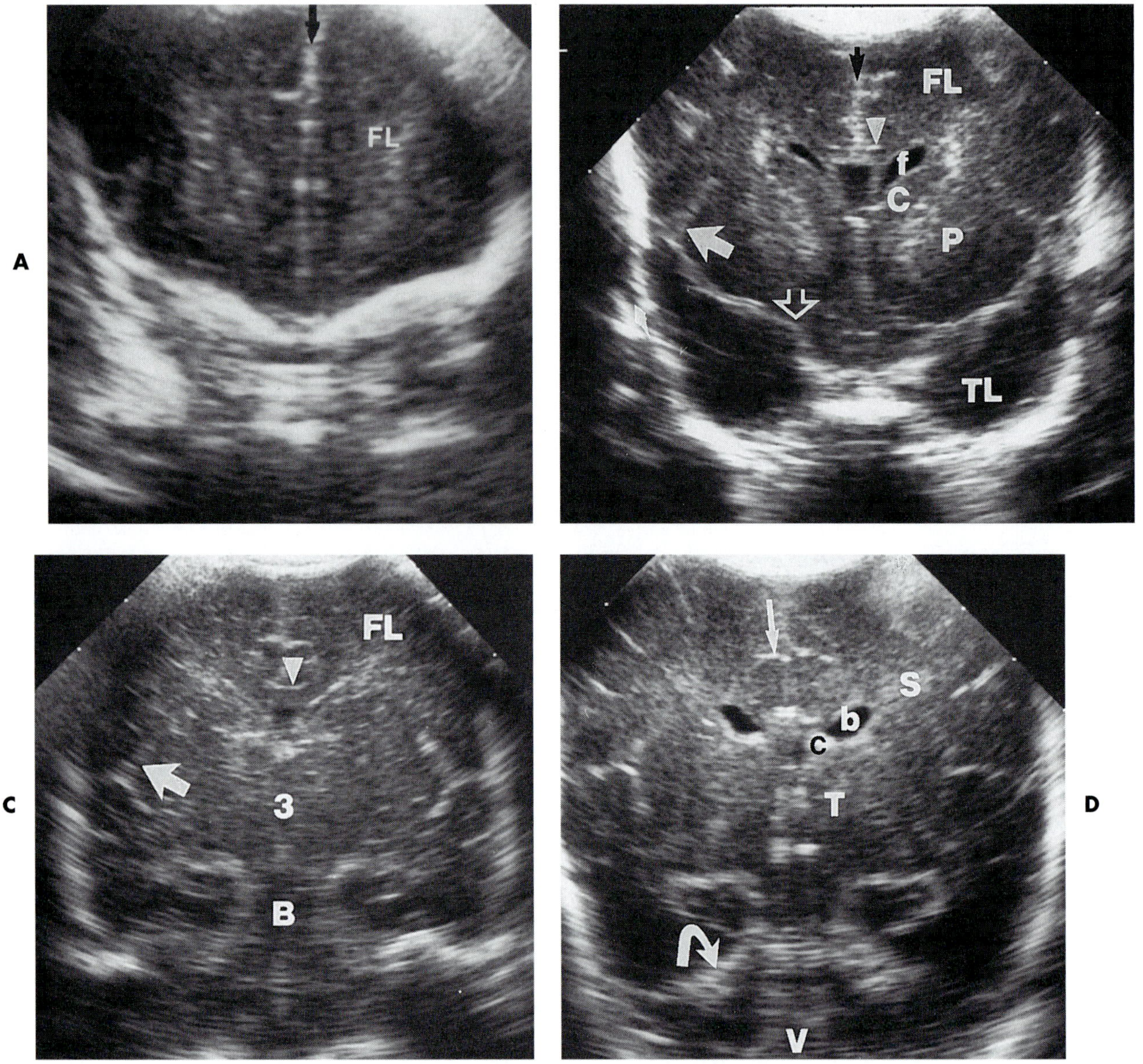

FIG. 52-2. Coronal brain scans of a normal full-term infant. Anterior to posterior corresponds to sections in Figure 52-1, **A** to **F. A,** FL—Frontal lobes. **B,** f—Frontal horns of lateral ventricles; C—caudate nucleus; TL—temporal lobe; Arrowhead—corpus callosum; Closed arrow—sylvian fissure; Open arrow—bifurcation of internal carotid artery, P—putamen. **C,** B—brain stem; 3—location of third ventricle (third and fourth ventricles are difficult to see in normal patients on coronal cuts). (On images **A** through **C,** straight black arrow represents interhemispheric fissure.). **D,** S—Centrum semiovale; b—body of lateral ventricle; c—choroid plexus; T—thalamus; V—vermis of cerebellum; Curved arrow—tentorium cerebelli; Straight white arrow—cingulate sulcus.

Continued.

E
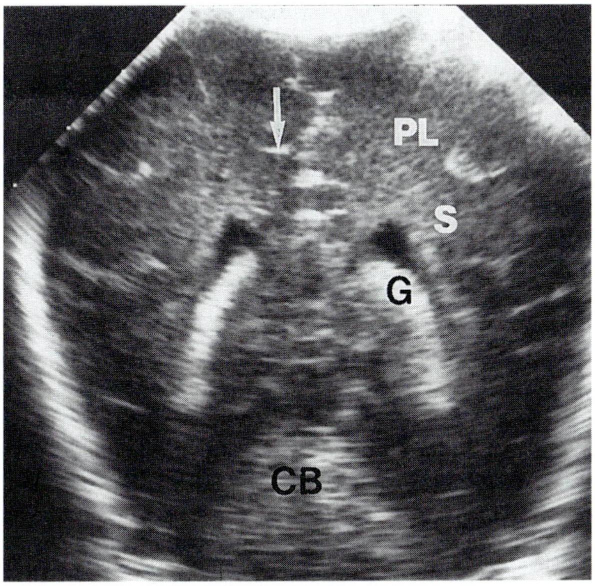

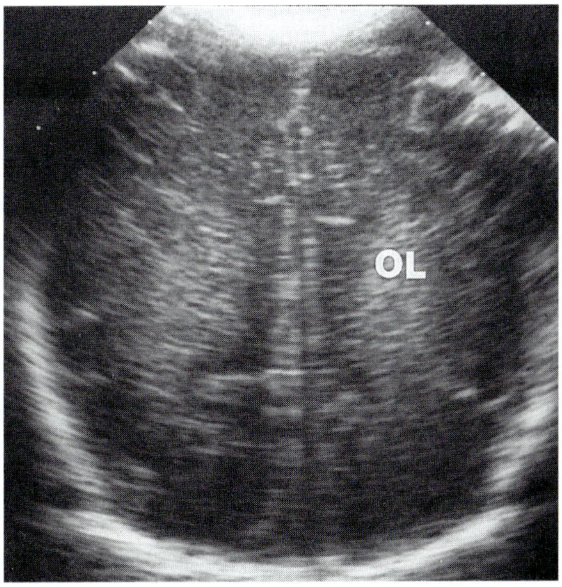

F

FIG. 52-2, cont'd. **E**, PL—parietal lobe; G—glomus of choroid plexus. **F**, OL—occipital lobe; CB—cerebellum. (*B and C*, from Rumack CR, Horgan JG, Hay TC, et al: *Pocket Atlas of Pediatric Ultrasound*, Philadelphia, 1990, Lippincott-Raven.)

heads within the concave lateral border. Structures visualized from superior to inferior in the midline include: (1) the interhemispheric fissure; (2) the cingulate sulcus; (3) the genu and anterior body of the corpus callosum; and (4) the septum pellucidum between the ventricles. Moving laterally from the midline the caudate nucleus is separated from the putamen by the internal capsule. Lateral to the putamen, the Sylvian fissure is echogenic because it contains the middle cerebral artery (MCA). It separates the frontal from the temporal lobe. Inferiorly, the internal carotid arteries bifurcate to form the echogenic anterior and middle cerebral arteries.

Progressing further posteriorly (Fig. 52-2, *C*) more of the body of the lateral ventricles is seen on either side of the cavum septi pellucidi. The thalami lie on either side of the third ventricle which is usually too thin to visualize in normal infants. Deep to the thalami, the brain stem begins to be visualized. Lateral to the midline, the thalami are separated from the lentiform nuclei by the internal capsule. Lateral to the lentiform nuclei is the deep white matter region of brain called the *centrum semiovale*. Again, the Sylvian fissures are seen.

At a slightly more posterior transducer angulation the body of the lateral ventricle becomes somewhat more rounded as the size of the caudate nucleus decreases once posterior to the foramen of Monro (Fig. 52-2, *D*). Echogenic material in the floor of the lateral ventricles is the choroid plexus. At this level in the midline the body of the corpus callosum is deep to the cingulate sulcus and the third ventricle is located between the anterior portions of the thalami. Echogenic choroid plexus may be seen in the roof of the third ventricle. The thalami are now more prominent on either side of the third ventricle. Midline structures are unchanged except that deep to the thalami the tentorium covering the cerebellum is visualized. In the posterior fossa, the vermis is the echogenic structure in the midline surrounded by the more hypoechoic cerebellar hemispheres. When the septum pellucidum is cystic posteriorly, it is called the *cavum vergae*. Because the cystic center of the septum pellucidum closes from posterior to anterior as the brain matures, late gestation neonates often have only the more anterior cavum septi pellucidi. The lentiform nuclei may no longer be seen at this level. The temporal horns of the lateral ventricles may be seen lateral and inferior to the thalami, but are usually not seen unless there is hydrocephalus.

Further posterior, the trigone or atrium of the lateral ventricles is visualized (Fig. 52-2, *E*). The extensive echogenic glomus of the choroid plexus nearly obscures the lumen of the cerebrospinal fluid (CSF)–filled ventricle in this area. In the midline—the visualized portion of the corpus callosum deep to the cingulate sulcus—is the splenium. Inferiorly, the cerebellum is separated from the occipital cortex by the tentorium cerebelli.

The most posterior section (Fig. 52-2, *F*) visualizes predominantly occipital lobe cortex and the most posterior aspect of the occipital horns of the lateral ventricles. This section is angled posterior to the cerebellum.

CORONAL BRAIN SCANS: NORMAL STRUCTURES

Midline
Interhemispheric fissure
Cingulate sulci
Corpus callosum
Cavum septi pellucidi
Cavum vergae (when present)
Third ventricle
Fourth ventricle
Brain stem
Vermis of cerebellum

Paramedian
Frontal lobe
Parietal lobe
Occipital lobe
Frontal horn of lateral ventricle
Body of lateral ventricle
Temporal horn of lateral ventricle
Trigone of lateral ventricle
Choroid plexus
Glomus of choroid plexus
Caudate nucleus
Internal capsule
Thalamus
Lentiform nucleus
Tentorium cerebelli
Cerebellar hemisphere
Sylvian fissure

Sagittal Brain Scans

The **sagittal** images are obtained by placing the transducer longitudinally across the anterior fontanelle and angling it to each side (Fig. 52-3). The midline is first identified through the interhemispheric fissure by recognition of the curving line of the corpus callosum, above the cystic cavum septi pellucidi, the third and fourth ventricles, and the highly echogenic cerebellar vermis (Fig. 52-4, *A and B*). Shallow angulation to each side of about 10 degrees will show the normally small lateral ventricles (Fig. 52-5, *A*). The ventricles are not located in a perfectly straight plane anterior to posterior. The technologist must angle the probe so that the anterior portion of the sector is directed more medially, and the posterior portion of the sector more laterally to include the entire lateral ventricle in a single-image plane.[11,12,14,15]

Above the lateral ventricle is the cerebral cortex and below it is the cerebellar hemisphere. The caudate nucleus and the thalamus are within the arms of the ventricle (Fig. 52-5, *B*). The caudothalamic groove is an important area to recognize, because this is the most common site of germinal matrix hemorrhage (GMH).

SAGITTAL BRAIN SCANS: NORMAL STRUCTURES

Midline structures
Frontal lobe
Parietal lobe
Occipital lobe
Cingulate sulcus
Corpus callosum
Cavum septi pellucidi
Cavum vergae
Third ventricle
Fourth ventricle
Tentorium
Pericallosal artery
Choroid plexus
Massa intermedia
Aqueduct
Occipitoparietal fissure
Brain stem
Vermis of cerebellum

Paramedian structures
Frontal lobe
Parietal lobe
Occipital lobe
Frontal horn of lateral ventricle
Body of lateral ventricle
Atrium of lateral ventricle (trigone)
Temporal horn of lateral ventricle
Occipital horn of lateral ventricle
Choroid plexus
Caudate nucleus
Thalamus
Caudothalamic groove
Cerebellum

More pronounced lateral angulation will demonstrate the peripheral aspect of the ventricles and more lateral cerebral hemisphere, including the temporal lobes (Fig 52-5, *C*).[10]

In actual practice, one must learn to cope with the normal shadowing caused by the midline falx on sagittal cuts. This is easily achieved and only requires that the scan be performed slightly laterally to the falx. Problems arise only when the disruptive shadowing that causes loss of resolution is not recognized.

Sagittal sonography almost always reveals a normal hyperechoic "blush" just posterior and superior to the ventricular trigones on parasagittal views. It is probably caused by the interface of numerous parallel fibers that are nearly perpendicular to the longitudinal axis of a sonography beam passing through the anterior fontanelle. The same echogenicity is not seen on sonograms obtained through the posterior fontanelle,

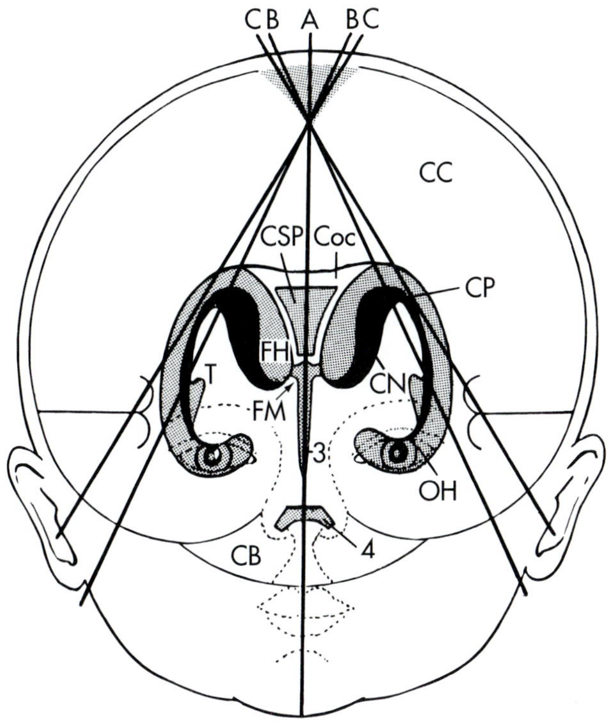

FIG. 52-3. Schematic representation of sagittal planes used in brain scanning through anterior fontanelle. A to C correspond to midline to lateral. CB—Cerebellum; CC—cerebral cortex; Coc—corpus callosum; CN—caudate nucleus; CP—choroid plexus; CSP—cavum septi pellucidi; FH—frontal horn; FM—foramen of Monro; OH—occipital horn; T—temporal horn; 3—third ventricle; 4—fourth ventricle. (Modified from Rumack CM, Johnson ML: *Perinatal and Infant Brain Imaging*, St. Louis, 1984, Mosby–Year Book.)

A

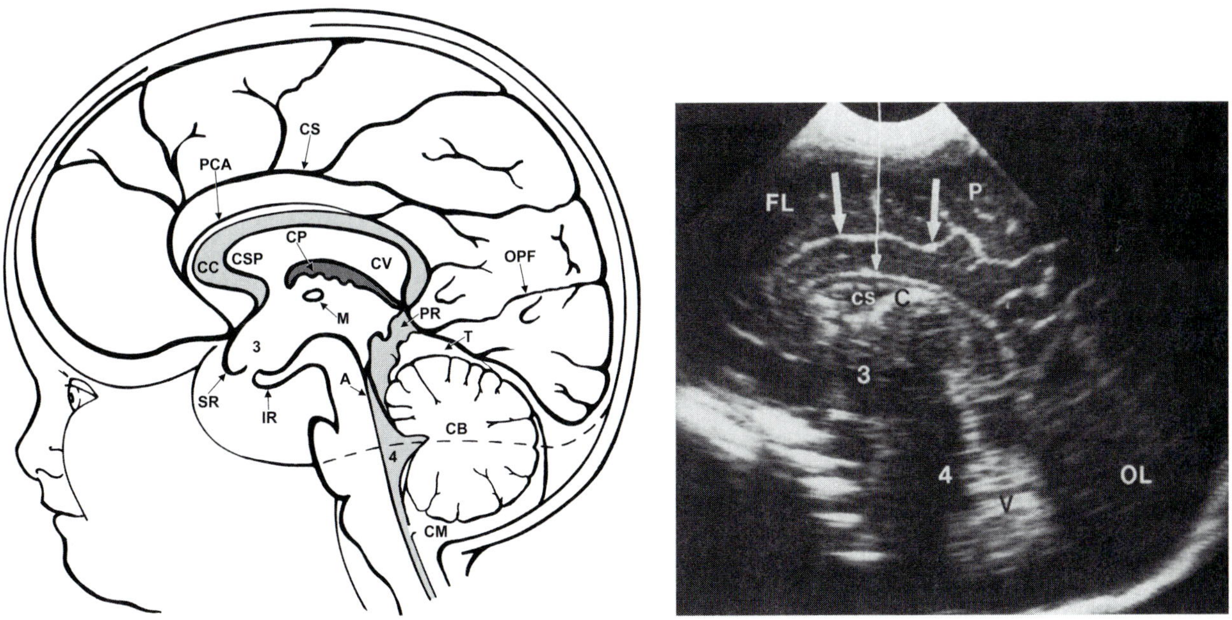

B

FIG. 52-4. Normal midline sagittal. **A, Drawing.** CC—Corpus callosum; CSP—cavum septi pellucidi; CP—choroid plexus; CV—cavum vergae; PR—pineal recess; SR—supraoptic recess; IR—infundibular recess; 3—third ventricle; 4—fourth ventricle; A—aqueduct; CB—cerebellum (vermis); CM—cisterna magna; PCA—pericallosal artery; CS—cingulate sulcus; M—massa intermedia; T—tentorium; OPF—occipito-parietal fissure. **B, Normal midline sagittal brain scans,** corresponding to images in Fig. 52-3: midline (**A**). FL—Frontal lobe; P—parietal lobe; OL—occipital lobe; long thin arrow—corpus callosum; cs—cavum septi pellucidi; C—choroid plexus; 3—third ventricle; 4—fourth ventricle; V—cerebellar vermis; shorter thick arrows—cingulate sulcus. (*B* from Rumack CM, Manco-Johnson ML: Neonatal brain ultrasonography. In Sarti DA, editor: *Diagnostic Ultrasound: Text and Cases*, ed 2, St. Louis, 1987, Mosby–Year Book.)

A

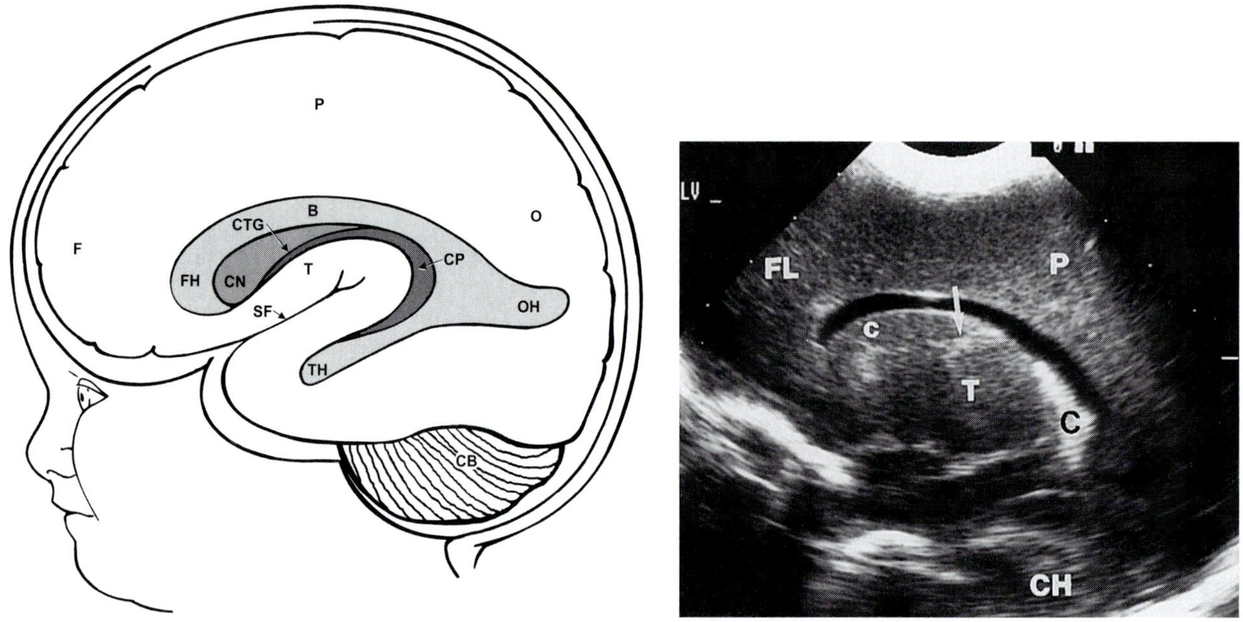

B

FIG. 52-5. Normal parmedian sagittal anatomy. A, **Schematic drawing.** F—Frontal lobe; P—parietal lobe; O—occipital lobe; FH—frontal horn; CTG—caudothalamic groove (arrow on *B*)—body of lateral ventricle; OH—occipital horn; TH—temporal horn; SF—sylvian fissure; T—thalamus; CB—cerebellum; CP—choroid plexus. **B, Sagittal sonogram,** paramedian view. FL—frontal lobe; P—parietal lobe; T—thalamus; c—caudate nucleus; C—choroid plexus; CH—cerebellar hemisphere. (*B* from Rumack CR, Horgan JG, Hay TC, et al.: *Pocket Atlas of Pediatric Ultrasound*, Philadelphia, 1990, Lippincott-Raven.)

because with that angulation, the long axis of the sonographic beam and the fiber tracts are nearly parallel. Sonographic-pathologic correlations demonstrated the normal peritrigonal hyperechogenicity.[16]

DEVELOPMENTAL ANATOMY

Brain Sulcal Development

In the very premature infant, the brain sulci are not fully developed and the brain appears quite smooth (Fig. 52-6). Sulcal development begins with the calcarine fissure as simple straight lines in the fifth gestational month (20 weeks).[17] By 24 weeks' gestation, only the parieto-occipital fissure is present. By 28 weeks of gestation, the callosomarginal and cingulate sulci are seen (Fig. 52-7, *A*), and by 30 weeks of gestation, the cingulate sulcus is also branched (Fig 52-75, *B*). During the eighth and ninth months of gestation, sulci bend, branch, and anastomose so that a full-term infant has many peripheral branches over the brain surface (Fig. 52-7, *C*).

Cavum Septi Pellucidi and Cavum Vergae

There is one continuous cystic midline structure in the septum pellucidum during fetal life. Anterior to the foramen of Monro (Fig. 52-7) is the cavum septi pellucidi, and posterior is the cavum vergae. Both parts are normally present early in gestation, but they close from back to front, starting at approximately 6 months' gestation (Fig. 52-8). By full-term, closure has occurred posteriorly in 97% of infants so that there is only a cavum septi pellucidi at birth. By 3 to 6 months after birth, this septum is completely closed in 85% of infants, although in some, the septum remains open into adulthood.[18]

Choroid Plexus

The choroid plexus is the site of CSF production in the ventricles (Fig. 52-9). The largest portion of the choroid plexus is the glomus, a highly echogenic structure attached to the trigone of each lateral ventricle. The choroid tapers as it extends anteriorly to the foramen of Monro. At this point, it continues through the foramen from each lateral ventricle and continues along the roof of the third ventricle. The choroid also tapers posteriorly as it extends into the temporal horn of the lateral ventricle. Choroid plexus is also present in the roof of the fourth ventricle. At no time does the normal choroid plexus extend into the frontal or occipital horn.

Germinal Matrix

The germinal matrix develops deep to the ependyma and consists of loosely organized, proliferating cells

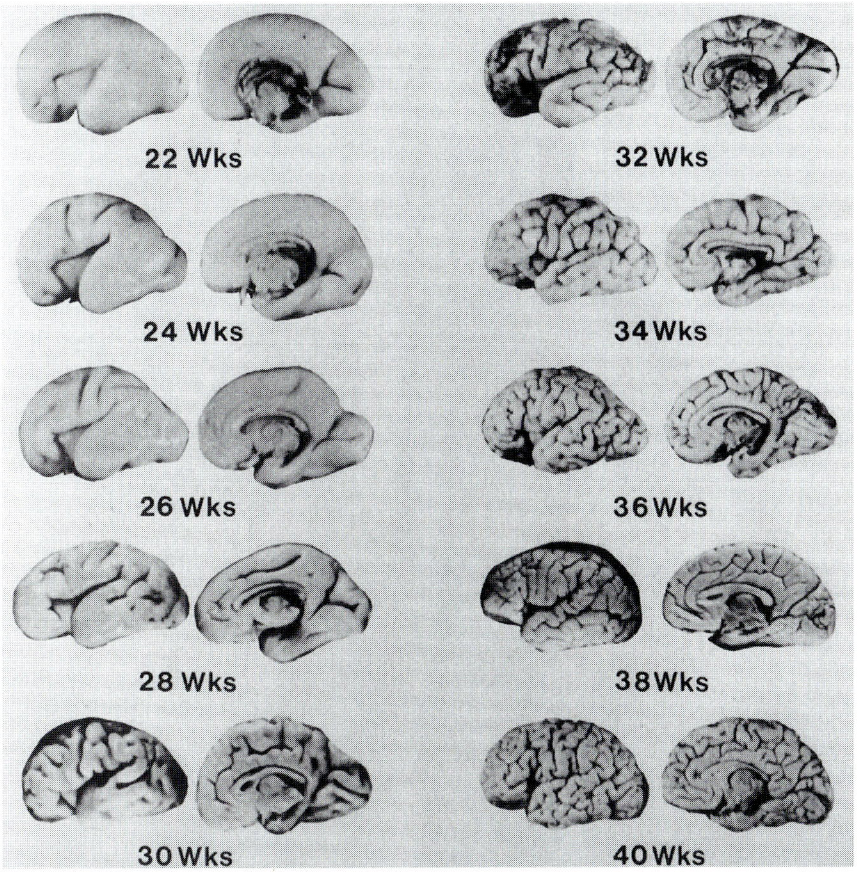

FIG. 52-6. Normal sulcal pattern development, at 22 to 40 weeks' gestation. (From Dolan CL, Dorovini ZIS: Gestational development of the brain, *Arch Pathol Lab Med,* 101:192-195, 1977.)

that give rise to the neurons and glia of the cerebral cortex and basal ganglia (Fig. 52-10). Its vascular bed is the most richly perfused region of the developing brain. Vessels in this region form an immature vascular rete of fine capillaries, extremely thin-walled veins, and larger irregular vessels.[19] The capillary network is best developed on the periphery of the germinal matrix and becomes less well developed toward the central glioblastic mass. Although the germinal matrix is not visualized on sonography, it is important as the typical anatomic site where hemorrhage occurs in premature infants.

Early in gestation, the germinal matrix forms the entire wall of the ventricular system. After the third month of gestation, the germinal matrix regresses, first around the third ventricle, then around the temporal and occipital horns and trigone. By 24 weeks' gestation, the germinal matrix persists only over the head of the caudate nucleus and to a lesser extent over the body of the caudate. This regression continues until 40 weeks' gestation, when it ceases to exist as a discrete structure and the immature vascular rete has been remodeled to form adult vascular patterns.[14,15]

CONGENITAL BRAIN MALFORMATIONS

Classification

Congenital brain malformations are extremely common—they represent the most common anomalies in humans.[19,23-25] Malformations can be classified based on brain development and the types of anomalies that result when development is altered (see box on p. 1452).

Brain development can be divided into three stages: (1) cytogenesis; (2) histogenesis; and (3) organogenesis (see box on p. 1452).[26] Cytogenesis involves the formation of cells from molecules. Histogenesis is the formation of cells into the tissues and involves neuronal proliferation and differentiation. Organogenesis is the formation of tissues into organs.

Organogenesis can be further divided into stages (Fig. 52-11).[20] The first stage is that of **neural tube formation and closure**, which occur at 3 to 4 weeks' gestation. The neural plate folds in on itself, fusing dorsally and giving rise to the earliest recognizable brain and spinal cord. In the next step, segmentation and **diverticulation** of the forebrain occur at approx-

A

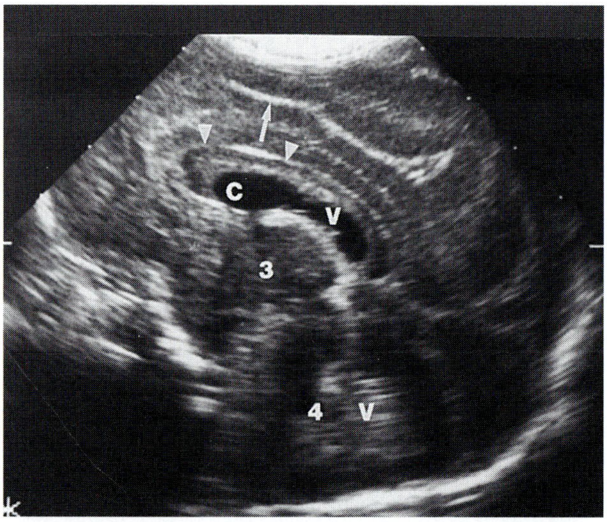

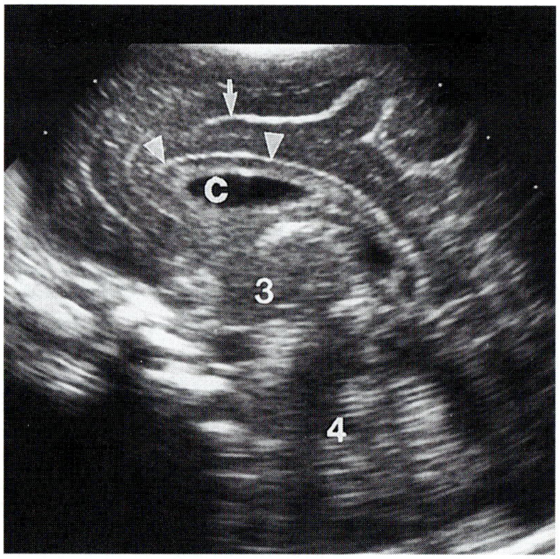

B

C

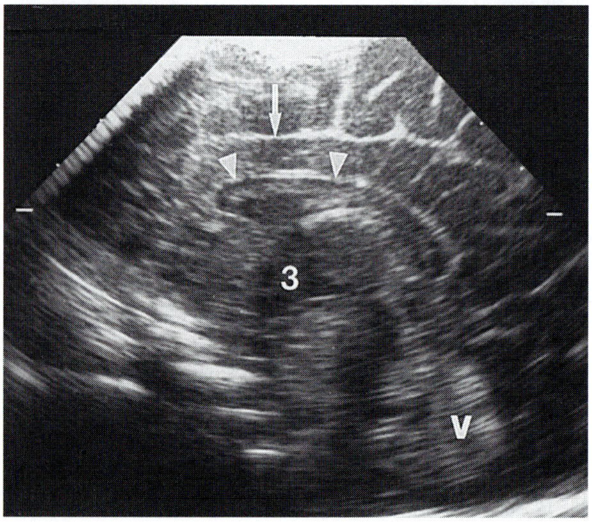

FIG. 52-7. Normal premature infant brain at 28 to 40 weeks' gestation. Sagittal images **A,** cingulate sulcus (*arrow*) is just developed, and cavum septi pellucidi (*C*) and cavum vergae (*V*) are readily visible. **B,** 30 weeks' gestation. Cingulate sulcus has a few branches. **C,** 40 weeks' gestation. Cingulate sulcus has many branches. The septum pellucidum is no longer cystic. 3—third ventricle; 4—fourth ventricle; V—cerebellar vermis; Arrowheads—corpus callosum.

CONGENITAL BRAIN MALFORMATIONS

- Disorders of Organogenesis
  - Disorders of Neural Tube Closure
    - Chiari malformations
    - Agenesis of the corpus callosum
    - Lipoma of the corpus callosum
    - Dandy-Walker malformation/variant
    - Posterior fossa arachnoid cyst
    - Teratoma
  - Disorders of Diverticulation and Cleavage
    - Septo-optic dysplasia
    - Holoprosencephaly
      - Alobar, Semilobar, and Lobar
  - Disorders of Sulcation/Cellular Migration
    - Lissencephaly
    - Schizencephaly
    - Heterotopias
    - Pachy-polymicrogyria
- Disorders of Size
- Disorders of Myelination
- Destructive Lesions
- Disorders of Histogenesis
  - Neurocutaneous Syndromes (Phakomatoses)
    - Tuberous sclerosis
    - Neurofibromatosis
  - Congenital Vascular Malformations
- Disorders of Cytogenesis
  - Congenital Neoplasms

DeMeyer classification of anomalies.[20-22]
Modified from Rumack CM, Johnson ML: *Perinatal and Infant Brain Imaging,* St. Louis, 1984, Mosby–Year Book.

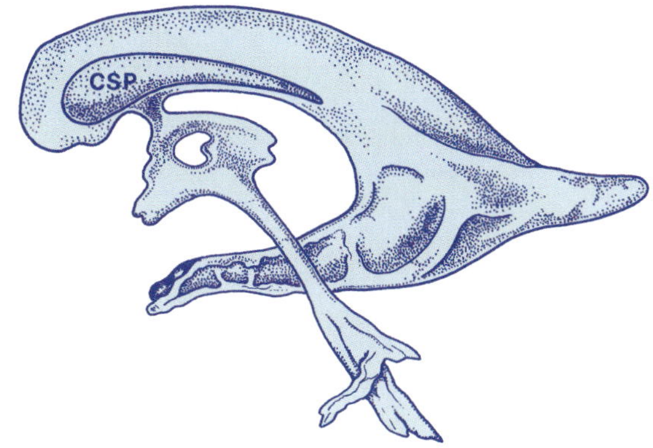

FIG. 52-8. Cava septi pellucidi and vergae (CSP) as it projects on the medial surface of the lateral ventricles. (From Rumack CM, Johnson ML: *Perinatal and Infant Brain Imaging*, St. Louis, 1984, Mosby–Year Book.)

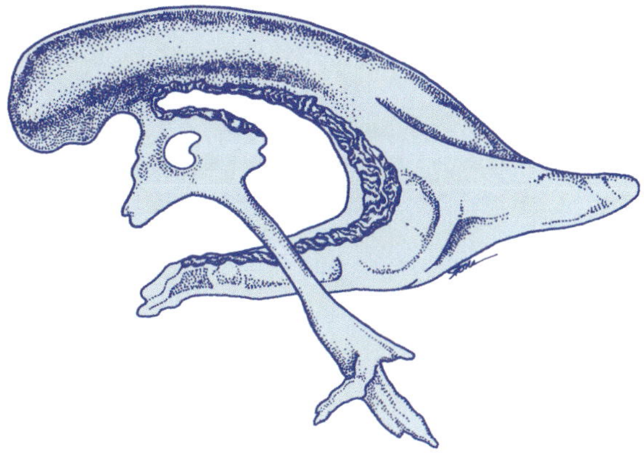

FIG. 52-9. Choroid plexus as it courses through the lateral and third ventricle. (From Rumack CM, Johnson ML: *Perinatal and Infant Brain Imaging*, St. Louis, 1984, Mosby–Year Book.)

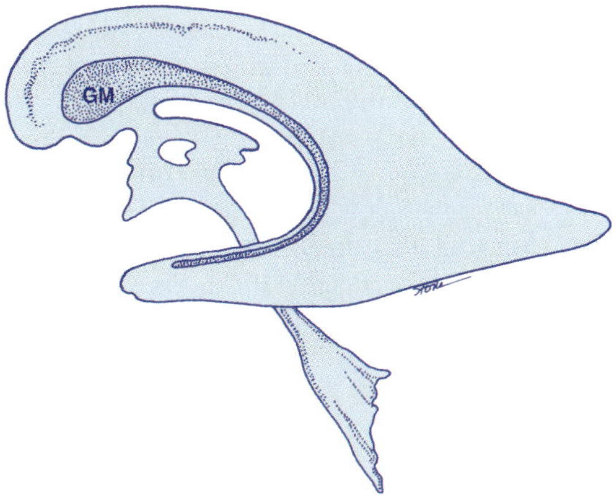

FIG. 52-10. Geminal matrix at 30 to 32 weeks' gestation with largest amount near the caudate nucleus. (From Rumack CM, Johnson ML: *Perinatal and Infant Brain Imaging*, St. Louis, 1984, Mosby–Year Book.)

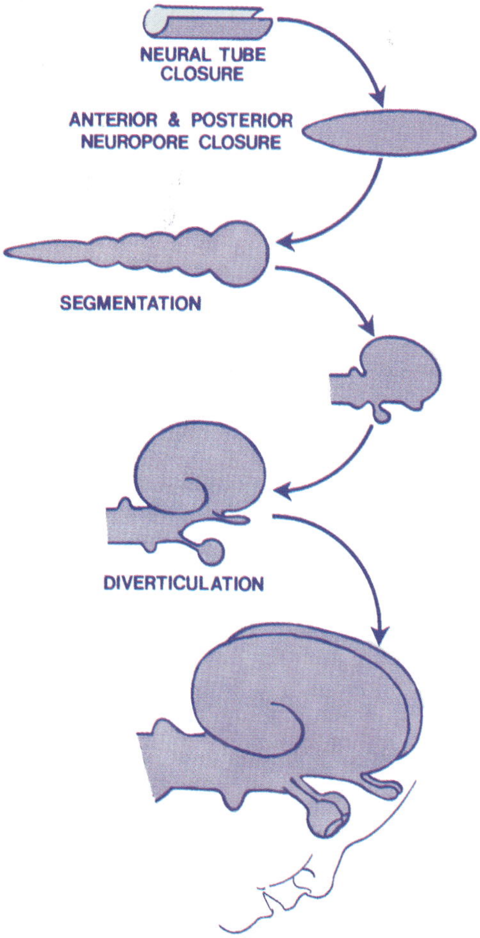

FIG. 52-11. Stages of organogenesis. The neural tube closes at 3 to 4 weeks' gestation, including closure of the anterior and posterior neuropores. At 5 to 6 weeks' gestation, the brain segments and five types of diverticula form. First the paired olfactory tracts, optic tracts, and cerebral ventricles develop, then the unpaired pineal and pituitary. Neural proliferation, migration, organization, and myelination occur after these stages. (From DeMyer W, Zeman W, Gardella Palmer C: The face predicts the brain: diagnostic significance of median facial anomalies for holoprosencephaly (arrhinencephaly). *Pediatrics*, 34:256-263, 1964.)

imately 5 to 6 weeks. The single central fetal ventricle separates into two lateral ventricles, and the brain divides into two cerebral hemispheres. Anteriorly, diverticulation results in the formation of the olfactory bulbs, optic vesicles, and the induction of facial development. The pituitary and pineal gland also develop by diverticulation from the ventricle in this stage.

Neuronal proliferation and **migration** occur at 8 to 24 weeks' gestation. Tremendous cellular proliferation is necessary to provide a growing brain with the necessary building blocks to form properly. Finally, millions of cells must migrate into the organized functional structure that is recognized as a normal brain. **Myelination** occurs from approximately the second trimester to adulthood, but is most active from directly after birth until approximately 2 years of age.[23,24] Migration and myelination defects are best evaluated by MRI and will not be discussed in this chapter.

Destructive lesions can occur at any point in brain development. Congenital malformations of the brain are often diagnosed *in utero* and neonatal sonographic imaging may be needed to confirm and/or further evaluate the prenatal diagnosis. CT or MRI may be required to further characterize the ultrasound findings.

STAGES OF BRAIN DEVELOPMENT

Cytogenesis: Development of molecules into cells
Histogenesis: Development of cells into tissues
Organogenesis: Development of tissues into organs
- Neural tube closure (dorsal induction: 3-4 weeks' gestation)
- Diverticulation (ventral induction: 5-6 weeks' gestation)
- Neuronal proliferation (8-16 weeks' gestation)
- Neuronal migration (24 weeks' gestation to years)
- Organization (6 months' gestation to years after birth)
- Myelination (birth to years after birth)

*Stages overlap in time but may be individually abnormal. Modified from Volpe JJ: Normal and abnormal human brain development, *Clin Perinatol* 4(1):3-30, 1977.

SONOGRAPHIC FINDINGS IN CHIARI II MALFORMATION

Anterior and inferior pointed frontal horns
- Batwing configuration

Enlarged lateral ventricles with occipital horns larger than frontal horns
- Colpocephaly

Third ventricle appearing only slightly enlarged
- Enlarged massa intermedia fills third ventricle

Elongation and caudal displacement of the fourth ventricle, pons, medulla, and vermis
Nonvisualized fourth ventricle due to compression
Partial absence of the septum pellucidum
Interhemispheric fissure
- Wide, especially after shunting
- Interdigitation of gyri causes serrated appearance

DISORDERS OF NEUTRAL TUBE CLOSURE

Chiari Malformations

Chiari malformations have been classified into four groups. **Chiari I malformation** is simply the down-

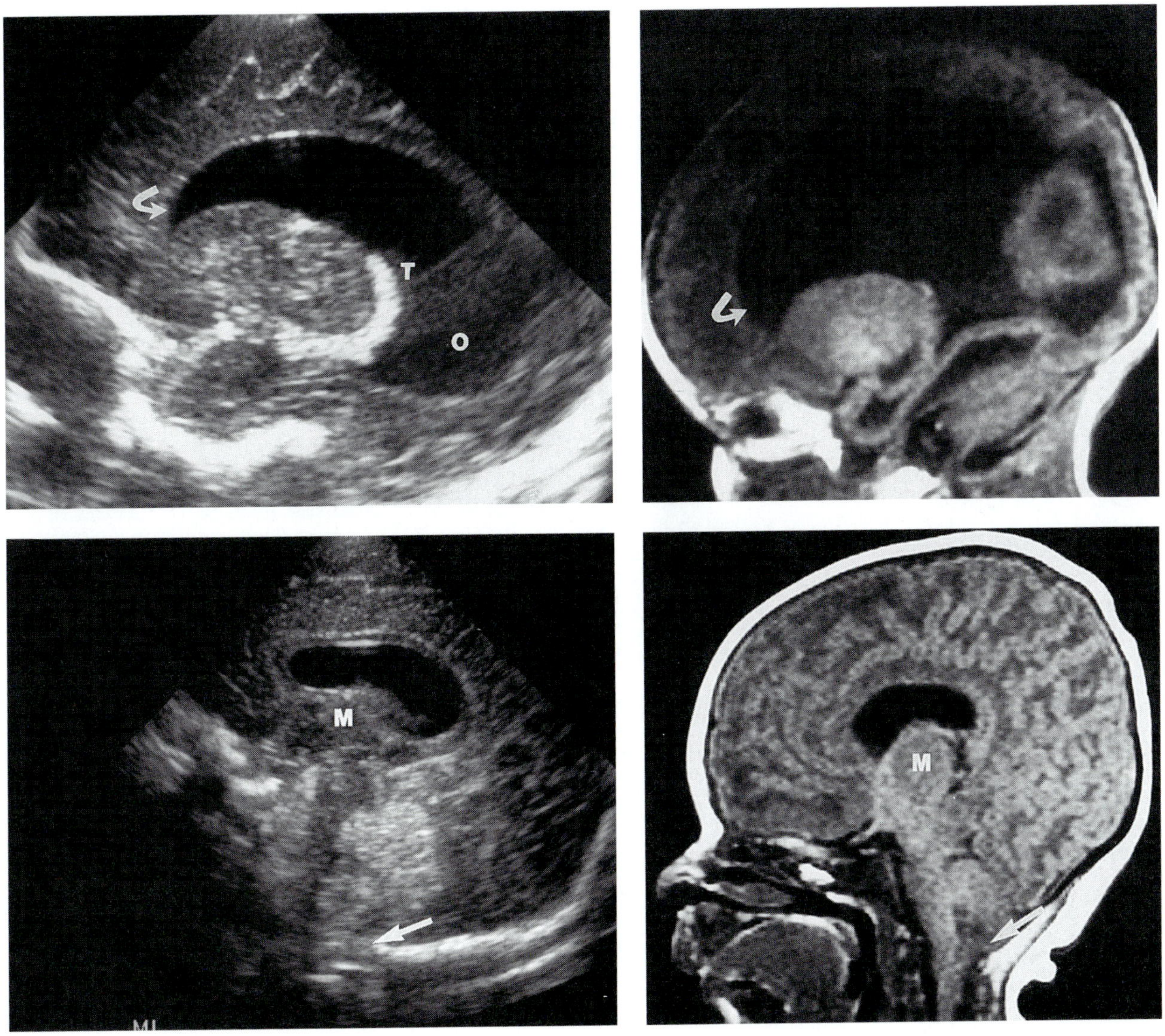

FIG. 52-12. Chiari II malformation. **A,** Lateral parasagittal sonogram and **B,** magnetic resonance imaging show pointing of frontal horn (curved arrow) and colpocephaly. O—Occipital horn; T—trigone of lateral ventricle. **C,** Midline sagittal sonogram and **D,** midline sagittal magnetic resonance imaging show enlargement of massa intermedia (*M*) and tonsillar herniation through foramen magnum (*arrow*). (From Rumack CM, Johnson ML: *Perinatal and Infant Brain Imaging*, St. Louis, 1984, Mosby–Year Book.)

ward displacement of the cerebellar tonsils, without displacement of the fourth ventricle or medulla. **Chiari II malformation** is the most common and of the greatest clinical importance because of its nearly universal association with meningomyelocele. **Chiari III malformation** is a high cervical encephalomeningocele in which the medulla, fourth ventricle, and virtually all of the cerebellum reside. **Chiari IV malformation** is severe hypoplasia of the cerebellum without displacement. Many authors do not consider this malformation to be part of the Chiari deformity spectrum but rather include it with cerebellar disorders.[22,27-29]

Classic Sonographic Findings of the Chiari II Malformation. Present theories propose that a failure in neural tube closure results in a small posterior fossa.[30] In early brain development, abnormal neural tube closure may result in a spinal defect such as a myelomeningocele. This decompresses the ventricles and leads to underdevelopment of the posterior fossa bony structures. The intracranial findings are the result of the small posterior fossa.[31-34] The tentorial attachment is low and the combined effect causes compression of the upper cerebellum by the tentorium. The inferior cerebellum is compressed and displaced into the foramen magnum. The cerebellar tonsils and vermis herniate into the spinal canal through an enlarged foramen magnum. The pons and medulla are inferiorly displaced, as is the elongated fourth ventricle (Figs. 52-12 and 52-13).

A

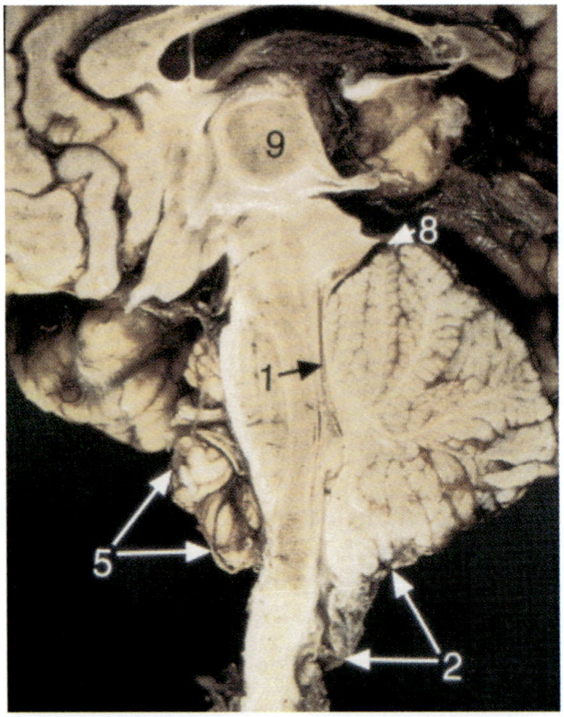

B

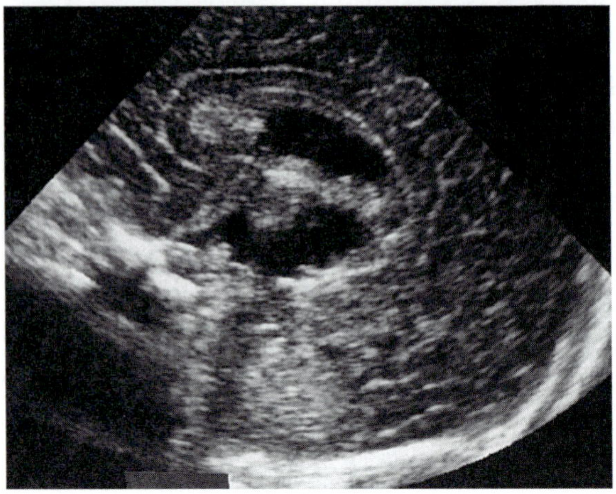

C

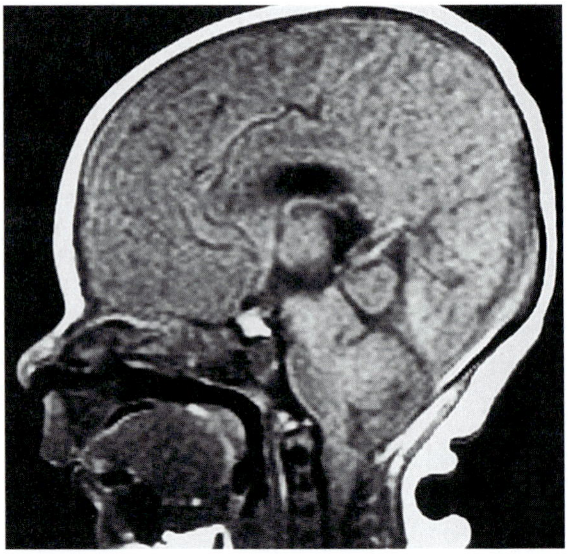

FIG. 52-13. Chiari II, midline images show large massa intermedia and tonsellar herniation, A, midsagittal path, B, ultrasound and C, magnetic resonance imaging. 9—massa intermedia; 2—tonsillar herniation; 1—compressed fourth ventricle. (From Osborn AG: *Diagnostic Neuroradiology*, St. Louis, 1994, Mosby–Year Book.)

There may be marked enlargement of the massa intermedia on the coronal and midline sagittal scans. Although the third ventricle is often enlarged and the aqueduct is kinked, the enlarged massa intermedia may fill the third ventricle causing it to appear only slightly larger than normal (Fig. 52-12). The fourth ventricle is often not visualized because it is thin, elongated, compressed, and displaced into the upper spinal canal. The frontal horns are typically small, with the posterior horns of the lateral ventricles often disproportionately large in a configuration similar to fetal ventricles called *colpocephaly*. The anterior and inferior pointing of the frontal horns has often been referred to as a "*batwing configuration*" (Figs. 52-13 and 52-14). The septum pellucidum may be completely or partially absent (Fig. 52-15). The interhemispheric fissure usually appears to be widened on coronal scans, particularly after shunting (Fig. 52-14). There may also be gyral interdigitation. The posterior fossa is usually small, and the tentorium appears relatively low and hypoplastic. Hydrocephalus resulting from the Chiari II malformation is frequently mild *in utero* and becomes more severe at birth after repair of the meningomyelocele. CSF circulation no longer can decompress into the myelomeningocele so hydrocephalus typically worsens.

Routine prenatal screening of maternal serum for alpha fetoprotein that is elevated with a neural tube de-

A B

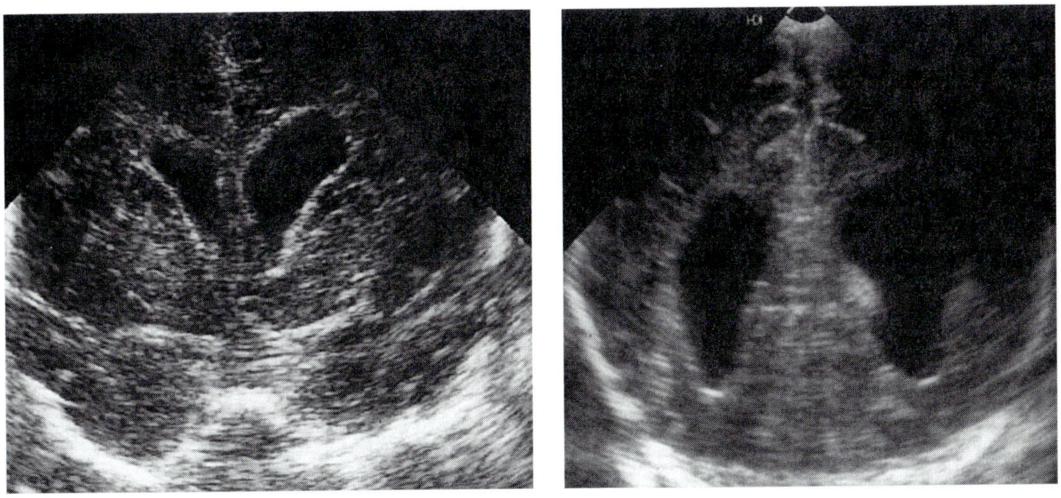

FIG. 52-14. Chiari II, coronal sonograms. A, Frontal horns and B, occipital horns show inferior pointing of frontal horns (batwing configuration) and widened interhemispheric fissure.

A B C

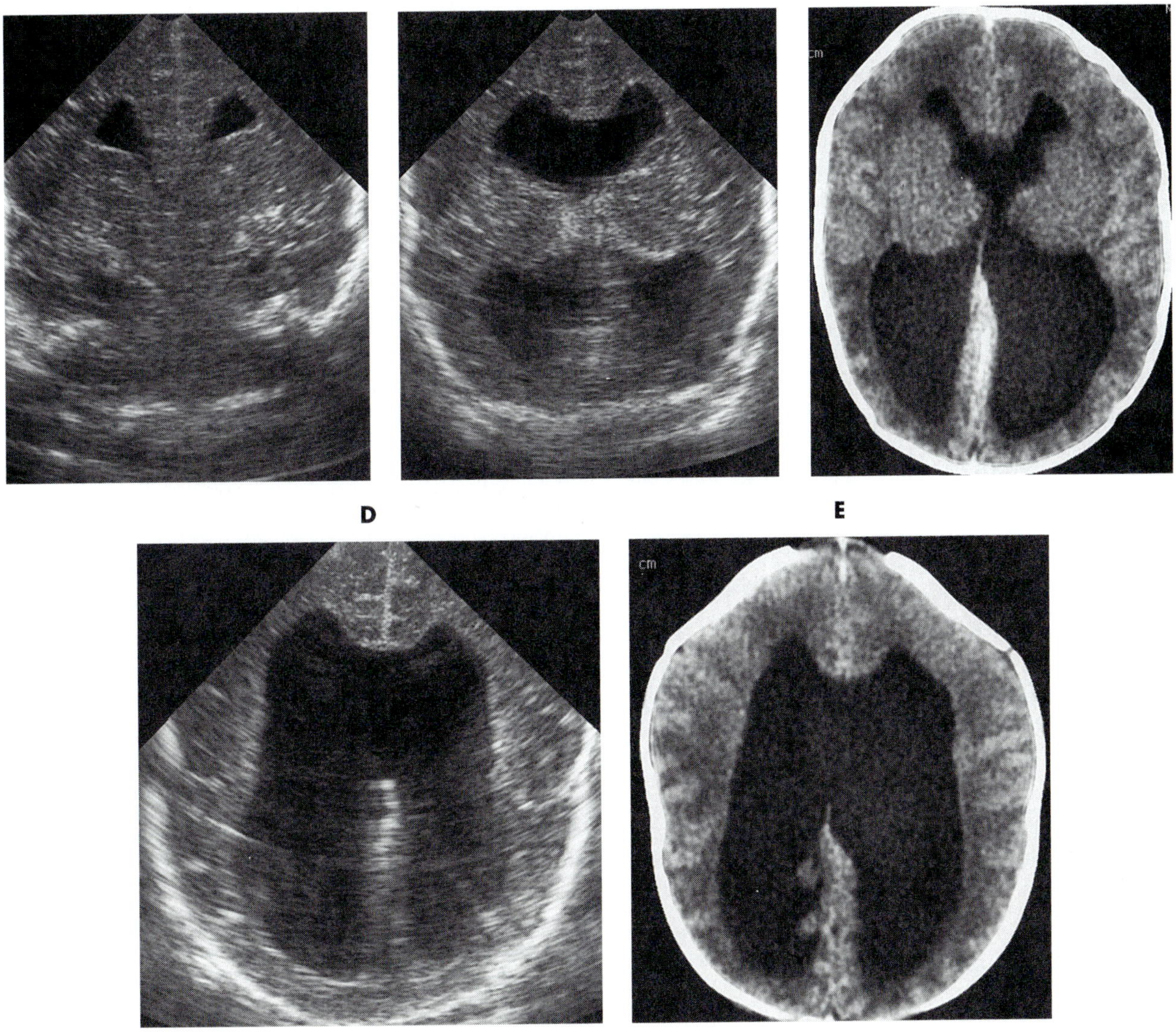

FIG. 52-15. Chiari II and absence of septum pellucidum. A, B, D, Coronal sonograms. C, E, Computed tomography scans.

fect, and widespread use of ultrasonography in pregnancy, allow for the prenatal diagnosis of the majority of Chiari malformations.[35] CT or MRI may be used initially in the neonatal period to document the severity of the process; however, sonography has been a reliable imaging method for follow-up of shunting procedures and evaluation of hydrocephalus in the first year of life.

Agenesis of the Corpus Callosum

The corpus callosum forms broad bands of connecting fibers between the cerebral hemispheres. Development of the corpus callosum occurs between the eighth and eighteenth week of gestation, beginning ventral and extending dorsal.[22,36,37] Recent review of this development by Kier and Truwit[38] suggests the anterior body of the corpus callosum develops earlier than the genu, and development proceeds both anteriorly and posteriorly.[38] Therefore, depending on the timing of the intrauterine insult, development can be partially arrested or complete agenesis may occur. If partial, then the genu or the dorsal aspect, the splenium, and the rostrum are absent. Because an insult causing anomalies of the corpus callosum must occur very early in development (between 8 and 18 weeks' gestation), it is not surprising that there are other associated CNS anomalies in up to 80% of cases.[38-41] These other anomalies include Chiari II and Dandy-Walker malformations, holoprosencephaly, encephaloceles, lipomas, arachnoid cysts, migrational abnormalities, and Aicardi syndrome (e.g., women with agenesis of the corpus callosum, ocular abnormalities, and infantile spasms). Isolated agenesis of the corpus callosum may have a normal prognosis.

Sonographic Findings.[36,40,42-44] The key diagnostic clues are the widely spaced, parallel oriented lateral ventricles that have extremely narrow frontal horns (often slitlike). Coronally, the frontal horns and ventricular bodies have sharply angled lateral peaks. There may be relative enlargement of the posterior horns (colpocephaly) (Fig. 52-16). Probst bundles—longitudinal callosal fibers that failed to decussate or cross to the other cerebral hemisphere—bulge into the ventricles along the superomedial aspect of the lateral ventricles. These are best seen coronally as the concave medial border to the lateral ventricles. The third ventricle is dilated and elevated so that its roof extends superiorly between the lateral ventricles and into the interhemispheric fissure and may be associated with a dorsal midline cyst (Fig. 52-17). The medial cerebral sulci are often radially arranged, perpendicular to the expected course of the corpus callosum, causing a "sunburst sign" on sagittal midline images (Fig. 52-18). The pericallosal sulcus is missing, and the cingulate sulcus is absent or present only as unconnected segments.

SONOGRAPHIC FINDINGS IN AGENESIS OF THE CORPUS CALLOSUM

- Absent corpus callosum
- Absent cingulate gyrus and sulcus
- Radial arrangement of medial sulci above the third ventricle ("sunburst sign")
- Widely spaced, parallel lateral ventricles
- Extremely narrow frontal horns (slitlike)
- Concave or straight medial borders secondary to Probst bundles
- Colpocephaly (dilated atria and occipital horns)
- Elevated third ventricle extending between the lateral ventricles, continuous with the interhemispheric fissure with or without dorsal cyst
- Absent septum pellucidum

Corpus Callosum Lipoma

Maldevelopment of embryonic neural crest tissues may result in lipomas of the interhemispheric fissure. These lipomas account for 30% to 50% of intracranial lipomas and are associated with dysgenesis of the corpus callosum (Fig. 52-19).[22,37]

Dandy-Walker Malformation

Dandy-Walker malformation presents as a dilated fourth ventricle in direct communication with the cisterna magna (Fig. 52-20). The posterior fossa is enlarged with elevation of the tentorium cerebelli, straight sinus, and torcula herophili. The vermis of the cerebellum is variably hypoplastic to absent, and the cerebellar hemispheres are variably hypoplastic and displaced laterally by the enlarged fourth ventricle. The brain stem may be compressed or hypoplastic. Generalized obstructive hydrocephalus occurs in up to 80% of cases. If there is also agenesis of the corpus callosum, colpocephaly is typically present.[7,22,45,46]

SONOGRAPHIC FINDINGS IN DANDY-WALKER MALFORMATION

- Enlarged fourth ventricle connects to cisterna magna
- Large posterior fossa
- Hypoplastic cerebellar vermis
- Hypoplastic cerebellar hemispheres displaced laterally by fourth ventricle
- Small brain stem
- Hydrocephalus of ventricles (80%)
  - Obstruction above and below fourth ventricle
- Absent corpus callosum (70%)

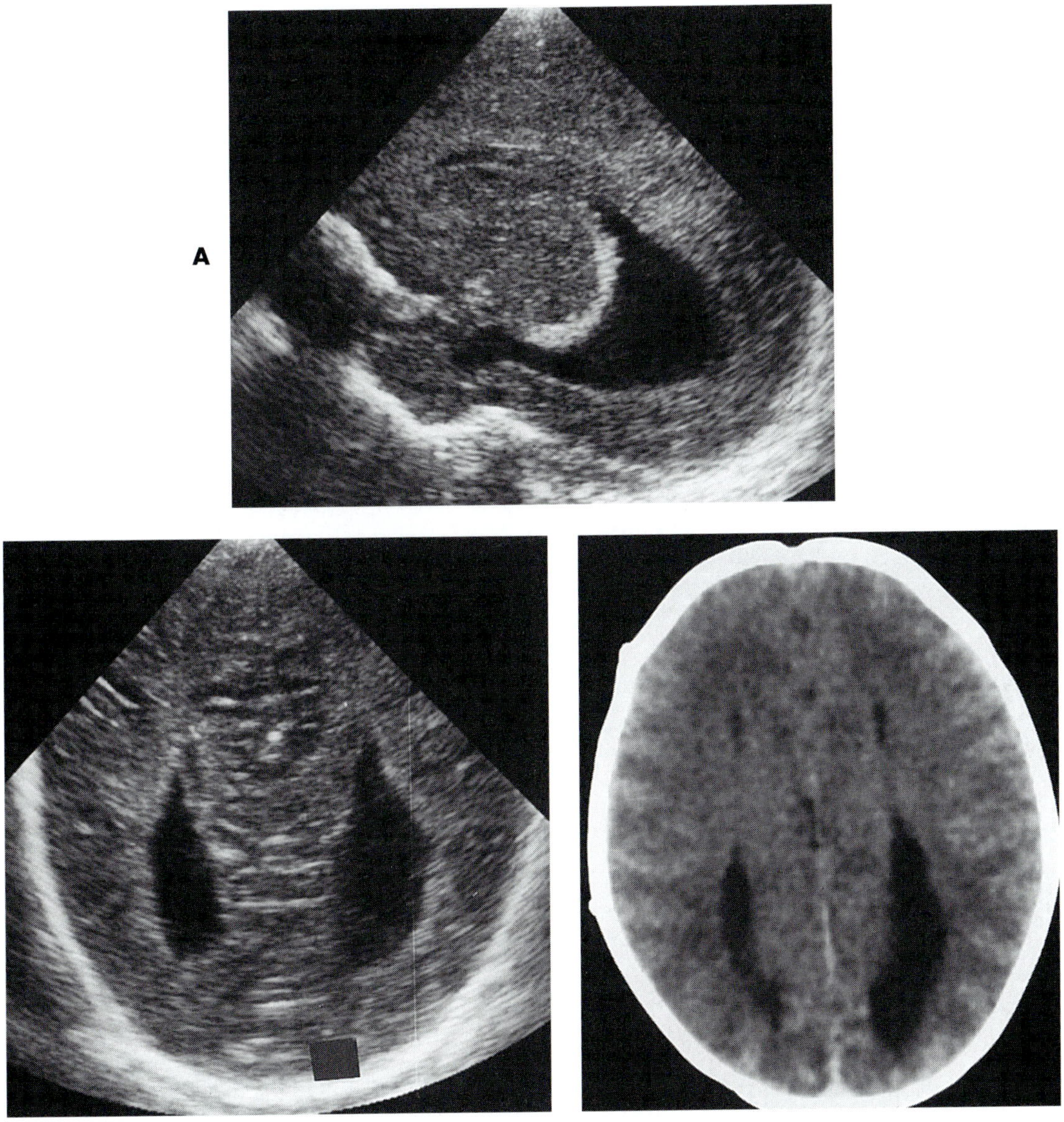
A
B
C

FIG. 52-16. Agenesis of the corpus callosum. A, Sagittal and B, coronal sonograms and C, computed tomography show marked tapering of the frontal horns with larger occipital horns (colpocephaly).

A B C

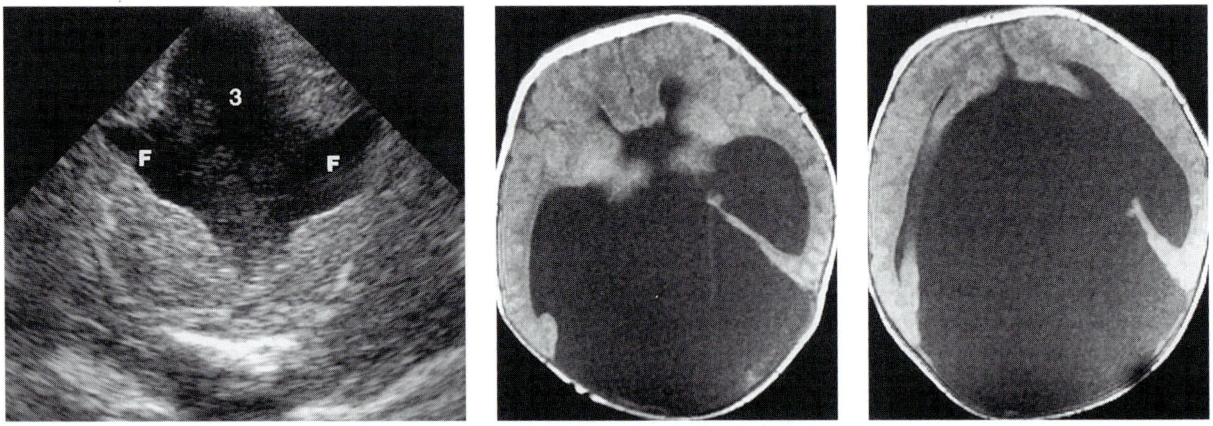

FIG. 52-17. Agenesis of the corpus callosum with elevation of third ventricle and continuation into a large dorsal cyst. **A**, Coronal sonogram and **B** and **C**, computed tomography scans show widely separated frontal horns, a large third ventricle.

A

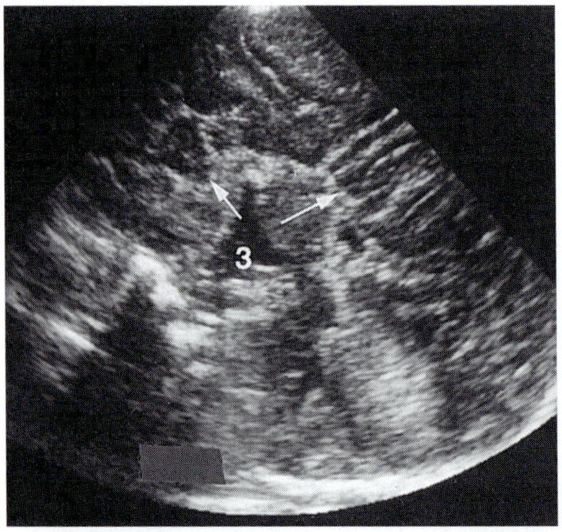

FIG. 52-18. "Sunburst" or radial arrangement of the sulci in agenesis of the corpus callosum. **A**, Midline sagittal sonogram, **B**, midline sagittal magnetic resonance imaging, and **C**, sagittal pathological specimen. Third ventricle (*3*) is elevated and lacks the normal parallel corpus callosum and cingulate sulcus. Radial array of sulci (*arrows*). (*B* from Osborn AG: *Diagnostic Neuroradiology*, St. Louis, 1994, Mosby–Year Book; *C* from Friede R: *Developmental Neuropathology*, ed 2, New York, 1975, Springer-Verlag.)

B

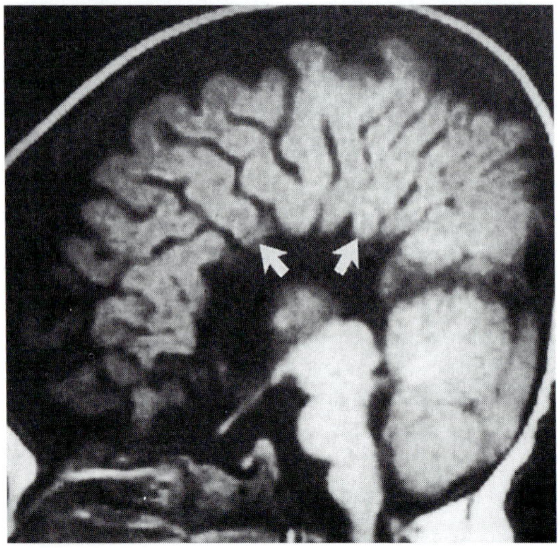

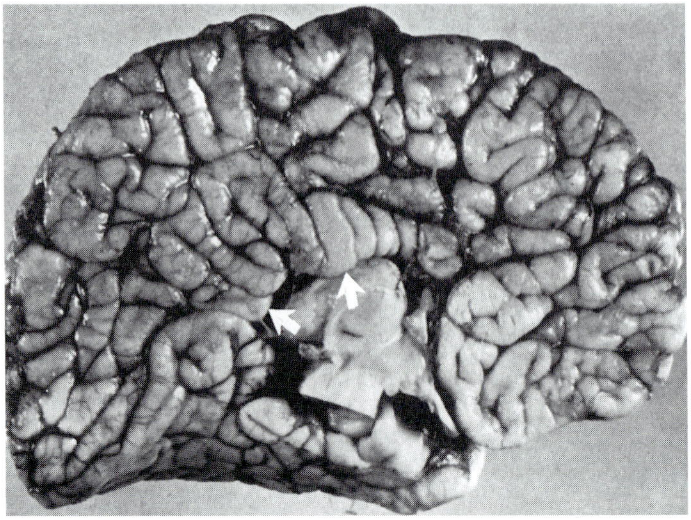

C

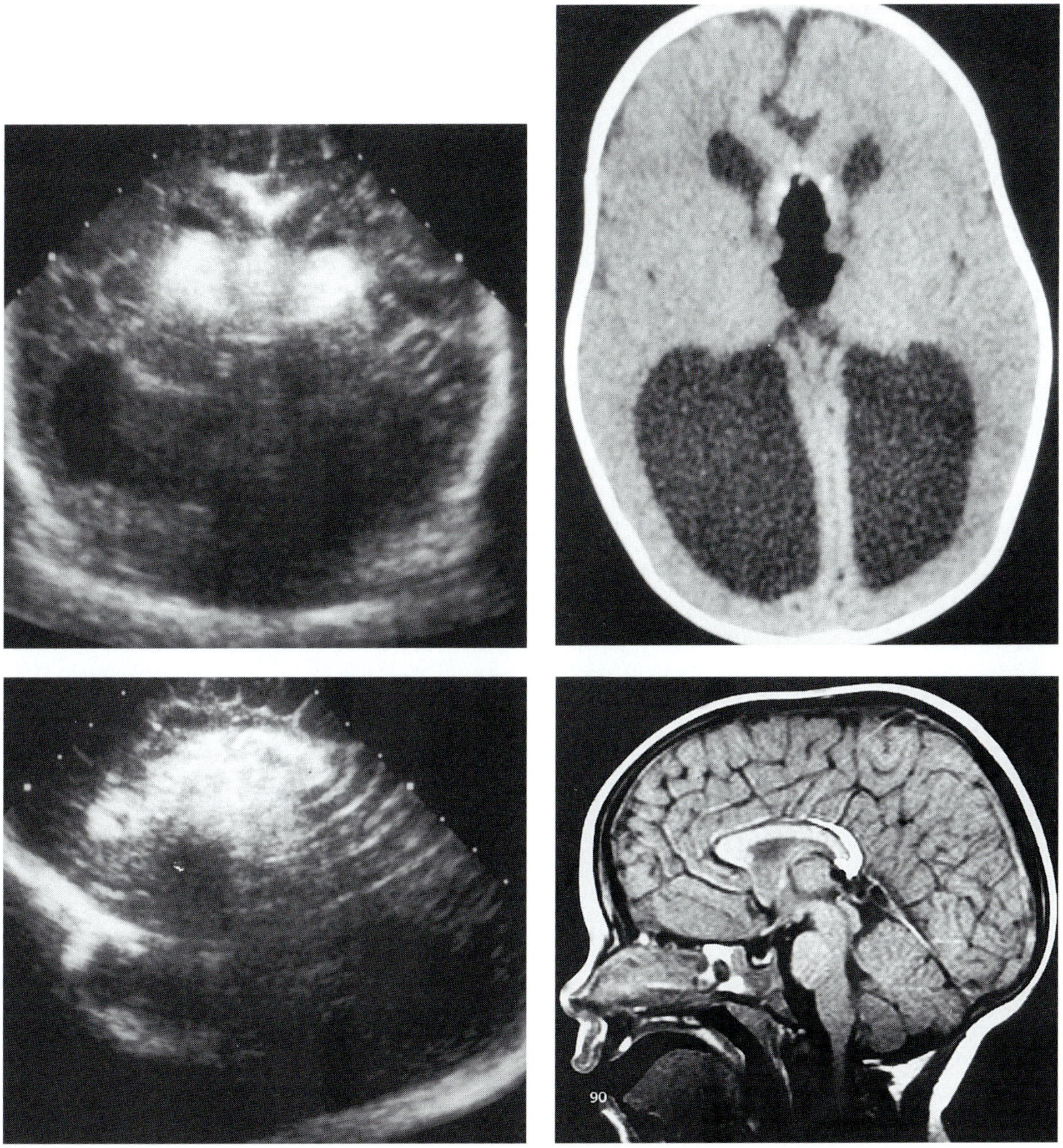

FIG. 52-19. Lipoma of the corpus callosum. **A,** Coronal and **B,** sagittal sonograms show highly echogenic fat surrounded by calcification. Both are causing major acoustic shadowing. **C,** Computed tomography scan shows black central fat surrounded by white flecks of calcium, and **D,** sagittal magnetic resonance imaging shows fat (bright white on T_1) extending over the corpus callosum.

The etiology of Dandy-Walker malformation is not definitively known. Theories to explain this malformation include agenesis of the foramina of Luschka and Magendie in the first trimester, malformation of the roof of the fourth ventricle, or delayed opening of the foramina of Magendie.[22] The prenatal diagnosis of Dandy-Walker malformation, with the differentiation between Dandy-Walker variant, a posterior fossa arachnoid cyst and mega cisterna magna, is usually possible with high-resolution equipment. It can be diagnosed after 17 weeks' gestation when the inferior vermis has normally completely formed.[47-51]

The Dandy-Walker malformation is associated with other CNS anomalies in up to 70% of cases. These include dysgenesis or agenesis of the corpus callosum, encephalocele, holoprosencephaly, microcephaly, heterotopia, and gyral malformations. Chromosomal abnormalities are described in up to 20% to 50% of cases and include trisomy 13, 18, and 21. Other associated anomalies include: gastrointestinal (GI), genitourinary

A

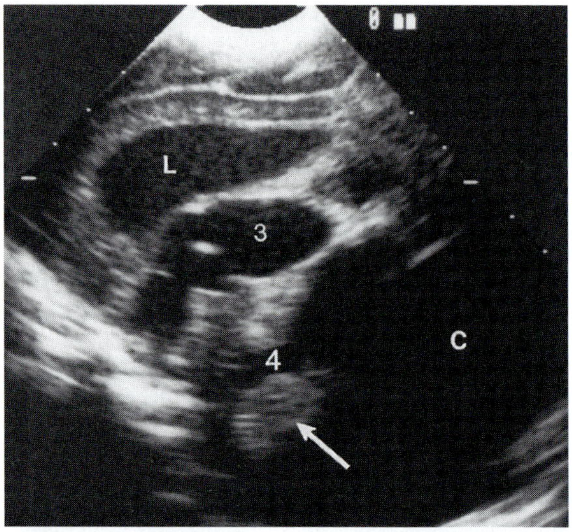

FIG. 52-20. Dandy-Walker malformation. **A,** Sagittal, **B,** coronal, and **C,** posterior coronal images. Third ventricle (*3*), fourth ventricle (*4*), Dandy-Walker posterior fossa cyst (*C*), hypoplastic cerebellum (*thin arrows*), thin septum pellucidum (*arrowhead*), dilated lateral ventricles (*L*), and elevated tentorium cerebelli (*thick arrow*). Internal echoes in the ventricles represent blood in the cerebrospinal fluid. The curved arrow shows resorbing parenchymal and intraventricular hemorrhage.

B C

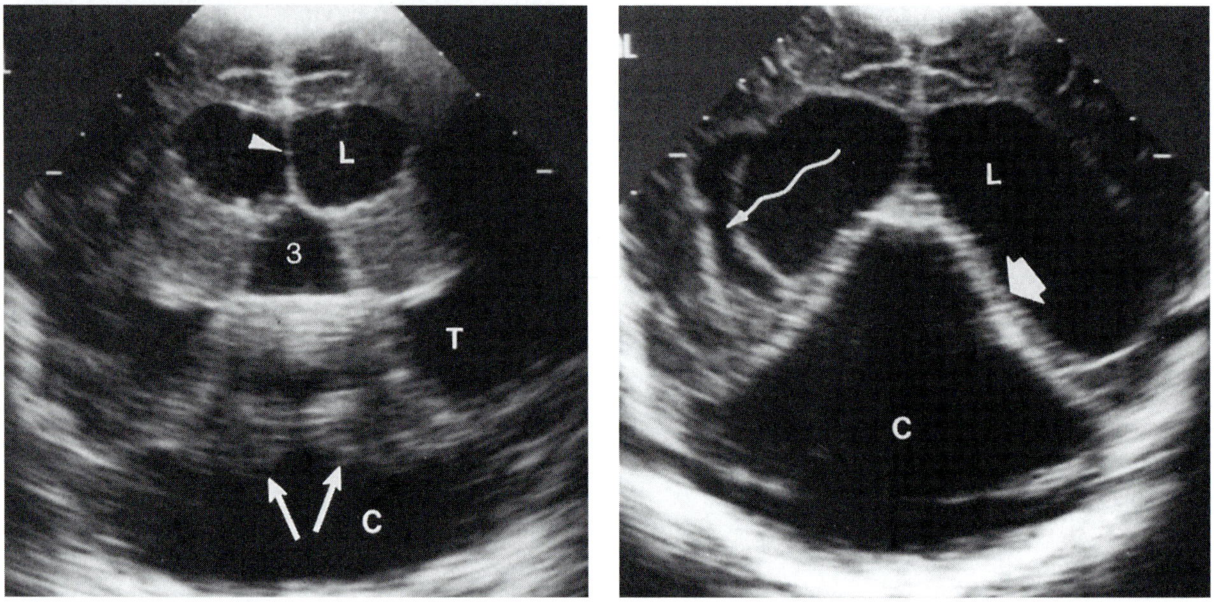

(GU), cardiac, musculoskeletal and pulmonary malformations including congenital diaphragmatic hernia and cystic hygroma.[28,34,45-47,51-53]

Therapy for the Dandy-Walker malformation includes ventriculoperitoneal shunting, which will decompress the lateral ventricles but may not decompress the posterior fossa cyst (Fig. 52-21). The cyst may require a separate shunt for decompression. Sonography can be used to follow these procedures until the infant is approximately 1.5 years of age, but this method is rarely used after the first few months of life.

In **Dandy-Walker variant** (Fig. 52-22), there again is variable hypoplasia of the posterior inferior vermis and communication between the fourth ventricle and cisterna magna. The fourth ventricle is slightly to moderately enlarged. In the Dandy-Walker variant, the posterior fossa is normal in size and although the vermis is small, the cerebellar hemispheres are normal. There is no associated hydrocephalus. There are chromosomal abnormalities in up to 30% of these infants and associated CNS or extra CNS anomalies, which may have more of an impact on the outcome of the infant[22,45,48,50] than the Dandy-Walker variant anomaly.

Differential of posterior fossa cystic lesions which mimic Dandy-Walker syndrome. A **mega cisterna magna** (Fig. 52-23) is a normal variant that is not associated with the development of hydrocephalus and has a normal cerebellar vermis, fourth ventricle, and cerebellar hemisphere.[22] A **posterior fossa subarachnoid cyst** can be differ-

A

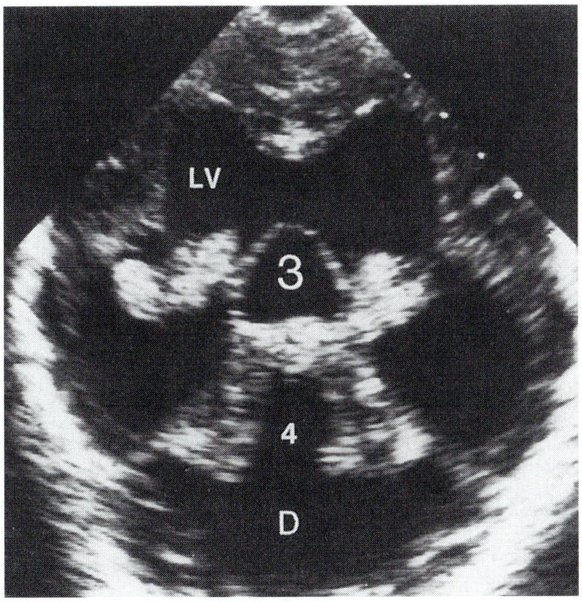

B

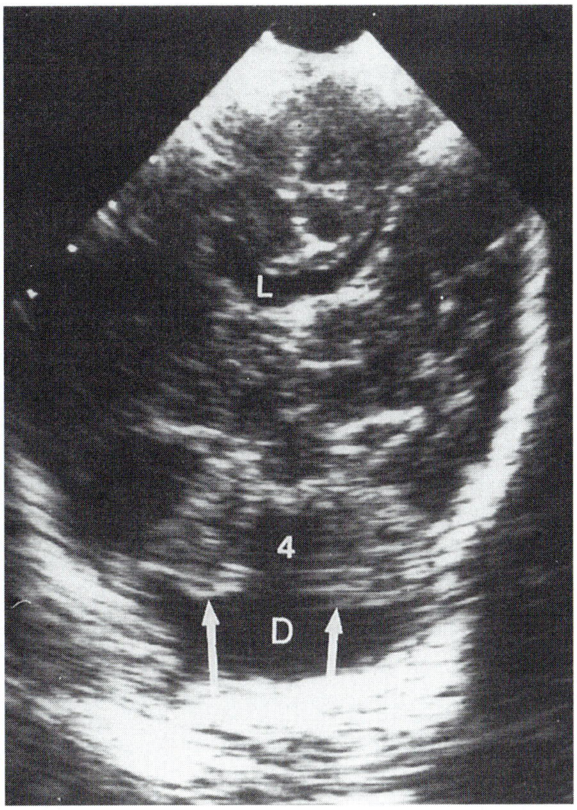

FIG. 52-21. Dandy-Walker malformation. **A,** Initially, marked hydrocephalus was present. LV—Lateral ventricle; 3—third ventricle; 4—fourth ventricle; D—Dandy-Walker cyst. **B,** Later, lateral (*L*) and third ventricles (*3*) have collapsed, but the Dandy-Walker cyst (*D*) remains dilated. Frequently, posterior fossa cysts require additional shunt for decompression. (From Rumack CM, Johnson ML: *Perinatal and Infant Brain Imaging*, St. Louis, 1984, Mosby–Year Book.)

POSTERIOR FOSSA CYSTIC LESIONS

Dandy-Walker syndrome
Mega cisterna magna
  Normal variant
Posterior fossa subarachnoid cyst
  Cyst does not connect with the fourth ventricle

entiated from Dandy-Walker malformation or variant by the lack of communication of the cyst with the fourth ventricle. The normal fourth ventricle, vermis, and cerebellum are displaced by the arachnoid cyst.[28,46,49]

Another syndrome associated with vermian agenesis is **Joubert's syndrome,** which includes vermian dysgenesis, episodic hyperpnea, ataxia, abnormal eye movements, and mental retardation.[22]

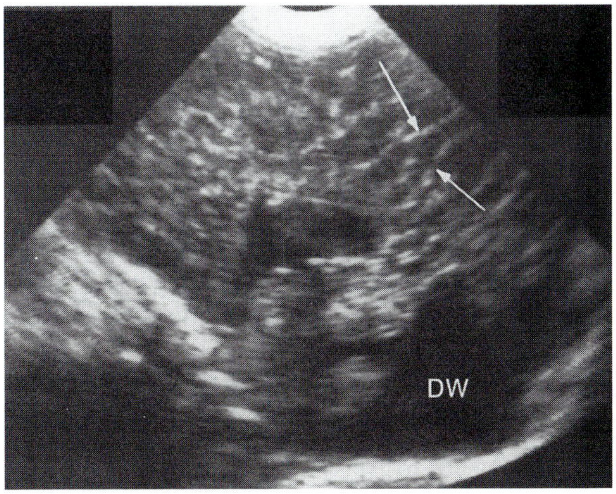

FIG. 52-22. Agenesis of corpus callosum and Dandy-Walker variant. Midline sagittal image shows no identifiable corpus callosum or cingulate gyrus. Medial gyri and sulci are radially arranged (*arrows*) above third ventricle. DW—Dandy-Walker cyst.

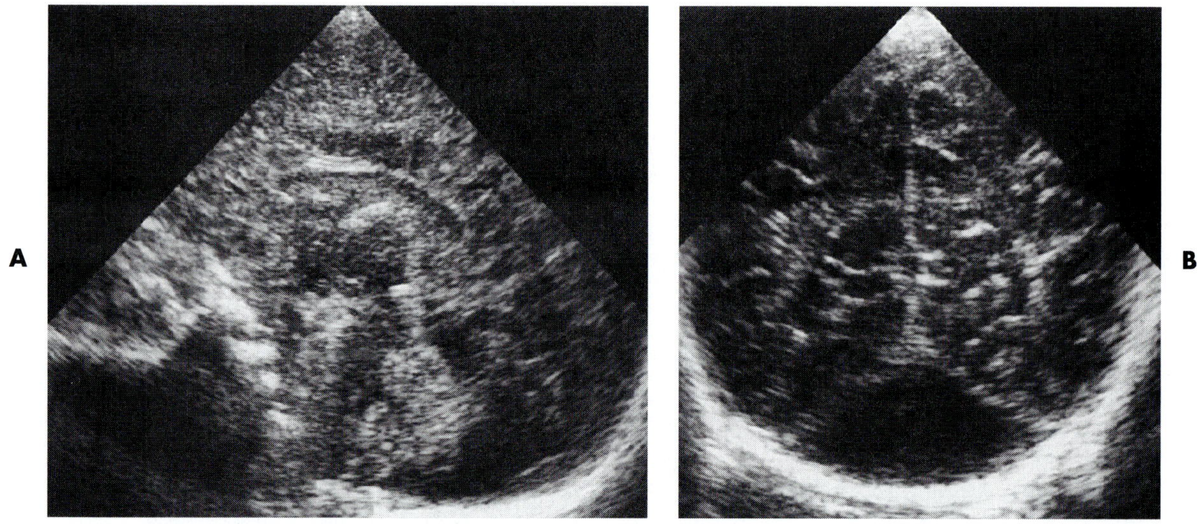

FIG. 52-23. Mega cisterna magna. **A,** Sagittal and **B,** coronal sonograms show an enlarged cisterna magna behind the vermis on *A* and below the tentorium on *B* with no communication to the fourth ventricle and no hydrocephalus.

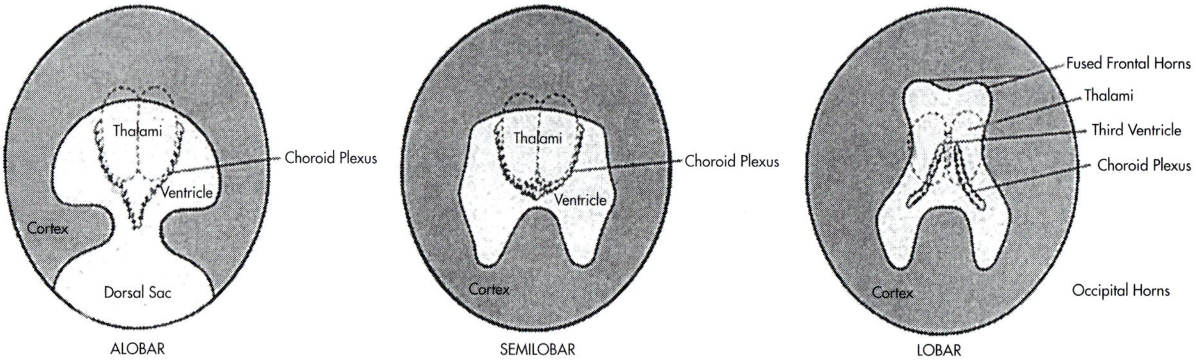

FIG. 52-24. Types of holoprosencephaly.

DISORDERS OF DIVERTICULATION AND CLEAVAGE

Holoprosencephaly

Holoprosencephaly results from a failure of diverticulation when the primitive prosencephalon does not divide into the telencephalon and the diencephalon between the fourth and eight weeks of gestation.[27] The telencephalon develops into the cerebral hemispheres, ventricles, putamen, and caudate nuclei. The diencephalon becomes the third ventricle, thalami, hypothalamus and the lateral globus pallidus. Holoprosencephaly represents a spectrum of malformations that form a continuum from most severe with no separation of the telencephalon (alobar) to least severe with partial separation of the dorsal aspects of the brain (lobar) (Fig. 52-24). The mildest form is **septo-optic dysplasia** (Fig. 52-25), in which there is absence of the septum pellucidum and optic nerve hypoplasia. A third classification of intermediate severity between alobar and lobar is semilobar holoprosencephaly. Anomalies of the face and calvarium accompany and help predict the severity of the brain malformation, because the face develops at the same time as the brain during diverticulation. Cases of holoprosencephaly are usually suspected as a result of the accompanying facial anomalies, with more severe facial anomalies predicting more severe intracranial anomalies. Brain sonographic examination can confirm the diagnosis.[54,55]

A

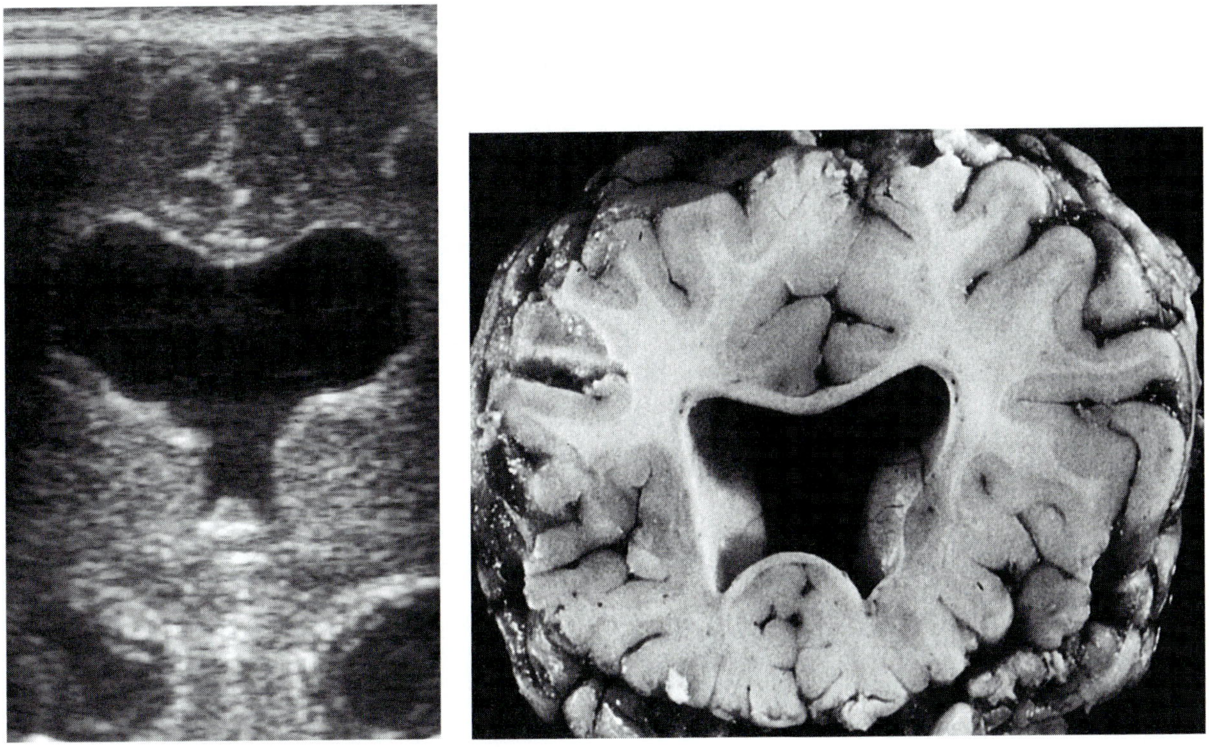

B

FIG. 52-25. Septo-optic dysplasia. **A,** Coronal sonogram and **B,** pathological specimen show absence of septum pellucidum with relative flattening of the frontal horns across the midline.

Alobar Holoprosencephaly

Alobar holoprosencephaly is the most severe form of this disorder, and infants with this form usually die within the first months of life or are stillborn. Facial features may include cebocephaly (Fig. 52-26), cyclopia, and ethmocephaly (cyclopia or hypotelorism with a midline proboscis above the eyes).[55] The brain surrounds a single midline horseshoe- or crescent-shaped ventricle with a surrounding thin, primitive cerebral cortex (Fig. 52-26).[28] The hemispheres and thalami are fused, and there is no falx, corpus callosum, or interhemispheric fissure between them. Midline, moderately echogenic, fused thalami are seen anterior to the fused hyperechogenic choroid plexus. The third ventricle is usually absent, so that the large single ventricle then communicates directly with the aqueduct.[56,57] Pachygyria may be seen. There is often a large dorsal cyst. Posterior fossa structures may be normal.

SONOGRAPHIC FINDINGS IN ALOBAR HOLOPROSENCEPHALY

- Single midline crescent-shaped ventricle
- Thin layer of cerebral cortex
- No falx
- No interhemispheric fissure
- No corpus callosum
- Fused thalami and basal ganglia
- Fused echogenic choroid plexus
- Absent third ventricle
- Large dorsal cyst

Semilobar Holoprosencephaly

In semilobar holoprosencephaly, there is more brain parenchyma, but the single ventricle persists. There may be separate occipital and temporal horns. A small portion of the falx and interhemispheric fissure develops in the occipital cortex posteriorly. The splenium of the corpus callosum is often formed and may be seen on midline sagittal sections. The thalami are partially separated and the third ventricle is rudimentary. Facial anomalies are less severe than in alobar holoprosencephaly, usually with only mild hypotelorism and median or lateral cleft lip.

Lobar Holoprosencephaly

Lobar holoprosencephaly is the least severe form of this disorder. There is nearly complete separation of hemispheres with development of a falx and inter-

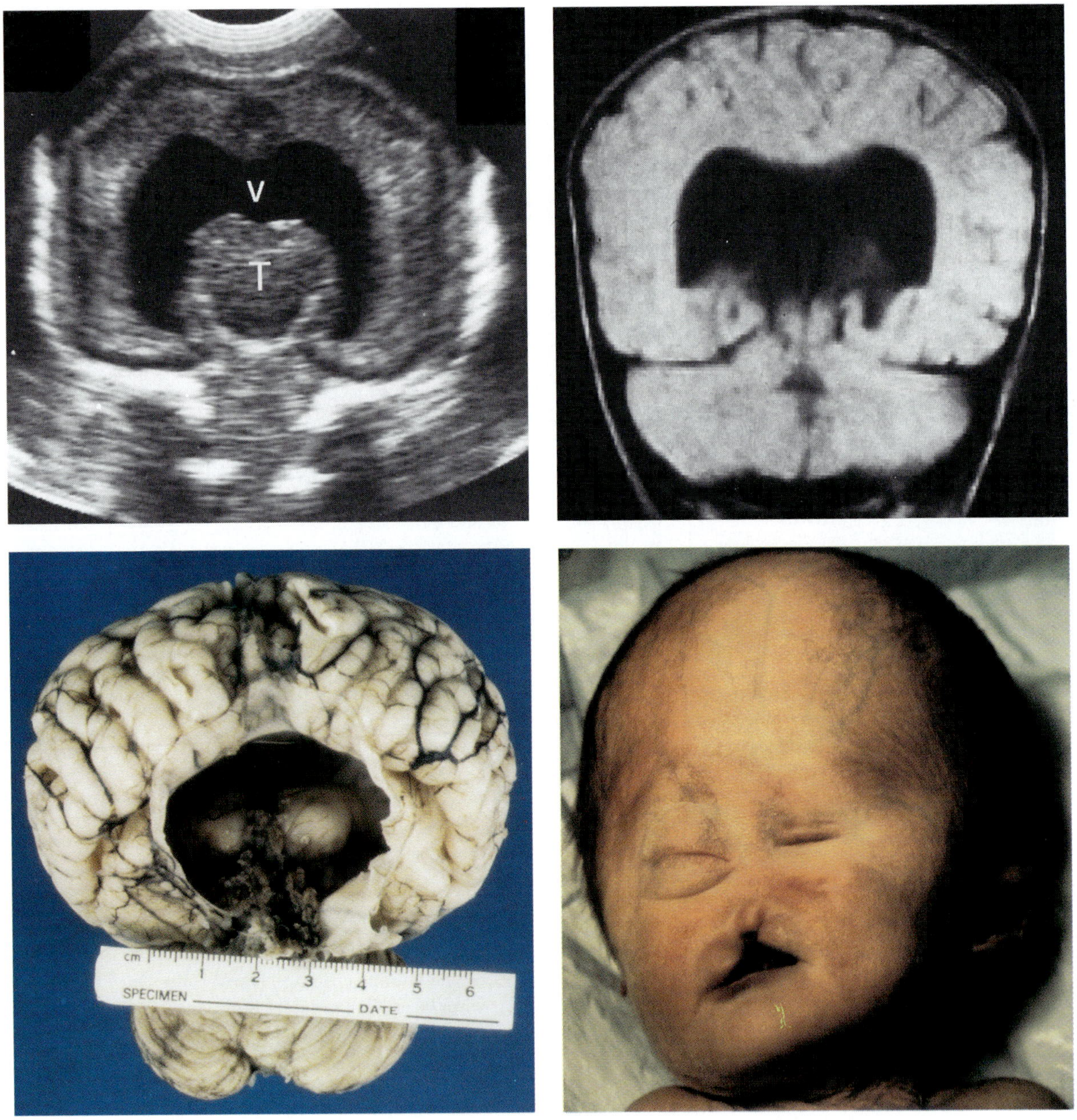

FIG. 52-26. Alobar holoprosencephaly with single central ventricle (*V*) and fused thalami (*T*). **A, Coronal sonogram.** No falx or interhemispheric fissure is present. **B,** Magnetic resonance imaging and **C,** pathological specimen show single central ventricle and fused thalami. **D,** Autopsy specimen shows cebocephaly (severe hypotelorism and malformed nose).

hemispheric fissure, but they may be shallow anteriorly and the frontal lobes are fused. The septum pellucidum is absent. The anterior horns of the lateral ventricles are fused and square shaped, but the occipital horns are separated. The third ventricle is usually present, separating the thalami. The splenium and body of the corpus callosum are often present with the absence of the genu and rostrum. Facial anomalies are mild and similar to the semilobar form or absent.

DISORDERS OF SULCATION AND CELLULAR MIGRATION

Schizencephaly

Believed to be caused by a destructive process *in utero*, these are gray-matter lined clefts that extend through the entire hemisphere from the ependymal lining of the lateral ventricles to the pial covering of the cortex. The clefts may be bilateral or unilateral

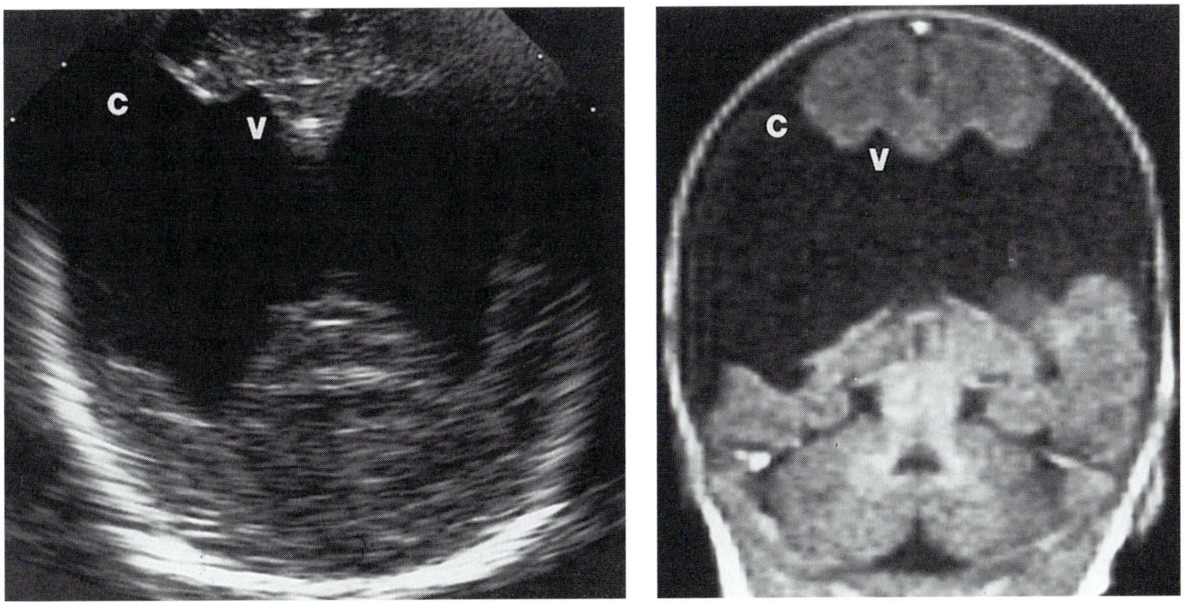

FIG. 52-27. Schizencephaly. **A,** Coronal sonogram and **B,** coronal magnetic resonance imaging show bilateral clefts with wide openings to the ventricular system (open-lip schizencephaly).

(Fig. 52-27). There may be wide openings of the clefts (open-lip schizencephaly). In some cases, the cleft is closed (closed-lip type) and will require MRI for diagnosis, because gray-white matter differentiation is not well demonstrated on sonography.

DESTRUCTIVE LESIONS

Porencephalic Cyst

Focal brain destruction prior to 26 weeks' gestation will typically heal with dysplastic gray matter and result in schizencephaly usually associated with migrational defects.[19] A porencephalic cyst is an area of normally developed brain that has been damaged and heals with a lining of gliotic white matter. By definition, porencephalic cysts always connect with the ventricular system but do not extend to the surface cortex. They typically occur after birth secondary to hemorrhage, infection, or trauma.

Hydranencephaly

Classically, hydranencephaly is believed to be the result of bilateral occlusion of the internal carotid arteries during fetal development, but it may result from any number of intracranial destructive processes (Fig 52-28).[58] This disorder could be thought of as the severest form of porencephaly—that is, there is almost total destruction of the cerebral cortex.[59-61] These infants may appear surprisingly normal at birth, but are developmentally delayed from an early age and frequently die within the first year of life.

The sonographic findings include a calvarium filled with CSF, but little else (Fig. 52-28). Structures that receive a blood supply from the posterior cerebral artery and vertebral artery, such as the thalamus, cerebellum, brain stem, and posterior choroid plexus, are spared and are usually identifiable. Doppler flow imaging in the carotid arteries is absent. An incomplete or complete falx may be identifiable even *in utero* (Fig. 52-29). The presence of the falx helps differentiate this lesion from alobar holoprosencephaly in which the falx does not form. It can be difficult to differentiate hydranencephaly from severe hydrocephalus, but a thin rim of cortex should be visualized by sonography in hydrocephalus.[59-61] If there is an enlarging head circumference, ventriculo-peritoneal shunting may be indicated, regardless of the actual diagnosis to control growth.

Cystic Encephalomalacia

Encephalomalacia is an area of focal brain damage which pathologically has astrocytic proliferation and glial septations. In diffuse brain damage, there may be large areas of cystic encephalomalacia. The location of the damage depends on the type of insult. Typically, there is no connection to the ventricular system. In neonates, infection or anoxia can cause widespread damage, whereas a thrombus may cause very focal damage.

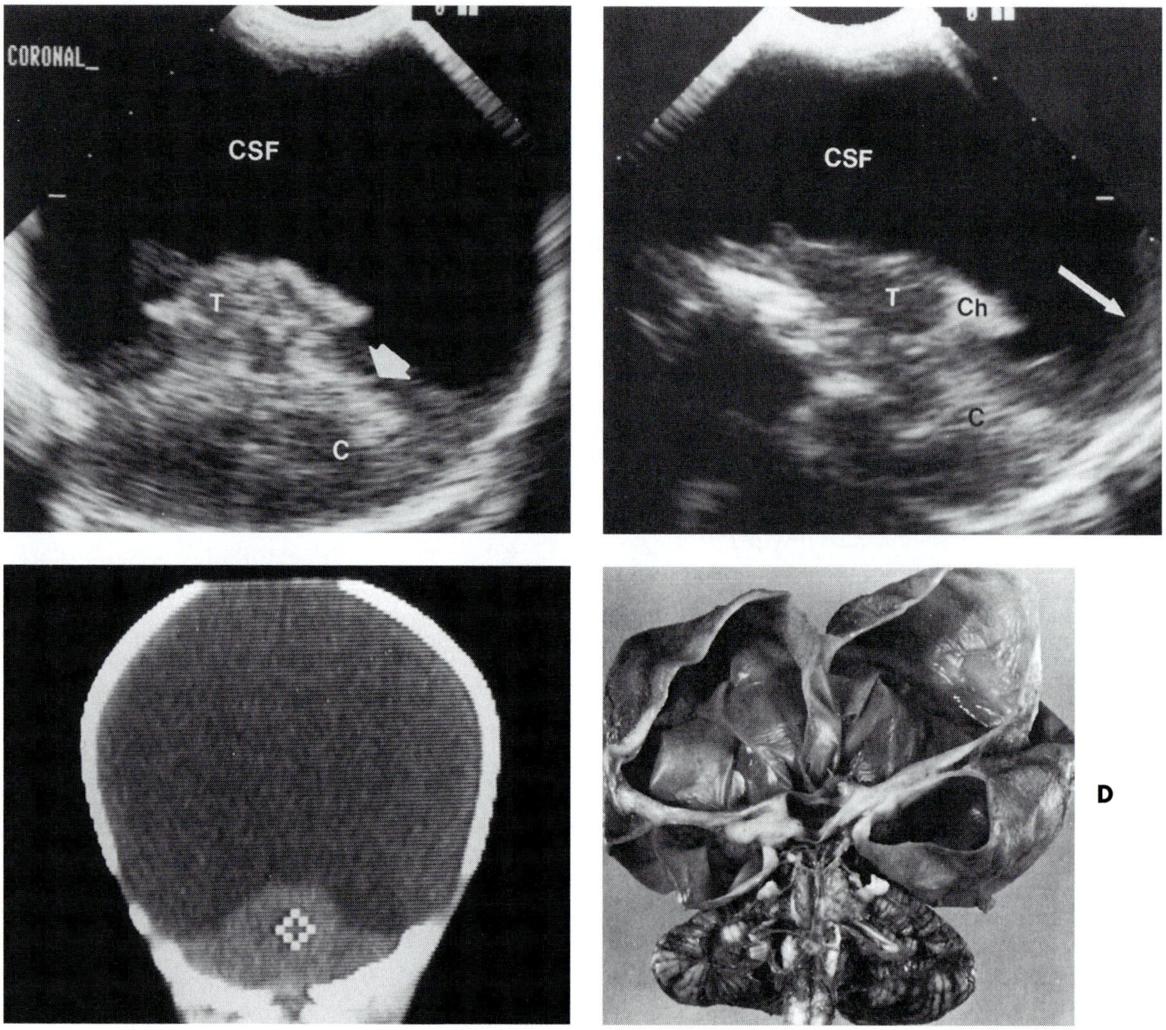

FIG. 52-28. Hydranencephaly. **A,** Coronal, and **B,** sagittal sonograms. **C,** Computed tomography scan. Note that only anechoic cerebrospinal fluid is seen above thalamus (*T*). Tentorium cerebelli (*thick arrow*), cerebellum (*C*), choroid plexus (*Ch*) and thin remnant of cerebral cortex posteriorly (*thin arrow*). Posterior fossa is usually normal. **D,** Pathological specimen with a complete falx and relatively normal posterior fossa structures. (*D* from Friede R: *Developmental Neuropathology*, ed 2, New York, 1975, Springer-Verlag.)

HYDROCEPHALUS

Hydrocephalus occurs in approximately 5% to 25% per 10,000 births. It results when there is an imbalance between the production of CSF and its drainage by the arachnoid villi. Three mechanisms account for the development of hydrocephalus. These include obstruction to outflow, decreased absorption, or overproduction (e.g., a choroid plexus tumor).

Normal CSF Production and Circulation

CSF provides a chemically controlled protective environment that continually bathes and circulates around the CNS. The majority of CSF is produced by the choroid plexus, but it is also produced by the ventricular ependyma, the intracranial subarachnoid lining, and the spinal subarachnoid lining. CSF normally flows from the lateral ventricles, through the foramina of Monro, the third ventricle, the aqueduct of Sylvius, the fourth ventricle, the lateral foramina of Luschka or medial foramen of Magendie, and into the basal cisterns. From there, a small quantity circulates down into the spinal subarachnoid space. CSF flows upward around the brain anteriorly and posteriorly to reach the vertex, where it is resorbed by the arachnoid granulations into the superior sagittal sinus.

A

B

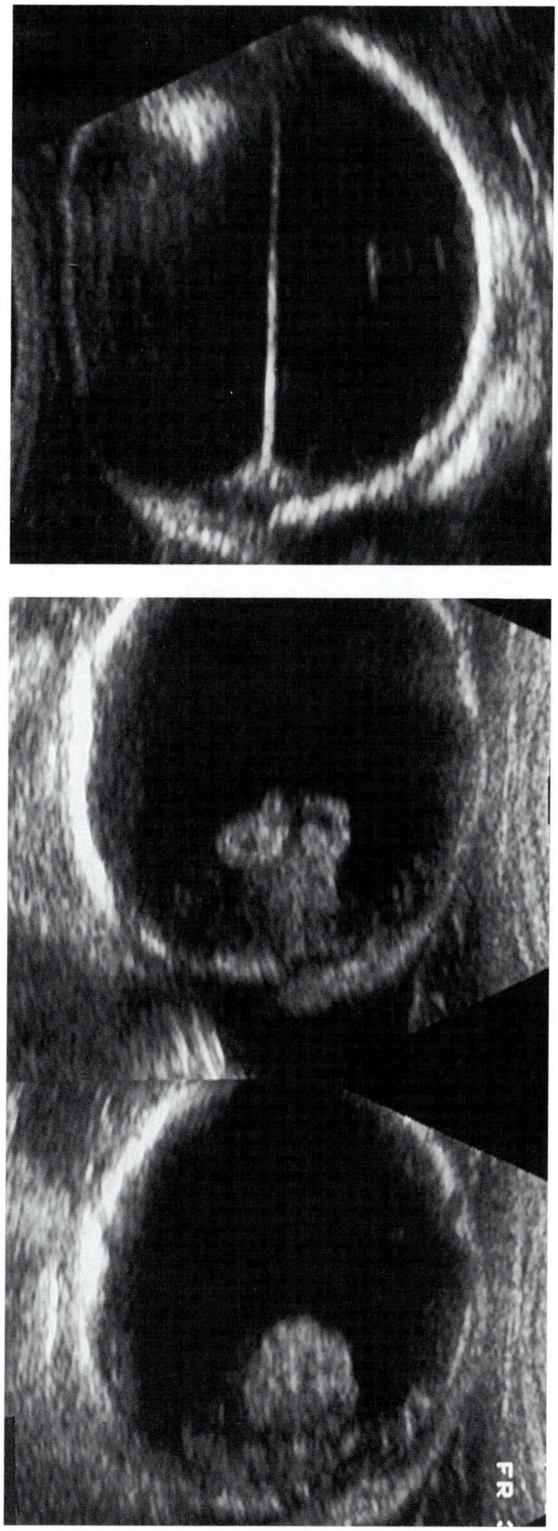

FIG. 52-29. Hydranencephaly *in utero*. **A**, Axial, and **B**, coronal sonograms show a falx, no cerebral cortex, midline structures only in posterior fossa region.

Diagnosis

Often hydrocephalus can be diagnosed *in utero* by 15 weeks' gestation. The size of the atrium of the ventricle and the glomus of the choroid plexus remains constant in the second and third trimester in the transaxial plane. *In utero*, an upper limit of 10 mm for the ventricular atrium has been established and well reviewed.[62-64] Once hydrocephalus is recognized, close inspection for spinal dysraphism, other CNS, or extra CNS anomalies is warranted, because these findings will affect outcome. Chromosome evaluation is necessary if other anomalies are recognized.[65-67] Hydrocephalus diagnosed *in utero* has a variable course making counseling of the family difficult. Often, especially if other anomalies or chromosome abnormalities are diagnosed, the family chooses to terminate the pregnancy.

With a little experience, neonatal hydrocephalus is easily recognized by routine coronal and sagittal imaging.[6,62-64] Ventricular size is slightly larger in newborns than in older children. Progression of hydrocephalus can best be estimated by comparison with previous studies. Sonography is also helpful in following ventricular decompression in patients shunted for hydrocephalus. A word of caution is in order about following ventricular size in cases of hydrocephalus. Care must be taken so that changes in ultrasound sector depth do not result in apparent enlargement or decompression of the ventricles related to magnification differences when different depth scales are used. Failure to do so may result in a false impression of changing hydrocephalus.

Level of Obstruction

Asymmetry of the lateral ventricles can cause one to be slightly larger as a normal variant. Evaluation of the entire ventricular system should be obtained so that the level is identified at which there is a transition from a large to a small ventricle.[68] Dilatation of the lateral and third ventricles indicates an aqueduct of Sylvius obstruction most often caused by intraventricular hemorrhage (IVH) and also often an x-linked recessive trait. In rare cases, there may be isolated dilatation of the fourth ventricle, and thus each part of the ventricular system requires evaluation. Dilatation of all ventricles should lead to an extraventricular source.

Neonatal hydrocephalus can also be evaluated by Doppler to assess (indirectly) intracranial pressure and help determine the need for shunt placement.[69] Regional CSF flow imaging with color Doppler has also been investigated as a method to exclude obstructive hydrocephalus.[70]

Etiologies

Hydrocephalus can be a result of intraventricular obstruction (IVOH), which is when flow is obstructed

A

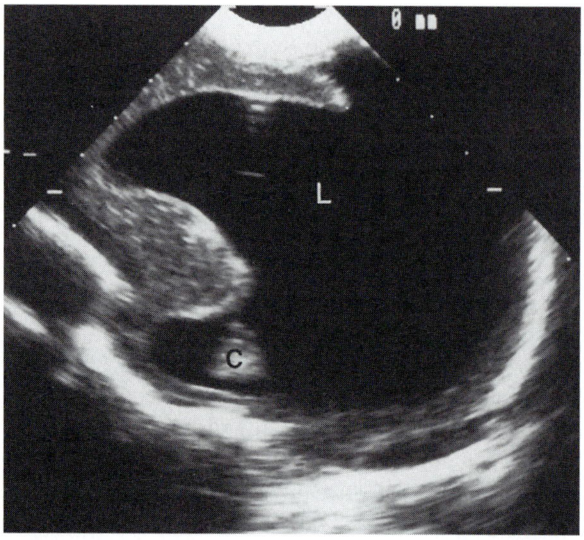

B

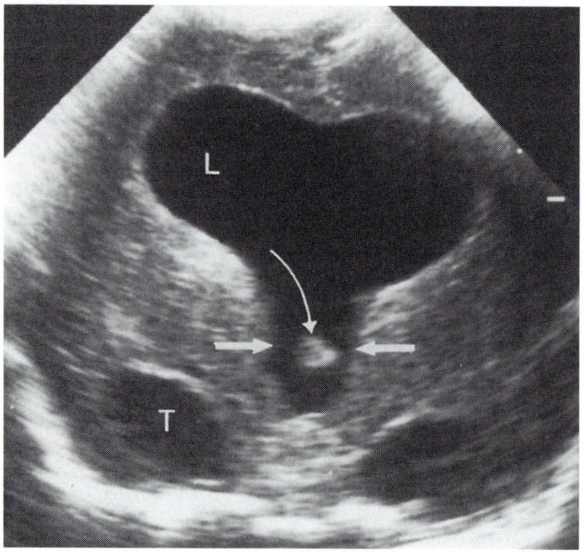

FIG. 52-30. Aqueductal stenosis. **A**, Parasagittal, and **B**, coronal scans. Marked lateral *(L)* and third (*straight arrows*) ventricular dilation demonstrated, but fourth ventricle is small and not identifiable. Massa intermedia is in third ventricle (*curved arrow*). T—Temporal horns; C—choroid plexus.

CAUSES OF HYDROCEPHALUS

Intraventricular obstruction	**Posthemorrhagic** Aqueductal obstruction Fourth ventricle obstruction Posterior fossa subdural hematoma Chiari II malformation Dandy-Walker malformation Aqueductal stenosis Postinfectious Vein of Galen malformation Tumor or cyst
Extraventricular obstruction	**Posthemorrhagic** Postinfectious Achondroplasia Absence or hypoplasia of arachnoid granulations Venous obstruction
Overproduction	Choroid plexus papilloma

within the ventricular system (noncommunicating) or extraventricular obstruction (EVOH) to CSF circulation (communicating), which is obstruction to flow occurring within the subarachnoid spaces and cisterns or secondary to decreased absorption at the arachnoid villi. Overproduction of CSF from a choroid plexus papilloma is an unusual cause. Other causes include venous obstruction or vascular malformations. In many cases, the cause of hydrocephalus is never found. The most common causes of **intraventricular obstructive hydrocephalus** include infection or hemorrhage (causing obstruction to the exiting foramina of the third or fourth ventricle), congenital anomalies (Fig. 52-30) (stenosis of the aqueduct of Sylvius), tumor, and fibrosis of the foramina of Monro. The most common causes of **extraventricular obstruction** are hemorrhage and infection with fibrosis at the basal cisterns, incisura, convexity cisterns, or parasagittal region.

HYPOXIC-ISCHEMIC EVENTS

Hypoxic-ischemic events in the neonate can be divided into maternal causes and causes attributable to the neonate. Maternal causes include chronic cardiac or pulmonary lung disease, placental insufficiency, shock, abruptio of the placenta, and cardiorespiratory arrest. These can all cause severe birth asphyxia. An uncommon cause is maternal cocaine use.[71] Some therapeutic maneuvers in these very sick hypoxic neonates have also been associated with an increased risk for germinal matrix hemorrhage (GMH) and may do so by causing increased venous obstruction.[72] Increased venous pressure has been demonstrated in infants breathing out of sequence with a mechanical ventilator, during endotracheal tube suctioning and with high peak inspiratory pressure.[73] Other factors including tension pneumothorax, exchange transfusions, rapid infusions of colloid, and myocardial injury caused by asphyxia may greatly affect hemodynamics and venous pressure.[73-75]

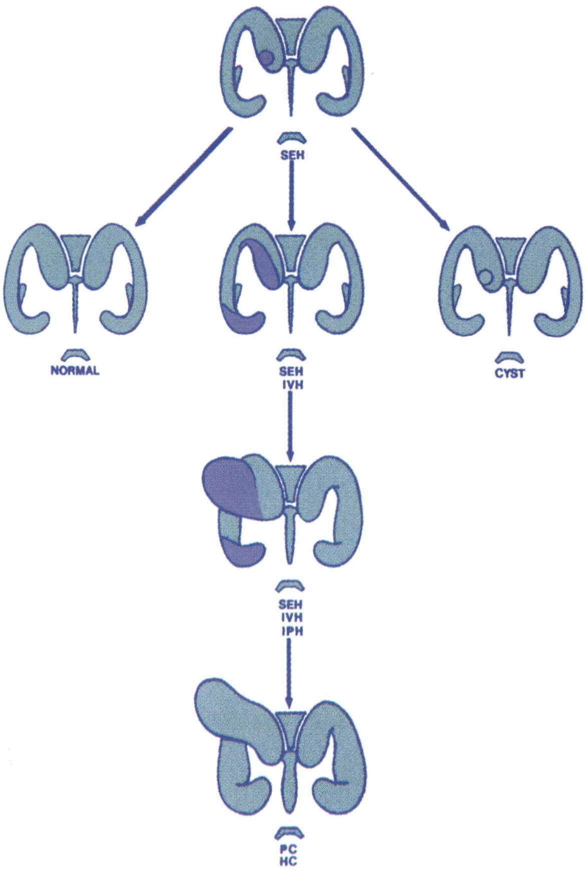

FIG. 52-31. Sequelae of sulrependymal hemorrhage. Subependymal hemorrhage (SEH) may resolve, leaving a normal scan; may resolve, leaving a small subependymal cyst; may progress, rupturing into the ventricle, causing interventricular hemorrhage, or extending into the parenchyma, causing intraparencymal hemorrhage. Hydrocephalus and porencephaly are common sequelae of SEH. (From Rumack CM, Johnson ML: *Perinatal and Infant Brain Imaging*, St. Louis, 1984, Mosby–Year Book.)

Arterial Watershed Determines the Region of Brain Damage

The sonographic findings are varied depending on the cause and the age of the neonate when the event occurs, because the watershed areas of the brain change in location during the last trimester. In premature infants, the watershed is in the immediate periventricular region, and thus GMH and periventricular leukomalacia (PVL) are common pathological findings. In full-term infants, damage tends to occur more in the cortical or subcortical regions, because the watershed moves to these areas more toward the brain surface in a parasagittal distribution.

Lack of autoregulation of cerebral blood pressure, which commonly occurs in premature infants and less often in asphyxiated full-term infants, will cause cerebral perfusion to be directly affected by hypertensive or hypotensive episodes. This pressure passive system can result in sudden focal hemorrhage or with hypotension, diffuse or focal infarction.

The neurologic manifestations of brain injury in the premature infant include the less severe motility and cognitive deficits to major spastic motor deficits including spastic diplegia and spastic quadriplegia with more profound intellectual deficits. In the full-term infant, the hypoxic-ischemic events may manifest as seizures, movement disorders including arching and fisting, altered tone, absent suck, and depending on the severity, intellectual deficits.

Germinal Matrix Hemorrhage

Germinal matrix hemorrhage is a common event occurring primarily in premature infants who are less than 32 weeks' gestational age. Although the incidence once was as high as 55%, most nurseries have experienced a significant drop in GMH in the past few years. Infants at greatest risk are those at gestational ages of less than 30 weeks, of a birth weight of less than 1500 grams, or both.[76-78]

Multiple factors have been studied as causes for this hemorrhage. Although no single cause has been identified, frequently associated events include prematurity with complications such as hypoxia, hypertension, hypercapnia, hypernatremia, rapid volume increase, and pneumothorax.[73-75,78,79] Full-term infants rarely experience this type of hemorrhage.

Germinal matrix hemorrhage may occur in **subependymal** (SEH), **intraventricular** (IVH), or **intraparenchymal** (IPH) regions.[79,80] However, it originates predominantly as an extension of hemorrhage from the germinal matrix in the subependymal layer and may be contained by the ependyma or may rupture into the ventricular system or less often into the adjacent parenchyma (Fig. 52-31). The germinal matrix is a fine network of blood vessels and primitive neural tissue that lines the ventricular system in the subependymal layer during fetal life. As the fetus matures, the germinal matrix regresses toward the foramen of Monro so that, by full-term, only a small amount of germinal matrix is present in the caudothalamic groove between the thalamus and the caudate nucleus. This fine network of blood vessels is highly susceptible to pressure and metabolic changes which can lead to rupture of the vessels. The germinal matrix is rarely a site of hemorrhage after 32 weeks' gestation because it has nearly disappeared.

The classification of GMH most widely used was proposed by Burstein and Papile (see box). There are other systems as well, but the anatomic description of the brain damage is more important than the classification. The key causes of poor neurological outcome relate to hydrocephalus and parenchymal extension into the descending white matter tracks.

Sonography is the most effective method for detecting this hemorrhage in the newborn period and for follow-up in the subsequent weeks. Most hemorrhage (90%) occurs in the first 7 days of life, but only one third of these occur in the first 24 hours.[81] Screening for GMH has usually been performed at the end of the patient's first week of life. The optimal cost-effective timing of screening has been questioned by Boal et al.[82] They suggest that screening premature infants at 2 weeks of age would capture patients with significant hemorrhage as well as those who are developing hydrocephalus.[3] Small subependymal hemorrhages (Grade 1) might be missed when screening late if they resolve quickly but these have not been clinically important. To screen for both hemorrhage and late signs of PVL, we are now screening patients between 1 and 2 weeks of life as the first planned evaluation of the brain. A second scan is then performed later at 1 month to search for the cystic changes of PVL. Of course, an examination should be performed earlier if the patient's condition requires it.

Severe grades of hemorrhage with hydrocephalus (Grade III) and intraparenchymal hemorrhage (Grade IV), are becoming less prevalent in the neonatal intensive care unit. Many factors probably contribute to this fact. Included is the increasing use of perinatal steroids[83,84] and the improvement of neonatal respiratory technology, including surfactant therapy. Because a pneumothorax has been proven to be associated with a higher incidence of GMH, the effective use of high-frequency ventilators, oscillators, and surfactant, which decrease pressure to the lung, is a likely cause for the decreasing incidence of GMH. A controversial issue is the use of antenatal vitamin K and phenobarbital. This therapy is still under investigation, and its benefit in the reduction of IVH yet to be established.[85]

GRADES OF GERMINAL MATRIX HEMORRHAGE

Grade I: Subependymal hemorrhage
Grade II: Intraventricular extension without hydrocephalus
Grade III: Intraventricular hemorrhage with hydrocephalus
Grade IV: Intraparenchymal hemorrhage with or without hydrocephalus

Complications of SEH and IVH are intraventricular obstructive hydrocephalus (usually at the foramina of Monro or the sylvian aqueduct) and extraventricular obstructive hydrocephalus (at the arachnoid granulations). Complications of IPH are permanent areas of damaged brain that can become necrotic, leading to porencephalic cysts.

Subependymal Hemorrhage. On sonographic examination, **acute subependymal** (Fig. 52-32) **hemorrhage** presents as a homogeneous, moderately to highly echogenic mass. The echogenic clot may cause focal enlargement of the choroid in the caudothalamic groove.[86] The choroid plexus is normally quite thick at the trigone of the lateral ventricle and tapers progressively anteriorly, descending between the head of the caudate and the thalamus just above the foramen of Monro. As the hematoma ages, the clot becomes less echogenic with its center becoming sonolucent (Fig. 52-33). The aging of the clot can often be followed up to 6 weeks or more, depending on its initial size. The clot retracts, and necrosis occurs with complete resolution of hemorrhage or development of a subependymal cyst. It may persist as a linear echo adjacent to the ependyma.

Intraventricular Hemorrhage. IVH appears sonographically as hyperechoic material that fills a portion of the ventricular system or all of a ventricle when the clot forms a cast of the ventricle (Fig. 52-34). The clot itself may obscure the ventricle due to complete filling of the lumen. The normally thick echogenic choroid plexus may appear asymmetrically thick and be difficult to define within the ventricle separate from the densely echogenic hemorrhage. As the clot matures it becomes echolucent centrally and more well defined and separable from the more echogenic choroid plexus. Low level echoes floating in a ventricle may occur in IVH as the clot breaks apart (Fig. 52-34, *C*). Use of the posterior fontanelle or axial views may increase the detection of IVH in normal sized ventricles as at times there are only small clots or CSF-blood fluid levels in the occipital horn.[8]

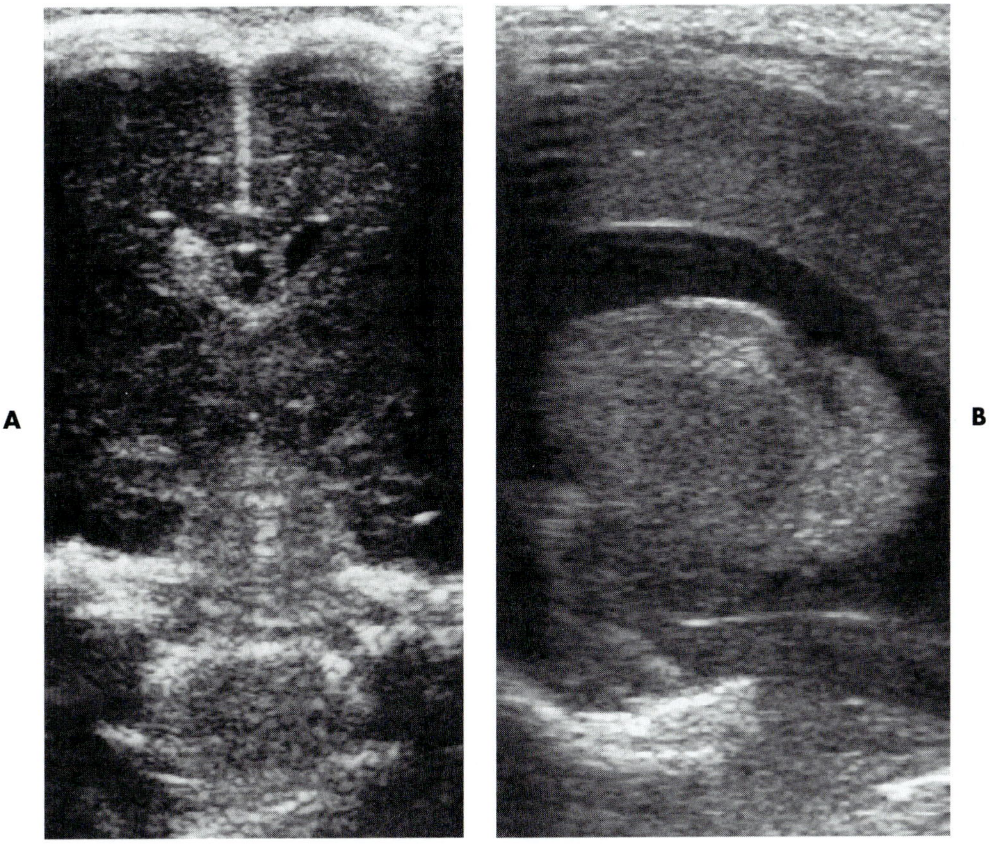

FIG. 52-32. Subependymal hemorrhage (SEH). **A,** Coronal and **B,** sagittal sonograms show SEH in the region of the caudate nucleus (near the caudothalamic groove on sagittal). This echogenicity is close to the choroid so it most likely occurred several days prior to this scan.

SIGNS OF IVH

Hyperechoic material that fills a portion of the ventricular system
Clot forms a cast of the ventricle
 May obscure the ventricle due to complete filling of the lumen
Thick echogenic choroid plexus
Echolucent centrally late
Low level echoes floating in a ventricle
CSF-blood fluid levels

Intraventricular Hemorrhage with Hydrocephalus (Fig. 52-35). Because IVH causes hydrocephalus, the clot and then the choroid plexus may be more defined. Echogenic clot may be adherent to various ventricular walls or become dependent within the ventricle. A change in the head position while scanning will demonstrate clot movement in some cases (Fig. 52-36). Posterior fossa and sometimes axial views may show IVH in the occipital horn in more subtle cases. As with subependymal hemorrhage, in time the echogenic clot will become more echolucent centrally and may eventually resolve (Fig. 52-36). A chemical ventriculitis as a response to blood in the CSF typically causes thickening of the subependymal lining of the ventricle.[87] Hydrocephalus may require shunting if it is progressive. Follow-up scans should be obtained at weekly intervals unless the head size grows rapidly or another crisis intervenes.

Intraparenchymal Hemorrhage. Intraparenchymal hemorrhage is usually located in the frontal or parietal lobes because it often extends from the subependymal layer over the caudothalamic groove (Fig. 52-37). Recent studies suggest that IPH is caused by hemorrhagic venous infarction.[73,74] Taylor[75] has shown obstruction of terminal veins by SEH or IVH is often seen with secondary IPH or periventricular white matter hemorrhage. **Periventricular hemorrhagic infarction** (PHI) is believed to be venous infarction secondary to a large subependymal hemorrhage

Text continued on p. 1477.

A
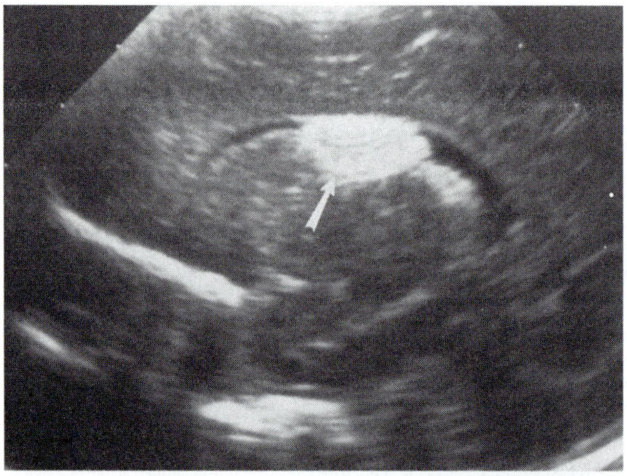
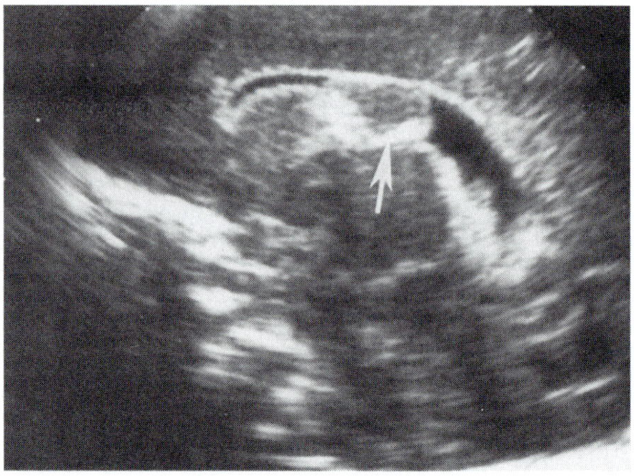
B

C
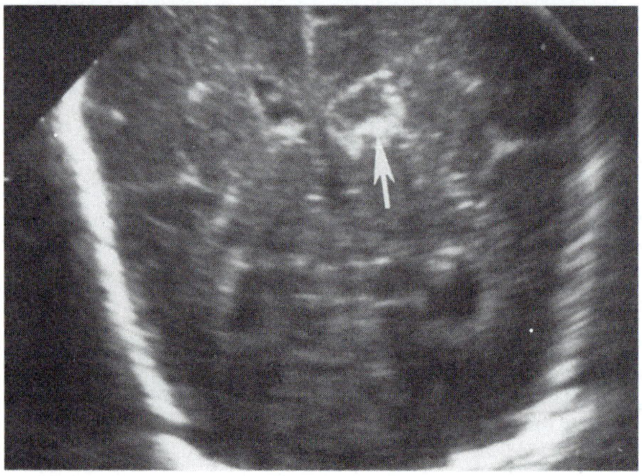

FIG. 52-33. Subependymal hemorrhage (changes with time). A, Sagittal section shows highly echogenic hematoma (*arrow*) in caudothalamic groove. **B,** Sagittal and **C,** coronal sections 1 week later show hematoma is becoming less echogenic centrally, which is consistent with aging hemorrhage.

A
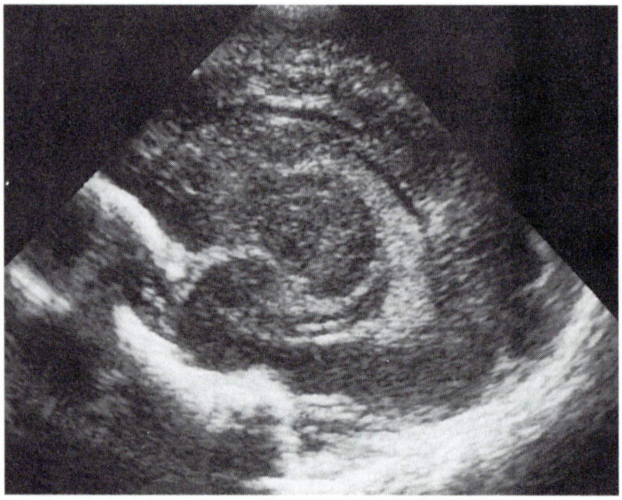
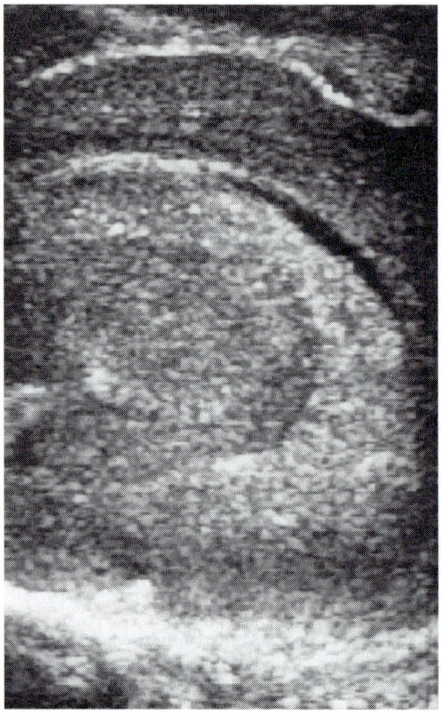
B

FIG. 52-34. Subependymal (SEH) and intraventricular hemorrhage (IVH). A, Sagittal and **B,** sagittal magnified sonograms show SEH in the caudothalamic groove. The occipital horn in both cases is filled with echogenic clot (IVH).

Continued.

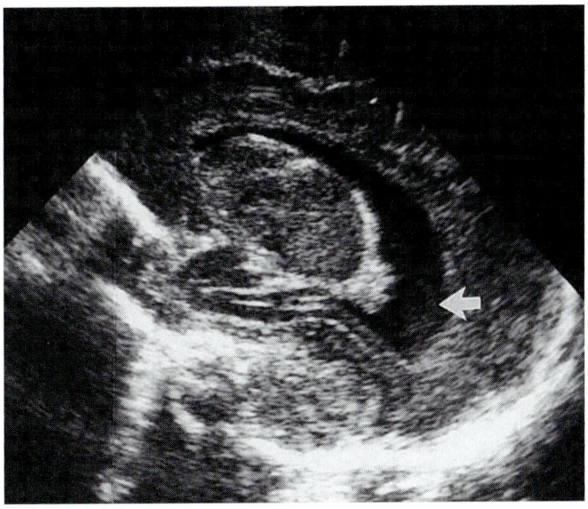

C

FIG. 52-34, cont'd. **C,** Two weeks later, lateral ventricle shows low level echoes (*arrow*) from IVH.

A

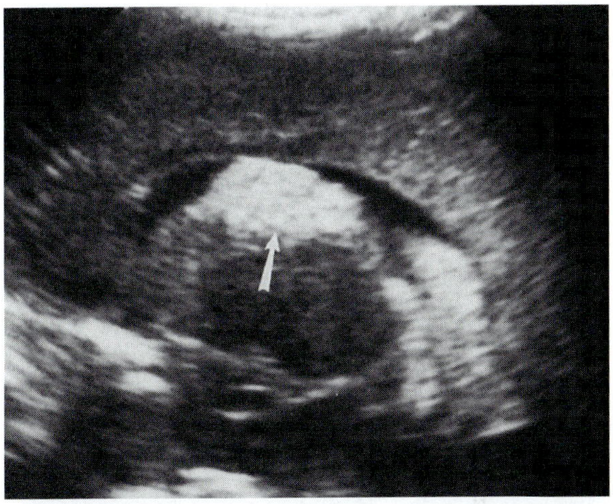

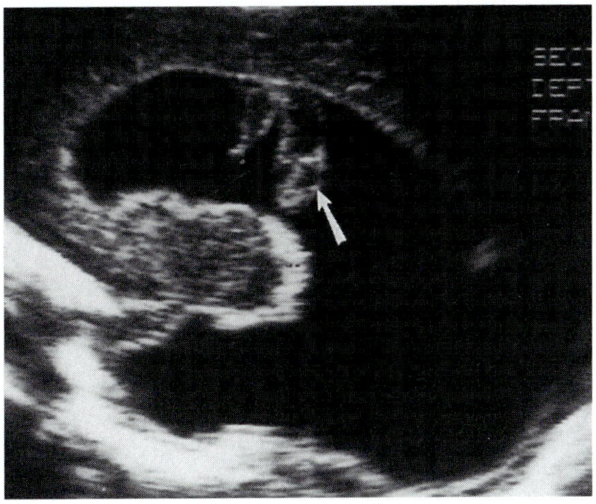

B

C

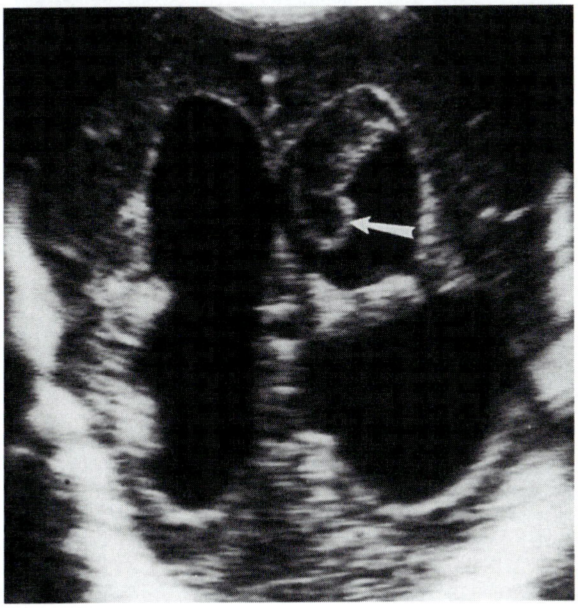

FIG. 52-35. Intraventricular hemorrhage and hydrocephalus. **A,** Sagittal scan shows echogenic clot (*arrow*) in slightly dilated lateral ventricle. **B,** Posthemorrhagic hydrocephalus has developed. **C,** Coronal scan shows clot fragments attached to roof of ventricle (*arrow*).

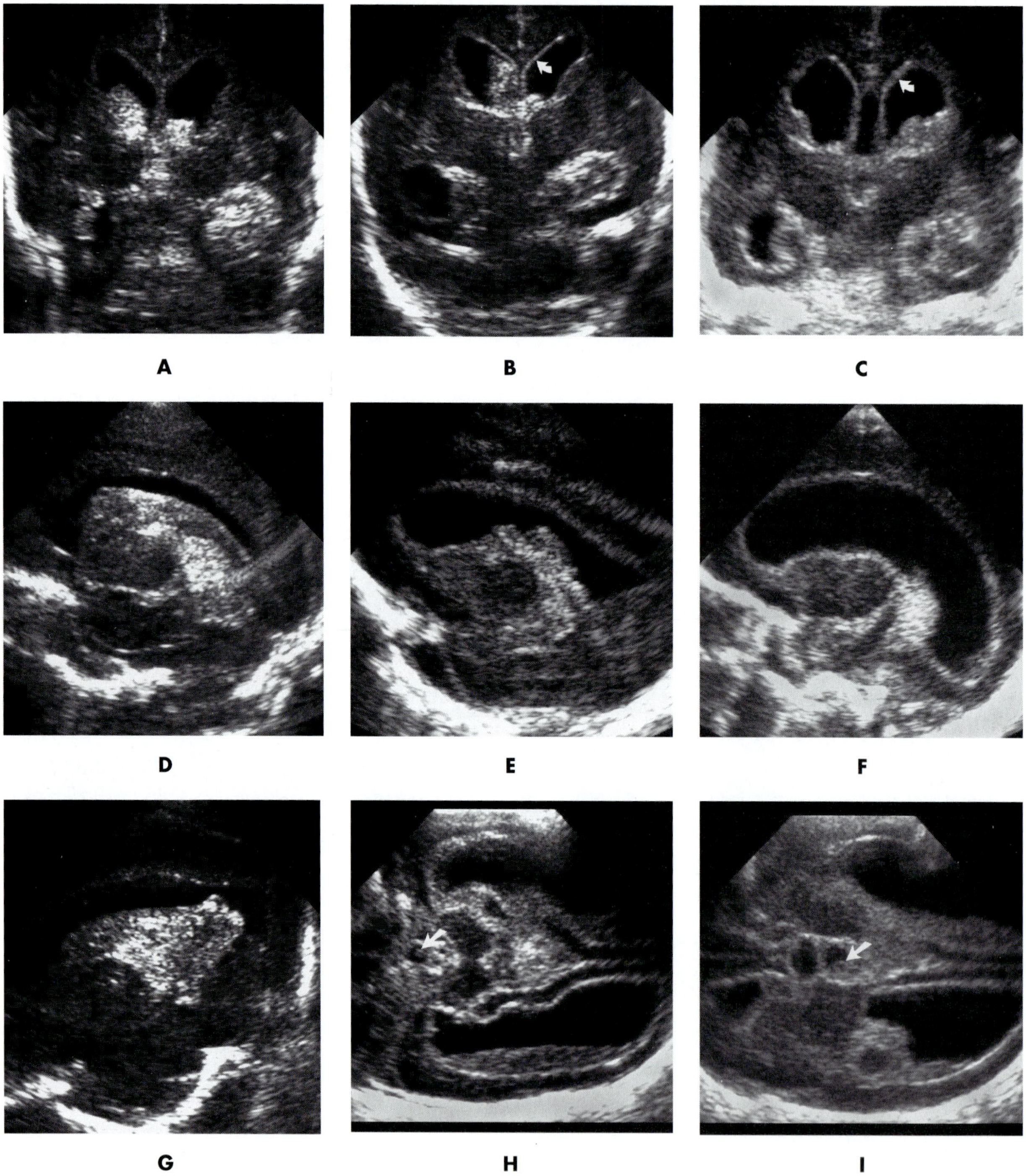

FIG. 52-36. Ventricular enlargement, hemorrhage, and ventriculitis. A, B, C, Coronal sonograms show echogenic clot in frontal and temporal horns of the lateral ventricle and the third ventricle. **B and** C show echogenic ependyma (arrows) caused by ventriculitis. **D, E, F,** Sagittal sonograms show progressive enlargement of lateral ventricle over two weeks. Blood fills the occipital horn in **D**, causes a CSF-blood level in **E**, and low-level echos in **F**. **G,** Posterior fossa angled view shows an echogenic clot in occipital horn. **H and I**, Axial views show CSF blood levels in enlarged third (arrows) and lateral ventricles.

A

B

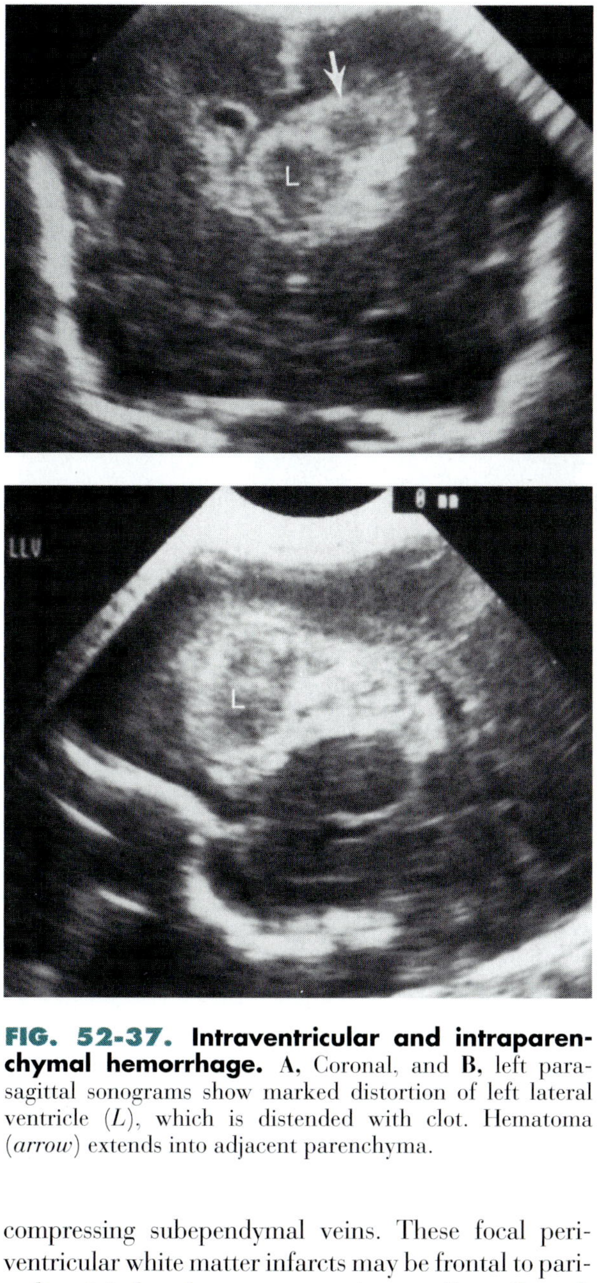

FIG. 52-37. Intraventricular and intraparenchymal hemorrhage. **A**, Coronal, and **B**, left parasagittal sonograms show marked distortion of left lateral ventricle (*L*), which is distended with clot. Hematoma (*arrow*) extends into adjacent parenchyma.

A

B

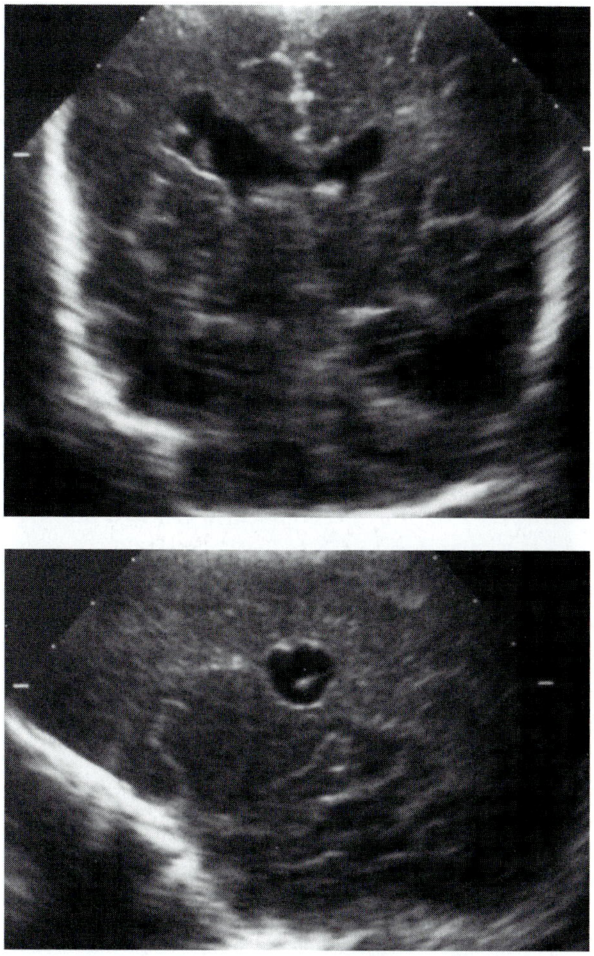

FIG. 52-38. Posthemorrhagic hydrocephalus and porencephaly. **A**, Coronal, and **B**, right sagittal sections show cystic area caused by resolution of intraparenchymal hematoma. It communicates with right lateral ventricle so it is termed *porencephaly*.

compressing subependymal veins. These focal periventricular white matter infarcts may be frontal to parietal-occipital and are asymmetric, usually unilateral, and if bilateral then asymmetric in size. These infarcts typically cause spastic hemiparesis.[88] In this lesion, the venous infarction caused by the initial subependymal hemorrhage leads to intraparenchymal damage. Later, necrosis may lead to porencephaly in this region.

Acutely, IPH appears as an echogenic homogeneous mass extending into the brain parenchyma. As the clot retracts, the edges form an echogenic rim around the center, which becomes sonolucent. The clot may move to a dependent position, and by 2 to 3 months following the injury, an area of porencephaly (if there is communication with the ventricle) or encephalomalacia develops (Fig. 52-38).[86,89]

Unusual sites of IPH may occur as a result of hemorrhage into PVL, secondary to infarction or thromboembolism, from a bleeding diathesis (such as vitamin K deficiency), and from alloimmune thrombocytopenia or RH immune incompatibility (Fig. 52-39).[90]

Extracorporeal membrane oxygenation (ECMO) complications include IPH secondary to infarction, ischemia, and thromboembolism. Germinal matrix or IVH is less common after ECMO because premature infants are at high risk for these types of hemorrhage and thus almost never undergo this procedure. These complications may be from the hypoxic brain damage secondary to the underlying lung disease even prior to initiation of ECMO therapy. The complications from ECMO are also caused by heparinization and transient hypertension.[91-93]

Ultrasound is used to evaluate the newborn on ECMO on a daily basis. The portability and ease of use in the critically ill infant without the need for transport, are the main advantages. Sonography can

A B C D

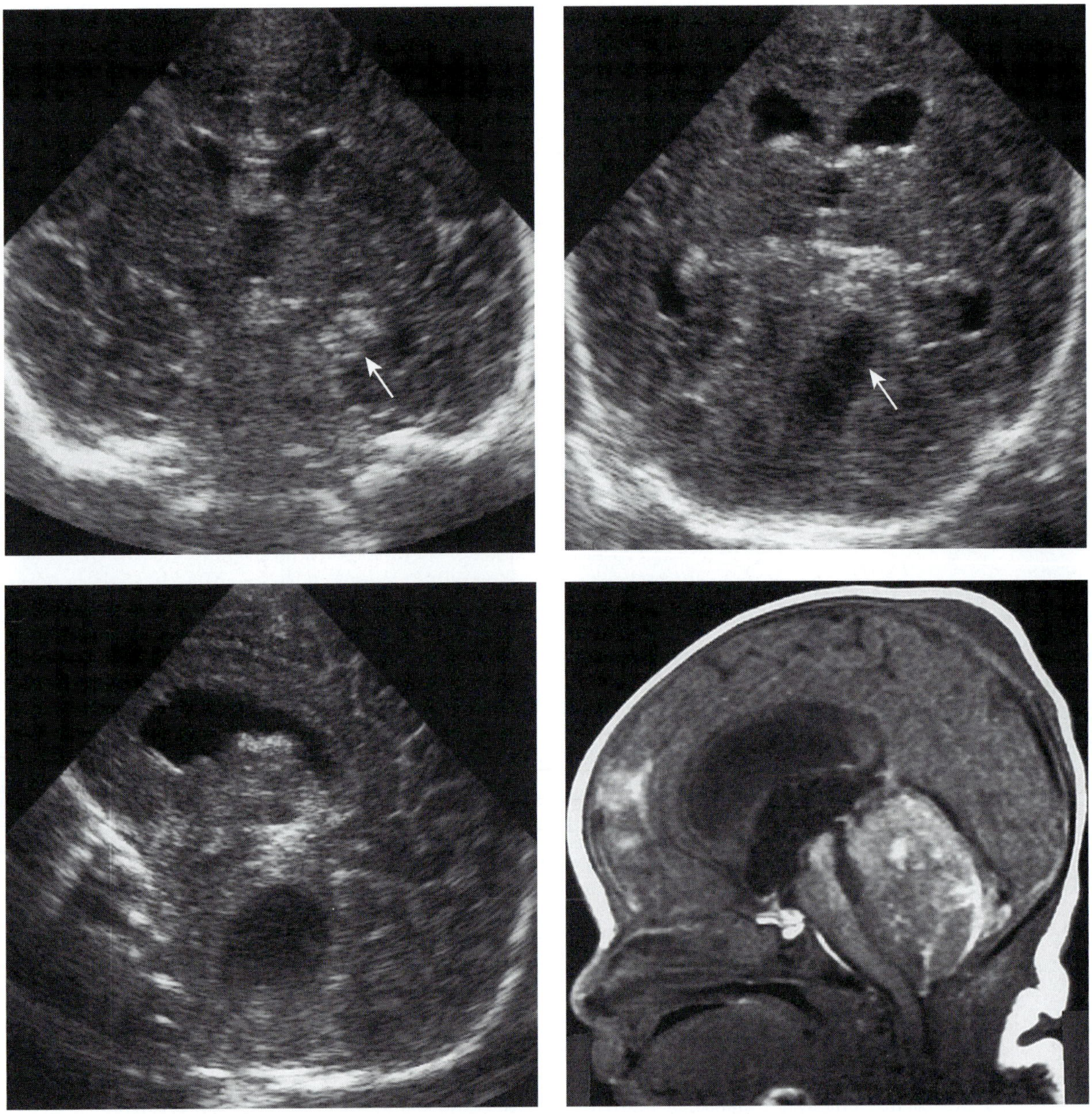

FIG. 52-39. Cerebellar hemorrhage. **A** and **B**, Coronal sonograms show the progression of hemorrhage in the left side of the cerebellum from echogenic to cystic in just a few days (*arrow*). The echogenic phase is quite subtle. **C**, Sagittal sonogram and **D**, sagittal T_1-weighted magnetic resonance imaging show the hemorrhage is compressing the fourth ventricle and obstructing the third and lateral ventricles causing hydrocephalus.

alert the clinician to intracranial hemorrhage and the consideration can be made to stop ECMO therapy.[92-98]

Subarachnoid Hemorrhage. The presence of enlarged interhemispheric and Sylvian fissures with thickened sulci and increased echogenicity can suggest the diagnosis of subarachnoid hemorrhage.[96] Subarachnoid hemorrhage may occur in neonates who have experienced asphyxia, trauma, or disseminated intravascular coagulation and may be the only hemorrhage in full-term infants who are not at risk for GMH. Cisternal subarachnoid hemorrhage may be a predictor of IVH but a difficult diagnosis on ultrasound. Subarachnoid hemorrhage is poorly demonstrated with ultrasound but easily demonstrated by CT or MRI.

Cerebral Edema and Infarction

Periventricular Leukomalacia. Periventricular leukomalacia—the principal ischemic lesion of the premature infant—is infarction and necrosis of the periventricular white matter. In some cases, there is a history of cardiorespiratory compromise, resulting in hypotension and severe hypoxia and ischemia. The prevalence of PVL in the very-low birth weight infant (< 1000 g) is approximately 25% to 40%.[99] The white

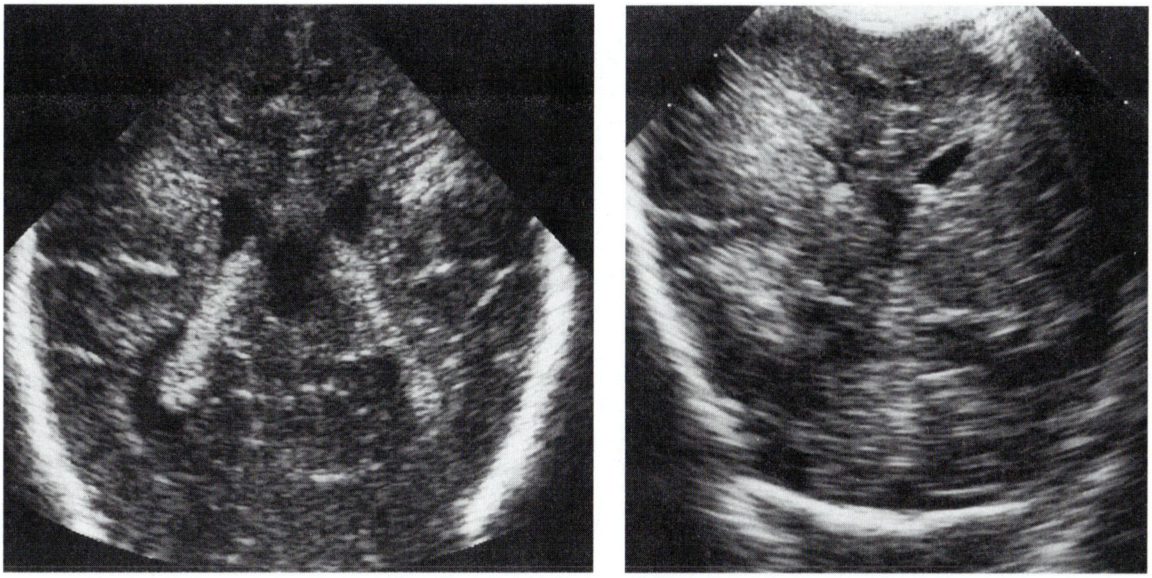
A B

FIG. 52-40. Periventricular leukomalacia (early findings). Coronal sonograms of two different patients. **A,** Bilateral increased echogenicity just lateral and superior to lateral ventricles. **B,** Coronal unilateral right-sided increased echogenicity.

matter most affected is in the arterial border zones at the level of the optic radiations adjacent to the trigones of the lateral ventricles and the frontal cerebral white matter near the foramina of Monro. The prevalence of PVL has been noted to increase with the duration of survival in premature infants. Therefore, the possibility of cumulative postnatal insults (i.e., circulatory compromise, apneic spells, sepsis) has been raised.[80,99-101]

Clinically, the patients may be initially asymptomatic. However, developmental delay and symmetric spastic diplegia involving both legs are common sequelae and are often noticeable by 6 months of age. Spastic diplegia occurs because the pyramidal tracts from the motor cortex that innervate the legs pass through the internal capsule and travel close to the lateral ventricular wall. Severe cases of PVL will also affect the arms, resulting in spastic quadriplegia and cause vision and intellectual deficits.[99,102-105]

Pathologically, the periventricular white matter undergoes coagulation necrosis followed by phagocytosis of the necrotic tissue. Most commonly, this occurs in the white matter adjacent to the external angles of the lateral ventricles. This results in decreased myelination in these areas and focal dilated lateral ventricles. In more severe cases of PVL, cystic cavities develop.[103,105,106] Petechial hemorrhages can complicate PVL.

Sonographically, the initial examination in PVL may be normal. However, within 2 weeks, the periventricular white matter increases in echogenicity until it is greater than the adjacent choroid plexus. This increased echogenicity is usually caused by edema from infarction and occasionally by hemorrhage (Fig. 52-40).[100,107] Two to three weeks following the insult, cystic changes may develop in the area of abnormal echogenic parenchyma (Fig. 52-41). The cysts can be single or multiple and are parallel to the ventricular border in the deep white matter and often lateral and/or superior to the top of the ventricles. These cysts measure from millimeters to 1 to 2 cm in diameter. The cystic changes are usually bilateral and often symmetric. A recent pathologic study suggests that sonography actually underestimates the incidence of PVL.[107] CT and MRI have even less ability to resolve the early edema from normal brain water or the later cystic areas, because the cysts are so small. This seems to be because the cysts are so tiny that they are not resolved by present equipment. Newer techniques, such as quantitative sonographic imaging, recently reported by Barr et al.[108] may allow the diagnosis of these subtle findings in more infants.

On subsequent sonograms, the cystic lesions may enlarge or resolve.[105] Therefore, normal-appearing white matter on either ultrasound or CT examinations performed several weeks to months following the insult does not exclude the occurrence of PVL.[109,110] MRI becomes more sensitive than either CT or ultrasound for long-term follow-up of parenchymal injury, because when myelination progresses, glial scarring from damaged white matter can be diagnosed (Fig. 52-41). Because the initial ultrasound examination is often normal in infants who have sustained a significant hypoxic/ischemic event, late sonograms should be obtained at least 3 weeks after birth to exclude evolving PVL. The characteristic distribution of lesions that are clearly separated from the ventricle in

A

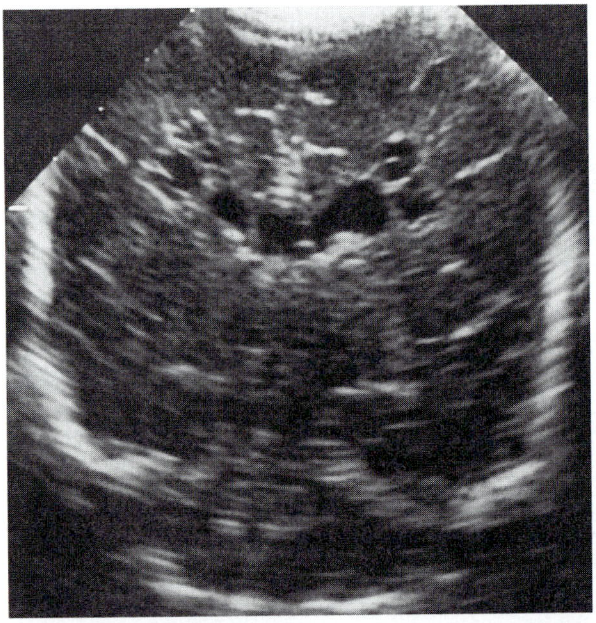

FIG. 52-41. Cystic changes of periventricular leukomalacia (late findings). **A**, Coronal and **B**, sagittal sonograms show multiple cysts above and lateral to the ventricles. **C**, Computed tomography scan shows marked cystic areas where individual cysts are not resolved. **D and E**, Coronal T_2 magnetic resonance imaging scans show highly intense white matter caused by gliosis and defective myelination in the periventricular region.

B

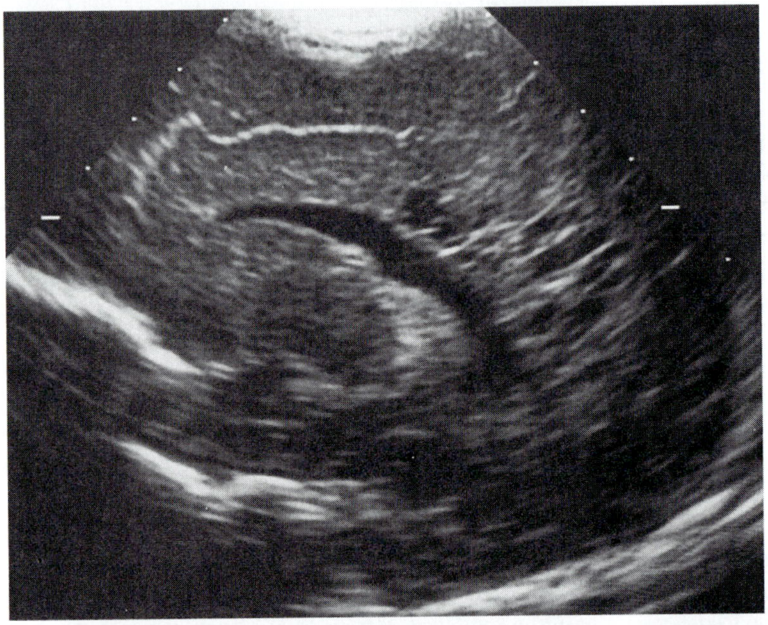

C

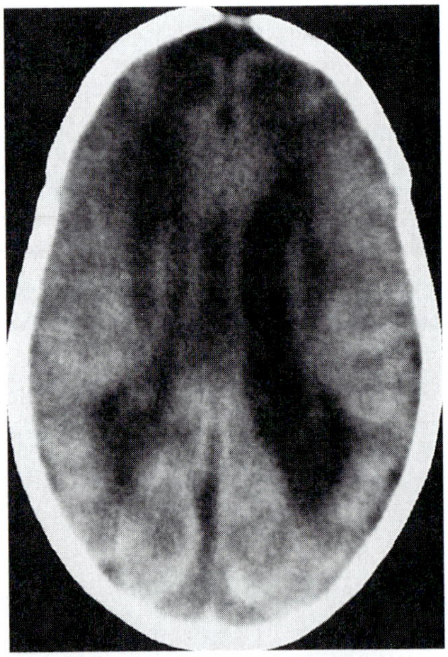

D

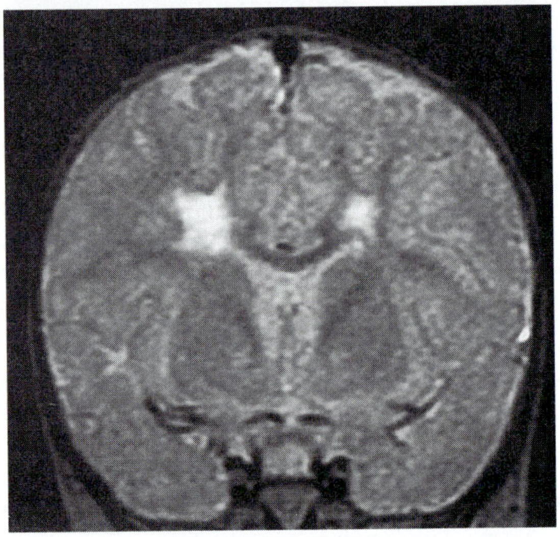

E

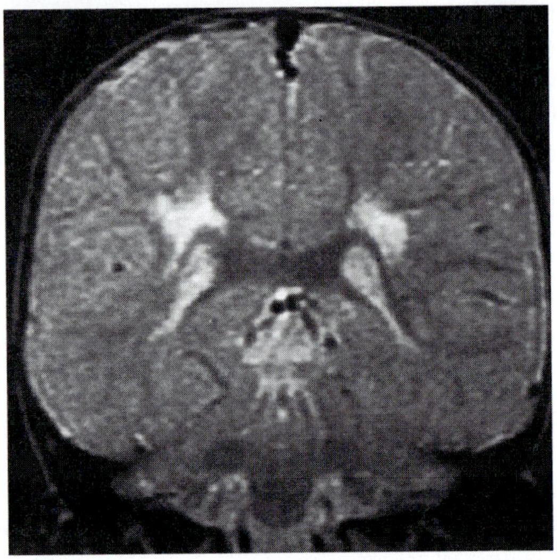

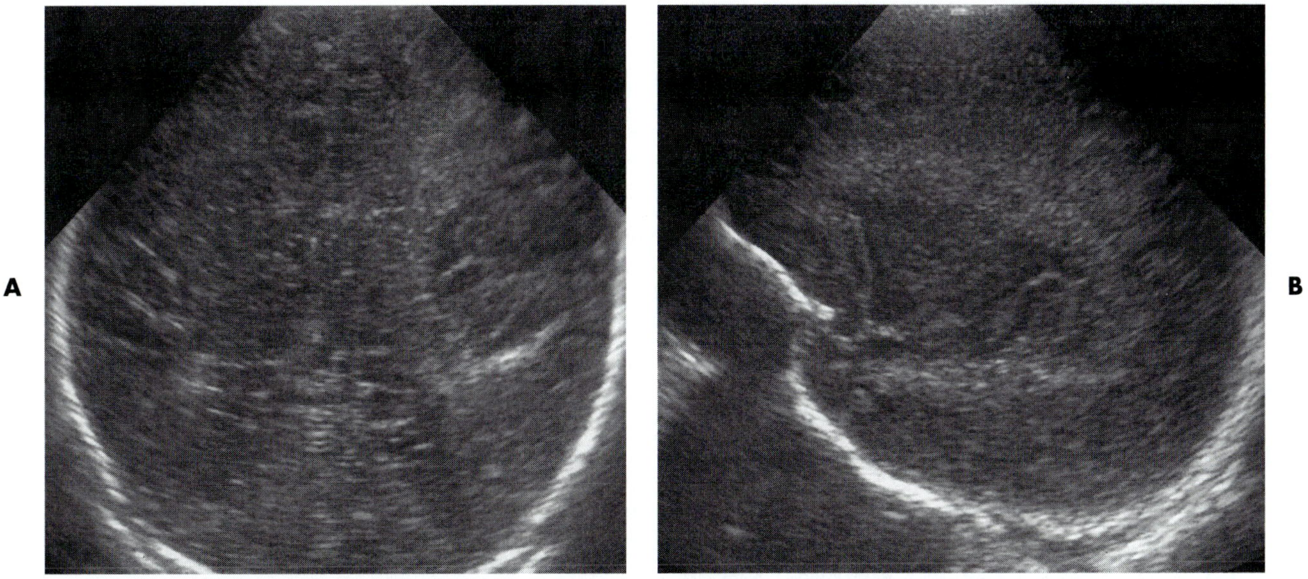

FIG. 52-42. Diffuse cerebral edema with silhouetting of the sulci. **A,** Coronal and **B,** sagittal sonograms show cerebral edema that is slightly worse on the left than right. The ventricles were so small that they were not visualized. Sulci are observed—even the interhemispheric and sylvian fissures are hard to find.

PVL should distinguish them from the parenchymal hemorrhage which occurs in grade IV GMH. However, PVL and GMH can occur simultaneously.[111-113]

Diffuse Edema. Diffuse cerebral edema with or without subarachnoid hemorrhage is a common result of hypoxic ischemic events in full-term infants. Initially, the brain edema will cause slitlike ventricles in a diffusely echogenic brain with poorly defined sulci. This may cause **silhouetting of the sulci** so that the sulci seem to disappear (Fig. 52-42). The brain parenchyma appears echogenic in the distribution of the injury and the sulci are difficult to appreciate because of surrounding echogenic edematous brain. The mechanism of the increased echogenicity of the brain parenchyma from cerebral edema is not understood completely. One possibility is that the increased intracellular fluid causes more interfaces, which accounts for the hyperechoic appearance. Doppler evaluation of severely asphyxiated infants has demonstrated earlier and at times more focal abnormalities than on gray scale alone. Several investigators have used Doppler either to classify brain edema[114] or to predict outcome.[115] A few studies show MRI changes early in neonatal life from asphyxia but most neonatologists resist moving a very unstable newborn to MRI.[116] If the ischemic event was severe enough to lead to infarction, then within 2 weeks diffuse brain volume loss occurs with ventricular enlargement secondary to atrophy. Enlarged extra-axial fluid spaces also develop as a consequence of the atrophic changes. The head circumference is very helpful to distinguish diffuse atrophy from hydrocephalus, because the head circumference is normal to small in patients who have undergone diffuse brain atrophy. Depending upon the type of insult, generalized brain atrophy may result or focal areas of porencephaly or encephalomalacia. Sonography can detect these complications of hypoxic-ischemic events, but MRI is more sensitive to the full extent of the insult near the cortical surface.[37,117-127]

Focal Infarction. Cerebral infarction in the neonate, aside from PVL, is uncommon. Risk factors are prematurity, severe birth asphyxia, congenital heart disease (resulting in a left-to-right shunt), meningitis, emboli (from the placenta or systemic circulation), polycythemia, and trauma. Symptoms can vary, ranging from asymptomatic to seizures with lethargy and coma. The initial physical examination often does not indicate lateralized findings. These develop later and often are first noted at 6 months of age, as the infant's neurologic system matures. The middle cerebral artery distribution is the most frequent site, although the anterior and posterior circulation have been reported.[23] Single areas of infarction are more commonly seen in full-term infants, whereas premature infants often demonstrate multiple sites of injury.

Cerebellar infarction is much less common than cerebral infarction but 6 cases were recently reported in 3 years at Hammersmith Hospital in London, diagnosed by MRI in patients at several years of age who were born prematurely.[128] All of these patients also had IVH, and thus cerebellar damage was likely a result of diffuse ischemic injury. Only one of six was diagnosed on ultrasonography as having cerebellar damage by

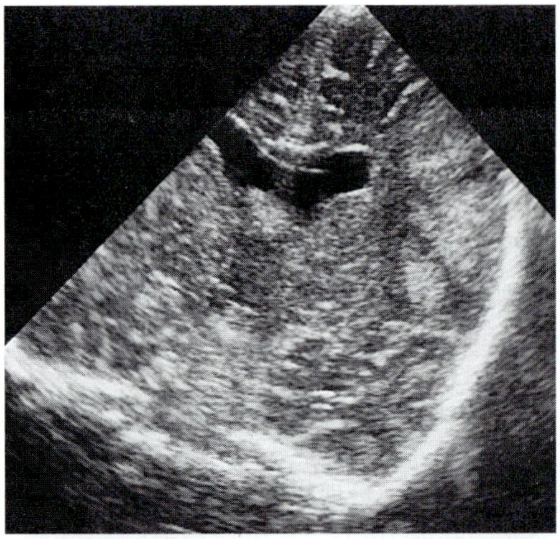

A

FIG. 52-43. Focal infarction in a term infant. **A,** Coronal sonogram shows early focal echogenicity in the left temporoparietal region in the region of the middle cerebral artery vascular distribution. **B,** CT scan performed several days later shows evolving infarction seen as large areas of hypodensity on both sides of the brain—a typical parasagittal distribution. **C,** Coronal pathological specimen in a different patient shows a typical focal infarction extending to the brain surface in a parasagittal distribution. (*C* from Friede R: *Developmental Neuropathology*, ed 2, New York, 1975, Springer-Verlag.)

B

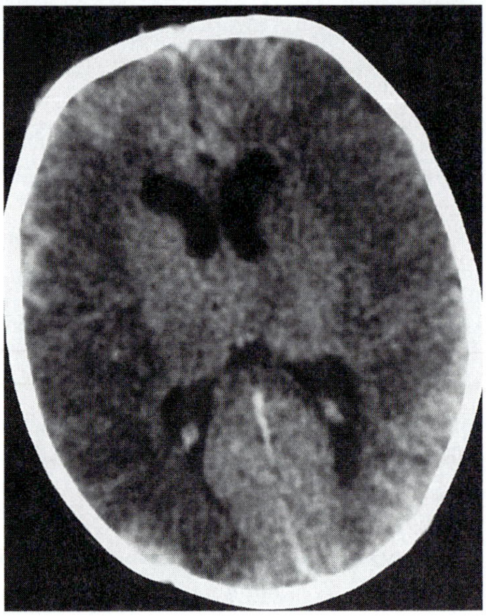

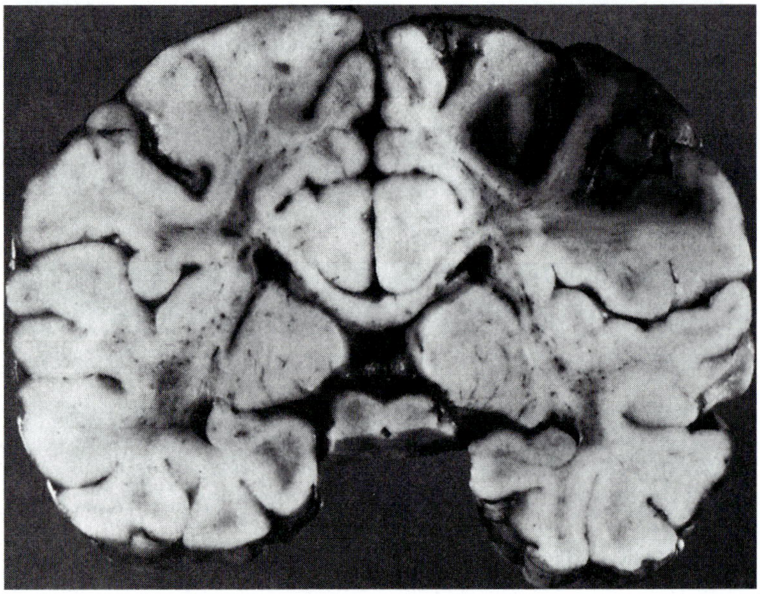

C

sonography. Because the vermis is so echogenic, edema or hemorrhage can be a difficult diagnosis in this region (Fig. 52-39).

Sonographically (Fig. 53-43), the affected brain parenchyma demonstrates some of the following findings within the first 2 weeks: echogenic parenchyma, lack of arterial pulsation, lack of a Doppler signal or Doppler flow, mass effect from edema, arterial territorial distribution of injury, decreased sulcal definition, and increased pulsation in the periphery of the infarcted section (see Chapter 53).[129-132]

After 2 weeks, the echogenic lesions begin to show cystic changes and ipsilateral ventricular enlargement from evolving atrophy (hydrocephalus ex vacuo), as well as a gradual return of arterial pulsations in the major branches from proximal to peripheral distribution. Taylor has demonstrated luxury perfusion within hours of a focal vascular insult, both experimentally and in newborn infants.[130-132]

SONOGRAPHIC SIGNS OF CEREBRAL INFARCTION

- Echogenic parenchyma
- Lack of arterial pulsation at real-time examination
- Lack of a vascular waveform on pulsed Doppler
- Lack of flow on color Doppler
- Mass effect from edema
- Arterial territorial distribution of injury
- Decreased sulcal definition
- Increased pulsation in the periphery of the infarcted section
- Early collateral arterial vessels within hours of the insult

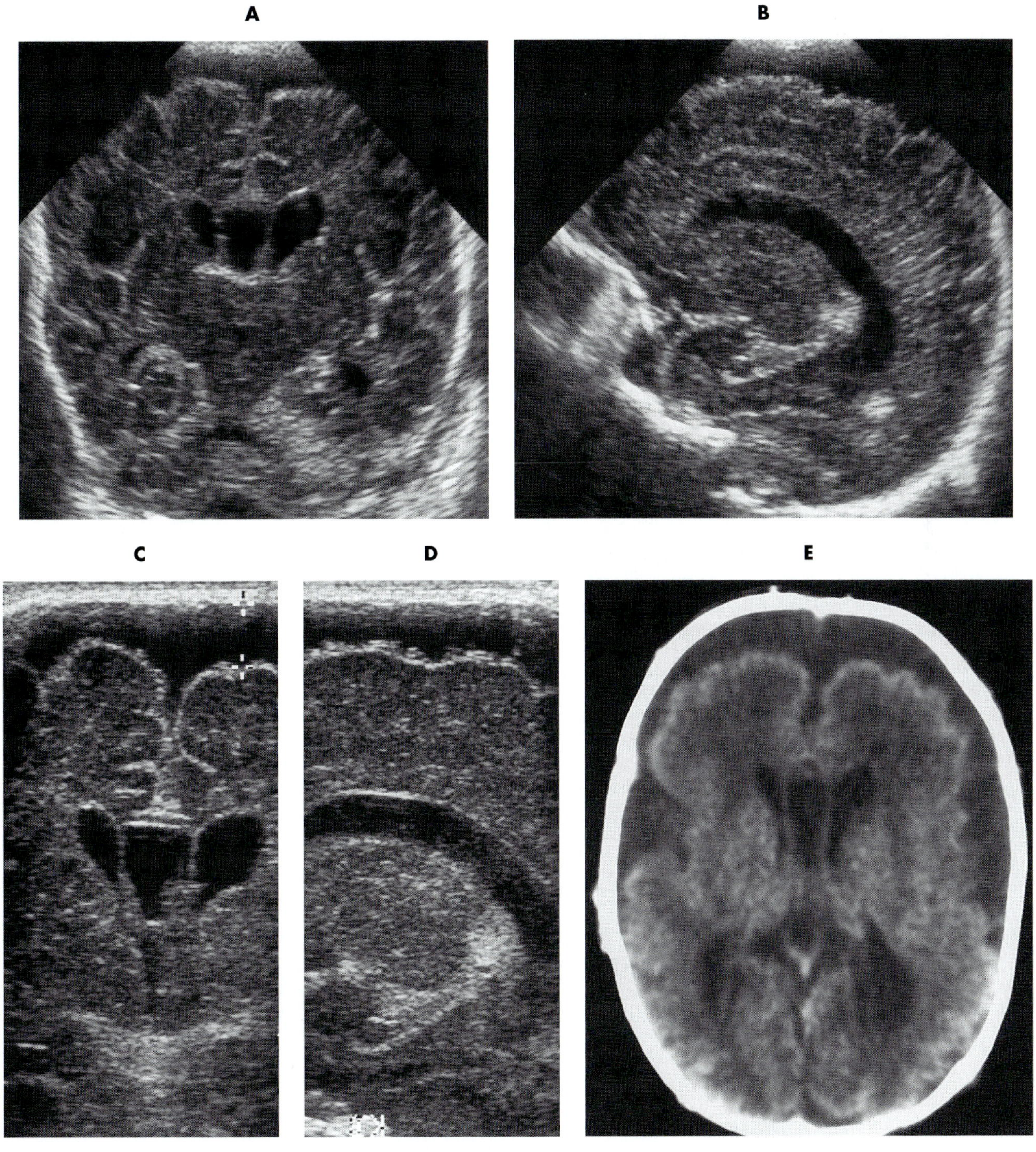

FIG. 52-44. Subdural hematoma. **A**, Coronal and **B**, sagittal sonograms show fluid over the surface of the brain (surface sulci are usually not imaged because the initial transducer artifact obscures the first 1 cm below the fontanelle). **C and D**, Magnified, high-resolution sonograms show sulci more clearly. **E**, Computed tomography scan shows extracerebral fluid.

POSTTRAUMATIC INJURY

Subdural and Epidural Hematomas

Subdural and epidural hemorrhage can be a difficult diagnosis on sonography compared with CT or MRI.[7,133] On sonographic examinations, they present as unilateral or bilateral hypoechoic fluid collections surrounding the brain parenchyma (Fig. 52-44). The fluid must be near 1 cm thick to be detected on sonographic equipment as a result of the approximately 1-cm nearfield artifact from most transducers. The nearfield artifact is less of a problem with newly developed, very high-frequency transducers (prototypes in 10 to 12 mHz range). Interposing an acoustic gel pad between the transducer and the fontanelle can assist in eliminating the nearfield artifact by moving it superiorly out of the brain. Magnified coronal sections are best for appreciating the epidural and subdural collections in the supratentorial space. Imaging through the foramen magnum or posterior fontanelle can assist in diagnosing infratentorial extra-axial fluid collections.

Cheng Yu Chen[9] reported that color Doppler sonography has been shown to separate subarachnoid and subdural fluid and/or hemorrhage based on displacement of vessels on the brain surface (see Chapter 53) (Fig. 52-45). Whether this method can always reliably predict atrophy in subarachnoid collections from the excess fluid under pressure in subdural fluid collections is yet to be proven. This may prove a reliable diagnostic tool to determine which patients may be simply observed and which require MRI for a more specific diagnosis of hemorrhage.

After the neonatal period when birth trauma may cause hemorrhage, the presence of new subdural fluid collections should raise the possibility of preexisting **meningitis** (most often from *Haemophilus influenzae*) or of **nonaccidental trauma.**[9,134,135] Infant's head circumference increases after the first 2 weeks of life, a CT examination should be used in most cases to search for extra-axial fluid, because the most common cause is subdural hemorrhage, not hydrocephalus. If a sonographic examination is performed, one should carefully search the nearfield with magnified views for extracerebral fluid and cerebral tears, as well as neomembranes seen in chronic subdural fluid collections.[9,136]

INFECTION

Congenital Infections

Congenital infections can have serious consequences for the developing fetus. Death of the fetus, congenital malformations, mental retardation or developmental delay, spasticity or seizures may result from infection at critical times during gestation.[137] Ultrasound plays an important role in identifying and following both antenatal and neonatal complications from congenital infections.

The most frequent congenital infections are commonly referred to by the acronym *TORCH.* This refers to the infections *Toxoplasma gondii*, rubella virus, cytomegalovirus (CMV), and herpes simplex type 2. The O stands for "other," such as syphilis. Syphilis causes acute meningitis, uncommonly resulting in parenchymal lesions in the newborn.[13]

Cytomegalovirus and Toxoplasmosis. Of the TORCH group, congenital infection by CMV is the most common, occurring in approximately 1% of all births.[137-139] CMV may be acquired at or after birth with little or no consequences, but prenatal infections may result in serious damage to the developing brain. Toxoplasmosis is the second common congenital infection and is caused by the unicellular parasite

A

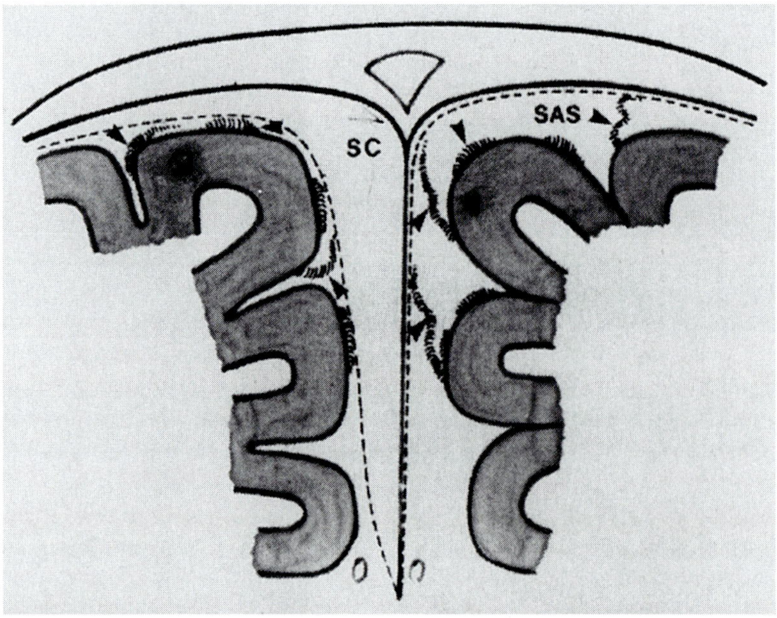

FIG. 52-45. Subdural versus subarachnoid fluid collections. A, Drawing shows vessels are compressed onto the surface of the brain in subdural fluid collections (*SC*) and vessels transverse the fluid in subarachnoid fluid (*SAS*). *Continued.*

B

C

D

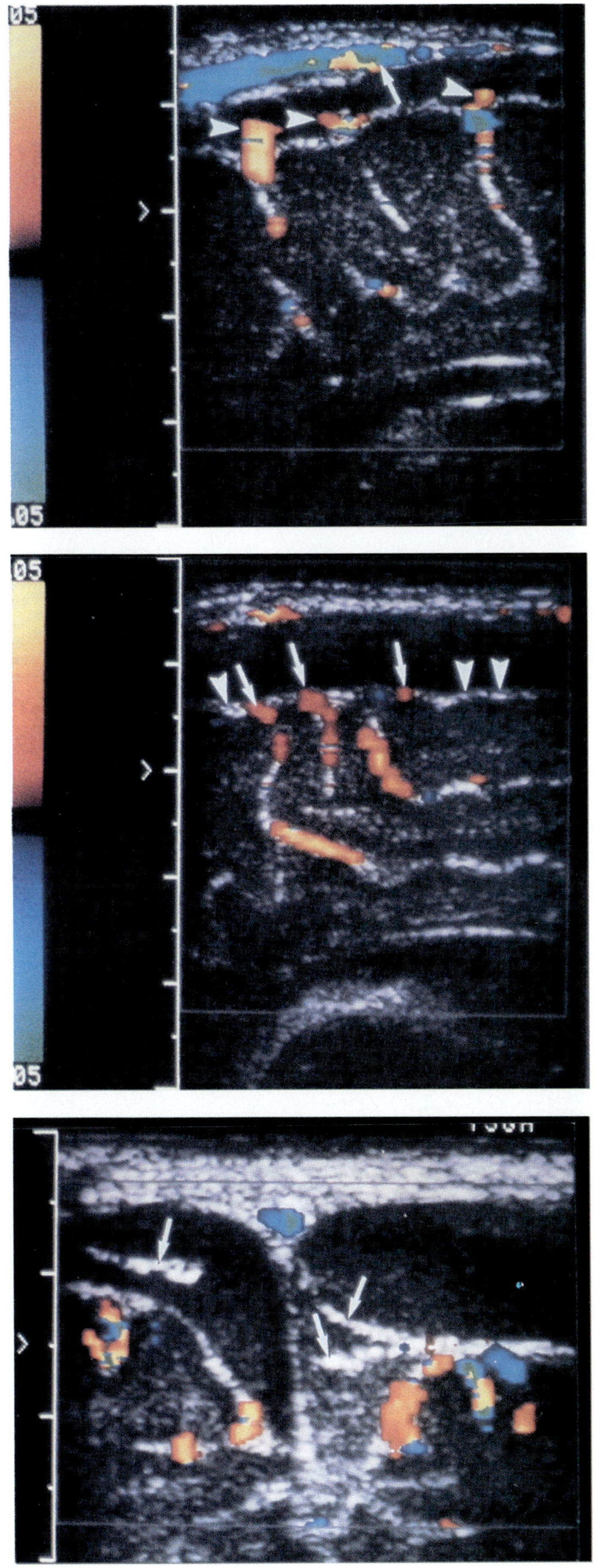

FIG. 52-45, cont'd. B, Color Doppler shows vessels crossing into SA subarachnoid fluid. **C,** Color Doppler shows vessels compressed in subdural. **D,** Shows "neomembrane" formed in subdural fluid collections. (From Cheng-Yu C, Chou TY, Zimmerman RA, et al. Pericerebral fluid collection: differentiation of enlarged subarachnoid spaces from subdural collections with color Doppler, *Radiology* 201(2):389-392, 1996.)

A

B

C

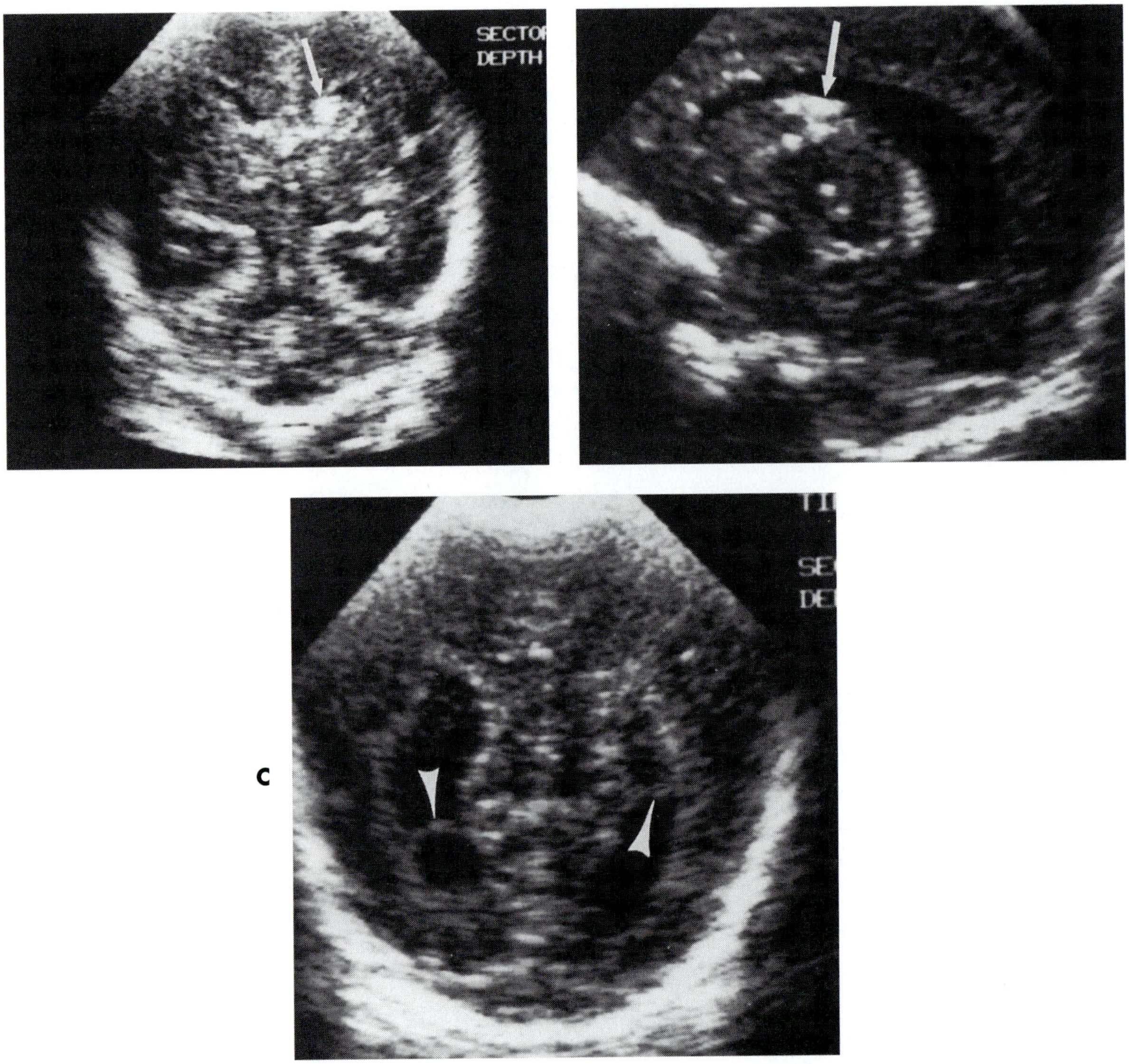

FIG. 52-46. Cytomegalovirus encephalitis. **A,** Coronal, and **B,** sagittal sonograms show diffusely echogenic brain and classic focal echogenic periventricular calcifications (*arrows*), which do not always shadow. **C,** Coronal image shows ventricular septations (*arrowheads*), which may occur in any form of ventriculitis. (From Rumack CM, Manco-Johnson ML: Neonatal brain ultrasonography. In: Sarti DA, editor: *Diagnostic ultrasound: Text and Cases*, ed 2, St. Louis, 1987, Mosby–Year Book.)

Toxoplasma gondii.[137,140,141] Maternal infection is usually subclinical.

The severity of the infection with either CMV or toxoplasmosis depends on the timing of the infection during gestation. Earlier infection, before 20 to 24 weeks, results in more devastating outcomes. These include microcephaly, lissencephaly with abnormal myelination and hypoplastic cerebellum, polymicrogyria and cortical dysplasias, porencephaly, and multicystic encephalomalacia. Ventriculomegaly results from brain volume loss. Later infection will result in less severe neurologic damage. Clinical outcomes correlate with the severity of CNS damage. Perinatal or neonatal death is expected with the more severe and earlier insults. Mental retardation, developmental delay, spasticity, and seizures are all potential outcomes. To differentiate CMV from toxoplasmosis serum titers for antibodies against these organisms are useful.[142] Other differentiating hints include the petechial skin lesions and hepatomegaly associated with CMV and chorioretinitis associated with toxoplasmosis. Intracranial calcifications have been described in both infections.[143,144] CMV classically causes periventricular calcifications (Figs. 52-46 and 52-47). Toxoplasmosis causes more scattered calcifications with a predilection for the basal ganglia. However, both patterns have been

A

B

C

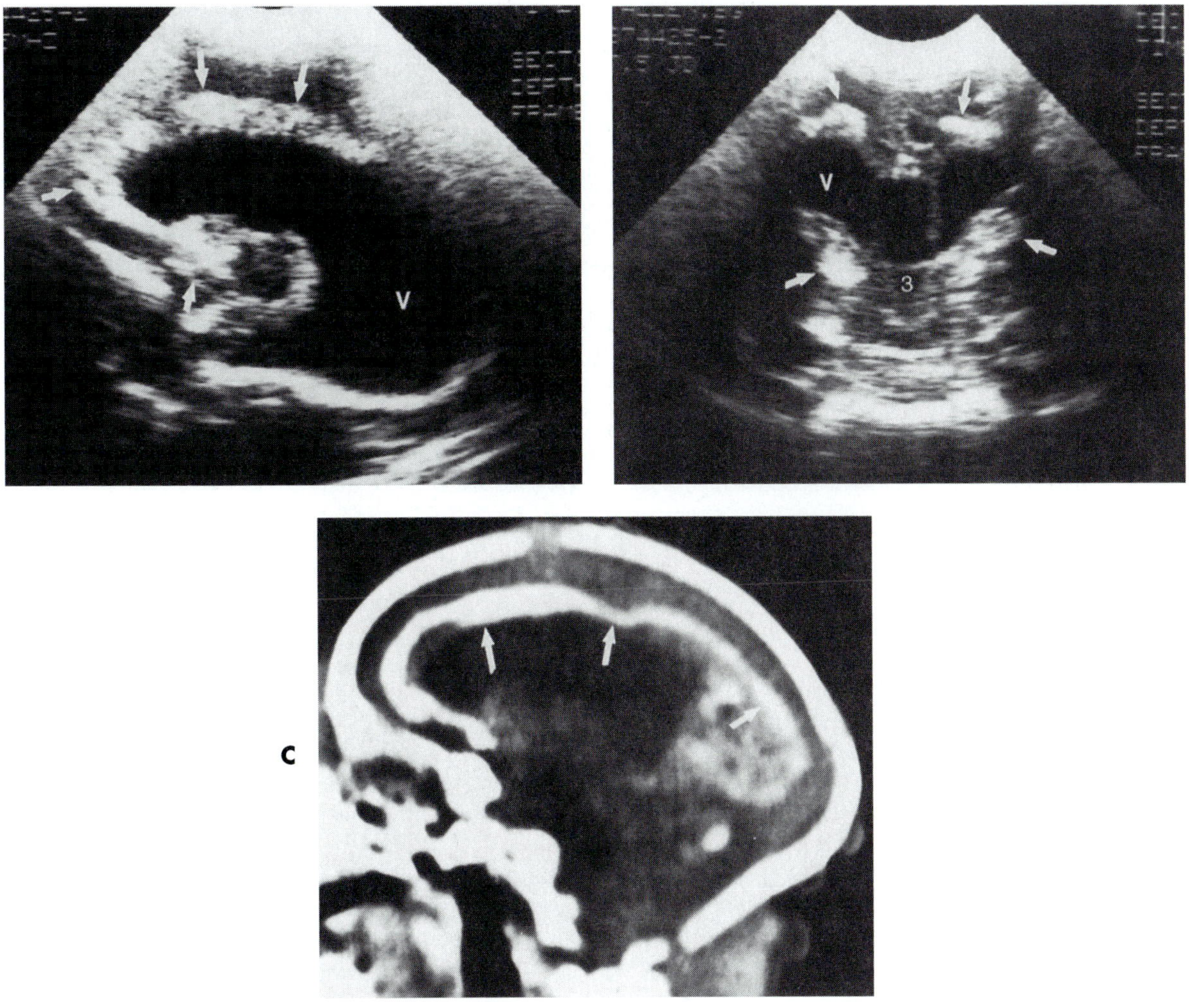

FIG. 52-47. Cytomegalovirus infection. **A,** Sagittal and coronal sonograms show ventriculomegaly probably caused by diffuse brain damage and periventricular calcification (*arrows*). V—Lateral ventricle. **B,** Third ventricle (*3*). **C,** Computed tomography. (From Rumack CM, Johnson ML: *Perinatal and Infant Brain Imaging*, St. Louis, 1984, Mosby–Year Book.)

seen in the other infection.[13,140-146] Resolution of intracranial calcification has been reported after treatment of congenital toxoplasmosis, consistent with improved neurologic outcome.[147]

Sonography can demonstrate the periventricular or scattered cerebral calcifications as echogenic foci with or without acoustic shadowing. The brain parenchyma may appear disorganized with poorly defined sulci. CT will demonstrate the calcification better, but MRI will demonstrate abnormal myelination or cortical dysplasias most reliably.[109]

Herpes Virus. There are two recognized types of herpes virus, herpes simplex virus types 1 and 2. Either may cause disease of the CNS, although type 2 is more common in the neonate and type 1 occurs primarily in older children and adults.[137,148-150]

Herpes type 2 may be acquired either transplacentally or by vaginal exposure during birth. The resulting encephalitis is typically diffuse resulting in loss of gray white differentiation. (This differs from the temporal lobe disease seen in older children and adults with HSV type I.) Cystic encephalomalacia of periventricular white matter and/or hemorrhagic infarction with scattered parenchymal calcifications frequently results.[151] Relative sparing of the lower neural axis including the basal ganglia, thalamus, cerebellum, and brain stem is typical.[152,153] Infections acquired *in utero* may lead to microcephaly, intracranial calcifications, and retinal dysplasias.[154]

Rubella. Since the widespread availability of rubella vaccine after 1967, congenital rubella has fortunately become extremely uncommon in the Western world. Unfortunately, it remains a significant problem in many other parts of the world. Rubella is not known to cause cerebral malformations. A case described by Levene[152] showed echogenic calcifications

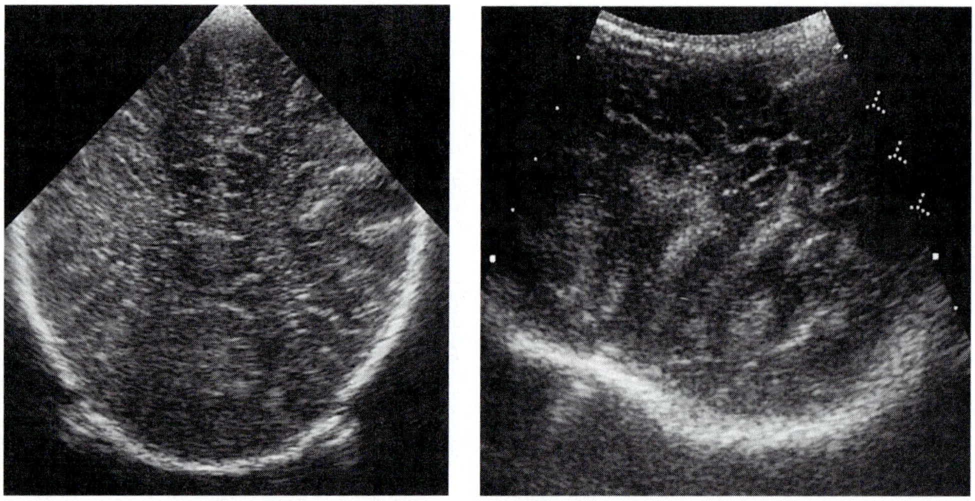

A B

FIG. 52-48. Group B streptococcal meningitis. A, Coronal and B, sagittal sonogram show diffusely echogenic sulci which appear thicker than normal.

in the basal ganglia confirmed at autopsy. Subependymal cysts are also described.[155] Microcephaly, vasculopathy,[155] and massive calcification of the brain that are detectable on a plain radiograph have been described in an infant who died at 9 days of age.[153]

Neonatal Acquired Infections

Meningitis and Ventriculitis. Despite the development of antibiotics for the treatment of bacterial infections in the latter half of this century, bacterial meningitis remains a serious concern for infants and children. During the first month of an infant's life, the two most common infections result from *Escherichia coli* and group B streptococcus. Between 4 to 12 weeks *E. coli* and *Streptococcus pneumoniae* are the most common, and from 3 months to 3 years, *Haemophilus influenzae* is the most frequent.[154] This is usually a clinical diagnosis. Imaging is only needed to evaluate for complications or when the patient's clinical situation deteriorates.[155-160]

Complications of meningitis include subdural empyemas or fluid collections (Fig. 52-44), cerebritis, abscess formation, and venous sinus thrombosis. Infarctions can occur from either arterial vasculitis or venous obstruction, as a result of venous sinus thrombosis. Sonography can identify these complications, but is not specific. Areas of increased or decreased echogenicity of brain parenchyma or sulci may represent edema, cerebritis (Figs. 52-48 and 52-49), or evolving infarction (Fig. 52-50).

Ventriculitis, another complication of meningitis, seen in 60% to 95% of cases, is suggested by the sonographic findings of hydrocephalus, echogenic debris within the ventricles, increased echogenicity, or a shaggy ependymal lining or fibrous septa within the ventricles (Fig. 52-51).[87,157,160] Ultrasound is best for identifying intraventricular septa formation as compared to CT or MRI. These septations can result in shunt failure or allow bacteria to escape antibiotic exposure. MRI and CT with enhancement are more sensitive for localizing the complications of infection, such as infarcts, venous sinus thrombosis, and extra-axial fluid collections.[137]

INTRACRANIAL MASSES

Brain Tumors

Only 11% of children with brain neoplasms present before 2 years of age. Tumors that do present before 2 years of age are usually congenital.[161] Brain tumors can be difficult to diagnosis in the neonate. If the neoplasm causes hydrocephalus, then signs and symptoms of increased ICP such as enlarging head size, vomiting, or behavior alteration may be recognized. More specific signs and symptoms may be recognized depending upon the location of the tumor, such as cranial nerve findings or pituitary gland/hypothalamic functions. MRI or CT is generally the first imaging modality of choice in these infants.[162] However, with nonspecific signs and symptoms including an enlarging head from hydrocephalus, ultrasound may be the first imaging performed. Sonography can delineate the tumor site and size and evaluate cystic and solid components.

Tumors may present initially as hemorrhage, and it may be extremely difficult to differentiate a simple

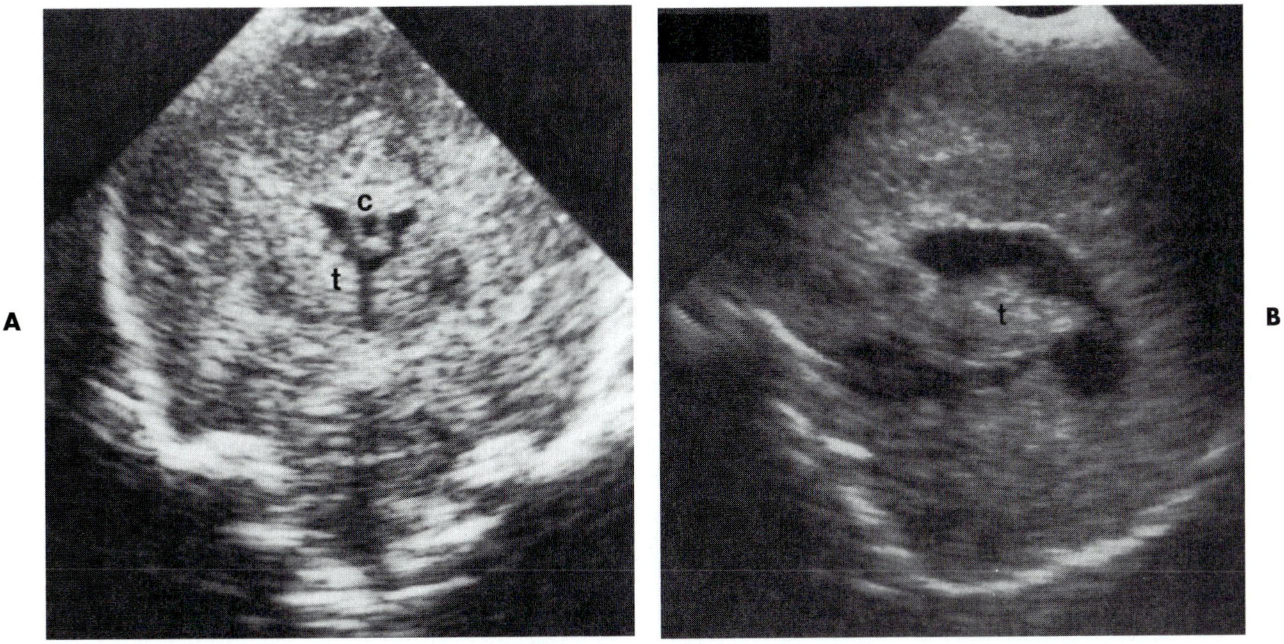

FIG. 52-49. Salmonella meningitis. **A**, Coronal, and **B**, sagittal sonograms show diffusely echogenic brain. Sulci are obliterated by edematous brain. Corpus callosum (*c*) and thalamus (*t*) are quite echogenic but normally should be hypoechoic.

hematoma from a tumor. We have seen at least three cases of congenital tumor presenting as hemorrhage. Any hemorrhage presenting in unusual circumstances or in an unusual location should be investigated by contrast-enhanced CT or contrast-enhanced MRI, searching for an occult tumor.[7] Follow-up scans also can be most helpful, because clotting from the hemorrhage will resolve over time, allowing the tumor to be visualized alone.

Doppler imaging can evaluate vascular components of the tumor. Follow-up with MRI or CT is then performed to evaluate the full extent of the neoplasm, assist with differential diagnosis, and evaluate for therapeutic approaches. Differentiating the histologic type of the neoplasm is not possible, but localizing the tumor usually allows for determining a differential diagnosis.

Tumor location in infants who are **less than 1 year of age** differs from that in older children.[162-167] Supratentorial neoplasms are more common than infratentorial tumors by approximately 2.5 to 1. Astrocytomas are the most frequent neoplasms reported in the first year of life (Fig. 52-52), and usually arise from the optic chiasm and nerves or the hypothalamus (Fig. 52-53). Other neoplasms include choroid plexus papilloma (Fig. 52-54 on page 1494), primitive neuroectodermal tumor (PNET), and ependymoma.[168-174] Sporadic cases of oligodendrogliomas, hemangioblastomas, hemangiomas, dermoid cysts, lipomas, primary neuroblastoma, teratomas, and meningiomas are also reported.

The ultrasound appearance is variable and nonspecific. Not enough data are available in the ultrasound evaluation of neoplasms as the majority are evaluated with MRI or CT. A tumor may present initially as hemorrhage; differentiating a simple hematoma from a tumor can be difficult.

Cystic Lesions

Cystic intracranial lesions are quite common and ultrasound is the best method for evaluating such lesions (short of surgical proof). Fortunately, most cystic masses of the brain are quite benign, so it is important to recognize them for what they are.[175,176]

Cystic intracranial lesions (see box on p. 1494) are defined by Harwood, Nash, and Fitz[177] as "a fluid-filled cavity within or adjacent to the brain, which has mass effect." A large cisterna magna is not a true cyst. Ventricular cysts include choroid plexus, subependymal, porencephalic, and colloid varieties. Congenital cysts other than arachnoid cysts are discussed in detail in the section on malformations. Cysts associated with tumors and infections are also discussed in their respective sections.

Text continued on p. 1494

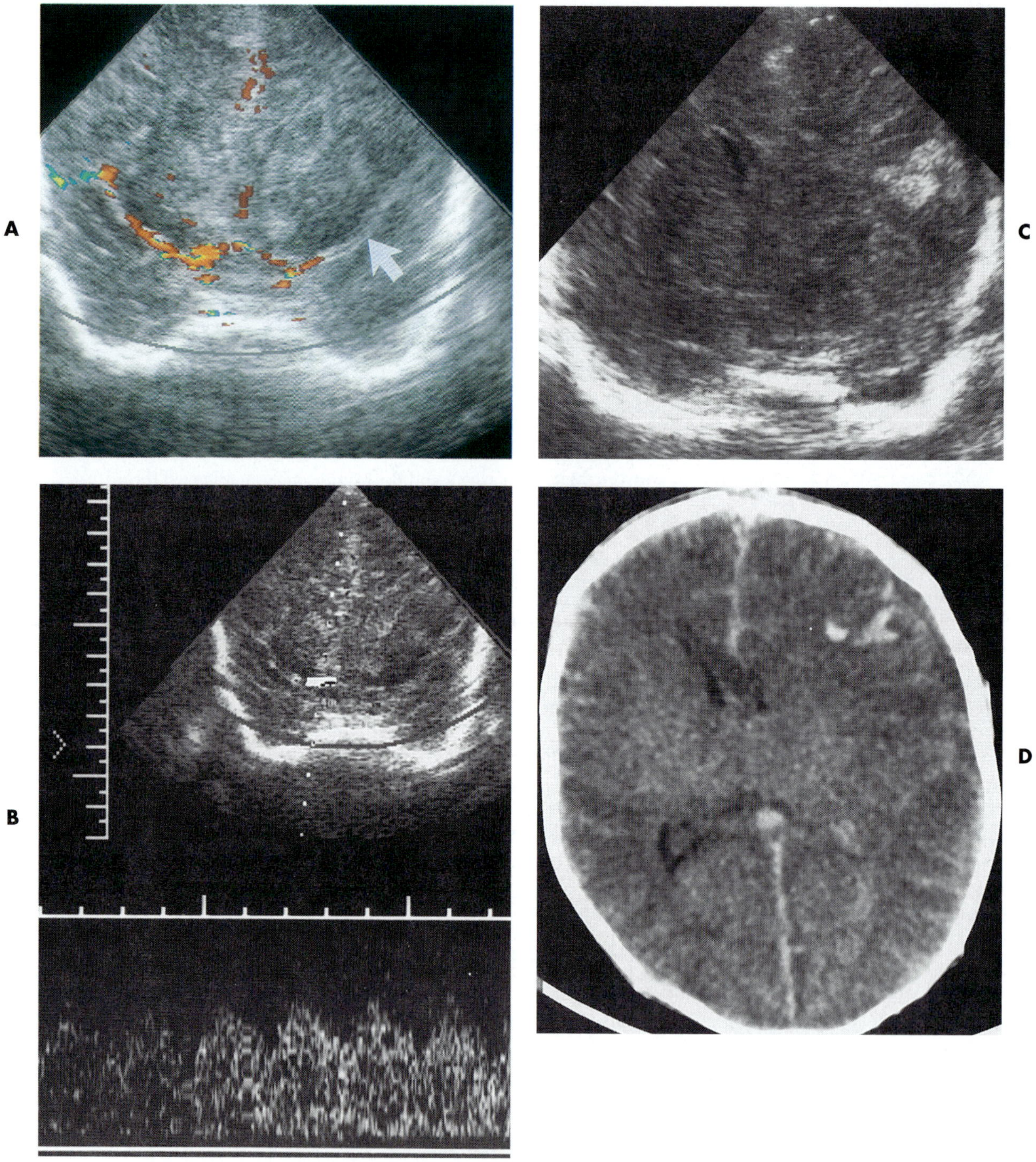

FIG. 52-50. Group B streptococcal meningitis with focal infarction. **A,** Coronal sonogram with color Doppler shows lack of flow in the left middle cerebral artery (*arrow*); gray scale alone showed symmetric increased echogenicity. **B,** Pulsed Doppler in the right middle cerebral artery (*opposite side*) shows greatly increased diastolic flow. **C,** Coronal sonogram and **D,** computed tomography scan later show hemorrhage (*arrow*) into an infarction with midline shift from left to right.

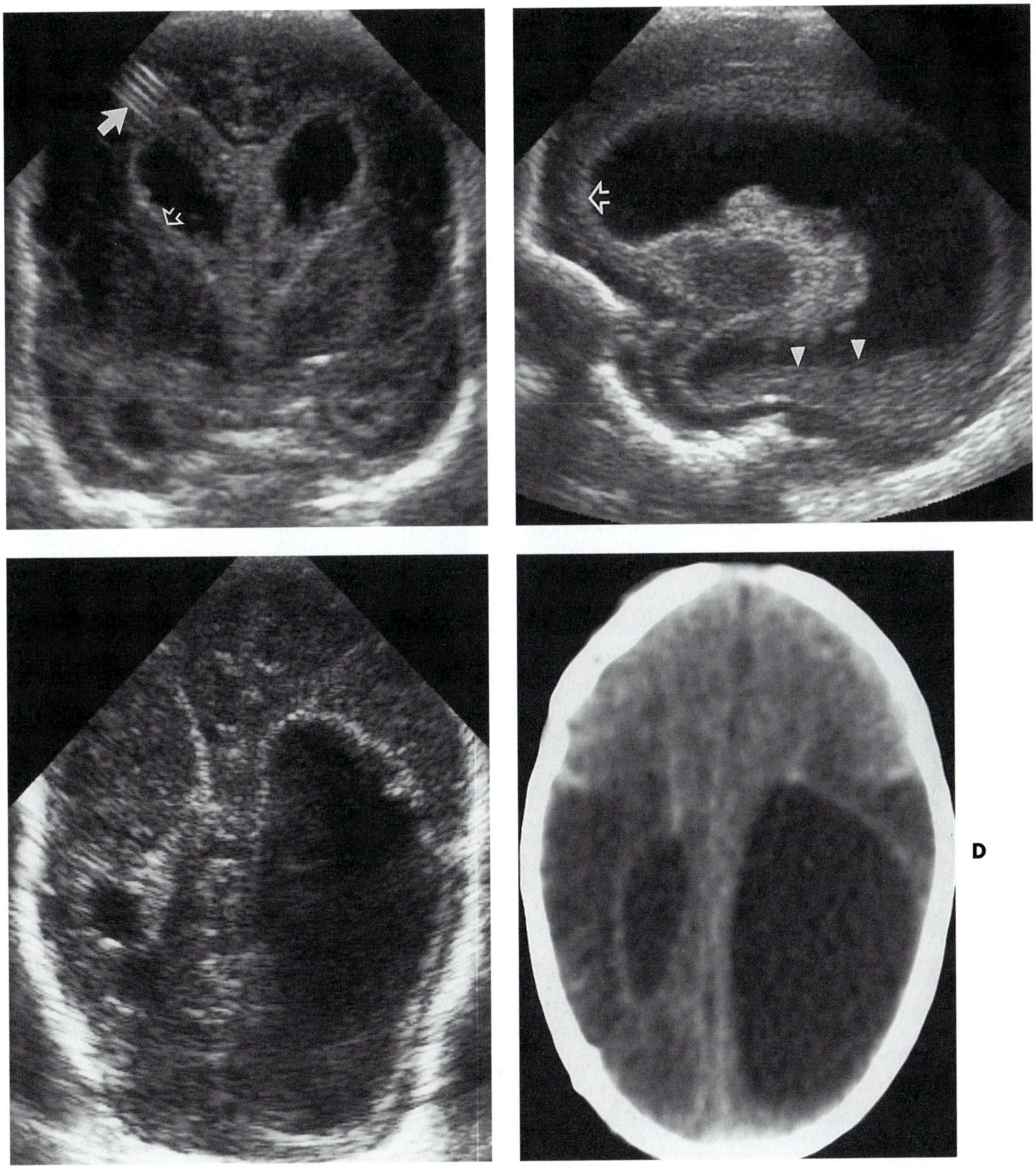

A C B D

FIG. 52-51. Ventriculitis. **A,** Coronal sonogram in premature infant who had a ventriculoperitoneal shunt (*arrow*) inserted for progressive hydrocephalus. After intraventricular hemorrhage, the ventricles are often lined by echogenic material (*open arrows*)—a chemical ventriculitis from blood (and rarely as here from infection). **B,** Sagittal sonogram shows cerebrospinal fluid debris level (*arrowheads*) (leukocytes) that looks similar to cerebrospinal fluid blood (erythrocytes) levels. **C,** Coronal sonogram and **D,** computed tomography scan show later asymmetry of ventricles.

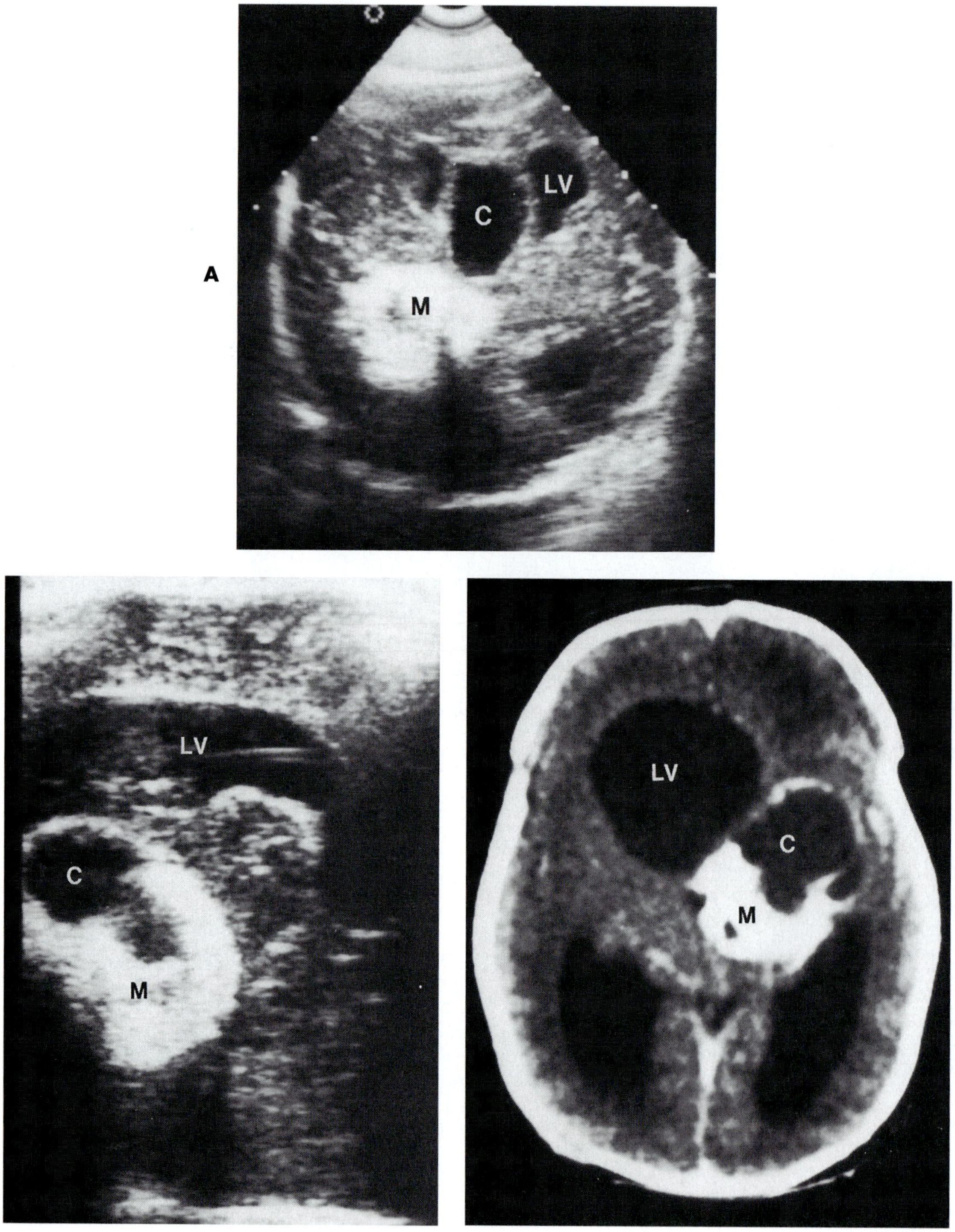

FIG. 52-52. Glioma. **A,** Coronal, and **B,** sagittal scans show echogenic mass (*M*) with cystic component (*C*) extending superiorly between lateral ventricles (*LV*). **C,** Axial enhanced computed tomography scan. (Courtesy of T. Stoeker, MD, Roanoke, Virginia)

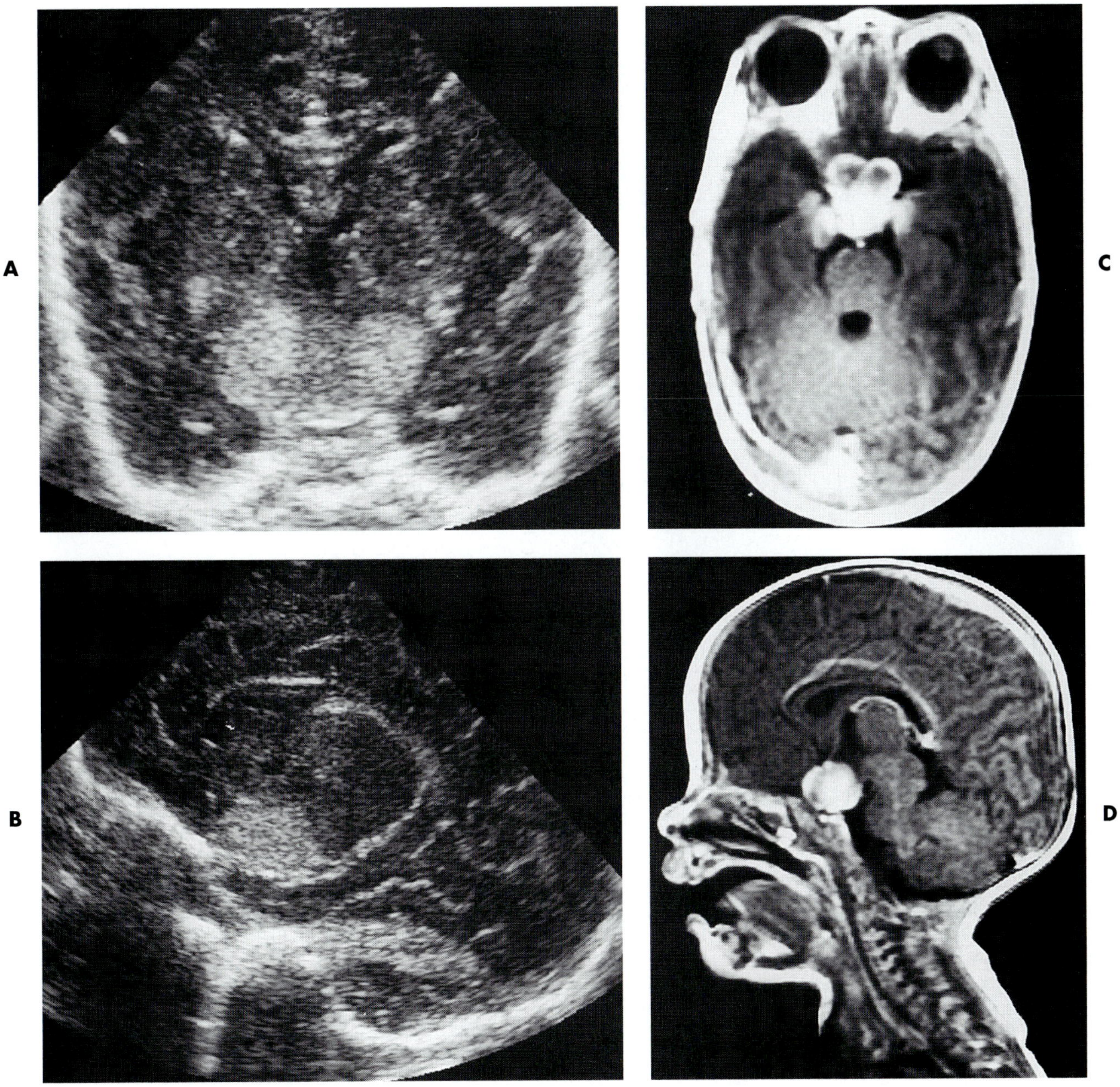

FIG. 52-53. Optic glioma. A, Coronal and **B,** sagittal sonograms show midline echogenic mass. **C,** Computed tomography scan and **D,** sagittal T_1 magnetic resonance imaging with contrast show enhancement of midline optic glioma.

A

B

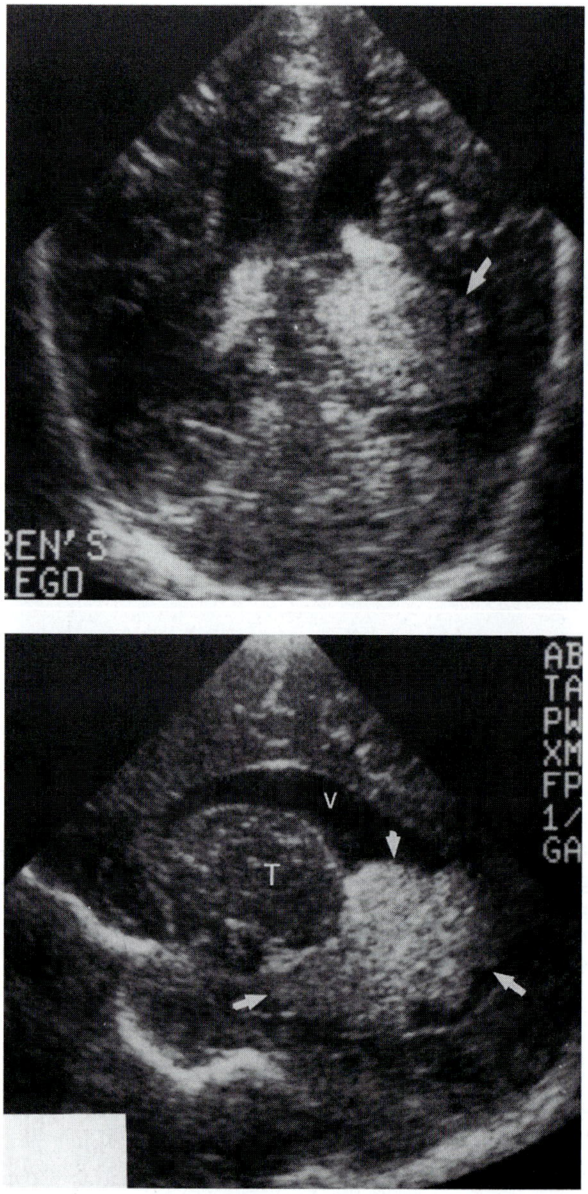

FIG. 52-54. Choroid plexus papilloma (*arrows*) in left lateral ventricle. **A,** Coronal, and **B,** sagittal sonograms. T—Thalamus, V—lateral ventricle. (Courtesy of D. Pretorius, MD, University of California at San Diego.)

CYSTIC BRAIN LESIONS

Congenital cysts	Primary arachnoid cyst Dandy-Walker malformation Hydranencephaly Holoprosencephaly
Ventricular cysts	Porencephalic cyst Choroid plexus cyst Hydranencephaly Subependymal cyst Colloid cyst
Neoplastic cysts	Cerebellar astrocytoma (cystic type) Craniopharyngioma Teratoma
Inflammatory cysts	Abscess Subdural empyema
Other cysts	Secondary arachnoid cysts Vein of Galen malformation

SITES OF ARACHNOID CYSTS IN DECREASING ORDER OF FREQUENCY

Anterior portions of the middle cranial fossa
Suprasellar region
Posterior fossa
Quadrigeminal region
Cerebral convexities
Interhemispheric fissure

Arachnoid Cysts. Arachnoid cysts are the most common true cysts of the brain, but they make up only 1% of all space-occupying lesions in children.[37] They are CSF-containing spaces between two layers of arachnoid. Primary and secondary cysts are believed to develop by different mechanisms. Primary cysts are believed to result from abnormal splitting of the arachnoid and from CSF collecting between the two layers. Secondary arachnoid cysts may develop by CSF trapped between arachnoid adhesions.

Arachnoid cysts, particularly those in the midline, may grow and cause obstruction of the ventricular system.[175-178] The arachnoid cyst most commonly presents as hydrocephalus in infancy. The ultrasound appearance of an arachnoid cyst is an anechoic area with discrete walls (Fig. 52-55).

Midline cysts are frequently associated with other brain anomalies. With agenesis of the corpus callosum, midline cysts are frequently continuous with an elevated third ventricle. In alobar holoprosencephaly, a dorsal cyst may be continuous with the single central ventricle.

Porencephalic Cysts. Porencephalic cysts are a result of brain necrosis and cavitation, which is continuous with the ventricular system (Fig. 52-38). They are usually a result of parenchymal hemorrhage, infection, or surgery.[7]

Choroid Plexus Cysts. Choroid plexus cysts are common and usually asymptomatic.[179-182] They occur in all age groups and are found in 34% of fetuses and

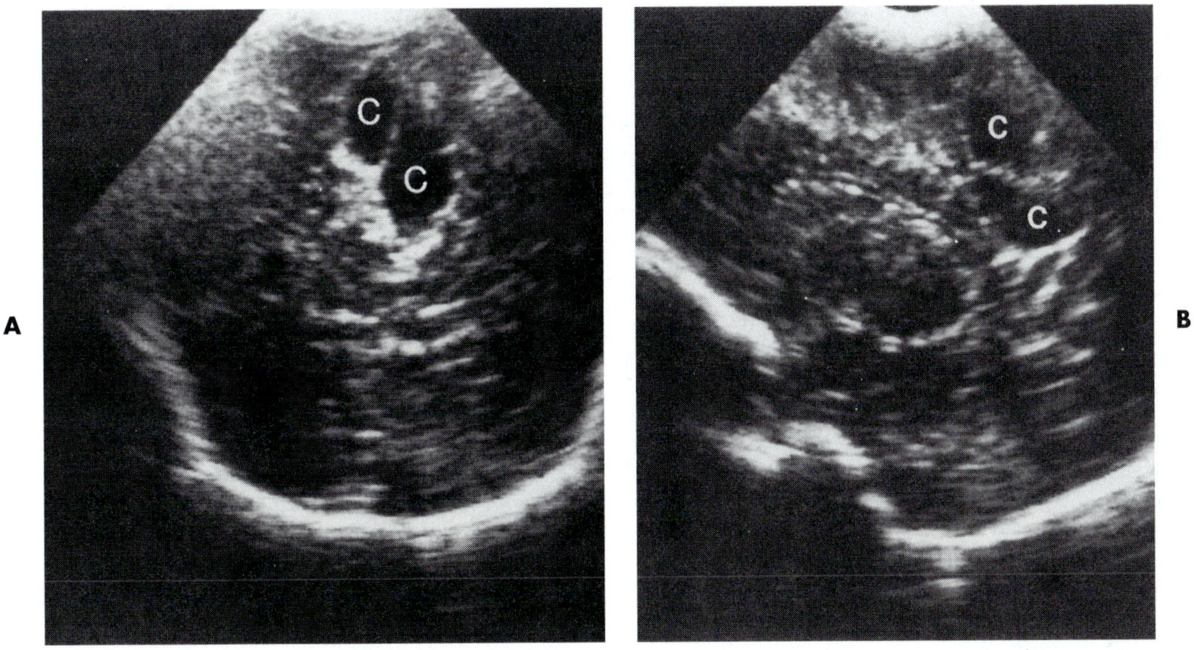

FIG. 52-55. Midline arachnoid cyst. **A,** Coronal, and **B,** sagittal scans show two arachnoid cysts (*C*) in interhemispheric fissure, just above lateral ventricle. (From Rumack CM, Johnson ML: *Perinatal and Infant Brain Imaging*, St. Louis, 1984, Mosby–Year Book.)

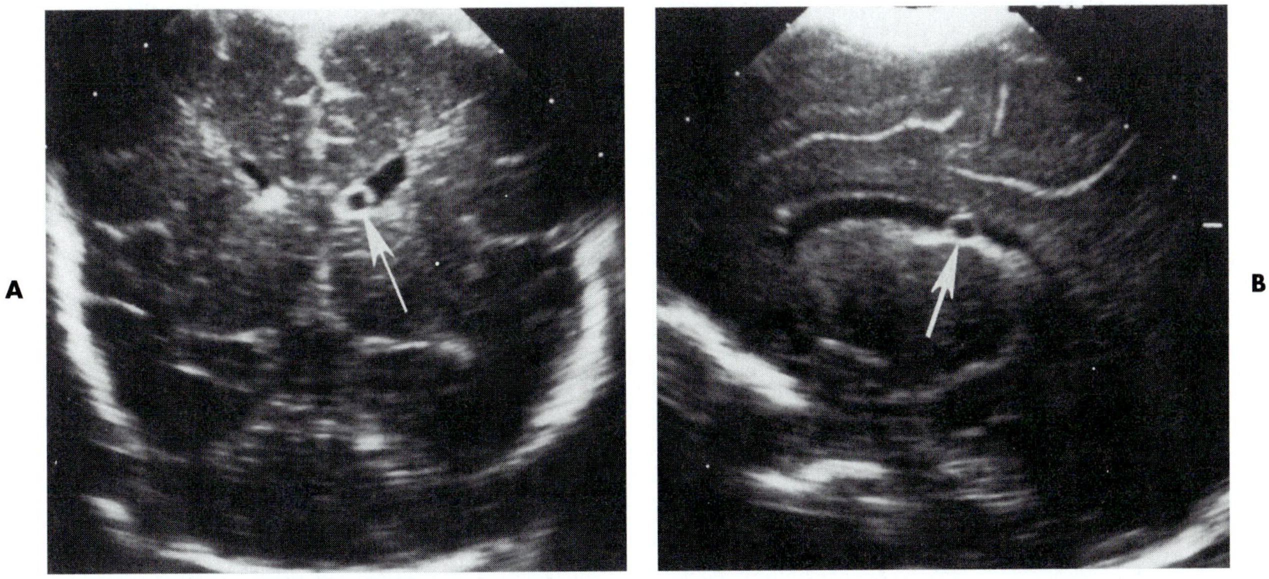

FIG. 52-56. Choroid plexus cyst (*arrows*). **A,** Coronal, and **B,** sagittal images show a single cyst in the choroid.

infants at autopsy.[135] However, prenatal and neonatal ultrasound reports have identified these cysts in only approximately 1% of the populations studied. They are distinctly different from and should not be confused with subependymal cysts. Choroid plexus cysts tend to be an isolated finding, not associated with other CNS abnormalities or chromosomal abnormalities.[183]

A choroid plexus cyst appears as a cystic mass with well-defined walls within the choroid plexus (Fig. 52-56). They range in size from less than 4 millimeters to 7 millimeters and are usually unilateral, left greater than right, and situated in the dorsal aspect of the choroid plexus. Rare cases of symptomatic choroid cysts causing obstructive hydrocephalus have been re-

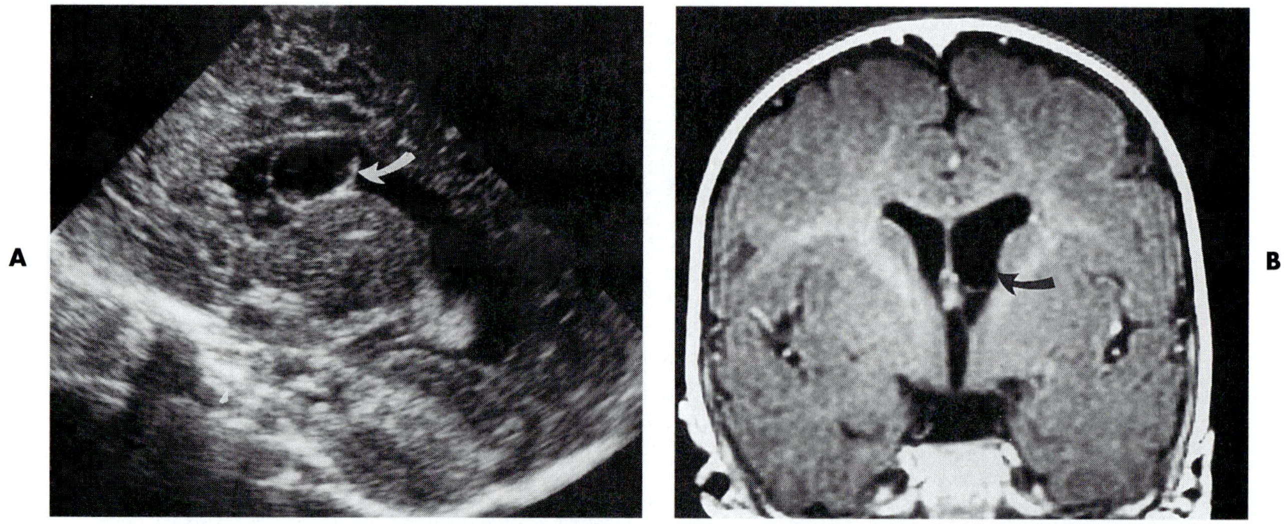

FIG. 52-57. Subependymal cyst. **A,** Sagittal sonogram and **B,** coronal T_1-weighted magnetic resonance imaging show a smooth-walled spherical subependymal cyst (*arrows*) in the lateral ventricle. This is so large it could also be called an *intraventricular cyst.*

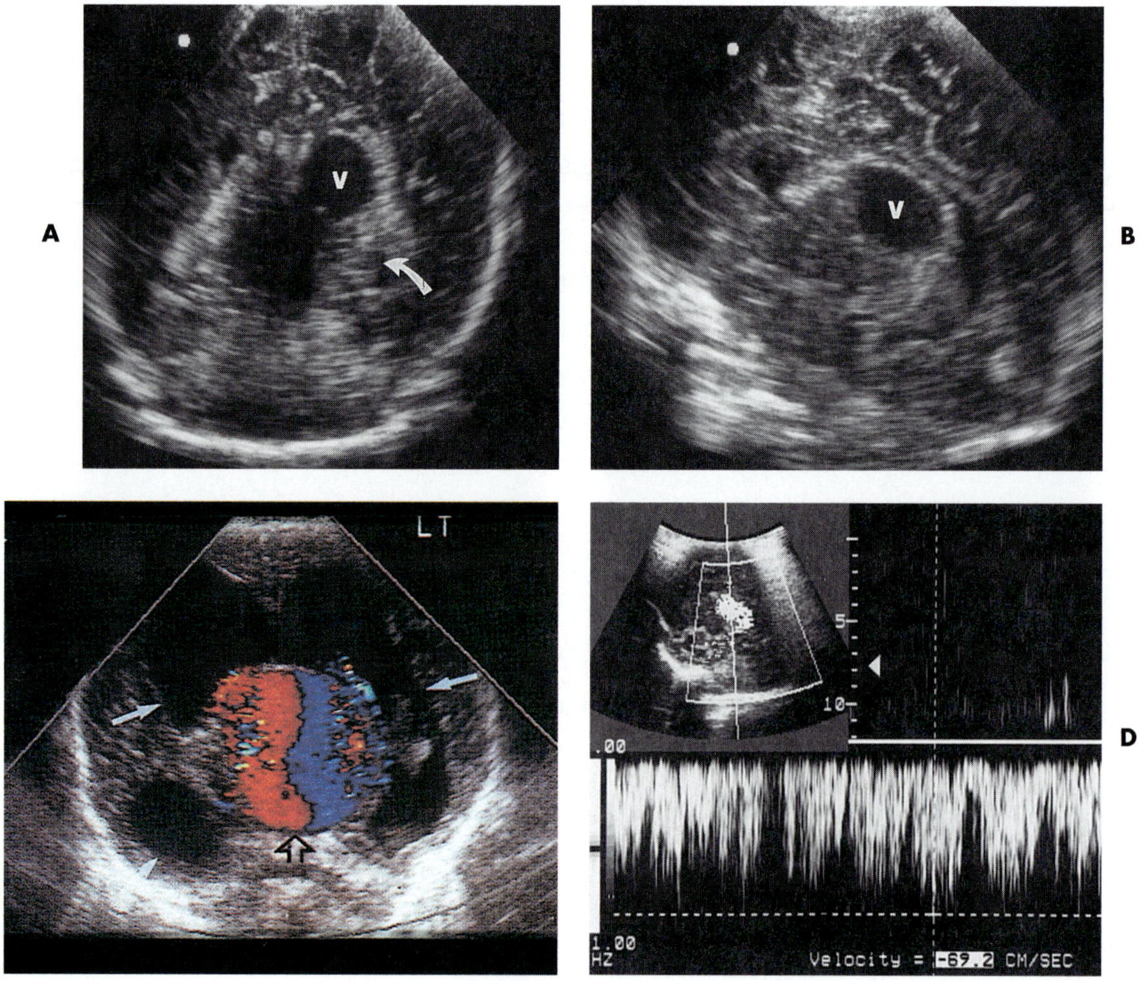

FIG. 52-58. Galenic venous malformation. **A,** Coronal, and **B,** sagittal sonograms show enlarged vein of Galen (*V*) and straight sinus. Echogenic arterial feeding vessels below and anterior to dilated vein of Galen (*curved arrow*). **C,** Color and **D,** duplex Doppler scans show turbulent flow, which clearly defines this cystic-appearing mass as vascular.

E

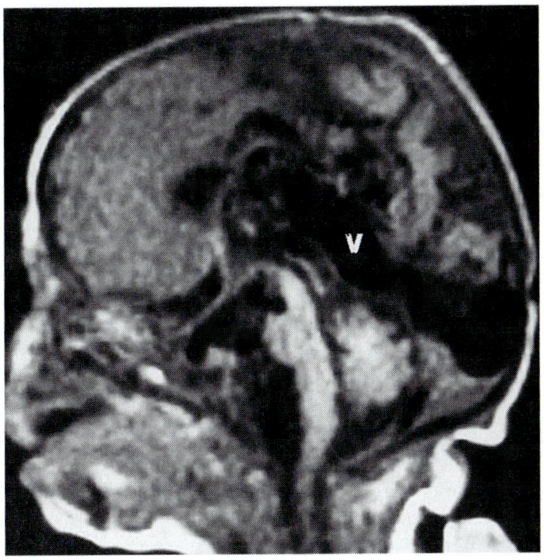

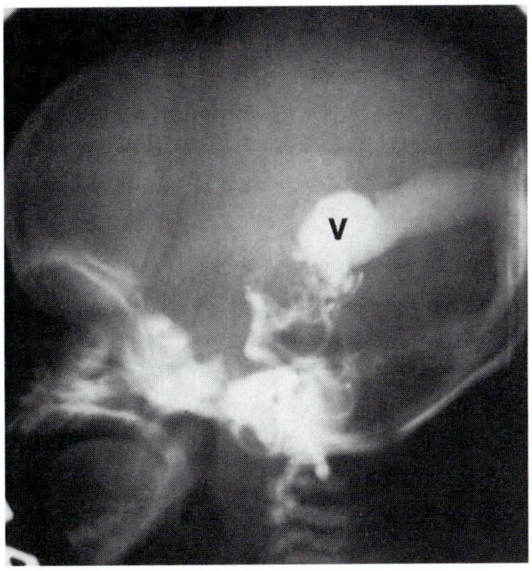

F

FIG. 52-58, cont'd. **E,** Sagittal magnetic resonance imaging scan and **F,** angiogram (different patient) show the echogenic region is tortuous tangle of abnormal feeding vessels and cystic mass is dilated vein of Galen (*V*).

ported but are probably related to some specific cause rather than a normal variant.[182] Many choroid plexus "cysts" are actually vessels in the choroid,[184] which can be recognized with color flow Doppler even *in utero.*

Subependymal Cysts. Subependymal cysts present as discrete cysts in the lining of the ventricles (Fig. 52-57). They are most commonly the result of the sequela of GMH in premature infants.[185-188] Other causes include infection, including CMV and rubella, and a rare syndrome known as *cerebrohepatorenal syndrome* (Zellweger syndrome).[189-191] Subependymal cysts can also be an isolated finding with no apparent predisposing event.[181]

Galenic Venous Malformations

Galenic venous malformations are frequently referred to as vein of Galen aneurysms, but this is a misnomer because they are not true aneurysms. They actually represent dilation of the vein of Galen caused by a vascular malformation that is fed by large arteries off the anterior or posterior cerebral artery circulation.[192] Infants with this disorder usually present with congestive heart failure.[193-195] In later childhood, the presentation includes seizure, cranial bruit, hydrocephalus, and cardiomegaly.

Sonographically, a galenic malformation appears as an anechoic, cystic mass between the lateral ventricles (Fig. 52-58). It lies posterior to the foramen of Monro, superior to the third ventricle and primarily in the midline.[196-198] These malformations, however, should be easily differentiated from other cystic masses by identification of the large feeding vessels. Pulsed or color Doppler images can be used to confirm the diagnosis.[199] Hydrocephalus may or may not be present and calcification may occur, especially if there is thrombosis in the malformation.[200] If treatment is considered with embolization, angiography may be performed (Fig. 52-58).[201]

REFERENCES

1. DiPietro MA, Faix RG, Donn SM: Procedural hazards of neonatal ultrasonography *J Clin Ultrasound* 1986;14:361-366.
2. Mitchell DG, Merton D, Desai H, et al: Neonatal brain: color doppler imaging, II: altered flow patterns from extracorporeal membrane oxygenation, *Radiology* 1988;167:307-310.
3. Babcock DS: Sonography of the brain in infants: role in evaluating neurologic abnormalities, *AJR* 1995;165:417-423.
4. Cohen HL, Haller JO: Advances in perinatal neurosonography, *AJR* 1994;163:801-810.
5. Bezinque SL, Slovis TL, Touchette AS, et al: Characterization of superior sagittal sinus blood flow velocity using color flow Doppler in neonates and infants, *Pediatr Radiol* 1995;25:175-179.
6. Soboleski D, McCloskey D, Mussari B, et al: Sonography of normal cranial sutures, *AJR* 1997;168:819-821.

Equipment

7. Rumack CM, Johnson ML: *Perinatal and infant brain imaging*, St. Louis, 1984, Mosby–Year Book.
8. Anderson N, Allan R, Darlow B, Malpas T: Diagnosis of intraventricular hemorrhage in the newborn: Value of sonography via the posterior fontanelle. *AJR* 1994;163:893-896.

Sonographic Technique

9. Cheng-Yu C, Chou TY, Zimmerman RA, et al: Pericerebral fluid collection: Differentiation of enlarged subarachnoid spaces from subdural collections with color Doppler, *Radiology* 1996;201(2):389-392.
10. Mack LA, Ellsworth CA Jr: Neonatal cranial ultrasound: normal appearances, *Semin Ultrasound* 1982;3(3):216-230.
11. Pigadas A, Thompson JR, Grube GL: Normal infant brain anatomy: Correlated real-time sonograms and brain specimens, *AJR* 1981;137:815-820.

12. Yousefzadeh DK, Naidich TP: Ultrasound anatomy of the posterior fossa in children: correlation with brain sections, *Radiology* 1985;156(2):353-361.
13. Frank JL: Sonography of intracranial infections in infants and children. In Naidich TP, Quencer RM, editors: *Clinical neurosonography*, Berlin, 1987, Springer-Verlag.
14. Schuman WP, Rogers JV, Mack LA, et al: Real-time sonographic sector scanning of the neonatal cranium: technique and normal anatomy, *AJNR* 1981;2:349-356.
15. Rumack CM, Manco-Johnson ML: Neonatal brain ultrasonography. In Sarti DA, editor: *Diagnostic ultrasound: Text and cases*, ed 2, Chicago, 1987, Year Book Medical Publishers.
16. DiPietro MA, Brody BA, Teele RL: Peritrigonal echogenic "blush" on cranial sonography: Pathologic correlates, *AJR* 1986;146:1067-1072.

Developmental Anatomy

17. Worthen NJ, Gilbertson V, Lau C: Cortical sulcal development seen on sonography: Relationship to gestational parameters, *J Ultrasound Med* 1986;5:153-156.
18. Shaw CM, Alvord EC Jr: Cava septi pellucidi et Vergae: Their normal and pathological states, *Brain* 1969;92:213-224.
19. Friede R: *Developmental neuropathology*, ed 2, New York, 1975, Springer-Verlag.

Congenital Brain Malformations

20. DeMeyer W: Classification of cerebral malformations, *Birth Defects* 1971;7:78-93.
21. Harwood-Nash DC, Fitz CR: *Neuroradiology in infants and children*, St Louis, 1976, CV Mosby.
22. Osborn AG: *Diagnostic neuroradiology*, St. Louis, 1994, CV Mosby.
23. Volpe JJ: *Neurology of the newborn*, Philadelphia, 1995, WB Saunders.
24. Gilles FH, Leviton A, Dooling EC: *The developing human brain*, Boston, 1983, John Wright-PSG.
25. Diebler C, Dulac O: *Pediatric neurology and neuroradiology*, Berlin, 1987, Springer-Verlag.
26. Volpe JJ: Normal and abnormal human brain development, *Clin Perinatol* 1977;4(1):3-30.

Disorders of Neural Tube Closure

27. Byrd SE, Osborn RE, Radkowski MA, et al: Disorders of midline structures: Holoprosencephaly, absence of the corpus callosum and Chiari malformations, *Semin Ultrasound* 1988; 9(3):201-215.
28. Babcock DS: Sonography of congenital malformations of the brain. In Naidich TP, Quencer RM, editors: *Clinical neurosonography*, Berlin, 1987, Springer-Verlag.
29. Babcock DS, Han BK: Cranial sonographic findings in meningomyelocele, *AJNR* 1980;1:493-499.
30. McLone DG, Naidich T: Developmental morphology of the subarachnoid space, brain vasculature, and contiguous structures, and the cause of Chiari II malformation, *AJNR* 1992; 13:463-482.
31. Naidich TP, Pudlowski RM, Naidich JB: Computed tomographic signs of Chiari II malformation, II: Midbrain and cerebellum, *Radiology* 1980;134:391-398.
32. Naidich TP, Pudlowski RM, Naidich JB: Computed tomographic signs of Chiari II malformation, III: Ventricles and cisterns, *Radiology* 1980;134:657-663.
33. Zimmerman RD, Breckbill D, Dennis MW, et al: Cranial CT findings in patients with meningomyelocele, *AJR* 1980;132: 623-629.
34. Fitz CR: Disorders of ventricles and CSF spaces, *Semin Ultrasound* 1988;9(3):216-230.
35. Babcock CJ, Goldstein RB, Berth RA, Damato NM, Callan PW, Filly RA: Prevalence of ventriculomegaly in association with myelomeningocele: Correlation with gestational age and severity of posterior fossa deformity, *Rad* 1994;190:703-707.
36. Babcock DS: The normal absent and abnormal corpus callosum: Sonographic findings, *Rad* 1984;151(2):450-453.
37. Barkovich AJ: *Pediatric neuroimaging*, ed 2, Raven Press 1995.
38. Kier EL, Truwit CL: The normal and abnormal genu of the corpus callosum, *AJNR* 1996;17:1631-1641.
39. Parrish ML, Roessmann U, Levinsohn MV: Agenesis of the corpus callosum: A study of the frequency of associated malformations, *Ann Neurol* 1979;6(4):349-354.
40. Larsen PD, Osborn AG: Computed tomographic evaluation of corpus callosum agenesis and associated malformations, *CT* 1982;6:225-230.
41. Guibert-Tranier F, Piton J, Billerey J, et al: Agenesis of the corpus callosum, *J Neuroradiol* 1982;9:135-160.
42. Jinkins JR, Whittemore AR, Bradley WG: MR imaging of callosal and corticocallosal dysgenesis, *AJNR* 1989;10:339-344.
43. Hernanz-Schulman M, Dohan FC Jr, Jones T, et al: Sonographic appearance of callosal agenesis: Correlation with radiologic and pathologic findings, *AJNR* 1985;6:361-368.
44. Atlas SW, Shkolnik A, Naidich TP: Sonographic recognition of agenesis of the corpus callosum, *AJNR* 1985;6:359-375.
45. Nyberg DA, Cyr DR, Mack LA, et al: The Dandy-Walker malformation prenatal sonographic diagnosis and its clinical significance, *J Ultrasound Med* 1988;7:65-71.
46. Taylor GA, Sanders RC: Dandy-Walker syndrome: Recognition by sonography, *AJNR* 1983;4:1203-1206.
47. Nyberg DA, Mahony BS, Hegge FN, et al: Enlarged cisterna magna and the Dandy-Walker malformation: Factors associated with chromosomal abnormalities, *Obstet Gynecol* 1991; 77:436-442.
48. Bromley B, Nadel AS, Pauker S, et al: Closure of the cerebellar vermis: Evaluation with second trimester ultrasound, *Rad* 1994;193:761-763.
49. Estroff JA, Parad RB, Barnes PD, et al: Posterior fossa arachnoid cyst: An in utero mimicker of Dandy-Walker Malformation, *J Ultrasound Med* 1995;14:787-790.
50. Chang MC, Russell SA, Callen PW, et al: Sonographic detection of inferior vermian agenesis in Dandy-Walker malformations: Prognostic implications, *Rad* 1994;193:765-770.
51. Keogan MT, DeAtkine AB, Hertzberg BS: Cerebellar vermian defects: Antenatal sonographic appearance and clinical significance, *JUM* 1994;13(8):607.
52. Hart MN, Malamud N, Ellis WG: The Dandy-Walker syndrome: A clinicopathologic study based on 28 cases, *Neurology* 1972;22(8):771-779.
53. Warkany J, Lemire RJ, Cohen MM Jr: *Mental retardation and congenital malformations of the central nervous system*, Chicago, 1981, Year Book Medical Publishers.

Disorders of Diverticulation and Cleavage

54. DeMyer W, Zeman W, Gardella Palmer C: The face predicts the brain: Diagnostic significance of median facial anomalies for holoprosencephaly (arrhinencephaly), *Pediatrics* 1964; 34:256-263.
55. Fitz CR: Holoprosencephaly and related entities, *J Neuroradiol* 1983;25:225-238.
56. Altman NR, Altman DH, Sheldon JJ, et al: Holoprosencephaly classified by computed tomography, *AJNR* 1984;5:433-437.
57. Fitz CR: Midline anomalies of the brain and spine, *Radiol Clin North Am* 1982;20(1):95-104.

Destructive Lesions

58. Grant EG, Tessler F, Perrella R: Infant cranial sonography, *Radiol Clin North Am* 1988;26(5):1089-1110.
59. Pretorius DH, Russ PD, Rumack CM, et al: Diagnosis of brain neuropathology *in utero*. In Naidich TP, Quencer RM, editors: *Clinical Neurosonography*, Berlin, 1987, Springer-Verlag.

60. Dublin AB, French BN: Diagnostic image evaluation of hydranencephaly and pictorially similar entities with emphasis on computed tomography, *Radiology* 1980;137:81-91.
61. Diebler C, Dulac O: *Pediatric neurology and neuroradiology*, Berlin, 1987, Springer-Verlag.

Hydrocephalus

62. Farrell TA, Hertzberg BS, Kliewer MA, et al: Fetal lateral ventricles: Reassessment of normal values for atrial diameter at ultrasound, *Rad* 1994;193:409.
63. Filly RA, Goldstein RB: The fetal ventricular atrium: Fourth down and 10 mm to go, *Rad* 1994;193:315.
64. Alagappan R, Browning PD, Laorr A, McGahan JP: Distal lateral ventricular atrium: Reevaluation of the normal range, *Rad* 1991;193:405.
65. Rosseau GL, McCullough DC, Joseph AL: Current prognosis in fetal ventriculomegaly, *J Neurosurg* 1992;77:551-555.
66. Nicolaides KH, Berry S, Snijders RJM, et al: Fetal lateral cerebral ventriculomegaly: Associated malformations and chromosomal defects, *Fetal Diagn Ther* 1990;5:5-14.
67. Hudgins RJ, Edwards MSB, Goldstein R, et al: Natural history of fetal ventriculomegaly, *Pediatr* 1988;82:692-697.
68. Rosenfeld DL, DeMarco ELK: Transtentorial herniation of the fourth ventricle, *Pediatr Radiol* 1995;25:436-439.
69. Taylor GA, Madsen JR: Neonatal hydrocephalus: Hemodynamic response to fontanelle compression—correlation with intracranial pressure and need for shunt placement, *Radiology* 1996;201:685-689.
70. Winkler P: Cerebrospinal fluid dynamics in infants evaluated with echographic color-coded flow imaging, *Rad* 1994;192: 431-437.

Hypoxic-Ischemic Events

71. Dogra VS, Shyken JM, Menon PA, et al: Neurosonographic abnormalities associated with maternal history of cocaine use in neonates of appropriate size for gestational age, *AJNR* 1994; 15:697-702.
72. Dean LM, Taylor GA: The intracranial venous system in infants: Normal and abnormal findings on color and duplex Doppler sonography, *AJR* 1995;164:151-156.
73. Taylor GA: New concepts in the pathogenesis of germinal matrix intraparenchymal hemorrhage in premature infants, *AJNR* 1997;18:231-232.
74. Ghazi-Birry HS, Brown WR, Moody DM, et al: Human germinal matrix venous origin of hemorrhage and vascular characteristics, *AJNR* 1997;18:219-229.
75. Taylor GA: Effect of germinal matrix hemorrhage on terminal vein positions and patency, *Pediatr Radiol* 1995;25:S37-S40.
76. Bowerman RA, Donn SM, Silver TM, et al: Natural history of neonatal periventricular/intraventricular hemorrhage and its complications: Sonographic observations, *AJR* 1984;143:1041.
77. Kirks DR, Bowie JD: Cranial ultrasonography of neonatal periventricular/intraventricular hemorrhage: Who, why and when? *Pediatr Radiol* 1986;16:114.
78. Volpe JJ: Neonatal intraventricular hemorrhage, *N Engl J Med* 1981;304:886-891.
79. Hayden CK Jr, Swischuk LE: *Pediatric ultrasonography*, ed 2, Baltimore, 1992, Williams & Wilkins.
80. Burstein J, Papile L, Burstein R: Intraventricular hemorrhage and hydrocephalus in premature newborns: A prospective study with CT, *AJR* 1979;132:631.
81. Rumack CM, Manco-Johnson ML, Manco-Johnson MJ, et al: Timing and course of neonatal intracranial hemorrhage using real-time ultrasound, *Radiology* 1985;154:101.
82. Boal, Watterberg, Miles, et al: Optimal cost effective timing of cranial ultrasound in low birthweight infants, *Pediatr Radiol* 1995;25:425-428.
83. Shankaran S, Bauer C, Bain R, Wright LL, Zachary J: Antenatal steroids to reduce the risk of intracranial hemorrhage in the neonate, *Report of the Consensus Development Conference on the Effects of Corticosteroids for Fetal Maturation on Perinatal Outcomes*, NIH No. 95-3784, 1994.
84. Maher JE: Effects of corticosteroid therapy in the very premature infant, *Report of the Consensus Development Conference on the Effects of Corticosteroids for Fetal Maturation on Perinatal Outcomes*, NIH No. 95-3784, 1994.
85. Thorpe JA, Parriott J, Ferrette-Smith D, et al: Antepartum vitamin K and phenobarbital for preventing intraventricular hemorrhage in the premature newborn: A randomized double-blind, placebo-controlled trial, *Obstet Gynecol* 1994; 83:70-76.
86. Hay TC, Rumack CM, Horgan JG: Cranial sonography: Intracranial hemorrhage, periventricular leukomalacia, and asphyxia. In Babcock DS, editor: *Neonatal and pediatric ultrasonography: Clinics in diagnostic ultrasound*, New York, 1989, Churchill Livingstone.
87. Rypens F, Avni EF, Dussaussois L, et al: Hyperechoic thickened ependyma: Sonographic demonstration and significance in neonates, *Pediatr Radiol* 1994;24:550-553.
88. Levene MI, Wigglesworth JS, Dubowitz V: Hemorrhagic periventricular leukomalacia in the neonate: A real-time ultrasound study, *Pediatrics* 1983;71:794.
89. Schellinger D, Grant EG, Manz HS, et al: Intraparenchymal hemorrhage in preterm neonates: A broadening spectrum, *AJR* 1988;150:1109-1115.
90. Dean LM, McLeary M, Taylor GA: Cerebral hemorrhage in alloimmune thrombocytopenia, *Pediatr Radiol* 1995;25:444-445.
91. Babcock DS, Han BK, Weiss RG, et al: Brain abnormalities in infants on extracorporeal membrane oxygenation: Sonographic and CT findings, *AJR* 1989;153:571-576.
92. Taylor GA, Fitz CR, Kapur S, et al: Cerebrovascular accidents in neonates treated with extracorporeal membrane oxygenation: Sonographic-pathologic correlation, *AJR* 1989;153:355-361.
93. Slovis TL, Sell LL, Bedard MP, Klein MD: Ultrasonographic findings (CNS, thorax, abdomen) in infants undergoing extracorporeal membrane oxygenation therapy, *Pediatr Radiol* 1988;18:112-113.
94. Jarjour IT, Abdab-Barmada M: Cerebrovascular lesions in infants and children dying after extracorporeal membrane oxygenation, *Pediatr Neurol* 1994;10:13-19.
95. Bulas DT, Taylor GA, O'Donnel RM, et al: Intracranial abnormalities in infants treated with ECMO: Update in sonographic and CT findings, *AJNR* 1995;17:287-294.
96. Kazan E, Rudelli R, Rubenstein WA, et al: Sonographic diagnosis of cisternal subarachnoid hemorrhage in the premature infant, *AJNR* 1994;15:1009-1020.
97. Luisiri A, Graviss ER, Weber T, et al: Neurosonographic changes in newborns treated with extracorporeal membrane oxygenation, *JUM* 1988;7:429-438.
98. Taylor GA, Glass P, Fitz CR, et al: Neurologic status in infants treated with extracorporeal membrane oxygenation: correlation of imaging findings with developmental outcome. *Radiology* 1987;165:679-682.
99. Volpe JJ: Current concepts of brain injury in the premature infant, *AJR* 1989;153:243-291.
100. DeRenck J, Chattha AS, Richardson EP: Pathogenesis and evolution of periventricular leukomalacia in infancy, *Arch Neurol* 1972;27:229.
101. Lou HC, Lassen NA, Friis-Hansen B: Impaired auto regulation of cerebral blood flow in the distressed newborn infant, *J Pediatr* 1979;94:118-121.
102. Chow PP, Horgan JG, Taylor KJW: Neonatal periventricular leukomalacia: Real-time sonographic diagnosis with CT correlation, *AJR* 1985;145:155.
103. Stannard MW, Jimenez JF: Sonographic recognition of multiple cystic encephalomalacia, *AJNR* 1983;4:1111.

104. Schellinger D, Grant EG, Richardson JD: Cystic periventricular leukomalacia: Sonographic and CT findings, *AJNR* 1984; 5:439.
105. Dubowitz LMS, Bydder GM, Mushin J: Developing sequence of periventricular leukomalacia, *Arch Dis Child* 1985;60:349.
106. Bejar R, Coen RW, Merritt TA, et al: Focal necrosis of the white matter (periventricular leukomalacia): Sonographic, pathologic and electro-encephalographic features, *AJNR* 1986;7:1073.
107. Carson SC, Hertzberg BS, Bowie JD, Burger PC: Value of sonography in diagnosis of intracranial hemorrhage and periventricular leukomalacia: A postmortem study of 35 cases, *AJR* 1990;155:595-601.
108. Barr LL, McCullough PJ, Ball WS, et al: Quanitative sonographic feature analysis of clinical infant hypoxia: A pilot study, *AJNR* 1996;17(6):1025-1031.
109. Skranes JS, Nilsen G, Smevik O: Cerebral magnetic resonance (MRI) of very low birthweight infants at one year of age, *Pediatr Radiol* 1992;22:406-409.
110. Martin DJ, Hill A, Fitz CR, et al: Hypoxic/ischemic cerebral injury in the neonatal brain: A report of sonographic features with computed tomographic correlation, *Pediatr Radiol* 1983;13:307.
111. Manger MN, Feldman RC, Brown WJ, et al: Intracranial ultrasound diagnosis of neonatal periventricular leukomalacia, *J Ultrasound Med* 1984;3:59.
112. Grant EG, Schellinger D, Smith Y, et al: Periventricular leukomalacia in combination with intraventricular hemorrhage: Sonographic features and sequelae, *AJNR* 1986;7:443.
113. deVries LS, Dubowitz LMS, Pennock JM, et al: Extensive cystic leukomalacia: Correlation of cranial ultrasound, magnetic resonance imaging and clinical findings in sequential studies, *Clin Radiol* 1989;40:158.
114. Deeg KG, Rupprecht, Zeilinger G: Doppler sonographic classification of brain edema in infants, *Pediatr Radiol* 1990;20: 509-514.
115. Stark JE and Sibert JJ: Cerebral artery Doppler ultrasonography for prediction of outcome after perinatal asphyxia, *Ultrasound Med* 1994;13:595-600.
116. Rollins NK, Morriss MC, Evans D, et al: The role of early MR in the evaluation of the term infant with seizures, *AJNR* 1994;15:239-248.
117. Hernanz-Schulman M, Cohen W, Genieser NB: Sonography of cerebral infarction in infancy, *AJNR* 1988;9:131.
118. Levy SR, Abroms IF, Marshall PC, et al: Seizures and cerebral infarction in the full-term newborn, *Ann Neurol* 1985;17:366.
119. Ment LR, Duncan CC, Ehrenkranz RA: Perinatal cerebral infarction, *Ann Neurol* 1984;16:559.
120. Hill A, Martin DJ, Daneman A, et al: Focal ischemic cerebral injury in the newborn: Diagnosis by ultrasound and correlation with computed tomography scan, *Pediatrics* 1983;71:790.
121. Connolly B, Kelehen P, O'Brien N, et al: The echogenic thalamus in hypoxic ischemic encephalopathy, *Pediatr Radiol* 1994;24:268-271.
122. Babcock DS, Ball W Sr: Postasphyxial encephalopathy in full-term infants: Ultrasound diagnosis, *Radiology* 1983;148:417.
123. Volpe JJ: Value of MR in the definition of the neuropathology of cerebral palsy *in vivo*, *AJNR* 1992;13:79-83.
124. Truwit CL, Barkovich AJ, Koch TK, et al: Cerebral palsy: MR findings in 40 patients, *AJNR* 1992;13:76-78.
125. Barkovich AJ, Sargent SK: Profound hophyxia in the premature infant: Imaging findings, *AJNR* 1995;16:1837-1846.
126. Siegel MS, Shackelford GD, Perlman JM, et al: Hypoxic-ischemic encephalopathy in term infants: Diagnosis and prognosis evaluated by ultrasound, *Radiology* 1984;152:395.
127. Hay TC, Rumack CM, Horgan JG: Cranial sonography: Intracranial hemorrhage, periventricular leukomalacia and asphyxia, In Babcock DS, editor: *Neonatal and pediatric ultrasonography: Clinics in diagnostic ultrasound*, New York, 1989, Churchill Livingstone.
128. Mercuri E, He Julian, Curati WL, et al: Cerebellar infarction and atrophy in infants and children with a history of premature birth, *Pediatr Radiol* 1997;27:139-143.
129. Steventon DM, John PR: Power Doppler ultrasound appearances of neonatal ischaemic brain injury, *Pediatr Radiol* 1997;27:147-149.
130. Taylor GA: Alterations in regional cerebral blood flow on neonatal stroke: Preliminary findings with color Doppler sonography, *Pediatr Radiol* 1994;24:111-115.
131. Taylor GA: Regional cerebral blood flow estimates in newborn lamb using amplitude-mode color Doppler ultrasound, *Pediatr Radiol* 1996;26:282-286.
132. Taylor GA, Trescher WA, Traystman RJ, et al: Acute experimental neuronal injury in the newborn lamb: US characterization and demonstration of hemodynamic effects, *Pediatr Radiol* 1993;23:268-275.

Posttraumatic Injury

133. Luang LT, Lui CC: Tentorial hemorrhage associated with vacuum extraction in a newborn, *Pediatr Radiol* 1995;25: S230-S231.
134. Siegel M, et al: *Pediatric sonography*, ed 2, New York, 1995, Raven Press.
135. Kleinman PK: Diagnostic imaging in infant abuse, *AJR* 1990; 155:703-712.
136. Jaspan T, Narborough G, Punt JAG, et al: Cerebral contusional tears as a marker of child abuse—detection by cranial sonography, *Pediatr Radiol* 1992;22:237-245.

Infection

137. Shaw DWW, Cohen WA: Viral infections of the CNS in children: Imaging features, *AJNR* 1993;160:125-133.
138. Barkovich AJ, Lindan CE: Congenital cytomegalovirus infection of the brain: Imaging analysis and embryologic considerations, *AJNR* 1994;15:703-715.
139. Frank JL: Sonography of intracranial infection in infants and children, *Neuroradiology* 1986;28:440-451.
140. Diebler C, Dusser A, Dulac O: Congenital toxoplasmosis: Clinical and neuroradiological evaluation of the cerebral lesions, *Neuroradiology* 1985;27:125-130.
141. Collins AT, Cromwell LD: Computed tomography in the evaluation of congenital cerebral toxoplasmosis, *J Comput Assist Tomogr* 1980;4(3):326-329.
142. Virkola K, Lappalainen M, Valanne L, et al: Radiological signs in newborns exposed to primary Toxoplasma infection *in utero*, *Pediatr Radiol* 1997;27:133-138.
143. Graham D, Guidi SM, Sanders RC: Sonography features of *in utero* periventricular calcification due to cytomegalovirus infection, *J Ultrasound Med* 1982;1:171-172.
144. Molloy PM, Lowman RM: The lack of specificity of neonatal intracranial paraventricular calcifications, *Radiology* 1963; 80:98-102.
145. Ramsey RG: Central nervous system infections in the immunocompromised and immunocompetent patient, *RSNA Special Course in Neuroradiology* 1994;181-189.
146. Shaw CM, Alvord EC Jr: Subependymal germinolysis, *Arch Neurol* 1974;31:374-381.
147. Patel DV, Holfels EM, Vogel NP, et al: Resolution of intracranial calcifications in infants with treated congenital toxoplasmosis, *Radiology* 1996;199:433-440.
148. Florman AL, Gershon AA, Blackett PR, et al: Intrauterine infection with herpes simplex virus, *JAMA* 1973;225(2):129-132.
149. South MA, Tompkins WAF, Morris CR, et al: Congenital malformation of the central nervous system associated with genital type (type 2) herpes virus, *J Pediatr* 1969;75(1):13-18.

150. Benator RM, Magill HL, Gerald B, et al: Herpes simplex encephalitis: CT findings in the neonate and young infant, *AJNR* 1984;6:539-542.
151. Gray PH, Tudehope DI, Masel J: Cystic encephalomalacia and intrauterine herpes simplex virus infection, *Pediatr Radiol* 1992;22:529-532.
152. Levene MI, Williams JL, Fawer CL: *Ultrasound of the infant brain*, London, 1985, Spastics International Medical Publications.
153. Harwood-Nash DC, Reilly BJ, Turnbull I: Massive calcification of the brain in a newborn infant, *AJR* 1970;108(3):528-532.
154. Bell WE, McCormick WF: *Neurologic infections in children*, Philadelphia; 1981, WB Saunders.
155. Ben-Ami T, Yousezadeh D, Backus M, et al: Lenticulostriate vasculopathy in infants with infections of the central nervous system sonographic and Doppler findings, *Pediatr Radiol* 1990;20:575-579.
156. Han BK, Babcock DS, McAdams L: Bacterial meningitis in infants: Sonographic findings, *Radiology* 1985;154(3):645-650.
157. Reeder JD, Sanders RC: Ventriculitis in the neonate: Recognition by sonography, *AJNR* 1983;4:37-41.
158. Edwards MK, Brown DL, Chua GT: Complicated infantile meningitis: Evaluation by real-time sonography, *AJNR* 1982; 3:431-434.
159. Rosenberg HK, Levine RS, Stoltz K, et al: Bacterial meningitis in infants: sonographic features, *AJNR* 1983;4:822-825.
160. Hill A, Shackelford GD, Volpe JJ: Ventriculitis with neonatal bacterial meningitis: Identification by real-time ultrasound, *J Pediatr* 1981;99(1):133-136.

Intracranial Masses

161. Chuang S, Harwood-Nash DC: Tumors and cysts. In Naidich TP, Quencer RM, editors: *Clinical neurosonography*, Berlin, 1987, Springer-Verlag.
162. Ball WS Jr: Pediatric neuroradiology: Part I, *RSNA Special Course in Neuroradiology* 1994;113-126.
163. Tadmor R, Harwood-Nash DC, Savoiardo M, et al: Brain tumors in the first two years of life: CT diagnosis, *AJNR* 1980; 1:411-417.
164. Farwell JR, Dohrmann GJ, Flannery JT: Intracranial neoplasms in infants, *Arch Neurol* 1978;35:533-537.
165. Jooma R, Kendall BE: Intracranial tumors in the first year of life, *Neuroradiology* 1982;23:267-274.
166. Ambrosino MM, Hernanz-Schulman M, Genieser NB, et al: Brain tumors in infants less than a year of age, *Pediatr Radiol* 1988;19:6-8.
167. Jooma R, Hayward RD, Grant DN: Intracranial neoplasms during the first year of life: Analysis of one hundred consecutive cases, *Neurosurgery* 1984;14(1):31-41.
168. Chow PP, Horgan JG, Burns PN, et al: Choroid plexus papilloma: detection by real-time and Doppler sonography, *AJNR* 1986;7:168-170.
169. Han BK, Babcock DS, Ostreich AE: Sonography of brain tumors in infants, *AJR* 1984;143:31-36.
170. Smith WL, Menezes A, Franken EA: Cranial ultrasound in the diagnosis of malignant brain tumors, *J Clin Ultrasound* 1983; 11(2):97-100.
171. Babcock DS, Han BK: The accuracy of high resolution, real-time ultrasonography of the head in infancy, *Radiology* 1981;139:665-676.
172. Schellhas KP, Siebert RC, Heithoff KB, et al: Congenital choroid plexus papilloma of the third ventricle: Diagnosis with real-time sonography and MR imaging, *AJNR* 1988; 9:797-798.
173. Hopper KD, Foley LC, Nieves NL, et al: The interventricular extension of choroid plexus papillomas, *AJNR* 1987;8:469-472.
174. Shkolnik A: B-Mode scanning of the infant brain a new approach. Case report of craniopharyngioma, *J Clin Ultrasound* 1975;3(3):229-231.
175. Babcock DS, Han BK: *Cranial ultrasonography in infants*, Baltimore, 1981, Williams & Wilkins.
176. Maravilla KR, Kirks RR, Maravilla AM: CT diagnosis of intracranial cystic abnormalities in children, *CT* 1978;2:221-235.
177. Chuang S, Harwood-Nash DC: Tumors and cysts, *Neuroradiology*, 1986;28:463-475.
178. Armstrong EA, Harwood-Nash DC, Hoffman H, et al: Benign suprasellar cysts: The CT approach, *AJNR* 1983;4:163-166.
179. Fakhry J, Schechter A, Tenner MS, et al: Cysts of the choroid plexus in neonates: Documentation and review of the literature, *J Ultrasound Med* 1985;4:561-563.
180. Riebel T, Nasir R, Weber K: Choroid plexus cysts: A normal finding on ultrasound, *Pediatr Radiol* 1992;22:410-412.
181. Shuangshoti S, Netsky MG: Neuroepithelial (colloid) cysts of the nervous system, *Neurology* 1966;16:887-903.
182. Giorgi C: Symptomatic cyst of the choroid plexus of the lateral ventricle, *Neurosurgery* 1979;5(1):53-56.
183. Riebel T, Nasir R, Weber K: Choroid plexus cysts: A normal finding on ultrasound, *Pediatr Radiol* 1992;22:410-412.
184. Kurjak A, Schulman H, Predanic A, et al: Fetal choroid plexus vascularization assessed by color flow ultrasonography, *J Ultrasound Med* 1994;3:841-844.
185. Shackelford GD, Fulling KH, Glasier CM: Cysts of the subependymal germinal matrix: Sonographic demonstration with pathologic correlation. *Radiology* 1983;149:117-121.
186. Larcos G, Gruenewald SM, Lui K: Neonatal subependymal cysts detected by sonography: Prevalence, sonographic findings and clinical significance, *AJR* 1994;162:953-956.
187. Levene MI: Diagnosis of subependymal pseudocyst with cerebral ultrasound, *Lancet* 1980;2:210-211.
188. Horbar JD, Philip AGP, Lucey JF: Ultrasound scan in neonatal ventriculitis, *Lancet* 1980;1:976.
189. Danks DM, Tippett P, Adams C, et al: Cerebro-hepato-renal syndrome of Zellweger, *J Pediatr* 1985;86(3):382-387.
190. Sommer A, Bradel EJ, Hamoudi AB: The cerebro-hepato-renal syndrome (Zellweger's Syndrome), *Biol Neonate* 1974; 25:219-229.
191. Russel IMB, van Sonderon L, van Straaten HLM, Barth PG: Subependymal germinolytic cysts in Zellweger Syndrome, *Pediatr Radiol* 1995;25:254-255.
192. Litvak J, Yahr MD, Ransohoff J: Aneurysms of the great vein of Galen and midline cerebral arteriovenous anomalies, *Neurosurgery* 1960;17:945-954.
193. Long DM, Seljeskog EL, Chou SN, et al: Giant arteriovenous malformations of infancy and childhood, *J Neurosurg* 1974;40:304-312.
194. Lee SH, Rao KCVG: *Cranial computed tomography*, New York, 1983, McGraw-Hill.
195. Kangarloo H, Gold RH, Benson L, et al: Sonography of extrathoracic left-to-right shunts in infants and children, *AJR* 1983;141:923-926.
196. Cubberley DA, Jaffe RB, Nixon GW: Sonographic demonstration of galenic arteriovenous malformations in the neonate, *AJNR* 1982;3:435-439.
197. Soto G, Daneman A, Hellman J: Doppler evaluation of cerebral arteries in a galenic vein malformation, *J Ultrasound Med* 1985;4:673-675.
198. Tessler FN, Dion J, Vinuela F, et al: Cranial arteriovenous malformations in neonates: Color Doppler imaging with angiographic correlation, *AJR*, 1989;153:1027-1030.
199. Westra SJ, Curran JG, Duckwiler GR, et al: Pediatric intracranial vascular malformations: Evaluation of treatment results with color Doppler US, *Radiology* 1993;186:775-783.
200. Chapman S, Hockley AD: Calcification of an aneurysm of the vein of Galen, *Pediatr Radiol* 1989;19:541-542.
201. Hurst RW, Kagetsu NJ, Berenstein A: Angiographic findings in two cases of aneurysmal malformation of vein of Galen prior to spontaneous thrombosis: Therapeutic implications, *AJNR* 1992;13:1446-1450.

CHAPTER 53

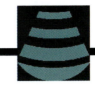

Doppler of the Neonatal and Infant Brain

George A. Taylor, M.D.

CHAPTER OUTLINE

Continuous and **pulsed wave** or **spectral Doppler** techniques have been in use for many years in the monitoring of intracranial hemodynamics in the newborn.[1-3] Although early Doppler studies were useful in attempting to understand the pathophysiology of cerebrovascular injury, they were limited by the inability to image the actual vessels. The introduction of **color flow Doppler** technology made identification of the origin of the Doppler signal and its orientation to the transducer easier to achieve. Further improvements in color sensitivity and transducer design now allow the imaging of the intracranial vasculature in newborns routinely possible, including the identification of flow in submillimeter arteries and in the main venous drainage pathways of the brain.[4] The extended dynamic range and increased sensitivity of **power mode Doppler** (amplitude mode color or color flow Doppler energy) can be used to improve depiction of low velocity and low amplitude flow and show potential for creation of regional cerebral blood flow maps[5,6] (Fig. 53-1). Although cranial Doppler sonography is not used as part of the routine screening examination of asymptomatic premature infants, it can be a helpful diagnostic and problem-solving tool in a variety of clinical situations.

TECHNIQUE

Transcranial Approaches

Three different scanning approaches have worked well, each with its own advantages.[7-11] The **anterior**

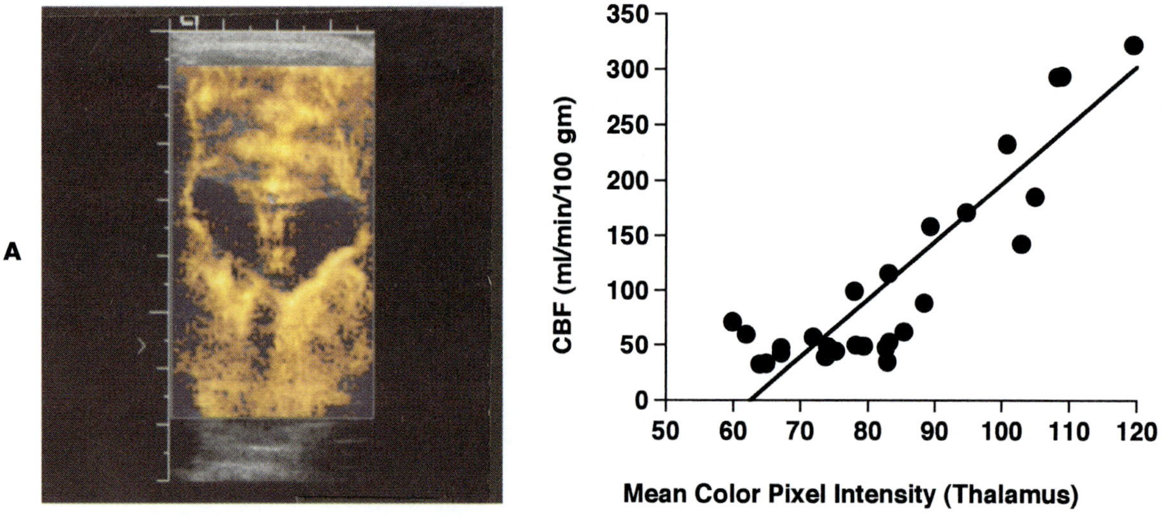

FIG. 53-1. Normal power mode Doppler cerebral blood flow map in premature infant. **A,** Coronal color amplitude (power mode Doppler) sonogram shows flow in submillimeter vessels throughout brain parenchyma. **B,** Graph comparing mean color flow Doppler pixel intensity with regional cerebral blood flow in thalamus of lambs shows good correlation between changes in regional color flow Doppler signal and cerebral blood flow measured by radiolabeled microspheres. (From Taylor GA. Regional cerebral blood flow estimates in newborn lamb using amplitude mode color Doppler ultrasound. *Pediatr Radiol* 1996;26:282-286.)

fontanelle approach is the easiest and most commonly used. The basilar, internal carotid, and anterior cerebral arteries as well as the internal cerebral veins, vein of Galen, and the superior sagittal and straight sinus can be routinely visualized on sagittal scans near the midline (Fig. 53-2, *A* and *B*). The inferior sagittal sinus is difficult to resolve as a separate vessel because its course is often superimposed on the posterior portion of the pericallosal artery. The smaller thalmostriate arteries and opercular branches of the middle cerebral artery may be seen on angled sagittal images (Fig. 53-2, *C*).

On coronal scans through the anterior fontanelle, the supraclinoid internal carotids, M1 segments of the middle cerebral arteries, thalmostriate arteries, A1 segments of the anterior cerebral arteries, and the cavernous sinus can almost always be visualized on anteriorly angled scans (Fig. 53-3, *A*). Paired terminal and internal cerebral veins, thalmostriate arteries, the basilar artery, straight sinus, and transverse sinuses can be seen on more posteriorly angled scans (Fig. 53-3, *B*).

A major drawback of the coronal plane is the near perpendicular angle between the middle cerebral arteries and the ultrasound beam such that measured frequency shifts from flowing red blood cells approach zero.

The **temporal bone approach** is best for the middle cerebral artery, as it is parallel to flow. The transducer is placed in axial orientation approximately 1 cm anterior and superior to the tragus of the ear. Using the thin temporal bone as an acoustic window, adequate penetration for imaging and Doppler studies can be achieved in most full-term neonates. This approach allows visualization of the major branches of the circle of Willis (Fig. 53-4). In most premature infants both middle cerebral arteries can be easily insonated from one side of the head.

The **posterolateral (mastoid) fontanelle approach** is an angled axial scan. This portal is located approximately 1 cm behind and superior to the concha of the ear. It is the preferred approach for imaging flow in the transverse venous sinuses (Fig. 53-5).

Doppler Optimization

For best visualization of the intracranial vascular system, the image should be **electronically magnified** and the **color region of interest restricted** to enhance color sensitivity and frame rate. **Color gain** should be adjusted to maximize vascular signal and minimize tissue motion artifacts, and the **lowest band pass filter** should be used to maximize low-flow sensitivity necessary for evaluating venous structures. A 7-MHz linear transducer with electronic beam steering is recommended for examining the superficially located superior sagittal sinus. Visualization of smaller arterial branches of the middle and anterior cerebral arteries can also be accomplished in the majority of normal premature and full-term infants, but often requires **higher-frequency** (5- or 7-MHz) vector or sector transducers capable of detecting lower velocity

A B C

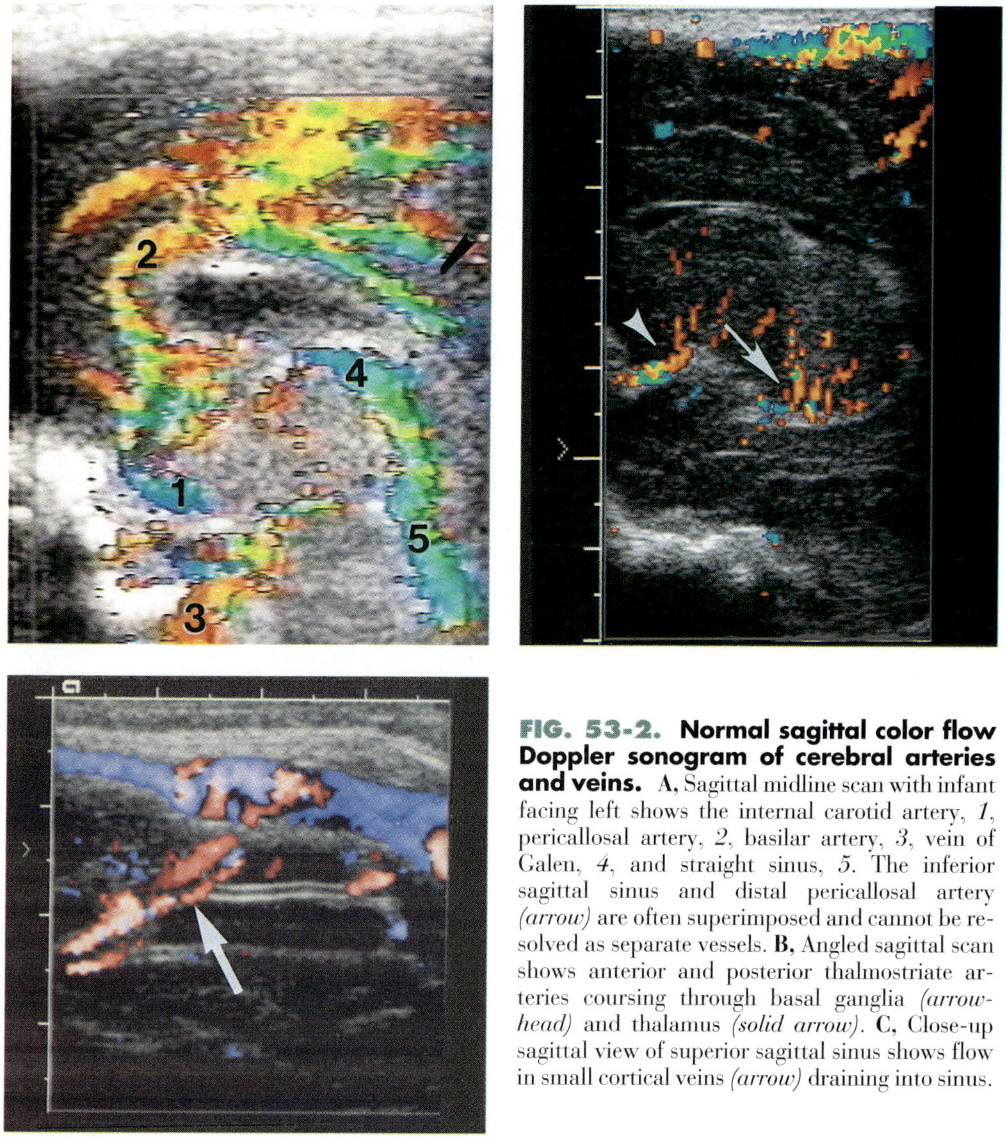

FIG. 53-2. Normal sagittal color flow Doppler sonogram of cerebral arteries and veins. **A,** Sagittal midline scan with infant facing left shows the internal carotid artery, *1*, pericallosal artery, *2*, basilar artery, *3*, vein of Galen, *4*, and straight sinus, *5*. The inferior sagittal sinus and distal pericallosal artery *(arrow)* are often superimposed and cannot be resolved as separate vessels. **B,** Angled sagittal scan shows anterior and posterior thalmostriate arteries coursing through basal ganglia *(arrowhead)* and thalamus *(solid arrow)*. **C,** Close-up sagittal view of superior sagittal sinus shows flow in small cortical veins *(arrow)* draining into sinus.

and amplitude signal. The use of **power mode Doppler** is recommended when directional information is of secondary importance and detection of flow is of primary importance.

For specific vessel evaluation, spectral or duplex pulsed wave Doppler imaging can be performed using 3.5- to 7.5-MHz probes, depending on the depth and location of the target vessel. Spectral Doppler imaging is essential for the evaluation of intracranial hemodynamics in both the arterial and venous systems.

Safety Considerations

During pulsed wave and color flow Doppler examinations, signal is obtained by imparting energy into tissues. Although intracranial Doppler ultrasound is safe, the possibility exists that biologic effects may be identified in the future. Thus, Doppler exposure

DOPPLER OPTIMIZATION

- Electronically magnify image
- Restrict color region of interest so that you can enhance color sensitivity and frame rate
- Color gain adjusted to maximize vascular signal and minimize tissue artifact
- Lowest band pass filter to maximize low-flow sensitivity and evaluate venous structures
- 7-MHz linear transducer for superior sagittal sinus
- Power mode Doppler for smallest vessels when flow direction not needed

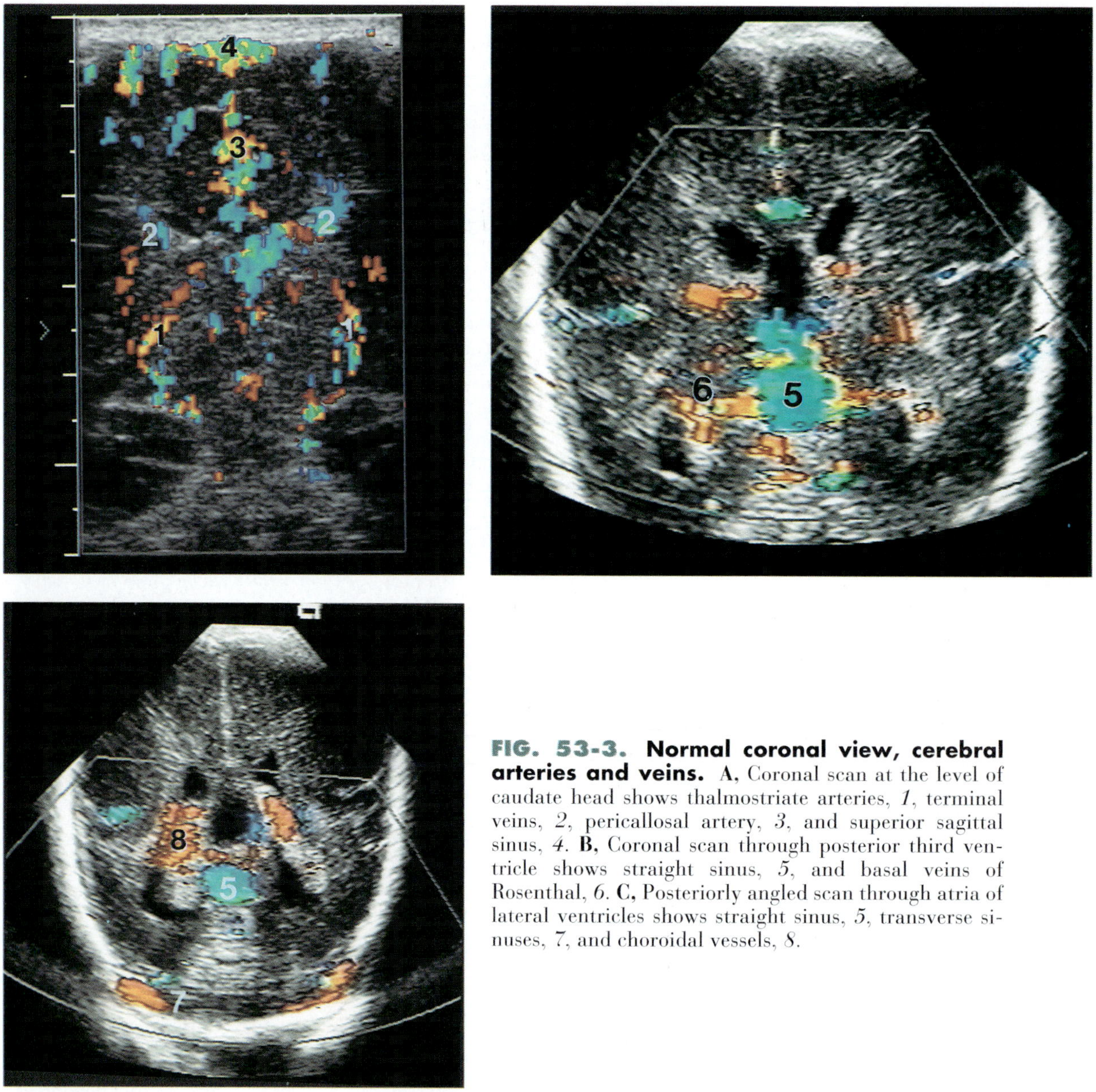

FIG. 53-3. Normal coronal view, cerebral arteries and veins. **A,** Coronal scan at the level of caudate head shows thalmostriate arteries, *1*, terminal veins, *2*, pericallosal artery, *3*, and superior sagittal sinus, *4*. **B,** Coronal scan through posterior third ventricle shows straight sinus, *5*, and basal veins of Rosenthal, *6*. **C,** Posteriorly angled scan through atria of lateral ventricles shows straight sinus, *5*, transverse sinuses, *7*, and choroidal vessels, *8*.

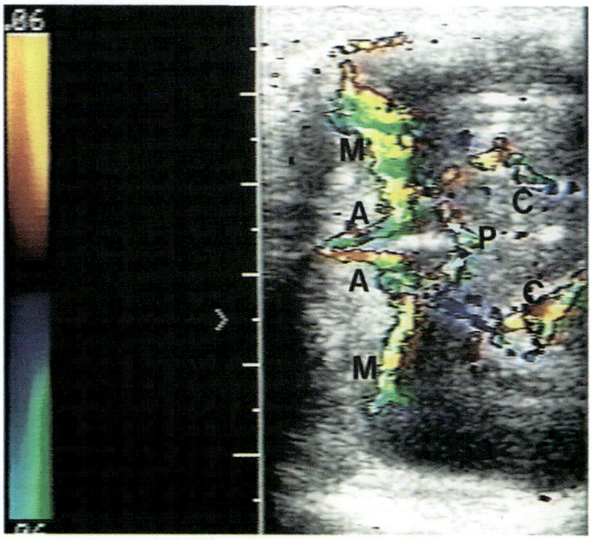

FIG. 53-4. Normal axial view, middle cerebral artery and circle of Willis. Axial scan obtained through left temporal bone shows major branches of the circle of Willis. The A1 segment of the left and right anterior cerebral artery, *A*, the middle cerebral arteries, *M*, posterior communicating artery, *P*, and posterior cerebral artery, *C*.

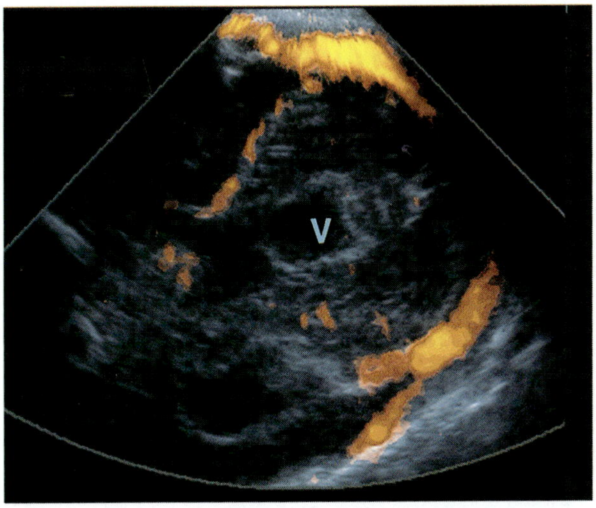

FIG. 53-5. Normal transverse sinus flow on power mode Doppler. Angled axial amplitude mode color flow Doppler image through mastoid fontanelle shows flow in both transverse sinuses. Note dilated fourth ventricle, *V*.

should be time limited, and the signal intensity should be maximized by increasing gain and not transducer power output settings. Current FDA guidelines for intracranial exposure (≤ 94 mW/cm^2 maximum *in situ* I_{SPTA} intensities in water) are equal to those recommended for fetal examinations and achievable by most recently manufactured units.[12]

Doppler Measurements

The **resistive index** (RI), **instantaneous peak systolic** and **end diastolic velocities**, and **mean blood flow velocity over time** (time averaged velocity) are the most commonly used spectral Doppler measures for monitoring intracranial hemodynamics. The easiest and most reproducible are measures of pulsatility (Fig. 53-6). They are relatively insensitive to differences in angle of insonation and correlate well with acute changes in intracerebral perfusion pressure.[13] However, many factors other than cerebrovascular resistance may affect the RI in an intracranial vessel[14-16] (Fig. 53-7). Common factors and their effects on RI are listed in Table 53-1.

The mechanism by which these factors modify RI is as follows: with **increasing filter settings**, lower velocities are not depicted, resulting in a falsely elevated RI. **Transducer pressure** on the anterior fontanelle may transiently increase intracranial pressure, which in turn preferentially reduces flow during diastole and increases RI. In infants with a symptomatic **patent ductus arteriosus**, resistance to flow in the cerebral vascular bed is higher than pulmonary vascular resistance. This results in shunting of blood away from the brain during diastole and an elevated intracranial RI. During **tachycardia**, there is less time for the arterial pressure wave to dissipate before another systolic ejection occurs. Intracranial RI is artificially lower because diastolic velocities are measured at middiastole when velocities are higher, rather than during end diastole. **Left ventricular dysfunction** (decreased cardiac output) results in a decreased systolic pressure wave, lowered systolic velocities, and a reduced RI.

In addition, the RI is only a weak predictor of cerebrovascular resistance under most physiologic conditions.[17] Mean blood flow velocity measures are the most informative indices of cerebral blood flow (CBF). Although accurate placement of the sample volume and angle of insonation are required, a strong correlation has been demonstrated between mean blood flow velocity and changes in global CBF under a variety of clinical and experimental conditions (Fig. 53-8).[17-20]

TABLE 53-1
FACTORS THAT CHANGE THE RESISTIVE INDEX

Factor	Effect on RI
High-pass filter settings	Increased
Scanning pressure	Increased
Patent ductus arteriosus	Increased
Elevated heart rate	Decreased
Decreased cardiac output	Decreased

NORMAL HEMODYNAMICS

Normal Arterial Blood Flow Patterns

Arterial hemodynamics in the cerebral circulation are affected by normal maturational events in the healthy newborn. The **resistive index** (RI) in the anterior cerebral artery decreases from a mean of 0.78 (range 0.5 to 1) in **preterm** infants to a mean of 0.71 (range 0.6 to 8) in **full-term** newborns.[2,3,21] This trend is associated with increasing diastolic flow velocities and may be related to peripheral changes in cerebrovascular resistance or to changes proximal to the site of recording such as a closing ductus arteriosus and a diminishing left-to-right shunt. In full-term infants, RI may also change over the first few days of life.[2] In a study of 476 normal newborns weighing over 2500 g at birth, anterior cerebral artery RI decreased from a mean of 70.6 ± 7 (range 51 to 87) to 68.3 ± 6 (range 51 to 83) within the first 24 hours.[22] The range of published peak systolic and end diastolic velocities and RI in several intracranial arteries is shown in Table 53-2. Although the range of published normal values is broad, variability within an individual patient should not be great. Changes of more than 50% from baseline values should be considered abnormal. There are no consistent differences in instantaneous

A

B

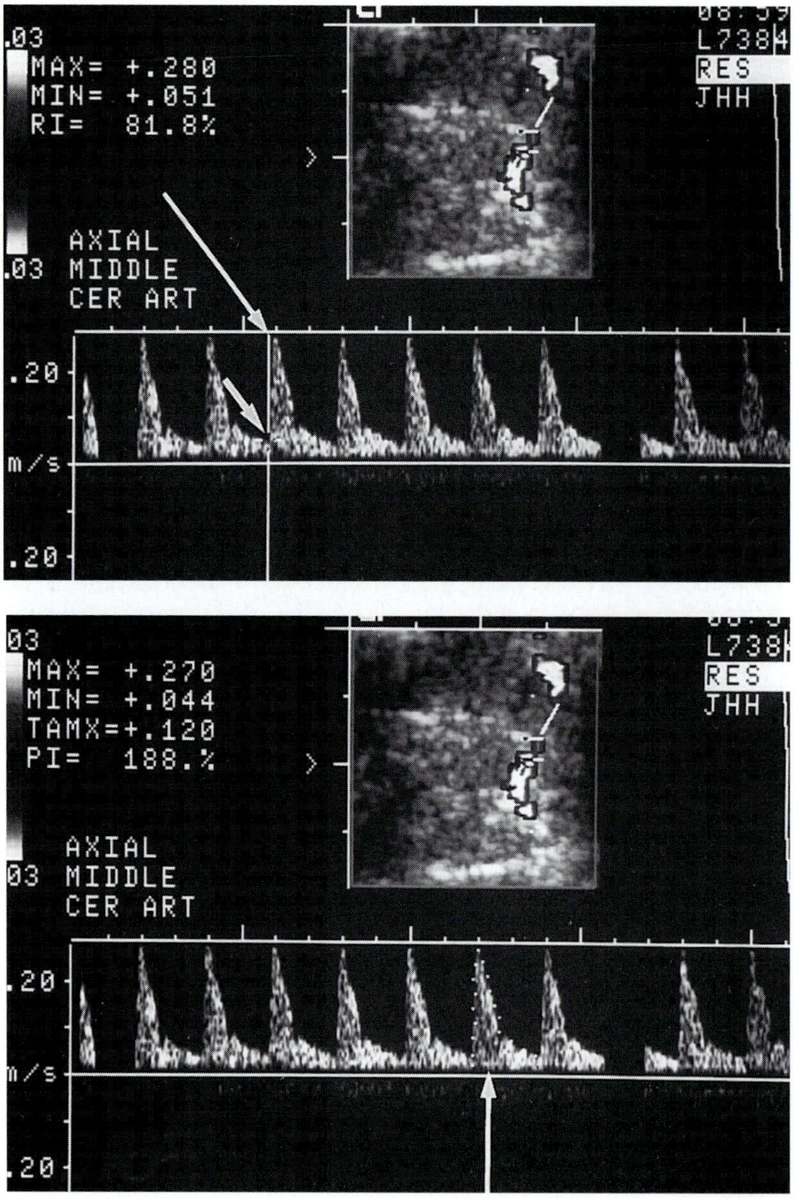

FIG. 53-6. Determination of resistive index (RI) and pulsatility index (PI). **A,** The RI of Pourcelot can be derived by placing the Doppler cursor at peak systolic velocity, *Vs*, or maximum velocity *(long arrow)* and at end diastolic velocity, *Ved*, or minimum velocity *(short arrow)*. The RI is calculated as Vs−Ved/Vs. **B,** PI of Gosling is derived by tracing the outer envelope of a single cardiac cycle *(arrow)* and calculating the time-averaged maximum velocity envelope (TAMX). The PI is calculated as Vs−Ved/TAMX.

A

B

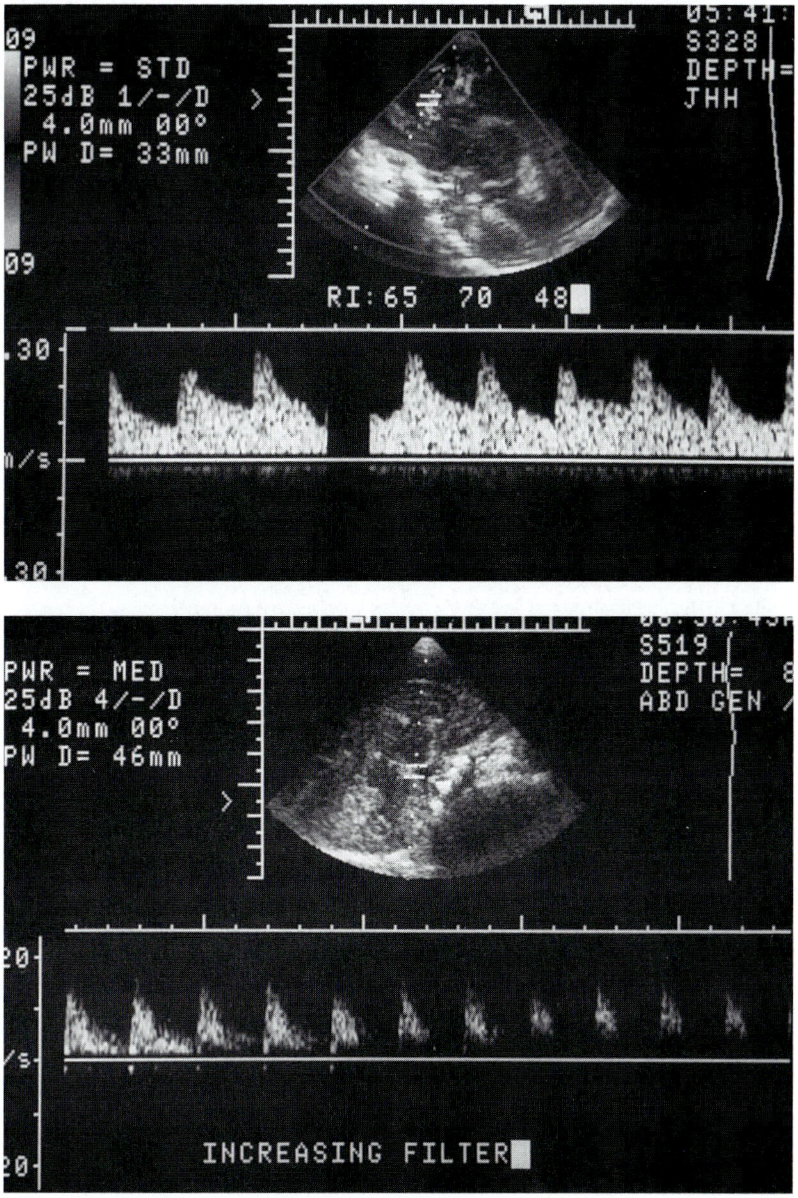

FIG. 53-7. Factors affecting intracranial RI. A, High variability in pulsatility of flow related to left ventricular dysfunction. Doppler tracing from the anterior cerebral artery in an infant with congenital heart disease. **B,** Progressively higher wall filter settings show what appears to be absent flow during diastole as the filter cuts out lower flow.

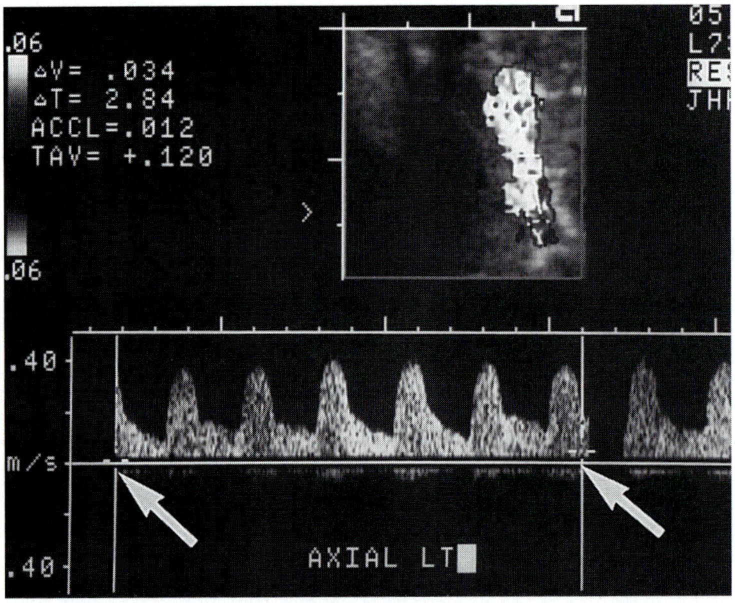

FIG. 53-8. Determination of mean blood flow velocity. Angle-corrected Doppler tracing obtained from the middle cerebral artery. Cursors are placed at the beginning and end of a continuous Doppler tracing *(arrows)*. The time-averaged mean blood flow velocity (TAV) is calculated by integrating all instantaneous mean blood flow velocities between both cursors. In this example, the TAV measured 0−.12 cm/s.

TABLE 53-2

ARTERIAL BLOOD FLOW VELOCITIES IN FULL-TERM INFANTS: RANGE OF PEAK SYSTOLIC, END DIASTOLIC FLOW VELOCITIES AND RESISTIVE INDEX*

	Peak Systolic Velocity (cm/s)	End Diastolic Velocity (cm/s)	Resistive Index
Internal carotid	12-80	3-20	0.5-0.8
Basilar	30-80	5-20	0.6-0.8
Middle cerebral	20-70	8-20	0.6-0.8
Anterior cerebral	12-35	6-20	0.6-0.8
Posterior cerebral	20-60	8-25	0.6-0.8

*Values modified from references 2, 21, and 23.

TABLE 53-3

VENOUS BLOOD FLOW VELOCITIES: MEAN BLOOD FLOW VELOCITIES IN FULL-TERM NEWBORNS*

Vessel	Mean TAV†(cm/s)
Terminal veins	3.0 ± 0.3
Internal cerebral veins	3.3 ± 0.3
Vein of Galen	4.3 ± 0.7
Straight sinus	5.9 ± 1.0
Superior sagittal sinus	9.2 ± 1.1
Inferior sagittal sinus	3.5 ± 0.3

*Values modified from reference 10.
†*TAV*, Time averaged mean blood flow *velocity* expressed in ± standard error of the mean.

blood flow velocity or pulsatility of flow among the major branches of the circle of Willis or between right- and left-sided structures.

Normal Venous Blood Flow Patterns

Venous blood flow is **continuous** in smaller intracerebral veins such as the terminal and internal cerebral veins. Low-amplitude **cardiac pulsations** are common in more central venous structures such as the vein of Galen and the sagittal sinuses (Fig. 53-9). High-amplitude or **"sawtooth" patterns** of pulsatility are not normal and may be seen in infants with elevated right-heart pressures or tricuspid regurgitation (Fig. 53-10). Although **respiratory**

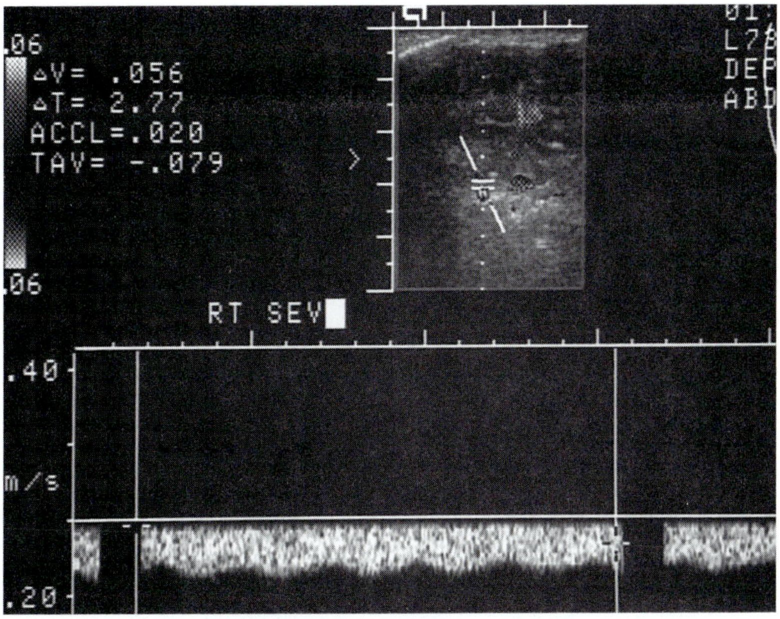

FIG. 53-9. Normal referred cardiac pulsations in veins. Low-amplitude pulsatility from referred cardiac pulsations in a Doppler tracing from terminal vein in a normal full-term infant.

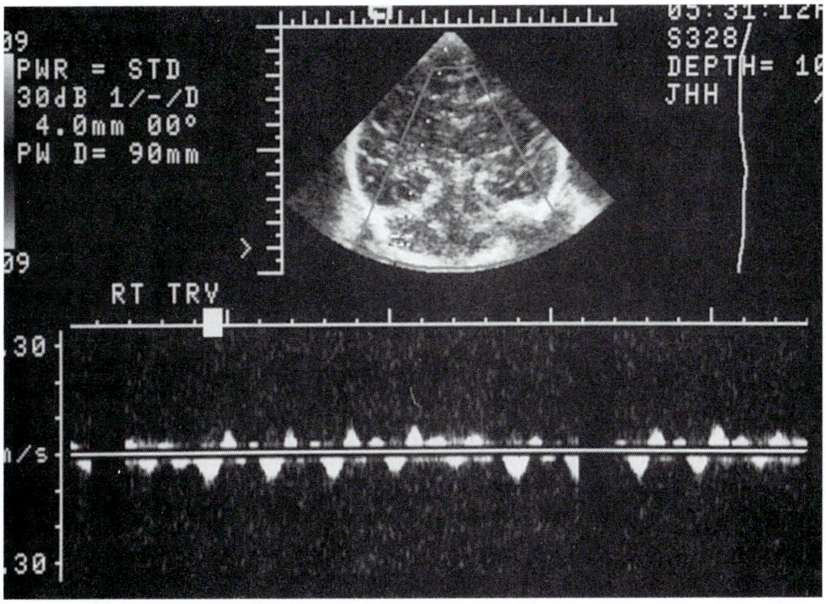

FIG. 53-10. Exaggerated venous pulsations from tricuspid regurgitation. Doppler tracing from transverse sinus in infant with tricuspid regurgitation shows an abnormal "sawtooth" pattern of flow due to referred right atrial pulsations.

changes are not usually observed during normal quiet respiration, marked changes in velocity can occur during forceful crying as a result of rapid changes in intrathoracic pressure.[10,24,25] Ranges for mean blood flow velocities in several intracranial veins and sinuses are shown in Table 53-3.

INTENSIVE CARE THERAPIES AND CEREBRAL HEMODYNAMICS

Mechanical Ventilation

Cerebral hemodynamics can be markedly affected by mechanical ventilation. Changes in venous return to

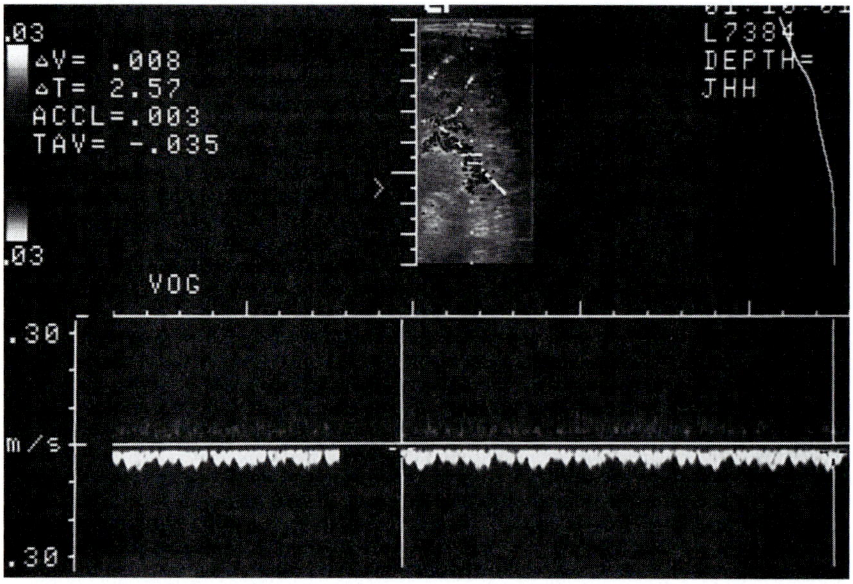

FIG. 53-11. Effect of high-frequency ventilation on venous hemodynamics. Vein of Galen pulsed wave Doppler tracing in a premature infant on high-frequency ventilation shows superimposed 15-Hz oscillations in flow.

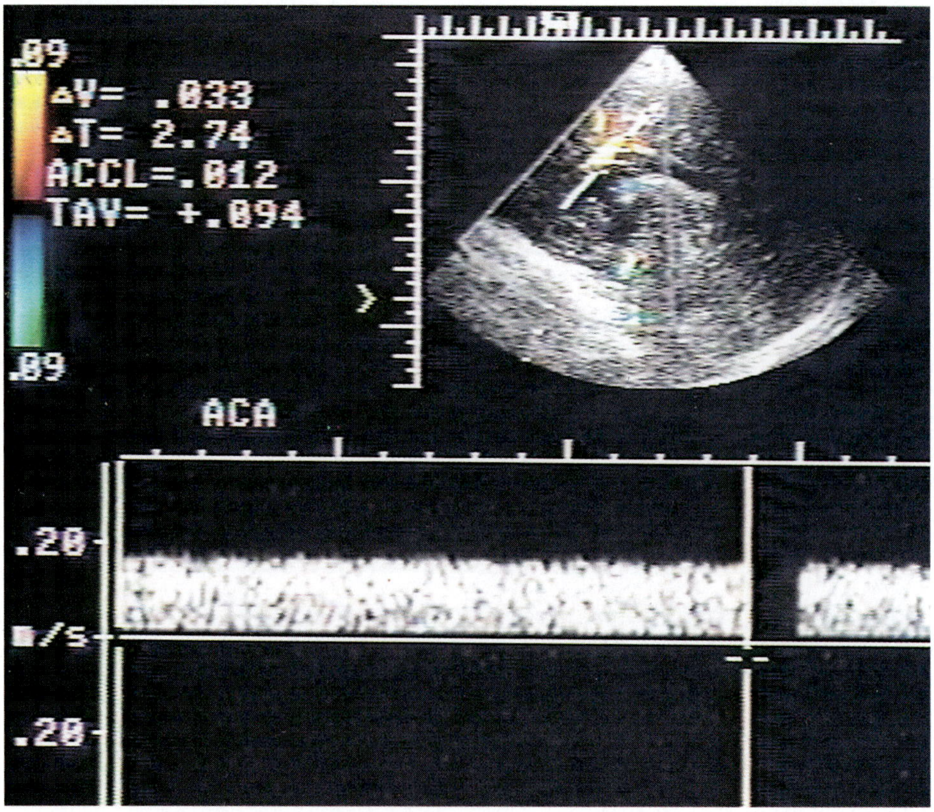

FIG. 53-12. Absent arterial pulsatility during ECMO. Continuous nonpulsatile flow on pulsed wave Doppler tracing from the anterior cerebral artery in an infant with congenital heart disease and severe cardiac dysfunction.

the heart associated with breathing out of synchrony with the ventilator may result in significant beat-to-beat variability in arterial waveforms.[26]

Similarly, high peak inspiratory pressures can impede venous return to the heart and result in reversal of flow in the intracranial veins. Treatment with high-frequency ventilation exerts its effects on venous hemodynamics in the form of short-amplitude oscillations at approximately 15 cycles per second (Fig. 53-11).[11] Endotracheal suctioning has been associated with marked increases in mean arterial blood pressure and arterial blood flow velocities in premature infants and has been attributed to the relative pressure-passive cerebral circulation (lack of autoregulation) in these patients.[27]

Extracorporeal Membrane Oxygenation

Extracorporeal membrane oxygenation (ECMO) is frequently used for the treatment of infants with severe respiratory failure who have not responded to maximal conventional ventilatory support. During venoarterial ECMO, infants undergo cannulation and ligation of the right common carotid artery and jugular vein for vascular access and are placed on nonpulsatile partial cardiopulmonary bypass. This results in significant alterations in intracranial hemodynamics[28,29] (Fig. 53-12). As the amount of flow through the ECMO bypass circuit increases, arterial pulsatility decreases proportionately and may disappear altogether, especially in association with severe cardiac dysfunction.[28] During bypass, flow to the right middle cerebral artery is typically achieved by shunting blood from the left internal carotid and A1 segment of the anterior cerebral artery across the anterior communicating artery. Flow then proceeds in retrograde fashion along the left A1 segment to the left middle cerebral artery (Fig. 53-13). Alterations in venous drainage may also occur during ECMO bypass as a result of jugular vein ligation and may be associated with a higher risk of hemorrhagic infarction[30] (Fig. 53-14).

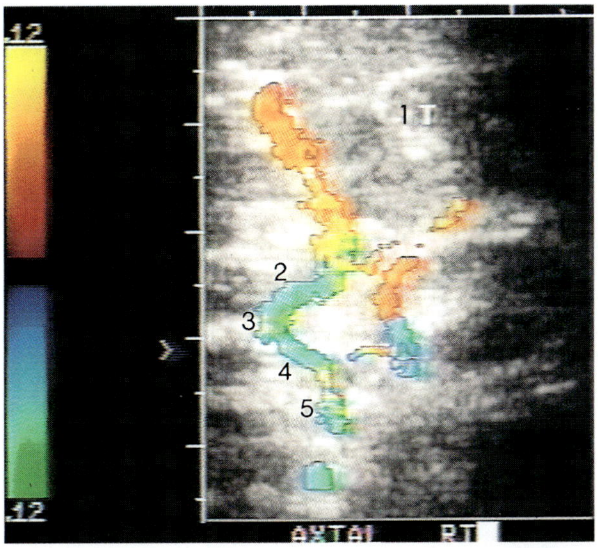

FIG. 53-13. Collateral flow via circle of Willis during ECMO. Left axial scan shows antegrade flow in left middle cerebral artery, *1*, and A1 segment, left anterior cerebral artery, *2*. Flow to right middle cerebral artery, *5*, is via retrograde flow through A1 segment, right anterior cerebral artery, *4*, and anterior communicating artery, *3*. Compare with normal appearance in Fig. 53-3. (From Taylor GA. Current concepts in neonatal cranial Doppler sonography. *Ultrasound Q* 1992;4:223-244.)

DIFFUSE NEURONAL INJURY

Asphyxia

The hemodynamic changes associated with asphyxia depend on the severity of the insult, ongoing hypercapnia and hypoxemia, and vary depending on the time from injury.

Infants with **mild degrees of asphyxia** will have normal cerebral hemodynamics throughout. In the setting of **severe or prolonged asphyxia,** tissue hypoxic injury results in the excessive release or diminished reuptake of endogenous excitatory amino acids such as glutamate and aspartate. This in turn results in the production of intracellular nitric oxide and subsequent cerebral vasodilatation.[31] As a consequence, increased mean blood flow velocities and decreased arterial pulsatility may be seen on spectral Doppler imaging during the first several days after the initial insult (Fig. 53-15).[32] This reflects the impaired autoregulation and elevated cerebral blood flow associated with diffuse hypoxic brain injury. In asphyxiated infants, a very low RI (< 60) in the first few days of life is associated with severe subsequent neurodevelopmental delay.[33] Persistent hypoxia or hypercapnia will also contribute to generalized vasodilatation and abnormal Doppler spectra, and fluctuation of systolic velocities may be present due to asphyxia-related cardiac ischemia.[34,35]

Cerebral Edema

Cerebral edema often accompanies hypoxic-ischemic brain injury. Edema begins during the course of hypoxia-ischemia and appears to be related to the formation of idiogenic osmoles (H+ ions and lactate) within cells combined with cellular energy failure and loss of transcellular ionic gradients. The more severe the brain injury, the more extensive and prolonged the associated edema.[36] As cerebral edema worsens, cerebrovascular resistance increases, resulting in dampening of diastolic blood flow velocities. Pulsed wave Doppler imaging typically shows progressive elevation of the RI and reversal of diastolic flow in the intracranial arteries.[35,37]

A

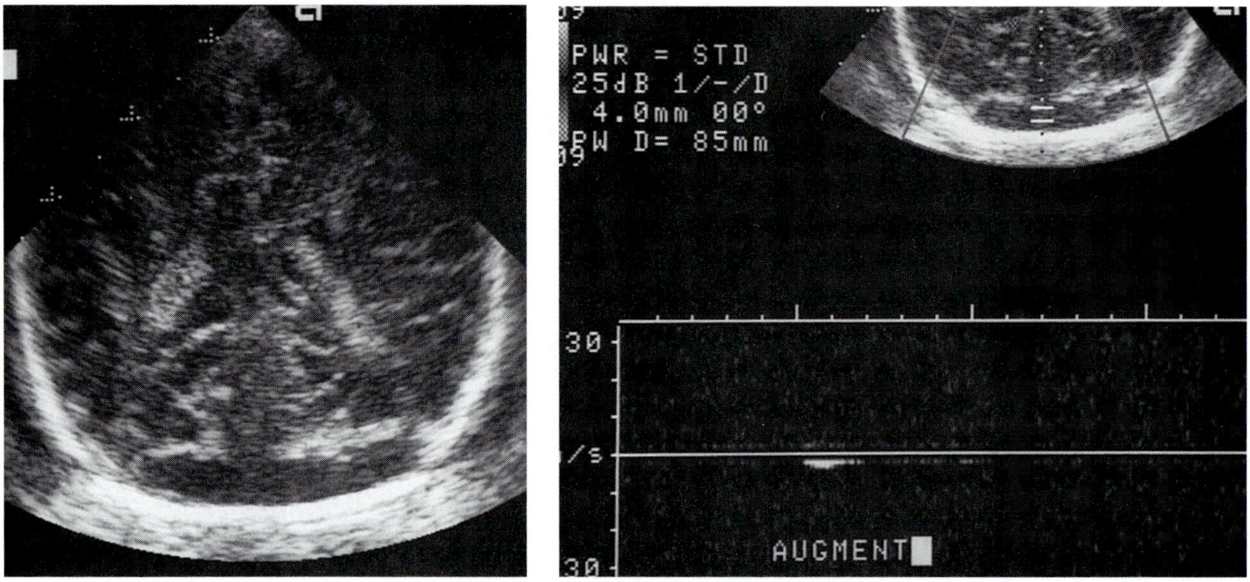

B

FIG. 53-14. Partial venous obstruction during ECMO. **A,** Posteriorly angled coronal scan shows dilated sinus confluence (see cursor on B). **B,** Flow only detectable during augmentation by gentle compression and release of left internal jugular vein. Infant developed signs of superior vena caval obstruction on day three of ECMO. (From Taylor GA, Walker LK. Intracranial venous system in newborns treated with extracorporeal membrane oxygenation: Doppler US evaluation after ligation of the right jugular vein. *Radiology* 1992;183:453-456.)

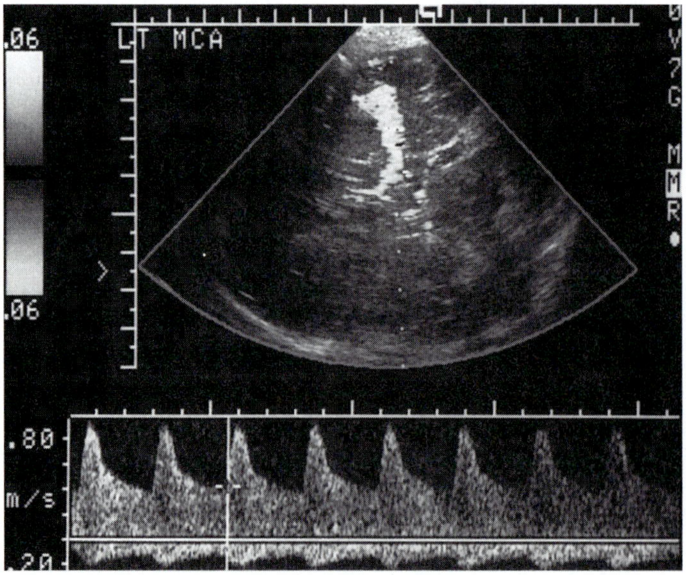

FIG. 53-15. Severe perinatal asphyxia. Middle cerebral artery Doppler shows elevated flow during diastole and a reduced pulsatility of flow. RI: 54.

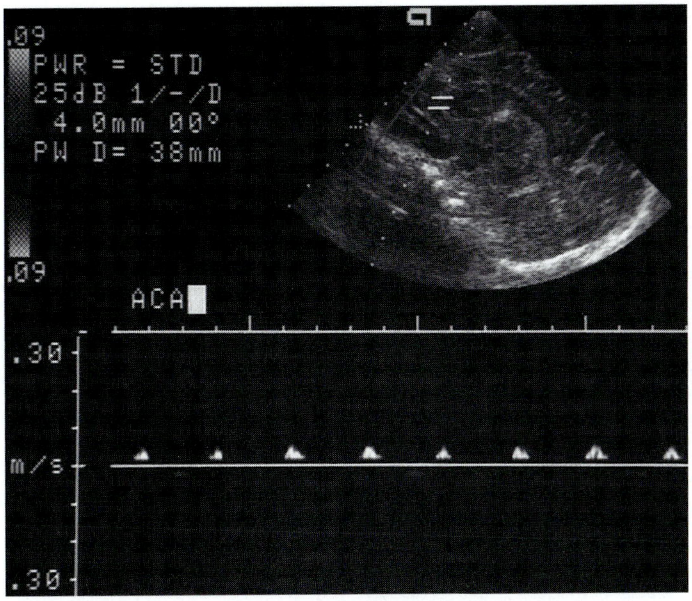

FIG. 53-16. Brain death with nonviable brain blood flow. Infant with diffuse cerebral edema. Pulsed wave Doppler tracing from anterior cerebral artery shows very low flow velocities during peak systole and reversal of flow during diastole.

Brain Death

Eventually, flow during systole becomes diminished and present only during a brief portion of the cardiac cycle. This represents **nonviable brain blood flow** (Fig. 53-16).[37] Although absence of intracranial flow by Doppler techniques is a reliable sign of absent cortical function, the presence of flow does not guarantee functional integrity, and brain death may be seen in the presence of preserved intracranial blood flow.[38]

INTRACRANIAL HEMORRHAGE AND STROKE

The periventricular white matter is drained primarily via the medullary veins into the terminal and internal cerebral veins. Obstruction of these small veins by germinal matrix hemorrhage and subsequent venous hypertension may play an important role in the pathogenesis of periventricular hemorrhagic infarction in the preterm infant.[39,40] Color flow Doppler imaging may be used to show initial displacement, gradual encasement, and **obstruction of the terminal veins by an enlarging germinal matrix hemorrhage** (Fig. 53-17). In one study, displacement or occlusion of the terminal vein could be demonstrated in 50% of germinal matrix hemorrhages and in 92% of periventricular white matter hemorrhages.[41] This finding may be useful in the early prediction of infants at risk for worsening intracranial hemorrhage.

Not all cerebral infarcts show alterations in regional blood flow. However, decreased arterial pulsations, increased size and number of visible vessels, and increased mean blood flow velocities can be demonstrated in the tissues surrounding larger cerebral infarcts (Fig. 53-18).[42,43] This pattern of vasodilatation has been well described on computed tomography (CT) and angiography and is thought to be caused by the uncoupling of cerebral blood flow from local metabolic demands ("luxury perfusion").[44,45]

HYDROCEPHALUS

As the intracranial pressure rises, arterial flow tends to be more affected during diastole than during systole, resulting in an elevated pulsatility of flow. Seibert et al. have shown that increasing RI correlates well with elevation in intracranial pressure (ICP) in an animal model of acute hydrocephalus.[13] They and others have also shown a significant drop in pulsatility following ventricular tapping and shunting in infants with hydrocephalus.[13,46] However, elevated ICP may not always be present in infants with ventricular dilatation, and the RI may be well within the normal range. Doppler examination of the anterior or middle cerebral artery during fontanelle compression may be useful in the early identification of infants with abnormal intracranial compliance prior to the development of increased ICP as shown by elevated baseline RI.[47] According to the Monro-Kellie hypoth-

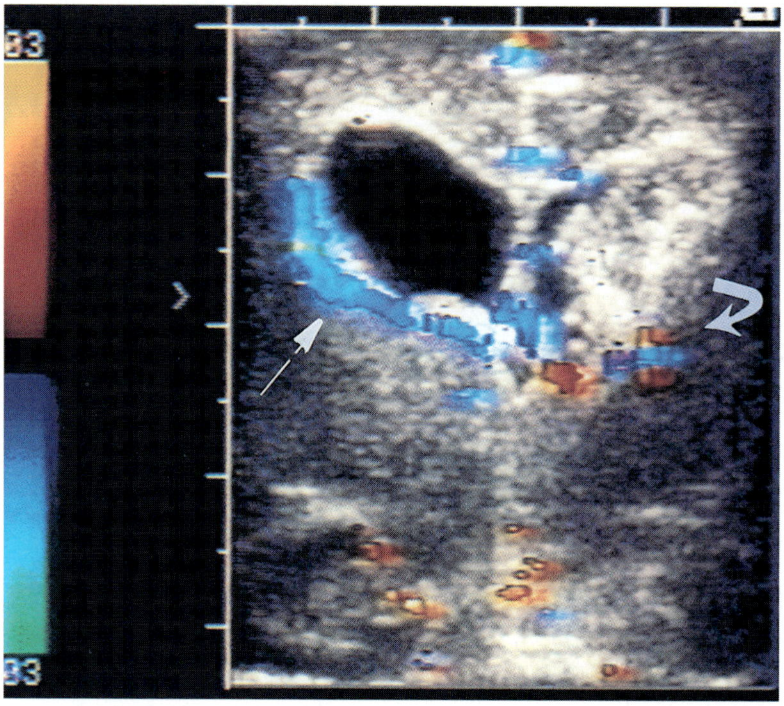

FIG. 53-17. Grade IV intracranial hemorrhage with obstruction of terminal vein. Flow in left subependymal vein *(curved arrow)* is obliterated by hematoma. Normal right subependymal vein is shown joining internal cerebral vein *(large arrow)*. (From Taylor GA. Effect of germinal matrix hemorrhage on terminal vein position and patency. *Pediatr Radiol* 1995;25:S37-S40.)

A

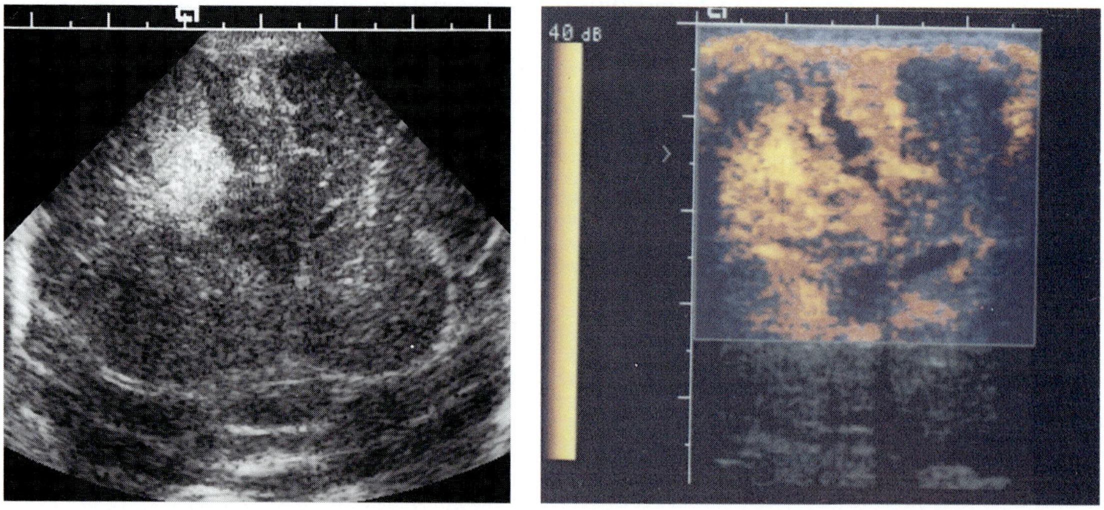

B

FIG. 53-18. Parasagittal infarct with luxury perfusion in full-term infant. **A,** Focal echogenic infarct in subcortical white matter of the right frontal lobe. **B,** Coronal power (color amplitude) Doppler image shows markedly increased blood flow to abnormal area consistent with luxury perfusion.

esis, the volume of brain, spinal fluid, blood, and other intracranial components is constant.[48] During graded fontanelle compression in normal infants, CSF or blood can be readily displaced to compensate for the small increase in volume delivered by compression of the anterior fontanelle, resulting in no increase in ICP. In infants with hydrocephalus, however, the **increase in intracranial volume with fontanelle compression** is translated into a transient increase in ICP and an acute increase in arterial pulsatility (Fig. 53-19). Serial examinations using this technique can also be used to follow an indi-

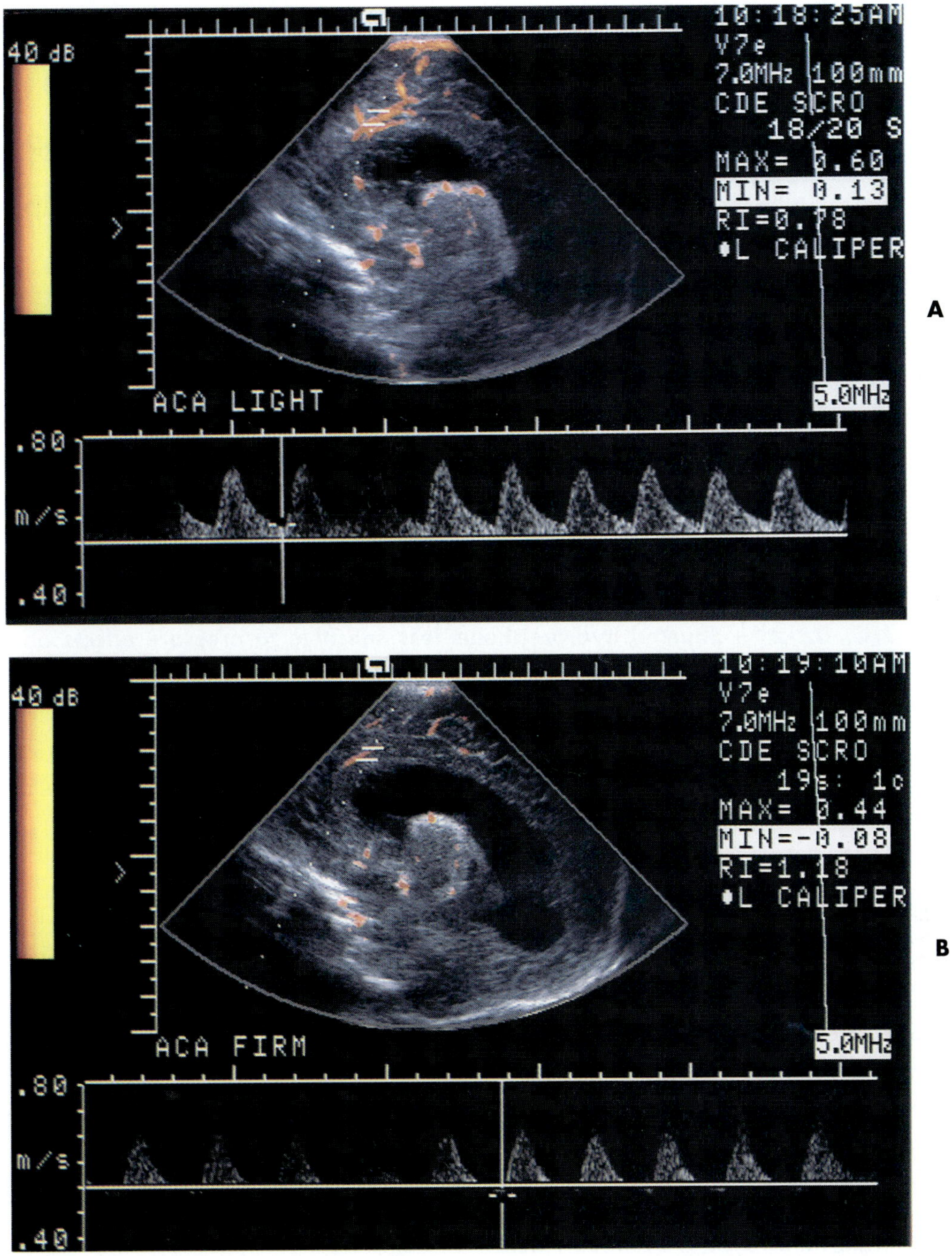

FIG. 53-19. Effect of increased fontanelle pressure on RI in infant with hydrocephalus. **A,** Pulsed wave Doppler tracing of the anterior cerebral artery with transducer held lightly over anterior fontanelle shows an RI of 0.78. **B,** Repeat tracing obtained a few seconds later with transducer firmly held over fontanelle. RI has increased to 1.18.

vidual infant's ability to compensate for minor changes in intracranial volume and thus can be used as a **noninvasive indirect measure of intracranial compliance** (Fig. 53-20).

Color flow Doppler techniques may also be helpful in evaluating cerebrospinal fluid dynamics in these infants. Winkler has shown that Doppler examination of the ventricular system during cranial or abdominal compression may induce movement of CSF detectable with color flow or duplex Doppler imaging.[49] These dynamic techniques can be used to demonstrate obstruction at the foramina of Monro and aqueduct of Sylvius (Fig. 53-21).

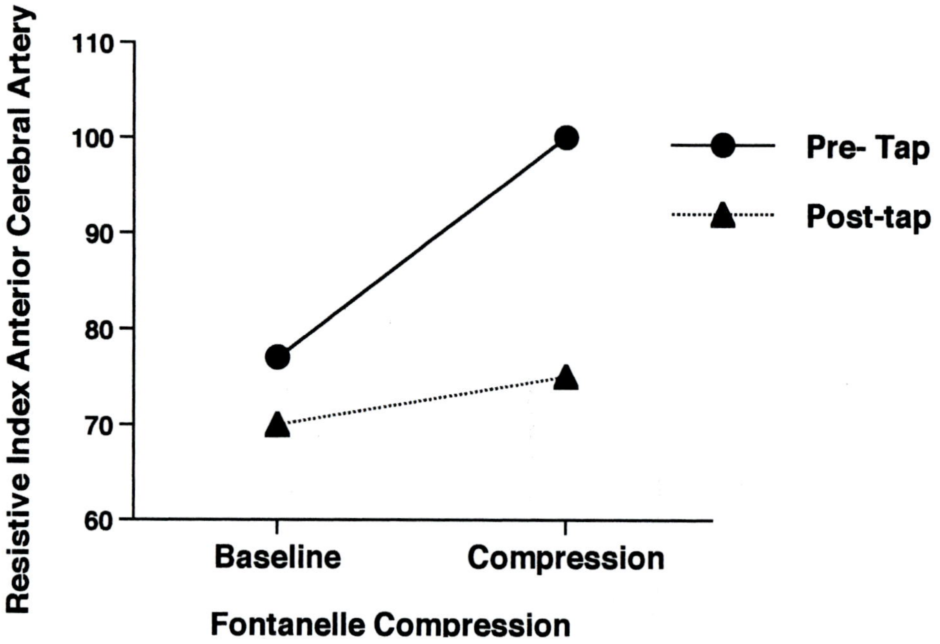

FIG. 53-20. Shunted hydrocephalus less sensitive to pressure effects on fontanelle. Graph of serial RI determinations in an infant with hydrocephalus before and after shunt shows markedly diminished hemodynamic response to fontanelle compression after ventricular drainage. Note similar RI without fontanelle compression.

VASCULAR MALFORMATIONS

The most common intracranial vascular malformation presenting in the neonatal period is the **vein of Galen malformation.** Color flow Doppler imaging can be useful in the identification of vein of Galen malformations and in distinguishing the two most common types.[50] The **choroidal type** is characterized by multiple abnormal feeding vessels arising in the midbrain with venous drainage via an aneurysmally dilated vein of Galen and straight sinus (Fig. 53-22). The **infundibular type** is an arteriovenous fistula with one or few arterial feeders draining directly into the vein of Galen (Fig. 53-23). Spectral Doppler imaging typically shows arterialization of venous flow and increased flow velocities with reduced pulsatility of the arterial feeders. Blood flow in the more peripheral portions of brain may show diminished or absent flow as a result of a "vascular steal" phenomenon away from the normal cerebral circulation via the low-resistance malformation.[51] Color flow Doppler imaging has also been used to monitor and quantify the hemodynamic effects of interventional procedures such as transcatheter embolization.[52] Occasionally, large facial or cervical arteriovenous malformations may have an intracranial component that can be suggested by abnormal intracranial hemodynamics (Fig. 53-24).

INTRACRANIAL TUMORS

Neonatal intracranial tumors are uncommon and thus experience with Doppler characterization of these lesions is limited.[53] We have found it helpful in characterizing the degree of intratumoral vascularity and in identifying its vascular supply (Fig. 53-25).

NEAR-FIELD STRUCTURES

Differentiation of Subarachnoid from Subdural Fluid Collections

Color flow Doppler ultrasound using high-frequency linear transducers can be used to characterize extracerebral fluid collections as subarachnoid, subdural, or combined. Because superficial cortical blood vessels lie within the pia-arachnoid, fluid in this (subarachnoid) space lifts the cortical vessels away from the brain surface. Fluid in the subdural space pushes cortical vessels toward the brain surface and is separated from these vessels by a thin membrane (Fig. 53-26).

Text continued on page 1524.

A

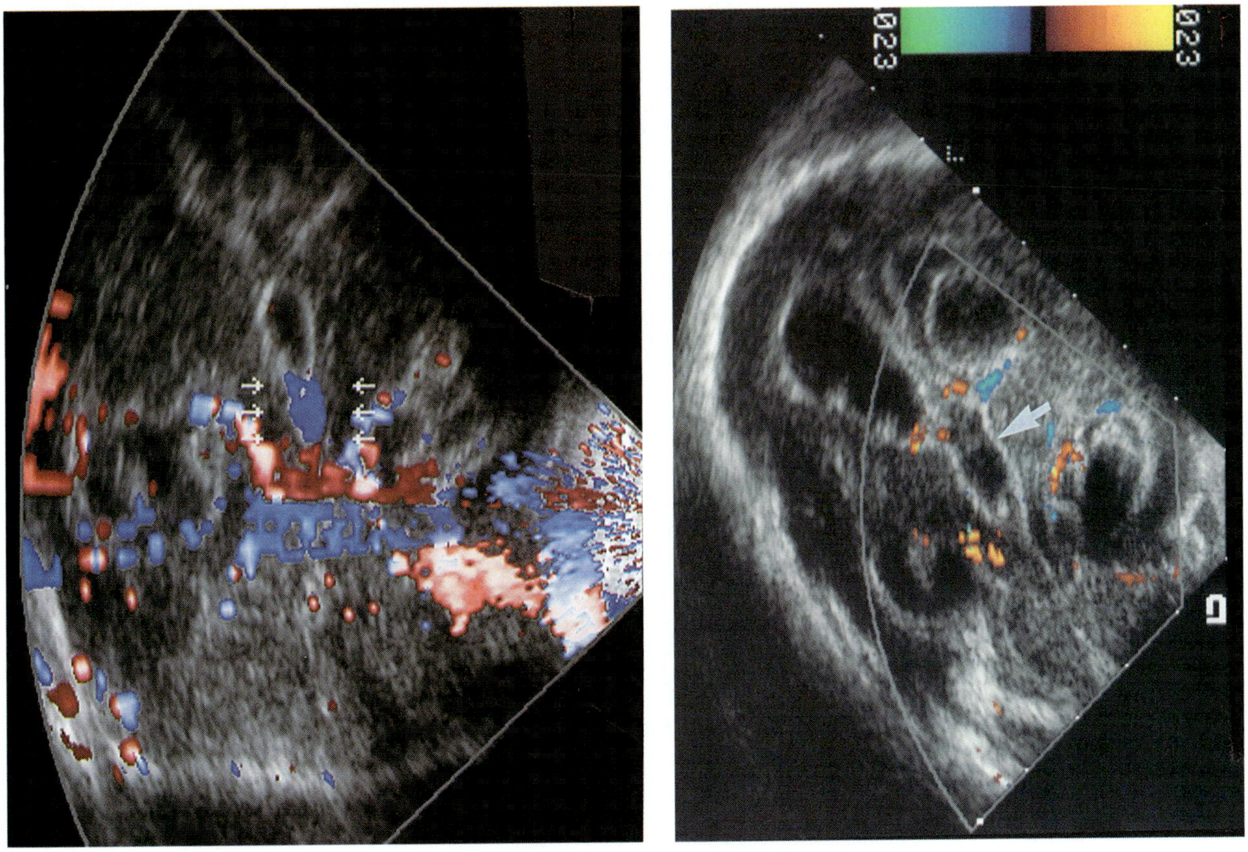

B

FIG. 53-21. Evaluation of aqueductal patency (angled axial color flow Doppler sonogram turned 90 degrees for ease of visualization). **A,** Communicating hydrocephalus (extraventricular obstruction) and patent aqueduct of Sylvius show blue color signal *(arrows)* in the third ventricle caused by normal retrograde flow of CSF from fourth ventricle obtained immediately after manual compression and rapid release of fontanelle. **B,** Intraventricular hemorrhage causing hydrocephalus. Clot obstructs the outlet of third ventricle *(arrow)* and allows no retrograde flow during rapid release of fontanelle compression.

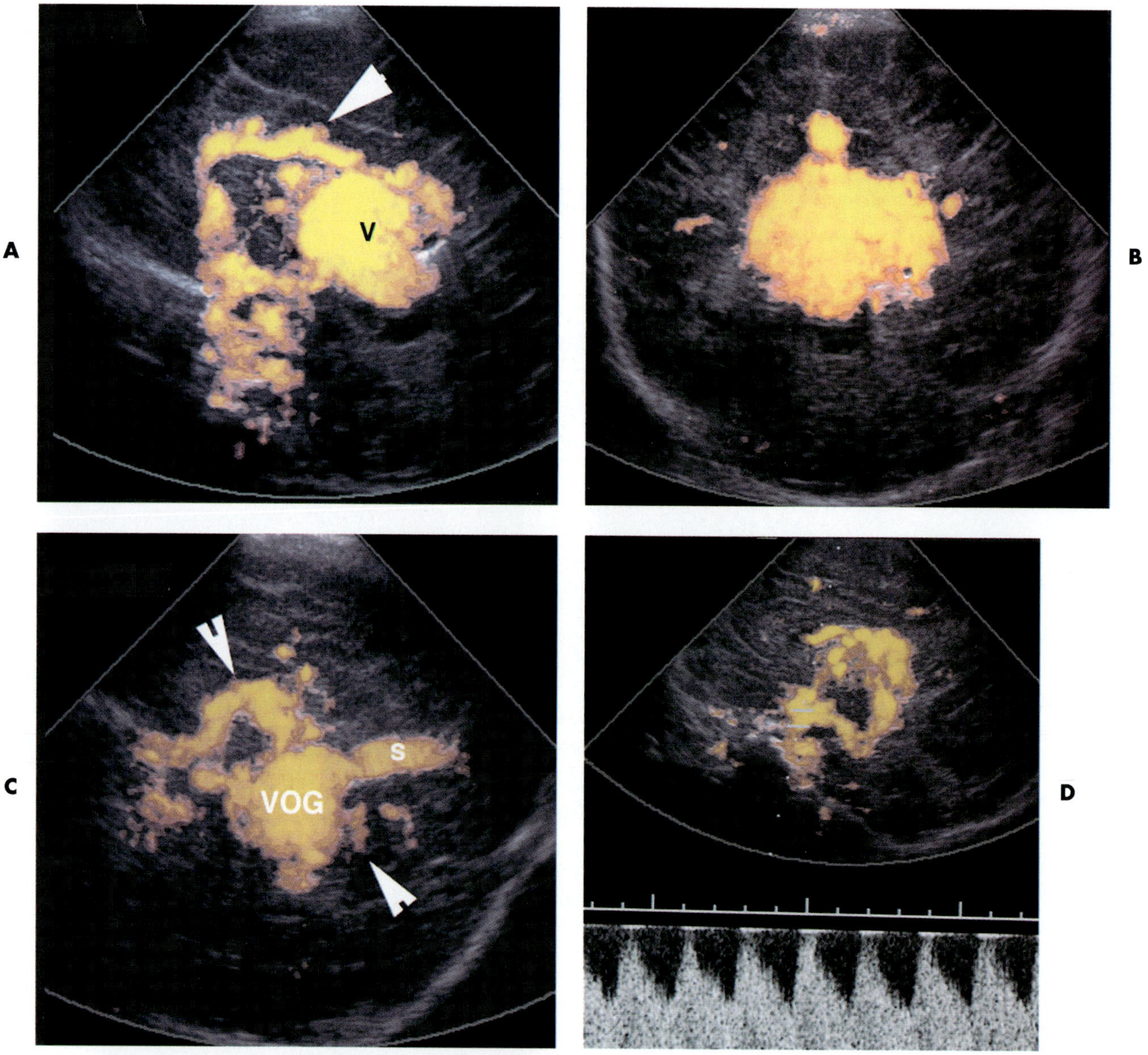

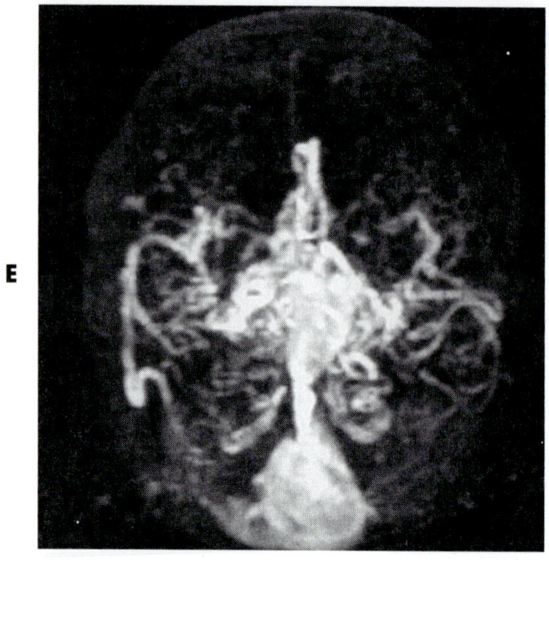

FIG. 53-22. Choroidal type vein of Galen aneurysm. **A,** Sagittal and, **B,** coronal amplitude mode (power) color flow Doppler images show large vein of Galen aneurysm, *V*, and dilated pericallosal artery *(arrowhead)*. **C,** Right posterior axial image shows multiple abnormal vessels arising from midbrain *(arrowheads)* and draining into an aneurysmally dilated vein of Galen aneurysm, *VOG*, and straight sinus, *S*. **D,** Pulsed wave Doppler tracing of the basilar artery shows markedly elevated flow velocities with dampened pulsatility. **E,** Axial time-of-flight magnetic resonance angiography confirms findings.

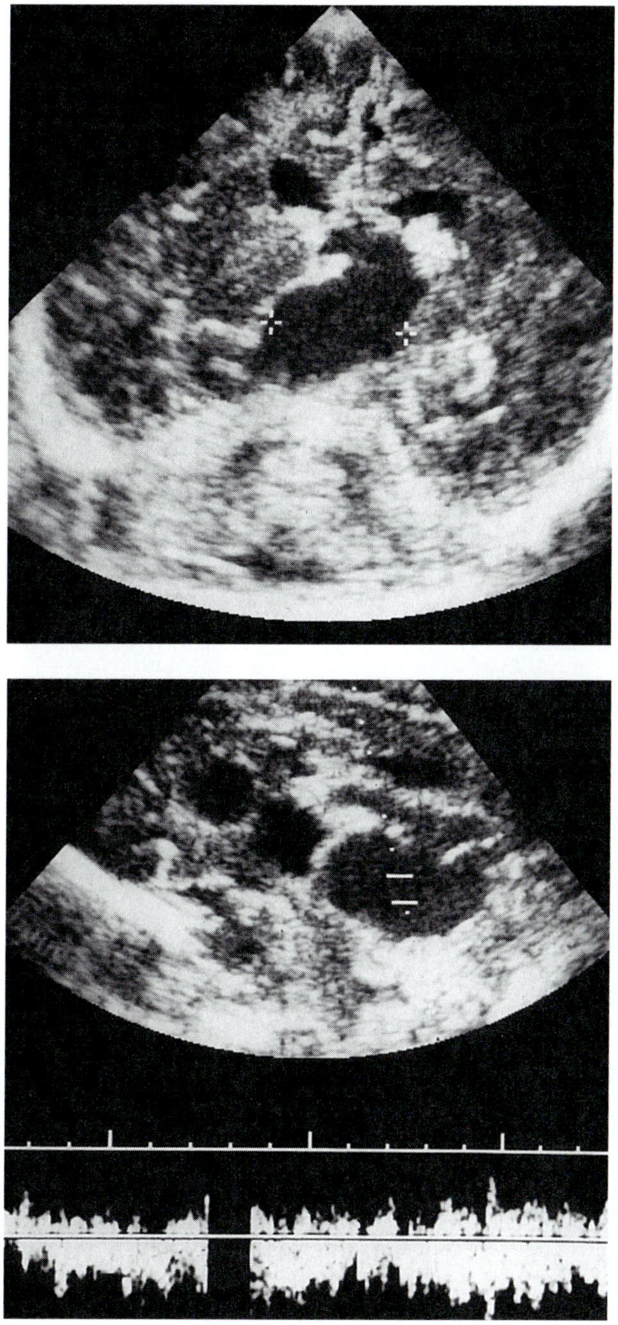

A

B

FIG. 53-23. Mural or infundibular type vein of Galen aneurysm. **A,** Dilated vein of Galen aneurysm *(between cursors)* with single feeding vessel entering superiorly *(arrow)*. **B,** Pulsed wave Doppler tracing from vein of Galen shows characteristic turbulent flow (posteriorly angled coronal image).

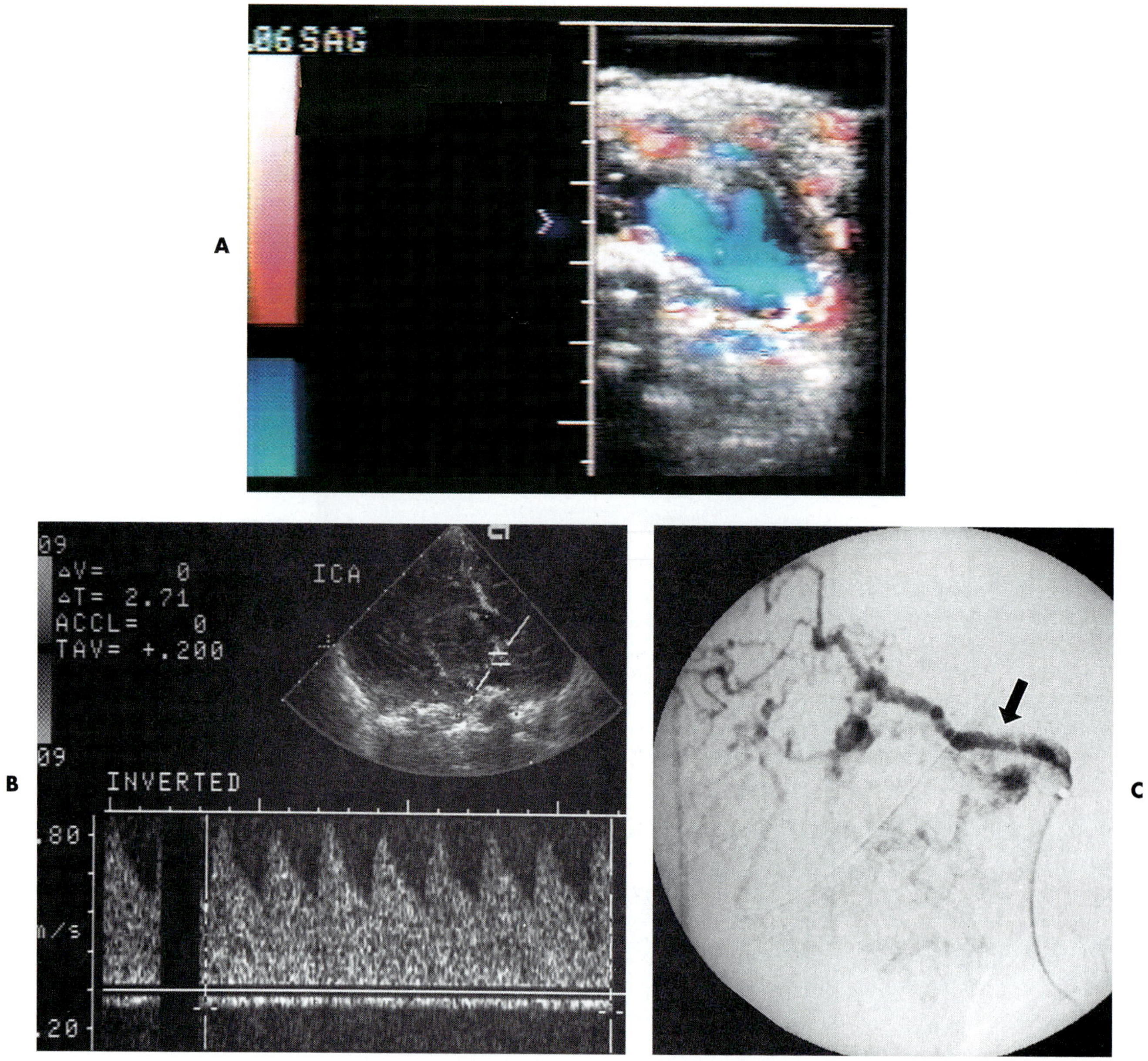

FIG. 53-24. Cervical vascular malformation with partial intracranial blood supply. **A,** Large vascular malformation of the neck and face sagittal. Color flow Doppler image. **B,** Supraclinoid internal carotid artery. **Inverted Doppler tracing** shows high-velocity, low-pulsatility flow in caudad (**reversed**) direction. **C,** Right internal carotid arteriogram shows multiple feeding vessels arising from a dilated ophthalmic artery *(arrow)*.

A

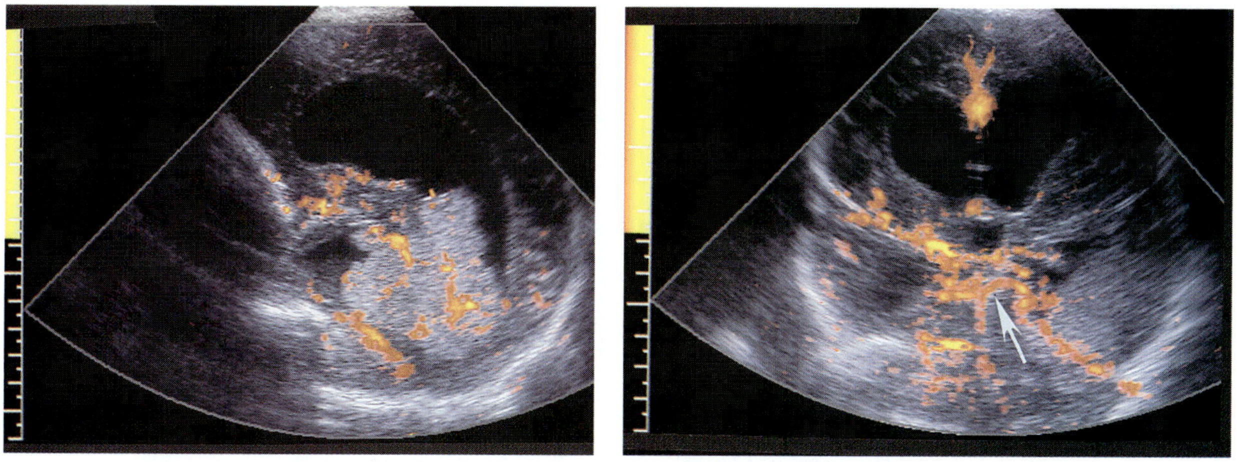

B

FIG. 53-25. Choroid plexus papilloma in 6-week-old infant. **A,** Angled sagittal and, **B,** coronal color amplitude (power) Doppler images show increased tumor vascularity within the echogenic mass, with arterial supply arising from a branch of the basilar artery *(arrow)*.

A

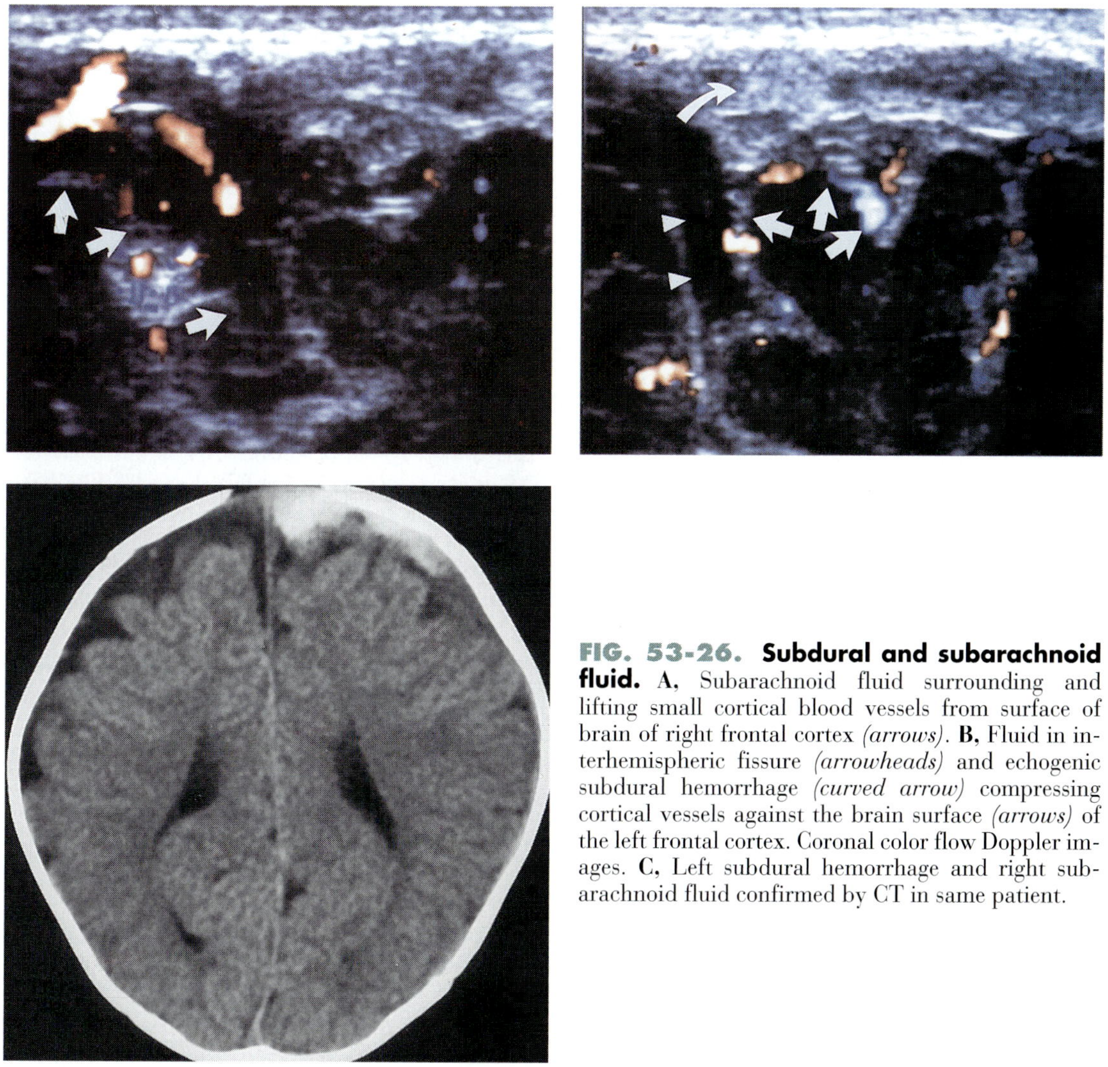

B

C

FIG. 53-26. Subdural and subarachnoid fluid. **A,** Subarachnoid fluid surrounding and lifting small cortical blood vessels from surface of brain of right frontal cortex *(arrows)*. **B,** Fluid in interhemispheric fissure *(arrowheads)* and echogenic subdural hemorrhage *(curved arrow)* compressing cortical vessels against the brain surface *(arrows)* of the left frontal cortex. Coronal color flow Doppler images. **C,** Left subdural hemorrhage and right subarachnoid fluid confirmed by CT in same patient.

A 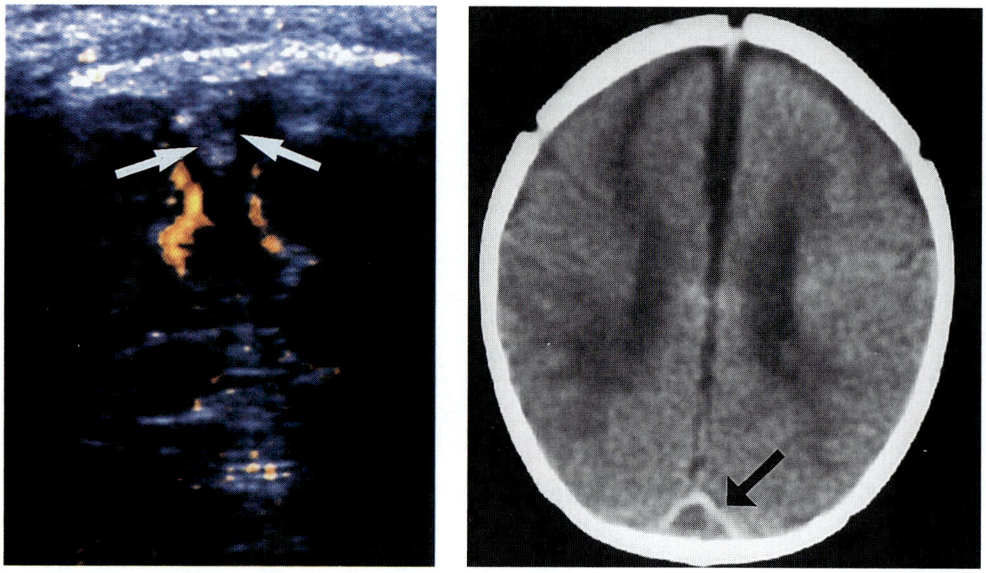 B

FIG. 53-27. Sagittal sinus thrombosis in 6-week-old infant. **A,** No flow present within the superior sagittal sinus *(arrows)*. Coronal color amplitude Doppler image. **B,** Clot in superior sagittal sinus confirms no flow *(arrow)*. Axial postcontrast CT.

Correlation with magnetic resonance imaging and CT suggests that color flow Doppler imaging is reliable in making this differentiation.

Venous Thrombosis

Thrombosis of the intracranial venous sinuses may occur in the neonate as the result of dehydration and as a complication of meningitis. Color flow Doppler ultrasound can be used as a noninvasive tool for initial identification and monitoring of these infants[11] (Fig. 53-27).

REFERENCES

1. Bada HS, Hajjar W, Chua C et al. Noninvasive diagnosis of neonatal asphyxia and intraventricular hemorrhage by Doppler ultrasound. *J Pediatr* 1979;95:775-779.
2. Archer LNJ, Evans DH, Levene MI. Doppler ultrasound examination of the anterior cerebral arteries of normal newborn infants: the effect of postnatal age. *Early Hum Dev* 1985;10:255-260.
3. Grant EG, White EM, Schellinger D et al. Cranial duplex sonography of the infant. *Radiology* 1987;163:177-185.
4. Taylor GA. Current concepts in neonatal cranial Doppler sonography. *Ultrasound Q* 1992;4:223-244.
5. Rubin JM, Bude RO, Carson PL et al. Power Doppler: a potentially useful alternative to mean-frequency based color Doppler sonography. *Radiology* 1994;190:853-856.
6. Taylor GA. Regional cerebral blood flow estimates in newborn lamb using amplitude mode color Doppler ultrasound. *Pediatr Radiol* 1996;26:282-286.

Technique

7. Wong WS, Tsuruda JS, Liberman RL et al. Color Doppler imaging of intracranial vessels in the neonate. *AJR* 1989; 152:1065-1070.
8. Mitchell DG, Merton D, Needleman L et al. Neonatal brain: color Doppler imaging. Part I. Technique and vascular anatomy. *Radiology* 1988;167:303-306.
9. Mitchell DG, Merton D, Mirsky PJ et al. Circle of Willis in newborns: color Doppler imaging of 53 healthy full-term infants. *Radiology* 1989;172:201-205.
10. Taylor GA. Intracranial venous system in the newborn: evaluation of normal anatomy and flow characteristics with color Doppler US. *Radiology* 1992;183:449-452.
11. Dean LM, Taylor GA. The intracranial venous system in infants: normal and abnormal findings on duplex and color Doppler sonography. *AJR* 1995;164:151-156.
12. 510(k) *Guide for Measuring and Reporting Acoustic Output of Diagnostic Medical Devices.* Rockville, Md: US Food and Drug Administration, 1985.
13. Seibert JJ, McCowan TC, Chadduck WM et al. Duplex pulsed Doppler US versus intracranial pressure in the neonate: clinical and experimental studies. *Radiology* 1989;171:155-159.
14. Perlman JM, Hill A, Volpe JJ. The effect of patent ductus arteriosus on flow velocity in the anterior cerebral arteries: ductal steal in the premature infant. *J Pediatr* 1981;99:767-771.
15. Taylor GA. Effect of scanning pressure on intracranial hemodynamics during transfontanellar duplex US. *Radiology* 1992;185:763-766.
16. Taylor GA, Martin G, Short BL. Cardiac determinants of cerebral blood flow during ECMO. *Invest Radiol* 1989;24:511-516.
17. Taylor GA, Short BL, Walker LK et al. Intracranial blood flow: quantification with duplex Doppler and color Doppler flow US. *Radiology* 1990;176:231-236.
18. Greisen G, Johansen K, Ellison PH et al. Cerebral blood flow in the newborn infant: comparison of Doppler ultrasound and 133 xenon clearance. *J Pediatr* 1984;104:411-418.
19. Hansen NB, Stonestreet BS, Rosenkrantz TS et al. Validity of Doppler measurement of anterior cerebral artery blood flow velocity: correlation with brain blood flow in piglets. *Pediatrics* 1983;72:526-531.
20. Lundell BP, Lindstrom DP, Arnold TG. Neonatal cerebral blood flow velocity. I. An in vitro validation of the pulsed Doppler technique. *Acta Pediatr Scand* 1984;73:810-815.

Normal Hemodynamics

21. Horgan JG, Rumack CM, Hay T et al. Absolute intracranial blood-flow velocities evaluated by duplex Doppler sonography in asymptomatic preterm and term neonates. *AJR* 1989;152: 1059-1064.
22. Agoestina T, Humphrey JH, Taylor GA et al. Safety of one 52 mmol (50,000 IU) oral dose of vitamin A administered to neonates. *Bull World Health Organ* 1994;72:859-868.
23. Raju TNK, Ikos E. Regional cerebral blood velocity in infants. A real-time transcranial and fontanellar pulsed Doppler study. *J Ultrasound Med* 1987;6:497-507.
24. Winkler P, Helmke K. Duplex-scanning of the deep venous drainage in the evaluation of blood flow velocity of the cerebral vascular system in infants. *Pediatr Radiol* 1989;19:79-90.
25. Cowan F, Thoresen M. Changes in superior sagittal sinus blood velocities due to postural alterations and pressure on the head of the newborn infant. *Pediatrics* 1985;75:1038-1047.

Intensive Care Therapies and Cerebral Hemodynamics

26. Rennie JM, South M, Morley CJ. Cerebral blood flow velocity variability in infants receiving assisted ventilation. *Arch Dis Child* 1987;62:1247-1251.
27. Perlman JM, Volpe JJ. Suctioning in the preterm infant: effects on cerebral blood flow velocity, intracranial pressure, and arterial blood pressure. *Pediatrics* 1983;72:329-334.
28. Taylor GA, Short BL, Glass P et al. Cerebral hemodynamics in infants undergoing extracorporeal membrane oxygenation: further observations. *Radiology* 1988;1968:163-167.
29. Mitchell DG, Merton D, Desai H et al. Neonatal brain: color Doppler imaging. Part II. Altered flow patterns from extracorporeal membrane oxygenation. *Radiology* 1988;167:307-310.
30. Taylor GA, Walker LK. Intracranial venous system in newborns treated with extracorporeal membrane oxygenation: Doppler US evaluation after ligation of the right jugular vein. *Radiology* 1992;183:453-456.

Diffuse Neuronal Injury

31. Taylor GA, Trescher WH, Johnston MV et al. Experimental neuronal injury in the newborn lamb: a comparison of N-Methyl-D-Aspartic acid receptor blockade and nitric oxide synthesis inhibition on lesion size and cerebal hyperemia. *Pediatr Res* 1995;38:644-51.
32. van Bel F, van de Bor M, Stijnen T et al. Cerebral blood flow velocity pattern in healthy and asphyxiated newborns: a controlled study. *Eur J Pediatr* 1987;146:461-467.
33. Stark JE, Seibert JJ. Cerebral artery Doppler ultrasonography for prediction of outcome after perinatal asphyxia. *J Ultrasound Med* 1994;13:595-600.
34. van Bel F, van de Bor M, Baan J et al. The influence of abnormal blood gases on cerebral blood flow velocity in the preterm newborn. *Neuropediatrics* 1988;19:27-32.
35. Deeg KH, Rupprecht TH, Zeilinger G. Doppler sonographic classification of brain edema in infants. *Pediatr Radiol* 1990;20:509-514.
36. Vannucci RC. Mechanisms of perinatal hypoxic-ischemic brain damage. *Semin Perinatol* 1993;17:330-337.
37. McMenamin JB, Volpe JJ. Doppler ultrasonography in the determination of neonatal brain death. *Ann Neurol* 1983;14:302-307.
38. Glasier CM, Seibert JJ, Chadduck WM et al. Brain death in infants: evaluation with Doppler US. *Radiology* 1989;172:377-380.

Intracranial Hemorrhage and Stroke

39. Gould SJ, Howard S, Hope PL et al. Periventricular intraparenchymal cerebral haemorrhage in preterm infants: the role of venous infarction. *J Pathol* 1987;151:197-202.
40. Volpe JJ. Current concepts of brain injury in the premature infant. *AJR* 1989;153:243-251.
41. Taylor GA. Effect of germinal matrix hemorrhage on terminal vein position and patency. *Pediatr Radiol* 1995;25:S37-S40.
42. Hernanz-Schulman M, Cohen W, Genieser NB. Sonography of cerebral infarction in infancy. *AJR* 1988;150:897-902.
43. Taylor GA. Alterations in regional cerebral blood flow in neonatal stroke: imaging with color Doppler. *Pediatr Radiol* 1994;24:111-115.
44. Savoiardo M. CT scanning. In: Barnett HJM, Stein BM, Mohr JP et al, eds. *Stroke, Pathophysiology, Diagnosis and Management. Vol I.* New York: Churchill Livingstone; 1986:189-219.
45. Taylor GA, Trescher WH, Traystman RJ et al. Acute experimental neuronal injury in the newborn lamb: US characterization and demonstration of hemodynamic effects. *Pediatr Radiol* 1993;23:268-275.

Hydrocephalus

46. Bada HS, Miller JE, Menke JA et al. Intracranial pressure and cerebral arterial pulsatile flow measurements in neonatal intraventricular hemorrhage. *J Pediatr* 1982;100:291-296.
47. Taylor GA, Phillips MD, Ichord RN et al. Intracranial compliance in infants: evaluation with Doppler US. *Radiology* 1994;191:787-791.
48. Bruce DA, Berman WA, Schut L. Cerebrospinal fluid pressure monitoring in children: physiology, pathology and clinical usefulness. *Adv Pediatr* 1977;24:233-290.
49. Winkler P. Colour-coded echographic flow imaging and spectral analysis of cerebrospinal fluid (CSF) in infants. Part II. CSF-dynamics. *Pediatr Radiol* 1992;22:31-42.

Vascular Malformations

50. Tessler FN, Dion J, Vinuela F et al. Cranial arteriovenous malformations in neonates: color Doppler imaging with angiographic correlation. *AJR* 1989;153:1027-1030.
51. Soto G, Daneman A, Hellman J. Doppler evaluation of cerebral arteries in a galenic vein malformation. *J Ultrasound Med* 1985;4:673-675.
52. Westra SJ, Curran JG, Duckwiler GR et al. Pediatric intracranial vascular malformations: evaluation of treatment results with color Doppler US. *Radiology* 1993;186:775-783.

Intracranial Tumors

53. Chow PP, Horgan JG, Burns P et al. Choroid plexus papilloma: detection by real-time and Doppler sonography. *AJR* 1986;7:168-170.

CHAPTER 54

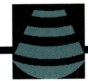

Doppler of the Brain in Children

Joanna J. Seibert, M.D.

CHAPTER OUTLINE

Transcranial Doppler (TCD) sonography is a noninvasive emerging technique that uses a 2- to 2.5-MHz pulsed wave Doppler transducer to measure the velocity and pulsatility of blood flow within the intracranial arteries of the circle of Willis and the vertebrobasilar system through the thin temporal bone, the orbits, or the foramen magnum. Duplex Doppler with color flow imaging through the anterior fontanelle has proven useful in the neonate to evaluate abnormalities of cerebral blood flow in the neonate and young child.[1-4] Continuous wave and nonimaging pulsed wave Doppler techniques insonating specific vessels using criteria for vessel identification based primarily on depth and direction of flow for intracranial vessels were developed through the temporal bone in adults in the early 1980s.[5-6] The blinded technique requires meticulous skill and ability to maintain the mental image of the circle of Willis. Its greatest advantages are the small size of the units, lower purchase price, Doppler sensitivity, and window maneuverability. Duplex sonography with color imaging is readily available in radiology departments, which allows positive vessel identification and more reliable and reproducible information.[7]

TECHNIQUE

Three naturally occurring cranial windows (in addition to burr holes and surgical defects) can be used routinely after fontanelle closure in children to insonate the intracranial circulation: (1) **the temporal bone**, (2) **the orbit,** and (3) **the foramen magnum.**[8] The **transtemporal approach** is through the thin suprazygomatic portion of the temporal bone with a 2-MHz transducer. We have also used a 2.5-MHz transducer to insonate this plane before the 2-MHz transducer was available. The transtemporal window is usually found on the temporal bone cephalad to the zygomatic arch and anterior to the ear. The intracranial anatomic window in this plane is the heart-shaped cerebral peduncles (Fig. 54-1, *A*). Just anterior to the peduncles is the star-shaped echogenic interpeduncular or suprasellar cistern. Anteriorly and laterally from this basilar cistern lies the echogenic fissure for the middle cerebral artery (MCA). Color imaging (Fig. 54-1, *B*) and spectral analysis (Fig. 54-1, *C*) of this vessel will show flow toward the transducer. Insonating the vessel deeper toward the midline directs the operator into the bifurcation of the A1 segment of the anterior cerebral artery (ACA) and the MCA. Spectral analysis at this bifurcation landmark will show flow in the MCA toward the

A B C

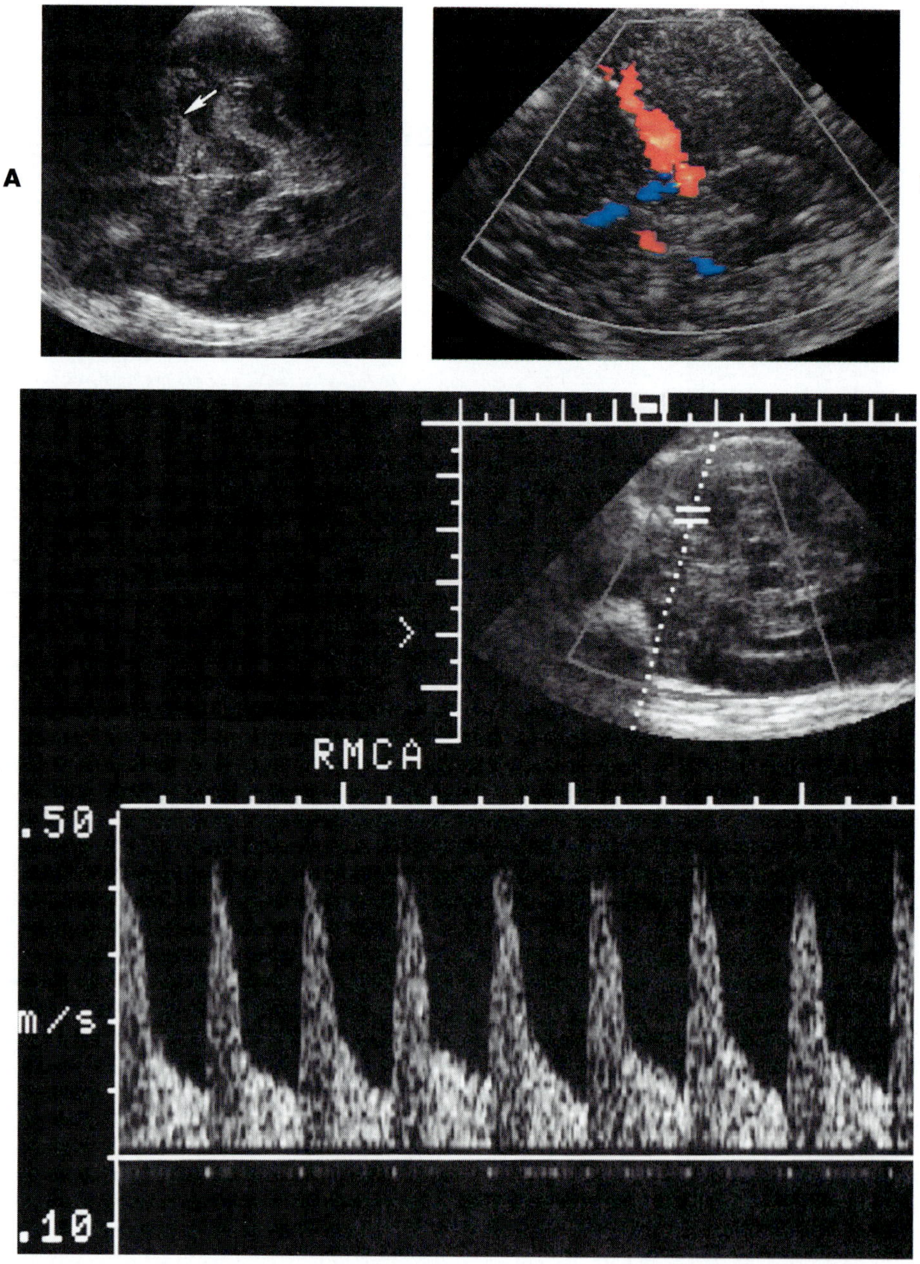

FIG. 54-1. Temporal window. A, Transtemporal transcranial Doppler scan with normal landmarks. Note the heart-shaped cerebral peduncles with the echogenic suprasellar cistern. Anteriorly and laterally from this basilar cistern is the echogenic fissure for the MCA *(arrow)*. **B,** Transtemporal color flow Doppler scan again shows landmark of heart-shaped cerebral peduncles. Flow is directed toward the transducer in red in the MCA in the middle cerebral fissure just anterior to the cerebral peduncles. Flow in the ACA on that side is in blue away from the transducer. Flow is also seen in blue in the PCA on the opposite side as it courses around the cerebral peduncle. **C,** Doppler waveform shows the right MCA with flow directed toward transducer.

Continued.

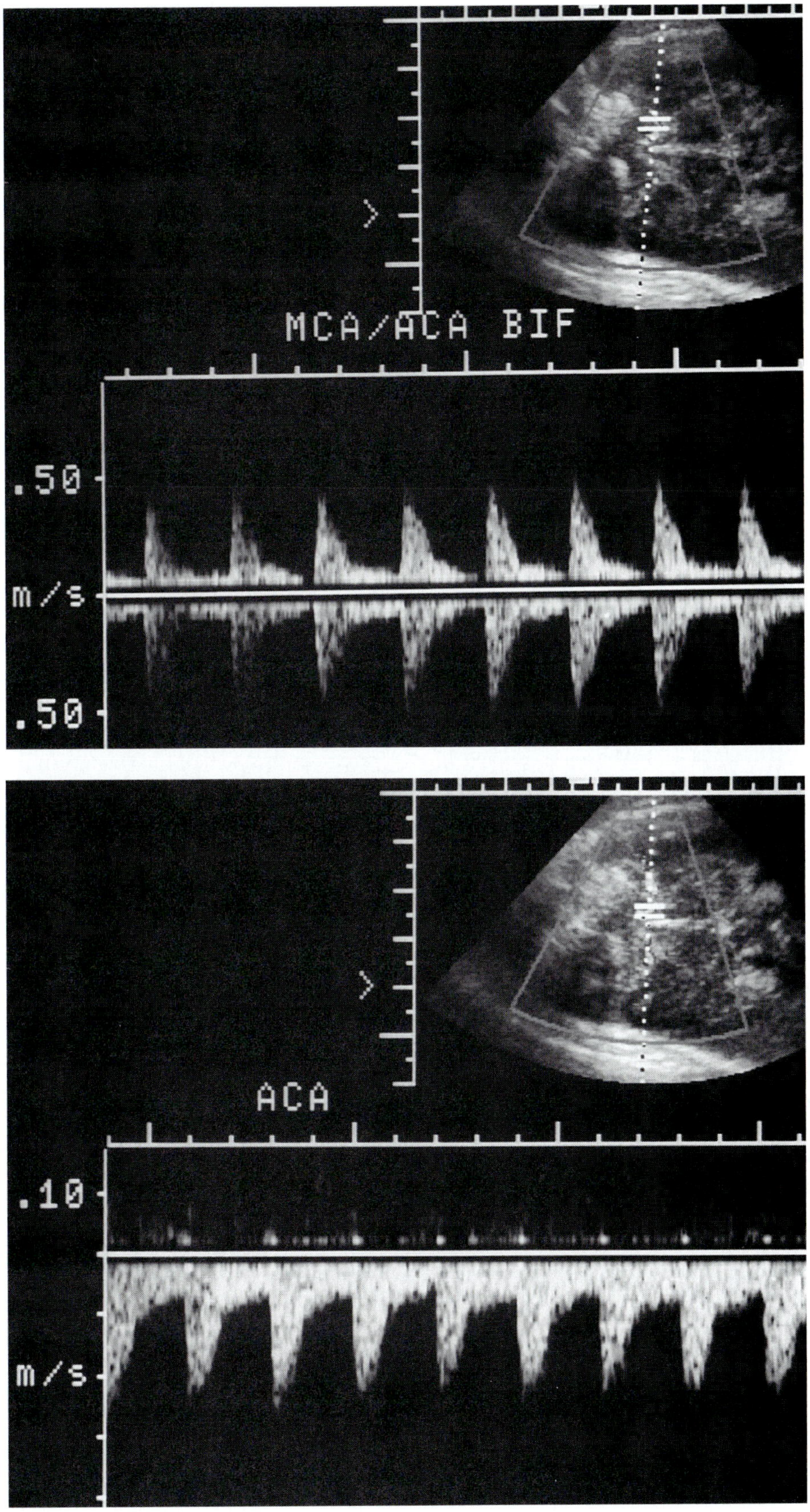

FIG. 54-1, cont'd. **D,** Doppler waveform shows bifurcation of MCA and ACA with flow toward transducer in MCA and away from transducer in ACA. **E,** Doppler waveform shows ACA with flow away from transducer.

transducer and flow in the ACA away from the transducer (Fig. 54-1, *D*). As the cursor is moved more medially, flow is seen entirely in the ACA away from the transducer (Fig. 54-1, *E*). The MCA should be studied from its most peripheral location to the point of bifurcation, and the ACA should be studied as medially as possible. The posterior cerebral artery (PCA) can be visualized as it circles around the cerebral peduncles. Flow in this vessel may be away or toward the transducer. Often the MCA, ACA, and the PCA on the opposite side may also be evaluated. Angle correction with color flow in the vessel should be attempted but is often difficult because of the size of these vessels. Angle correction is felt to be less necessary with the MCA, ACA, and ophthalmic (OA) artery since these vessels are coursing almost directly toward or away from the transducer.

The vertebral and basilar arteries can be studied through the foramen magnum with a 2-MHz transducer. If the patient lies on one side and the head is bowed slightly so the chin touches the chest, the gap between the cranium and the atlas is enlarged. The transducer is placed midline in the nape of the neck and angled through the foramen magnum toward the eye. The normal landmark is the rounded hypoechoic medulla just anterior to the echogenic clivus (Fig. 54-2, *A*). The vertebral arteries appear in a V-shaped fashion as they rise to the medullopontine junction to form the basilar artery between the hypoechoic medulla-pons junction and the echogenic clivus (Fig. 54-2, *B*). From this posterior view, flow in the vertebral and basilar arteries should be directed away from the transducer (Fig. 54-2, *C*).

The ophthalmic artery (OA) is evaluated through the orbit with the eyes closed with a 3-, 5-, or 7.5-MHz transducer (Fig. 54-3) on its lowest power setting. Flow in the OA should be toward the transducer (see Fig. 54-3, *A*). The ophthalmic artery enters the optic foramen to lie lateral and slightly inferior to the optic nerve. It then usually crosses superior to the optic nerve and proceeds anteriorly on the medial side of the orbit. The central retinal artery branch of the ophthalmic artery is the easiest branch interrogated by color flow Doppler imaging just posterior to the retina (see Fig. 54-3). Since visualization of this central retinal artery entails directing sound waves through the lens, the lowest power setting is recommended. Current recommended FDA guidelines suggest limiting spatial peak temporal average to 17 mW/cm^2 for orbital imaging.[9,10] However, a large branch of the ophthalmic artery proceeds along the nasal or medial wall of the orbit. Since interrogating this vessel does not involve directing the sound beam through the lens, a higher power setting may be used.

On spectral analysis of the waveform, the maximum, minimum, and mean velocities (mean of the maximum velocity envelope) can be measured as well as the index of pulsatility. We have used the **Pourcelot or RI** (systolic velocity minus diastolic velocity divided by systolic velocity). A few other investigators have used the **pulsatility index (PI)** (systolic velocity minus diastolic velocity divided by mean velocity). Both of these pulsatility indices, the RI and PI, are ratios that minimize the effect of our difficulty in angle correcting in these intracranial vessels. Since the RI is a ratio, it may be expressed as a whole number (70 to 80), representing a percentage (%), or as a fraction (0.7 to 0.8). An RI greater than 1, 100%, 100 means that diastolic flow is reversed or in the opposite direction to systolic flow. At least two readings should be made for each vessel. The highest velocity obtained may be taken as the truest velocity, as it is believed to be the velocity obtained at the best insonating angle to the vessel.[11]

Normal mean velocity in the MCA in adults is 50 to 80 cm/s, in the ACA 35 to 60 cm/s, in the PCA 30 to 50 cm/s, and in the basilar artery 25 to 50 cm/s. The velocity in the OA is normally approximately one fourth the velocity in the MCA. The velocity in the PCA and vertebral and basilar arteries should be approximately one half the velocity in the MCA. **Normal RI after fontanelle closure** should be 0.50 to 0.59, except in the OA, which has a higher RI (usually 0.70 to 0.79) and less diastolic flow because it supplies a muscular bed (see Fig. 54-3, *B*).[8] Velocities up to 150 cm/s have been described in patients with sickle cell disease secondary to anemia.[12-13]

ULTRASOUND DOSAGE

The American Institute of Ultrasound and Medicine (AIUM) and the federal guidelines of the **spatial peak time averaged intensity (I_{SPTA}) for the pediatric head should not exceed 94 mW/cm^2**. For evaluating vessels in the eye, the limit is 17 mW/cm^2.[14] The power settings of transducers of various manufacturers are different for each piece of equipment and each probe.[15] With Acuson equipment, the energy levels for the eye are within the guidelines for the 2-MHz probe if a low or medium setting is used for Doppler imaging. This is also true for the 3-MHz transducer.[16] The other transducers are only within the guidelines on the low power setting with Acuson. However, when the transtemporal approach is used, at least 65% (and probably much more) of the energy is attenuated by the skull. These higher settings may therefore be used in the transtemporal approach but should not be exceeded in using the eye or foramen magnum.[17]

A

B

C

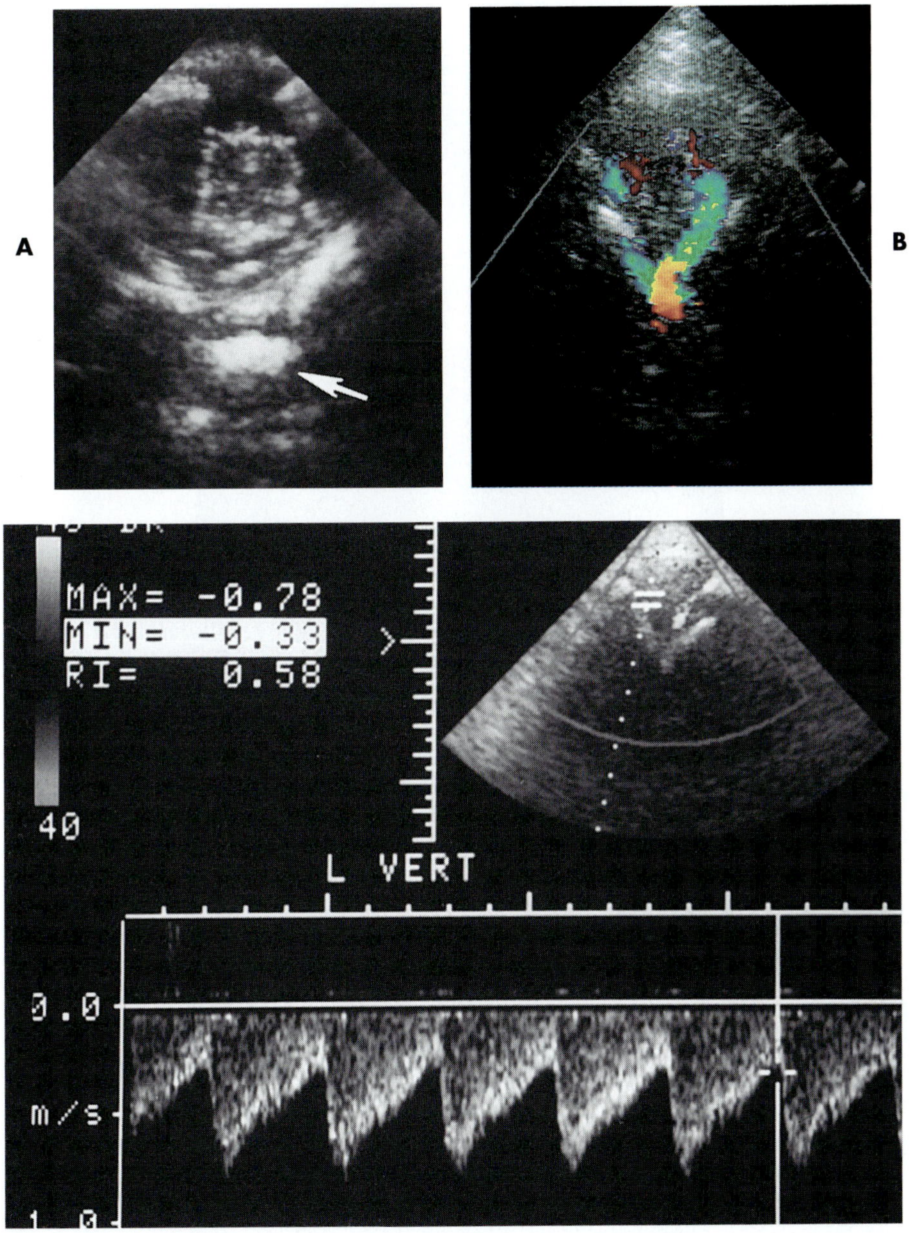

FIG. 54-2. Occipital view through the foramen magnum. **A,** Normal landmark in the transforamen magnum view shows rounded medulla just anterior to the very echogenic clivus *(arrow)*. **B,** With color imaging the V-shaped vertebral arteries join to form the basilar artery at the medulla-pons junction. **C,** Doppler waveform in vertebral artery shows flow away from transducer.

A

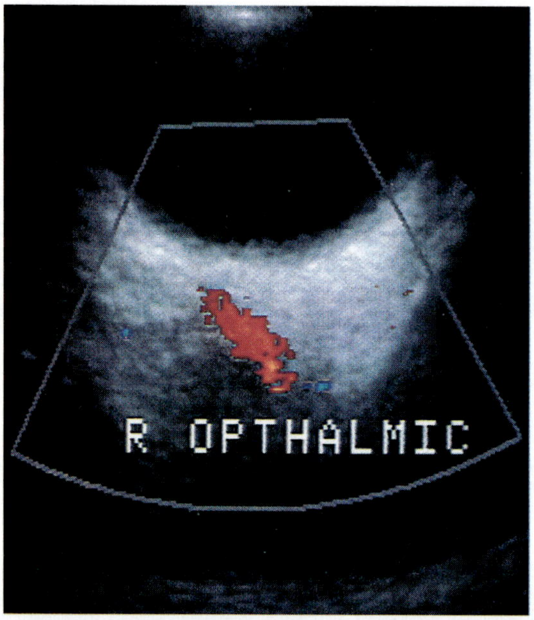

B

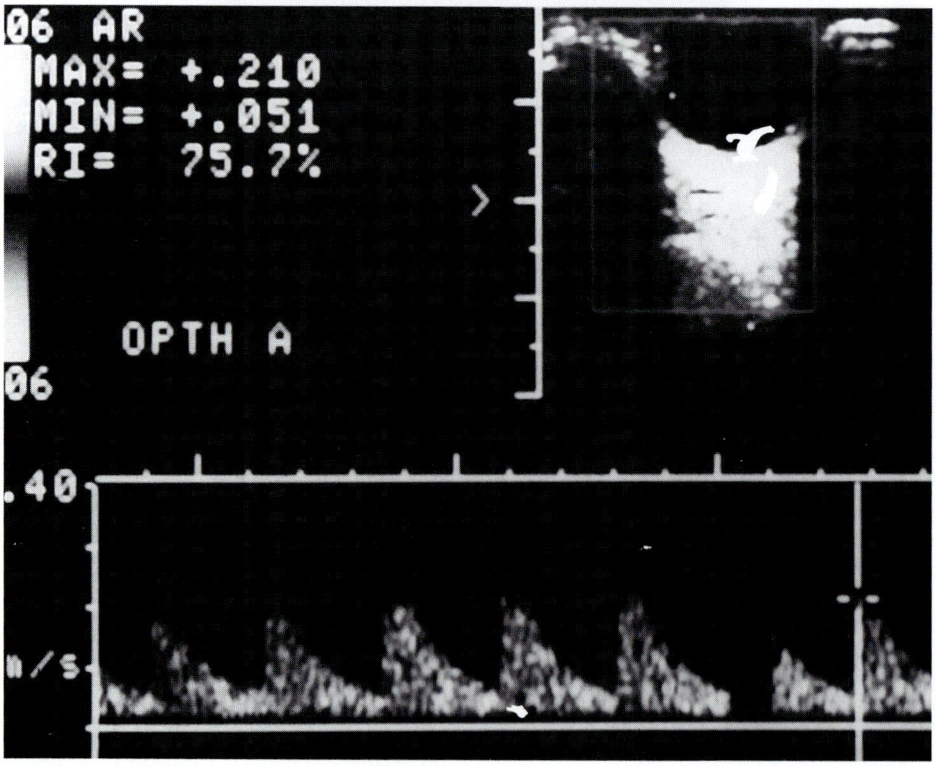

FIG. 54-3. Normal TCD through eye. **A,** Color flow visualizing the OA posterior to the globe with flow directed toward the transducer in red. **B,** Normal waveform of OA with RI of 75.

PITFALLS IN DOPPLER INVESTIGATIONS

Winkler et al.[18-19] have described many pitfalls to Doppler examination in children. Pitfalls may be avoided by using low wall filter adjustment, high Doppler frequency, and critical assessment of velocity spectral analysis. One artery should not be used to represent the entire cerebral circulation.

INDICATIONS FOR TRANSCRANIAL DOPPLER

ESTABLISHED INDICATIONS FOR TCD IN ADULTS

Detection of severe (>65%) stenosis in a major basal intracranial artery
Evaluating patterns and extent of collateral circulation in patients with known severe stenosis or occlusion
Evaluating and following patients with *vasospasm* or *vasoconstriction*, especially after subarachnoid hemorrhage
Detection of arteriovenous malformations and study of their feeding arteries and effects of treatment
Confirmation of the clinical diagnosis of brain death[20]

POTENTIAL OTHER APPLICATIONS FOR TCD IN ADULTS

Monitoring during cerebral endarterectomy, cardiopulmonary bypass, and other cerebrovascular/cardiovascular interventional and surgical procedures
Evaluating patients with dilated vasculopathies such as fusiform aneurysms
Assessing autoregulation, physiologic, and pharmacologic responses of the cerebral arteries
Evaluation of patients with migraine headaches[21-23]

INDICATIONS FOR TCD IN CHILDREN

Evaluating children with various vasculopathies such as sickle cell disease and moyamoya
Evaluating children with arteriovenous malformations
Confirmation of clinical brain death
Evaluation of children with asphyxia, cerebral edema, and their treatment, including hyperventilation therapy
Following children with hydrocephalus and subdural effusions
Monitoring children during cerebrovascular and cardiovascular interventional and surgical procedures
Evaluating patients with migraine headaches[8,21,24-27]

VASOSPASM

A major clinical value of TCD in adults is in diagnosing vasospasm that may occur after subarachnoid hemorrhage due to rupture of an intracranial aneurysm or other pathologic condition.[22,23] Patients with persistent severe vasospasm may develop permanent deficits due to cerebral infraction. The vasospasm develops in the first few days following subarachnoid hemorrhage, gradually increases for a week, and then peaks between 11 and 17 days before gradually decreasing. TCD is highly specific (98% to 100%)[28,29] in diagnosing vasospasm, which is manifested as increased blood flow velocity due to a decrease in the luminal cross-sectional area of the affected vessels. TCD can be used to optimize the timing of surgery and to evaluate the effects of therapies. TCD is more accurate in predicting vasospasm of the MCA. TCD cannot be used to assess the ACA beyond its A1 segment or to evaluate the distal branches of the MCA. MCA mean velocities of 100 to 140 cm/s correlate with mild vasospasm demonstrated by angiography. Moderate vasospasm is defined as velocities ranging from 140 to 200 cm/s, and severe vasospasm is considered if velocities are >200 cm/s. A steep increase (>25 cm/s per day) in velocity in the first few days after subarachnoid hemorrhage is associated with a poor prognosis. **Sources of error** in the detection of vasospasm by TCD (compared with arteriography) are distal branch vasospasm, increased intracranial pressure, and reduction in volume flow.[6]

MIGRAINE HEADACHES

Evaluating patients with vascular headaches is a new clinical application for TCD.[6] Thie et al.[30] found a significant increase in mean velocity in migraine patients versus controls in the headache-free period. Thie et al.[31] also found that patients during headache attack with common migraines had decreased intracranial velocities and increased pulsatility whereas symptomatic patients with classic migraines demonstrated an increase in velocities and a decrease in pulsatility. Thie et al.[31]

TABLE 54-1
CEREBRAL DOPPLER CHANGES

	RI	Systolic Velocity
Intracranial Abnormalities		
Intracranial bleed	Increased	(Beat-to-beat variation, risk factor for IVH)
PVL	Increased	
Asphyxia	Decreased acutely	
Brain edema	Increased	
Hydrocephalus	Increased, reverses after drainage	
Subdural	Increased	
Brain death	Increased	Decreased, reverse diastolic
ECMO	Decreased	
Vascular malformation stenoses	Decreased	Increased, turbulence
Extracranial Abnormalities		
Pco_2	Inverse relationship	
Heart rate	Inverse relationship	
Shock		Decreased systolic/diastolic
PDA	Increased	
Pneumothorax	Increased	
Cardiac ischemia	Increased	
GI bleed	Increased	
Polycythemia, hyperviscosity	Increased	Decreased
Drugs		
Indomethacin	Increased	Decreased
Maternal cocaine		Increased
Exogenous surfactant		Increased

PVL, Periventricular leukomalacia; *RI*, resistive index; *IVH*, intraventricular hemorrhage; *ECMO*, extracorporeal membrane oxygenation; *PDA*, patent ductus arteriosus; *GI*, gastrointestinal.

concluded that TCD may have a potential to aid in the differential diagnosis of headaches of unknown etiology and possibly assist in therapeutic interventions.

BRAIN DEATH

Volpe described a characteristic sequence of deterioration of the flow velocity waveform in the ACA in neonatal brain death.[32] First there is loss of forward diastolic flow followed by reversal of diastolic flow, followed by a decrease in systolic flow, and finally, no detectable flow. With this loss of forward diastolic flow, the RI increases, becoming >100 as the diastolic flow is reversed. As is evident in Table 54-1, many factors can increase the RI above 100 in the neonate—increased intracranial pressure with or without hydrocephalus and a PDA are the most common.[4,33] **A markedly elevated RI (100 to 200)** in a term infant with no evidence of hydrocephalus or a PDA is strongly suggestive of brain death.[34] Brain death in the neonate is more difficult to determine than in the older child. Occasionally, the neonate who is clinically brain dead will have normal or decreased RI as well as intracranial perfusion by nuclear medicine scan.[34] **After fontanelle closure,** an RI >100 or absence of any forward diastolic flow in the MCA or ACA in a child with no evidence of hydrocephalus is a reliable predictor of brain death (Figs. 54-4 and 54-5).[35,36] In two independent studies of a total of 91 comatose patients, Petty et al.[35] and Feri et al.[37] found a TCD waveform of absent or complete reversed diastolic flow or small early systolic spikes in at least 2 intracranial arteries in all 43 brain-dead patients but in none of other patients with coma. The age range of the patients was from 2 to 88 years. Bulas et al. reported a study in 19 children (4 to 14 years) who sustained severe closed head injury.[38] All 7 children with complete retrograde diastolic flow on the initial examination met brain death criteria within 24 hours of that study. Feri et al.[37] and Shiogai et al.[36] described 3 very unstable pa-

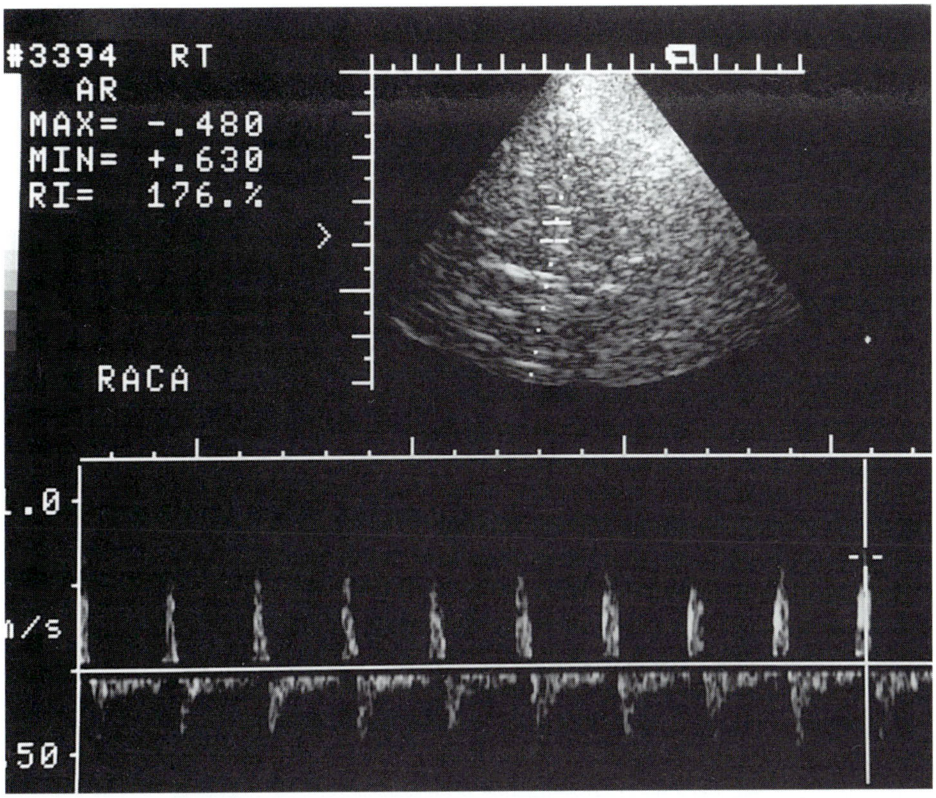

FIG. 54-4. Brain death. Spectral waveform from the right ACA in a 3-year-old with acute encephalopathy, clinically brain dead with RI of 176 with reverse of diastolic flow. (From Seibert JJ. Doppler evaluation of cerebral circulation. In: Dieckmann RA, Fiser DHB, Selbst SM. *Illustrated Textbook of Pediatric Emergency and Critical Care Procedures*. St Louis: Mosby–Year Book; 1997.)

tients who briefly showed diastolic reversal followed by a forward diastolic flow in the same waveform who improved; but of the patients observed by Feri et al., none with complete reversal of diastolic flow survived. Shiogai et al. reported one 80-year-old survivor at 1 month with a Glasgow Coma Scale of 8 in a patient with complete reversal of diastolic flow in the MCA who sustained forward diastolic flow in the PCA.

Undetectable flow in the brain has also been described by Feri et al.,[37] Bulas et al.,[38] Shiogai et al.,[36] and Hasseler et al.[39] in brain death. The occurrence of undetectable middle cerebral flow, however, could sometimes be due to technical factors and therefore should probably not be used unless multiple other exams in the patient showed previous flow in the MCA.

Some investigators have studied simultaneously both the extracranial and the intracranial carotid circulation in their evaluation of brain death. Feri et al.[37] described three waveform patterns in the MCAs as well as in the extracranial internal carotid and vertebral arteries as specific for brain death: (1) diastolic reverse flow without diastolic forward flow, (2) brief systolic forward flow, and (3) undetectable flow. Feri et al.[37] found the absence of middle cerebral flow on TCD with a simultaneous recording of complete reversal of diastolic flow in the extracranial internal carotid artery as a reliable sign of cerebral circulatory arrest. Some investigators have studied only the extracranial carotid circulation in the neck. Jalili et al. reported 100% specificity for brain death with bilateral reversal of diastolic flow in the internal carotid artery of children with brain death.[40]

Some investigators have advocated continuous TCD monitoring. Powers et al. showed that a mean velocity in the MCA of less than 10 cm/s for longer than 30 minutes was not compatible with survival.[41]

TCD may be very helpful also in proving the absence of brain death, especially in patients with a flat EEG secondary to phenobarbital coma (Fig. 54-6).

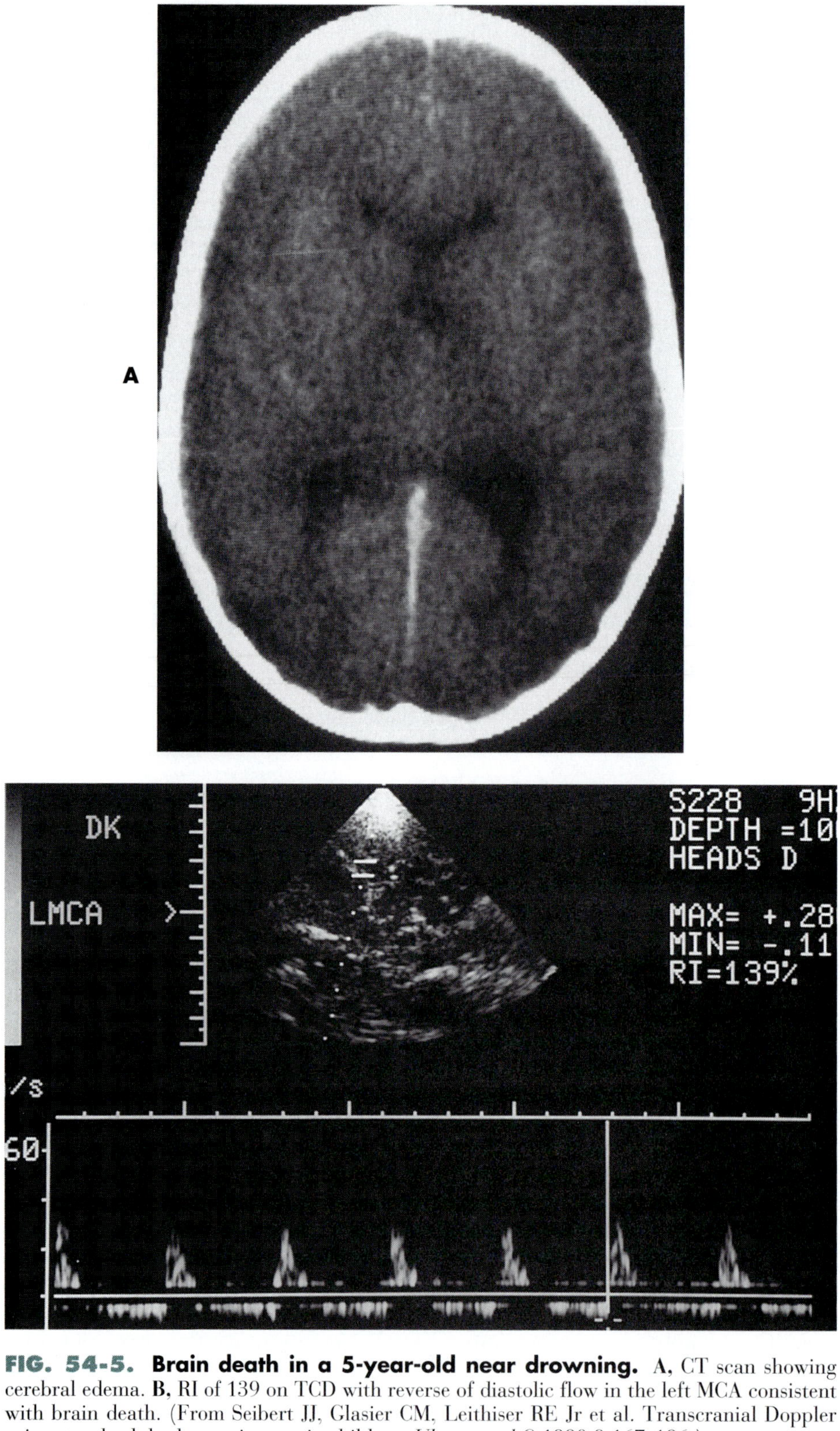

FIG. 54-5. Brain death in a 5-year-old near drowning. **A**, CT scan showing cerebral edema. **B**, RI of 139 on TCD with reverse of diastolic flow in the left MCA consistent with brain death. (From Seibert JJ, Glasier CM, Leithiser RE Jr et al. Transcranial Doppler using standard duplex equipment in children. *Ultrasound Q* 1990;8:167-196.)

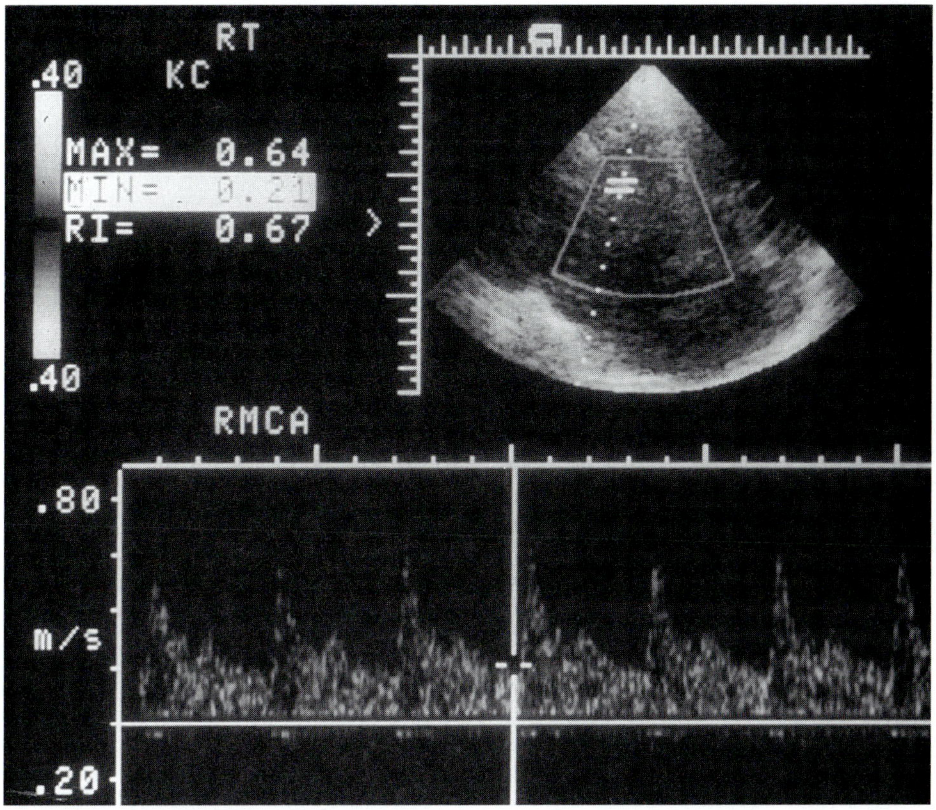

FIG. 54-6. Not brain death. Teenager in status epilepticus with flat EEG in phenobarbital coma with a P_{CO_2} of 27. TCD shows good diastolic flow in the right MCA with slightly elevated RI of 67 but no evidence of brain death. Patient recovered without sequella.

TCD CRITERIA FOR BRAIN DEATH AFTER FONTANELLE CLOSURE

- Absent or complete reversal of diastolic flow with no forward diastolic flow
- Small early systolic spikes
- No flow in the MCA, especially with complete reversal of diastolic flow in the extracranial internal cerebral artery
- Mean velocity in the MCA of <10 cm/s for longer than 30 minutes

ASPHYXIA

Intracranial Doppler imaging in the neonate has been extremely helpful in predicting the presence of significant hypoxic-ischemic brain injury.[42-44] Archer et al.[44] found 100% sensitivity of a **low RI with increased diastolic flow** in the ACA and MCA and an adverse neurologic outcome when performed within the first 48 hours of the asphyxic insult in the neonate. Stark and Seibert[42] reported 10 of 13 neonates with initial low RIs developed severe neurodevelopmental handicaps.

This finding of increased diastolic flow can also be useful in evaluating the older child after head injury or cardiac arrest to predict significant cerebral injury before computed tomography (CT) findings (Fig. 54-7). The increased diastolic flow is postulated to be due to an impairment in cerebral autoregulation during asphyxia, producing an increased diastolic blood flow and a decrease in cerebrovascular resistance.[2]

CEREBRAL EDEMA AND HYPERVENTILATION THERAPY

Initially, with significant cerebral hypoxic insult there is an increase in diastolic flow velocity with a reduced RI during this early hyperemic phase. As intracranial pressure increases, however, the diastolic flow velocity decreases and the systolic peaks become more spiky.[2] Just as there is a direct relationship between an increase in RI with a decrease in diastolic flow in pa-

A

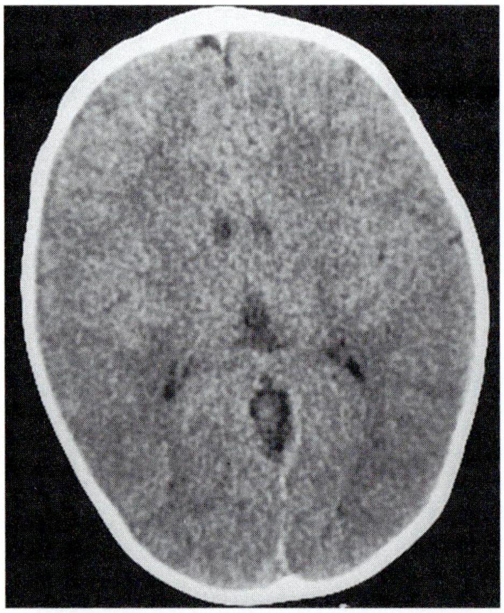

FIG. 54-7. Asphyxia. **A,** A 1-year-old with postrespiratory arrest with a normal CT scan but, **B,** an abnormal Doppler evaluation with a low RI of 43 (50 to 60 normal for age) in the left posterior cerebral artery. **C,** A CT scan 2 days later shows cerebral edema. **D,** A CT scan 1 month later shows marked atrophy. (From Seibert JJ. Doppler evaluation of cerebral circulation. In: Dieckmann RA, Fiser DHB, Selbst SM. *Illustrated Textbook of Pediatric Emergency and Critical Care Procedures*. St Louis: Mosby–Year Book; 1997.)

B

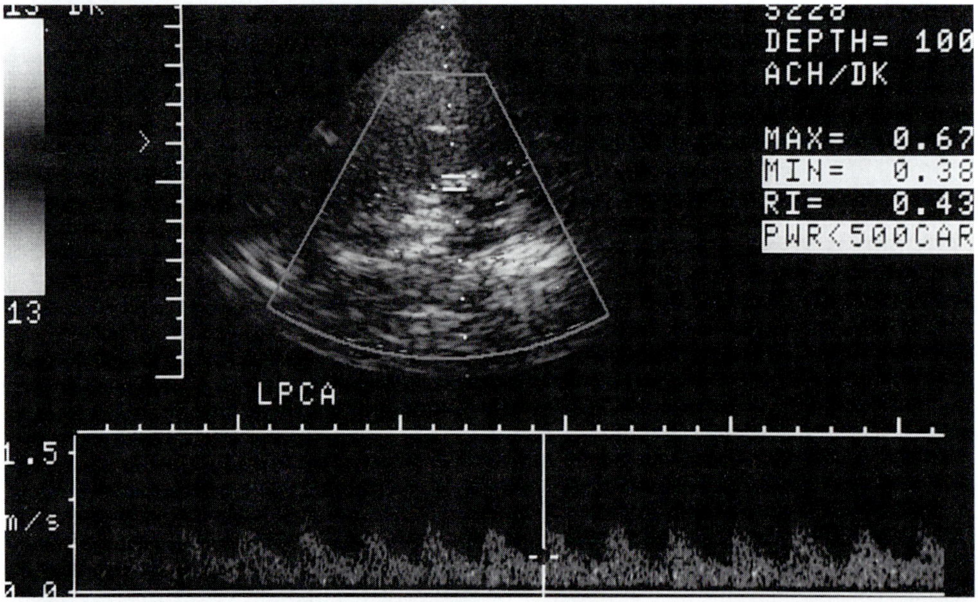

C

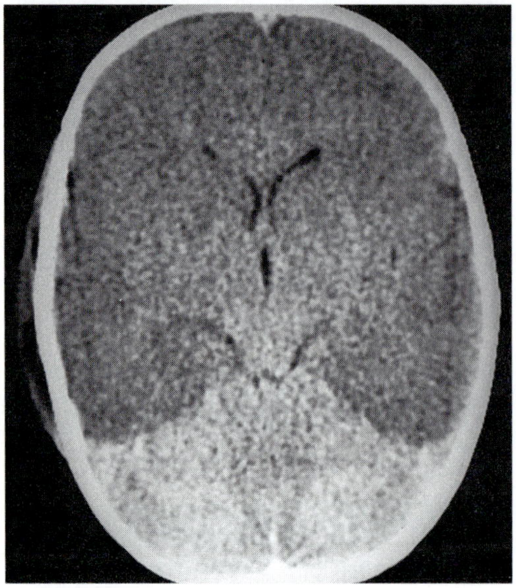

D

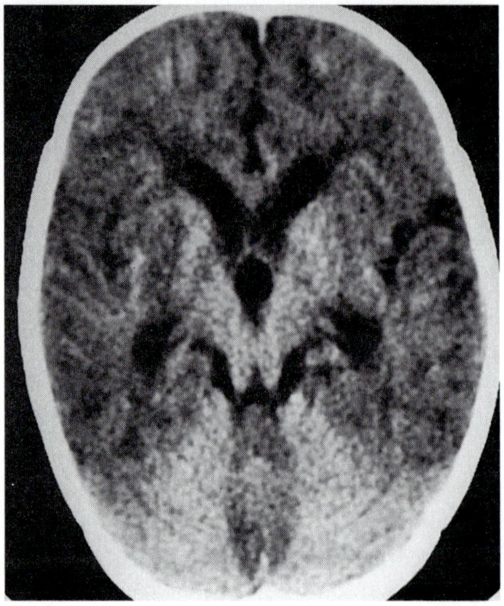

tients with increased intracranial pressure with hydrocephalus, there is an increase in RI with loss of forward diastolic flow in patients with increased intracranial pressure secondary to cerebral edema from a variety of other causes.[45] As cerebral edema develops, the RI increases. Continuous and intermittent TCD readings may be helpful in evaluating the presence of edema and following the course of treatment of the patient with edema, especially from head trauma (Fig. 54-8).

Hyperventilation is a frequent treatment for cerebral edema. There is an inverse relationship between $P\text{CO}_2$ and the RI. The higher the $P\text{CO}_2$, the greater the diastolic flow and the lower the RI. This is probably due to the vasodilatory effect of CO_2. When the $P\text{CO}_2$ is lowered, there is vasoconstriction with a decrease in diastolic flow with an elevation of the RI. In fact, CO_2 reactivity can be measured using the RI. The cerebral blood flow should rise 4% per mm Hg rise in CO_2.[26,45-47] The absence of change in the RI as the patient's hyperventilation is increased is an absent CO_2 reactivity test and is a sign of severe brain injury.[48]

The RI can also be used to monitor hyperventilation therapy[2,48] in cerebral edema associated with head trauma. As hyperventilation decreases the $P\text{CO}_2$, the RI will increase with the concomitant vasoconstriction of cerebral vessels. Of course, increasing cerebral edema will also increase the RI. Therefore, this measurement should be closely correlated with other clinical and laboratory findings. For example, a patient who is on hyperventilation treatment whose RI increases in the face of no change in intracranial pressure may benefit from a decrease in the hyperventilation. The hyperventilation may be producing too much cerebral vasoconstriction.

HYDROCEPHALUS

Hill and Volpe first described a decrease in the pulsatility of the cerebral arterial flow velocity with decrease in diastolic to systolic flow ratio in 11 hydrocephalic infants.[49] Because of its noninvasive and repeatable nature, Doppler imaging has been increasingly used to assess changes in cerebral hemodynamics in hydrocephalus through the anterior fontanelle in infants or transcranially through the temporal bone in older children.[4,50,51] There is general agreement that a direct correlation exists between the intracranial pressure (from experimental, fontanometric, and direct measurement evidence) and the RI, and that the increasing index has been predominantly due to a reduction in the end diastolic velocity.[45,51] Stable ventriculomegaly is associated with normal pulsatility. The two pulsatility indices most commonly applied in hydrocephalic patients have been the Pourcelot RI, which is the peak systolic velocity minus the end diastolic velocity divided by peak systolic velocity, and the Gosling PI, which is the peak systolic velocity minus the end diastolic velocity divided by the mean velocity. Both indices, being ratios, minimize the error in estimating true velocity due to a varying angle of insonation. This may be more important in hydrocephalus as Finn et al. have shown that vascular anatomy may be significantly distorted by ventricular enlargement, and a small angle of insonation cannot be assumed.[52] Difficulties with using the RI[53] have occurred because of two main problems:

1. **There are many other intracranial and extracranial factors that can change the RI** other than increased intracranial pressure (see Table 54-1). Therefore, the RI must be correlated closely with the clinical condition of the patient ($P\text{CO}_2$, heart rate, presence of PDA, etc.).
2. **There is a wide range of normal values** (0.65 to 0.85 in the neonate, 0.60 to 0.70 in the child before fontanelle closure, 0.50 to 0.60 in older children and adults through temporal window after fontanelle closure).[8]

Goh et al. uses an RI of >0.8 as a sign of increased pressure in the neonate and an RI >0.65 in children.[51] Because of this wide variation of normal and an overlap between normal and abnormal values, we have found the RI most useful on an individual basis following a patient's course to determine whether clinical changes and/or ventricular dilatation are secondary to increased pressure or atrophy (Figs. 54-9 to 54-12).

VASCULAR MALFORMATIONS

Intracranial Doppler imaging is exquisitely sensitive for detecting vascular malformations at the bedside in the distressed neonate through the fontanelle or transcranially.[3,54] The vascular malformation may be imaged with color. Spectral analysis of the involved vessels will show high velocity, low pressure with low pulsatility with increased diastolic flow. These hemodynamic qualities result in the characteristic TCD findings of higher than normal mean and peak systolic velocities in conjunction with turbulence and lower than normal RIs (Fig. 54-13). TCD can correctly diagnose arteriovenous malformations with a sensitivity of 87% to 95%.[55-57] Because magnetic resonance imaging (MRI) affords an even higher sensitivity than TCD in diagnostic screening, Doppler imaging is used more often to quantitate the hemodynamics of arteriovenous malformations and to monitor the effects of surgical or endoluminal interventions.[58] After surgical or embolization treatment, TCD can substantiate the increase in RI and decrease in systolic velocity in the feeding arteries.

Text continued on page 1546.

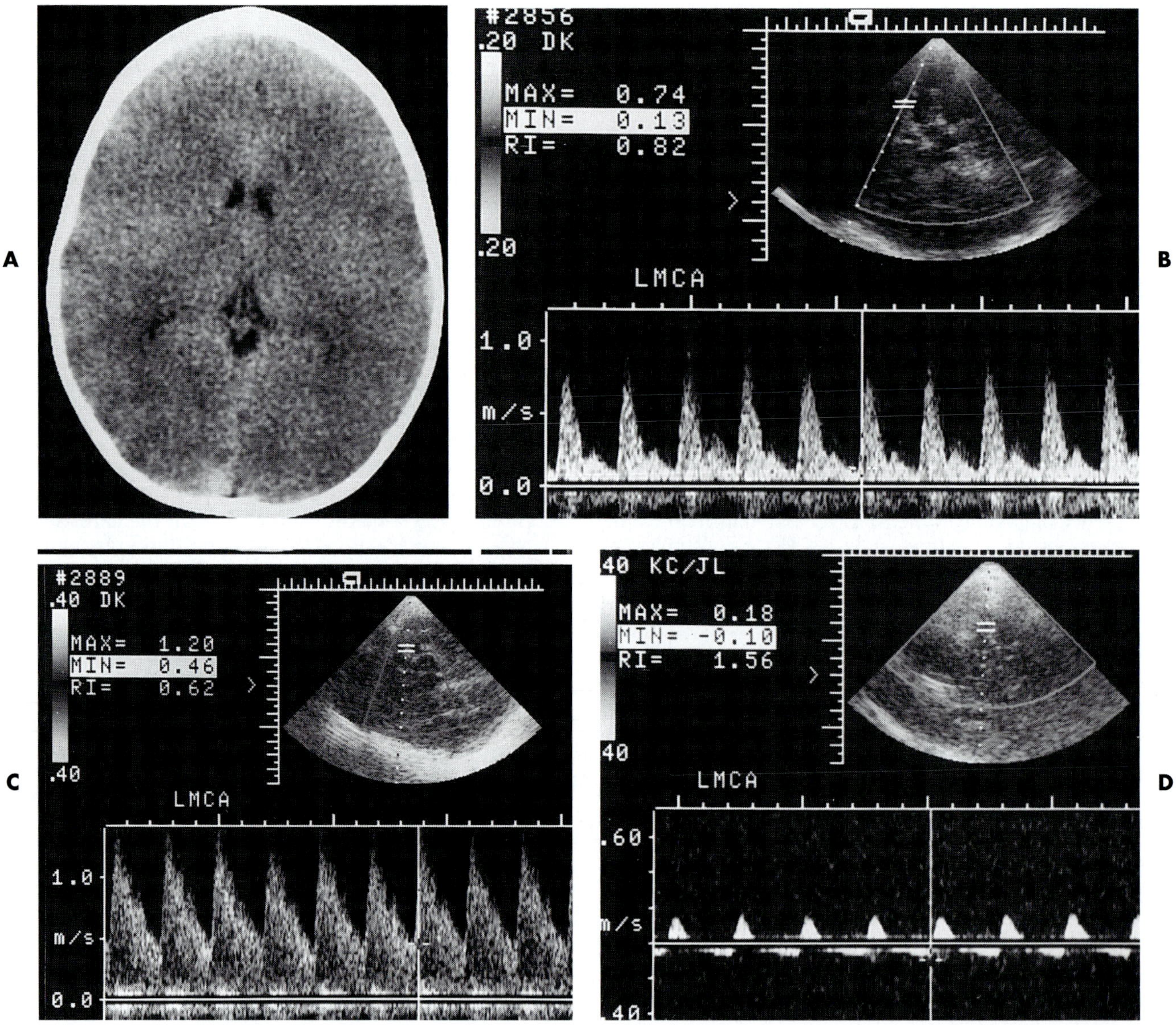

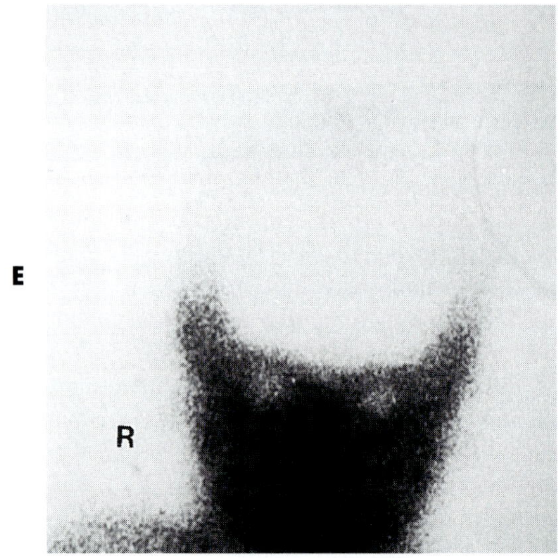

FIG. 54-8. Cerebral edema. Brain death. A, 1½ -year-old child with near drowning. **A,** CT scan shows cerebral edema. **B,** Doppler evaluation shows an elevated RI of 82 from the MCA. **C,** Doppler evaluation of the MCA 2 days later shows that the RI has decreased to 62 with treatment. **D,** MCA Doppler evaluation 4 days later shows brain death with decreased velocity and reverse of diastolic flow with an RI of 156. **E,** Technetium Tc 99m-DTPA brain scan done at this time also shows brain death with no cerebral perfusion. (From Seibert JJ. Doppler evaluation of cerebral circulation. In: Dieckmann RA, Fiser DHB, Selbst SM. *Illustrated Textbook of Pediatric Emergency and Critical Care Procedures*. St Louis: Mosby–Year Book; 1997.)

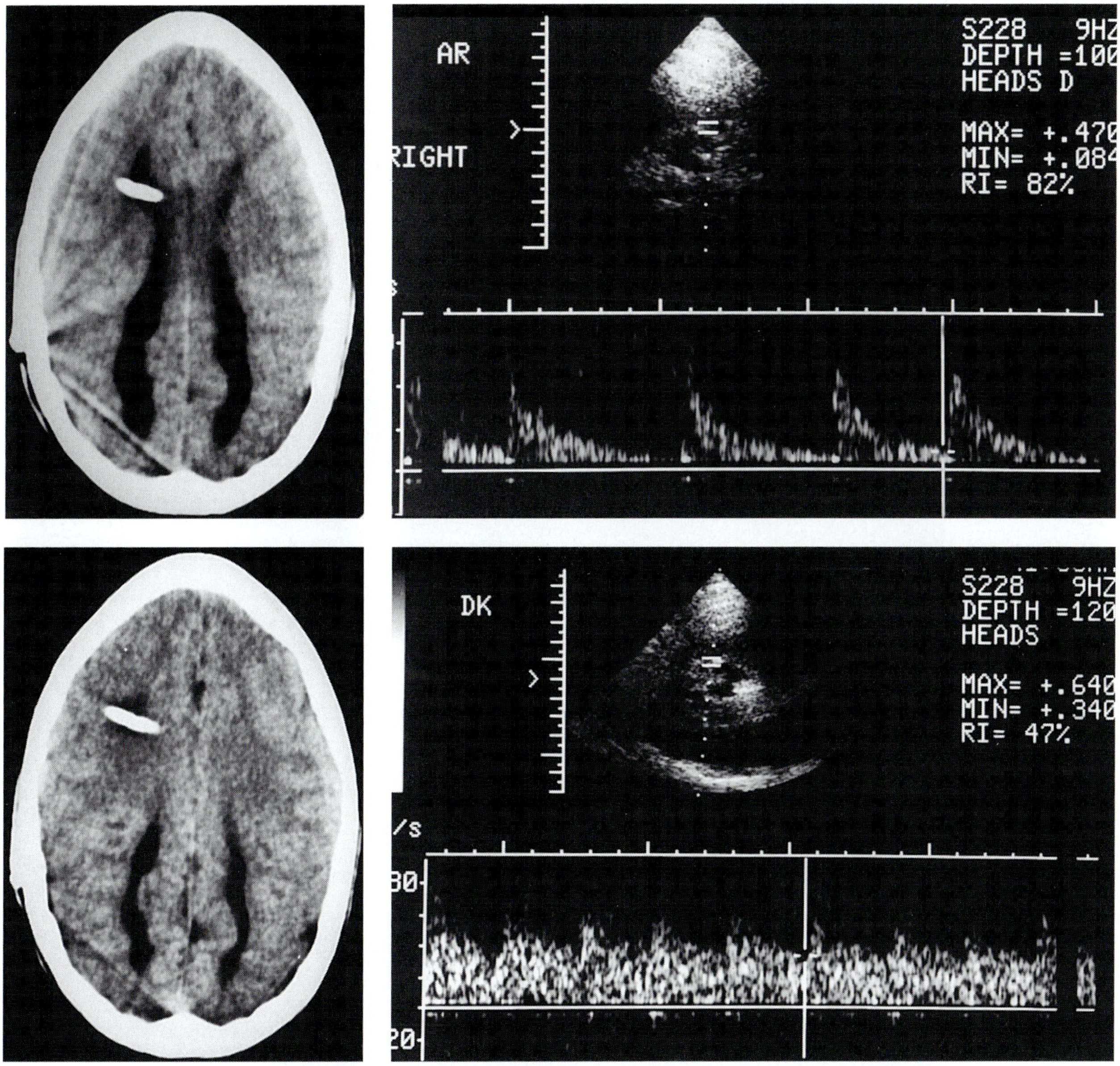

FIG. 54-9. Shunt dysfunction in an 8-year-old. A, CT scan in a patient with very mildly dilated ventricles. **B,** Transcranial Doppler imaging through the temporal window shows increased RI of 82 in an MCA. **C,** CT scan postshunt revision shows decrease in ventricular size. **D,** TCD through the temporal window shows decrease in RI to 47 (normal about 50 after fontanelle closure). (From Seibert JJ, Glasier CM, Leithiser RE Jr et al. Transcranial Doppler using standard duplex equipment in children. *Ultrasound Q* 1990;8:167-196.)

A

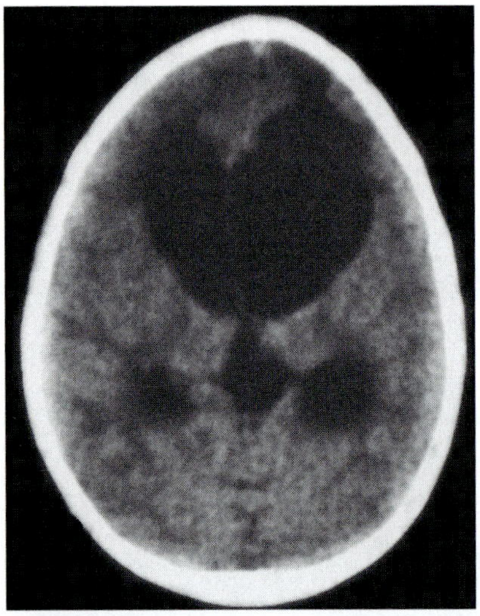

FIG. 54-10. Shunt malfunction. **A,** A 3-year-old with hydrocephalus with increasing signs of shunt malfunction. **B,** TCD through the temporal window shows elevated RI of 70 in an MCA. **C,** TCD postshunt revision shows a normal RI of 55. (From Seibert JJ, Glasier CM, Leithiser RE Jr et al. Transcranial Doppler using standard duplex equipment in children. *Ultrasound Q* 1990;8:167-196.)

B

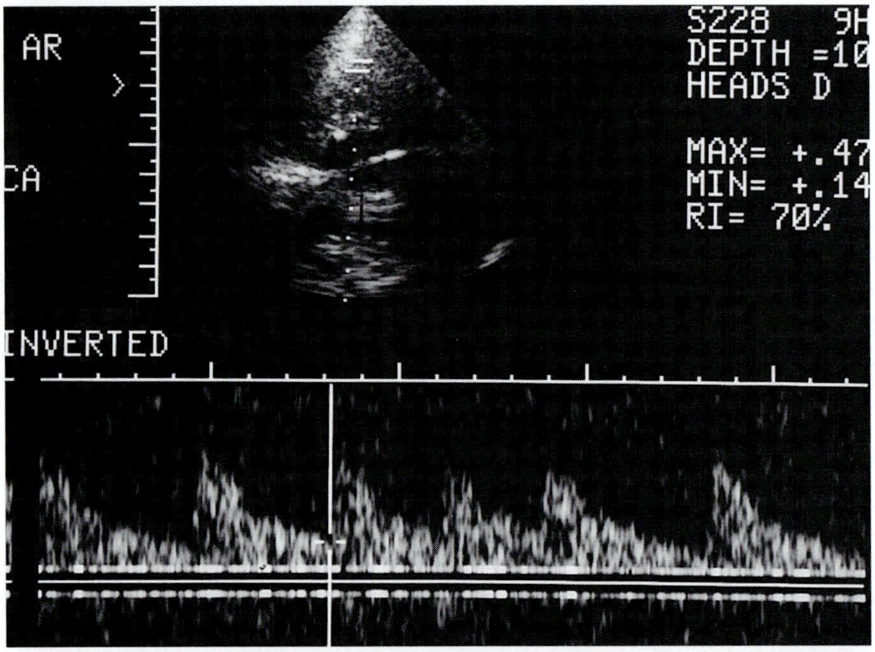

C

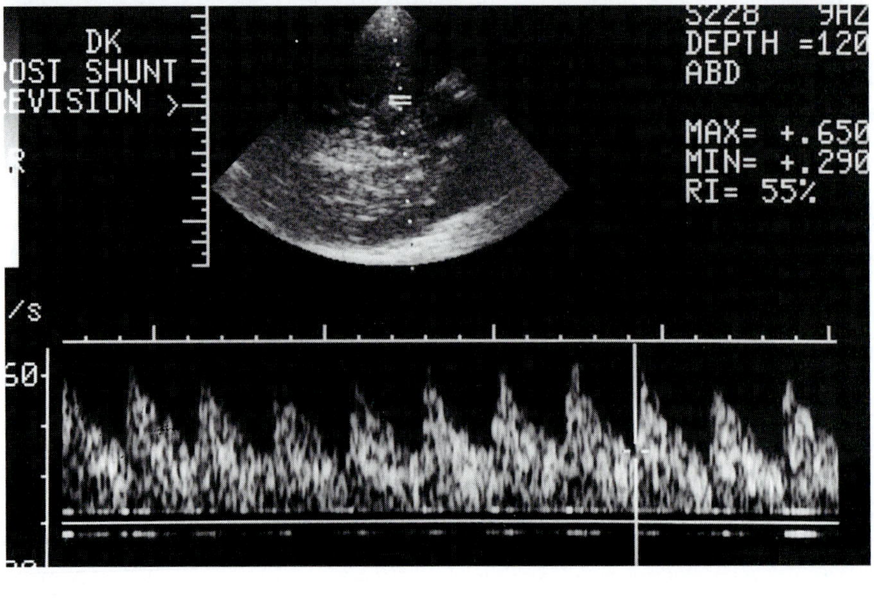

A

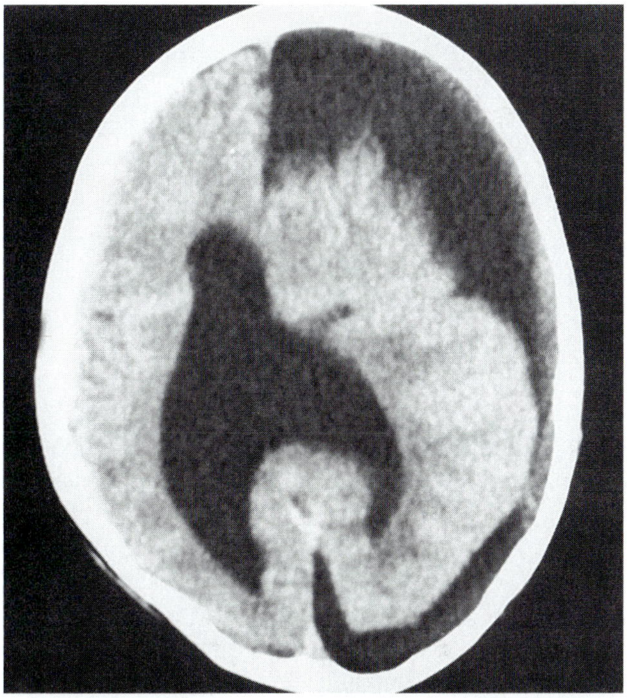

B

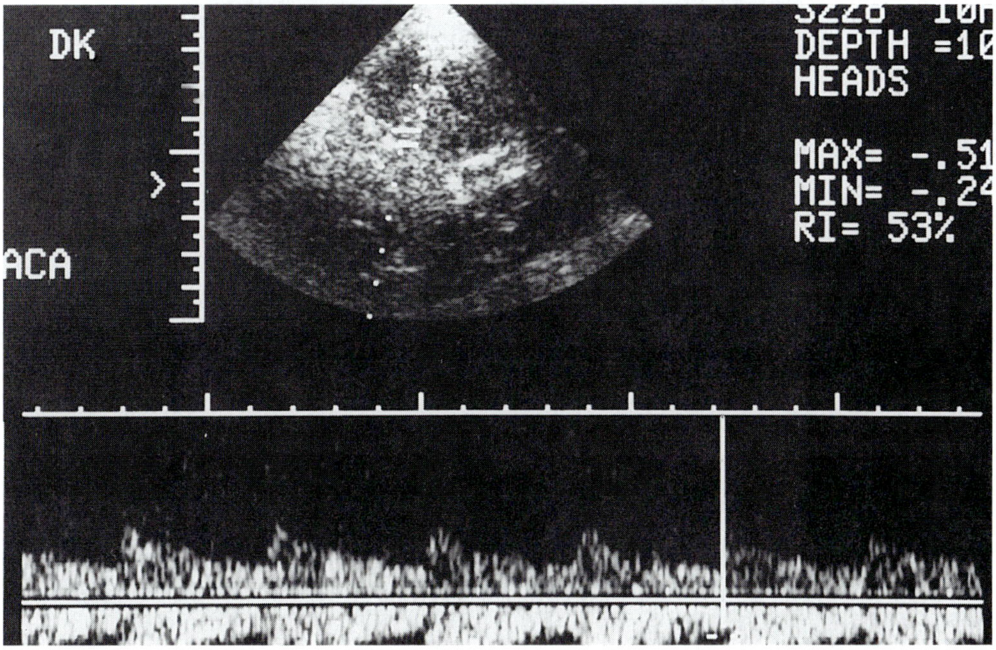

FIG. 54-11. Atrophy. **A,** CT scan shows extraaxial fluid on the left and dilated ventricles in this 9-year-old with increasing seizure activity. **B,** Normal bifurcation landmark on Doppler imaging with flow toward the transducer in the MCA *(above the line)* and flow away from the transducer in the ACA *(below the line)*. The RI is 53, which is normal in this 9-year-old with atrophy. (From Seibert JJ, Glasier CM, Leithiser RE Jr et al. Transcranial Doppler using standard duplex equipment in children. *Ultrasound Q* 1990;8:167-196.)

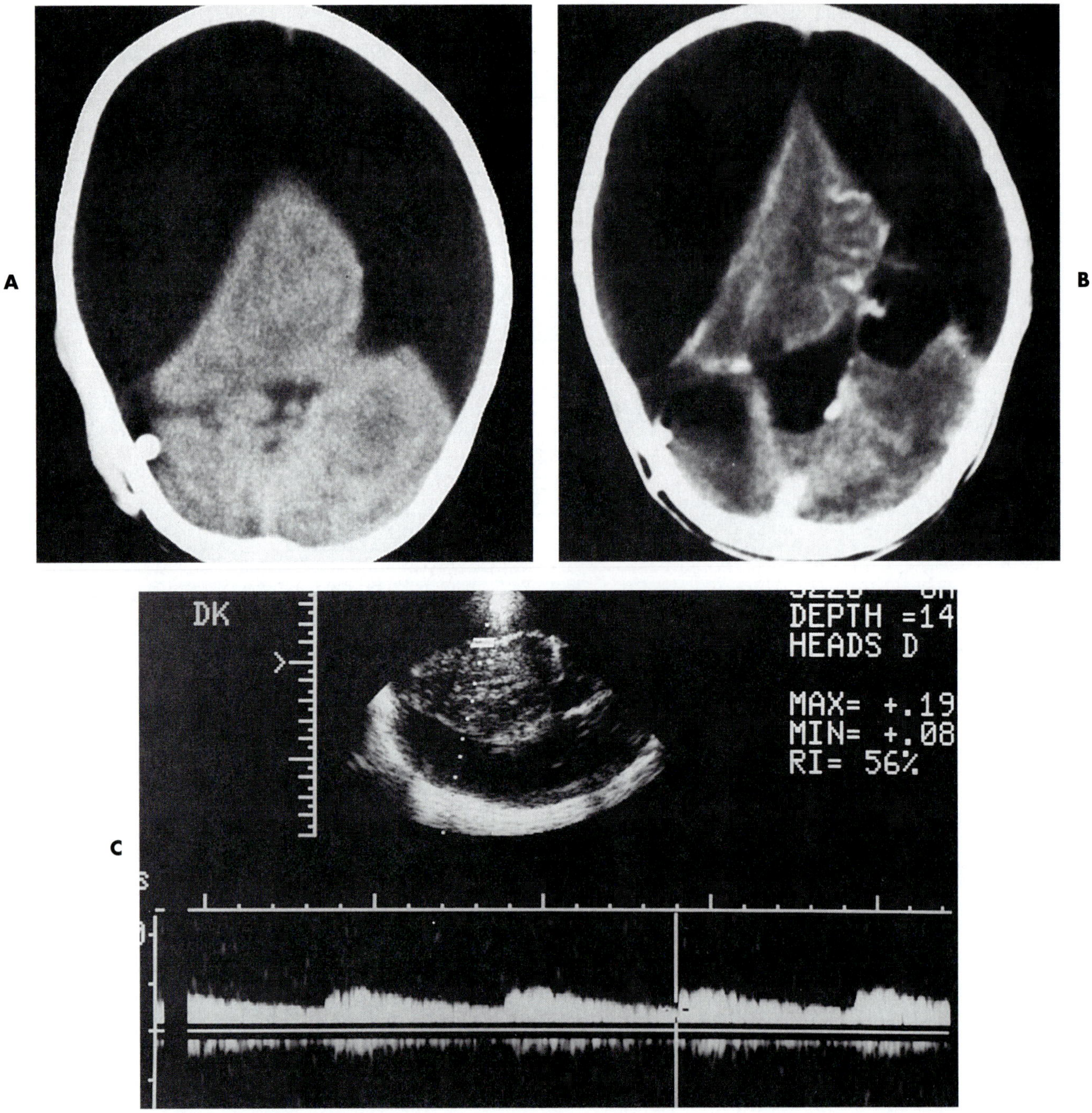

FIG. 54-12. Atrophy. **A,** CT scan at 7 years shows dysmorphic brain with a large amount of extraaxial fluid. **B,** Repeat CT at 10 years for increasing seizures shows increasing ventricular dilatation. **C,** TCD through temporal window shows a normal RI of 56, which is consistent with atrophy. (From Seibert JJ, Glasier CM, Leithiser RE Jr et al. Transcranial Doppler using standard duplex equipment in children. *Ultrasound Q* 1990;8:167-196.)

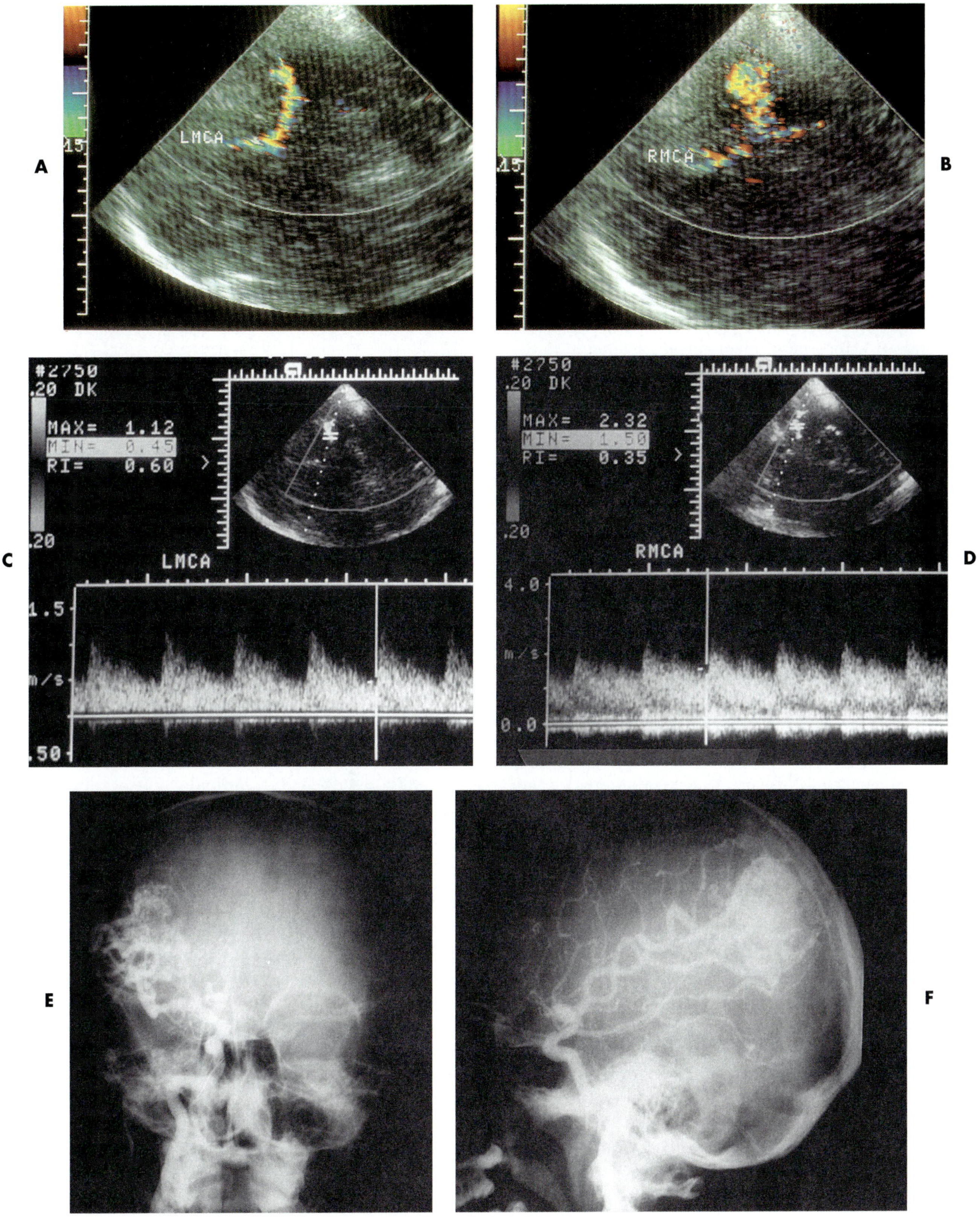

FIG. 54-13. Teenager with AV malformation. A, Normal color image in left MCA. **B,** Increased vessels in region of arteriovenous (AV) malformation in right MCA. **C,** TCD of left MCA shows normal maximum velocity of 112 cm/s. **D,** Increased maximum velocity in right MCA of 232 cm/s. **E,** Frontal and, **F,** lateral arteriograms showing AV malformation.

TCD may also be used to evaluate children with suspected cerebrovascular disease such as moyamoya or cerebrovascular disease of sickle cell anemia.

INTRAOPERATIVE NEURORADIOLOGIC PROCEDURES

Intraoperative TCD monitoring of the velocity in the MCA during carotid endarterectomy is an accepted clinical application in adults.[23] Intraoperative complications of carotid endarterectomy relate mainly to ischemia during cross-clamping, hyperemic phenomena, or embolization of atheromatous or gaseous materials. Hyperemic phenomena secondary to ischemia are depicted by a sudden increase in flow velocity. Solid or gaseous microemboli as small as 30 to 50 μm can be documented by TCD as high-amplitude spikes on spectral waveform and a characteristic auditory "chirping" sound.[59] Ischemia during cross-clamping is a classic complication that may occur in up to 10% of patients and is caused by incompetent intracranial collateral circulation, mainly the anterior and posterior communicating arteries and the leptomeningeal vessels. TCD can be used to assess the effect of carotid cross-clamping on the MCA in both children and adults (Fig. 54-14). TCD monitoring during cardiopulmonary bypass for cardiac surgery is an area of current research. TCD can demonstrate emboli showers that occur during aortic cannulation, cardiac manipulation, or other surgical maneuvers.[60]

The use of TCD during diagnostic and therapeutic neuroangiographic procedures is another area of current research.[61] TCD has shown that asymptomatic microemboli enter the cerebral circulation in large numbers during "routine" carotid angiography.

STROKE IN SICKLE CELL PATIENTS

Cerebral infarction secondary to occlusive vasculopathy is a major complication of patients with sickle cell disease (hemoglobin SS) with a prevalence ranging from 5.5%[62] to 17%.[63] The stenotic lesions involve large vessels in the intracranial internal, middle, and anterior artery circulation and progress for months and years before symptoms develop. Prevention of stroke symptoms by hypertransfusion therapy is theoretically possible in patients at risk.[11] Bone marrow transplantation has also proven curative in young patients with symptomatic sickle cell disease and has led to stabilization of nervous system vasculopathy as documented by MRI.[64] TCD is the most cost-effective screening method for children at risk.

CEREBROVASCULAR DISEASE INDICATIONS IN CHILDREN

- Maximum velocity, OA >35 cm/s
- Mean velocity, MCA >170 cm/s
- Resistive index in OA <50 cm/s
- Velocity in OA greater than velocity in MCA (ipsilateral)
- Maximum velocity in PCA, vertebral, or basilar arteries >MCA
- Turbulence
- PCA or ACA visualized without MCA
- ANY RI <30
- Maximum MCA velocity >200 cm/s

Adams et al. first showed the effectiveness of nonduplex Doppler imaging in screening for cerebrovascular disease in sickle cell disease.[11-13,65,66] Using the transtemporal and suboccipital approach, Adams et al. screened 190 asymptomatic sickle cell patients and found in clinical follow-up that a mean flow velocity in the MCA = or >170 cm/s was an indicator of a patient at risk for development of stroke.[11] Adams et al. then compared TCD to cerebral angiography in 33 neurologically symptomatic patients and found five criteria for cerebrovascular disease: (1) mean velocity of 190 cm/s, (2) low velocity in the MCA (<70 cm/s), (3) MCA ratio (lower or higher) of 0.5 or less, (4) ACA/MCA ratio > 1.2 on the same side, and (5) inability to detect an MCA in the presence of a demonstrated ultrasound window.[66] Using duplex Doppler imaging, MRA, and MRI, Seibert et al. (see box above) originally described **five indicators of cerebrovascular disease in sickle cell patients:** (1) maximum velocity in the OA of more than 35 cm/s (Fig. 54-15); (2) mean velocity in the MCA of more than 170 cm/s (Fig. 54-16); (3) RI in the OA <50 (Fig. 54-17); (4) velocity in the OA greater than that of the ipsilateral MCA; and (5) maximum velocity in the PCA, vertebral, or basilar arteries greater than maximum velocity in the MCA.[25] An 8-year follow-up of 27 neurologically symptomatic and 90 asymptomatic sickle cell patients showed all five original TCD indicators of disease still significant.[67] Four additional factors were also significant: (1) turbulence, (2) PCA or ACA visualized without seeing the MCA (Figs. 54-18 and 54-19), (3) any RI <30, and (4) maximum MCA velocity >200 cm/s. Siegel et al. compared transtemporal TCD using duplex equipment to neurologic examination and found also a maximum flow in the MCA of >200 cm/s or <100 cm/s (including no flow) as significant for disease.[68] Verlhac et al. studied sickle cell patients with duplex Doppler imaging with a 3-MHz transducer transtemporally and suboccipitally, as well as with MRA and MRI.[69] Arteriography was performed in cases where a stenosis was suspected on TCD. This

Text continued on page 1553.

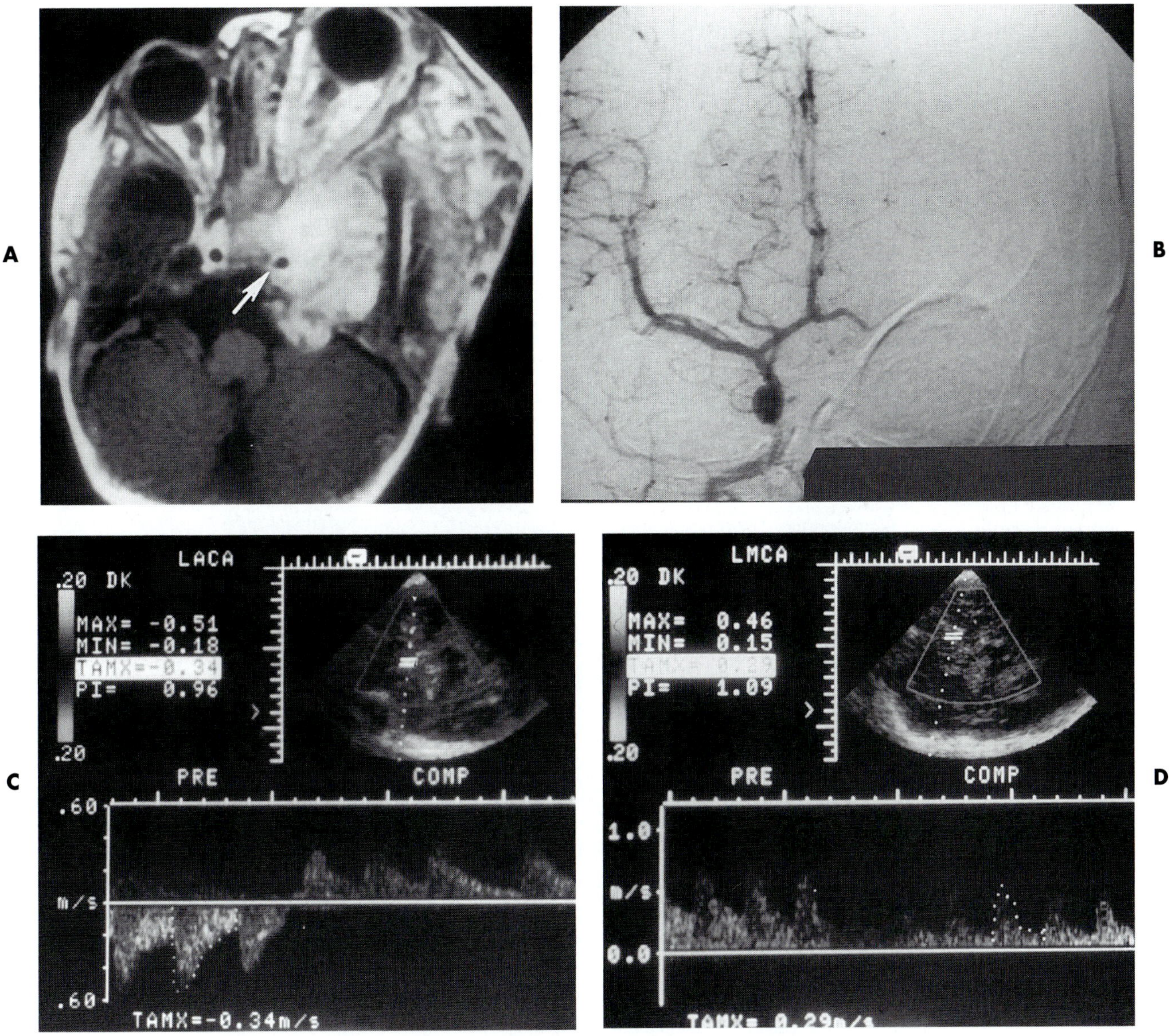

FIG. 54-14. Preoperative evaluation for possible ligation of carotid. **A,** Patient with plexiform neurofibroma surrounding the left internal carotid artery on MRI *(arrow)*. **B,** Compression of left carotid artery at arteriography shows cross filling from right side into left ACA. **C,** TCD at time of compression also shows good filling of left ACA from right side (reverse flow in the left ACA) and, **D,** good filling of left MCA.

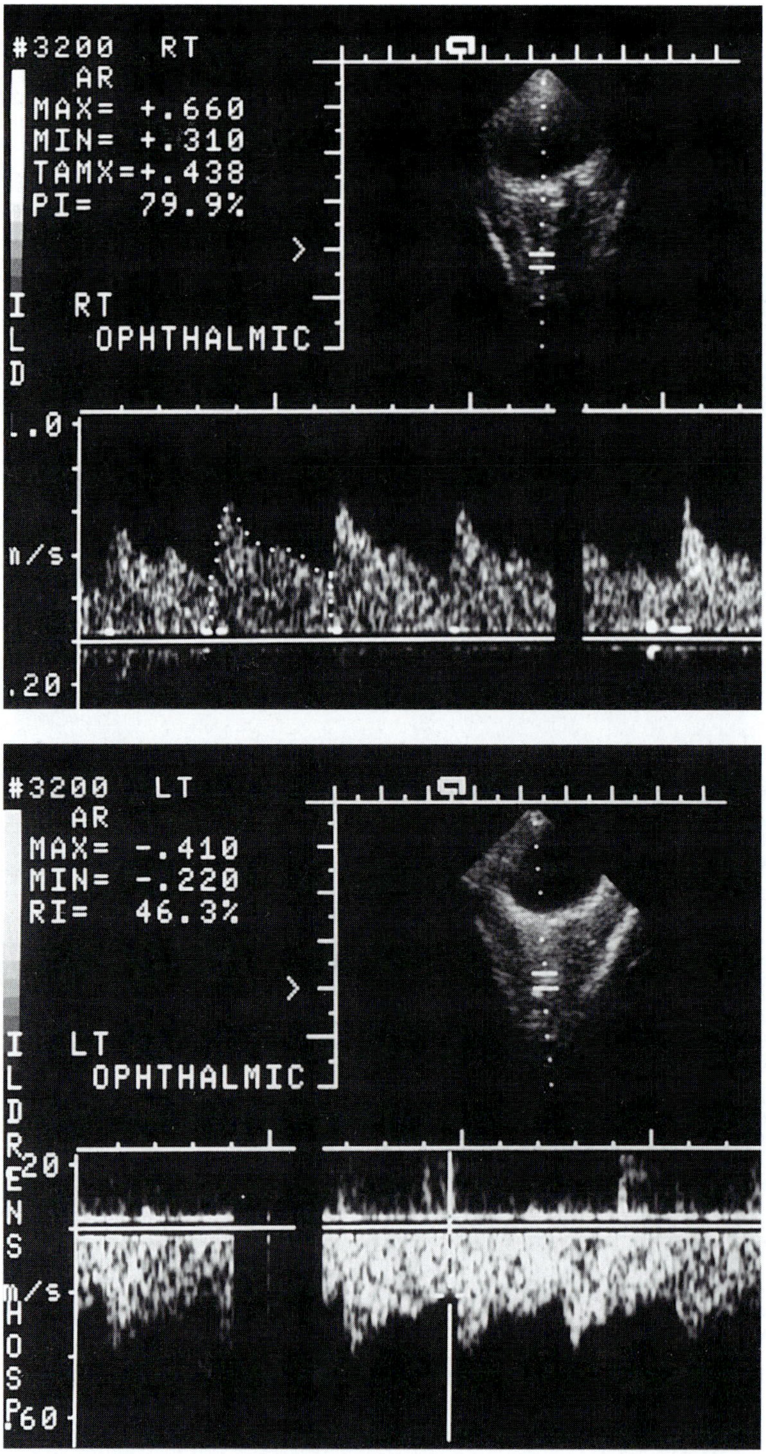

FIG. 54-15. Abnormal OA TCD. A 16-year-old boy with first cerebrovascular accident at age 7. Doppler waveforms through the eye show increased diastolic flow in both OAs. **A,** Increased velocity in the right OA with a maximum velocity of 66 cm/s and with, **B,** reversed flow in the left OA. (From Seibert JJ, Miller SF, Kirby RS et al. Cerebrovascular disease in symptomatic and asymptomatic patients with sickle cell anemia: screening with duplex transcranial Doppler US—correlation with MR imaging and MR angiography. *Radiology* 1993;189:457-466.)

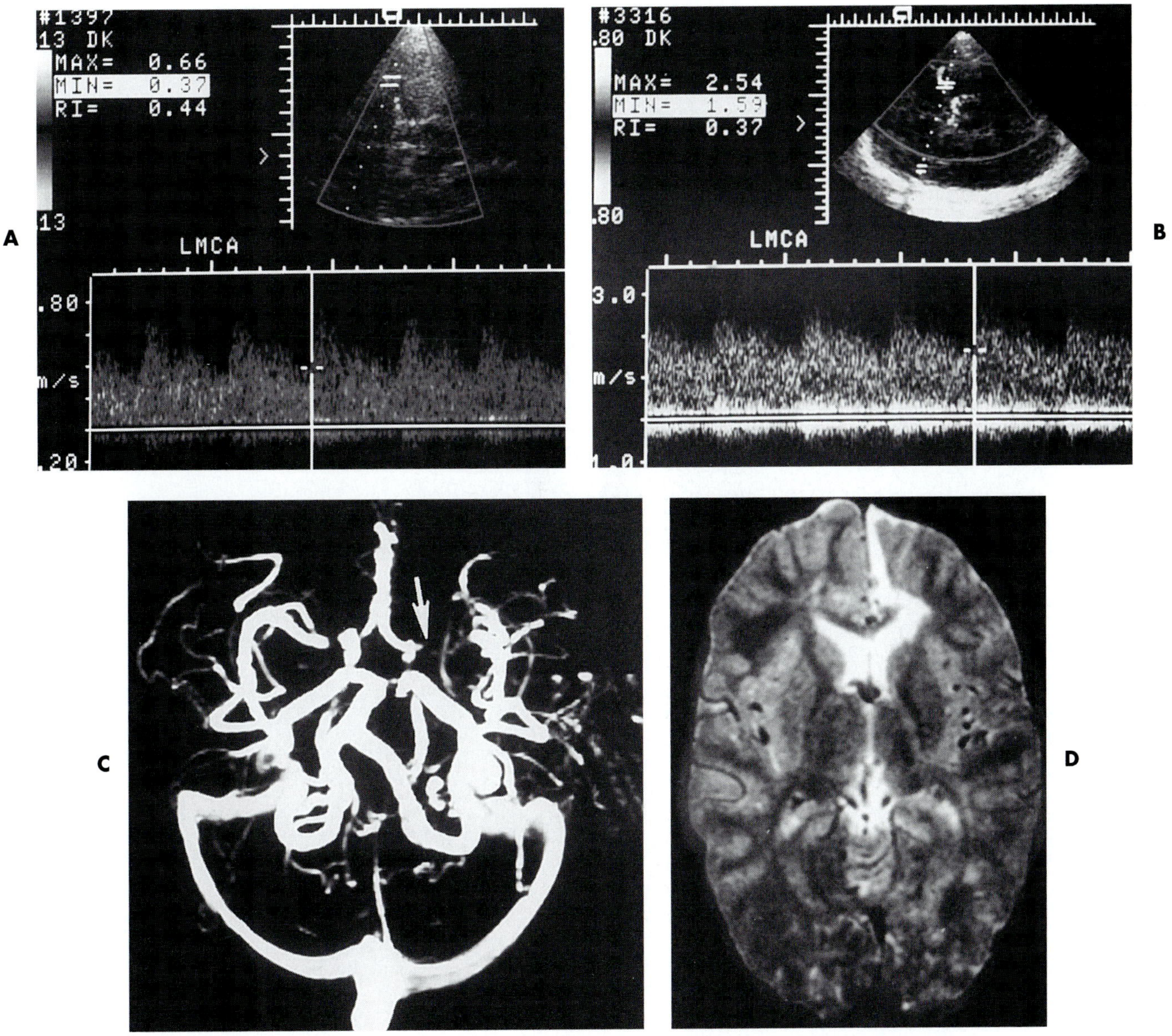

FIG. 54-16. MCA stenosis. Images of a 10-year-old girl with left hemisphere stroke at age 7. **A,** TCD in distal left MCA shows low velocity of 66 cm/s. **B,** TCD in more proximal MCA proximal to stenosis shows increased velocity of 254 cm/s. **C,** Axial collapsed image from three-dimensional phase-contrast MRA with velocity encoding of 60 cm/s shows stenosis of the left MCA *(arrow)* with small internal carotid arteries bilaterally. **D,** Axial T2-weighted image (2500/90, with three-fourths signal averaged) shows encephalomalacia in the left frontal lobe from previous infarction of the ACA. (From Seibert JJ, Miller SF, Kirby RS et al. Cerebrovascular disease in symptomatic and asymptomatic patients with sickle cell anemia: screening with duplex transcranial Doppler US—correlation with MR imaging and MR angiography. *Radiology* 1993;189:457-466.)

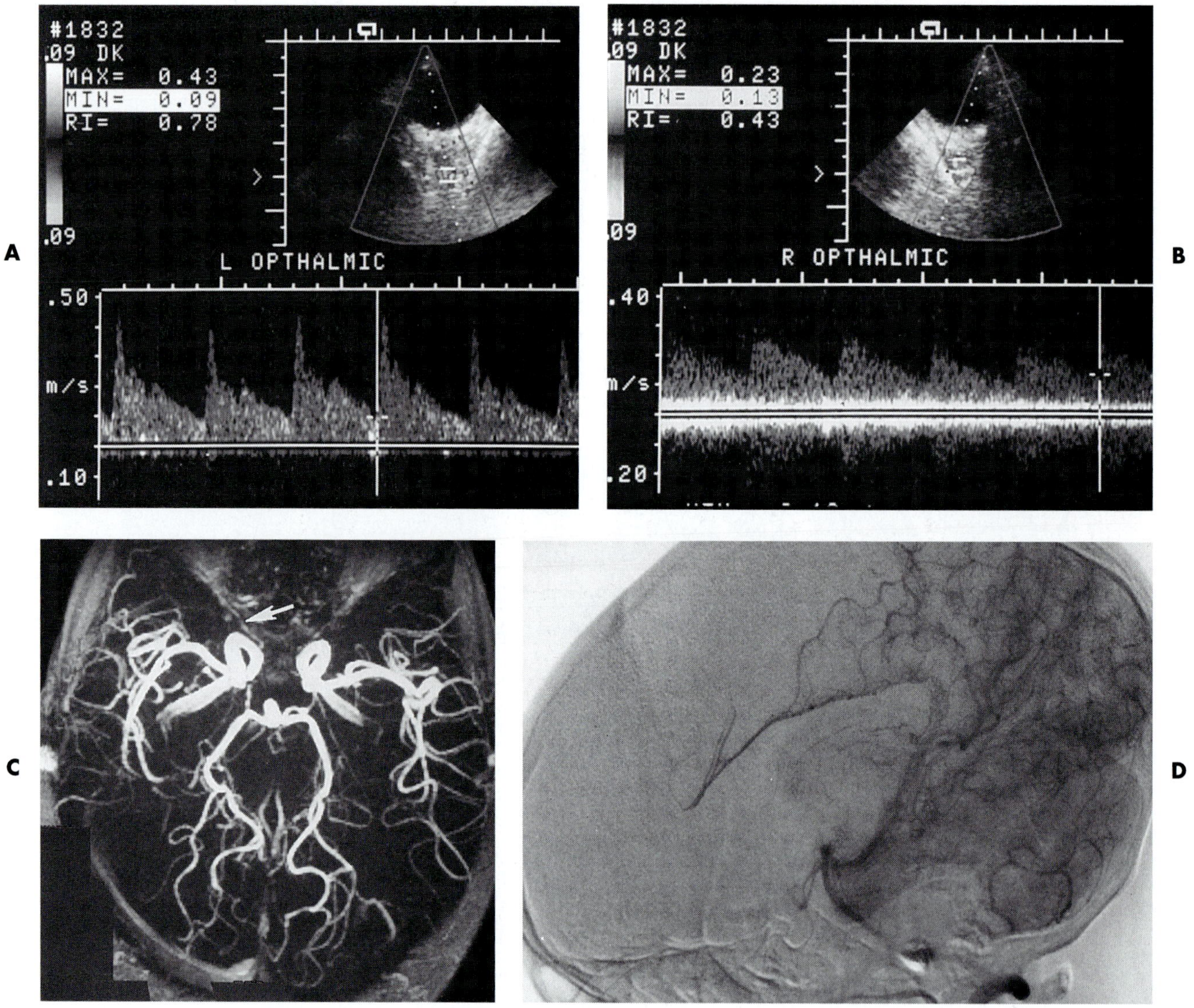

FIG. 54-17. Developing stroke in an asymptomatic 13-year-old boy with sickle cell anemia. **A,** TCD through the left eye shows relatively normal ophthalmic waveform with normal RI of 78 but increased flow with a maximum velocity of 43 cm/s. **B,** TCD through the right eye shows more abnormal waveform with increased diastolic flow in the right OA with a low RI of 43. **C,** Collapsed image from axial three-deminsional time-of-flight MRA shows absent ACAs bilaterally with prominent right OA *(arrow)*. **D,** Vertebral arteriogram demonstrates retrograde filling of the ACA. *Continued.*

E

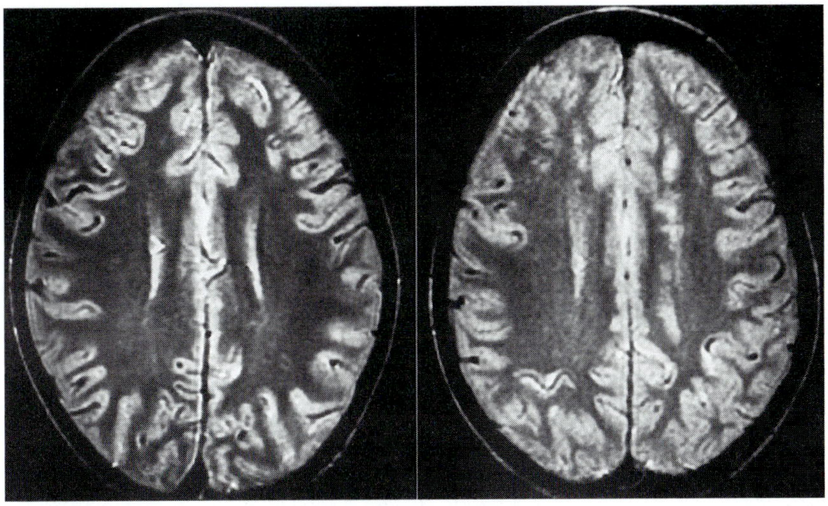

FIG. 54-17, cont'd. **E,** Initial image *(on left)* obtained at time of MRA is normal. Six months later, patient suffered acute stroke, and second MRA now shows bilateral spotty hyperintense areas in the ACA distribution. Both images are axial proton-density-weighted (2500/30, with three-fourths signal averaged). (From Seibert JJ, Miller SF, Kirby RS et al. Cerebrovascular disease in symptomatic and asymptomatic patients with sickle cell anemia: screening with duplex transcranial Doppler US—correlation with MR imaging and MR angiography. *Radiology* 1993;189:457-466.)

A

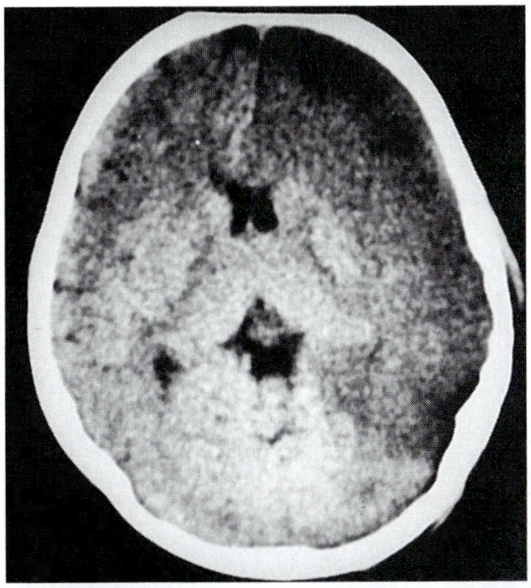

B

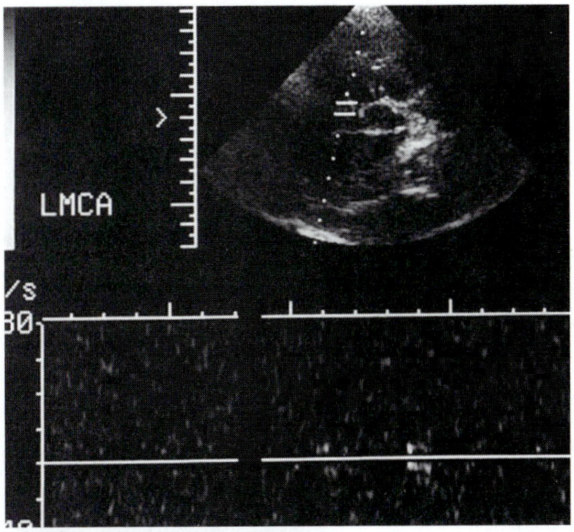

C

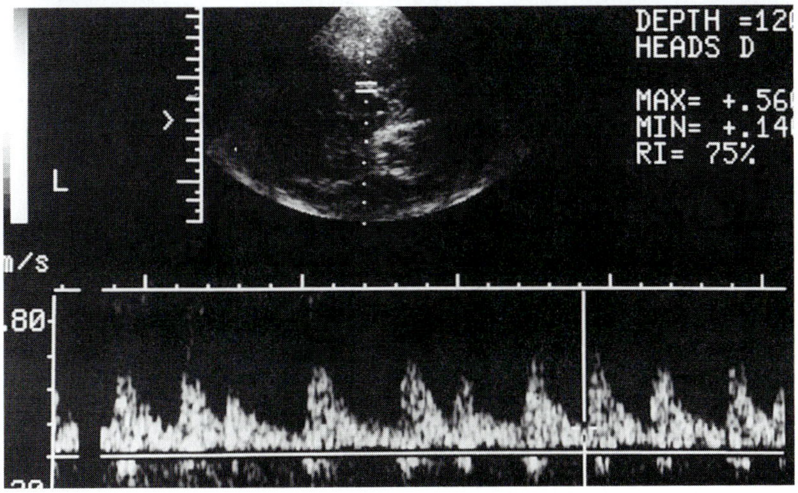

FIG. 54-18. Acute stroke. A 2-year-old with cerebral vascular accident. **A,** CT scan shows low density in the distribution of the left ACA and MCA. **B,** TCD through the temporal bone on the left demonstrates no flow in the ACA or MCA. **C,** Flow could be obtained through the temporal window in the PCA on the left as it circled the cerebral peduncle. (From Seibert JJ, Glasier CM, Leithiser RE Jr et al. Transcranial Doppler using standard duplex equipment in children. *Ultrasound Q* 1990;8:167-196.)

A B C D E

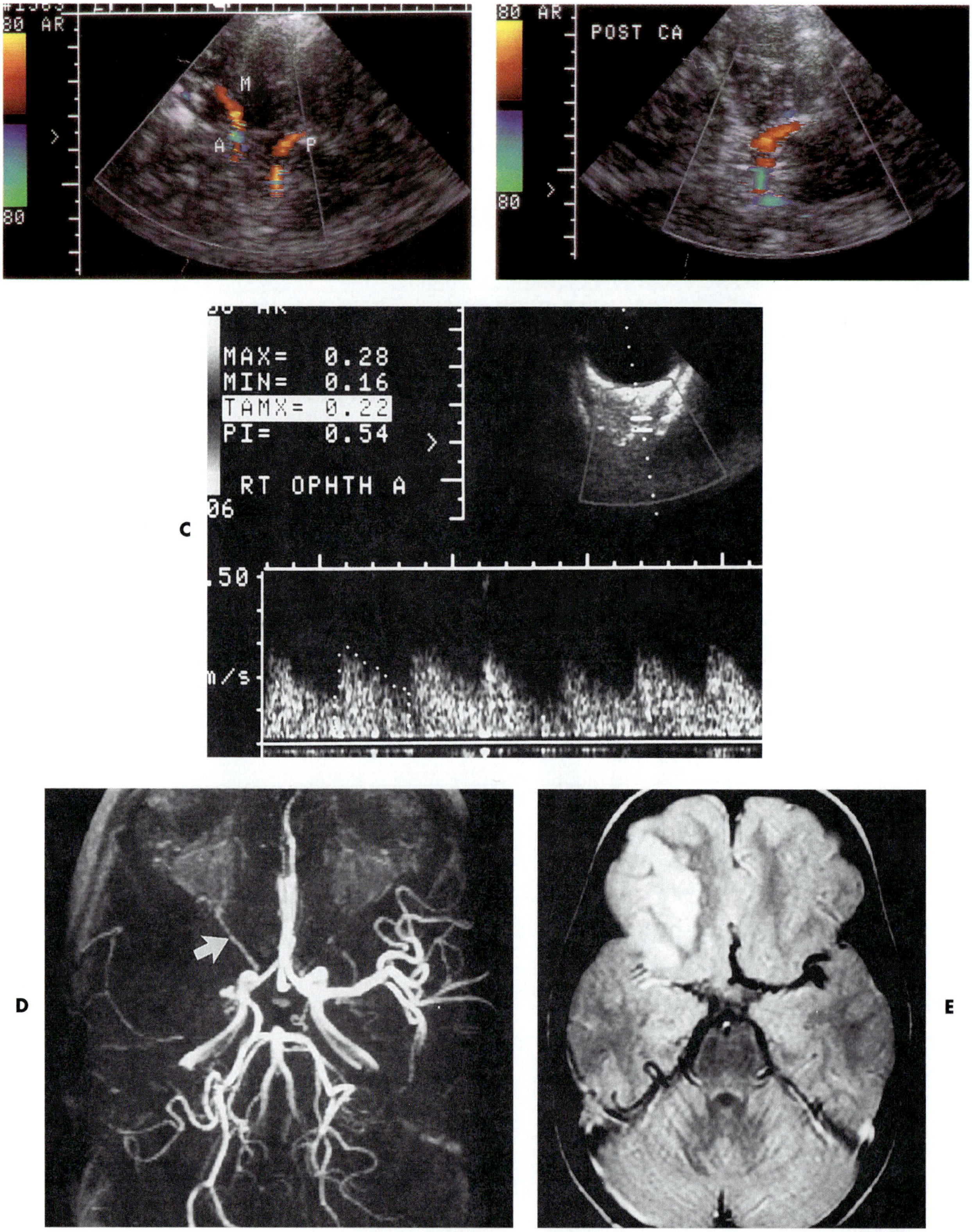

FIG. 54-19. Acute stroke. A 3-year-old boy with acute slurred speech and left-sided weakness. **A,** Normal TCD color flow through temporal bone of left MCA, *M*, left ACA, *A*, and left PCA, *P*. **B,** Right temporal TCD shows no right MCA while the normal right PCA is depicted in orange and the normal left PCA is shown in blue. **C,** Doppler waveform of the right OA shows increased diastolic flow. **D,** Axial collapsed image from three-dimensional time-of-flight MRA shows absent flow in the right MCA and a prominent right OA *(arrow)*. **E,** Axial proton-density-weighted image (2500/30, with three-fourths signal averaged) shows absent M1 segment of the right MCA and hyperintense area in the right frontal lobe compatible with acute infarction. (From Seibert JJ, Miller SF, Kirby RS et al. Cerebrovascular disease in symptomatic and asymptomatic patients with sickle cell anemia: screening with duplex transcranial Doppler US—correlation with MR imaging and MR angiography. *Radiology* 1993;189:457-466.)

group found patients with a mean velocity of > 190 cm/s had stenoses by arteriography. Kogutt et al.[70] also evaluated symptomatic sickle cell patients with duplex Doppler imaging, MRI, and MRA and found 91% sensitivity and 22% specificity of TCD using MRA as the standard. Abnormal TCD values were (1) VMax and VMean >2 standard deviations from these normal values reported by Adams et al. in sickle cell patients: VMax MCA >168 ± 38 cm/s and VMean MCA 115 ± 31 cm/s, VMax ACA 138 ± 34 cm/s and VMean ACA 94 ± cm/s; (2) RI <40; and (3) VMax MCA <VMax ACA.

Our recommendation for screening sickle cell patients with duplex Doppler imaging involves scanning the patient transtemporally to evaluate the MCA, ACA, and PCA. The ophthalmic artery should also be evaluated through the eye. This vessel was more sensitive for detecting cerebrovascular abnormality than the MCA in our series. The basilar and vertebral arteries can be evaluated from the occipital approach. This third plane is probably not necessary in routine screening and may be only necessary when a good transtemporal window cannot be obtained. The maximum, minimum, and mean velocities, as well as the RI in each of these vessels, should be measured at least twice. The highest velocity obtained can be taken as the truest velocity obtained at the best insonating angle. We use the nine factors described above as indicators of cerebrovascular disease and recommend that if at least two of these factors are present, the patient be evaluated by MRA for stenosis. The sensitivity of Doppler ultrasound as a predictor of stroke from our investigation was 94% with a specificity of 51%.

REFERENCES

1. Raju TNK. Cranial Doppler applications in neonatal critical care. *Crit Care Clin* 1992;8(1):93-111.
2. Saliba EM, Laugier J. Doppler assessment of the cerebral circulation in pediatric intensive care. *Crit Care Clin* 1992;8(1):79-92.
3. Taylor GA. Current concepts in neonatal cranial Doppler sonography. *Ultrasound Q* 1992;(4):223-244.
4. Seibert JJ, McCowan TC, Chadduck WM et al. Duplex pulsed Doppler US versus intracranial pressure in the neonate. Clinical and experimental studies. *Radiology* 1989;171:155-159.
5. Lupetin AR, Davis DA, Beckman I et al. Transcranial Doppler sonography. Part 1. Principles, technique, and normal appearances. *RadioGraphics* 1995;15:179-191.
6. Katz ML, Comerota AJ. Transcranial Doppler: a review of technique, interpretation and clinical applications. *Ultrasound Q* 1991;8:241-265.
7. Byrd SM. An overview of transcranial Doppler color flow imaging: a technique comparison. *Ultrasound Q* 1996;13(4):197-210.

Technique

8. Seibert JJ, Glasier CM, Leithiser RE Jr et al. Transcranial Doppler using standard duplex equipment in children. *Ultrasound Q* 1990;8:167-196.
9. Erickson SJ, Hendrix LE, Massaro BM et al. Color Doppler flow imaging of the normal and abnormal orbit. *Radiology* 1989;173:511-516.
10. Baxter GM, Williamson TH. Color Doppler imaging of the eye: normal ranges, reproducibility, and observer variation. *J Ultrasound Med* 1995;14:91-96.
11. Adams R, McKie V, Nichols F et al. The use of transcranial ultrasonography to predict stroke in sickle cell disease. *N Engl J Med* 1992;326(9):605-610.
12. Adams RJ, Nichols FT, McKie VC et al. Transcranial Doppler: influence of hematocrit in children with sickle cell anemia without stroke. *J Cardiovasc Tech* 1989;8:97-101.
13. Adams RJ, Nichols FT III, Aaslid R et al. Cerebral vessel stenosis in sickle cell disease: criteria for detection by transcranial Doppler. *Am J Pediatr Hematol Oncol* 1990;12:277-282.
14. Lizzi R, Mortimer A, Cartensen E et al. Bioeffects considerations for the safety of diagnostic ultrasound. *J Ultrasound* 1988;7(suppl):1-38.
15. Rabe H, Grohs B, Schmidt RM et al. Acoustic power measurements of Doppler ultrasound devices used for perinatal and infant examinations. *Pediatr Radiol* 1990;20:277-281.
16. Acuson 128 Systems Manual. Doppler Section. Appendix C. Transducer Power Values. 1987.
17. Aaslid R. *Transcranial Doppler Sonography.* New York: Springer-Verlag; 1986:10-21.
18. Winkler P, Helmke K. Major pitfalls in Doppler investigations with particular reference to the cerebral vascular system. Part I. Sources in error, resulting pitfalls, and measures to prevent errors. *Pediatr Radiol* 1990;20:219-228.
19. Winkler P, Helmke K, Mahl M. Major pitfalls in Doppler investigations. Part II. Low flow velocities and colour Doppler applications. *Pediatr Radiol* 1990;20:304-310.
20. American Academy of Neurology, Therapeutics and Technology Subcommittee. Assessment: transcranial Doppler. *Neurology* 1990;40:680-681.
21. Allan PL. Transcranial colour Doppler imaging. Acuson International Clinical Notes.
22. Petty GW, Wiebers DO, Meissner I. Transcranial Doppler ultrasonography: clinical applications in cerebrovascular disease. *Mayo Clin Proc* 1990;65:1350-1364.
23. Lupetin AR, Davis DA, Beckman I et al. Transcranial Doppler sonography. Part II. Evaluation of intracranial and extracranial abnormalities and procedural monitoring. *RadioGraphics* 1995;15:193-209.
24. Seibert JJ. Doppler evaluation of cerebral circulation in the critical care patient. In: Dieckmann R, Fiser D, Selbst S, eds. *Illustrated Textbook of Pediatric Emergency & Critical Care Procedure.* St Louis: Mosby-Year Book; 1995:87-102.
25. Seibert JJ, Miller SF, Kirby RS et al. Cerebrovascular disease in symptomatic and asymptomatic patients with sickle cell anemia: screening with duplex transcranial Doppler US—correlation with MR imaging and MR angiography. *Radiology* 1993;189:457-466.
26. Bode H. *Pediatric Applications of Transcranial Doppler Sonography.* New York: Springer-Verlag; 1988:44-75.
27. Fischer AQ, Truemper EJ. Pediatric applications. In: Newell DW, Aaslid R, eds. *Transcranial Doppler.* New York: Raven Press; 1992:245-268.
28. Lennihan L, Petty GW, Mohr JP et al. Transcranial Doppler detection of anterior cerebral artery vasospasm (abstract). *Stroke* 1989;20:151.
29. Sloan MA, Haley EC Jr, Kassell NF et al. Sensitivity and specificity of transcranial Doppler ultrasonography in the diagnosis of vasospasm following subarachnoid hemorrhage. *Neurology* 1989;39:1514-1518.
30. Thie A, Fuhlendorf A, Spitzer K et al. Transcranial Doppler evaluation of common and classic migraine. Part I. Ultrasonic

features during the headache-free period. *Headache* 1990; 30:201-208.
31. Thie A, Fuhlendorf A, Spitzer K et al. Transcranial Doppler evaluation of common and classic migraine. Part II. Ultrasonic features during attacks. *Headache* 1990;30:209-215.
32. McMenamin JB, Volpe JJ. Doppler ultrasonography in the determination of neonatal brain death. *Ann Neurol* 1983;14:302-307.
33. Chui NC, Shen EY, Lee BS. Reversal of diastolic cerebral blood flow in infants without brain death. *Pediatr Neurol* 1994; 11:337-340.
34. Glasier CM, Seibert JJ, Chadduck WM et al. Brain death in infants: evaluation with Doppler US. *Radiology* 1989;172:377-380.
35. Petty GW, Mohr JP, Pedley TA et al. The role of transcranial Doppler in confirming brain death: sensitivity, specificity, and suggestions for performance and interpretation. *Neurology* 1990;40:300-303.
36. Shiogai T, Sato E, Tokitsu M et al. Transcranial Doppler monitoring in severe brain damage: relationships between intracranial haemodynamics, brain dysfunction, and outcome. *Neurol Res* 1990;12:205-213.
37. Feri M, Ralli L, Felici M et al. Transcranial Doppler and brain death diagnosis. *Crit Care Med* 1994;22(7):1120-1126.
38. Bulas DJ, Chadduck WM, Vezina GL. Pediatric closed head injury: evaluation with transcranial Doppler US. Presented at the Eighty-First Scientific Assembly and Annual Meeting, Radiological Society of North America; Nov 26-Dec 1, 1995; Chicago, Ill.
39. Hassler W, Steinmetz H, Gawlowski J. Transcranial Doppler ultrasonography in raised intracranial pressure and in intracranial circulatory arrest. *J Neurosurg* 1988;68:745-751.
40. Jalili M, Crade M, Davis AL. Carotid blood-flow velocity changes detected by Doppler ultrasound in determination of brain death in children: a preliminary report. *Clin Pediatr* 1994;33:669-674.
41. Powers AD, Graeber MC, Smith RR. Transcranial Doppler ultrasonography in the determination of brain death. *Neurosurgery* 1989;24:884-889.
42. Stark JE, Seibert JJ. Cerebral artery Doppler ultrasonography for prediction of outcome after perinatal asphyxia. *J Ultrasound Med* 1994;13:595-600.
43. Gray PH, Tudehope DI, Massel JP et al. Perinatal hypoxic-ischaemic brain injury: prediction of outcome. *Dev Med Child Neurol* 1993;35:965-973.
44. Archer LNJ, Levene ME, Evans DH. Cerebral artery Doppler ultrasonography for prediction of outcome after perinatal asphyxia. *Lancet* 1986;2:1116.
45. Klingelhofer J et al. Evaluation of intracranial pressure from transcranial Doppler studies in cerebral disease. *J Neurol* 1988; 235:159-162.
46. Raju TNK. Cerebral Doppler studies in the fetus and newborn infant. *J Pediatr* 1991;119(2):165-174.
47. Raju TNK. Cranial Doppler applications in neonatal critical care. *Crit Care Med* 1992;8(1) 93-111.
48. Newell DW, Seiler RW, Aaslid R. Head injury and cerebral circulatory arrest. In: Newell DW, Aaslid R, eds. *Transcranial Doppler.* New York: Raven Press; 1992:109-121.
49. Hill A, Volpe JJ. Decrease in pulsatile flow in the anterior cerebral arteries in infantile hydocephalus. *Pediatrics* 1982;69:4-7.
50. Goh D, Minns RA. Intracranial pressure and cerebral arterial flow velocity indices in childhood hydrocephalus: current review. *Child Nerv Syst* 1995;11:392-396.
51. Goh D, Minns RA, Hendry GMA et al. Cerebrovascular resistive index assessed by duplex Doppler sonography and its relationship to intracranial pressure in infantile hydrocephalus. *Pediatr Radiol* 1992;22:246-250.
52. Finn JP, Quinn MW, Hall-Craggs MA et al. Impact of vessel distortion on transcranial Doppler velocity measurements: correlation with magnetic resonance imaging. *J Neurosurg* 1990; 73:572-575.
53. Hanlo PW, Gooskens RHJM, Nijhuis IJM et al. Value of transcranial Doppler indices in predicting raised ICP in infantile hydrocephalus. *Child Nerv Syst* 1995;11:595-603.
54. Westra SJ, Curran JG, Duckwiler GR et al. Pediatric intracranial vascular malformations: evaluation of treatment results with color Doppler US. *Radiology* 1993;186:775-783.
55. Grolimund P, Seiler RW, Aaslid R et al. Evaluation of cerebrovascular disease by combined extracranial and transcranial Doppler sonography: experience in 1,039 patients. *Stroke* 1987;18:1018-1024.
56. Lindegaard KF, Aaslid R, Nornes H. Cerebral arteriovenous malformations. In: Aaslid R, ed. *Transcranial Doppler Sonography.* New York: Springer-Verlag; 1986:86-105.
57. Lindegaard KF, Grolimund P, Aaslid R et al. Evaluation of cerebral AVM's using transcranial Doppler ultrasound. *J Neurosurg* 1986;65:335-344.
58. Petty GW, Massaro AR, Tatemichi TK et al. Transcranial Doppler ultrasonographic changes after treatment for AVMS. *Stroke* 1990;21:260-266.
59. Albin MS, Bunegin BS, Garcia C et al. Transcranial Doppler can image microaggregates of intracranial air and particulate matter. *J Neurosurg Anesth* 1989;1:134-135.
60. Pugsley W. The use of Doppler ultrasound in the assessment of microemboli during cardiac surgery. *Perfusion* 1986;4:115-122.
61. Dagirmanjian A, Davis DA, Rothful WE et al. Silent cerebral microemboli occurring during carotid angiography: frequency as determined with Doppler sonography. *AJR* 1993;161:1037-1040.
62. Powars D, Wilson B, Imbus C et al. The natural history of stroke in sickle cell disease. *Am J Med* 1978;65:461-471.
63. Huttenlocher PR, Moohr JW, Johns I et al. Cerebral blood flow in sickle cell cerebrovascular disease. *Pediatrics* 1984;73:615-621.
64. Waters MC, Patience M, Leisenring W et al. Bone marrow transplantation for sickle cell disease. *N Engl J Med* 1996; 335(6):369-376.
65. Adams RJ, Aaslid R, Gammal TE et al. Detection of cerebral vasculopathy in sickle cell disease using transcranial Doppler ultrasonography and magnetic resonance imaging: case report. *Stroke* 1988;19:518-520.
66. Adams RJ, Nichols FT, Figueroa R et al. Transcranial Doppler correlation with cerebral angiography in sickle cell disease. *Stroke* 1992;23:1073-1077.
67. Seibert JJ, Glasier CM, Allison JW et al. Transcranial Doppler (TCD), MRA, and MRI as a screening examination for cerebral vascular disease in patients with sickle cell anemia: a four-year follow-up. Presented at Third Conjoint Meeting, International Pediatric Radiology; May 1996; Boston, Mass.
68. Siegel MJ, Luker GD, Glauser TA et al. Cerebral infarction in sickle cell disease: transcranial Doppler US versus neurologic examination. *Radiology* 1995;197:191-194.
69. Verlhac S, Bernaudin F, Tortrat D et al. Detection of cerebrovascular disease in patients with sickle cell disease using transcranial Doppler sonography: correlation with MRI, MRA, and conventional angiography. *Pediatr Radiol* 1995;25:S14-S19.
70. Kogutt MS, Goldwag SS, Gupta KL et al. Correlation of transcranial Doppler ultrasonography with MRI and MRA in the evaluation of sickle cell disease patients with prior stroke. *Pediatr Radiol* 1994;24:204-206.

CHAPTER 55

Pediatric Head and Neck Masses*

Joanna J. Seibert, M.D.
Robert W. Seibert, M.D.

CHAPTER OUTLINE

High-resolution ultrasound has become extremely useful in evaluation of head and neck masses.[1-5] The absence of ionizing radiation or need for sedation make ultrasound the ideal initial examination in children.[6] Accurate anatomic localization of the mass can be determined with a knowledge of the normal anatomy of the region.[2] Sonographic tissue characteristics of the mass can often classify the lesion as inflammatory, neoplastic, congenital, traumatic, or vascular, and can be diagnostic in 40% of cases.[7] Ultrasound is also an excellent tool for use in following progression or regression of the lesion.[8] The complete extent of the lesion is better evaluated with computed tomography (CT) or magnetic resonance imaging (MRI)[7,9-16]

The neck can be divided into three anatomic areas: the face and upper neck, the lateral neck, and the thyroid and parathyroid glands. Normal anatomy and landmarks of the area are important to understand the characteristic sonographic findings of pathologic conditions.

FACE AND UPPER NECK

Normal Anatomy and Technique

Salivary Glands. The salivary glands are divided into three groups: the parotid glands, the submandibular glands, and the sublingual glands.

Parotid gland. The parotid gland is the largest of the salivary glands. It is located within a triangle bounded by the tip of the mastoid process, the mid-

*We wish to acknowledge that much of this original chapter, "Head and Neck Masses in Children," was based on the original article titled "Ultrasonography of Pediatric Neck and Masses" written by Gregory J. Lewis, M.D., Richard E. Leithiser Jr., M.D., Charles M. Glasier, M.D., Vaseem Iqbal, M.D., Carol A. Stephenson, and Joanna J. Seibert, M.D., and published by *Ultrasound Quarterly* 1989;7(4):315-335.

portion of the zygomatic arch, and the angle of the mandible. It is made up of acini connected by ducts that drain into Stensen's duct. The approximate location of Stensen's duct in the adolescent can be obtained by placing the index finger on the inferior margin of the zygomatic arch. The duct will be located on the lower surface of the finger.[17] The parotid gland also contains lymphoid tissue, vessels, and nerves. In particular, the seventh cranial nerve exits the stylomastoid foramen and passes into the parotid gland.[18] Here, it divides into five major branches, which predominantly supply the facial muscles. It divides the parotid gland into the deep and superficial lobes.[15] The deep lobe accounts for approximately 20% of the gland and is located adjacent to the parapharyngeal space.[19]

This gland is best evaluated in the axial and coronal planes using a high-frequency, linear, small-parts transducer with or without a stand-off pad. For the axial images, the transducer should be placed perpendicular to the ear with its superior margin touching the lobule (Fig. 55-1). In this position, the mastoid tip is seen posteriorly as an echogenic line with posterior acoustic shadowing (Fig. 55-2, *A*). As the transducer is moved inferiorly, the sternocleidomastoid muscle can be seen originating from the mastoid. Anteriorly, the mandible is identified as an echogenic line with posterior acoustic shadowing (Fig. 55-2, *B*). The masseter muscle is seen superficial to the mandible. The muscle mass deep to the mastoid tip is the posterior belly of the digastric muscle. This muscle originates from the base of the skull, just medial to the mastoid tip. The styloid process can be identified as an echogenic area superior and deep to the posterior belly of the digastric muscle. These two structures pass inferiorly and anteriorly toward the angle of the mandible. They are located deeper than the mandibular ramus. The parotid gland is seen as a homogeneous mass located just beneath the skin surface. It extends anteriorly over the masseter muscle, medially behind the posterior aspect of the mandible, and posteriorly to the mastoid tip and sternocleidomastoid muscle. It is more echogenic and homogeneous than the adjacent muscles and fat.[19,20] This is probably because it contains fatty glandular tissue. The retromandibular or posterior facial vein is identified within the substance of the parotid gland, just posterior to the mandible.

The vascular anatomy of the parotid gland can be well evaluated with color flow Doppler imaging.[21] The terminal branch of the external carotid artery can be seen just medial to the superior aspect of the posterior facial vein. The internal jugular vein and internal and external carotid arteries are often well visualized deep to the styloid process and posterior belly of the digastric muscle. The internal jugular vein is posterior and

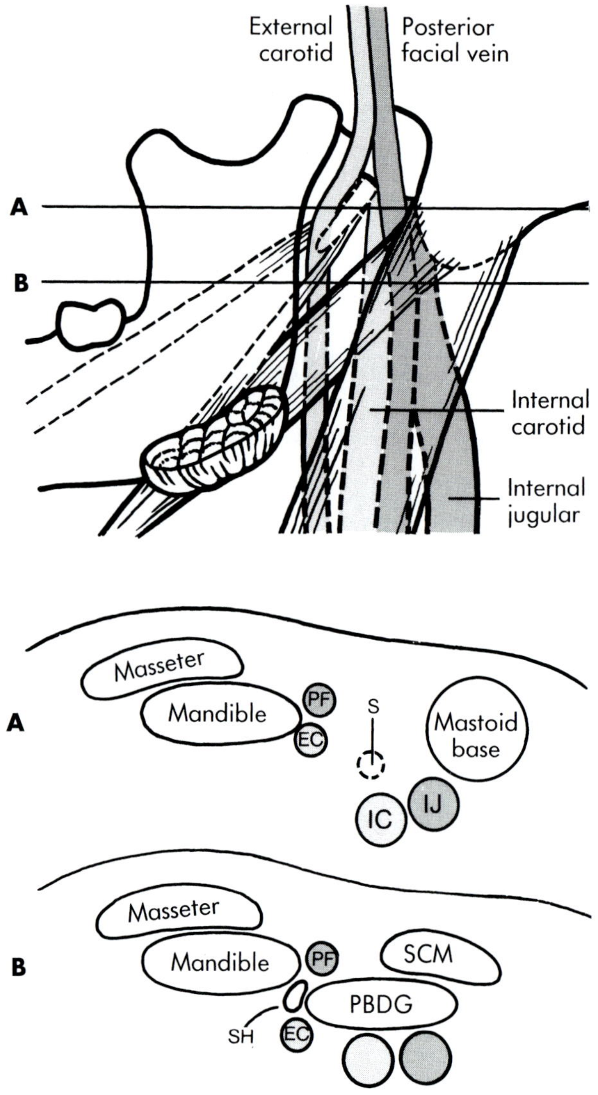

FIG. 55-1. Normal parotid gland diagram in axial or perpendicular scans. Normal landmarks such as the sternocleidomastoid muscle, *SCM*, posterior belly of the digastric muscle, *PBDG*, styloid process, *S*, internal carotid artery, *IC*, internal jugular vein, *IJ*, external carotid artery, *EC*, posterior facial vein, *PF*, and stylohyoid muscle, *SH*, can be seen. The parotid gland lies between the sternocleidomastoid muscle and mastoid tip posteriorly and the masseter muscle and mandible anteriorly. (From Lewis GJS, Leithiser RE Jr, Glasier GM et al. Ultrasonography of pediatric neck masses. *Ultrasound Q* 1989;7:315-355.)

lateral to the internal carotid artery. Because of the surgical importance of localizing tumors in the deep or superficial lobes,[18] the course of the facial nerve can be estimated by drawing a line from the upper aspect of the posterior belly of the digastric muscle to the posterior facial vein and then to the lateral aspect of the mandibular ramus.[11,19]

The coronal images are obtained by placing the transducer just anterior and parallel to the ear (Fig. 55-3). The transducer is then angled anteriorly and

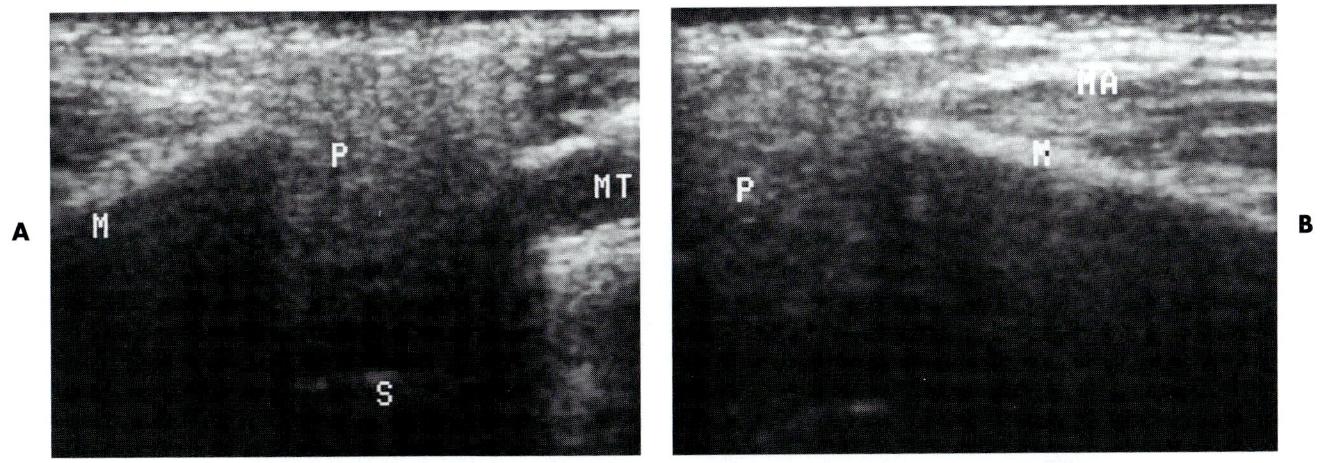

FIG. 55-2. Normal parotid gland ultrasound. **A,** Axial view of the parotid gland, showing mastoid tip, *MT*. Between the mastoid tip, *MT*, and the mandible, *M*, is the echogenic styloid process, *S*. **B,** Axial scan of the parotid gland, *P*, with the masseter muscle, *MA*, and the mandible, *M*, anterior to it.

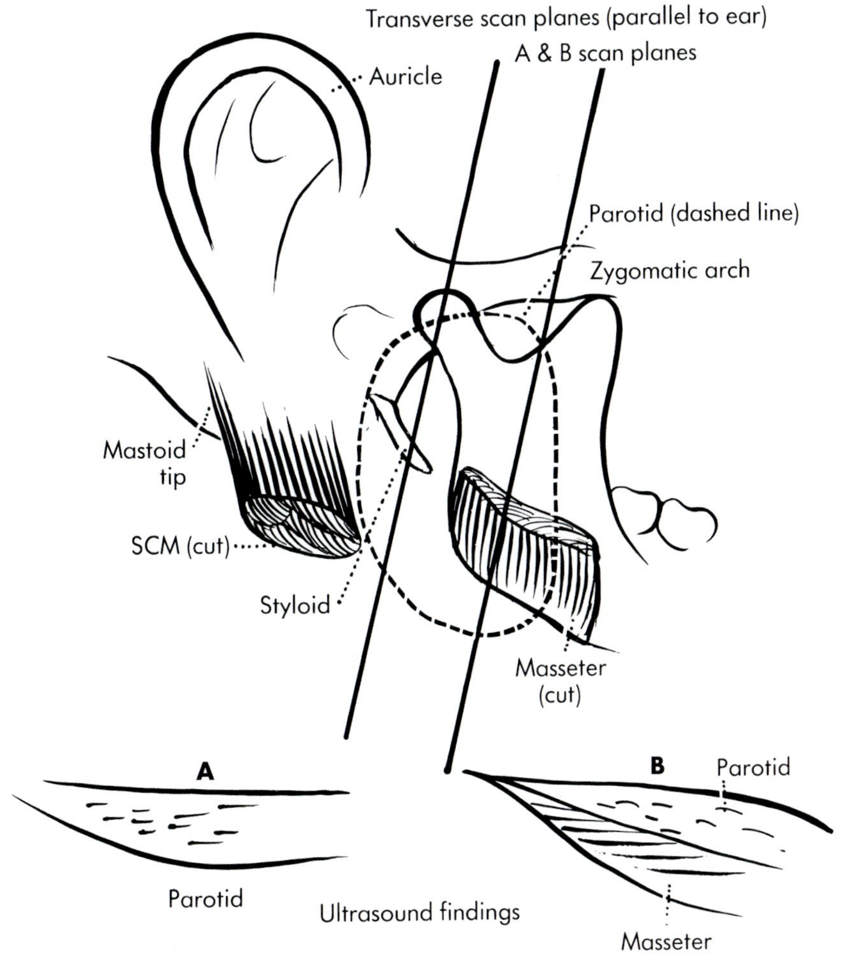

FIG. 55-3. Normal parotid gland. Transverse scan planes, **A,** parallel and just anterior to the ear show the elliptical parotid gland. **B,** The second plane, slightly more anterior on the mandible, shows the parotid gland with the masseter muscle medial and inferior to it. (From Seibert RW, Seibert JJ. High-resolution ultrasonography of the parotid gland in children. Part I. *Pediatr Radiol* 1986;16:374-379.)

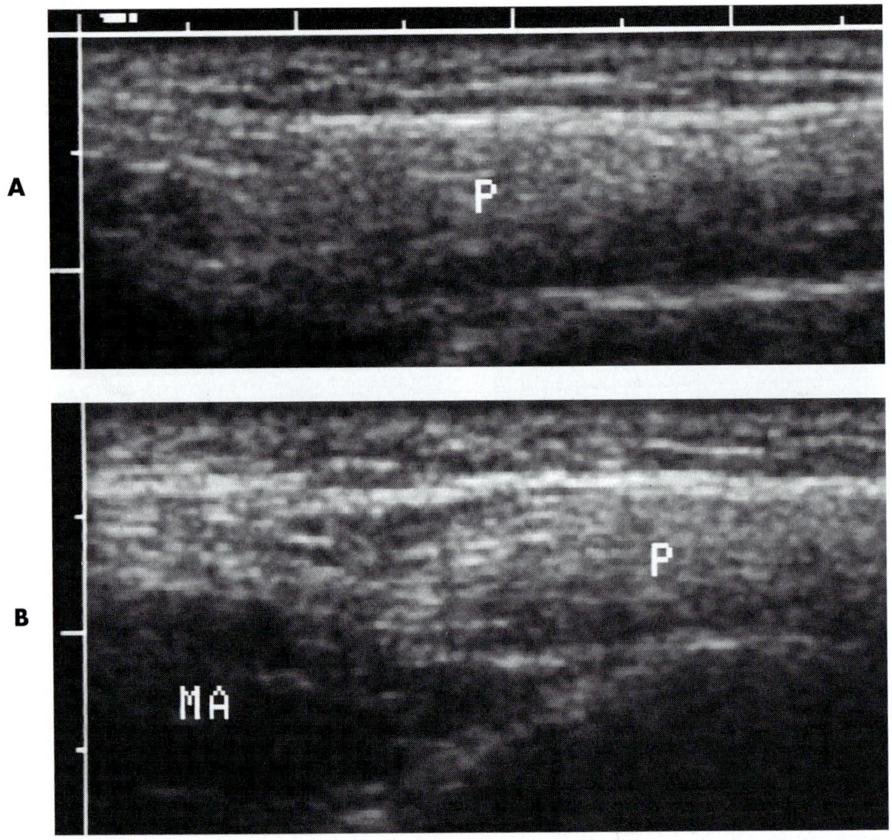

FIG. 55-4. Normal parotid gland. **A,** Transverse scan of the parotid gland just anterior to the ear shows the elliptical echogenic parotid gland, *P*. **B,** Scanning more anteriorly, the masseter muscle, *MA*, is noted medial to the parotid gland, *P*.

posteriorly. The parotid gland is seen as an elliptical, homogeneous, echogenic area just beneath the skin (Fig. 55-4).

Submandibular gland. The submandibular gland predominantly lies in the submandibular space, which is bounded laterally by the body of the mandible and superiorly and medially by the mylohyoid muscle. A small portion of this gland may pass posterior to the back of the mylohyoid muscle and lie within the sublingual space.[14] It is drained by Wharton's duct, which passes between the lateral mylohyoid muscle and medial hyoglossus muscle.[22]

The submandibular gland is best evaluated by sonography from a submental position with the transducer angled in both the sagittal and coronal planes. The submandibular gland is located medial to the body of the mandible and superficial to the anterior belly of the digastric and mylohyoid muscles. Its posterior aspect may wrap around the back of the mylohyoid muscle to lie in the sublingual space. The position of Wharton's duct can be seen by having patients move their tongue. This reveals the plane between the mylohyoid and hyoglossus muscles where the duct runs.[22]

Sublingual glands. There are multiple sublingual glands that lie in the floor of the mouth. These are located deep to the mylohyoid muscle and superficial to the hyoglossus muscle[22] and the intrinsic muscles of the tongue. The sublingual glands are difficult to see sonographically.[20]

Inflammation

Inflammatory processes of the salivary glands are considerably more frequent than neoplasms and developmental abnormalities and account for approximately one third of all salivary gland pathology in one series.[23] Inflammation can be either acute or chronic.

Acute inflammation may be secondary to a generalized **parotitis,** usually of viral etiology (Fig. 55-5). Ultrasound shows diffuse enlargement of the gland with an associated irregular decrease in the gland's echotexture.[20,24,25] **Focal abscesses** can form, especially in the neonate between 7 and 14 days after birth. ***Staphylococcus aureus*** is the most common organism

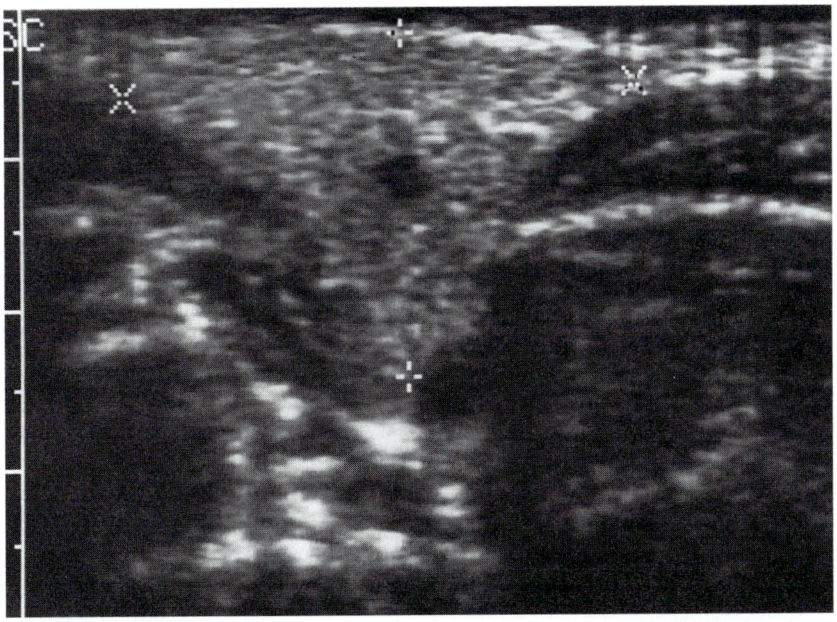

FIG. 55-5. Viral parotitis. A diffusely enlarged gland (bounded by *X* and +). The echogenic line of the mandible is anterior with the hypoechoic masseter muscle superficial to it. Note the normal posterior facial vein posterior to the mandible. (From Seibert RW, Seibert JJ. High-resolution ultrasonography of the parotid gland in children. Part II. *Pediatr Radiol* 1988;19:13-18.)

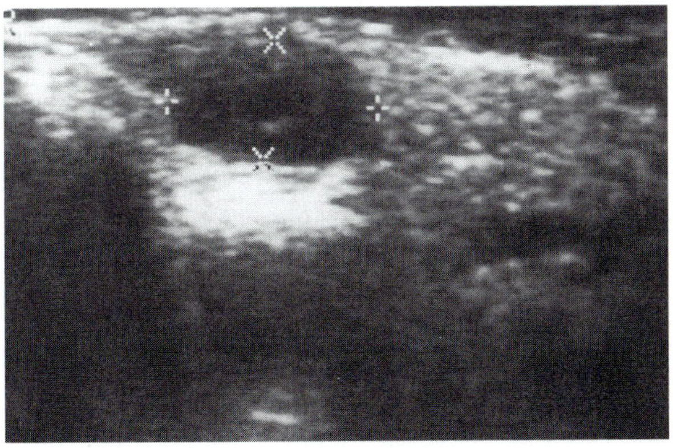

FIG. 55-6. Intraparotid lymph node. A hypoechoic mass bounded by *X* and + is located within the homogeneous echogenic parotid gland. (From Lewis GJS, Leithiser RE Jr, Glasier GM et al. Ultrasonography of pediatric neck masses. *Ultrasound Q* 1989;7:315-355.)

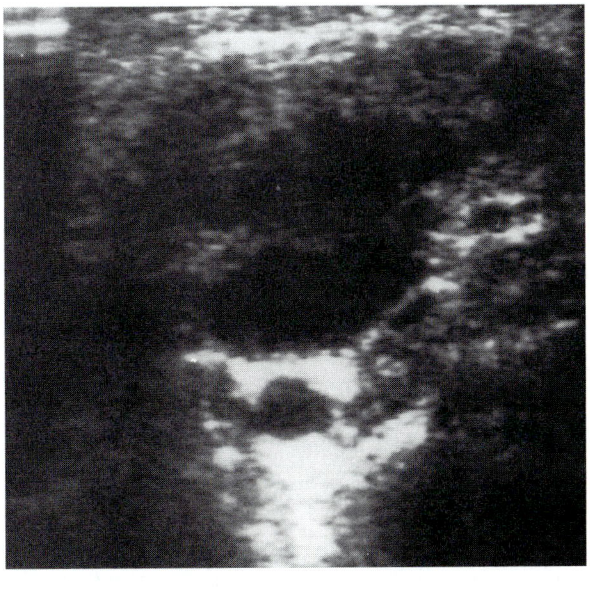

FIG. 55-7. Parotid abscess in the left neck just below the parotid gland. This abscess has the typical findings of a hypoechoic center with irregular walls. (From Lewis GJS, Leithiser RE Jr, Glasier GM et al. Ultrasonography of pediatric neck masses. *Ultrasound Q* 1989;7:315-355.)

and is seen in 60% of cases.[26] These abscesses are predominantly seen in the parotid gland.[27] When a focal abscess has formed, ultrasound-guided drainage can be performed.[28] The parotid gland may also be diffusely enlarged secondary to trauma.[29]

Inflammatory lymph node enlargement in the parotid gland is often associated with neck adenopathy and is sometimes difficult to distinguish from acute parotitis clinically. However, ultrasound shows discrete hypoechoic masses within the gland that represent intraparotid nodes (Fig. 55-6).

Intraparotid adenopathy associated with conjunctivitis is a distinct entity called **Parinaud's syndrome.** Lymph node involvement from sarcoidosis has also been described.[30] Sonography is also useful in separating adenopathy from masses in the submandibular and sublingual glands (Fig. 55-7).

A

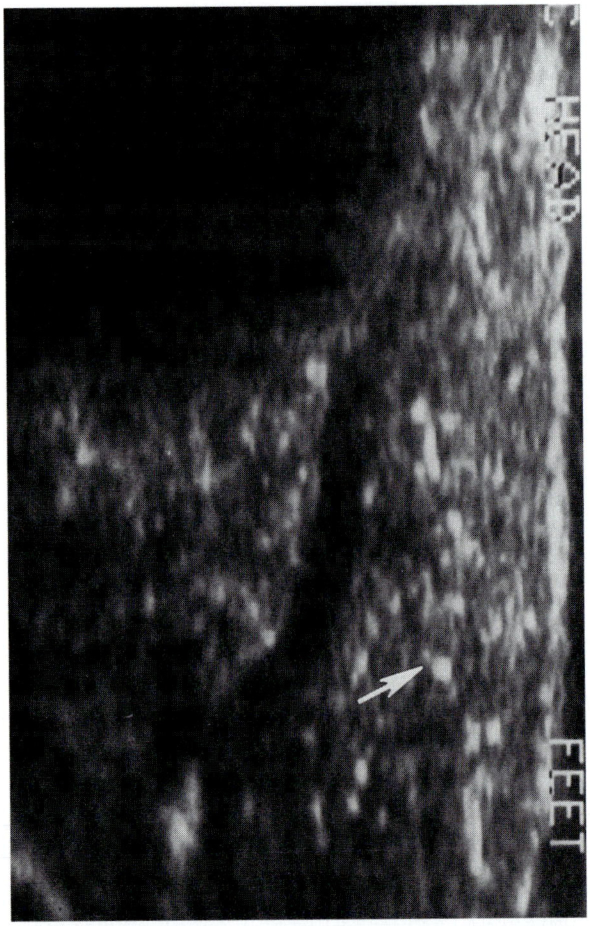

B

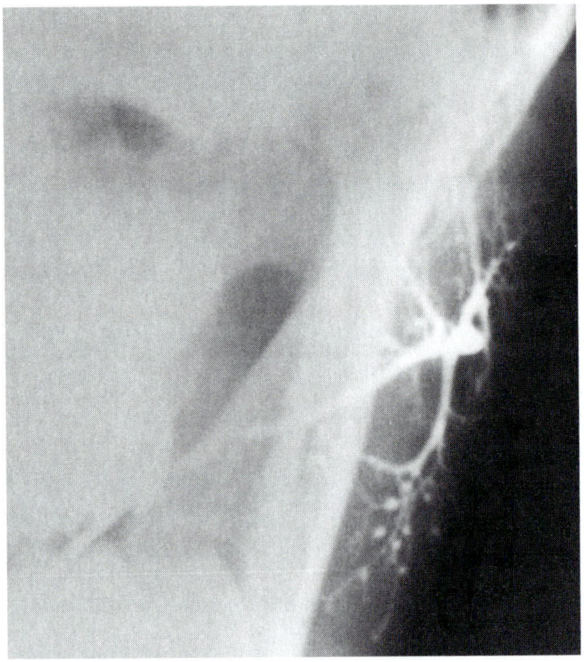

FIG. 55-8. Chronic parotitis. **A,** Transverse sonogram shows multiple, small, punctate, echogenic, but nonshadowing, densities throughout the parotid gland *(arrow)*, probably representing mucus within the dilated ducts. **B,** Sialogram shows retention of contrast within the dilated ducts. (From Seibert RW, Seibert JJ. High-resolution ultrasonography of the parotid gland in children. Part II. *Pediatr Radiol* 1988;19:13-18.)

Chronic parotitis often presents as intermittent, unilateral, painless swelling of the gland.[23] It may be associated with **sialectasis,** which has a typical sonographic appearance of small, punctate, echogenic densities scattered through the gland (Fig. 55-8). We have also seen one patient with sialectasis who had an inhomogeneous gland with multiple hypoechoic areas.[29] If there is chronic painful swelling of the gland, then benign lymphosialadenopathy or **Sjögren's syndrome** should be considered.[23] This may be part of **Mikulicz's disease,** which is similar to Sjögren's syndrome except that Mikulicz's disease has no systemic component.[31,32] Differentiation between chronic inflammation and autoimmune disease by ultrasound is not possible, according to some authors.[20] However, Bradus et al.[33] and Rubaltelli et al.[34] believe that this area has not been fully explored by sonography and that Sjögren's syndrome may have a distinct pattern of "multiple, scattered cystic changes of variable complexity throughout the parotid gland presumably caused by sialectasis."[33]

Parotid enlargement can be seen in children who are HIV positive with **AIDS-related complex,** especially those with lymphocytic interstitial pneumonitis (LIP) and diffuse cervical lymphadenopathy.[35] The enlargement is typically bilateral, and on sonography the gland is filled with multiple hypoechoic masses having the appearance of cysts but often without back wall enhancement (Fig. 55-9). Sialography reveals generalized acinar dilatation consistent with sialectasis, and pathology reveals lymphocyte infiltration and lymphoepithelial cysts.[36] The lymphocytic hyperplasia in the parotid gland probably mirrors the process in other areas with the development of epithelial-lined clefts in the parotid gland surrounded by hyperplastic lymphoid tissue with prominent germinal centers.

Sialolithiasis is rarely seen in children but may be associated with **cystic fibrosis.**[23] Most stones are seen in the submandibular gland (80%) and are calcified.[37] Plain radiographs should first be obtained. If no stone is identified, sonography is useful in discovering the noncalcified stones or concretions (Fig. 55-10).[20,34,37,38]

Obstruction of a sublingual salivary gland duct can result in a cystic mass known as a **ranula.** The mass is located deep to the mylohyoid muscle,[20] but can have a diving (plunging) component, yielding a cystic mass located medial to the angle of the mandible and superficial to the mylohyoid muscle (i.e., in the submandibular space).

Neoplasms

Salivary gland tumors are uncommon, especially in children less than 16 years old.[39] Excluding vascular

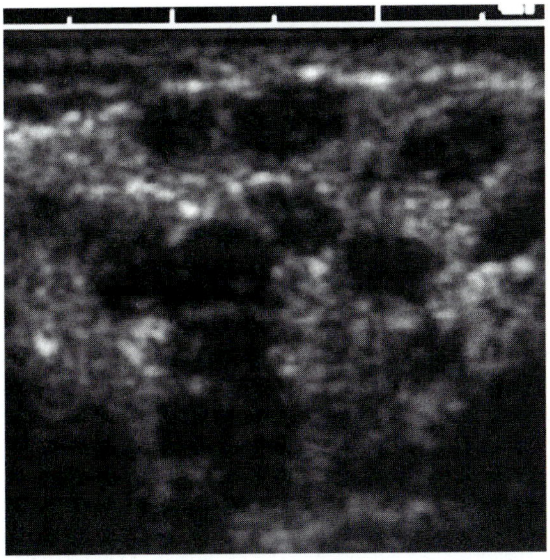

FIG. 55-9. Parotid gland enlargement in child with HIV infection. Both parotid glands were enlarged with multiple hypoechoic lesions without back wall enhancement.

FACIAL AND UPPER NECK MASSES

Vascular
- Hemangioendotheliomas
- Hemangioma
- Lymphangioma

Nonvascular
- Pleomorphic adenomas of the parotid gland
- Mucoepidermoid carcinomas
- Undifferentiated sarcoma
- Neurofibroma

Cysts
- Branchial pouch or cleft
- Mucous retention cyst
- Vallecular cyst
- Abscess
- Hematoma
- Pseudoaneurysm

lesions, 50% of parotid masses are malignant.[40] Overall, angiomas are the most common type of tumors, especially hemangiomas.[41,42]

In the neonate, **hemangioendotheliomas** are the most common neoplasm.[19,23] These masses present predominantly in the female, with a 4:1 predominance. Clinically, they are painless, enlarging masses in the region of the parotid gland. Approximately 50% have a sentinel bluish or red stain of the skin overlying the mass.[42] Recent experience suggests that there is a high rate of spontaneous resolution, which precludes the use of surgery.[23] Steroids have been noted to be beneficial in their treatment.[42]

Other angiomas include lymphangiomas or cystic hygromas and hemangiomas. **Hemangiomas** appear to infiltrate between the salivary glands, particularly the parotid gland. Unlike the hemangioendothelioma, hemangiomas are rarely entirely localized to the parotid gland and often extend into the lateral neck. They also have a marked female predominance. Sonography is useful in evaluating hemangiomas and demonstrating calcifications and compression of the vascular spaces (Fig. 55-11).[20]

Color flow Doppler evaluation will reveal the presence and type of vascular flow in a vascular malformation (see Fig. 55-11).[43,44] Hemangiomas show nonspecific echogenicity with high flow pattern. Spectral analysis reveals arterial and venous flow without shunting. Venous malformations exhibit heterogeneous echogenicity with a hypoechoic lacunar pattern. Color flow Doppler imaging shows either no flow or low venous flow. Arteriolocapillary malformations have

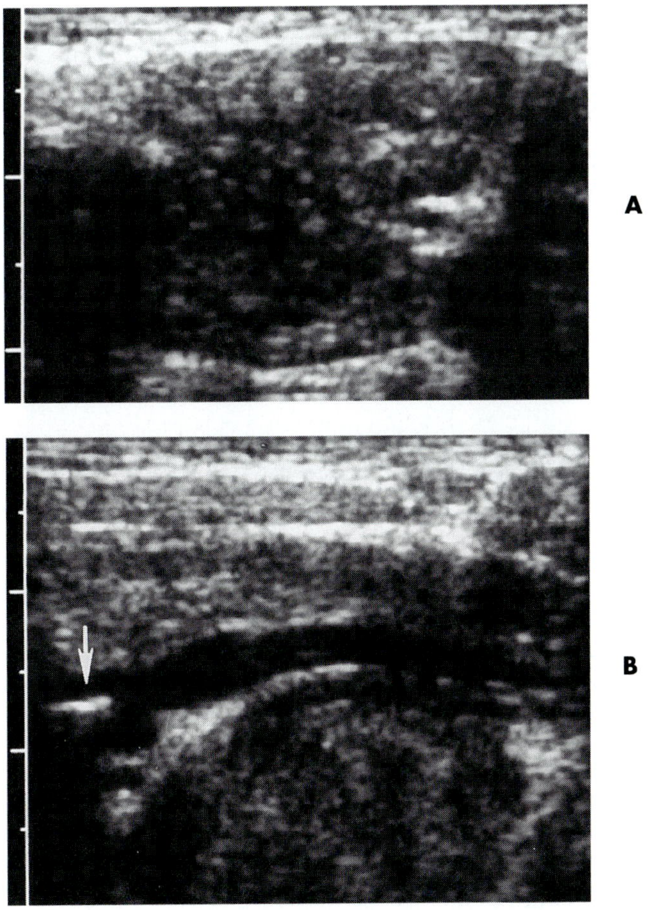

FIG. 55-10. Submandibular duct obstruction. **A,** Enlarged submandibular gland. **B,** Dilated submandibular duct secondary to stone *(arrow)*.

A

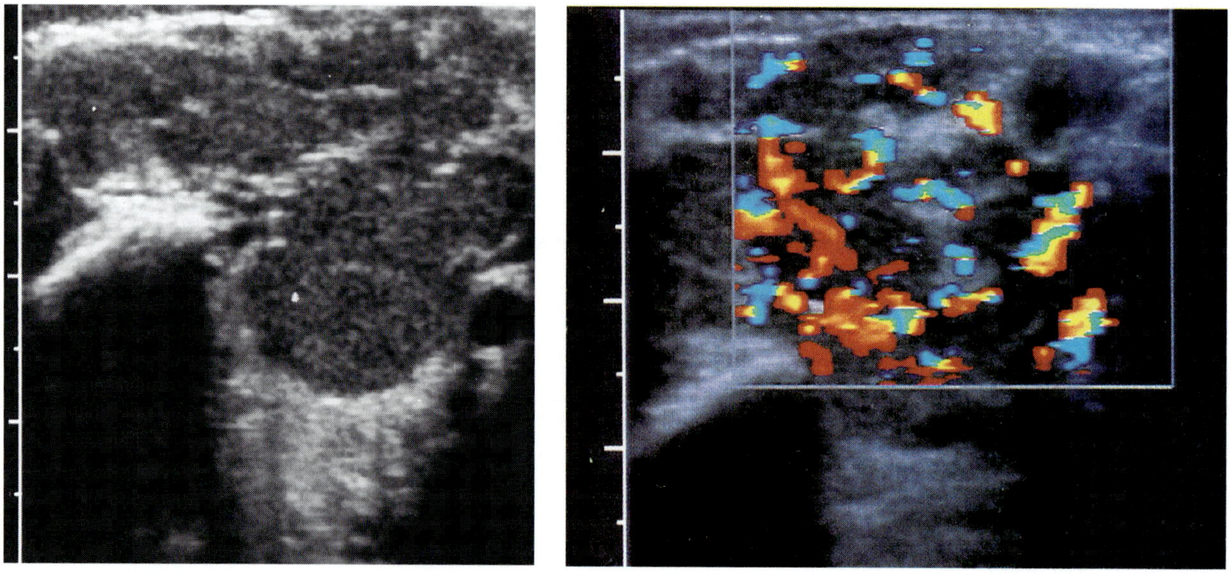

B

FIG. 55-11. Hemangioma. **A,** Ultrasound of young girl with an enlarged parotid gland shows diffusely enlarged gland with multiple small, hypoechoic areas. **B,** Color flow Doppler imaging demonstrates markedly vascular parotid gland. Spectral analysis demonstrated arterial and venous flow without shunting. The parotid gland enlargement responded to steroid treatment.

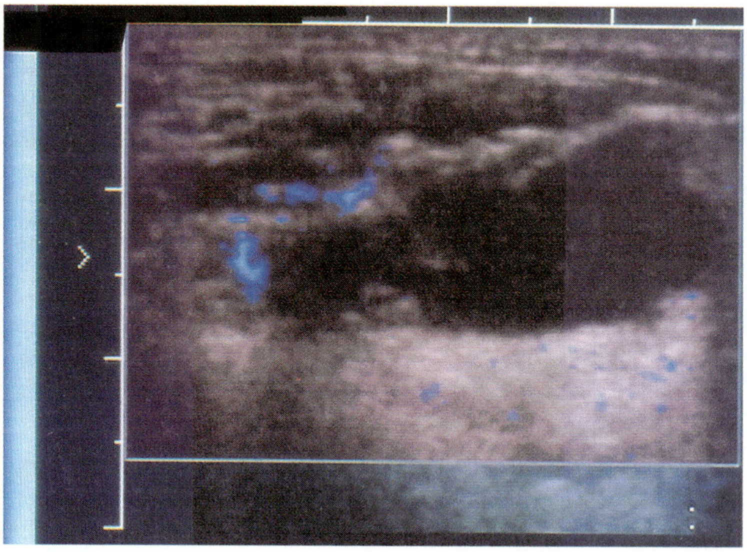

FIG. 55-12. Lymphangioma. Power mode Doppler imaging of cystic neck mass with no increased flow.

homogeneously echogenic, low-flow lesions with arterial and venous patterns without shunting. Arteriovenous (AV) malformations are heterogeneously echogenic, high-flow lesions with typical arteriovenous shunting. Mixed and microcystic lymphangiomas show variable echogenicity. Macrocystic lymphangiomas present with either anechoic or hypoechoic homogeneous lesions. No flow is usually detected within **lymphangiomas** (Fig. 55-12).

In the older child and adolescent, mixed tumors or **pleomorphic adenomas of the parotid gland** are the most common epithelial neoplasm.[19,23,39] Rarely, they can invade and develop late metastatic lesions.[39] No definite sex predominance is noted in children.[23] They most frequently occur in the parotid gland (90%)[39] and are rarely seen in the submandibular gland. There is a high rate of recurrence (20%).[39] These tumors are slightly hypoechoic with respect to the parotid gland.[20,29,30] Other authors have described them as anechoic at normal gain settings with a few echoes at higher gain settings.[25,45] They can have cystic areas and small calcifications within them.

A

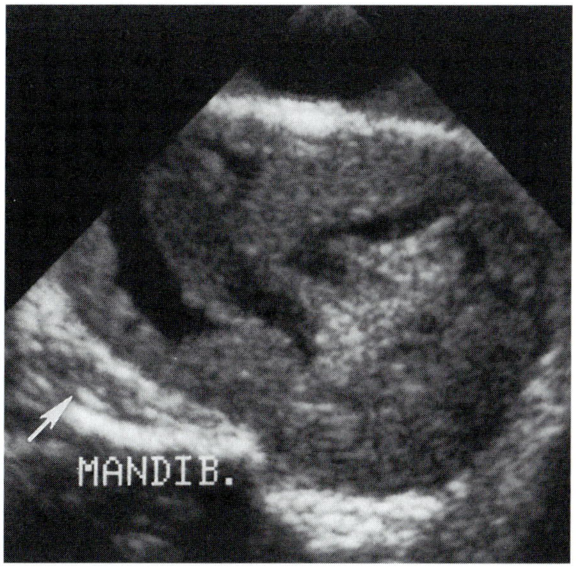

B

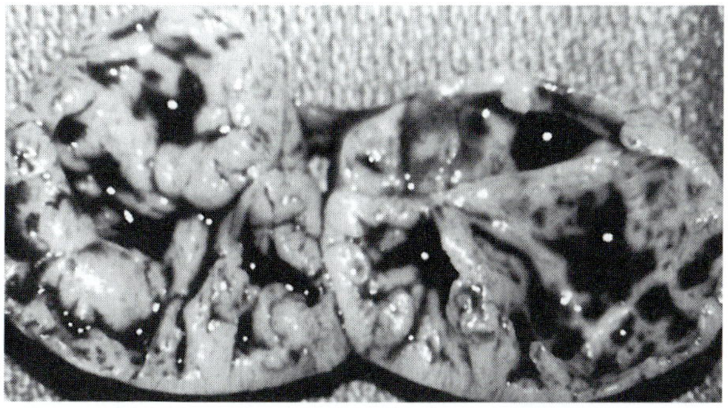

FIG. 55-13. Undifferentiated carcinoma. **A,** Thin rim of parotid tissue noted anteriorly *(arrow)* to mandible. The remainder of the parotid gland is replaced by a mixed mass with hypoechoic central areas. **B,** Cut surface of the tumor, showing blood-filled cavities centrally. (From Seibert RW, Seibert JJ. High-resolution ultrasonography of the parotid gland in children. Part II. *Pediatr Radiol* 1988; 19:13-18.)

A

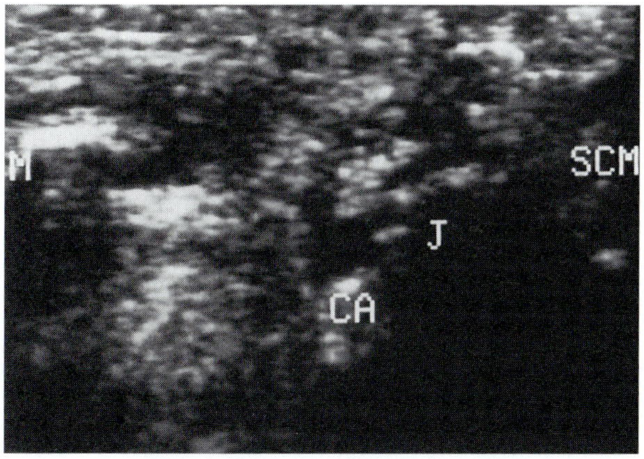

B

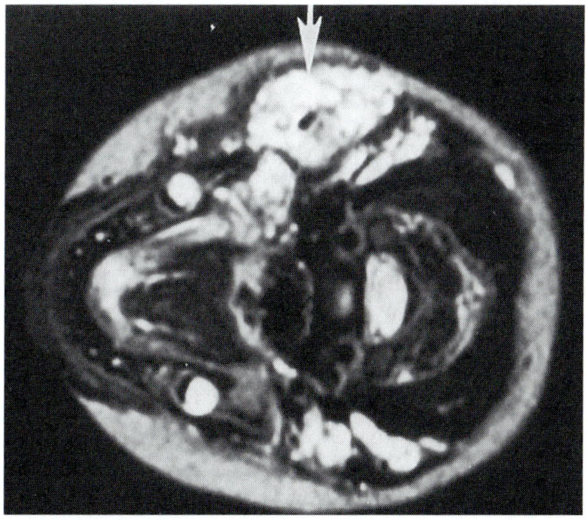

FIG. 55-14. Neurofibromas. **A,** Ultrasound of the left parotid gland shows inhomogeneous hypoechoic areas scattered throughout the parotid gland. **B,** T2-weighted axial MRI of the upper neck (turned to same position as ultrasound) shows diffuse increased signal infiltrating the left parotid gland *(arrow)*. *SCM,* Sternocleidomastoid muscle; *J,* jugular vein; *CA,* carotid artery; *M,* mandible. (From Lewis GJS, Leithiser RE Jr, Glasier GM et al. Ultrasonography of pediatric neck masses. *Ultrasound Q* 1989;7:315-355.)

Among the primary malignant tumors that occur in children, **mucoepidermoid carcinomas** are the most common.[23] These have a good prognosis[39] and are followed in incidence by undifferentiated carcinomas and undifferentiated sarcomas,[23] which have poorer prognoses.[39] **Undifferentiated sarcomas** tend to occur in children under 5 years of age (Fig. 55-13).[23] On sonography, malignant tumors tend to have ill-defined borders, but can have well-defined smooth or lobulated edges. Most benign tumors have well-defined smooth or lobulated margins.[11,25,30,45]

Neurofibromas can involve the parotid gland. Sonography shows multiple hypoechoic areas throughout the gland (Fig. 55-14). When neurofibromas are plexiform, neurofibromatosis should be considered.[46]

Congenital Lesions

Cysts of the parotid gland may be derived from the **branchial clefts** or **branchial pouches** (Fig. 55-15).[23,47] A **mucous retention cyst** of the parotid gland has also been described by ultrasound in a 13-year-old girl.[48]

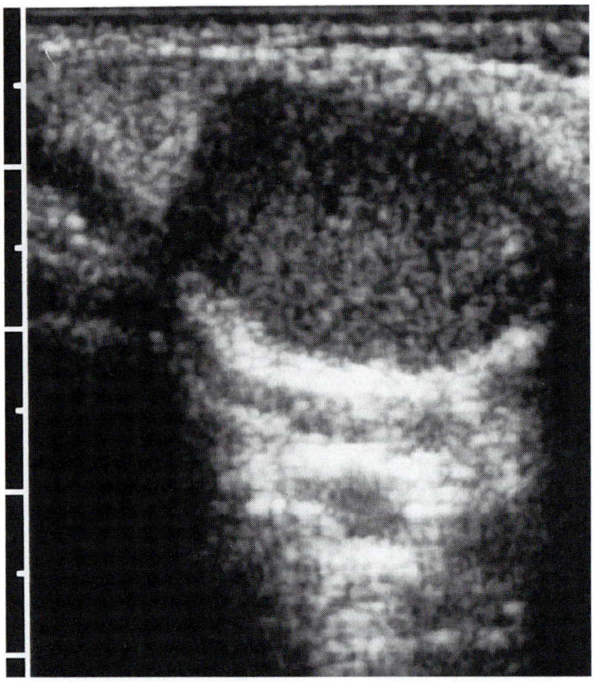

FIG. 55-15. Parotid gland cyst. Ultrasound of enlarged parotid gland in a child shows echogenic mass with through transmission. At surgery, a parotid gland cyst was found filled with debris.

A 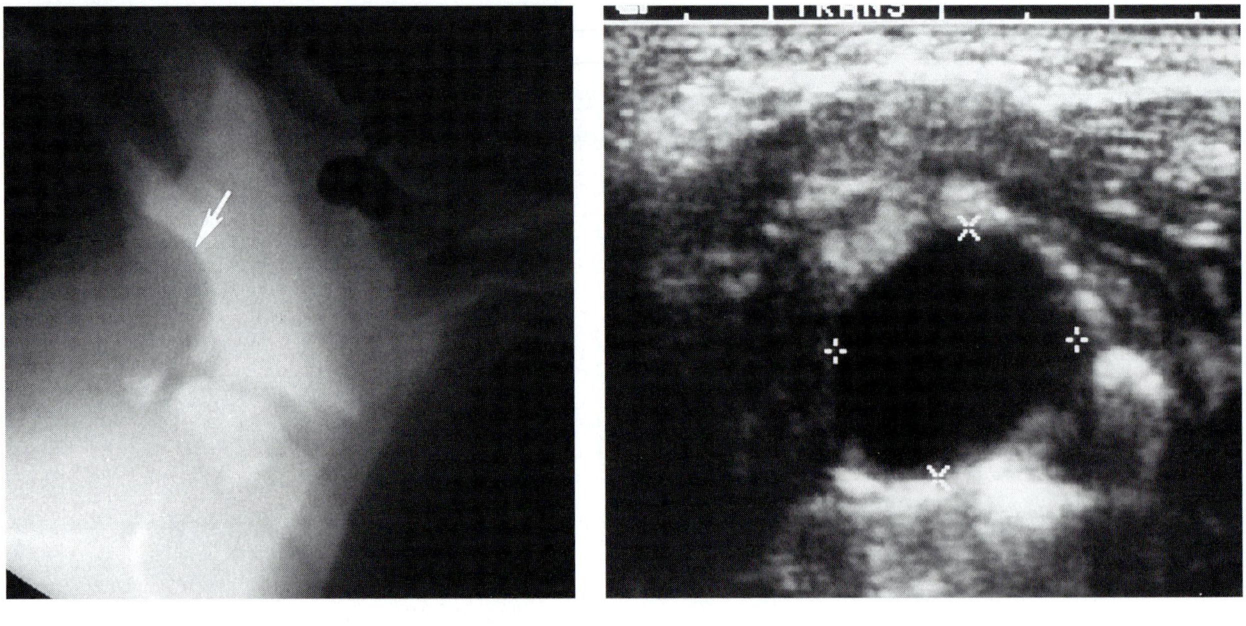 B

FIG. 55-16. Cyst of vallecula. **A,** Lateral neck scan demonstrating vallecular mass *(arrow)* in an infant with stridor *(black and white reversed)*. **B,** Transverse ultrasound of upper neck demonstrates the cystic nature of the mass.

Other Facial and Upper Neck Masses

Children with **cysts of the vallecula** may present with stridor. Sonography is helpful to demonstrate the cystic nature of this mass in the vallecula (Fig. 55-16).

The premasseteric space is superficial to the masseter muscle and is a frequent site for trauma and infections. Clinically, it is difficult to differentiate swelling in this area from swelling in the parotid gland, lymph nodes, or masseter muscle. Ultrasound is helpful in characterizing the pathology and demonstrating whether there is parotid gland involvement. A **hematoma** of the masseter should present as a hy-

A
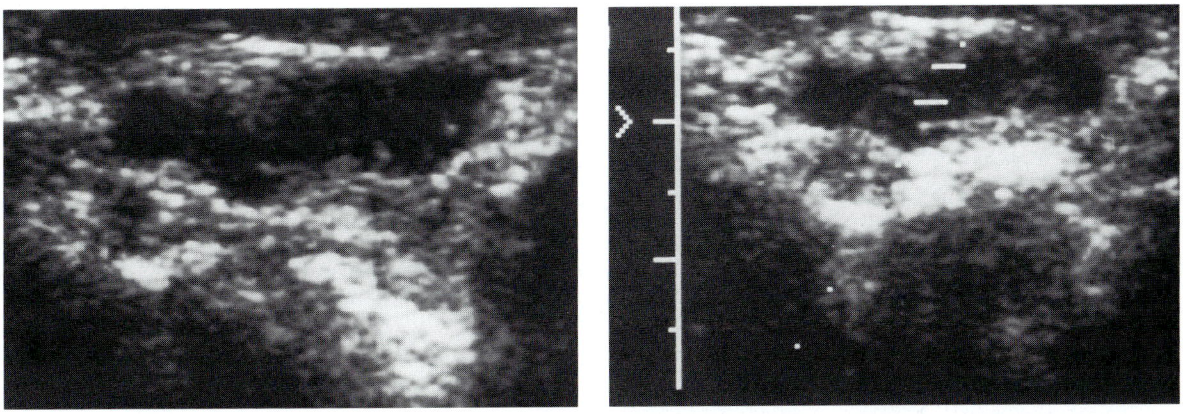
B

FIG. 55-17. Posttraumatic hematoma of the masseter muscle (13-year-old). **A,** Ultrasound shows a hypoechoic mass with irregular walls. **B,** Doppler ultrasound shows no flow within this area. (From Lewis GJS, Leithiser RE Jr, Glasier GM et al. Ultrasonography of pediatric neck masses. *Ultrasound Q* 1989;7:315-355.)

A
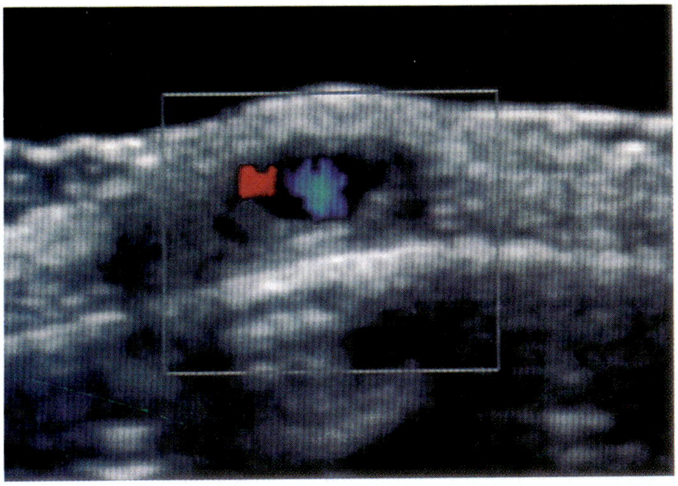

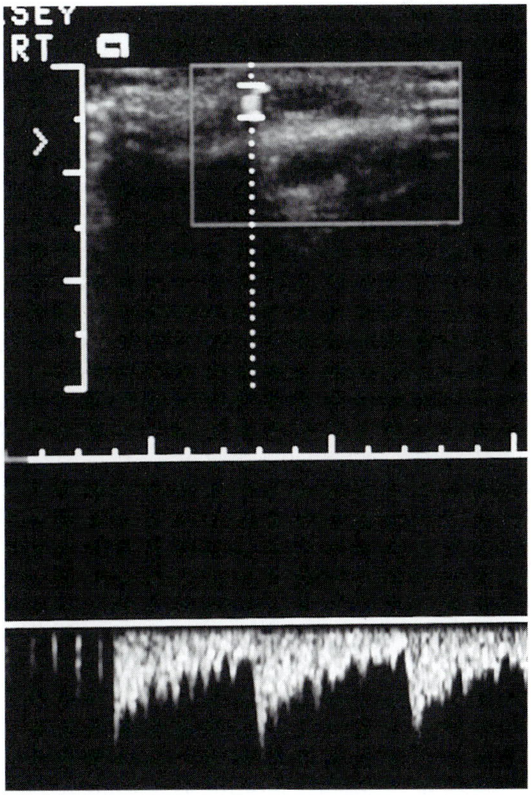

B

FIG. 55-18. Posttraumatic aneurysm. **A,** Color flow Doppler ultrasound of a pulsatile scalp lesion in a 14-year-old after trauma shows a hypoechoic superficial mass with swirling flow. **B,** Spectral analysis shows arterial flow in the pseudoaneurysm.

poechoic mass (Fig. 55-17)[49] and may appear similar to an **abscess** of the premasseteric space. During resolution, it may have a mixed echotexture with the suggestion of septations.[7,29,50,51]

Another facial mass is a posttraumatic **pseudoaneurysm.** Doppler imaging is extremely valuable in demonstrating that this cystic mass is vascular (Fig. 55-18).

Benign hypertrophy of the masseter muscle has been described by CT and ultrasound (Fig. 55-19).[11,52]

Sonography also has been used for localization of **foreign bodies** in the extremities and should be useful for this purpose in the face and neck (Fig. 55-20).[53]

Ultrasound has recently been used to evaluate the larynx.[54] It has particular application for children with laryngeal papillomatosis.[55]

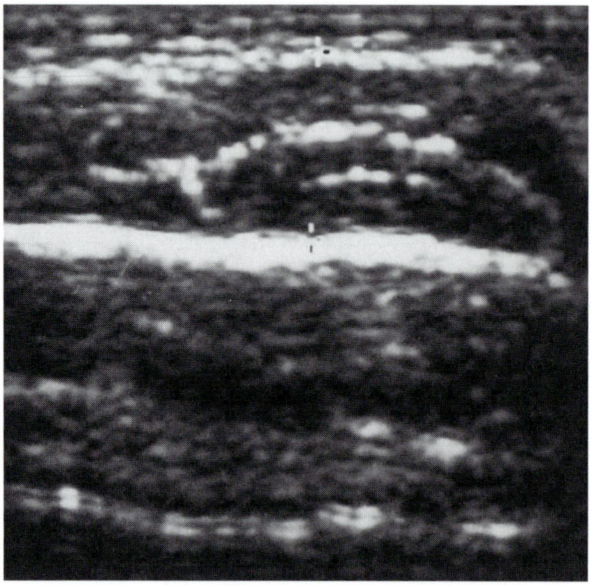

FIG. 55-19. Masseter muscle hypertrophy. Young girl with prominent cheek masses bilaterally, which by ultrasound were enlarged masseter muscles.

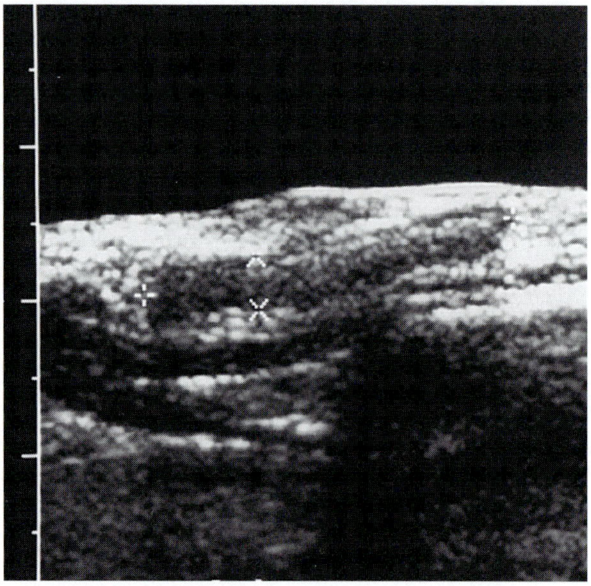

FIG. 55-20. Foreign body (2-year-old). Post-operative removal of branchial cleft cyst with chronic drainage from the neck. Ultrasound shows a foreign body just beneath the patient's hypertrophic scar *(cursors)*.

LATERAL NECK

Normal Anatomy

The neck is divided into the posterior and anterior triangles anatomically. The division is made by the sternocleidomastoid muscle, which extends from the mastoid tip anteriorly and inferiorly. This muscle has two heads inferiorly, a clavicular head and a sternal head. The sternal head is located medially. The posterior aspect of the posterior triangle is bounded by the trapezius muscle. This muscle extends from the occiput inferiorly and laterally to insert into the spinous process of the scapula. The anterior aspect of the anterior triangle is the midline.[17,56] The common carotid artery and internal jugular vein lie just deep to the sternocleidomastoid muscle. In the upper neck, the internal jugular vein lies lateral and posterior to the carotid artery. In the lower neck, this vessel lies anterior and lateral to the common carotid artery. The cervical lymph node chains are divided into four or five major groups. However, for the purposes of sonography, two major groups should be considered: those located in the anterior triangle and those located in the posterior triangle. As a general rule, posterior triangle lymphadenopathy tends to be benign.[23]

Normal cervical nodes are oval and hypoechoic, with an echogenic linear hilus.[57] Power mode Doppler imaging will often identify a **central vessel in the hilum of the normal node** (Fig. 55-21). Ying et al.

studied cervical nodes in normal patients older than 14 years and found nodes in all 100 subjects.[57]

Inflammation

The majority of pediatric neck masses are secondary to acute lymphadenitis, which should resolve with appropriate medical treatment.[6] The most common organisms identified are ***Staphylococcus aureus***; in fewer instances, group A beta-hemolytic ***Streptococcus*** is seen.[23] Sonography is useful in following acute inflammatory processes. **Lymphadenitis** initially presents as homogeneous hypoechoic masses. Inflammatory nodes may be highly vascular on color flow Doppler imaging (see Fig. 55-21, *D* and *E*). If these develop into **abscesses,** the ultrasound picture shows development of a central lucency with a surrounding irregular wall (Fig. 55-22).[6,7,58,59] Lymph nodes also tend to **coalesce** in abscess formation (Fig. 55-23).[9] Nodes with **thick pus may appear echogenic** rather than echolucent (Fig. 55-24). **Sonographic signs of the liquefied nature of the abscessed nodes** (see box, top of right column) are present through transmission, movement of necrotic material in the abscessed node[60] with compression and release dynamic imaging, absence of the central hilar stripe on imaging, and absence of the central hilar vessel on power mode Doppler imaging (Fig. 55-25). Echogenic gas bubbles in a neck mass may be diagnostic of the unusual but life-threatening anaerobic infections of the neck.[61] Rarely, mycobacterial or fungal infections occur. In the case of granulomatous disease, **calcifications** may be seen (Fig. 55-26).

Sonography is also useful in the evaluation of **retropharyngeal abscesses.**[62] Because the retropharyngeal lymph nodes atrophy after 4 years of age, retropharyngeal abscesses are a disease of young children.[63] Lateral neck radiography and contrast CT identify and localize retropharyngeal inflammatory masses, but ultrasound is superior to CT in distinguishing between adenitis and abscess formation.[62] We have used intraoperative ultrasound guidance for transoral drainage of retropharyngeal and peripharyngeal abscesses. This is important because the great vessels are often located just lateral to the abscess (Fig. 55-27).

Mucocutaneous lymph node syndrome (Kawasaki's disease) also tends to present with cervical adenopathy and should be considered in the differential diagnosis. No distinguishing characteristic has been noted between this and other causes of lymph node enlargement (Fig. 55-28).

Neoplasms

Neuroblastomas may present in the head and neck region in approximately 5% of cases.[23] They originate from the sympathetic chain ganglia. As a whole, they have a better prognosis than neuroblastomas originating in the abdomen.[23] The small, echogenic microcalcifications seen in these solid tumors are their hallmarks ultrasonographically (Fig. 55-29).[6,64]

Primary **rhabdomyosarcomas** of the head and neck generally occur in the orbit, nasopharynx, and middle ear. Rarely, they arise from the parotid gland.[23] Rhabdomyosarcomas generally present as metastatic lesions involving lymph nodes. On sonography, they are solid and may have a high arterial Doppler signal (Fig. 55-30). This is opposed to lymphoma and neuroblastoma, which have moderate Doppler signals (20 to 50 cm/s).[58]

The majority of **Hodgkin's lymphomas** are unilateral and involve supraclavicular nodes. Non-Hodgkin's lymphoma tends to present bilaterally.[23,56] Typically, lymphoma presents as multiple hypoechoic masses and cannot be distinguished from inflammatory adenopathy (Fig. 55-31).[2,9,52] Color flow Doppler imaging may be helpful in differentiation of malignant from reactive lymphadenopathy.[65] Criteria of malignancy are avascular intranodal regions, displacement of intranodal vessels, aberrant course of central vessels, and accessory peripheral vessels.

Ultrasound guidance of cutting-needle biopsy of neck masses has proven effective and safe when malignancy is being considered.[66]

Text continued on page 1574.

SONOGRAPHIC SIGNS OF ABSCESSED NODES

Increased through transmission
Movement of echogenic material (with compression and release)
Absence of hilar stripe
Absence of central hilar vessel (on color flow Doppler imaging)
Central lucency with echogenic wall

LATERAL NECK MASSES

Lymphadenitis
Abscess
Neoplasms
- Neuroblastoma
- Rhabdomyosarcoma
- Lymphoma
- Aggressive fibromatosis
- Teratoma

Fibromatosis coli
Cystic hygroma

A

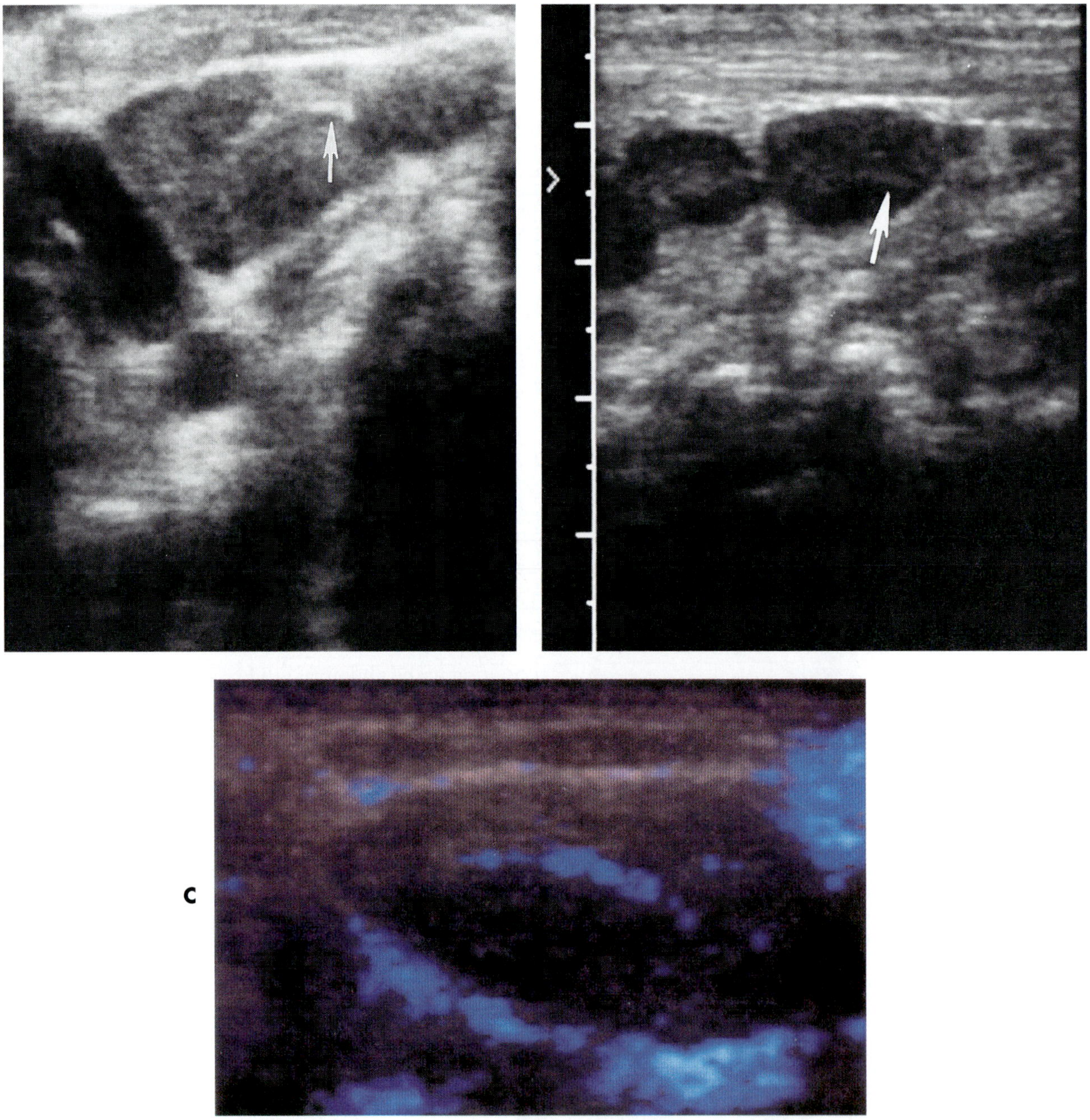

B

C

FIG. 55-21. Node. A and **B,** Enlarged neck nodes in patient with mononucleosis with central linear hilar stripe *(arrow)*. **C,** Color flow Doppler imaging shows vessel in central hilum.

Continued.

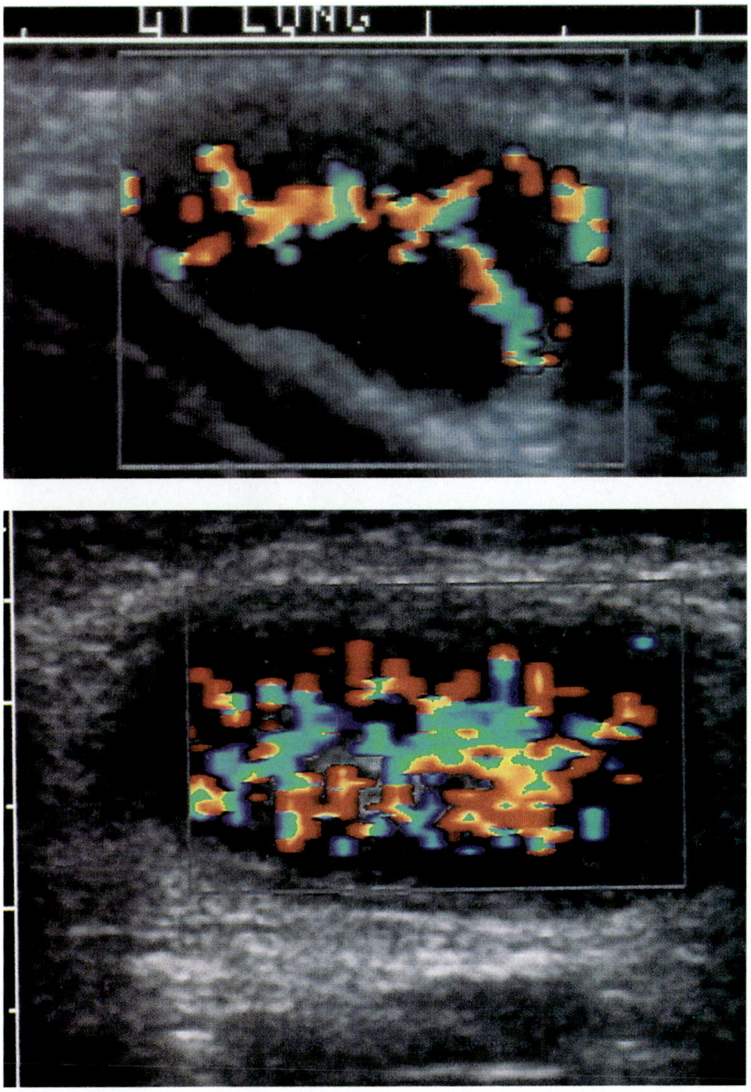

D

E

FIG. 55-21, cont'd. D and E, Two other patients with inflammatory nodes with diffuse vascularity on color flow Doppler imaging.

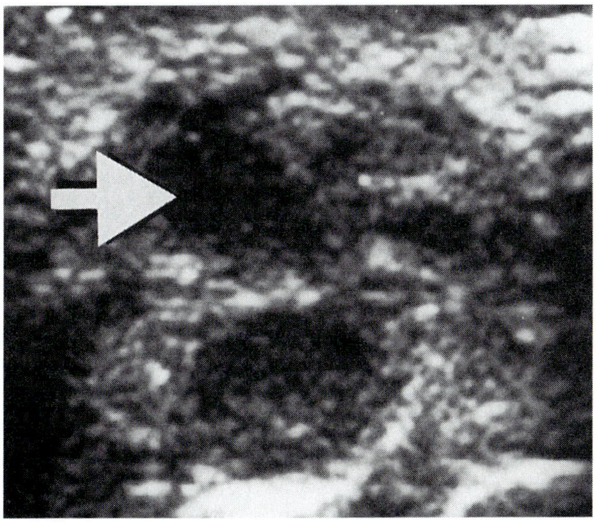

FIG. 55-22. Submental abscess in lymphadenitis. Node with irregular walls and hypoechoic center *(arrow)* representing early abscess formation.

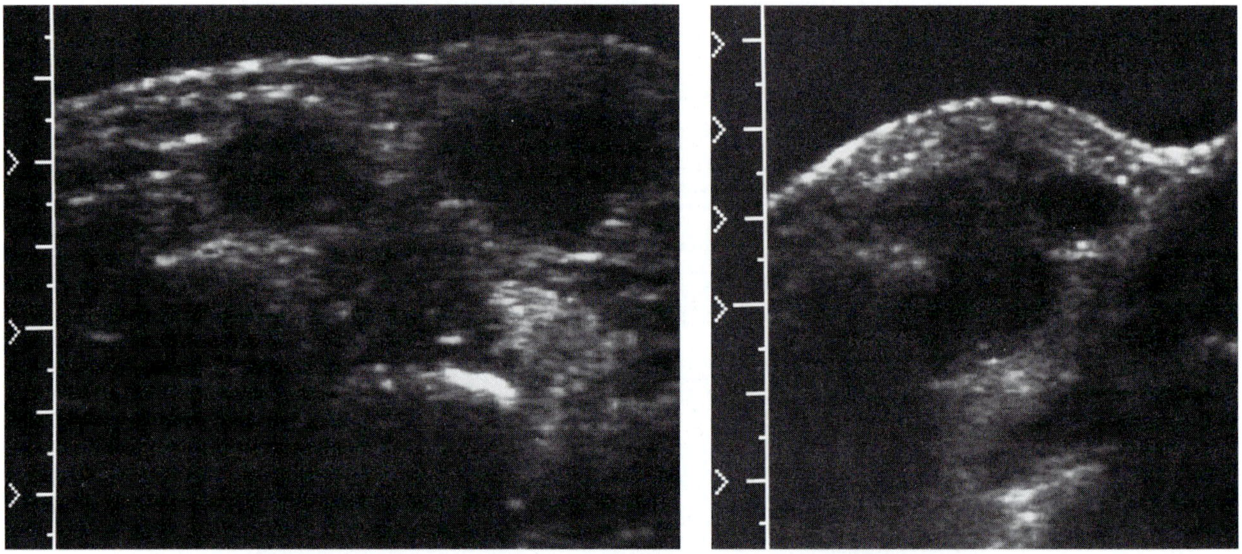

A B

FIG. 55-23. Lymphadenitis with coalescence. **A,** Multiple, discrete, hypoechoic masses in the neck are thought to represent lymph nodes. **B,** A repeat sonogram 5 days later shows coalescence of the lymph nodes with development of more hypoechoic centers, which are associated with irregular walls. (From Lewis GJS, Leithiser RE Jr, Glasier GM et al. Ultrasonography of pediatric neck masses. *Ultrasound Q* 1989;7:315-355.)

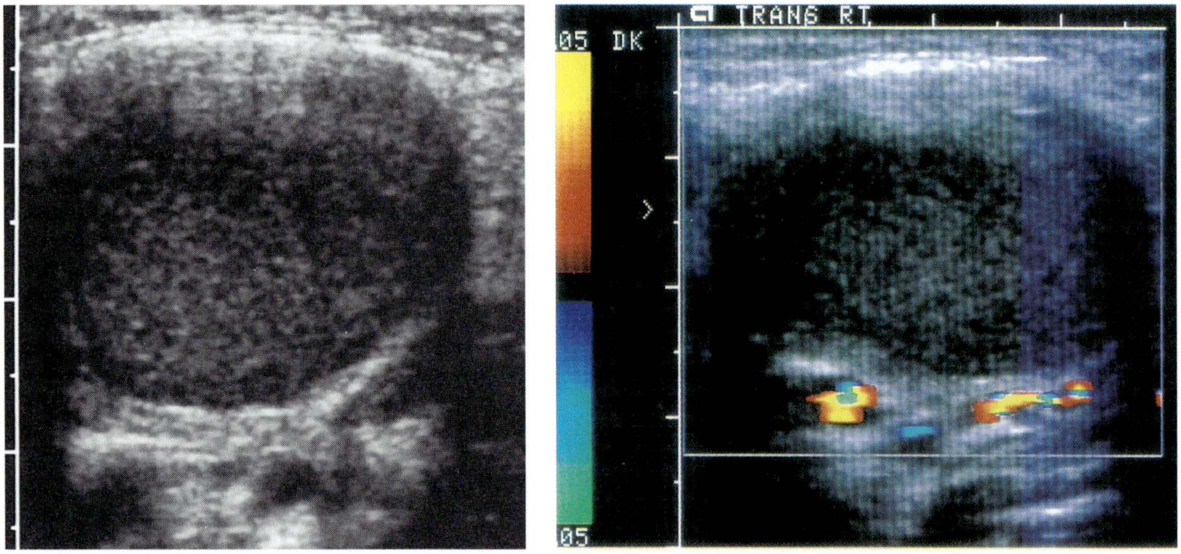

A B

FIG. 55-24. Abscess. **A,** Tender, rounded, enlarged, echogenic, submandibular node with no central stripe. **B,** Color flow Doppler imaging shows no central vessel, suggesting node has undergone abscess formation. At surgery, a necrotic node with pus was found.

A 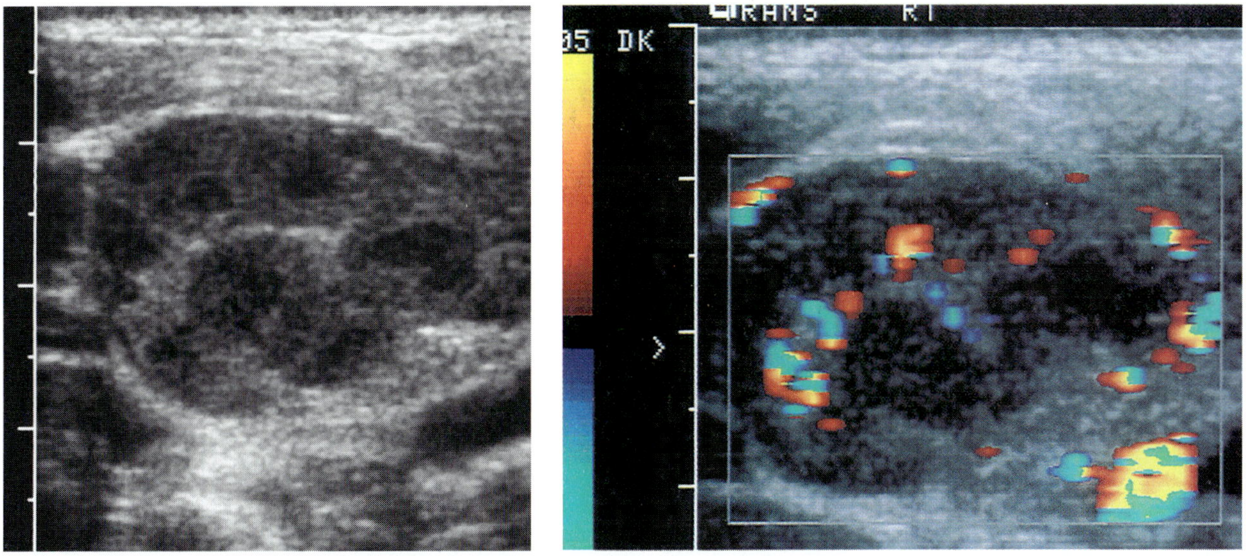 B

FIG. 55-25. Node with multiple small abscesses. **A,** Enlarged neck node with multiple, hypoechogenic, small abscesses. **B,** Doppler imaging demonstrates increased vascularity around the abscesses.

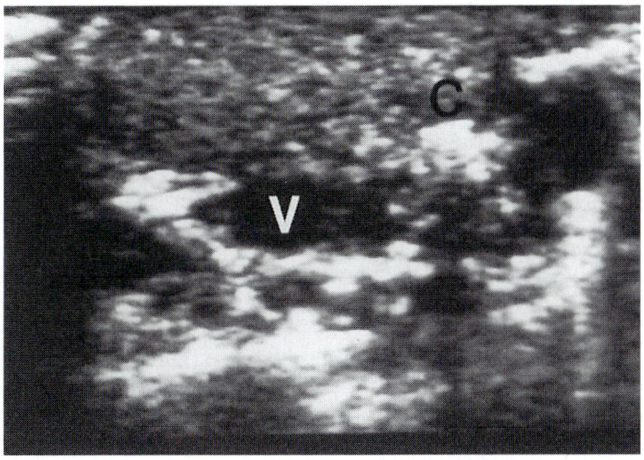

FIG. 55-26. Lymph node calcification. An oval, enlarged lymph node is seen just anterior to the jugular vein, *V.* Some calcification, *C,* with posterior acoustic shadowing, is seen on its medial aspect. (From Lewis GJS, Leithiser RE Jr, Glasier GM et al. Ultrasonography of pediatric neck masses. *Ultrasound Q* 1989;7:315-355.)

A

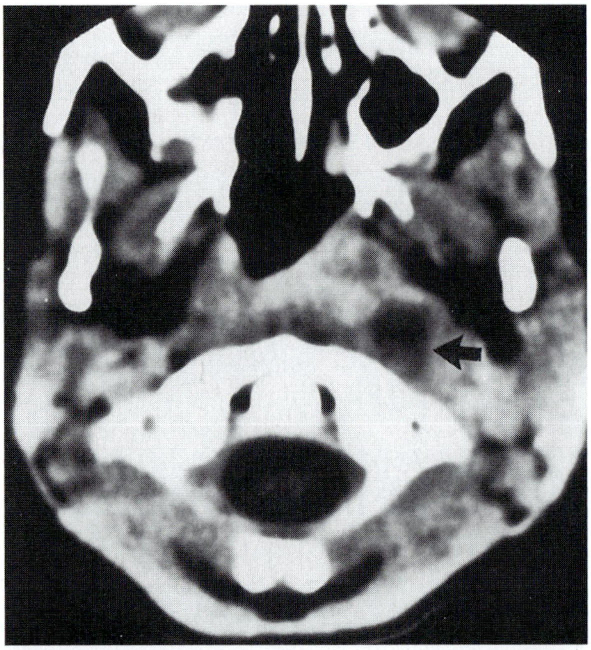

FIG. 55-27. Retropharyngeal abscess. A, Contrasted CT shows a round area of decreased attenuation in the left retropharyngeal area *(arrow)*. **B,** Intraoperative ultrasound of the lateral neck shows the carotid artery *(small arrow)* lateral to the abscess *(large arrow)*. **C,** Sonogram shows a transorally placed needle *(arrow)* within the abscess. (From Lewis GJS, Leithiser RE Jr, Glasier GM et al. Ultrasonography of pediatric neck masses. *Ultrasound Q* 1989;7:315-355.)

B

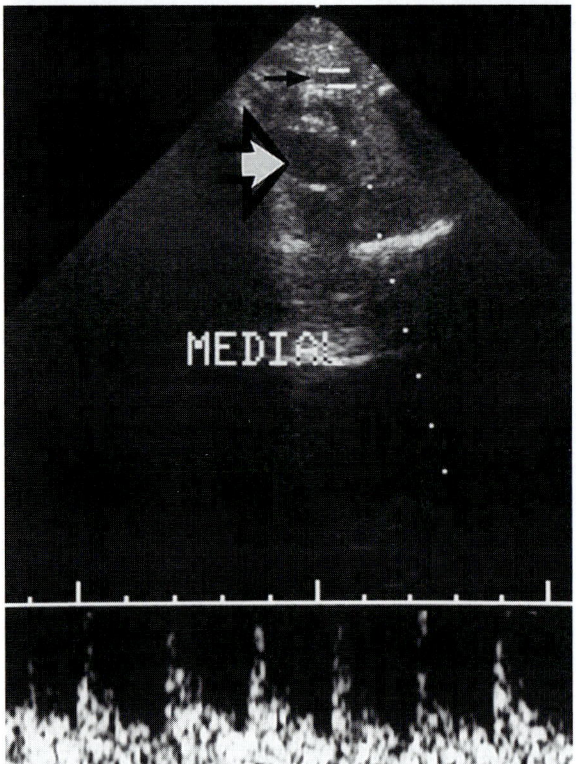

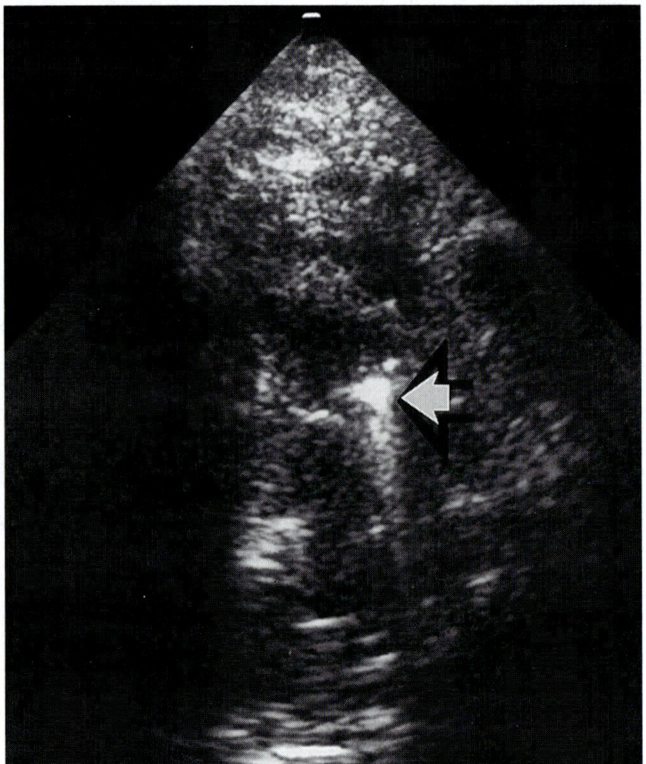

C

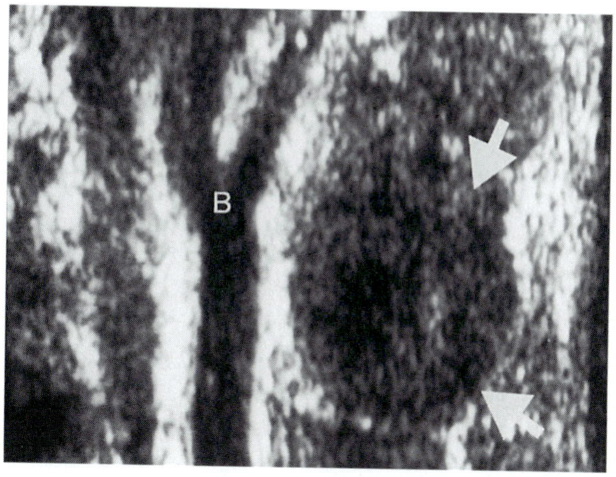

FIG. 55-28. Kawasaki's disease. Longitudinal scan of the carotid artery shows adenopathy *(arrows)* just anterior to the carotid bifurcation, *B*. (From Lewis GJS, Leithiser RE Jr, Glasier GM et al. Ultrasonography of pediatric neck masses. *Ultrasound Q* 1989;7:315-355.)

A

B

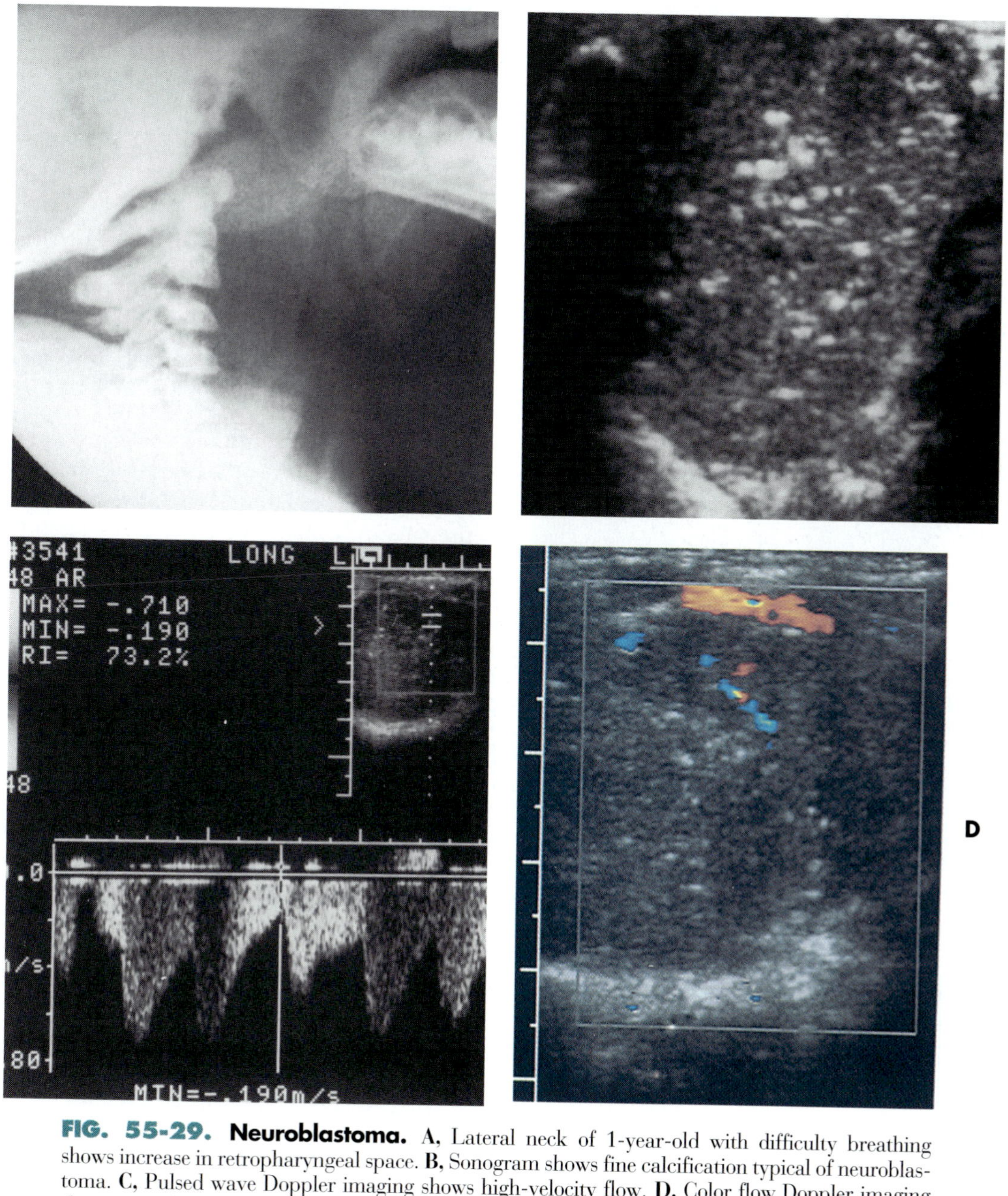

C

D

FIG. 55-29. Neuroblastoma. **A,** Lateral neck of 1-year-old with difficulty breathing shows increase in retropharyngeal space. **B,** Sonogram shows fine calcification typical of neuroblastoma. **C,** Pulsed wave Doppler imaging shows high-velocity flow. **D,** Color flow Doppler imaging shows vascularity around the periphery of the mass.

A

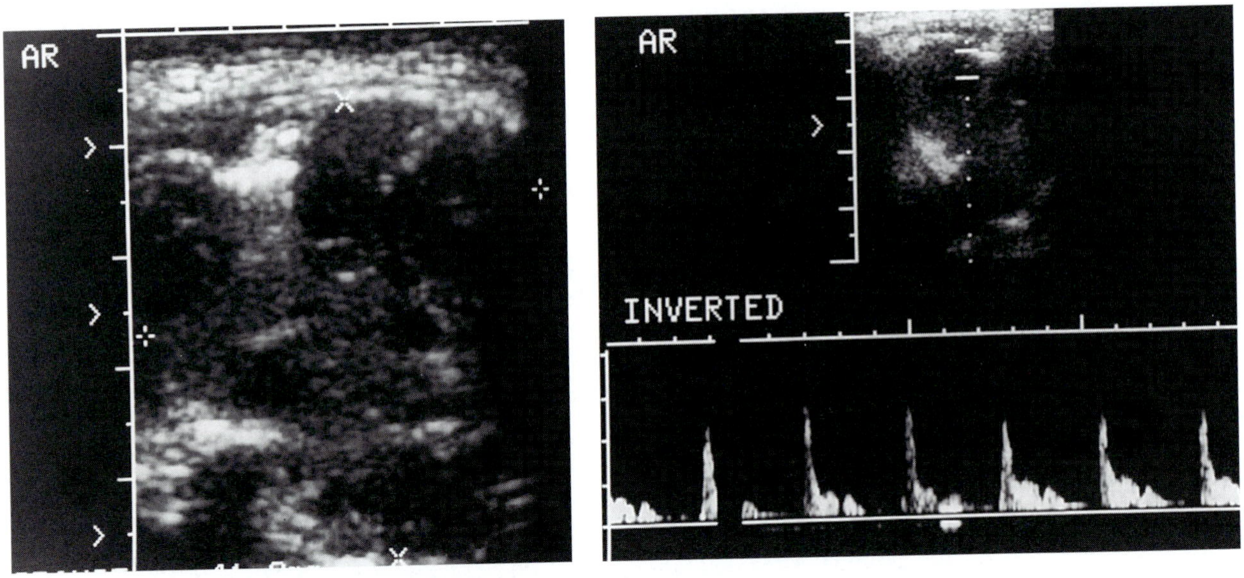

B

FIG. 55-30. Rhabdomyosarcoma. **A,** Sonogram of the right neck shows a mass of mixed echogenicity. **B,** Doppler ultrasound shows arterial flow with velocities greater than 1 m/s. (From Lewis GJS, Leithiser RE Jr, Glasier GM et al. Ultrasonography of pediatric neck masses. *Ultrasound Q* 1989;7:315-355.)

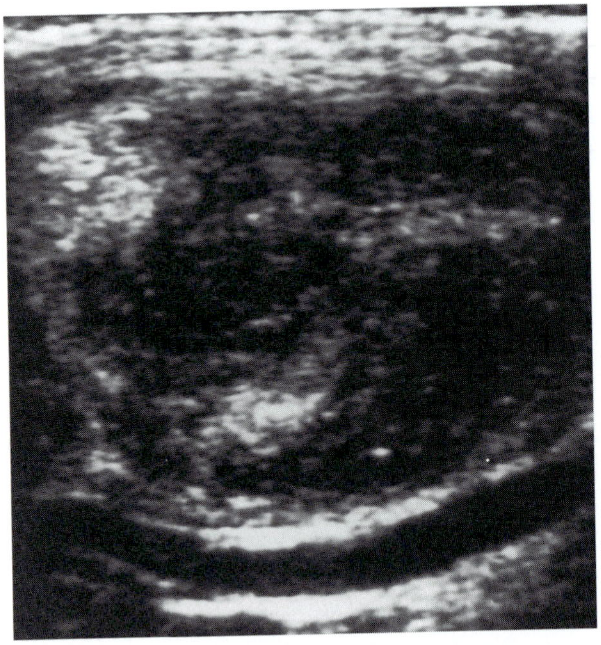

FIG. 55-31. Lymphoblastic lymphoma. Sonogram shows a large, inhomogeneous lymphoma node located anterior to the carotid artery. (From Lewis GJS, Leithiser RE Jr, Glasier GM et al. Ultrasonography of pediatric neck masses. *Ultrasound Q* 1989;7:315-355.)

Aggressive fibromatosis may present as a neck mass. This can invade the mandible, larynx, trachea, and tongue (Fig. 55-32).[23]

Sternocleidomastoid Muscle

Fibromatosis colli is a mass that predominantly involves the sternal head of the **sternocleidomastoid muscle.** It is thought to be related to birth trauma. It presents by 1 month of age and resolves in 1 year in the majority of cases.[23] Sonography is extremely helpful by demonstrating the typical appearance of fibromatosis colli and avoiding unnecessary surgery.[56] Typically, the mass is elliptical and slightly hypoechoic, and blends with the sternocleidomastoid muscle (Fig. 55-33).[7,9,64] It may be bilateral. Atypical patterns have been observed that were similar to lymph node enlargement.

Since this muscle courses obliquely, transverse cuts may suggest the mass is a lymph node. It is key to orient the longitudinal scans along the oblique long arcs of the sternocleidomastoid muscle.

Thymus

The normal thymus may intermittently herniate into the neck, producing a midline, suprasternal, anterior neck mass.[67] The cervicothoracic trachea is buckled posteriorly and to the right on forced exhalation (crying). Sonography can be very useful in demonstrating the intermittent cephalic movement of the homogeneous echotextured thymus from the anterior mediastinum into the neck.

A

B

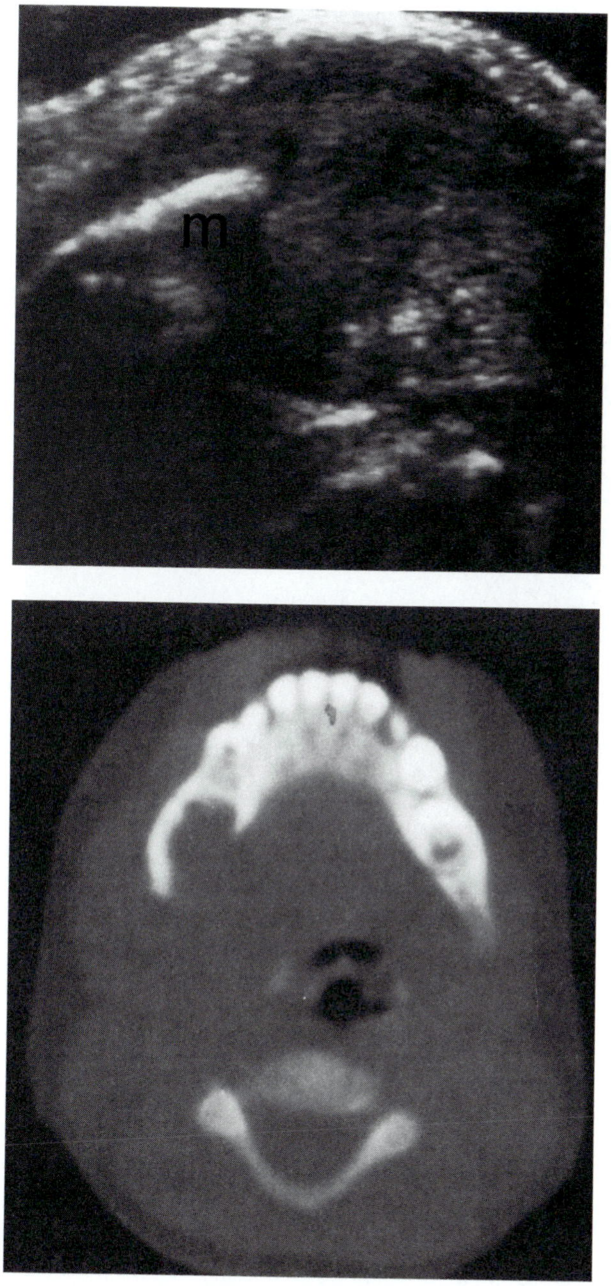

FIG. 55-32. Aggressive fibromatosis. **A,** Transverse ultrasound at the level of the angle of the mandible shows a hypoechoic mass surrounding the posterior aspect of the mandible, *M.* **B,** CT scan (bone windows) shows bone destruction of the mandible by the aggressive fibromatosis. (From Lewis GJS, Leithiser RE Jr, Glasier GM et al. Ultrasonography of pediatric neck masses. *Ultrasound Q* 1989;7:315-355.)

Congenital Lesions

Branchial cleft cysts or sinuses are the more common noninflammatory pediatric lateral neck masses. Clinically, they present as unilateral masses or draining sinuses in children between birth and 15 years. The mean age is 5 years.[23] The majority arise from the second branchial cleft and are found just anterior to the lower third of the sternocleidomastoid muscle,[48,68] lateral to the thyroid, and anterolateral to the common carotid artery.[2] The posterior medial extent of second branchial cleft cysts generally passes between the internal and external carotid arteries.[69] They can become infected. Sonographically, they appear complex and can contain fluid with scattered debris, which may be secondary to infection.[70] The debris may change with position.[6] Back wall enhancement will help to differentiate complex cysts from lymph nodes.

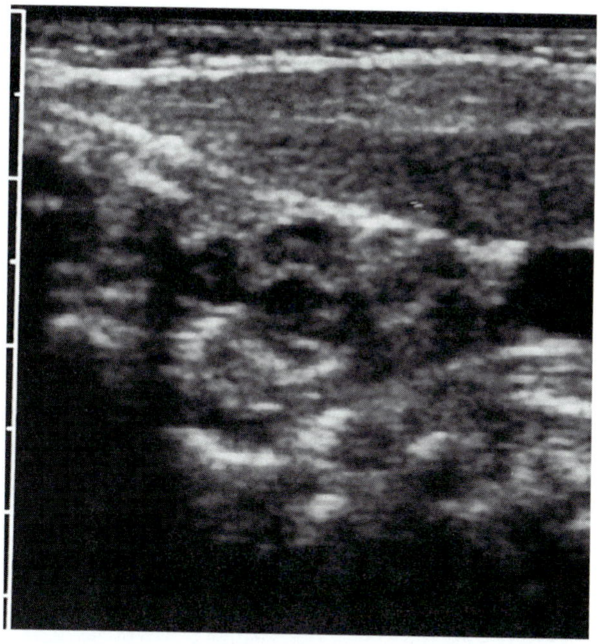

FIG. 55-33. Fibromatosis colli. An ovoid mass blends with the body of the sternocleidomastoid muscle.

Cystic hygromas or lymphangiomas are generally recognized in the neonatal period.[53] The majority are found in the neck in the posterior triangle area.[23,71] They can extend into the mediastinum or axillae. They are associated with Turner's syndrome, especially when they present in the nuchal area.[23] Sonographically, they are unilocular or multiseptated cystic structures with occasional incomplete echogenic septae (Fig. 55-34).[52,64,71] When they contain blood or are infected, they will have a mixed pattern (Fig. 55-35).[9,64] Doppler evaluation of the cystic masses will show no venous or arterial flow (see Fig. 55-12).

When **teratomas** originate in the neck region, they are most commonly seen slightly to one side of the midline.[72] They generally present at birth. No sex predominance is noted. Calcification and cystic areas are typically seen sonographically (Figs. 55-36

A

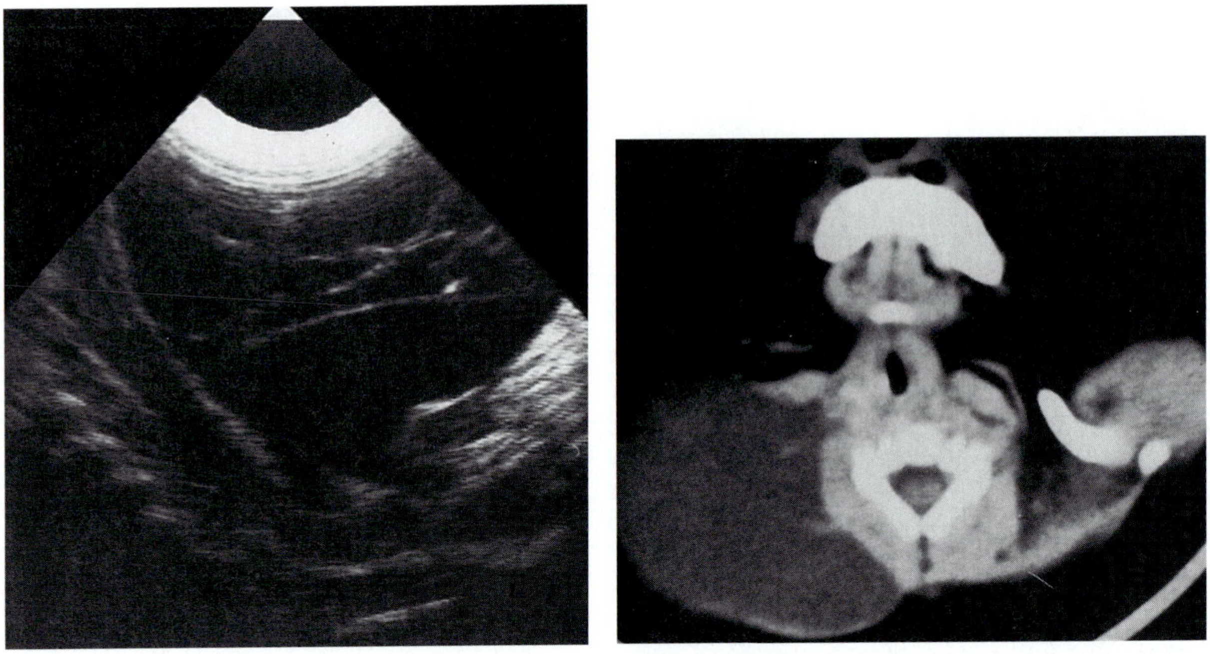

B

FIG. 55-34. Cystic hygroma. **A,** A multiseptated, hypoechoic mass in the right posterior neck. **B,** The septations are not as well seen on the CT. (From Lewis GJS, Leithiser RE Jr, Glasier GM et al. Ultrasonography of pediatric neck masses. *Ultrasound Q* 1989;7:315-355.)

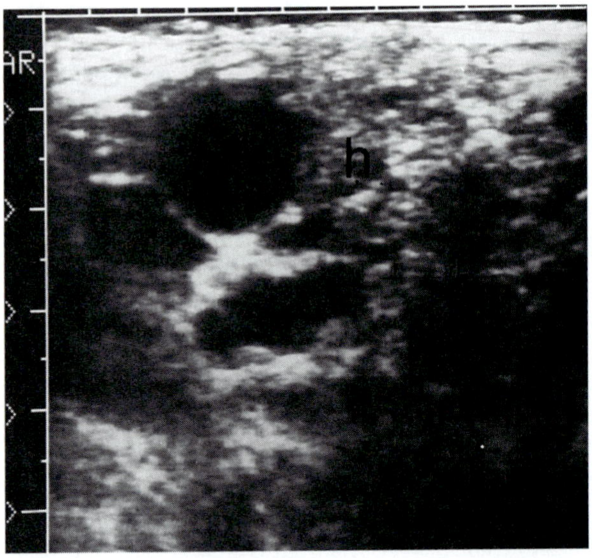

FIG. 55-35. Cystic hygroma with hemorrhage. Transverse scan of the right neck shows multiple cystic areas. A hemorrhagic cyst, *H*, presents as a hyperechoic mass. (From Lewis GJS, Leithiser RE Jr, Glasier GM et al. Ultrasonography of pediatric neck masses. *Ultrasound Q* 1989;7:315-355.)

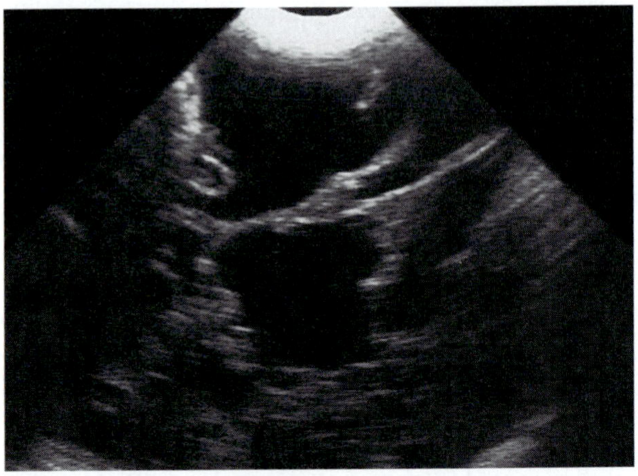

FIG. 55-36. Teratoma. Newborn with a large, soft-tissue neck mass. Ultrasound shows multiple cystic areas between thick septae.

and 55-37).[9,64] Cystic areas would be more typical of teratoma than neuroblastoma, which could present as a calcified neck mass.

When a cystic midline mass is seen posteriorly, a **pedunculated encephalocele**[2] or **cervical myelomeningocele** should be considered.[7,52] If the mass has an echogenic component, then a **lipomeningocele** should be considered.[73]

Vascular Lesions

Doppler imaging can be extremely valuable, demonstrating the vascular nature of neck masses that may be normal vessels such as an **ectatic carotid artery** (Fig. 55-38).

Sonography can be useful in pediatrics for evaluation of patency of the jugular and subclavian veins for

A

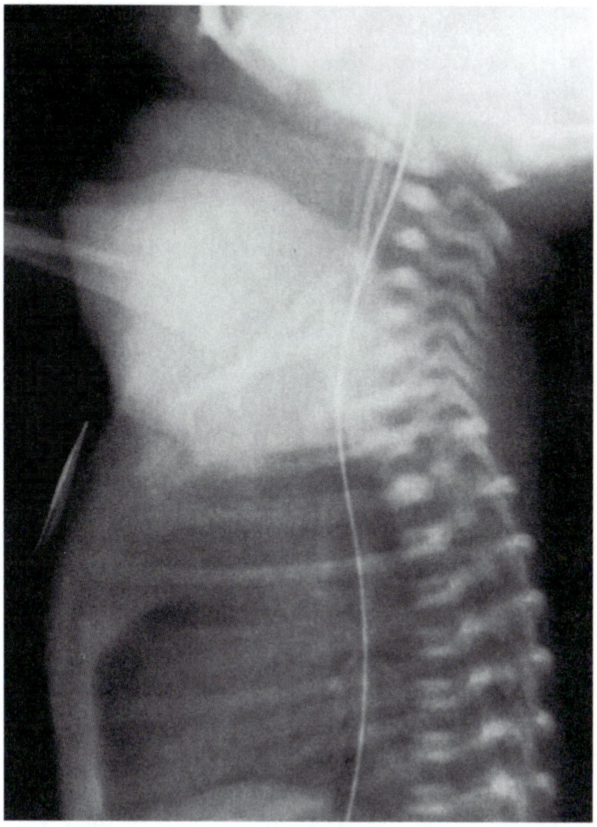

B

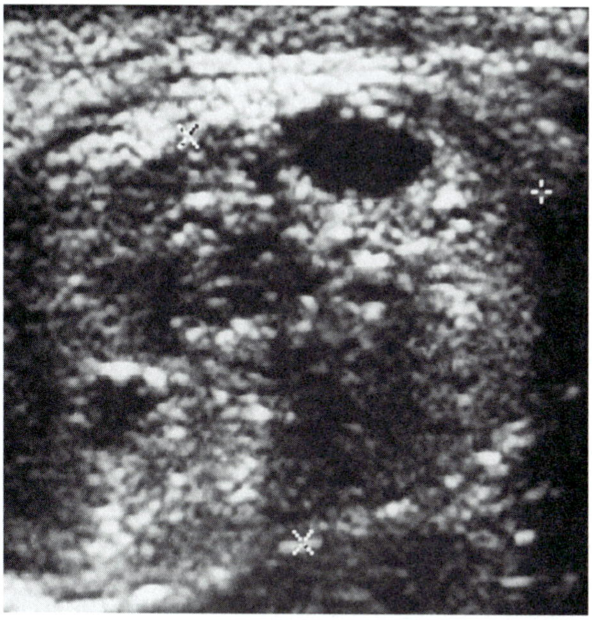

FIG. 55-37. Teratoma. **A,** Lateral chest radiograph (newborn) with large neck mass anterior to the trachea. **B,** Ultrasound shows solid mass with cystic components, *C*, and small calcifications *(curved arrow)*. (From Lewis GJS, Leithiser RE Jr, Glasier GM et al. Ultrasonography of pediatric neck masses. *Ultrasound Q* 1989; 7:315-355.)

A B

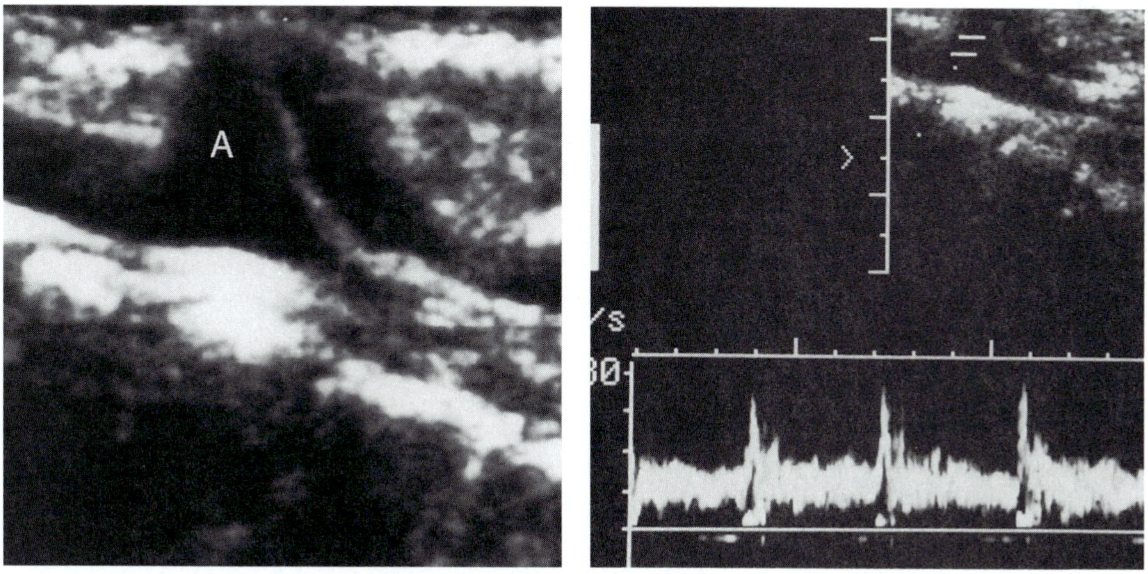

FIG. 55-38. Ectatic carotid artery. **A,** Longitudinal scan of the left carotid artery bifurcation shows an ectatic carotid artery, *A*, at its bifurcation in this patient with a pulsatile neck mass. **B,** Doppler examination shows arterial flow. (From Lewis GJS, Leithiser RE Jr, Glasier GM et al. Ultrasonography of pediatric neck masses. *Ultrasound Q* 1989;7:315-355.)

central venous access.[74,75] (See also Chapter 57.) Rand et al. observed that 25% of neonates who had central jugular vein catheterization as newborns had **jugular thrombosis** in a 2- to 4-year follow-up.[74] Sonography may also be used to guide the choice of site for insertion of a catheter to decrease complications. Cassey et al. has shown that previous access of a conventional venous site should not be considered an automatic contraindication to reuse of that site, and image-directed Doppler ultrasonography can be used as a noninvasive assessment of venous patency.[75]

Color flow Doppler imaging may also be used to evaluate the fate of **the reconstructed common carotid artery in neonates after ECMO** (extracorporeal membrane oxygenation) therapy.[76] The common carotid artery can be imaged (Fig. 55-39), and a velocity ratio of the peak systolic velocity above the level of the anastomosis to the peak systolic velocity below the anastomosis can be measured to assess the degree of stenosis at the repair site. Merton et al. found that the examination done between 2 and 12 months predicted the status of the vessel at a 4-year follow-up better than predischarge examinations.[77]

Doppler imaging can also be very helpful in evaluating **vascular tumors** and **AV malformations** (Fig. 55-40).

THYROID AND PARATHYROID GLANDS

Normal Anatomy and Technique

During development, the thyroid diverticulum migrates inferiorly to below the larynx, where it develops into the thyroid gland. The remnant of the thyroid diverticulum is known as the thyroglossal duct.[78,79] The right and left lobes of the thyroid gland are homogeneous echogenic masses located on either the larynx or the trachea (which are seen as markedly echogenic areas, with shadowing, in the midline of the lower neck). The great vessels are seen on the posterolateral aspects of both lobes. Generally, the parathyroid

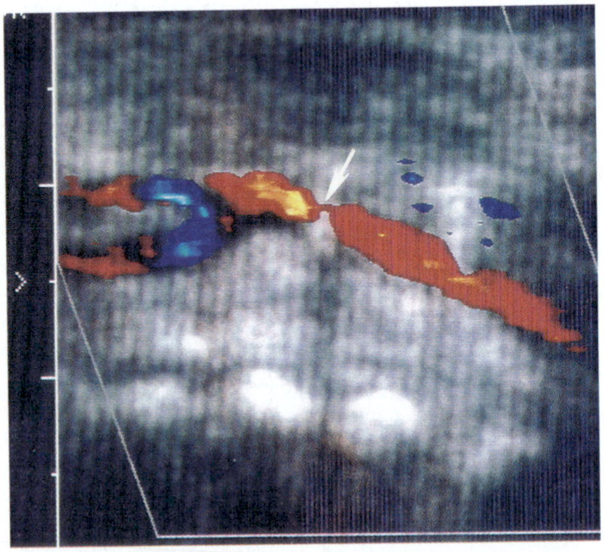

FIG. 55-39. Carotid artery narrowing. Longitudinal scan of the neck in a 2-month-old post-ECMO shows narrowing at the anastomotic site in the common carotid artery *(arrow)* just below the carotid bifurcation. The ratio of flow velocity above to below the anastomosis was 2, indicating at least a 50% narrowing.

A

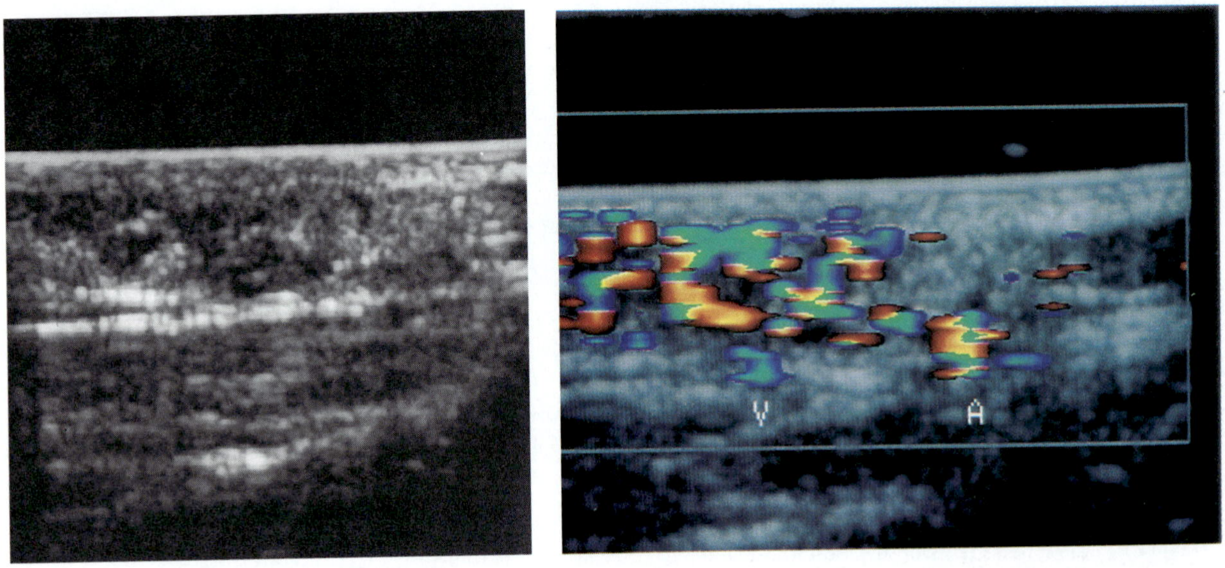

B

FIG. 55-40. AV malformation. Fourteen-year-old with skin lesion that has increased in size since birth. **A,** Superficial skin lesion with heterogeneous echotexture with multiple hypoechoic areas. **B,** Color flow Doppler imaging shows the lesion is very vascular.

Continued.

C

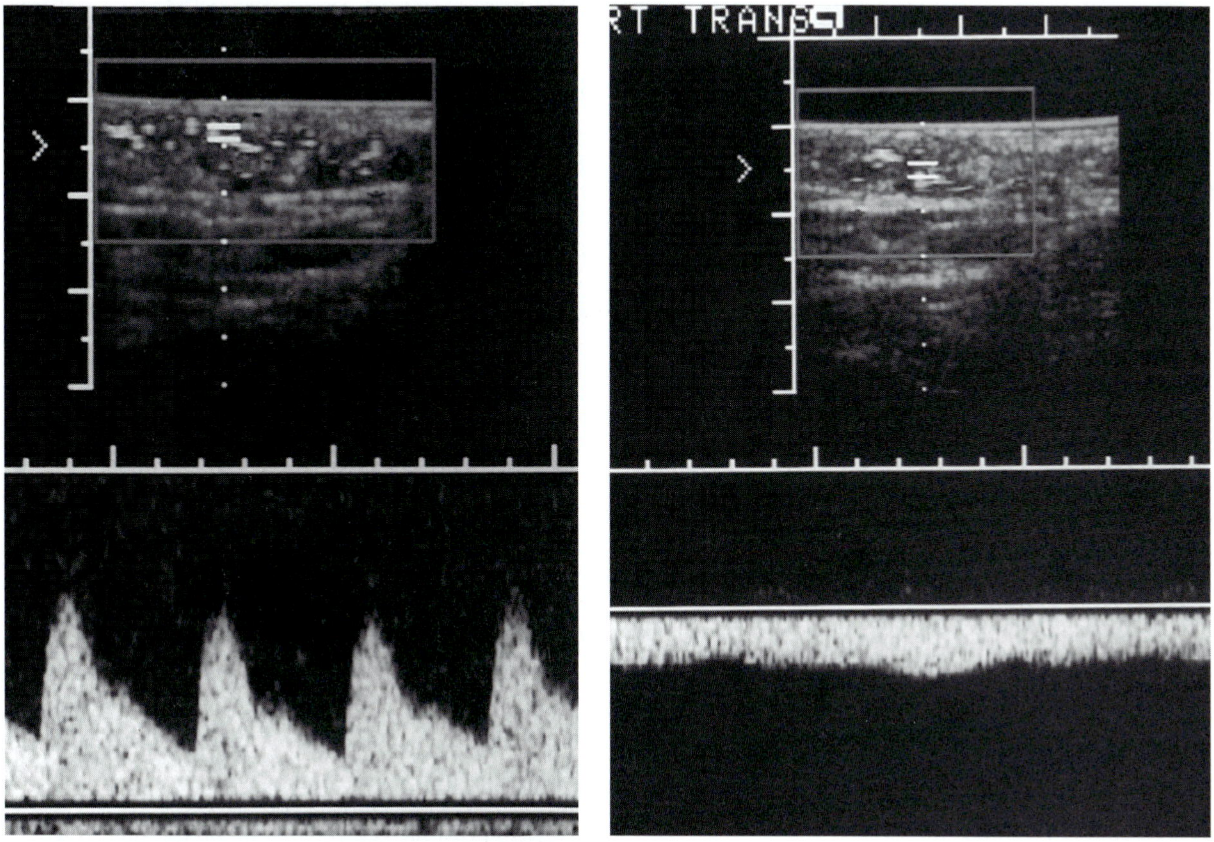

D

E

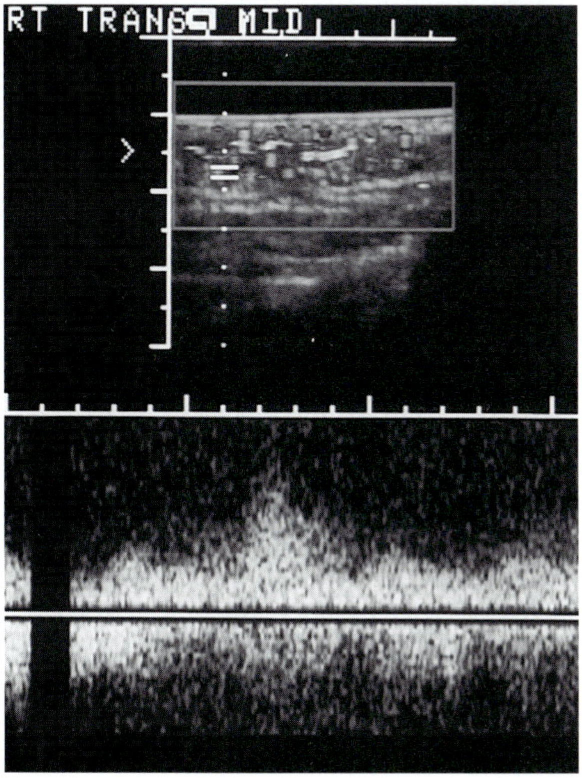

FIG. 55-40, cont'd. Spectral Doppler, **C,** arteries, **D,** veins, and, **E,** vessels with arterial waveforms with high diastolic flow, suggesting AV shunts.

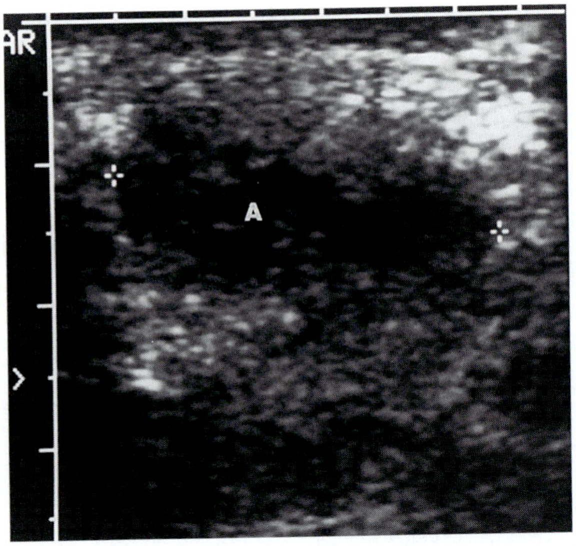

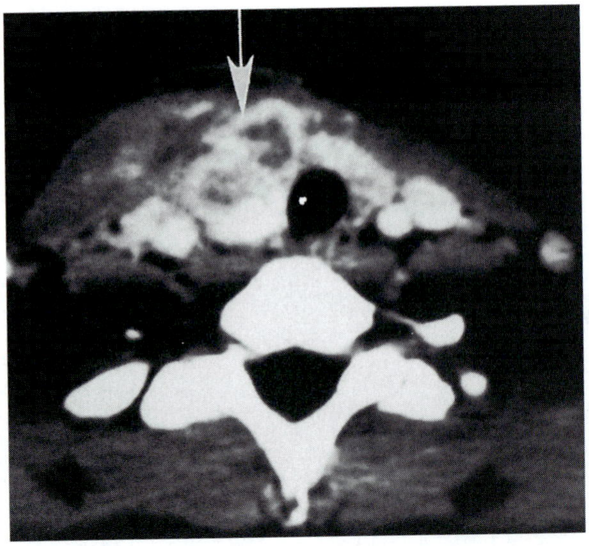

FIG. 55-41. Thyroid gland abscess. **A,** Longitudinal ultrasound of the right thyroid gland shows a poorly defined abscess, *A*, with hypoechoic center and an irregular wall. **B,** CT of the neck shows an enlarged right thyroid gland with enhancement around multiple low-attenuation areas of the abscess *(arrow)*. (From Lewis GJS, Leithiser RE Jr, Glasier GM et al. Ultrasonography of pediatric neck masses. *Ultrasound Q* 1989;7:315-355.)

THYROID MASSES

- Acute suppurative thyroiditis
- Neoplasms
  - Papillary carcinoma
  - Follicular carcinoma
  - Medullary carcinoma
- Multinodular goiters
- Thyroglossal duct cysts
- Congenital goiter

glands are not identified, but occasionally they can be seen as hypoechoic masses along the posteromedial aspects of the thyroid lobes.[7,80]

Inflammation

Inflammatory disorders of the thyroid include acute (suppurative), subacute, and chronic thyroiditis. When a complex mass is seen sonographically in the clinical setting of thyroiditis, **acute suppurative thyroiditis** with abscess formation should be considered (Fig. 55-41).[64] The most common organisms are *Staphylococcus* and *Streptococcus*; anaerobic infections have also been found.[23,81,82] When the left lobe of the thyroid is involved, the possibility of a remnant of the left third pharyngeal pouch, which results in a fistula between this lobe and the ipsilateral pyriform sinus, should be considered. When acute symptoms have subsided, a barium swallow should be performed.[83,84]

Patients with **acute hyperthyroidism** will demonstrate a diffusely enlarged gland bilaterally, which may be very vascular on Doppler imaging (Fig. 55-42).

Subacute thyroiditis is rarely seen in the pediatric population[23]; however, we have seen one case as unilateral enlargement of the right lobe with an associated decrease in tracer activity on thyroid scan (Fig. 55-43). The majority of patients in the pediatric age group have chronic lymphocytic thyroiditis (Hashimoto's thyroiditis) as a presenting symptom.[23,85] There is a 4:1 or 5:1 female-to-male predominance.[23] Most patients are older children with painless enlargement of the thyroid gland. This condition can be associated with Turner's syndrome, Noonan's syndrome, Down's syndrome, phenytoin (Dilantin) therapy, juvenile diabetes mellitus, and treated Hodgkin's disease.[23,86] The majority of these patients will have spontaneous resolution.[23] Sonographically, the thyroid gland shows diffuse enlargement with a homogeneous[52,64] or heterogeneous[6] appearance.[85] If the echotexture of the thyroid is less than that of adjacent muscles, severe follicular degeneration from Hashimoto's thyroiditis should be considered.[87]

Neoplasms

In one series, one third of pediatric neck masses were located in the thyroid gland.[6] In general, diffuse enlargement of the thyroid is a benign process whereas a solitary nodule must be more fully evaluated.[23] Whenever thyroid pathology is present, a thyroid scan

A

B

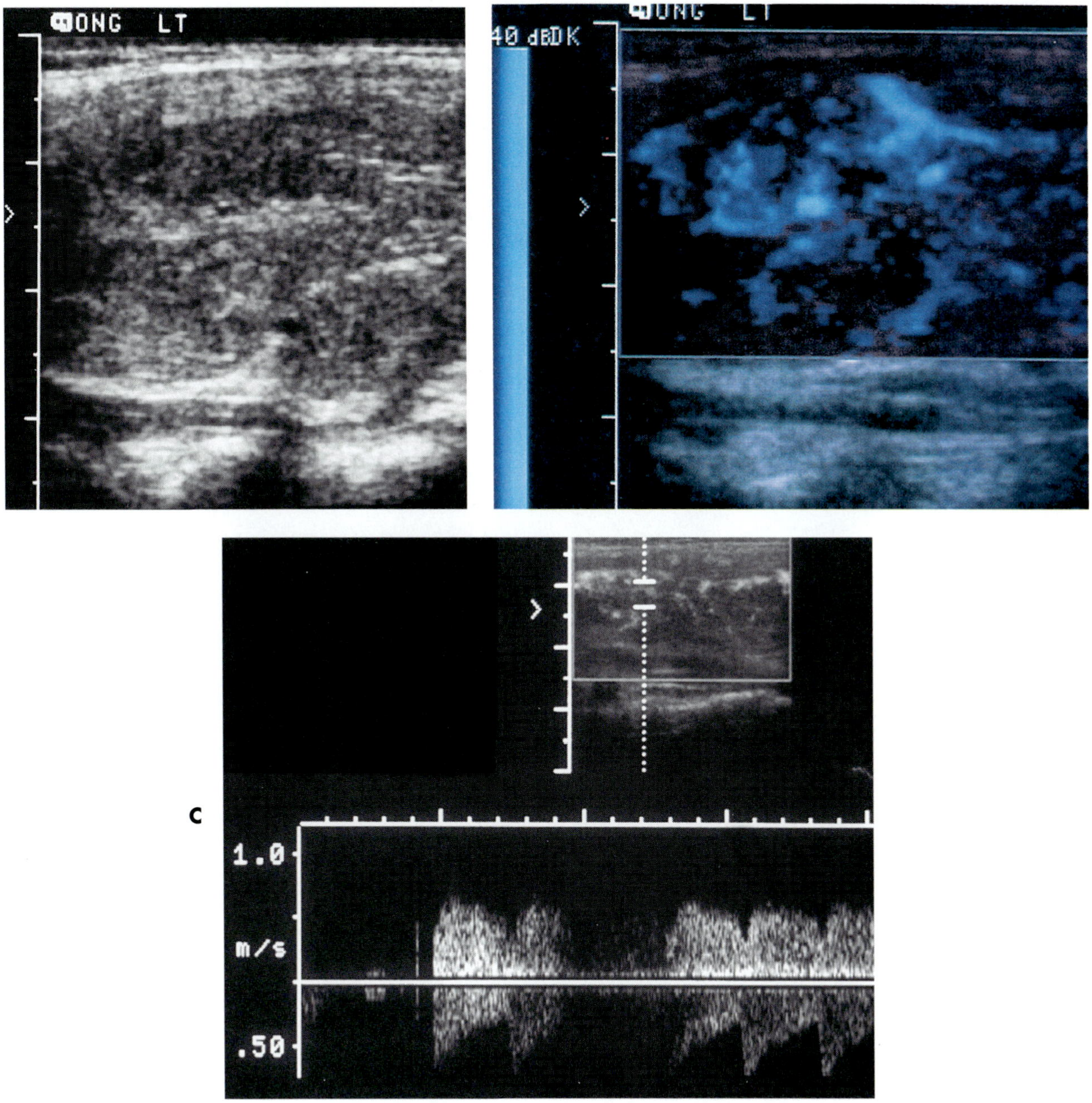

C

FIG. 55-42. Hyperthyroidism in 18-year-old with multinodular toxic goiter. **A,** Enlarged gland bilaterally with multiple nodules. **B,** Power mode Doppler imaging demonstrates markedly increased flow. **C,** Spectral analysis demonstrates high diastolic flow.

A
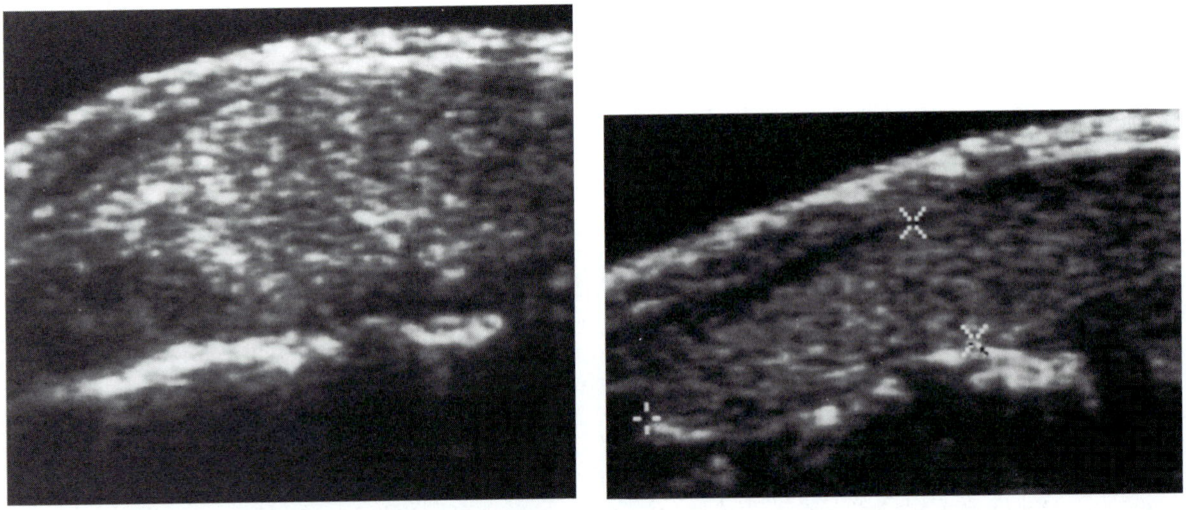
B

FIG. 55-43. Subacute thyroiditis. **A,** Longitudinal sonogram through the enlarged and homogeneously hyperechoic right lobe of the thyroid gland. **B,** Normal left lobe of the thyroid gland. (Thyroid nuclear scan showed thyroiditis as a diffusely enlarged right lobe with decreased activity.) (From Lewis GJS, Leithiser RE Jr, Glasier GM et al. Ultrasonography of pediatric neck masses. *Ultrasound Q* 1989;7:315-355.)

A
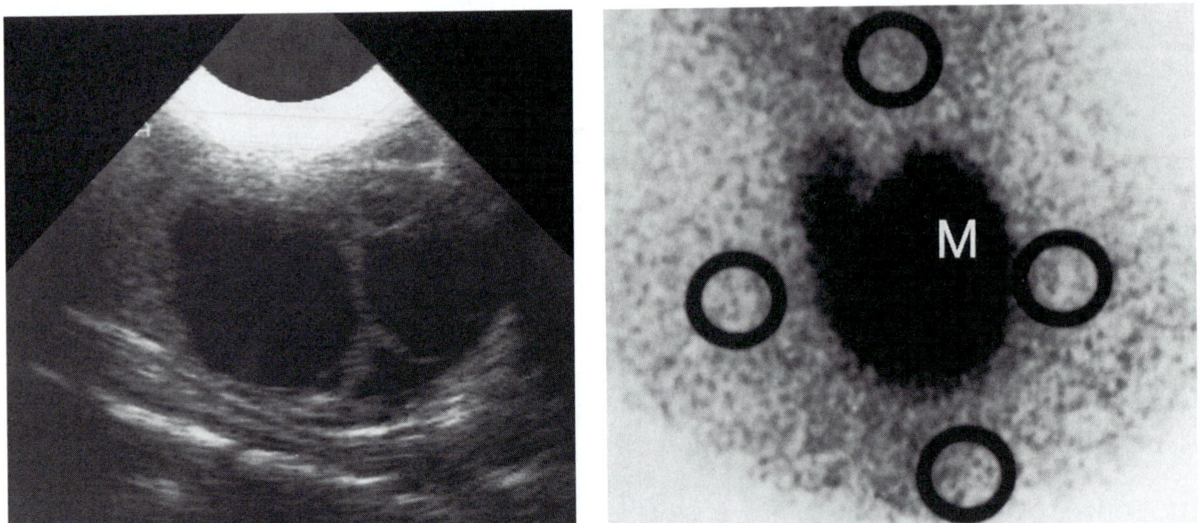

B

FIG. 55-44. Cystic adenoma of the thyroid gland. **A,** Sonogram shows large, multiseptated, inferior cystic mass. **B,** Mass, *m*, accumulates tracer on technetium scan. (From Lewis GJS, Leithiser RE Jr, Glasier GM et al. Ultrasonography of pediatric neck masses. *Ultrasound Q* 1989;7:315-355.)

is indicated.[88] Discrete thyroid nodules are uncommon in children, especially in the prepubescent child.[6] In the case of a cold nodule, a malignancy of the thyroid should be considered, especially if there is a history of previous irradiation[89-91] or the patient is a male.[6,92,93] Ultrasound can determine whether these masses are cystic or solid.

Adenomas present as hyperechoic or hypoechoic masses. They may have cystic, hypoechoic necrotic centers (Fig. 55-44).[80] Ultrasound is useful in following the size of thyroid masses that are being treated with hormonal therapy.[94]

Papillary carcinoma is the most common thyroid malignancy in children.[23,95] Seventy-five percent of papillary carcinomas have metastatic cervical disease at presentation. Metastases tend to spread to cervical lymph nodes. **Follicular carcinomas,** on the other hand, have associated hematogenous spread.[82] Children, like adults, have a low incidence of follicular carcinomas (Fig. 55-45).[23,96,97] Sonographically, most

A

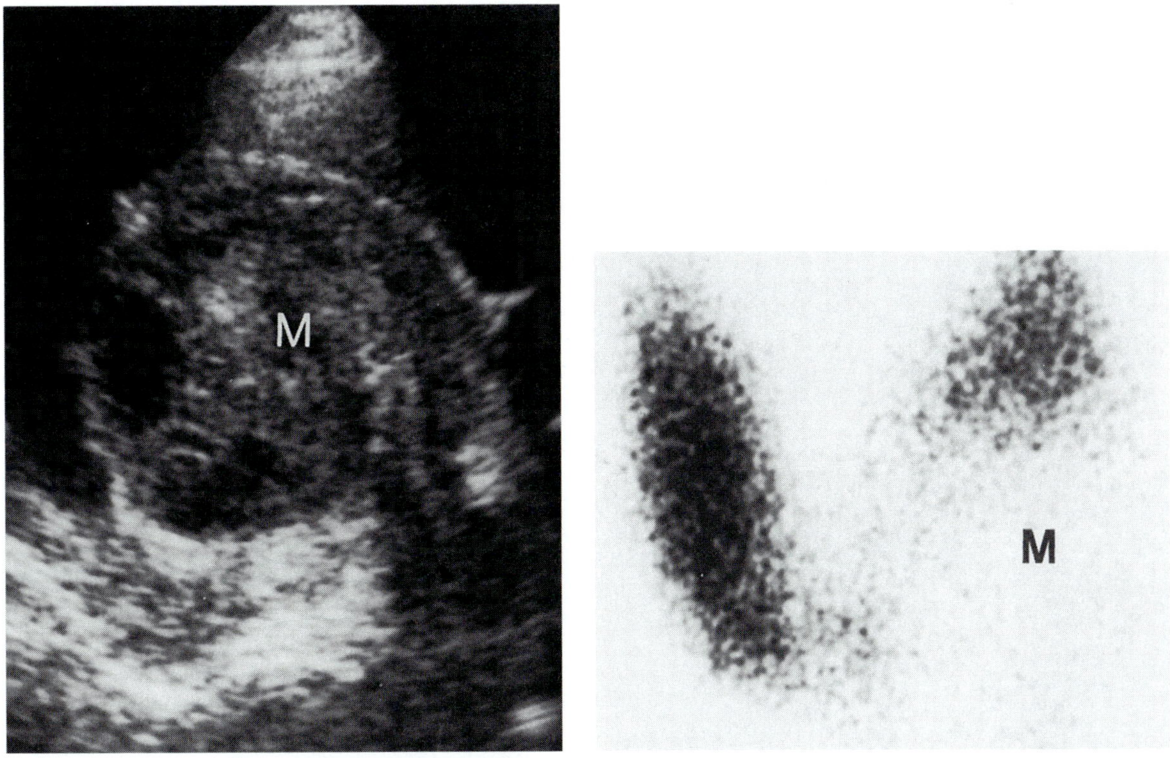

B

FIG. 55-45. Follicular carcinoma. **A,** Sonogram shows a large, complex mass, *M,* containing cystic areas in the left lobe of the thyroid gland. **B,** An I 123 thyroid scan shows the mass was not functioning. (From Lewis GJS, Leithiser RE Jr, Glasier GM et al. Ultrasonography of pediatric neck masses. *Ultrasound Q* 1989;7:315-355.)

SONOGRAPHIC SIGNS OF THYROID MALIGNANCY

Hypoechogenicity
Nodular calcifications
Origin in upper half of thyroid

carcinomas are hypoechoic compared with the gland and do not contain large cystic areas.[93] However, they may have small cystic components.[80] When local metastases are present, extensive cystic degeneration within the lymph nodes has been observed.[23,80] Because of the overlap of the ultrasound findings with those of adenomas, biopsy of solid or mixed thyroid lesions has been recommended.[85,94,98]

Medullary carcinoma of the thyroid is uncommon in childhood. When present, there is a higher association with multiple endocrine neoplasia syndromes than in adults.[23,93,99]

Multinodular goiters present as multiple hypoechoic masses causing unilateral or bilateral thyroid lobe enlargement.[52,98] These goiters have a significantly lower incidence of malignancy as cold nodules.[94] Hypoechogenicity, nodular calcifications, and location in the upper half of the thyroid are sonographic features associated with a higher risk for malignancy. Fine-needle aspiration biopsy should be considered in multinodular goiters with these features.[100]

Sonography is very helpful in differentiation of multinodular goiters from single thyroid nodules and diffuse thyroid disease without discrete nodules.[101] Multinodular thyroid disease in children is often associated with other disorders, such as renal and digital anomalies, McCune-Albright syndrome, and Hashimoto's thyroiditis. Garcia et al. reported that one fourth of children may have thyroid carcinoma, especially with a history of previous radiation therapy.[101]

Multiple thyroid cysts, with associated thyrotoxicosis, have been seen in patients with clinical findings of the McCune-Albright syndrome.[85]

Congenital Lesions

Seventy percent of congenital anomalies in the neck are **thyroglossal duct remnants or cysts.**[23,64,102,103] Fistulas may develop with infection and should be evaluated with fistulograms.[104] Cysts can be located anywhere from the base of the tongue to the thyroid isthmus.[64] The majority of them present in the young child as a firm, classically midline mass located at or below the level of the hyoid bone (Figs. 55-46 and 55-47).[23,78,102,105] Some present in parasagittal loca-

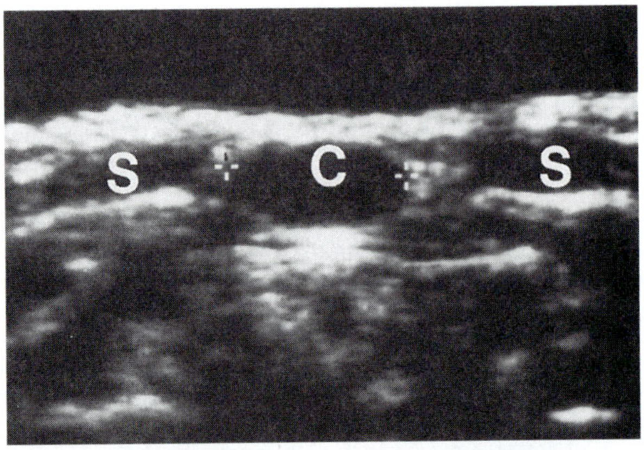

FIG. 55-46. Thyroglossal duct cyst. A cystic mass, *C*, in the midline of the upper neck with increased through transmission. The strap muscles, *S*, are located on each side of it. (From Lewis GJS, Leithiser RE Jr, Glasier GM et al. Ultrasonography of pediatric neck masses. *Ultrasound Q* 1989;7:315-355.)

A

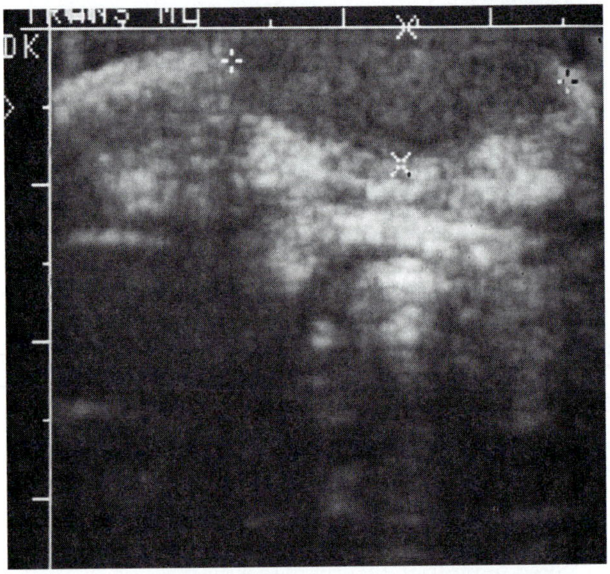

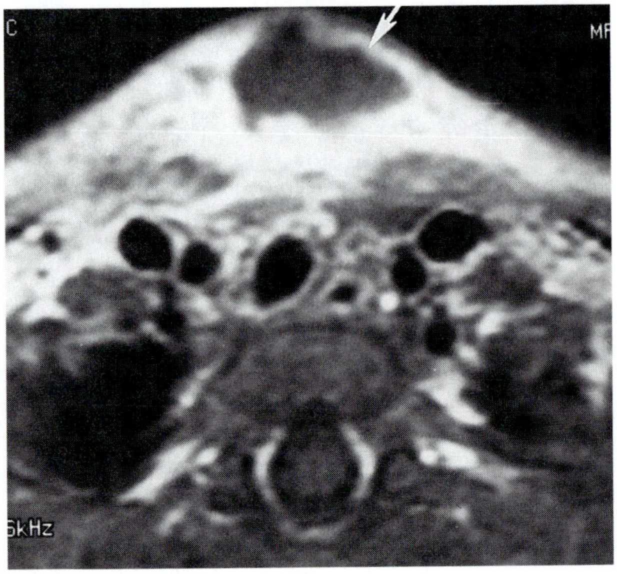

B

C

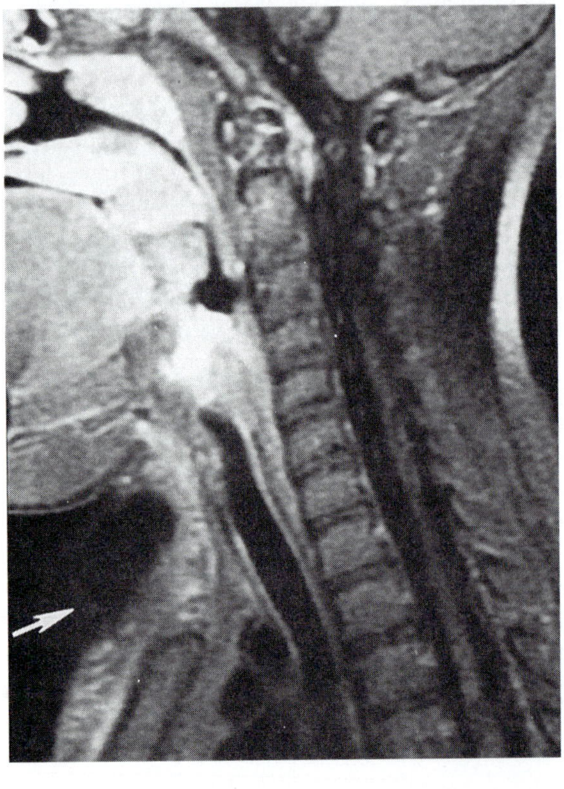

FIG. 55-47. Infected thyroglossal duct cyst. **A,** Axial ultrasound shows cyst with debris with back wall enhancement. **B,** Sagittal and, **C,** axial MRI scans show anterior midline cystic mass *(arrow)* with increased signal in relationship to blood.

tions, especially if they are at the level of the larynx.[64,102] They can have the sonographic characteristics typical of cysts (hypoechoic, good through transmission with posterior acoustic enhancement, and smooth walls)[52] or present as complex midline masses containing solid and cystic areas, especially if they are infected.* Ultrasound is also helpful in documenting the presence of the normal thyroid gland. CT may be useful in evaluating infected cysts.[102]

Congenital goiters may be secondary to a number of diseases. Goiters secondary to enzyme deficiencies[23,107] may be present at birth. However, most of these develop in the early months and years of extrauterine life.[107] Infants born to mothers with thyrotoxicosis secondary to long-acting thyroid-stimulating hormone that can cross the placenta can have goiters.[108] Other causes include maternal prenatal ingestion of iodine, antithyroid medication, lithium,[109] and other goitrogens.[108]

Newborns presenting with hypothyroidism may be studied with ultrasound for the presence of normal thyroid tissue.[110] Radioisotope scanning should be the next step to investigate for functioning ectopic thyroid tissue.

Rarely, **congenital cysts** of the thyroid are seen. When these occur, they are predominantly located in the upper pole.[23]

Other congenital cysts of this area are **thymic cysts.** One of these thymic cysts has been associated with hemithyroid agenesis.[111]

Parathyroid Lesions

Hyperplasia and adenomas of the parathyroid glands are rarely seen in children. They can be difficult to visualize by ultrasound because their echotexture may be similar to the thyroid and they can be buried within it.[79,112-119] High-resolution ultrasound with color flow Doppler imaging, however, now has proven more effective and has identified these small lesions in 67% of the cases in one series.[120,121] Most of the adenomas were solid, oval, and hypoechoic with a vascular ring or arc around the mass. MRI should be performed when no adenoma is identified with ultrasound, and the patient then undergoes either planned or exploratory surgery.[121]

ACKNOWLEDGEMENTS

We would like to acknowledge the tremendous competence of Rochelle Graves in preparing this manuscript.

REFERENCES

1. Chodosh PL, Silbey R, Oen KT. Diagnostic use of ultrasound in diseases of the head and neck. *Laryngoscope* 1980;90:814-821.
2. Friedman AP, Haller JO, Goodman JD et al. Sonographic evaluation of noninflammatory neck masses in children. *Radiology* 1983;147:693-697.
3. Lewis GJS, Leithiser RE Jr, Glasier CM et al. Ultrasonography of pediatric neck masses. *Ultrasound Q* 1989;7:315-355.
4. Scheible FW. Recent advances in ultrasound: high-resolution imaging of superficial structures. *Head Neck Surg* 1981;4:58-63.
5. Scheible FW, Leopold GR. Diagnostic imaging in head and neck disease: current applications of ultrasound. *Head Neck Surg* 1978;1:1-11.
6. Sherman NH, Rosenberg HK, Heyman S et al. Ultrasound evaluation of neck masses in children. *J Ultrasound Med* 1985;4:127-134.
7. Glasier CM, Seibert JJ, Williamson SL et al. High-resolution ultrasound characterization of soft tissue masses in children. *Pediatr Radiol* 1987;17:233-237.
8. Oestreich AE. Ultrasound imaging of musculoskeletal and superficial tissues in infants and children. *Appl Radiol* 1984;13(1):83-93.
9. Casselman JW, Mancusa AA. Major salivary gland masses: comparison of MR imaging and CT. *Radiology* 1987;165:183-189.
10. McGahan JP, Walter JP, Bernstein L. Evaluation of the parotid gland. *Radiology* 1984;152:453-458.
11. Rabinov K, Kell T Jr, Gordon PH. CT of the salivary glands. *Radiol Clin North Am* 1984;22(1):145-159.
12. Radecki PD, Arger PH, Arenson RL et al. Thyroid imaging: comparison of high-resolution, real-time ultrasound and computed tomography. *Radiology* 1984:153:145-147.
13. Som PM, Biller HF. The combined CT-sialogram. *Radiology* 1980;135:387-390.
14. Tabor EK, Curtin HD. MR of the salivary glands. *Radiol Clin North Am* 1989;27(2):379-392.
15. Teresi LM, Kolin E, Lufkin RB et al. MR imaging of the intraparotid facial nerve: normal anatomy and pathology. *AJR* 1987;148:995-1000.
16. Vincent LM. Ultrasound of soft tissue abnormalities of the extremities. *Radiol Clin North Am* 1988;26(1):131-143.

The Face and Upper Neck

17. Moore KL. *Clinically Oriented Anatomy*. Baltimore: Williams & Wilkins; 1980.
18. Beahrs OH. The facial nerve in parotid surgery. *Surg Clin North Am* 1963;43(4):973-977.
19. Seibert RW, Seibert JJ. High-resolution ultrasonography of the parotid gland in children. Part I. *Pediatr Radiol* 1986;16:374-379.
20. Gritzmann N. Sonography of the salivary glands. *AJR* 1989;153:161-166.
21. Martinoli C, Derchi LE, Solbiati L et al. Color Doppler of salivary glands. *AJR* 1994;163:933-941.
22. Bartlett LJ, Pon M. High-resolution real-time ultrasonography of the submandibular salivary gland. *J Ultrasound Med* 1984;3:433-437.
23. Dehner LP. *Pediatric Surgical Pathology*. 2nd ed. Baltimore: Williams & Wilkins; 1987.
24. Gooding GAW. Gray scale ultrasound of the parotid gland. *AJR* 1980;134:469-472.
25. Kralj Z, Pichler E. Ultrasonic diagnosis of parotid gland tumors. *Acta Med Iugosl* 1984;38:111-118.
26. Lundeberg D. Non-neoplastic disorders of the parotid gland. *Western J Med* 1983;138(4):589-595.
27. Wells DH. Suppuration of the submandibular salivary glands in the neonate. *AJDC* 1975;129:630-638.
28. Magaram D, Gooding GAW. Ultrasonic guided aspiration of parotid abscess. *Arch Otolaryngol* 1981;107:549.

*References 6, 64, 94, 105, 106.

29. Seibert RW, Seibert JJ. High-resolution ultrasonography of the parotid gland in children. Part II. *Pediatr Radiol* 1988; 19:13-18.
30. Rothberg R, Noyek AM, Goldfinger M et al. Diagnostic ultrasound imaging of parotid disease: a contemporary clinical perspective. *J Otolaryngol* 1984;13(4):232-240.
31. Som PM, Shugar JMA, Train JS et al. Manifestations of parotid gland enlargement: radiographic, pathologic and clinical correlations. Part I. The autoimmune pseudosia-lectasis. *Radiology* 1981;141:415-419.
32. Som PM, Shugar JMA, Train JS et al. Manifestations of parotid gland enlargement: radiographic, pathologic and clinical correlations. Part II. The diseases of Mikulicz syndrome. *Radiology* 1981;141:421-426.
33. Bradus RJ, Hybarger P, Gooding GAW. Parotid gland: ultrasound findings in Sjögren syndrome. Work in progress. *Radiology* 1988;169:749-751.
34. Rubaltelli L, Sponga T, Candiani F et al. Infantile recurrent sialectatic parotitis: the role of sonography and sialography in diagnosis and follow-up. *Br J Radiol* 1987;60:1211-1214.
35. Goddart D, Francois A, Vermylen C et al. Parotid gland abnormality found in children seropositive for the human immunodeficiency virus (HIV). *Pediatr Radiol* 1990;20:355-357.
36. Tao LC, Gullane PJ. HIV infection-associated lymphoepithelial lesions of the parotid gland: aspiration biopsy cytology, histology, and pathogenesis. *Diagn Cytopathol* 1991;7(2): 158-62.
37. Rabinov K, Weber AL. *Radiology of the Salivary Glands.* Boston: G.K. Hall Medical Publishers; 1985.
38. Bellina PV Jr. Diagnostic use of ultrasound in sialolithiasis of the parotid gland. *J L State Med Soc* 1982;134(3):79-82.
39. Bianchi A, Cudmore RE. Salivary gland tumors in children. *J Pediatr Surg* 1978;13(6):519-522.
40. Schuller DE, McCabe BF. The firm salivary mass in children. *Laryngoscope* 1977;87:1891-1898.
41. Hebert G, Quimet-Oliva D, Ladouceur J. Vascular tumors of the salivary glands in children. *AJR* 123(4):815-819.
42. Ravitch MM, Welch KJ, Benson CD et al. *Pediatric Surgery.* 3rd ed. Chicago: Yearbook Medical Publishers, Inc; 1979:1.
43. Paltiel HJ, Patriquin HB, Keller MS et al. Infantile hepatic hemangioma: Doppler US. *Radiology* 1992;182:735-742.
44. Guibaud L, Dubois J, Garel LA et al. Hemangiomas and vascular malformations in 86 pediatric cases: evaluation with gray-scale and color Doppler imaging. Presented at the Eighty-First Scientific Assembly and Annual Meeting, Radiological Society for North America; Nov 26–Dec 1, 1995; Chicago, Ill.
45. Ballerini G, Mantero M, Sbrocca M. Ultrasonic patterns of parotid masses. *J Clin Ultrasound* 1984;12:273-277.
46. Aoki S, Barkovich AJ, Nishimura K et al. Neurofibromatosis types 1 and 2: cranial MR findings. *Radiology* 1989;172:527.
47. Work WP. Cysts and congenital lesions of the parotid gland. *Otolaryngol Clin North Am* 1977;10(2):339-342.
48. Ward-Booth RP, Williams EA, Faulkner TPJ et al. Ultrasound: a simple non-invasive examination of cervical swellings. *Plast Reconstr Surg* 1984;73(4):577-581.
49. Wicks JD, Silver TM, Bree RL. Gray scale features of hematomas: an ultrasonic spectrum. *AJR* 1978:131:977-980.
50. Giyanani VL, Grozinger KT, Gerlock AJ Jr et al. Calf hematoma mimicking thrombophlebitis: sonographic and computed tomographic appearance. *Radiology* 1985;154: 779-781.
51. Lovern RE, Bosse DA, Hartshorne MF et al. Organizing hematoma of the thigh: multiple imaging technique. *Clin Nucl Med* 1987;12(8):661-664.
52. Gianfelice D, Jequier S, Patriquin H et al. Sonography of neck masses in children: is it useful? *Int J Pediatr Otorhinolaryngol* 1986;11:247-256.
53. Fornage BD, Schernberg FL. Sonographic diagnosis of foreign bodies of the distal extremities. *AJR* 1986;147:567-569.
54. Grunert D, Schoning M, Stier B. Sonographic evaluation of the larynx in children. New perspectives by application of computed sonography. Part I. Anatomy and method. *Klin Padiatr* 1989;201:201-205.
55. Grunert D, Schoning M, Stier B et al. Sonographic evaluation of the larynx in children. New perspectives by application of computed sonography. Part II. Sonographic findings in a case of laryngeal papillomatosis. *Klin Padiatr* 1989;201:206-208.

Lateral Neck

56. Zitelli BJ. Neck masses in children: adenopathy and malignant disease. *Pediatr Clin North Am* 1981;28(4):813-821.
57. Ying M, Ahuja A, Brook F et al. Sonographic appearance and distribution of normal cervical lymph nodes in a Chinese population. *J Ultrasound Med* 1996;15:431-436.
58. Kreutzer EW, Jafek BW, Johnson ML et al. Ultrasonography in the preoperative evaluation of neck abscesses. *Head Neck Surg* 1982;4:290-295.
59. Sandler MA, Alpern MB, Madrazo BL et al. Inflammatory lesions of the groin: ultrasonic evaluation. *Radiology* 1984; 151:747-750.
60. Loyer EM, Kaur H, David CL et al. Importance of dynamic assessment of the soft tissues in the sonographic diagnosis of echogenic superficial abscesses. *J Ultrasound Med* 1995;14: 669-671.
61. Tovi F, Barki Y, Hertzanu Y. Imaging case study of the month: ultrasound detection of anaerobic neck infection. *Ann Otol Rhino Laryngol* 1993;102:157-158.
62. Glasier CM, Stark JE, Jacobs RF et al. CT and ultrasound imaging of retropharyngeal abscesses in children. *AJNR* 1992;13:1191-1195.
63. Ramilo J, Harris VJ, White H. Empyema as a complication of retropharyngeal and neck abscesses in children. *Radiology* 1978;126:743-746.
64. Kraus R, Han BK, Babcock DS et al. Sonography of neck masses in children. *AJR* 1986;146:609-613.
65. Tschammler A, Ott G, Kumpflein P et al. Differentiation of malignant from reactive lymphadenopathy using color Doppler flow imaging. Presented at the Fortieth Annual Convention, American Institute of Ultrasound in Medicine; March 17-20, 1996; New York, NY.
66. Bearcroft PWP, Berman LH, Grant J. The use of ultrasound-guided cutting needle biopsy in the neck. *Clin Radiol* 1995; 50:690-695.
67. Mandell GA, Bellah RD, Boulden MEC et al. Cervical trachea: dynamics in response to herniation of the normal thymus. *Radiology* 1993;186:383-386.
68. Remine WH. Branchial-cleft cysts and sinuses: their embryologic development and surgical management. *Surg Clin North Am* 1963;43(4):1033-1039.
69. Proctor B. Lateral vestigial cysts and fistulas of the neck. *Laryngoscope* 1955;65(6):355-401.
70. Badami JP, Athey PA. Sonography in the diagnosis of branchial cysts. *AJR* 1981;137:1245-1248.
71. Lynn HB. Cystic hygroma. *Surg Clin North Am* 1963; 43(4):1157-1163.
72. Goodwin BD, Gay BB Jr. The roentgen diagnosis of teratoma of the thyroid region. A review of the literature. *AJR* 1965; 95(1):25-31.
73. Ymaguchi M, Takeuchi S, Matsuo SS. Ultrasonic evaluation of pediatric superficial masses. *J Clin Ultrasound* 1987; 15:107-113.
74. Rand T, Kohlhauser C, Popow C et al. Sonographic detection of internal jugular vein thrombosis after central venous catheterization in the newborn period. *Pediatr Radiol* 1994; 24:577-580.

75. Cassey J, Hendry M, Patel J. Evaluation of long-term central venous patency in children with chronic venous catheters using image-directed Doppler ultrasonography. *J Clin Ultrasound* 1994;22:313-315.
76. Taylor BJ, Seibert JJ, Glasier CM et al. Evaluation of the reconstructed carotid artery following extracorporeal membrane oxygenation. *Pediatrics* 1992;90(4):568-573.
77. Merton DA, Needleman L, Desai SA et al. The fate of the reconstructed common carotid artery: a four-year follow-up in children post-ECMO. Presented at the Fortieth Annual Convention, American Institute of Ultrasound in Medicine; March 17-20, 1996; New York, NY.

Thyroid and Parathyroid Glands

78. Judd ES. Thyroglossal-duct cysts and sinuses. *Surg Clin North Am* 1963;43(4):1023-1031.
79. Moore KL. *The Developing Human—Clinically Oriented Embryology*. 2nd ed. Philadelphia: WB Saunders; 1977.
80. Leopold GR. Ultrasonography of superficially located structures. *Radiol Clin North Am* 1980;18(1):161-173.
81. Bussman YC, Wong ML, Bell MJ et al. Suppurative thyroiditis with gas formation due to mixed anaerobic infection. *J Pediatr* 1977;90(2):321-322.
82. Wojtowycz M, Duck SD, Lipton M et al. Acute suppurative thyroiditis: denouement and discussion. *AJDC* 1981;135: 1063-1064.
83. Abe K, Fujita H, Matsuura N et al. A fistula from pyriform sinus in recurrent acute suppurative thyroiditis. *AJDC* 1981; 135:178.
84. Miller D, Hill JL, Sun CC et al. The diagnosis and management of pyriform sinus fistulae in infants and young children. *J Pediatr Surg* 1983;18(4):377-381.
85. Bachrach LK, Daneman A, Martin DJ. Use of ultrasound in childhood thyroid disorders. *J Pediatr* 1983;103(4):547-552.
86. Winter RJ, Green OC. Carbohydrate homeostasis in chronic lymphocytic thyroiditis: increased incidence of diabetes mellitus. *J Pediatr* 1976;89(3):401-405.
87. Hayashi N, Tamaki N, Konishi J et al. Sonography of Hashimoto's thyroiditis. *J Clin Ultrasound* 1986;14:123-126.
88. Freitas JE, Gross MD, Riplet S et al. Radionuclide diagnosis and therapy of thyroid cancer: current status report. *Semin Nucl Med* 1985;15(2):106-131.
89. Beahrs OH. Workshop on late effects of irradiation to the head and neck in infancy and childhood. *Radiology* 1976; 120:733-734.
90. Beahrs OH et al. Information for physicians on irradiation-related thyroid cancer. *CA* 1976;26(3):150-159.
91. Favus MJ, Schneider AB, Stachura ME et al. Thyroid cancer occurring as a late consequence of head-and-neck irradiation. *N Engl J Med* 1976;294(19):1019-1025.
92. Desjardins JG, Khan AH, Montupet P et al. Management of thyroid nodules in children: a 20-year experience. *J Pediatr Surg* 1987;22(8):736-739.
93. Hung W, August GP, Randolph JG et al. Solitary thyroid nodules in children and adolescents. *J Pediatr Surg* 1982; 17(3):225-229.
94. Cole-Beuglet C, Goldberg BB. New high-resolution ultrasound evaluation of diseases of the thyroid gland. A review article. *JAMA* 1983;249(21):2941-2944.
95. Silverman SH, Nussbaum M, Rausen AR. Thyroid nodules in children: a ten year experience at one institution. *Mt Sinai J Med* 1979;46(5):460-463.
96. Theros EG, Harris JR Jr. *Nuclear Radiology (Third Series) Syllabus*. Chicago: American College of Radiology; 1983.
97. Withers EH, Rosenfeld L, O'Neill J et al. Long-term experience with childhood thyroid carcinoma. *J Pediatr Surg* 1979; 14(3):332-335.
98. Katz JF, Kane RA, Reyes J et al. Thyroid nodules: sonographic-pathologic correlation. *Radiology* 1984;151:741-745.
99. Graze K, Spiler IJ, Tashjian AH Jr et al. Natural history of familial medullary thyroid carcinoma: effect of a program for early diagnosis. *N Engl J Med* 1978;229(18):980-985.
100. Brkljacic B, Cuk V, Tomic-Brzac H et al. Ultrasonic evaluation of benign and malignant nodules in echographically multinodular thyroids. *J Clin Ultrasound* 1994;22:71-76.
101. Garcia CJ, Daneman A, Thorner P et al. Sonography of multinodular thyroid gland in children and adolescents. *AJDC* 1992;146:811-816.
102. Reede DL, Bergeron RT, Som PM. CT of thyroglossal duct cysts. *Radiology* 1985;157:121-125.
103. Wadsworth DT, Siegel MJ. Thyroglossal duct cysts: viriability of sonographic findings. *AJR* 1994;163:1475-1477.
104. Rabinov K, Van Orman P, Gray E. Radiologic findings in persistent thyroglossal tract fistulas. *Radiology* 1979;130:135-139.
105. Solomon JR, Rangecroft L. Thyroglossal-duct lesions in children. *J Pediatr Surg* 1984;19(5):555-561.
106. Miller JH. Lingual thyroid gland: sonographic appearance. *Radiology* 1985;156:83-84.
107. Fisher DA, Kleink AH. Thyroid development and disorders of thyroid function in the newborn. *N Engl J Med* 1981;304(12): 702-712.
108. Hardwick DF, Cormode EJ, Riddell DG. Respiratory distress and neck mass in a neonate. *J Pediatr* 1976;89(3):501-505.
109. Nars PW, Girard L. Lithium carbonate intake during pregnancy leading to large goiter in a premature infant. *AJDC* 1977;131:924-925.
110. De Bruyn R, Ng WK, Taylor J et al. Neonatal hypothyroidism: comparison of radioisotope and ultrasound imaging in 54 cases. *Acta Paediatr Scand* 1990;79:1194-1198.
111. Lopez-Perez GA, Camacho F, Unda A et al. Case report: hemithyroid agenesis associated with a cervical thymic cyst. *J Pediatr Surg* 1979;14(4):468-470.
112. Law WM Jr, James EM, Charboneau JW et al. High-resolution parathyroid ultrasonography in familial benign hypercalcemia (familial hypocalciuric hypercalcemia). *Mayo Clin Proc* 1984;59:153-155.
113. Peck WW, Higgins CB, Fisher MR et al. Hyperparathyroidism: comparison of MR imaging with radionuclide scanning. *Radiology* 1987;163:415-420.
114. Rodriguez-Cueto G, Manzano-Sierra C, Villalpando-Hernandez S. Preoperative ultrasonographic diagnosis of a parathyroid adenoma in a child. *Pediatr Radiol* 1984;14:47-48.
115. Simeone JF, Meuller PR, Ferrucci JT et al. High-resolution real-time sonography of the parathyroid. *Radiology* 1981; 141:745-751.
116. Spritzer CE, Gefter WB, Hamilton R et al. Abnormal parathyroid glands: high-resolution MR imaging. *Radiology* 1987; 162:487-491.
117. Takebayashi S, Matsui K, Onohara Y et al. Sonography for early diagnosis of enlarged parathyroid glands in patients with secondary hyperparathyroidism. *AJR* 1987;148:911-914.
118. Winzelberg GG, Hydovitz JD. Radionuclide imaging of parathyroid tumors: historical perspectives and newer techniques. *Semin Nucl Med* 1985;15(2):161-169.
119. Winzelberg GG, Hydovitz JD, O'Hara KR et al. Parathyroid adenomas evaluated by Tl-201/Tc-99m pertechnetate subtraction and high-resolution ultrasonography. *Radiology* 1985;155:231-235.
120. Wolf RJ, Cronan JJ, Monchik JM. Color Doppler sonography: an adjunctive technique in assessment of parathyroid adenomas. *J Ultrasound Med* 1994;13:303-308.
121. Weinberger MS, Robbins KT. Diagnostic localization studies for primary hyperparathyroidism: a suggested algorithm. *Arch Otolaryngol Head Neck Surg* 1994;120:1187-1189.

CHAPTER 56

The Pediatric Spinal Canal

Michael A. DiPietro, M.D.

CHAPTER OUTLINE

Sonography of the intact spinal canal has been performed for the past 15 years.[1-8] This application is unique to pediatrics because of the incomplete ossification of the posterior vertebral elements in children. The spinal canal and its contents are best visualized in the neonate, the age group in which spinal sonography is most widely used. Usually the spinal canal and its contents (the cord, the cauda equina, or an intracanalicular mass) and not the spine per se are studied. However, osseous anomalies of the sacrum, posterior elements, and vertebral bodies are sometimes noted (Fig. 56-1). The ability of spinal sonography to display normal anatomy and pathology extends beyond the neonate to the infant and young child. Sonography and magnetic resonance imaging (MRI) findings correlated well in infants who were evaluated for congenital anomalies of the lower spine. In this series, sonography depicted the same pathology as MRI, or at least the main abnormality, and no patient with a normal sonogram had an abnormal MRI.[9] The absence of any false-negative sonography study supports its use as a screening examination in infants. In the older child, sonography can provide useful, although limited, information.

Spinal sonography is most often used to determine the level of the conus medullaris, looking for a tethered spinal cord. The tip of the conus is normally at or above the L2-L3 interspace.[10,11] A position lower than L3 almost always indicates a tethered cord. Babies with assorted midline back abnormalities, including hair tufts (hypertrichosis), hemangiomas, skin defects such as aplasia cutis, skin tags, nevi, subcutaneous masses (lipomas), dermal sinuses, and dimples, are routinely screened with spinal sonography for an associated occult tethered cord.[3,7,12,13] Other abnormalities that can be associated with a tethered spinal cord include neurogenic bladder, anomalous sacrum, spina bifida with widened spinal canal (increased interpediculate distance), and anorectal malformations.[14-18]

The spinal cord can also be studied in cases of obvious dysraphism, such as myelomeningocele or myeloschisis.[2,19,20] Imaging in affected newborns is

A

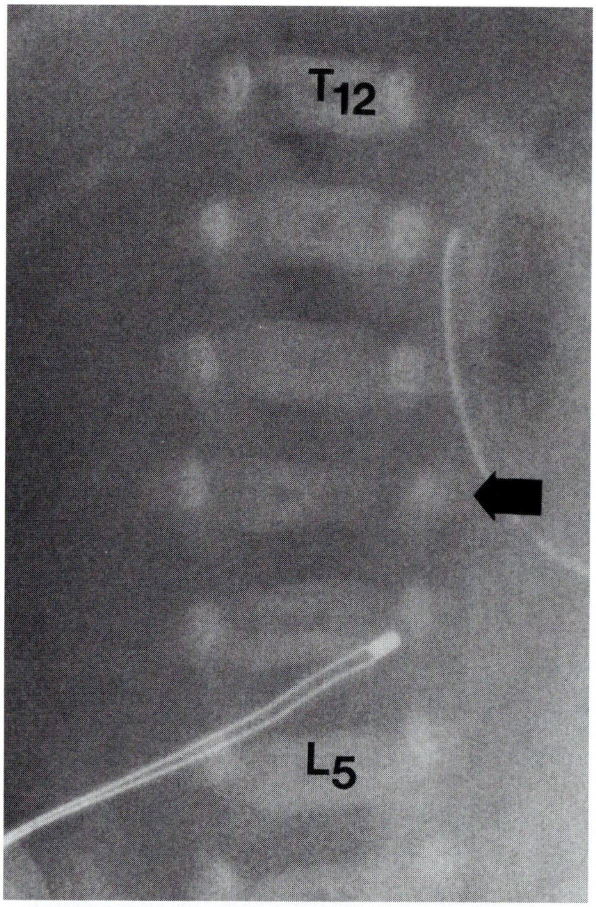

B

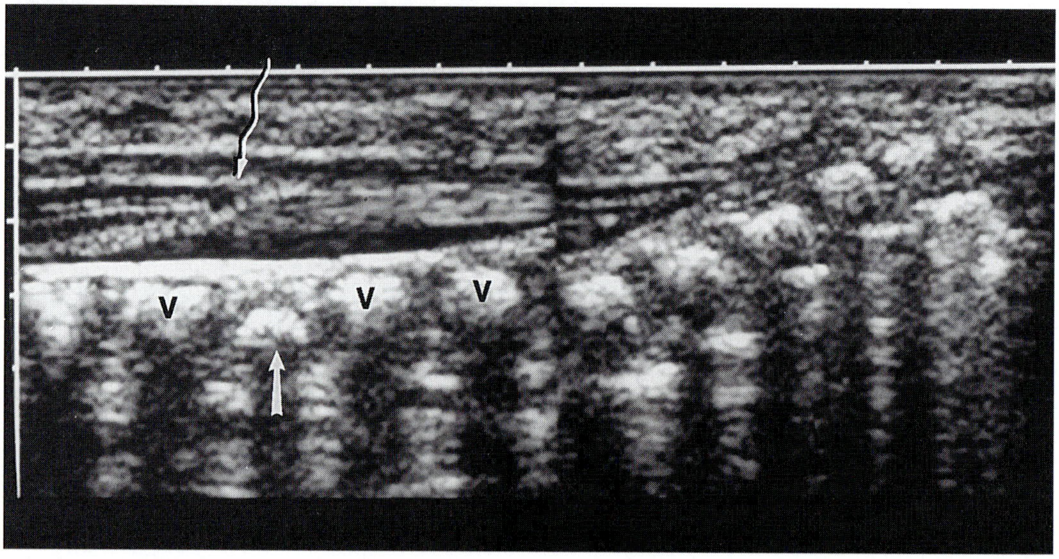

FIG. 56-1. Hypoplastic vertebral body. **A,** AP radiograph showing the hypoplastic left portion of L3 vertebral body *(arrow)*. **B,** Split-screen composite longitudinal sonogram of the lumbosacral canal. The hypoplastic midlumbar vertebral body *(small straight arrow)* is noted in relation to other lumbar vertebral bodies, *V*. *Wavy arrow*, Tip of normal conus. (From DiPietro MA, Garver KA. Sonography of the neonatal spinal canal. In: Haller J. *Textbook of Neonatal and Perinatal Ultrasound Diagnosis.* New York: Parthenon; 1997.)

primarily to find other associated malformations of the cord, such as hydromyelia or diastematomyelia.[19] Sonography of older patients with myelomeningocele is usually to look for retethering of the cord, the myelomeningocele having already been repaired at birth.[1,5,21]

TECHNIQUE

Scanning is performed along the back, usually with the patient prone or in a lateral decubitus position. The baby can also be scanned in sitting posture or while being held upright. The thoracolumbar spine should be

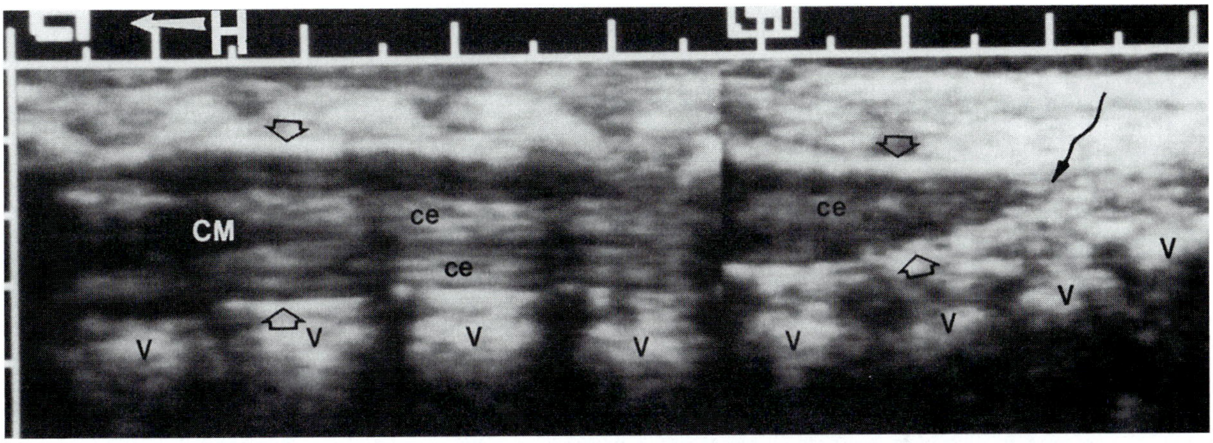

FIG. 56-2. Normal lumbosacral canal (5-week-old). Longitudinal composite scan made by adjoining two split screens. *CM*, Conus medullaris; *ce*, roots of cauda equina; *open arrowheads*, dura; *V*, vertebral bodies; *wavy arrow*, caudal end of thecal sac. (From DiPietro MA. Pediatric musculoskeletal and spinal sonography, In: van Holsbeeck M, Introcaso JH. *Musculoskeletal Ultrasound.* St Louis: Mosby-Year Book, Inc; 1991.)

SPINAL SONOGRAPHY TECHNIQUE

Scan midline between spinous processes (neonate)
Scan lateral and parallel to spinous process (older child)
Split screen for longitudinal view length
Find level of conus and place a metal marker over it
Use metal marker on plain film for accurate level
Start scan at sacrum
Look for oscillation of nerve roots
- Neonate at respiratory rate
- Older infant and child at heart rate

flexed to separate the spinous processes and thus widen the acoustic window to the spinal canal. Placing the patient prone over a pillow or blanket roll will facilitate flexing the spine. Adequate flexion is crucial, but care should be taken not to compromise respiratory excursion, especially in the neonate. Slight elevation of the head might help distend the caudal aspect of the thecal sac.[3,4] Use the highest-frequency transducer that provides adequate tissue penetration, which is usually 5 MHz or 7.5 MHz, although 10 MHz or 12 MHz works well in smaller patients. Linear array transducers are preferred over sector transducers for progressing along the longitudinal axis of the spinal canal in the sagittal plane. **Neonates** and young, small infants are scanned over the midline **between the spinous processes.** Their posterior vertebral elements are so unossified that a broad longitudinal view of the spinal canal is obtained over several segments. This can be maximized by using a **split screen** and combining the two aligned half screens to give one, long, panoramic, longitudinal view (Fig. 56-2). The spinal canal in the **older infant** and

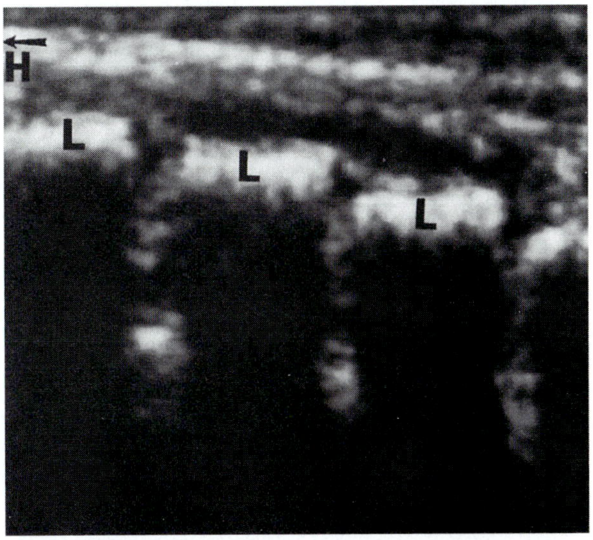

FIG. 56-3. Laminae, *L.* Longitudinal scan off midline (parasagittal) resembles overlapping roof tiles.

larger child is usually better viewed longitudinally from a slightly different approach.[1] The transducer is placed slightly **lateral and parallel to the spinous processes.** From this parasagittal position the transducer is aimed medially into the spinal canal. Access is limited to the spaces between the vertebral laminae (Fig. 56-3). This interlaminar approach provides a more limited, segmental view of the spinal canal, yet it is often adequate. Access is more limited as the child gets older and bigger and ossification advances. However, we have been able to identify the **level of the conus** in chldren up to 10 years of age with intact spines (Fig. 56-4). In these older children, limited visualization has prevented ascertaining much else, but the conus level was the information that was needed.

A

B

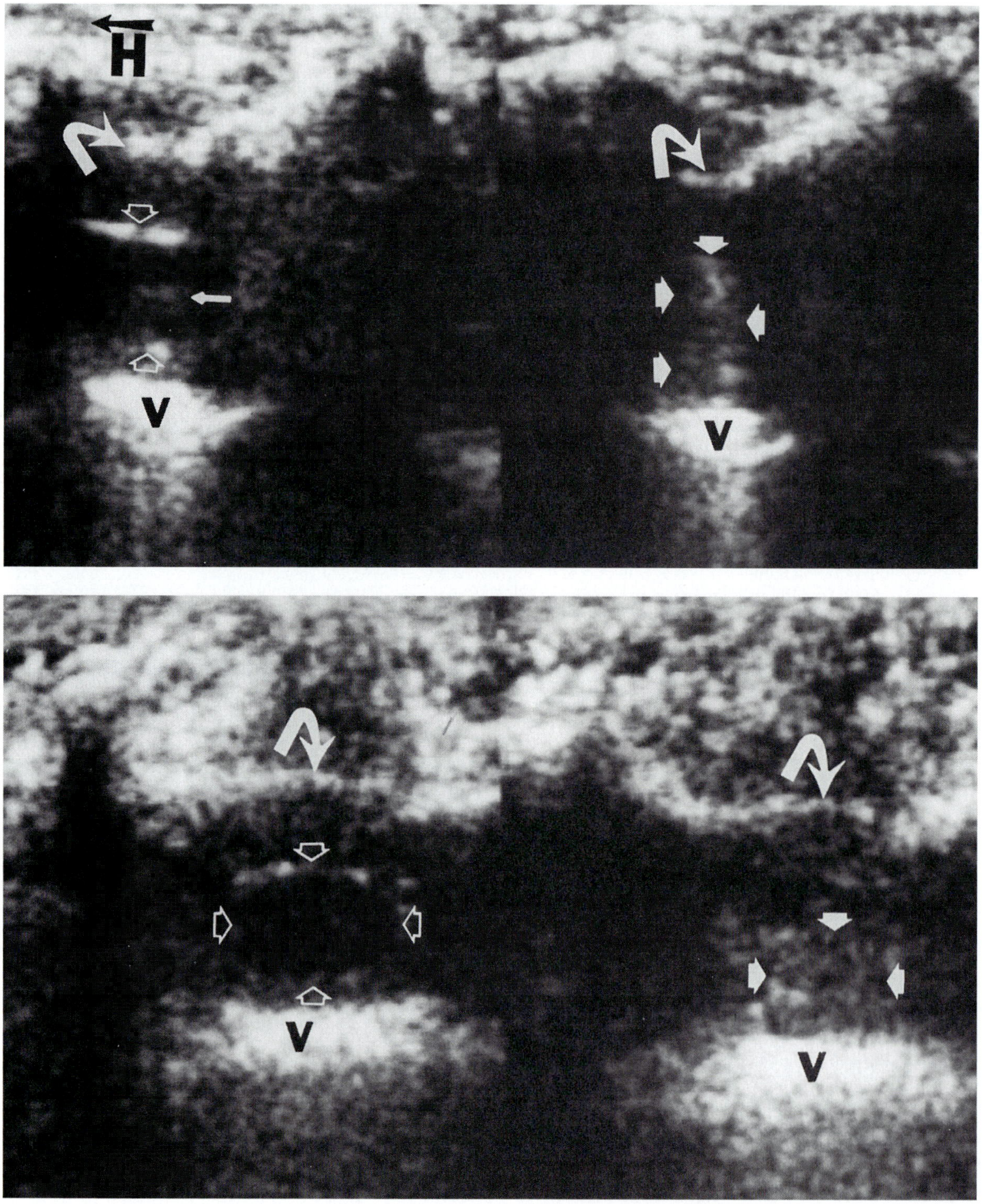

FIG. 56-4. Normal 9-year-old conus in the high lumbar canal. **A,** Parasagittal and, **B,** transverse scans (displayed on split screens) show the cord *(open arrowheads)* in the high lumbar canal, but the next lower vertebral level (to the right of the split screen) showed only nerve roots (i.e., cauda equina; outlined by closed arrowheads); therefore the conus was somewhere between these two levels. *Curved arrows*, Dorsal dura; *straight arrows*, central echo; *v*, vertebral bodies.

A problem with correctly judging scale and depth sometimes occurs with the novice examiner scanning either too shallowly or too deeply. In those cases, it helps to **start scanning over the sacrum** where the spinal canal is easily found, and to then scan cephalad, following the spinal canal from there. The spinal cord and roots of the cauda equina are not static.[1,7,8,22] They move rhythmically with respirations and, especially beyond the neonatal period, oscillate briskly in dorsoventral and cephalocaudal directions at the heart rate.[1] Cord and root motion is better appreciated when frame averaging or persistence is minimal, although this causes the image to appear grainier (i.e., less smooth). Some authors have advocated routine use of a standoff pad for improved near-field resolution.[5,23] We use it primarily to study the subcutaneous tissues, looking for a sinus tract.

NORMAL CORD ANATOMY

The spinal cord appears relatively hypoechoic, slightly more echogenic than the surrounding anechoic cerebrospinal fluid (CSF) (see box below). The surface of the spinal cord is echogenic, with its dorsal and ventral surfaces each demarcated by a bright line (Fig. 56-5). The center of the spinal cord contains 1 or 2 echogenic dots in the transverse plane and correspondingly 1 or 2 echogenic lines in the longitudinal plane (see Fig. 56-5; Figs. 56-6 to 56-8), which are referred to as the **central echo complex**. The cause of these lines (dots) and what they represent have been debated. One study with sonographic-anatomic correlation in a spinal cord specimen suggested that the central echo complex is generated by the central canal or glial fibrils immediately surrounding it.[24] However, another study of spinal cord specimens, also with sonographic correlation, demonstrated convincingly that the central echo complex is produced by the interface between myelinated ventral white commissure and the central end of the anterior median fissure.[25] This interface is ventral to the central canal. The authors of that study transected a cord specimen in the coronal plane so that the central canal remained in the dorsal segment and the ventral white commissure and anterior median fissure remained in the ventral segment. Sonography of the separate segments in a water bath demonstrated no central echo in the dorsal segment (containing the central canal) and a typical central echo in the ventral segment.

In our experience, the central echo complex in normal neonates sometimes appears as slightly separated double dots (transverse view) or parallel lines (longitudinal view) in a dorsoventral relationship. A prospective study of 103 neurologically asymptomatic neonates showed 9% with such a widened central echo complex in the conus medullaris.[26] Variations in the shape of the central echo complex could reflect varying

NORMAL CORD ANATOMY

Echogenic cord surface
Central echo complex
Slightly echogenic cord
Very echogenic nerve roots

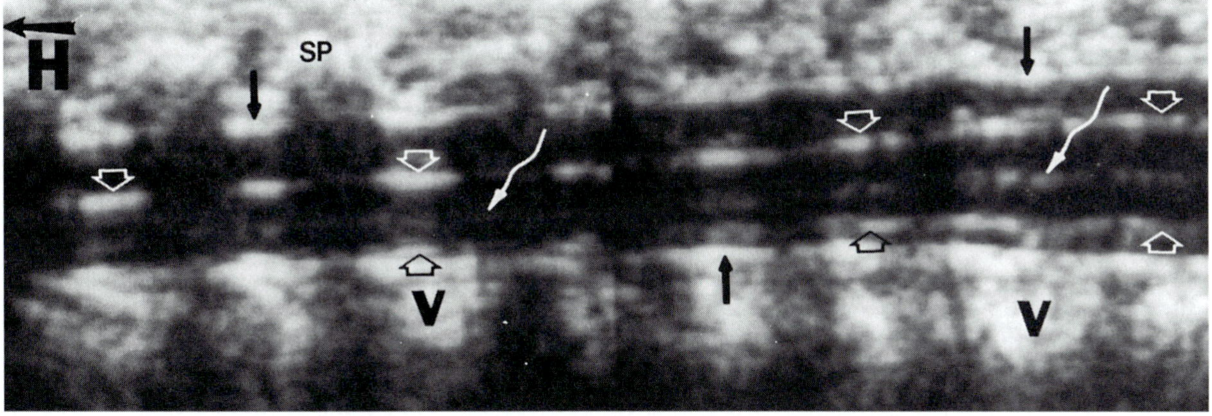

FIG. 56-5. Midthoracic—high lumbar canal in a normal 5-day-old. Longitudinal composite scan shows the cord *(open arrowheads)* at the thoracic level, where it is more ventral in the canal and becomes thicker and more centrally positioned in the lumbar canal. *V*, Vertebral bodies (only two are labeled); *black arrows*, dura; *wavy arrows*, central echo complex; *sp*, spinous process; *H*, patient's head.

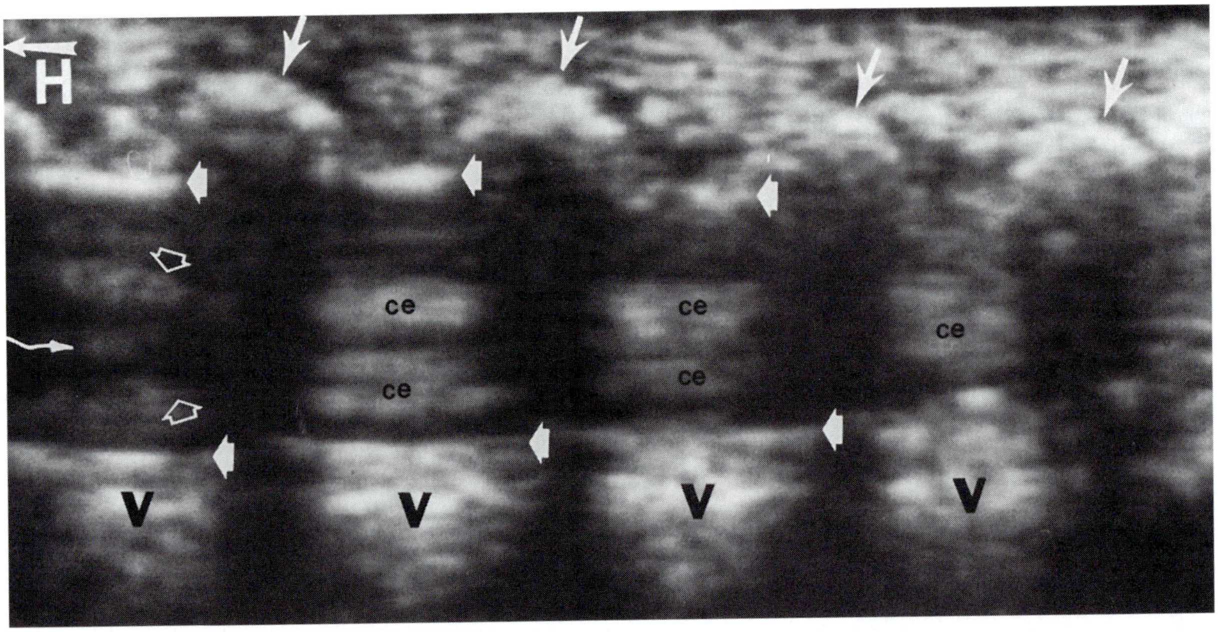

FIG. 56-6. Normal conus *(open arrowheads)* **and cauda equina,** *ce* **(2-month-old).** Longitudinal scan. *Closed arrowheads,* Dura; *wavy arrow,* central echo; *straight arrows,* spinous processes with shadowing; *V,* vertebral bodies.

CORD ANATOMY VARIATION BY LEVEL

Oval cervical cord
Circular thoracic cord and dentate ligaments
Larger thoracolumbar cord
Conus medullaris tapers
Conus usually ends above L2
Cauda equina roots ventral and dorsal
Anterior spinal artery
Epidural veins

degrees of flaring of the central end of the anterior median fissure.[25] Even if the echoes do not represent the dorsal and ventral walls of the central canal per se, they separate progressively with worsening hydromyelia.

The size and shape of the spinal cord vary with respect to vertebral level.[23,27-29] The **cervical cord** has an oval shape (the major axis is horizontal) (Fig. 56-7) that becomes more circular at the thoracic level. The **thoracic cord** appears as a relatively small circle in the transverse plane (Fig. 56-8, *A*). It expands to a larger circle at the **thoracolumbar junction and upper lumbar levels** because of the large number of neurons supplying the lower extremities (Fig. 56-8, *B*).

The **conus medullaris** appears as a diminishing circle in the transverse plane on sequential caudal scanning, but with its surrounding nerve roots it sometimes has the illusion of a triangular shape (Fig. 56-9). In the longitudinal view the conus is tapered,

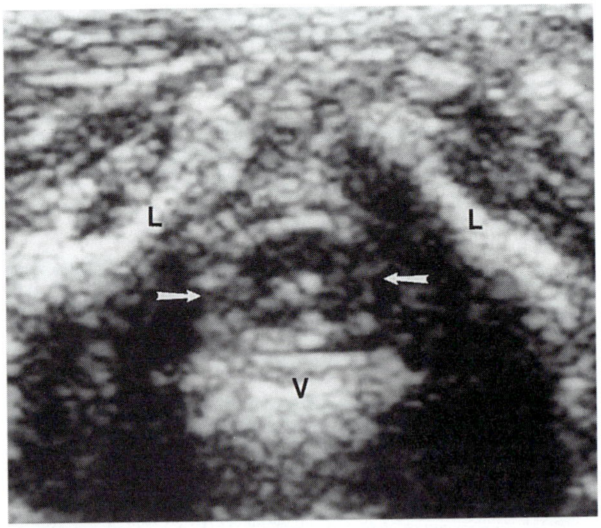

FIG. 56-7. The normal cervical spinal cord, transverse view. *Arrows,* cord; *L,* lamina; *V,* vertebral body. (From DiPietro MA, Garver KA. Sonography of the neonatal spinal canal. In: Haller J. *Textbook of Neonatal and Perinatal Ultrasound Diagnosis.* New York: Parthenon; 1997.)

appearing like a horizontally oriented carrot (see Figs. 56-2 and 56-6). In contrast with the normally tapered conus, a blunt, **"wedge-shaped" conus** can be seen on longitudinal views in cases of caudal regression.[30]

The most common request for sonography is to determine the level of the tip of the conus medullaris. The **normal cord usually ends above L2,** although it can

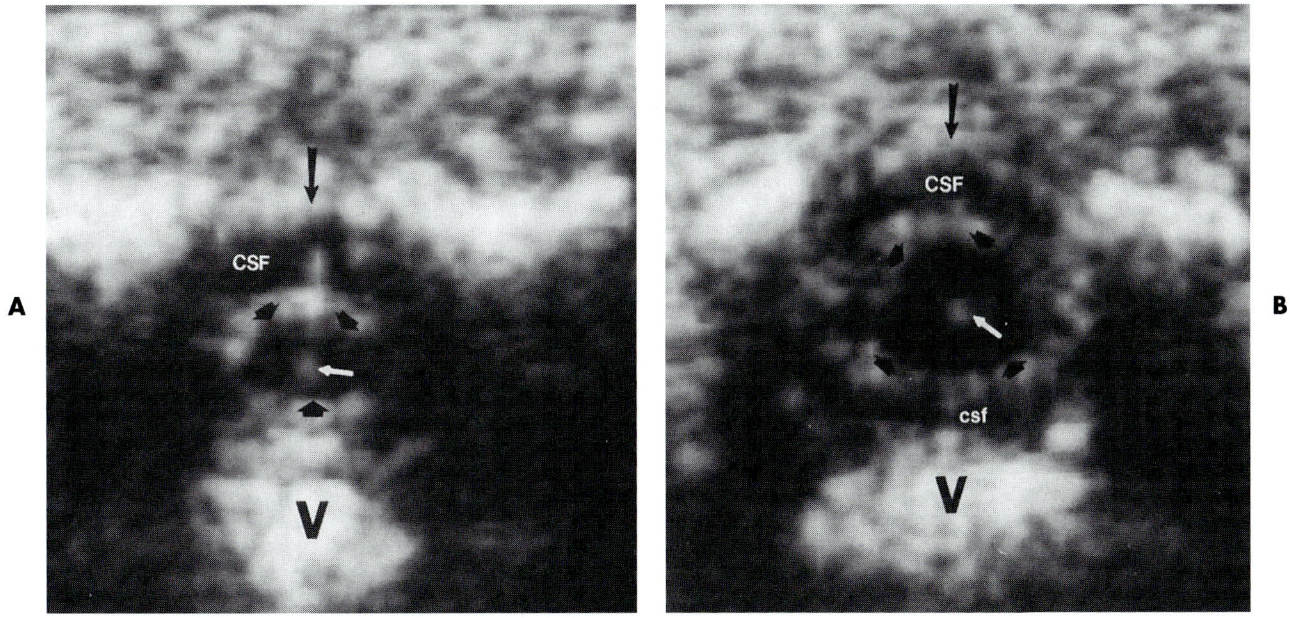

FIG. 56-8. Normal 5-day-old cord. A, Thoracic and, B, lumbar. Transverse scans. The degree of magnification is constant and shows that the cord is smaller at thoracic than at lumbar levels. Hypoechoic CSF surrounds the cord *(black arrowheads). Black arrow*, dorsal dura; *white arrow*, central echo complex; *V*, vertebral body.

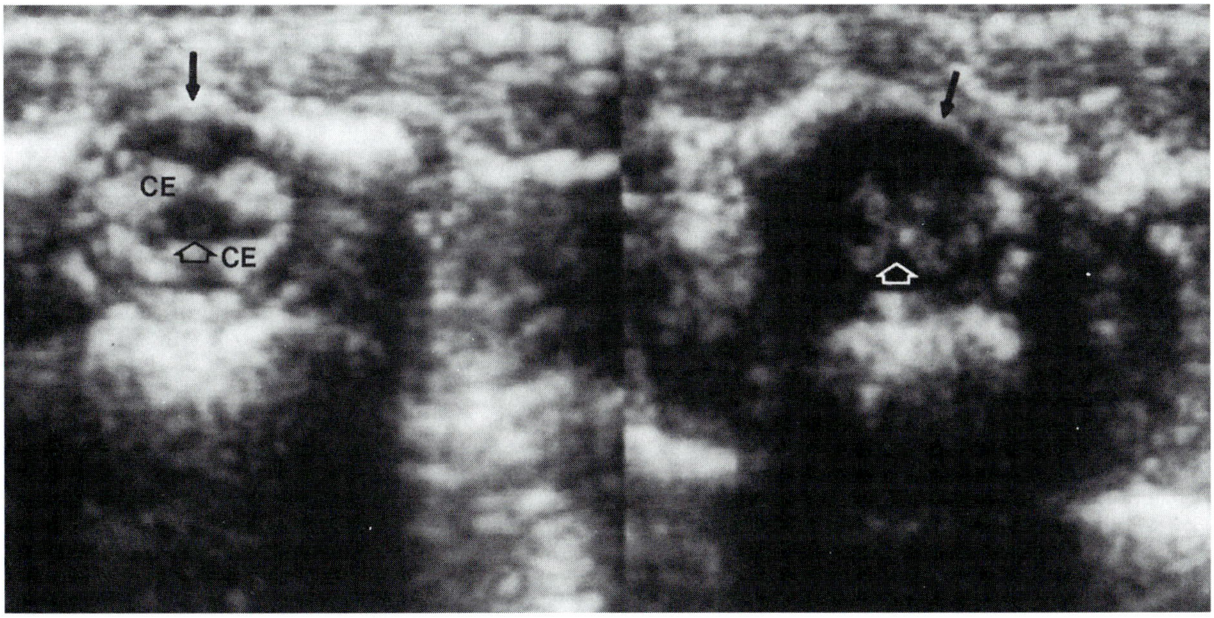

FIG. 56-9. Hypoechoic conus with surrounding echogenic cauda equina, *CE*, in a normal 5-day-old. Transverse views (left screen, *open black arrowhead*). The dorsal and ventral roots of the cauda equina form an "X" (right screen, *open white arrowhead*) at the tip of the conus. *Black arrow*, Dorsal dura.

occasionally extend to the superior endplate of L3.[11] Cross-section population studies using MRI[10] and sonography[11] showed that normal conus levels are the same throughout infancy and childhood. A study that included premature neonates indicated that the normal conus has ascended by the fortieth postmenstrual week.[31] Between 30 and 39 postmenstrual weeks a few conus tips were at L3,4; 77.8% were L2-L4; and 22.2% were T12-L1,2. In contrast, between 40 and 63 postmenstrual weeks the lowest conus tip was at L2,3;

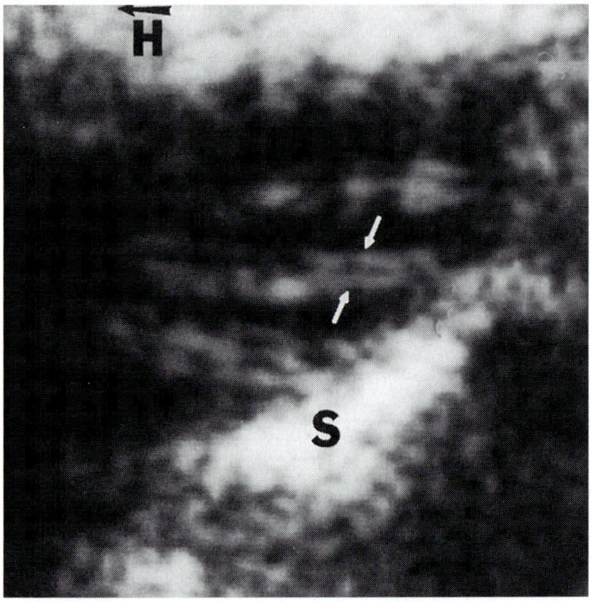

FIG. 56-10. Sacral canal nerve roots. Longitudinal magnification view shows them as double echogenic lines *(arrows)*. *S*, Sacrum.

15.7% were L2-L4; and 84.3% were T12-L1,2.[31] The low thoracic and lumbar cord is relatively easy to see, even in the nonobese older child who has been properly positioned. Although the actual tip of the conus might be obscured by lamina or spinous processes, the level of the conus can be inferred to lie between the lowest level showing cord and the next caudal level showing only cauda equina. This should be verified in both longitudinal and transverse views. The low thoracic and upper lumbar cord is relatively easy to see. It occupies the midportion of the spinal canal when the spine is straight. This is in contrast with the upper and midthoracic cord, which is difficult to see well after early infancy due to the marked overlap of the posterior spinal elements at those levels, which obscures visibility. The natural, slight, upper and midthoracic, spinal kyphosis is accentuated when the patient is positioned for scanning. At those levels the cord is ventral in the spinal canal where it "hugs" the posterior surface of the vertebral bodies (see Fig. 56-5).

The roots of the **cauda equina** appear as echogenic strands on longitudinal views or dots on transverse views (see Figs. 56-2, 56-6, and 56-9). The nerve roots are sometimes seen as double lines in high-resolution scans, similar to their appearance on intraoperative sonography (Fig. 56-10). Dorsal and ventral roots can be identified separately on transverse views (see Fig. 56-9; Fig. 56-11, *A*). Nerve roots are often clustered together, and this appearance, especially close to the conus, where there are many roots, could be mistaken for an echogenic intracanalicular mass (see Figs. 56-4, *B* and 56-9; Fig. 56-11, *B*). However, undulating movement within "the mass" helps to identify it as a cluster of nerve roots. In addition to nerve roots, **dentate ligaments** can be noted in the thoracic cord. They extend horizontally from the cord at the 9- and 3-o'clock positions (Fig. 56-12). The **anterior spinal artery** and **epidural veins** are apparent with color flow Doppler imaging. The latter are noted best in the lower lumbar canal (Figs. 56-13 and 56-14).

The spinal cord and cauda equina oscillate in dorsoventral and cephalocaudal directions syn-

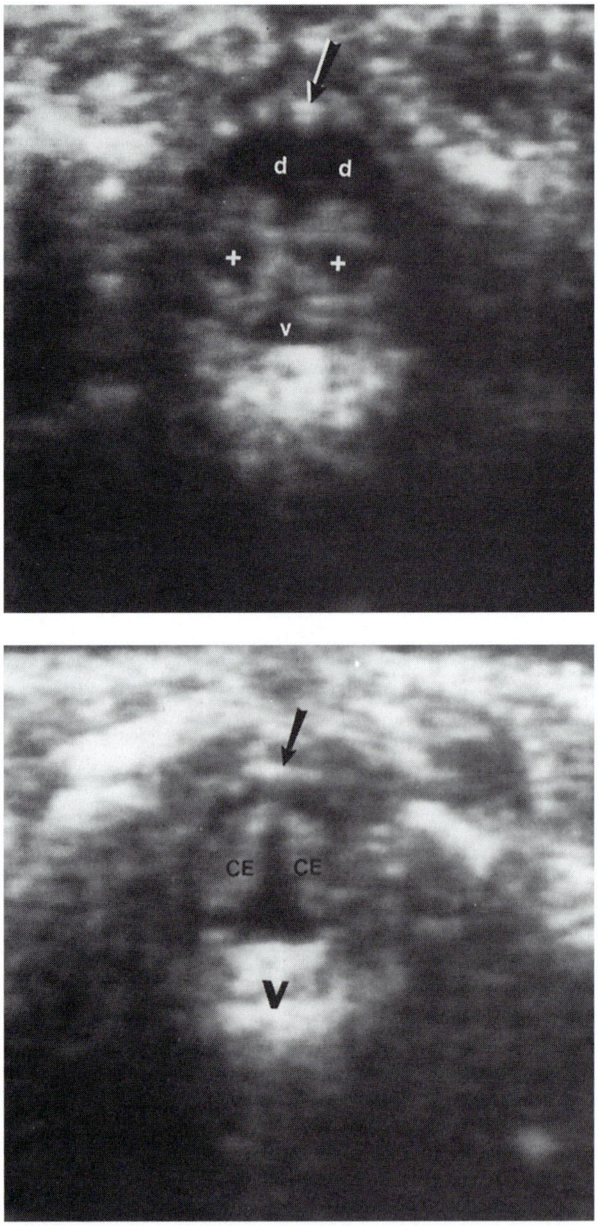

A

B

FIG. 56-11. Tip of cauda equina in normal 2-month-old. Transverse scans. A, The "X"-shaped echogenic cauda equina surrounds anechoic CSF (+). *d*, Dorsal CSF; *v*, ventral CSF; *arrow*, dorsal dura. **B,** Lower in the lumbar canal the cauda equina has formed two nerve root clusters, *CE*. *Arrow*, Dorsal dura; *V*, vertebral body.

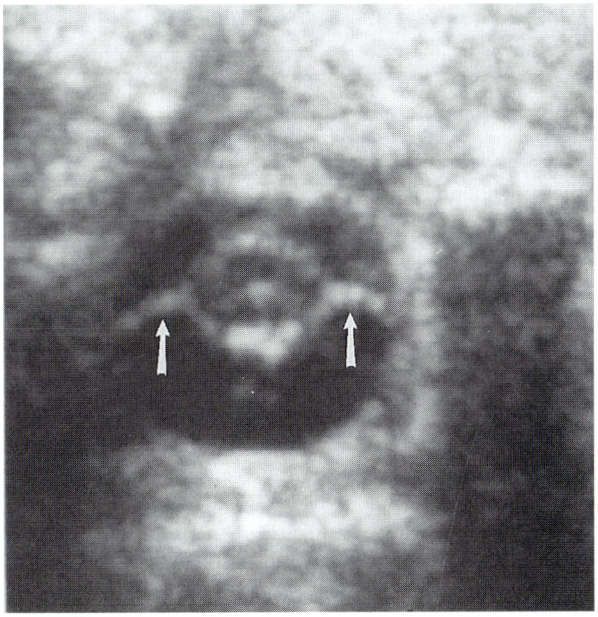

FIG. 56-12. Dentate ligaments. Transverse view of thoracic cord with dentate ligaments *(arrows)*. (From DiPietro MA, Garver KA. Sonography of the neonatal spinal canal. In: Haller J. *Textbook of Neonatal and Perinatal Ultrasound Diagnosis.* New York: Parthenon; 1997.)

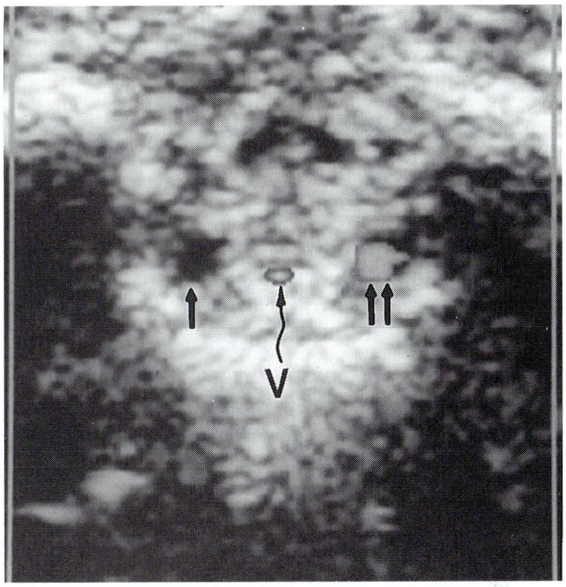

FIG. 56-13. Normal color flow Doppler imaging at conus. Epidural veins (*straight arrows*) without *(single arrow)* and with *(dual arrows)* color signal. *Wavy arrow,* Color signal in anterior spinal artery; *V*, vertebra.

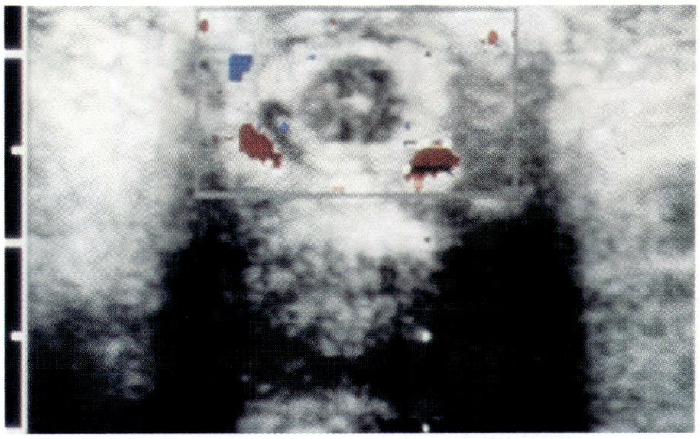

FIG. 56-14. Normal color flow Doppler imaging of lumbar cord shows epidural veins in color.

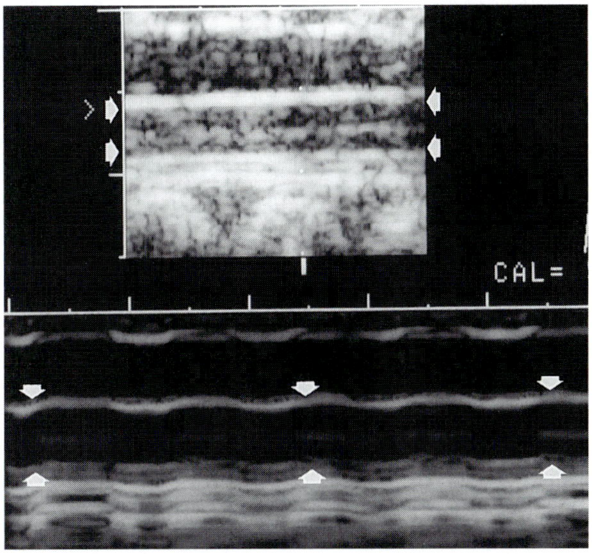

FIG. 56-15. Normal spinal cord M-mode ultrasound. Dorsal and ventral aspects of cord are demarcated by arrows; note oscillations on M-mode scan.

chronously with the heart beat. This motion is usually brisk in the child beyond a few months of age. **Cord and root oscillation** synchronous with the heart rate has been documented on MRI[32] and with M-mode sonography[8,22] (Fig. 56-15). In our opinion, M-mode sonography is not necessary to appreciate the oscillatory motion, but it can document it. In the neonate, this brisk oscillation is usually subtle or absent. However, the neonate's cord is not completely motionless. One usually sees some cord and root motion with breathing, crying, or moving.[1]

Anatomic detail is remarkable in the neonate and young infant but less so in the older child. However, with experience, even in the older child sonographic visualization can be sufficient to answer the particular clinical question, which is most often to determine the level of the conus medullaris. The examiner's overall appreciation of sonographic anatomy, especially where it is less clearly seen in the older child, can be enhanced by gaining some experience with intraoperative spinal sonography. Radiologists with an interest in spinal sonography should try to be present during intraoperative scanning where it is performed through a saline-

CAUSES OF TETHERED CORD

Lipomeningocele
Intraspinal lipoma
Thick filum terminale
Diastematomyelia
Dermal sinus

TETHERED CORD FINDINGS

Conus below L3
Conus often eccentric, especially dorsal
Cord oscillations decreased
May be normal motion in newborn until tethered later or distant from end of cord

filled laminectomy. Anatomy and pathology are clearly seen, unimpeded by overlying bone or soft tissues.[28,33]

THE TETHERED SPINAL CORD

The tethered spinal cord is "a pathologic fixation of the spinal cord in an abnormal caudal location, so that the cord suffers mechanical stretching, distortion, and ischemia with daily activities, growth, and development."[34] The child might be neurologically intact at birth (typical of lipomyelomeningocele) but develops a deficit that progresses with growth spurts. Neurologic deficits include reflex changes, sensory loss, muscle wasting, power loss, and sphincter problems.[35] An occult tethered cord can present with a lower-extremity deformity or abnormal gait as the patient's major complaint.[36,37] Of 29 patients with tethered cords caused by congenital intraspinal lipoma, 17 had cavus (8) or equinovarus (9) foot deformities.[37] Orthopedic procedures done for foot deformity were more successful when the tethered cord had been previously released than when it remained tethered.[37]

Spinal cord tethering can have a variety of pathologic causes, including **intraspinal lipoma, thick filum terminale, diastematomyelia,** and **dermal sinus** (see box at top of this column). The progressive neurologic impairment results from stretching of the cord as the child grows. Evidence of impaired oxidative metabolism has been noted in the distal tethered spinal cord.[38]

Terminology regarding **tethered cord** and types of lipomas associated with tethered cord is confusing. The "tethered spinal cord" has been used to mean a tethered, low cord due to a thickened filum terminale. In this chapter, "tethered cord" is used in a more generic sense. A conus terminating low in the spinal canal below the superior aspect of L3 is probably a tethered cord (see box at top of next column). However, in the child who has had a myelomeningocele repaired in the past the cord remains low and is not necessarily still tethered. Therefore the diagnosis of retethering in a myelomeningocele patient (postclosure) is more difficult and depends on criteria other than solely the level of the cord (vide infra).

One can estimate the **vertebral level of the conus** on sonography by using sonographic landmarks. The lumbosacral junction is usually apparent on the longitudinal view where the line tangent to the posterior borders of the lumbar vertebral bodies intersects the line tangent to the sacrum, forming an angle similar to that seen on a lateral radiograph.[39] The coccyx is mostly or completely unossified in the neonate,[40] and the caudal tip of the thecal sac often corresponds to S2[41] (see Fig. 56-2). These landmarks allow counting of the vertebral segments to the conus tip and thereby establish its level. In addition, the lowest rib can usually be palpated close to the spine or it can be visualized sonographically and traced medially to its vertebral body (Fig. 56-16). Since a patient might have 11 or 13 sets of ribs instead of 12, a margin of error of plus or minus one vertebral level must be considered. Ribs should be identified by sonography far enough lateral (usually over the kidneys) from the vertebral column so that transverse processes are not mistaken for ribs (Fig. 56-17). As rough estimates, the tip of the lowest rib often corresponds to L2 and the top of the iliac crest to L5.[11] If the vertebral level of conus termination remains questionable, careful placement of a **radiopaque marker on the skin at the level of the conus tip** followed by a radiograph will usually verify the level. The confirmatory radiograph has usually not been necessary in our experience because most tethered cords have been unquestionably low, extending to the low lumbar or sacral canal. In addition to being low, the tethered lumbar cord is usually eccentric, often dorsal, within the spinal canal (Fig. 56-18). Hence, the expression "the low-down stuck-up" spinal cord seems appropriate. **Cord oscillations** are often diminished or absent at or above the point of tethering.[5-7] However, oscillations can persist distant from the tethered site.[1,6,22,32] Therefore cord oscillations might persist normally at thoracic levels but become dampened in the lower lumbar canal toward the site of tethering. We have observed that brisk cord oscillations are often not apparent in the first 2 postnatal months; therefore their absence has less significance than in older infants and children. In addition, we have found that tethered cords might not lose oscillations until the child grows and the cord is stretched.[34,38]

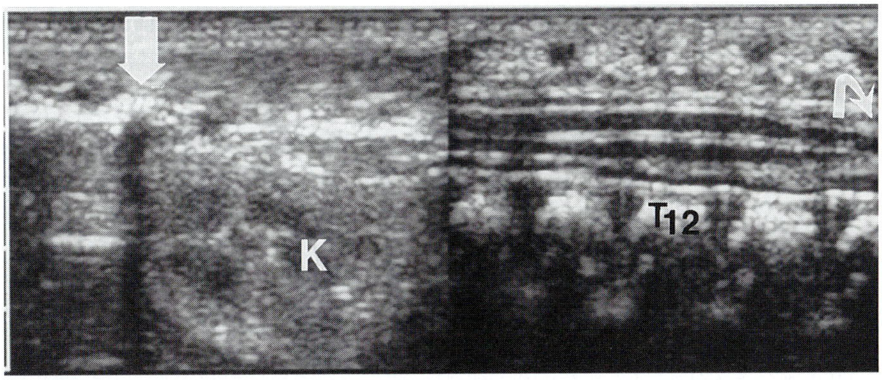

FIG. 56-16. Estimating the vertebral level of the conus tip. Longitudinal split screen with lowest rib *(straight arrow)* over the kidney, *K*, in the left frame. In the right frame the rib was sonographically followed back to the vertebral column to presumably locate T12. *Curved arrow*, Conus tip. (From DiPietro MA, Garver KA. Sonography of the neonatal spinal canal. In: Haller J. *Textbook of Neonatal and Perinatal Ultrasound Diagnosis.* New York: Parthenon; 1997.)

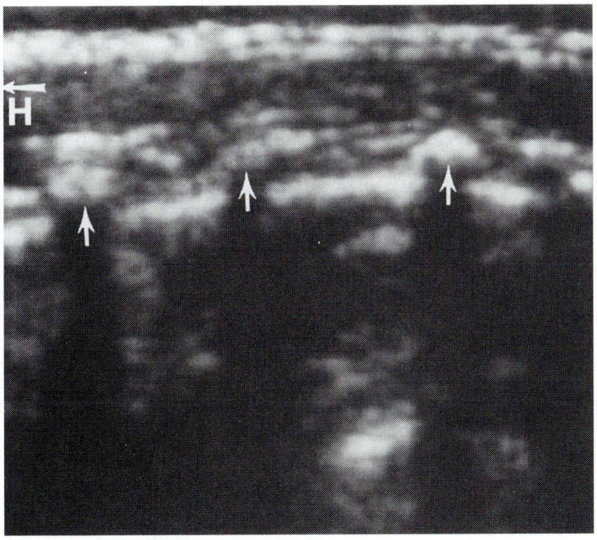

FIG. 56-17. Transverse processes *(arrows)*, **not to be confused with ribs.**

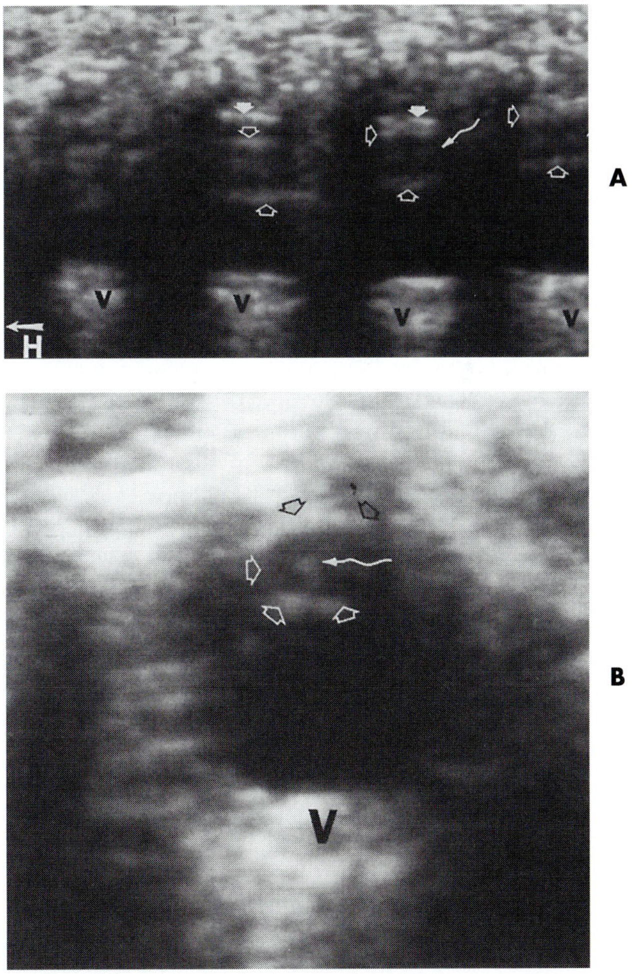

FIG. 56-18. Cord tethered by a lipomyelomeningocele. **A,** Longitudinal and, **B,** transverse scans (7-month-old child) of low lumbar canal. The too caudal cord *(open arrowheads)* is dorsal instead of centrally located in the canal. *Closed arrowheads*, Dorsal dura; *wavy arrow*, central echo; *v*, vertebral bodies.

Cutaneous Markers

Midline, lumbosacral, skin abnormalities can herald an occult tethered spinal cord while the child is still neurologically intact (see box on p. 1600). **Subcutaneous lipoma, hair tuft, sinus tract, dimple, skin defect** (i.e., aplasia cutis[42] or scarlike white patch), **hemangioma, skin tag or appendage**, or **pigmented nevi,** alone or in combination, are **cutaneous markers** often associated with an **occult spinal dysraphism** (spina bifida occulta) and a **tethered cord.**[43,44] It is not surprising that skin and central nervous system (CNS) (spinal) defects occur together since the neural tube is closing and the overlying ectoderm is differentiating into neural and epithelial tissues in the embryo's first gestational month.[44]

RISK FACTORS FOR TETHERED CORD

- Atypical sacral dimples
- Subcutaneous lipoma
- Hair tuft
- Skin defect
- Hemangioma
- Skin tag
- Pigmented nevi
- Occult spinal dysraphism
- Dermal sinus
- Anorectal malformations
- Lipomeningomyelocele
- Leptomyelolipoma
- Lipomyeloschisis

Failure to recognize the possible association of these cutaneous abnormalities with an occult tethered cord could result in a formerly neurologically intact child developing such problems as foot and lower extremity deformities, decreased sensation, scoliosis, weakness, abnormal gait, and bladder dysfunction with age.[44,45] Children with **hemangiomas** of the lower back should be screened for a tethered cord. In one report, seven consecutive children with hemangiomas crossing the midline of the lower back were neurologically intact, yet all had tethered cords.[43] They were discovered by MRI in that study, but we have diagnosed similar cases using sonography. The published hemangiomas were large, between 4 and 20 cm across, but small hemangiomas can also be seen with a tethered cord. Since hemangiomas tend to involute with age, this cutaneous marker might disappear and the tethered cord will go unnoted until neurologic signs and symptoms develop.[43] Therefore **screening in the newborn period or infancy** is recommended. In addition, sonographic visualization is optimal then because the acoustic window continues to get smaller as the child grows. Patients with progressively symptomatic occult dysraphism are often found to have lumbosacral skin markers. However, regarding the converse, the question of how often children with these cutaneous abnormalities have CNS pathology has not been answered.[44,46] In a study of 73 cases of occult spinal dysraphism, plain radiography demonstrated laminar defects, increased interpediculate distance (i.e., widened spinal canal), and sacral deformities.[36] The lesions were varied and included dermal sinuses (some with epidermoid inclusion cysts), lipomas, and thick fila terminale. Of 70 children, 11 had spine radiographs that were read as normal, even in retrospect,[36] which illustrates the limitation of plain radiography as a screening tool for occult spinal dysraphism. However, the ages of those 11 patients or their lesions were not reported by the authors. Interpretation of neonatal spine radiographs can be difficult because of normal incomplete ossification.

The most common reason for performing newborn spine sonography has been to investigate the significance of **lumbosacral dimples,** most of which are in the low sacrococcygeal region. Most low sacrococcygeal dimples, without other skin or subcutaneous abnormalities, are usually insignificant.[12,44,47] Those within the gluteal cleft are less significant than those above.[12] Such small indentations or shallow cutaneous pits at the level of the coccyx (pilonidal dimples) are commonly present in 2% to 4.3% of newborns.[46,48] A total 7.3% of 1997 consecutive newborns had congenital midline dermal abnormalities at or below the lumbar level.[46] Approximately 4.3% were shallow pilonidal dimples or deep gluteal creases with intact skin at the base, probably normal variants, and 3% had one or more of the following findings:

- Deep dimples requiring magnification or retraction to visualize the bottom (1.4%);
- Presumed sinuses in which the bottom could not be seen (1.2%); and
- Skin tags (0.3%).

No difference in the incidence of abnormality by race or sex was apparent.[46] Of 57, 36 (63%) had "roentgenographic abnormalities," not specified in this report, that predated the availability of sonography.

In one study of sacrococcygeal dimples, 43 newborns had their spinal canals studied sonographically and their dimples photographed.[47] Of the 43, 33 had typical pilonidal dimples, and sonography was normal. Of 43, 8 had atypical dimples with normal sonography, but 2 with atypical dimples had tethered cords. One of the 2 also had an **imperforate anus,** an entity that has an association with occult tethered cord.[17] The other newborn with a tethered cord had an atypical "craterlike" dimple.[47]

The dimple should be scanned using a high-frequency, small-parts transducer and/or a standoff pad. Both will improve near-field resolution to show the soft-tissue interfaces, normally appearing as continuous echogenic lines between skin, subcutaneous fat, muscle, and fascia. The **dermal sinus** will appear as a hypoechoic band extending through and interrupting these echogenic soft-tissue interfaces[12,49] (Figs. 56-19 and 56-20). The sinus might be seen extending to the dural sac, but whether it penetrates the dura cannot be determined on sonography.[12,49] The **normal, hypoechoic, unossified coccyx** must not be mistaken for a cyst deep to a dimple (Fig. 56-21). Although the simple, low, intergluteal, coccygeal, pilonidal dimple is not usually associated with spinal pathology, it could still cause problems later in life as a pilonidal sinus or cyst.[12] Interestingly, one sonographic study of 29 newborns with pilonidal dimples

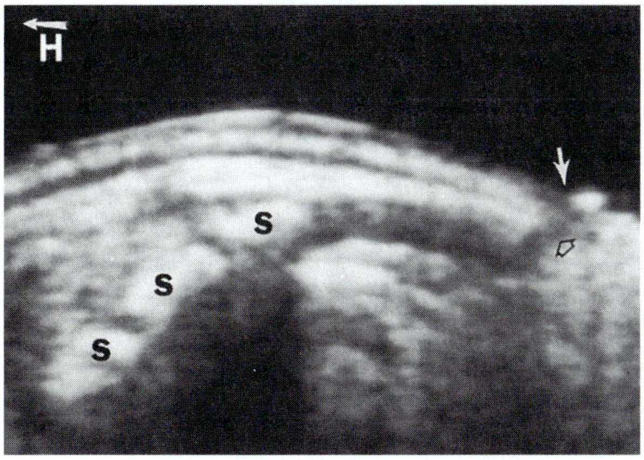

FIG. 56-19. Sacral dimple *(arrow)*. Longitudinal scan over the lower portion of the sacrum, *S* (6-month-old girl). The standoff allows definition of the superficial soft tissues, showing tissue planes interrupted by a pilonidal sinus *(open arrowhead)*. (From DiPietro MA. Pediatric musculoskeletal and spinal sonography. In: van Holsbeeck M, Introcaso JH. *Musculoskeletal Ultrasound.* St Louis: Mosby-Year Book, Inc; 1991.)

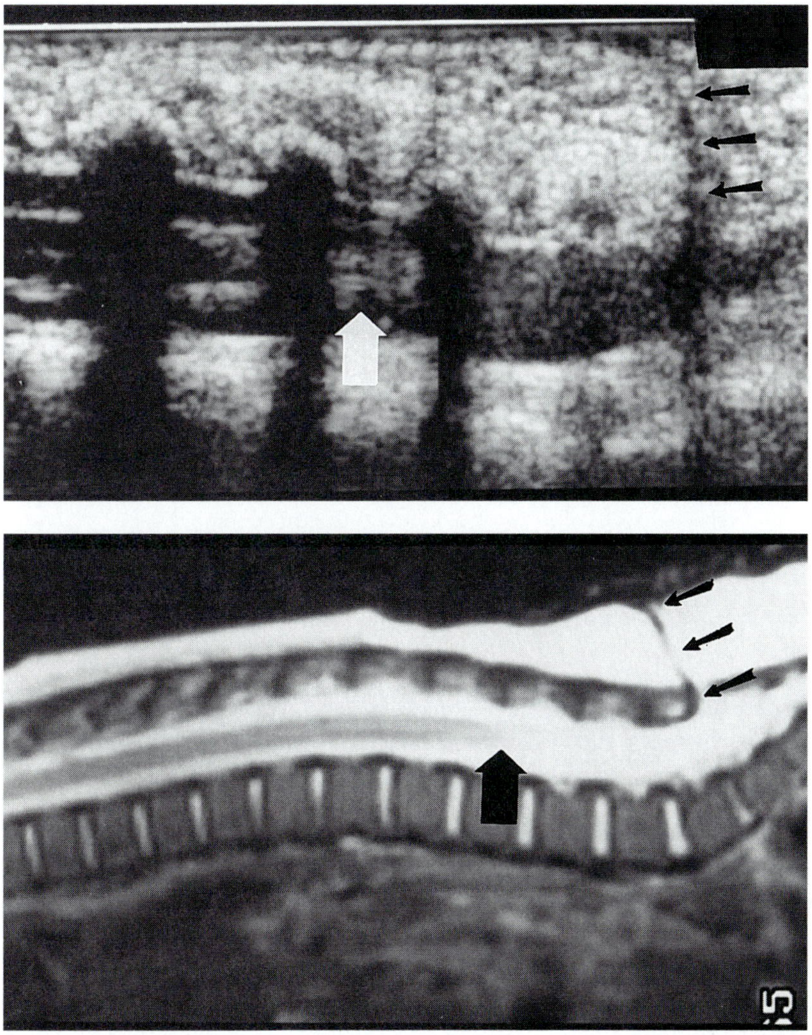

FIG. 56-20. Sinus tract extending to the dorsal aspect of the sacral canal. **A,** Sagittal sonogram and, **B,** MRI. *Arrows,* Sinus tract; *broad arrow,* tip of the conus medullaris. (From DiPietro MA, Garver KA. Sonography of the neonatal spinal canal. In: Haller J. *Textbook of Neonatal and Perinatal Ultrasound Diagnosis.* New York: Parthenon; 1997.)

A

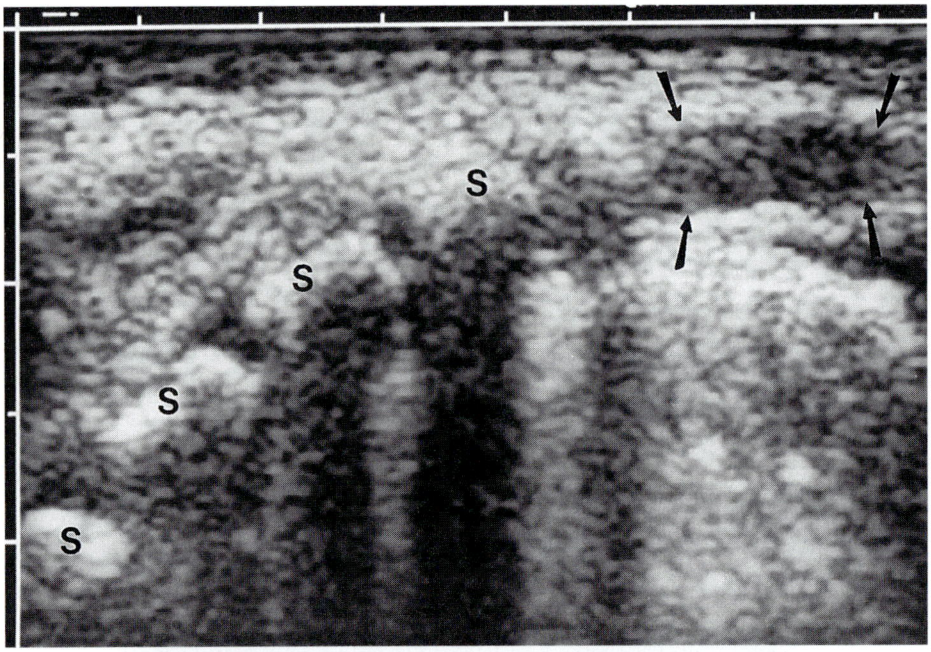

B

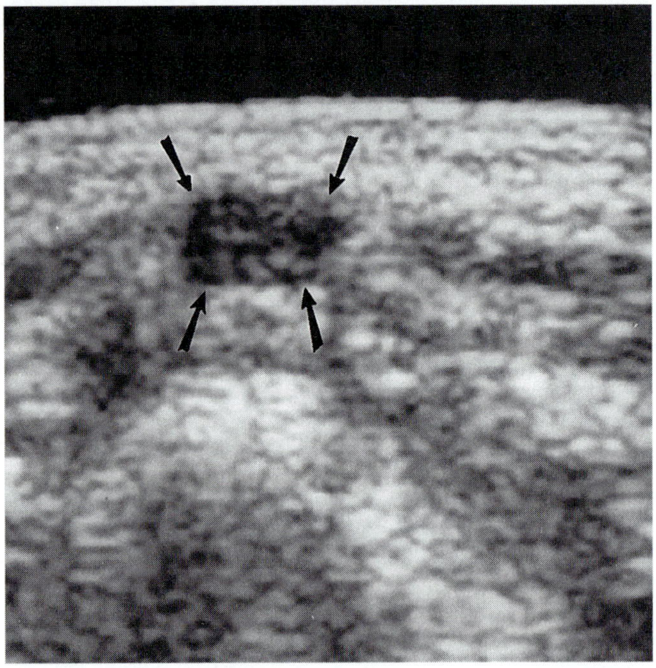

FIG. 56-21. Normal unossified coccyx *(arrows)* in, **A,** sagittal and, **B,** transverse views. *S,* Ossified sacral vertebral bodies. (From DiPietro MA, Garver KA. Sonography of the neonatal spinal canal. In: Haller J. *Textbook of Neonatal and Perinatal Ultrasound Diagnosis.* New York: Parthenon; 1997.)

discovered 5 (all girls) with sinus tracts. They extended to the periosteum of the coccyx, not to the spinal canal.[48] In all 5 the spinal cord was normal. Surgery revealed an epidermoid and a dermoid, both presumably "retained cutaneous elements, left behind at the failure of closure of the neuropore and dysjunction of the cutaneous and neuroectoderm."[48] However, 2 benign sacrococcygeal teratomas were also found. This was unexpected because the frequency of sacrococcygeal teratoma in infancy is 1 per 40,000 and there is no known association of sacrococcygeal teratoma and cutaneous dimples.[48] The authors queried whether this was coincidence or whether sonography could have detected clinically inapparent,

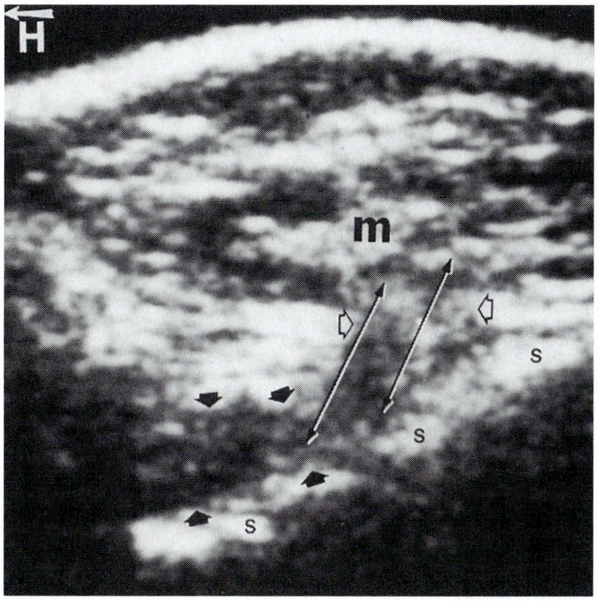

FIG. 56-22. Sacral lipoma. Longitudinal sacral scan (18-month-old girl) shows the sacral intracanalicular extension of a subcutaneous mass, *m.* Transmitted movement of the mass through the defect was seen on real-time sonography *(double headed arrows). Open arrowheads,* Dorsal sacral defect; *closed arrowheads,* sacral canal; *s,* sacrum. (From DiPietro MA. Pediatric musculoskeletal and spinal sonography. In: van Holsbeeck M, Introcaso JH. *Musculoskeletal Ultrasound.* St Louis: Mosby-Year Book, Inc; 1991.)

normal involution of remnants of the caudal cell mass,[48] an early developmental stage of the tip of the conus and filum terminale.

Lipomas

Subcutaneous soft-tissue lumps in the lumbosacral area (masses of fat and fibrous tissue) may sometimes be associated with dermal sinuses, hemangiomas, nevi, and hairy tufts. In one series of 97 children with lipomyelomeningoceles, all had a subcutaneous lipoma, and more than half the cases had other skin lesions.[35] These collections of connective tissue and fat can be attached to one or more of the meninges, cord, conus, or filum terminale. The various types of intraspinal lipomas are described on the basis of their sites of insertion in the spinal canal. **Lipomas** extend from the subcutaneous tissues to the spinal canal through focal midline defects in dura, bone, muscle, and fascia (Fig. 56-22). In a **lipomyelomeningocele,** the subarachnoid space and cord bulge through the spina bifida into subcutaneous tissues. In a **lipomyelocele,** the cord remains intracanalicular and the meninges do not bulge. The lipoma, appearing echogenic, tethers the cord, which is low and often eccentrically positioned within the spinal canal (see Fig. 56-18; Fig. 56-23). The relationship of the

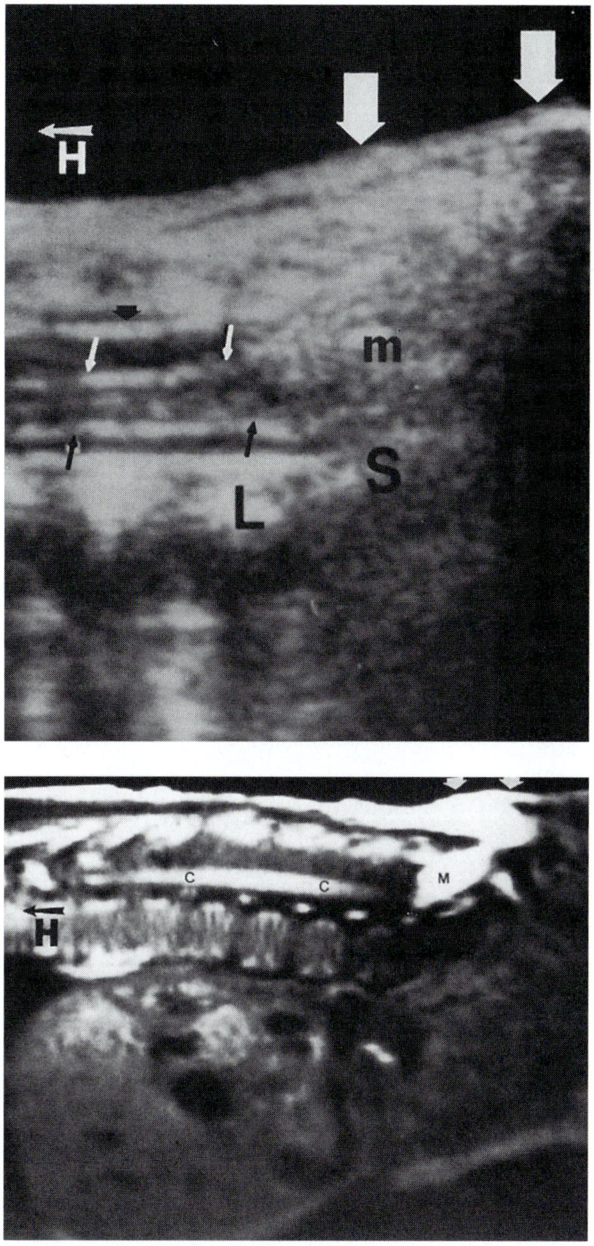

A

B

FIG. 56-23. Leptomyelolipoma. A, Longitudinal sonogram and, **B,** MRI (8-week-old). The cord (*arrows* in **A**; *c* in **B**) extends to the lumbosacral, *LS,* junction, where it is tethered by the mass, *M.* A lipoma, *M,* that extends to the subcutaneous soft tissues forms a visible bump *(white arrowheads)* on the lower back. *Black arrowhead* in **A,** Dorsal dura. (From DiPietro MA. Pediatric musculoskeletal and spinal sonography. In: van Holsbeeck M, Introcaso JH. *Musculoskeletal Ultrasound.* St. Louis: Mosby-Year Book, Inc; 1991.)

lipoma to the cord is often "intimate"; the two are not merely juxtaposed, but the lipoma grows into the cord, precluding safe, complete surgical excision.[5,50] It can grow into the central canal and along the cord[51] (Fig. 56-24). Unless the lipoma or fibrolipoma is limited to the filum or dura, an attempt at complete ex-

A

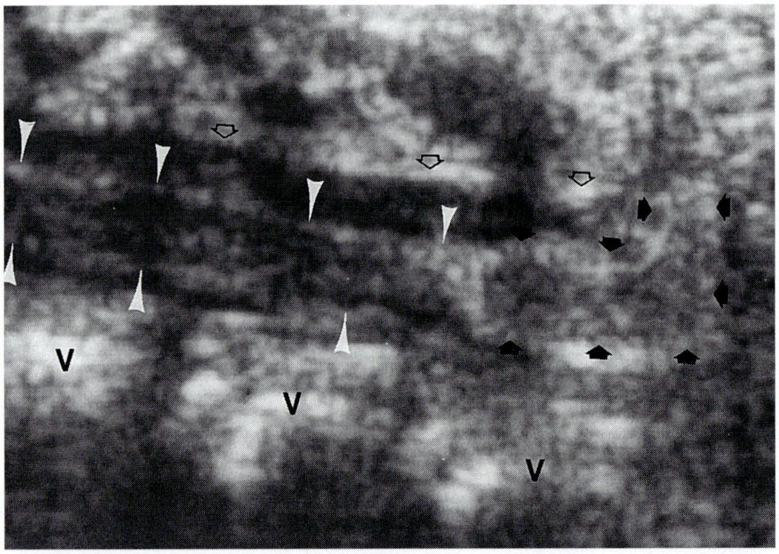

B

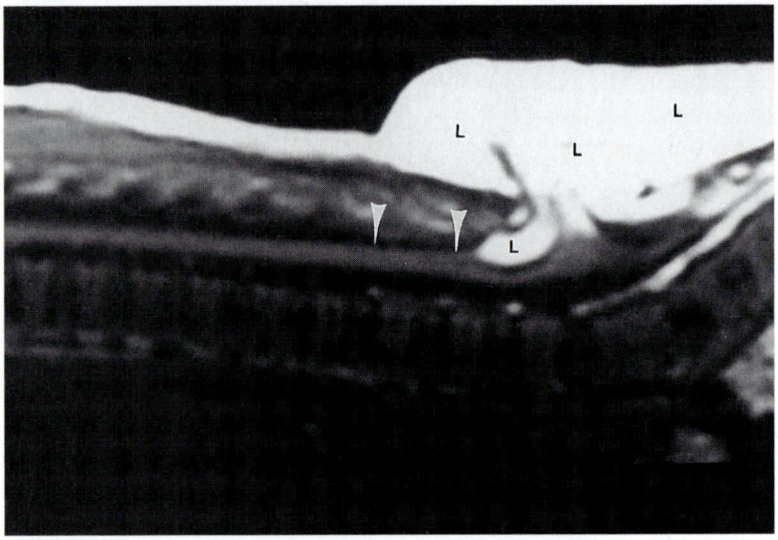

C

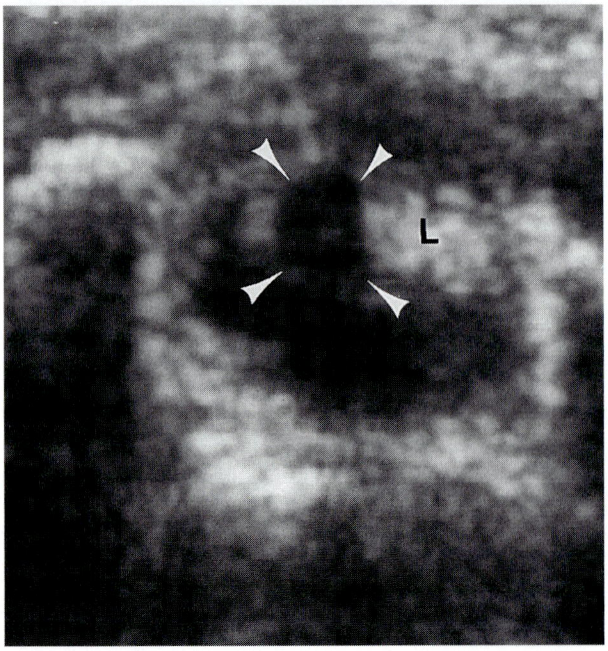

D

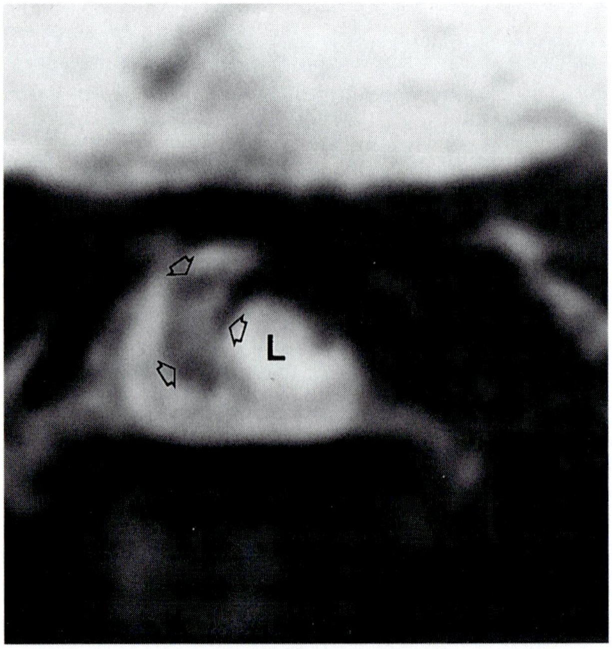

FIG. 56-24. Spinal cord tethered by a lipoma in the low lumbar canal. **A,** Sagittal sonogram of the cord *(white arrowheads)* tethered in the low lumbar canal by the lipoma *(black solid arrowheads)*. *V*, Vertebrae; *open arrowheads*, dorsal dura. **B,** Sagittal MRI of cord *(arrows)* tethered at the lumbosacral junction by the lipoma, *L*, which extends from the subcutaneous tissues to the spinal cord. **C,** Transverse sonogram and, **D,** transverse MRI of the low lumbar canal showing the cord *(arrows)* tethered dorsally and caudally by an intracanalicular lipoma, *L*, on its right (image inverted to match the prone sonogram). (From DiPietro MA, Garver KA. Sonography of the neonatal spinal canal. In: Haller J. *Textbook of Neonatal and Perinatal Ultrasound Diagnosis.* New York: Parthenon; 1997.)

cision carries a high risk of cord or nerve root damage. The relationship between the lipoma and cord, roots, and leptomeninges is often complex. The lipoma with a large area of direct interface with the spinal cord is termed a **leptomyelolipoma.**[50,52] Leptomyelolipomas commonly have a subcutaneous component and in one series were the most common form of occult spinal dysraphism.[50] They have been reported more often in females than in males. In three series the female-to-male ratios varied from 1.6:1 to 3.7:1.[35,50,51] Another term, **"lipomyeloschisis,"** emphasizes, as the three roots of the word indicate, dorsal dysraphism with attachment of the subcutaneous lipoma on the dorsal half of the partially cleft spinal cord.[51] Similar to leptomyelolipoma, it includes intradural lipoma and lipomyelomeningocele.

Combined forms of cord tethering can coexist. In one series of 97 patients with lipomyelomeningocele, 14 (45%) of the 32 with lipomas attached to the dorsal aspect of cord also had a thick filum terminale, which had to be sectioned to completely untether the cord.[35] Lipomas can also coexist with myelomeningoceles. Of 100 cases of myelomeningocele, 67 were found at autopsy to have a fibrolipoma of the filum terminale, intrathecal, extrathecal, or combined.[52] In this same series, 26 dural fibrolipomas and 8 leptomyelolipomas were discovered.[52] Various lipomatous lesions coexisted in the same cord, and of the 100 autopsy cord specimens, only 26 showed no fibrofatty inclusion.[52] Although the analysis of this series does not define the incidence of lipomas in living patients with myelomeningocele, it does emphasize the possible coexistence of the two entities in individual patients.

Postoperatively, residual echogenic leptomyelolipoma is often seen attached to the cord. This is expected because the goal of surgery is to free and untether the cord and not necessarily to completely resect the lipoma per se[35] (Fig. 56-25). Postoperatively, the untethered cord should be in a more central, less eccentric position within the spinal canal, and it should now oscillate freely. The cord in lipomyelomeningocele is also **tethered by a thick, fibrovascular band** that joins the laminae of the most cephalic vertebra with widely bifid laminae. It kinks and notches the superior surface of the spinal cord and meningocele and is resected at the time the cord is untethered.[51] Sonography can also show when a soft-tissue mass on the back is isolated and does not extend to the spinal canal (Fig. 56-26).

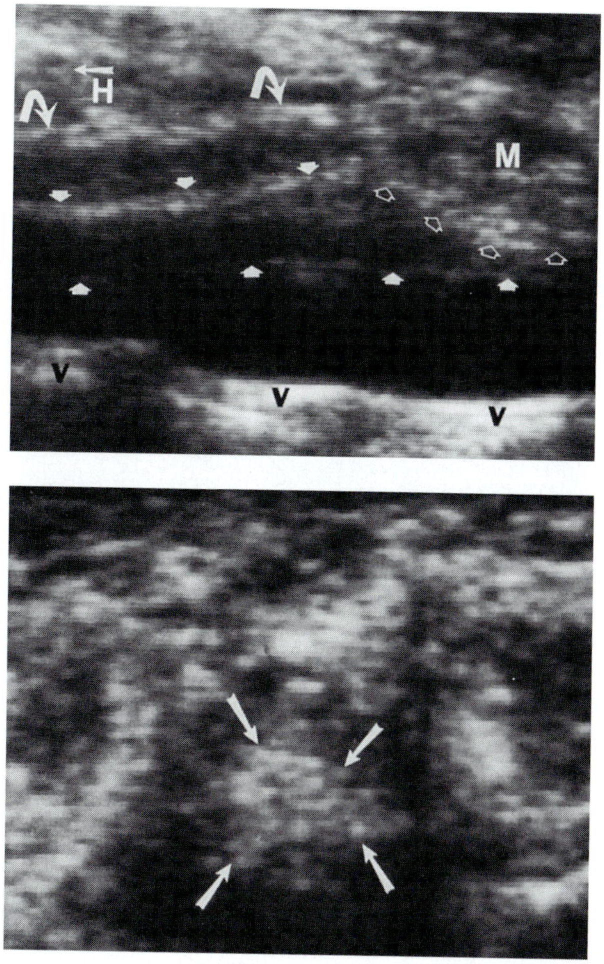

FIG. 56-25. Repaired lipomyelomeningocele. **A,** Longitudinal scan (3-year-old girl) shows the lower cord *(closed arrowheads)* contains residual echogenic lipoma, *M,* on its dorsal surface. *Open arrowheads,* Cord-lipoma interface; *curved arrows,* dorsal dura. **B,** Transverse scan shows the residual lipoma as an echogenic mass *(arrows).*

Anorectal Malformations

Children with anorectal malformations, including **imperforate anus, anorectal atresia, caudal regression,** and **cloacal exstrophy,** exhibit neurologic deficits attributable to defective sacral nerve root development. However, these children are also at an increased risk for having an **occult tethered cord** (Fig. 56-27). Progressive bowel, bladder, and lower extremity neurologic dysfunction that worsens with age is suggestive of a tethered cord that might be prevented if the tethered cord is detected and repaired early. **Therefore sonographic screening of the spinal canal in neonates with anorectal malformations is recommended.**[14-17] A series of 21 infants with anorectal malformations was evaluated for tethered cords with plain radiography, sonography, and MRI.[15] In the authors' experience, intraspinal pathology was unlikely with normal radiographs but was highly likely if the spine was abnormal. Sonography was used to evaluate the cartilaginous distal aspect of the spine. The authors' opinion was that the presence of skeletal abnormalities is more important for the prediction of intraspinal pathology than whether the imperforate anus is of the high, intermediate, or low

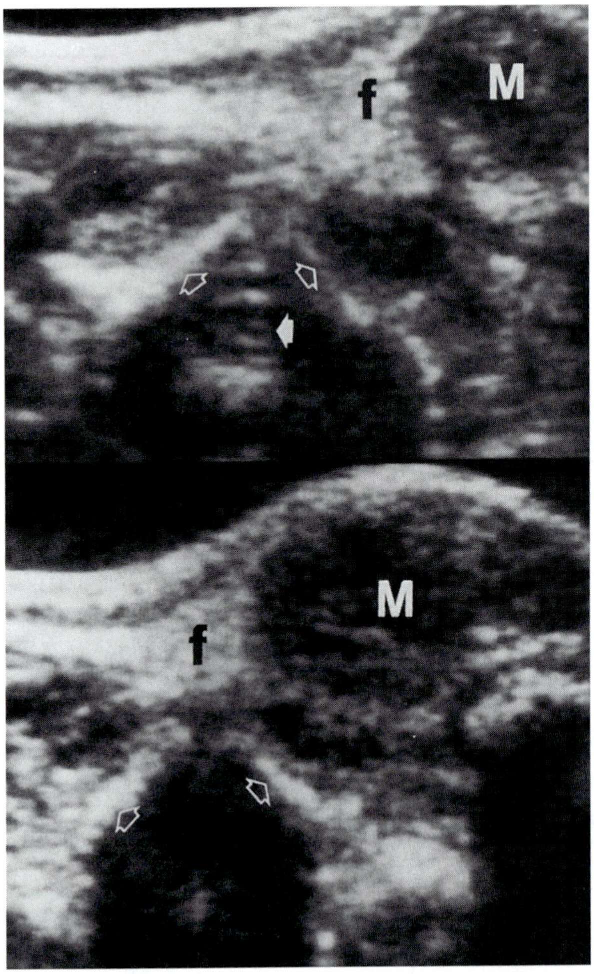

FIG. 56-26. Hemangiopericytoma. Transverse scans of a subcutaneous mass, *M* (5-day-old), on the upper back that did not extend into the thoracic spinal canal. *f*, Fat; *open arrowhead*, lamina; *closed arrowhead*, thoracic cord. (From DiPietro MA. Pediatric musculoskeletal and spinal sonography. In: van Holsbeeck M, Introcaso JH. *Musculoskeletal Ultrasound*. St. Louis: Mosby-Year Book, Inc; 1991.)

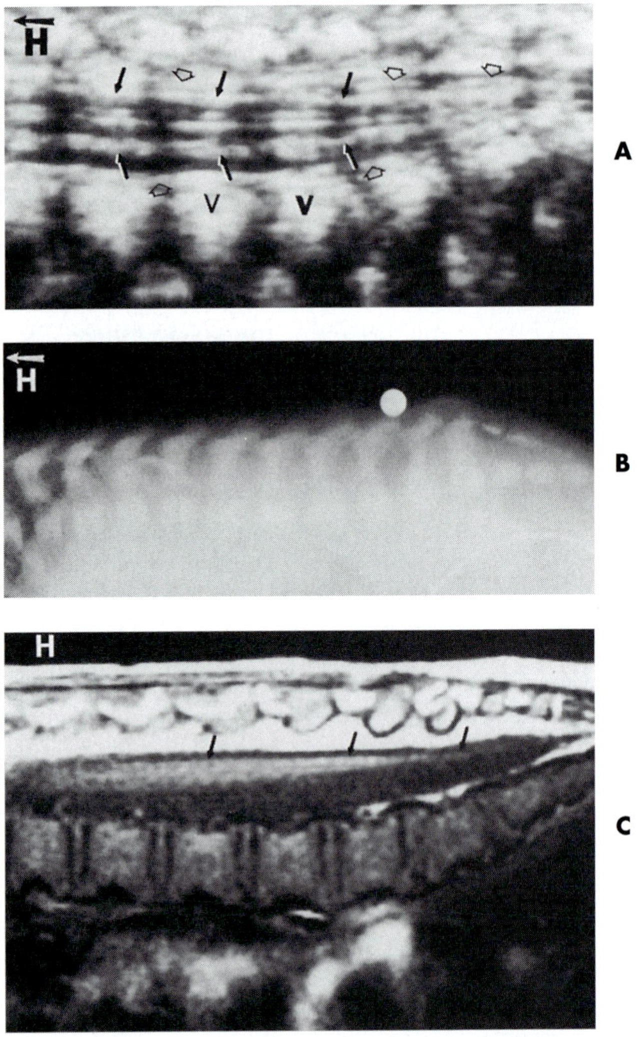

FIG. 56-27. Imperforate anus with tethered cord *(arrows)* **(1-week-old). A,** Longitudinal scan shows the cord extends into the sacral canal. The central echo complex appears as double lines. *Open arrowheads*, Dura; *V*, vertebral bodies. **B,** Lateral radiograph with a marker shows the low level of the conus (at L5) on sonography and the wide sacral canal. **C,** Sagittal MRI confirms the low, tethered cord *(arrows)*.

type.[15] Another series of 86 patients with imperforate anus and spine MRI showed that tethered cord can occur with either high or low imperforate anus and even with normal spine radiographs.[18] Of all patients with high, intermediate, and low imperforate anus, the occurrences of tethered cords were 44%, 33%, and 27%, respectively.[18] Of all the patients with tethered cords, 52% were asymptomatic and 26% had no vertebral anomaly.[18] Another study of spine MRI in 92 children with imperforate anus complex, cloacal malformation, and cloacal exstrophy revealed occult dysraphic myelodysplasia in all groups but with different frequencies of occurrence and types.[14] Imperforate anus (17% of low and 34% of high) was most commonly associated with tethered cord and a filar or intradural lipoma. Of patients with cloacal malformations and cloacal exstrophy, 46% and 100%, respectively, had tethered cords with more complex lipomatous lesions such as lipomyelomeningocele.[14]

Presacral Anomalies

Osseous **sacral anomalies** occur in 35% of patients with anorectal anomalies.[53] The **Currarino's triad** of associated lesions[54] includes anorectal malformations (stenotic, ectopic, or imperforate anus), crescentic or scimitar-shaped sacral defects or segmentation anomalies, and a presacral mass (anterior meningocele, teratoma, or enteric cyst). This entity has also been reported in association with tethered

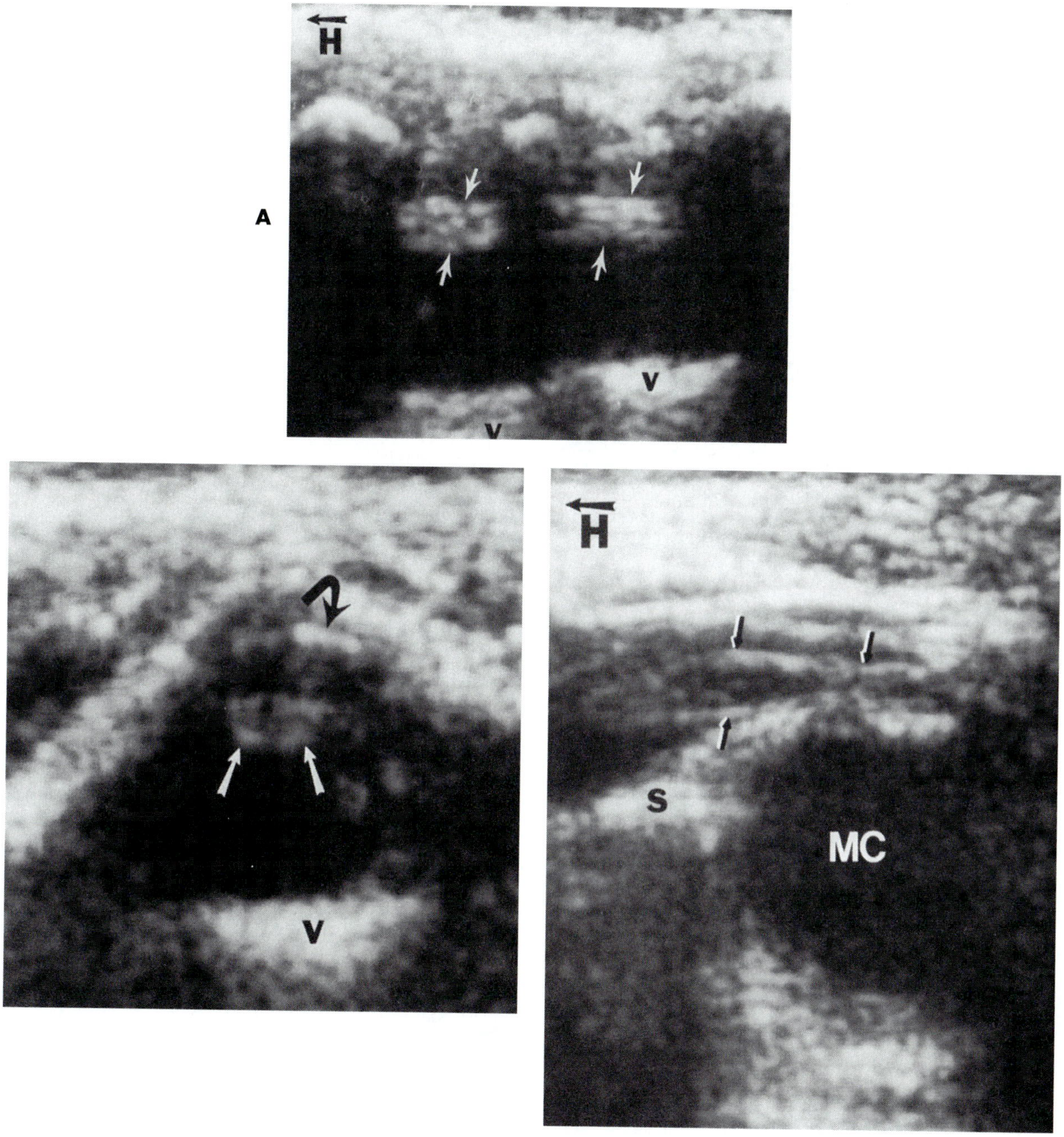

FIG. 56-28. Cord tethered by a thick filum *(white arrows)*. **A,** Longitudinal and, **B,** transverse scans of the low lumbar canal (6-year-old) with a sacral defect. *Curved arrow,* Dorsal dura; *v,* vertebrae. **C,** Longitudinal scan of the sacral canal shows the thick filum *(arrows)* attached to an anterior meningocele, *MC. S,* Sacrum.

spinal cords and intradural lipomas[55] (Fig. 56-28). A familial occurrence has been described in at least half the cases in the literature,[55] although its expression might be incomplete in some family members.[54] The familial transmission of anterior sacral meningocele or presacral teratoma and a sacral bony defect is thought to follow an autosomal dominant pattern.[56]

HYDROMYELIA

Hydromyelia, dilation of the cord's central canal, can be seen with myelomeningocele,[21] Chiari I and II malformations,[57] lipomyelomeningocele,[35] and diastematomyelia.[58,59] The entire cord may be involved, but focal involvement can exist, especially in the segments just cephalad to the tethering lesion. The cord's cen-

A

B

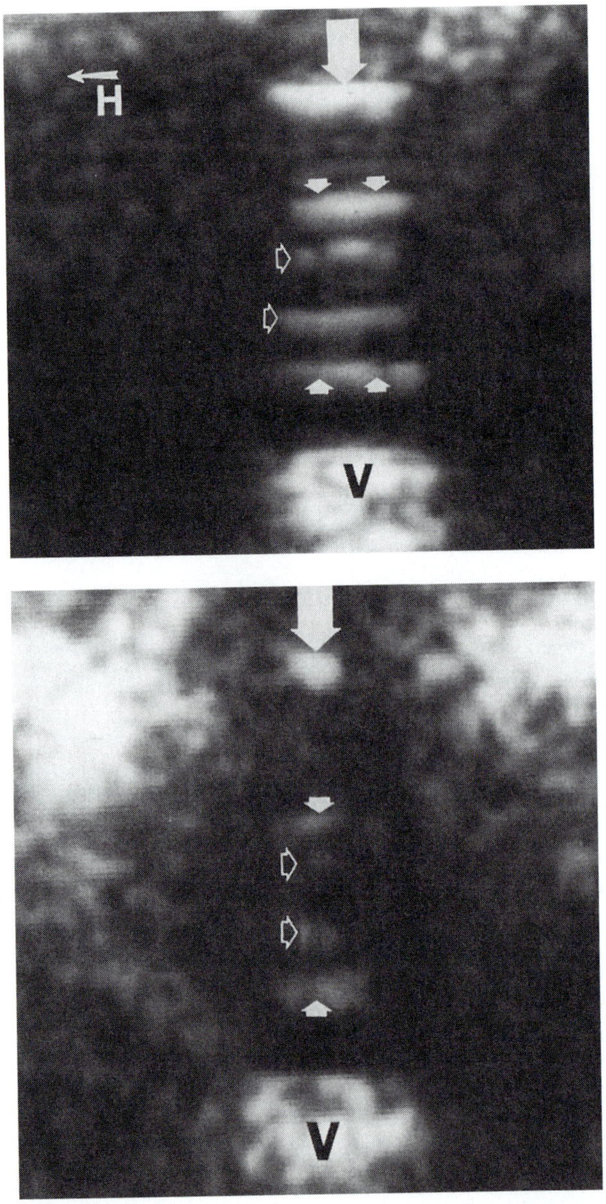

FIG. 56-29. Hydromyelia. A, Longitudinal and, B, transverse scans of the lumbar cord show widely separated central echoes *(open arrowheads)*. The dorsal and ventral margins of the cord are demarcated by closed arrowheads. *Large arrow,* Dorsal dura; *v,* vertebral body.

tral echogenic lines separate as the central canal distends with hydromyelia[1] (Fig. 56-29). **Syrinx, syringomyelia,** or **syringohydromyelia** signify cystic degeneration of a part of the cord and often follow trauma or accompany intramedullary neoplasms. The terms are usually used interchangeably, and because it is often difficult to distinguish between them and hydromyelia on imaging, and because both conditions can coexist, they are even used interchangeably with hydromyelia in many cases. Slight separation of the central echoes can occur normally, especially near the conus in neonates.[60] A more bulbous focal distention of the caudal central canal, a **terminal ventricle** can be seen occasionally in otherwise normal spinal cords[26,60-62] or in conjunction with a cord anomaly.[15] **Small cysts** in the cauda equina, often just caudal to the tip of the conus, occur in normal children and could be thin arachnoid cysts.[26] In some cases they seem to be in the filum terminale. Perhaps these **filar cysts** are remnants of the caudal cell mass from early embryonic development, a "terminal ventricle" caudal to the conus in the filum? These arachnoid or filar cysts are usually small and are found incidentally in normal children. However, they can accompany tethered cords and other abnormalities (Fig. 56-30).

DIASTEMATOMYELIA

Split or cleft cord (**diastematomyelia**) can sometimes be seen sonographically in the young patient.[49] It is a partial or complete sagittal cleft of the cord, conus medullaris, or filum terminale that may be associated with hydromyelia.[58,59] Of 13 cases of diastematomyelia in one series, 6 had concomitant hydromyelia.[59] Each hemicord has a central canal, and hydromyelia can extend from the more cephalad single cord (holocord) into either or both hemicords.[5,59] Diastematomyelia has also occurred with meningocele or myelomeningocele.[19,59] A **septum** (osseous, fibrous, or cartilaginous) often lies between the hemicords, which may be asymmetric and which may rejoin caudal to the cleft. The two portions of the cord are best demonstrated sonographically in cross section on the axial view[19,63] (Fig. 56-31). They are usually side by side, but they can also acquire some degree of a ventral-dorsal alignment, especially if scoliosis is present.[5] The sonographic appearance is pathognomonic,[63] but care must be taken not to misinterpret a normal conus and its draping dorsal and ventral nerve roots, which can superficially mimic a split cord (Fig. 56-32). Scanning along the cord should easily identify the true diastematomyelia. The vertebral column is virtually always abnormal in diastematomyelia.[5] Spina bifida is common and provides an acoustic window. However, this advantage is offset by intersegmental laminar fusion, which is also common and obscures visualization of the spinal canal.[5]

MYELOMENINGOCELE

When segments of the neural groove along the dorsal aspect of the embryo fail to close and form a tube (i.e., spinal cord) in the first gestational month, the result is a myelocele or a myelomeningocele. In the **myelocele** the exposed flat plate of neural tissue (i.e., **placode,**

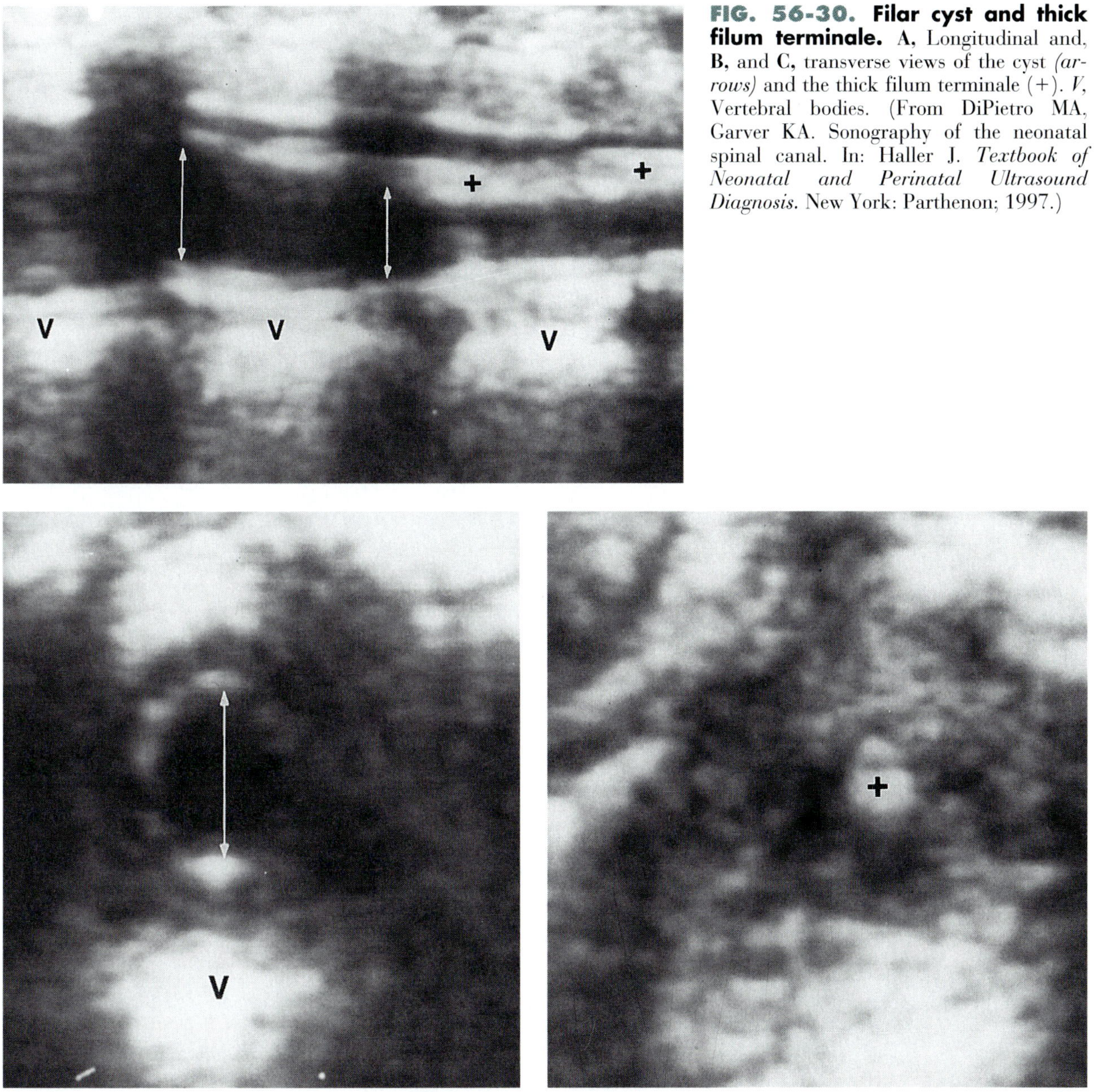

FIG. 56-30. Filar cyst and thick filum terminale. A, Longitudinal and, **B,** and **C,** transverse views of the cyst *(arrows)* and the thick filum terminale (+). *V,* Vertebral bodies. (From DiPietro MA, Garver KA. Sonography of the neonatal spinal canal. In: Haller J. *Textbook of Neonatal and Perinatal Ultrasound Diagnosis.* New York: Parthenon; 1997.)

plaque) is flush with the back. In the **myelomeningocele** the placode is pushed above the surface by a distended ventral subarachnoid space.[5] The pathology is visible and, therefore, some conclude that there is little reason to study the patient preoperatively.[5] Surgical closure of the defect is usually performed within the first few days after birth before infection sets in. Occasionally, the performance of sonography over a sac might be needed to distinguish a meningocele from a myelomeningocele. Nerve roots can be seen extending between the sac and dysraphic spinal canal in the myelomeningocele[20] (Fig. 56-33). In contrast, **meningoceles** will appear as empty sacs (Fig. 56-34) or as containing strands of thin, lacelike membranes, randomly oriented **"filmy arachnoid trabeculae"**[64] (Fig. 56-35). Scanning over the sac must be performed gently and carefully so as not to disrupt or contaminate it. Unless it is skin covered, it should not be in direct contact with the transducer. The membranous sac itself can be scanned when it is covered by a clear plastic wrap or drape. Scanning along the spinal canal from cephalad to the defect will show spinal cord entering a **myelomeningocele** (Fig. 56-36). In one series,[19] the thoracolumbar cord was thin, more than 2 standard deviations below normal values.[27] Those babies with markedly diminished lower-extremity function often had a distal echogenic cord less than 2 mm in diameter.

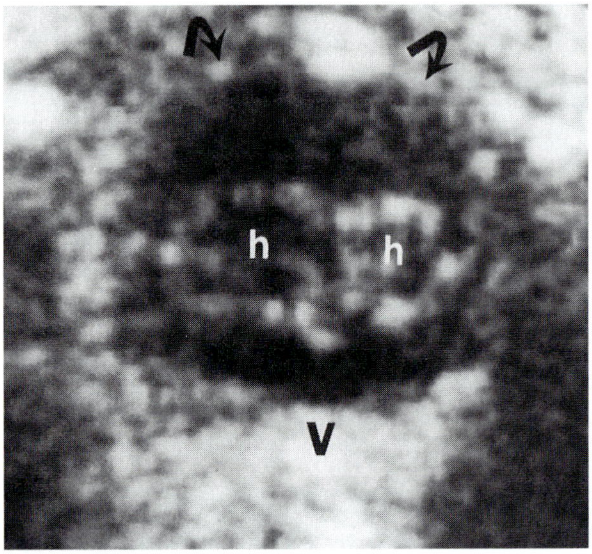

FIG. 56-31. Diastematomyelia. Transverse scan (3-year-old girl) of lumbar canal shows two hemicords, *h*, confirmed on MRI and at surgery. *V*, Vertebral body; *curved arrows*, dorsal dura.

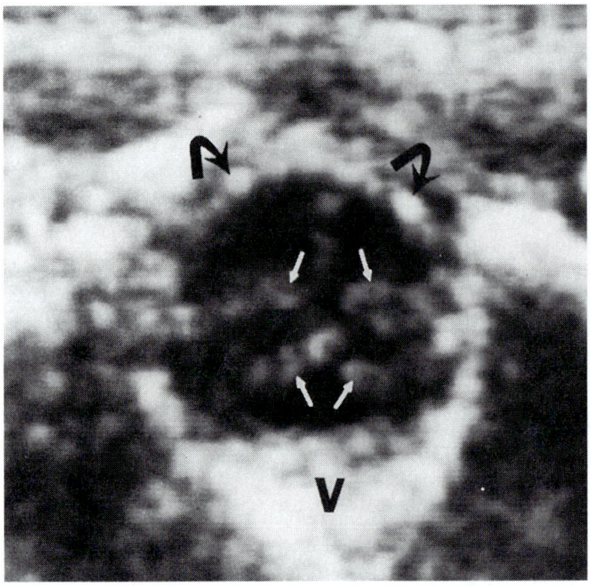

FIG. 56-32. Normal cauda equina. Transverse view at the tip of the conus where the dorsal and ventral roots form an "X." The echogenic roots *(arrows)* surrounding CSF in this normal 5-day-old superficially resemble the hemicords of diastematomyelia. *Curved arrows*, Dorsal dura; *v*, vertebral body.

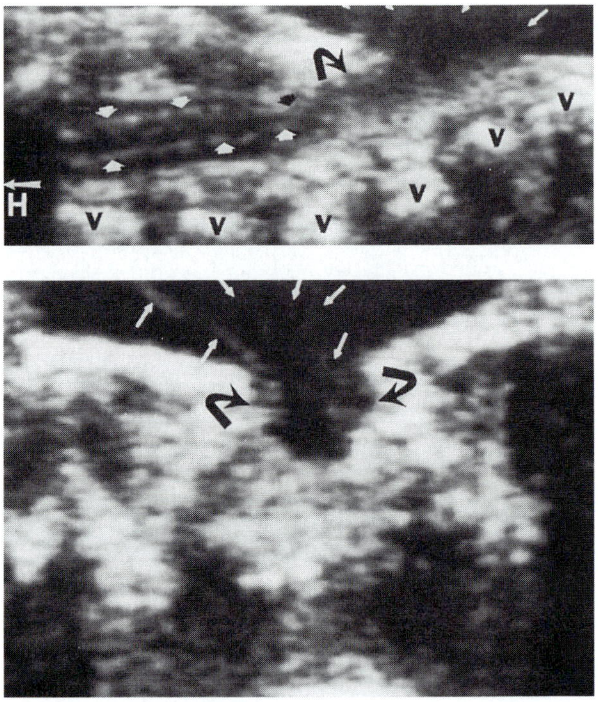

A

B

FIG. 56-33. Sacral myelomeningocele. **A**, Longitudinal and, **B**, transverse scans of a newborn. *Curved arrow*, Dorsal defect. *Arrowheads* outline the low cord extending to the defect. Nerve roots *(arrows)* emanate from the neural placode in the sac. *V*, Vertebra.

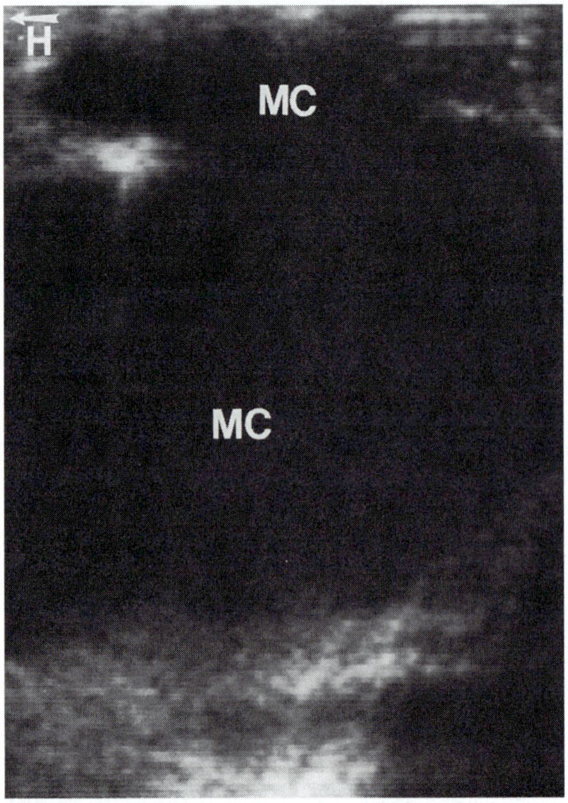

FIG. 56-34. Lumbar meningocele, *MC*. Longitudinal scan shows an empty sac.

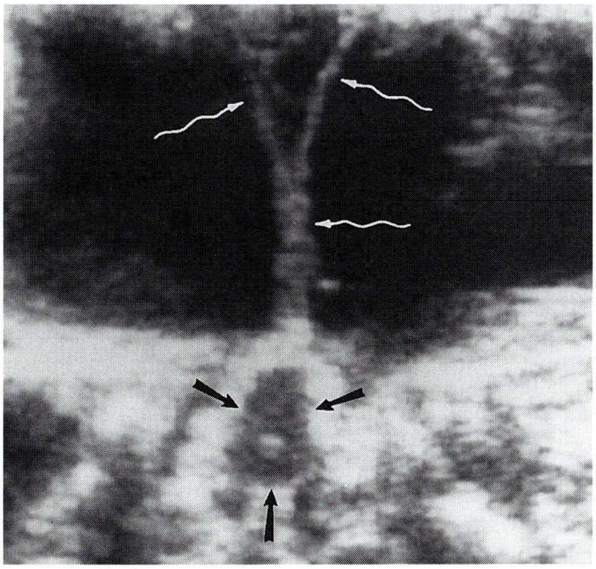

FIG. 56-35. Unrepaired meningocele in a newborn. Transverse view of the lumbar cord *(black arrows)*, which remains within the spinal canal. The dorsal aspect of the cord is distorted by strands of lacelike arachnoid *(white arrows)*, which extend into the meningocele. (From DiPietro MA, Garver KA. Sonography of the neonatal spinal canal. In: Haller J. *Textbook of Neonatal and Perinatal Ultrasound Diagnosis.* New York: Parthenon; 1997.)

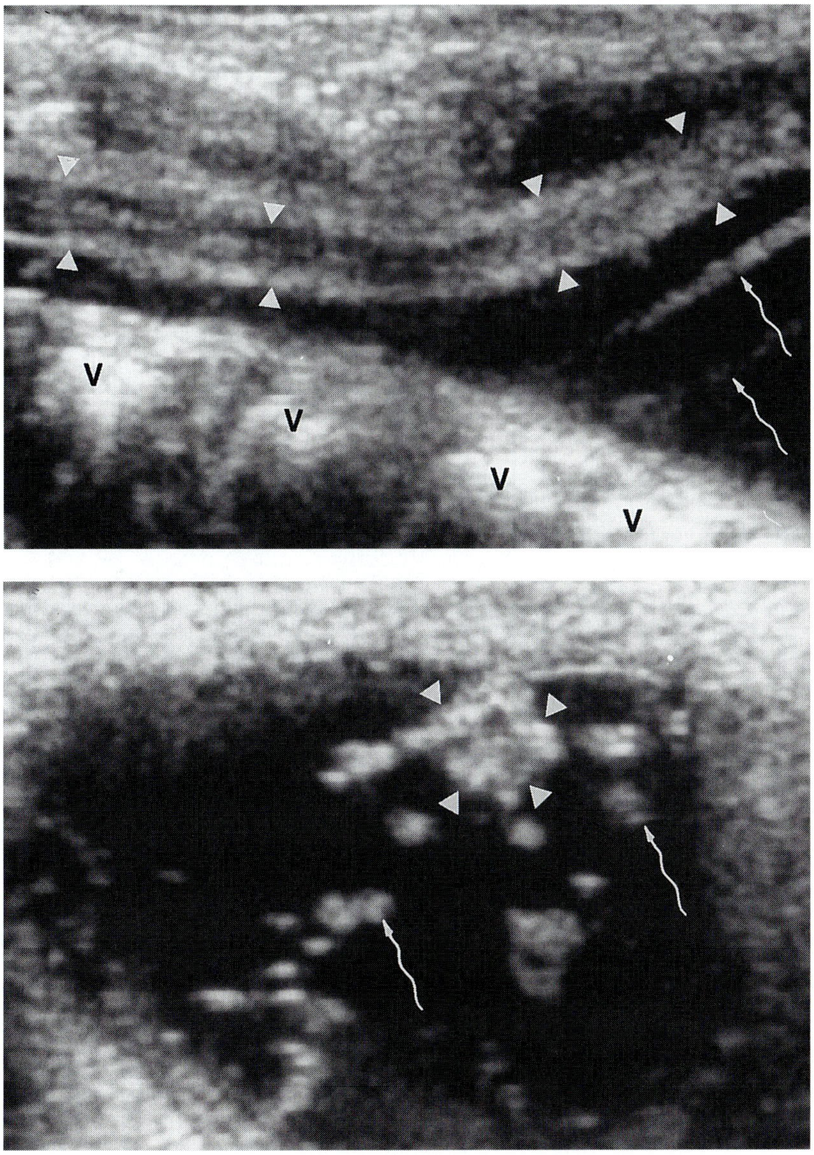

A

B

FIG. 56-36. Newborn with an unrepaired myelomeningocele. **A,** Longitudinal and, **B,** transverse views of lower cord *(arrowheads)* entering the dorsal sac. *Wavy arrows,* Nerve roots; *V,* vertebral bodies. (From DiPietro MA, Garver KA. Sonography of the neonatal spinal canal. In: Haller J. *Textbook of Neonatal and Perinatal Ultrasound Diagnosis.* New York: Parthenon; 1997.)

Advocates of preoperative sonography[2,19] in myelocele and myelomeningocele have recommended examining the remainder of the cord for associated anomalies: hydromyelia, diastematomyelia, lipoma, and thick filum terminale. Associated lipomas (dural and filum fibrolipomas and leptomyelolipomas) occur with myelomeningocele.[52] Failure to recognize and correct abnormalities distal or proximal to the placode at the time of initial repair will often result in late symptomatic retethering of the cord.[65]

Retethered Cord Following Myelomeningocele Repair

Neurologic function should not deteriorate in the patient with a repaired myelomeningocele. Progressive deterioration can be insidious and may be caused by retethering of the cord, hydrocephalus, hydromyelia, and/or brainstem-cervical dysfunction from Chiari II malformation. "Delineation of the specific offending abnormality is often difficult."[66] The incidence of progressive neurologic deterioration in children with repaired myelomeningocele was 15% in one series.[67] In another series, the common presenting symptoms of a retethered cord were progressive scoliosis (50%), motor loss (51%), and spasticity (40%).[21] The untethered repaired cord should lie toward the central or ventral portion of the spinal canal when the patient is prone, the usual posture during sonography. The cord remains low (i.e., caudal) in myelomeningocele patients so that a low cord per se cannot be used as evidence of retethering. The entire length of the repaired, untethered cord and its roots should oscillate normally. The **retethered cord** had scarred, usually to the site of closure, in all myelomeningocele patients operated on for retethered cord in one large series.[21] In another series, **dense adhesions** were present at the previous repair site and also at the level of the lowest nondysraphic lamina in patients with signs and symptoms of cord retethering.[67] The retethered cord was tightly adherent to the posterior wall of the spinal canal with no CSF between the roof of the canal and the cord at that level. However, in that same series most patients **without** clinical signs and symptoms of cord retethering had dorsal adhesion of the cord ***only*** at the site of previous repair but not also more cephalad as in the symptomatic patients.[67] The MR images in all patients in this series[67] and in 89% of patients in another series[68] showed a low-lying conus fixed dorsally at the site of previous repair, and no relation to the presence or absence of clinical retethering. Because all cords in patients who had undergone myelomeningocele repair might thus appear "retethered," the length of the dorsally fixed segment,[67] the mobility of the lower cord segments,[1] or both might be useful to separate clinically "significant" from "insignificant" fixation.

Oscillations of the lower retethered cord will be dampened or absent, and the lower cord will move little, if at all, with crying.[5] **Cord motion might be normal distant from the site of tethering** as has been observed during scanning on the skin surface and intraoperatively scanning directly on the dura.[1,6] Therefore scanning must be done over several segments toward the operative site. Cord oscillations at a few or more segmental levels rostral to the point of tethering are maintained. For example, normal oscillations of the thoracic cord will not exclude a retethered low lumbar myelomeningocele, but oscillations will likely appear dampened as one scans closer to the point of retethering. A retethered cord may move passively with general pulsations of the thecal sac, especially in the region of the laminar defects. Such movement of the cord with dural pulsations should not be mistaken for the free oscillation of an untethered cord. Spinal cord oscillation in 46 children with repaired meningomyelocele but without major neurologic deficits was prospectively evaluated using M-mode sonography over 15 to 18 months. Pulse-induced oscillations of the cord and cauda equina appeared to diminish first with retethering of the cord, also known as **secondary tethered cord syndrome.** Later, respiratory-induced, slow undulations were also lost, and the caudal cord was motionless.[22] Dermoids, epidermoids, or lipomas included with the closure can also retether the cord in a repaired myelomeningocele (Fig. 56-37). Of patients with retethered cords in one large series, 16% had **inclusion dermoids** that resulted from epithelial tissue that was not removed at initial closure or was trapped in the surgical scar.[21] An untreated, **thick filum terminale** or **diastematomyelia** accompanying a myelomeningocele can cause persistent cord tethering. **Hydromyelia**

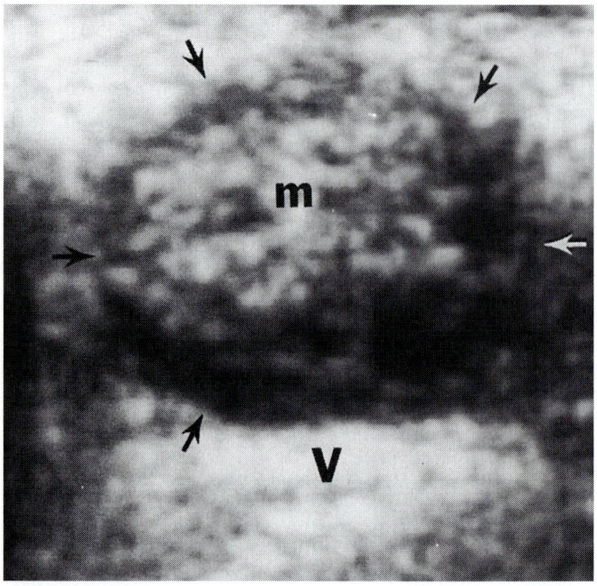

FIG. 56-37. Repaired myelomeningocele. Transverse scan (2-year-old boy) shows a retethered cord, which had no oscillation of its caudal portion and a large, dorsal, echogenic mass, *m*. *Arrows*, Spinal canal; *V*, vertebra.

can also result in progressive deterioration (especially scoliosis, weakness, or spastiity) and was present in 38% of retethered cords[21] (Fig. 56-38).

Chiari II Malformation

The cervical canal and foramen magnum can be scanned from the posterior aspect of the neck. In the newborn, resolution is good, and a **Chiari II malformation** is distinguishable from normal anatomy. In contrast with the normal, clear cisterna magna and dorsal cervical subdural space (Fig. 56-39), the newborn with myelomeningocele will usually demonstrate echogenic soft tissue dorsal to the upper cervical cord[2,13,69,70] (Fig. 56-40). This echogenic soft tissue is a caudally displaced, dysplastic peg of cerebellar

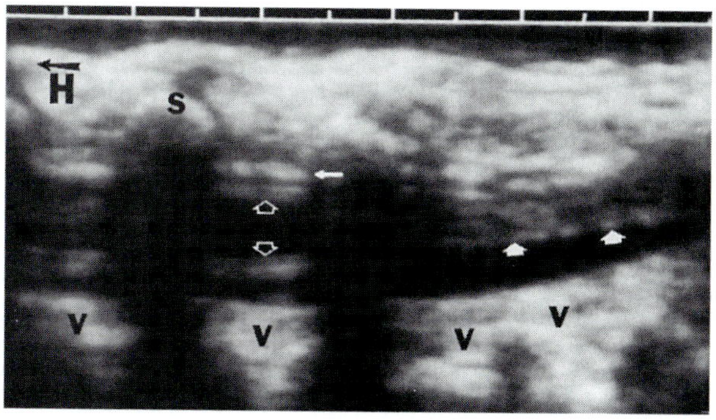

FIG. 56-38. Repaired myelomeningocele. Longitudinal scan (3-month-old boy) shows the cord extends to the sacral canal. The distal cord *(closed arrowheads)* is small and echogenic, and there is marked hydromyelia *(open arrowheads)* of the low lumbar cord. *Arrow*, Dorsal dura; *S*, spinous process with shadow; *V*, vertebral bodies.

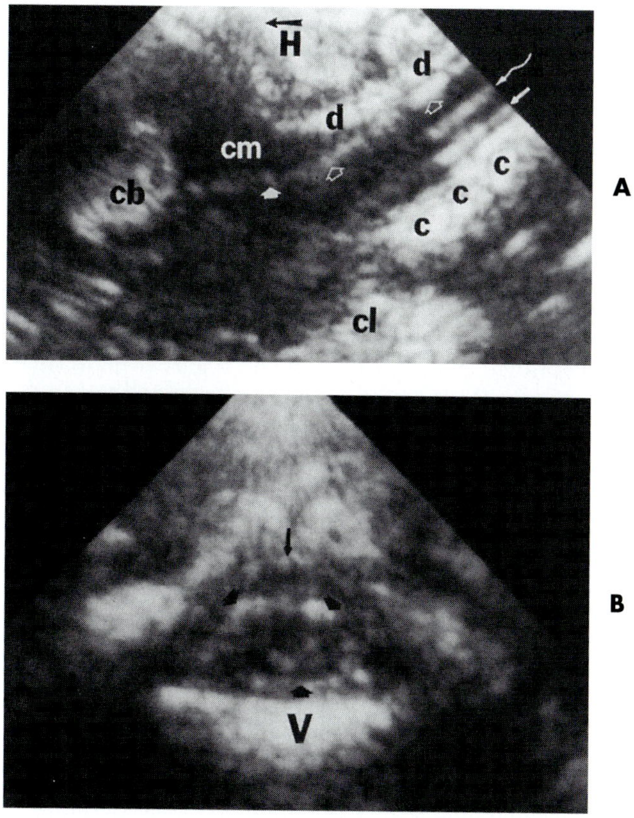

FIG. 56-39. Normal neonate, lower brainstem *(closed arrowhead)* **and cervical cord** *(open arrowhead)*. **A,** Longitudinal sonogram shows clear CSF dorsal to the brainstem and cervical cord. *cb*, Cerebellum; *cl*, clivus; *c*, cervical vertebral bodies; *cm*, cisterna magna; *d*, dura; *arrow*, ventral surface of cervical cord; *wavy arrow*, central echo. **B,** Transverse scan shows clear CSF dorsal to the upper cervical cord, which is outlined by arrowheads. *Arrow*, Dorsal dura; *V*, vertebral body.

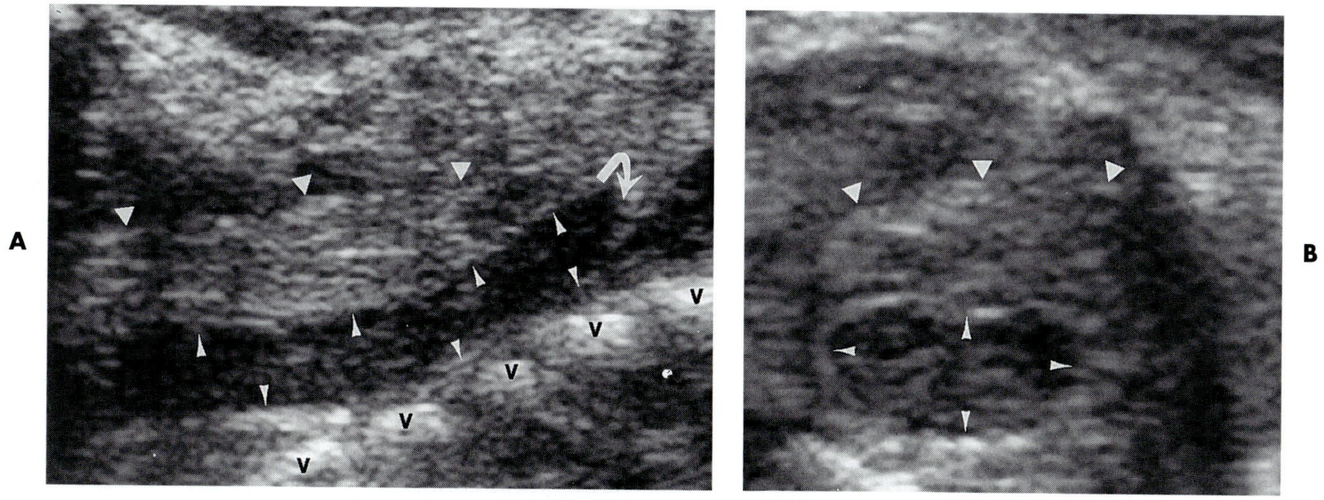

FIG. 56-40. Chiari II malformation with caudally displaced thick vermian peg. **A,** Sagittal and, **B,** transverse views of the cervical spinal canal in a patient with Chiari II malformation. Caudally displaced, thick, vermian peg is outlined by thick arrowheads. *Thin arrowheads*, Caudally displaced medulla and cervical cord; *curved arrow*, cervicomedullary kink; *V*, cervical vertebral bodies. (From DiPietro MA, Garver KA. Sonography of the neonatal spinal canal. In: Haller J. *Textbook of Neonatal and Perinatal Ultrasound Diagnosis.* New York: Parthenon; 1997.)

vermis (**vermian peg**), part of the hindbrain anomaly of the Chiari II malformation. The caudally displaced midbrain and cervical cord can overlap to varying degrees (**cervicomedullary kink**) and be visible on sonography (see Fig. 56-40). The Chiari II malformation is present to some degree in almost all patients with myelomeningocele. As the child grows, other hindbrain and cervical complications, such as **fourth ventricular dilation, cyst development, and hydromyelia,** may occur, but by then sonographic visualization through the intact spine and soft tissues will be limited. Familiarity with the Chiari II malformation from MRI or intraoperative sonographic experience will greatly enhance the sonographer's ability to recognize the findings during sonography through the intact skin[71,72] (see Chapter 52). The normal cervical cord usually oscillates briskly at the heart rate. Cervical cord oscillations can be dampened with severe impaction of herniated structures: cerebellum, fourth ventricle, and medulla in the cervical canal of patients with the Chiari II malformation.

Spinal cord oscillation, the loss of which can indicate spinal cord tethering or retethering, is more easily assessed with real-time sonography than with MRI. This fact and the relative ease of performing a screening sonographic examination for occult tethered cord in newborns and infants continue to maintain a role for sonography.

REFERENCES

1. DiPietro MA, Venes JL. Real-time sonography of the pediatric spinal cord. Horizons and limits. In: Marlin AE, ed. *Concepts in Pediatric Neurosurgery*. Basel: Karger; 1988;8:120-132.
2. Jequier S, Cramer B, O'Gorman AM. Ultrasound of the spinal cord in neonates and infants. *Ann Radiol* 1985;28:225-231.
3. Naidich TP, Fernbach SK, McLone DG et al. Sonography of the caudal spine and back: congenital anomalies in children. *AJR* 1984;142:1229-1242.
4. Naidich TP, McLone DG, Shkolnik A et al. Sonographic evaluation of caudal spine anomalies in children. *AJNR* 1983; 4:661-664.
5. Naidich TP, Radkowski MA, Britton J. Real-time sonographic display of caudal spinal anomalies. *Neuroradiology* 1986;28: 512-527.
6. Raghavendra BN, Epstein FJ, Pinto RS et al. The tethered spinal cord: diagnosis by high-resolution real-time ultrasound. *Radiology* 1983;149:123-128.
7. Scheible W, James HE, Leopold GR et al. Occult spinal dysraphism in infants: screening with high-resolution real-time ultrasound. *Radiology* 1983;146:743-746.
8. Zieger M, Dorr U. Pediatric spinal sonography. Pt I. Anatomy and examination technique. *Pediatr Radiol* 1988;18:9-13.
9. Rohrschneider WK, Forsting M, Darge K et al. Diagnostic value of spinal US: comparative study with MR in pediatric patients. *Radiology* 1996;200:383-388.
10. Wilson DA, Prince JR. MR imaging determination of the location of normal conus medullaris throughout childhood. *AJR* 1989;152:1029-1032.
11. DiPietro MA. The conus medullaris: normal US findings throughout childhood. *Radiology* 1993;188:149-153.
12. Nelson Jr MD, Segall HD, Gwinn JL. Sonography in newborns with cutaneous manifestations of spinal abnormalities. *Am Fam Physician* 1989;40:198-203.
13. Zieger M, Dorr U, Schulz RD. Pediatric spinal sonography. Part II. Malformations and mass lesions. *Pediatr Radiol* 1988; 18:105-111.
14. Appignani BA, Jaramillo D, Barnes PD et al. Dysraphic myelodysplasias associated with urogenital and anorectal anomalies: prevalence and types seen with MR imaging. *AJR* 1994;163:1199-1203.
15. Beek FJA, Boemers TML, Witkamp TD et al. Spine evaluation in children with anorectal malformations. *Pediatr Radiol* 1995;25:S28-S32.
16. Carson JA, Barnes PD, Tunell WP et al. Imperforate anus: the neurologic implication of sacral abnormalities. *J Pediatr Surg* 1984;19:838-842.
17. Karrer FM, Flannery AM, Nelson Jr MD et al. Anorectal malformations: evaluation of associated spinal dysraphic syndromes. *J Pediatr Surg* 1988;23:45-48.
18. Long FR, Hunter JV, Mahboubi S, et al. Tethered cord and associated vertebral anomalies in children and infants with imperforate anus: evaluation with MR imaging and plain radiography. *Radiology* 1996;200:377-382.
19. Glasier CM, Chadduck WM, Leithiser Jr, RE, et al. Screening spinal ultrasound in newborns with neural tube defects. *J Ultrasound Med* 1990;9:339-343.
20. Jacobs NM, Grant EG, Dagi TF et al. Ultrasound identification of neural elements in myelomeningocele. *J Clin Ultrasound* 1984;12:51-53.
21. Nelson Jr MD, Bracchi M, Naidich TP et al. The natural history of repaired myelomeningocele. *RadioGraphics* 1988;8:695-706.

Technique

22. Schumacher R, Kroll B, Schwarz M et al. M-mode sonography of the caudal spinal cord in patients with meningomyelocele: work in progress. *Radiology* 1992;184:263-265.
23. Gusnard DA, Naidich TP, Yousefzadeh DK et al. Ultrasonic anatomy of the normal neonatal and infant spine: correlation with cryomicrotome sections and CT. *Neuroradiology* 1986; 28:493-511.

Normal Anatomy

24. St. Amour TE, Rubin JM, Dohrmann GJ. The central canal of the spinal cord: ultrasonic identification. *Radiology* 1984; 152:767-769.
25. Nelson Jr MD, Sedler JA, Gilles FH. Spinal cord central echo complex: histoanatomic correlation. *Radiology* 1989;170:479-481.
26. Rypens F, Avni EF, Matos C, et al. Atypical and equivocal sonographic features of the spinal cord in neonates. *Pediatr Radiol* 1995;25:429-432.
27. Kawahara H, Andou Y, Takashima S, et al. Normal development of the spinal cord in neonates and infants seen on ultrasonography. *Neuroradiology* 1987;29:50-52.
28. Quencer RM, Montalvo BM. Normal intraoperative spinal sonography. *AJR* 1984;143:1301-1305.
29. Resjo IM, Harwood-Nash DC, Fitz CR, et al. Normal cord in infants and children examined with computed tomographic metrizamide myelography. *Radiology* 1979;130:691-696.
30. Barkovich AJ, Raghavan N, Chuang SH. MR of lumbosacral agenesis. *AJNR* 1989;10:1223-1231.
31. Wolf S, Schneble F, Troger J. The conus medullaris: time of ascendence to normal level. *Pediatr Radiol* 1992;22:590-592.

32. Brunelle F, Sebag G, Baraton J, et al. Lumbar spinal cord motion measurement with phase-contrast MR imaging in normal children and in children with spinal lipomas. *Pediatr Radiol* 1996;26:265-270.
33. Quencer RM, Montalvo BM, Naidich TP, et al. Intraoperative sonography in spinal dysraphism and syringohydromyelia. *AJR* 1987;148:1005-1013.

The Tethered Spinal Cord

34. Reigel DH. Tethered spinal cord. *Concepts Pediatr Neurosurg* 1983;4:142-164.
35. Hoffman HJ, Taecholarn C, Hendrick EB, et al. Management of lipomyelomeningoceles: experience at the Hospital for Sick Children, Toronto. *J Neurosurg* 1985;62:1-8.
36. Anderson FM. Occult spinal dysraphism: a series of 73 cases. *Pediatrics* 1975;55:826-835.
37. Lhowe D, Ehrlich MG, Chapman PH, et al. Congenital intraspinal lipomas: clinical presentation and response to treatment. *J Pediatr Orthop* 1987;7:531-537.
38. Yamada S, Zinke DE, Sanders D. Pathophysiology of the 'tethered cord syndrome.' *J Neurosurg* 1981;54:494-503.
39. Beek FJA, van Leeuwen MS, Bax NMA, et al. A method for sonographic counting of the lower vertebral bodies in newborns and infants. *AJNR* 1994;15:445-449.
40. Beek FJA, Bax KMA, Mali WPTM. Sonography of the coccyx in newborns and infants. *J Ultrasound Med* 1994;13:629-634.
41. Koroshetz AM, Taveras JM. Anatomy of the vertebrae and spinal cord. In: Taveras JM, ed. *Radiology-Diagnosis-Imaging-Intervention.* Philadelphia: JB Lippincott Co; 1986:5.
42. Higginbottom MC, Jones KL, James HE, et al. Aplasia cutis congenita: a cutaneous marker of occult spinal dysraphism. *J Pediatr* 1980;96:687-689.
43. Albright AL, Gartner JC, Wiener ES. Lumbar cutaneous hemangiomas as indicators of tethered spinal cords. *Pediatrics* 1989;83:977-980.
44. Hall DE, Udvarhelyi GB, Altman J. Lumbosacral skin lesions as markers of occult spinal dysraphism. *JAMA* 1981;246: 2606-2608.
45. Till K. Spinal dysraphism: a study of congenital malformations of the back. *Dev Med Child Neurol* 1968;10:470-477.
46. Powell KR, Cherry JD, Hougen TJ, et al. A prospective search for congenital dermal abnormalities of the craniospinal axis. *J Pediatr* 1975;87:744-750.
47. Radkowski MA, Byrd SE, McLone DG. Unpublished data, 1990. Clinical and sonographic correlation of sacrococcygeal dimples. Presented at the Thirty-Third Annual Meeting of the Society for Pediatric Radiology; April 19-22, 1990.
48. Storrs BB, Walker ML. Sacral dermal sinus—occult sacral masses discovered by routine ultrasound. *Concepts Pediatr Neurosurg* 1987;7:172-178.
49. Korsvik HE, Keller MS. Sonography of occult dysraphism in neonates and infants with MR imaging correlation. *RadioGraphics* 1992;12:297-306.
50. Chapman PH. Congenital intraspinal lipomas: anatomic considerations and surgical treatment. *Child's Brain* 1982;9:37-47.
51. Naidich TP, McLone DG, Mutluer S. A new understanding of dorsal dysraphism with lipoma (lipomyeloschisis): radiologic evaluation and surgical correction. *AJR* 1983;140:1065-1078.
52. Emery JL, Lendon RG. Lipomas of the cauda equina and other fatty tumours related to neurospinal dysraphism. *Dev Med Child Neurol* Suppl 1969;20:62-70.
53. Tunell WP, Austin JC, Barnes PD, et al. Neuroradiologic evaluation of sacral abnormalities in imperforate anus complex. *J Pediatr Surg* 1987;22:58-61.
54. Currarino G, Coln D, Votteler T. Triad of anorectal, sacral, and presacral anomalies. *AJR* 1981;137:395-398.
55. Kirks DR, Merten DF, Filston HC, et al. The Currarino triad: complex of anorectal malformation, sacral bony abnormality, and presacral mass. *Pediatr Radiol* 1984;14:220-225.
56. Yates VD, Wilroy RS, Whitington GL, et al. Anterior sacral defects: an autosomal dominantly inherited condition. *J Pediatr* 1983;102:239-242.

Hydromyelia

57. Hoffman HJ, Neill J, Crone KR, et al. Hydrosyringomyelia and its management in childhood. *Neurosurgery* 1987;21:347-351.
58. Brühl K, Schwarz M, Schumacher R, et al. Congenital diastematomyelia in the upper thoracic spine. Diagnostic comparison of CT, CT-myelography, MRI and US. *Neurosurg Rev* 1990;13:77-82.
59. Schlesinger AE, Naidich TP, Quencer RM. Concurrent hydromyelia and diastematomyelia. *AJNR* 1986;7:473-477.
60. Kriss VM, Kriss TC, Babcock DS. The ventriculus terminalis of the spinal cord in the neonate: a normal variant on sonography. *AJR* 1995;165:1491-1493.
61. Avni EF, Matos C, Grassart A et al. Sinus pilonidaux neonatals et echographie medullaire de depistage: resultats preliminaires. *Pediatrie* 1991;46:607-611.
62. Sigal R, Denys A, Holimi P, et al. Ventriculus terminalis of the conus medullaris: MR imaging in four patients with congenital dilatation. *AJNR* 1991;12:733-737.

Diastematomyelia

63. Raghavendra BN, Epstein FJ, Pinto RS, et al. Sonographic diagnosis of diastematomyelia. *J Ultrasound Med* 1988;7:111-113.

Myelomeningocele

64. Naidich TP, McLone DG. Congenital pathology of the spine and spinal cord. In: Taveras JM, ed. *Radiology-Diagnosis-Imaging-Intervention.* Philadelphia: JB Lippincott Co; 1986:18.
65. Venes JL, Stevens EA. Surgical pathology in tethered cord secondary to myelomeningocele repair. *Concepts Pediatr Neurosurg* 1983;4:165-185.
66. Levy LM, DiChiro G, McCullough DC, et al. Fixed spinal cord: diagnosis with MR imaging. *Radiology* 1988;169:773-778.
67. Tamaki N, Shirataki K, Kojima N, et al. Tethered cord syndrome of delayed onset following repair of myelomeningocele. *J Neurosurg* 1988;69:393-398.
68. Just M, Ermert J, Higer H-P, et al. Magnetic resonance imaging of post repair—myelomeningocele—findings in 31 children and adolescents. *Neurosurg Rev* 1987;10:47-52.
69. Cramer BC, Jequier S, O'Gorman AM. Sonography of the neonatal craniocervical junction. *AJR* 1986;147:133-139.
70. Storrs BB, Reid BS, Walker ML. Ultrasound evaluation of the Chiari II malformation in infants. *Concepts Pediatr Neurosurg* 1985;6:172-180.
71. DiPietro MA, Venes JL. Intraoperative sonography of Arnold-Chiari malformations. In: Rubin JM, Chandler WF. *Ultrasound in Neurosurgery.* New York: Raven Press; 1990:183-199.
72. DiPietro MA, Venes JL, Rubin JM. Arnold-Chiari II malformation: intraoperative real-time sonography. *Radiology* 1987; 164:799-804.

CHAPTER 57

The Pediatric Chest

Joanna J. Seibert, M.D.
Charles M. Glasier, M.D.
Richard E. Leithiser, Jr., M.D.

CHAPTER OUTLINE

INDICATIONS FOR CHEST SONOGRAPHY

Initially, it was thought that sonography would have little beneficial use in the evaluation of the chest because the major organ of the chest contained air, which does not transmit sound, and the surrounding echogenic rib cage blocks sound from entering the chest. However, ultrasound has developed into an invaluable tool in evaluating the abnormal chest in which fluid and solid densities interpose between the chest wall and lung, which becomes an excellent medium for the transmission of sound waves. Originally, sonography was used to detect the presence of pleural fluid. With the advent of real-time ultrasound, higher-resolution scanners, and the ingenuity of sonographers, the chest applications of sonography have skyrocketed. High-resolution ultrasound in children can also be performed through the thymus to evaluate mediastinal and pulmonary structures. Lung lesions can be assessed using the liver or spleen as an acoustic window. Any radiographically opaque-appearing chest is often initially evaluated by sonography to determine whether there is fluid, a chest mass, atelectasis, or lung hypoplasia. Ultrasound can also be used therapeutically as a guide to thoracentesis, pleural biopsy, and lung biopsy.

SONOGRAPHIC SIGNS OF PLEURAL FLUID

The most frequent use of sonography is for the determination of pleural opacification on the chest radiograph to determine whether there is **pleural fluid** or pleural thickening,[2] or if there is an underlying pneumonia or mass (Fig. 57-1). Chest ultrasound examinations have proved to be significantly superior to decubitus radiographs alone for detecting small amounts of effusion.[3] Sonographic signs of a pleural effusion include detection of an **echo-free space immediately deep to the chest wall** (Fig. 57-2). Because pleural effusions transmit sound, structures deep to the effusion that normally cannot be seen by ultrasound become visible when an effusion is present.

INDICATIONS FOR CHEST SONOGRAPHY[1]

Diagnostic for:
Pleural effusions
Diaphragmatic paralysis
Cystic vs. solid masses
Diaphragmatic hernia (e.g., liver, bowel)
Diaphragm defect
Subpulmonic vs. subphrenic fluid
Pericardial effusion
Vascular thrombi (e.g., cardiac, SVC, IVC)
Tumor vs. large or persistent pleural effusion
Chest wall mass vs. pleural fluid
Catheter position in vessels
Mediastinal masses
Thymus relationship to masses
Extension of neck masses into the chest

Ultrasound guidance for:
Thoracentesis
Needle biopsy of masses
Endotracheal tube placement

A

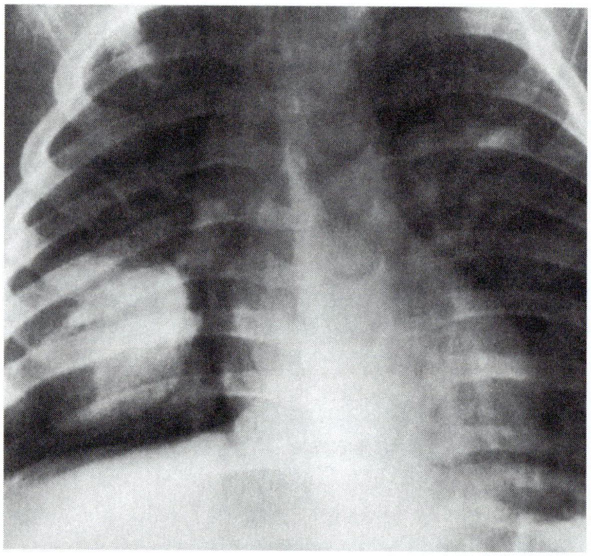

B

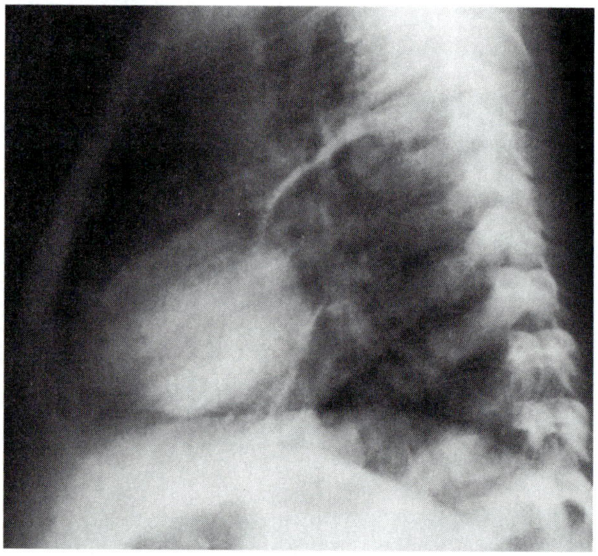

C

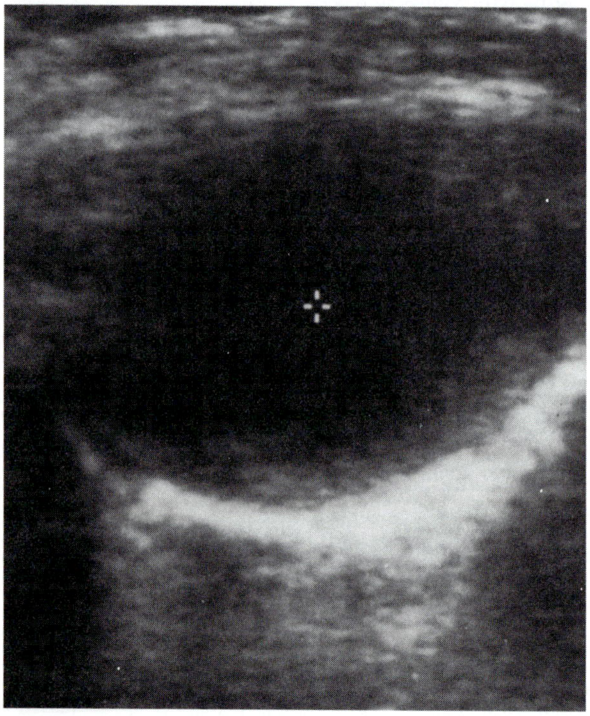

FIG. 57-1. Loculated fluid in chest—minor fissure of right middle lobe. **A**, Posteroanterior and, **B**, lateral radiographs show round mass. **C**, Sonography shows rounded mass is hypoechoic, loculated fluid collection.

Normally, when scanning through the liver, the chest wall behind the liver is not visible because aerated lung stops the sound beam. However, when a pleural effusion is present, the posterior **chest wall becomes visible.**[4]

Access to the pleural space is obtained by using either subcostal or intercostal scans. The spleen or liver may be used as windows to the pleural space because they are relatively homogeneous, solid, parenchymal organs and provide good through transmission. A pleural effusion appears as a hypoechoic collection just above the diaphragm and adjacent to it. Underlying consolidated lung can be separated from the effusion because the **consolidated lung is denser** and contains multiple echogenic areas of air (bronchograms) within it (Fig. 57-3). An uncomplicated effusion is totally anechoic whereas a complex collection such as a **hemothorax** or **empyema** has **thicker fluid with septations** (Fig. 57-4).

A

B

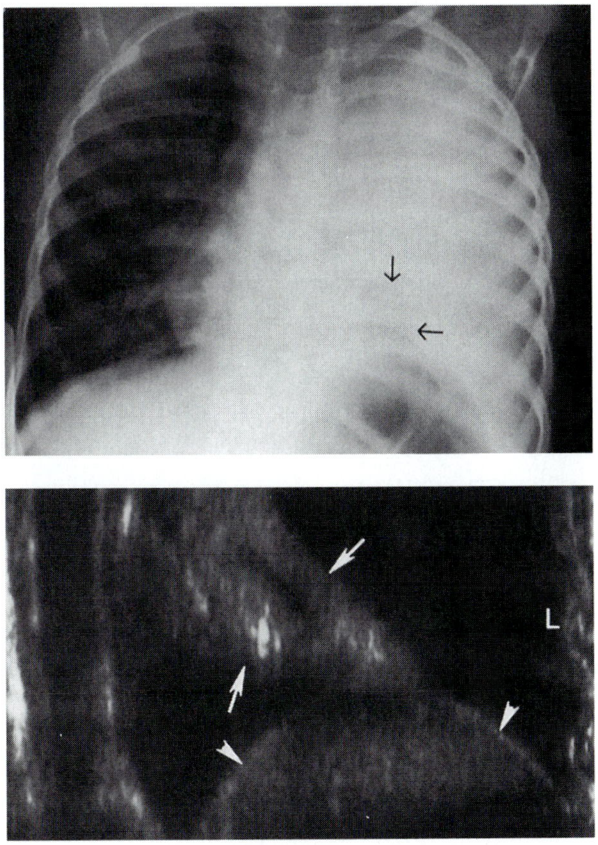

FIG. 57-2. Pleural fluid caused by streptococcal pneumonia (18-month-old boy). A, Chest radiograph shows totally opacified left hemithorax with possible pneumatocele *(arrows)*. **B,** Left coronal sonogram (turned same way as chest radiographic film) shows large, clear fluid collections surrounding compressed left lower lung *(arrows)* above left hemidiaphragm *(arrowheads)*. *L,* Left lateral chest wall. (From Glasier CM, Leithiser RE Jr, Williamson SL et al. Extracardiac chest ultrasonography in infants and children: radiographic and clinical implications. *J Pediatr* 1989;114(4):540-544.)

Free fluid changes position with changes in the patient's position. When the patient is supine, fluid moves behind the liver and lung (Fig. 57-5). When the patient is upright, the fluid moves between the lung and diaphragm.

Initial reports found that almost 20% of echo-free pleural lesions did not yield free fluid on thoracentesis.[5] The same authors later reported two observations, which have proved to be **more predictive of pleural fluid:** (1) the presence of a **definite change in shape of a pleural density with inspiration and expiration** and (2) the presence of **moving septations within the pleural lesion.**[6] The septations are presumably fibrin strands. This to-and-fro motion is unequivocal evidence that the fluid has a relatively low viscosity. With real-time scanners, the detection of fluid is not difficult.

Color flow Doppler ultrasound may also aid in distinguishing pleural effusion from pleural thickening.[7-8] When a **free pleural effusion** is present, there is a color signal between the visceral and parietal pleura or near the costophrenic angle, which is related to respiratory movement. The spectral waveform analysis shows a chaotic, to-and-fro turbulent flowlike signal related to the respiratory and cardiac cycle. The movable cells, cell debris, and fibrinlike materials may scatter the sound and produce the color flow Doppler signals. **Organized pleural thickening** will appear as a colorless pleural lesion with no Doppler signal.

The liver and spleen are also excellent acoustic windows to evaluate pleural-based masses.[9-14] The same criteria as those used in computed tomography (CT) apply to the sonographic evaluation of lower chest masses; the added information supplied by sagittal or longitudinal plane sonographic imaging is not available on CT, except by reconstruction.[4,12] Chest sonography

SONOGRAPHIC SIGNS OF PLEURAL FLUID

- Hypoechoic fluid collection under chest wall
- Septations if loculated
- Hyperechoic lung beneath fluid
- Posterior chest wall visualized below fluid
- Hypoechoic fluid above diaphragm
- Free fluid moves with respiration
- Septations move if loculated fluid
- Color signal between visceral and parietal pleura
- Color signal at costophrenic angle
- Diaphragm sign (fluid outside or peripheral to diaphragm)
- Displaced crus sign
- Bare area sign

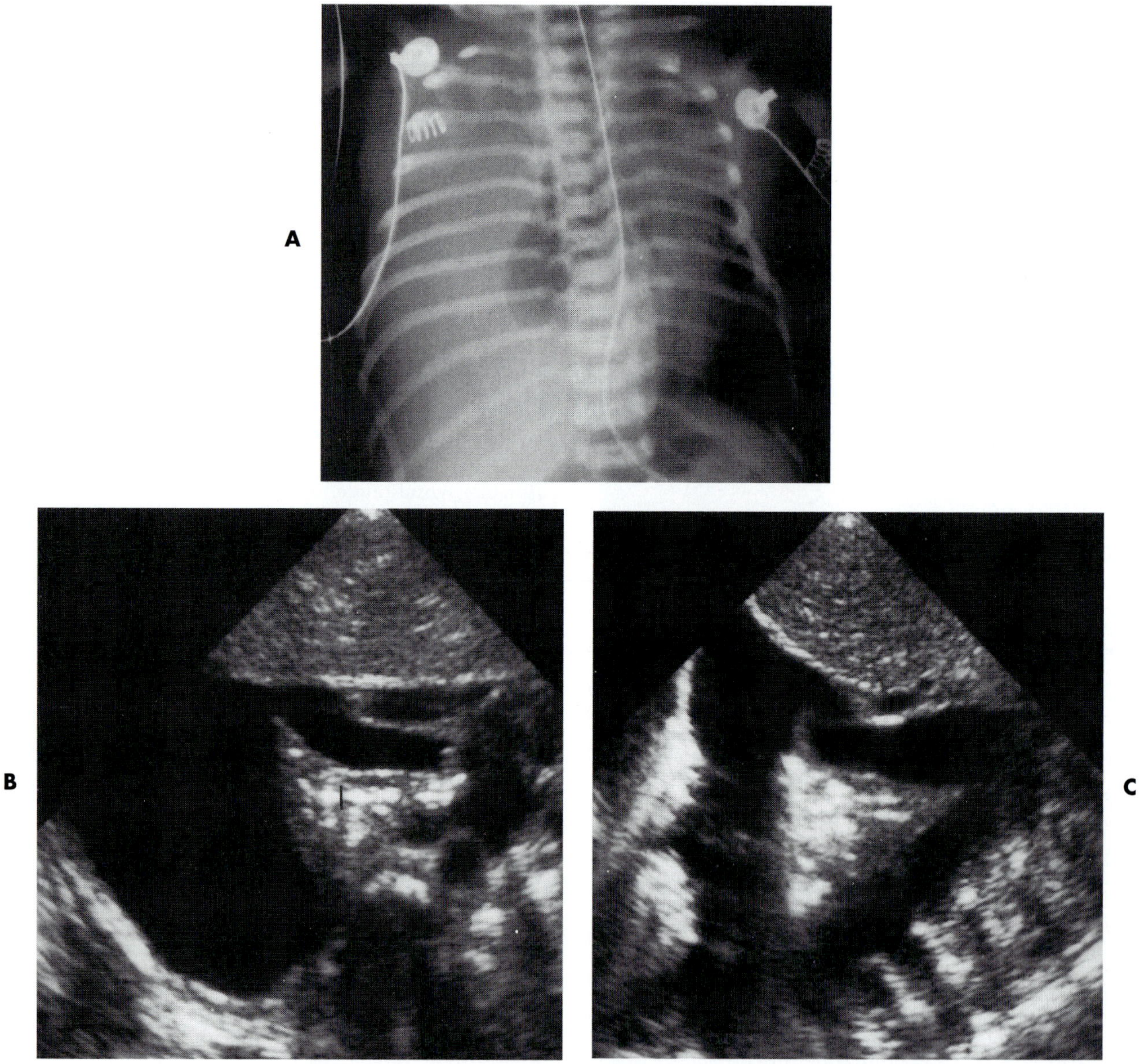

FIG. 57-3. Neonatal chylothorax. **A,** Anteroposterior chest radiograph in 2-week-old infant shows opacified right chest and shift of heart and mediastinum to left. **B,** Transverse sonograms through liver show that mass is large accumulation of fluid and that collapsed lung, *l*, is surrounded by fluid. **C,** Multiple air shadows (air bronchograms) are within lung.

A

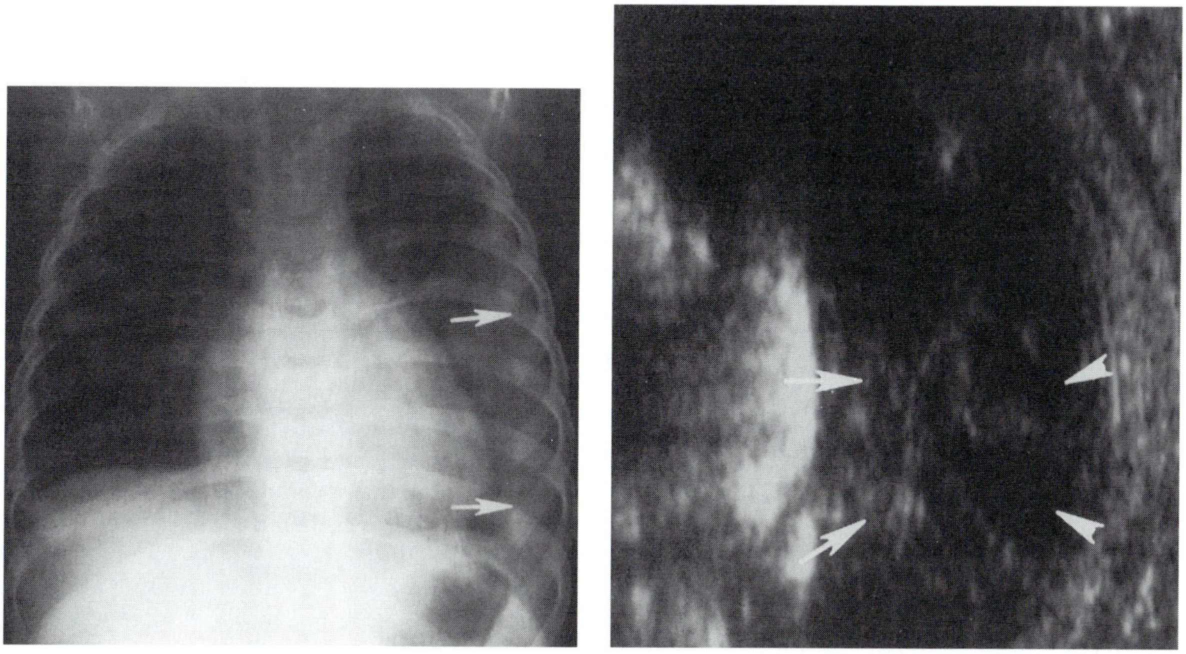

B

FIG. 57-4. Pleural thickening. **A,** Supine chest radiograph in 3-year-old girl with treated *Haemophilus pneumoniae* and recurrent fever shows left pleural density *(arrows)*. **B,** Left coronal sonogram (reoriented as chest radiographic film) shows echogenic pleural fluid *(arrows)* with multiple loculated pockets of clear fluid *(arrowheads)*. (From Glasier CM, Leithiser RE Jr, Williamson SL et al. Extracardiac chest ultrasonography in infants and children: radiographic and clinical implications. *J Pediatr* 1989;114(4):540-544.)

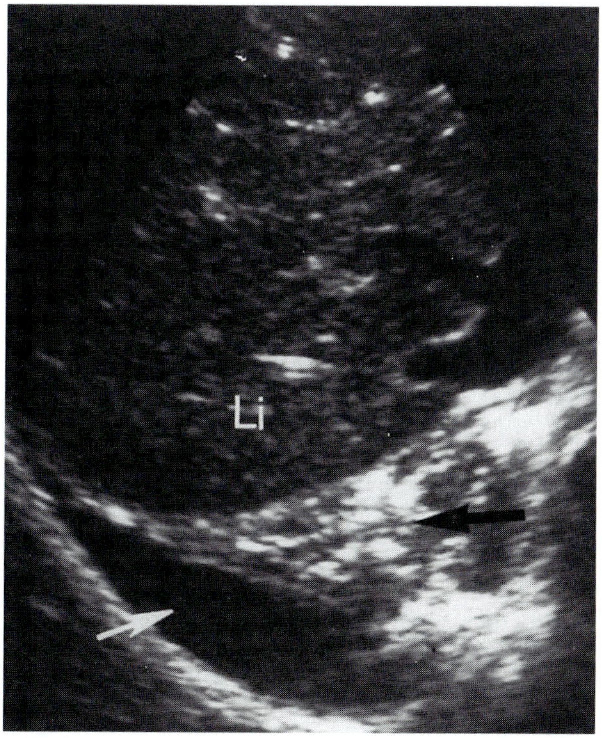

FIG. 57-5. Posterior pleural fluid over bare area of liver. Transverse scan through liver with patient in supine position shows liver, triangular consolidated lung (air bronchograms) behind it *(black arrow)*, and fluid *(white arrow)* posterior to lung and liver, *Li*.

through the abdomen is clearly superior on the right side as a result of the larger acoustic window of the liver.

Diaphragm Sign

When the liver or spleen is used as an acoustic window and fluid is seen adjacent to them, the location of the fluid is determined in reference to the diaphragm's position. If the fluid is inside the diaphragm and more centrally located, it is **ascites.** If the fluid is outside the diaphragm and more peripherally located, it is in the **pleural space.**[4]

Displaced Crus Sign

The fluid is in the pleural space if there is interposition of the **fluid between the crus and the vertebral column,** displacing the crus away from the spine.[4]

Bare-Area Sign

The posterior aspect of the right lower lobe of the liver is directly attached to the posterior diaphragm without peritoneum. Thus ascitic fluid in the subhepatic or subphrenic space cannot extend behind the liver at the level of the bare area. Pleural fluid can be seen to extend **behind the liver at the level of the bare area** (see Fig. 57-5).

A

B

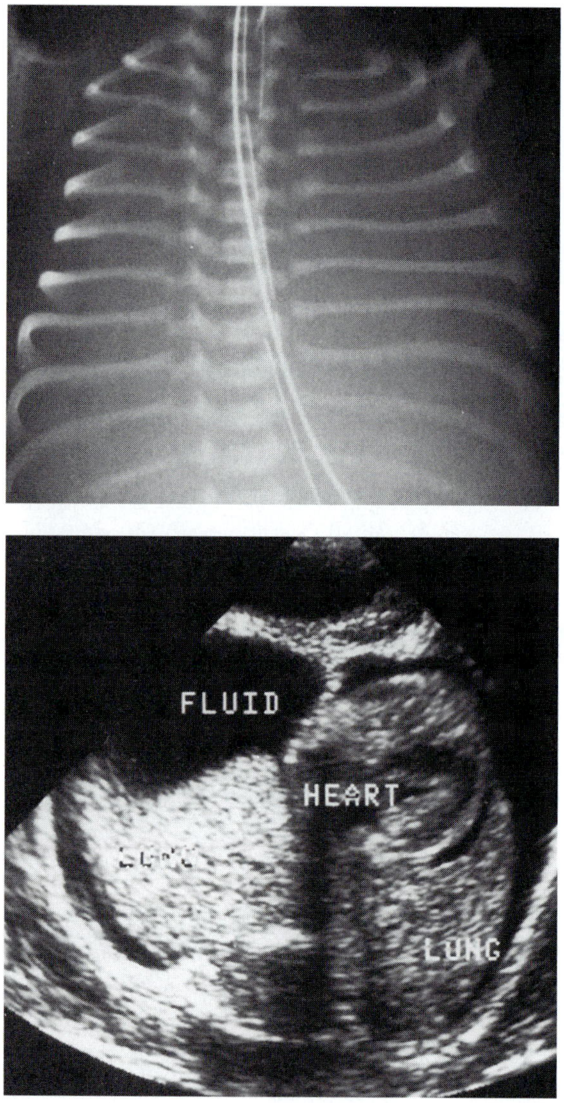

FIG. 57-6. Bilateral pleural fluid and pericardial fluid. **A,** Chest radiograph of infant on extracorporeal membrane oxygenation (ECMO) shows complete lung opacification. **B,** Transverse sonogram shows collapsed lung bilaterally with small amount of pericardial fluid.

Advantages and Disadvantages of Sonography

Sonography has an advantage over CT in that the inverted diaphragm can be detected on the longitudinal or sagittally oriented scan, which is not possible on CT, except on reconstruction. In CT scans, pleural fluid sometimes appears to be ascites, but this confusion does not occur with ultrasound. Sonography can also detect fluid behind the inferior vena cava (IVC), which would suggest pleural fluid. Ultrasound also has the advantage over CT of being a bedside portable technique, which makes it useful for studying critically ill infants (Fig. 57-6) when lung opacification may be confused with pleural effusions.

A limitation of chest sonography is that very homogeneous, **solid lesions may at times appear fluid-filled** (Fig. 57-7).[4] Below the diaphragm, the criteria for fluid-filled structures are (1) lack of internal echoes, (2) a sharp posterior wall, and (3) increased through transmission of sound deep to the collection of fluid. The lack of echogenicity is a relative phenomenon that is judged by the echogenicity of the surrounding structures. In the chest, there is no referenced solid or cystic structure for comparison to assist in making this observation. The increased transmission of sound is called **acoustic enhancement** and may be difficult to judge in the chest. Deep to a pleural effusion is an air-containing lung; the air interfaced with lung tissue is strongly echogenic, regardless of what the pleural lesion contains. Therefore free fluid, organized lung tissue, and solid pleural masses may produce apparently increased transmission of sound. Observing the pleural fluid change in shape on inspiration and expiration and observing the movement of septations are two additional signs to detect thick pleural fluid: (1) the **presence of air or fluid bronchograms** in the lung parenchyma can be used to differentiate **lung as the area of increased transmission** (Fig. 57-3); and (2) collapsed or consolidated lung tissue often has the appearance of liver or spleen.

Another pitfall in the sonographic evaluation of the chest is the **acoustic shadow** cast by a dense rib **(rib shadowing),** which may trap the unwary sonographer into believing that a mass is anechoic. To overcome this, the controls on the equipment should be set by scanning between the lower ribs over the liver. This enables the sonographer to become familiar with the acoustic shadows cast by the ribs. The echogenicity of the mass or pleural density can be compared with that of the liver.[7]

ABSCESS AND EMPYEMA

An **empyema or lung abscess** adjacent to the chest wall or to acoustic windows such as the liver or spleen usually appears as a complex collection with fluid-debris levels and septations (Fig. 57-8). Abscesses and empyemas usually **exhibit different types of motion** when visualized under ultrasound. An abscess demonstrates expansion of the entire circumference with inspiration whereas with an empyema, only the internal wall adjacent to the lung shows slight motion.[2] Lung abscesses may be difficult to differentiate from empyema when the empyema contains multiple, loculated air collections caused by thoracentesis. Movement of the air collections with positioning may distinguish the empyema (Figs. 57-9 and 57-10).

A

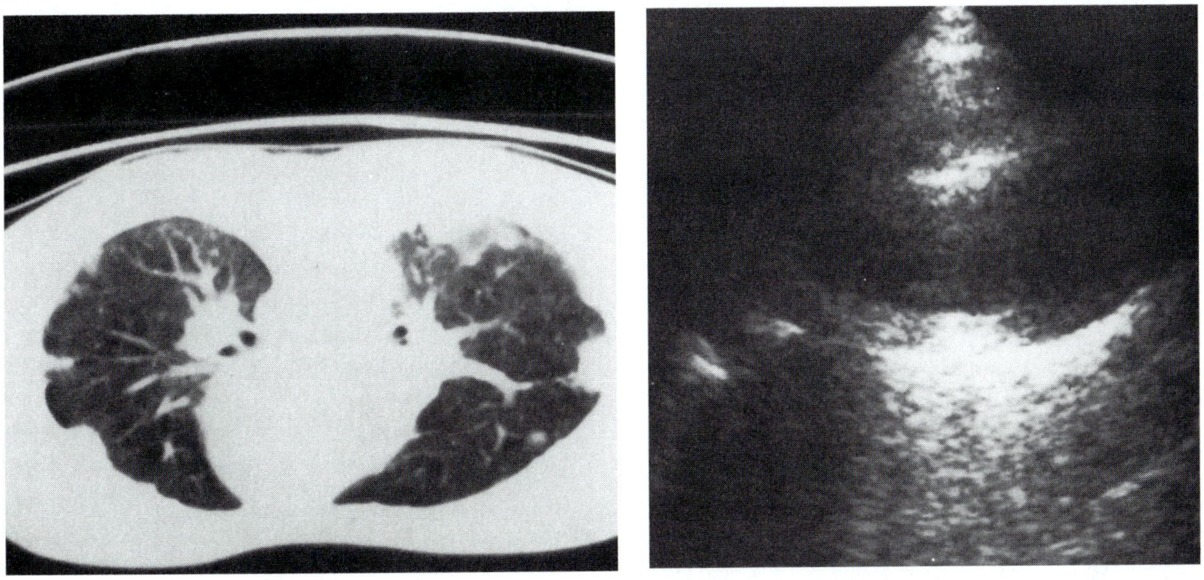

B

FIG. 57-7. Metastases from renal cell carcinoma. **A,** CT scan (teenager) shows multiple metastases. **B,** Sonogram shows large pleural mass is relatively hypoechoic.

A

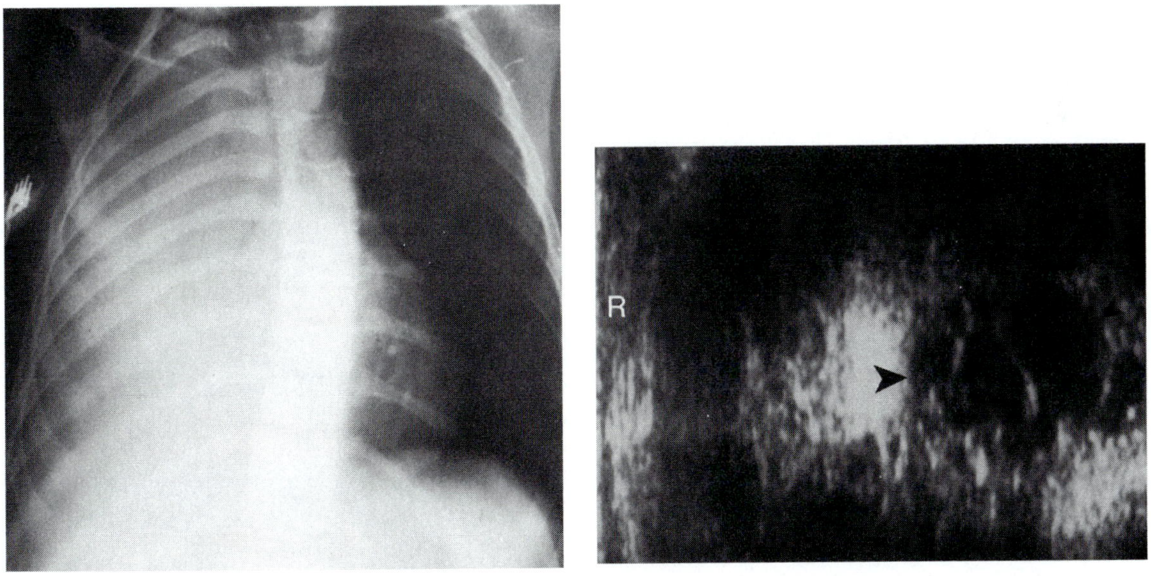

B

FIG. 57-8. Loculated abscess. **A,** Chest radiograph of 7-year-old boy with cough, fever, and pneumococcal sepsis shows opaque right hemithorax. Multiple thoracenteses were unsuccessful. **B,** Right coronal sonogram (in same orientation as chest radiograph film) shows consolidated echogenic lung with multilocular cystic areas *(arrowheads)* from early abscess formation (purulent fluid was aspirated under ultrasound guidance.) *R,* Right lateral chest wall.

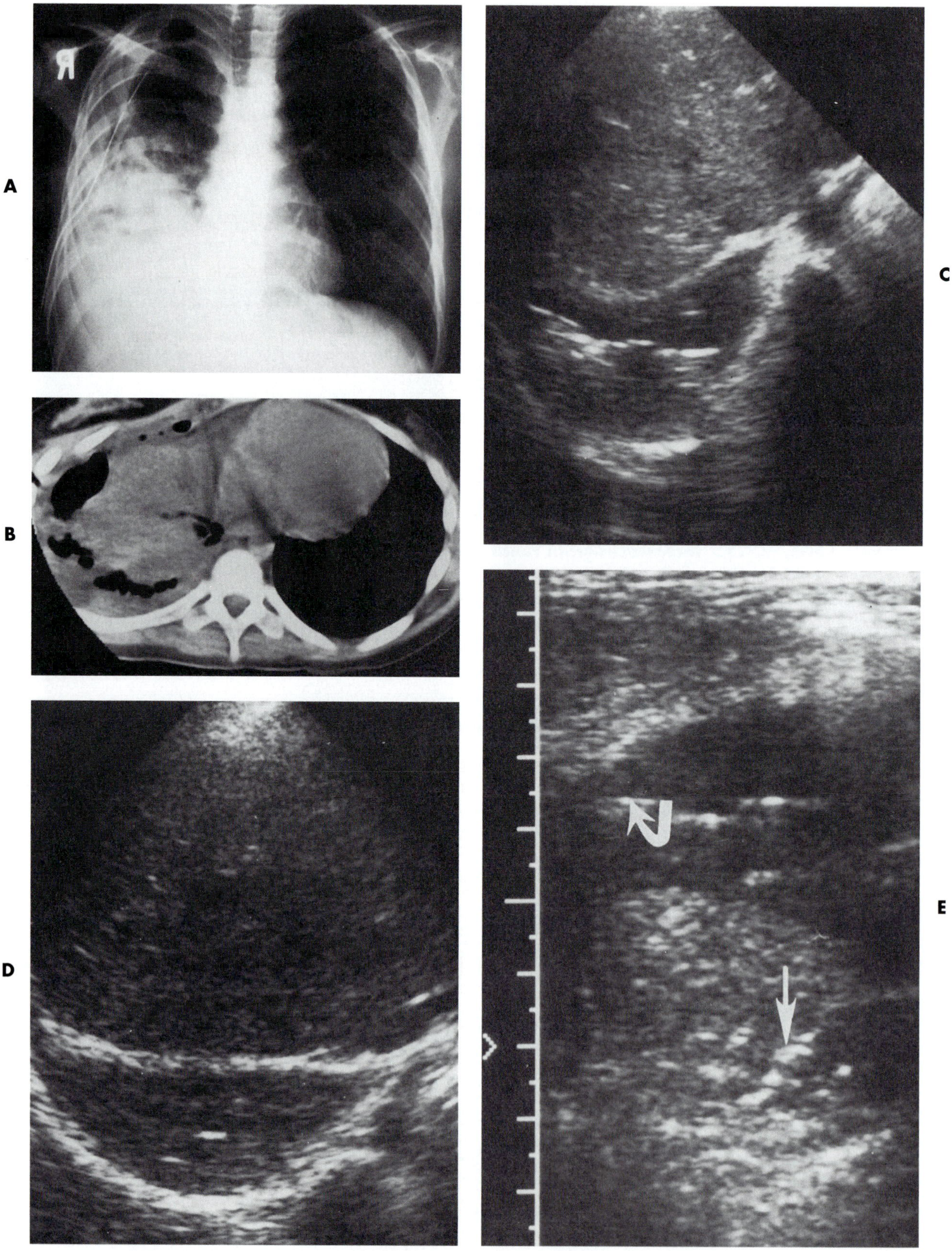

FIG. 57-9. Air-fluid levels in complex empyema. **A**, Chest radiograph shows multiple air-fluid levels in lung abscess or empyema. Multiple air-fluid levels in empyema on **B**, CT and, **C**, sonogram through liver. **D**, Upright sonogram. Air-fluid levels change when patient is erect (air moved up and out of this transverse scan through lower chest). **E**, Transverse intercostal scan through anterior chest wall shows both the linear lines of bronchi *(arrow)* at random pattern and linear lines of air *(curved arrow)* in the pleural fluid all at one level.

A

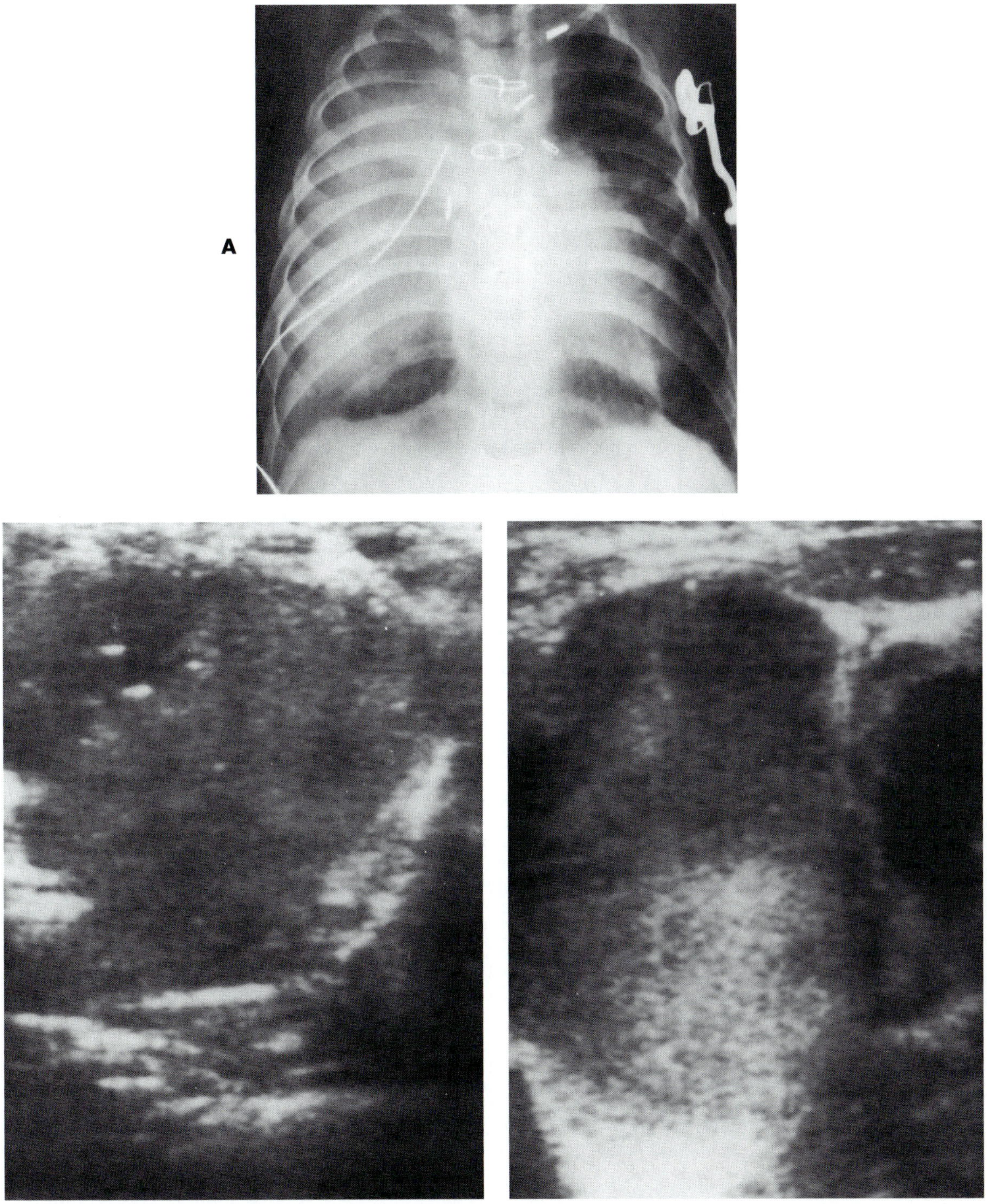

B

C

FIG. 57-10. Thick pleural fluid with changing appearance. A, Chest radiograph shows pneumonia that is not draining by chest tube. **B,** Transverse sonogram shows very thick fluid in chest with no air bronchograms within the thick density. **C,** Differential thick fluid/fluid level with change in position.

LUNG PARENCHYMA

Consolidated lung is relatively hypoechoic in relation to the highly reflective normal surrounding lung.[13] Strong, nonpulsatile, linear echoes produced by air-filled bronchi can be seen converging toward the root of the lung. This linear pattern of bright echoes can be observed when scanning parallel to the long axis of the bronchi. When the scanning is done at different angles, scattered echoes of variable lengths produced by the **air bronchograms** can be observed (Fig. 57-11). Posterior reverberation and acoustic shadowing can be seen and are related to the large, proximal, air-filled bronchi. If there is adjacent pleural fluid, the hypoechoic consolidated lung can be differentiated from the hypoechoic to anechoic pleural effusion by identification of these air bronchograms (Fig. 57-12). **Consolidated lung** may have an echogenicity similar to the liver (Fig. 57-13), but the air bronchograms can differentiate it from liver. **Atelectatic lung** may be more echogenic than the liver (Fig. 57-14). Occasionally, the bronchi may be filled with fluid rather than with air.[15-17] The echogenic, parallel, branching walls again can be seen but without the acoustic shadowing and reverberation artifacts normally seen with air. Parenchymal lesions adjacent to the heart have been mistaken for pericardial effusion.[18] Ultrasound can be used to demonstrate that an opacified chest contains very little lung tissue (Fig. 57-15) in a hypoplastic lung.

A

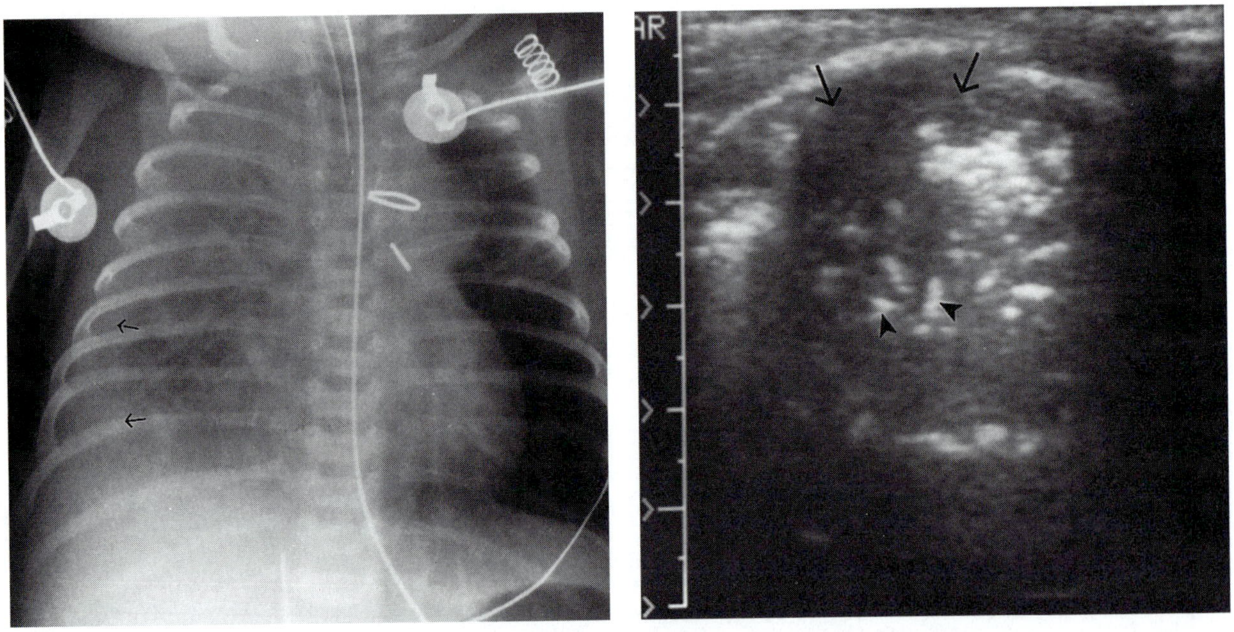

B

FIG. 57-11. Pneumonia without effusion in 2-week-old girl with persistent fever and purulent endotracheal drainage after coarctation repair. **A,** Chest radiograph shows right parenchymal infiltrates and possible pleural fluid *(arrows)*. **B,** Transverse sonogram shows consolidated lung parenchyma *(arrows)* with echogenic, branching, tubular structures *(arrowheads)* suggestive of air-filled bronchi. No pleural fluid was seen. At autopsy, necrotizing pneumonia was found throughout right lung without evidence of empyema.

A

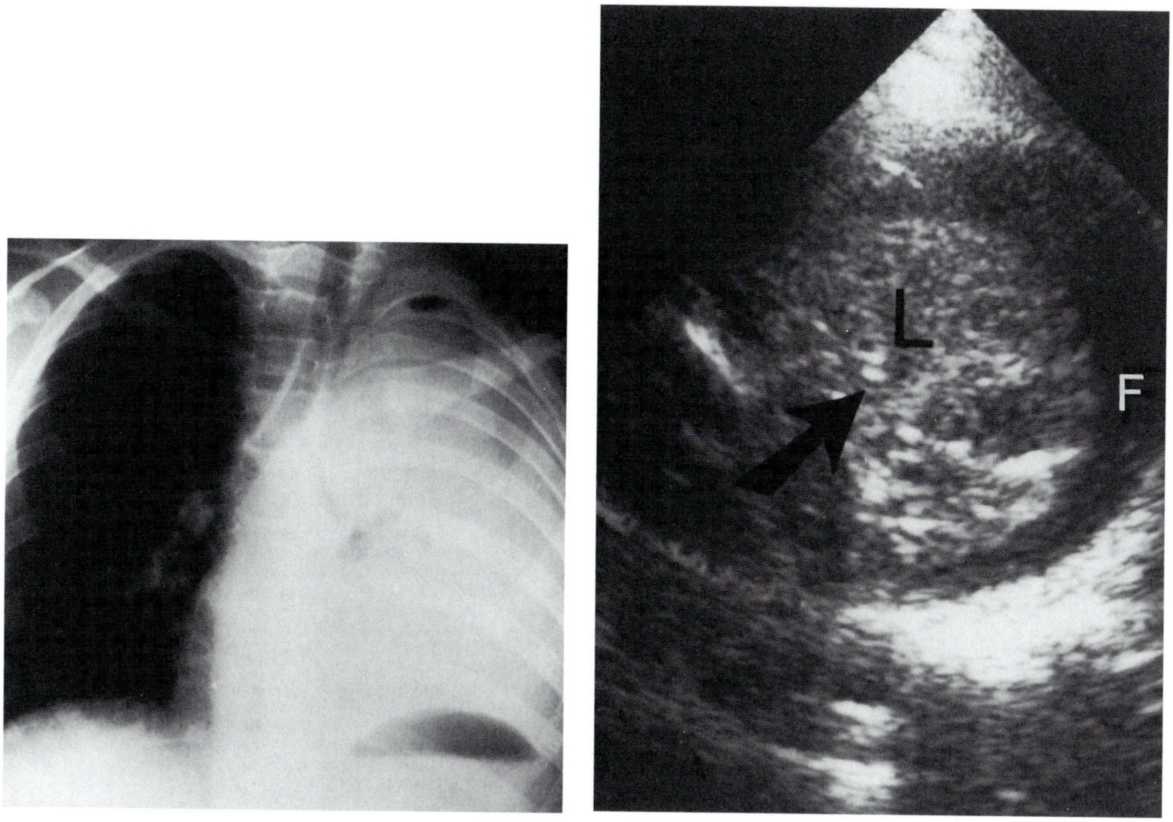

B

FIG. 57-12. Pneumonia with fluid in 6-year-old child. **A,** Chest radiograph shows opacified left side of chest with some air bronchograms within density. **B,** Transverse scan through chest shows fluid, *F,* around lung, *L,* with air bronchograms within lung *(arrow)*.

A

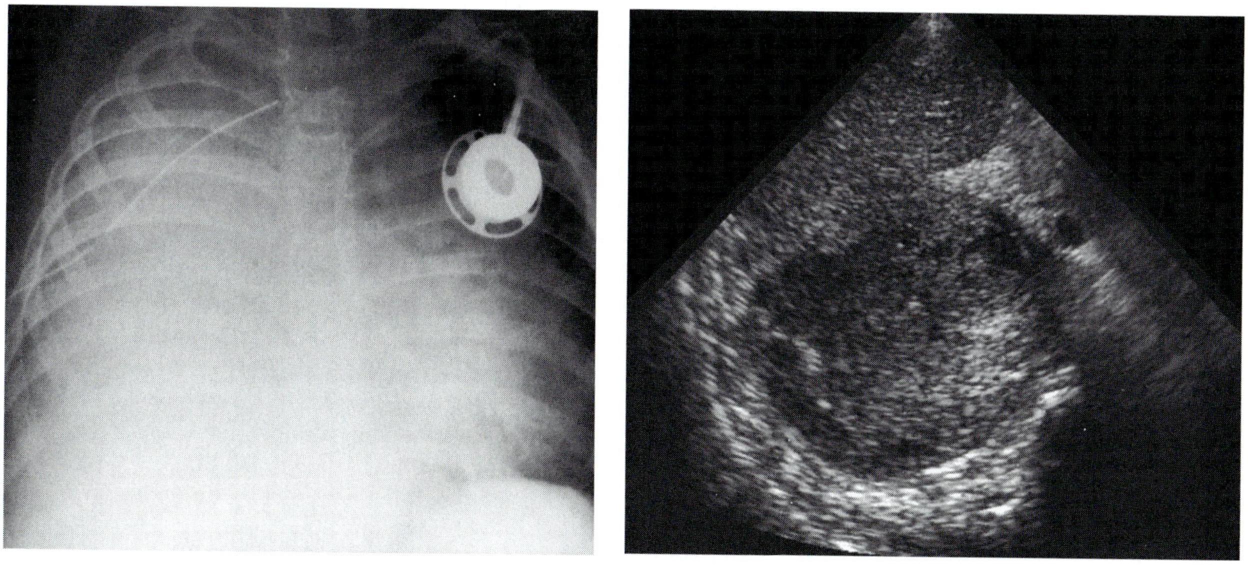

B

FIG. 57-13. Consolidated lung without effusion. **A,** Right chest opacification with shift of heart to left side, suggesting fluid in right side of chest. No drainage, however, was obtained from chest tube. **B,** Right chest is filled with solid tissue *(arrow)*, which at surgery was infected with aspergillosis extending from liver, *L*. Ultrasound through liver.

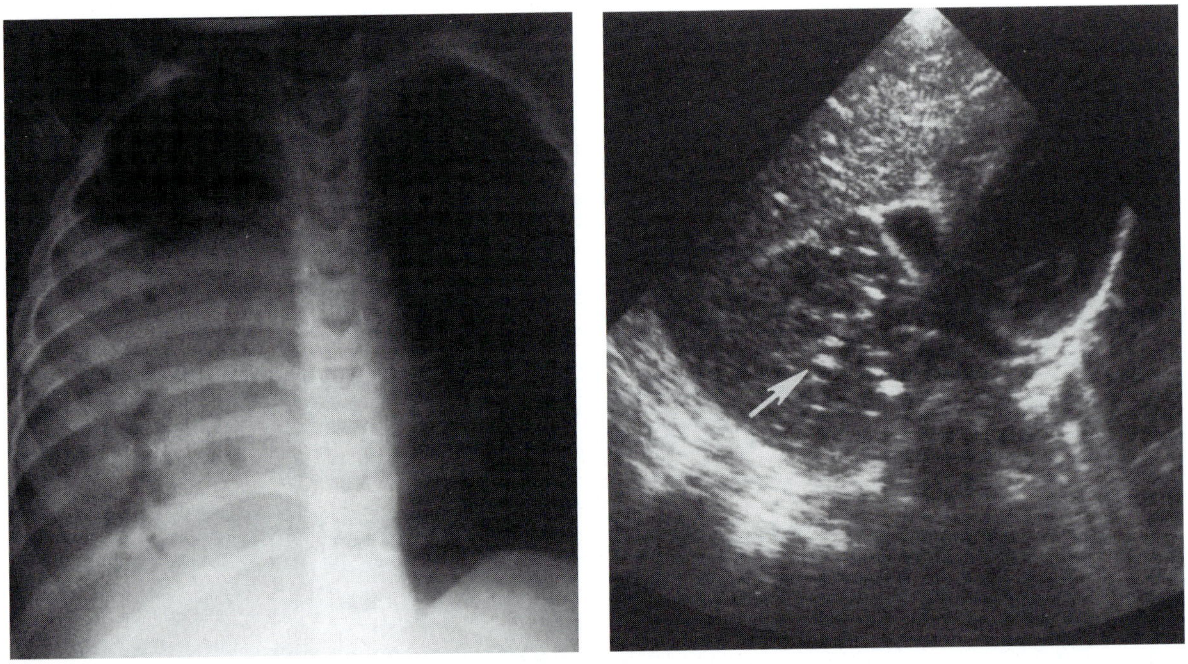

A B

FIG. 57-14. Atelectasis from foreign body. **A,** Chest radiograph shows air bronchograms in opacified right side of chest with shift of heart to right, suggesting volume loss. **B,** Transverse sonogram through liver shows no fluid in chest. Multiple air bronchograms *(arrow)* within collapsed lung. At endoscopy, foreign body was found in right mainstem bronchus. (From Seibert RW, Seibert JJ, Williamson SL. The opaque chest: when to suspect a bronchial foreign body. *Pediatr Radiol* 1986;16:193-196.)

MEDIASTINUM

In children the normal thymus is an excellent acoustic window to view normal mediastinal structures and mediastinal masses.[18] The **thymus** is located anterior to the great vessels and extends down to the upper portion of the heart (Fig. 57-16). The thymus can be used as a window to visualize these vessels. The echogenicity of the thymus is usually less than that of the liver, spleen, and thyroid.[19] The **great vessels,** the superior vena cava, the aorta, and the pulmonary artery can be well-imaged through the thymus. These vessels are especially more evident with Doppler ultrasound (see Fig. 57-16, *C*).[20] The left innominate vein runs transversely from left to right through the thymus to enter the SVC. This can be extremely useful in evaluating children for **central venous catheter placement** to determine catheter position and the **presence of a clot** (Figs. 57-17 to 57-19).

Superior Vena Caval Thrombosis

The Doppler waveform will be abnormal when there is **thrombus or obstruction of the SVC** (see box). There will be (1) loss of biphasic SVC waveform, (2) continuous forward flow rather than distinct systolic and diastolic peaks, (3) a turbulent flow profile, (4) increased velocity downstream, and (5) decreased velocity upstream.[21]

SIGNS OF SVC THROMBOSIS

Loss of biphasic waveform
Continuous forward flow (no systolic or diastolic peaks)
Turbulent flow
Increased downstream velocity
Decreased velocity upstream

Mediastinal Masses

Sonography may be useful in evaluating a mediastinal mass to determine whether it is normal, enlarged, or an ectopic thymus.[22] Mediastinal ultrasound can also determine whether chest masses extend into the neck (Fig. 57-20).

Three longitudinal planes can be identified in the mediastinum (Fig. 57-21 on p. 1634)—one laterally on the right through the SVC, one in the midline through the aortic root, and one laterally on the left at the level of the pulmonary outflow tract. Two distinct transverse planes through the mediastinum can be identified (Fig. 57-22 on p. 1635)—the superior plane where the left innominate vein joins the superior vena cava and a lower transverse plane where the SVC, aorta, and pulmonary outflow tract may be visualized in one plane.

Text continued on p. 1635.

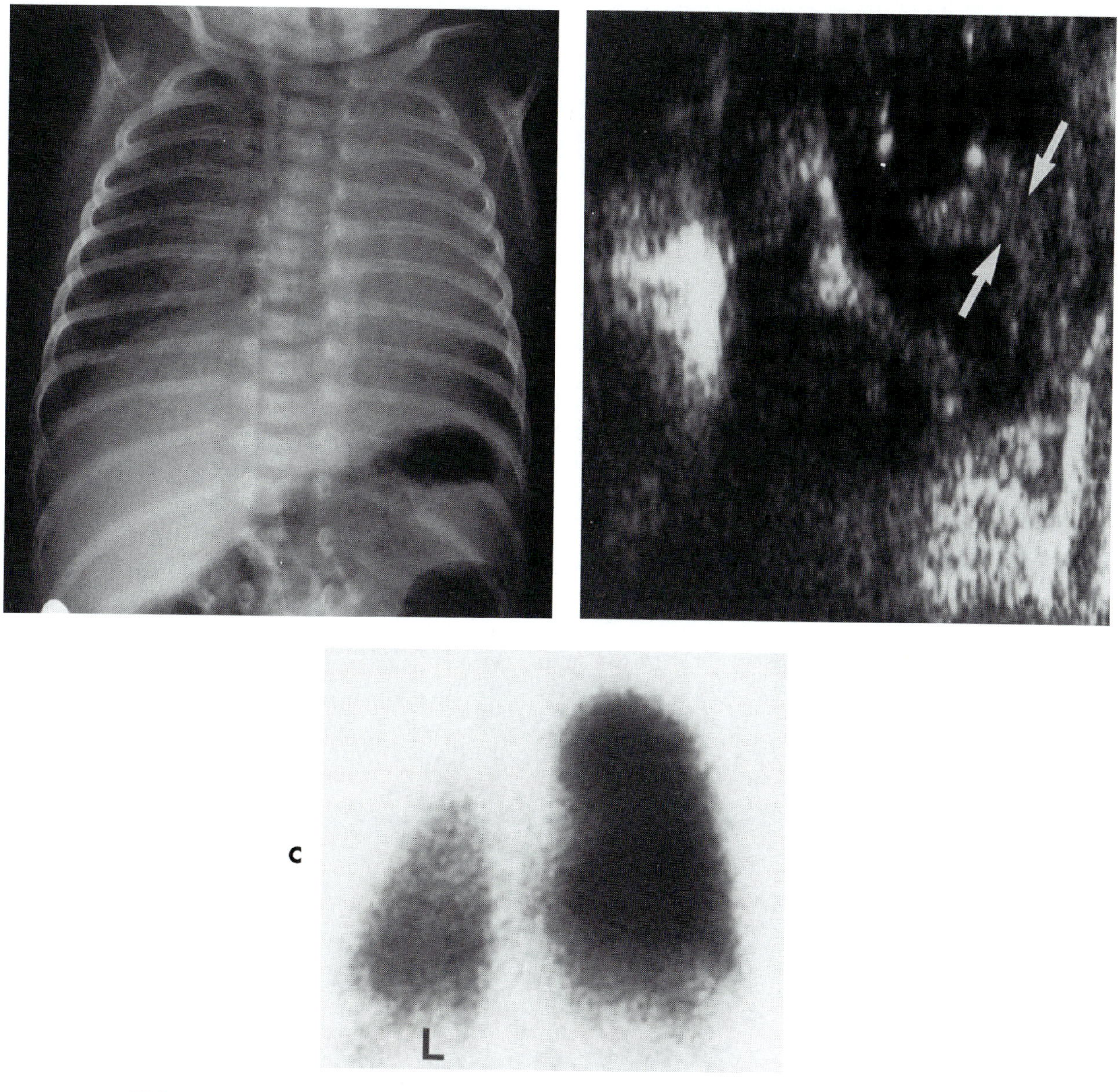

FIG. 57-15. Hypoplastic left lung in neonate. **A**, Chest radiograph shows left shift of the heart and mediastinum. **B**, Left coronal sonogram shows heart in the left lower chest with small amount of lung parenchyma *(arrows)*. **C**, Perfusion lung scan shows hypoplastic left lung.

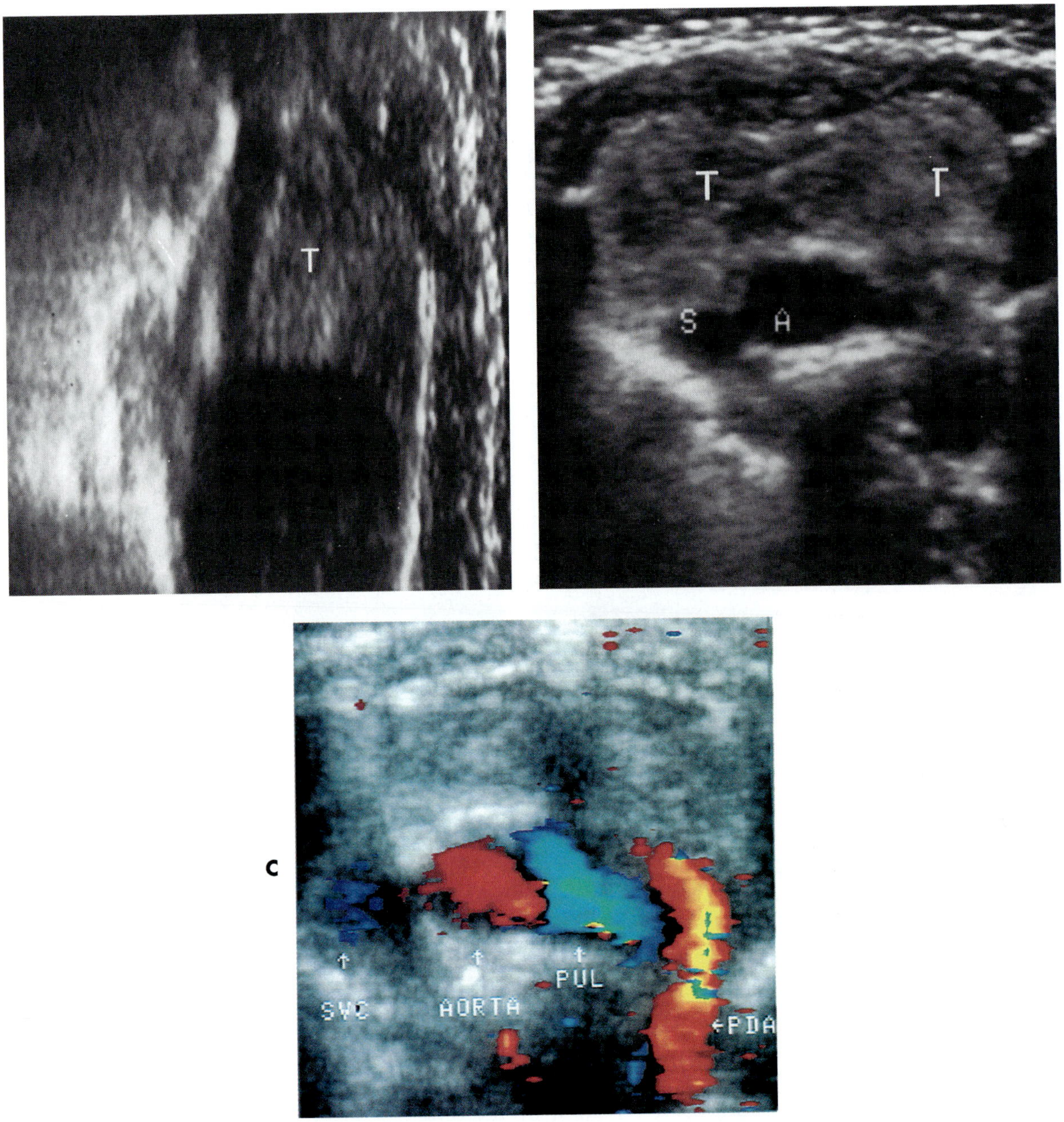

FIG. 57-16. Normal thymus in neonate. **A,** Longitudinal and, **B,** transverse sonograms show superior vena cava, *S*, aorta, *A*, and thymus, *T*. **C,** Color flow Doppler imaging of normal great vessels in chest seen in transverse scan through the thymus. *SVC*, Superior vena cava; *PUL*, pulmonary artery.

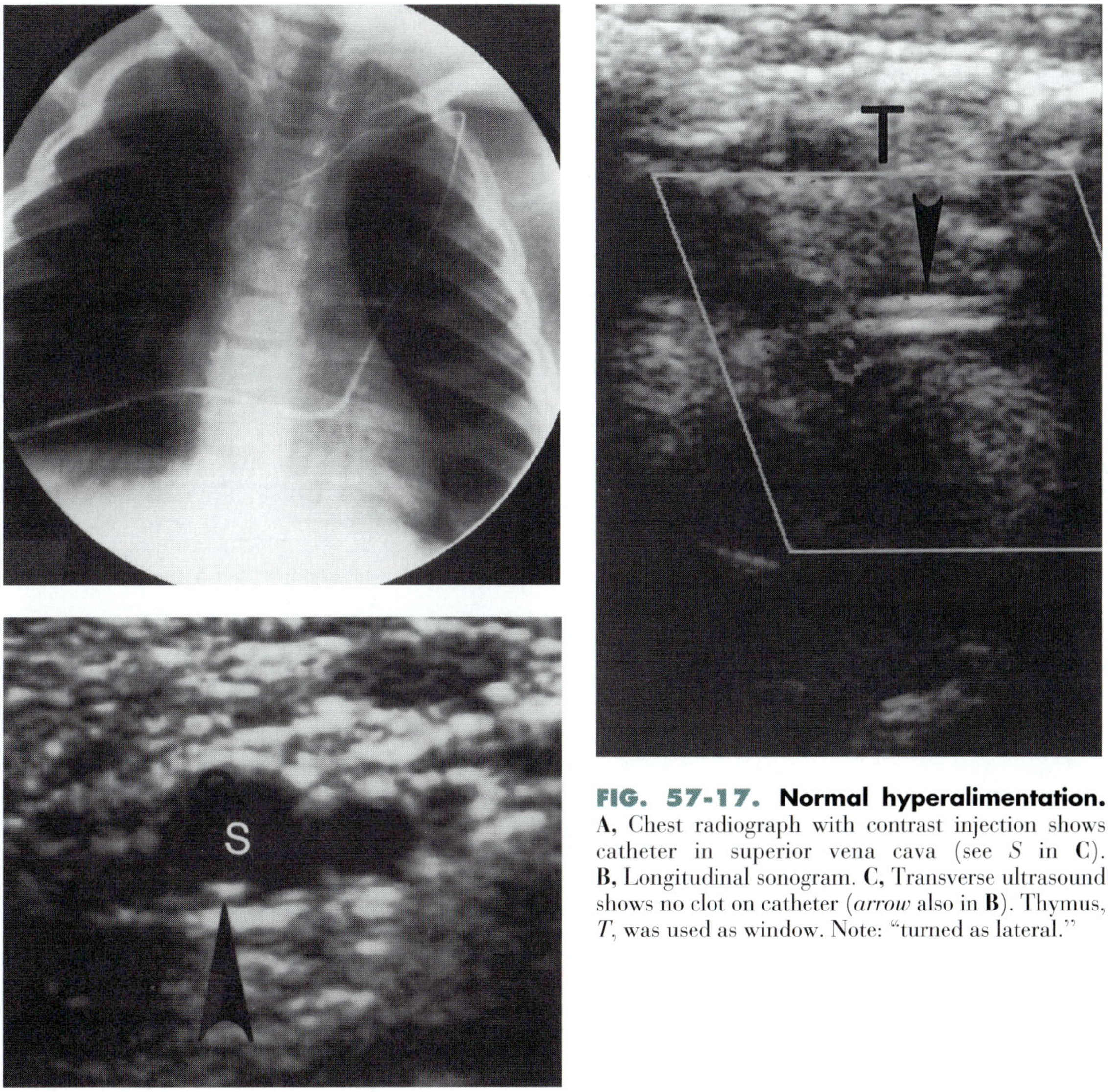

FIG. 57-17. Normal hyperalimentation. **A,** Chest radiograph with contrast injection shows catheter in superior vena cava (see *S* in **C**). **B,** Longitudinal sonogram. **C,** Transverse ultrasound shows no clot on catheter (*arrow* also in **B**). Thymus, *T*, was used as window. Note: "turned as lateral."

A
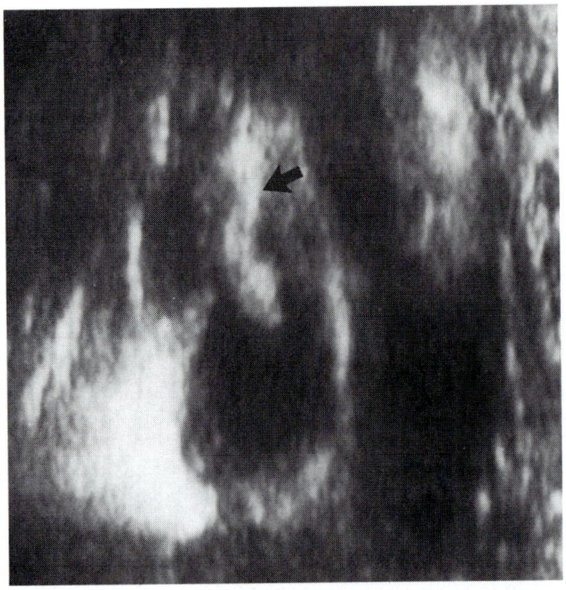
B
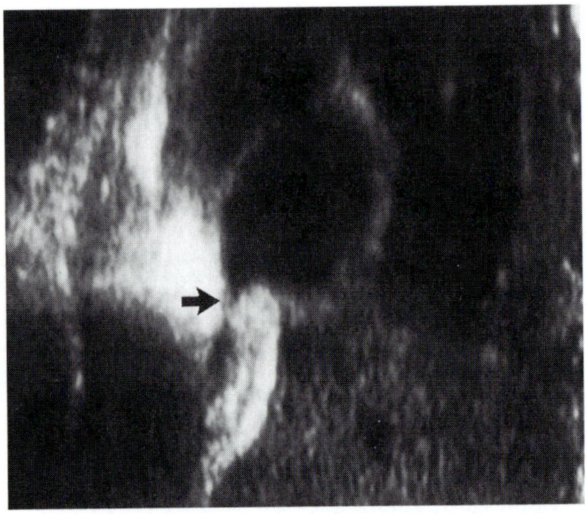

FIG. 57-18. Clot on catheter. **A,** Clot in superior vena cava extending into right atrium. **B,** Clot on inferior vena caval catheter *(arrow)* in patient with superior vena caval syndrome. Sonograms turned to anatomic position.

A
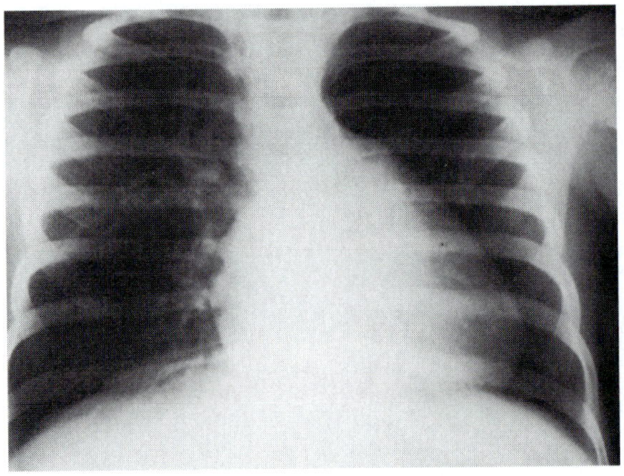
B
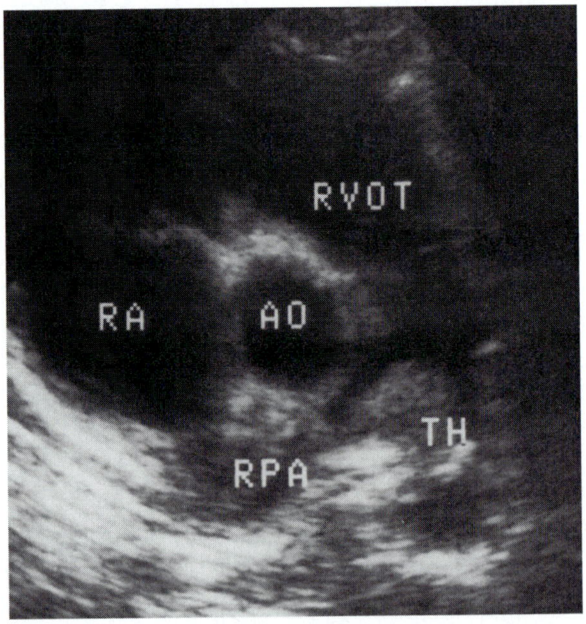

C
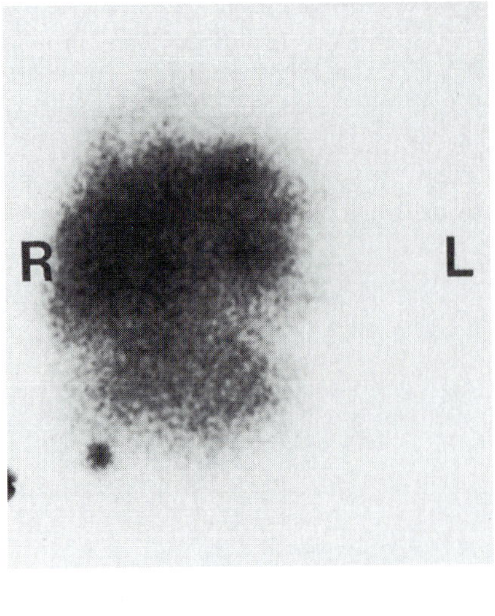

FIG. 57-19. Pulmonary embolus. **A,** Chest radiograph shows hyperlucent left lung in 4-year-old child. **B,** Pulmonary perfusion scan shows no perfusion to left lung. **C,** Transverse sonogram through heart shows saddle embolus in main pulmonary artery. *TH,* Thrombus; *RVOT,* right ventricular outflow tract; *AO,* aorta; *RA,* right atrium; *RPA,* right pulmonary artery.

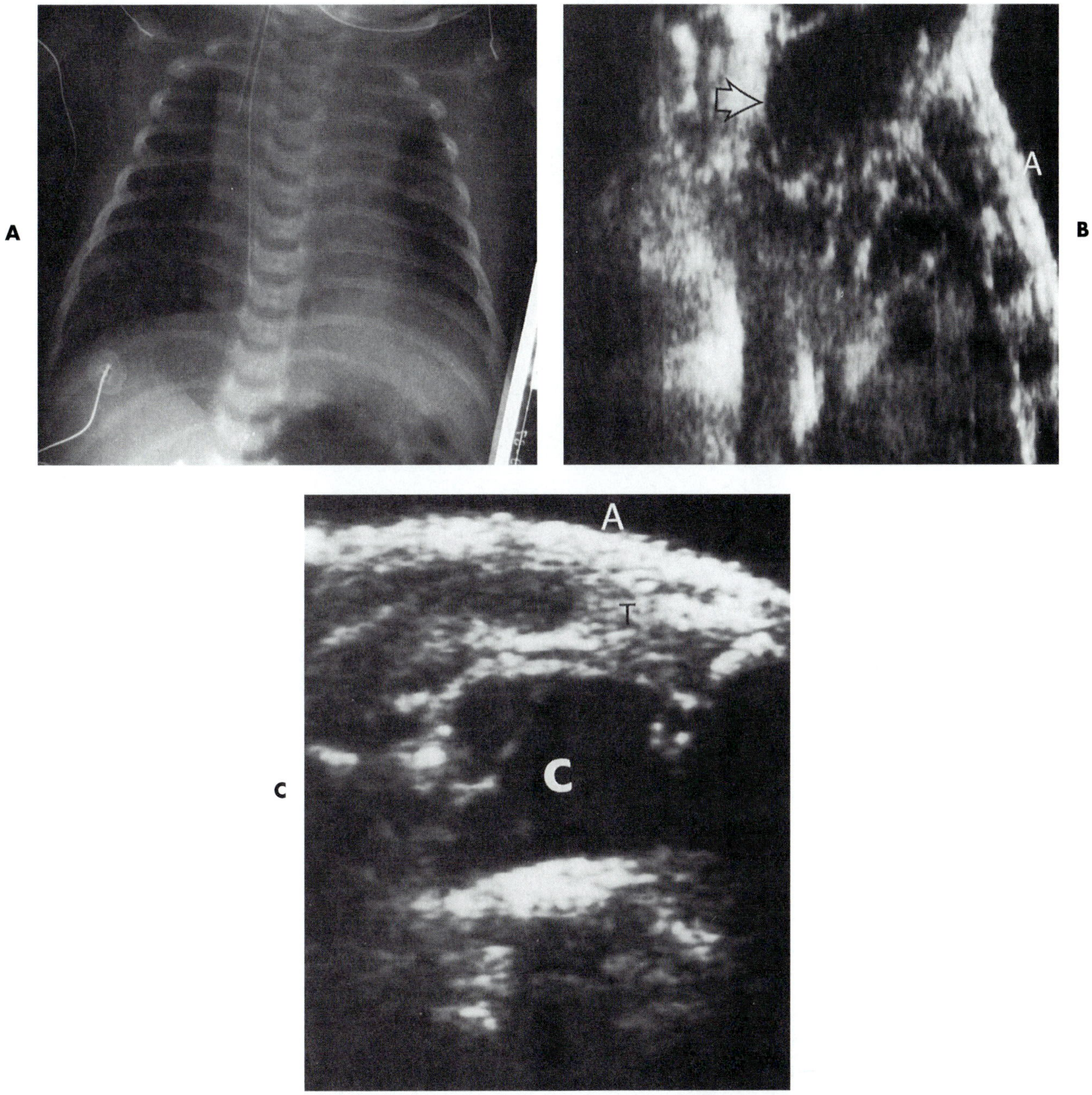

FIG. 57-20. Cystic hygroma extending into chest. **A,** Chest radiograph of neonate with large left neck mass that might extend into chest. **B,** Cystic hygroma extending into chest *(arrow)*. Longitudinal sonogram (turned anatomically) through upper neck and sternum. **C,** Transverse sonogram through the upper chest shows cystic hygroma, *C*, extending into chest behind thymus, *T*. *A*, Anterior chest wall.

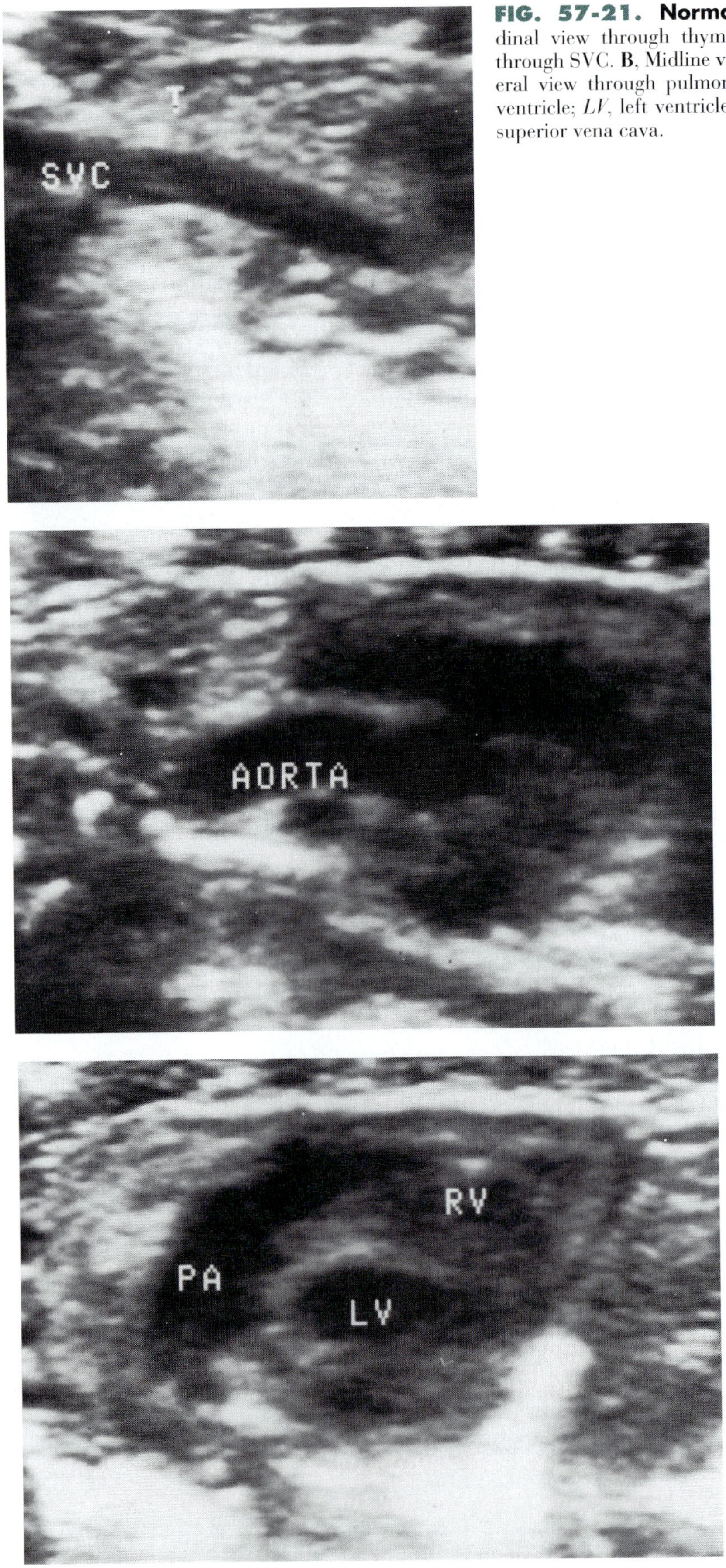

A

B

C

FIG. 57-21. Normal mediastinum. Longitudinal view through thymus, *T*. **A**, Right lateral view through SVC. **B**, Midline view through aorta. **C**, Left lateral view through pulmonary outflow tract. *RV*, Right ventricle; *LV*, left ventricle; *PA*, pulmonary artery; *SVC*, superior vena cava.

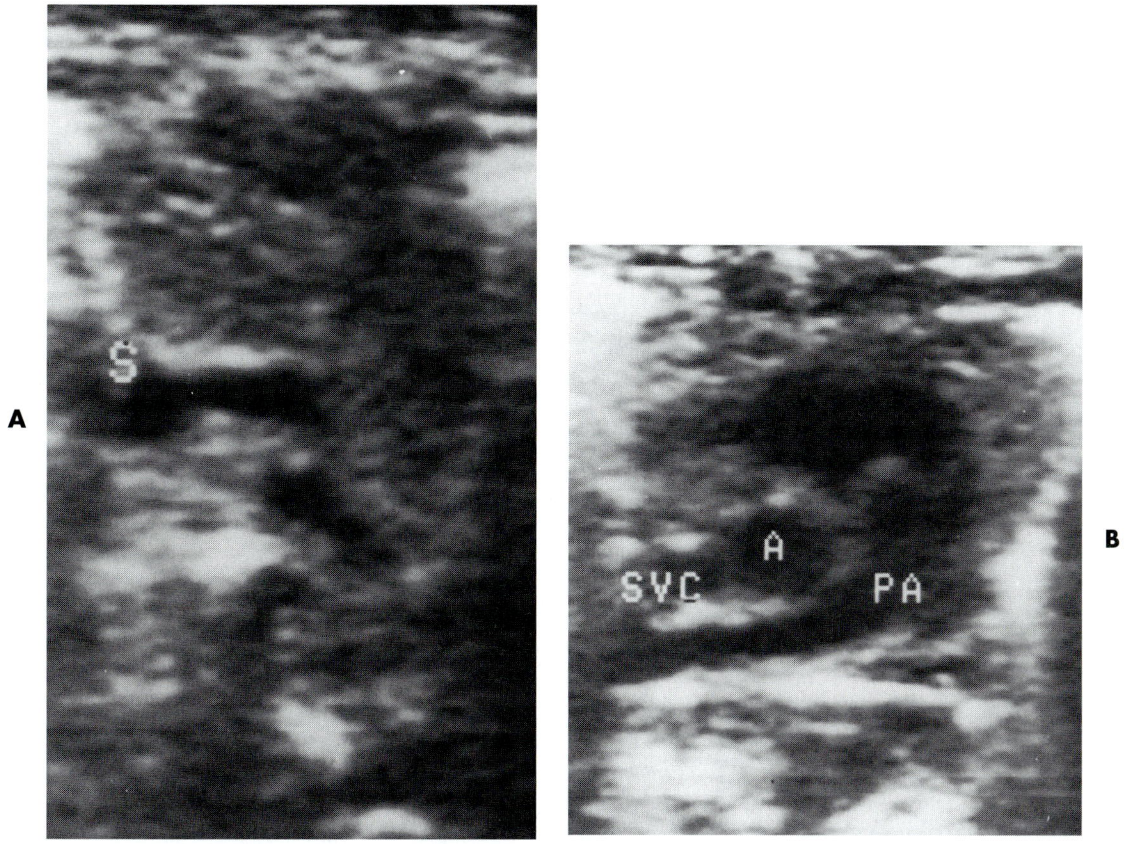

FIG. 57-22. Normal mediastinum, transverse view. **A,** Superior plane with innominate vein running through thymus to superior vena cava, *S*. **B,** Inferior plane through superior vena cava, *SVC*, aorta, *A*, and pulmonary artery, *PA*.

Suprasternal sonography can also be useful for detecting small and large mediastinal masses, particularly lymphoma in both children and adults.[23-26] When evaluating the mediastinum, one should **always try to include in the field of view a major blood vessel or cardiac chamber for direct comparison of the echogenicity of the mass** with that of the great vessels. Otherwise, the operator is tempted to turn down the gain controls because of the highly echogenic adjacent lung. This will give the mass a hypoechoic appearance when it may be more solid (see Fig. 57-7).[14]

EXTRACARDIAC CHEST MASSES

Chest sonography is also an excellent way to evaluate chest masses outside of the mediastinum if they are adjacent to the pleura or to an acoustic window such as the liver or spleen.[27-29] Any patient with persistent pleural fluid not responding to drainage should be evaluated by ultrasound for a **possible underlying tumor** (Figs. 57-23 and 57-24). It is important to compare the echogenicity of the mass with adjacent structures such as the liver, spleen, or heart. Ultrasound has three distinct advantages over CT in these instances—besides its ability to visualize masses in the sagittal or longitudinal plane, it also can often visualize masses adjacent to the diaphragm more clearly than can CT. Doppler imaging may be helpful in evaluating whether a chest mass is vascular in origin.[29] Doppler spectral analysis has also proven useful in distinguishing between benign and malignant chest masses.[30] Malignant chest masses will demonstrate a low-impedance, high-diastolic-flow Doppler signal.

Sonography is particularly valuable in **evaluating a paradiaphragmatic mass,** which may be an eventration of the diaphragm, a diaphragmatic hernia (Figs. 57-25 and 57-26), or an intrathoracic kidney.[31] Ultrasound is helpful in this situation because the infant may be experiencing respiratory compromise, and the bedside portable technique of sonography makes it the study of choice. Ultrasound may also be useful in the diagnosis of pulmonary sequestration[32-34] by demonstrating an echogenic mass with an abnormally enlarged vessel from the abdominal or thoracic aorta to it.[35] Chest sonography may also demonstrate that the mass has the appearance typical of the air seen on air bronchogram of a parenchymal lesion (Fig. 57-27).

Text continued on p. 1640.

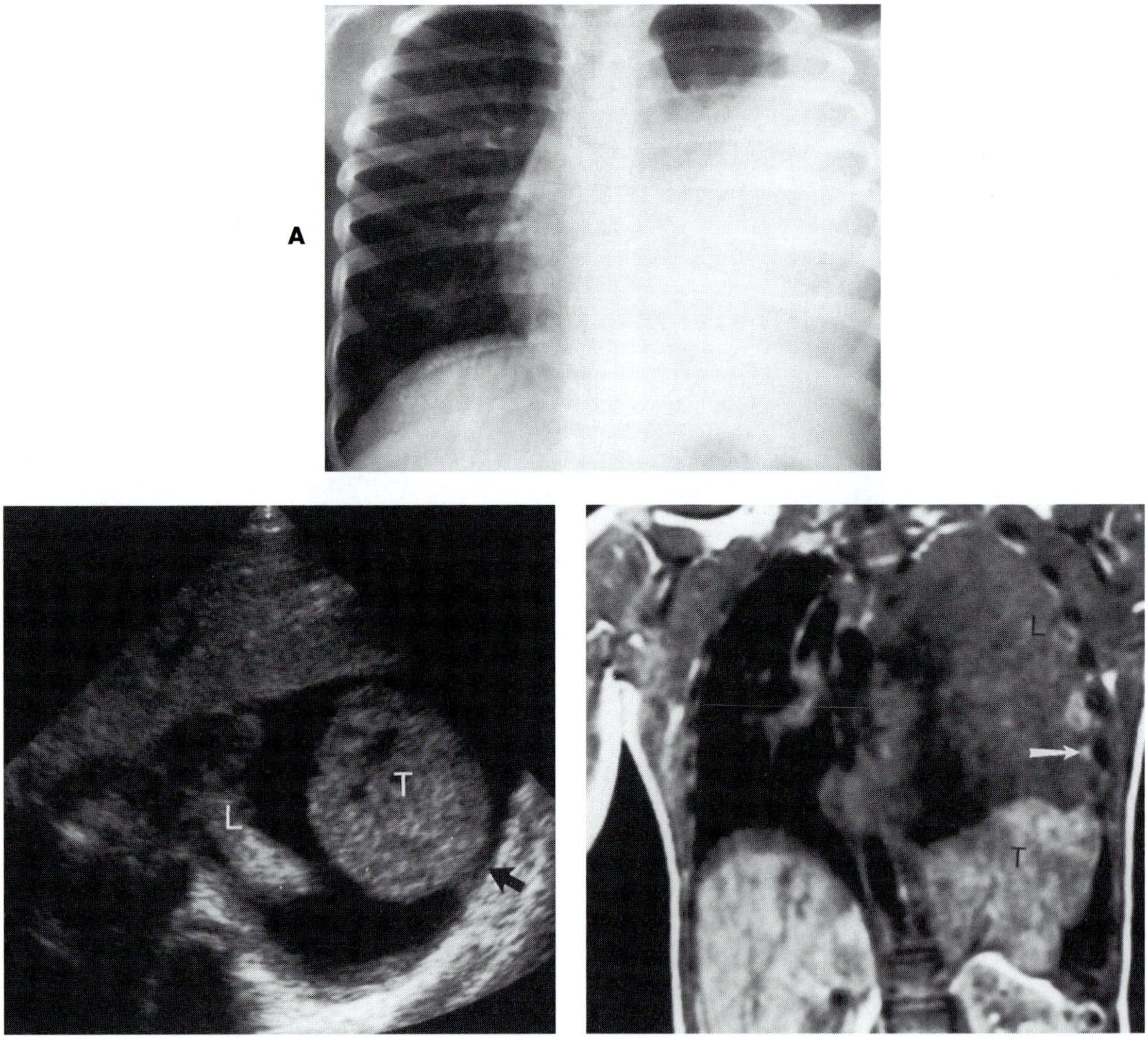

FIG. 57-23. Mesothelioma. **A,** Radiograph of young girl with opacified left chest. **B,** Transverse left side of chest sonogram and, **C,** MRI shows fluid with multiple echogenic pleural nodules *(arrow)*. *T,* Tumor; *L,* lung.

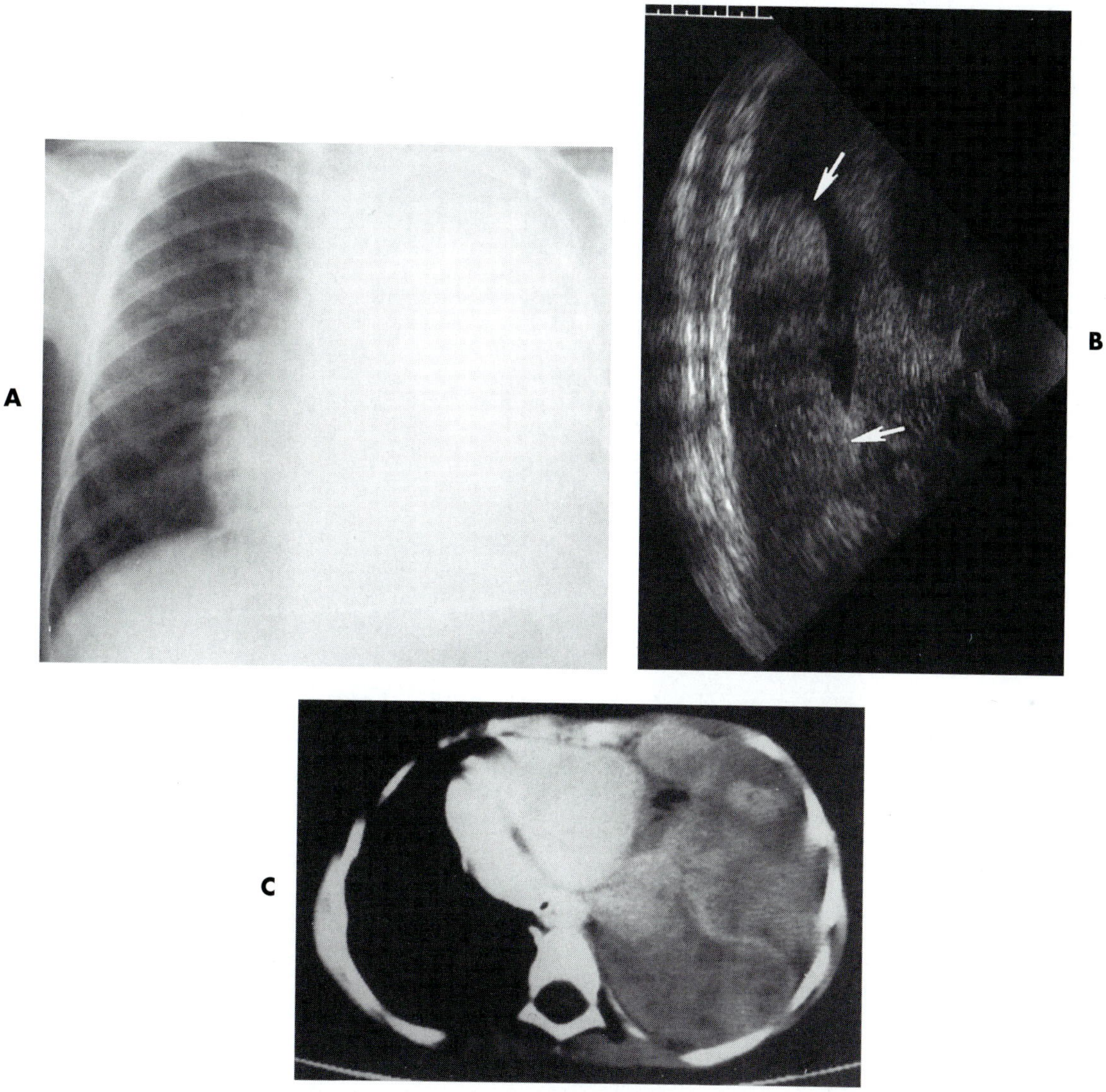

FIG. 57-24. Metastatic lung disease from Wilms' tumor in 7-year-old boy. **A,** Chest radiograph shows opaque left hemithorax with mediastinal shift to right. **B,** Longitudinal left chest sonogram (turned to compare with chest radiograph film) shows pleural fluid surrounding consolidated lung with multiple, echogenic, pleural, metastatic densities *(arrows)*. **C,** CT of thorax shows massive pleural and parenchymal metastases and malignant effusion that was surgically proven.

A

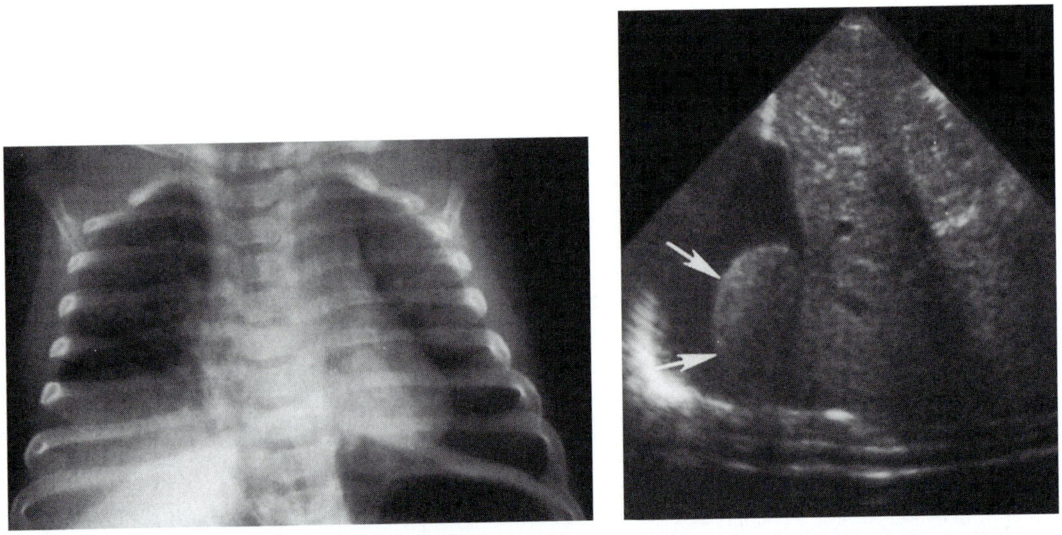

B

FIG. 57-25. Diaphragmatic hernia in 3-month-old child with right chest mass and history of cough and fever. **A,** Posteroanterior and chest radiograph shows increased density in right lung base and elevation of right hemidiaphragm. **B,** Longitudinal sonogram of right chest (turned to compare with chest radiograph film) shows posterior portion of liver herniating into chest *(arrows)*. Anechoic space was a fluid-filled sac surrounding herniated liver at surgery. (From Glasier CM, Leithiser RE Jr, Williamson SL et al. Extracardiac chest ultrasonography in infants and children: radiographic and clinical implications. *J Pediatr* 1989;114(4):540-544.)

A

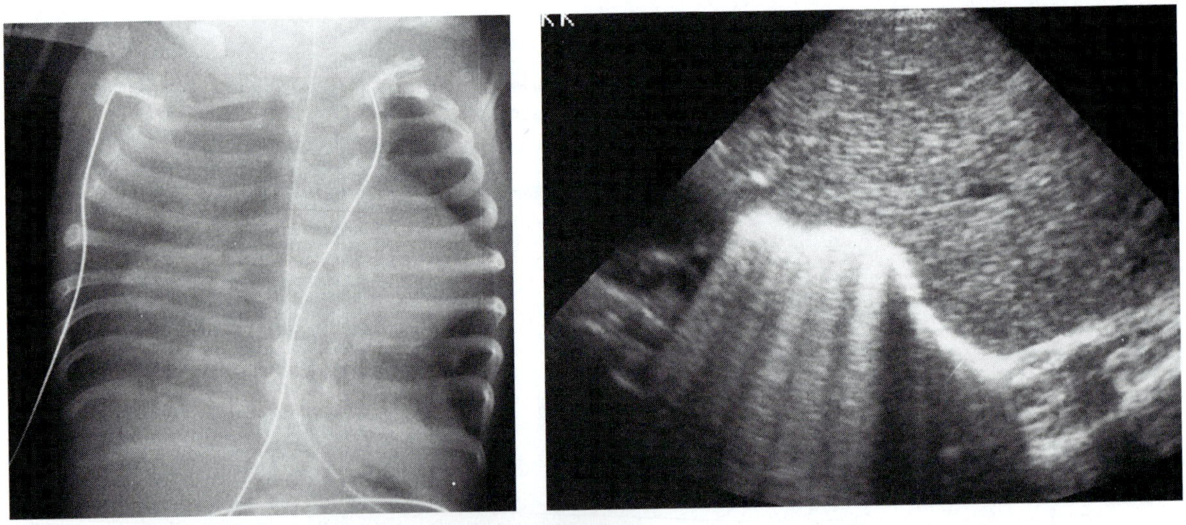

B

C

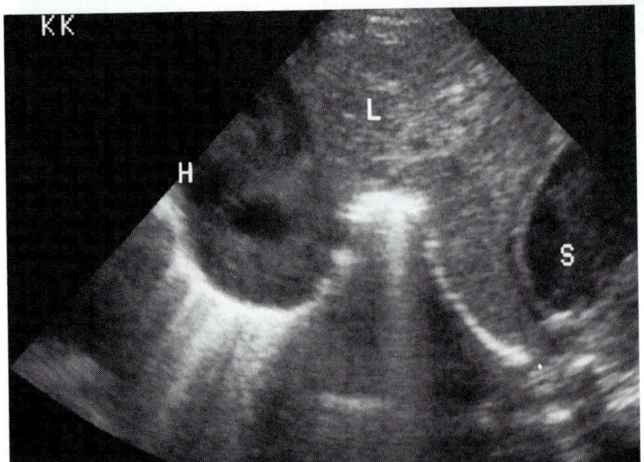

FIG. 57-26. Morgagni's hernia. **A,** Anteroposterior radiograph of the chest demonstrates a mass adjacent to the heart on the right. **B,** Longitudinal scan over the liver demonstrates liver extending into the chest. **C,** Transverse midine scan over the lower chest demonstrates liver extending into the chest between the heart and stomach.

A

B

C

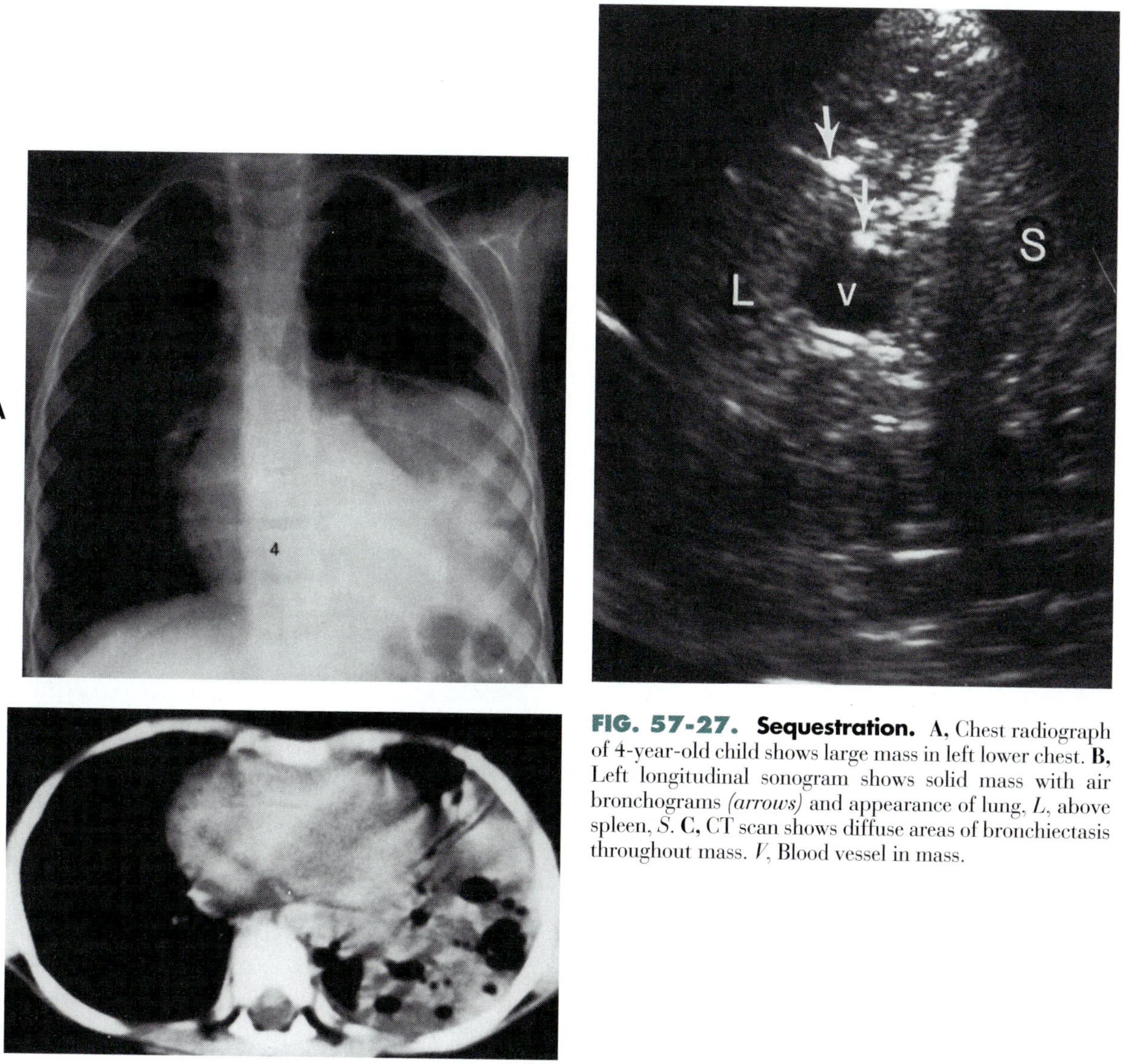

FIG. 57-27. Sequestration. A, Chest radiograph of 4-year-old child shows large mass in left lower chest. **B,** Left longitudinal sonogram shows solid mass with air bronchograms *(arrows)* and appearance of lung, *L*, above spleen, *S*. **C,** CT scan shows diffuse areas of bronchiectasis throughout mass. *V*, Blood vessel in mass.

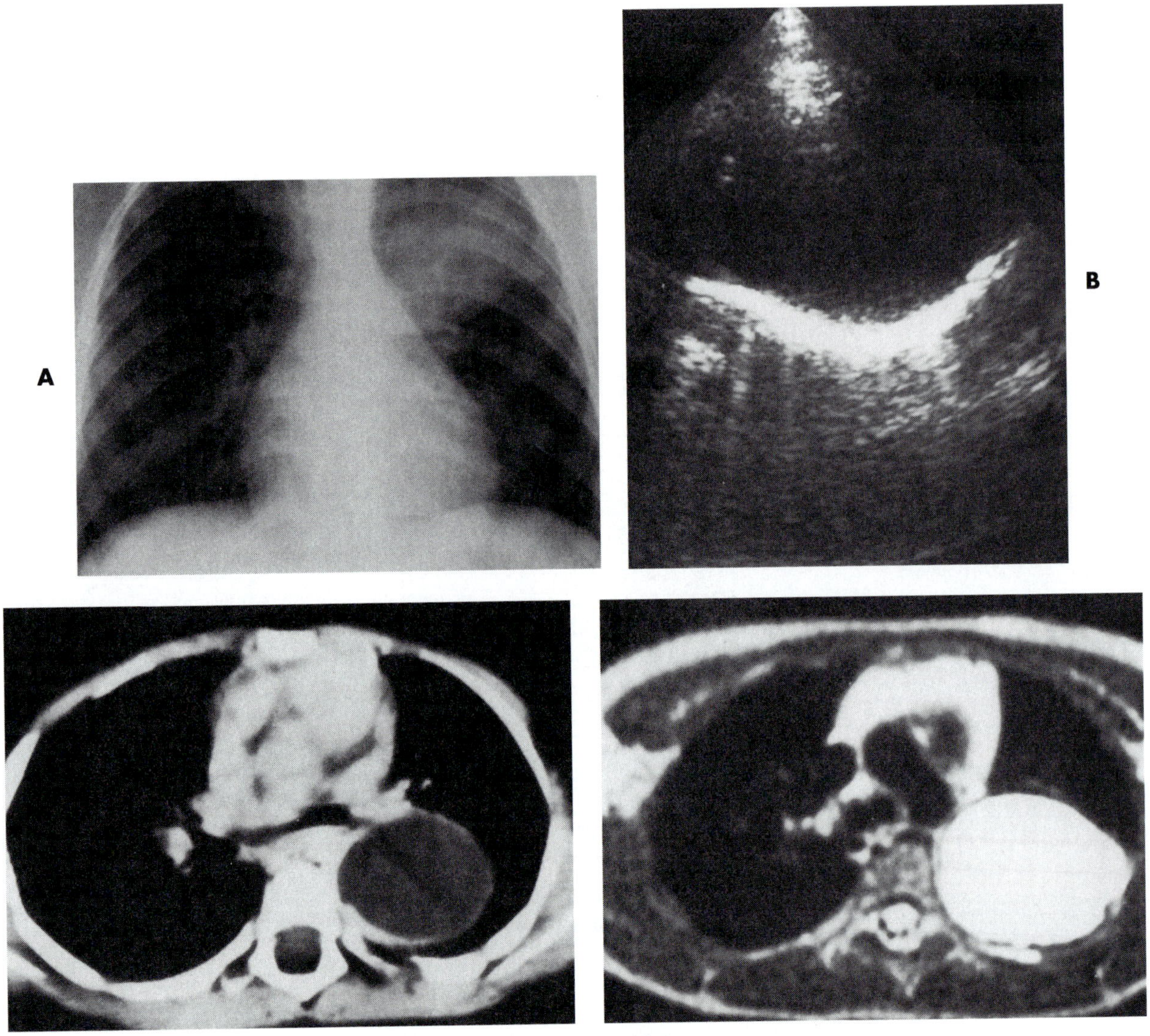

FIG. 57-28. Bronchopulmonary foregut malformation (duplication cyst). **A,** Posteroanterior radiograph shows round mass in left upper lung. **B,** Posterior sonogram shows fluid-filled cyst with "back-wall enhancement." **C,** CT and, **D,** MRI show fluid-filled chest mass.

Multiple cysts within the dysplastic lung of pulmonary sequestration have been demonstrated by ultrasound.[34] These cystic structures have likewise been described with cystadenomatoid malformation.[36] Bronchogenic cysts or **bronchopulmonary foregut malformations** may similarly be identified by chest ultrasound if they are adjacent to the chest wall (Fig. 57-28).[37] Other diaphragmatic structures, such as localized eventration, loculated fluid, subphrenic abscesses, pericardial cysts, and pericardial fat pads, can also be visualized adjacent to the diaphragm using the liver or spleen as a window.

Chest wall masses may be evaluated by sonography.[38-40] In particular, ultrasound may be used to demonstrate the soft-tissue swelling associated with osteomyelitis of the ribs. The ultrasound demonstration of thickening around the ribs may be the first sign of periosteal edema associated with early osteomyelitis before the radiographic changes of bone destruction are present.[38]

SONOGRAPHIC-GUIDED ASPIRATION/ BIOPSY OF PULMONARY LESIONS

Sonography is an excellent method for localization before aspiration of pleural fluid and biopsy of chest wall lesions.[41-44] Ultrasound can be used to mark the position of fluid, and the needle can be visualized during the procedure using ultrasound guidance if necessary. **Marking for fluid aspiration** is usually

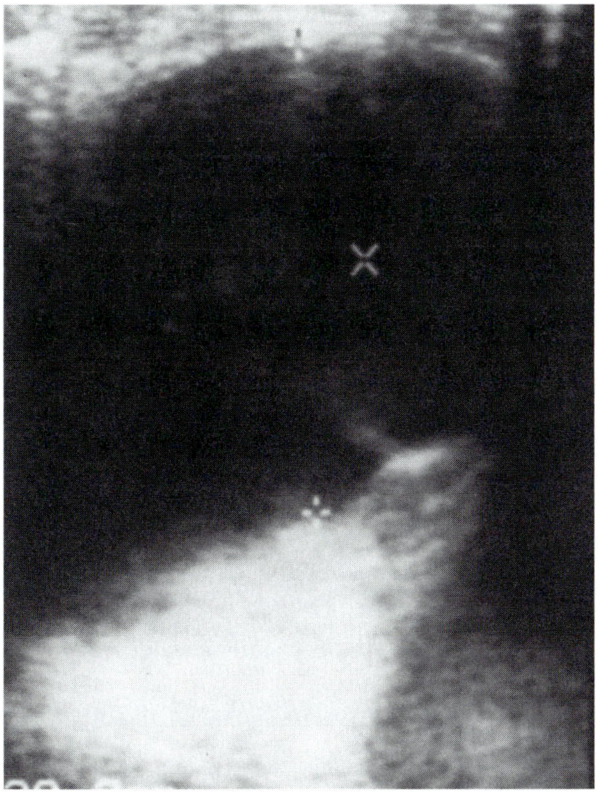

FIG. 57-29. Streptococcal pneumonia in 18-month-old child with fluid containing no debris. Cursor marks depth to which fluid extends. Thoracentesis yielded copious straw-colored fluid. (From Glasier CM, Leithiser RE Jr, Williamson SL et al. Extracardiac chest ultrasonography in infants and children: radiographic and clinical implications. *J Pediatr* 1989;114(4):540-544.)

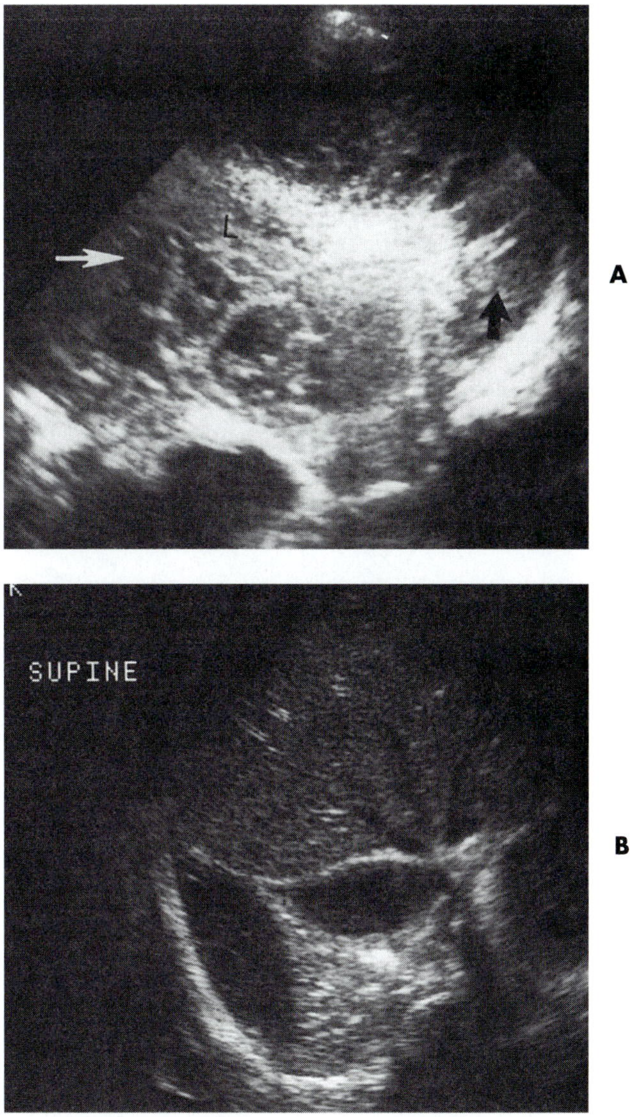

FIG. 57-30. Empyema requiring surgical decortication. A, Patient with sickle cell anemia and pneumonia with very thick fluid *(black arrow)* surrounding lung, *L*, with multiple loculations. Thick, putty rind was found at surgery. Lung also initially appeared to have intraparenchyma abscesses *(white arrow)* when patient underwent transverse scanning through intercostal space in upright position. **B,** When patient underwent scanning in supine position using liver as window to angle into chest, it was obvious that there was no parenchymal abscess but only empyema surrounding lung, *L*.

done with the patient in the upright position at the bedside (Fig. 57-29). Ultrasound is particularly helpful in determining whether the pleural effusion will respond to simple drainage or will require surgical decortication.[45] If the fluid is relatively anechoic or clear, simple drainage with thoracentesis or chest tube drainage is an adequate treatment. If the fluid is **thick with multiple septations** (Fig. 57-30), and if the patient does not respond promptly to antibiotic therapy, decortication may be recommended.

On sonography what appears to be an intraparenchymal abscess may be empyema surrounding the lung. Changing the patient's position and the viewing planes may distinguish an **empyema from a parenchymal abscess** (see Fig. 57-29). An abscess should be visualized in two planes.

Ultrasound has also proven useful in the evaluation of pulmonary consolidation. It can be used for needle aspiration guidance for etiologic diagnosis in patients with complicated pneumonia as well as aspiration of microabscesses in necrotizing pneumonia.[46]

Sonography promises also to be a method of detecting pneumothoraces after thoracentesis.[47] Before and after thoracentesis, the ipsilateral pulmonary apex and adjacent lung should be examined in the upright position for normal pleural respiratory movement. If the pleural respiratory motion is absent, then a pneumothorax should be suspected.[47]

DIAPHRAGM

Sonography has become an excellent imaging modality for the evaluation of **juxtadiaphragmatic masses.** Ultrasound has also become the bedside examination of choice for evaluation of suspected **abnormalities of diaphragmatic motion.**[48-50] Real-time sonography is the only imaging procedure that can simultaneously evaluate the paradiaphragmatic spaces, the hemidiaphragms, and their motion.

When the transducer is placed in the subxiphoid position in a transverse orientation and angled upward toward the posterior leaflets of the hemidiaphragms, motion on the sides can be compared (Fig. 57-31). Such comparison can be done with transverse sonographic scanning in infants, but in older children, unilateral

A B C

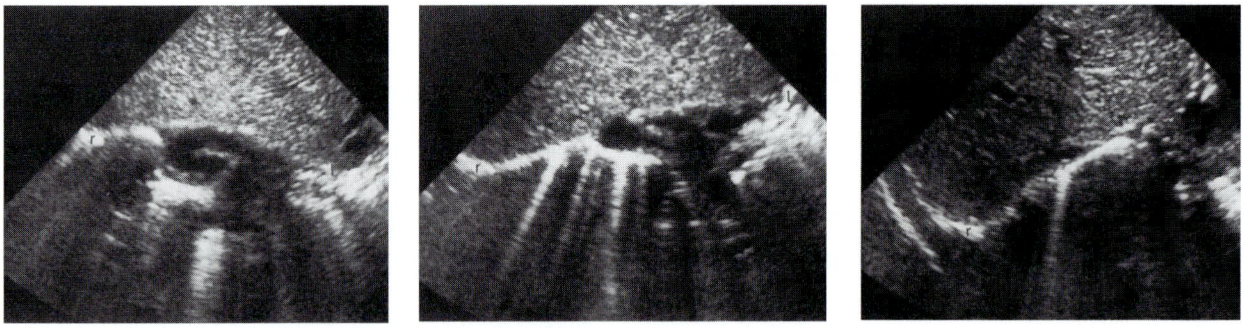

FIG. 57-31. Paralyzed left diaphragm. Note change in position and shape of hemidiaphragm, *R*, on **A, B,** and **C,** but no change on left.

A B

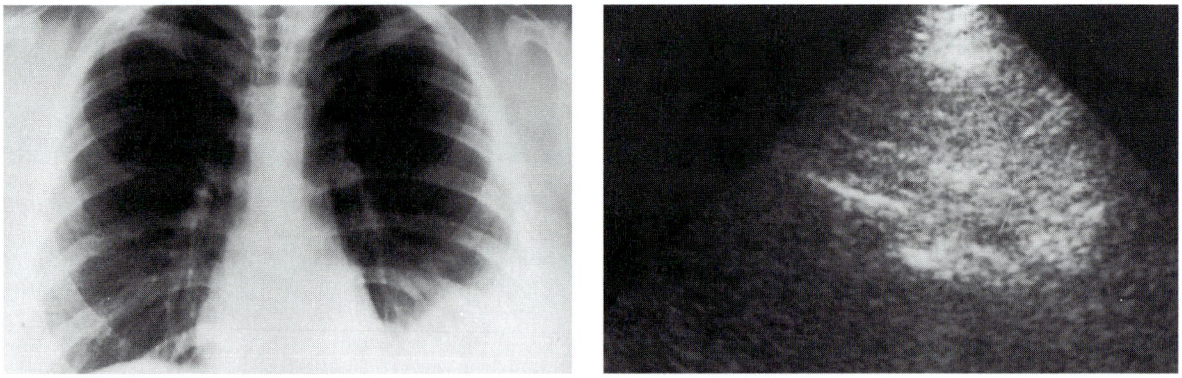

C

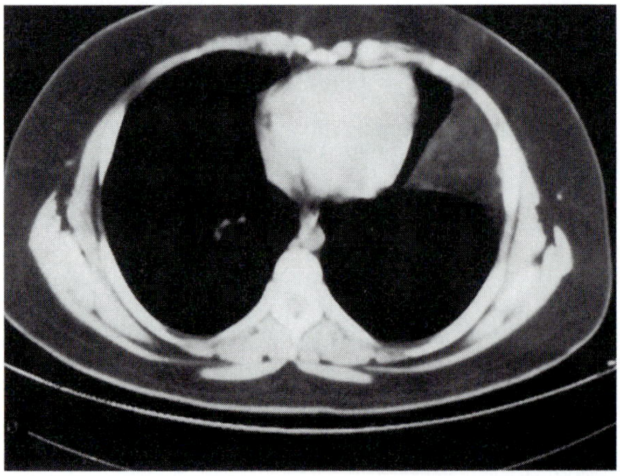

FIG. 57-32. Intrathoracic fat with traumatic rupture of diaphragm. **A,** Chest radiograph shows round mass in left lower lung adjacent to left cardiophrenic border. **B,** Transverse sonogram shows echogenic mass. **C,** CT shows mass with fat density. During chest-tube drainage of empyema 4 years earlier, chest tube had ruptured through diaphragm, and omental fat filled defect at surgery.

sagittal scanning of each diaphragm will be necessary. A comparison of the maximal excursion of the diaphragm for each side has proven even more accurate than fluoroscopy in demonstrating diaphragmatic movement abnormality.[51] If the patient is using artificial ventilation, the respirator must be disconnected for approximately 5 to 10 seconds to observe unassisted respiration. With paralysis, there is typically absent or paradoxical motion on one side, with exaggerated excursions on the opposite side. However, severe eventration and a diaphragmatic hernia may also show this paradoxical motion. In addition, sonography can be used to demonstrate **rupture of the diaphragm** (Fig. 57-32).[50]

POTENTIAL USES OF CHEST SONOGRAPHY

Sonography can often be used to detect the **endotracheal tube position** in intubated children and adults.[52,53] In theory, this technique can replace chest radiographs ordered only for tube position and therefore can reduce the exposure of infants to radiation. The nonintubated airway produces a broken, linear, dense echo whereas the endotracheal tube produces a continuous linear density. The distal tip of the tube can be reliably identified when motion is produced by a gentle oscillation of the tube tip up and down in the airway. Optimum tube position is obtained when the tip is 1 cm above the aortic arch. In practice it is difficult to justify the time spent in the nursery when sonography is needed for other diagnostic problems that will not be solved by a chest film.

Another possible use of chest sonography in the neonate is in the diagnosis of **hyaline membrane disease.**[54] Infants with hyaline membrane disease display a specific sonographic pattern with retrohepatic hyperechogenicity on abdominal ultrasound. The pattern is thought to represent an ultrasound artifact of a summation of multiple aerated airways surrounded by collapsed alveoli.

REFERENCES

Indications for Chest Sonography

1. Ablin DS, Newell JD II. Diagnostic imaging for evaluation of the pediatric chest. *Clin Chest Med* 1987;8(4):641-660.

Sonographic Signs of Pleural Fluid

2. Simeone JF, Mueller PR, vanSonnenberg E. The uses of diagnostic ultrasound in the thorax. *Clin Chest Med* 1984;5(2):281-290.
3. Kohan JM, Poe RH, Israel RH, et al. Value of chest ultrasonography versus decubitus roentgenography for thoracentesis. *Am Rev Respir Dis* 1986;133:1124-1126.
4. Halvorsen RA Jr, Thompson WM. Ascites or pleural effusion? CT and ultrasound differentiation. *CRC Crit Rev Diagn Imag* 1986;26(3):210-240.
5. Laing FC, Filly RA. Problems in the application of ultrasonography for the evaluation of pleural opacities. *Radiology* 1978;126:211-214.
6. Marks WM, Filly RA, Callen PW. Real-time evaluation of pleural lesions: new observations regarding the probability of obtaining free fluid. *Radiology* 1982;142:163-164.
7. Wu RG, Yang PC, Kuo SH et al. A fluid color sign: a useful indicator for discrimination between pleural thickening and pleural effusion. *J Ultrasound Med* 1995;14:767-769.
8. Wu RG, Yuan A, Liaw YS et al. Image comparison of real-time gray-scale ultrasound and color Doppler ultrasound for use in diagnosis of minimal pleural effusion. *Am J Resp Crit Care Med* 1994;150:510-514.
9. Baron RL, Lee JKT, Melson GL. Sonographic evaluation of right juxtadiaphragmatic masses in children using trans-hepatic approach. *J Clin Ultrasound* 1980;8(2):156-159.
10. Rosenberg HK. The complementary roles of ultrasound and plain film radiography in differentiating pediatric chest abnormalities. *RadioGraphics* 1986;6(3):427-455.
11. Miller JH, Reid BS, Kemberling CR. Water-path ultrasound of chest disease in childhood. *Radiology* 1984;152:401-408.
12. Haller JO, Schneider M, Kassner EG et al. Sonographic evaluation of the chest in infants and children. *AJR* 1980;134:1019-1027.
13. Bedi DG, Fagan CJ, Hayden CK Jr. The opaque right hemithorax: identifying the diaphragm with ultrasound. *Tex Med* 1985;81:37-42.
14. Goddard P. Indications for ultrasound of the chest. *J Thorac Imag* 1985;1(1):899-997.

Lung Parenchyma

15. Weinberg B, Diakoumakis EE, Seife B, et al. The air bronchogram: sonographic demonstration. *AJR* 1986;147:595-598.
16. Dorne HL. Differentiation of pulmonary parenchymal consolidation from pleural disease using the sonographic fluid bronchogram. *Radiology* 1986;158:41-42.
17. Seibert RW, Seibert JJ, Williamson SL. The opaque chest: when to suspect a bronchial foreign body. *Pediatr Radiol* 1986;16:193-196.
18. Erasmie U, Lundell B. Pulmonary lesions mimicking pericardial effusion on ultrasonography. *Pediatr Radiol* 1987;17:447-450.

Mediastinum

19. Han BK, Babcock DS, Oestreich AE. Normal thymus in infancy: sonographic characteristics. *Radiology* 1989;170:471-474.
20. Babcock DS. Sonographic evaluation of suspected pediatric vascular diseases. *Pediatr Radiol* 1991;21:486-489.
21. Hammerli M, Meyer RA. Doppler evaluation of central venous lines in the superior vena cava. *J Pediatr* 1993;122(6):S104-S108.
22. Lemaitre L, Arconi V, Avni F, et al. The sonographic evaluation of normal thymus in infants and children. *Eur J Radiol* 1987;7:130-136.
23. Wernecke K, Peters PE, Galanski M. Mediastinal tumors: evaluation with suprasternal sonography. *Radiology* 1986;159:405-409.
24. Claus D, Coppens JP. Sonography of mediastinal masses in infants and children. *Ann Radiol* 1984;27(2/3):150-159.
25. Ries T, Currarino G, Nikaidoh H, et al. Real-time ultrasonography of subcarinal bronchogenic cysts in two children. *Radiology* 1982;145:121-122.
26. Marx MV, Cunningham JJ. Sonographic findings in mediastinal embryonal carcinoma. *J Ultrasound Med* 1986;5:41-43.

Extracardiac Chest Masses

27. Glasier CM, Leithiser RE Jr, Williamson SL, et al. Extracardiac chest ultrasonography in infants and children: radiographic and clinical implications. *J Pediatr* 1989;114(4):540-544.
28. Hudson TD, Lesar M, Blei L. Ultrasound diagnosis of a middle mediastinal mass. *J Clin Ultrasound* 1982;10:183-185.
29. O'Laughlin MP, Huhta JC, Murphy DJ Jr. Ultrasound examination of extracardiac chest masses in children: Doppler diagnosis of a vascular etiology. *J Ultrasound Med* 1987;6:151-157.
30. Yuan A, Chang D-B, Yu C-J, et al. Color Doppler sonography of benign and malignant pulmonary masses. *AJR* 1994;163:545-549.
31. Sumner TE, Volberg FM, Smolen PM. Intrathoracic kidney: diagnosis by ultrasound. *Pediatr Radiol* 1982;12:78-80.
32. West MS, Donaldson JS, Shkolnik A. Pulmonary sequestration: diagnosis by ultrasound. *J Ultrasound Med* 1989;8:125-129.
33. Kaude JV, Laurin S. Ultrasonographic demonstration of systemic artery feeding extrapulmonary sequestration. *Pediatr Radiol* 1984;14:226-227.
34. Thind CR, Pilling DW. Case report: pulmonary sequestration—the value of ultrasound. *Clin Radiol* 1985;36:437-439.
35. Smart LM, Hendry GMA. Imaging of neonatal pulmonary sequestration including Doppler ultrasound. *Br J Radiol* 1991;64:324-329.
36. Hartenberg MA, Brewer WH. Cystic adenomatoid malformation of the lung: identification by sonography. *AJR* 1983;140:693-694.
37. Rodgers BM, Harman PK, Johnson AM. Broncho-pulmonary foregut malformations: the spectrum of anomalies. *Ann Surg* 1986;203(5):517-524.
38. Bar-Ziv J, Barki Y, Maroko A, et al. Rib osteomyelitis in children: early radiologic and ultrasonic findings. *Pediatr Radiol* 1985;15:315-318.
39. Birnholz J. Chest wall and lung surface viewing with ultrasound. *Chest* 1988;94(6):1275-1276.
40. Dershaw DD. Actinomycosis of the chest wall: ultrasound findings in empyema necessitants. *Chest* 1984;86(5):779-780.

Sonographic-Guided Aspiration/Biopsy of Pulmonary Lesions

41. Yang PC, Luh KT, Sheu JC, et al. Peripheral pulmonary lesions: ultrasonography and ultrasonically guided aspiration biopsy. *Radiology* 1985;155:451-456.
42. Mace AH, Elyaderani MK. Ultrasonography in the diagnosis and management of empyema of the thorax. *South Med J* 1984;77(3):294-296.
43. Elyaderani MK, Gabriele OF. Aspiration of thoracic masses and fluid collections under guidance of ultrasonography. *South Med J* 1982;75(5):536-539.
44. Harnsberger HR, Lee TG, Mukuno DH. Rapid, inexpensive real-time directed thoracentesis. *Radiology* 1983;146:545-546.
45. Golladay ES, Wagner CW. Management of empyema in children. *Am J Surg* 1989;158:618-621.
46. Yang PC, Luh KT, Chang DB, et al. Ultrasonographic evaluation of pulmonary consolidation. *Am J Respir Dis* 1992;146:757-762.
47. Hashimoto BE, Hubler BE, Gass MA. Promising new application: ultrasound diagnosis of pneumothorax after thoracentesis. Presented at the Fortieth Annual Convention, American Institute of Ultrasound; May 17-20, 1996; New York City, NY.

Diaphragm

48. Diament MJ, Boechat MI, Kangarloo H. Real-time sector ultrasound in the evaluation of suspected abnormalities of diaphragmatic motion. *J Clin Ultrasound* 1985;13:539-543.
49. Oyen RH, Marchal GJ, Verschakelen JA et al. Sonographic aspect of hypertrophic diaphragmatic muscular bundles. *J Clin Ultrasound* 1984;12:121-123.
50. Ammann AM, Brewer WH, Maull KI et al. Traumatic rupture of the diaphragm: real-time sonographic diagnosis. *AJR* 1983;140:915-916.
51. Houston JG, Fleewt M, Cowan MD, et al. Comparison of ultrasound with fluoroscopy in the assessment of suspected hemidiaphragmatic movement abnormality. *Clin Radiol* 1995;50:95-98.

Potential Uses of Chest Sonography

52. Slovis TL, Poland RL. Endotracheal tubes in neonates: sonographic positioning. *Radiology* 1986;160:262-263.
53. Raphael DT, Conard FU III. Ultrasound confirmation of endotracheal tube placement. *J Clin Ultrasound* 1987;15:459-462.
54. Avni EF, Braude P, Pardou A et al. Hyaline membrane disease in the newborn: diagnosis by ultrasound. *Pediatr Radiol* 1990;20:143-146.

CHAPTER 58

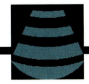

The Pediatric Liver and Spleen

Heidi B. Patriquin, M.D., F.R.C.P.(C)

CHAPTER OUTLINE

ANATOMY

The anatomy of the liver can be explored in many planes with sonography. The usual course of intrahepatic vessels and their normal variants can be traced. There is a simple sonographic approach to the segmental anatomy of the liver based on the nomenclature of the French surgeon Couinaud,[1,2] who described the segments according to the distribution of the portal and hepatic veins. Each segment has a branch (or a group of branches) of the portal vein at its center and a hepatic vein at its periphery. Each lobe of the liver contains four segments; the segments are numbered counterclockwise: 1 through 4 comprising the left lobe and 5 through 8 the right. Segment 1 is the caudate or Spiegel lobe. The right and left lobes are separated by the main hepatic fissure, a line connecting the gallbladder and the left side of the inferior vena cava (IVC) (Fig. 58-1).[2]

The segmental branches of the portal vein (each one of which leads into a segment) can be outlined in the form of two Hs turned sideways, one for the left lobe (segments 1 through 4) and one for the right lobe (segments 5 through 8) (Fig. 58-2).

Portal Vein Anatomy

Left Lobe of Liver. The H of the left lobe is visualized with an oblique, upwardly tilted subxiphoid view. The H is formed by the left portal vein, the branch entering segment 2, the umbilical portion of the left portal vein, and the branches to segments 3 and 4 (Fig. 58-2). To this recumbent H are attached two ligaments, the ligamentum venosum (also called

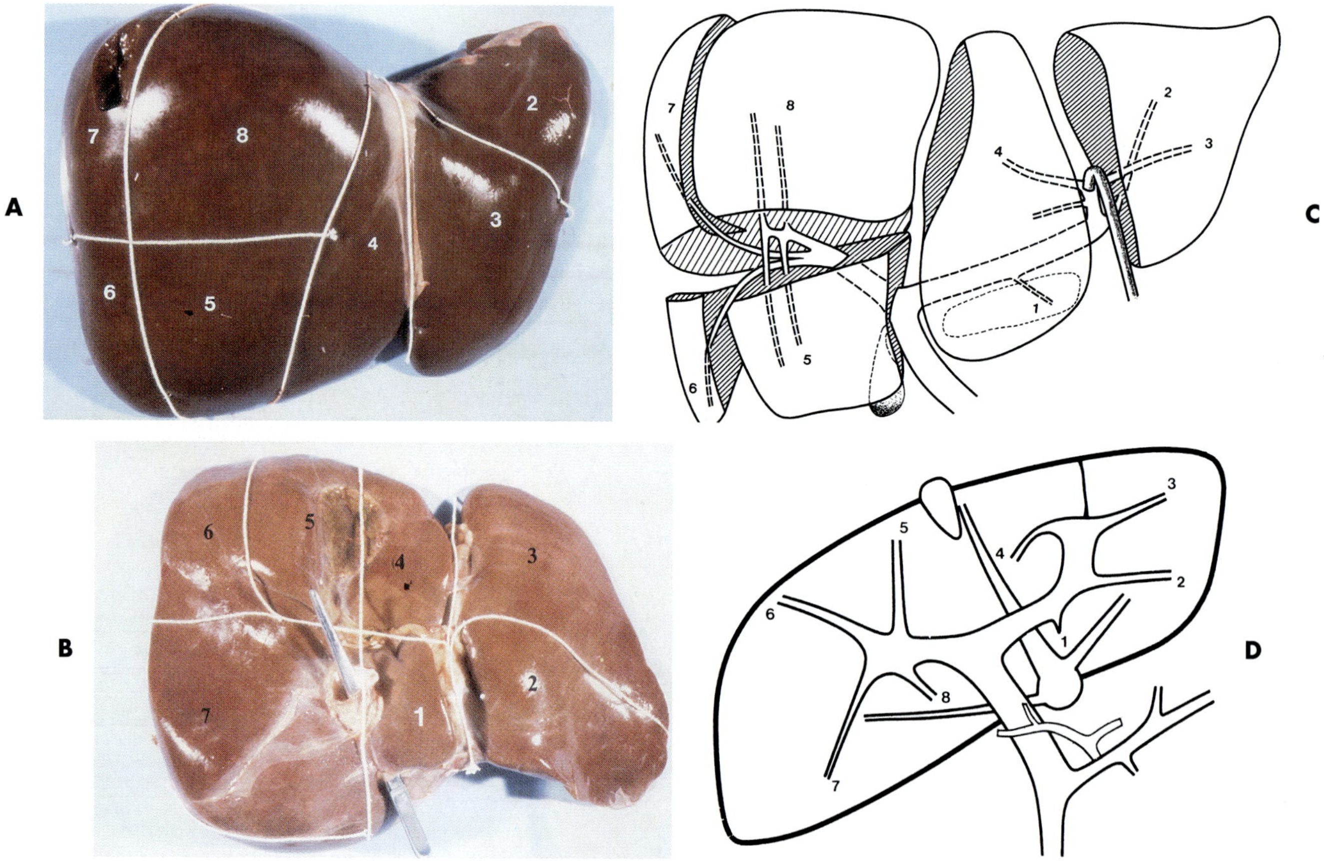

FIG. 58-1. External segmental anatomy of the liver.[2] Segments are numbered in a counterclockwise direction. Their borders are marked with string. **A,** Upper and anterior surface: note the whitish falciform ligament that separates segments 3 and 4. **B,** Lower surface: the forceps are in the main portal vein; the gallbladder has been removed from its bed, which separates segments 4 and 5. The vertical string between segments 4 and 5 and between 1 and 7 follows the gallbladder-middle hepatic vein axis and marks the main hepatic fissure, the division between right and left lobes. Segment 1, the caudate lobe, is to the right of the forceps. Segments 3 and 4 are separated by the falciform ligament; 1 and 2 by the ligamentum venosum. **C,** Schema of the hepatic segments with their portal venous branches upper, anterior, viewed as A. **D,** Diagram of the portal and hepatic veins and their relationship to the segments (lower liver surface, viewed as B). (From Lafortune M et al. *Radiology* 1991;181:443-448.)

the lesser omentum or the hepatogastric ligament) and the falciform ligament. The ligamentum venosum separates segment 1 from segment 2 (Figs. 58-1, *B* and 58-2, *A*). The falciform ligament is seen between the umbilical portion of the left portal vein[1] and the outer surface of the liver (Figs. 58-1, *A*, *B* and 58-2, *A*, *C*). It separates segment 3 from segment 4.

Segment 1 (the caudate lobe) is bordered posteriorly by the IVC, laterally by the ligamentum venosum, and anteriorly by the left portal vein (Fig. 58-1, *B*). Unlike the other segments of the liver, it may receive branches of the left and right portal veins. The portal veins to segment 1 are usually small and are rarely seen sonographically. The caudate lobe has one or more hepatic veins that drain directly into the IVC, separately from the three main hepatic veins.[3] This special vascularization is a distinctive characteristic of segment 1.

The portal vein leading to segment 2 is a linear continuation of the left portal vein, completing the lower horizontal limb of the H. Segmental branches to segments 3 and 4 form the other horizontal limb (Fig. 58-2). Segments 2 and 3 are thus located to the left of the umbilical portion of the left portal vein, the ligamentum venosum, and the falciform ligament. Segment 4 (the quadrate lobe) is situated around the right anterior limb of the portal venous H, to the right of the umbilical portion of the left portal vein and the falciform ligament (Fig. 58-2). Segment 4 is separated from segment 5 by the main fissure (a line between the neck of the gallbladder and the IVC) (Fig. 58-1, *B*) and from 5 and 8 by the middle hepatic vein. It is separated from segment 1 by the left portal vein.

Right Lobe of Liver. The right portal vein and its branches are best seen with a sagittal or oblique mid-

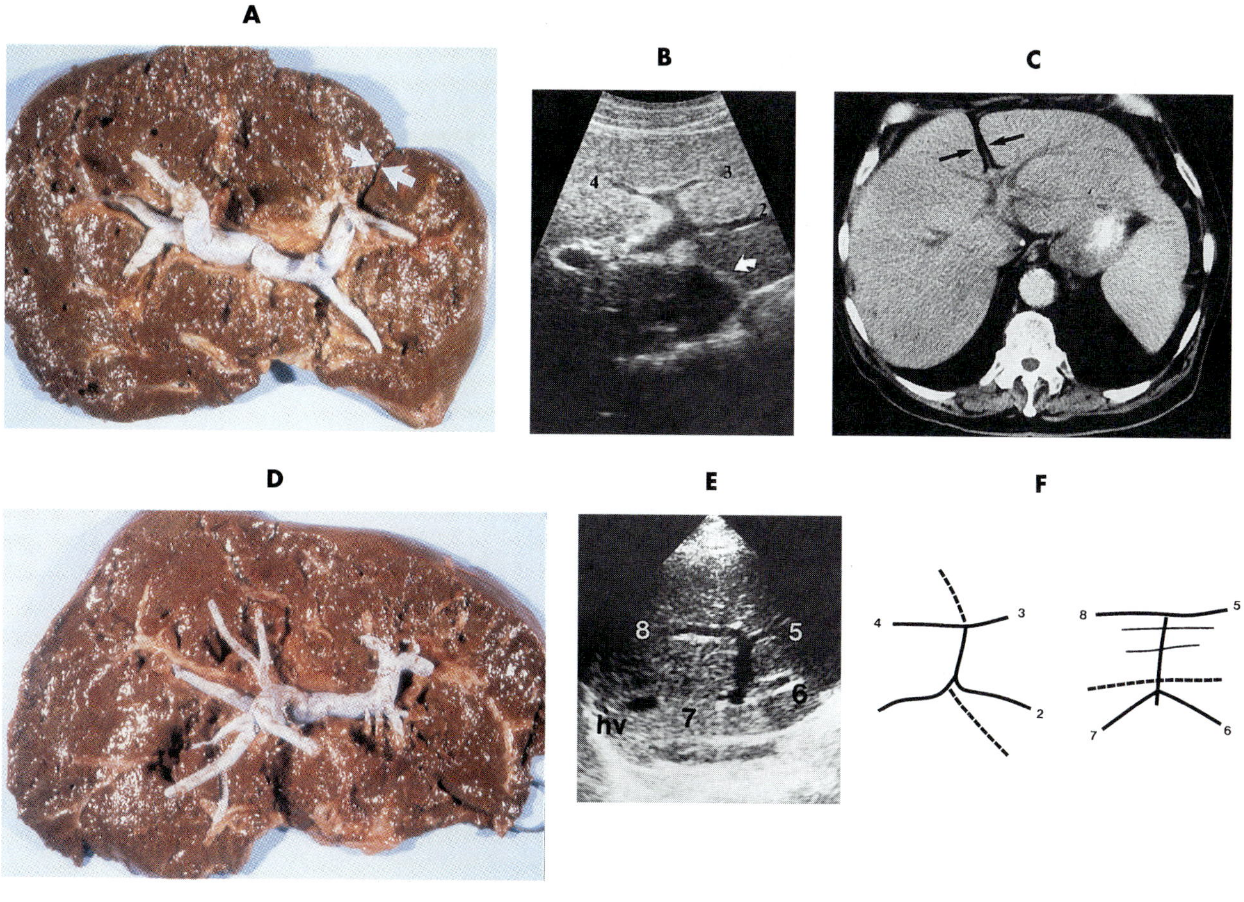

FIG. 58-2. Anatomy of the segmental portal veins (PVs): one H for each lobe. **A,** Left lobe, shown on a dissected specimen (with pale blue dye in the portal vein), **B,** on a subxiphoid transverse sonogram, and **C,** on computed tomography. The left portal vein, with branches to segments 2, 3, and 4, forms a horizontally placed H. The umbilical portion of the left PV forms the crossbar of the H. Falciform ligament (*arrows*) is an extension of the umbilical part of the left PV. Ligamentum venosum (*curved arrow*). **D,** Right hepatic lobe of a dissected specimen and **E,** on a sagittal-oblique, intercostal sonogram obtained at the midaxillary line. PV branches to segments 5 through 8 and 6 and 7 form the main limbs of the H, and the right PV forms its crossbar. Once again the H is turned horizontally. **F,** Diagram of the PV branches to the left and right lobes. (From Bismuth H. Surgical anatomy and anatomical surgery of the liver. *World J Surg* 1982:6:3-9.)

axillary intercostal approach. In some subjects, a subcostal approach is also useful. The right portal vein follows an oblique or vertical course, directed anteriorly.

The branches leading to the segments of the right lobe of the liver are also distributed in the shape of a sideways H. The right portal vein forms the crossbar of the H. The branches to segments 5 and 8 form the upper limb of the H (Fig. 58-2), while the branches to segments 6 and 7 form its lower portion. The branches of segments 6 and 7 are more obliquely oriented, and the transducer should be rotated slightly upward for segment 7 and downward in the direction of the right kidney for segment 6.

The middle hepatic vein separates segments 5 and 8 from segment 4. The right hepatic vein separates segments 5 and 8 from the segments 6 and 7 (Fig. 58-3).

Segment 5 is bordered medially by the gallbladder and the middle hepatic vein and laterally by the right hepatic vein. The right portal vein serves as a landmark for the separation of segment 5 from segment 8

A B C

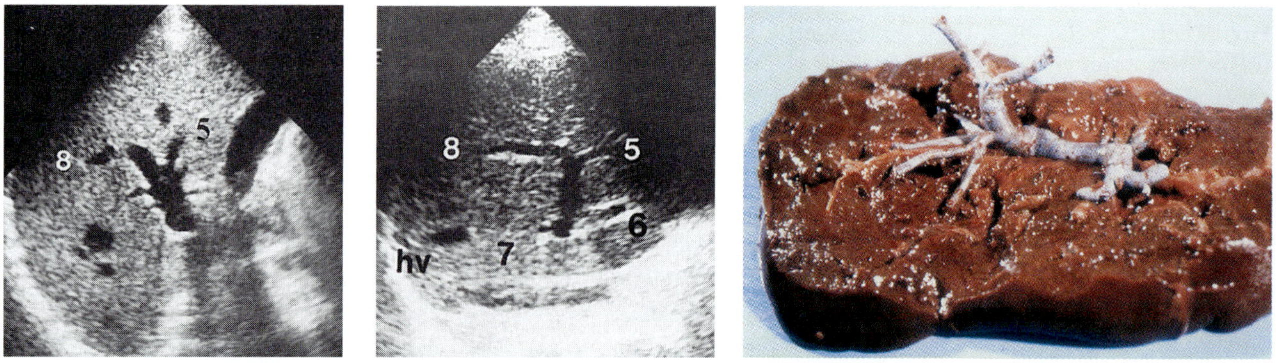

FIG. 58-3. The right portal vein (RPV) and its branches.[2] Intercostal midaxillary sonograms with varying obliquity show the RPV, the crossbar of the right H: **A,** The anterior extreme of the RPV shows its bifurcation into branches to segments 5 and 8. (In this patient there are two small additional branches to each of segments 5 and 8). **B,** By tracing the crossbar of the H to its root posteriorly, the segmental branch 7 is found. Segmental branch 6 is directed toward the right kidney. **C,** The right portal vein and its branches: a dissected specimen shows the segmental branches and their oblique course. (From Bismuth H. Surgical anatomy and anatomical surgery of the liver. *World J Surg* 1982:6:3-9.)

A

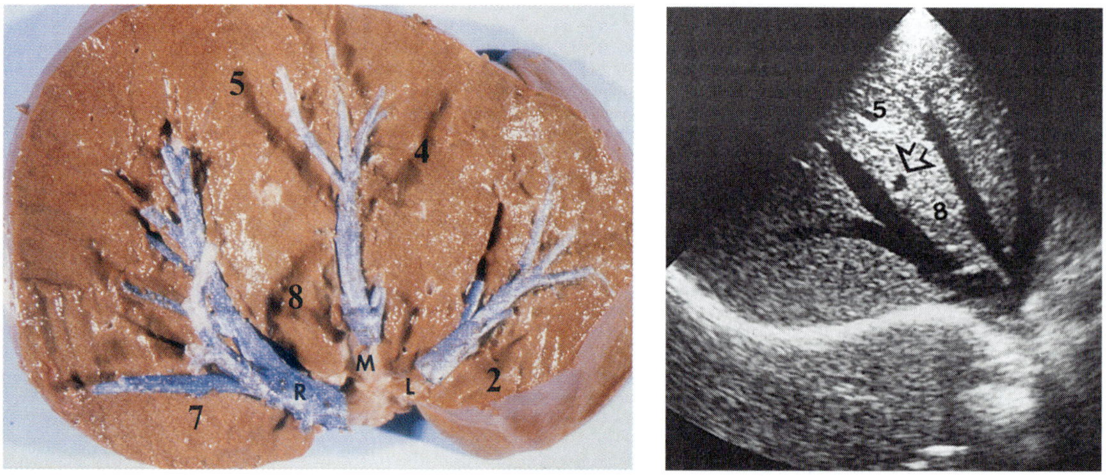

B

FIG. 58-4. The peripheral borders of the segments: the hepatic veins. **A,** A dissected specimen shows the left, middle, and right hepatic veins (L, M, R). The position of the segments is indicated by numbers. **B,** Subxiphoid, oblique sonogram at a similar plane as *A* shows the three hepatic veins. The middle hepatic vein joins the left just before emptying into the left part of the IVC. The right portal vein (*arrowhead*) divides segment 5 from 8 before giving birth to segmental branches. (From Bismuth H. Surgical anatomy and anatomical surgery of the liver. *World J Surg* 1982:6:3-9.)

(Fig. 58-3). Segment 8 is separated from segment 7 by the right hepatic vein, and from segment 4 by the middle hepatic vein (Fig. 58-3).

Segments 6 and 7 are separated from segments 5 and 8 by the right hepatic vein. Segment 6 is the part of the liver closest to the kidney; its lateral border is the rib cage. Segment 7 is separated from segment 8 by the right hepatic vein and is bordered laterally by the rib cage and cephalically by the dome of the diaphragm.

Hepatic Vein Anatomy

When seen with an oblique coronal subxiphoid view, the three hepatic veins form a W, with its base on the IVC. The left and middle hepatic veins join the left anterior part of the IVC (Fig. 58-4). The hepatic veins separate the following segments: the left hepatic vein separates segment 2 from segment 3; the middle hepatic vein separates segment 4 from segments 5 and 8; and the right hepatic vein separates segments 5 and 8 from segments 6 and 7 (Fig. 58-1, *D*). With the oblique subxiphoid view, the right portal vein is seen en face, which helps separate the superficial segment 5 from the more deeply situated segment 8.

The sonographic examination of the child's liver should include visualization of the right and left portal vein and their segmental branches, as well as the hepatic veins. Not only can focal lesions be identified and accurately localized, but thrombosis, compression, or tumor invasion of vessels can be outlined. Doppler sonography is added when the presence and direction of blood flow within these veins need to be assessed. Exploring the liver through its vessels is an excellent way to insure that the sonographic examination is complete and not just an arbitrary glance at this otherwise homogeneous organ with variable contours and few landmarks except for its veins. Since the branches of the hepatic artery and the bile ducts are neighbors of the portal veins, the examination of the lobar and segmental portal veins assures a complete look at these structures as well.

NEONATAL JAUNDICE

The cause of persistent jaundice in the newborn is often difficult to define because clinical and laboratory features may be similar in hepatocellular and obstructive jaundice. If bile obstruction, biliary atresia, or metabolic diseases such as galactosemia and tyrosinemia are to be treated effectively with surgery or specific diet and medication, the diagnosis must be made early (in the first 2 to 3 months), before irreversible cirrhosis has occurred.

Sonography plays an important role in defining causes of **extrahepatic obstruction to bile flow** that may be effectively treated with early surgery: choledochal cyst, biliary atresia, and spontaneous perforation of the bile ducts. (Other causes of bile duct obstruction, such as cholelithiasis, tumors of the bile ducts or pancreas, and congenital stenosis of the common bile duct, usually appear later in childhood.)

Intrahepatic causes of neonatal jaundice include hepatitis (bacterial, viral, or parasitic) and metabolic diseases (galactosemia, tyrosinemia, fructose intolerance, alpha-1 antitrypsin deficiency, cystic fibrosis, paucity of interlobular bile ducts, North American Indian cirrhosis, and so forth). **Systemic diseases** that cause cholestasis include heart failure, shock, sepsis, neonatal lupus, histiocytosis and severe hemolytic disease (see box below).

The baby with jaundice is usually screened with sonography. When dilatation of the bile ducts is found, percutaneous cholangiography or cholecystography may be performed if the cause and anatomy of

CAUSES OF NEONATAL JAUNDICE

- Obstruction of Bile Ducts
  - Choledochal cyst
  - Biliary atresia
  - Spontaneous perforation of the bile ducts
  - Paucity of interlobular bile ducts (Alagille's syndrome)
- Hepatocellular Damage (Cholestasis)
  - Hepatitis
    - Bacterial
      - Syphilis
      - Listeria
      - Staphylococcus
    - Viral
      - Hepatitis B
      - Hepatitis C
      - CMV
      - HIV
      - Rubella
      - Herpes
      - Epstein-Barr
    - Parasitic
      - Toxoplasma
  - Systemic diseases
    - Shock
    - Sepsis
    - Heart failure
    - Neonatal lupus
    - Histiocytosis
    - Hemolytic diseases
  - Metabolic liver diseases
    - Galactosemia
    - Tyrosinemia
    - Fructose intolerance
    - Alpha-1 antitrypsin deficiency
    - Cystic fibrosis

the obstruction are unclear. If sonography fails to outline an anatomic abnormality, DISIDA scintigraphy may define patency of the common bile duct, unless hepatocyte damage is extensive. If no radionuclide reaches the gut, liver biopsy is generally performed. Both scintigraphy and the sonographic search for the gallbladder seem to be enhanced by the bile-stimulating effect of phenobarbital administered for 3 to 5 days prior to the test.[4] (A truly absent gallbladder favors the diagnosis of biliary atresia, although some affected babies have a small but visible gallbladder.)

Choledochal Cyst

Dilatation of varying lengths and severity of the common bile duct, termed choledochal cyst, has been detected *in utero* and usually presents as jaundice in infancy, clinically mimicking neonatal hepatitis and biliary atresia (Fig. 58-5). Tondani's classification,[5] a modification of that proposed by Alonson-Lej, describes five types. **Cylindrical or saccular dilatation of the common bile duct** (CBD) (type I) is most common (80% to 90%) and is thought to be due to an abnormal insertion of the CBD into the pancreatic duct, forming a common channel and facilitating reflux of enzymes into the bile duct, with consequent inflammation. Because choledochal cysts have been detected in 15-week old fetuses, when amylase is not yet present, and because cysts operated on in the newborn period show little inflammation, there must be causative factors (as yet unknown) other than the common-channel theory. Two rare but well documented causes of bile duct dilatation (choledochal cyst) in the newborn are localized atresia of the CBD and multiple intestinal atresias in which the CBD empties into a blind pouch of bowel.[6] The wall of the CBD is devoid of elastic fibers in the fetus and newborn, for the fibers do not begin to develop until 1 year after birth. This may explain why a greatly dilated common bile duct (the choledochal cyst) is seen in infants and not in adults.[7] A choledochal cyst presenting later in childhood may have a different pathogenesis. It is usually complicated by cholangitis and classically causes abdominal pain, obstructive jaundice, and fever. Sometimes the cyst is palpable as a mass.

Choledochal cyst (type II) consists of one or more diverticula of the CBC (2% of cysts). **Choledochocele** (type III) is a dilatation of the intraduodenal part of

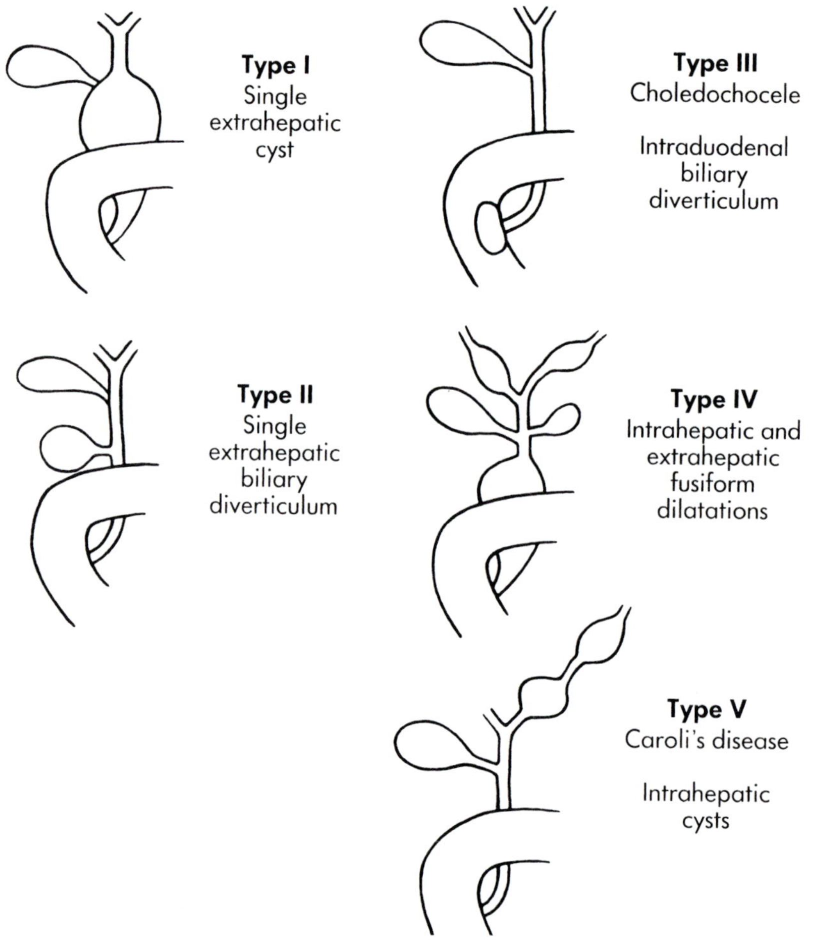

FIG. 58-5. Choledochal cyst classification.

the CBC (1% to 5%). **Multiple intrahepatic and extrahepatic cysts** make up type IV (10%). Caroli disease, type V, affects intrahepatic bile ducts.

Sonography, used to screen the jaundiced baby, shows one or several thin-walled cysts at the liver hilum or within the liver (Fig. 58-6). The gallbladder is identified separately. Dilatation of intrahepatic ducts, as well as stones, may occur later as a result of bile stasis and cholangitis. Scintigraphy is used to document bile flow into the cyst, and percutaneous cholecysto/cholangiography or ERCP is performed if detailed mapping of the bile system is deemed necessary prior to surgery.

Caroli disease (type V choledochal cyst) consists of nonobstructive dilatation of intrahepatic bile ducts[8,9] and is often associated with congenital hepatic fibrosis and infantile polycystic disease.[10] The cause of bile duct ectasia is unknown. Patients tend to seek medical attention later than with other types of choledochal cysts, usually after cholangitis and stones have formed later in childhood (Fig. 58-7). At sonography, the

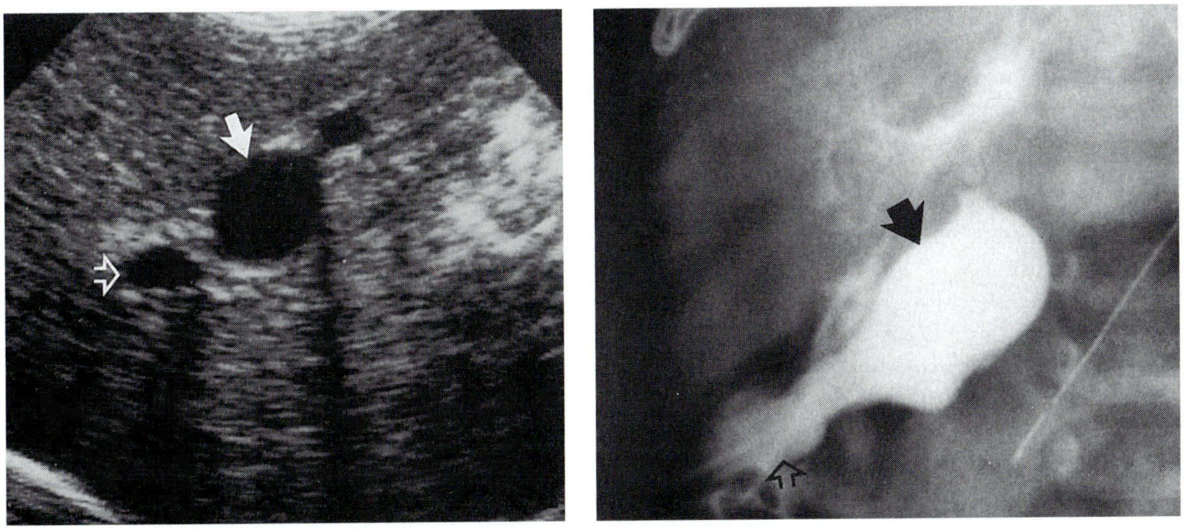

FIG. 58-6. Choledochal cyst in a 6-week-old girl with jaundice. **A,** Transverse sonogram. A large cyst (*arrow*), a greatly dilated common bile duct, displaces the gallbladder (*open arrow*). **B,** Intraoperative cholangiogram shows choledochal cyst (*arrow*) and gallbladder (*open arrow*). (Courtesy of Carol M. Rumack, M.D., Denver, Colorado.)

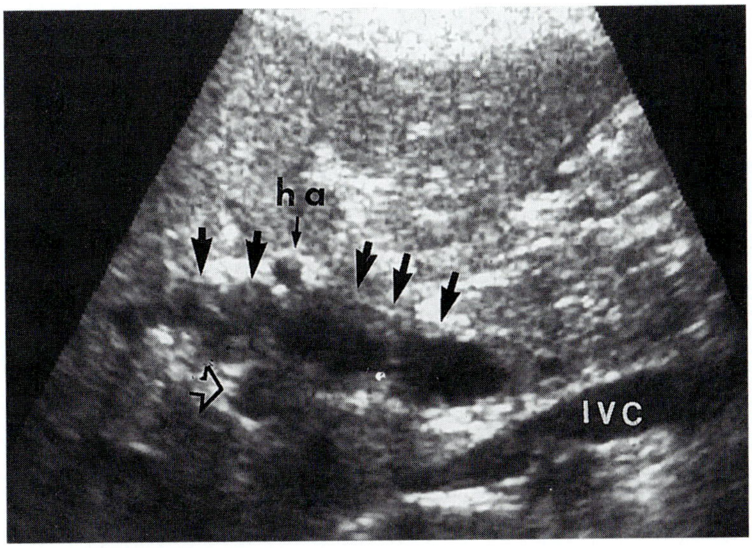

FIG. 58-7. Caroli disease. Cholangitis, caused by obstruction of the bile ducts or by ascending infection, leads to dilatation of the intrahepatic and common bile ducts. Note an irregularly dilated CBD (*arrows*) with an edematous wall in a 7-year-old girl with Crohn's disease. Portal vein, open arrow, IVC, inferior vena cava, ha, hepatic artery.

dilated ducts surround branches of the portal vein.[9] Sludge and stones are often visible within the dilated ducts. Abscesses complicating cholangitis are seen as cavities with walls thicker than those of the ducts and filled with heterogeneous material. The kidneys, when abnormal, are another clue to the diagnosis.

Spontaneous Rupture of the Bile Duct

Rupture of the bile duct is rare. When it occurs in newborns, it leads to jaundice, abdominal distention, and death unless it is repaired. The cause is unknown. Since the site of rupture is usually the junction of the cystic and common bile ducts, it is believed that a developmental weakness at this site leads to the rupture. The biliary system is undilated, but there are ascites and/or loculated fluid collections around the gallbladder.[11]

Paucity of Interlobular Bile Ducts and Alagille's Syndrome

Presenting with chronic cholestasis, usually within the first 3 months of life, these diseases are diagnosed histologically by noting a reduced number of intralobular bile ducts in comparison to the total number of portal areas. Because of cholestasis, the gallbladder may be very small (disuse). The liver is usually enlarged, especially the left lobe. Portal hypertension ensues, with splenomegaly and esophageal varices. In children with arteriohepatic dysplasia (**Alagille's syndrome**) paucity of bile ducts is associated with a particular facies, pulmonary stenosis, butterfly vertebrae, posterior embryotoxon, and, infrequently, renal abnormalities (renal tubular acidosis).[12] Alagille's syndrome appears to be inherited as an autosomal dominant disease with variable penetrance.

Biliary Atresia

The incidence of biliary atresia varies from 1 in 8000 to 1 in 10,000 births. Boys and girls are equally affected and are usually born at term. Biliary cirrhosis occurs early and is often present in the first weeks after birth.

Characterized by absence or obliteration of the lumen of the extrahepatic and/or intrahepatic bile ducts, this disease was once thought to be caused by faulty development of the bile system. It is associated with the polysplenia syndrome (biliary atresia, situs inversus, polysplenia, symmetrical liver, interrupted inferior vena cava, and preduodenal portal vein) in about 20% of patients,[13] as well as with trisomy 17 or 18. Because the disease is extremely rare in fetuses and stillborn or newborn babies, and because the pancreatic duct, which develops in concert with the bile ducts, is normal in affected children, it is now believed that biliary atresia develops after the bile ducts have been formed. There is probably an *in utero* insult to the hepatobiliary system, either infectious, immunologic, or vascular, which results in a progressive sclerosis of the extrahepatic and/or intrahepatic bile ducts. Infection with renovirus type 3 was thought to be a cause of biliary atresia; however, there has been no conclusive serologic evidence of *in utero* infection with this agent in affected children.[14]

Jaundice classically develops gradually, 2 to 3 weeks after birth. The diagnosis is readily made if there are radiologic or sonographic signs of the polysplenia syndrome (Fig. 58-8). Because the flow of bile is inter-

A

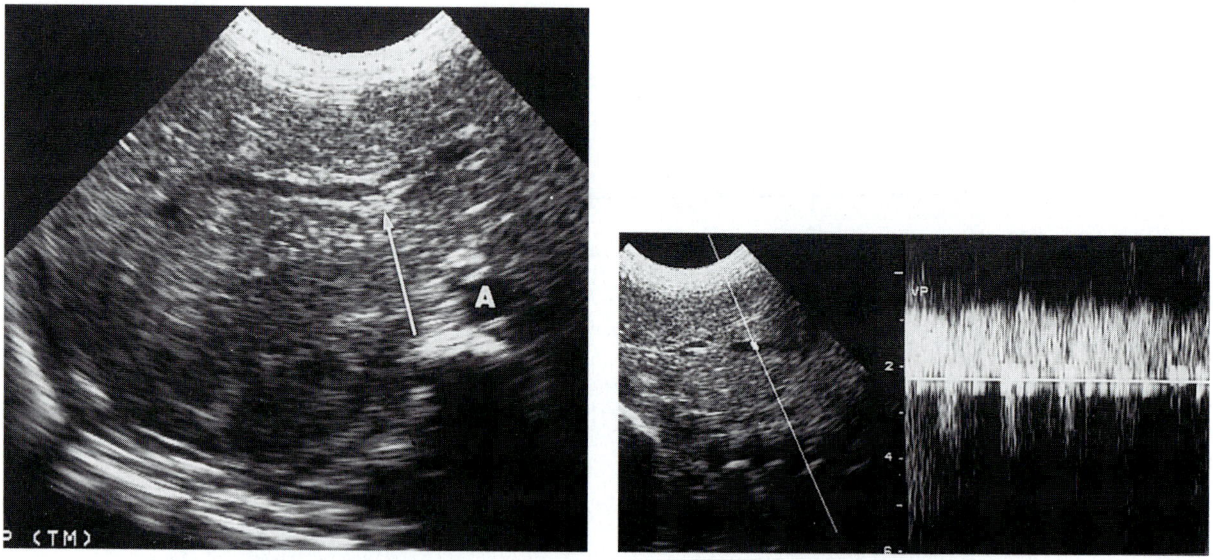

B

FIG. 58-8. Preduodenal portal vein and interruption of the inferior vena cava are signs of the polysplenia syndrome. **A,** Transverse liver sonogram shows aorta (A) anterior and left of the spine (3-month-old girl). The bifurcation of the portal vein (*arrow*) is more anterior than usual. **B,** Right sagittal sonogram. Doppler cursor in the portal vein shows normal hepatopetal flow, but is located far anteriorly. The inferior vena cava is missing on both views.

rupted, the gallbladder is very small or absent in the majority of patients.[13] After having the infant fast for 4 to 6 hours, a specific search with a 7.5 or 10.0 HMz transducer will demonstrate a very small gallbladder in about 20% of cases. Any intrahepatic bile duct remnants may dilate and be visible at sonography as bile duct dilation or small cysts. In addition, the cholangitis that complicates biliary atresia may result in cystic areas within the liver.[15]

Surgical treatment creates contact between a loop of jejunum (transposed to the liver after a Roux-en-Y anastomosis) and any patent bile "ductules" at the liver hilum. This is the classic hepatoporto-enterostomy described by Kasai in 1959.[16] Even if there is no mucosal contact between intestine and the bile ducts, the procedure permits bile drainage with complete clinical remission in 30% and partial drainage in 30% of affected children. The prognosis becomes much more guarded when the Kasai operation is delayed to more than 60 days after birth.[16,17]

Neonatal Hepatitis

Defined as an infection of the liver occurring before the age of 3 months, neonatal hepatitis is now considered an entity distinct from toxic or metabolic diseases affecting the neonate. The causative agent (bacteria, virus, or parasite) reaches the liver through the placenta, via the vagina from infected maternal secretions, or through catheters or blood transfusions. Transplacental infection occurs most readily during the third trimester of pregnancy, and syphilis, toxoplasma, rubella, and cytomegaloirus (CMV) are the most common agents.[14]

Neonatal bacterial hepatitis is usually secondary to upward spread of organisms from the vagina, infecting endometrium, placenta, and amniotic fluid. (In twin pregnancies, the fetus nearest the cervix is the one most frequently affected.) *Listeria* and *E. coli* are the usual organisms. During vaginal delivery, direct contact with the viruses of herpes, CMV, human immunodeficiency virus (HIV), and *Listeria* may lead to hepatitis. Blood transfusions may contain the hepatitis viruses B or C, CMV, Epstein-Barr, and HIV. Infected umbilical vein catheterization usually results in bacterial hepatitis or abscesses.[14] With the exception of diffuse hepatomegaly, there are no specific sonographic signs of hepatitis, unless abscesses (usually bacterial in origin) occur. The gallbladder wall may be thickened, probably secondary to hypoalbuminemia (Fig. 58-9).[18,19]

Neonatal Jaundice and Urinary Tract Infection/Sepsis

The association of these two entities occurs more commonly in newborn boys than girls. Jaundice, hepatomegaly, and vomiting are common clinical signs. Urinary tract symptoms are uncommon, as are shock and fever. A thorough examination of the kidneys, ureters, and bladder should, therefore, accompany sonography of the liver in the baby with jaundice. Similarly, the diaphragm and lung bases should be examined to look for pleural effusions and pneumonia

A

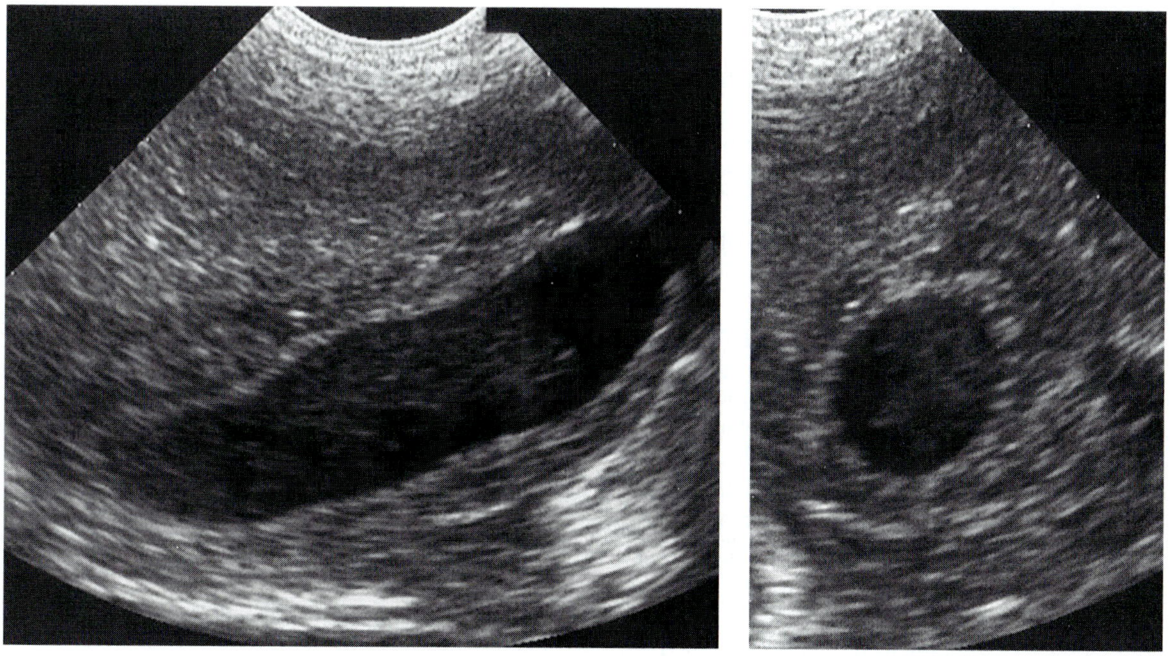

B

FIG. 58-9. Acute hepatitis (6-year-old girl). **A,** Sagittal and **B,** coronal views of the gallbladder show edema of the wall and thick bile within the lumen.

INBORN ERRORS OF METABOLISM

- Hepatocyte Injury Consistently
  - Glycogen storage type IV
  - Galactosemia
  - Fructose intolerance
  - Tyrosinemia
  - Wolman disease
  - Zellweger syndrome
  - Neonatal iron storage disease
  - Wilson's disease
- Hepatocyte Injury Sometimes
  - Alpha 1-antitrypsin deficiency
  - Cystic fibrosis
  - Glycogen storage disease (I and III)
- No Hepatocyte Damage (Store Metabolites)
  - Mucopolysaccharidoses
  - Gaucher's disease

which may be accompanied by sepsis and jaundice in the newborn.

Inborn Errors of Metabolism

Because these disorders cause liver damage in the newborn, some of them rapidly destroying the liver if untreated, and because several of them can be treated effectively with diet or drugs once the diagnosis is known, pediatricians and radiologists should be well acquainted with them (see box). Liver damage is caused by storage of a hepatotoxic metabolite or by absence of an essential enzyme that impairs the liver's detoxification process.

Steatosis (fatty degeneration or infiltration) is especially prominent in the glycogen storage diseases, galactosemia, tyrosinemia, and cystic fibrosis. **Cirrhosis** eventually develops in all the diseases that cause liver damage, and portal hypertension then follows. The risk of **hepatocellular carcinoma** is significantly increased in alpha-1 antitrypsin deficiency, in tyrosinemia, and in glycogen storage disease type I. **Liver adenomas** also develop in the latter two, as does **renal tubular disease,** usually characterized by acidosis and nephrocalcinosis.[14]

Tyrosinemia is now best treated by transplantation. Until drug therapy became available for the treatment of the acute neurologic crises in babies with acute tyrosinemia, transplantation was performed as a life-saving procedure as soon as surgically feasible. Now transplantation is done once liver nodules appear (Fig. 58-10) because hepatocarcinoma develops in about 30% of children with tyrosinemia who survive the neonatal period. In a recent review of livers dissected at the time of liver transplantation, we found that our preoperative sonograms and CT scans were not accurate in the distinction between regeneration nodules, adenomas, and carcinomas (Fig. 58-10), and neither was alpha-fetoprotein analysis.[20]

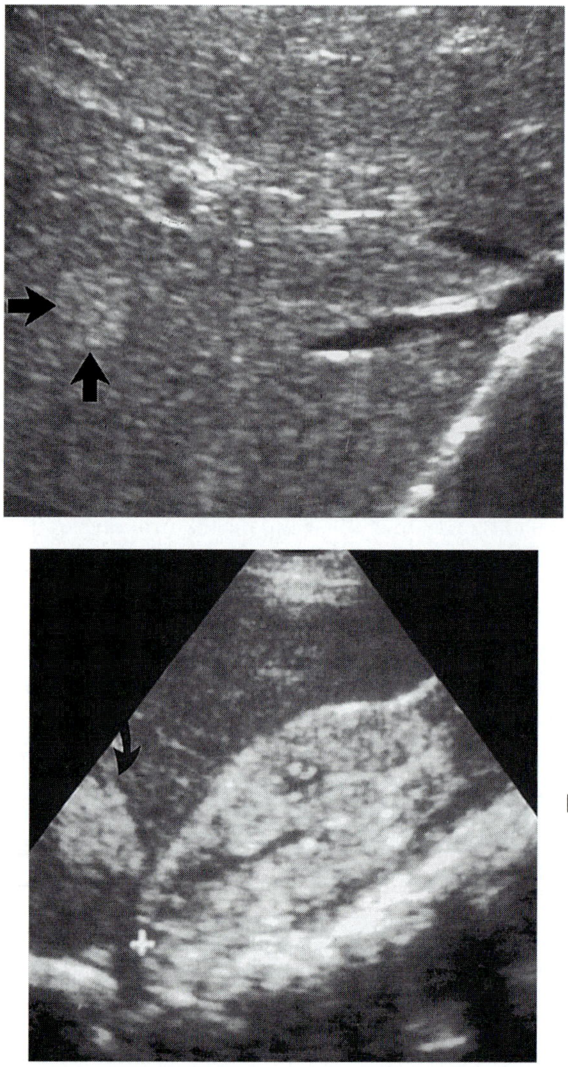

A

B

FIG. 58-10. Tyrosinemia. A, Hyperechogenic nodule (*arrows*) in the right lobe of the liver in a 1-year-old child. Sonography and CT could not determine if it was adenoma or hepatocellular carcinoma. At histology after transplantation, an adenoma was found. **B,** The kidney of another child shows that it is hyperechogenic. Both cortex and medulla are involved. Also note nodule in the adjacent liver (*curved arrow*).

The sonographic examination of children with possible metabolic disease includes a careful analysis of liver size and architecture, searching for steatosis, cirrhosis, and nodules; an analysis of renal architecture (Fig. 58-10), searching for increased size and nephrocalcinosis; and a Doppler examination of the abdomen searching for signs of portal hypertension.

STEATOSIS (FATTY DEGENERATION OR INFILTRATION)

Fat accumulates in hepatocytes following cellular damage (fatty degeneration) through the overloading of previously healthy cells with excess fat (fatty infiltration) or,

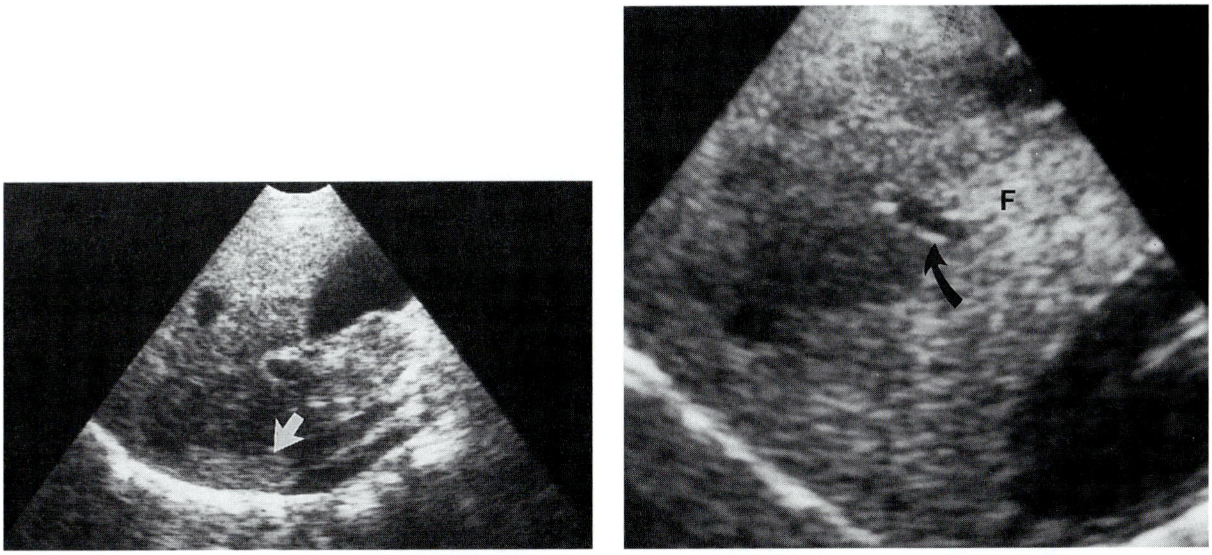

FIG. 58-11. Fatty infiltration of the liver (steatosis) in two patients with cystic fibrosis. **A,** Sagittal view includes the gallbladder and shows a region of normal parenchyma surrounded by hyperechogenic, fatty liver (*arrow*). **B,** Dark zones of focal sparing are surrounded by hyperechogenic areas of fatty infiltration. Note the wall of the portal vein (*arrow*) visible near the normal parenchyma but obscured by adjacent, very echogenic fat (F) steatosis on the opposite side. The cortex of the right kidney is much less echogenic than the fatty liver. (From Patriquin HB, Roy CC, Weber AM et al. Liver disease and portal hypertension. *Clin Diagn Ultrasound* 1989;24:103-127.)

in certain enzyme deficiency syndromes, through the inability of fat to be mobilized out of the liver. Drugs (acetylsalicylic acid, tetracycline, valproate, warfarin) and toxins (aflatoxin, hypoglycine) as well as alcohol abuse lead to fatty degeneration of liver cells. Steatosis is also seen in metabolic liver disorders such as galactosemia, fructose intolerance, and Reye's syndrome. Obesity, steroid therapy, hyperlipidemia, and diabetes are examples of increased fat mobilization and its entry into the liver. In malnutrition, nephrotic syndrome, and cystic fibrosis not only does excess fat enter the liver, but in addition, there is deficient mobilization of fat out of the hepatocyte. When parenteral nutrition does not include lipids, steatosis occurs because of a deficiency of essential fatty acids. Most of the inherited disorders of the liver mentioned previously involve an enzyme deficiency and result in steatosis. Fatty changes are reversible, may be diffuse or focal, and are often detected by ultrasonography before clinically suspected.[21] Areas of steatosis are highly echogenic, blurring vessel walls. The nearby kidney cortex appears much less echogenic. When focal, steatosis usually has smooth, geometric, or finger-like borders (Fig. 58-11). Intervening normal liver may appear hypoechogenic and masquerade as mass lesions (metastases or abscesses), especially if the ultrasound gain is adjusted by using the fatty areas as a normal reference.[22] Segments 4 and 5 are often spared in steatosis, perhaps because of favorable blood supply by the gallbladder and its vessels.[23] Nodules of steatosis may mimic metastases on CT. We follow our doubtful ultrasonographic studies with CT and have found the two modalities complementary in this situation. In spite of sophisticated imaging, ultrasound- or CT-guided biopsy is sometimes necessary.

CIRRHOSIS

The usual forms of cirrhosis in childhood are biliary and postnecrotic. Morphologically, the cirrhotic liver consists of regenerating nodules devoid of central veins and surrounded by variable amounts of connective tissue. Hepatic architecture is sufficiently distorted to disturb hepatic circulation and hepatocellular function. Increased resistance to blood flow through the liver leads to portal hypertension.

The sonographic appearance of the liver depends on the severity of the cirrhosis. With progressive replacement of hepatocytes by fibrous tissue, the liver attenuates sound increasingly, and sound penetration of the liver, even with low-frequency (2 or 3 MHz) transducers, becomes difficult. The macronodules of advanced cirrhosis become visible sonographically at the surface of the liver (contrasted against the neighboring lesser omentum, peritoneum, or ascites, if present) or within its substance (nodular architecture, increased hyperechogenic fibrous tissue around portal vein branches and the ligamentum teres).[22] The caudate lobe is often prominent (Fig. 58-12). Parts of segment 4 of the right lobe of the liver may atrophy in advanced disease.

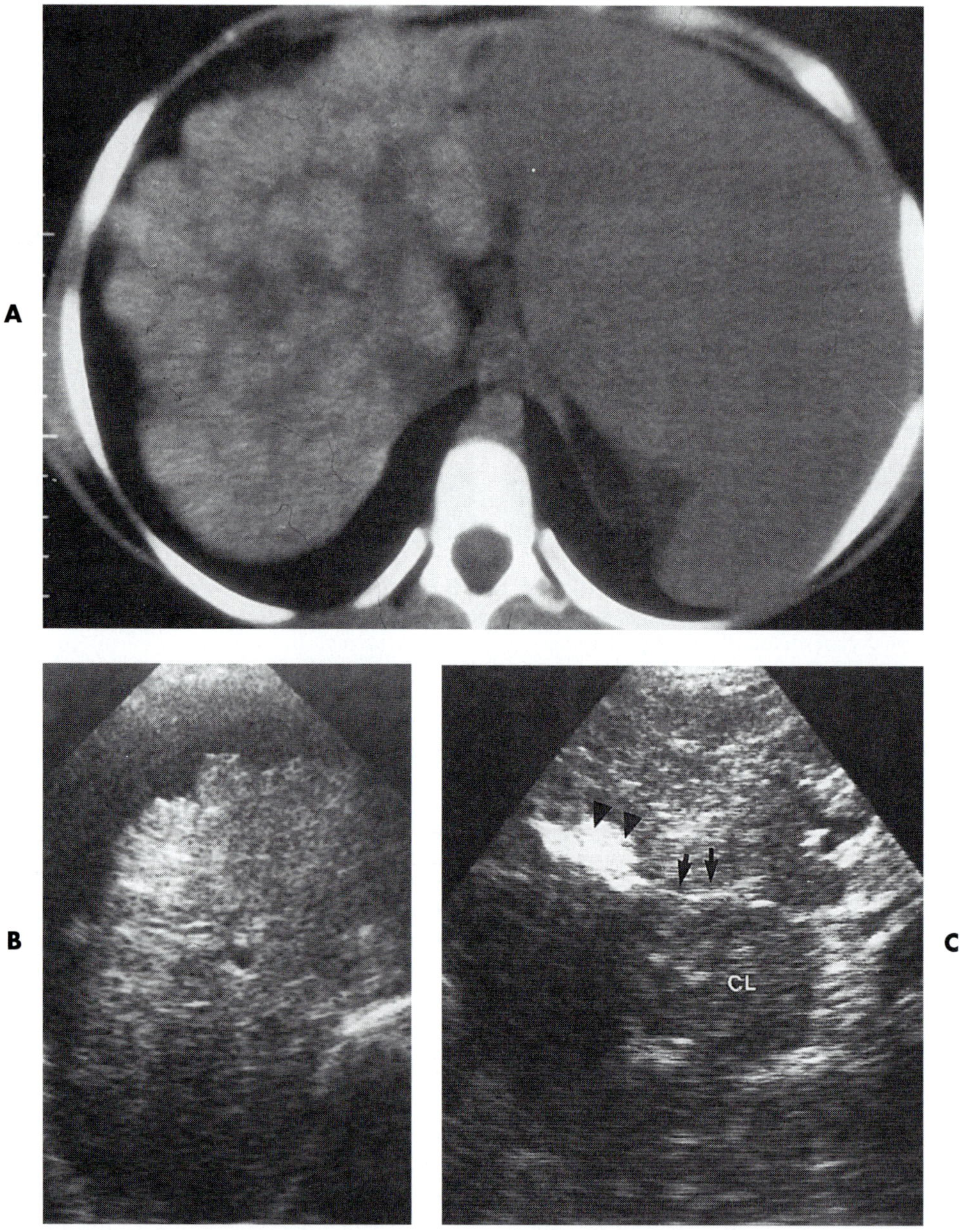

FIG. 58-12. Cirrhosis. A and B, tyrosinemia. A, CT scan of the upper abdomen (6-year-old child) shows a small liver with multiple nodules visible both on the contour and within the liver. Microscopy of the native liver after transplantation showed regenerating nodules and severe cirrhosis (portal hypertension). **B, Macronodules of cirrhosis** at the surface of the liver outlined by ascitic fluid (sonogram of another child). **C, Cystic fibrosis and cirrhosis** with increased echogenic fibrous tissue around the ligamentum venosum (*arrows*) and the round ligament (*arrowheads*). Note the nodular inferior surface of the liver and the larger caudate lobe (CL) (liver sonogram of a 12-year-old child). (From Patriquin HB, Roy CC, Weber AM et al. Liver disease and portal hypertension. *Clin Diagn Ultrasound* 1989;24:103–127.)

CHOLELITHIASIS

Gallstones are less common in children than in adults and are usually related to an associated disease (see box on next page). Their composition can be mixed or of calcium bilirubinate. The "adult" cholesterol stone is rare except in children with cystic fibrosis.[24] Gallstones are mobile and hyperechogenic, and they cast acoustic shadows only if they are of appropriate size and composition.

In some children, especially those receiving total parenteral nutrition, thick bile can be observed to form sludge, loosely formed "bile balls" and, finally, stones, when serial sonograms are performed over sev-

DISEASES ASSOCIATED WITH GALLSTONES IN CHILDREN

Hematopoietic
- Hemolytic anemias or hemolysis (artificial heart valve)
- Rh incompatibility
- Blood transfusions
- Sickle cell anemia

Gastrointestinal
- Cystic fibrosis
- Bile duct anomalies
- Ileal dysfunction (Crohn's disease, short bowel)
- Total parenteral nutrition (TPN)
- Metabolic liver diseases

Other
- Immobilization (scoliosis surgery)
- Dehydration
- Sepsis

eral weeks (Fig. 58-13). Stasis of bile flow is the probable cause of sludge and stone formation, which is also seen *in utero* and in premature babies, and which usually regresses spontaneously.[25]

The wall of the gallbladder thickens in children with acute hepatitis, hypoalbuminemia, obstructed hepatic venous return, and ascites.[18,19] The classic signs of impacted gallstone, thick gallbladder wall, and fluid around the gallbladder seen in adults with acute cholecystitis are rare in children. The gallbladder becomes dilated and rounded (rather than the normal oval shape) in fasting children (especially babies on TPN), children with sepsis (especially streptococcal), and those in the acute phase of Kawasaki disease. When distended, the gallbladder may become tender and painful. It heals with the underlying disease. Acalculous cholecystitis in children is rare and should be diagnosed only if no disease causing gallbladder distention or wall edema is found.[26] The distinction between gallbladder atony and obstruction cannot always be made with iminodiacetic acid scintigraphy.

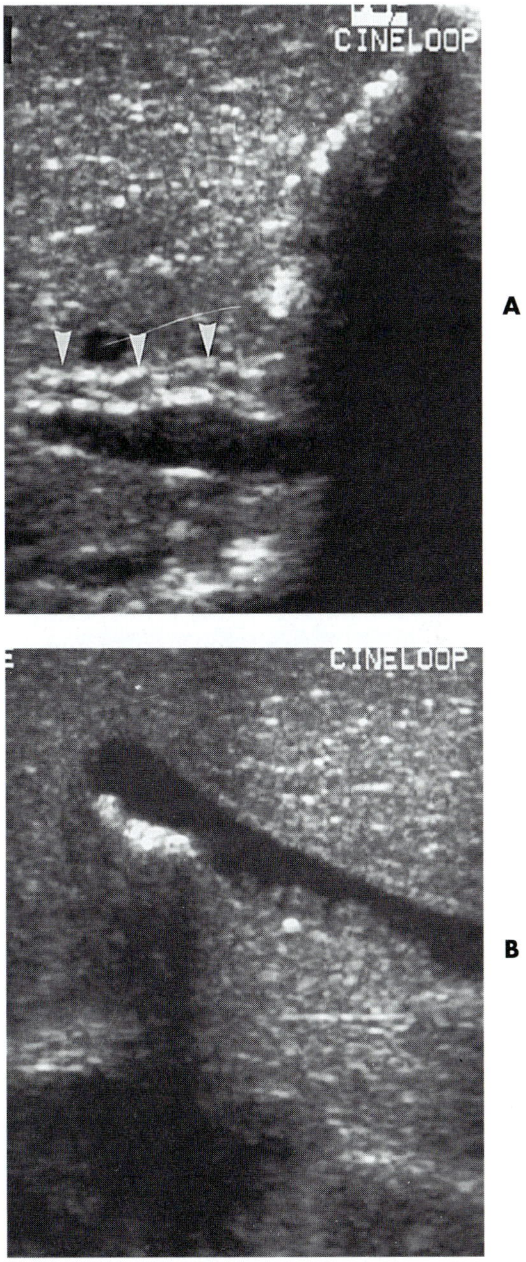

FIG. 58-13. Thick bile and stones. Three-month-old boy on total parenteral nutrition for intractable diarrhea. **A,** Stones (with acoustic shadowing) and sludge in the common bile duct (*arrowheads*). **B,** Stones and thick bile are seen within the gallbladder.

LIVER TUMORS

Identification

It is sometimes difficult to define the origin of an abdominal mass, especially when it is large. The following questions are helpful in tracing a mass to hepatic origin (see box on p. 1658).

1. **Vascular anatomy:**
   Can a feeding hepatic vessel be identified by means of Doppler sonography? Are segmental portal veins displaced or invaded by the tumor?[27] What liver segments are involved? Is the main hepatic artery enlarged? (This usually signals the presence of a highly vascular hemangioendothelioma.)
2. **Biliary anatomy:**
   Are the bile ducts normal? Has the gallbladder been identified?
3. **Anatomy of the abdomen:**
   Does the mass move with the liver during respiration? Is the liver parenchyma normal or cirrhotic?

LIVER MASSES IN CHILDREN

Solid
- Hemangioendothelioma (single or multiple)
- Adenoma, hamartoma
- Focal nodular hyperplasia
- Regeneration nodules in cirrhosis
- Hepatoblastoma
- Hepatocellular carcinoma
- Lymphoma
- Metastasis

Cysts In or Near the Liver
- Congenital cysts
- Congenital hepatic fibrosis
- Choledochal cysts
- Duodenal duplication cyst
- Hydatid cyst ("sand," daughter cysts)
- Caroli disease
- Hamartoma

Is there ascitic fluid available for cytology? Is there another abdominal, retroperitoneal, para-aortic, or pelvic mass that could be a primary tumor?

Benign Liver Tumors

About 40% of primary liver tumors in children are benign. Hemangiomas are by far the commonest. Mesenchymal hamartomas, adenomas, and focal nodular hyperplasia together constitute about one half of benign liver tumors in the child.

Hemangiomas. **Hemangiomas** are vascular, mesenchymal masses that are characterized by initial active endothelial growth (angiogenesis). At this stage, the tumor is highly vascular and may cause sufficient arteriovenous shunting to result in high-output heart failure. This lesion is usually called hemangioendothelioma and it presents in the newborn baby or infant. As the tumor matures, vessel growth slows. Existing vessels may enlarge and form "lakes" with little blood flow. This is the cavernous hemangioma typically seen in adults and rare in children.[28]

Infantile Hemangioendotheliomas. **Infantile hemangioendotheliomas** are single or multiple solid masses of varying echoginecity, often containing foci of calcium.[29] Doppler sonography shows blood flow in multiple tortuous vessels both within and at the periphery of the mass (Fig. 58-14). Doppler shifts exceed those seen in normal intrahepatic arteries. When arteriovenous shunting is severe, the celiac axis, hepatic artery, and veins are dilated and the infraceliac aorta is small. Doppler shifts from hemangioendothelioma vessels may resemble those from malignant tumors.[30] The vascular nature of these lesions is confirmed by bolus-injection CT and the search for rapid filling and rapid washout in these masses. Angiography is usually reserved for patients for whom embolization is considered.

Mesenchymal Hamartomas. **Mesenchymal hamartomas** are vascular, usually multiseptate cystic masses derived from periportal mesenchyma. Calcifications are rare. They typically present as an asymptomatic mass in the right lobe of the liver in children of under two years.[31]

Adenomas. **Adenomas** are rare except in association with metabolic liver disease (especially glycogen storage disease type I),[32] with oral contraceptive therapy or anabolic steroid therapy for aplastic anemia. (The latter may develop hepatocellular carcinoma). Serum alpha-fetoprotein levels are normal. Sonographic appearance varies from hyper- to hypoechogenic and is nonspecific. Malignant degeneration is rare. The distinction between adenoma and a malignant mass is difficult with sonography, CT, and MR because imaging findings vary and are nonspecific.

Focal Nodular Hyperplasia. **Focal nodular hyperplasia** typically shows a central scar, which may be visible sonographically or at CT. The normal or increased uptake of ^{99m}Tc sulfur colloid by the mass helps to distinguish it from malignant masses, which typically fail to take up the isotopic contrast material.[33]

Malignant Liver Tumors

Most solid liver tumors are malignant and are derived from epithelium.

Hepatoblastoma. **Hepatoblastoma,** the most common primary liver tumor in childhood, which presents in children under 5 years, is sometimes considered the infantile form of hepatocellular carcinoma. There is an association with the Beckwith-Wiedemann syndrome, hemihypertrophy, and the 11p13 chromosome.[34] Serum alpha-fetoprotein levels are almost always elevated. Some tumors secrete gonadotropins and lead to precocious puberty.

The tumor is usually single, solid, large, of mixed echogenicity, and poorly marginated, with small cysts and rounded or irregularly shaped deposits of calcium (Fig. 58-15). (The latter are quite different from the fine, linear calcifications seen in hemangioendotheliomas.)[35] The remaining liver is usually normal, although sometimes metastases are found at the time of diagnosis. Intrahepatic vessels are displaced and/or amputated by the mass. Tumor thrombi are less common than in hepatocellular carcinoma. Doppler sonography is helpful in diagnosing vessel invasion and in detecting flow in malignant neovasculature.[36,37] Complete resection of the tumors results in a 50% to 60% cure rate. Resectability depends on the number of segments and vessels involved and is best determined with MRI.[38]

A B C D

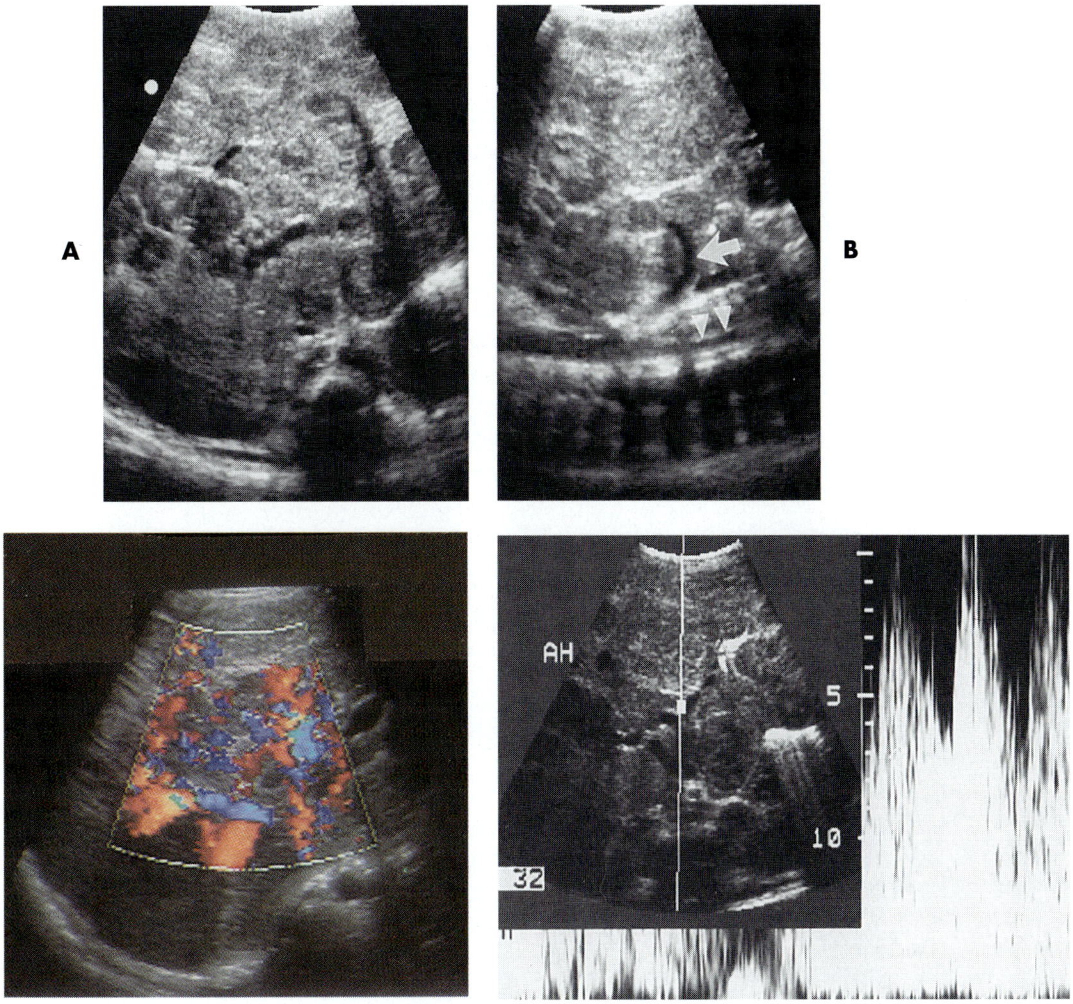

FIG. 58-14. Hemangioendothelioma. **A,** Transverse and **B,** longitudinal sonogram of 4-month-old girl with a greatly enlarged liver containing multiple nodules. The celiac axis is dilated (*arrow*) and the aorta distal to its origin is narrow (*arrowheads*). **C,** The hepatic artery within the liver is dilated. **D,** Low-resistance flow of great velocity is noted in the hepatic artery (Doppler shift 6 kHz, 5 MHz transducer), resembling malignant tumor flow. AH, cursor in hepatic artery.

Hepatocellular Carcinoma. **Hepatocellular carcinoma,** the malignant tumor second in frequency, has its peak incidences at 4 to 5 and 12 to 14 years. About one half of affected children have preexisting liver disease, especially tyrosinemia, glycogen storage type I, alpha-1 antitrypsin deficiency, or posthepatitis B or C cirrhosis or biliary cirrhosis following biliary atresia, Byler disease, or the Alagille syndrome. Serum alpha-fetoprotein levels are usually elevated. The tumor is often multicentric; masses are solid, they rarely calcify, and they are of variable echogenicity. Portal venous invasion is common and easily detected with Doppler sonography, as is the high-velocity flow in peripheral neovasculature.[36,37,39]

Undifferentiated Embryonal Sarcoma. **Undifferentiated embryonal sarcoma** (malignant mesenchymoma) is considered the malignant counterpart of the hamartoma. It is rare, occurs in children that are older than those with hamartomas, grows rapidly, and develops central necrosis and cysts. Serum alpha-fetoprotein levels are normal.

Metastases. Metastases to the liver usually arise from neuroblastoma, Wilms' tumor, leukemia, or lymphoma. Diffuse infiltration of the liver (or multiple nodules) in stage 4S neonatal neuroblastoma is remarkable for its good prognosis.

Detection of Tumor Angiogenesis

Hepatoblastoma and hepatocellular carcinoma very commonly produce a network of microscopic, parasitic tumor vessels at their periphery. Flow in these vessels, which lack a normal muscularis, produces Doppler shifts greater than 3.5 kHz (3 MHz transducer), which are greater than shifts expected in the aorta.[37,39]

A

B

C

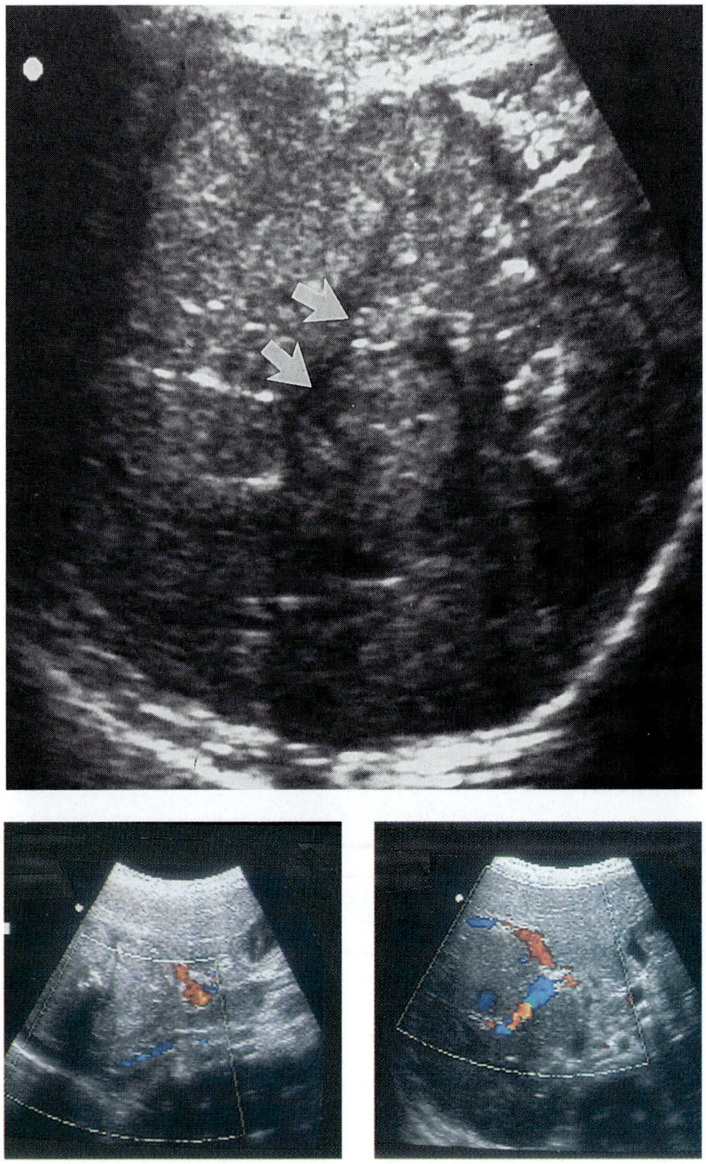

FIG. 58-15. Hepatoblastoma. Palpable abdominal mass in a 1-year-old girl. **A,** Right lobe of the liver contains a multinodular mass (*arrows*) with central calcifications. **B** and **C,** Surrounding portal veins are displaced around the mass.

LIVER ABSCESS AND GRANULOMAS

Pyogenic Abscess

Pyogenic liver abscesses are very rare in the normal child. They generally occur in association with sepsis, in children with depressed immunity (leukemia, drugs), in those with primary immune defects (chronic granulomatous disease, dysgammaglobulinemia), or in association with contiguous infection (appendicitis, cholangitis). At sonography, abscesses are generally well-defined masses, with or without heterogeneous fluid content and small air bubbles signaled by ring-down artifacts. They displace but do not invade neighboring vessels. A Doppler examination may be used to confirm the patency of nearby portal venous branches. Fluid in the pleural space or in Morison's pouch should be sought in the supine position. Aspiration, with or without drainage of abscesses, under sonographic or CT guidance is becoming the preferred treatment in many centers. Some abscesses, especially those accompanying chronic granulomatous disease, gradually calcify during medical treatment.[40] Multiple small abscesses, usually seen in the immunosupressed child, may result in an enlarged, painful liver. Distinguishing these tiny hypoechogenic lesions from normal liver parenchyma is a challenge to the resolution of the equipment and the skill of the examiner. Scanning the anterior surface of the liver with a high-frequency (7.5 MHz) transducer often outlines some of the multiple lesions otherwise missed. We routinely complement the ultrasound examination with high-resolution CT in these children because small abscesses are often better seen with CT.

Parasitic Abscesses

Amoebic Infection. The incidence of parasitic abscesses in children, although low, is increasing because of expanding travel and immigration. Amoebic infection is endemic in the tropics and spreads through person-to-person contact. The protozoan *Entamoeba histolytica* is ingested, invades the colonic mucosa, enters intestinal veins, and spreads into portal venous branches. The organism secretes proteolytic enzymes, and hepatic abscess formation occurs rapidly. It is the most frequent extraintestinal complication of amoebic infection. In children, abscesses are usually multiple and occur most often in babies under 1 year of age, in whom they are life-threatening. Fever spikes and hepatomegaly without jaundice are the usual forms of presentation. Diagnosis is made by serologic testing, but that is not always positive in babies. Both sonographic and CT imaging are highly sensitive but fail to differentiate amoebic from pyogenic abscesses. The sonographic pattern of hypoechogenic, homogeneous, or heterogeneous target masses may mimic that of hematoma or neoplasm. Abscess rupture into the thorax, although rare in childhood, is pathognomonic for amoebic abscess. (Extension into subphrenic or perihepatic spaces, peritoneum, and nearby abdominal organs is more frequent.) Diagnostic puncture is disappointing because of the low yield of organisms. Since pyogenic abscesses usually occur in the immunodeficient child, an abscess occurring in an otherwise healthy baby should be considered amoebic until proven otherwise. In the past, high mortality rates (60% in babies) have been due to late diagnosis. They have been reduced to near zero with early detection through the use of refined imaging techniques (scintigraphy, ultrasonography, and CT).[41]

Echinococcus Infection. The adult tapeworm, *Echinococcus*, lives in the jejunum of the dog, where it lays its eggs, which are spread through feces and then swallowed by the intermediate host (usually sheep but sometimes humans). Endemic areas include the Middle East, the southern United States, and northern Canada. Embryos, freed in the duodenum, invade the mucosa to enter a mesenteric vein, which flows to the liver where a slowly growing cyst composed of an acellular outer layer and an endothelialized inner layer may develop. Compressed surrounding liver tissue forms a third layer. The inner layer forms freely floating embryos (scolices), or "hydatid sand," which are visible with ultrasonography. Daughter cysts form within the main

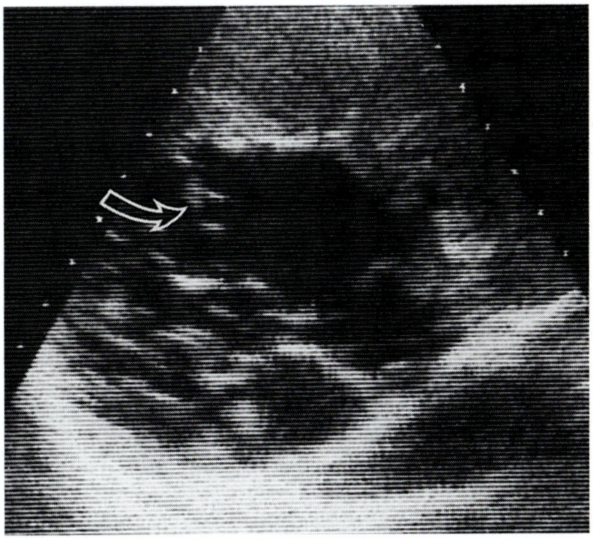

FIG. 58-16. Hydatid cyst. A sagittal sonogram of the liver shows a cyst with multiple septa. There are several small (daughter) cysts in the center (*arrow*).

cyst under certain circumstances and, when seen sonographically, suggest the diagnosis of hydatid cyst (Fig. 58-16). Ruptured daughter cysts form floating membranes. A dead cyst decreases in size and gradually calcifies.[42,43]

Schistosomiasis Infection. Invasion of the portal vein by the ova of *Schistosoma* leads to portal hypertension without cirrhosis. Liver disease progresses so slowly that portal hypertension is very rarely seen in a child.

Granulomas of the Liver

Granulomas are circumscribed, focal, inflammatory lesions that may be of bacterial (*Mycobacterium tuberculosis*, other mycobacteria, *Listeria*, spirochetes), fungal (*Candida, Histoplasma, Aspergillus*), parasitic (*Toxocara, Ascaris*), or malignant (lymphoma) origin. Clinical features are those of the underlying disease, and the liver is usually enlarged. Confluent granulomas or abscesses may be recognized as distinct masses at sonography.

LIVER DISEASES AND PORTAL HYPERTENSION: ASSESSMENT WITH DOPPLER SONOGRAPHY

Basic Principles

The physics of Doppler ultrasound and the details of instrumentation have been well described by Taylor et al.[44,45] and by Burns and Jaffe[46] in their review articles. There are a few principles essential to the performance of a successful clinical examination with real-time ultrasound coupled to a Doppler display, either spectral or color. The Doppler shift depends on the following factors, expressed in the Doppler equation:

$$fd = (2\ fv \cos\Theta)/c$$

where **fd** = Doppler shift (in Hz), **v** = velocity of moving blood (in meters per second), **f** = the frequency of ultrasound (in Hertz), **c** = the velocity of sound in (human) tissue, and Θ = the angle between the axis of the vessel studied and the ultrasound Doppler beam. Since **c** is constant and **f** is determined by the frequency of the transducer being used, the main factors that affect the Doppler shift in the clinical situation are (**v**) **the velocity** and (Θ) **the vessel-transducer angle.** Commercial machines express the Doppler shift in kilohertz or in centimeters per second. It must be remembered that true velocity calculations require a vessel beam-angle measurement. When the Doppler beam is perpendicular to the vessel axis, the **cos 90° is 0,** and flow will not be registered. At that angle there is no motion either toward or away from the transducer. Therefore, the vessel beam angle to detect blood flow should be small, ideally less than 60°. There is a conflict between the ultrasound image, which is best when the transducer is perpendicular to a structure, and the Doppler angle, which is best at up to 60°. The art of performing abdominal Doppler ultrasound consists of placing the transducer at a location where the angle between the Doppler beam and the axis of the vessel is optimal.

The basic technique of the **duplex Doppler** examination consists of visualizing the vessel with real-time or color Doppler and then placing a Doppler beam with a small "aperture," the sample volume, within the vessel. The sample volume size can be adjusted and should be slightly less than the diameter of the vessel. The transducer alternately sends and receives sound waves from the aperture. If there are cells moving within the vessel, a Doppler shift will result. The audible signal is translated into a spectral display on the screen. The multiple dots displayed represent the different velocities of the moving red cells.

Most of the abdominal vessels studied in children have a low-flow velocity. Therefore, the wall filter should be as low as possible, preferably at 50 Hz or less. The pulse repetition frequency should be as low as possible for the same reason, unless aliasing (projection of a "cut off" spectral image on the opposite side of the reference line or a very light and reverse-color image) occurs. The direction of flow is displayed on the screen according to whether the Doppler shift is higher or lower than the originally transmitted beam frequency. Thus, flow approaching the transducer is seen above the reference line, and flow receding from the transducer is seen below the reference line.

In this way the presence or absence of flow in a vessel can be determined, as can the direction of that flow. If the vessel beam angle q can be measured, velocity of flow can be estimated. When the diameter of the vessel can be determined accurately, an estimate of flow volume can be made (with some limitations of accuracy).[46]

Color Doppler ultrasound is another method of displaying the Doppler shift arising from moving blood cells within a vessel.[47] Instead of interrogating a small volume within a vessel, the Doppler receiver detects signals from many scan lines. The resultant numerous Doppler signals are displayed as color signals: high-frequency shifts are light-colored (yellow or white) and, by convention, flow toward the transducer is red and flow away from it is blue. Turbulent flow is displayed as a mosaic of shades of red and blue. The basic principles are identical to those already described, and a knowledge of duplex Doppler ultrasound is essential for intelligent analysis of the color Doppler image. There are great advantages to color mapping because entire segments of vessels are seen at a glance (for example, portosystemic collateral veins in portal hypertension or stenoses of vessels). The limitations of the vessel/beam angle remain, and no flow may be detected in that part of the vessel perpendicular to the transducer. Flow in tortuous vessels may be difficult to understand because it will obviously have both red and blue segments. When examining small vessels in children, motion may produce flashes or dots of color artifacts. Pulsed Doppler sampling of such doubtful signals distinguishes these artifacts from flow signals. Color Doppler displays direction of flow (blue or red) and an estimate of velocity (a lighter color represents faster flow) but does not indicate the force (or power) of the Doppler signal. The latter is a reflection of the number of moving blood cells within the area of tissue being tested. Pulsed Doppler indicates direction and estimates velocity in the small sample volume examined. The power of the Doppler signal is estimated by the number of pixels seen in the spectral display.

Power Doppler sonography measures the force (power) of the Doppler signal but gives no indication of direction or velocity. It is much less angle-dependent than color or pulsed Doppler and is more sensitive to slowly flowing blood. It is most useful in detecting slow flow in small vessels or in vessels perpendicular to the ultrasound beam. Arterial and venous flow cannot be distinguished, but a pulsed Doppler examination can be made at any point in the vessel identified with power Doppler. Because of their small body size and ready access to the Doppler beam, children are particularly suited to color, power, and pulsed Doppler abdominal examinations.

Doppler Sonography of Normal Flow Patterns in Splanchnic Vessels

Arteries to the liver and spleen supply a low-resistance vascular bed and normally show forward flow throughout the cardiac cycle (systole and the entire duration of diastole). Blood flow in the superior mesenteric is of low resistance. Flow in the inferior mesenteric artery shows few or no diastolic Doppler shifts. The superior mesenteric artery in the fasting person has very little forward flow during diastole. Shortly after a meal, its diastolic flow increases considerably.[48] The Doppler profile of the abdominal aorta changes throughout its course. Continuous forward diastolic flow in the upper abdominal aorta is no longer seen beyond the origins of the low-resistance branches to the liver, spleen, intestine, and kidneys. In the distal abdominal aorta, flow reverses during diastole. Taylor et al. outlined typical Doppler curves for abdominal arteries. Figure 58-17 shows curves of some arteries and veins pertinent to this discussion.[49]

The **systemic veins of the abdomen** (inferior vena cava, hepatic, and renal veins) show a pulsatile flow pattern that reflects cardiac motion: two flow peaks toward the heart occur during atrial and ventricular diastole. A short spurt of reversed flow occurs in the hepatic veins and proximal IVC. This reversed flow accompanies atrial systole (the P wave of the electrocardiogram). In addition, the phase of respiration will influence the flow pattern of the systemic intra-abdominal veins (with increasing velocity in expiration). Consequently, the Doppler sonographic characteristics of these veins are variable in the breathing child.

Flow in splanchnic veins is more steady, with only gentle undulations that mirror cardiac motion (Fig. 58-17).[49] Blood is constantly directed toward the portal vein and into the liver. Flow velocity in the portal vein increases markedly after a meal and decreases with exercise.[50,51]

Possibilities and Pitfalls of Doppler Sonography

Doppler sonography is an excellent complement to splanchnic angiography and MRI. It provides answers to the queries left by an examination that depends on injection of contrast medium with or without pharmaceutical manipulation. Sometimes doubts remain regarding direction of flow or whether a vessel is obstructed or simply inaccessible to the contrast medium (such as reversed flow in the portal vein). The Doppler examination is a reliable indicator of direction of flow and assesses the splanchnic system in its physiologic state. The hepatic veins, difficult to outline with angiography, are easily identified with sonography and their flow pattern outlined. The major splanchnic vessels, such as the splenic, mesenteric, and portal veins, are readily opacified with arterioportography, but small vessels are hard to explore. This is particularly true of the branches of the left portal vein, which often are not opacified. The intrahepatic portal circulation can be readily studied with Doppler sonography, both in health and in disease. Each segmental branch of the portal vein is usually accessible to the Doppler beam. Regional flow patterns and the result of compression, obstruction of flow, reversal of flow, or arteriovenous fistulas can be assessed. With angiography and magnetic resonance, to-and-fro flow in a splanchnic vein is difficult to perceive. The Doppler examination yields clear signals of to-and-fro flow motions both on spectral display (a signal above and then below the reference line) and with color (alternating red and blue signals). If there is any doubt about details of the examination or when the patient's condition changes, the Doppler examination can be repeated without danger.

These advantages are counterbalanced by certain limitations, most of which are identical to those of real-time sonography. The examination is operator-dependent and requires some training not only in sonography, but also in the physics of Doppler and in the normal anatomy and physiology of the liver and splanchnic circulation. Doppler sonography is subject to the same physical laws as is real-time ultrasound. It is wishful thinking to expect a good Doppler examination in a patient in whom a poor real-time sonogram has just been obtained. The child's cirrhotic liver may be enlarged and have increased sound attenuation. To penetrate all this tissue with a real-time or Doppler beam sonogram may be a challenge to present instrumentation.

Quantitative analysis of splanchnic blood flow with Doppler instrumentation is a fascinating possibility because physiologic flow as well as portal hypertension and response to various drugs could be studied more intensively. However, because the technique depends on exact vessel beam angle and vessel diameter measurements, it is currently fraught with inaccuracies.[46,52]

In the present state of the art, in spite of the above-mentioned limitations, the Doppler examination of the splanchnic circulation is valuable. If a noninvasive test can answer such questions as whether the patient has portal hypertension, where the level of obstruction to blood flow is, and whether esophageal varices exist, it is a very useful clinical tool indeed. For this reason, the Doppler examination is rapidly becoming the screening method of choice for children with liver disease and potential portal hypertension.

Technique

Children over 5 years of age are usually examined after a 4-hour fast. Normally, their cooperation can be obtained if the procedure is explained to them. Sedation is rarely necessary. Whenever possible, respiration is stopped during the Doppler examination of a vessel so as to minimize its movement. The usual Doppler frequency is 3.0 or 5.0 MHz, even though the appropriate real-time frequency for the examination may vary from 3.0 to 7.5 MHz.

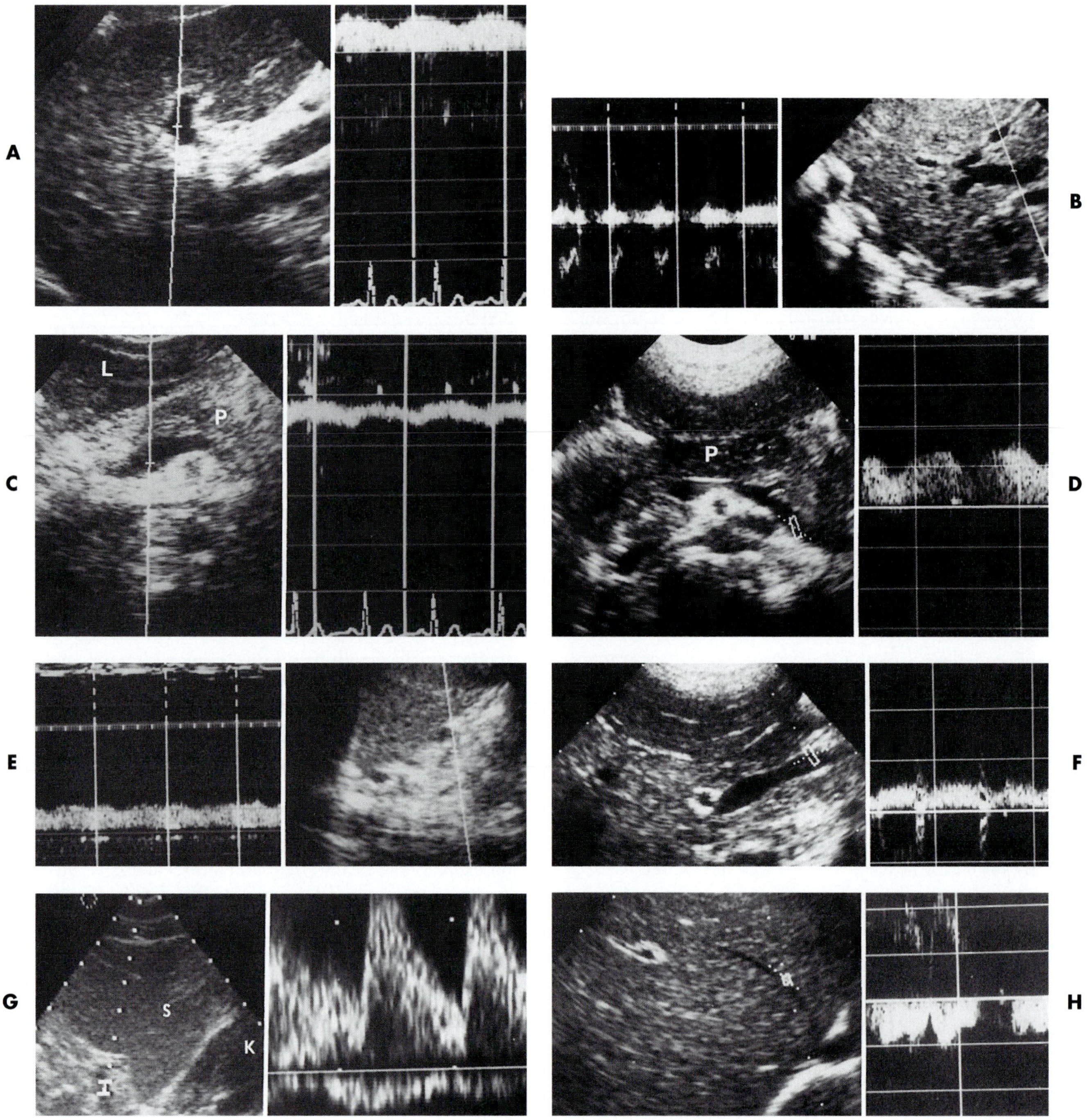

FIG. 58-17. Typical duplex Doppler images of splanchnic vessels of various patients. **A, Normal portal vein** examined through a longitudinal, paramedian, subcostal approach. Flow fluctuates slightly with cardiac systole. **B, Normal right branch of portal vein** seen from an oblique right subcostal approach in a 2-day-old neonate. (Wall motion artifacts originate from nearby hepatic artery.) **C, Normal splenic vein.** Doppler sample volume is in vein near splenomesenteric confluence and in its middle third. **D, Normal splenic vein** with cardiac-related modulation of flow. P, pancreas. **E, Enlarged left gastric vein** in a 17-year-old boy with cirrhosis. Left paramedian longitudinal view shows a thickened lesser omentum and a tortuous vein. Flow is directed anteriorly and superiorly toward esophagus. **F, Normal superior mesenteric vein** in 1-month-old boy, right paramedian longitudinal view. Flow modulation is synchronous with wall pulsations from adjacent superior mesenteric artery. Flow is directed toward the transducer Doppler sampler and superiorly toward the liver. **G, Normal splenic vein at hilum** (Doppler sample) in 2-year-old boy, seen from a left intercostal approach. Adjacent splenic artery (not seen) is shown with Doppler mode. Flow in artery (above the line) and vein (below the line) are in opposite directions, as expected normally. S, spleen. K, kidney. **H, Normal hepatic vein** in 1-week-old girl, transverse subcostal view, with flow away from transducer and modulated by pulsations of nearby right atrium. (From Patriquin HB, Lafortune M, Burns PN et al. Duplex Doppler examination in portal hypertension: technique and anatomy. *AJR* 1987;149:71-76.)

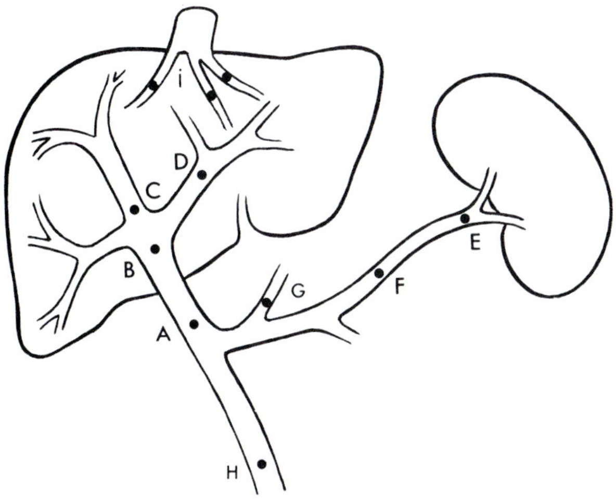

FIG. 58-18. Essential splanchnic vein reference points for Doppler sampling for possible portal hypertension in children with liver disease. A, Main portal vein. B, Intrahepatic portal vein. C, Right portal vein. D, Left portal vein. E, Splenic vein at hilum. F, Splenic vein. G, Left coronary vein. H, Superior mesenteric vein. I, Hepatic veins. Evaluation of the hepatic artery and IVC should be done as well. (From Patriquin HB, Lafortune M, Burns PN et al. Duplex Doppler examination in portal hypertension: technique and anatomy. *AJR* 1987;149:71-76.)

Because a small or upset child will not stop his or her rapid respiration, the examiner must be familiar with the Doppler equipment so as to be able to manipulate it quickly. All technical settings are adjusted beforehand. The vessel to be examined is outlined with real-time sonography. Color Doppler may be used to guide the placement of the sample volume. A spectral display of the Doppler shift is usually quite easily obtained even though it may disappear during part of the respiratory cycle.

Doppler Examination of the Child with Liver Disease for Portal Hypertension. The aim of the exam is to assess the presence and direction of flow in splanchnic veins, the main portal vein and its segmental intrahepatic branches, the hepatic veins, and the inferior vena cava (Fig. 58-18).[53,54] In addition, the presence of flow in the main hepatic artery and its intrahepatic branches is to be determined. When the clinical or basic Doppler examination raises the suspicion of portal hypertension, a systematic search for portosystemic collateral veins follows. The usual sites for spontaneous portosystemic shunts are outlined in Figure 58-19.[55] The lesser omentum[56] (from the splenomesenteric junction to the esophagus) and the renal, splenic, and hepatic hila as well as the pelvis are screened for the presence of dilated, tortuous veins. If hepatofugal (reversed) flow is found in a splanchnic vein, this vein is then traced to the recipient systemic vessel. The left gastric vein drains blood into the inferior esophageal vein; the splenic vein drains into the renal (or pararenal) veins; the superior

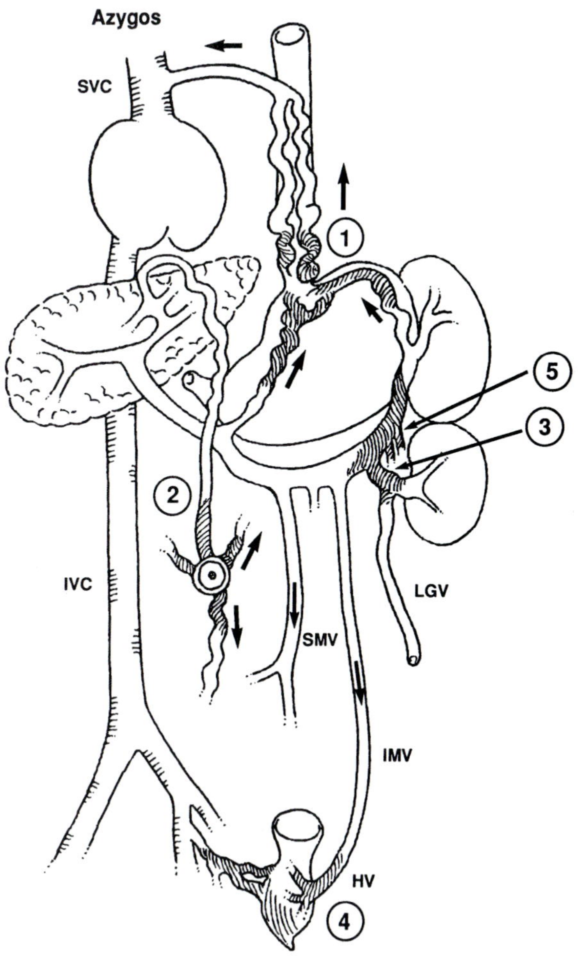

FIG. 58-19. Diagram of common spontaneous portosystemic collateral routes. SVC, superior vena cava. IVC, inferior vena cava. SMV, IMV, superior, inferior mesenteric vein. LGV, left gonadal vein. HV, hemorrhoidal vein. 1, Left gastric-azygos route (esophageal varices). 2, Paraumbilical-hypogastric/internal mammary route (caput medusa). 3, Spleno-renal route. 4, IMV-hemorrhoidal route. 5, Spleno-retroperitoneal-gonadal route. (From Patriquin HB, Lafortune M. Society for Pediatric Radiology Syllabus in Pediatric Radiology; 1994.)

and inferior mesenteric veins drain into gonadal, retroperitoneal, or hemorrhoidal veins; and the paraumbilical veins follow the round and falciform ligaments to drain into the anterior abdominal and iliac veins to form the classic caput medusae or into veins of the anterior chest wall and the internal mammary vein.

Direction of flow in one or several veins comprising the portal venous system may change in portal hypertension, and it is essential to record the flow direction accurately. One must carefully check that the orientation of the spectral or color display is normal and not inverted before starting the examination. The Doppler sample volume should be placed in the center of the vessel lumen. If the direction of flow within a vessel is difficult to ascertain, a nearby vessel with known flow direction can be used as a reference (e.g., the splenic or hepatic artery or their adjacent veins). During the Doppler recording, a simultaneous ECG tracing is useful for the understanding of certain flow fluctuations or pulsations within the system.

The **main portal vein and its right hepatic branches** are best studied through a right intercostal approach. Sometimes the superior mesenteric vein is also clearly seen from this position. **The left portal vein and three of its four branches** (the portal branch to the caudate lobe is rarely seen) and the **hepatic veins** are best seen through an oblique subcostal approach. The **splenic vein** is explored through a transverse approach over the spleen. The **superior mesenteric and main portal vein** are best visualized through a sagittal right paramedian approach (Fig. 58-17). The **left gastric vein** usually ends near the splenoportal junction and when enlarged, is easily observed through a sagittal left paramedian view (Fig. 58-17). The **inferior mesenteric vein,** when normal, can rarely be outlined. When enlarged, it may be traced through a left axillary approach to its junction with the splenic or superior mesenteric vein.

The various possible origins of the **hepatic artery** are sometimes difficult to recognize; we usually look for the artery at its usual origin from the celiac axis and also as it passes between the portal vein and the common bile duct. When the left hepatic artery arises from the superior mesenteric artery, it passes through the ligamentum venosum. The intrahepatic arterial branches accompany branches of the portal vein and can be detected with a slightly enlarged Doppler sample volume placed over a portal venous branch, even if the arterial branch cannot be seen with real-time ultrasound. Flow in the arteries to the right lobe of the liver (especially segments 5, 7, and 8) is usually easy to identify in this manner. The hepatic arterial branch accompanying the umbilical portion of the left portal vein (to segment 4) is especially easy to examine with Doppler because of the almost ideal vessel beam angle, which can be obtained through an anterior abdominal approach (Fig. 58-20). For this reason, we routinely look for arterial Doppler signals at this site in children who have undergone liver transplantation (Figs. 58-2 and 58-20).

A

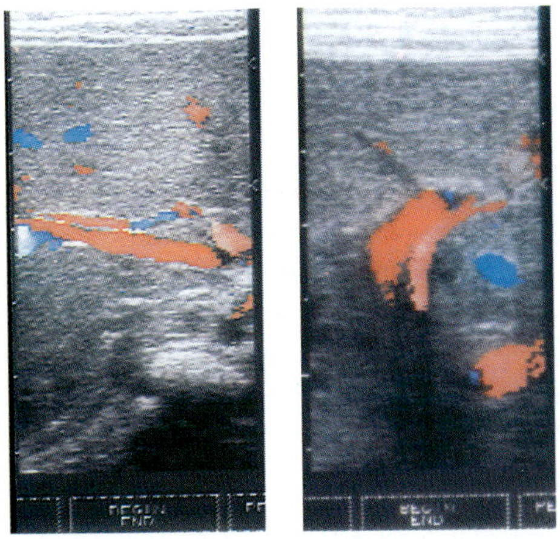

B

FIG. 58-20. Normal liver in a 2-month-old baby, oblique subcostal color Doppler sonogram. **A,** Right portal vein. **B,** Ascending or umbilical branch of the left PV is shown. Hepatic arterial (HA) branches lie close to the veins. Doppler shifts from both HA and PV are red because direction of flow is identical.

Abnormal Flow Patterns within the Portal System

Absent Doppler Signal. Proof of absence of a Doppler signal is much more difficult to establish than is its presence (see box). When the examiner fails to obtain a Doppler signal from a given vessel, one usually doubts the sensitivity of the machine and tests other nearby vessels. Failure to obtain a pulsed, color, or power Doppler signal from a splanchnic vein examined at an angle of less than 60°, full Doppler gain, low pulse repetition frequency with a 50 Hz wall filter and a restricted Doppler window means that blood is flowing at a velocity of less than 4 cm/sec. This is extremely slow. Thus, absence of a Doppler signal in this situation generally means absence of flow or a prethrombotic state.

Arterialized Flow Patterns Within the Portal System. The normal gently undulating flow within a portal vein is replaced by systolic peaks and high diastolic Doppler shifts. This pattern may signal the presence of an arterioportal fistula.[57]

Reversed or To-and-Fro Flow. Reversed flow in a splanchnic or intrahepatic portal vein is the most reliable Doppler sign of portal hypertension (PHT). However, hepatofugal flow in the portal vein occurs late and relatively rarely in patients with liver disease. To-and-fro flow in the portal vein also suggests the presence of PHT. Highly pulsatile or to-and-fro flow in the portal vein may also be seen in right heart failure (Fig. 58-21) or tricuspid insufficiency.

Abnormal Hepatic Arterial Doppler Patterns. Absence of a hepatic artery Doppler signal

CAUSES OF ABSENT DOPPLER SIGNAL

Doppler angle > 60°
Low Doppler gain
Low PRF
High filter (best is 50 Hz)
Small sample volume
PV flow decreases if fasting
HA flow decreases if eating

suggests arterial thrombosis or reduced flow in prethrombotic states.[58] Locally increased systolic Doppler shifts or peripheral tardus-parvus curves may be the result of stenosis of the hepatic artery, as at any other arterial site.

The portal vein and hepatic artery act in concert to nourish the liver. Changes in flow volumes in one affect the other. After a meal, portal venous flow increases and hepatic arterial flow diminishes, probably by vasoconstriction. Hepatic arterial diastolic flow is decreased and systolic peaks are lower when measured at the same sites in the same person.[59] Arterial signals within the liver may be difficult to find after a meal. (This is particularly disturbing in the patient who has received a liver transplant, in whom a false diagnosis of thrombosis may be made.)

Portal Venous Hypertension

Portal venous hypertension is a pathologic condition characterized by increased pressure in the portal vein or one of its tributaries. The normal pressure in the portal vein is between 5 and 10 mm Hg. When the pressure in the portal vein is more than 5 mm Hg above inferior vena caval pressure, portal hypertension is present.

The sequelae of portal hypertension are numerous. They include splenomegaly, collateral vein formation, and a thickened lesser omentum. In children, the lesser omentum is observed between the left lobe of the liver and the aorta on sagittal images. Its thickness should not exceed the diameter of the aorta (Fig. 58-22).[59,60] In PHT, it is thickened by lymphatic stasis and an engorged left gastric vein. Morphologic changes of the liver architecture are usually present also.

An increased caliber of the portal vein and a lack of variation in the caliber of the splenic and mesenteric veins have been described in portal hypertension in adults. The accuracy of these findings in the assessment of portal hypertension in children has not been established. Indeed, in our experience of children with biliary cirrhosis, portal venous caliber has decreased as cirrhosis has progressed.

The hemodynamic information gleaned from the Doppler examination usually answers the following questions: Is portal hypertension present? What is the level of obstruction? What is the direction of flow within the system? Are there portosystemic collaterals?

Hepatofugal flow in a portosystemic collateral vein establishes the diagnosis of portal hypertension. Clinically, the most significant route is via the **left gastric vein,** which supplies esophageal varices. The left gastric vein is rarely visible sonographically in the normal child. When it dilates to a diameter of greater than 2 to 3 mm, it can be traced from the splenic vein near the splenomesenteric junction through the lesser omentum (behind the left lobe of the liver and anterior to the aorta) to the esophagus (Fig. 58-17, *E* and Fig. 58-22). A venous Doppler flow pattern makes it possible to distinguish the vein from the nearby left gastric or hepatic arteries. Flow direction is determined at the same time. The caliber of the left gastric vein is usually related to the size of esophageal varices and probably to the likelihood of bleeding.[61]

The **paraumbilical vein** classically shunts blood from the left portal vein to the periumbilical venous network. It follows a vertical, right paramedian course to enter the falciform ligament through the left lobe of the liver (Fig. 58-23). With a high-frequency transducer (7.5 MHz), its subcutaneous course is easily seen sonographically from the lower tip of the left lobe of the liver to the umbilicus (Fig. 58-23). Other spontaneous portosystemic collateral veins should be sought near the spleen, left kidney, and flanks, where splenorenal shunts (Fig. 58-24 on p. 1670) or dilated

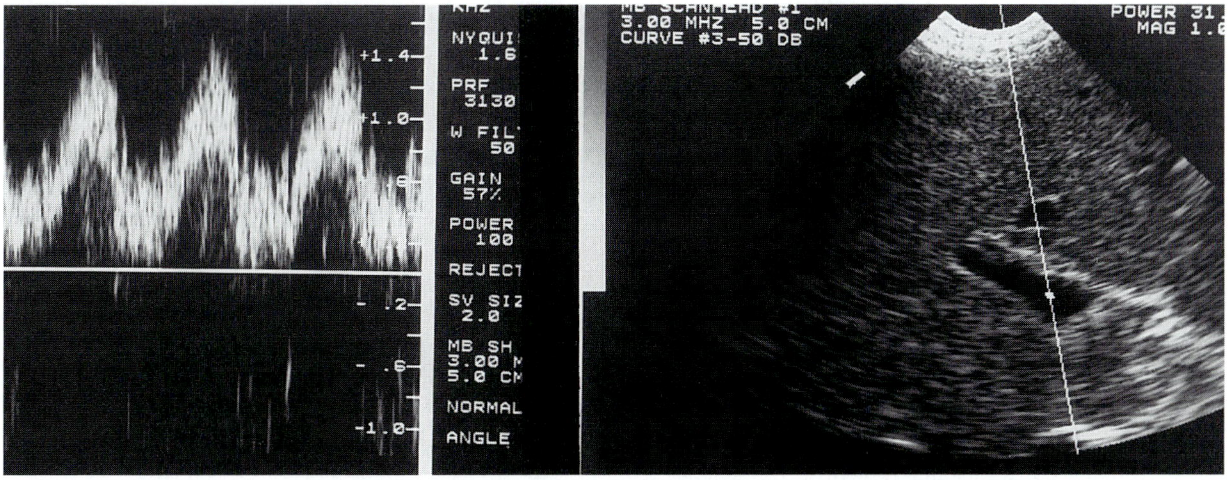

FIG. 58-21. Highly pulsatile portal venous flow in a child with right heart failure. Compare to the gently undulating flow in Fig. 58-17.

A

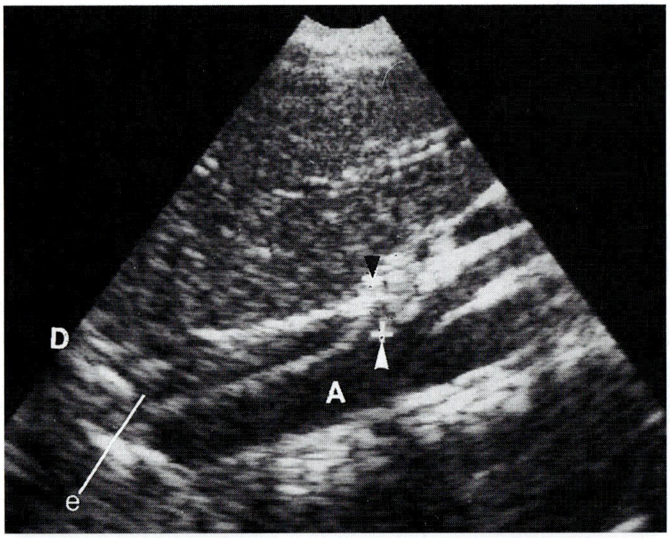

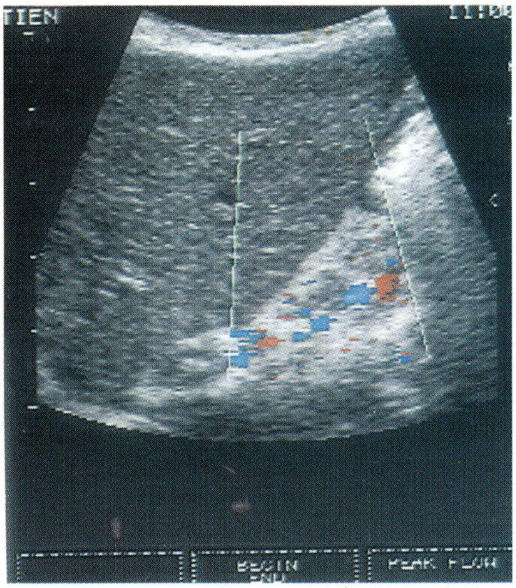

C

B

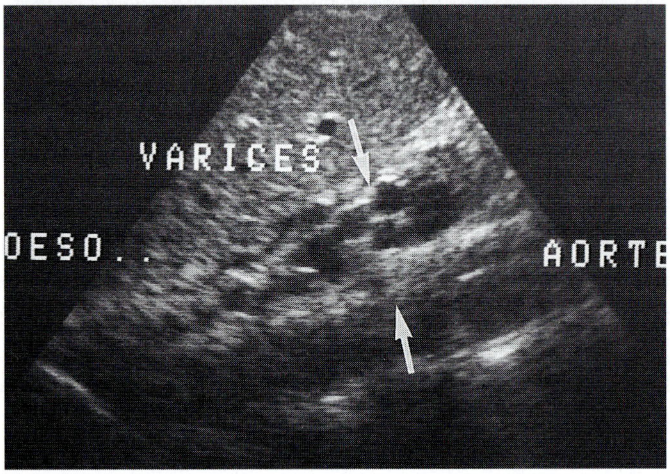

FIG. 58-22. A, Normal lesser omentum (on sagittal left paramedian sonogram of a 9-year-old boy), seen between the left lobe of the liver and the aorta, measured between the arrowheads, and smaller than the aorta. e, Esophagus; D, diaphragm. **B, Abnormal lesser omentum** (*arrows*) **thickened by a tortuous, dilated left gastric vein in a child with cirrhosis. C,** Color Doppler image of the abnormal left gastric vein showing flow signals mainly directed toward the esophagus (blue).

perirenal, retroperitoneal (Fig. 58-25), or gonadal veins receive blood from the splenic or mesenteric veins; in the pelvis (Fig. 58-26 on p. 1672), around the right kidney; and near the porta hepatis and gallbladder (Fig. 58-27 on p. 1673 and Fig. 58-28 on p. 1674), where portocaval, paraduodenorenal, or veins of Sappey may shunt the blood between portal and hepatic veins. The variety of spontaneous portosystemic collaterals is almost limitless.

All portosystemic collaterals should be traced to their recipient systemic vein, which is usually dilated where the shunt enters (Fig. 58-25). The "donor" splanchnic vein is also dilated. When portal hypertension decreases after shunt surgery or transplantation, portosystemic collaterals decrease in size (as do the enlarged spleen and lesser omentum).

If a spontaneous (or surgical) portosystemic shunt is large, hepatic encephalopathy may ensue. The Doppler examination, being "physiologic," may at times reveal unusual portosystemic collateral routes difficult to demonstrate with arterioportographic studies (locally inverted flow in intrahepatic portal venous branches, new "neo" veins leading from portal veins to the abdominal wall, or hepatofugal flow in the splenic vein).

Prehepatic Portal Hypertension

Prehepatic portal hypertension results from obstruction of the splenic, mesenteric, or portal vein. As with other venous thromboses, predisposing factors involve the vessel wall (trauma, catheters), stagnant blood flow, and abnormal clotting factors. Principal causes of **thrombosis of the portal vein** include **(a)** trauma such as umbilical venous catheterization, **(b)** dehydration or shock, **(c)** pyelophlebitis following appendicitis or abdominal sepsis, **(d)** coagulopathy, with protein C deficiency being recognized with increasing frequency, **(e)** portal vein invasion by adjacent tumors, **(f)** compression of the vein by pancreatitis, lymph nodes, or tumor, and **(g)** increased resistance to portal venous flow into the liver in cirrhosis or the Budd-Chiari syndrome (see box on p. 1670).

Recanalization of portal venous thrombi usually occurs rapidly in children. In addition, paraportal venous channels and the cystic veins draining the gall-

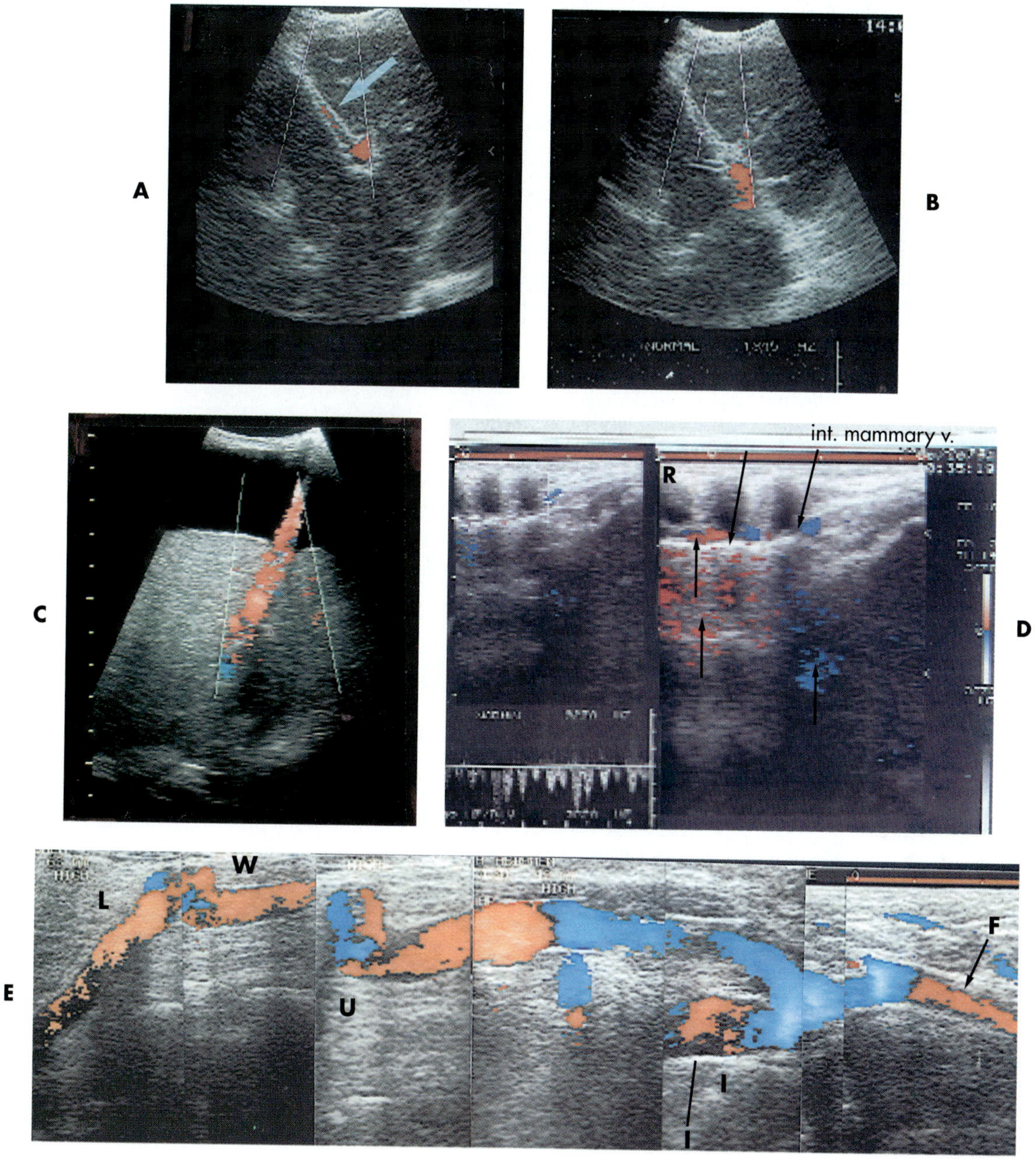

FIG. 58-23. Paraumbilical collateral route. A and B, **Cirrhosis and portal hypertension.** Oblique subcostal and sagittal paramedian Doppler sonograms of a 10-year-old boy. Left lobe of liver: venous flow signals are directed into the liver through the left portal vein (B-red) and into a vein within the round ligament (arrow in A and sample volume in B) leading to the anterior surface of the liver. (From Patriquin HB. RSNA publications: *Current Concepts in Pediatric Radiology*; 1994.) **C, Cystic fibrosis and ascites.** Blood flow leaves the liver through a patent paraumbilical vein that enters the falciform ligament which is surrounded by fluid (sagittal color Doppler abdominal sonogram). **D,** Another child **with cirrhosis and portal hypertension** in the parasternal region: pulsed and color Doppler images show pulsatile flow in cephalad direction in the internal mammary veins, originating from a paraumbilical vein. R, rib. Arrows, flash color artifacts from moving lungs. **E, Same child** as D, a composite sagittal sonogram (7.5 MHz transducer) of the abdominal wall (W) shows the paraumbilical vein leaving the liver (L), surrounding the umbilicus (U), and entering the iliac vein (I). F, femoral vein. (From Patriquin HB. In: Taylor KJW, Burns PN, Wells PNT, eds. *Clinical Applications of Doppler Ultrasound*. Philadelphia: Lippincott-Raven; 1996.)

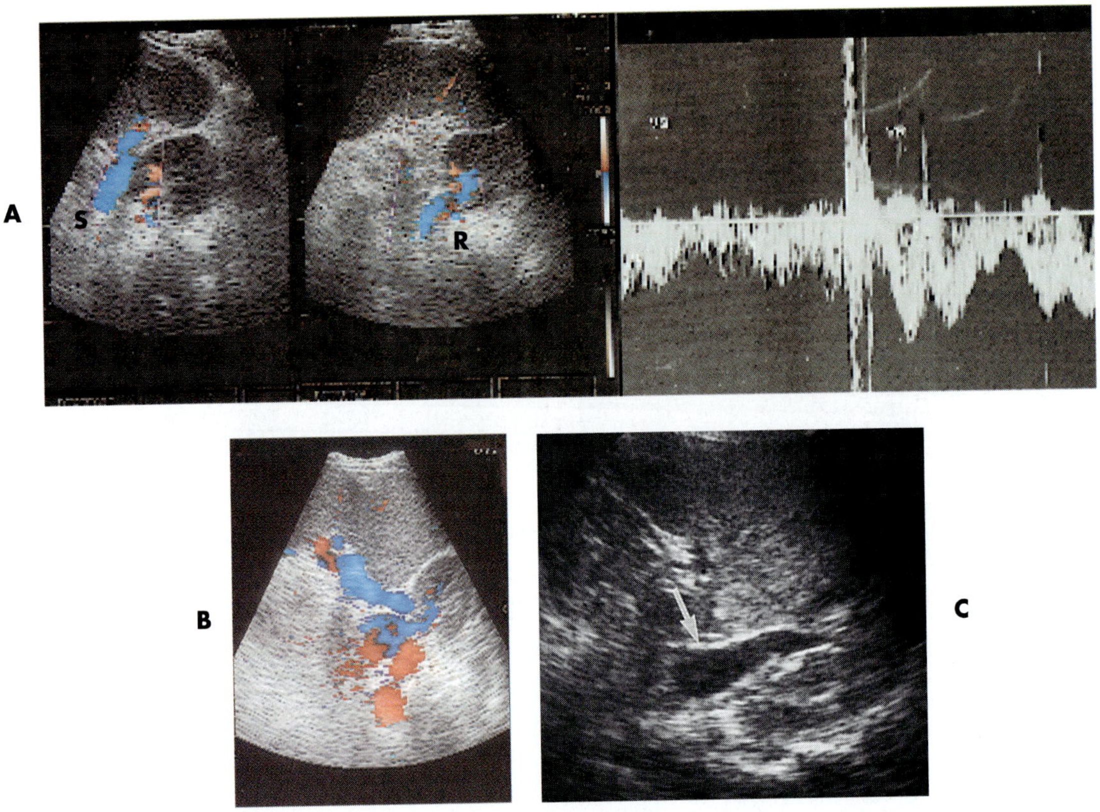

FIG. 58-24. Normal splenic (S) and renal veins (R). **A,** Coronal views are close together near the left renal hilum. Pulsed Doppler images show gently undulating flow in the splenic V (VS) and triphasic flow in the renal V (VR). This difference implies that the two veins are not connected by a shunt. **Spontaneous splenorenal shunt in an 8-year-old boy with cirrhosis. B,** Color Doppler sonogram shows blood flow leaving the spleen toward the dilated renal vein (blue). Flow is circular at the site of communication (red and blue). **C,** In another child with a splenorenal shunt, the left renal vein is dilated (*arrow*).

bladder dilate and channel blood into the liver if there is no obstruction at this site (in cirrhosis or hepatic vein thrombosis). The resultant collection of tortuous veins is called a **cavernoma** (Fig. 58-29 on p. 1674). Hepatopetal flow in these vessels is easily detected with Doppler sonography. In spite of these collateral channels, portal hypertension follows and esophageal varices occur frequently.[62]

Following thrombosis of the portal vein, the peripheral intrahepatic portal veins become small and threadlike. The lumen may not be visible. Careful examination of these vessels with Doppler sonography usually shows hepatopetal venous flow, likely the result of shunting through the vessels at the porta hepatis which constitute the "cavernoma." (Because the obstruction to venous flow occurs at the porta hepatis, it is not surprising that children with portal venous thrombosis do not have enlarged paraumbilical veins and a caput medusa; this portosystemic route relies on abundant flow in the left portal vein.)[62]

Another cause of prehepatic (or intrahepatic "presinusoidal") portal hypertension in children is **congenital hepatic fibrosis.** It is an inherited, autosomal recessive disease characterized by fibrosis at the portal triad where terminal branches of the portal vein and small bile ducts are compressed. Hepatocytes are found to be normal, as is liver function.[10] Liver architecture is disturbed by linear or cyst-like structures representing variable bile duct ectasia as well as paraportal collaterals (cavernoma)[63,64] (Fig. 58-28). The children usually present with bleeding esophageal

CAUSES OF PORTAL VEIN THROMBOSIS

Trauma
Catheters
Dehydration
Shock
Pyelophlebitis
Coagulopathy, especially protein C deficiency
Portal vein invasion
Portal vein compression
Cirrhosis
Budd-Chiari syndrome

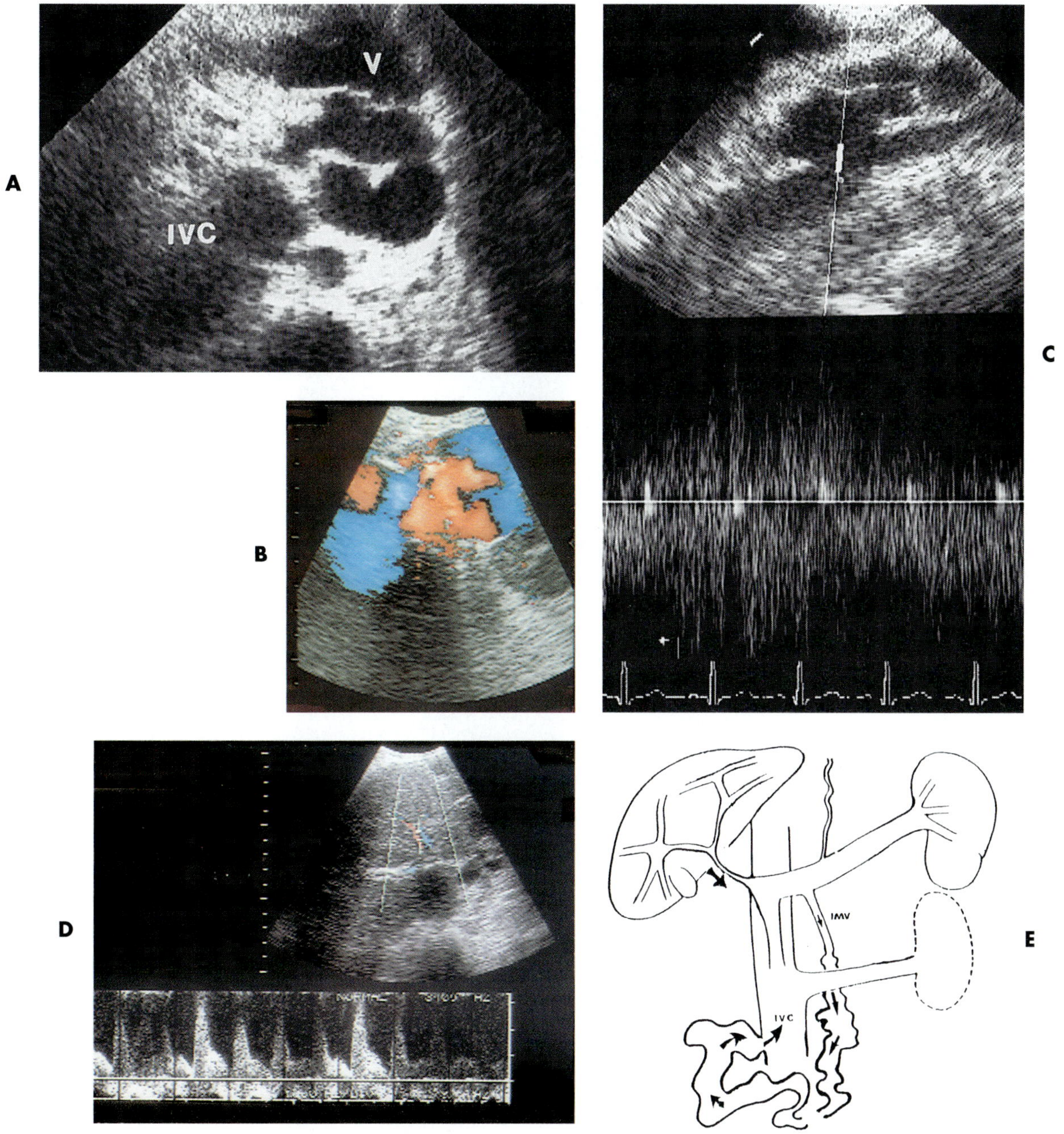

FIG. 58-25. Retroperitoneal portosystemic shunt (10-year-old boy with biliary cirrhosis). **A,** Coronal, periumbilical sonogram shows tubular structures. **B,** Vessels with color Doppler sonography. V, veins. IVC, inferior vena cava. **C,** Sagittal pulsed Doppler examination shows highly turbulent venous flow at the site where the collateral veins enter the IVC. Note the increase in caliber of the IVC cephalad to the shunt entry (to the left of the cursor). **D,** Color and spectral Doppler image of the liver shows hepatofugal (reversed) flow in the PV. **E,** Drawing of the shunt to IVC as perceived with Doppler sonography. IMV, inferior mesenteric vein.

varices. Sonography shows hallmarks of portal hypertension: splenomegaly and a thick lesser omentum in which a dilated tortuous left gastric vein is visible, with hepatofugal flow detected with Doppler sonography (Fig. 58-22). Congenital hepatic fibrosis is usually associated with **recessive polycystic kidney disease** (Fig. 58-28). The dilatation of renal collecting ducts in these children is variable and less severe than it is in the neonatal form, and renal impairment is less marked. However, renal architecture is greatly disturbed. The pyramids are hyperechogenic and may contain calcium; small cysts are sometimes seen; the kidneys are usually enlarged. These features enable informed sonologists to find the cause of upper intestinal bleeding

A
B
C

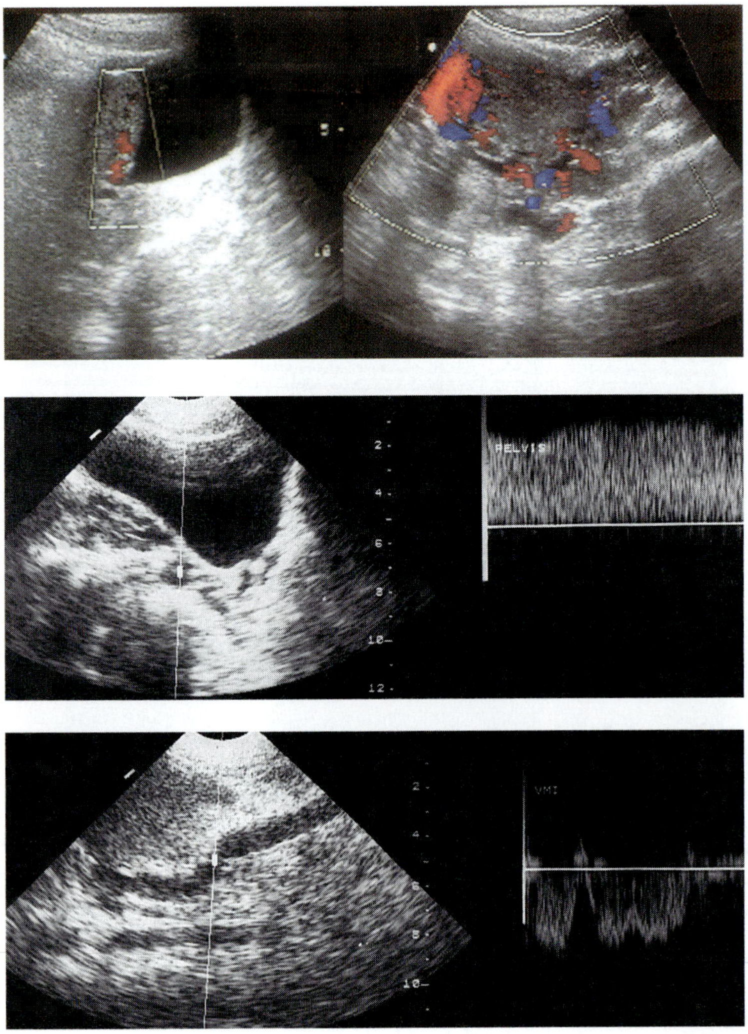

FIG. 58-26. Pelvic varices. 17-year-old girl with portal vein cavernoma. **A,** Sagittal and coronal views of the uterus show dilated vessels around the uterus. **B,** Pulsed Doppler image shows paraovarian venous varices. **C,** Left flank (axillary view): a dilated vein with triphasic flow is the left gonadal (ovarian) vein shunting blood toward the renal vein.

in these children during their first abdominal sonogram. (A description of the kidneys in this disease is found in the chapter on renal diseases in children.)

Intrahepatic Portal Hypertension

Serious insult to the hepatocyte results in necrosis. Unless necrosis is overwhelming, scarring and the formation of multiple regenerating nodules follow. The process of cirrhosis results in scarred and obstructed sinusoids and abnormal portal venous blood flow through the regenerated nodules. In children, cirrhosis follows:

- hepatitis;
- destruction of the hepatocyte by toxins accumulated in inherited metabolic diseases such as tyrosinemia, some forms of glycogenosis, and Wilson's disease; and
- bile stasis such as biliary atresia and cystic fibrosis.

Although different types of cirrhosis form their initial obstruction at presinusoidal (schistosomiasis, biliary cirrhosis), sinusoidal (Laennec's cirrhosis), and postsinusoidal levels, progressive scarring usually spreads to the entire sinusoid. As intrahepatic portal venous flow stagnates, portosystemic collaterals open. Portal blood flow decreases. Total hepatic blood supply is usually maintained by an increase of blood flow in the hepatic artery.

CAUSES OF CIRRHOSIS IN CHILDREN

Hepatitis
Toxins accumulated in inherited metabolic diseases
Biliary atresia
Cystic fibrosis

Sonographically, these changes in hemodynamics are signaled by decreasing diameter of the portal vein and its segmental branches to the point where they are reduced to thread-like structures. Flow velocity, when measurable, is reduced. Conversely, branches of the hepatic artery (normally very difficult to see in children) may become visible with gray scale sonography. Doppler sonography mirrors the increased hepatic ar-

A

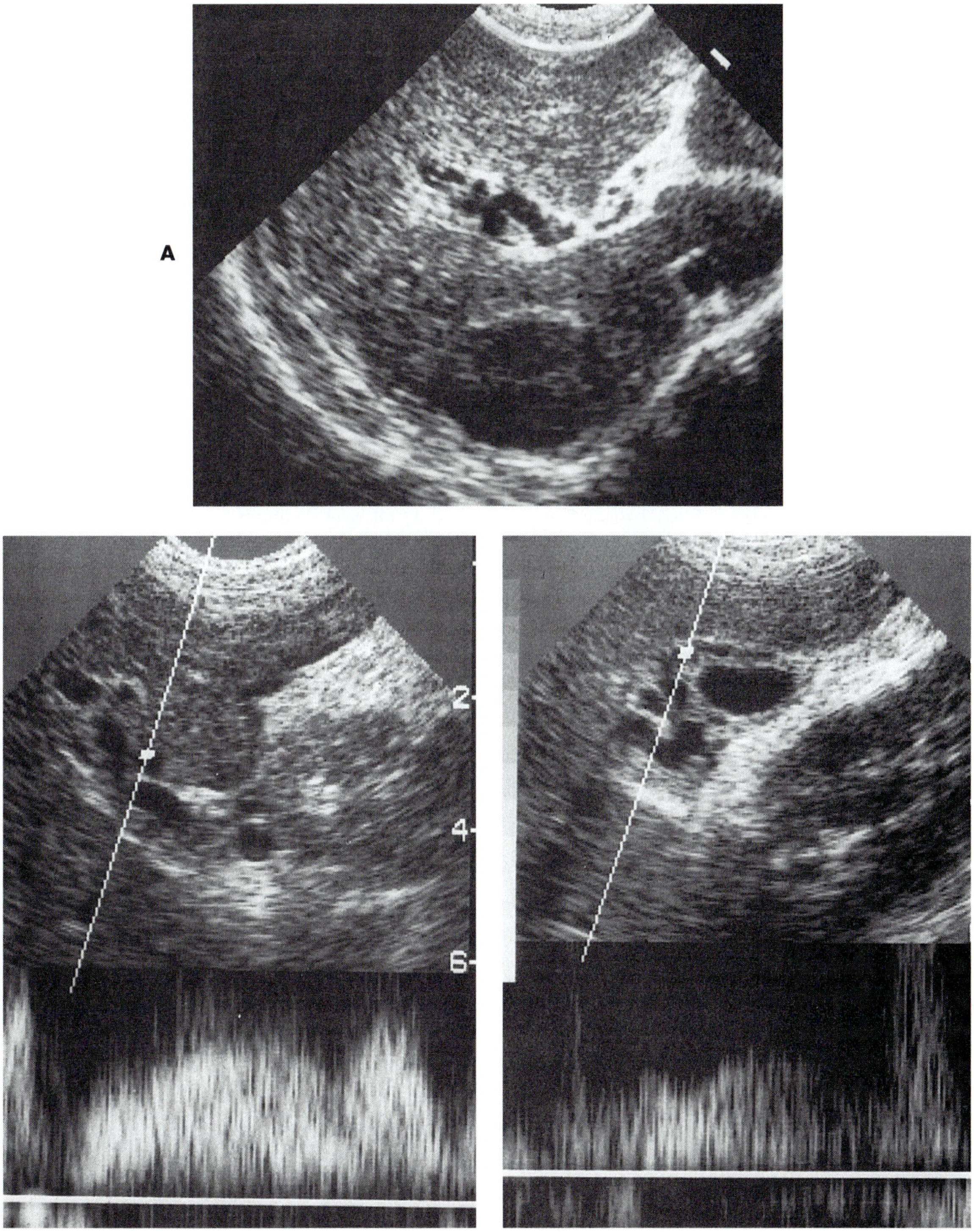

B

C

FIG. 58-27. Portal vein cavernoma in a 2-year-old girl following severe gastroenteritis in infancy. **A,** Oblique sonogram of the liver shows several tortuous tubular veins. **B,** Hepatopetal venous flow at pulsed Doppler examination. **C,** The gallbladder is surrounded by dilated cholecystic veins. In spite of the venous collaterals transporting blood into the liver around the thrombosed portal vein, the child had esophageal varices. (B and C from Patriquin HB. In: Taylor et al. *Clinical Doppler Sonography*. Philadelphia: Lippincott-Raven, 1995.)

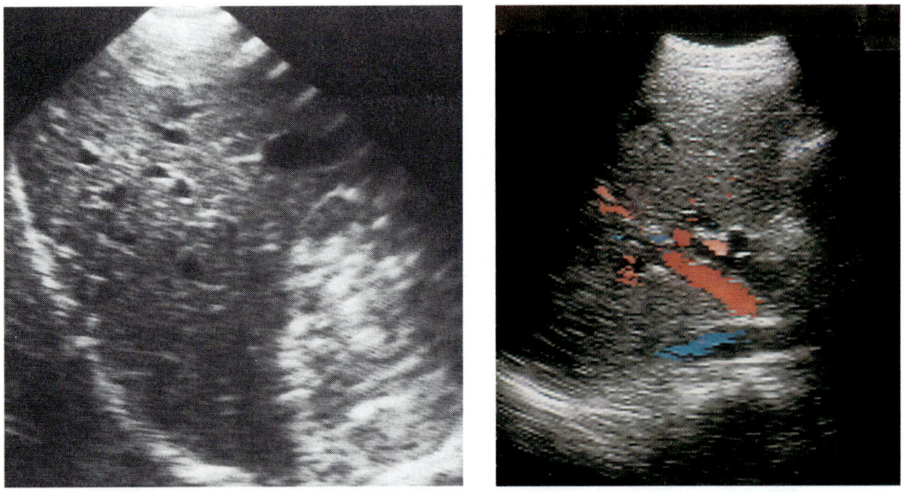

FIG. 58-28. Congenital hepatic fibrosis causes portal vein and biliary obstruction (portal cavernoma and bile duct ectasia). **A,** A sagittal view shows multiple small cystic structures in the right lobe of the liver. The adjacent kidney is large and contains multiple hyperechoic foci throughout the cortex and medulla due to recessive polycystic kidney disease. **B,** The liver hilum in a 12-year-old girl contains three tubular structures: two "portal veins" and a dilated bile duct (devoid of color flow signals). (From Patriquin HB. In: Pediatric Diseases Test and Syllabus, vol. 35. American College of Radiology.)

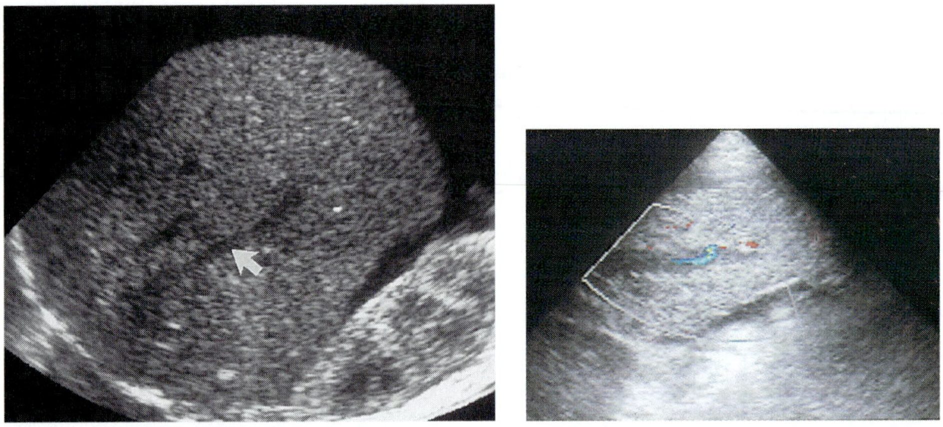

FIG. 58-29. Budd-Chiari syndrome. **A,** Acute: the liver is surrounded by ascitic fluid. The diagonal course of a hepatic vein is shown. The lumen is filled with echogenic clot (*arrow*). **B,** Several days later, color Doppler image shows almost complete absence of flow within the hepatic vein (blue). (Courtesy of M. Lafortune, M.D., Montreal.)

terial caliber and flow seen angiographically. Doppler shifts from segmental arteries are increased in comparison to their portal venous neighbors.

Two hemodynamic mechanisms appear to operate in patients with portal hypertension, especially in those with cirrhosis. The **backward-flow** theory explains portal hypertension by the increased resistance to portal venous flow caused by the intrahepatic block described above. In response to stagnating intrahepatic flow, portosystemic collaterals form and drain blood away from the liver, finally resulting in hepatofugal flow in some or all segmental branches and in the main portal vein, which is easily demonstrated with Doppler sonography. Why does the portal pressure remain elevated despite the presence of such a decompression mechanism? This question may be answered by the forward-flow theory. In the backward-flow theory, portal blood flow is unchanged or even diminished. The **forward-flow** theory proposes that splanchnic arterioles dilate in patients with cirrhosis. The resultant decreased splanchnic resistance leads to increased flow in the intestinal arteries and veins with subsequently increased portal venous blood flow. This would explain why portal hypertension is maintained despite extensive portosystemic shunting.

Because the obstruction to portal blood flow in cirrhosis is within the liver, periportal and cystic venous collaterals rarely develop. However, blood is often shunted from the left portal vein through one or several tortuous paraumbilical veins to veins of the anterior wall of the abdomen and thorax. Documenting hepatofugal flow in such a vein situated within the falciform ligament is an easy way to establish the diagnosis of portal hypertension in children. The superficial abdominal (thoracic) wall collaterals are readily traced with color Doppler sonography if one uses a high-frequency transducer (Fig. 58-23).

The left gastric vein, shunting blood from the liver to esophageal varices, although dilated, becomes increasingly difficult to detect sonographically in children with advanced cirrhosis; atrophy of the left lobe of the liver abolishes the acoustic window through which the lesser omentum is normally explored.

All the other portosystemic shunts described in Fig. 58-19 are possible in children with cirrhosis. Thus, the entire abdomen and pelvis should be explored sonographically in order to find them. The principle of shunting is constant in all portosystemic collaterals; a dilated, often tortuous splanchnic vein with reversed (hepatofugal) flow shunts blood into a systemic vein that is equally dilated at the site of the shunt. Rapid venous blood flow produces high, steady Doppler shifts. Turbulence and bidirectional flow often occur at the shunt site. A diagram that summarizes the Doppler findings is extremely helpful in visualizing the entire shunt route as well as the intrahepatic circulation (Fig. 58-25). A minority of patients with severe portal hypertension develop reversal of flow in the main portal vein, sometimes because of the proximity of a large shunt near the porta hepatis (Fig. 58-26). **If one were to depend on reversed portal venous flow to make the diagnosis of PHT, one would miss the diagnosis in the majority of such patients.**[65]

Suprahepatic (Posthepatic) Portal Hypertension

The clinical quartet of ascites, abdominal pain, jaundice, and hepatomegaly that follows obstruction of the hepatic veins is called the **Budd-Chiari syndrome.** It is rare in children. Doppler sonography is particularly useful in excluding the diagnosis, since the four clinical signs that make up the syndrome are quite common in children with other forms of portal hypertension. The first patients with thrombosis of the hepatic veins described by Budd (1846), Fredrichs, Lange, and Chiari (1899) were thought to have hepatic phlebitis secondary to sepsis or syphilis, with primary involvement of small branches of the hepatic veins. Since then, other causes have been recognized and they are now classified as obstruction of the central and sublobular veins, the major hepatic veins, or the inferior vena cava near the hepatic vein ostia.[66] **Small-vessel hepatic venous occlusive disease** is due to the following: toxins, especially pyrolizidine alkaloids contained in ragwort or Jamaican bush tea; chemotherapy; bone marrow transplantation; lupus erythematosus; hepatic irradiation; and the use of oral contraceptives. This disease involves primarily small hepatic venous radicles, although the major branches may be secondarily involved. **Thrombosis of the main hepatic veins** is usually due to coagulation abnormalities or to congenital malformations of the hepatic vein ostia. Obstruction of the hepatic portion of the IVC may result in thrombosis of the hepatic veins. Congenital membranes of the IVC resulting from faulty embryologic fenestration of its lumen can also lead to obstruction of hepatic veins.[67] The most common position for such a membrane is below an obstructed left hepatic vein and above a patent right hepatic vein, probably a result of an obstructing fibrous remnant of the left umbilical vein and ductus venosus.

CAUSES OF HEPATIC VENOUS OCCLUSIVE DISEASE

Toxins
- Ragwort or Jamaican bush tea

Chemotherapy
Bone marrow transplantation
Lupus erythematosus
Hepatic irradiation
Oral contraceptives
Coagulation abnormalities
Congenital malformations of the hepatic vein ostia
Obstruction of the hepatic portion of the IVC
Congenital membranes of the IVC

Following any obstruction of the hepatic veins, the liver becomes enlarged and congested. Because the caudate lobe has its own hepatic vein which drains into the IVC below the others, it is often spared and serves as the only initial venous drainage route for the entire liver. It enlarges quickly and often compresses the IVC. This is followed by ascites, often pleural effusions, splenomegaly, and the formation of portosystemic collaterals. These findings can be confirmed sonographically. Doppler sonography shows absence or reversal of flow in the hepatic veins (Fig. 58-29). Areas of high-velocity flow near stenoses of hepatic veins are easily detected with color-guided, pulsed Doppler sonography. In the absence of hepatic venous drainage, arterial blood may be shunted into the portal vein through microscopic shunts at the portal triad or through larger intrahepatic shunts. Portal venous flow may reverse. Alternately, the portal vein may thrombose when liver congestion is severe. All these changes can be detected with Doppler sonography; wedge hepatic venography, which shows a spiderweb network of intrahepatic veins instead of the usual hepatic venous lumens, is now rarely performed.

The patient with acute Budd-Chiari syndrome rarely has time to form portosystemic collateral routes. If there are shunt routes, they are similar to those seen in cirrhosis. (Periportal and cystic veins do not usually serve as shunt routes because they drain into the segmental branches of the right portal vein, which are highly congested in response to hepatic vein obstruction.) Extensive intrahepatic shunts may form and can be demonstrated with color Doppler sonography.

The treatment of hepatic vein occlusion is anticoagulant therapy, the ablation of obstructive webs, or emergency portocaval shunting. The recanalization of hepatic veins, the regression of portal hypertension (decreased caliber and flow velocity in portosystemic shunts, smaller spleen, absorption of ascites), and the patency of therapeutic shunts can be assessed with Doppler sonography.

Surgical Portosystemic Shunts

At one time the definitive treatment of children with bleeding esophageal varices was surgical portosystemic shunts. These shunts are now created only when sclerotherapy of varices has failed or transplantation is not feasible. Children with healthy livers and prehepatic portal hypertension are still candidates for shunt procedures. **Transjugular intrahepatic portosystemic shunts (TIPS)** are being performed as an alternate to classical surgical shunts in adults. Their use in children is beginning to grow. The patency of transjugular shunts is being monitored with Doppler sonography, which shows blood flowing from the "donor" right portal vein through the intrahepatic stent and into the right (or another) hepatic vein. Shunt stenoses, thrombosis, and flow around the stent are readily visible with Doppler sonography.

Surgical portosystemic shunts can be total or partial. Total shunts direct the entire venous blood flow from the congested splanchnic system into a systemic vein, as in the end-to-side portocaval shunt in which the main portal vein is redirected. The hepatic end is ligated and the splanchnic end is connected to the IVC. In this situation, there is little portal venous perfusion of the liver. Partial shunts divert only some of the splanchnic blood into a systemic vein, thereby yielding better liver perfusion and reducing the incidence of hepatic encephalopathy: the distal splenorenal (Warren) shunt connects the splenic vein to the left renal vein; the side-to-side, or H-type portocaval shunt, connects the portal vein to the IVC at the porta hepatis.

The Doppler examination of portosystemic shunts includes study of the shunt site and the splanchnic and hepatic venous system. The site of a shunt may vary with the surgical technique; if the veins used for a standard shunt are not suitable, the surgeon may use the nearest available vein, for example, the superior mesenteric vein. If the shunt is patent, it is quite often visible sonographically,[68,69] and Doppler signals are usually easily discerned at the site itself. Color Doppler is particularly useful in this situation. Blood flow often accelerates at and near the site of a patent shunt and there may be some turbulence. Flow direction is hepatofugal, toward the systemic vein. Poststenotic signs of stenosis include rapid flow (high Doppler shifts) at the shunt site and poststenotic turbulence (bidirectional or reversed Doppler flow signals). Should angioplasty be considered, direct visualization of the shunt by contrast venography is necessary.

In our experience, a Doppler study of the intrahepatic portal veins is invaluable in the assessment of portocaval shunt patency. In the majority of patent shunts, flow in the intrahepatic portal veins is hepatofugal.[70] It is easy to understand why this should be so in latero-lateral portocaval shunts where high-pressure intrahepatic venous blood flows through the shunt into the low-pressure vena cava. It is more difficult to explain hepatofugal flow in the intrahepatic portal veins in patients with an end-to-side portocaval shunt, in whom the hepatic end of the portal vein has been ligated and cut. Blood may leave the liver through a system of collateral veins between intrahepatic branches of the portal vein and low-pressure systemic veins. This phenomenon has been demonstrated angiographically.[71]

Signs of shunt obstruction include the following:

- The shunt site is difficult or impossible to detect, and no Doppler signals can be obtained;
- blood in the splanchnic vein feeding the shunt no longer flows toward the shunt;
- the direction of intrahepatic portal venous flow returns to normal; and
- spontaneous portosystemic shunts and other signs of portal hypertension reappear.

SIGNS OF SHUNT OBSTRUCTION

Shunt site has no Doppler signals
Blood in the splanchnic vein no longer flows toward the shunt
Intrahepatic portal venous flow returns to normal
Signs of portal hypertension reappear

DOPPLER SONOGRAPHY IN THE CHILD RECEIVING A LIVER TRANSPLANT

Pretransplantation Evaluation

Before transplantation can be considered, the caliber and patency of the main portal vein and inferior vena cava must be assessed. This can usually be done with Doppler sonography.[72,73] If the portal vein diameter is less than 4 mm (as it may be in advanced cirrhosis) or if Doppler flow studies are equivocal, MRI or angiography may be performed. Children with biliary atresia sometimes have an associated **polysplenia syndrome** (Fig. 58-8), which includes intestinal malrotation, bilaterally symmetrical patterns of the major bronchi, abnormal location of the portal vein anterior to the duodenum, and interruption of the IVC.[13,74] Liver transplantation may be more difficult in these children. It is essential that the surgeon be aware of this anatomic abnormality before transplantation.

In addition, portocaval or mesenteric-caval shunts, whether created surgically or occurring naturally, change both the flow pattern and the caliber of the main portal vein and may alter the surgical approach to transplantation. The anatomic variants of the hepatic artery are not always demonstrated sonographically, but angiography is rarely performed for the purpose of outlining the anatomy of the hepatic artery. (The examination of the child before transplantation includes several organs outside of the liver: the kidneys, lungs, heart, and intestinal tract.)[72]

During liver transplantation in the child, the donor hepatic artery is sometimes removed with a cuff of aorta and anastomosed to the recipient's abdominal aorta or iliac artery. An adult liver is usually divided prior to being transplanted into a small child. Although the left lobe, or segments 2 and 3, are preferred, an adult liver may be divided and used for two recipients. A transient fluid collection often forms around the cut surface of the transplanted lobe or segments, even though the cut is packed with hemostatic material such as gelfoam. Because the anatomy involved in segmental or lobar liver transplantation differs considerably from the normal anatomy and from the anatomy involved in whole-organ transplantation, a diagram of the operative procedure is a useful guide for the sonologist assessing patency of anastomosed vessels.

Posttransplantation Evaluation

The most common complication in the immediate postoperative period is **hepatic artery thrombosis.** Although collateral vessels may form in the child and shunt arterial blood into the liver, bile duct necrosis usually occurs, followed by the formation of bile lakes and recurrent infection. Retransplantation is almost invariably necessary.

We usually perform an initial Doppler examination at the child's bedside soon after the operation and daily for 7 days thereafter, in order to confirm patency of the anastomosed vessels, before clinical or biochemical liver examinations become abnormal. The hepatic arterial anastomosis is usually difficult to see, so we examine the intrahepatic arterial branches adjacent to intrahepatic portal veins, where they are rarely seen at gray scale sonography, even though flow is readily discerned with Doppler techniques. We have found that the following sites are optimal for the detection of hepatic arterial Doppler signals: adjacent to the umbilical branch of the left portal vein and adjacent to the branch to segments 3 and 4, and alongside the right portal vein and the branches to segments 6 and 7 (Fig. 58-20). The presence of arterial signals at these sites usually establishes patency of the hepatic artery. (We have seen two children with clinically undetected, chronic obstruction of the hepatic artery in whom intrahepatic arterial flow was detected with Doppler sonography. Angiography showed obstruction of the hepatic artery. The liver was perfused through extensive arterial collaterals around the site of a previous Kasai operation at the porta hepatis.)

In patients who are well enough to eat or receive gastric tube feedings, it must be remembered that hepatic arterial Doppler shifts are difficult to detect following a meal.[59] A repeat examination after a fast may show much stronger signals. Failure to detect intrahepatic arterial Doppler shifts signals thrombosis or a prethrombotic state. We perform arteriography in doubtful situations. Although hepatic artery interrogation is the most important part of the examination, the Doppler study is also helpful in assessing the patency of the venous anastomosis—the portal and hepatic veins and the IVC. The sites of venous anastomosis are clearly visible with gray scale sonography and should be demonstrated (Fig. 58-30). **Portal venous thrombosis** at the anastomosis may occur but is less frequent than arterial occlusion. Turbulence may be expected at the anastomotic site of the portal vein (Fig. 58-31). Stenosis or compression of the portal vein is accompanied by locally increased Doppler shifts. Portal hypertension may follow. Poststenotic dilatation of the portal vein may occur without serious sequelae.

Thrombosis of the IVC is usually asymptomatic in the child, because collateral flow through the paravertebral venous system is quickly established. The sonographic diagnosis of an IVC thrombus in a child with lobar transplantation can be quite difficult. The IVC lumen is obliterated by thrombus, and the vessel becomes very difficult to find (Fig. 58-32). However, even a patent IVC can be hard to find, since anatomical relationships are greatly altered in these children. At Doppler sonography, flow in a hemiazygous vein is quite easily mistaken for flow in the IVC.

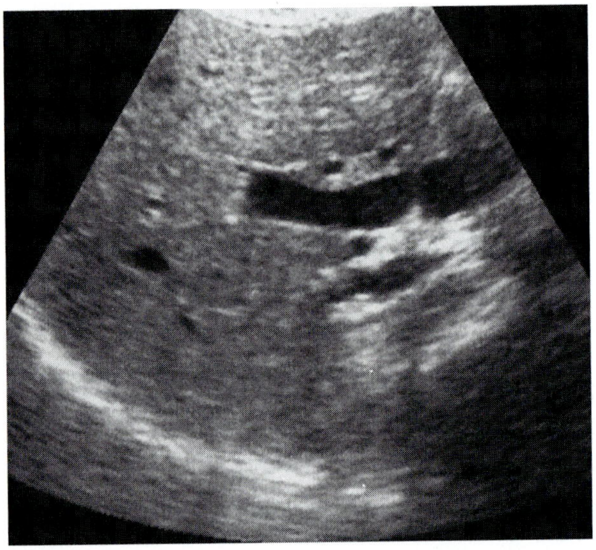

FIG. 58-30. Portal venous anastomosis following transplantation. Normal in a 10-year-old girl. The caliber of the pre- and postanastomotic segments is constant.

During segmental transplantation, the recipient's IVC is left intact and the hepatic vein(s) are directly anastomosed to the IVC or right atrium. Both the hepatic vein and IVC may thrombose, starting at the anastomosis. The immediate postoperative examination outlines the surgical anatomy in these children and serves as a useful standard for comparison in assessing the continued patency of the anastomosed vessels.

Graft rejection does not result in predictable flow alterations of the hepatic artery (unlike the increased intrarenal resistance to flow noted in acute renal allograft rejection). The Doppler examination is as yet unsatisfactory in assessing the possibility of liver graft rejection.

THE SPLEEN

Examination of the spleen is an integral part of the sonographic assessment of the child with liver or pancreatic disease or with infection or trauma.

Congenital abnormalities (polysplenia or asplenia) usually coexist with those of the heart. Polysplenia is associated with biliary atresia, anomalous venous return, preduodenal portal vein, and interrupted vena cava, and may be associated with abnormal abdominal situs.[13,74] The diagnosis of asplenia is best established with scintigraphy, as the sonographic diagnosis is difficult. Splenic parenchyma fused *in utero* with primitive liver, kidney, or gonadal tissue may persist in these locations after birth. After splenic rupture, small "seedlings" of splenic tissue may survive throughout the peritoneum. Small, round accessory spleens located in the splenic hilum are a frequent variation of normal (10% of autopsies) and should not be mistaken for lymph nodes or masses.

Cysts of the spleen are congenital (epithelial lined),[75] posttraumatic (pseudocyst without lining), or hydatid (unilocular and later daughter cysts).[43] Splenic cysts associated with polycystic kidney disease are rare in childhood. Splenic **abscesses** are found most frequently in immunosuppressed or leukemic children with candidiasis. The abscesses within the enlarged spleen usually become visible long after the diagnosis of candidal sepsis has been made. Cat scratch disease is another cause of multiple splenic abscesses. Splenic **calcifications** may be the result of granulomatous infections (histoplasma, tuberculosis) or chronic granulomatous disease of childhood.

Enlargement of the spleen accompanies many systemic infections (infectious mononucleosis and other viral infections, typhoid fever, fungal infections). Both the length and width of the spleen enlarge. The lower tip of the spleen becomes rounded. Other causes of enlargement include congestion in portal hypertension and infiltration with leukemic or lymphomatous tissue (usually impossible to distinguish from normal splenic parenchyma sonographically). These conditions underline the importance of examining the spleen in the context of the entire abdomen (e.g., for liver disease and portosystemic collaterals or for lymphadenopathy).[76]

The spleen is one of the most frequently injured organs when abdominal trauma has occurred. **Splenic hematomas** are usually hypoechoic lesions, often located under the capsule. Fresh hematomas may be isoechoic or hyperechoic and some linear lacerations are difficult to see sonographically. Hemoperitoneum is almost always present. Sonography has been used at St. Justine Hospital in Montreal as the initial screening examination in children with abdominal trauma for the past 15 years.[77] CT is used there only in doubtful cases or when there is concomitant spinal trauma. In spite of underdiagnosing some pancreatic and exceptional splenic hematomas as well as some mesenteric tears, the surgical management of their children was not affected and no child died because lesions were missed at the initial examination. In their cases, CT was performed if sonography was difficult because of rib fractures or if there was doubt or increasing unexplained hemoperitoneum.

Spontaneous rupture of the spleen occurs in the enlarged fragile organ in infectious mononucleosis[78] and is heralded by hemoperitoneum.

Splenic infarcts occur frequently in children with sickle cell anemia, and also in children suffering from various forms of vasculitis. Lesions are usually triangular and hypoechoic.

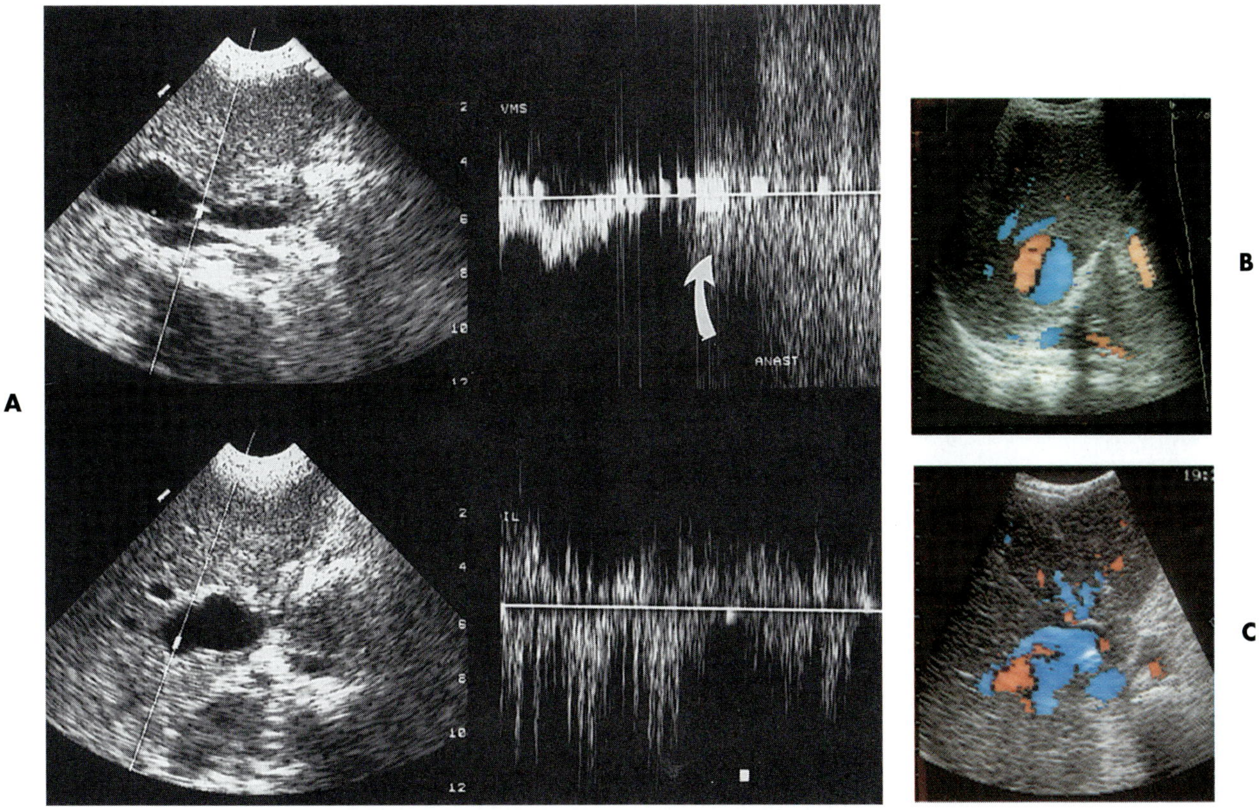

FIG. 58-31. Portal vein stenosis after transplantation (4-year-old boy). **A**, Subcostal oblique sonogram and pulsed Doppler tracing show a narrowed segment of the portal vein at the anastomotic site (*top cursor*), with poststenotic dilatation of the vein (*bottom cursor*). Pulsed Doppler tracing at the site of stenosis (*curved arrow*) shows turbulent, high-velocity bidirectional flow. Superior mesenteric vein flow obtained before the stenosis shows normal hepatopetal flow (*left of curved arrow*). Beyond the stenosis, flow is bidirectional (*bottom*). **B** and **C,** Color sonograms of the same region show **B,** circular, bidirectional flow in the dilated portal vein, **C,** less disturbed, hepatopetal flow into the right lobe. (From Patriquin HB. In: Taylor, et al. *Clinical Doppler Sonography*. Philadelphia: Lippincott-Raven; 1995)

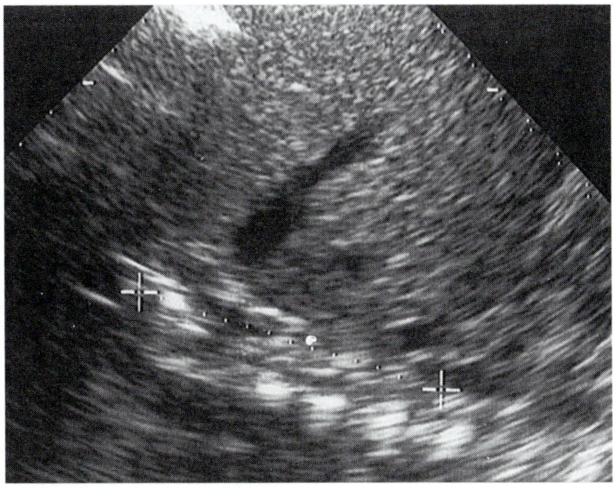

FIG. 58-32. Thrombosis of the inferior vena cava (between + cursors) following bisegmental liver transplantation in a 2-year-old child. The lumen is filled with echogenic clot (in contrast to the hypoechoic lumen of a nearby patent hepatic vein).

REFERENCES

Anatomy

1. Couinaud C. Le foie: études anatomiques et chirurgicales. Paris: Masson; 1957.
2. Bismuth H. Surgical anatomy and anatomical surgery of the liver. *World J Surg* 1982;6:3-9.
3. Todds WJ, Erickson SJ, Taylor AJ, Lawson TL, Stewart ET. Caudate lobe of the liver: anatomy, embryology and pathology. *AJR* 1990;154:87-93.

Neonatal Jaundice

4. Ikeda S, Sera Y, Yamamoto H, Ogawa M. Effect of phenobarbital on serial ultrasonic examination in the evaluation of neonatal jaundice. *Clin Imaging* 1994;18:146-148.
5. Todani T, Watanabe Y, Narusue M. Congenital bile duct cyst. *Am J Surg* 1977;134:263.
6. McHugh K, Daneman A. Multiple gastrointestinal atresias: sonography of associated biliary abnormalities. *Pediatr Radiol* 1991;21:355.
7. Garel L, Filiatrault D, Grignon A, Dubois J, Russo P, Pariente D, Avni F. Pathogenesis of choledochal cysts: the fetus' opinion. *Pediatr Radiol*; in press.
8. Caroli J, Soupault R, Kossakowski J et al. La dilatation polykystique congénitale des foies biliaires intrahépatiques: essai de classification. *Sem Hop* 1958;34:488.
9. Toma P, Lucigrai G, Pelizza A. Sonographic patterns of Caroli's disease: report of 5 new cases. *J Clin Ultrasound* 1991;19:155.
10. Davies CH, Stringer DA, Whyte H et al. Congenital hepatic fibrosis with saccular dilatation of intrahepatic bile ducts and infantile polycystic kidneys. *Pediatr Radiol* 1986;16:302.
11. Haller JO, Condon VR, Berdon WE et al. Spontaneous perforation of the bile duct in children. *Radiology* 1989;172:621.
12. Alagille D, Estrada A, Hadchouel M et al. Syndromic paucity of interlobular bile ducts (Alagille syndrome or arteriohepatic dysplasia): review of 80 cases. *J Pediatr* 1987;110:195.
13. Abramson SJ, Berdon WE, Altman RP, Amodio JB, Levy J. Biliary atresia and noncardiac polysplenic syndrome: US and surgical considerations. *Radiology* 1987;163:377-379.
14. Roy CC, Silverman A, Alagille D. *Pediatric Clinical Gastroenterology*. 4th ed. St. Louis: Mosby; 1994:620-635.
15. Betz BW, Bisset GS 3rd, Johnson ND, Daugherty CC, Balistreri WF. MR imaging of biliary cysts in children with biliary atresia: clinical associations and pathologic correlation. *AJR* 1994;162:167-171.
16. Kasai M, Susuki H, Ohashi E et al. Technique and results of operative management of biliary atresia. *World J Surg* 1978;2: 571-580.
17. Otte JB, de Ville de Goyet J; Reding R, Hausleithner V, Sokal E, Chardot C, Debande B. Sequential treatment of biliary atresia with Kasai portoenterostomy and liver transplantation: a review. *Hepatology* 1994;20(1Pt2):41S-48S.
18. Patriquin HB, DiPietro M, Barber FE, Littlewood Teele R. Sonography of thickened gallbladder wall: causes in children. *AJR* 1983;141:57-60.
19. Maresca G, De Gaetano AM, Mirk P et al Sonographic patterns of the gallbladder in acute viral hepatitis. *JCU* 19;12:141,184.
20. Dubois J, Garel L, Patriquin H et al. The liver in tyrosinemia: a radiologic-pathologic comparison. *Pediatr Radiol*, in press.
21. Henschke CI, Goldman H, Teele RL. The hyperechogenic liver in children: cause and sonographic appearance. *AJR* 1982; 138:841.
22. Patriquin HB, Roy CC, Weber AM et al. Liver disease and portal hypertension. *Clin Diagn Ultrasound* 1989;24:103-127.
23. Aubin B, Denys A, Lafortune M et al. Focal sparing of liver parenchyma in steatosis: role of the gallbladder and its vessels. *J Ultrasound Med* 1995;14:77.
24. Henschke CI, Teele RL. Cholelithiasis in children: recent observations. *J Ultrasound Med* 1983;2:481-484.
25. Keller MS, Markle BM, Laffey PA et al. Spontaneous resolution of cholelithiasis in infants. *Radiology* 1985;157:345-458.
26. Littlewood Teele R, Chrestman Share J. *Ultrasonography of Infants and Children*. Philadelphia: WB Saunders Co; 1991: 431-433.

Liver Tumors

27. Brunelle F, Chaumont P Hepatic tumors in children: ultrasonic differentiation of malignant from benign lesions. *Radiology* 1984;150:695-699.
28. Mulliken JB, Glowacki J. Hemangiomas and vascular malformations in infants and children: a classification based on endothelial characteristics. *Plast Reconstr Surg* 1982;69:412-420.
29. Dachman AH, Lichtenstein JE, Friedman AC et al. Infantile hemangioendothelioma of the liver: a radiologic-pathologic clinical correlation. *AJR* 1983;140:1091-1096.
30. Paltiel HJ, Patriquin HB, Keller MS, Babcock DS, Leithiser RE. Infantile hepatic hemangioma: Doppler US[1]. *Radiology* 1992; 182:735-742.
31. Ros PR, Goodman ZD, Ishak KG et al. Mesenchymal hamartoma of the liver: radiologic-pathologic correlation. *Radiology* 1986;159:619-624.
32. Brunelle F, Tamman S, Odievre M et al. Liver adenomas in glycogen storage disease in children: ultrasound and angiographic study. *Pediatr Radiol* 1984;14:94-101.
33. D'Souza VJ, Summer TE, Watson NE et al. Focal nodular hyperplasia of the liver imaging by differing modalities. *Pediatr Radiol* 1983;13:77-81.
34. Koufos A, Hansen MF, Copeland NG et al. Loss of heterozygosity in three embryonal tumours suggests a common pathogenic mechanism. *Nature* 1985;316:330-334.
35. Dachman AH, Pakter RL, Ros PR, Fishman EK, Goodman ZD, Lichtenstein JE. Hepatoblastoma: radiologic-pathologic correlation in 50 cases. *Radiology* 1987;183:815-819.
36. Bates SM, Keller MS, Ramos IM, Carter D, Taylor KJW. Hepatoblastoma detection of tumor vascularity with duplex Doppler US. *Radiology* 1990;176:505-507.
37. Van Campenhout I, Patriquin H. Malignant microvasculature in abdominal tumors in children: detection with Doppler sonography. *Radiology* 1992;183:445-448.
38. Boechat MI, Hooshang K, Ortega J, Hall T, Feig S, Stanley P, Gilsanz V. Primary liver tumors in children: comparison of CT and MR imaging. *Radiology* 1988;169:727-732.
39. Taylor KJ, Ramos I, Morse SS, Fortune KL, Hammers L, Taylor CR. Focal liver masses: differential diagnosis with pulsed Doppler US. *Radiology* 1987;164:643-647.

Liver Abscess and Granulomas

40. Garel LA, Pariente DM, Nezelof C et al. Liver involvement in chronic granulomatous disease: the role of ultrasound in diagnosis and treatment. *Radiology* 1984;153:117.
41. Merten DF, Kirks DR. Amoebic liver abscess in children: the role of diagnostic imaging. *AJR* 1984;143:13-25.
42. Lewall DB, McCorkell SJ. Hepatic echinococcal cysts: sonographic appearance and classification. *Radiology* 1985;155: 773.
43. Beggs I. The radiology of hydatid disease. *AJR* 1985;145:639-648.

Liver Diseases and Portal Hypertension: Assessment with Doppler Sonography

44. Taylor KJW, Burns PN, Woodcock JP et al. Blood flow in deep abdominal and pelvic vessels: ultrasonic pulsed Doppler analysis. *Radiology* 1985;154:487-493.

45. Taylor KJW, Burns PN. Duplex scanning in the pelvis and abdomen. *Ultrasound Med Biol* 1985;4:643-658.
46. Burns PN, Jaff CC. Quantitative measurements with a Doppler ultrasound: technique, accuracy and limitations. *Radiol Clin North Am* 1985;23:641-657.
47. Nelson TR, Pretorius DH. The Doppler signal: where does it come from and what does it mean? *AJR* 1988;151:439-447.
48. Sato S, Ohnishi K, Sujita S et al. Splenic artery and superior mesenteric artery blood flow: nonsurgical Doppler ultrasound measurement in healthy subjects and patients with chronic liver disease. *Radiology* 1987;164:347-352.
49. Patriquin HB, Paltiel H. Abdominal Doppler ultrasound in children: clinical applications. *Pediatric Radiology Categorical Course Syllabus* RSNA, 1989:185-196.
50. Ohnishi K, Saito M, Nakayama T et al. Portal venous hemodynamics in dynamics in chronic liver disease: effects of posture change and exercise. *Radiology* 1985;155:757-761.
51. Madjar H, Gill RW, Griffiths KA et al. Liver function tested by pulsed Doppler measurements of portal venous flow and fasting following a standard meal. In: Gill RW, Dadd MJ, eds. *Proceedings of the Fourth Meeting WFUMB*. Sidney, Australia: Pergamon Press; 1985.
52. Burns PN, Taylor KJW, Blei AT. Doppler flowmetry and portal hypertension. *Gastroenterology* 1987;92:824-826.
53. Lafortune M, Madore F, Patriquin H, Braton G. Segmental anatomy of the liver: a sonographic approach to the Couinaud nomenclature. *Radiology* 1991;181:443-448.
54. Vanleeuwen MS. Doppler ultrasound in the evaluation of portal hypertension. *Clin Diag Ultrasound* 1989;26:53-76.
55. Subramanyam BR, Balthazar EJ, Madamba MR et al. Sonography of porto-systemic venous collaterals in portal hypertension. *Radiology* 1983;146:161-166.
56. Patriquin HB, Tessier G, Grignon A et al. Lesser omental thickness in normal children: baseline for detection of portal hypertension. *AJR* 1985;145:693-696.
57. Lafortune M, Breton G, Charlebois S. Arterioportal fistula demonstrated by pulsed Doppler ultrasonography. *J Ultrasound Med* 1986;5:105-106.
58. Siegel MC, Zajko AB, Bowen A et al. Hepatic artery thrombosis after liver transplantation: radiologic evaluation. *AJR* 1986;146:137-141.
59. Lafortune M, Dauzat M, Pomier-Layrargues G et al. Hepatic artery: effect of meal in normal persons and in transplant recipients. *Radiology* 1993;187:391-394.
60. Brunelle F, Alagille D, Pariente D et al. An ultrasound study of portal hypertension in children. *Ann Radiol* 1981;24:121-124.
61. Lebrec D, De Fleury P, Rueff D et al. Portal hypertension size of oesophageal varices and risk of gastrointestinal bleeding in alcoholic cirrhosis. *Gastroenterology* 1980;79:1139-1144.
62. De Gaetano AM, Lafortune M, Patriquin H, De Franco A, Aubin B, Paradis K. Cavernous transformation of the portal vein: patterns of intrahepatic and splanchnic collateral circulation detected with Doppler sonography. *AJR* 1995;165:1135-1140.
63. Besnard M, Pariente D, Hadchouel M et al. Portal cavernoma in congenital hepatic fibrosis: angiographic reports of 10 pediatric cases. *Pediatr Radiol* 1994;24:61.
64. Odievre M, Chaumont P, Montagne JP, Alagille D. Anomalies of the intra-hepatic portal venous system in congenital hepatic fibrosis. *Radiology* 1977;122:427-430.
65. Bolondi L, Gandolfi L, Arienti V et al. Ultrasonography in the diagnosis of portal hypertension diminished response of portal vessels to respiration. *Radiology* 1982;142:172-176.
66. Stanley P. Budd-Chiari syndrome. *Radiology* 1989;170:625-627.
67. Hosoki T, Kuroda C, Tokunaga K, Murakawa T, Masuike M, Kozuka T. Hepatic venous outflow obstruction: evaluation with pulsed duplex sonography. *Radiology* 1989;170:733-737.
68. Rodgers BM, Kaude JV. Real-time ultrasound in determination of portosystemic shunt patency in children. *J Pediatr Surg* 1981;16:968-971.
69. Forsberg L, Holmin T. Pulsed Doppler and B-mode ultrasound features of interposition meso-caval and porta-caval shunt. *Acta Radiol* 1983;24:353-357.
70. Lafortune M, Patriquin HB, Pomier-Layrargues G et al. Hemodynamic changes of portal circulation following porto-systemic shunts: a study of 45 patients using duplex ultrasonography. *AJR* 1987;149:701-706.
71. Nova D, Butzow GH, Becker K. Hepatic occlusion venography with a balloon catheter in patients with end-to-side porto-caval shunts. *AJR* 1976;127:949-953.

Doppler Sonography in the Child Receiving a Liver Transplant

72. Ledesma-Medina J, Dominguez R, Bowen A et al. Pediatric liver transplantation, I: standardization of preoperative diagnostic imaging. *Radiology* 1985;157:335-338.
73. Longley DG, Skolnick ML, Zajko AB et al. Duplex Doppler sonography in the evaluation of adult patients before and after liver transplantation. *AJR* 1988;151:687-696.
74. Hernanz-Schulman M, Ambrosino MM, Genieser NB et al. Current evaluation of the patient with abnormal visceroatrial situs. *AJR* 1990;154:797-802.

The Spleen

75. Daneman A, Martin DJ. Congenital epithelial splenic cysts in children: emphasis on sonographic appearances and some unusual features. *Pediatr Radiol* 1982;12:119-125.
76. Littlewood Teele R, Chrestman Share J. *Ultrasonography of infants and children*, p. 405.
77. Filiatrault D, Longpre D, Patriquin H et al. Investigation of childhood blunt trauma: a practical approach using ultrasound as the initial diagnostic modality. *Pediatr Radiol* 1987;17:373-379.
78. Johnson MA, Cooperberg PL, Boisvert J, Stoller JL, Winrob H. Spontaneous splenic rupture in infectious mononucleosis: sonographic diagnosis and follow-up. *AJR* 1981;136:111-114.

CHAPTER 59

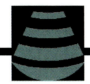

The Pediatric Kidney and Adrenal Glands

Diane S. Babcock, M.D., F.A.C.R.
Heidi B. Patriquin, M.D., F.R.C.P.(C)

CHAPTER OUTLINE

CHAPTER OUTLINE, cont'd.

PEDIATRIC RENAL SONOGRAPHY

Improvement in resolution of ultrasound equipment and the development of higher-frequency transducers have resulted in the widespread use of sonography for diagnosing and studying diseases of the kidney and adrenal gland in the pediatric patient. Sonography has the advantages of requiring no contrast material and of using nonionizing radiation; and it has replaced the excretory urogram as the primary imaging modality of the pediatric urinary tract.

Technique

The examination of the urinary tract in the pediatric patient should include images of the kidneys, ureters if visualized, and urinary bladder. The child's parents are asked to bring the patient for the study with a full urinary bladder. The child may be given fluid to drink and asked not to void for several hours before the examination. For a young child who is not yet toilet-trained, the examination may be timed to bladder filling, with the patient being given fluids to drink while in the ultrasound department. The bladder must be checked first and frequently, as the patient may fill and void suddenly.

Although children vary in their ability to hold still for a sufficient period of time, sedation is rarely needed. Infants under 3 months of age can be fed or given a pacifier during the examination and immobilized with sandbags and wraps. If sedation is necessary, it may be given in the ultrasound department and the patient can be monitored during the procedure and before going home. The patient older than 3 years of age can be distracted and/or entertained during the examination by watching video tapes on a VCR, playing with toys, or reading a book. The addition of cine loop often compensates for the movement of the child.

A variety of ultrasound equipment can be used. The highest-frequency transducer that will penetrate the area being examined is optimal. In an infant, this is usually a 7.5 MHz transducer, and in a child, a 5.0 MHz transducer. Different types of transducers are used for different parts of the body. Scans of the kidneys from the back are best performed with a linear or convex transducer, whereas frontal scans of the kidney are best performed with a sector or convex transducer that gets between the ribs. Views of the bladder are performed with a sector or convex transducer. The ureters are evaluated as they leave the renal pelvis and enter the bladder. The images are recorded on hard-copy film or digital storage.

Routine examination includes longitudinal and transverse views of both kidneys. Scans are performed with the patient in both the prone and the supine positions. Prone views of the kidney from the back show optimal detail of the lower poles and overall renal size. Coronal views in the supine position, using the liver and spleen as windows, allow optimal visualization of the upper poles and comparison of renal parenchymal echogenicity to the adjacent liver and spleen. Scans of the bladder are performed with the bladder comfortably full so that abnormalities including wall thickening and trabeculation can be seen. Dilatation of the distal ureters and ureteroceles is also sought. Postvoid views of the bladder and kidneys may be helpful in patients with neurogenic bladders and/or dilated upper collecting systems. Doppler is used in selected clinical situations.

Renal size should be measured and compared to charts (Fig. 59-1).[1] In patients with chronic problems, such as recurrent urinary tract infections, reflux, or a neurogenic bladder, renal growth should be plotted on follow-up examinations.[2]

Normal Renal Anatomy

Throughout the second trimester, the kidney consists of a collection of renunculi (small kidneys), each composed of a central large pyramid with a thin peripheral rim of cortex. As the renunculi fuse progressively, their adjoining cortices form a column of Bertin. The former renunculi are then called lobes. Remnants of these lobes with somewhat incomplete fusion are recognized by a lobulated surface of the kidney. This "renal lobulation" (sometimes called fetal lobulation) should not be confused with renal scars[3] and may persist into adulthood (Fig. 59-2). At birth, the pyramids are still very large in comparison to the thin rim of cortex that surrounds them. Glomerular filtration rate shortly after birth is low and increases rapidly after the first week postpartum. Throughout childhood, there is a significant growth of the cortex, and the pyramids gradually become proportionately smaller.

The renal anatomy of the pediatric patient varies depending upon the age of the patient. The anatomy in the teenager and older child is similar to that in the adult (Fig. 59-3). The renal parenchyma consists of the **cortex,** which is peripheral, contains the

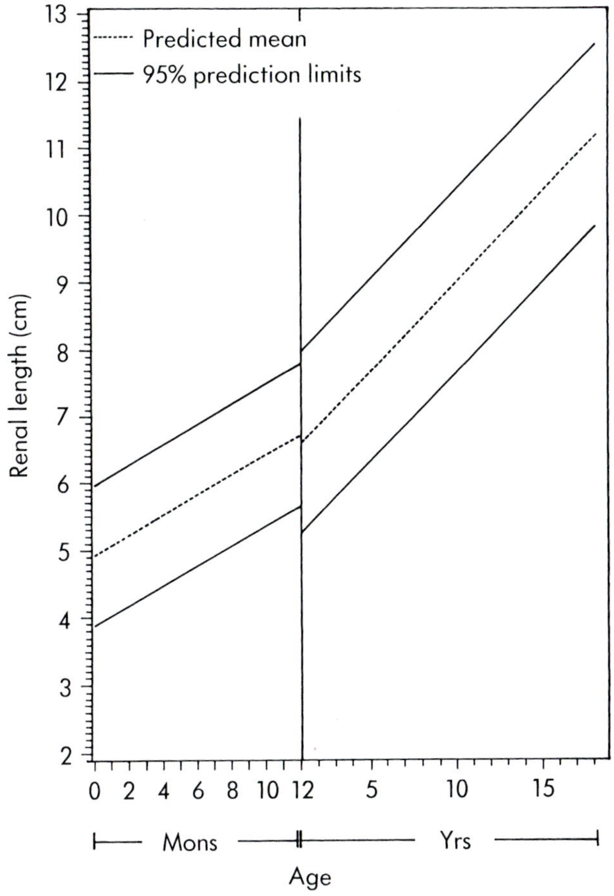

FIG. 59-1. Normal renal length versus age.

glomeruli, and has several extensions to the edge of the **renal sinus** (the septa of Bertin), and the **medulla** (containing the renal pyramids), which is more central and adjacent to the calices. The normal cortex produces low-level, back-scattered echoes. The medullary pyramids are relatively hypoechoic and arranged around the central, echo-producing **renal sinus.** The **arcuate vessels** can be demonstrated as intense specular echoes at the **corticomedullary junction.**[4] This corticomedullary differentiation can be identified in most children but occasionally is not seen in those in whom resolution is diminished by increased overlying soft tissues. The central echo complex consists of strong specular echoes from the renal sinus including the renal collecting system, calices and infundibula, arteries, veins, lymphatics, peripelvic fat, and part of the renal pelvis. With distention of the renal collecting system, these echoes become separated and small degrees of hydronephrosis can be demonstrated. Mild degrees of distention can be seen in normal children, particularly after recent high intake of fluids or diuretics. A normally distended urinary bladder can also cause obstruction and mild distention of the renal collecting systems. Rescanning when the bladder is empty will resolve this question.

In the **infant,** the normal kidney has several features that differ from those of the kidney in the normal adult patient (Fig. 59-3).[5] The **central echo complex** is much less prominent as compared to the renal parenchyma because there is less peripelvic fat in the infant than in the adult. **The echogenicity of the renal cortex** in the normal infant is often **the same echogenicity as the adjacent normal liver,** whereas in the older child and adult, the renal cortex is less echogenic than the liver. The renal cortex echogenicity can occasionally be increased in the very premature infant. The medullary pyramids in the infant are relatively larger and tend to appear more prominent. **The corticomedullary differentiation** is greater in the infant kidney than in the adult, possibly because of increased resolution from higher-frequency transducers and less overlying body fat tissue. It may also be due to differences in the cellular composition of the renal parenchyma in the infant. These prominent pyramids in the infant kidney can easily be mistaken for multiple cysts by those not familiar with the differences; normal pyramids line up around the central echo complex in a characteristic pattern and can therefore be differentiated from cysts. Also, the position of the arcuate artery at the corticomedullary junction can help to identify a structure as a pyramid.

Normal Bladder Anatomy

The normal urinary bladder is thin-walled in the distended state (< 3 mm). When empty, the wall thickness increases but is still less than 5 mm.[6] The distal ureters may be visible at the bladder base, especially if the child is well hydrated (Fig. 59-4).

CONGENITAL ANOMALIES OF THE URINARY TRACT

Renal Duplication

A common congenital anomaly of the urinary tract is duplication of the collecting system, which may be partial or complete. In complete duplication, two pelves and two separate ureters drain the kidney. The lower-pole collecting system usually inserts into the bladder at the normal site; however, the intramural portion may be shorter than usual, and vesicoureteral reflux frequently results. The upper-pole system often inserts ectopically, inferior and medial to the site of the normal ureteral insertion (the Weigert-Meyer rule).[2] Its orifice may be stenotic and obstructed. Ballooning of the submucosal portion of this upper-pole ureter causes a ureterocele. The upper-pole ureter may have an insertion entirely outside of the bladder, in the urethra, above, at, or

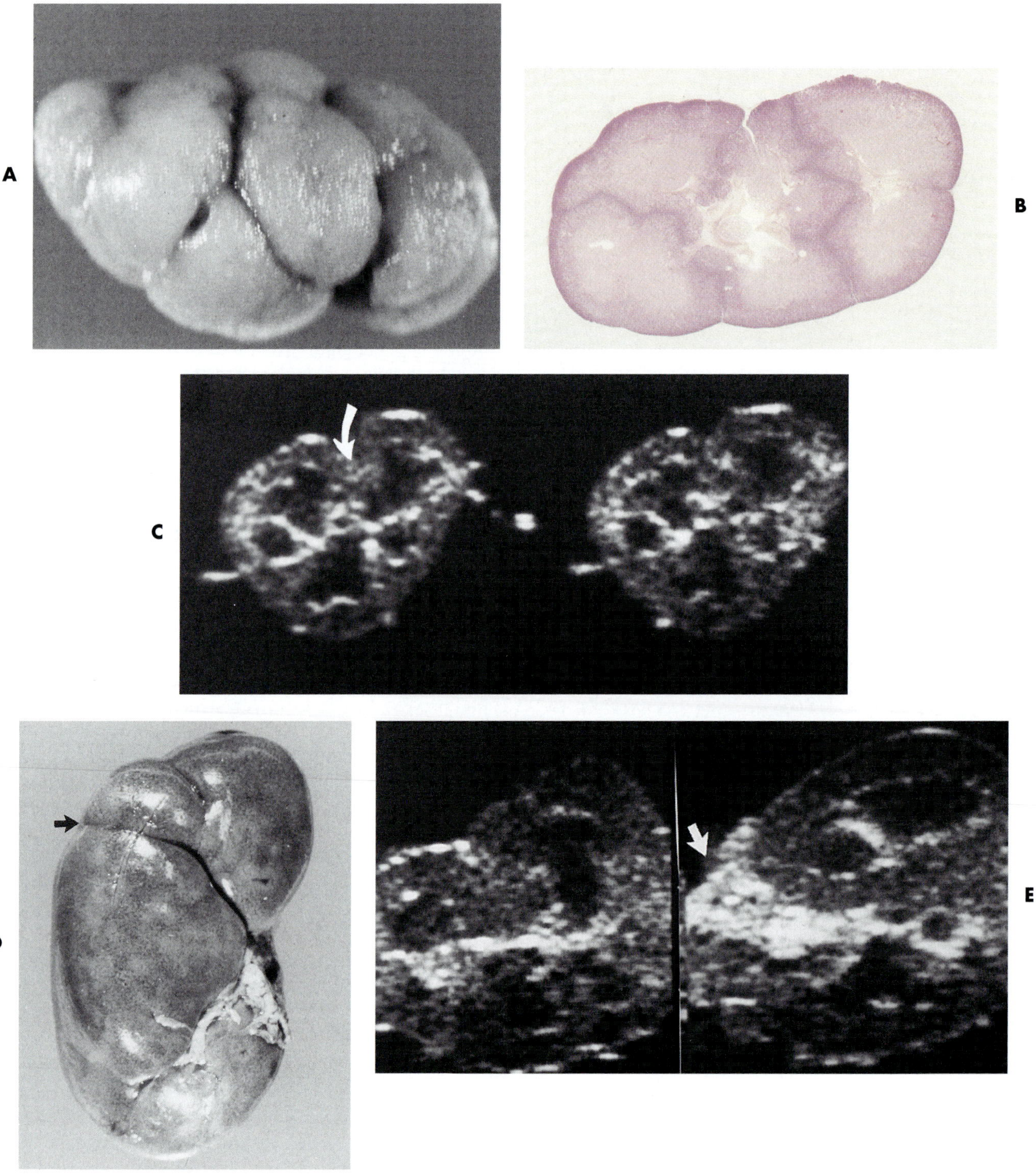

FIG. 59-2. Renal lobulation changes with maturation. **A,** Fetal kidney of 16 weeks' gestation. The external surface shows individual lobes, or renunculi, separated by deep grooves. **B,** Microscopic section of a whole kidney (hematoxylin and eosin stain) at 23 weeks' gestation. Individual renunculi, each composed of a central pyramid and a thin peripheral eosinophilic cortex are visible. **C,** Kidney at 1 month after birth (in vitro sonogram). The lobes are well seen, each with a central pyramid and a thin rim of cortex. A line of fusion *(arrow)* is faintly seen in the center of a column of Bertin. **D,** Renal lobes are fused and the external surface of a cadaver kidney is smooth except for three grooves; the most prominent is the interrenicular junction or junctional parenchymal defect, which extends from the hilum to the cortex *(arrow)*. **E,** In vitro longitudinal and transverse sonographic cuts of the same kidney; as in D, it shows the junctional parenchymal defect extending from the hilum to the cortex *(arrow)*.

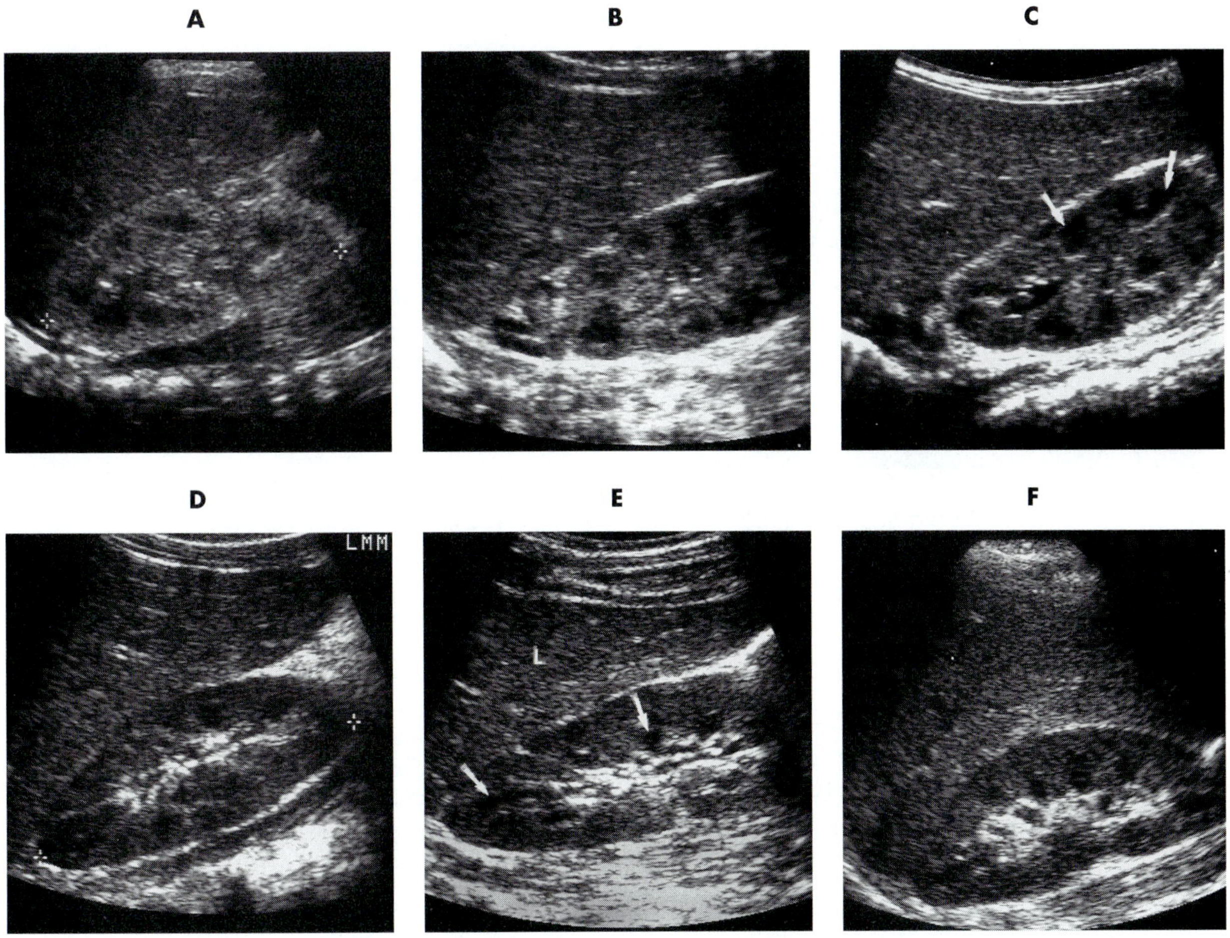

FIG. 59-3. Normal renal appearances at different ages. **A, Premature infant:** cortex is prominent and more echogenic than the liver. **B, Term infant:** normal fetal lobulations of renal cortex are isoechoic or slightly hyperechoic to liver and spleen. Prominent renal pyramids are hypoechoic. **C,** In the **infant,** the central echo complex is less prominent because of less peripelvic fat, the renal cortex equals the liver in echogenicity, and the medullary pyramids (*arrows*) are relatively larger and appear more prominent. **D, 2-year-old child:** renal cortex is slightly less echogenic than liver. Renal sinus fat begins to develop central echogenicity around vessels. **E, 10-year-old child:** normal cortex produces low-level echoes, whereas the medullary pyramids (*arrows*) are relatively hypoechoic and are arranged around the central echo complex consisting of strong specular echoes. The renal cortex is equally or less echogenic than the adjacent liver (L). **F, 14-year-old child:** renal cortex is less echogenic than liver or spleen. Pyramids are much less prominent. Renal sinus fat is increased.

below the external urinary sphincter, into the uterus or vagina, or into the ejaculatory duct, seminal vesicle, or vas deferens.[7]

Patients with unobstructed duplications do not have more clinical problems than their normal counterparts. Patients with complicated renal duplications may present with urinary tract infections, failure to thrive, abdominal mass, hematuria, or symptoms of bladder outlet obstruction from a ureterocele. Females with urethral insertions of the upper-pole ureter below the external urinary sphincter or with vaginal or uterine insertions may present with chronic constant incontinence or dribbling.

Duplication of the renal collecting system is diagnosed on sonography when the central echo complex separates into two parts with an interposed column of normal renal parenchyma termed a column of Bertin (Fig. 59-5). It is usually impossible to distinguish a partial, uncomplicated duplication from a complete one because the normal ureter is difficult to visualize sonographically.[8]

With **obstruction of an upper-pole moiety,** dilatation of the upper-pole collecting system and its entire ureter is seen (Fig. 59-6). The renal parenchyma may be thinned over this upper-pole collecting system. If the obstruction is associated with a **simple ureterocele,** views of the bladder may demonstrate the ureterocele as a curvilinear structure within the bladder, in addition to the dilated distal ureter. A large ureterocele may cross the midline and obstruct the

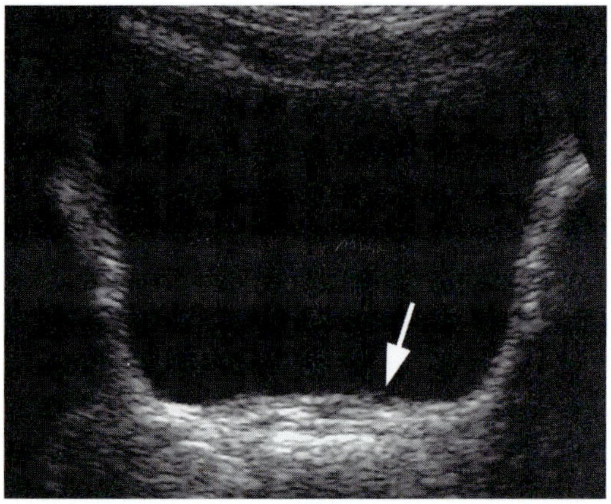

FIG. 59-4. Normal urinary bladder and ureter. Transverse sonogram of distended bladder with thin wall (< 3 mm). Distal ureteric insertion visible at trigone *(arrow)*.

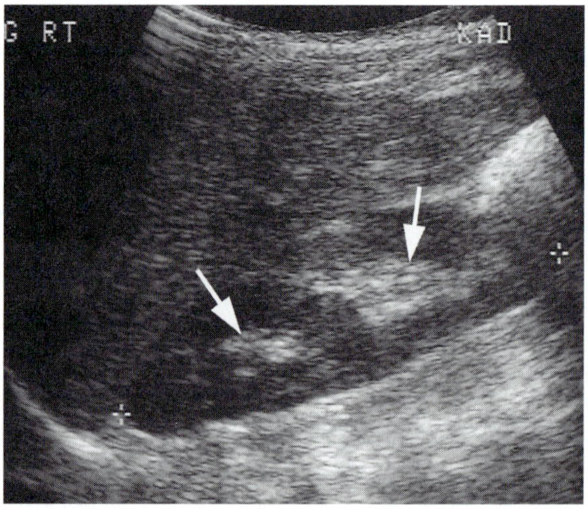

FIG. 59-5. Renal duplication. The central echo complex (*arrows*) is separated into two parts with an interposed column of normal renal parenchyma (column of Bertin).

A

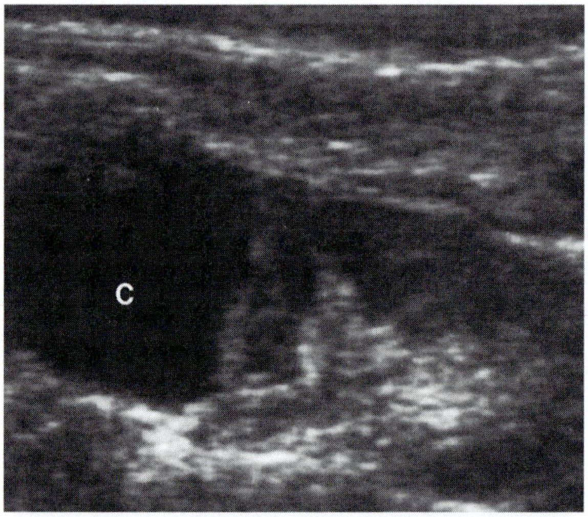

B

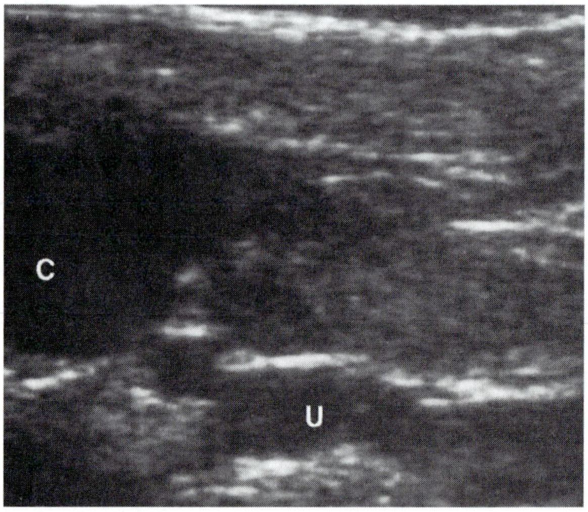

C

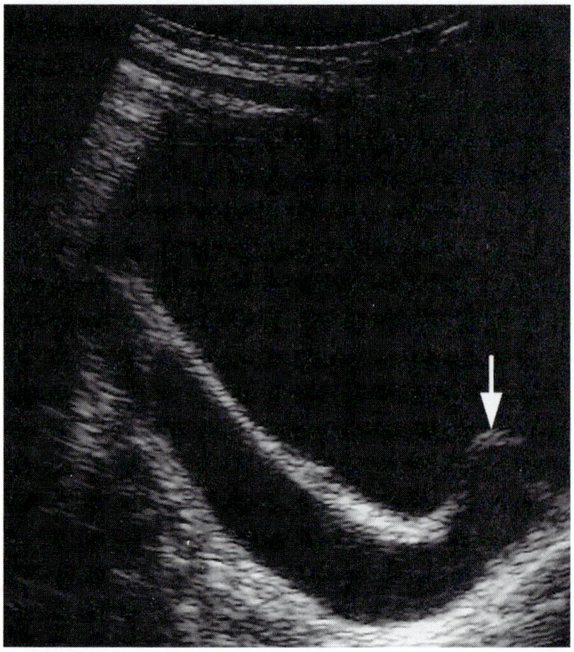

FIG. 59-6. Renal duplication with obstructing ureterocele. **A,** Longitudinal scan of the left kidney shows upper-pole cyst (C) representing dilated upper-pole collecting system. **B,** Medial longitudinal scan shows this dilated ureter (U) extending toward the bladder. **C,** Longitudinal scan of the bladder demonstrates ureterocele *(arrow)* projecting into the bladder.

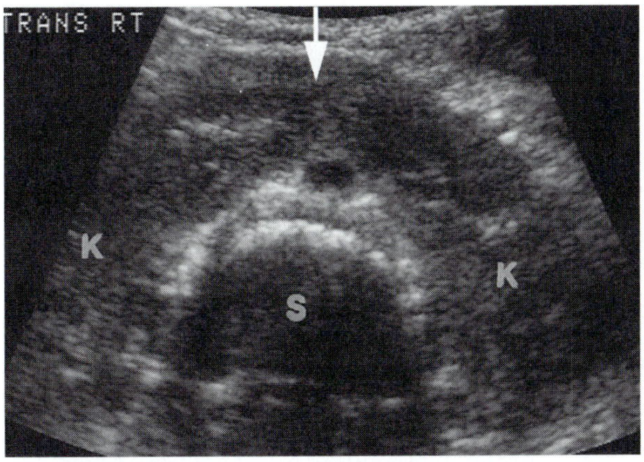

FIG. 59-7. Horseshoe kidney. Transverse supine scan demonstrates lower poles of kidneys (K) more medial than usual in the midline anterior to the spine (S). Fusion is by band of renal parenchyma *(arrow)*.

contralateral ureter or bladder outlet and cause bilateral hydronephrosis.

With **reflux into the lower-pole moiety,** the lower-pole collecting system and its ureter will be dilated to varying degrees. If reflux is mild, there may be no lower-pole dilatation.

Other Renal Anomalies

Other renal anomalies include **congenital absence of the kidney,** abnormal position of the kidney, such as a **pelvic kidney** or a **cross-fused ectopia,** and **horseshoe kidney,** with fusion of the lower poles in the midline. Absence of the kidney is suspected when no renal tissue can be identified on sonography. Care must be taken to search for the kidney not only in its usual position in the renal fossa, but also in the lower abdomen or pelvis. The contralateral kidney, when healthy, shows compensatory hypertrophy when one kidney is absent or severely damaged. Nuclear renal scan may be helpful in identifying a small functioning kidney not visualized by ultrasound.

With a **horseshoe kidney,** the longitudinal axis of the kidneys is abnormal, with the lower poles located more medially than usual and fusing in the midline anterior to the spine (Fig. 59-7). The fusion may be a fibrous band or actual fusion of the renal parenchyma. The lower poles of the kidneys are usually rotated medially and may be positioned somewhat lower than usual. In **cross-fused ectopy,** both kidneys are located on the same side of the abdomen and are fused inferior to the ipsilateral kidney. They can also be fused in an L-shaped configuration. The ureters insert into each side of the bladder normally.[9] A horseshoe kidney may be missed easily if the abnormal axis of the kidney is not recognized. The central renal tissue may also be thin and easy to miss, particularly if it is only fibrous tissue.

HYDRONEPHROSIS

Dilatation of the renal collecting system—hydronephrosis—is a fairly common problem in the pediatric patient. It is frequently but not always associated with obstruction; ultrasound is particularly sensitive for its detection. Small amounts of fluid may be detected in the normal renal pelvis. Dilatation of the renal calyces is abnormal and suggests significant pathology. In order to make a more precise diagnosis and estimate severity, information concerning the degree of dilatation, whether unilateral or bilateral, if ureters and bladders are dilated, and status of the renal parenchyma should be obtained with sonography. Dilatation may be due to obstruction, reflux, or abnormal muscle development.

Ureteropelvic Junction Obstruction

The most common neonatal abdominal mass is hydronephrosis,[10] and obstruction is most common at the level of the ureteropelvic junction (UPJ), secondary to a functional stricture, which results in a functional disturbance in either the initiation or the propagation of the normal peristaltic activity within the ureter. The obstruction produces proximal dilatation of the collecting system, whereas the ureter is normal in caliber. There is an increased incidence of abnormalities of the contralateral kidney.[2] The investigation of a child with suspected hydronephrosis usually begins with sonography to evaluate the anatomy of the kidneys, ureters, and bladder. The typical appearance of a hydronephrotic kidney is that of a cystic mass in the renal fossa, which maintains its reniform shape (Fig. 59-8). With a UPJ obstruction, a larger cyst medially represents a dilated medial pelvis, whereas smaller cysts arranged around the periphery of the pelvis represent the dilated renal calices. A variable amount of renal parenchymal tissue can be visualized. With obstruction at the ureteropelvic junction, the ureter is normal in size and is usually not visualized by ultrasound.

Ureteral Obstruction

The ureter can be obstructed anywhere along its course by extrinsic compression by a mass such as a lymphoma or abscess. The exact site of obstruction may be difficult to visualize by ultrasound because of overlying bowel gas. The ureter is more commonly obstructed by intrinsic abnormalities such as stones, blood clot, and fungus balls.

Obstruction can occur at the **ureterovesical junction** because of primary megaureter, atresia, or an ectopically inserted ureter. With **primary megaureter,** the juxtavesicular segment of the ureter near the bladder is narrowed by an increase in fibrous tissue or by circumferential tissue that is devoid of muscle.

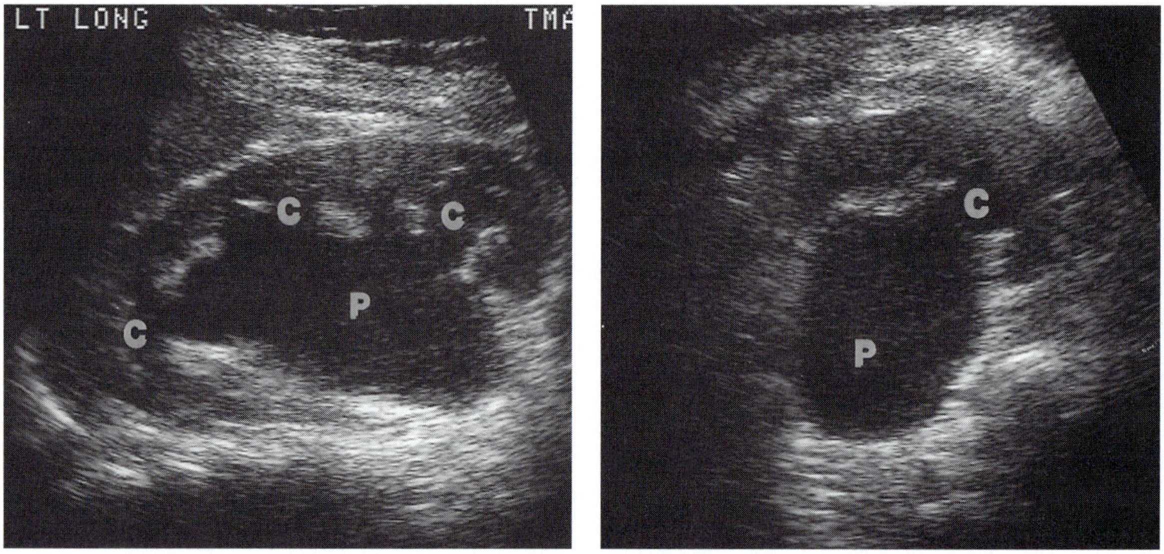

A B

FIG. 59-8. Hydronephrosis with ureteropelvic junction obstruction. **A,** Longitudinal and **B,** transverse scans show marked dilatation of the collecting system with a larger cyst (P) medially representing a dilated renal pelvis and smaller connecting cysts representing dilated renal calices (C). The ureter is normal in size and not visualized.

There is a variable degree of dilatation of the intrarenal collecting system and the ureter proximal to the narrowing. Sonography[11] typically shows hydronephrosis and hydroureter with a narrow segment of the distal ureter behind the bladder (Fig. 59-9). Increased peristalsis in the ureter may be detected with real-time sonography. Doppler sonography often shows a diminished or **abnormal ureteric jet on the side of obstruction** (Fig. 59-9).[12]

Ectopic insertion of a ureter can occur with or without a ureterocele and result in dilatation of the more proximal collecting system and ureter. As discussed previously, this is usually associated with a duplication.

Bladder Outlet Obstruction

Bilateral hydronephrosis is frequently caused by obstruction at the level of the bladder or bladder outlet. A **neurogenic bladder** (e.g., with meningomyelocele) can result in a thickened and/or dilated bladder and bilateral dilatation of the collecting systems and ureters. The bladder and bladder outlet may be obstructed by congenital anomalies such as **posterior urethral valves** or **polyps,** or it may be obstructed by a **pelvic mass** such as a tumor distorting the bladder base. In either case, the bladder will be enlarged and have a thickened irregular wall.[13] Congenital anomalies of the spine should be searched for with radiographs and spinal ultrasound in neonates, if not obvious clinically. **Posterior urethral valves** can sometimes be diagnosed by ultrasound with demonstration of a dilated posterior urethra (Fig. 59-10).[13] Voiding cystography should be performed for optimal visualization of the posterior urethral valves.

Dilatation of the renal collecting system is not always caused by obstruction, and other abnormalities such as **vesicoureteral reflux** should be considered. In a patient with hydronephrosis detected by ultrasound, the bladder and urethra should be further evaluated with a voiding cystourethrogram. Bladder size, contractility, and the urethra can be evaluated. In addition, vesicoureteral reflux can be assessed and may even be the cause of the urinary tract dilatation.

Prune-Belly Syndrome

Eagle-Barrett, prune-belly, or **abdominal muscle deficiency syndrome** includes congenital absence or deficiency of the abdominal musculature, large hypotonic dilated tortuous ureters, a large bladder, a patent urachus (see section on urachal anomalies), bilateral cryptorchidism, and dilated prostatic urethra. There are decreased muscular fibers throughout the urinary tract and prostate, resulting in dilatation and hypoperistalsis. Renal dysplasia and hydronephrosis can occur to varying degrees. There may be associated pulmonary hypoplasia, leading to Potter's syndrome and death.[14]

Megacystic Microcolon Malrotation Intestinal Hypoperistalsis Syndrome

This rare syndrome occurs in girls who are born with a grossly distended abdomen. An enlarged bladder, hydronephrosis, and hydroureter are demonstrated sonographically. Microcolon, malrotation, and dimin-

A
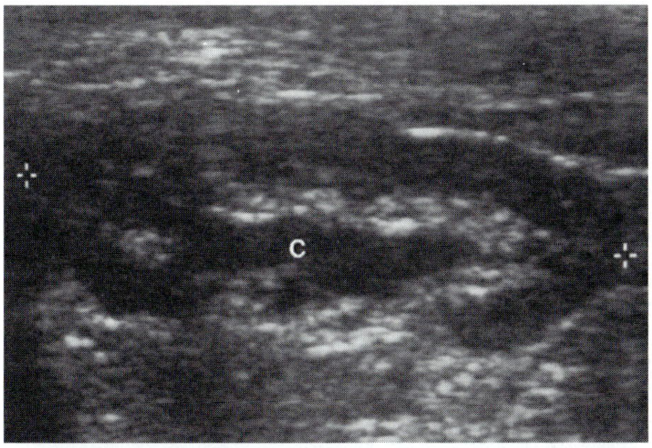

B
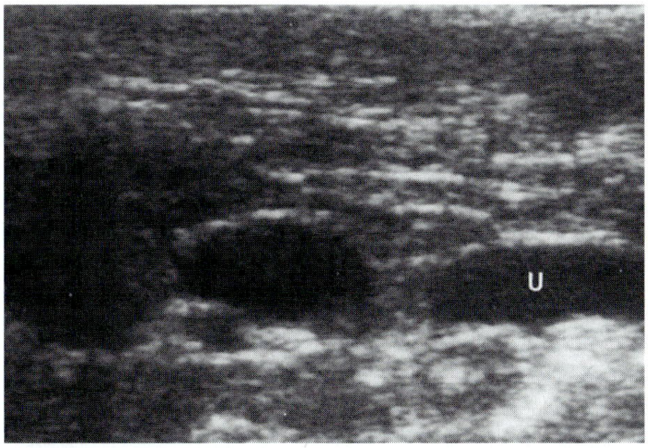

C
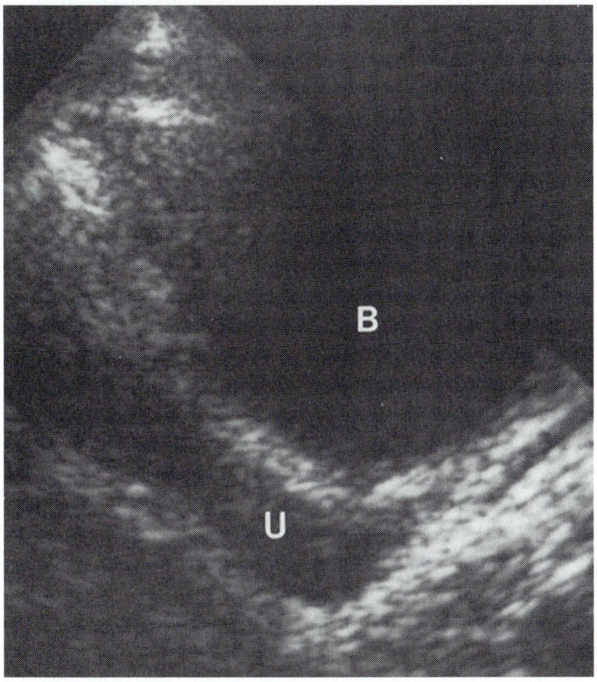

D
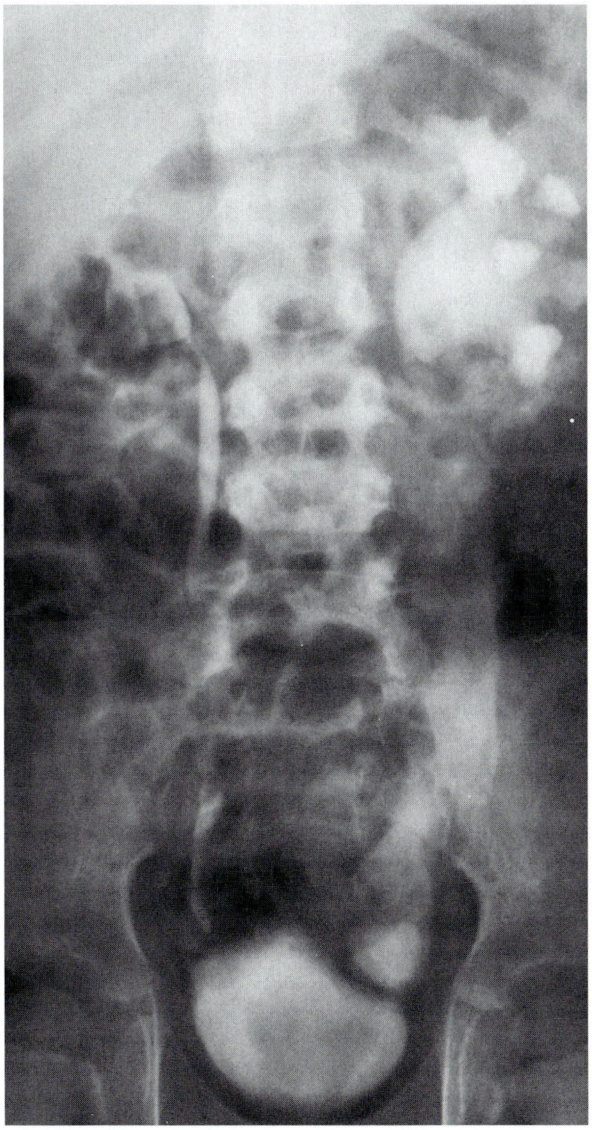

E
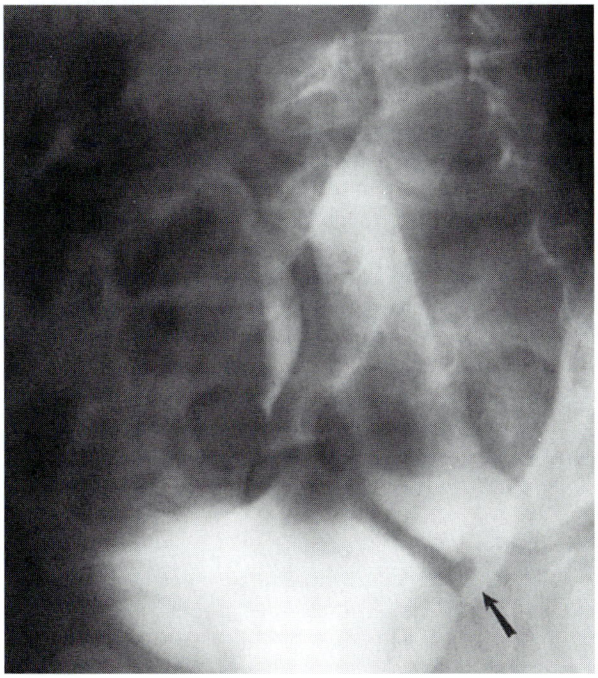

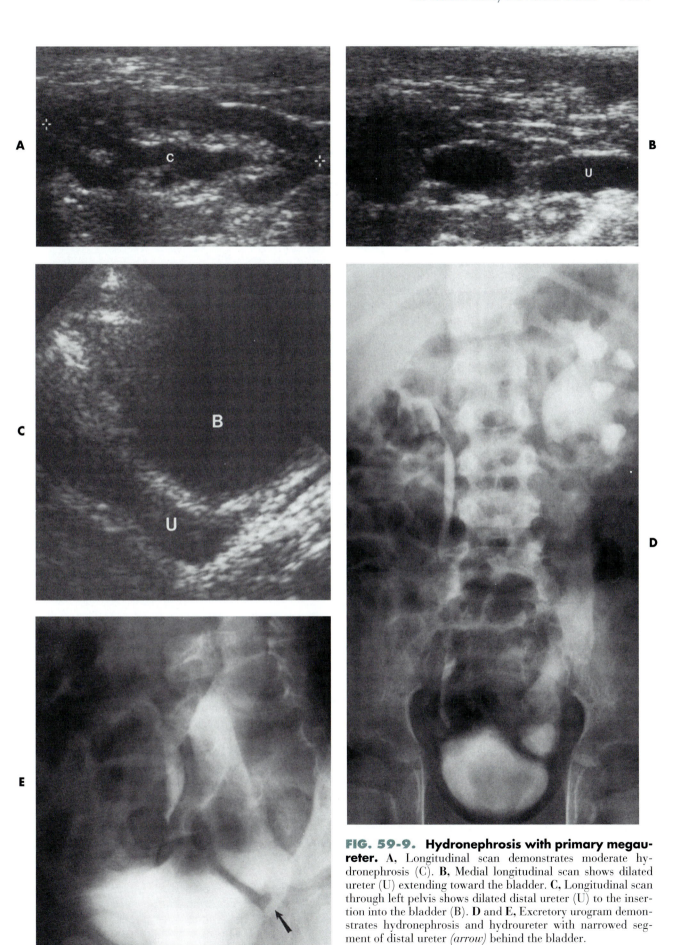

FIG. 59-9. Hydronephrosis with primary megaureter. **A,** Longitudinal scan demonstrates moderate hydronephrosis (C). **B,** Medial longitudinal scan shows dilated ureter (U) extending toward the bladder. **C,** Longitudinal scan through left pelvis shows dilated distal ureter (U) to the insertion into the bladder (B). **D** and **E,** Excretory urogram demonstrates hydronephrosis and hydroureter with narrowed segment of distal ureter *(arrow)* behind the bladder.

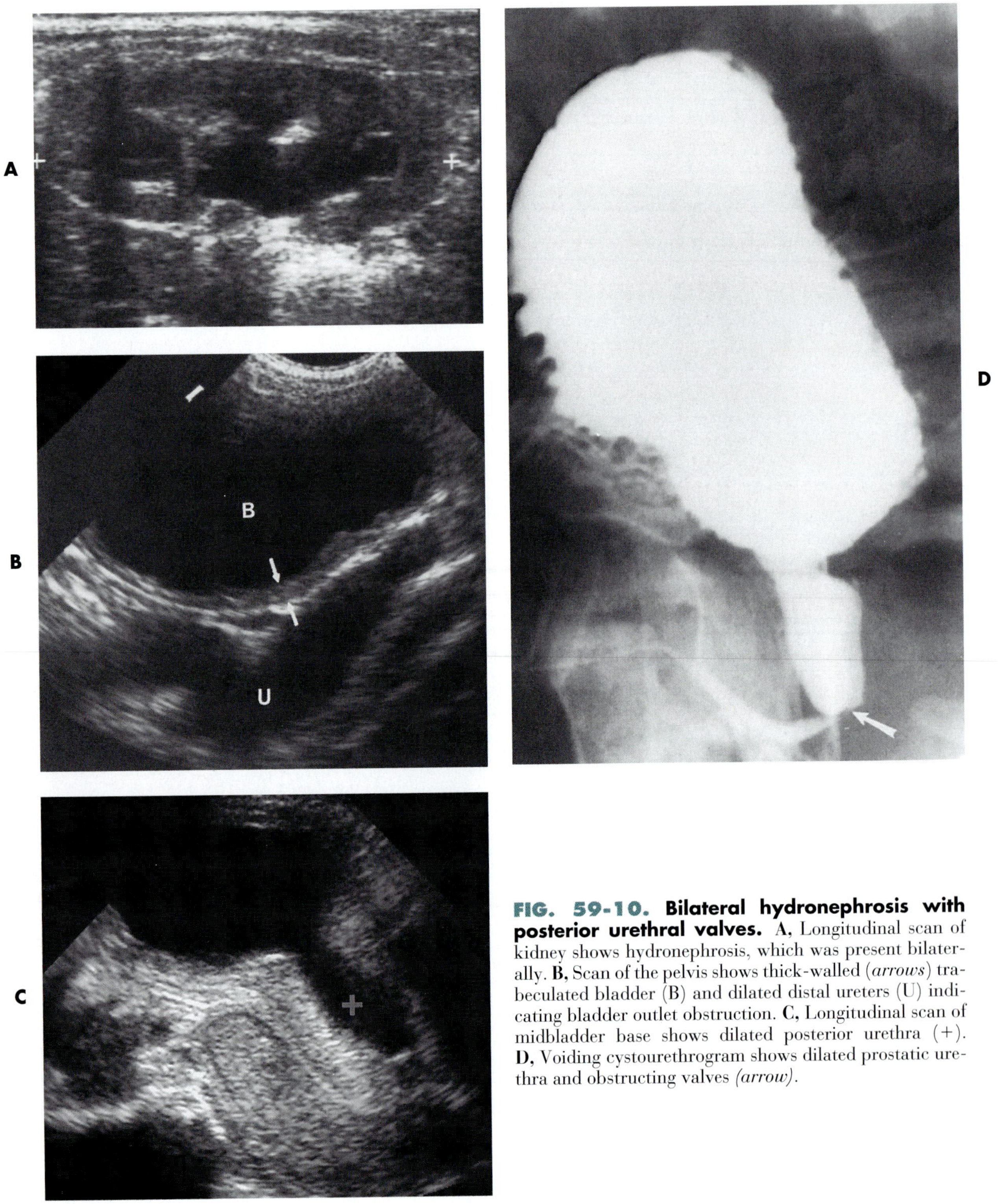

FIG. 59-10. Bilateral hydronephrosis with posterior urethral valves. **A,** Longitudinal scan of kidney shows hydronephrosis, which was present bilaterally. **B,** Scan of the pelvis shows thick-walled *(arrows)* trabeculated bladder (B) and dilated distal ureters (U) indicating bladder outlet obstruction. **C,** Longitudinal scan of midbladder base shows dilated posterior urethra (+). **D,** Voiding cystourethrogram shows dilated prostatic urethra and obstructing valves *(arrow)*.

ished-to-absent peristalsis of the bowel are seen with contrast radiography. The condition is fatal unless the patient can be maintained with total parenteral hyperalimentation.[14]

Exstrophy of the Bladder

This a rare anomaly in which the pubic bones are far apart and the bladder and urethral mucosa are exposed. The kidneys and ureters are usually normal. After surgical repair of the bladder, there may be hydronephrosis secondary to poor bladder emptying. After surgical repair, the bladder is usually small and irregularly shaped[15] and is readily visualized sonographically.

Urachal Anomalies

The fetal urachus is a tubular structure extending from the umbilicus to the bladder. It normally closes by birth; if it remains patent, urine may leak from the umbilicus. If part of the urachus closes, patent parts may form urachal cysts. These may become infected. The proximal portion of the urachus may remain open, producing a diverticulum-like structure from the dome of the bladder.[15] These anomalies are sometimes associated with prune-belly syndrome. Urachal abnormalities are evaluated with cystography in the lateral projection and with sonography. The latter is particularly useful in demonstrating urachal cysts and masses near the abdominal wall along the site of the urachal tract (Fig. 59-11).[16,17]

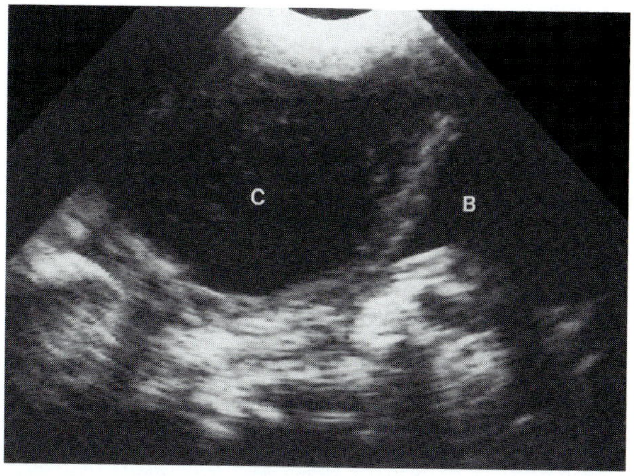

FIG. 59-11. Urachal cyst. Midline longitudinal scan of the pelvis shows compression of the bladder dome (B) by a thick-walled cystic mass containing low-level echoes (C). The patient had sepsis and an infected cyst.

RENAL CYSTIC DISEASE

Autosomal Recessive Polycystic Kidney Disease

Renal cystic disease is a complex subject, with several confusing overlapping classifications. This is a summary of the most common forms.

Autosomal recessive polycystic kidney disease (Potter type 1) (ARPKD) is characterized by dilated collecting ducts, seen as radially arranged, fusiform "cysts" that are most prominent in the medullary portions of the kidney.[18] This disease has a spectrum of severity and a reciprocal relationship with liver involvement (periportal fibrosis, often with proliferation and variable dilatation of the bile ducts).[19,20] Severe renal involvement can be diagnosed in the second trimester of pregnancy by enlarged hyperechogenic kidneys followed by oligohydramnios. In the third trimester, the kidneys occupy almost the entire abdomen and cause it to enlarge. At this time, the kidneys resemble those of the newborn with ARPKD: They are hyperechogenic and greatly enlarged, often with a hypoechogenic outer rim which probably represents the cortex compressed by the greatly expanded pyramids (Fig. 59-12).[21] Intravenous urography outlines a little

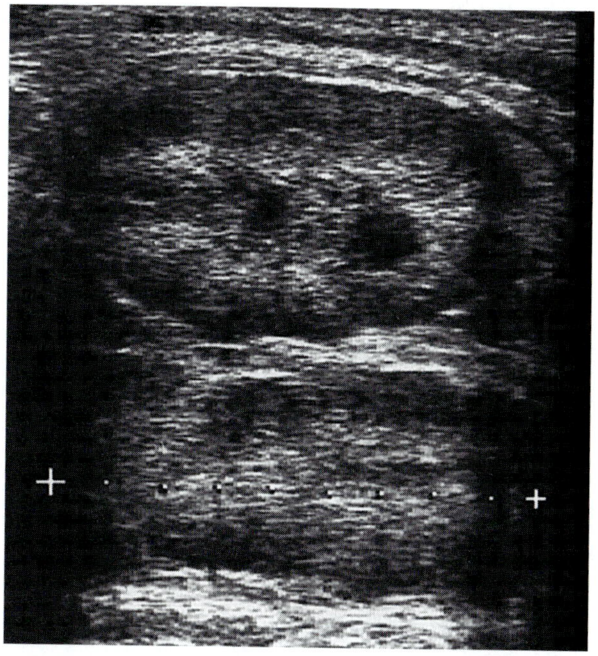

FIG. 59-12. Autosomal recessive polycystic kidney disease (ARPKD). Longitudinal sonogram of the abdomen of a 38-week-old fetus shows two symmetrically enlarged kidneys almost entirely filling the abdomen. The kidneys retain their normal shape. The entire medulla is very echogenic, representing dilated collecting tubules; the subcapsular region is relatively hypoechoic, reflecting compressed cortex. Pyramids are no longer recognizable. (From Siegel BA, Proto AV. *Pediatric Disease Test and Syllabus*, 4th series. Reston, Va: American College of Radiology; 1993.)

of the stagnation of urine that occurs within the tubules; the enlarged kidneys show a striated, increasingly dense nephrogram and poor visualization of the collecting system. These children generally succumb to their renal failure and no clinical liver disease is noted.

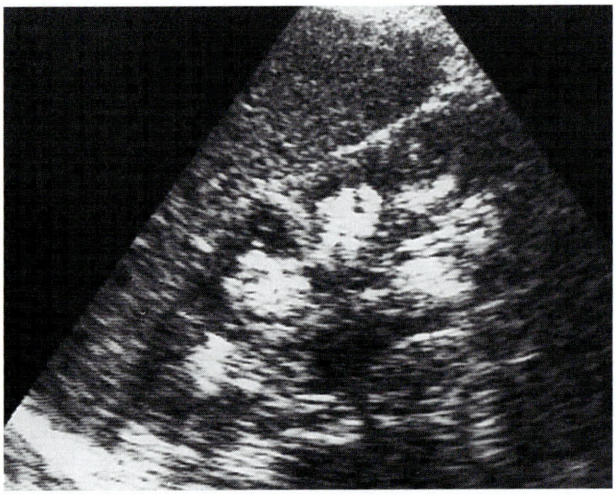

FIG. 59-13. ARPKD and congenital hepatic fibrosis. A 2-year-old boy with enlarged kidneys (and liver) due to congenital hepatic fibrosis and recessive polycystic kidney disease. Note the hyperechogenic pyramids, likely representing calcium in dilated collecting ducts.

Autosomal Recessive Polycystic Kidney Disease with Severe Hepatic Fibrosis

At the other end of the spectrum is the teenager who presents with bleeding esophageal varices due to portal hypertension secondary to congenital hepatic fibrosis. In these children, approximately 10% of kidney tubules are cystic and renal failure presents much later in life. The kidneys in these children are often slightly to moderately enlarged with echogenic pyramids (Fig. 59-13). The latter often contain calcium. At intravenous urography, the pattern resembles that of adult medullary sponge kidney with pooling of contrast medium in the dilated collecting ducts. In more advanced cases, the entire kidney may be replaced by tiny cysts.

Autosomal Dominant Polycystic Kidney Disease

Although more than 90% of patients with autosomal dominant polycystic kidney disease (ADPKD) (Potter type 3) have a gene locus on the short arm of chromosome 16, and although penetrance is complete, there is a great variation in the severity of the disease. It has been diagnosed in utero and in early childhood but the typical presentation is between the ages of 30 and 40, at which time hypertension or azotemia is present. At the extreme end of the spectrum, the disease has been discovered incidentally in otherwise healthy persons in the seventh or eighth decade. Twenty-five percent of patients have a negative family history. This disease is characterized by a weakness in basement membranes, likely because of a generalized defect in collagen formation. All parts of the nephron are affected, although only 5% to 10% of the nephrons are involved. Cysts can therefore occur anywhere and are usually macroscopic and of varying size (Fig. 59-14).[22,23] The incidence of cysts in other organs depends on the stage and severity of the disease. About 10% of patients with ADPKD have hepatic cysts and there is a much lower incidence of splenic, pancreatic, and pulmonary cysts. There are also cerebral aneurysms, colonic diverticulosis and cysts in the ovaries, seminal vesicles, and brain. Extrarenal cysts are rare in children.

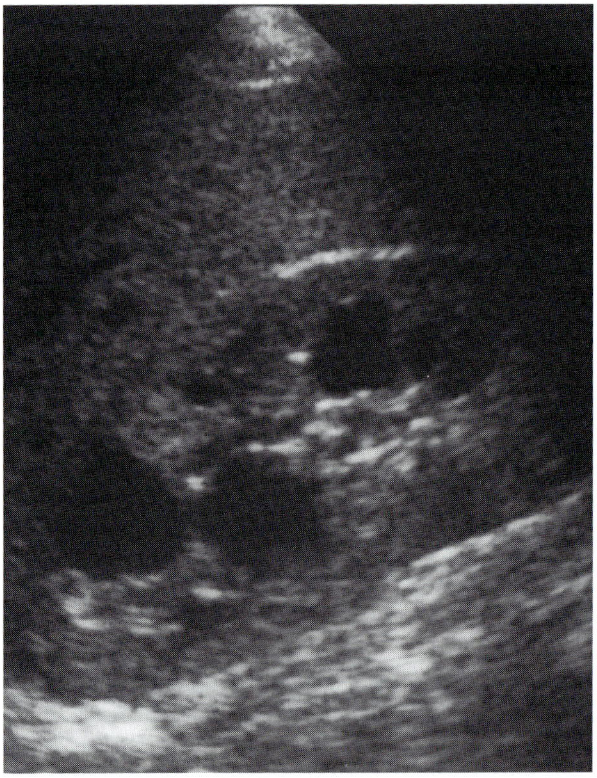

FIG. 59-14. Autosomal dominant polycystic kidney disease (ADPKD) in an 18-year-old. Longitudinal scan of the left kidney demonstrates cysts of varying size. The kidneys are mildly enlarged.

Multicystic Renal Dysplasia

Multicystic renal dysplasia (Potter type 2) (MCDK) is the most common form of cystic disease in infants and is associated with an increased incidence of abnormalities in the contralateral kidney, including ureteral pelvic junction (UPJ) stenosis, multicystic dysplastic kidney (in which case the disease is fatal), primary megaureter and vesicoureteral reflux. Multicystic dysplastic kidney is now usually detected sonographically in utero; large cysts of varying sizes are arranged like a bunch of grapes and there is no recognizable renal pelvis (Fig. 59-15). Ureteral obliteration causes renal function to diminish and then cease. In cases where the cysts of the multicystic dysplastic kidney resemble

A

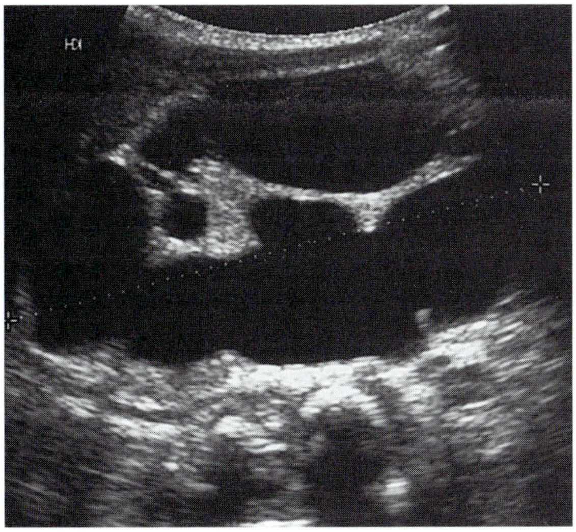

B

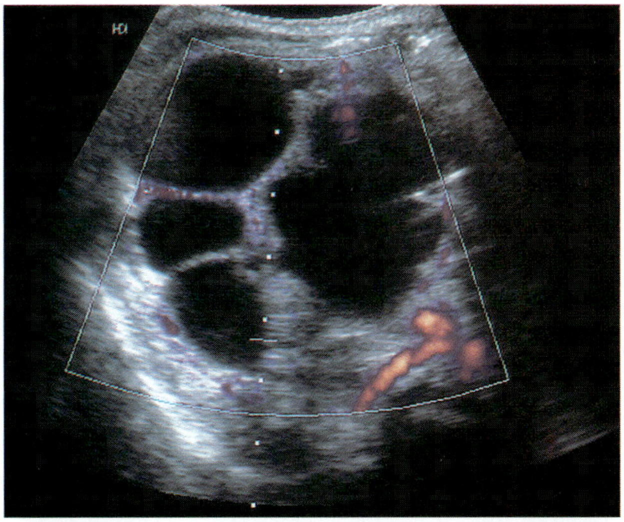

C

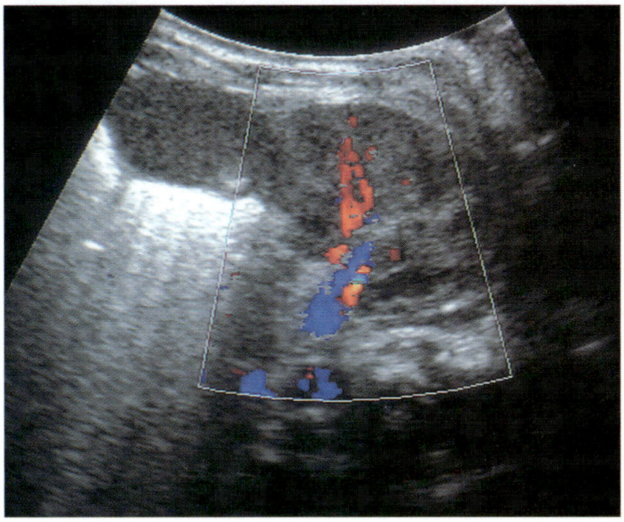

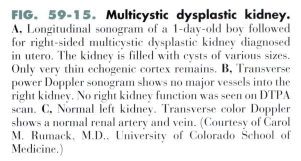

FIG. 59-15. Multicystic dysplastic kidney. **A,** Longitudinal sonogram of a 1-day-old boy followed for right-sided multicystic dysplastic kidney diagnosed in utero. The kidney is filled with cysts of various sizes. Only very thin echogenic cortex remains. **B,** Transverse power Doppler sonogram shows no major vessels into the right kidney. No right kidney function was seen on DTPA scan. **C,** Normal left kidney. Transverse color Doppler shows a normal renal artery and vein. (Courtesy of Carol M. Rumack, M.D., University of Colorado School of Medicine.)

the dilated calyces of severe ureteropelvic junction stenosis, scintigraphy is useful to detect any remaining renal function. The calyces in severe hydronephrosis due to UPJ stenosis communicate, whereas the cysts in the multicystic dysplastic kidney do not.[24] Surgery of multicystic dysplastic kidney is usually not necessary unless the kidney is massively enlarged.[25] Periodic follow-up sonography shows decrease in the size of the cysts as urine production stops to the point where the kidney may no longer be visible.

Medullary Cystic Disease and Juvenile Nephronophthisis

Medullary cystic disease and juvenile nephronophthisis; these two entities are morphologically indistinguishable. Both cause chronic renal failure in adolescents or young adults. At sonography, the kidneys are small, echogenic, and contain cysts of variable sizes at the cortico-medullary junction and elsewhere (Fig. 59-16). Medullary cystic disease is inherited in autosomal dominant, juvenile nephronophthisis in autosomal recessive fashion.

Cysts and Syndromes

Cysts of various sizes and location occur in a variety of syndromes, including tuberous sclerosis and in von Hippel-Lindau disease.

Tuberous Sclerosis. Tuberous sclerosis is an autosomal dominant disease consisting of mental retardation, epilepsy, adenoma sebaceum, multiple ectodermal lesions, and mesodermal hamartomas. Renal lesions are present in more than 40% of cases and include cysts, which can be multiple and resemble adult-type polycystic kidney disease with renal enlargement. **Angiomyolipomas** can occur and may be multiple. They vary in their echogenicity depending upon the type of tissue contained and can be markedly echogenic when they contain considerable fat (Fig. 59-17).[26] In **von Hippel-Lindau disease,** there are cysts and increased incidence of renal cell carcinoma which is often bilateral.

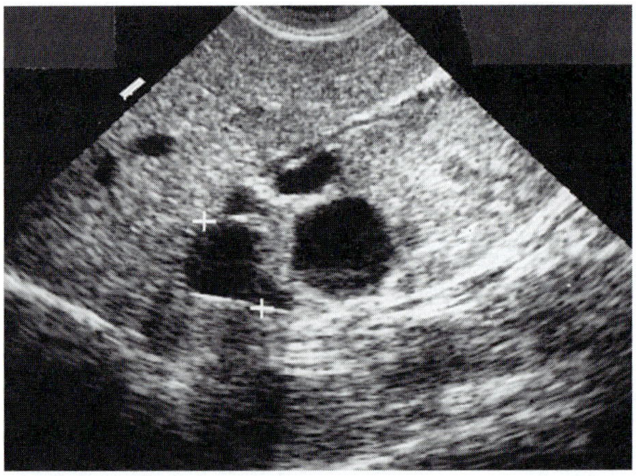

FIG. 59-16. Nephronophthisis. A 17-year-old girl with hypertension. The kidneys contain several cysts of various sizes. Pyramids are no longer visible. The contours and size of the kidneys are normal.

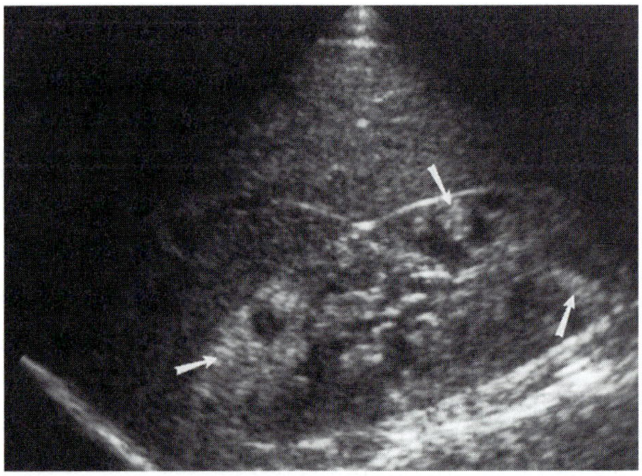

FIG. 59-17. Tuberous sclerosis. 16-year-old girl with hydrocephalus. Sagittal sonogram of the right kidney shows several small cysts and numerous hyperechogenic foci *(arrows)*, especially in the medulla. No acoustic shadowing is seen. (These echogenic deposits were confirmed to be fat at CT.)

Acquired Cysts

Patients with chronic renal failure, especially those receiving dialysis, often develop multiple small renal cysts. The kidneys usually remain small, and large cysts are rare. There is an increased incidence of formation of adenomas and a slightly increased incidence of adenocarcinoma in patients on long-term dialysis. Spontaneous hemorrhage may occur.

Simple cysts are much less common in children than in adults. They have the typical appearance of a single cystic mass arising from the kidney and are clinically important only in that they can be associated with hematuria or infection.

URINARY TRACT INFECTION

Urinary tract infection is a common clinical problem in children and a common indication for renal sonography. The imaging work-up of the child with a urinary tract infection is usually performed **after the first culture has documented infection in a male or female infant or child.** The purpose of the work-up is to identify congenital anomalies, obstructions, and other abnormalities that may predispose the patient to infections. In the past, excretory urography (EU) was used, but **renal sonography has now replaced excretory urography for initial screening.** The lower urinary tract, the bladder, and the urethra are evaluated by radiographic cystography, and either nuclear or radiographic cystography can be used to evaluate vesicoureteral reflux. Our current approach is to perform a radiographic cystogram in males, in whom it is important to visualize the urethral anatomy, and in girls if abnormalities are seen at sonography. The nuclear cystogram is associated with a lower radiation dose to the gonads and is used in females with normal renal and bladder sonograms and those in whom urethral abnormalities are rare and as well as for follow-up examinations for reflux in both males and females. If abnormalities that require further investigation are detected on the renal sonogram or the cystogram, renal nuclear scintigraphy with DTPA or MAG 3 is performed. Renal nuclear scintigraphy with Tc 99m glucoheptonate or dimercaprol succinate acid is extremely sensitive for demonstrating focal areas of inflammation and parenchymal scars. Mild scars may be missed with sonography. At the present time, it is thought that mild scars are of little practical importance and do not alter the course of therapy; therefore, the radiation dose of a renal cortical scan is not warranted.[27-29]

Acute Pyelonephritis

Acute pyelonephritis, or infectious interstitial nephritis, is usually diagnosed by the clinical features of sudden fever, flank pain, and costovertebral-angle tenderness with microscopic evidence of infection in the urine. The infection usually occurs as an ascending infection from the bladder via reflux but can occur by hematogenous spread.[30] The findings on sonography or excretory urography are usually few but include swelling of the infected kidney, altered renal parenchymal echogenicity due to edema,[2] or triangular areas of increased echogenicity (Fig. 59-18). There may be thickening of the wall of the renal pelvis and ureter, also caused by edema and inflammation (Fig. 59-19).[31] Scintigraphy, CT and Doppler sonography may show absent or decreased perfusion in a diffuse or lobar distribution, especially at the upper or lower poles (Fig. 59-18).[32-34]

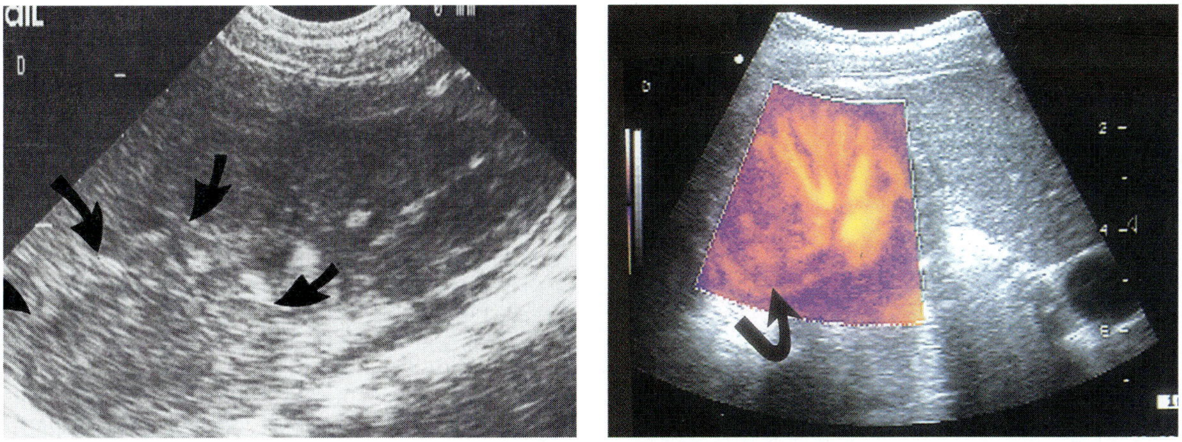

FIG. 59-18. Acute pyelonephritis in a 1-year-old boy. **A,** Sagittal sonogram of the right kidney shows a swollen, hyperechogenic upper pole *(arrow)*. **B,** On power Doppler sonography, this area *(arrow)* is devoid of flow signals.

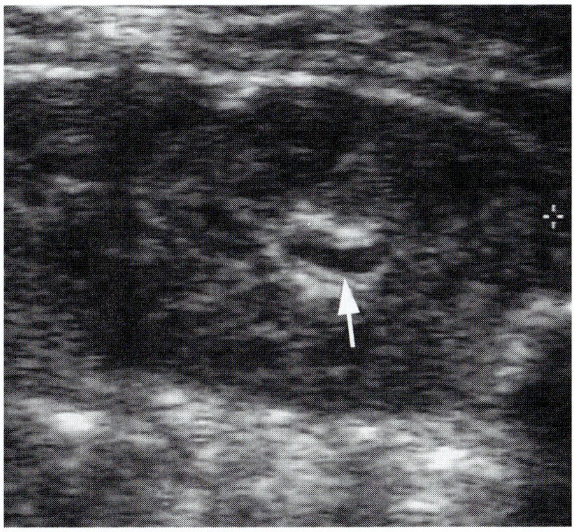

FIG. 59-19. Thickening of the wall of the renal pelvis. Edema of the wall of the renal pelvis and ureter can occur with inflammation and/or reflux. The wall *(arrow)* is thickened with medium-level echoes less than the adjacent sinus fat.

Pyelonephritis may involve one portion of the kidney more than others.[30] Sonography may demonstrate a localized renal mass with altered echogenicity compared to the remainder of the kidney but containing low-level echoes that disrupt the corticomedullary definition of the kidney in that area.[34] Sequential examinations will demonstrate a rapid change, with resolution of the mass in response to antibiotic therapy. If response to antibiotic therapy is inadequate, the mass may liquefy centrally and become a renal abscess that requires drainage. **Sonography of an abscess** shows a focal mass with an echogenic wall and a hypoechoic central area representing liquefied pus. On long-term follow-up, focal scarring and clubbed calices may result from the focal infection (Fig. 59-20). Another complication that requires drainage is **pyonephrosis,** identified sonographically as echogenic material filling a dilated collecting system (Fig. 59-21). When patients with urinary tract infections do not respond rapidly to antibiotic therapy, repeat sonographic and/or CT examinations are indicated in order to search for these complications that require drainage.

Chronic Pyelonephritis

Chronic pyelonephritis is the result of repeated episodes of acute pyelonephritis and results in a small, scarred kidney, indicative of end-stage renal disease. The kidney is usually irregular in outline owing to focal parenchymal loss. The renal cortex becomes more echogenic than the liver parenchyma. The pyramids are difficult to outline sonographically. These findings are not specific and can also be seen in chronic glomerulonephritis, dysplastic kidneys, and hypertensive or ischemic disease.[2]

Neonatal Candidiasis

Candida albicans is a saprophytic fungus that usually infects immunocompromised patients, particularly neonates on broad-spectrum antibiotics with indwelling catheters. Systemic candidiasis leads to infection of multiple organs, including the kidneys, and may present in the neonate with anuria, oliguria, a flank mass, or hypertension. Sonography may show diffuse enlargement of the kidney with loss of normal architecture and presence of abnormal parenchymal echogenicity. Mycelial clumping (fungus ball formation) may occur in the collecting system causing hydronephrosis and echogenic filling defects within the

A

B

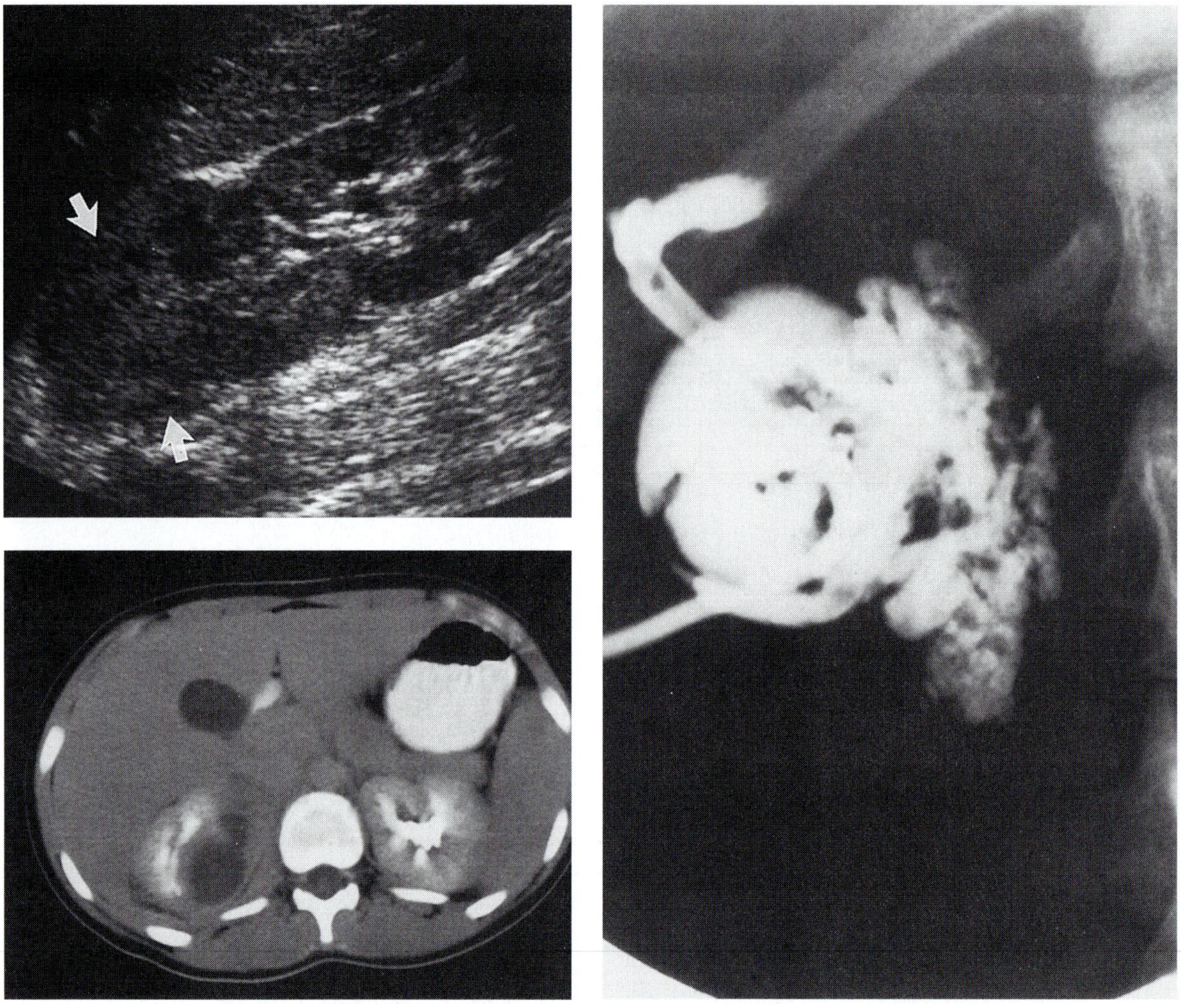

C

FIG. 59-20. Renal abscess. **A,** Longitudinal scan demonstrates a localized renal mass (*arrowheads*) and destruction of the cortical medullary definition by an area of focal bacterial nephritis. **B,** CT scan 5 days later shows central liquefaction and abscess formation. **C,** Abscess drained with a percutaneously placed catheter.

A

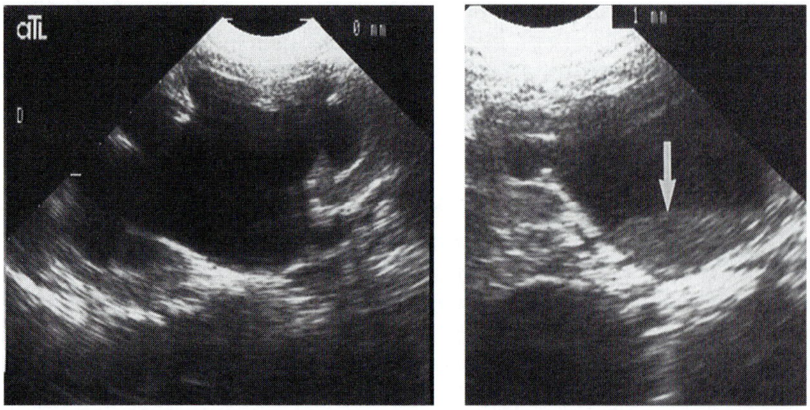

B

FIG. 59-21. Pyonephrosis. Three-month-old boy with bilateral ureteropelvic junction stenosis. Sagittal sonograms of the **A,** right, and **B,** left, kidneys showing bilateral hydronephrosis. Urine in the pelvis of the right kidney appears anechoic; in contrast, there is a dependent layer of pus in the pelvis of the left kidney *(arrow)*.

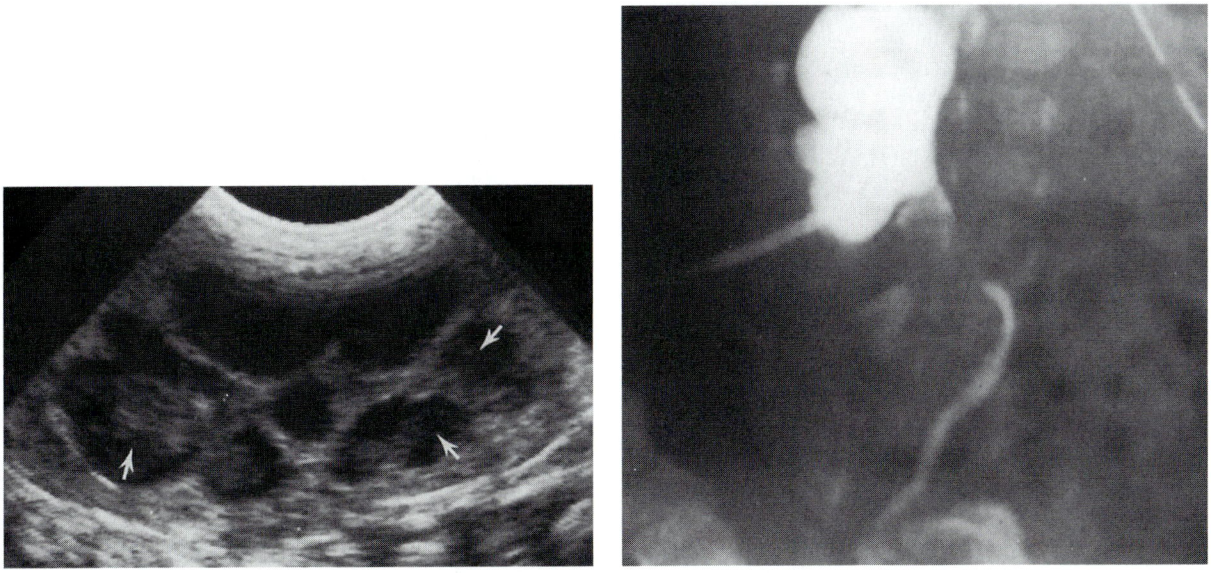

FIG. 59-22. Neonatal candidiasis. **A,** Longitudinal scan of the right kidney shows hydronephrosis with echogenic filling defects (*arrows*) representing fungus ball formation. **B,** Nephrostomy was performed under ultrasound guidance to drain obstructed system.

collecting system (Fig. 59-22). The filling defects may obstruct the collecting system and require drainage procedures such as a nephrostomy.[35,36]

Cystitis

Inflammation of the urinary bladder may occur in children as a result of infection or drug therapy (Cytoxan). The bladder wall becomes thickened (> 3 mm) and irregular. Echogenic debris or blood clot may be seen in the urine (Fig. 59-23).[17]

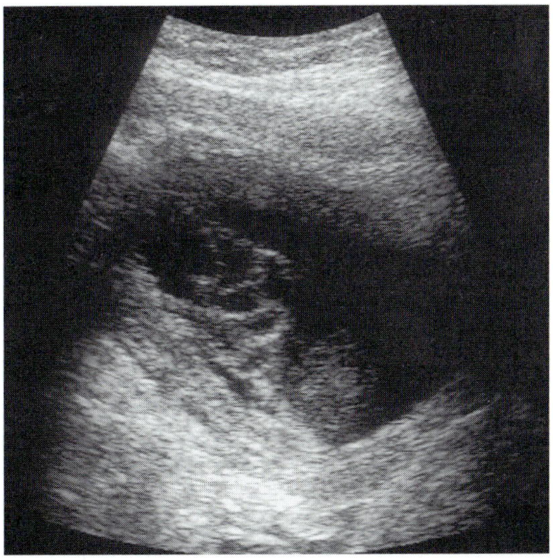

FIG. 59-23. Cystitis in patient on Cytoxan. Longitudinal scan of pelvis shows thick-walled bladder and echogenic debris and blood clot within urine.

MEDICAL RENAL DISEASE

Glomerulonephritis

The glomerulonephritides include lesions resulting from glomerular reaction to immunologic injury. In acute poststreptococcal glomerulonephritis, the kidneys are moderately swollen and have cellular infiltrate in the glomerular tufts. There may be interstitial edema followed by atrophy. Sonographic findings include normal or bilaterally enlarged kidneys with diffuse increase in the echogenicity of the renal cortex (Fig. 59-24). The renal cortical echogenicity may be greater than that of the adjacent liver, and the medullary pyramids appear prominent in contrast to the hyperechoic cortex. The echogenicity of the renal cortex decreases with regression of the acute disease, and sonography can be used to demonstrate this, obviating the need for serial renal biopsies. The findings in acute glomerulonephritis are those of type I medical renal disease as described by Rosenfield[37] and are nonspecific, being also seen in **amyloidosis, nephrosclerosis, acute tubular necrosis, leukemia, Goodpasture's syndrome, Henoch-Schönlein purpura,** and the **nephrotic syndrome.** In chronic glomerulonephritis, the kidneys are small, diffusely hyperechogenic, and show loss of corticomedullary differentiation. These findings are also nonspecific and identical to those of end-stage renal disease of any cause.[37]

Nephrocalcinosis

Causes of the deposition of calcium within the kidney in childhood include hypervitaminosis D, milk alkali

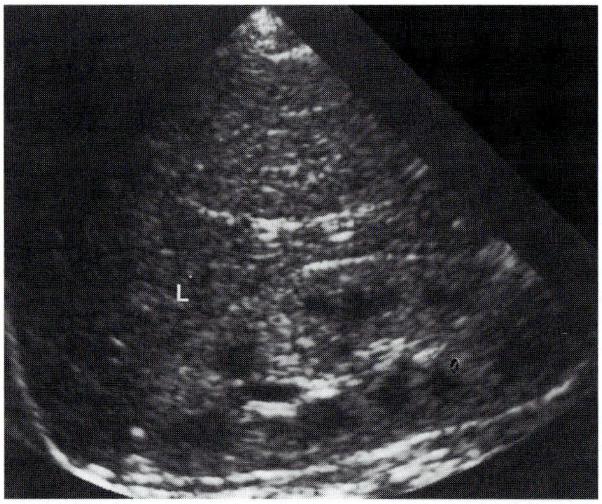

FIG. 59-24. Acute glomerulonephritis. Longitudinal scan of the kidney demonstrates renal enlargement with diffuse increase in renal cortical echogenicity greater than adjacent liver (L).

> **CAUSES OF NEPHROCALCINOSIS**
>
> Hypervitaminosis D
> Milk alkali syndrome
> Renal tubular acidosis
> Hyperparathyroidism
> Hyperoxaluria
> Sarcoidosis
> Cushing's syndrome
> Williams syndrome
> Chronic treatment with furosemide or lasix

syndrome, renal tubular acidosis, hyperparathyroidism, hyperoxaluria, sarcoidosis, Cushing's syndrome, Williams syndrome, and chronic treatment with furosemide or lasix (in premature babies). In these conditions, an increased load of calcium is presented to the kidney. The mineral content within the kidney increases progressively from the glomerulus to the collecting ducts and thus the greatest concentration of calcium is found in the pyramids, especially at their tips. Randall, Anderson, and Carr described calcareous deposits at the tips or sides of pyramids at microscopy in normal pediatric and adult cadaver kidneys. Bruwer outlined identical deposits in cadaver kidney slices using high-resolution radiography.[38] These authors postulate that the concentration of calcium is high in fluids about the renal tubules and that calcium is normally removed from this area by lymphatic flow. If the calcium load exceeds the lymphatic capacity, microscopic calcium aggregates occur in the medulla, mainly at the tips of the fornix and at the margins. They may fuse to form plaques such as Randall's plaque and migrate toward the caliceal epithelium, finally perforating through it. A nidus for urinary stones is provided. Bruwer termed this process the Anderson-Carr-Randall progression of calculus formation.

Sonography is more sensitive than radiography in detecting calcium deposits within the kidney. We found four patterns of calcium deposition within the kidney (Fig. 59-25)[39] and were able to show the progression from nephrocalcinosis to the formation of macroscopic plaques of calcium near the calyx; they later perforated into the calyx and formed a ureteral stone.

Any form of urinary stasis predisposes not only to infection but also to calcium formation. Thus, the tubular ectasia encountered in **medullary sponge kidney**[40] and also in **autosomal recessive polycystic kidney disease** associated with congenital hepatic fibrosis often shows deposits of calcium, once again in the pyramids, at the site of the dilated tubules. Similarly, milk of calcium may deposit in caliceal diverticula or in ureteropelvic junction obstruction (Fig. 59-26).[41]

The finely branching calcifications within the cortex and medulla of the kidney found after renal vein thrombosis are actually calcified microthrombi in the intrarenal veins.[42] Chronic infections such as mycoses and tuberculosis, tumors and tubular or papillary necrosis, or infection cause dystrophic calcification at the renal site affected.[43]

RENAL TRAUMA

Because the child's kidneys are relatively larger and less protected than the adult's, they are quite frequently affected when the abdomen is injured. Preexisting and often clinically silent renal abnormalities such as hydronephrosis may make the kidney more suspectible to injury by minor trauma. Renal trauma is often associated with other organ injury, particularly of the liver and spleen. CT has become the primary imaging modality for suspected multiorgan blunt abdominal trauma in the pediatric patient.[44] There is a role for ultrasound and nuclear medicine, primarily in the follow-up of the injuries found on CT.[45] Sonography in renal trauma shows distortion of the normal renal architecture. Renal hematoma can vary but is usually echogenic at first and becomes hypoechoic as it liquefies. There may be extravasation of urine around the kidney, which can be difficult to distinguish from hypoechoic blood. Injuries to the vascular renal pedicle are uncommon but constitute a surgical emergency. Doppler sonography can demonstrate both arterial and venous patency. Absent flow signals in part or all of the kidney (when signals are detected elsewhere in the abdomen)

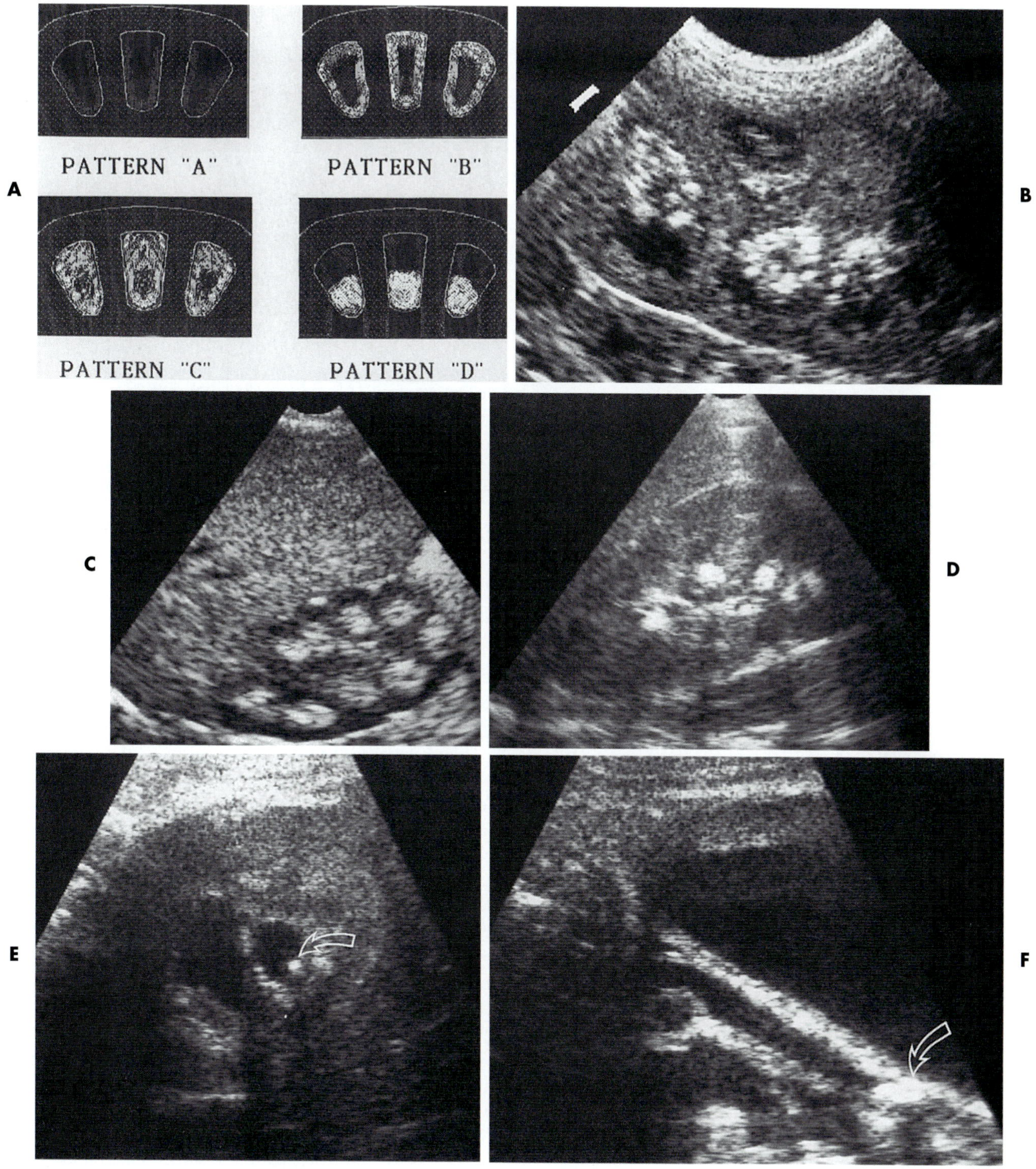

FIG. 59-25. Nephrocalcinosis. A, Diagram of four patterns of renal medullary calcium deposition seen at sonography. Patterns A through C represent increasing stages of calcium deposition beginning in the periphery of the renal pyramids. Pattern D shows stone formation at fornices. **B,** Type B nephrocalcinosis in a 3-week-old boy with renal tubular acidosis. Calcium deposits are at the periphery of the pyramids. **C,** Type C pattern in a 7-month-old boy with glycogenosis. Sonogram of the right kidney shows pyramids virtually completely filled with calcium deposits. **D,** Pattern D in an 11-year-old boy with hypercholesterolemia and a portocaval shunt. Sonogram of right kidney shows hyperechoic foci with acoustic shadows in the tips of the pyramids (fornices), suggesting presence of calcium. **E** and **F,** The spectrum of nephrocalcinosis is demonstrated on the sonogram of a 7-year-old boy with vitamin-D-resistant rickets treated with Rocaltrol and type B nephrocalcinosis (not shown). Sonogram of the right kidney shows a small stone at edge of dilated calyx *(arrow)*. Longitudinal sonogram shows a stone impacted in dilated distal right ureter *(arrow)*. (From Patriquin H, Robitaille P. Renal calcium deposition in children: sonographic demonstration of the Anderson-Carr progression. *AJR* 1986;146:1253-1256.)

A

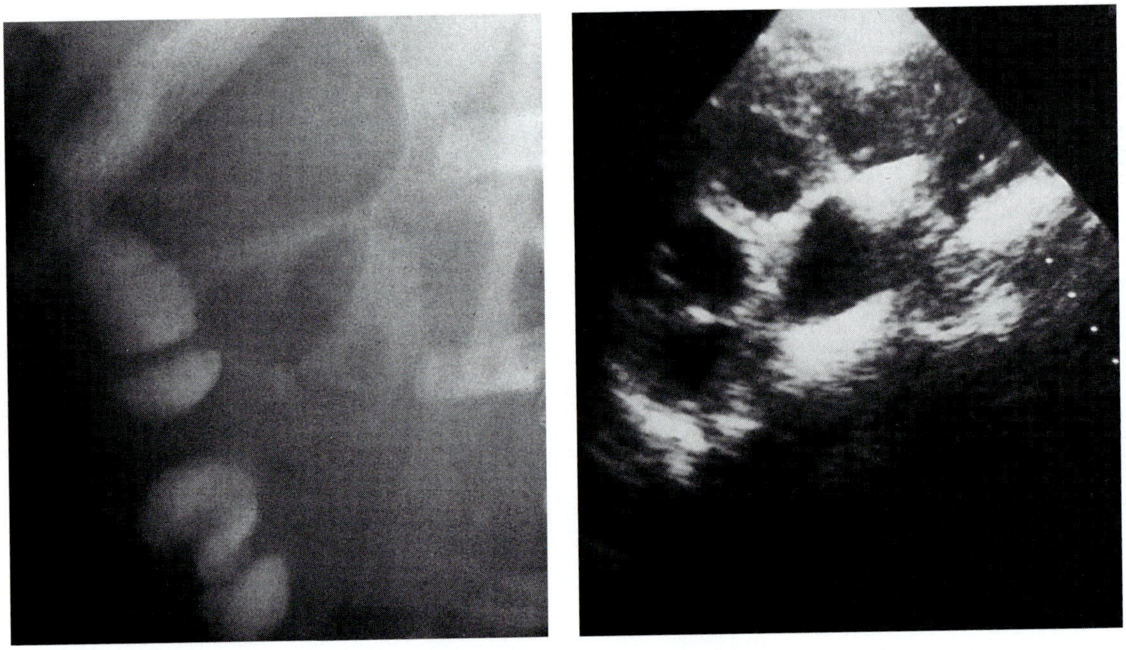

B

FIG. 59-26. Urinary calculi. A 17-year-old girl with repeated UTI and ureteropelvic junction stenosis. **A,** Supine abdominal film suggests several large stones or staghorn calculus. **B,** Supine sonogram with horizontal beam shows urine-milk of calcium levels in dependent part of dilated calices. The milk of calcium moved with change in patient position. (From Patriquin H, Lafortune M, Filiatrault D. Urinary milk of calcium in children and adults: use of gravity-dependent sonography. *AJR* 1985;144:407-413.)

herald arterial obstruction. The sonographic gray scale apearance of the kidney acutely deprived of its arterial blood supply is normal.

RENAL AND ADRENAL TUMORS

The most common abdominal masses in the child are of renal origin: hydronephrosis and multicystic dysplasia.[10] Solid tumors are less common. Initial imaging includes sonography and often a plain film of the abdomen. The site of origin of the mass, its architecture (cystic or solid), and vascularization can usually be outlined with sonography. Metastases and tumoral invasion of the renal vein or inferior vena cava are sought during the sonographic survey of the abdomen. If the mass is cystic and arises from the kidney, the most likely differential diagnosis is between a hydronephrotic kidney and a multicystic dysplastic kidney. The configuration of the cysts on sonography as well as the presence of function on nuclear renogram help to distinguish between these two entities. If the mass is solid and related to the kidney, then Wilms' tumor is the most likely diagnosis. Staging of the tumor is usually done with CT or MRI. If the kidney is normal and the mass is related to another organ, then the work-up continues with imaging that is optimal for that organ.

Several types of renal tumors occur in the pediatric patient. The most common renal neoplasm is the Wilms' tumor. When large, it may be difficult to differentiate from neuroblastoma, which frequently arises from the adrenal gland and occurs in a similar age group.

Wilms' Tumor

Wilms' tumor, or nephroblastoma, is the most common intra-abdominal malignant tumor to occur in the child. Its incidence peaks between 2 and 5 years of age.[46] The tumor is usually bulky and expands within the renal parenchyma, resulting in distortion and displacement of the collecting system and capsule. It is usually sharply marginated. Typically, a large solid mass distorting the sinus, pyramids, cortex, and contour of the kidney (Fig. 59-27) is outlined with sonography. Echogenicity is usually quite hyperechoic and homogeneous, although there may be hypoechoic areas that represent hemorrhage and necrosis.[47,48] From 5% to 10% of patients have bilateral tumors, and nephroblastomatosis may be present in both kidneys in children with unilateral Wilms' tumors. Specific malformations associated with Wilms' tumors include **congenital hemihypertrophy, Beckwith-Wiedemann syndrome, sporadic aniridia, neurofibromatosis,** and **cerebral gigantism.**[46]

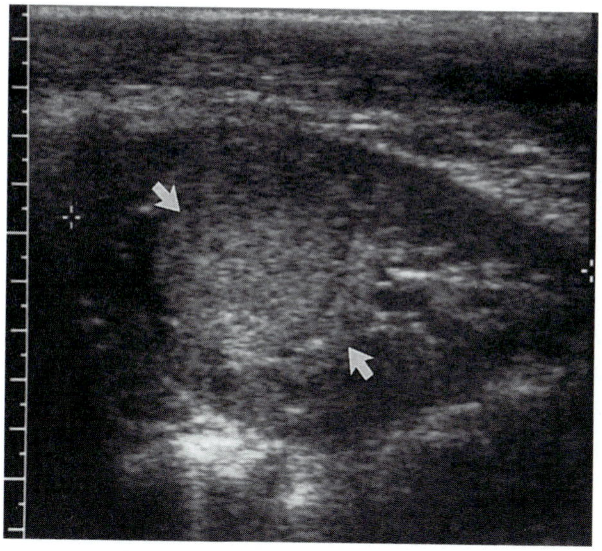

FIG. 59-27. Wilms' tumor. Longitudinal scan demonstrates large echogenic solid mass *(arrows)* within the kidney.

MALFORMATIONS ASSOCIATED WITH WILMS' TUMORS

Congenital hemihypertrophy
Beckwith-Wiedemann syndrome
Sporadic aniridia
Neurofibromatosis
Cerebral gigantism

Wilms' tumor spreads through direct extension into the renal sinus and peripelvic soft tissues, the lymph nodes in the renal hilum, and the para-aortic areas. Because extension is possible into the renal vein, inferior vena cava, right atrium, and liver, they should also be examined for the presence of tumor. Color and spectral Doppler sonography is useful in detecting residual flow around a tumor clot as well as tumor arterial signals both from the periphery of the tumor[49] and from within the tumor thrombus. The opposite kidney should be carefully examined for the presence of bilateral tumor. CT and MRI are usually performed for further work-up and staging. Spiral or helical CT is often favored, as the chest can also be evaluated for metastases,[50] which most commonly involve the lungs.

Neuroblastoma

The second most common abdominal tumor of childhood, occurring mainly between the age of 2 months and 2 years, neuroblastoma arises from the adrenal gland or the sympathetic nervous chain. Its extrarenal origin displaces and compresses the kidney without otherwise distorting the internal renal architecture. Neuroblastoma spreads early and widely, so the majority of patients have metastases at presentation. Its spread around the aorta and celiac and superior mesenteric arteries occurs early and helps to distinguish neuroblastoma from Wilms' tumor at sonography. Wilms' tumor is usually well defined and relatively homogeneous, whereas neuroblastoma is usually quite poorly defined and heterogeneous, with irregular hyperechogenic areas caused by calcifications (Fig. 59-28).[51,52] Syndromes associated with neuroblastoma include **Beckwith-Wiedemann syndrome, Klippel-Feil syndrome, fetal alcohol** and **phenylhydantoin syndromes,** and **Hirschsprung's disease.** Sonography is followed by CT or MRI for staging of the disease. MRI is particularly useful because the tumor can extend into the spinal canal and cause neurologic symptoms. It is critical to know if this extension has occurred before the tumor is surgically removed because the child may develop neurologic symptoms postoperatively if the tumor is not carefully resected.

Mesoblastic Nephroma

Mesoblastic nephroma or fetal renal hamartoma (congenital Wilms' tumor) is the most common neonatal renal neoplasm to occur within the first few months of life, and it is sometimes detected in the fetus. It is a benign tumor but can spread by local invasion and is usually treated by simple nephrectomy. Sonography demonstrates a mass arising within the kidney with an appearance similar to that of a Wilms' tumor. The tumor is solid but may have cystic-appearing areas of hemorrhage and necrosis. The young age of the patient, the tumor's benign biologic behavior, and its more favorable outcome help to differentiate it from the classic Wilms' tumor.[53]

Renal Cell Carcinoma

Renal cell carcinoma, rare in childhood, occurs later (at a mean age of 12 years) than Wilms' tumor. Its presentation and sonographic appearance are similar to those in adults.

Angiomyolipoma

Angiomyolipoma is a form of hamartoma that can cause symptoms related to hemorrhage and rupture. In children, these tumors are usually multiple and are associated with tuberous sclerosis.[26] Sonography typically shows multiple masses of varying echogenicity because of the fat content; some masses may be hyperechogenic (Fig. 59-17). There may be associated cysts within the kidney, and the kidneys may be enlarged.

Multilocular Renal Cyst

Sometimes called a cystic nephroma, this is a rare lesion that is generally considered benign. It can occur at any age but is not common under the age of 2 years.

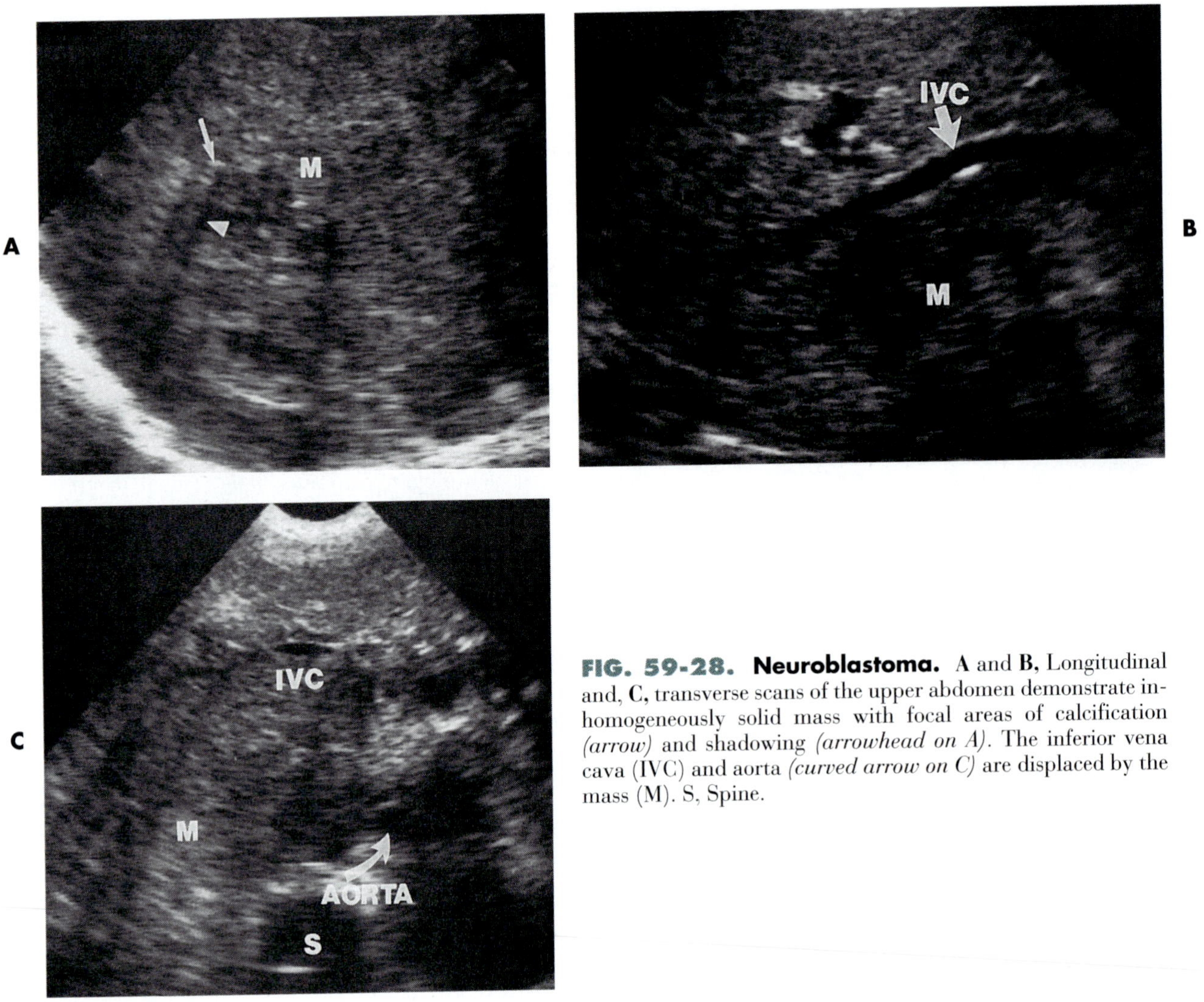

FIG. 59-28. Neuroblastoma. **A** and **B**, Longitudinal and, **C**, transverse scans of the upper abdomen demonstrate inhomogeneously solid mass with focal areas of calcification *(arrow)* and shadowing *(arrowhead on A)*. The inferior vena cava (IVC) and aorta *(curved arrow on C)* are displaced by the mass (M). S, Spine.

The mass is composed of multiple cysts of varying size that are connected by connective tissue septa. It may be difficult to distinguish from cystic, well-differentiated Wilms' tumor with nephroblastoma components in the walls of the cysts. Sonography demonstrates a well-circumscribed, multiloculated cystic mass with septations.[54] Some authors have suggested a malignant potential for these lesions and recommend nephrectomy.

Renal Lymphoma

Lymphomatous involvement of the kidney is usually a secondary process and can be seen on sonography as single or multiple relatively hypoechoic or weakly echogenic masses within the kidney. The kidney may be enlarged and lobulated in outline. Diffuse infiltration of the kidney can also occur, and the appearance in the pediatric patient is similar to that in the adult.[55,56]

Bladder Tumors

Primary tumors of the lower urinary tract are uncommon in children. Sarcoma botryoides is a rhabdomyosarcoma arising in the bladder base in males and it presents with bladder outlet obstruction. In girls, this rare tumor typically occurs in the uterus or vagina. Polyps can occur in the urethra.[17]

RENAL VASCULAR DISEASES IN CHILDREN: ASSESSMENT WITH DOPPLER SONOGRAPHY

Technique of Doppler Examinations of the Kidney

Babies and small children are examined without special preparation, but may be given juice or milk to drink during the examination in order to calm them, to increase hydration, and to provide an acoustic window through the fluid-filled stomach. Sedation is very rarely necessary. The older child is examined after a 4- to 6-hour fast (in order to reduce intestinal gas) only if a detailed examination of the main renal artery is planned. Color and pulsed Doppler examinations are performed. Power Doppler may also be useful to evaluate the presence of vascular flow.

A 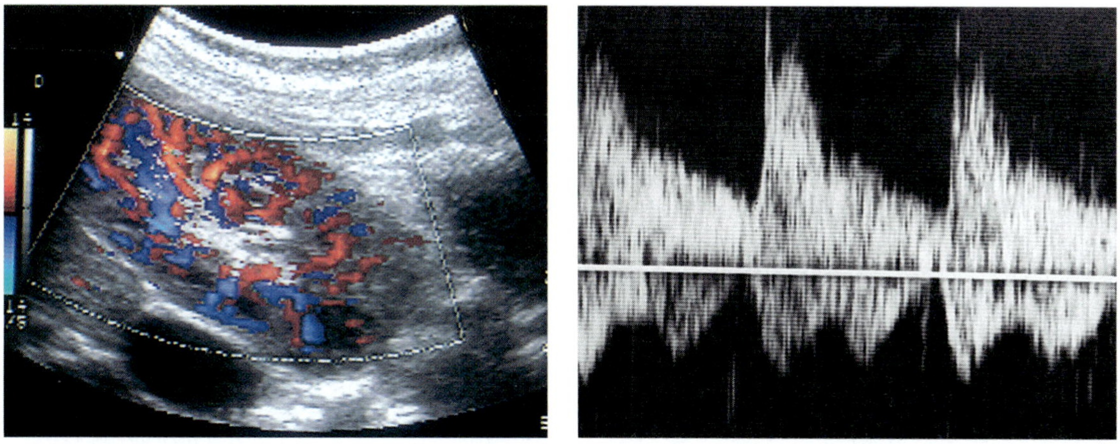 B

FIG. 59-29. Normal intrarenal circulation. A, Color Doppler sonogram of a newborn baby shows the position of intrarenal vessels at the hilum (segmental) alongside the pyramids (interlobar) and at the inner edge of the cortex (arcuate). **B,** Spectral display from a normal segmented artery (parabolic, low-resistance allowing high diastolic flow) and vein (triphasic flow reflecting right atrial pulsations).

OPTIMIZE DOPPLER FOR SLOW FLOW

Highest transducer frequency
Restriction of color area of interest
Low pulse repetition frequency (PRF)
Aliasing corrected by increasing PRF
Small sample volume
Lowest vessel/beam angle

Doppler settings are adjusted for maximal detection of slow flow: highest possible transducer frequency, relatively small color area of interest, low pulse repetition frequency, and low wall filter. Pulse repetition frequency is augmented if aliasing occurs. A small sample volume and the lowest possible vessel/beam angle are used.

The aorta and main renal arteries are examined by means of an anterior left paramedian as well as a left axillary approach with longitudinal and transverse views. The color mode is used to trace the renal arteries which are then examined with serial pulsed Doppler samples, especially in areas of high-velocity flow. Even if the entire renal artery cannot be outlined because of overlying intestinal gas, the retrocaval portion of the right renal artery and the hilar arteries can usually be analyzed. A segmental or interlobar artery in each third of the kidney (upper, middle, and lower) is then studied with pulsed Doppler and the resistive (Pourcelot) index or pulsatility index is calculated.

Normal Vascular Anatomy and Flow Patterns

The intrarenal arteries and veins and their relationship to the renal cortex, pyramids, and calices are exceptionally well outlined with color Doppler technology. The **main renal artery(ies)** divides in the renal hilum to form several pairs (anterior and posterior) of **segmental arteries.** These course toward the pyramids and there divide into interlobar branches, which follow the periphery of the pyramids. At the outer edge of the pyramids, interlobar arteries give rise to **arcuate arteries,** which follow the outer contour of the pyramids. **Cortical arteries** arise from the arcuate arteries and radiate into the cortex, following a direction similar to that of interlobar vessels. The venous circulation follows that of the arteries and simultaneous adjacent signals are often visible both with color Doppler and on spectral analysis (Fig. 59-29).

The renal arterial bed normally has low resistance, and there is a constant flow into the kidney throughout the cardiac cycle. The normal resistive index in adults is estimated at 0.65 ± 0.10. In the neonatal period, probably concurrent with the physiologic low glomerular filtration rate, the resistance of the renal arterial bed is somewhat higher: RI = 0.7 to 0.8. Because there is a range of normal values of the resistive index, the diagnosis of abnormal intrarenal resistance is much more reliably made by comparing waveforms from the pathologic kidney to those of the normal kidney or tracings from one day to the next of the pathlogic one.

Pulsed Doppler tracings from the normal intrarenal and main renal veins are somewhat variable: in some children the pulsations from right atrial diastole and systole are clearly visible, while in others the flow is steadier (Fig. 59-29, *B*). To-and-fro venous flow throughout the cardiac cycle may be seen in right heart failure or in the absence of arterial perfusion of end-stage renal disease.

Causes of Increased Resistance to Intrarenal Arterial Flow

Any increase in intrarenal arterial pressure results in decreased flow. Diastolic flow occurs at the lowest pressure during the cardiac cycle, so it will decrease or disappear before systolic Doppler flow curves are affected appreciably. The causes of increased intrarenal resistance to flow can be classified as intravascular, perivascular, and perirenal (Fig. 59-30). Any decrease in the size of the lumen of small intrarenal arteries or arterioles (spasm as in shock, or endothelial inflammation as in the hemolytic uremic syndrome (HUS)) leads to increased resistance to arterial inflow. However, compression of small vessels by intrarenal edema (e.g., renal vein thrombosis) may result in identical arterial Doppler tracings. Back pressure from an acutely obstructed ureter has the same result. Finally, significant compression from hematomas, lymphangiomas, or the tight abdominal wall around an adult kidney transplanted into a small child may have the same effect.

The successful Doppler examination of intrarenal arteries, therefore, comprises two steps:

- Comparison of the resistive index, either to the other side or to a previous examination; and
- Review of the pertinent pathophysiologic factors involved in a patient whose resistive index is high.

CAUSES OF INCREASED RI IN RENAL ARTERIES

- Intravascular
  - Vascular spasm in shock
  - Endothelial inflammation in HUS
- Perivascular
  - Intrarenal edema
    - Renal vein thrombosis
    - Acutely obstructed ureter
- Perirenal Compression
  - Hematoma
  - Lymphangioma
  - Tight abdominal wall

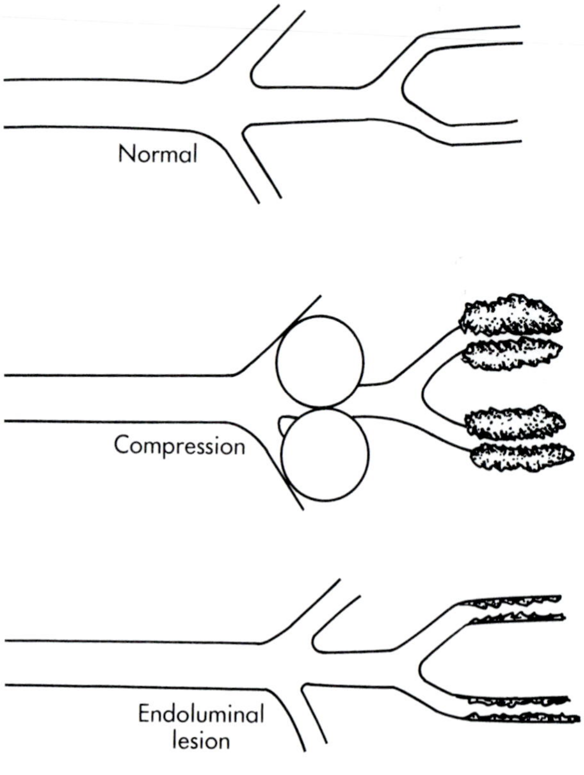

FIG. 59-30. Causes of increased resistance to intrarenal arterial flow. Diagram of intrarenal circulation.

Clinical Applications of Renal Doppler

Vessel Patency. The Doppler examination is a reliable indicator of the patency of the renal arteries, of the veins, and of the presence of intrarenal perfusion. The examination is, therefore, particularly useful in the evaluation of allograft perfusion immediately following surgery. It is also useful in the exclusion of arterial injury following trauma, especially when the renal architecture is sonographically normal and other, more invasive examinations are not indicated. Color Doppler is especially valuable in the search for postbiopsy A-V fistulas and aneurysms.[57]

Acute Renal Vein Thrombosis. Acute renal vein thrombosis may occur following shock, after the nephrotic syndrome, in abnormal coagulation, or in the presence of a nearby malignant mass such as Wilms' tumor. In the neonate it is usually associated with dehydration, decreased renal perfusion and oxygenation, and polycythemia. It is more prevalent in infants of diabetic mothers (IDM). The clinical presenta-

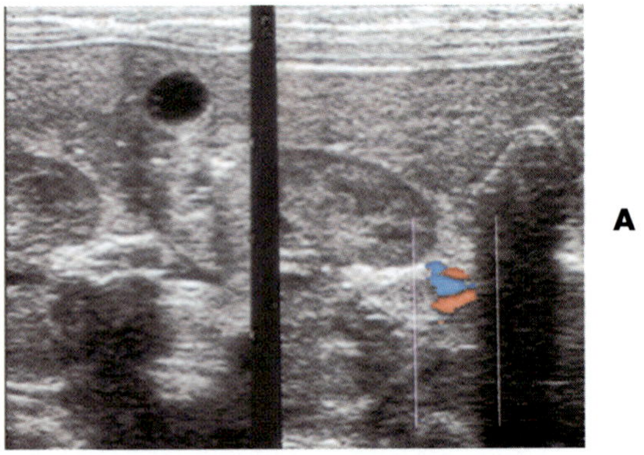

FIG. 59-31. Renal vein thrombosis. A, Supine coronal sonograms of the right renal hilum in a 12-day-old infant show a calcified thrombus dilating the renal vein, and there are color Doppler signals around the clot.

Continued.

B

C

D

E

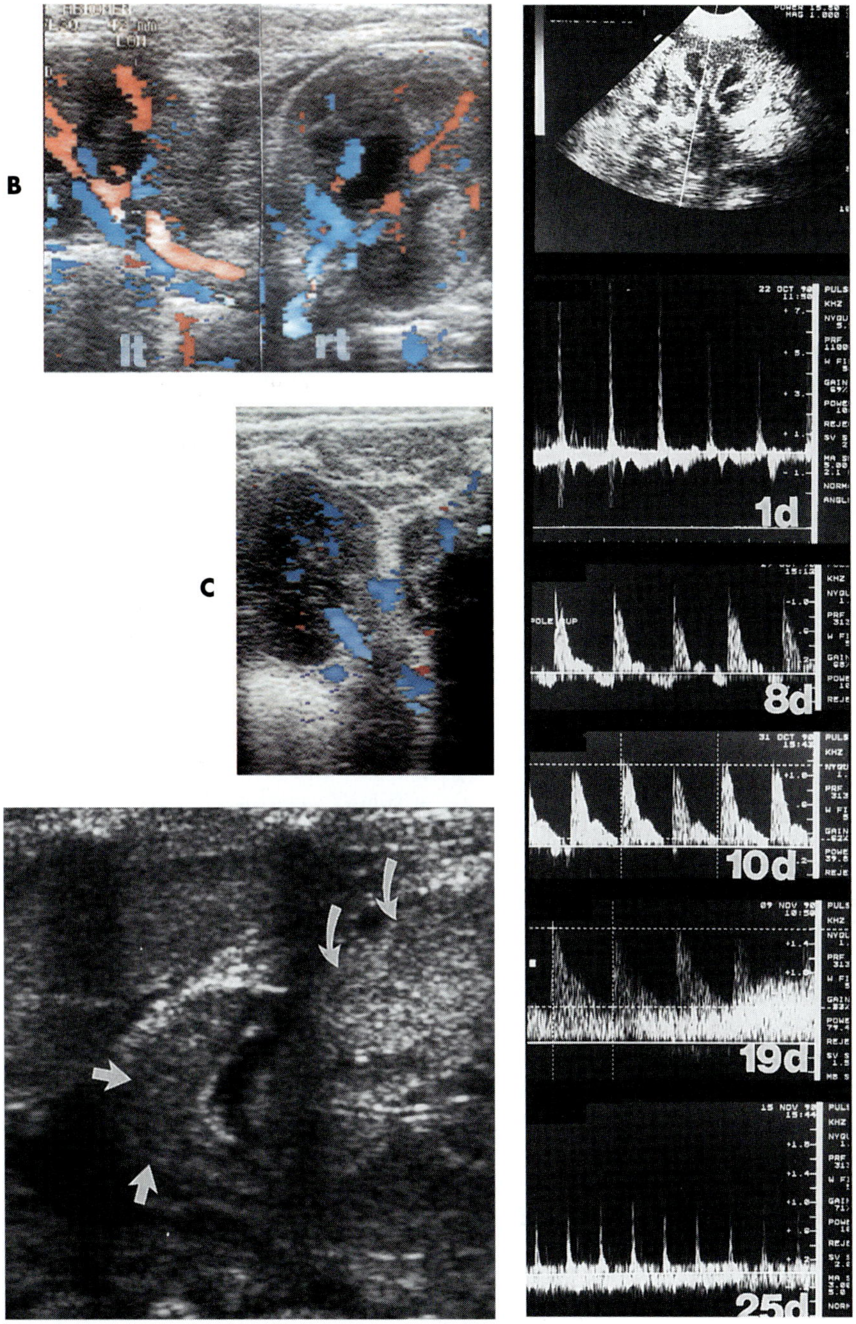

FIG. 59-31, cont'd. B, Prone coronal sonograms of the normal left (lt) and thrombosed right (rt) kidneys showing arterial and venous flow signals in both kidneys. There is venous flow around the renal vein clot at the right hilum. **C,** Left renal vein thrombosis in a 1-year-old infant (prone sonogram): Note tiny calcifications, mainly in the medulla, and numerous collateral renal veins at the hilum and near the spine. **D,** Left renal vein thrombosis associated with adrenal hemorrhage in a 2-week-old premature baby of 28 weeks' gestation. A longitudinal sonogram of the left kidney shows an enlarged hemorrhagic adrenal *(arrows)* and an echogenic edematous kidney *(curved arrows)*. **E,** Renal vein thrombosis following renal transplantation. Pulsed Doppler tracings from a segmental artery were obtained 1 day after onset of symptoms (top). In first tracing (day 1) there is pulsatile, reversed diastolic flow. Systolic peaks are narrow. Intrarenal resistance is very high. In second tracing (day 8) early orthograde diastolic flow has returned, but end diastolic flow remains reversed. Systolic peaks are less narrow. In third tracing (day 10) normal diastolic flow is seen except at end diastole, where it is still absent. In fourth tracing (day 19) there is further increase in diastolic flow. (Signals from an adjacent segmental vein are superimposed on the arterial tracing.) In last tracing (day 25) intrarenal impedance has once again increased. There is no diastolic flow, and systolic peaks are narrow. (There is a steady low-noise artifact on either side of the reference line.) Biopsy on this day showed severe, acute rejection. (From Laplante S, Patriquin HB, Robitaille P et al. Renal vein thrombosis in children: evidence of early flow recovery with Doppler US. *Radiology* 1993;189:37-42.)

CAUSES OF ACUTE RENAL VEIN THROMBOSIS

Shock
Nephrotic syndrome
Coagulopathy
Adjacent tumors, e.g. Wilms' tumor
Neonatal dehydration, especially IDM

tion includes hematuria, palpable flank mass, proteinuria, and decreased renal function. Sonography typically shows an enlarged kidney with altered parenchymal echogenicity (Fig. 59-31 on pages 1706 and 1707). The normal cortical medullary differentiation is obliterated. There are patchy areas of decreased and increased echogenicity secondary to edema and parenchymal hemorrhage.[58] Sonography may demonstrate echogenic thrombus within the renal vein and inferior vena cava. Thrombi start in small venules and propagate toward the hilum. (In the renal allograft, thrombosis usually starts at the anastomosis.)

Doppler sonography has shown decreased or absent flow in the renal veins as well as a significantly increased resistive index in the involved kidney. This decreased diastolic flow is due to edema and obstruction to outflow of arterial blood entering the kidney. In babies, these signs are far less reliable. There is **rapid reestablishment of flow in the main renal vein** as well as within intrarenal veins. Diastolic flow, although affected in the early stages of the process, is rapidly reestablished to 80% or 90% of that of the opposite kidney. There appears to be an increased number of collateral veins around the hilum of the kidney and around the vertebral column (Fig. 59-31). This reestablishment of venous flow occurs not only in native kidneys but also in renal transplants, although the process takes much longer (up to 3 weeks in the transplanted kidney).[58,59]

Renal Artery Stenosis. The main causes of the narrowing of a child's renal artery are fibromuscular hyperplasia, neurofibromatosis, and radiation arteritis (see box at top of right column). However, the renal artery ostia may be narrowed in diseases affecting the aorta, such as abdominal aortic coarctation, neurofibromatosis, and Takayasu's disease. Prior to detailed examination of the renal arteries, sonography of the abdominal aorta and of renal size and architecture is useful. The **classic signs of stenosis** include increased resistance to flow proximally (decreased or absent diastolic or even systolic flow), high velocity at the site of narrowing (> 180 cm/sec), turbulence immediately distally, and flow possibly returning to normal at some distance from the stenosis.

CAUSES OF RENAL ARTERY STENOSIS

Fibromuscular hyperplasia
Neurofibromatosis
Radiation arteritis
Coarctation of the aorta
Takayasu's disease

SIGNS OF RENAL ARTERY STENOSIS

Increased resistance to flow proximally
Decreased or absent diastolic or even systolic flow
High velocity at the site of narrowing (> 180 cm/sec)
Turbulence immediately distally
Downstream circulation showing parvus–tardus curve

Unfortunately, the renal arteries are not always entirely seen sonographically. The following renal arterial Doppler criteria have been found to suggest **significant stenosis:** flow velocity measurements exceeding 180 cm/sec and velocity ratio between renal artery and abdominal aorta of > 3.5 to 1.[54] In addition, the effects of severe arterial stenosis on the downstream circulation can be used to diagnose stenosis. These **downstream effects,** due to a loss of kinetic energy and the normal high elastic recoil of renal arteries, include:

- Decreased flow velocity;
- Dampened systolic wave; and
- Slowed acceleration of systolic upstroke.[60,61]

Because the intrarenal arteries are almost always accessible to Doppler interrogation, the secondary effects of severe (> 75%) renal arterial stenosis may well be reflected here (Fig. 59-32).[60,61] Doppler curves return to normal immediately after repair of stenosis. It must be remembered that the parvus-tardus curve (described in the downstream circulation) reflects any stenosis occurring upstream, including Takayasu's disease or coarctation of the aorta.

Intrarenal Arterial Disease. The **hemolytic-uremic syndrome,** consisting of anemia, thrombocytopenia, and acute renal failure, usually follows gastroenteritis, especially *E. coli* 0 157:H7 infection and its resultant toxins. It is a major cause of acute renal failure in children and leads to multiple glomerular thrombi and vasculitis affecting arterioles in the kidney. These lesions cause increased resistance to arterial flow of blood into the kidney. At sonography, the renal cortex is uniformly hyperechogenic, and the

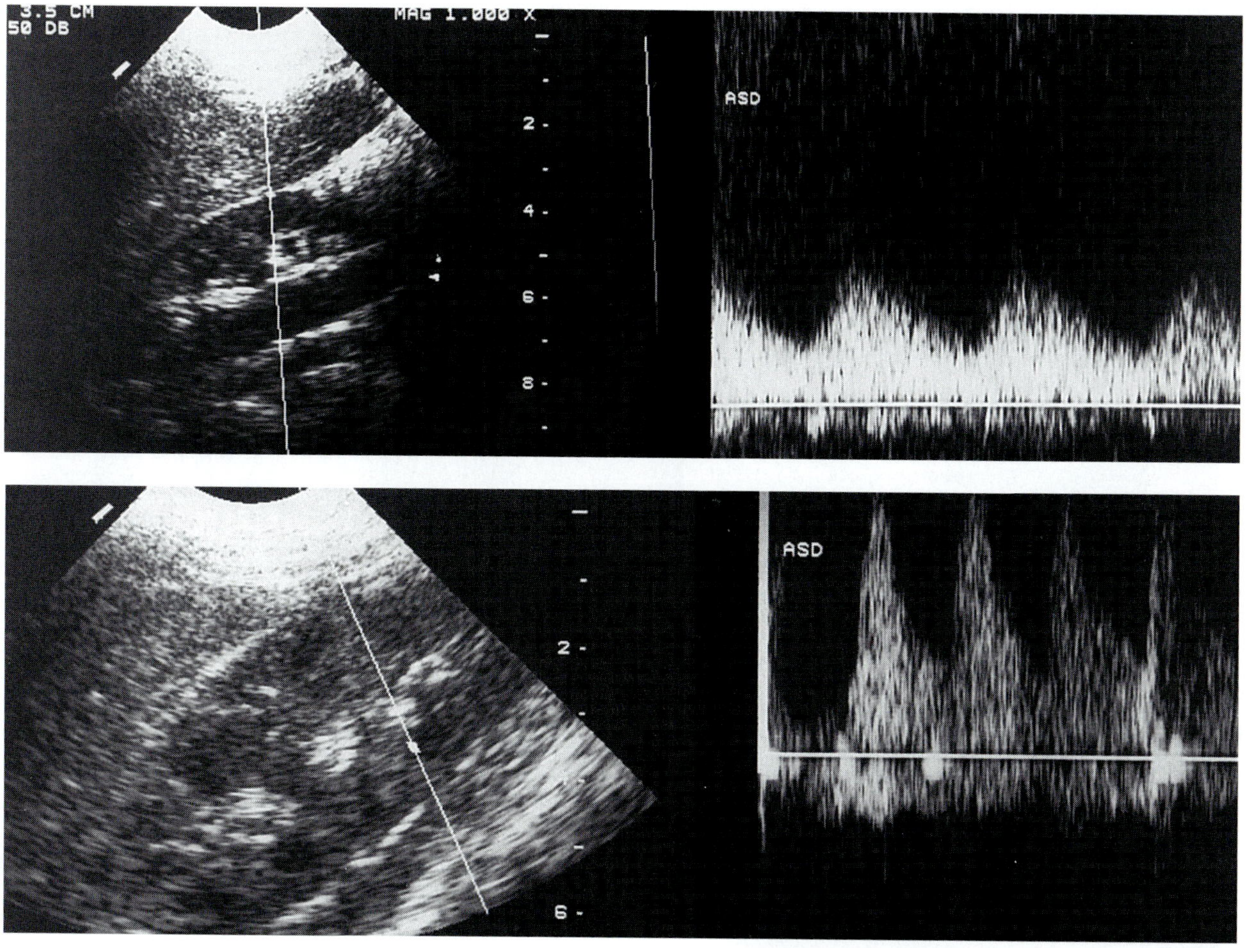

A

B

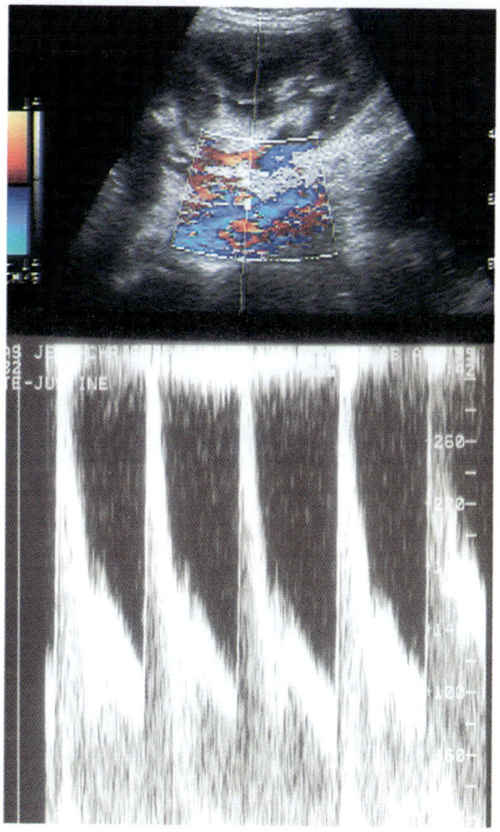

C

FIG. 59-32. Renal artery stenosis. A, Fibromuscular dysplasia with severe renal artery stenosis proven by arteriography. Segmental artery pulsed Doppler tracings of a 6-year-old hypertensive boy (blood pressure = 180/110mm Hg). There is a diagonal upsweep and a dampened systolic wave. **B, Normal** same patient, 48 hours following surgical repair of the stenosis, the waveform has returned to normal. **C, Posttransplantation renal artery stenosis with high velocity flow at the iliorenal anastomosis:** A 13-year-old boy 3 months after renal transplantation. A sagittal color Doppler image of the graft shows high velocity (yellow) turbulent flow (Doppler cursor). The spectral display shows velocity of 280 cm/sec (angle 60°). (From Patriquin HB, Lafortune M, Jequier JC et al. Stenosis of the renal artery: assessment of slowed systole in the downstream circulation with Doppler sonography. *Radiology* 1992;184:479-485.)

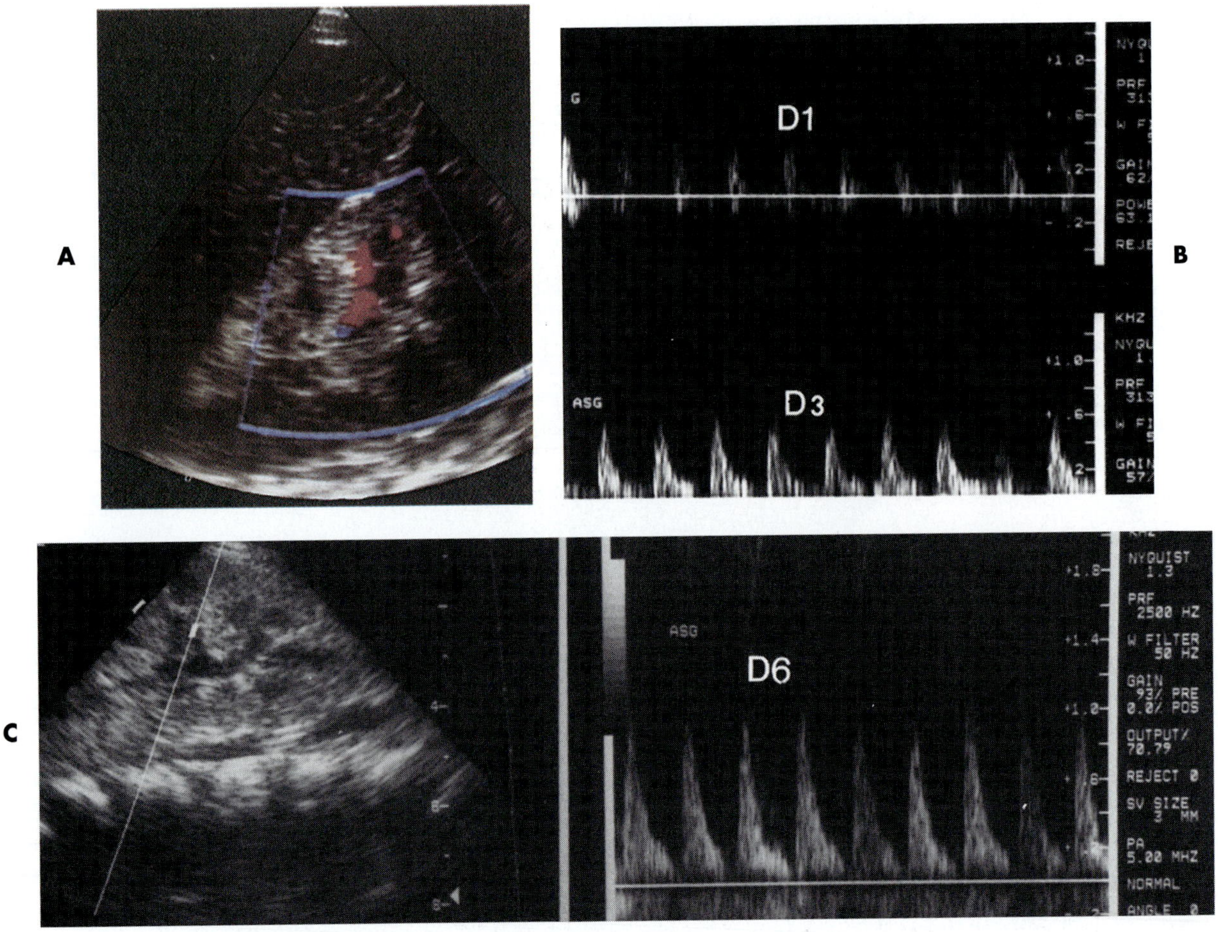

FIG. 59-33. Hemolytic uremic syndrome (2-year-old girl). **A,** Color Doppler shows patent segmental and interlobar artery *(red)* outlined against the side of a pyramid, well seen because of the intensely hyperechoic cortex. **B,** Spectral Doppler display from a segmental artery during the anuric phase. Top, day 1: systole is very short; there is no diastolic flow; the resistive index is therefore 1. Bottom, day 3: systole has lengthened and there is some diastolic flow. **C,** Spectral Doppler, day 6: diastolic flow is much improved even though end diastolic flow is not yet normal.

pyramids are sharply demarcated (Fig. 59-33). The kidneys may greatly enlarge. During a study of 20 children with hemolytic uremic syndrome, we found that during the phase of anuria there was no diastolic flow.[62] As the acute vascular lesions healed, diastolic flow returned, followed by diuresis within 24 to 48 hours. Because the Doppler examinations predicted the onset of diuresis, the duration of peritoneal dialysis was kept to a minimum, thus reducing the risk of complications.

Hydronephrosis. Not all dilated renal collecting systems in children are obstructed, and an acutely obstructed ureter can go into spasm and not dilate at all. DTPA lasix scintigraphy and the Whitaker test are being used to distinguish dilated from truly obstructed ureters, with incomplete success.

Because at this time, no single reliable distinguishing test exists, the possibilities of the Doppler examination in this field are being watched with interest, especially in pediatric urology. Acute ureteral obstruction causes immediate intrarenal vasodilatation followed several hours later by vasoconstriction. During days or weeks, this vasoconstriction lessens either because pressure is relieved by forniceal rupture or because of adaptation mediated by hormones.[63] The effect of acute vasoconstriction has been shown angiographically in animals in which ureteral ligation was followed by absence of arteriolar filling after injection of contrast material into the renal artery.[64] Platt et al.[65] have shown decreased diastolic flow, reflecting increased arterial resistance, on Doppler sonography in adults with acute ureteral obstruction. The RI measurements are best compared to the patient's own norm: the normal kidney in unilateral disease (Fig. 59-34) or a preoperative baseline examination in the case of a single kidney or a renal allograft. Keller et al.[65] have shown that the RI in the obstructed kidney of children exceeds that from the healthy side by 0.08 or more.

Increased resistance appears to be detectable only in the acutely obstructed kidney. In an ongoing study of 110 children with unilateral urinary obstruction,

A

B

C

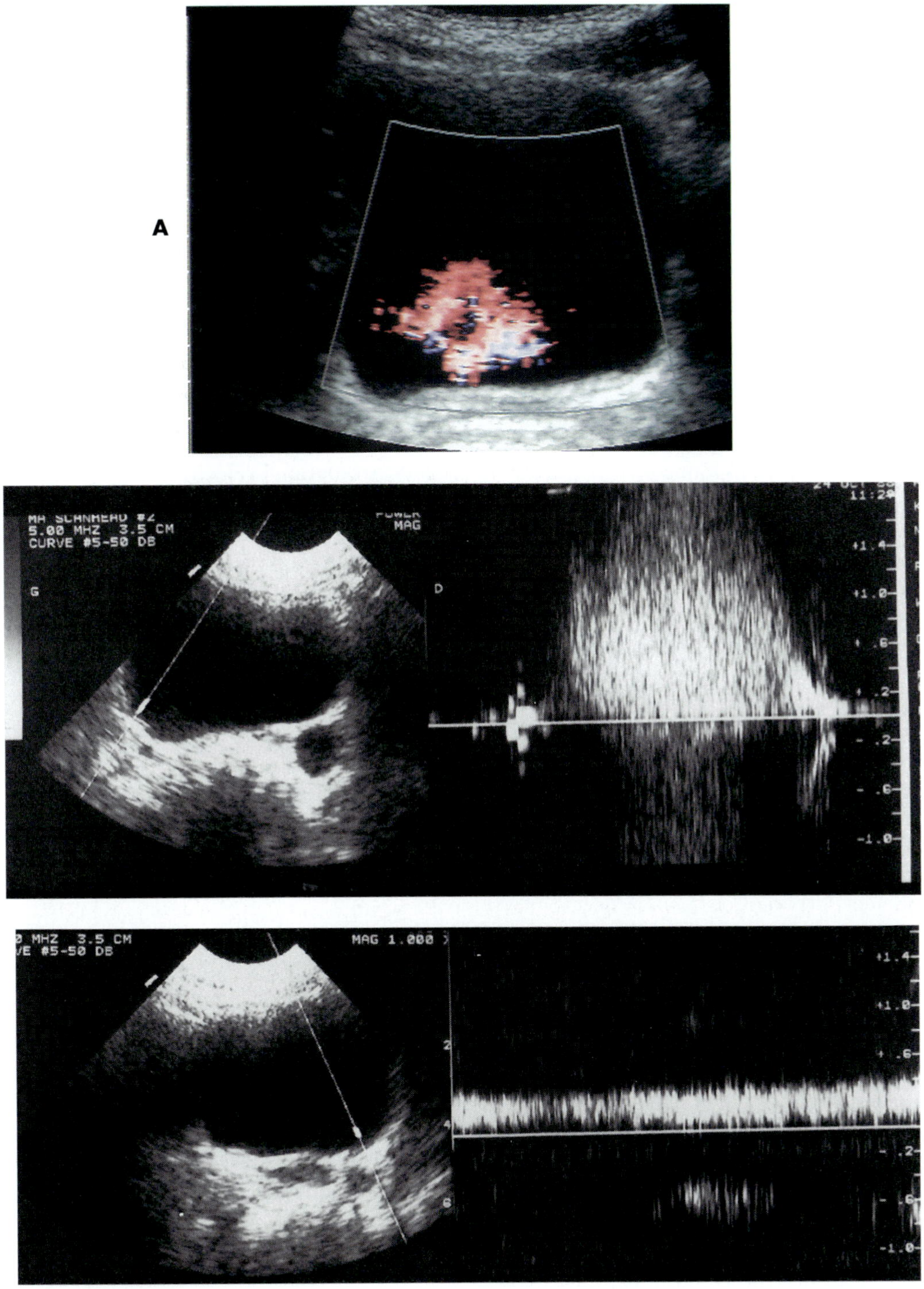

FIG. 59-34. Ureteral jets. Transverse sonogram of tne bladder base (8-year-old boy). **A,** Color Doppler aids in locating jet. **B,** Normal Bell curve jet from the normal right ureter. **C,** Bottom: constant Doppler signal from the dilated obstructed left ureter. Urine appears to be reaching the bladder in a more or less constant dribble. (From Patriquin HB, Paltiel H. *Pediatric Radiology Categorical Course Syllabus*, RSNA, 1989.)

we have found no significant alterations in the RIs from chronically obstructed kidneys such as in-utero-detected ureteropelvic junction stenosis.

Ureteral Jets. Visible at both urography and vesical sonography, these jets are easily perceptible with Doppler imaging.[66] The jet is measured within the bladder, near the ureterovesical junction, in transverse section. It has a near vertical upsweep, a short peak, and a rapid downsweep. In partial ureteral obstruction the normal jet is replaced by a slow, almost constant dribble of urine entering the bladder (Fig. 59-34). Reflux cannot be diagnosed by ureteral jet flow pattern.[12]

However, abnormally located ureteral orifices can be outlined with this method, as the more lateral the orifice, the greater the probability of vesicoureteral reflux.

Renal Transplantation

Common causes of malfunction of a renal allograft soon after operation include dehydration, obstruction of the renal artery, vein, or ureter, acute tubular necrosis, acute rejection, cyclosporine toxicity, and infection (pyelonephritis). Sonography is the screening examination of choice in the search for anatomic abnormalities. The hemodynamic information obtained with Doppler is useful in several ways. The Doppler examination is a reliable indicator of the patency of the newly anastomosed renal artery and vein, and of flow in the intrarenal (segmental, interlobar, arcuate) arteries and veins[67] as well as into postbiopsy arteriovenous shunts.[57] The renal artery and its anastomosis to the iliac artery are usually seen with real-time and Doppler ultrasound; the detection of renal artery stenosis in a graft is much easier than in the native kidney (Fig. 59-32, *C*). The renal artery is traced from the hilum to the iliac artery. The Doppler pattern changes from pandiastolic flow in the renal artery to the typical high-resistance pattern with reversed early diastolic flow in the iliac artery distal to the graft. Stenosis is signaled by a zone of high-frequency Doppler shift. The flow pattern beyond the stenosis and within the kidney may be normal or may show a pulsus parvus-tardus waveform as in Figure 59-32.

Rejection of the Renal Allograft. Histocompatibility difference between donor and recipient (unless they are monozygotic twins) leads to rejection of the renal allograft. There are two types: interstitial or cellular, mediated by T cells, and vascular or humoral, mediated by B cells. In the **interstitial type of rejection**, T cells activated by graft antigens stimulate the production of inflammatory cells which, in turn, cause cellular infiltration of the cortex, edema of the interstitium, and tubular necrosis. Inflammatory cells are found within interlobular capillaries, venules, and lymphatics, but arterioles and glomeruli are usually spared. Interstitial rejection resembles tubulointerstitial nephritis histologically. Vessel lumina are not reduced in caliber, and thus renal impedance and diastolic flow are not primarily affected. In the **vascular type of rejection** there is activation of B cells, and these produce antigraft antibodies directed against the endothelium of arterioles and capillaries. The result is swelling and inflammation of the endothelium which leads to vessel wall damage. Stasis of blood flow is greatly increased, which leads to decreased, absent, or reversed diastolic flow.[67]

Timing of Rejection. **Acute rejection** occurs mainly between week 3 and week 12 following transplantation, but may recur later. Because T or B cells must be stimulated, the rejection response usually takes a week or more to occur. **Hyperacute rejection** occurs during or within hours of transplantation and is the result of antibodies against the graft tissue that are already present in the host prior to transplantation. Hyperacute rejections are rare with modern assays for presensitization. **Accelerated rejection** occurs on days 1 through 7 in poorly matched living donor grafts. It is also caused by presensitization. Other causes of graft dysfunction in the first days or week after transplantation include acute tubular necrosis (ATN), obstructive uropathy, large perirenal fluid collections, cyclosporine toxicity, acute renal vein thrombosis, and pyelonephritis. Clinical findings in all are similar: decreasing urine output, rising

CAUSES OF RENAL TRANSPLANT DYSFUNCTION

Hyperacute rejection: hours after transplant
- Due to antibodies from presensitization

Accelerated rejection: 1 to 7 days after transplant
- Due to poorly matched donors; presensitization

Acute rejection: 3 to 12 weeks after transplant
- Due to antibodies newly formed

Graft dysfunction: 1 to 7 days
- Acute tubular necrosis (ATN)
- Obstruction of collecting system
- Large perirenal fluid collection
- Cyclosporine toxicity
- Acute renal vein thrombosis
- Pyelonephritis

Chronic rejection: months to years
- Due to repeated acute rejection

TABLE 59-1
INTRARENAL ARTERIAL RESISTANCE POSTTRANSPLANT

	RI Early	RI Late	Renal Length
Normal	↑	Baseline after 10 days	↑ slightly
ATN	↑	Baseline after 10 days	↑ slightly
Cyclosporine toxicity	No change	No change	No change
Acute rejection	↓ RI	↑ RI after 5 days	↑

serum creatinine, abdominal pain, fever, and leukocytosis. Hydronephrosis and perirenal fluid collections are easily detected with gray scale sonography.

Doppler sonography is a sensitive indicator of the increasing intrarenal impedance that accompanies acute vascular rejection; if serial measurements can be obtained by performing a baseline study shortly after operation, then the patient's RI can be compared to his own rather than to population norms (Fig. 59-35). Single measurements have been disappointing in distinguishing ATN and cyclosporine toxicity from acute rejection. Sonography is used for an initial investigation of a failing graft. The diagnosis of rejection is established by biopsy.

To assess alterations in intrarenal arterial resistance in conditions commonly encountered in the transplanted kidney, Pozniak et al.[68] studied four groups of dog allografts with pulsed Doppler: normal, ATN, cyclosporine-toxicity, and rejection (Table 59-1). In the normal and **ATN groups**, the RI rose immediately after surgery and returned to baseline levels after 10 days. Renal length also increased slightly. No significant change in RI or renal length was noted in the **cyclosporine toxicity** group. The **acute rejection group** showed an initial slight decrease in the RI and then a rapid and progressive rise in the RI after day 5. Renal length also increased steadily. This study is an elegant demonstration of the temporal changes in renal impedance in three of the most common diseases affecting the recent renal allograft. It also illustrates the difficulty in attempting to diagnose a specific disease process from a single RI or renal length measurement and emphasizes the importance of serial examinations and their correlation with clinical findings.

When acute vascular rejection is effectively treated (with cyclosporine, which prevents proliferation of T cells, or with polyclonal or monoclonal antibodies, which "blind" the T cells to graft antigens), the decrease in intrarenal resistance is dramatic and is well demonstrated with pulsed Doppler sonography (Fig. 59-35). **Chronic rejection** occurs months to years after transplantation and is the result of many episodes of unsuccessfully treated acute rejection. Chronic rejection may start as early as the first few months after transplantation and is characterized by sclerosing arteritis and tubular atrophy. The glomeruli are small or hyalinized, and there is vascular intimal proliferation, especially of interlobar and arcuate arteries. The resultant decreased diameter of small intrarenal vessels leads to increased vascular impedance and low or absent diastolic flow.

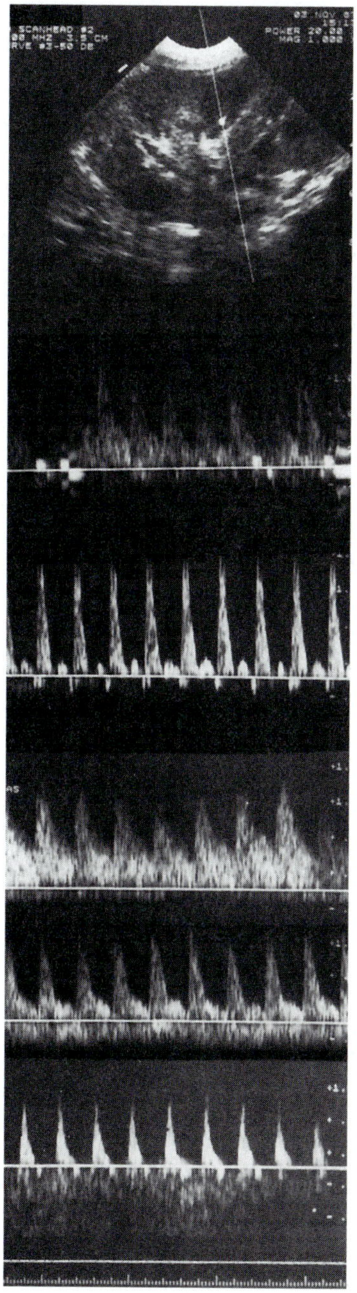

A B C D E

FIG. 59-35. Renal allograft rejection and treatment. **A,** Doppler cursor adjacent to a pyramid (within an interlobar artery) records a normal flow pattern 2 days after transplantation. **B,** One week later, normal diastolic flow has disappeared; flow reverses at the end of diastole. The serum creatinine level had risen and there was oliguria. **C,** 12 hours after completion of a course of antirejection therapy with monoclonal antibodies, normal intrarenal flow has resumed (urine flow and creatinine level had returned to nearly normal levels). **D,** Within 1 week, creatinine level rose again. Diastolic flow diminished. **E,** 2 days later, during oliguria, reversal of diastolic flow heralded another severe episode of rejection. (From Patriquin HB, Paltiel H. *Pediatric Radiology Categorical Course Syllabus,* RSNA 1989:185-196.)

PEDIATRIC ADRENAL SONOGRAPHY

Normal Anatomy

The success of sonographic visualization of the normal adrenal gland varies with the age and size of the pa-

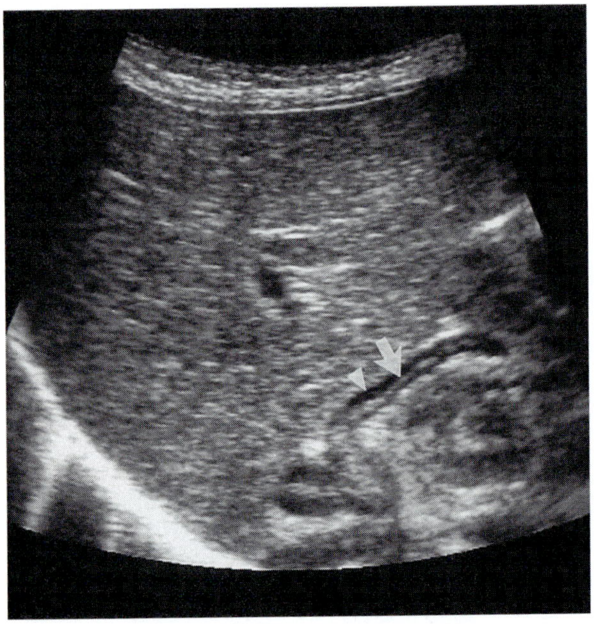

FIG. 59-36. Normal adrenal gland in the infant. Longitudinal scan of the right kidney and adrenal gland shows a Y-shaped gland with an echogenic central area *(arrow)* representing the adrenal medulla and a less echogenic peripheral rim representing the fetal adrenal cortex *(arrowhead)*.

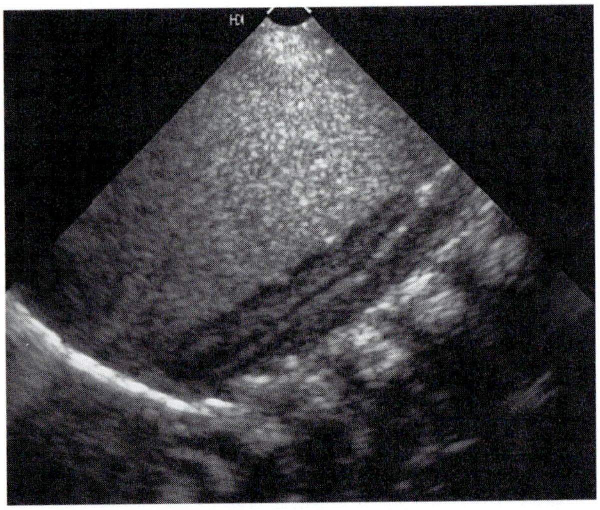

FIG. 59-37. "Lying-flat adrenal" in a newborn infant with renal agenesis. Longitudinal sonogram with only an adrenal in the right renal fossa, typical hypoechoic cortex, echogenic medulla, and a flat shape to the adrenal.

tient. In the **neonatal period** the normal adrenal gland can be readily visualized because it is relatively large, there is relatively little perirenal fat to obscure the gland, and high-frequency transducers can be used. Normal adrenal glands are readily identified in the suprarenal location and have a V-, Y-, or Z-shaped configuration (Fig. 59-36). The gland has a thin echogenic core that represents the adrenal medulla. This is surrounded by a less echogenic rim that represents the adrenal cortex.[69] In the neonate, there is a thick fetal zone that occupies about 80% of the cortex of the gland. After birth, the fetal zone of the adrenal cortex undergoes involution.

At birth, vascular congestion is present throughout the fetal zone, involution occurs by hemorrhagic necrosis, and the fetal zone gradually shrinks and is replaced by connective tissue by 1 year of age. Values for the normal size of the **adrenal gland in the infant** are available. Adrenal length ranges between 3.6 and 0.9 cm (mean = 1.5 cm)[68]; width ranges between 0.5 and 0.2 cm (mean = 0.3 cm). The mean adrenal length increases with gestational age. The adrenal gland in the older child and teenager is not easily seen by ultrasound, and other imaging modalities are preferable for its evaluation. If there is renal agenesis, the neonatal adrenal will be seen as a long linear structure (lying flat) still recognizable by the normal cortex and medulla (Fig. 59-37).

Congenital Adrenal Hyperplasia

Infants with deficiency of 21-hydroxylase, which is necessary for adrenal production of cortisol, have an excessive accumulation of androgenic precursors, with enlarged adrenal glands[70] and virilization of the genitalia in female infants. The width of the adrenal gland was enlarged in 4 of 6 patients reported by Sivit[71] (greater than 5 mm), with preservation of the normal architecture. However, a normal-sized gland does not exclude the diagnosis.

Neonatal Adrenal Hemorrhage

Hemorrhage into the adrenal gland occurs in the neonate and is associated with **stress, trauma at birth, anoxia, sepsis, bleeding disorders,** and **diabetes in the mother.** It occurs most frequently between the second and seventh day of life and presents as an abdominal mass, hyperbilirubinemia, and, occasionally, hypovolemic shock. Sometimes a hemorrhage is completely asymptomatic. If there is a palpable abdominal mass, an adrenal hemorrhage must be differentiated from a tumor of the adrenal gland or kidney. Sonography demonstrates a suprarenal mass that is variable in its echogenicity.[72,73] In the acute phase, the hemorrhage is usually echogenic, representing clot formation. Over several weeks, the hemorrhage becomes echo-free as the clot lyses and becomes liquefied (Fig. 59-38). The hemorrhage gradually decreases in size and may result in adrenal calcification. Differentiation from a neonatal neuro-

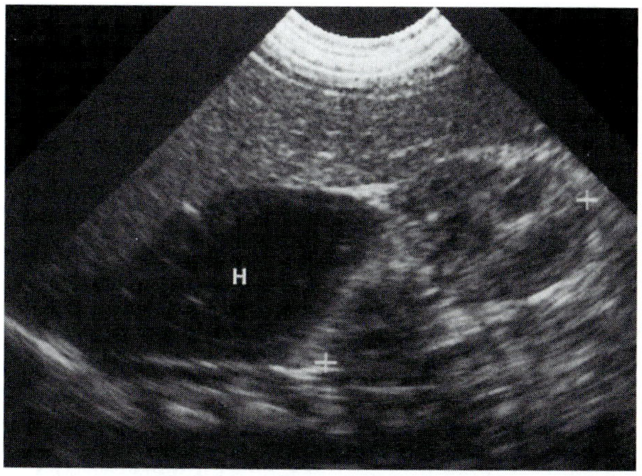

FIG. 59-38. Neonatal adrenal hemorrhage. Longitudinal scan of the right upper abdomen shows inferior displacement of the right kidney (+) by a suprarenal mass. The adrenal gland is enlarged secondary to hemorrhage with hypoechoic hematoma (H).

blastoma is important and follow-up examinations that demonstrate the mass decreasing in size and eventually resolving confirm the diagnosis of an adrenal hemorrhage.

REFERENCES

Pediatric Renal Sonography

1. Han BK, Babcock DS. Sonographic measurements and appearance of normal kidneys in children. *AJR* 1985;145: 611-616.
2. Slovis TL, Sty JR, Haller JO. *Imaging of the Pediatric Urinary Tract* Philadelphia: WB Saunders Co; 1989.
3. Patriquin H, Lefaivre J-F, Lafortune M et al. Fetal lobation: an anatomo-ultrasonographic corelation. *J Ultrasound Med* 1990; 9:191-197.
4. Rosenfield AT, Taylor KJW, Crade M et al. Anatomy and pathology of the kidney by gray scale ultrasound. *Radiology* 1978;128:737-744.
5. Hricak H, Slovis TL, Callen CW et al. Neonatal kidneys: sonographic anatomic correlation. *Radiology* 1983;147:699-702.
6. Jequier S, Rousseau O. Sonographic measurements of the normal bladder wall in children. *AJR* 1987;149:563-566.

Congenital Anomalies of the Urinary Tract

7. Mackie GG, Awange H, Stephens F. The ureteric orifice: the embryologic key to radiologic status of duplex kidneys. *J Pediatr Surg* 1975;10:473-481.
8. Schaffer RM, Shik YN, Becker JA. Sonographic identification of collecting system duplications. *J Clin Ultrasound* 1983;11: 309-312.
9. Hayden CK Jr, Swischuk LE. *Pediatric Ultrasonography*. Baltimore: Williams & Wilkins Co; 1987:263-345.

Hydronephrosis

10. Brown T, Mandell J, Lebowitz RL. Neonatal hydronephrosis in the era of sonography. *AJR* 1987;148:959-963.
11. Wood BP, Ben-Ami T, Teele RL et al. Ureterovesical obstruction and megaureter: diagnosis by real-time ultrasound. *Radiology* 1985;156:79.
12. Jequier S, Paltiel H, Lafortune M. Ureterovesical jets in infants and children: duplex and color Doppler US studies. *Radiology* 1990;175:349-353.
13. Gilsanz V, Miller JH, Reid BS. Ultrasonic characteristics of posterior urethral valves. *Radiology* 1982;145:143.
14. Silverman FN. *Caffey's Pediatric X-ray Diagnosis*. 8th ed. Chicago: Year Book Medical Pub; 1985:1885-1934.
15. Duckett JW, Caldamon AA. Bladder and urachus. In: Kelakis PP, King LR, Belman AB, eds. *Clinical Pediatric Urology*. Philadelphia: WB Saunders Co; 1985:726-751.
16. Cacciarelli AA, Kass EJ, Yang SS. Urachal remnants: sonographic demonstration in children. *Radiology* 1990;174:473-475.
17. Fernbach SK, Feinstein KA. Abnormalities of the bladder in children: imaging findings. *AJR* 1994;162:1143-1150.

Renal Cystic Disease

18. Osathanondk V, Potter EL. Pathogenesis of polycystic kidneys. *Arch Pathol* 1964;77:459-512.
19. Blyth H, Ockenden BG. Polycystic disease of the kidneys and liver presenting in childhood. *J Med Genet* 1971;8:257-284.
20. Premkumar A, Berdon WE, Levy J et al. The emergence of hepatic fibrosis and portal hypertension in infants and children with autosomal recessive polycystic kidney disease: initial and follow-up sonographic and radiographic findings. *Pediatr Radiol* 1988;18:123-129.
21. Melson GL, Shackelford GD, Cole BR et al. The spectrum of sonographic findings in infantile polycystic kidney disease with urographic correlations. *J Clin Ultrasound* 1985;13:113-119.
22. Rosenfield AT, Lipson MH, Wolf B et al. Ultrasonography and nephrotomography in the presymptomatic diagnosis of dominantly inherited (adult onset) polycystic kidney disease. *Radiology* 1980;135:423-427.
23. Kaariainen H, Jaaskelainen J, Kivisaari L et al. Dominant and recessive polycystic kidney disease in children: classification by intravenous pyelography, ultrasound, and computed tomography. *Pediatr Radiol* 1988;18:45-50.
24. Stuck KJ, Koff SA, Silver TM. Ultrasonic features of multicystic dysplastic kidney: expanded diagnostic criteria. *Radiology* 1982;143:217-221.
25. Gordon AC, Thomas DFM, Arthur RJ et al. Multicystic dysplastic kidneys: is nephrectomy still appropriate? *J Urol* 1988; 140:1231-1234.
26. Narla LD, Slovis TL, Watts FB et al. The renal lesions of tuberosclerosis (cysts and angiomyoliposis): screening with sonography and computerized tomography. *Pediatr Radiol* 1988;18:205-209.

Urinary Tract Infection

27. Lebowitz RL, Mandell J. Urinary tract infection in children: putting radiology in its place. *Radiology* 1987;165:1-9.
28. Jequier S, Forbes PA, Nogrady MB. The value of ultrasonography as a screening procedure in a first documented urinary tract infection in children. *J Ultrasound Med* 1985;4:373-400.
29. Mason WG. Urinary tract infections in children: renal ultrasound evaluation. *Radiology* 1984;153:109-111.
30. Talner LB, Davidson AJ, Lebowitz RL et al. Acute pyelonephritis: can we agree on terminology? *Radiology* 1994;192: 297.
31. Babcock DS. Sonography of wall thickening of the renal collecting system: a nonspecific finding. *J Ultrasound Med* 1987; 6:29-32.
32. Majd M, Rushton HG. Renal cortical scintigraphy in the diagnosis of acute pyelonephritis. *Sem Nucl Med* 1992;22:98-111.
33. Dacher J-N, Pfister C, Monroc M et al. Power Doppler sonographic pattern of acute pyelonephritis in children: comparison with CT. *AJR* 1996;166:1451-1455.
34. Rosenfield AT, Glickman MG, Taylor KJW et al. Acute focal bacterial nephritis (acute lobar nephronia). *Radiology* 1979; 132:553-561.
35. Cohen HL, Haller JO, Schechter S et al. The management of the infant: ultrasound evaluation. *Urol Radiol* 1986;8:17-21.

36. Robinson PJ, Pocock RD, Frank JD. The management of obstructive renal candidiasis in the neonate. *Br J Urol* 1987; 59:380-382.

Medical Renal Disease

37. Rosenfield AT, Siegel NJ. Renal parenchymal disease: histopathologic-sonographic correlation. *AJR* 1981;137:793-798.
38. Bruwer A. Primary renal calculi: Anderson-Carr-Randall progression? *AJR* 1979;132:751-758.
39. Patriquin H, Robitaille P. Renal calcium deposition in children: sonographic demonstration of the Anderson-Carr progression. *AJR* 1986;146:1253-1256.
40. Patriquin H, O'Regan S. Medullary sponge kidney in childhood. *AJR* 1985;145:315-319.
41. Patriquin H, Lafortune M, Filiatrault D. Urinary milk of calcium in children and adults: use of gravity-dependent sonography. *AJR* 1985;144:407-413.
42. Jayogapal S, Cohen HL, Brill PW et al. Calcified neonatal renal vein thrombosis demonstration by CT and US. *Pediatr Radiol* 1990;20:160-162.
43. Gilsanz V, Fernal W, Reid BS et al. Nephrolithiasis in premature infants. *Radiology* 1985;154:107-110.

Renal Trauma

44. Stalker P, Kaufman RA, Stedje K. The significance of hematuria in children after blunt abdominal trauma. *AJR* 1990; 154:569-571.
45. Furtschegger A, Egender G, Jakse G. The value of sonography in the diagnosis and follow-up of patients with blunt renal trauma. *Br J Urol* 1988;62:110-116.

Renal and Adrenal Tumors

46. Byrd RL. Wilms' tumor: medical aspects. In: Broecher BH, Klein FA, eds. *Pediatric Tumor of the Genitourinary Tract.* New York: Alan R. Liss; 1988:61-73.
47. Jaffe MH, White SJ, Silver TM et al. Wilms' tumor: ultrasonic features, pathologic correlation, and diagnostic pitfalls. *Radiology* 1981;140:147-152.
48. De Campo JF. Ultrasound of Wilms' tumor. *Pediatr Radiol* 1986;16:21-24.
49. Van Campenhout I, Patriquin H. Malignant microvasculature in abdominal tumors in children: detection with Doppler US. *Radiology* 1992;183:445-448.
50. White KS. Helical/spiral CT scanning: a pediatric radiology perspective. *Pediat Radiol* 1996;26:5-14.
51. Bousvaros A, Kirks DR, Grossman H. Imaging of neuroblastoma: an overview. *Pediatr Radiol* 1986;16:39-106.
52. Hartman DS, Sanders RC. Wilms' tumor versus neuroblastoma: usefulness of ultrasound differentiation. *J Ultrasound Med* 1982;1:117-122.
53. Hartman DS, Lesar MSL, Madewell JE et al. Mesoblastic nephroma: radiologic-pathologic correlation of 20 cases. *AJR* 1981;136:69-74.
54. McAlister WH, Seigel MJ, Askin FB et al. Multilocular renal cysts. *Urol Radiol* 1979;1:89-92.
55. Hartman DS, Davis CJ Jr, Goldman SM. Renal lymphoma: radiologic-pathologic correlation of 21 cases. *Radiology* 1982;144:759-766.
56. Heiken JP, McClennan BL, Gold RP. Renal lymphoma. *Semin Ultrasound,* CT & MR 1986;7:58-66.

Renal Vascular Diseases in Children: Assessment with Doppler Sonography

57. Hubsch PJS, Mostbeck G, Barton PP et al. Evaluation of arteriovenous fistulas and pseudoaneurysms in renal allografts following percutaneous needle biopsy. *J Ultrasound Med* 1990; 9:95-100.
58. Rosenfield AT, Zeman RK, Cronan JJ et al. Ultrasound in experimental and clinical renal vein thrombosis. *Radiology* 1980;137:735-741.
59. Laplante S, Patriquin HB, Robitaille P et al. Renal vein thrombosis in children: evidence of early flow recovery with Doppler US. *Radiology* 1993;189:37-42.
60. Stavros AT, Parker SH, Yakes WF et al. Segmental stenosis of the renal artery: pattern recognition of tardus and parvus abnormalities with duplex sonography. *Radiology* 1992;184:487.
61. Patriquin HB, Lafortune M, Jequier JC et al. Stenosis of the renal artery: assessment of slowed systole in the downstream circulation with Doppler sonography. *Radiology* 1992;184: 479-485.
62. Patriquin HB, O'Regan S. Hemolytic-uremic syndrome: intrarenal arterial Doppler patterns as a useful guide to therapy. *Radiology* 1989;172:625-628.
63. Tublin ME, Dodd GD, Verdile VP. Acute renal colic: diagnosis with duplex Doppler US. *Radiology* 1994;193:697-701.
64. Ryan PC, Maher KP, Murphy B et al. Experimental partial ureteric obstruction: pathophysiologic changes in upper tract pressures and renal blood flow. *J Urol* 1987;138:674-678.
65. Platt JF, Rubin JM, Ellis JH et al. Duplex Doppler US of the kidney: differentiation of obstructive from nonobstructive dilatation. *Radiology* 1989;171:515-517.
66. Keller MS, Korsvik HE, Piccolello ML et al. Comparison of diuretic Doppler sonography with diuretic renography in children with hydronephrosis. *Am Acad Pediatr*, San Francisco: 1992:80.
67. Taylor KJW, Morse SS, Rigsby CM et al. Vascular complications in renal allografts: detection with duplex Doppler ultrasound. *Radiology* 1987;162:31-38.
68. Pozniak MA, Kelcz F, D'Alessandro A et al. Sonography of renal transplants in dogs: the effect of acute tubular necrosis, cyclosporine nephrotoxicity, and acute rejection on resistive index and renal length. *AJR* 1992;158:791.

Pediatric Adrenal Sonography

69. Oppenheimer DA, Carroll BA, Yousem S. Sonography of the normal neonatal adrenal gland. *Radiology* 1983;146:157-160.
70. Bryan PJ, Caldamone AA, Morrison SC et al. Ultrasound findings in the adreno-genital syndrome (congenital adrenal hyperplasia). *J Ultrasound Med* 1988;7:675-679.
71. Sivit CJ, Kushner DC, Hung W. Sonography in neonatal congenital adrenal hyperplasia. *J Ultrasound Med* 1990;9:S69.
72. Mittelstaedt CA, Volberg FM, Merten D et al. The sonographic diagnosis of neonatal adrenal hemorrhage. *Radiology* 1979; 131:453-457.
73. Heij HA, Taets van Amerongen AHM, Ekkelkamp S et al. Diagnosis and management of neonatal adrenal hemorrhage. *Pediatr Radiol* 1989;19:391-394.

CHAPTER 60

The Pediatric Gastrointestinal Tract

•

Susan D. John, M.D.
Leonard E. Swischuk, M.D.

CHAPTER OUTLINE

ESOPHAGUS AND STOMACH

Normal Anatomy and Technique

Sonography has become an important diagnostic imaging modality in the observation of the gastrointestinal (GI) tract of children. Its ability to discern the various mural layers of the gastrointestinal tract has added a new dimension to the imaging of this body system. The use of ultrasound in the gastrointestinal tract continues to increase, and in the areas where it is already firmly established, refinement of both imaging and diagnosis continues.

Esophagus

Imaging of the esophagus with sonography is difficult; however, it is possible to visualize the gastroesophageal junction by examining the patient with sagittal images in the supine or right-side-down decubitus position.[1,2] This technique permits observation of function of the gastroesophageal junction and can be used to detect gastroesophageal reflux. **Reflux** is noted when fluid is regurgitated into the retrocardiac portion of the esophagus (Fig. 60-1). **Hiatal hernias** can also be detected with sonography, which may be more sensitive than barium studies for detecting small degrees of herniation, especially if color Doppler is also used.[3,4] However, the sonographic techniques required are operator-dependent and have not gained much popularity. On a practical basis, esophageal abnormalities are usually assessed with other imaging modalities or endoscopy.

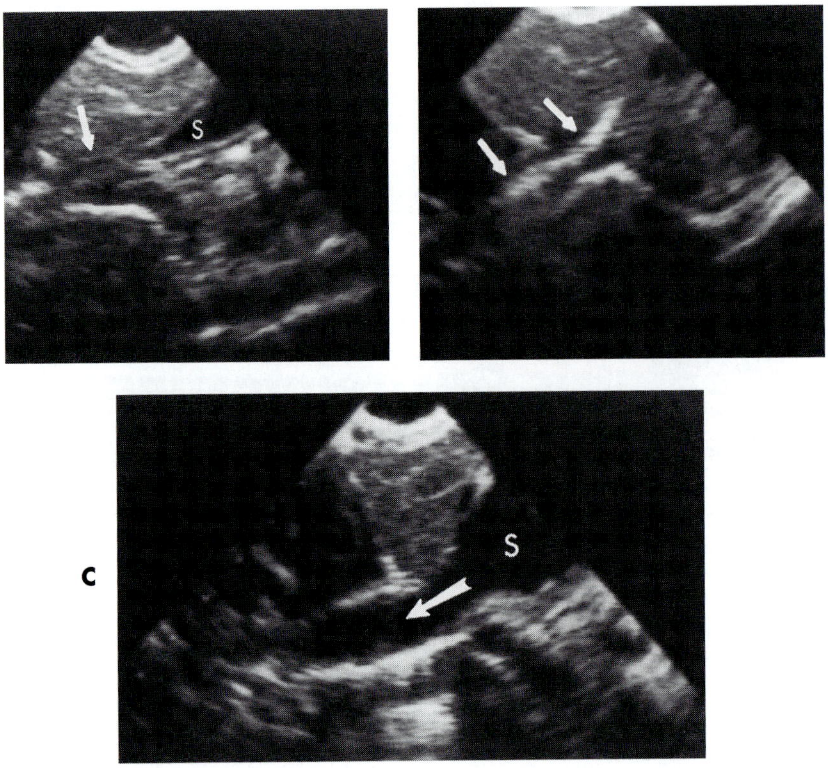

FIG. 60-1. Gastroesophageal reflux. **A,** Normal gastroesophageal junction (*arrow*); S, stomach. **B,** Gastroesophageal reflux (*arrows*). **C,** Gross gastroesophageal reflux (*arrow*). S, stomach.

STOMACH: OPTIMAL MEASUREMENTS

Normal pyloric muscle thickness ≤ 2 mm
Normal gastric mucosa thickness ≤ 2–3 mm
Peristalsis through pylorus

Stomach

Most abnormalities of the stomach in infants and children involve the gastric antrum or, at least, the distal third of the stomach. This is fortunate, for with the liver as an acoustical window, it is easy to examine this portion of the stomach.[4] The stomach should be examined after it has been distended with clear fluid (e.g., glucose water). In this way, the **gastric lumen, mucosa, muscularis mucosa, submucosa,** and **outer circular muscle layer** can be identified with clarity (Fig. 60-2). Furthermore, gastric peristalsis and emptying can be evaluated.

Normal gastric mucosa, including the muscularis mucosae and submucosal layers, measures 2 to 3 mm, whereas the outer circular muscle layer measures between 1 and 2 mm in thickness.[5,6] These measurements should be obtained with the stomach fully distended with fluid, and the scan should be performed in the midlongitudinal plane of the stomach or, on cross-section, proximal to the pyloric canal. On cross-sectional imaging, if the image obtained is too close to the contracted pyloric canal, thickening of the pyloric muscle can be suggested erroneously (Fig. 60-3, *A–C*). Similarly if tangential images are obtained on the longitudinal plane, the muscle may erroneously appear thickened (Fig. 60-3, *D–F*). Such **imaging pitfalls,** in our opinion, are the major factors leading to the **incorrect concept that normal muscle can measure up to 3 mm in thickness.**[7] This same phenomenon is also seen with the echogenic mucosal layer.

Hypertrophic Pyloric Stenosis

During the past decade, sonography has almost completely replaced the radiographic upper gastrointestinal series for the diagnosis of infantile hypertrophic pyloric stenosis (HPS). The diagnosis of this condition has been greatly improved by ultrasound because, although the upper GI series demonstrates secondary antral deformity, the ultrasound study unequivocally delineates the gastric muscle thickening that is the hallmark of the disease. Although a few pitfalls in the sonographic diagnosis of hypertrophic pyloric stenosis exist, the technique is relatively easily mastered and results in greatly

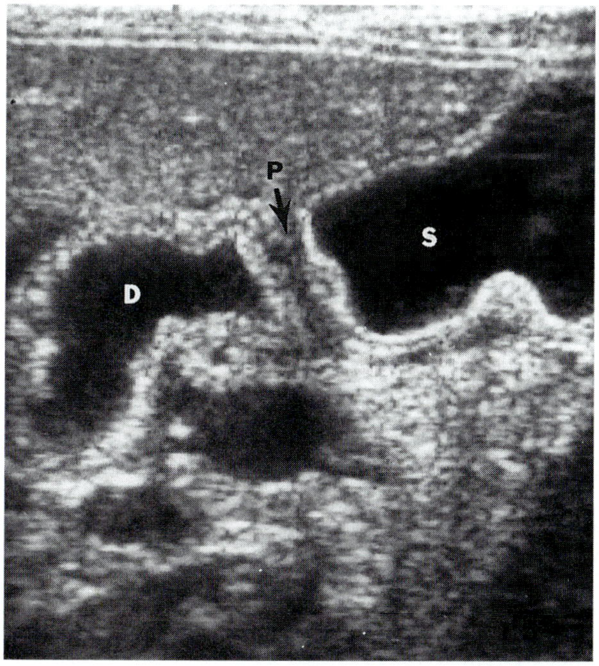

FIG. 60-2. Normal stomach. Normal antrum of stomach (S), pyloric canal (P), and proximal duodenum (D). Four gastric wall layers are visible (from inside out): echogenic mucosa, hypoechoic muscularis mucosae, echogenic submucosa, and hypoechoic outer circular muscle.

HYPERTROPHIC PYLORIC STENOSIS (HPS)

Muscle width ≥ 3 mm
Pyloric canal length ≥ 1.2 cm
No peristalsis through pylorus

improved accuracy of diagnosis of this condition.[7] Indeed, the accuracy approaches 100%[8-10] and ultrasonography is now the procedure of choice for the detection of pyloric stenosis.

After the initial documentation of the sonographic detection of the hypertrophied pyloric muscle in pyloric stenosis by Teele and Smith,[11] a plethora of articles ensued[5,6,12-18] describing the characteristic findings of this condition. Increased pyloric muscle thickness and canal length, increased transverse diameter of the pylorus, estimation of degree of gastric outlet obstruction, and calculation of pyloric muscle volume have all been used to diagnose pyloric stenosis, but of these criteria, thickening of the pyloric muscle and elongation of the pyloric canal have emerged as the most useful. Blumhagen[12] originally used 4 mm as the thickness diagnostic of hypertrophic pyloric stenosis, but more recent studies have suggested 3 mm as the cut-off point for the abnormal muscle thickness.[19] Pyloric canal length of 1.5 cm was originally considered diagnostic of pyloric stenosis when considered in conjunction with thickened pyloric muscle. In practice, however, normal canal length is much shorter than this and is often impossible to measure. Measurement of canal length is more difficult than is measurement of muscle thickness, and in many cases it is not performed because subjective observation of the enlarged muscle mass usually suffices. In borderline cases in which muscle thickness and canal length are less than classic, calculation of the pyloric volume may be helpful.[20]

In the classic case of **hypertrophic pyloric stenosis**, the thickened muscle mass is seen as a hypoechoic layer just superficial to the more echogenic mucosal layer of the pyloric canal (Fig. 60-4, *A*). In cross-section, this "**olive**," on clinical palpation, resembles a **sonolucent "doughnut"** medial to the gallbladder and anterior to the right kidney (Fig. 60-4, *B*). Often, small amounts of fluid can be seen to be trapped between the echogenic mucosal folds, corresponding to the "**string**" (elongated canal) and "**double-tract**" (folded mucosa) signs seen on radiographic upper GI series.[14] In longitudinal section, sonography also permits evaluation of functional alterations at the pylorus. Active gastric peristalsis that ends abruptly at the margin of the hypertrophied muscle along with the absence of a normal opening of the pylorus, with diminished passage of fluid from the stomach into the duodenum, are useful adjunctive findings in pyloric stenosis.

Ultrasound also is extremely useful for the evaluation of persistent vomiting in the postoperative patient.[21] The radiographic upper GI series is of limited value in such cases because it tends to show persistent deformity and narrowing of the canal even in asymptomatic patients. Sonography, however, can definitively identify persistently thickened muscle. After successful pyloromyotomy, the muscle mass should gradually regress, and by 6 to 8 weeks the muscle thickness should return to normal.[22]

Pylorospasm and Minimal Muscular Hypertrophy

In some vomiting infants, sonography shows a persistently contracted and elongated canal, but the degree of muscular thickening is below the criterion of 3 mm for surgically correctible hypertrophic pyloric stenosis. With prolonged observation, it is possible to see that eventually the canal opens and fluid passes into the duodenum, but the periods of spasm predominate. In the vast majority of cases, there is no thickening of the

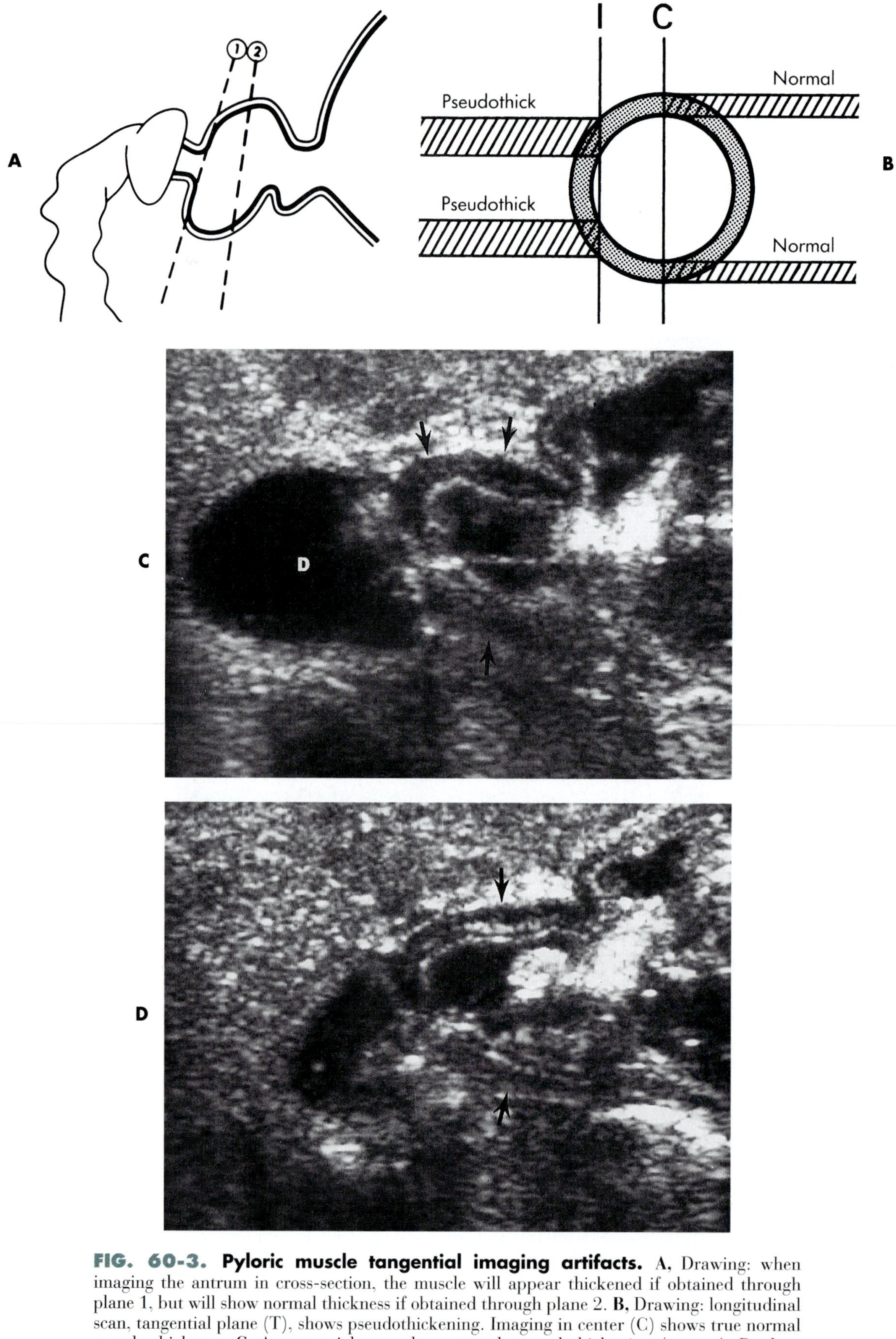

FIG. 60-3. Pyloric muscle tangential imaging artifacts. **A,** Drawing: when imaging the antrum in cross-section, the muscle will appear thickened if obtained through plane 1, but will show normal thickness if obtained through plane 2. **B,** Drawing: longitudinal scan, tangential plane (T), shows pseudothickening. Imaging in center (C) shows true normal muscle thickness. **C,** A tangential scan shows muscle pseudothickening (*arrows*). D, duodenum. **D,** Antrum distended with fluid shows normal muscle (*arrows*).

A

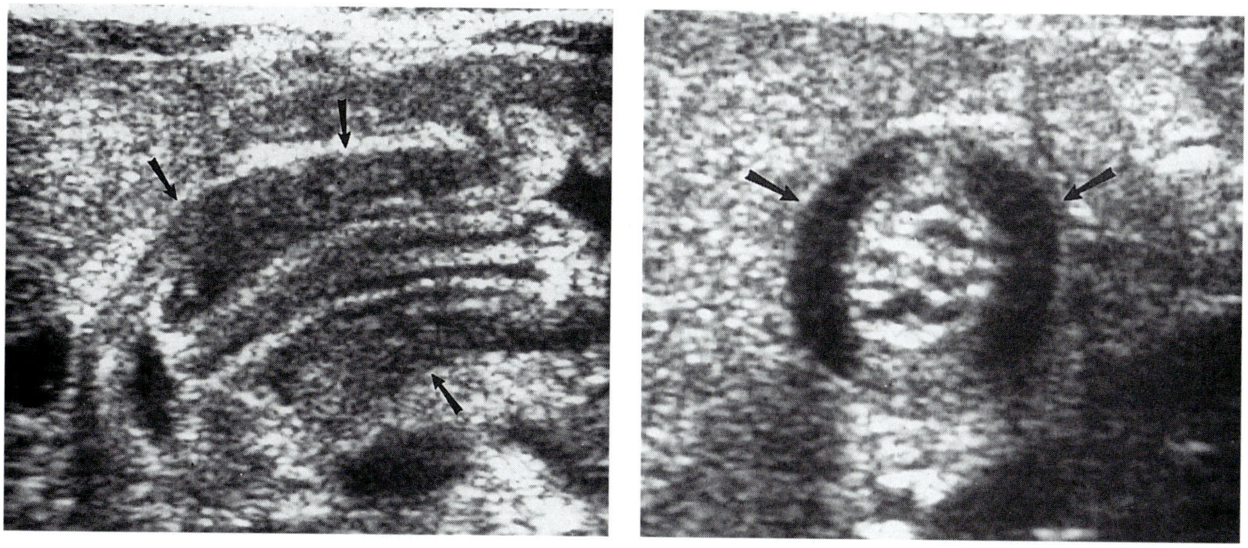

B

FIG. 60-4. Hypertrophic pyloric stenosis. **A,** Longitudinal scan shows markedly thickened, hypoechoic gastric antral muscle (*arrows*). Elongated canal is nearly 2 cm in length. **B,** Transverse scan shows typical hypoechoic doughnut (*arrows*). Central echogenic mucosa with anechoic fluid-filled crevices.

A

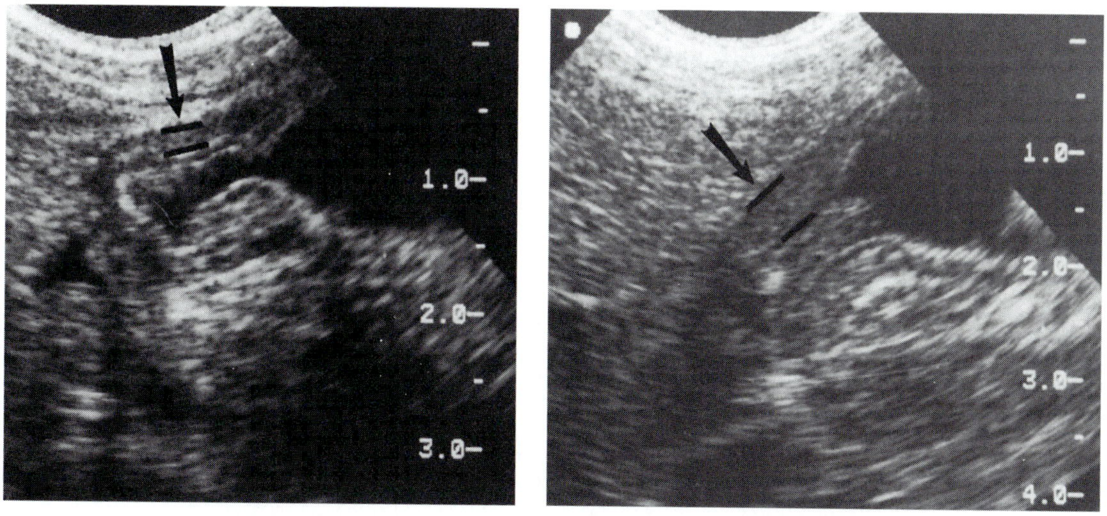

B

FIG. 60-5. Early pyloric stenosis: minimal muscle thickening. **A,** Longitudinal scan of pyloric muscle (*arrow*) is under 3 mm. **B,** One week later, the muscle measures 5 mm (*arrow*).

pyloric muscle or mucosa and the problem is primarily one of nonspecific **pylorospasm (antral dyskinesia).** This condition can sometimes accompany milk allergy or other forms of gastritis.

In some cases, the pyloric muscle will be mildly thickened, measuring 2 to 3 mm.[19] Such patients should be distinguished from those with normal muscle thickness (less than 2 mm) because some patients with minimal muscle hypertrophy can eventually progress to classic pyloric stenosis (Fig. 60-5). However, many, if not most, of these infants will respond to medical therapy (e.g., metoclopramide) and, therefore, such therapy is probably worthwhile when borderline muscular thickening is encountered (Fig. 60-6). In other infants, minimal muscle thickening will resolve spontaneously, but such patients should be followed closely with ultrasound until the muscle regresses to a normal thickness.

A

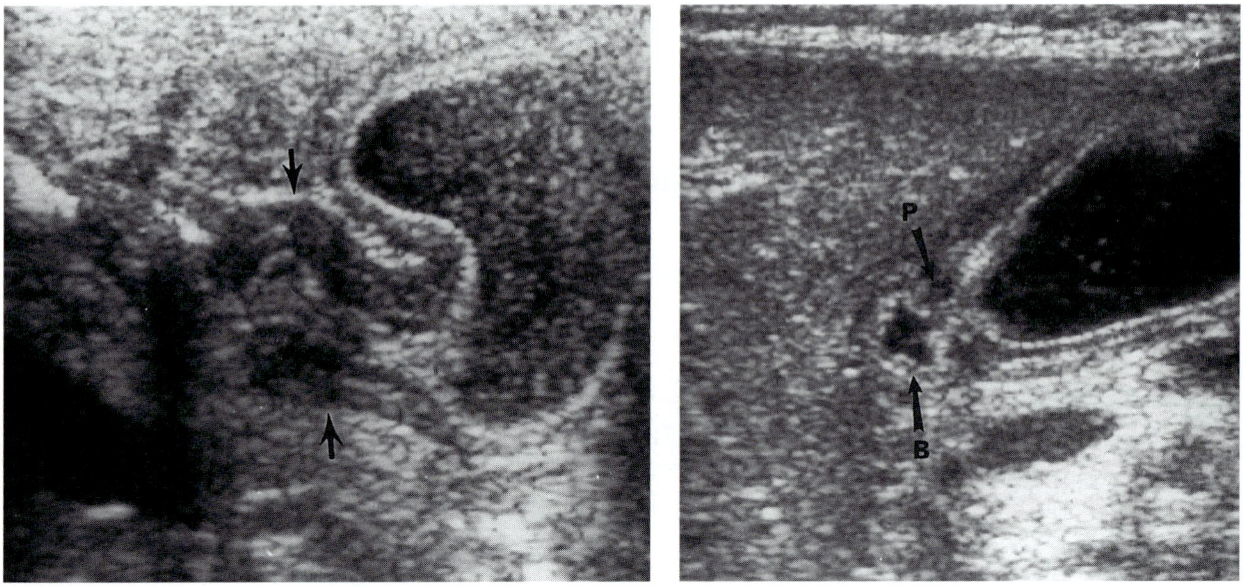

B

FIG. 60-6. Minimal pyloric muscle thickening treated with medical therapy. **A,** Longitudinal scan shows contracted pyloric canal and 2-mm-thick gastric muscle (*arrows*). **B,** After medical therapy, the pyloric muscle returned to a normal thickness. P, pylorus. B, duodenal bulb.

PITFALLS IN HPS DIAGNOSIS

- Echogenic muscle at 90° to beam (anisotropic effect)
- Posteriorly oriented antropyloric canal (overdistended stomach)
- Prostaglandin-induced HPS (mucosal, not muscular thickening)

Pitfalls in the Sonographic Diagnosis of Hypertrophic Pyloric Stenosis

One of the most common pitfalls in the sonography of hypertrophic pyloric stenosis is the absence of the classic sonolucency of the hypertrophied muscle when imaged in the midlongitudinal plane. This alteration of echogenicity is due to an artifact called the **anisotropic effect**[23] which occurs at approximately the **6- and 12-o'clock positions** of the muscle, where the ultrasound beam is perpendicular to the muscle fibers. The artifact, because it results in echogenicity, decreases the visibility of the hypertrophied muscle on the longitudinal plane but is not a significant problem in cross-section (Fig. 60-7). The other major imaging pitfall occurs when the **antropyloric canal is posteriorly directed.** This is most apt to occur when the stomach is overdistended, and a clue to the presence of pyloric stenosis is a squared-off configuration of the gastric antrum (Fig. 60-8, *B*). In such cases, one may be able to locate the pylorus by cephalad angulation of the transducer or by imaging from a more lateral position on the abdomen (Fig. 60-8). If these maneuvers fail, it may be necessary to aspirate some of the fluid from the stomach, allowing the antropyloric canal to rotate back to a more easily accessible position. Despite these occasional pitfalls, the sonographic diagnosis of pyloric stenosis is rather straightforward.

Gastric Diaphragm

The **gastric diaphragm**, or **web**, consists of a congenital membrane that extends across the gastric antrum. These diaphragms most often lie less than 2 cm from the pylorus and are, therefore, quite accessible through ultrasound examination.[24] Complete diaphragms are considered one form of gastric atresia, but many diaphragms are incomplete and cause variable degrees of obstruction. On sonography, the web appears as an echogenic band across the distal gastric antrum (Fig. 60-9, *A*). Care must be taken to image such webs in the true midlongitudinal plane, for if an incomplete diaphragm is imaged at its periphery, a complete diaphragm may be erroneously suggested (Fig. 60-9, *B*).

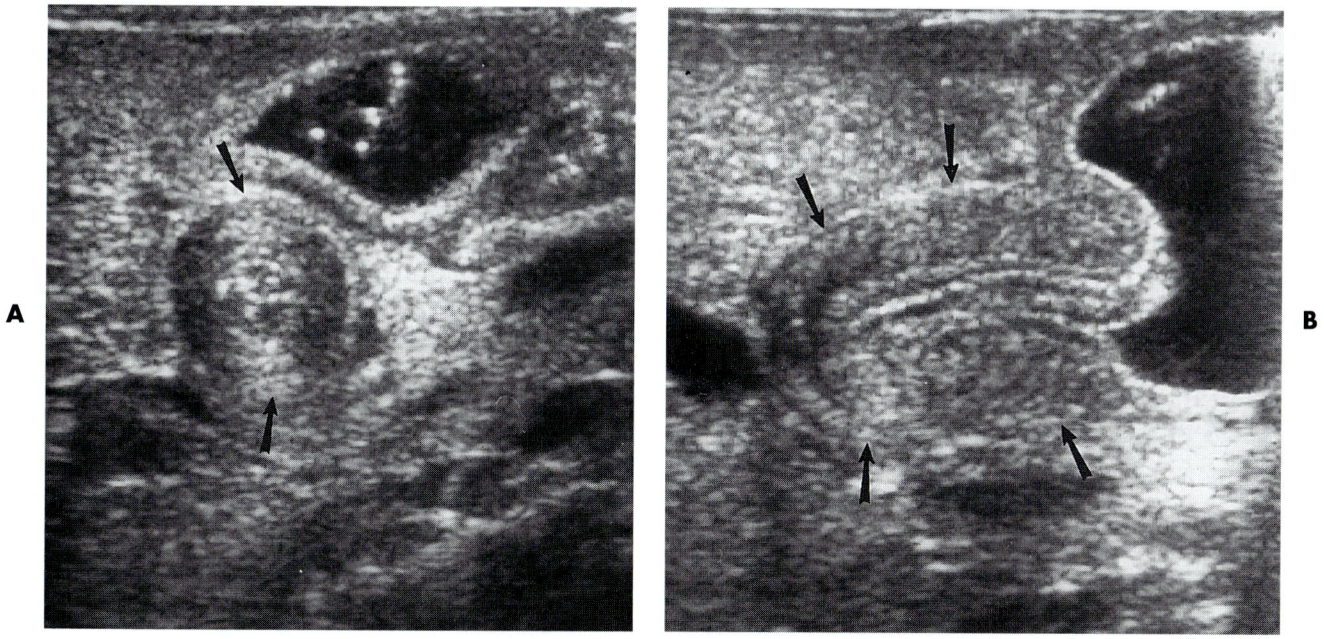

FIG. 60-7. Hypertrophic pyloric stenosis: echogenicity artifact at 6- and 12-o'clock positions (anisotropic effect). **A,** Cross-sectional image through the pylorus shows the thickened muscle with increased echogenicity at 6- and 12-o'clock positions (*arrows*). **B,** Longitudinal section taken through the midline clearly shows the elongated canal; however, the anisotropic effect causes the muscle to be echogenic (*arrows*), making it more difficult to discern.

Gastritis and Ulcer Disease

Peptic ulcer disease in pediatric patients is probably more common than generally is appreciated,[25,26] and in the newborn and young infant, the stomach is more commonly involved than is the duodenum. Barium radiographic studies often reveal nothing more than persistent deformity or spasm of the antropyloric region. However, sonography of the fluid-filled stomach in these patients permits direct visualization of the thickened gastric mucosa and submucosa,[27] which often is accompanied by loss of definition of the individual layers of the gastric wall (Fig. 60-10). The ulcer crater itself is not commonly visualized sonographically. Ultrasound can also be used to follow therapy, showing a return of the normal gastric wall layers as the ulcer heals (Fig. 60-11). Thickening of the gastric mucosa is by no means a specific finding; it can be seen with other conditions, such as **eosinophilic gastritis, inflammatory pseudotumor,**[28] **chronic granulomatous disease, Ménétrier's disease,**[29] **milk allergy,** and **prostaglandin-induced antral foveolar hyperplasia.**[30,31]

Bezoar

Lactobezoars are the most common form of bezoar in children, occurring predominantly in infants who are fed improperly reconstituted powdered formula. In older children, trichobezoars are more common; they are caused by the ingestion of hair. Both types of bezoars can be easily identified with ultrasound, especially if the patient is given clear fluid to help outline the mass. **Lactobezoars** appear as a solid, heterogeneous, echogenic intraluminal mass.[32] With **trichobezoars,** air tends to be trapped in and around the hair fibers, which causes a characteristic arc of echogenicity that obscures the mass but conforms to the shape of the distended stomach.[33]

DUODENUM AND SMALL BOWEL

Normal Anatomy and Technique

Normally, intestinal gas interferes with the use of sonography to examine the duodenum and small bowel. However, if the stomach is filled with fluid, it is often possible to identify the duodenal bulb and descending duodenum (see Fig. 60-2). In addition, as the abdomen is scanned, fleeting images of loops of normal fluid-filled intestine can sometimes be identified. The mucosa, submucosa, and muscular layers can be delineated,[34] particularly in more superficial loops that are accessible with higher frequency linear transducers (Fig. 60-12).

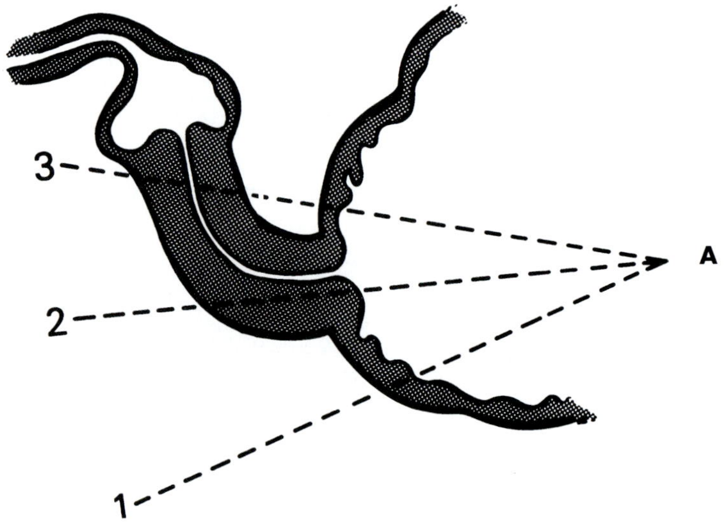

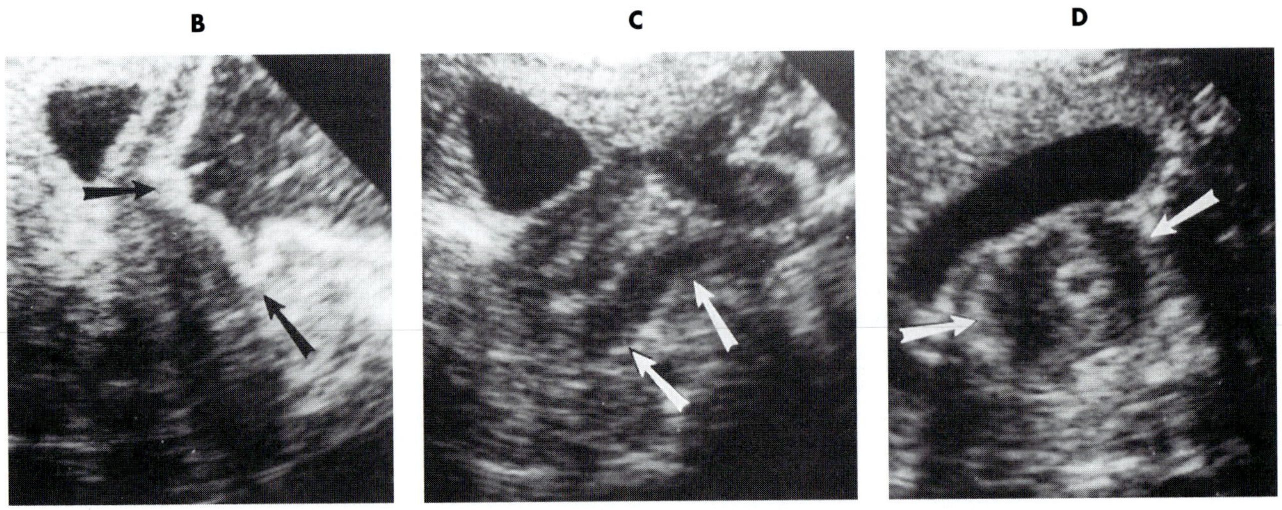

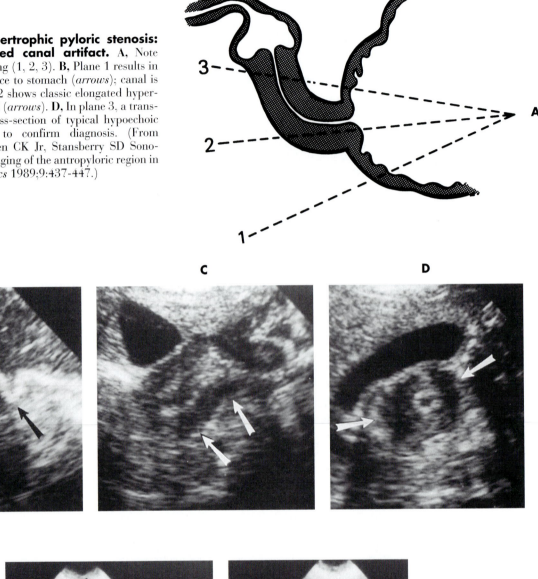

FIG. 60-8. Hypertrophic pyloric stenosis: posteriorly directed canal artifact. **A,** Note three planes of imaging (1, 2, 3). **B,** Plane 1 results in squared-off appearance to stomach (*arrows*); canal is not visible. **C,** Plane 2 shows classic elongated hypertrophied pyloric canal (*arrows*). **D,** In plane 3, a transverse scan shows cross-section of typical hypoechoic doughnut (*arrows*) to confirm diagnosis. (From Swischuk LE, Hayden CK Jr, Stansberry SD Sonographic pitfalls in imaging of the antropyloric region in infants. *RadioGraphics* 1989;9:437-447.)

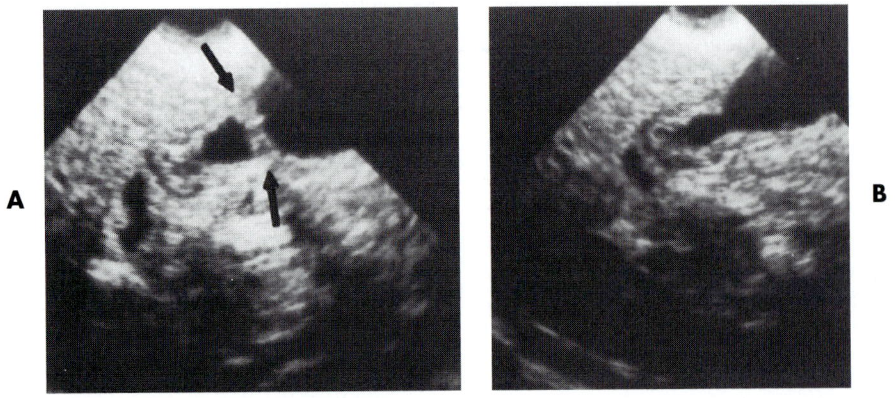

FIG. 60-9. Gastric diaphragm. **A,** Pitfall: apparent diaphragm scanned to side of pyloric canal caused the diaphragm to appear complete. **B,** Midline image shows diaphragm is partial and nonobstructing.

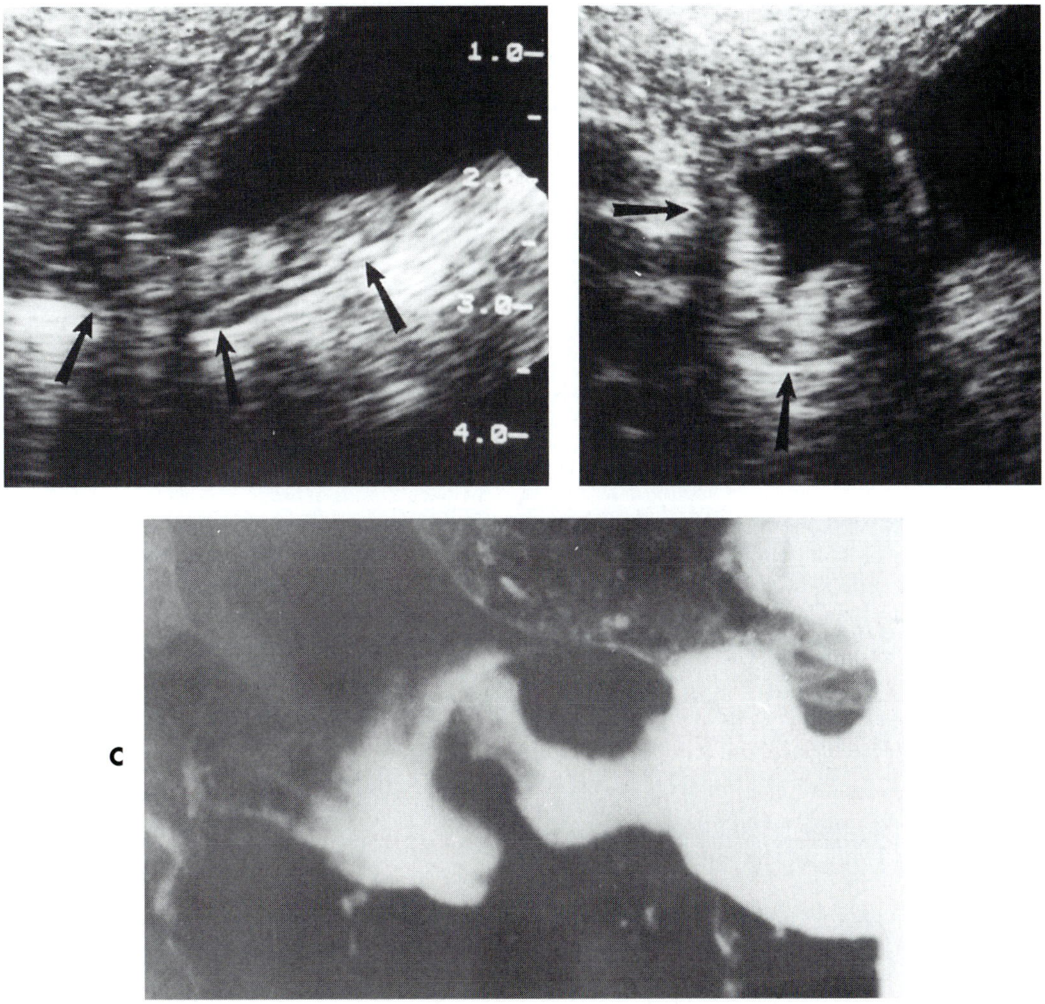

FIG. 60-10. Gastric ulcer disease. **A**, Longitudinal scan. Markedly thickened mucosa with disrupted and indistinguishable mural layers (*arrows*). **B**, Transverse scan shows focal wall thickening (*arrows*). **C**, Radiographic upper gastrointestinal series shows marked antral deformity.

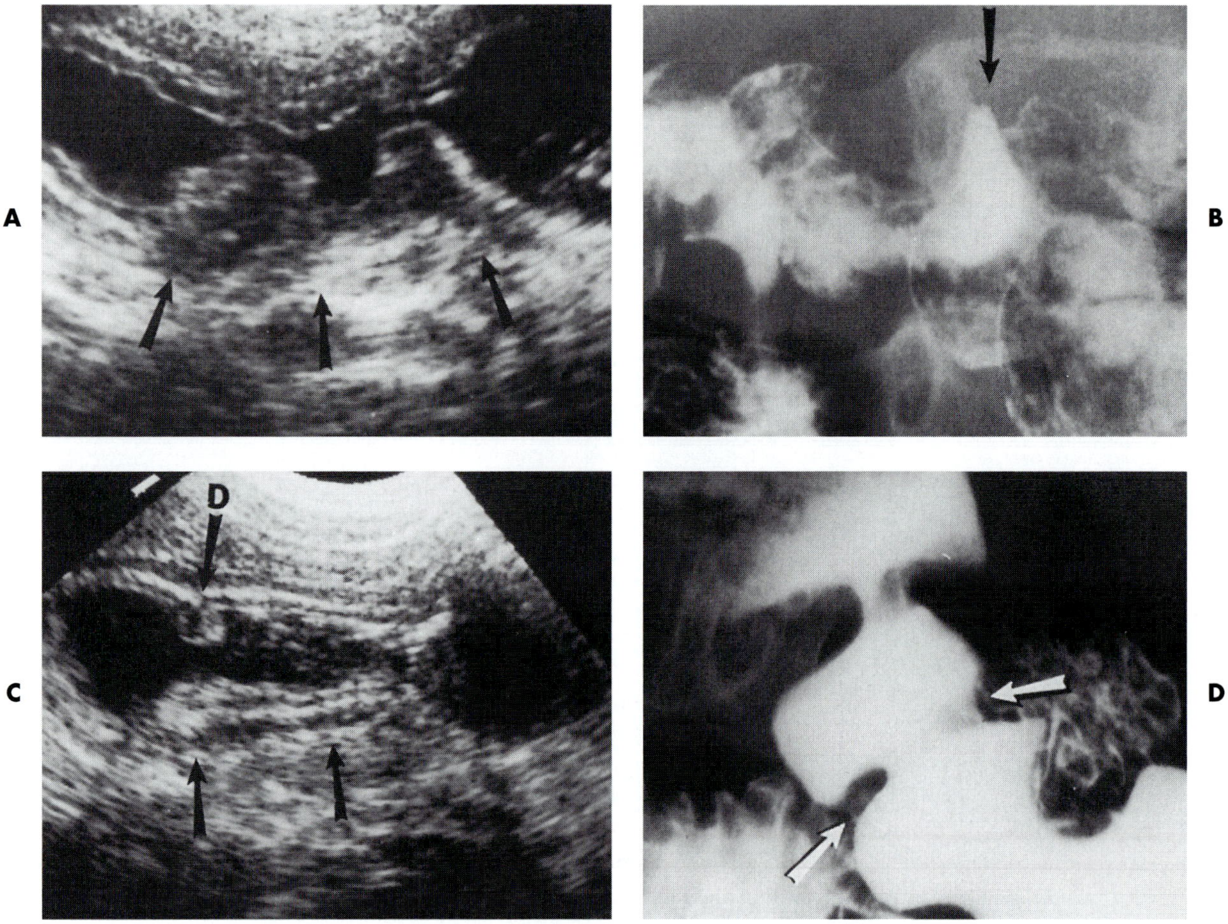

FIG. 60-11. Gastric ulcer disease. **A,** Longitudinal ultrasound image of antrum. Note markedly thickened gastric wall with poorly defined mural layers (*arrows*). An ulcer crater is suggested. **B,** Contrast study shows a large gastric ulcer (*arrow*). **C,** After medical therapy, only minimal antral wall thickening remains (*arrows*). An acquired, partial antral diaphragm has developed in the area (D). **D,** Contrast study shows the diaphragm (*arrows*).

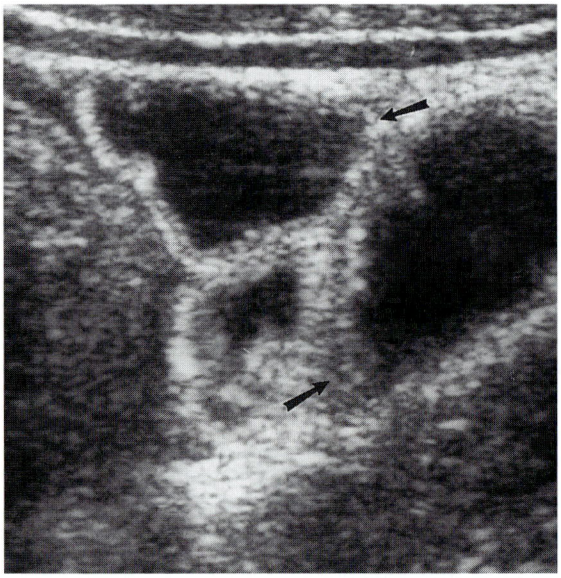

FIG. 60-12. Normal small bowel. Note the thin-walled, fluid-distended loops (*arrows*).

Congenital Duodenal Obstruction

Sonography can readily identify an obstructed, fluid-filled, distended duodenum, and frequently the level of obstruction can be determined. Of course, preliminary radiographs should always be obtained and, if the diagnosis is clearly apparent from the study, sonography can be omitted. However, radiographic findings are often nonspecific, and in such cases, ultrasound can be quite useful.

Proximal duodenal obstruction resulting in the classic **double-bubble sign** occurs with **duodenal atresia,** with or without associated annular pancreas (Fig. 60-13). Plain radiograph findings usually are diagnostic, showing two air-filled bubbles representing the dilated stomach and proximal duodenum. Similar findings can be seen with **severe duodenal stenosis** and **duodenal diaphragms** or webs, but in general sonography is not needed to identify obstructions in this portion of the duodenum. However, when **duodenal atresia is associated with esophageal**

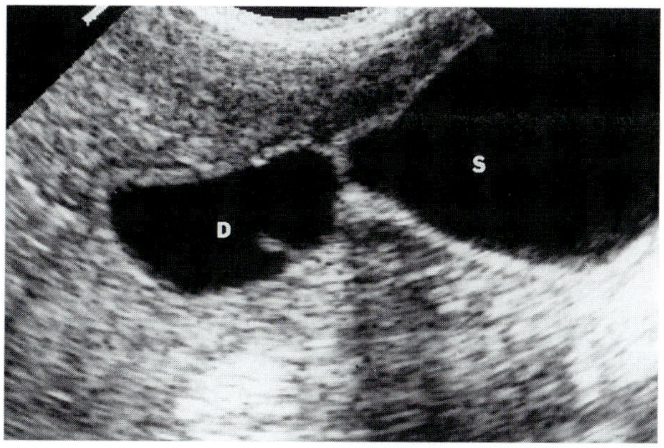

FIG. 60-13. Duodenal atresia. Note the grossly distended duodenal bulb (D) and stomach (S).

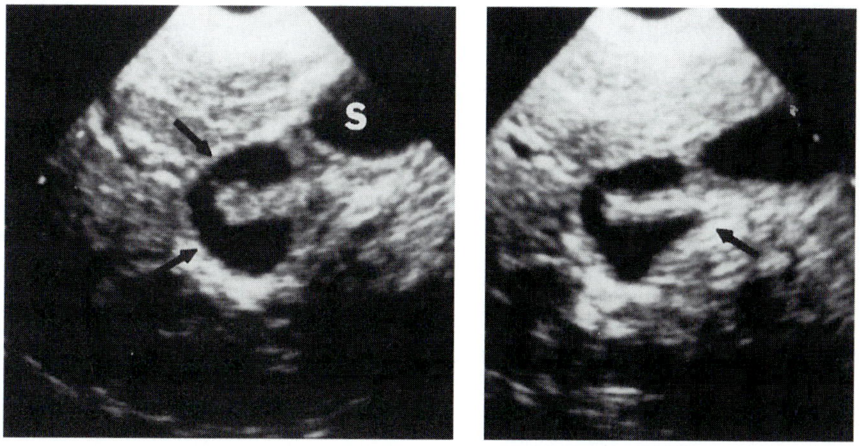

FIG. 60-14. Midgut volvulus. **A,** Distended duodenal C-loop (*arrows*). S, stomach. **B,** Vigorous peristaltic activity fails to empty duodenum, and the third portion of the duodenum has beak deformity (*arrow*).

atresia, air cannot reach the stomach and duodenum, making radiographic diagnosis more difficult. Sonography is diagnostic in such infants by demonstrating the grossly distended, fluid-filled duodenal bulb, stomach, and distal esophagus.[35-38]

Sonography can also be used to diagnose **intestinal malrotation with midgut volvulus** in an infant with bilious vomiting, although it has not yet replaced the radiographic upper gastrointestinal series for this purpose. With volvulus, vigorous peristalsis of the obstructed duodenal C-loop is seen, and often characteristic tapering of the distal, twisted end can be visualized (Fig. 60-14).[39] Above all, it is the location of the obstruction (i.e., the third or fourth portion of the duodenum) that most strongly suggests the diagnosis of midgut volvulus. Obstruction due to **peritoneal (Ladd's) bands,** which also accompanies rotational anomalies of the intestine, can have an identical appearance. In addition to these findings, an abnormal position of the superior mesenteric vein and artery (Fig. 60-15) can be seen in patients with intestinal malrotation, with or without volvulus. **Failure of normal embryologic bowel rotation leaves the superior mesenteric vein anterior and to the left of the superior mesenteric artery,**[40,41] as opposed to its normal position to the right of the artery. It is probably worthwhile to observe the relationship of these vessels in any child who is undergoing sonography for the evaluation of vomiting. When color Doppler is used, the twisted mesenteric vessels are seen swirling in a clockwise direction (**the "whirlpool sign**), and this finding is highly specific for midgut volvulus (Fig. 60-15, *C*).[42] A final cause of distal duodenal obstruction is a **duodenal diaphragm** that has stretched into a "windsock" configuration. The distal end of the obstructed duodenum will have a rounded shape in this condition, as opposed to the tapered end that is more often seen with midgut volvulus (Fig. 60-16).

A

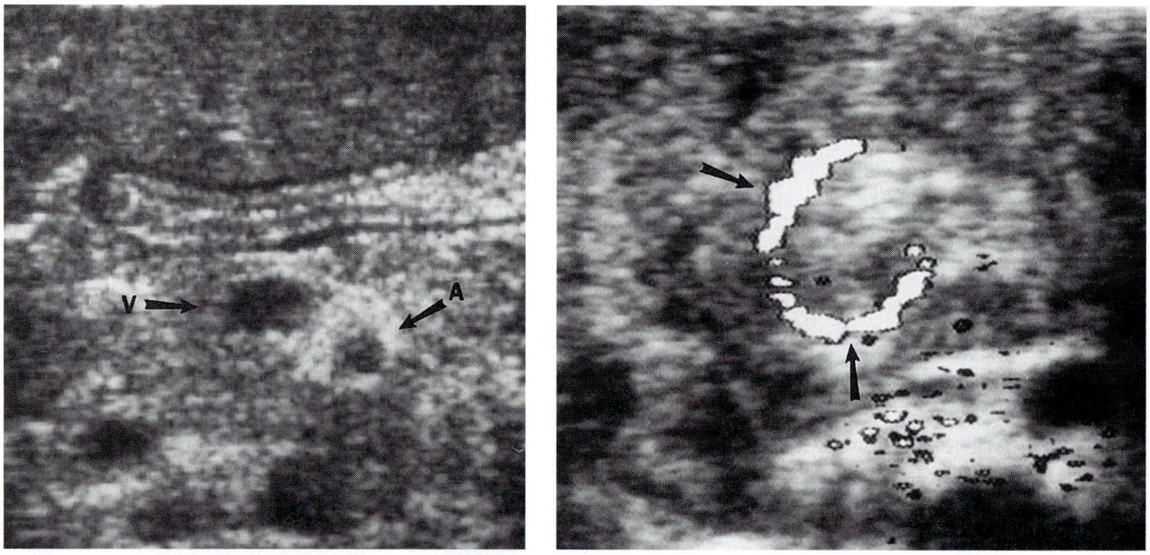

C

B

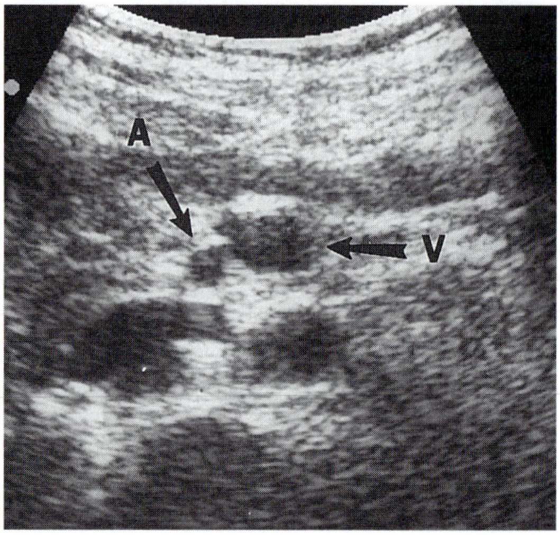

FIG. 60-15. Midgut volvulus: altered relationship of mesenteric vessels. **A,** Normal superior mesenteric vein (V) lies to the right of the superior mesenteric artery (A). **B,** Intestinal malrotation and midgut volvulus, the vein (V) lies to the left of the artery (A). **C,** Color Doppler shows a clockwise "whirlpool" of vessels (*arrows*) around a volvulus. (Courtesy of Kenneth Martin, M.D., Oakland Children's Hospital, Oakland, Calif.)

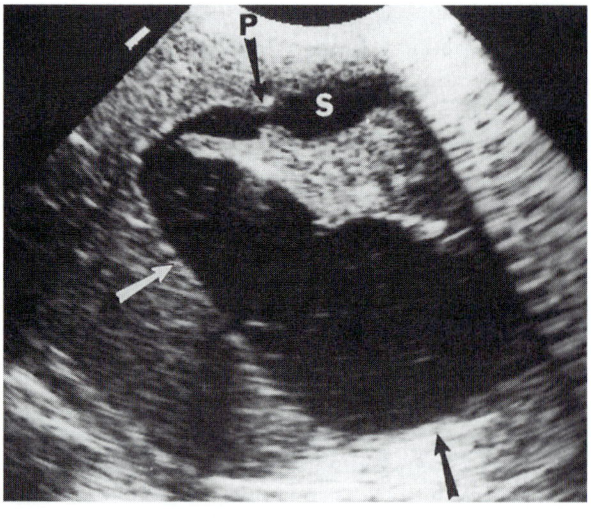

FIG. 60-16. Duodenal diaphragm. Grossly distended, obstructed descending duodenum (*arrows*). P, pyloric canal. S, stomach.

Duodenal Hematoma

Duodenal hematoma is a common complication of blunt abdominal trauma in children, including the battered child syndrome. Sonography can demonstrate the dilated, obstructed duodenum and, more specifically, can show evidence of an **intramural hematoma.**[43-45] The intramural hemorrhage initially causes echogenic thickening of the wall of the duodenum (Fig. 60-17, *A*), but as time passes, the hematoma undergoes liquefaction and the thickened wall becomes hypoechoic. Similar hematomas can occur with Henoch-Schönlein purpura (Fig. 60-17, *B*).[46-48]

Duodenal Ulcer Disease

The sonographic findings of duodenal ulcer disease are similar to those seen with gastric ulcer disease, but ultrasound is not a sensitive method for screening for duodenal ulcer disease.[49] The study is aided significantly by filling the stomach and duodenum with

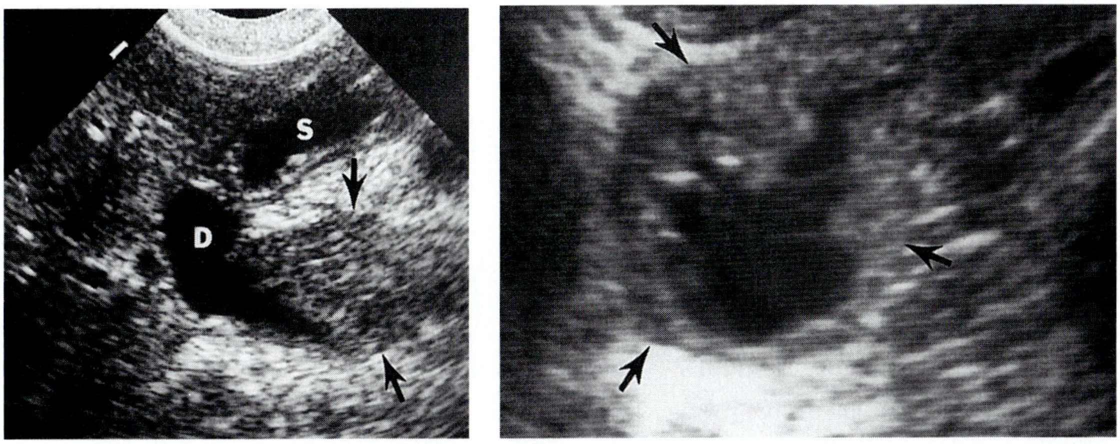

FIG. 60-17. Duodenal hematoma. **A,** Large echogenic hematoma (*arrows*), compressing and obstructing duodenum (D), due to blunt abdominal trauma. S, stomach. **B,** Asymmetric thickening of the duodenal wall (*arrows*) due to intramural hemorrhage in a patient with Henoch-Schönlein purpura. (Courtesy of C.K. Hayden, Jr., M.D., Ft. Worth, Tex.)

fluid, and although the ulcer crater itself is more difficult to visualize in the duodenum, mucosal thickening due to the inflammation can sometimes be demonstrated. In general, contrast studies of the duodenum remain the preferred method for identifying duodenal ulcers.

Small Bowel Obstruction

The diagnosis of small bowel obstruction is usually accomplished with plain radiographs. At times, however, ultrasound can be used to help determine the site or cause of a small bowel obstruction (e.g., **intussusception, intestinal hematoma).** In such cases, the obstructed, fluid-distended, hyperperistaltic small bowel loops may be seen.

In neonates with congenital causes of small bowel obstruction (e.g., ileal atresia, meconium ileus), in utero gastrointestinal perforation can occur, releasing variable amounts of meconium into the peritoneal cavity. In some of these fetuses the perforation heals in utero, and the only clues that remain after birth are scattered calcifications in the peritoneal cavity. However, in cases in which larger amounts of meconium have leaked or in which an active leak remains after birth, cystic masses can be found in the peritoneal cavity, giving rise to the term **"cystic meconium peritonitis."** Sonographically, these cysts appear as variably sized, fairly well-defined cystic collections, often with very heterogeneous cystic fluid.[50,51] The highly echogenic calcifications can also be found with ultrasound (Fig. 60-18).

Small bowel obstruction due to **intestinal hematomas** usually occurs as a result of Henoch-Schönlein purpura, blunt abdominal trauma, or coagulopathies. In any of these conditions, the mural hemorrhage can be detected sonographically as asymmetric or circumferential areas of intestinal wall thickening that can vary from echogenic to hypoechoic in texture.[46,47]

Intussusception

Intussusception is the most common cause of small bowel obstructions in children between the ages of 6 months and 4 years, with the peak incidence occurring between about 18 months and 3 years of age. Clinical findings of crampy, intermittent abdominal pain, vomiting, and "currant jelly" stools are virtually classic, and patients with these symptoms probably do not require ultrasound diagnosis prior to attempted enema reduction. However, many children present with less than classic findings, and in this situation, sonography can be very helpful to confirm or exclude intussusception. At our institution, the surgeons have come to rely on ultrasound for the confident diagnosis of this condition, which we now perform on all suspected intussusception patients. At many sites, sonography is not routinely done for intussusception.

Recent studies have suggested that ultrasound is highly sensitive and specific for the diagnosis of intussusception,[52-55] and this has also been our experience. Indeed, if an intussusception is not demonstrated sonographically, we feel confident that one is not present, and an enema need not be performed unless clinical suspicion is very high.

The sonographic appearance of **intussusceptions** can vary slightly depending on the type of ultrasound transducer that is used for the examination (see box on p. 1730). When a 5 MHz sector scanner is used, the intussusception appears as an oval, hypoechoic mass

A 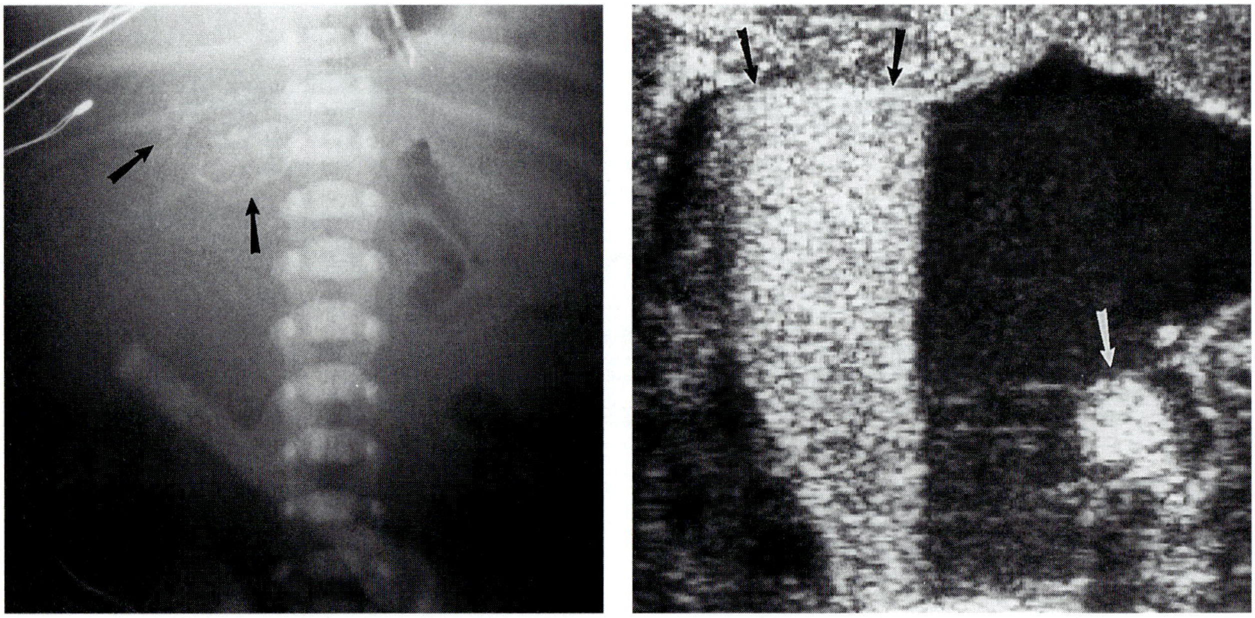 B

FIG. 60-18. Cystic meconium peritonitis. **A,** Curvilinear calcifications in the right upper quadrant (*arrows*) of a distended abdomen. **B,** Sonography revealed large loculated areas of fluid with echogenic debris (*black arrows*). Echogenic calcifications were also noted (*white arrow*).

US SIGNS OF INTUSSUSCEPTION

- Oval hypoechoic mass
  - (pseudokidney or doughnut sign)
- Hypoechoic rim with central echogenicity
- Multiple layers and concentric rings
- Small amount of peritoneal fluid
  - Large amount suggests perforation

with bright central echoes on longitudinal imaging (i.e., a **pseudokidney**) and a **hypoechoic doughnut,** or target configuration, on cross-sectional imaging.[56-60] The **hypoechoic rim** represents the edematous wall of the intussusceptum (Fig. 60-19, *A*) and the **central echogenicity** represents compressed mesentery, mucosa, and intestinal contents. Linear array transducers, however, display the intussusceptum with greater clarity, showing **multiple layers and concentric rings** (Fig. 60-19, *B*) representing the bowel wall, mesentery, and even **lymph nodes that have been drawn into the intussusception** (Fig. 60-19, *C*).[61] In some cases, anechoic fluid is also seen trapped within the incompletely compressed head of the intussusception.

Once an intussusception has been documented by sonography, the patient usually proceeds to nonsurgical reduction, unless clinical or radiographic evidence of perforation is found. Currently, air reduction is the most popular method of treatment, although many radiologists still prefer hydrostatic reduction using various types of contrast. Ultrasound-guided hydrostatic reduction has been used successfully in several centers,[62-65] but this technique has not been received with universal enthusiasm. Consequently, the primary role of ultrasound continues to be the diagnosis of intussusception. Ultrasound can also be used to identify postoperative ileo-ileal intussusception[66] or ileo-ileal intussusception that sometimes remains after the successful hydrostatic reduction of the ileocolic portion of an intussusception. Occasionally, an intussusception will be transient and will resolve spontaneously. In such patients, when symptoms subside between the time the diagnosis is made and the time a reduction procedure is begun, ultrasound can verify resolution of the intussusception and spare the patient an unnecessary enema procedure.[67]

The only absolute contraindications to nonsurgical reduction of an intussusception are radiographic evidence of free intraperitoneal air or clinical signs of peritonitis. With ultrasound, a small amount of **free peritoneal fluid** is commonly seen in patients with intussusception, even in the absence of perforation.[68-69] Therefore, a small amount of ascites is not a contraindication to nonsurgical reduction; however, if a large amount of ascites is found, the possibility of perforation should be considered.

A

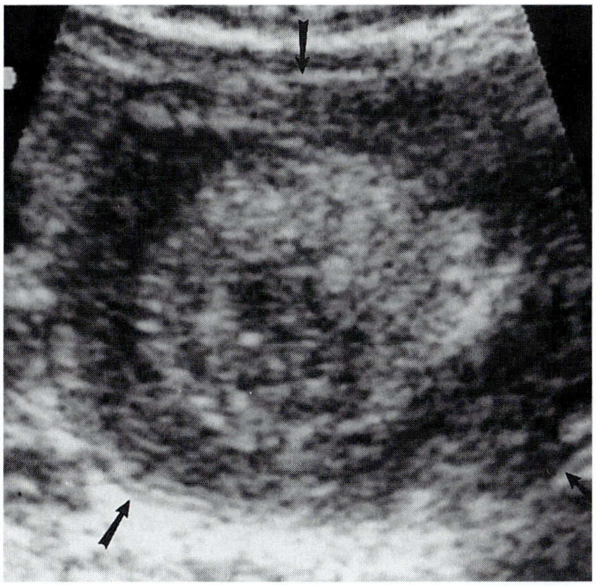

B

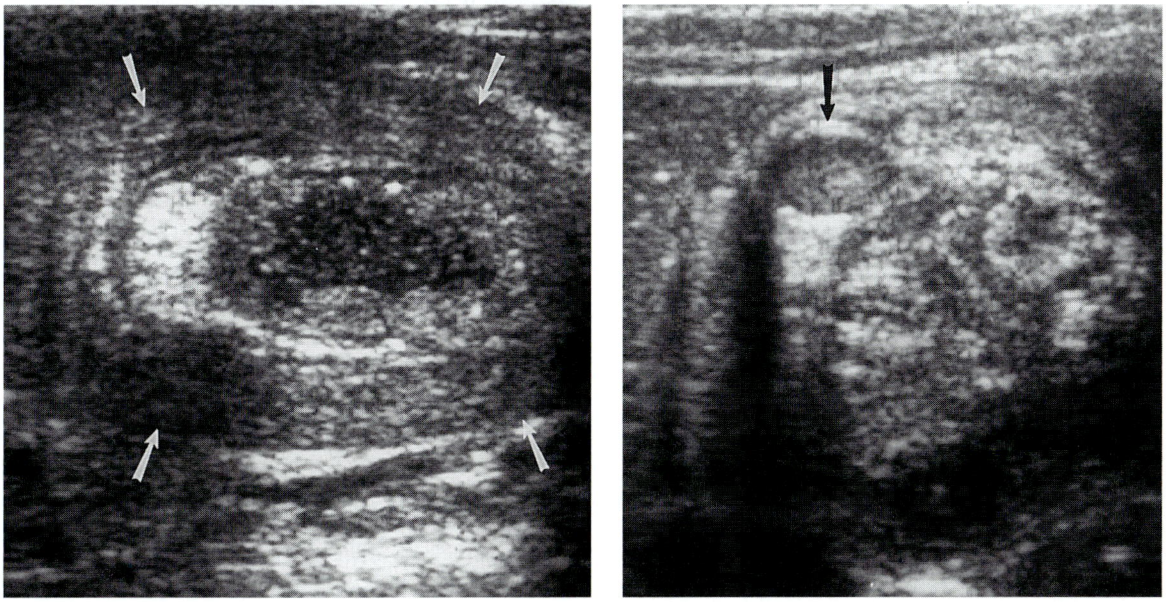

C

FIG. 60-19. Intussusception. **A,** Transverse image with a sector transducer shows hypoechoic rim and echogenic center (*arrows*). **B,** Linear transducers more clearly show the concentric rings of the edematous intussusceptum (*arrows*) with echogenic fat and hypoechoic fluid trapped in the center. **C,** Another intussusception demonstrating a trapped mesenteric lymph node (*arrow*).

Color Doppler assessment of blood flow to the intussusceptum (Fig. 60-20) has been used to try to predict those patients who have significant bowel ischemia and may be at greater risk of perforation during attempted nonsurgical reduction.[70,71] However, the true reliability of these findings has yet to be determined.

COLON

Normal Anatomy and Technique

Sonographic evaluation of the colon can be compromised by the gas and fecal material that are frequently present. However, when sufficient fluid is present within the colon, the characteristic haustral markings in the multilayered wall can be identified. When pathological wall thickening occurs, it tends to displace the gas and intestinal contents, and such abnormal areas of colon are often more easily visible than is the normal colon. The use of sonographic imaging in the colon, for the most part, is confined to imaging inflammatory disease and imperforate or ectopic anus.

Ectopic (Imperforate) Anus

In patients with ectopic, or imperforate, anus, it is important to determine where the distal end of the

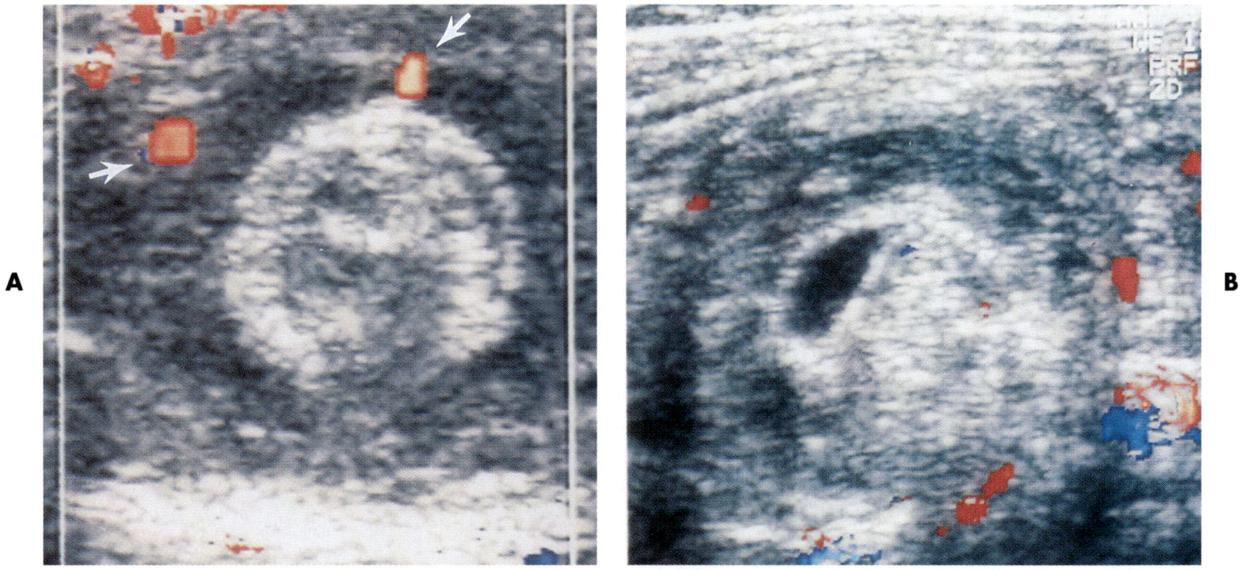

FIG. 60-20. Intussusception: color Doppler imaging. **A,** Color Doppler demonstrated substantial blood flow within the wall of the intussusceptum (*arrows*). Hydrostatic reduction was successful in this patient without complication. **B,** Another patient showing prominent blood flow in the tissue surrounding the intussusception, but no flow within the wall of the intussusceptum. At surgery, the bowel was necrotic.

hindgut terminates. There are well-known pitfalls in attempting to accomplish this with plain radiographs, including those that are taken in the inverted or cross-table prone position. Radiographically, the colon can erroneously appear to end in a high position if the air column fails to progress to the end of the colon because of impacted meconium. Sonography can directly **visualize the end of the hindgut pouch, and the corresponding sacral level** can be determined (Fig. 60-21). Thereafter, the level can be transferred to the plain radiographs and the M-line of Cremin[72] can be drawn. The M-line corresponds to the level of the puborectalis sling, and if the hindgut ends above the line, a **high fistula** is presumed. If the hindgut ends below this line, a **low fistula** should be present.

Ultrasound images can also be obtained from a perineal approach at the site of the anal dimple. In this way, the distance between the skin surface and the blind-ending hindgut can be measured, and a distance of less than 1.5 mm suggests a low pouch.[73,74] However, this procedure can be tricky to perform and it lacks precision. MRI can be performed if more precision is required. MRI can more accurately define the level of the pouch and, in addition, can directly evaluate the adequacy of the puborectalis muscle.[75]

Intestinal Inflammatory Disease

Although radiographic contrast studies are most often used for evaluating inflammatory conditions of the intestines, in some cases ultrasound can provide additional useful information. High-resolution linear array transducers allow direct and detailed evaluation of the intestinal wall, and areas of **intestinal wall thickening** can often be identified. Such thickening is nonspecific[76] and can be seen in a variety of inflammatory conditions, including regional enteritis,[77-79] ulcerative colitis,[78,79] pseudomembranous colitis,[80,81] neutropenic colitis (typhlitis),[82,83] bacterial ileocolitis,[84,85] necrotizing enterocolitis,[86] hemolytic-uremic syndrome,[87] and chronic granulomatous disease of childhood. Even **viral gastroenteritis** can produce mild mucosal thickening in fluid-filled loops with diminished peristalsis.

Sonography can sometimes differentiate **mucosal** from **transmural inflammation.** If the inflammatory process involves primarily the mucosa (e.g., ulcerative colitis, pseudomembranous colitis, typhlitis), the inner echogenic mucosal layer becomes thickened and sometimes nodular or irregular, but the outer muscular layer of the wall remains thin (Fig. 60-22). However, when the inflammation involves the entire intestinal wall (e.g., regional enteritis), thickening of the entire wall is seen (Fig. 60-23). Color Doppler sonography demonstrates increased blood flow to the thickened intestinal loops with most inflammatory bowel conditions,[88] but hypovascularity is more typical of hemolytic-uremic syndrome.[87] Ultrasound is indicated in most children with regional enteritis to identify distal right ureteral involvement by the inflammatory mass that can result in hydronephrosis.

A

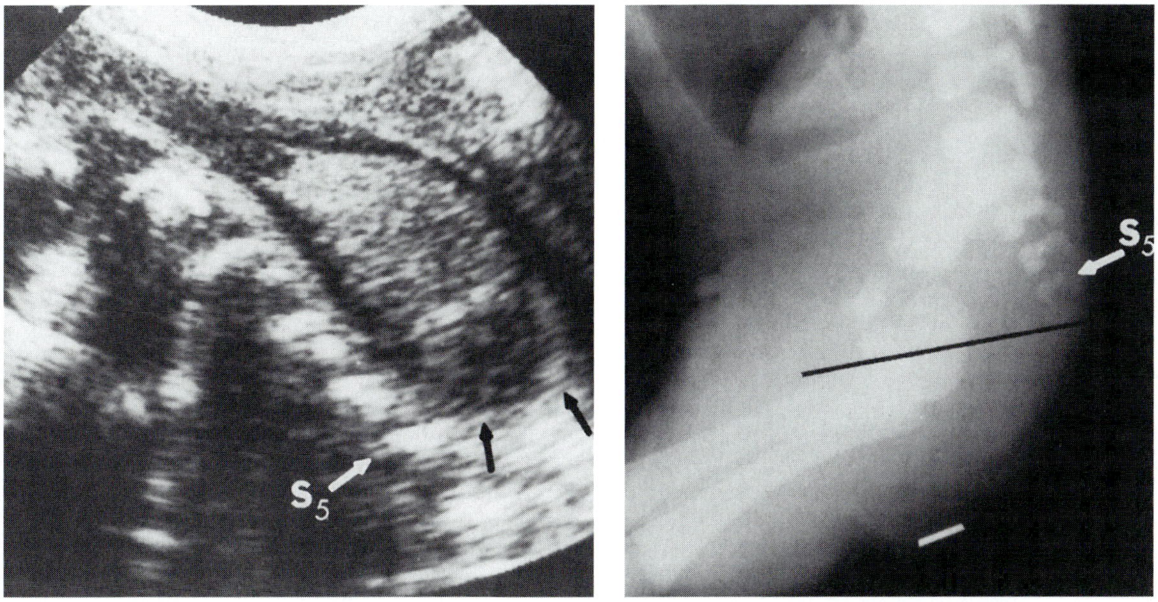

B

FIG. 60-21. Imperforate anus. **A,** Sagittal midline scan. Meconium-filled, distended distal hindgut (*arrows*) anterior to last vertebral body (S5). **B,** Inverted plain radiograph demonstrates no gas or meconium anterior to the sacrum and no air-filled pouch near the M-line (*line*). Radiograph suggests that the hindgut ends quite high, but ultrasound clearly demonstrates a low pouch filled with meconium.

A

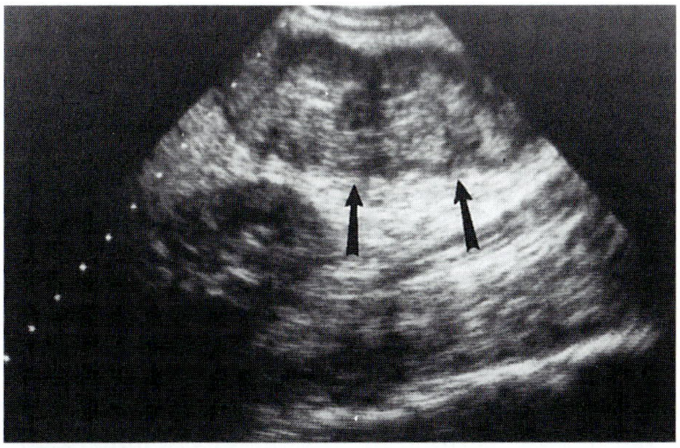

FIG. 60-22. Inflammatory disease: mucosal thickening. **A,** Markedly thickened, echogenic mucosa (*arrows*) due to ulcerative colitis. **B,** Echogenic thickening of the cecum (*arrows*) in a child with typhlitis. **C,** Echogenic thickening of small bowel mucosa (*arrows*) in a child with chronic granulomatous disease.

B

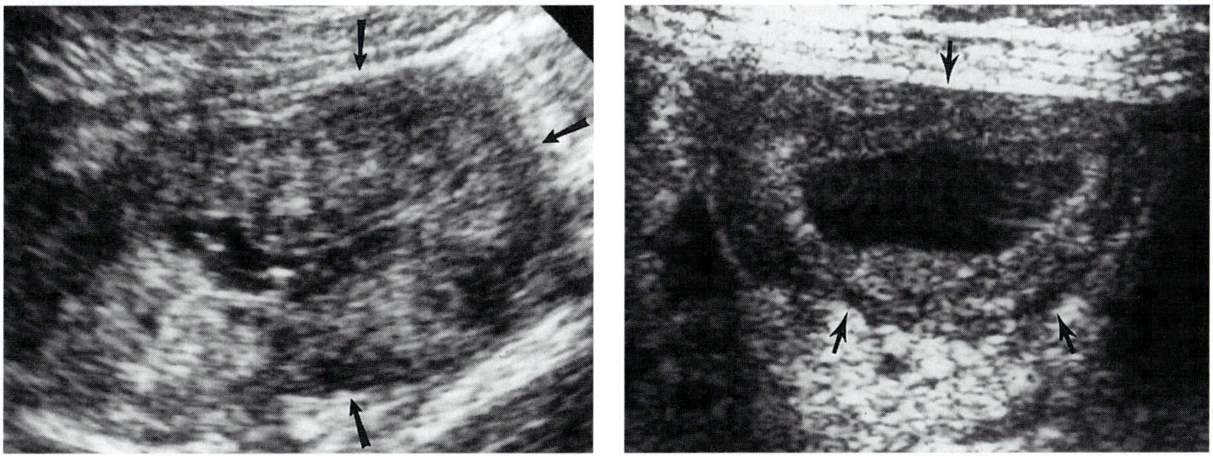

C

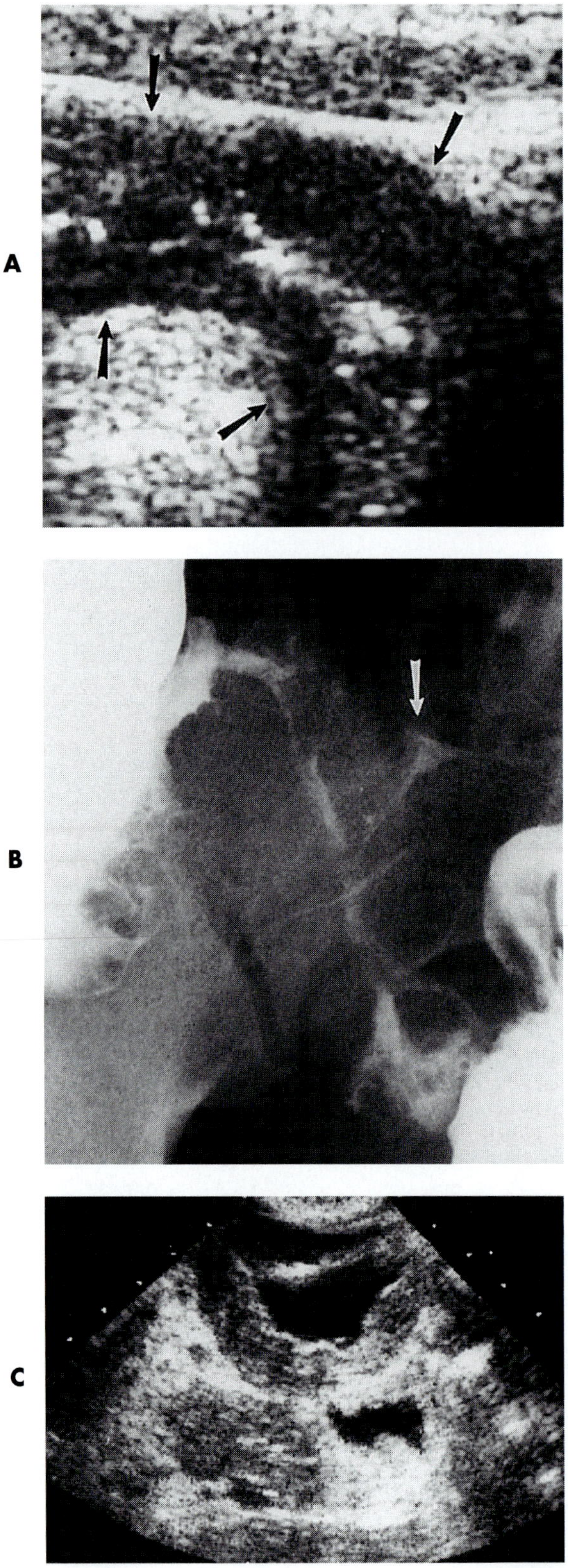

FIG. 60-23. Inflammatory disease: transmural thickening. A, Hypoechoic thickening of the entire wall of the terminal ileum (*arrows*) in a patient with regional enteritis. **B,** Markedly narrowed lumen and a small fistula (*arrow*) on a contrast study in the same patient. **C,** Marked thickening of the entire gastric wall in patient with chronic granulomatous disease (*arrows*). (Courtesy of W. McAlister, M.D.)

Although the fistulas and sinus tracts that develop in regional enteritis are usually not discernible sonographically, ultrasound can be used to identify resulting intra-abdominal abscesses.

Henoch-Schönlein purpura, a condition probably caused by an allergic vasculitis of small vessels in a variety of body systems, frequently involves the gastrointestinal tract. Of these patients, 50% to 60% develop abdominal pain due to intramural hemorrhage in the intestines, and this symptom may precede the development of the more characteristic purpuric skin rash. In such patients, sonography may detect the involved intestinal loops, which usually show circumferential, echogenic wall thickening, sometimes associated with small amounts of free abdominal fluid (Fig. 60-24).[46,47] Ultrasound also can be used to follow the resolution of the intestinal hemorrhage. Intussusception occasionally results as a complication of Henoch-Schönlein purpura, and sonography is highly useful to identify such intussusception,[89,90] which commonly involves only the small bowel and does not extend into the colon.

Necrotizing enterocolitis (**NEC**) in newborn infants is usually detected radiographically, but early in the disease, the classic findings of bowel dilatation and pneumatosis intestinalis may not be apparent (see box below). In such cases, sonography may detect early thickening of the intestinal loops. In addition, ultrasound can detect small amounts of gas within the portal venous system, which appear as small echogenic foci within the liver.[91,92] Pericholecystic hyperechogenicity has also been described in infants with necrotizing enterocolitis.[93] The most dreaded complication of this condition is bowel necrosis with perforation. Increased flow velocity in the splanchnic arteries, most likely due to vasoconstriction, has recently been suggested as a reliable early finding on Doppler sonography in infants with necrotizing enterocolitis.[94] Free intra-abdominal air may not be detectable in infants who have very little intestinal gas to escape through the perforation, but the sonographic demonstration of ascites with fluid/debris levels can suggest perforation in such patients.[95]

SONOGRAPHIC SIGNS OF NEC

Early thickening of the bowel loops
Small echogenic foci due to gas in liver
Pericholecystic hyperechogenicity
Increased flow in the splanchnic arteries
  SMA and celiac artery
Ascites with fluid/debris levels if perforation

Appendicitis

Sonography (see box below) is now accepted as a valuable diagnostic tool for the detection of appendicitis. Several recent studies have shown that ultrasound is both sensitive and specific.[96-100] Sonography is especially useful in those children with ambiguous clinical findings,[100] and when appendicitis is not found, frequently ultrasound can help to suggest or confirm an alternative diagnosis.[101] In the end, the diagnostic approach to the acute abdomen remains a surgical management decision, but enthusiasm continues to grow for the use of sonography to help diagnose appendicitis and to help manage postoperative complications.

> **SONOGRAPHIC SIGNS OF APPENDICITIS**
>
> Noncompressible, blind-ended tubular structure
> Diameter of tube measures 6 mm or greater
> Fluid trapped within nonperforated appendix
> Target appearance of echogenic mucosa around fluid center surrounded by hypoechoic muscle
> Fecalith: echogenic foci with pronounced posterior acoustic shadowing
> Lymphadenopathy: nonspecific
> Hypervascular appendix on color Doppler

Sonographically, the **acute inflamed appendix** appears as a blind-ending tubular structure that is noncompressible and measures 6 mm or greater in diameter.[102] Fluid is often seen trapped within a nonperforated appendix, and the surrounding echogenic mucosal layer and hypoechoic muscular layer of the appendiceal wall combined with the central anechoic fluid give the appendix a target appearance in cross-section (Fig. 60-25, *A*, *B*). **Fecaliths**, even those that are not calcified, can often be identified, and they appear as echogenic foci with pronounced posterior acoustic shadowing (Fig. 60-25, *C*, *D*). A small amount of fluid may be seen adjacent to the appendix, even in the absence of perforation. **Mesenteric lymphadenopathy** also frequently accompanies appendicitis, but isolated mesenteric lymphadenopathy is a nonspecific finding that can be seen with other types of abdominal inflammation (Fig. 60-26).[103]

A

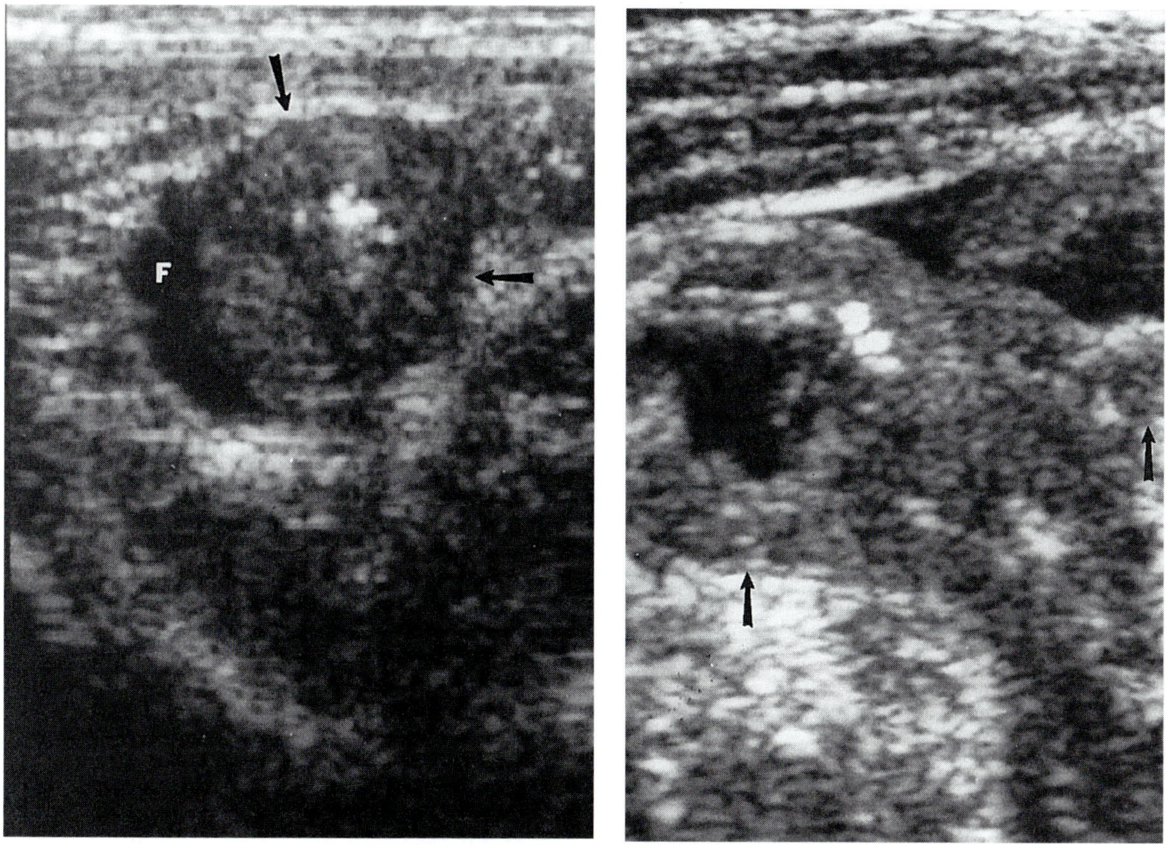

B

FIG. 60-24. Henoch-Schönlein purpura. **A,** Echogenic, circumferential wall thickening of a single intestinal loop (*arrows*), with a small amount of adjacent anechoic free fluid (F). **B,** Another patient showing adjacent loops with echogenic wall thickening (*arrows*) due to intramural hemorrhage.

A B C D

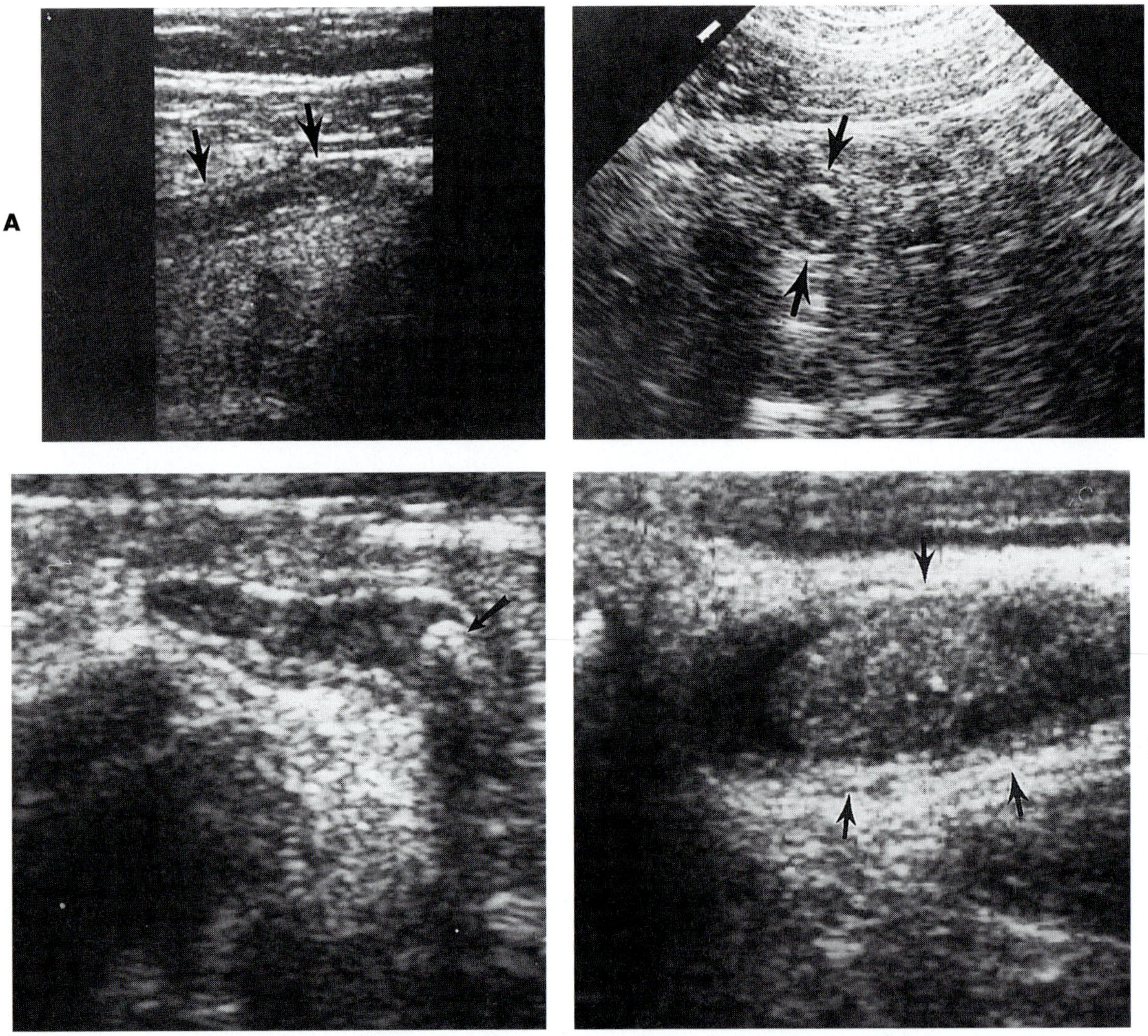

FIG. 60-25. Acute appendicitis. **A**, Longitudinal and **B**, transverse scans show a distended, fluid-filled appendix (*arrows*), which measured 7 mm in diameter. **C**, Note the echogenic fecalith with posterior shadowing (*arrow*) within a fluid-filled dilated appendix. **D**, Another dilated appendix (*arrows*) containing a large amount of fecal sludge.

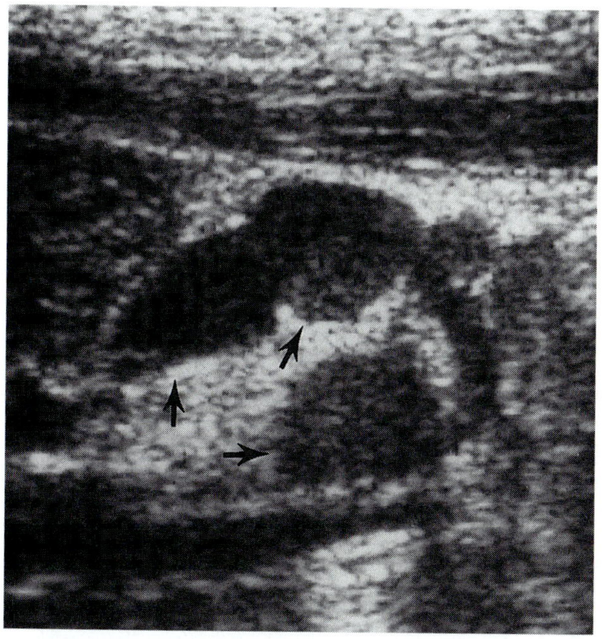

FIG. 60-26. Mesenteric adenitis. Enlarged lymph nodes in ileocecal region (*arrows*).

SONOGRAPHIC SIGNS OF APPENDICEAL PERFORATION

- Appendix hard to find
- Appendix decompressed
- Focal loops of paralyzed bowel
- Complex fluid collection in an abscess
- Loss of normal echogenic submucosal layer suggests gangrene
- Vascular flow may decrease as necrosis occurs in center of appendix

In cases of **perforated appendicitis,** the appendix itself is often more difficult to identify than in acute nonperforated appendicitis.[104] With perforation, the appendix becomes decompressed (Fig. 60-27, *A*), and increasing intestinal gas due to adynamic ileus and functional obstruction can interfere with the ultrasound examination. Nevertheless, a careful graded-compression technique may allow detection of focal loops of paralyzed bowel in the right lower quadrant or a complex fluid collection representing an abscess (Fig. 60-27, *B*).[105] Color Doppler can be a useful adjunct to the ultrasound exam in such patients, for the hypervascularity of the appendix and the surrounding inflamed tissues can draw the examiner's eye to otherwise subtle or partially obscured sonographic findings.[108] When the appendix is found with ultrasound, loss of the normal echogenic submucosal layer suggests a gangrenous appendix (Fig. 60-27, *C*)[105,108] which, for practical purposes, can be considered perforation.

Sonography of a child with acute abdominal pain is a procedure that requires patience and experience. The examination is facilitated by clinically localizing the pain, and even young children can help to guide the examination if asked to point with one finger to the site of maximal tenderness. The **normal appendix** occasionally can be visualized, and it should be easily compressible and smaller than the inflamed appendix (Fig. 60-28). When the appendix cannot be found sonographically, the study must be considered indeterminate; however, if no other abnormal abdominal findings are found, a prolonged ultrasound exam to try to localize the normal appendix is probably not worthwhile.

The value of color Doppler imaging for the diagnosis of appendicitis has yet to be definitively determined. However, recent studies have suggested that color Doppler imaging not only facilitates the identification of the inflamed appendix and increases confidence in the diagnosis,[106-108] but color Doppler may also provide clues to the presence of perforation. In **acute nonperforated appendicitis, the appendix itself is hypervascular** (Fig. 60-29), but as necrosis progresses, the amount of flow within the appendix decreases. After perforation, increasing flow may be seen in the soft tissues surrounding the appendix, and an abdominal fluid collection with peripheral hyperemia is a fairly reliable indicator of abscess formation.[107,108] It is vital to be aware that many inflammatory conditions of the intestine other than appendicitis can be associated with small amounts of free fluid surrounding the bowel loops. Therefore, small avascular collections of fluid without other definitive evidence of appendicitis should not necessarily suggest an appendiceal abscess.

Gastrointestinal Neoplasms and Cysts

The superior ability of ultrasound to distinguish solid from cystic masses makes this examination an excellent choice for the diagnosis of **gastrointestinal duplication cysts.** Characteristically, gastrointestinal duplications are filled with anechoic fluid and have a well-defined, double-layered wall that consists of an inner echogenic mucosal layer and a thin, outer hypoechoic muscular layer (Fig. 60-30, *A*). These two layers can usually be demonstrated to be continuous throughout the cyst wall,[109-111] helping to distinguish such cysts from other simple-walled cysts such as **mesenteric cysts or pseudocysts** (Fig. 60-30, *B*). We have observed one ovarian cyst that appeared to have a double-layered wall because of a fibrinous layer that was deposited along the inner cyst wall after intracystic bleeding, but this is probably a relatively rare occurrence. Duplication cysts frequently contain foci of ectopic gastric mucosa which can become inflamed and ulcerated. In such cases, intracystic hemorrhage may

A B C

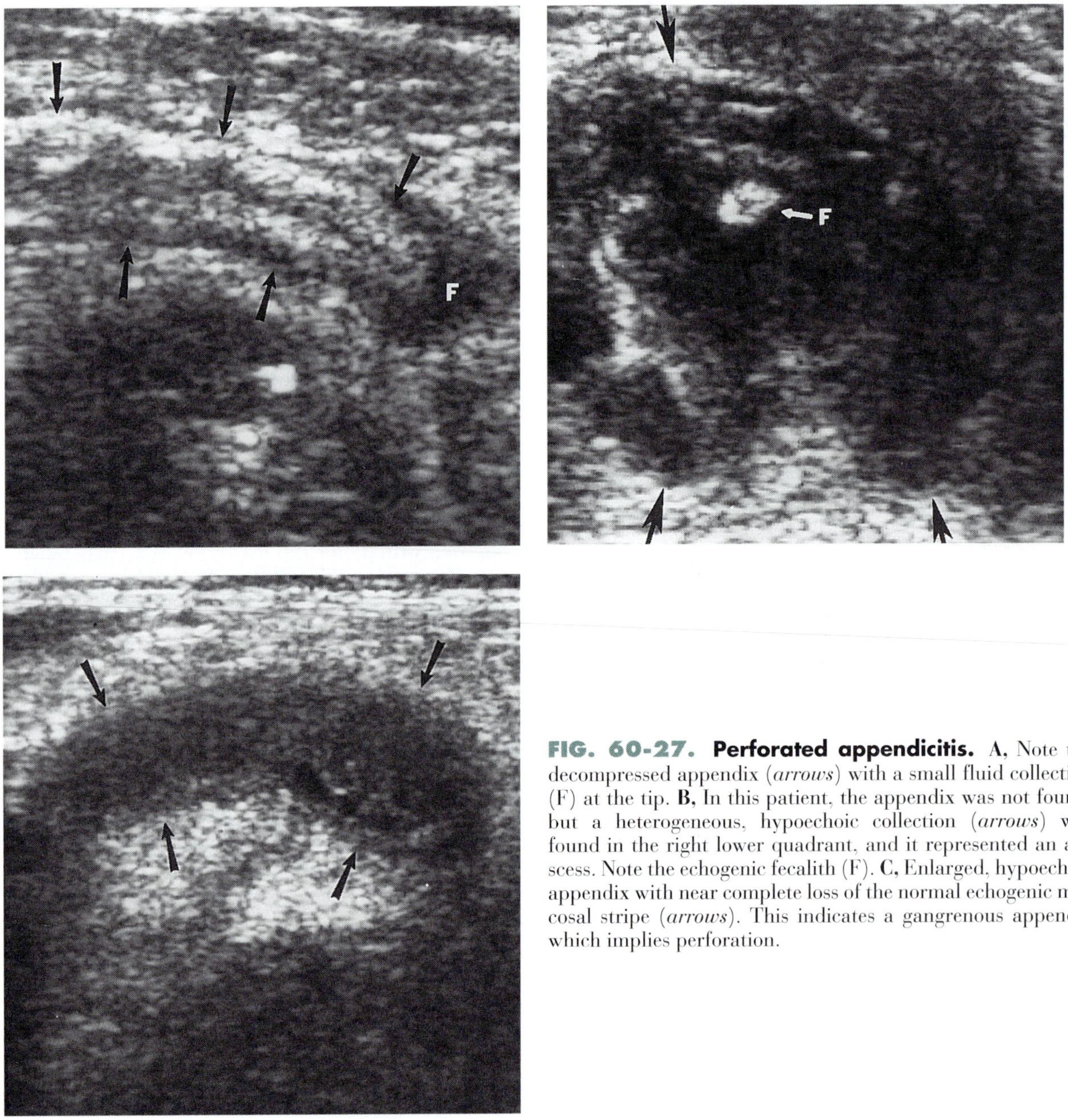

FIG. 60-27. Perforated appendicitis. **A,** Note the decompressed appendix (*arrows*) with a small fluid collection (F) at the tip. **B,** In this patient, the appendix was not found, but a heterogeneous, hypoechoic collection (*arrows*) was found in the right lower quadrant, and it represented an abscess. Note the echogenic fecalith (F). **C,** Enlarged, hypoechoic appendix with near complete loss of the normal echogenic mucosal stripe (*arrows*). This indicates a gangrenous appendix which implies perforation.

A

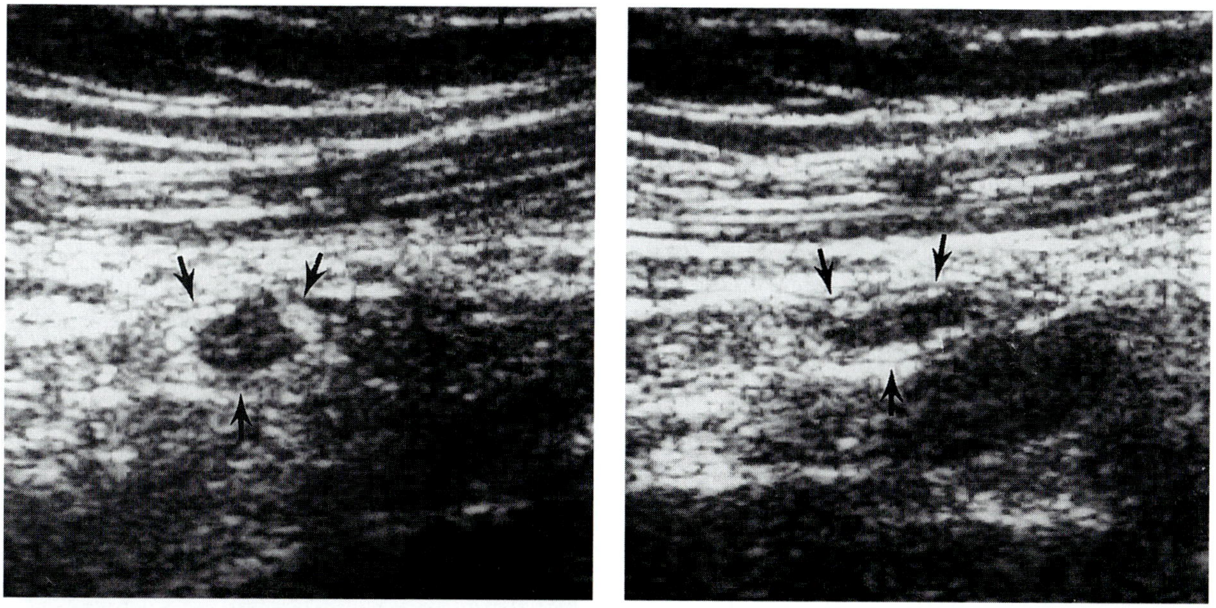

B

C

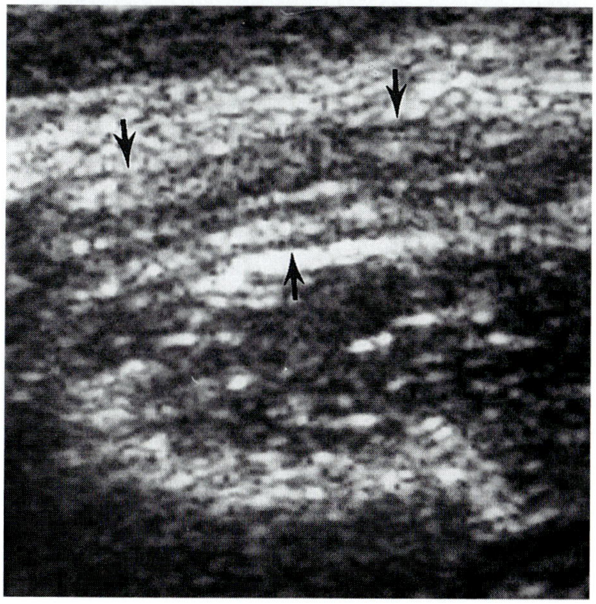

FIG. 60-28. Normal appendix. **A**, This fluid-filled appendix measured 4.5 mm in diameter (*arrows*). **B**, With compression, the appendix decreases to 3 mm (*arrows*). **C**, Another normal appendix with no intraluminal fluid, measuring 4 mm (*arrows*).

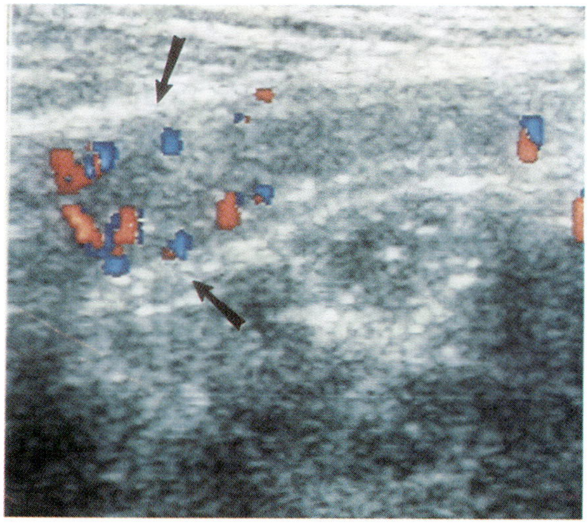

FIG. 60-29. Appendicitis: color Doppler imaging. Increased blood flow around the tip of this fluid-filled appendix (*arrows*).

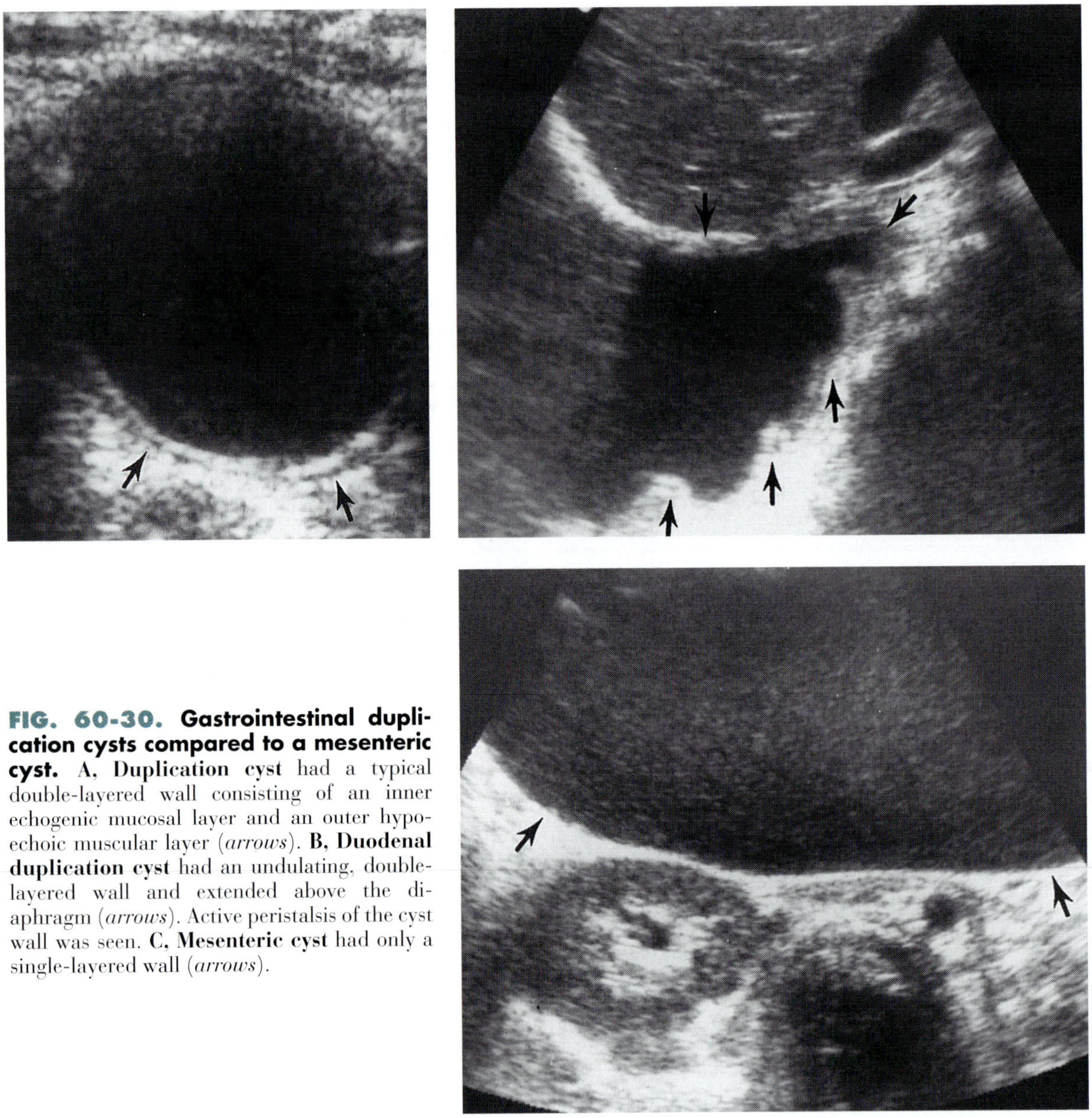

FIG. 60-30. Gastrointestinal duplication cysts compared to a mesenteric cyst. A, **Duplication cyst** had a typical double-layered wall consisting of an inner echogenic mucosal layer and an outer hypoechoic muscular layer (*arrows*). **B, Duodenal duplication cyst** had an undulating, double-layered wall and extended above the diaphragm (*arrows*). Active peristalsis of the cyst wall was seen. **C, Mesenteric cyst** had only a single-layered wall (*arrows*).

occur, and the resulting debris within the cyst fluid can cause the cyst to appear solid.[112] Some duplication cysts are **pedunculated**, and therefore they may be **located at a site remote** from the actual point of origin (Fig. 60-30, *C*). Occasionally, active peristalsis of the cyst wall can be seen in real-time ultrasound.

Ultrasound does not play a major role in the evaluation of **gastrointestinal neoplasms,** but masses or polyps can sometimes be identified when the bowel is filled with fluid.[113] More often, intraluminal gastrointestinal masses in children present with obstruction due to intussusception. The mass that acts as a lead point for the intussusception may not always be sonographically discernible. Most solid tumors present with a variably echogenic pattern and can not be reliably distinguished by their ultrasound characteristics.[114-117] In addition, areas of cystic degeneration may be seen. **Lymphoma** tends to be hypoechoic and may be associated with ulceration (Fig. 60-31). The tumors most likely to appear predominantly cystic are **teratomas** and **lymphangiomas.**[118-122] Abdominal lymphangiomas most commonly occur in the mesentery and can appear as solitary cysts or as multiloculated cystic masses (Fig. 60-32, *A*).[121] Gastrointestinal teratomas have large

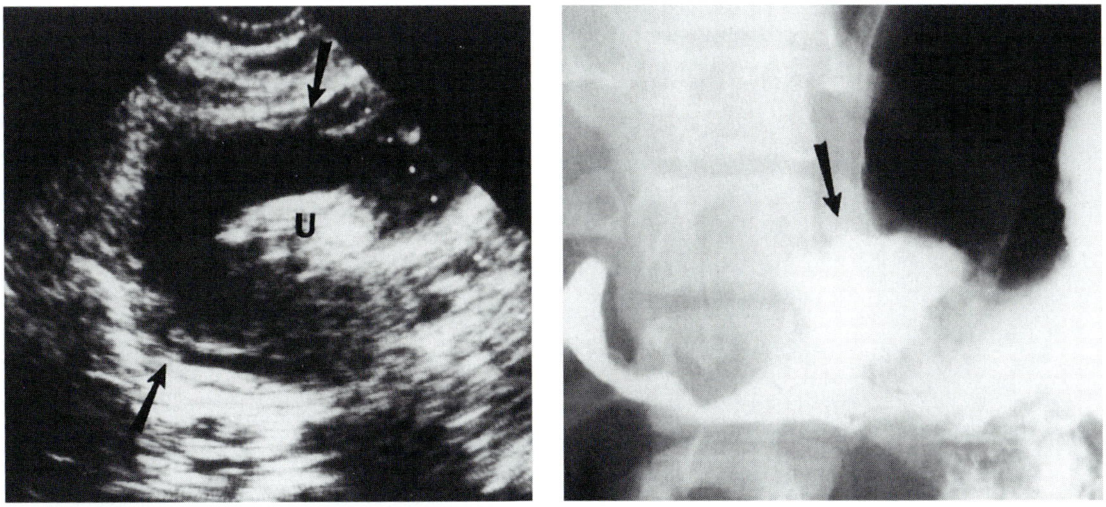

FIG. 60-31. Gastrointestinal neoplasms. **A,** Large hypoechoic lymphoma (*arrows*) with large, central, very echogenic ulcer crater (U). **B,** Radiographic upper gastrointestinal series shows large lymphoma with central ulcer (*arrow*).

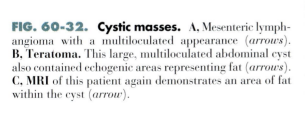

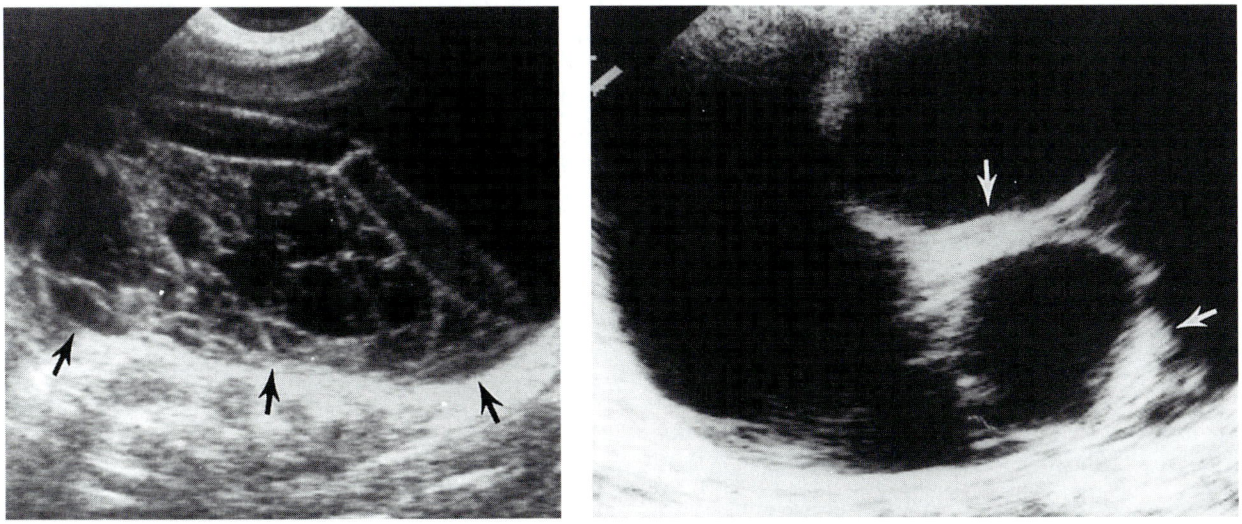

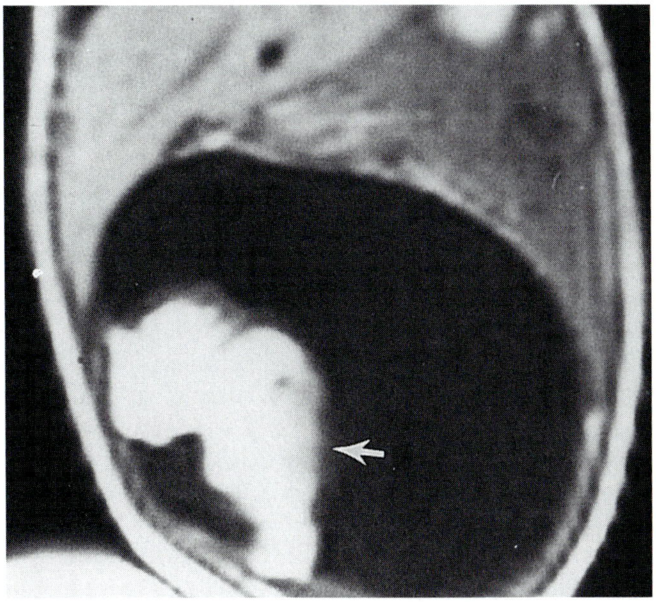

FIG. 60-32. Cystic masses. **A,** Mesenteric lymphangioma with a multiloculated appearance (*arrows*). **B, Teratoma.** This large, multiloculated abdominal cyst also contained echogenic areas representing fat (*arrows*). **C, MRI** of this patient again demonstrates an area of fat within the cyst (*arrow*).

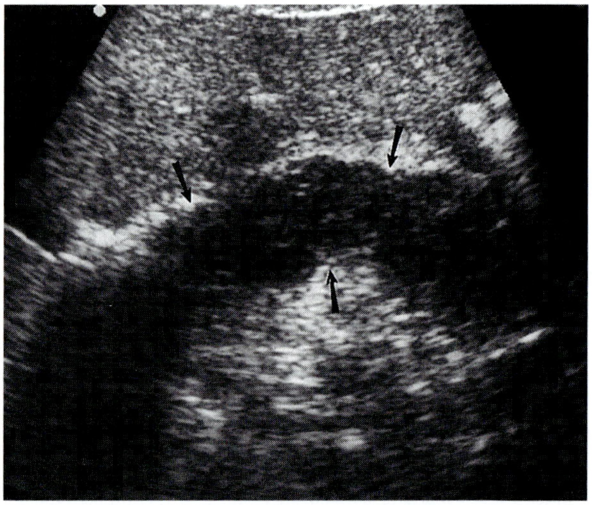

FIG. 60-33. Pancreatitis due to L-asparaginase toxicity. The pancreas is enlarged and hypoechoic as perceived through ultrasound (*arrows*).

cystic components, too, but echogenic fat and calcifications are also present (Fig. 60-32, *B, C*).[118,120]

PANCREAS

Normal Anatomy and Technique

The pancreas is easily imaged in children and normally appears relatively generous in size when compared to the pancreas of an adult. The normal echotexture of the pancreas in childhood is homogeneous and most often isoechoic or hyperechoic when compared to the liver. The normal pancreatic duct is usually not visible sonographically, unless a high-resolution linear transducer is used.

Pancreatitis

Pancreatitis is less common in children than in adults and is more likely to be acute rather than chronic. The most common causes of **acute pancreatitis** in children include blunt abdominal trauma (including the battered child syndrome), viral infection, and drug toxicity. Regardless of the cause, sonographic findings are usually sparse unless a complicating pseudocyst arises. The most common abnormal sonographic finding is pancreatic enlargement (Fig. 60-33), but a normal-sized pancreas does not exclude the diagnosis. Decreased echogenicity of the pancreas can occur with pancreatitis,[123,124] but this is a difficult finding to substantiate because of the variable echogenicity of the normal pancreas in children.[125] Occasionally, increased echogenicity of the pararenal space may be encountered; such a finding results from lipolysis of normal fat by pancreatic enzymes that have leaked into the hepatorenal space.[126] **Peripancreatic fluid collections** commonly accompany acute pancreatitis

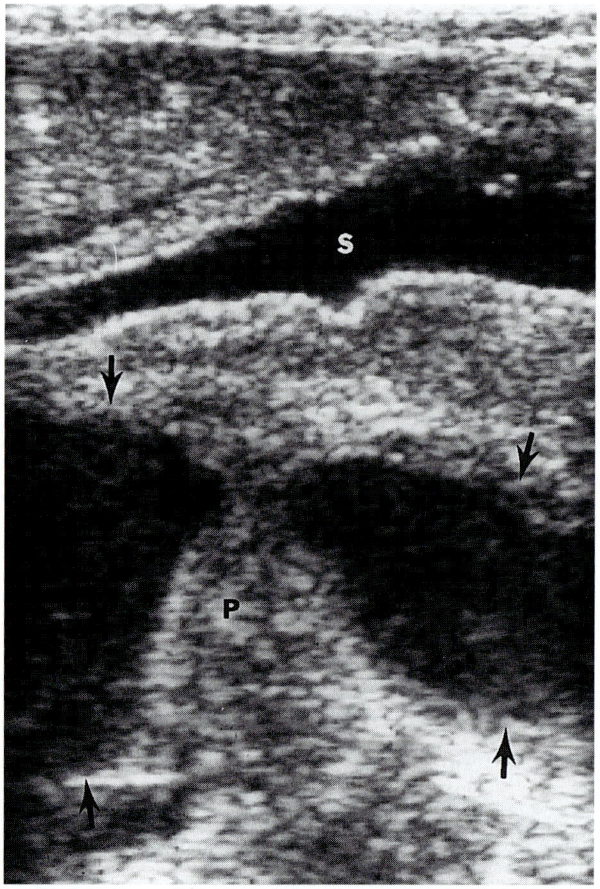

FIG. 60-34. Pancreatic pseudocyst in a battered child. Note the fluid collections (*arrows*) between the stomach (S) and the focally enlarged pancreas (P).

(Fig. 60-34), but such collections are not considered pseudocysts until they become chronic and are surrounded by a well-defined echogenic wall. Many pancreatic pseudocysts are now treated conservatively, and sonography is useful for following such patients to verify the spontaneous resolution of the fluid collection.[127] When the pseudocyst does not adequately resolve, ultrasound-guided percutaneous drainage has been successful in some cases.[128]

Chronic or recurrent pancreatitis in children is most likely to be secondary to congenital anomalies of the biliary tract (e.g., choledochal cysts, cystic fibrosis, or hereditary autosomal dominant pancreatitis). With cystic fibrosis, precipitation or coagulation of secretions in the small pancreatic ducts leads to ductal concretions and obstruction. Distention of the ducts and acini leads to degeneration and replacement by small cysts. This, along with atrophy of glandular elements and ensuing fibrosis, creates increased echogenicity of the pancreas.[129-131] Often, the gland is small, and calcifications may be seen as hyperechoic foci within the already hyperechoic pancreas. A similar appearance may be found in patients with hereditary pancreatitis.[132]

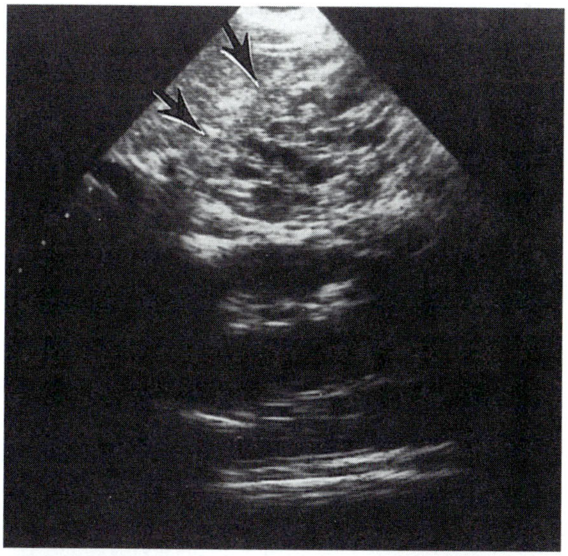

A

FIG. 60-35. Pancreatic masses. A, Lymphangioma of the head of the pancreas (*arrows*), showing multiple small cystic spaces. **B, Papillary-cystic neoplasm** of the pancreas in another patient with a large, heterogeneous but predominantly cystic mass in the region of the tail of the pancreas (*arrows*). **C.** CT also shows the predominantly cystic nature of this large, well-defined tumor (*arrows*).

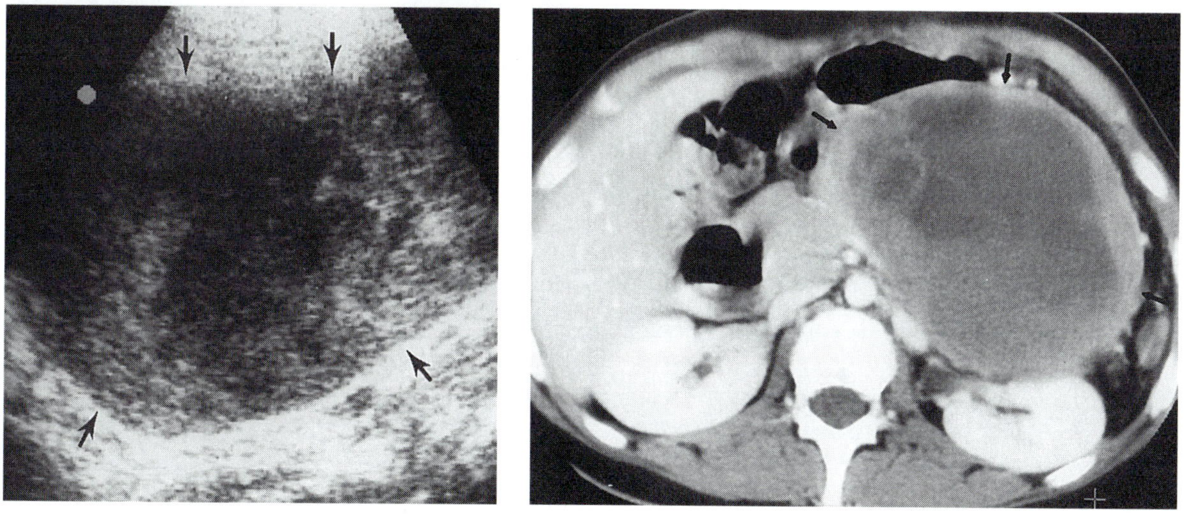

B

C

Pancreatic Masses

Tumors of the pancreas are extremely uncommon in children. The most common primary neoplasms are the benign insulinoma and adenocarcinoma.[133] Insulinomas are often difficult to detect sonographically, but intraoperative sonography has been used with more success. Carcinoma of the pancreas usually appears as an echogenic or complex pancreatic mass. Cystic masses of the pancreas include lymphangioma (Fig. 60-35, *A*), papillary-cystic neoplasm of the pancreas (Fig. 60-35, *B*),[134,135] and the rare congenital pancreatic cyst.[136,137]

Diffuse echogenic enlargement of the pancreas can be seen with **nesidioblastosis** (Fig. 60-36), a tumor-like condition of the pancreas characterized by diffuse proliferation and persistence of primitive ductal epithelial cells. The condition often is associated with hypoglycemia and the Beckwith-Wiedemann syndrome.

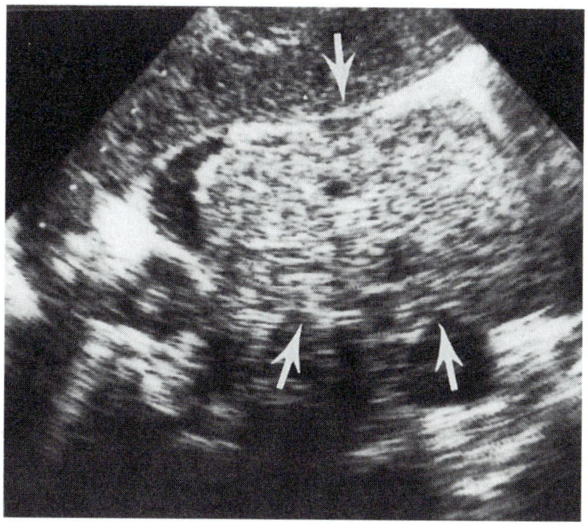

FIG. 60-36. Nesidioblastosis. The pancreas is markedly enlarged (*arrows*) in this child with Beckwith-Wiedemann syndrome.

Diffusely increased echogenicity of the pancreas can also occur with fatty infiltration in the Shwachman-Diamond syndrome, but in this condition the pancreas remains normal in size.[132]

REFERENCES

Esophagus and Stomach

1. Naik DR, Moore DJ. Ultrasound diagnosis of gastro-oesophageal reflux. *Arch Dis Child* 1984;59:366-367.
2. Wright LL, Baker KR, Meny RG. Ultrasound demonstration of gastroesophageal reflux. *J Ultrasound Med* 1988;7:471-475.
3. Gomes H, Lallenmand A, Lallemand P. Ultrasound of the gastroesophageal junction. *Pediatr Radiol* 1993;23:94-99.
4. Hirsch W, Kedar R, Preib U. Color Doppler in the diagnosis of the gastroesophageal reflux in children: comparison with pH measurements and B-mode ultrasound. *Pediatr Radiol* 1996;26:232-235.
5. Lambrecht L, Robberecht E, Deschynkel K, Afschrift M. Ultrasonic evaluation of gastric clearing in young infants. *Pediatr Radiol* 1988;18:314-318.
6. Gomes H, Menanteau B. Sonography of normal and hypertrophic pylorus. *Ann Radiol* 1983;26:154-160.
7. Hayden CK Jr, Swischuk LE, Lobe TE et al. Ultrasound: the definitive imaging modality in pyloric stenosis. *RadioGraphics* 1984;4:517-530.
8. Swischuk LE, Hayden CK Jr, Stansberry SD. Sonographic pitfalls in the imaging of the antrophyloric region in infants. *RadioGraphics* 1989;9:437-447.
9. Hernanz-Schulman M, Sells LL, Ambrosino MM, Heller RM, Stein SM, Neblett WW III. Hypertrophic pyloric stenosis in the infant without a palpable olive: accuracy of sonographic diagnosis. *Radiology* 1994;193:771.
10. Neilson D, Hollman AS. The ultrasonic diagnosis of infantile hypertrophic pyloric stenosis: technique and accuracy. *Clin Radiol* 1994;49:246-247.
11. Teele RL, Smith EH. Ultrasound in the diagnosis of idiopathic hypertrophic pyloric stenosis. *N Engl J Med* 1977;296:1149-1150.
12. Blumhagen JD, Maclin L, Krauter D, Rosenbaum DM, Weinberger E. Sonographic diagnosis of hypertrophic pyloric stenosis. *AJR* 1988;150:1367-1370.
13. Brambs HJ, Volk B, Spamer C, Holstege A. Diagnostic value of ultrasound in duodenal stenosis. *Gastrointest Radiol* 1986;11:135-138.
14. Cohen HL, Schechter S, Mestel AL, Eaton DH, Haller JO. Ultrasonic "double track" sign in hypertrophic pyloric stenosis. *J Ultrasound Med* 1987;6:139-143.
15. Haller JO, Cohen HL. Hypertrophic pyloric stenosis: diagnosis using ultrasound. *Radiology* 1986;161:335-339.
16. Lund-Kofoed PE, Host A, Elle B, Larsen C. Hypertrophic pyloric stenosis: determination of muscle dimensions by ultrasound. *Br J Radiol* 1988;61:19-20.
17. Stringer DA, Daneman A, Brunelle F, Ward K, Martin DJ. Sonography of normal and abnormal stomach (excluding hypertrophic pyloric stenosis) in children. *J Ultrasound Med* 1986;5:183-188.
18. Stunden RJ, LeQuesne GW, Little KE. The improved ultrasound diagnosis of hypertrophic pyloric stenosis. *Pediatr Radiol* 1986;16:200-205.
19. O'Keeffe FN, Stansberry SD, Swischuk LE, Hayden CK Jr. Antropyloric muscle thickness at US in infants: what is normal? *Radiology* 1991;178:827-830.
20. Westra SJ, de Groot CJ, Smits NJ, Steatman CR. Hypertrophic pyloric stenosis: use of the pyloric volume measurement in early ultrasound diagnosis. *Radiology* 1989;172:615-619.
21. Bowen A. The vomiting infant: recent advances and unsettled issues in imaging. *Radiol Clin North Am* 1988;26:377-392.
22. Okorie NM, Dickson JA, Carver RA, Steiner GM. What happens to the pylorus after pyloromyotomy? *Arch Dis Child* 1988;63:1339-1341.
23. Spevak MR, Ahmadjian JM, Kleinman PK, Henriquez G, Hirsh MP, Cohen IT. Sonography of hypertrophic pyloric stenosis: frequency and cause of nonuniform echogenicity of the thickened pyloric muscle. *AJR* 1992;158:129-132.
24. Cremin BJ, Solomon DJ. Ultrasonic diagnosis of duodenal diaphragm. *Pediatr Radiol* 1987;17:489-490.
25. Tomooka Y, Koga T, Shimoda Y, Kuroina T, Miyazaki S, Torisu M. The ultrasonic demonstration of acute multiple gastric ulcers in a child. *Br J Radiol* 1987;60:290-292.
26. Tomooka Y, Onitsuka H, Goy T, Koga T, Uchida S, Russell WJ, Torisu I. Ultrasonography of benign gastric ulcers: characteristics features and sequential follow-ups. *J Ultrasound Med* 1989;8:513-517.
27. Hayden CK, Jr., Swischuk LE, Rytting JE. Gastric ulcer disease in infants: ultrasound findings. *Radiology* 1987;164:131-134.
28. Maves CK, Johnson JF, Bove K, Malott RL. Gastric inflammatory pseudotumor in children. *Radiology* 1989;173:381-383.
29. Goldwag SS, Bellah RD, Ward KJ, Kogutt MS. Sonographic detection of Ménétrier's disease in children. *J Clin Ultrasound* 1994;22:567-570.
30. Mercado-Deane MG, Burton EM, Brawley AV, Hatley R. Prostaglandin-induced foveolar hyperplasia simulating pyloric stenosis in an infant with cyanotic heart disease. *Pediatr Radiol* 1994;24:45-46.
31. McAlister WH, Katz ME, Perlman JM, Tack ED. Sonography of focal foveolar hyperplasia causing gastric obstruction in an infant. *Pediatr Radiol* 1988;18:79-81.
32. Naik DR, Bolia A, Boon AW. Demonstration of a lactobezoar by ultrasound. *Br J Radiol* 1987;60:506-508.
33. Malpani A, Ramani SK, Wolverson MK. Role of sonography in trichobezoars. *J Ultrasound Med* 1988;7:661-663.

Duodenum and Small Bowel

34. Cohen HL, Haller JO, Mestel AL, Coren C, Schechter S, Eaton DH. Neonatal duodenum: fluid-aided ultrasound examination. *Radiology* 1987;164:805-809.
35. Boychuk RB, Lyons EA, Goodhand TK. Duodenal atresia diagnosed by ultrasound. *Radiology* 1978;127:500.
36. Crowe JE, Sumner TE. Combined esophageal and duodenal atresia without tracheoesophageal fistula: characteristic radiographic changes. *AJR* 1978;130:167-168.
37. Hayden CK Jr, Schwartz MZ, Davis M, Swischuk LE. Combined esophageal and duodenal atresia: sonographic findings. *AJR* 1983;140:225-226.
38. Jackson GH, Yiu-Chiu VS, Smith WL, Chiu LC. Sonography of combined esophageal and duodenal atresia. *J Ultrasound Med* 1983;2:473-474.
39. Hayden CK, Jr, Boulden TF, Swischuk LE, Lobe TE. Sonographic demonstration of duodenal obstruction with midgut volvulus. *AJR* 1984;143:9-10.
40. Loyer E, Eggli KD. Sonographic evaluation of superior mesenteric vascular relationship in malrotation. *Pediatr Radiol* 1989;19:173-175.
41. Zerin JM, DiPietro MA. Superior mesenteric vascular anatomy at US in patients with surgically proved malrotation of the midgut. *Radiology* 1992;183:693-694.
42. Shimanuki Y, Aihara T, Takano H, Moritani T, Oguma E, Kuroki H, Shibata A, Nozawa K, Ohkawara K, Hirata A,

Imaizumi S. Clockwise whirlpool sign at color Doppler US: an objective and definite sign of midgut volvulus. *Radiology* 1996;199:261-264.
43. Hayashi K, Futagawa S, Kozaki S, Hirao K, Hombo Z. Ultrasound and CT diagnosis of intramural duodenal hematoma. *Pediatr Radiol* 1988;18:167-168.
44. Hernanz-Schulman M, Genieser NB, Ambrosino M. Sonographic diagnosis of intramural duodenal hematoma. *J Ultrasound Med* 1989;8:273-276.
45. Orel SG, Nussbaum AR, Sheth S, Yale-Loehr A, Sanders RC. Case report: duodenal hematoma in child abuse—sonographic detection. *AJR* 1988;151:147-149.
46. John SD, Swischuk LE, Hayden CK Jr. Gastrointestinal sonographic findings in Henoch-Schönlein purpura. *Emerg Radiol* 1996;3:4-8.
47. Coutur A, Veyrac C, Baud C, Galifer RB, Armelin I. Evaluation of abdominal pain in Henoch-Schönlein syndrome by high-frequency ultrasound. *Pediatr Radiol* 1992;22:12-17.
48. Kagimoto S. Duodenal findings on ultrasound in children with Henoch-Schönlein purpura and gastrointestinal symptoms. *J Pediatr Gastroenterol* 1993;16:178-182.
49. Lim JH, Lee DH, Ko YT. Sonographic detection of duodenal ulcer. *J Ultrasound Med* 1992;11:91-94.
50. Carroll BA, Moskowitz PS. Sonographic diagnosis of a neonatal meconium cyst. *AJR* 1981;137:1262-1264.
51. Bowen A, Mazer J, Zarabi M, Fujioka M. Cystic meconium peritonitis: ultrasonographic features. *Pediatr Radiol* 1984; 14:18-22.
52. Verschelden P, Filiatrault D, Garel L, Grignon A, Perreault G, Boisvert J, Dubois J. Intussusception in children: reliability of US in diagnosis—a prospective study. *Radiology* 1992;184: 741-744.
53. Bhisitkul DM, Shkolnik A, Donaldson JS, Henricks BD, Feinstein KA, Fernbach SK, Listernick R. Clinical application of ultrasonography in the diagnosis of intussusception. *J Pediatr* 1992;121:182-186.
54. Shanbhogue RL, Hussain SM, Meradji M, Robben SG, Vernooij JE, Molenaar JC. Ultrasonography is accurate enough for the diagnosis of intussusception. *J Pediatr Surg* 1994;29:324-328.
55. Pracros JP, Tran-Minh VA, Morin de Finfe CH, Deffrenne-Pracros P, Louis D, Basset T. Acute intestinal intussusception in children: contribution of ultrasonography (145 cases). *Ann Radiol* 1987;30:525-530.
56. Swischuk LE, Hayden CK Jr, Boulden T. Intussusception: indications for ultrasonography and an explanation of the doughnut and pseudokidney signs. *Pediatr Radiol* 1985; 15:388-391.
57. Bowerman RA, Silver TM, Jaffe MH. Real-time ultrasound diagnosis of intussusception in children. *Radiology* 1982;143: 527-529.
58. Dinkel E, Dittrich M, Pister K, et al. Sonographic diagnosis of intussusception in childhood. *Z Kinderchild* 1983;38:220-223.
59. Morin ME, Blumenthal DH, Tan A et al. The ultrasonic appearance of ileocolic intussusception. *J Clin Ultrasound* 1981; 10:516-518.
60. Parienty RA, Lepreux JF, Gruson B. Sonographic and CT features of ileocolic intussusception. *AJR* 1981;136:608-610.
61. Del-Pozo G, Albillos JC, Trejedor D. Intussusception US findings with pathologic correlation—the cresence-in-doughnut sign. *Radiology* 1996;199:688-692.
62. Riebel TW, Nasir R, Weber K. US-guided hydrostatic reduction of intussusception in children. *Radiology* 1993;188:513-516.
63. Rohrschneider WK, Troger J. Hydrostatic reduction of intussusception under US guidance. *Pediatr Radiol* 1995;25:530-534.
64. Choi SO, Park WH, Woo SK. Ultrasound-guided water enema: an alternative method of nonoperative treatment for childhood intussusception. *J Pediatr Surg* 1994;29:498.
65. Woo SK, Kim JS, Suh SJ, Paik TW, Choi SO. Childhood intussusception: US-guided hydrostatic reduction. *Radiology* 1992;182:77-80.
66. Carnevale E, Graziani M, Fasanelli S. Postoperative ileo-ileal intussusception: sonographic approach. *Pediatr Radiol* 1994;23:161.
67. Swischuk LE, John S. Spontaneous reduction of intussusception: verification with US. *Radiology* 1994;192:269-271.
68. Swischuk LE, Stansberry SD. Ultrasonographic detection of free peritoneal fluid in uncomplicated intussusception. *Pediatr Radiol* 1991;21:350-351.
69. Feinstein KA, Myers M, Fernbach SK et al. Peritoneal fluid in children with intussusception: its sonographic detection and relationship to successful reduction. *Abdom Imag* 1993; 18:277.
70. Lam AH, Firman K. Value of sonography including color Doppler in the diagnosis and management of longstanding intussusception. *Pediatr Radiol* 1992;22:112-114.
71. Lim HK, Bae SH, Lee KH, Seo GS, Yoon GS. Assessment of reducibility of ileocolic intussusception in children: usefulness of color Doppler sonography. *Radiology* 1994;191:781.

Colon

72. Cremin BJ. The radiologic assessment of anorectal anomalies. *Clin Radiol* 1971;22:239-250.
73. Donaldson JS, Black CT, Reynolds M et al. Ultrasound of the distal pouch in infants with imperforate anus. *J Pediatr Surg* 1989;24:465-468.
74. Oppenheimer DA, Carroll BA, Shochat SJ. Sonography of imperforate anus. *Radiology* 1983;148:127-128.
75. Sata Y, Pringle KC, Bergman RA et al. Congenital anorectal anomalies: MR imaging. *Radiology* 1988;168:157-162.
76. Lim JH, Ko YT, Lee DH et al. Sonography of inflammatory bowel disease: findings and value in differential diagnosis. *AJR* 1994;163:343.
77. Dinkel E, Dittrich M, Peters H et al. Real-time ultrasound in Crohn's disease: characteristic features and clinical implications. *Pediatr Radiol* 1986;16:8-12.
78. Limberg B. Diagnosis of acute ulcerative colitis and colonic Crohn's disease by colonic sonography. *J Clin Ultrasound* 1989;17:25-30.
79. Worliceck H, Lutz H, Heyder N et al. Ultrasound findings in Crohn's disease and ulcerative colitis: prospective study. *J Clin Ultrasound* 1987;15:153-158.
80. Downey DB, Wilson SR. Pseudomembranous colitis: sonographic features. *Radiology* 1991;180:61.
81. Ros PR, Buetow PC, Pantograg-Brown L, Forsmark CE, Sobin LH. Pseudomembranous colitis. *Radiology* 1996;198: 1-9.
82. Alexander JE, Williamson SL, Seibert JJ et al. Ultrasonographic diagnosis of typhlitis (neutropenic colitis). *Pediatr Radiol* 1988;18:200-204.
83. Class-Royal MC, Choyke PL, Gootenberg JE et al. Sonography in the diagnosis of neutropenic colitis. *J Ultrasound Med* 1987;6:671-674.
84. Puylaert JBCM, Lalisang RI, van der Werf SDJ, Doornbos L. Campylobacter ileocolitis mimicking acute appendicitis: differentiation with graded-compression US. *Radiology* 1988; 166:737-740.
85. Matsumoto T, Iida M, Sakai T, Kimura Y, Fujishima M. Yersinia terminal ileitis: sonographic findings in eight patients. *AJR* 1991;156:965-967.
86. Kodroff MB, Hartenberg MA, Goldschmidt RA. Ultrasonographic diagnosis of gangrenous bowel in neonatal necrotizing enterocolitis. *Pediatr Radiol* 1984;14:168-180.

87. Friedland JA, Herman TE, Siegel MJ. *Escherichia coli* 0157:H7-associated hemolytic-uremic syndrome: value of colonic color Doppler sonography. *Pediatr Radiol* 1995; 25:S65-S67.
88. Quillin SP, Siegel MJ. Gastrointestinal inflammation in children: color Doppler ultrasonography. *J Ultrasound Med* 1994;13:751-756.
89. Hu SC, Feeney MS, McNicholas M, O'Halpin D, Fitzgerald FJ. Ultrasonography to diagnose and exclude intussusception in Henoch-Schönlein purpura. *Arch Dis Child* 1991;66:1065-1067.
90. Martinez-Frontanilla LA, Silverman L, Meagher DP Jr. Intussusception in Henoch-Schönlein purpura: diagnosis with ultrasound. *J Pediatr Surg* 1988;23:375-376.
91. Malin SW, Bhutani VK, Ritchie WW, Hall L, Paul D. Echogenic intravascular and hepatic microbubbles associated with necrotizing enterocolitis. *J Pediatr* 1983;103:637-640.
92. Meritt CRB, Goldsmith JP, Shary MJ. Conotraphic detection of portal venous gas in infants with NEC. *AJR* 1984;143: 1059.
93. Avni EF, Rypens F, Cohen E et al. Pericholecystic hyperechogenicities in necrotizing enterocolitis: a specific sonographic sign? *Pediatr Radiol* 1991;21:179-181.
94. Deeg D-H, Rupprecht T, Schmid E. Doppler sonographic detection of increased flow velocities in the celiac trunk and superior mesenteric artery in infants with necrotizing enterocolitis. *Pediatr Radiol* 1993;23:578.
95. Miller SF, Seibert JJ, Kinder DL, Wilson AR. Use of ultrasound in the detection of occult bowel perforation in neonates. *J Ultrasound Med* 1993;12:531-535.
96. Abu-Yousef MM, Bleicher JJ, Maher JW et al. High-resolution sonography of acute appendicitis. *AJR* 1987;149:53-58.
97. Ramachandran P, Sivit CJ, Newman KD, Schwartz MZ. Ultrasonography as an adjunct in the diagnosis of acute appendicitis: a 4-year experience. *J Pediatr Surg* 1996;31:164-169.
98. Vignault F, Ilitarault D, Brandt ML et al. Acute appendicitis in children: evaluation with US. *Radiology* 1990;176:501-504.
99. Rubin SZ, Martin DJ. Ultrasonography in the management of possible appendicitis in childhood. *J Pediatr Surg* 1990;25: 737-740.
100. Sivit CJ, Newman KD, Boenning DA, Nussbaum-Blask AR, Bulas DI, Bond SJ, Attorri R, Rebolo LC, Brown-Jones C, Garin DB. Appendicitis: usefulness of US in diagnosis in a pediatric population. *Radiology* 1992;185:549-552.
101. Siegel MJ, Carel C, Surratt S. Ultrasonography of acute abdominal pain in children. *JAMA* 1991;266:1087-1089.
102. Kao SC, Smith WL, Abu-Yousef MM et al. Acute appendicitis in children: sonographic findings. *AJR* 1989;153:375-379.
103. Puylaert JBCM. Mesenteric adenitis and acute terminal ileitis: ultrasound evaluation using graded compression. *Radiology* 1986;161:691-695.
104. Hayden CK, Jr. Kuchelmeister J, Lipscomb TS. Sonography of acute appendicitis in childhood: perforation versus nonperforation. *J Ultrasound Med* 1992;11:209.
105. Quillin SP, Siegel MJ, Coffin CM. Acute appendicitis in children: value of sonography in detecting perforation. *AJR* 1992;159:1265-1268.
106. Quillin SP, Siegel MJ. Appendicitis in children: color Doppler sonography. *Radiology* 1992;184:745.
107. Patriquin HB, Garcier J-M, Lafortune M, Yazbeck S, Russo P, Jequier S, Ouimet A, Filiatrault D. Appendicitis in children and young adults: Doppler sonographic-pathologic correlation. *AJR* 1996;166:629-633.
108. Quillin SP, Siegel MJ. Diagnosis of appendiceal abscess in children with acute appendicitis: value of color Doppler sonography. *AJR* 1995;164:1251-1254.
109. Barr LL, Hayden CK Jr, Stansberry SD et al. Enteric duplication cysts in children: are there ultrasonographic wall characteristic diagnostic? *Pediatr Radiol* 1990;20:326-328.
110. Kangarloo H, Sample WF, Hansen G et al. Ultrasonic evaluation of abdominal gastrointestinal tract duplication in children. *Radiology* 1979;131:191-194.
111. Moccia WA, Astacio JE, Kaude JV. Ultrasonographic demonstration of gastric duplication in infancy. *Pediatr Radiol* 1981;11:52-54.
112. Segal SR, Sherman NH, Rosenberg HK, Kirby CL, Caro PA, Bellah RD, Sagerman JE, Horrow MM. Ultrasonographic features of gastrointestinal duplications. *J Ultrasound Med* 1994;13:863-870.
113. Walter DF, Govil S, Korula A, William RR, Chandy G. Pedunculated colonic polyp diagnosed by colonic sonography. *Pediatr Radiol* 1992;22:148-149.
114. Cremin BJ, Brown RA. Carcinoma of the colon: diagnosis by ultrasound and enema. *Pediatr Radiol* 1987;17:319-320.
115. Schneider K, Dickerhoff R, Bertele RM. Malignant gastric sarcoma: diagnosis by ultrasound and endoscopy. *Pediatr Radiol* 1983;16:69-70.
116. Weinberg B, Rao PS, Shah KD. Ultrasound demonstration of an intramural leiomyoma of the gastric cardia with pathologic correlation. *J Clin Ultrasound* 1988;16:580-584.
117. Park JM, Yeon KM, Han MC, Kim IO, Choi BI. Diffuse intestinal arteriovenous malformation in a child. *Pediatr Radiol* 1991;21:314-315.
118. Bowen A, Ros PR, McCarthy MJ et al. Gastrointestinal teratomas: CT and US appearance with pathologic correlation. *Radiology* 1987;162:431-433.
119. Prieto ML, Casanova A, Delgado J et al. Cystic teratoma of the mesentery. *Pediatr Radiol* 1989;19:439.
120. Shah RS, Kaddu SJ, Kirtane JM. Benign mature teratoma of the large bowel: a case report. *J Pediatr Surg* 1996;31:701-702.
121. Steyaert H, Guitard J, Moscovivi J, Juricic M, Vaysse P, Jeskiewenski S. Abdominal cystic lymphangioma in children: benign lesions that can have a proliferative course. *J Pediatr Surg* 1996;31:677-680.
122. McCullagh M, Keen C, Dykes E. Cystic mesothelioma of the peritoneum: a rare cause of ascites in children. *J Pediatr Surg* 1994;29:1205-1207.

Pancreas

123. Coleman BG, Arger PH, Rosenberg HD et al. Gray-scale sonographic assessment of pancreatitis in children. *Radiology* 1983;146:145-155.
124. Fleischer AC, Parker P, Kirchner SG et al. Sonographic findings of pancreatitis in children. *Radiology* 1983;146:151-155.
125. Siegel MJ, Martin KW, Worthington JL. Normal and abnormal pancreas in children: US studies. *Radiology* 1987; 165:15-18.
126. Swischuk LE, Hayden CK Jr. Pararenal space hyperechogenicity in childhood pancreatitis. *AJR* 1985;145:1985-1986.
127. Slovis TL, VonBerg VJ, Mikelic V. Sonography in the diagnosis and management of pancreatic pseudocysts and effusions in childhood. *Radiology* 1980;135:153-155.
128. Criado E, De Stefano AA, Weiner TM et al. Long-term results of percutaneous catheter drainage of pancreatic pseudocysts. *Surg Gynecol Obstet* 1992;175:293-298.

129. Daneman A, Gaskin K, Martin DJ et al. Pancreatic changes in cystic fibrosis: CT and sonographic appearance. *AJR* 1983; 141:653-655.
130. Phillips HE, Cox KL, Reid MH et al. Pancreatic sonography in cystic fibrosis. *AJR* 1981;137:69-72.
131. Willi UV, Reddishm JM, Teele RL. Cystic fibrosis: its characteristic appearance on abdominal sonography. *AJR* 1980; 134:1005-1010.
132. Berrocal T, Prieto C, Pastor I, Gutierrez J, Al-Assir I. Sonography of pancreatic disease in infants and children. *RadioGraphics* 1995;15:301-313.
133. Hayden CK Jr, Siwschuk LE. *Pediatric Sonography*, 2nd ed. Baltimore: Williams & Wilkins; 1992:263.
134. Poustchi-Amin M, Leonidas JC, Valderrama E, Shende A, Paley C, Lanzkowsky P, Kutin N. Papillary-cystic neoplasm of the pancreas. *Pediatr Radiol* 1995;25:509-511.
135. Ward HC, Leake J, Spitz L. Papillary cystic cancer of the pancreas: diagnostic difficulties. *J Pediatr Surg* 1993; 28:89-91.
136. Auringer ST, Ulmer JL, Summer TE, Turner CS. Congenital cyst of the pancreas. *J Pediatr Surg* 1993;28:1570-1571.
137. Crowley JJ, McAlister WH. Congenital pancreatic pseudocyst: a rare cause of abdominal mass in neonate, report of two cases. *Pediatr Radiol* 1996;26:210-211.

CHAPTER 61

The Pediatric Pelvis

Henrietta Kotlus Rosenberg, M.D., F.A.C.R., F.A.A.P.
Cheryl L. Kirby, M.D.
Nancy H. Sherman, M.D.*

CHAPTER OUTLINE

*With great sadness, love, and respect, I dedicate this chapter to the memory of my dear friend and colleague, Nancy H. Sherman, M.D.
—Henrietta Kotlus Rosenberg, M.D.

TECHNIQUE

High-resolution, real-time sonography has become an indispensable imaging modality for the evaluation of the pelvis in infants, children, and adolescents. Using the distended bladder as an acoustic window, the lower urinary tract, uterus, adnexa, prostate gland, seminal vesicles, and pelvic musculature and vessels can be easily evaluated.[1,2]

Depending on the size of the child, a 3-, 5-, or 7.5-MHz real-time phased array or curvilinear broad bandwidth or sector scanhead is used to obtain scans in the transverse and sagittal planes. A 7.5- or 10-MHz transducer is usually necessary in the evaluation of the infant pelvis and scrotum.

Patients should be well hydrated with a full bladder before pelvic sonography. In infants and young children who are unable to maintain a full bladder despite drinking clear liquids, it may be necessary to catheterize and fill the bladder with sterile water via a no. 5 or 8 French feeding tube. The use of sterile water as a contrast agent to outline the vagina (hydrosonovaginography [water vaginography]) (Fig. 61-1), rectum (water enema) (Fig. 61-2),[3] or urogenital sinus may be very helpful in the evaluation of the pediatric patient with a pelvic mass or complex congenital anomalies of the genitourinary tract. Meticulous real-time scanning as these structures are filled retrograde is essential. Transvaginal scanning in mature, sexually active, teenage girls allows the examiner to be more accurate or specific in borderline or unclear transabdominal sonography of the pelvis and thus aids in the elucidation of the origin and characteristics of pelvic masses and complex adnexal lesions.[4]

The urinary bladder should have a smooth, thin wall. In the distended state, bladder wall thickness should measure less than 3 mm, with a mean of 1.5 mm.[5] In the empty or partially distended state, the normal bladder wall may appear thickened (5 mm or less) and irregular along the luminal surface. The distal ureters, with the exception of the submucosal intravesical portion, are not ordinarily visualized unless they are abnormally dilated.[6] The bladder neck and urethra can be demonstrated in both males and females by angling the transducer inferiorly (Fig. 61-3).[7] If a urethral abnormality is noted on suprapubic imaging, scans through the perineum or transrectally can confirm these findings via a different imaging plane.[8] Hydrosonourethrography may be used to detect anterior urethral abnormalities (strictures, calculi, anterior or posterior urethral valves, foreign bodies, bladder neck dyssynergia, diverticula, and trauma) by scanning the penis with a linear array transducer during real-time observation of a retrograde hand injection of saline into the urethra.[9] Postvoid scanning of the bladder can provide information about bladder function, differentiate the bladder from cystic masses or fluid collections in the pelvis, and evaluate the degree of drainage from dilated upper urinary tracts. When children cannot void, films taken after a Credé's maneuver or catheterization give an indication of the effectiveness of these bladder-emptying procedures. The authors measure the postvoid residual using the formula:

$$\text{Length} \times \text{Width} \times \text{Depth (in cm)} \div 2$$

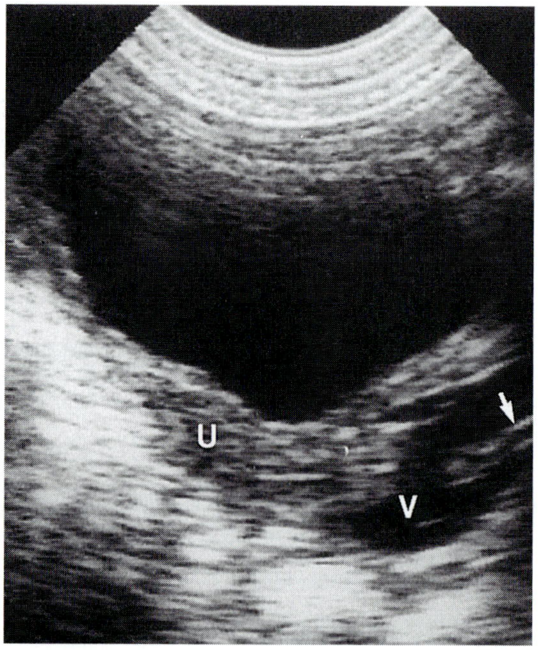

FIG. 61-1. Normal hydrosonovaginography in a prepubertal female. Sagittal sonogram demonstrates a catheter *(arrow)* in a fluid-distended vagina, *V*. A normal prepubertal uterus, *U*, is seen.

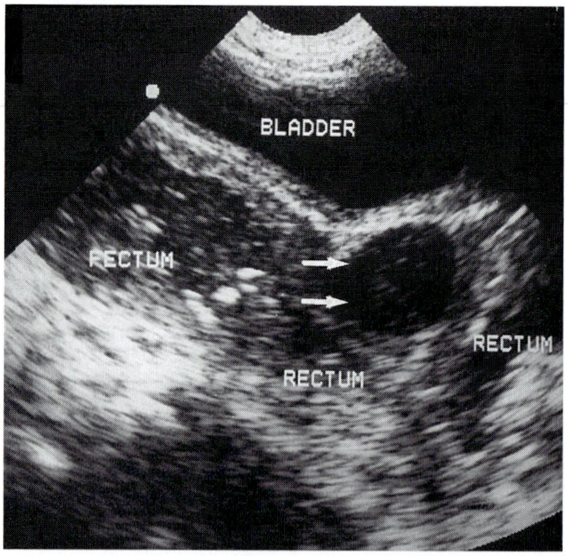

FIG. 61-2. Appendiceal abscess evaluated with water enema technique (5-year-old boy with diarrhea and fever for several days). Sagittal sonogram of a small, hypoechoic fluid collection *(arrows)* located posterior to the bladder and anterior to the water-filled rectum.

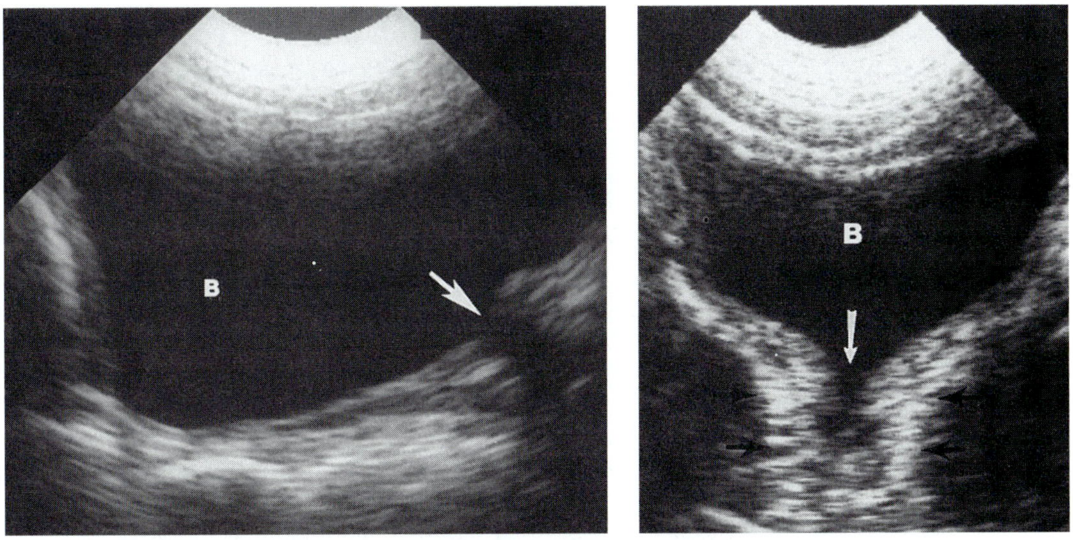

FIG. 61-3. A, Normal female urethra. Using bladder, *B*, as an acoustic window, urethra *(arrow)* may be seen. **B, Normal posterior urethra in young male child.** Transverse scan through moderately distended bladder, *B*, shows posterior urethra *(white arrow)* and prostate gland *(black arrows)* surrounding the urethra. (From Bush WH. *Urologic Imaging and Interventional Techniques*. Baltimore: Urban & Schwarzenberg; 1989.)

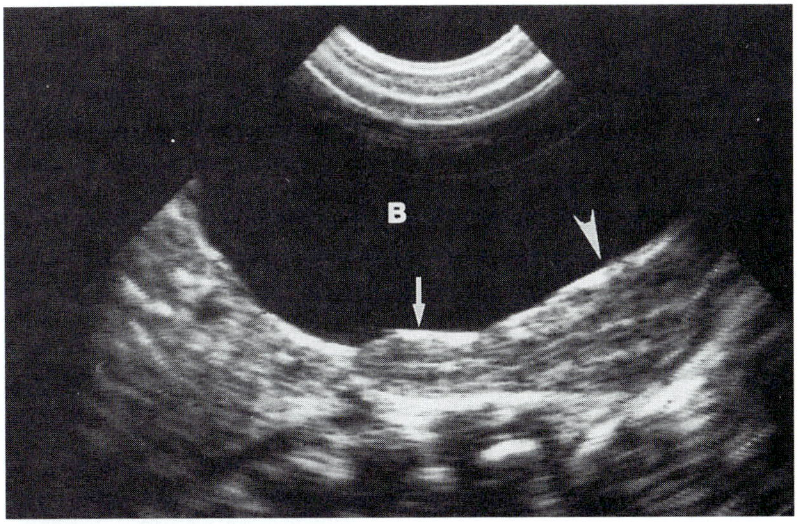

FIG. 61-4. Normal newborn uterus. Sagittal view shows the ratio of fundus *(white arrow)* to cervix *(white arrowhead)* length is 1:2, and thick endometrial lining is prominently echogenic as a result of *in utero* hormonal stimulation. *B*, Bladder. (From Bush WH. *Urologic Imaging and Interventional Techniques*. Baltimore: Urban & Schwarzenberg; 1989.)

NORMAL ANATOMY

The Uterus

The uterus and ovaries undergo a series of changes in size and configuration during normal growth and development.[10,11] In the newborn female, the uterus is prominent and thickened with a brightly echogenic endometrial lining caused by the *in utero* hormonal stimulation (Fig. 61-4).[12] The uterine configuration is spade-shaped, and the length is approximately 3.5 cm, with a fundus-to-cervix ratio of 1:2. At 2 to 3 months of age, the uterus regresses to a prepubertal size and tubular configuration (Fig. 61-5), with the length measuring 2.5 to 3 cm, the fundus-to-cervix ratio 1:1, and the endometrial stripe echoes are usually not visualized. This uterine configuration is maintained until puberty, at which time the uterine length gradually increases to 5 to 7 cm and the fundus-to-cervix ratio becomes 3:1 (Table 61-1).[10,12,13] The echogenicity and thickness of the endometrial lining then vary according to the phase of the menstrual cycle, as they do in adult women. The uterus is supplied by bilateral uterine arteries, which are

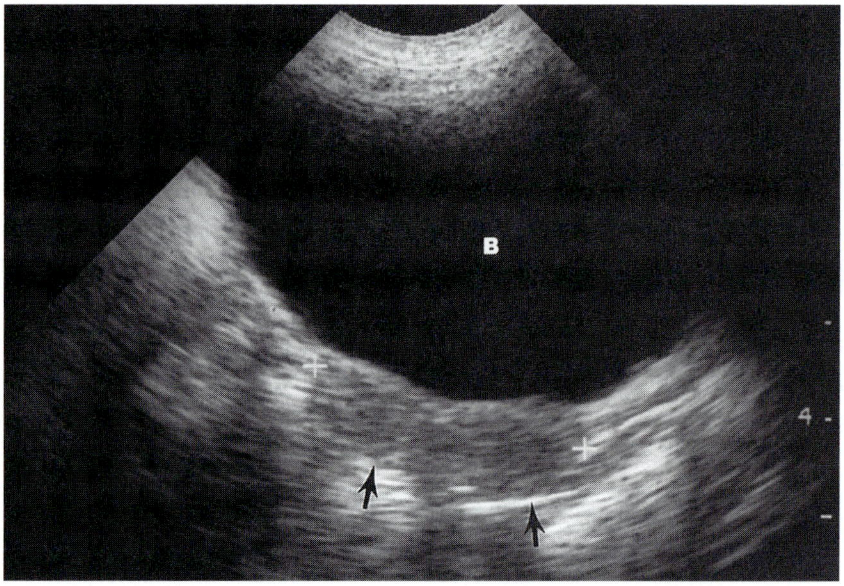

FIG. 61-5. Normal prepubertal uterus in a 2-year-old female. Sagittal sonogram through the bladder shows the uterus devoid of an endometrial stripe and a fundus-to-cervix ratio of 1:1.

TABLE 61-1
PEDIATRIC UTERINE MEASUREMENTS

Age	Uterine Length	Fundus-to-Cervix Ratio
Newborn	3.5 cm	1:2
Prepubertal*	2.5–3 cm	1:1
Postpubertal	5–8 cm	3:1

*Beginning at age 2 to 3 months.
Data from Comstock CH, Boal DK. Pelvic sonography of the pediatric patient. *Semin Ultrasound* 1984;5:54-67; Rosenberg HK. Sonography of the pediatric urinary tract. In: Bush WH, ed. *Urologic Imaging and Interventional Techniques.* Baltimore: Urban & Schwarzenberg; 1989:164-179.

branches of the internal iliac arteries. Color flow Doppler imaging generally demonstrates flow in the myometrium, with little or no flow in the endometrium.[14]

The Vagina

In children, digital and visual examination of the vagina is difficult. Often, physical examination of the vagina is performed under general anesthesia. High-resolution, real-time sonography can now obviate this need in many cases. In the infant or young girl presenting with an interlabial mass, sonography in conjunction with other imaging modalities can usually determine the cause.[15] The vagina is best visualized on midline longitudinal scans through the distended bladder. It appears as a long, tubular structure in continuity with the uterine cervix. The apposed mucosal surfaces cause a bright central echo. Hydrosonovaginography (water vaginography) under real-time sonography guidance can provide additional information about vaginal patency or confirm the presence or absence of a vaginal mass.

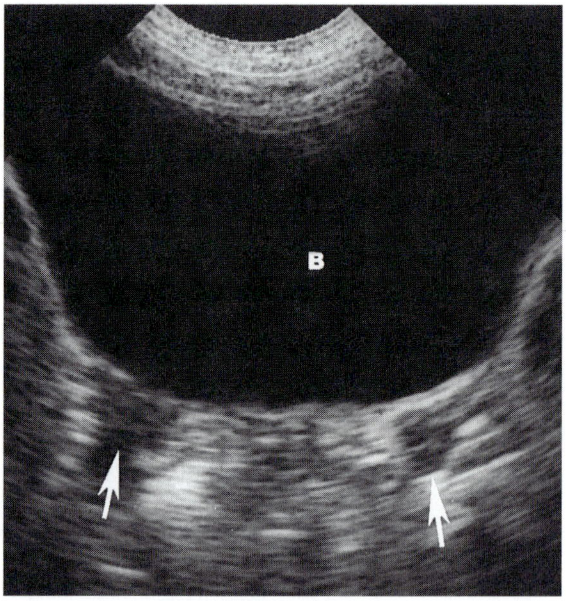

FIG. 61-6. Normal ovaries in a 2-year-old child. Ovaries *(arrows)* are small (less than 1 cm) in this young child transverse view. *B*, Bladder.

The Ovary

Sonographic visualization of the ovaries in children can be variable, depending on their location, size, and the age of the patient (Fig. 61-6). Because of a generally long pedicle and a small pelvis, the neonatal ovaries may be found anywhere between the lower pole of the kidneys and the true pelvis. Ovarian size is

TABLE 61-2
PEDIATRIC OVARIAN VOLUME MEASUREMENTS[17-19]

	Age	Mean Ovarian Volume cm^3 (+SD)
Premenarchal		
	0–5 yr	**≤1 cm^3**
	1 day–3 mo	1.06 (±0.96)
	4–12 mo	1.05 (±0.67)
	13–24 mo	0.67 (±0.35)
	3 yr	0.7 (±0.4)
	4 yr	0.8 (±0.4)
	5 yr	0.9 (±0.02)
	6–8 yr	**1.2 cm^3**
	6 yr	1.2 (±0.4)
	7 yr	1.3 (±0.6)
	8 yr	1.1 (±0.5)
	9–10 yr*	**2.1 cm^3**
	9 yr	2.0 (±0.8)
	10 yr	2.2 (±0.7)
	11 yr*	**2.5 cm^3 (±1.3)**
	12 yr*	**3.8 cm^3 (±1.4)**
	13 yr*	**4.2 cm^3 (±2.3)**
Menstrual		**9.8 cm^3 (±5.8)**

*Note that these measurements may differ, depending on degree of maturation and presence of menarche.
From Cohen HL, Shapiro MA, Mandel FS et al. Normal ovaries in neonates and infants: a sonographic study of 77 patients 1 day to 24 months old. *AJR* 1993;160:583-586. Also from references 18 and 19.

most reproducible and best described by measurement of the ovarian volume, which is calculated by a simplified prolate ellipse formula:

Length × Depth × Width × 0.523[16]

The mean ovarian volumes in neonates and girls of less than 6 years of age is usually less than or equal to 1 cm^3.[17] Ovarian volume gradually begins to increase at approximately age 6.[18] The mean ovarian volume measurement in premenarchal girls between ages 6 and 11 years ranges between 1.2 cm^3 and 2.5 cm^3 (Table 61-2).[18] There is marked enlargement in ovarian size postpuberty; thus ovarian sizes in menstruating females in late childhood will be larger than their premenarchal counterparts. Cohen et al. reported a mean ovarian volume of 9.8 cm^3 with a 95% confidence interval between 2.5 cm^3 and 21.9 cm^3 in menstruating females.[19]

Beginning in the neonatal period, the appearance of the typical ovary is heterogeneous secondary to small cysts. Cohen et al. reported observing ovarian cysts in 84% of children 1 day to 2 years of age and 68% of children 2 to 12 years of age. Macrocysts (cysts measuring greater than 9 mm) were more frequently seen in the ovaries of girls in their first year of life compared with those in their second year,

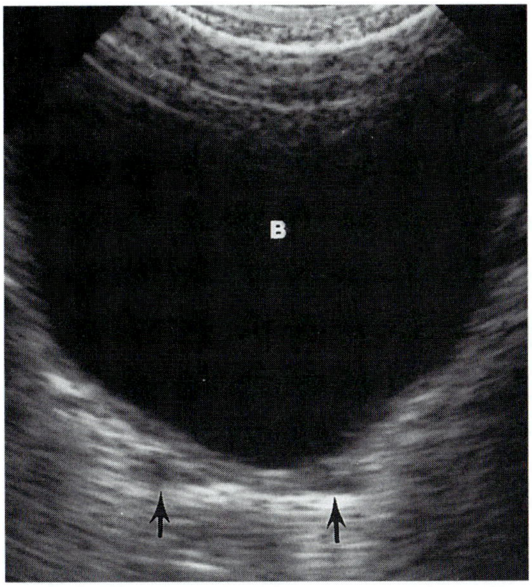

FIG. 61-7. Seminal vesicles. Through a well-distended bladder, *B*, the seminal vesicles *(arrows)* are seen as hypoechoic, bilaterally symmetric structures.

which probably accounts for the larger mean and top-normal ovarian volume measurements obtained in girls 0 to 3 months of age (mean ovarian volume of 1.06 cm^3 with range of 0.7 to 3.6 cm^3) versus those 13 to 24 months of age (mean ovarian volume 0.67 cm^3 with a range of 0.1 to 1.7 cm^3).[17] These findings are probably secondary to the higher residual maternal hormone level in younger infants. The blood supply of the ovary is dual, arising from the ovarian artery, which originates directly from the aorta, and from the uterine artery, which supplies an adnexal branch to each ovary.[14] Blood flow can be seen in 90% of the adolescent ovary, but Doppler imaging cannot distinguish between the two blood supplies. Typically, on color flow Doppler imaging, the intraovarian arteries appear as short, straight branches located centrally within the normal ovary.[20]

The Prostate

The configuration of the prostate is ellipsoid in boys compared with the more conical shape seen in adults. The prostatic echogenicity is hypoechoic and more homogeneous than in the adult prostate, which is frequently heterogeneous secondary to central gland nodules, calcifications, and corpora amylacea. Prostate volume may be calculated by using the formula for a prolate ellipsoid:

Length × Width × Depth × 0.523

Ingram et al. showed that in a group of 36 boys, aged 7 months to 13.5 years (mean 7.7 years), the prostatic volume ranged between 0.4 ml and 5.2 ml (mean 1.2).[21] The seminal vesicles may be identified in young boys and adolescents (Fig. 61-7) and are best seen in

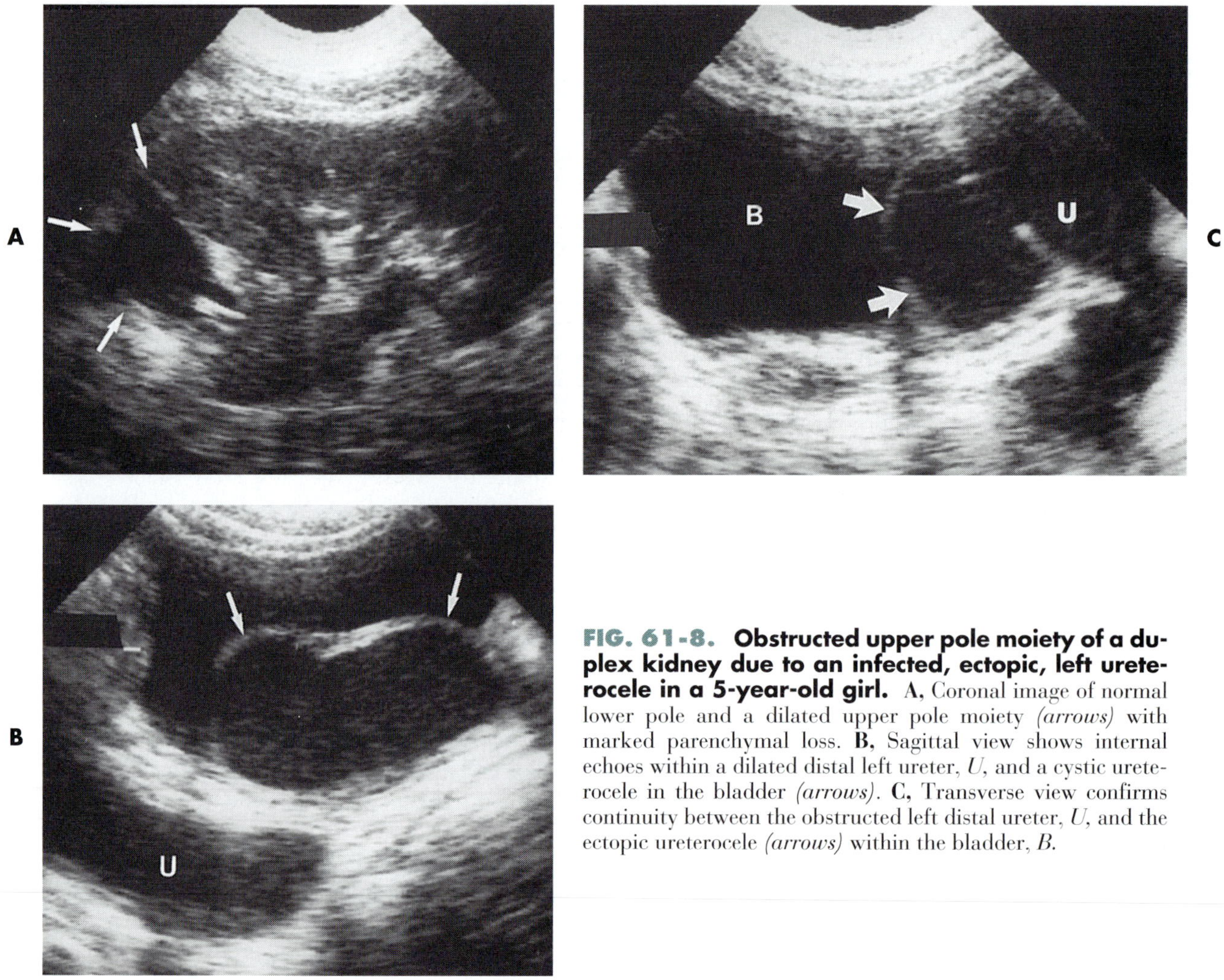

FIG. 61-8. Obstructed upper pole moiety of a duplex kidney due to an infected, ectopic, left ureterocele in a 5-year-old girl. **A,** Coronal image of normal lower pole and a dilated upper pole moiety *(arrows)* with marked parenchymal loss. **B,** Sagittal view shows internal echoes within a dilated distal left ureter, *U*, and a cystic ureterocele in the bladder *(arrows)*. **C,** Transverse view confirms continuity between the obstructed left distal ureter, *U*, and the ectopic ureterocele *(arrows)* within the bladder, *B*.

the transverse plane as small, hypoechoic structures giving an appearance similar to a seagull's wings.

LOWER URINARY TRACT

Congenital Anomalies

Duplication anomalies of the collecting systems and ureters are the most common congenital anomaly of the urinary tract. In complete ureteral duplication, the lower ureter inserts orthotopically into the trigone, often resulting in vesicoureteral reflux. The upper pole ureter usually inserts ectopically in the bladder (at the bladder neck) or in the trigone (inferomedial to the normal location). It can also insert into the urethra, vagina, or uterus in girls, resulting in urinary dribbling. In boys, the ectopic ureter can insert in the proximal urethra, seminal vesicle, vas deferens, or ejaculatory duct. Urinary incontinence is not a presenting symptom in boys because the ectopic insertion is always proximal to the external sphincter. Duplication anomalies are often asymptomatic; urinary tract infection is the most common initial presentation.[22] The upper pole moiety often becomes obstructed as a result of an **ectopic ureterocele.** Sonography demonstrates a dilated upper pole collecting system and ureter that ends distally as a well-defined, thin-walled cystic protuberance into the bladder base (Fig. 61-8). The lower pole system is often dilated secondary to reflux.[23,24] Less commonly, the lower pole moiety may be dilated as a result of obstruction of the ureteral orifice by the adjacent ectopic ureterocele. Ten to twenty percent of ectopic ureters are associated with a single collecting system (Fig. 61-9). The renal parenchyma associated with an ectopic ureter is often dysplastic (e.g., echogenic parenchyma, loss of corticomedullary junction, and variable-sized cysts).

Posterior urethral valves are a common cause of urinary tract obstruction (see box). Signs and symptoms at presentation include palpable flank masses caused by hydronephrosis or urinoma, poor urinary stream, urinary tract infection, and failure to thrive.

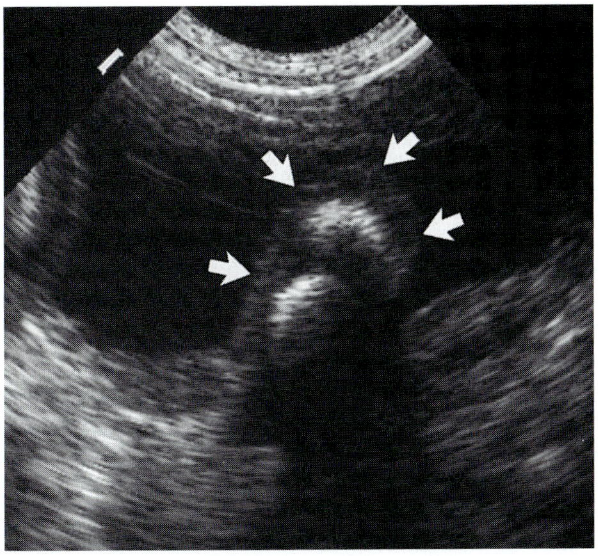

FIG. 61-9. Simple ureterocele with stones in a 7-year-old with recent mild trauma. Sagittal view of the left side of the bladder demonstrates a simple ureterocele *(arrows)* protruding into the bladder lumen containing two brightly echogenic, shadowing calculi.

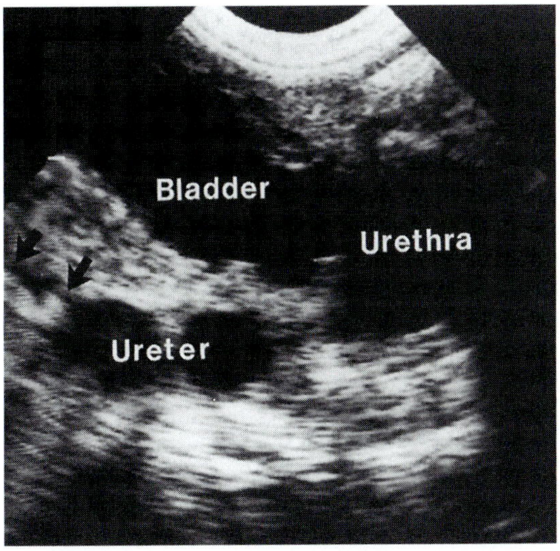

FIG. 61-10. Posterior urethral valves in a newborn boy. Midline sagittal scan shows irregularly thickened bladder wall (caused by obstruction), massively dilated posterior urethra, and moderately dilated tortuous distal ureter. *Arrows*, Serosal surface of the bladder wall. (From Rosenberg HK. Sonography of pediatric urinary tract abnormalities. Pt I. *Am Urol Assoc Weekly Update Series* 1986;35(5):1-8.)

CAUSES OF BLADDER OUTLET OBSTRUCTION

Posterior urethral valves
Prune-belly syndrome
Anterior urethral valves
Urethral duplication
Congenital urethral stricture
Anterior urethral diverticulum
Posterior urethral polyp

On sonography, the bladder has a thick, trabeculated wall, and the posterior urethra is dilated (Fig. 61-10).[2,8,25-27] There may be marked hydronephrosis with dilated, tortuous ureters secondary to vesicoureteral reflux. Occasionally, the reflux is unilateral, resulting in ipsilateral hydroureteronephrosis. The renal parenchymal echogenicity may be abnormally increased as a result of long-standing reflux or obstructive nephropathy. In many infants with posterior urethral valves, there is associated renal dysplasia manifested sonographically as brightly echogenic kidneys usually devoid of corticomedullary differentiation and often containing tiny cysts.[28] The appearance of the renal parenchyma has predictive value in infants with posterior urethral valves in regard to potential renal function.[29]

The **prune-belly syndrome** (abdominal muscle deficiency syndrome; Eagle-Barrett syndrome) is another common cause of urinary tract obstruction in infant boys. The syndrome is composed of a triad of absent abdominal musculature, bilateral hydroureteronephrosis, and cryptorchidism. There are three forms of urinary tract abnormality. In the most severe form, urethral atresia and renal dysplasia are present; these children have a very poor prognosis and die in infancy. Associated congenital anomalies are frequent and include intestinal malrotation or atresia, imperforate anus, Hirschsprung's disease, congenital heart defects, skeletal anomalies, and cystic adenomatoid malformation of the lung. In the less severe form of urinary tract abnormality, the bladder is large and atonic, and there is bilateral hydroureteronephrosis, impaired renal function, and no urethral obstruction. The changes are thought to be due to a neurogenic dysfunction rather than a mechanical obstruction. There are usually no associated congenital anomalies, and these infants have a better prognosis.[30,31] In the mildest type of prune-belly syndrome, the urinary tract is only mildly affected.

Other uncommon forms of bladder outlet obstruction include **anterior urethral valves, urethral duplication, congenital urethral stricture, anterior urethral diverticulum, posterior urethral polyp** (Fig. 61-11),[32] and **stones** (Fig. 61-12).[33] Voiding cystourethrography (VCUG), in addition to sonography, is usually necessary to identify the above entities.

The Ureter. Normally, the ureters cannot be visualized on ultrasound unless they are dilated. Real-time sonography can sometimes differentiate between

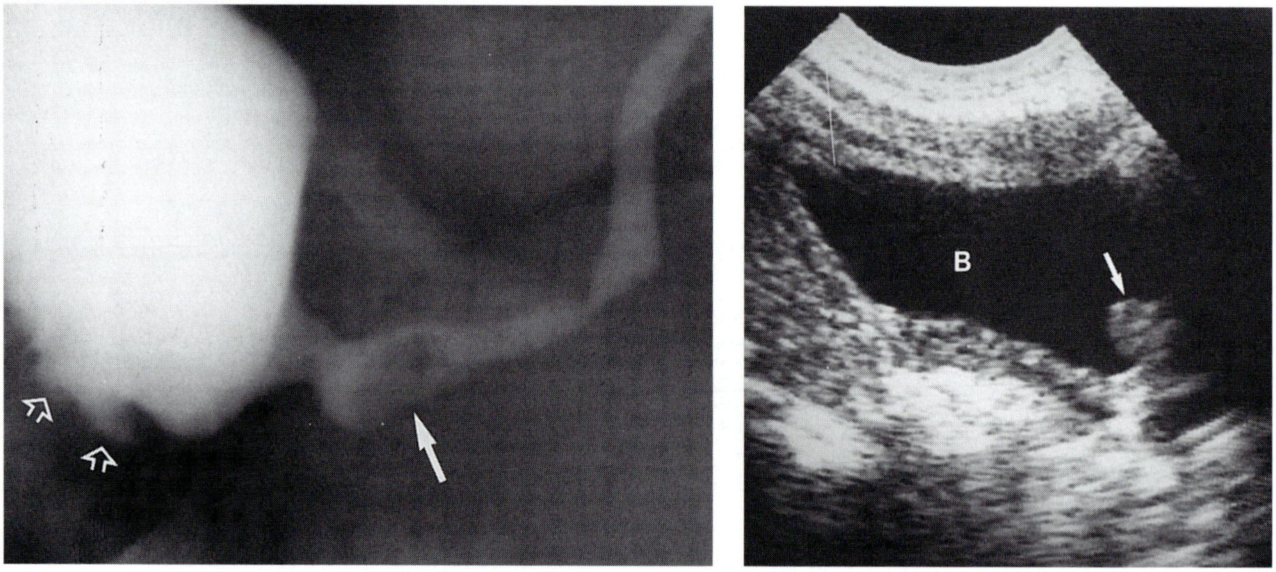

FIG. 61-11. Congenital urethral polyp that caused prenatal hydroureteronephrosis in a newborn boy. **A,** VCUG demonstrates an oval, polypoid mass in the posterior urethra *(solid arrow)* and posterior bladder wall thickening *(open arrows).* **B,** Sagittal sonogram of the bladder 4 months later shows a solid polypoid mass protruding from the bladder neck into the bladder lumen. (From Caro PA, Rosenberg HK, Snyder HM. Congenital urethral polyp. *AJR* 1986;147:1041-1042.)

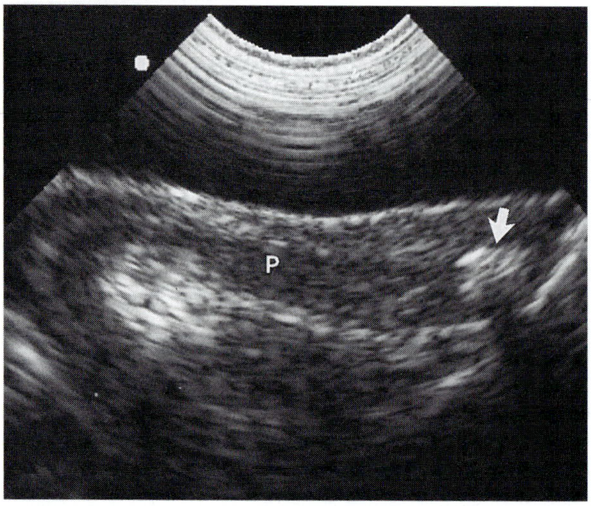

FIG. 61-12. Urethral stone in fossa navicularis. A 6-year-old boy with gross hematuria, dysuria, and suprapubic pain. Sagittal image of penis, *p,* via a stepoff pad, reveals a 7-mm calculus *(arrow)* in the distal urethra.

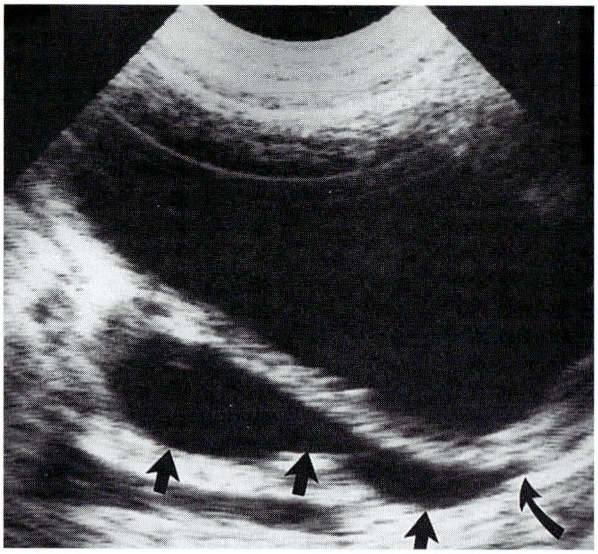

FIG. 61-13. Congenital ureterovesical junction (UVJ) obstruction in an infant with a urinary tract infection. Sagittal sonogram of the bladder shows the dilated ureter *(straight arrows)*, which tapers inferiorly at the UVJ *(curved arrow).*

mechanical obstruction and vesicoureteral reflux. In ureterovesical junction obstruction, the distal ureter is dilated but may taper, thus being difficult to visualize at the level of the bladder trigone, and at times ureteral peristalsis is absent (Fig. 61-13). With vesicoureteral reflux, the dilated distal ureter has a gaping or patulous insertion at the bladder, and active ureteral peristalsis is demonstrated (Fig. 61-14).[34,35]

In patients with a dilated tubular structure posterior to the bladder, duplex and/or color flow Doppler ultrasound can be used to differentiate between a ureter, artery, and vein. In addition, color flow Doppler ultrasonography allows reliable visualization of the ureteric jet phenomenon.[36] Marshall et al. noted that the distance

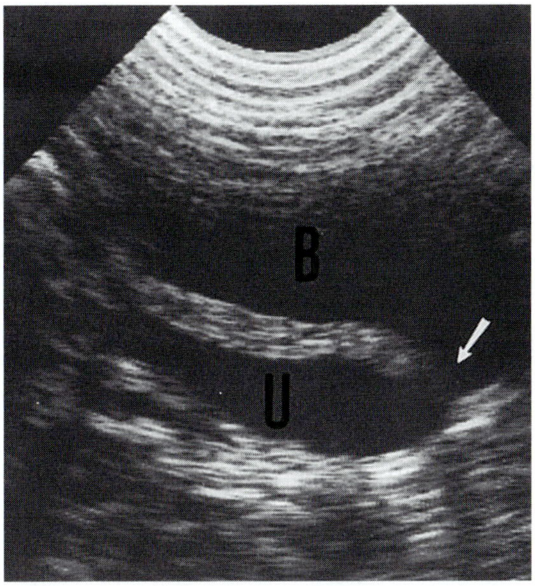

FIG. 61-14. Vesicoureteral reflux. Moderately distended ureter, *U*, can be traced to patulous ureterovesical junction (*arrow*). *B*, Bladder. (From Sherman NH, Boyle GK, Rosenberg HK. Sonography in the neonate. *Ultrasound Q* 1988;6:91-150.)

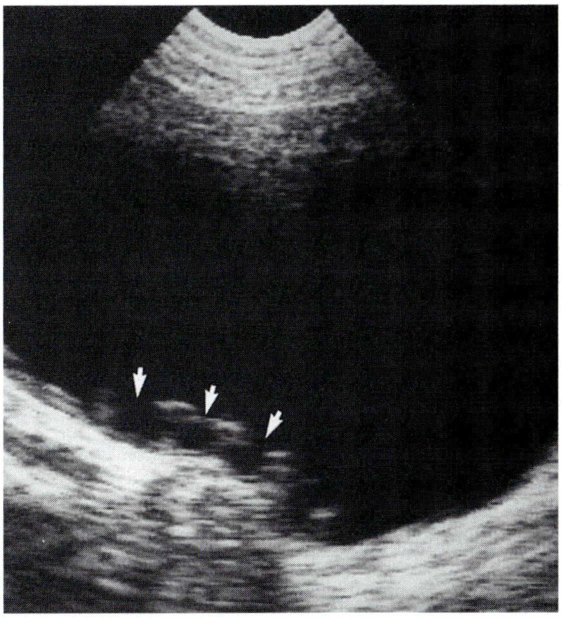

FIG. 61-15. Neurogenic bladder in a 14-year-old boy with spina bifida. Sagittal view of an overdistended bladder demonstrates multiple small diverticula *(arrows)*. (From Sherman NH, Rosenberg HK. Pediatric pelvic sonography. In: Fisher MR, Kricun ME, eds. *Imaging of the Pelvis*. Gaithersburg, MD: Aspen Publishers, 1989.)

of the ureteric orifice from the midline of the bladder was found to correlate with vesicoureteric reflux when the mean distance was 10.25 mm ± 2.40 SD.[36] Jequier et al. used color flow Doppler imaging to show that the duration of the ureteric jet varied from 0.4 sec to 7.5 sec and depended largely on fluid intake, that the direction of the normal jet was anteromedial and upward, that jets from refluxing ureters could appear normal, and that Doppler analyses of the ureteric jet do not allow either the diagnosis or exclusion of vesicoureteral reflux.[37]

The Bladder. Urinary tract sonography has become a routine screening procedure in children with **neurogenic or dysfunctional bladders.** The most common cause of neurogenic bladder in children is myelomeningocele. Other acquired forms of dysfunctional bladder include traumatic paraplegia, cerebral palsy, spinal cord tumor, and encephalitis or transverse myelitis. These children have a higher incidence of urinary tract infection, bladder stones, and reflux. Sonography of a neurogenic bladder demonstrates an irregularly thickened, trabeculated bladder wall, often with multiple diverticula (Fig. 61-15).[38] Echogenic material within the bladder lumen may represent complications of infection, hemorrhage, or stone formation. Ultrasound can also be used to assess the patient's ability to empty the bladder spontaneously or following Crede's maneuvers or catheterization. Residual urine volumes can be estimated as previously described.[39]

Urachal anomalies can be identified on ultrasound when there is persistence of the embryonic tract between the dome of the bladder and umbilicus. Cacciarelli et al. identified a normal urachal remnant in 62% of bladder sonograms in children.[40] A normal urachal remnant appears as a small (not > 6.2 mm depth × 13 mm length × 11.8 mm width), elliptical, hypoechoic structure located posterior to the rectus abdominis muscle and on the midanterosuperior surface of the distended bladder. There are four types of urachal anomalies: patent urachus (completely open urachal lumen associated with urinary drainage from the umbilicus), urachal sinus (opening to the umbilicus), urachal diverticulum (opening to the bladder), and urachal cyst (urachus obliterated at both ends with extraperitoneal position of isolated cyst) (Fig. 61-16, *A*). Two sonographic patterns have been described in urachal anomalies: (1) a cystic mass, often with internal echoes or septations caused by infection, and (2) an echogenic, thickened, tubular sinus tract (8 to 15 mm in diameter) (Fig. 61-16, *B*).[41]

Other anomalies of the lower urinary tract that can be identified on ultrasound include **ectopic pelvic kidney, seminal vesicle cysts, müllerian duct (prostatic utricle) cysts** (Fig. 61-17), and congenital or acquired **bladder diverticula** (Fig. 61-18).[42,43]

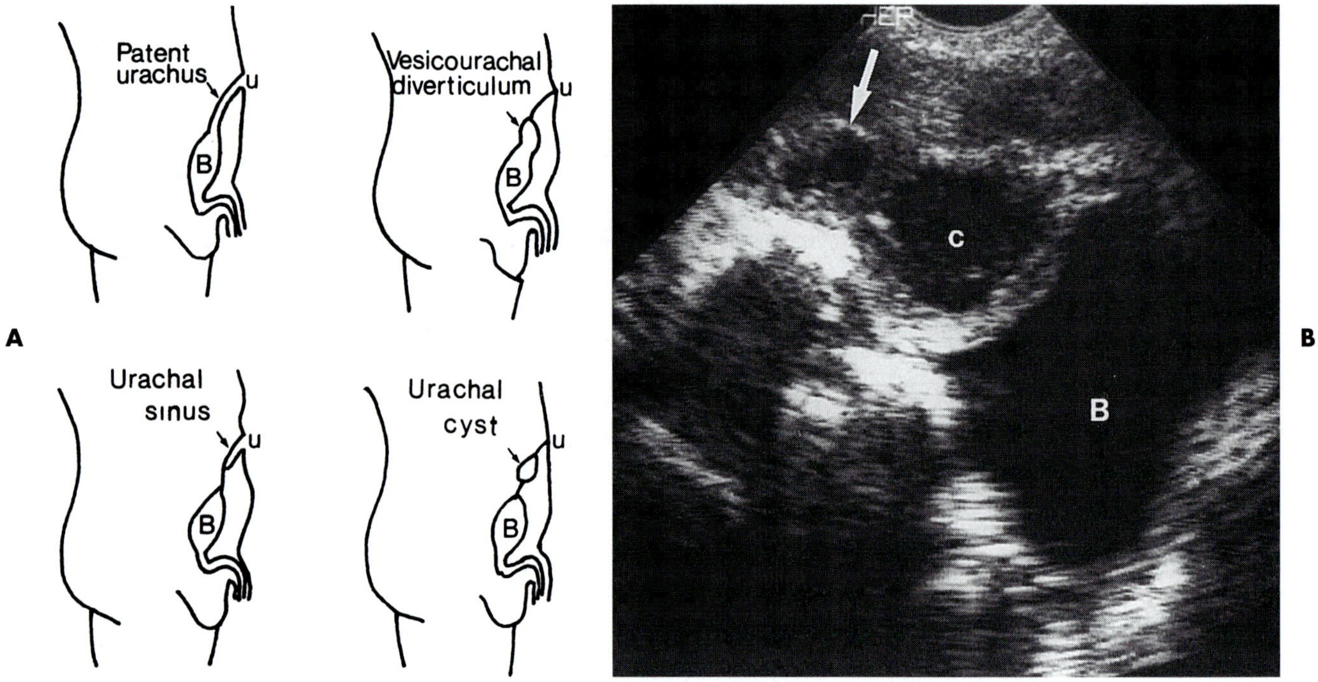

FIG. 61-16. A, Types of urachal abnormalities. Patent urachus (urachal lumen communicates with both the umbilicus and the bladder); vesicourachal diverticulum (urachal lumen communicates only with the bladder); urachal sinus (urachal lumen communicates only with the umbilicus); and urachal cyst (does not communicate with either the bladder or the umbilicus). **B, Infected urachal cyst.** This 6-year-old boy presented with lower abdominal pain, fever, intermittent diarrhea, polyuria, and dysuria. Sagittal midline scan of pelvis shows thick-walled cystic lesion, *C*, above bladder dome, *B*, containing internal echoes caused by infectious debris. Smaller hypoechoic area more superior *(arrow)* was caused by necrotic adenopathy. (**A** from Boyle G, Rosenberg HK, O'Neill J. An unusual presentation of an infected urachal cyst: review of urachal anomalies. *Clin Pediatr* 1988;27:130-134.)

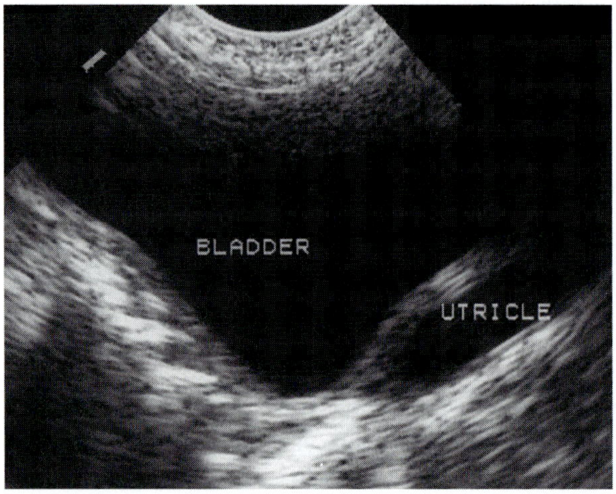

FIG. 61-17. Utricle in a 4-year-old true hermaphrodite raised as a boy after external genitalia reconstruction. Sagittal view of the bladder reveals a fluid-filled, tubular utricle posterior to the bladder base.

Infection

Urinary tract infections are common in children, especially girls, and are usually the result of cystitis. Clinically, these children may present with urinary frequency, incontinence, dysuria, and/or hematuria.[44-46] The infection is usually bacterial. **Hemorrhagic cystitis** can develop secondary to a viral infection, chemotherapy with cyclophosphamide, or indwelling catheters. Granulomatous cystitis in a patient with chronic granulomatous disease of childhood can be detected on ultrasound.[47] Sonographically, the bladder may appear normal in mild cases of cystitis. More specific signs of cystitis are diffuse or focal bladder wall thickening and irregularity (Fig. 61-19). Echogenic material in the bladder lumen may represent purulent or hemorrhagic urine. Bladder calculi are more common with *Proteus* or *Pseudomonas* infections.[48] With cystitis cystica or cystitis glandularis, rounded, isoechoic or hypoechoic, polypoid lesions may protrude into the lumen, mimicking a bladder tumor (Fig. 61-20). Rosenberg et al. reported that children with hematuria, dysuria, and frequency plus cystographic or sonographic demonstration of a bladder with reduced

A B C

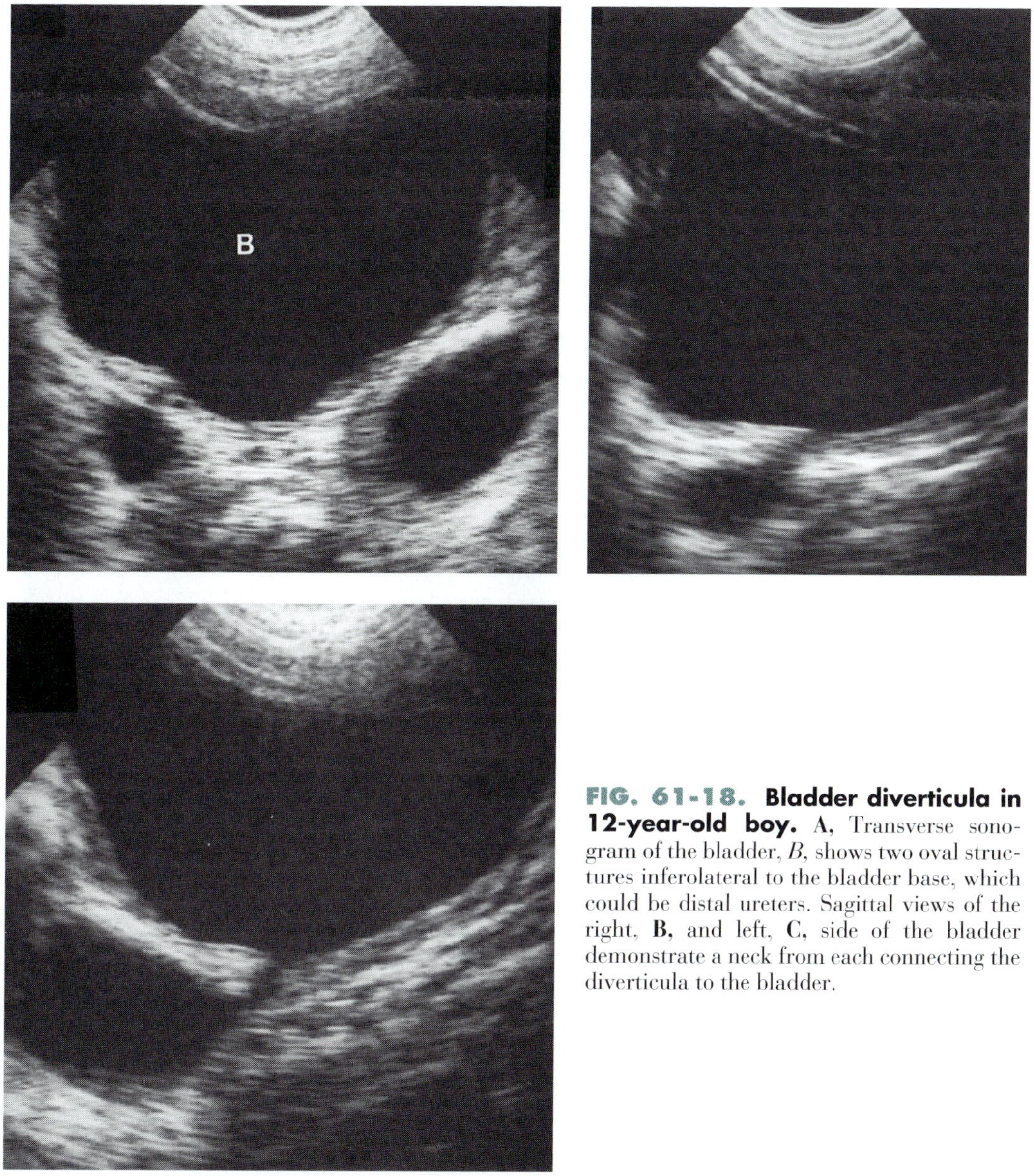

FIG. 61-18. Bladder diverticula in 12-year-old boy. **A,** Transverse sonogram of the bladder, *B*, shows two oval structures inferolateral to the bladder base, which could be distal ureters. Sagittal views of the right, **B,** and left, **C,** side of the bladder demonstrate a neck from each connecting the diverticula to the bladder.

capacity and circumferential wall thickening or sonographic findings of isoechoic bladder wall thickening (focal, multifocal, or circumferential distribution), intact mucosa, and bullous lesions should strongly suggest inflammation and not malignancy. In addition, changing mass contour and thickness with increasing bladder filling are particularly suggestive of inflammatory thickening (Fig. 61-21). When an inflammatory lesion is suspected, follow-up imaging should be performed in 2 weeks, which, if normal, will preclude biopsy.[49]

Neoplasm

Rhabdomyosarcoma is the most common tumor of the lower urinary tract in children. Twenty-one percent of rhabdomyosarcomas arise from the genitourinary tract. The most frequent primary site is the bladder trigone or prostate. Less frequent sites of origin are the seminal vesicles, spermatic cord, vagina, uterus, vulva, pelvic musculature, urachus, and paratesticular area.[50,51] There is a slight male predominance—1.6:1. The peak incidence occurs at 3 to 4 years of age; a second, smaller peak is seen in adolescence. The most common type of cell of rhabdomyosarcoma is the embryonal form, of which sarcoma botryoides is a subtype. The alveolar form is next in frequency; undifferentiated and pleomorphic types are uncommon. Tumors arising from the bladder, prostate, or both usually present early with symptoms from urinary tract obstruction and hema-

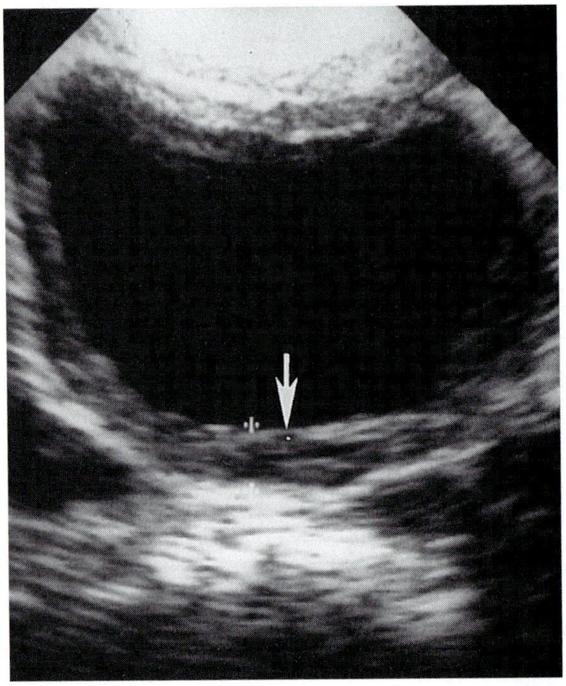

FIG. 61-19. Chronic bacterial cystitis. Transverse sonogram demonstrates diffuse bladder wall thickening *(arrow)*.

A

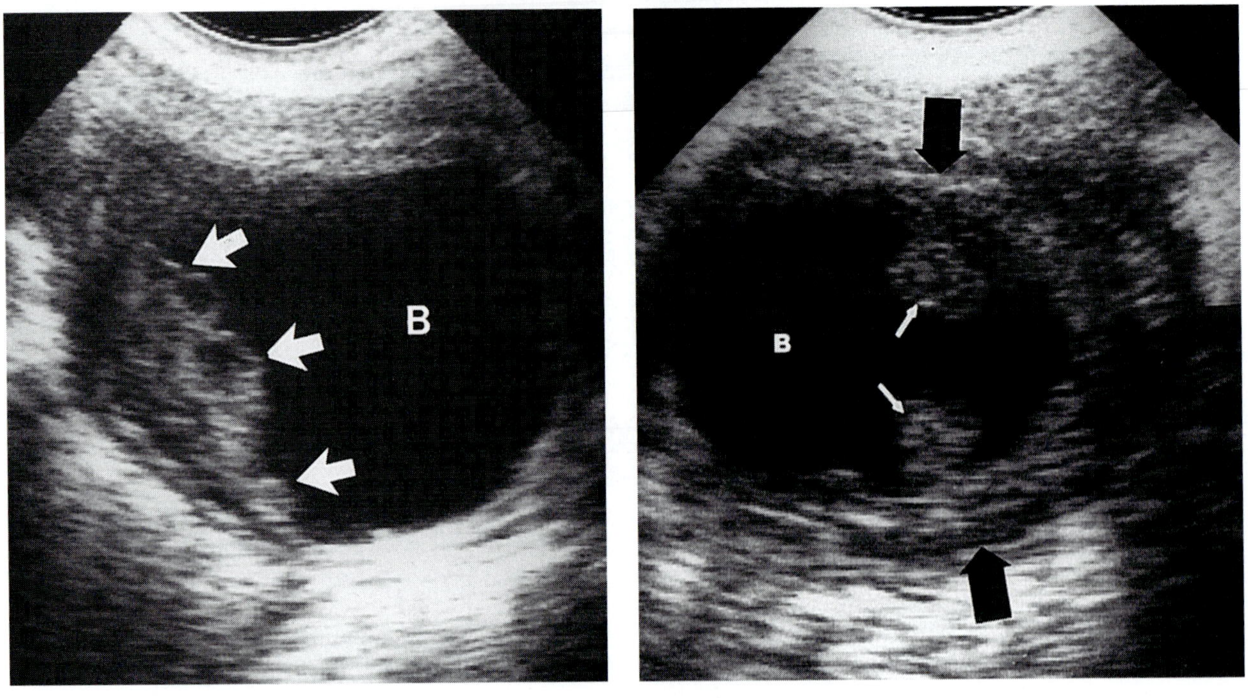

B

FIG. 61-20. A, Bullous, benign cystitis from cytomegalovirus after 24 hours of dysuria and hematuria. Sagittal sonogram of the bladder, *B*, shows a complex mass containing multiple, well-circumscribed, hypoechoic and anechoic, polypoid lesions arising from the dome and projecting into the lumen. **B, Hemorrhagic cystitis.** Transverse view of the bladder, *B*, showing asymmetric bladder wall thickening involving left half of bladder *(large black arrows)* with polypoid-like protrusions of thickened wall *(small white arrows)* into bladder lumen. (From Rosenberg HK, Zerin JM, Eggli KD et al. Benign cystitis in children mimicking rhabdomyosarcoma. *J Ultrasound Med* 1994;13:921-932.)

A

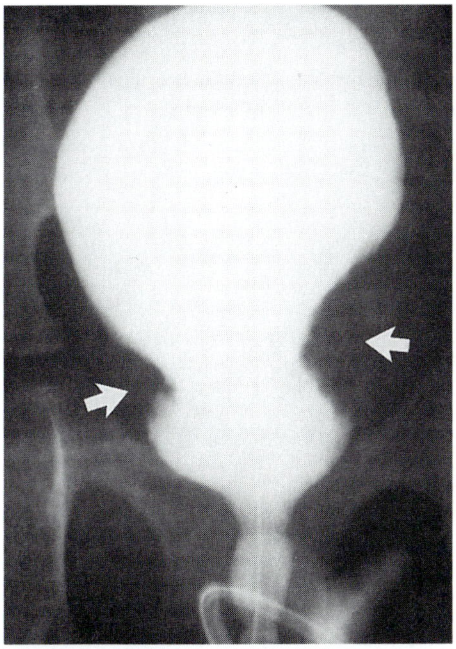

B

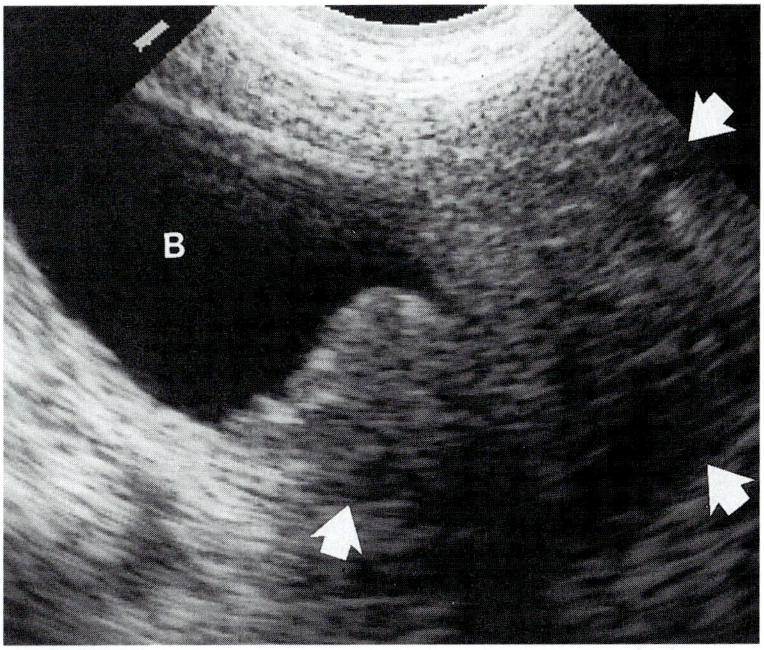

C

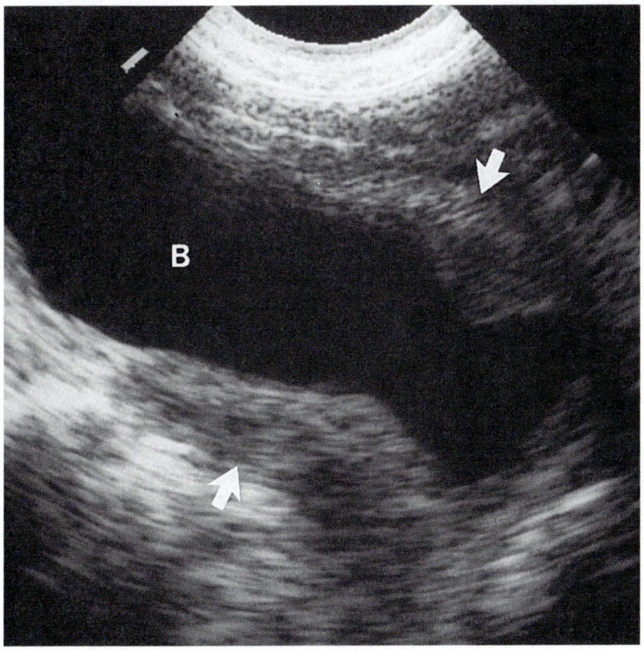

FIG. 61-21. Benign cystitis in a 4-year-old boy presenting with mild dysuria and gross hematuria 8 hours after a fall. Urinalysis showed no white blood cells or bacteria. **A,** Frontal image from a VCUG shows a large mass involving the posterior bladder wall narrowing the bladder circumferentially just above the base *(arrows)*. **B,** Sagittal sonogram with partial bladder, *B*, filling shows tremendous masslike thickening of the posteroinferior bladder walls *(arrows)*. **C,** Sagittal sonogram obtained after further bladder, *B*, filling shows a decrease in the size of the mass *(arrows)* with increased bladder distention. (From Rosenberg HK, Zerin JM, Eggli KD et al. Benign cystitis in children mimicking rhabdomyosarcoma. *J Ultrasound Med* 1994;13:921-932.)

turia. Rhabdomyosarcoma has been reported to be associated with neurofibromatosis, fetal alcohol syndrome, and basal cell nevus syndrome.

On sonographic examination, rhabdomyosarcoma appears as a homogeneous, solid mass with an echotexture similar to muscle. Anechoic spaces caused by necrosis and hemorrhage are occasionally seen (Fig. 61-22). Calcification is very uncommon. Bladder lesions originate in the submucosa, infiltrate the bladder wall, and produce polypoid projections into the lumen (sarcoma botryoides). Tumors arising in the prostate cause concentric or asymmetric enlargement of the prostate and often infiltrate the bladder neck, posterior urethra, and perirectal tissues (Fig. 61-23). Regional and retroperitoneal lymph node metastases are common.[52,53]

Benign tumors of the lower urinary tract are extremely rare. They include transitional cell papilloma (Fig. 61-24), neurofibroma, fibroma, hemangioma, and leiomyoma.[54,55] Neurofibromatosis can be invasive, with diffuse involvement of the pelvic organs.[56] Pheochromocytoma of the bladder is a rare tumor that probably arises in the paraganglia of the visceral (autonomic) nervous system and is located submucosally either in the dome or in the posterior wall close to the trigone. In children, 2% of bladder pheochromocytomas are malignant. Pheochromocytomas can be seen in the context of familial syndromes or diseases, which include neurofibromatosis, Hippel-Lindau disease, Sturge-Weber syndrome, tuberous sclerosis, type A multiple endocrine neoplasia (medullary thyroid carcinoma, hyperparathyroidism), and multiple endocrine neoplasia, type IIB (medullary thyroid carcinoma, mucosal neuromas, and pheochromocytoma). Pheochromocytomas of the bladder may cause headache, blurred vision, diaphoresis, palpitations, intermittent hypertension (70%), and hematuria (6%). Any of these symptoms may be seen with micturition.[57] Benign polyps in the male urethra can arise from a stalk near the verumontanum and cause urinary tract obstruction.

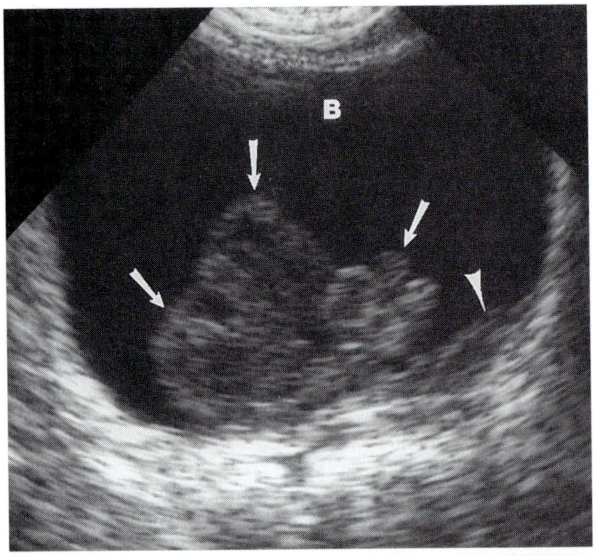

FIG. 61-22. Rhabdomyosarcoma of the bladder wall. Large, complex, polypoid-like mass *(arrows)* arises from base of the bladder, *B*, in this 9-year-old boy with painless hematuria. Asymmetric bladder wall thickening was noted posterolaterally on patient's left *(arrowhead)*.

Trauma

Trauma to the lower urinary tract in children most often is due to blunt trauma. Foreign bodies and complications of surgery are less frequent causes.[58] The bladder in children is in a more intraabdominal position than in adults, and therefore bladder rupture is usually intraperitoneal. Spontaneous bladder rupture is rare in children and is seen primarily in neonates with urinary ascites secondary to urethral obstruction or neurogenic bladder. Preexisting abnormalities of the vesical wall such as tumors, stones, tuberculosis, diverticula, and surgical scars can predispose a child to spontaneous rupture of the bladder.[59] Sonography can demonstrate urinary ascites in cases of intraperitoneal rupture or a loculated fluid collection (urinoma) in the retropubic or perivesical space in extraperitoneal rupture.

Postoperative Bladder

Sonography has assumed an important role in the evaluation of the postoperative bladder. **Ureteral reimplantation** is a common surgical procedure for the correction of persistent vesicoureteral reflux. The reimplanted ureteral segment is submucosal and contiguous to the bladder mucosa. Sonograms reveal an echogenic,

A

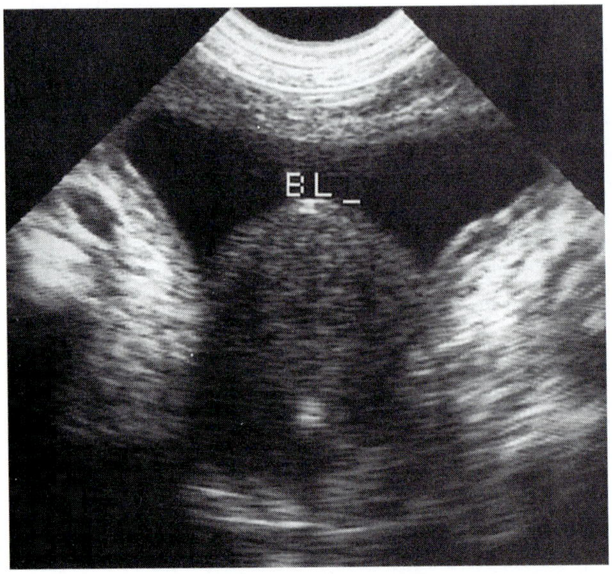

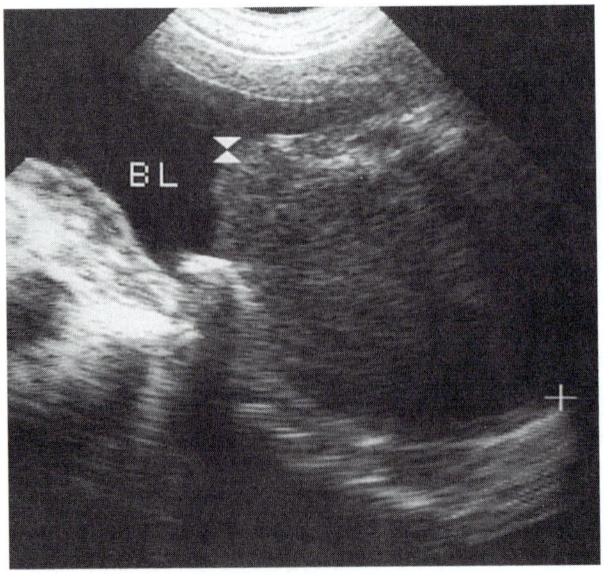

B

FIG. 61-23. Prostatic rhabdomyosarcoma with bladder invasion in an 11-month-old boy with pelvic pain. **A,** Transverse and, **B,** sagittal sonograms of the pelvis demonstrate a large, solid mass arising inferior to the bladder neck, *BL*, invading the bladder base.

nonacoustically shadowing, fixed, tubular, submucosal structure at or just above the trigone. Occasionally, the reimplanted ureter appears only as an area of focal thickening of the posterior bladder wall.[60]

Bladder augmentation is now a widely accepted surgical procedure for the reconstruction of small-capacity bladders caused by exstrophy, neurogenic bladder, or tumor. Segments of bowel, usually the sigmoid, cecum, ileum, or the ileocecal segment, are anastomosed to the bladder to increase the size of the urinary reservoir. Sonography of the augmented bladder reveals a thick or irregularly shaped bladder wall (Fig. 61-25). Pseudomasses within the bladder lumen, representing bowel folds, mucous collections, or bowel that was surgically intussuscepted into the reconstructed bladder to prevent reflux, are a common finding. Fine debris and linear strands often float within the urine and probably represent mucus. Active peristalsis within the bowel segment can be identified on real-time imaging. Complications of bladder reconstructive surgery can be detected on ultrasound and include enterocystic anastomotic strictures, ureteral reflux or obstruction, calculi, extravasation, abscess, urinoma, hematoma, and large amounts of residual urine after voiding.[61]

OVARY

Ovarian Cysts

Since the advent of sonography, simple ovarian cysts in children have been found to be more common than previously reported. Small cysts (1 to 7 mm) have been detected on sonograms in the third-trimester fetus and neonate and are secondary to maternal and placental chorionic gonadotropin. There is a higher incidence of larger ovarian cysts in infants of mothers with toxemia, diabetes, and Rh isoimmunization, all of which are associated with a greater than normal release of placental chorionic gonadotropin.[62] Large ovarian cysts in the fetus can cause mechanical complications during vaginal delivery.[63,64] As a result of the small size of the true pelvis in infants and young children, ovarian cysts are often intraabdominal in location and must be differentiated from mesenteric or omental cysts, gastrointestinal duplication cysts, and urachal cysts. Ovarian cysts are associated with cystic fibrosis,[65] congenital juvenile hypothyroidism,[63,66] McCune-Albright syndrome (fibrous dysplasia, patchy cutaneous pigmentation), and sexual precocity.[67] Autonomously functioning ovarian cysts can cause precocious pseudopuberty.[68] Although in the past neonatal ovarian cysts were surgically removed, recent reports have shown spontaneous resolution of some cysts as demonstrated on sonography (Fig. 61-26).[62] When a follicle continues to grow after failed ovulation or when it does not collapse after ovulation, follicular and corpus luteal cysts may result.[69] Most follicular cysts are unilocular, contain clear serous fluid, and range in size between 3 and 20 cm. **Corpus luteal cysts** can contain serous or hemorrhagic fluid and generally range in size from 5 to 11 cm. Theca-lutein cysts are thought to represent hyperstimulated follicles due to gestational trophoblastic disease or as a complication following the use of drugs

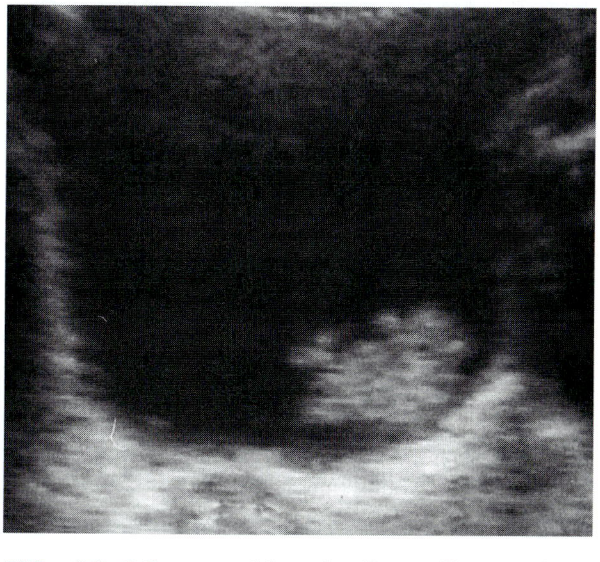

FIG. 61-24. Transitional cell papilloma of the bladder in a 7-year-old boy with hematuria. Transverse sonogram of the bladder reveals a polypoid, solid mass arising from the left posterior bladder wall.

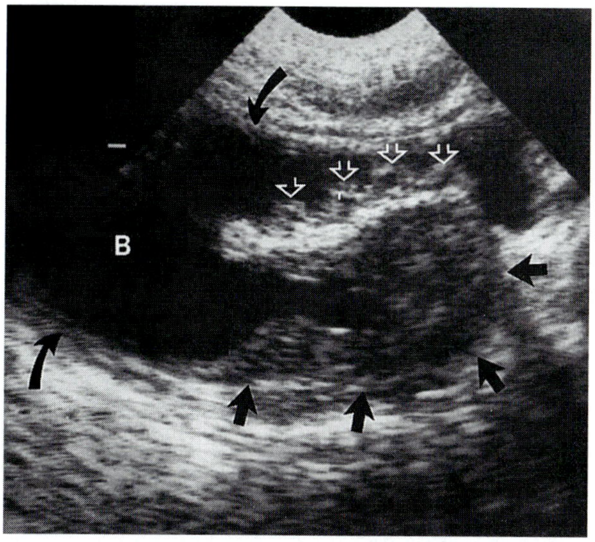

FIG. 61-25. Augmented bladder. Transverse view of the bladder, *B*, shows the thick wall of the anatomic bladder *(straight black arrows)* and the large augmentation *(curved arrows)*. *Open arrows*, Haustral markings. (From Rosenberg HK. Sonography of pediatric urinary tract abnormalities. Pt II. *Am Urol Assoc Weekly Update Series* 1986;36(5):1-8.)

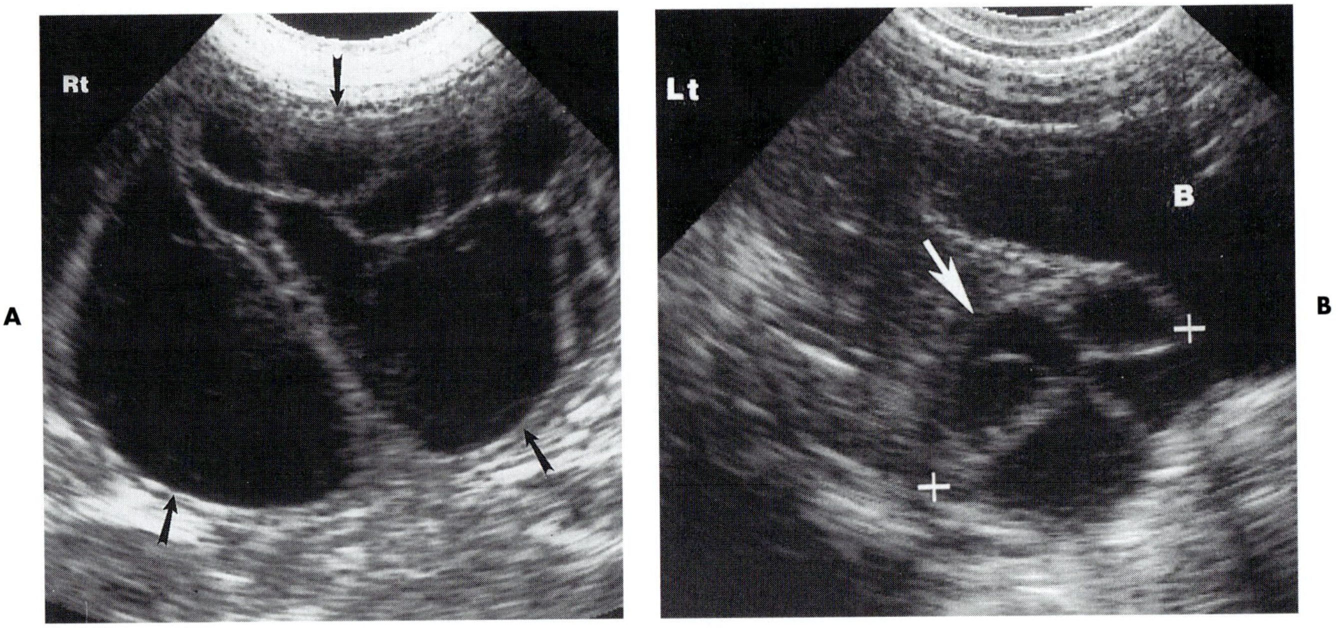

FIG. 61-26. Ovarian cysts in neonate. Female neonate presented with lower abdominopelvic mass. Multiple anechoic cystic areas with septations are noted in ovaries bilaterally *(arrows)*. **A,** Right ovary. **B,** Left ovary. Ovarian cysts were believed to be secondary to *in utero* hormonal stimulation. Follow-up studies showed complete regression. *B*, Bladder.

to stimulate ovulation.[70] Rarely, parovarian cysts are diagnosed in childhood. They are of mesothelial or paramesonephric origin and arise in the broad ligament or fallopian tubes.[71]

Complications of Ovarian Cyst: Torsion, Hemorrhage, or Rupture. Most ovarian cysts are asymptomatic. Symptoms of pain, tenderness, nausea, vomiting, and low-grade fever usually indicate complications of torsion, hemorrhage, or rupture. Torsion can occur in normal ovaries, but it is more commonly caused by an ovarian cyst or tumor (Figs. 61-27 to 61-29). The typical presentation is one of acute onset of acute lower abdominal pain often associated with nausea, vomiting, and leukocytosis.[72] Torsion of normal adnexa usually occurs in prepubertal girls and is thought to be related to excessive mobility of the adnexa, allowing torsion at the mesosalpinx with changes in intraabdominal pressure or body position.[73,74] **Torsion of the ovary and fallopian tube** results from partial or complete rotation of the ovary on its vascular pedicle. This results in compromise of arterial and venous flow, congestion of the ovarian parenchyma, and, ultimately, hemorrhagic infarction.[75] The **sonographic findings in acute ovarian torsion** are often nonspecific and include ovarian enlargement, fluid in the cul-de-sac,[76,77] and other adnexal pathologic findings such as cyst or tumor. A predominantly cystic or complex adnexal mass with a fluid-debris level or septa correlates with pathologic evidence of ovarian hemorrhage or infarction. The demonstration of multiple follicles (8 to 12 mm in size) in the cortical (peripheral) portion of a unilaterally enlarged ovary has been reported as a specific sonographic sign of torsion.[78] These cystic changes occur in up to 74% of twisted ovaries and are attributed to transudation of fluid into follicles secondary to vascular congestion.

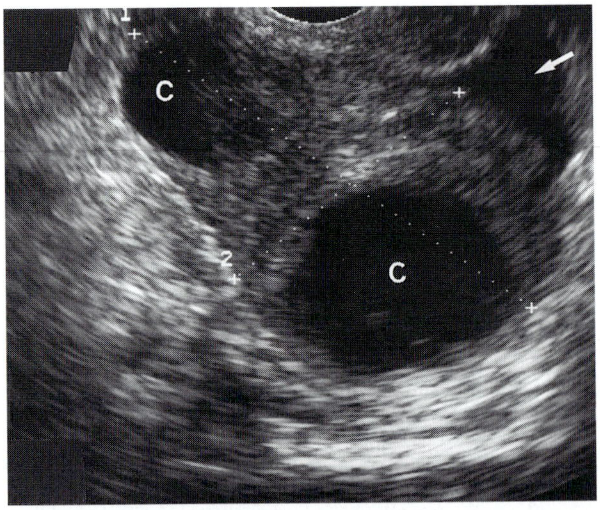

FIG. 61-27. Left ovarian torsion. Longitudinal ultrasound image reveals an enlarged left ovary *(calibers)* with prominent peripheral cysts, *C*, and a small amount of adjacent fluid *(arrow)*. *1*, 7.39 cm; *2*, 4.47.

Hemorrhagic ovarian cysts occur in adolescents and have a variety of sonographic patterns caused by

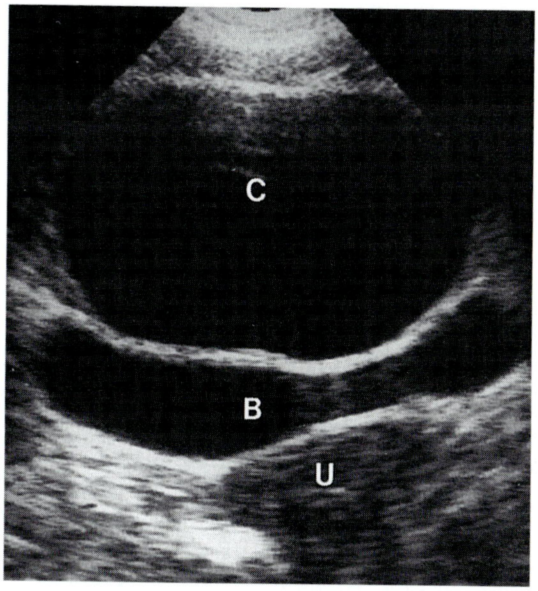

FIG. 61-28. Ovarian torsion complicating an ovarian cyst in a 16-year-old girl with pelvic pain. Transverse view of the pelvis shows an anterior cystic structure, *C*, compressing the bladder, *B*, representing an ovarian cyst at surgery. No ovarian parenchymal tissue was seen sonographically. The cystic ovary was found to be torsed at surgery. *U*, Uterus.

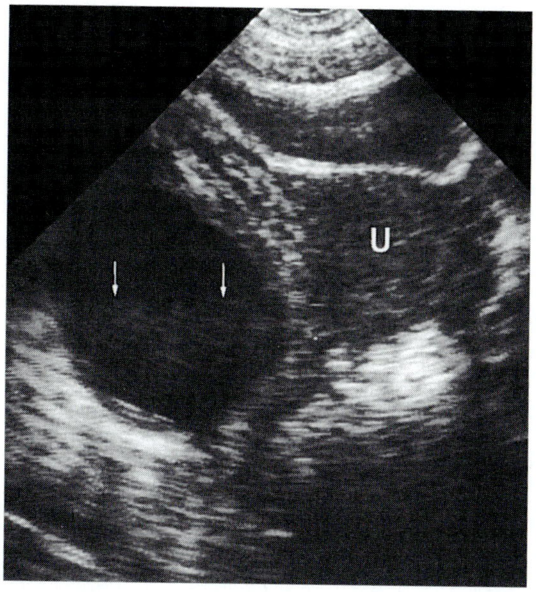

FIG. 61-30. Hemorrhagic ovarian cyst in a teenager with right pelvic pain. Transverse view of the pelvis reveals a large, round, cystic mass in the right adnexal region with a fluid-debris level *(arrows)* representing a hemorrhagic cyst. *U*, Uterus.

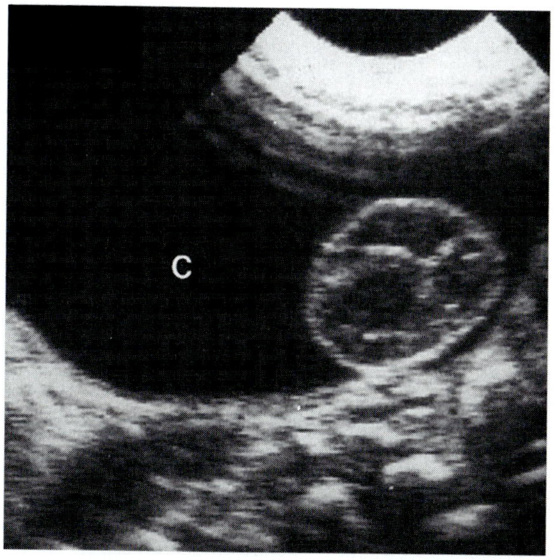

FIG. 61-29. Infarcted, encysted, ovarian torsion in a 6-day-old girl with an abdominal mass. Sonogram of the right lower abdomen and pelvis demonstrates an oval-shaped, complex structure within a larger cystic mass, *C*, proven at surgery to represent an infarcted, encysted, torsed ovary.

SONOGRAPHIC FINDINGS IN ACUTE OVARIAN TORSION

- Ovarian enlargement
- Fluid in cul-de-sac
- Adnexal mass (ovarian hemorrhage or infarction)
  - Cystic or complex
  - Fluid-debris level
  - Septated
- Peripheral, multiple follicles

internal blood clot formation and lysis (Fig. 61-30). The most common appearance is that of a heterogeneous mass, which is predominantly anechoic, containing hypoechoic material. Less commonly, hemorrhagic ovarian cysts are homogeneous, either hypoechoic or hyperechoic. Almost all hemorrhagic cysts (92%) have increased sound through transmission, indicating the cystic nature of the lesion. Additional sonographic features include a thick wall (e.g., 4 mm), septations, and fluid in the cul-de-sac. Although the sonographic findings are nonspecific, the changing appearance of hemorrhagic ovarian cysts over time, as a result of clot lysis, can help establish the diagnosis.[79,80] At times, though, the diagnosis can be confused with appendiceal abscess, dermoid cyst, or teratoma.

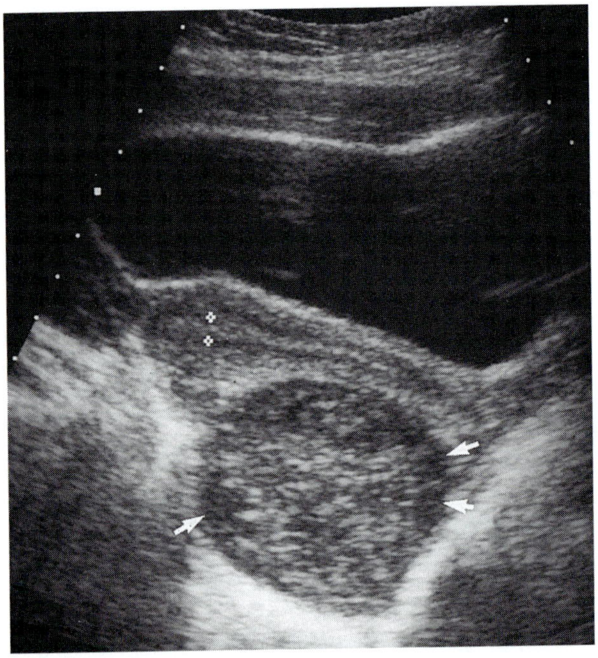

FIG. 61-31. Massive ovarian edema in a 13-year-old girl with masculinization and intermittent pelvic and abdominal pain. Sagittal sonographic image demonstrates a large, heterogeneous, primarily hypoechoic mass posterior and separate from the uterus. This mass contains marked through sound transmission and multiple tiny follicles *(arrows)*. *Calipers*, Endometrial stripe. (Case courtesy of Marilyn Goske, M.D.)

OVARIAN MASSES IN CHILDREN

Benign ovarian teratomas (nearly 60%)
Dysgerminoma
Embryonal carcinoma
Endodermal sinus tumor
Epithelial tumors of ovary (postpuberty)
Granulosa theca cell tumor (precocious puberty)
Arrhenoblastoma (rare, virilizing)
Gonadoblastoma (in dysplastic gonads, e.g., Turner's syndrome)
Acute leukemia

Polycystic Ovarian Disease: Stein-Leventhal Syndrome

Polycystic ovarian disease is characterized by amenorrhea, infertility, and hirsutism. The ovaries are bilaterally rounded and enlarged in 70% of affected patients with the mean ovarian volume 14 cm^3. The levels of follicle-stimulating hormone (FSH) are decreased while the luteinizing hormone (LH) levels are elevated. Sonographically, there are increased numbers of developing follicles seen as multiple, small (0.5 to 0.8 cm diameter) cysts throughout the ovaries in approximately 40% of patients, although maturing follicles are rare. Long-term follow-up is important in these patients because of the increased incidence of endometrial carcinoma due to long-term unopposed estrogen.[81]

Massive Ovarian Edema

Massive edema of the ovary, first described by Kalstone et al. in 1969,[82] is manifested by marked enlargement of the affected ovary due to accumulation of edema fluid in the stroma, separating normal follicular structures (Fig. 61-31). It is thought to result from partial or intermittent torsion that interferes with venous and lymphatic drainage. It affects patients during their second to third decade of life and presents with acute abdominal pain, palpable adnexal mass, menstrual disturbances at times, masculinization, and Meigs' syndrome. Two thirds of patients have right-sided ovarian edema, thought to be related to high pressure in the right ovarian vein due to direct drainage into the inferior vena cava (IVC), or to increased pressure secondary to uterine dextroposition. The ovaries may be massively enlarged with a diameter of up to 35 cm. Grossly, the external surface is soft and pearly white and appears similar to that seen in fibromatosis, a condition likely to occur in young women (25 years) in which primary proliferation of the ovarian stroma may result in torsion and ultimately in edema.[83] The sonographic features of ovarian edema include a solid, hypoechoic mass, enhanced through transmission, and cystic follicles within the lesion.[84] The masculinization is thought to be due to stromal luteinization that results from mechanical stretching of the stromal cells by the edema fluid.[85] In addition, human chorionic gonadotropic-like substance may accumulate in edema fluid and promote luteinization, and the level of 17-ketosteroids may be increased.[83]

Ovarian Neoplasms

Ovarian neoplasms account for 1% of all childhood tumors, and 10% to 30% of these are malignant (see box above). These neoplasms may develop at any age, but they most frequently occur at puberty. Abdominal pain or a palpable abdominal or pelvic mass is the usual presenting symptom. Symptoms may develop as a result of torsion or hemorrhage into the tumor. Ovarian torsion is more common in adolescents than in adults; however, ascites is less common in girls.[50]

Primary ovarian tumors can be classified into three types of cell origins: **germ cells, stromal cells, and epithelial cells.** In children, 60% of primary ovarian tumors are of germ cell origin, in contrast to adults, in whom 90% are epithelial in origin. Approximately 75% to 95% of germ cell tumors in childhood are be-

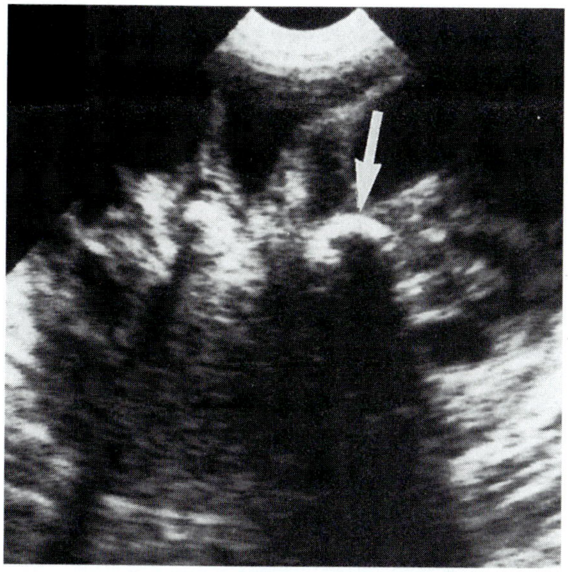

FIG. 61-32. Benign ovarian teratoma. Transverse sonogram of pelvis in 6-year-old girl with constipation and large abdominal mass revealed very large, complex mass filling pelvis and lower two thirds of abdomen, containing multiple, shadowing, echogenic foci *(arrows)* consistent with calcifications.

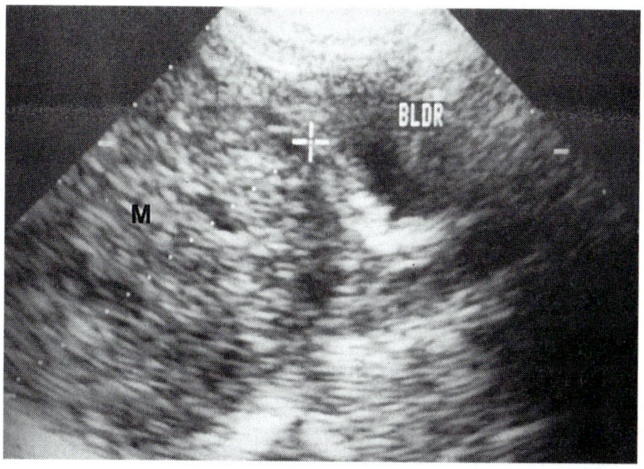

FIG. 61-33. Choriocarcinoma of the right ovary in an 11-year-old girl with right upper quadrant and midabdominal pain and vaginal bleeding. Sagittal transabdominal sonogram of the pelvis shows a very large, solid mass, *M*, which extends into the mid and upper abdomen and is located superior to the poorly distended bladder.

nign teratomas. However, there is a higher incidence of malignancy in younger patients. In girls who are less than 10 years of age, 84% of ovarian germ cell tumors are malignant. The presence of ascites suggests malignancy.[86,87]

Benign teratomas have a wide spectrum of sonographic characteristics (Fig. 61-32). They can be predominantly cystic, with or without a mural nodule. Solid masses and complex lesions with fat-fluid levels, hair-fluid levels, and calcification have been described.[88] Cystic teratomas are usually freely mobile on a pedicle; 10% are bilateral and 90% are less than 15 cm in diameter.[89,90]

Dysgerminoma is the most common malignant germ cell tumor of the ovary in childhood. They frequently occur before puberty, and 10% are bilateral. The tumor is usually a large, solid, encapsulated, rapidly growing mass containing hypoechoic areas as a result of hemorrhage, necrosis, and cystic degeneration. Retroperitoneal lymph node metastases are not uncommon. Dysgerminoma is more radiosensitive than the other malignant ovarian tumors.[86,87,91,92]

Embryonal carcinoma and endodermal sinus tumors are less common malignant germ cell tumors. Choriocarcinoma is rare in children (Fig. 61-33). They are all rapidly growing, highly malignant, solid neoplasms. Embryonal carcinoma is often associated with abnormal hormonal stimulation. All of these tumors tend to spread by direct extension to the opposite adnexa and retroperitoneal lymph nodes. Peritoneal seeding and hematogenous metastases to liver, lung, bone, and mediastinum are common.[93,94]

Epithelial tumors of the ovary, which include **serous and mucinous cystadenoma** or **cystadenocarcinoma,** represent 20% of ovarian tumors in children. They are rare before puberty. On sonography, they are predominantly cystic masses with septa of variable thickness. It is often difficult to differentiate benign from malignant and serous from mucinous cystadenomas or cystadenocarcinomas based only on sonographic criteria.[95-97]

Granulosa theca cell tumor is the most common stromal tumor in children. It is often associated with feminizing effects and precocious puberty as a result of estrogen production. Of these tumors, 10% are bilateral; only 3% are malignant. Their appearance on sonography is nonspecific, and they tend to be predominantly solid tumors.[86,98,99] Arrhenoblastoma (Sertoli-Leydig cell tumor) is rare but may result in virilization. Gonadoblastoma is composed of germ cells admixed with sex cell and stromal elements and usually arises in dysplastic gonads. Bilateral involvement occurs in one third of cases, and 50% contain dysgerminoma elements.[86]

Leukemic Infiltration. The ovaries, as well as the testes and central nervous system, are sanctuary sites for acute leukemia. Ovarian involvement in autopsy series ranges from 11% to 50%. In leukemia with ovarian relapse, most patients present with large, hypoechoic, pelvic masses with smooth, lobulated margins. The tumor can infiltrate the pelvic organs and bowel loops to such a degree that the uterus and ovaries cannot be separately identified. Secondary hy-

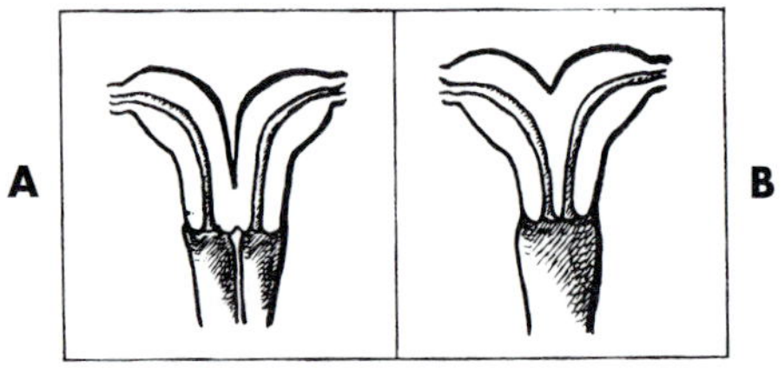

A, Uterus didelphys bicollis (septate vagina). B, Uterus bicornis bicollis (vagina simplex).

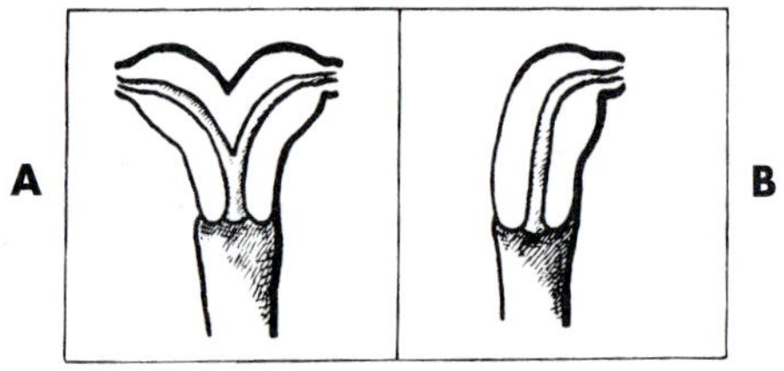

A, Uterus bicornis unicollis (vagina simplex). B, Uterus unicornis.

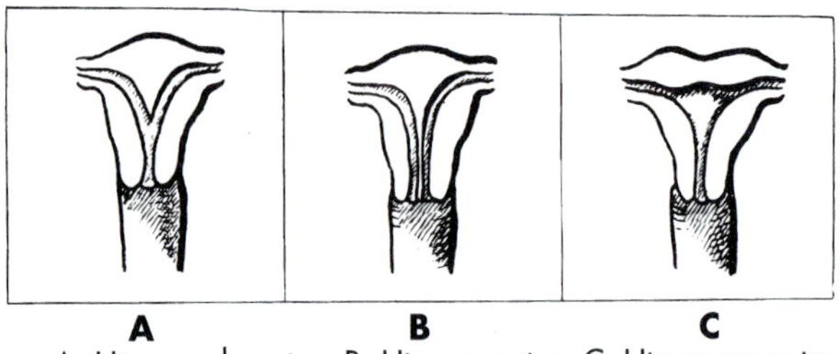

A, Uterus subseptus. B, Uterus septus. C, Uterus arcuatus.

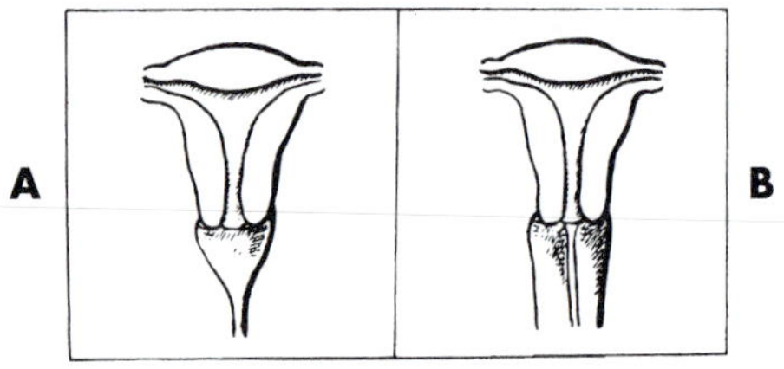

A, Congenital stricture of vagina. B, Septate vagina.

FIG. 61-34. Uterine anomalies. (From Wilson JR, Beecham CT, Carrington ER, eds. *Obstetrics and Gynecology*. 8th ed. St Louis: CV Mosby Co; 1987.)

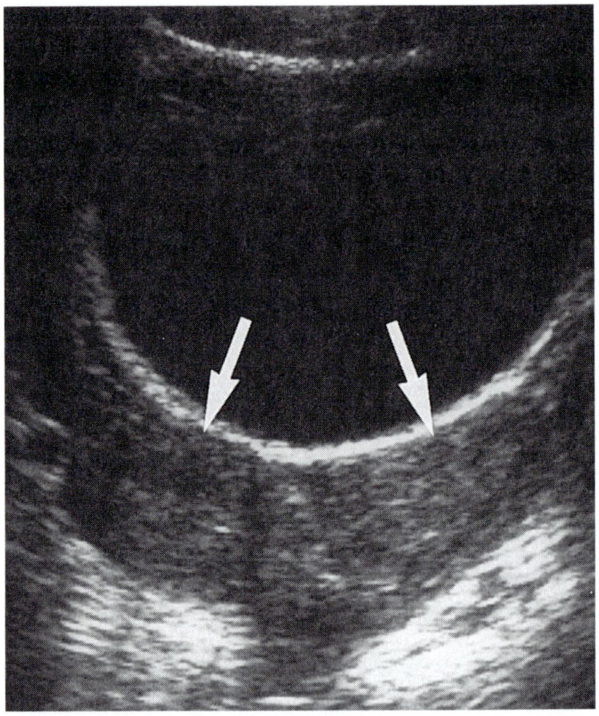

FIG. 61-35. Bicornuate uterus (Mayer-Rokitansky-Küster-Hauser syndrome) in a 15-year-old girl with right lower quadrant and right flank pain with left renal agenesis. Transverse image of the pelvis reveals two separate endometrial cavities *(arrows)* in the mid to fundal region of the uterus, representing a bicornuate uterus.

dronephrosis may develop.[100,101] Lane and Birdwell suggested that pelvic sonography should be used to monitor and detect early leukemic relapse in the ovaries of children in clinical remission.[102]

UTERUS AND VAGINA

Congenital Anomalies

Congenital anomalies of the uterus and vagina in children are uncommon and usually present as an abdominal or pelvic mass secondary to obstruction. There is a high incidence of associated renal anomalies (50%) and an increased incidence of skeletal anomalies (12%).[103-105] The uterus, cervix, and upper two thirds of the vagina are formed by the fused caudal ends of the müllerian (paramesonephric) duct. The paired fallopian tubes are formed by the unfused upper ends. The lower third of the vagina is derived from the urogenital sinus. Müllerian duct development into the uterus is dependent on the formation of the wolffian (mesonephric) duct. Therefore abnormal development of the müllerian duct, resulting in uterine and vaginal anomalies, is often associated with renal anomalies.

The **bicornuate uterus** is the most common congenital uterine anomaly. It results when the two müllerian ducts fuse only inferiorly (Fig. 61-34). The two separate uterine horns, which are joined at a variable level above the cervix, are best demonstrated on transverse sonograms through the superior portion of the uterus (Fig. 61-35). Only one cervix and vagina are identified. With complete duplication of the müllerian ducts, there is a septated vagina and duplicated cervix and uterus. In either anomaly, obstruction of one uterine horn can result in a pelvic mass as a result of unilateral hydrometra or hematometra. Other septation anomalies of the uterus can result from incomplete involution of the midline septum between the paired müllerian ducts. A unicornuate uterus is

A

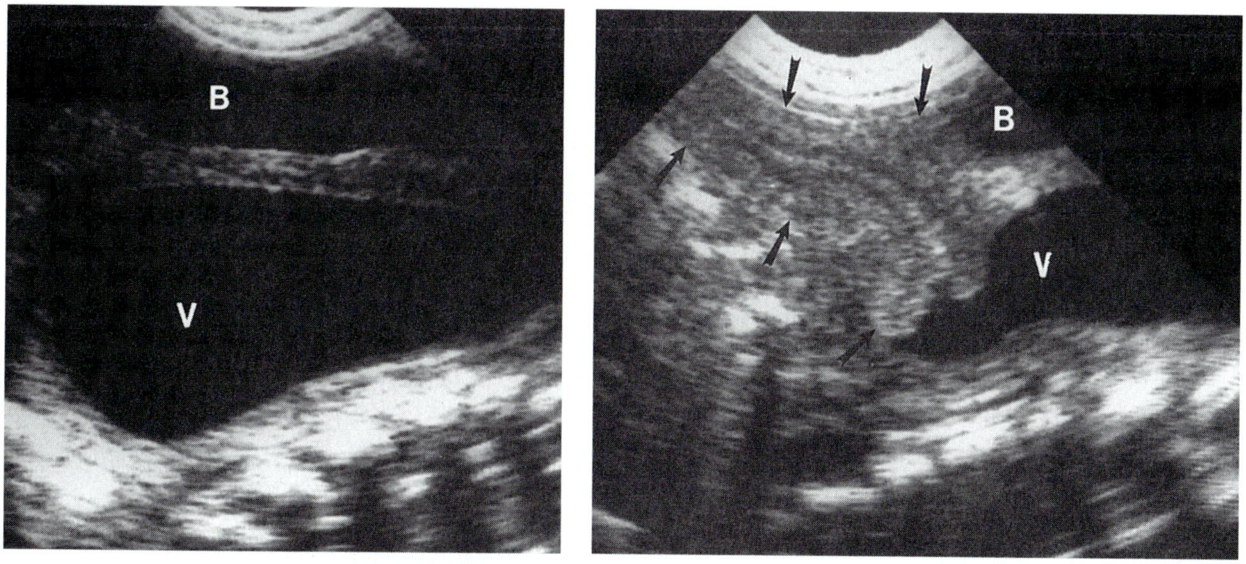

B

FIG. 61-36. Hydrocolpos. **A,** Sagittal scan of pelvis in newborn showing large, conical, fluid-filled mass representing obstructed vagina, *V*, behind bladder, *B*. **B,** Sagittal scan, angled higher than in **A,** shows uterus *(arrows)* with cervix projecting into dilated vagina, *V*. *B*, Bladder. (From Rosenberg HK. Sonography of pediatric urinary tract abnormalities. Pt I, *Am Urol Assoc Weekly Update Series* 1986;36(5):1-8.)

formed from the agenesis of one müllerian duct.[103] *In utero* exposure to diethylstilbestrol has been associated with development of a T-shaped uterus. Sonography shows a narrow uterus caused by absence of the normal, superior, bulbous expansion of the uterine fundus.[103,105]

Hydrocolpos or hydrometrocolpos, caused by obstruction of the vagina, accounts for 15% of abdominal masses in newborn girls (Fig. 61-36).[106,107] The obstruction is secondary to an imperforate hymen, a transverse vaginal septum, or a stenotic or atretic vagina. There is an accumulation of mucous secretions proximal to the obstruction. The secretions are secondary to intrauterine and postnatal stimulation of uterine and cervical glands by maternal estrogens. A simple **imperforate hymen** is not usually associated with other congenital anomalies. However, there is a high incidence of genitourinary, gastrointestinal, and skeletal anomalies associated with **vaginal atresia** or a **midtransverse or high-transverse vaginal septum.**[15] On sonographic examination, hydrocolpos appears as a large, tubular, cystic mass posterior to the bladder and extending inferior to the symphysis pubis. Low-level echoes within the fluid represent mucous secretions in neonates and blood in postpubertal girls (Fig. 61-37). There may be secondary urinary retention and hydronephrosis. Imperforate anus, cloacal exstrophy, and persistent urogenital sinus often have associated hydrometrocolpos.[108]

The Mayer-Rokitansky-Küster-Hauser syndrome, the second most common cause of primary amenorrhea, comprises vaginal atresia, rudimentary bicornuate uterus, normal fallopian tubes and ovaries, and broad and round ligaments.[104] There is a spectrum of uterine anomalies (hypoplasia or duplication), ranging from a partial lumen to a septate or bicornuate uterus with unilateral or bilateral obstruction. These girls have a normal female karyotype, sec-

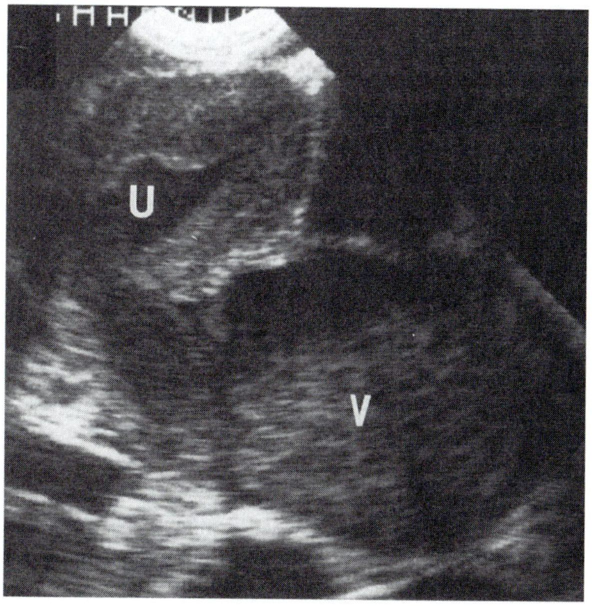

FIG. 61-37. Hematometrocolpos. Sagittal scan of pelvis shows dilated uterine cavity, *U*, filled with echogenic debris (blood). Fluid-debris level is seen in dilated, obstructed vagina, *V*. (From Fisher MR, Kricun ME, eds. *Imaging of the Pelvis*. Gaithersburg, Md: Aspen Publishers; 1989.)

ondary sexual development, and external genitalia. There is a high incidence of unilateral renal (50%) and skeletal (12%) anomalies. Unilateral renal agenesis or ectopia is the most common renal anomaly. The most common sonographic finding is uterine didelphys with unilateral hydrometrocolpos and ipsilateral renal agenesis. Water vaginography can help identify the septated vagina with unilateral vaginal obstruction.[104,109-112] The analogous genitourinary defects in the male result in duplicated müllerian duct remnants (müllerian cyst and dilated prostatic utricle) with unilateral renal agenesis.[113]

Neoplasm

Tumors of the uterus and vagina are uncommon in the pediatric patient. Malignant tumors are more common than benign tumors, and the vagina is a more common site than the uterus. **Rhabdomyosarcoma** is the most common primary malignant neoplasm.[114-116] It can arise from the uterus or vagina, although uterine involvement is more frequent by direct extension from a vaginal tumor. These children usually present at 6 to 18 months of age with vaginal bleeding or protrusion of a polypoid cluster of masses **(sarcoma botryoides)** through the introitus. Rhabdomyosarcoma most commonly arises from the anterior wall of the vagina near the cervix. It may also arise in the distal vagina or labia. Direct extension of the tumor into the bladder neck is common, but posterior invasion of the rectum is infrequent. Lymphadenopathy and distant metastases are uncommon at presentation. On sonographic examination, these tumors are solid, homogeneous masses that fill the vaginal cavity or cause enlargement of the uterus with an irregular contour.[1,117]

Endodermal sinus tumor is a less common genital neoplasm. It is a highly malignant germ cell tumor that can arise in the vagina. It has a similar clinical and sonographic presentation to that of rhabdomyosarcoma (Fig. 61-38).[114] Other malignant tumors of the uterus and vagina are rare. Adenocarcinoma of the cervix in adults arises from the endocervix whereas in children it is a polypoid lesion that originates from the ectocervix and upper vagina. Carcinoma of the vagina (usually clear cell adenocarcinoma) usually occurs in teenagers with a history of *in utero* exposure to diethylstilbestrol.[118] Leukemic infiltration of the uterus can occur secondary to contiguous extension from an ovarian relapse. Sonography shows a large, homogeneous, hypoechoic, pelvic mass incorporating the uterus and ovaries, which cannot be separately identified. There may be associated hydronephrosis caused by distal ureteral obstruction.[106]

Benign, solid neoplasms of the uterus and vagina are rare in children. However, benign cystic vaginal masses are not uncommon. The most common cystic lesion of the vagina is **Gartner's cyst.** A remnant of the distal wolffian (mesonephric) duct, Gartner's cysts may be single or multiple and typically arise from the anterolateral vaginal wall. They appear as fluid-filled cysts within the vagina on ultrasound.[114] Other cystic vaginal masses include paraurethral cysts, inclusion cysts, and paramesonephric (müllerian) duct cysts.[118]

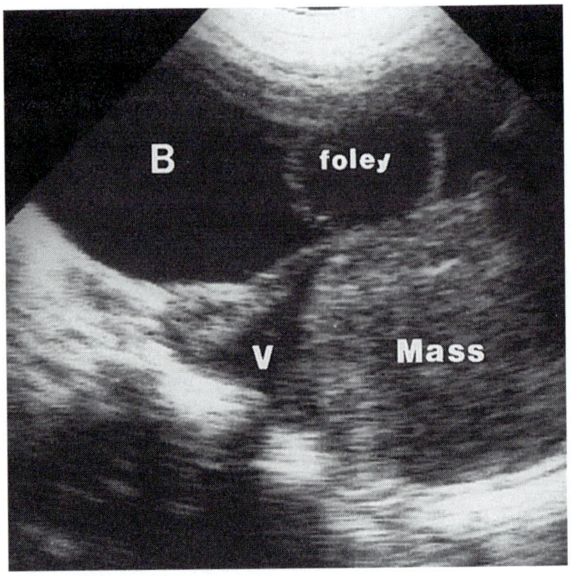

FIG. 61-38. Endodermal sinus tumor of the vagina. Sagittal scan of pelvis shows solid, homogeneous mass filling vagina, *V*. Foley catheter balloon is seen in bladder, *B*. (From Fisher MR, Kricun ME, eds. *Imaging of the Pelvis*. Gaithersburg Md: Aspen Publishers; 1989.)

Pregnancy

Intrauterine pregnancy must always be considered in the differential diagnosis of an abdominopelvic mass in girls 9 years of age or older. There is an increased incidence of complications related to pediatric pregnancy. These include toxemia, preeclampsia, placental abruption, lacerations, and cesarean sections. There is also an increase in prematurity and perinatal mortality among infants born of teenage mothers.[106] Although ectopic pregnancy is less common in young adolescents, the diagnosis should be considered in the presence of abdominal pain, a missed menstrual period, and irregular vaginal bleeding. Hypotension or overt shock suggest ruptured ectopic pregnancy.[119]

Infection

Pelvic inflammatory disease (PID) is an infection of the upper genital tract usually related to *Neisseria gonorrhoeae* and/or *Chlamydia trachomatis* infection. The serious sequelae of this disease include ectopic pregnancy, infertility, and chronic pelvic pain. Adolescent females are in a higher-risk group, and thus PID should be considered in sexually active females presenting with pelvic pain.

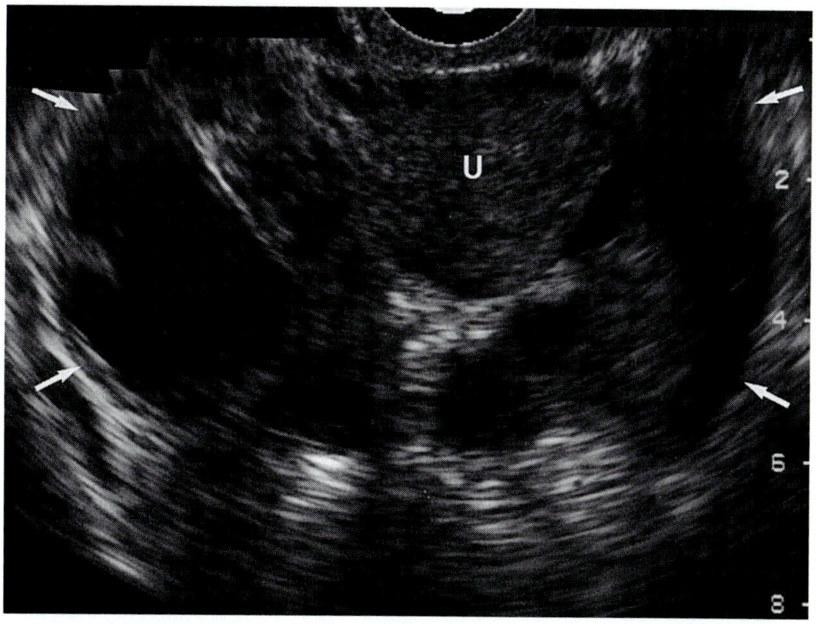

FIG. 61-39. Tuboovarian abscesses in adolescent girl with pelvic pain. Endovaginal axial image of the pelvis reveals bilateral, complex, cystic masses *(arrows)*. *U*, Uterus.

The ascending infection may affect the uterus, fallopian tubes, and ovaries, causing endometritis, salpingitis, oophoritis, pelvic peritonitis, and/or tuboovarian abscess.

In a study by Bulas et al., anatomic detail was improved with endovaginal scanning as compared with transabdominal scanning such that new abnormalities were seen in 71% of patients and the level of disease severity was changed in 33% of patients, which affected treatment decisions in many of these patients.[120]

Spectrum of Sonographic Findings in PID. Acutely, the pelvic sonogram may be normal.[120,121] In the endometritis stage of the disease, the uterus may be enlarged, more hyperechoic, contain a small amount of fluid in the endometrial canal, and/or have indistinct margins.[121]

The normal fallopian tube is usually not visualized sonographically. As the infection ascends, however, the fallopian tubes become thick-walled and fill with purulent material.[120,122] A pyosalpinx is a dilated occluded fallopian tube that contains echogenic purulent fluid. A residual hydrosalpinx is a tubular or round structure with anechoic fluid.

Ovarian changes from PID may include enlargement secondary to the production of inflammatory exudate and edema and the development of many tiny cysts, which may represent small follicles or abscesses.[121,122]

Periovarian adhesions may form, resulting in fusion of the ovary and thickened tube, forming a tuboovarian complex. Further progression leads to tissue breakdown and formation of a tuboovarian abscess. A **tuboovarian abscess** usually appears as a well-defined, heterogeneous, adnexal mass with enhanced sound through transmission. Most contain internal debris and septations (Fig. 61-39). Color flow Doppler evaluation of pelvic masses in patients with PID is not specific and overlaps with other entities. Flow in an abscess may be seen along its periphery; however, this pattern may be seen in other cystic lesions.[123]

In **extensive cases of PID** the pelvis is diffusely filled with a heterogeneous echo pattern containing cystic and/or solid components that obscure tissue planes and uterine margins (Fig. 61-40).[121]

A complication of PID includes gonococcal or chlamydial perihepatitis (Fitz-Hugh–Curtis syndrome) where the patient presents with right upper quadrant pain caused by localized peritonitis of the anterior liver surface and parietal peritoneum of the anterior abdominal wall. Sonographic findings include the presence of

SONOGRAPHIC FINDINGS IN PID

- Enlarged hyperechoic uterus
- Indistinct uterine margins
- Fluid in endometrial canal
- Hydrosalpinx with echogenic fluid
- Ovarian enlargement with tiny cysts
- Tuboovarian abscess (heterogeneous adnexal mass)

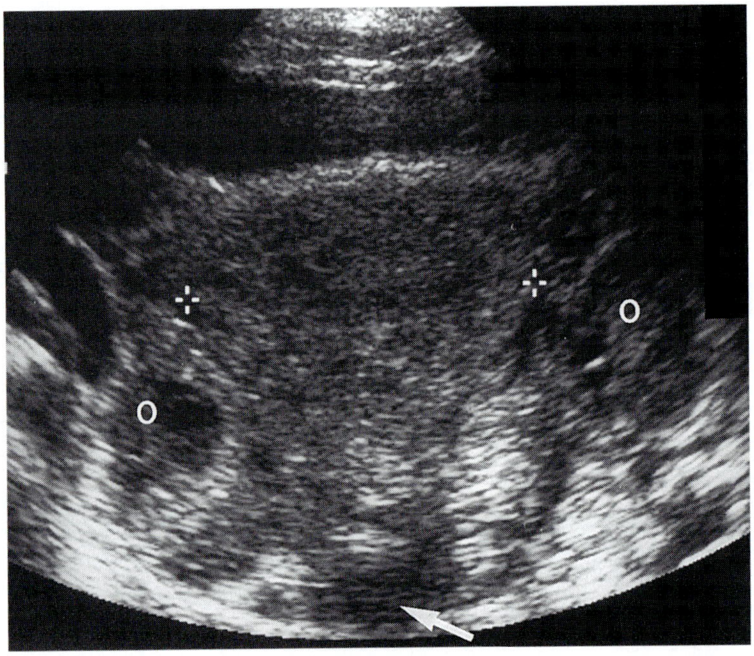

FIG. 61-40. Pelvic inflammatory disease. Transverse transabdominal image of the pelvis reveals increased, ill-defined, soft-tissue echogenicity representing inflammatory material causing indistinct uterine and ovarian margins and haziness in the parametrial area. A small amount of echogenic fluid is seen posteriorly *(arrow)*. Uterus is demarcated by calipers. *O*, Ovary.

ascitic fluid and/or thickening of the right anterior extrarenal tissue between the liver and right kidney.[124,125]

A vaginal discharge may be a sign of vaginal infection or trauma. **Foreign bodies in the vagina** are a cause of 4% of cases of vaginitis. A wad of toilet paper is the most common foreign body in the vagina.[105] Sonography, either transabdominal or transperineal, with or without water vaginography, can identify both radiopaque and nonradiopaque foreign bodies within the vagina as echogenic material with distal acoustic shadowing.

ENDOCRINE ABNORMALITIES

Ultrasound has become an integral part of the study in the evaluation of children with endocrine abnormalities. In the newborn infant with **ambiguous genitalia,** pelvic sonography can quickly determine the presence or absence of the uterus and vagina. Identification of the ovaries or testes is more difficult because normally the neonatal ovaries are not seen on ultrasound. Using a high-resolution transducer, preferably 10 MHz, the gonads may be found in the inguinal canal or in the ambiguous labioscrotal folds. Differentiation of the gonads between ovaries and testes may be possible because ovaries often have small, hypoechoic follicles and testes have a solid, homogeneous echotexture.[106,126]

Causes of Primary Amenorrhea

Sonographic assessment of the uterine size, shape, maturity, and ovarian development can provide a clue to the causes of primary amenorrhea. A small or absent uterus may be an indication of gonadal dysgenesis, chromosomal abnormalities, decreased hormonal states, testicular feminization, or isolated uterine hypoplasia or agenesis. In Turner's syndrome, the most common form of gonadal dysgenesis, there is delayed or absent puberty associated with short stature, webbed neck, renal anomalies, and coarctation of the aorta. Those girls with pure 45,XO karyotypes have nonvisualized ovaries and a prepubertal uterus on ultrasonic examination. In genetic mosaicism with 45,XO/46,XX karyotype, the ovaries can vary from nonvisualized streak ovaries to normal adult ovaries. The uterine configuration also varies from prepubertal to an intermediate length that is less than the normal adult female.[103]

Other forms of gonadal dysgenesis are also associated with nonvisualization of the ovaries as a result of absent or streak gonads. In pure gonadal dysgenesis (Swyer's syndrome), the patients have 46,XX or 46,XY karyotypes and normal height. Mixed gonadal dysgenesis is a genetic mosaic of karyotypes 45,XO/46,XY with a streak ovary and a contralateral intra-abdominal testicle. Both of these forms of gonadal dysgenesis have an increased risk of gonadal tumors as a result of the presence of the Y chromosome. Noonan's syndrome (pseudo-Turner's syndrome) is characterized by phenotypic changes of Turner's syndrome, normal ovarian function, and normal ovaries on ultrasound.[127]

Testicular feminization is another cause of primary amenorrhea. It is a sex-linked recessive abnormality, resulting in end-organ insensitivity to androgens. These patients are phenotypic females with a 46,XY karyotype. The uterus and ovaries are absent, the vagina ends blindly, and the testes are ectopic (usually pelvic).[1]

Precocious Puberty

Sonography is an important imaging modality in the evaluation of children with precocious puberty.[1,105] Precocious puberty is the development of secondary sexual characteristics, gonadal enlargement, and ovulation before the age of 8 years. In true precocious puberty, the endocrine profile is similar to that of normal puberty with elevated levels of estrogen and gonadotropins. The uterus has an enlarged, postpubertal configuration (fundus-to-cervix ratio is 2:1 to 3:1) with an echogenic endometrial canal. The ovarian volume is greater than 1 cm^3 and functional cysts are often present. More than 80% of these cases are idiopathic. Intracranial tumors, usually a hypothalamic glioma or hamartoma, account for 5% to 10% of cases.

In pseudoprecocious puberty, the endocrine profile is variable. Usually, the estrogen levels are elevated and the gonadotropin levels are low. The cause is outside the hypothalamic-pituitary axis and is usually caused by an ovarian tumor. Granulosa theca cell tumor is the most common lesion. Other less frequent causes are functioning ovarian cysts, dysgerminoma, teratoma, and choriocarcinoma. Ultrasound will identify the ovarian mass and a mature uterus. Although feminizing adrenal tumors are a rare cause of pseudoprecocious puberty, sonographic examination of the adrenal areas should also be performed in all patients with precocious puberty who are referred for pelvic ultrasound.[128,129] The liver should be examined as well because precocious puberty at times has been associated with hepatoblastoma.[130]

In isolated premature thelarche (breast development) or premature adrenarche (pubic or axillary hair development), sonography shows normal prepubertal uterus and ovaries.

SCROTUM

Technique

Prior to examining the scrotum sonographically, the examiner should carefully palpate the entire scrotum. The pediatric scrotum is examined sonographically with a 7.5- to 10-MHz linear array transducer equipped with gray-scale and duplex/color flow Doppler imaging. It is helpful to elevate and immobilize the testes by gently placing a rolled-up towel posterior to the scrotum in a vertical position between the legs. For accurate measurements of larger adolescent testes, a curvilinear, broad bandwidth probe and a step-off may be necessary. Both hemiscrota are routinely examined, and color flow Doppler imaging parameters are optimized for the best detection of low-velocity and low-volume blood flow typically seen in the scrotum (gain settings are increased and wall filter and pulse repetition frequencies are decreased). Power mode Doppler imaging, with its increased sensitivity for the detection of blood flow, is useful for examination of slow flow states in the cooperative patient.[131]

Normal

The **normal newborn's testes** have a homogeneous low- to medium-level echogenicity and are spherical or oval in shape with a diameter of 7 to 10 mm. The epididymis and mediastinum testis are usually not seen in the neonate. By puberty, the testis contains homogeneous medium-level echoes and an echogenic linear structure along its superoinferior axis, which represents the mediastinum testis. The testis measures 3 to 5 cm in length and 2 to 3 cm in depth and width after puberty.[132] Studies of testicular sizes during infancy and adolescence performed using orchidometers report the range of mean testicular volumes as 1.10 cm^3 (SD ±0.14) and 30.25 cm^3 (SD ±9.64).[133,134] The authors' personal experience as well as references to testicular sizes in more recent radiologic articles support the existence of normal testes smaller than 1 cm^3 in young infants and children.[135,136]

The normal color flow Doppler appearance of the testes also changes with age. Despite optimized slow-flow settings, it may not be possible to detect color flow in normal, small, prepubertal testes.[135-137] Atkinson et al. reported central arterial flow with color flow Doppler imaging in only 6 (46%) of 13 testes measuring less than 1 cm^3 and in all testes measuring greater than 1 cm^3.[135] When color flow is seen in prepubertal testes, it appears as pulsatile foci of color without the linear or branching pattern seen in adolescents or adults (Fig. 61-41).[135,138,139]

Luker and Siegel showed that power mode Doppler ultrasound improved depiction of intratesticular vessels in normal prepubertal and postpubertal testes, but there was still a lack of flow in several normal prepubertal testes.[137]

Normal pulsed wave Doppler testicular flow reflects its supply from the testicular artery, which has a low resistance pattern (low peak systolic velocities and relatively high diastolic velocities). Flow in extrates-

A

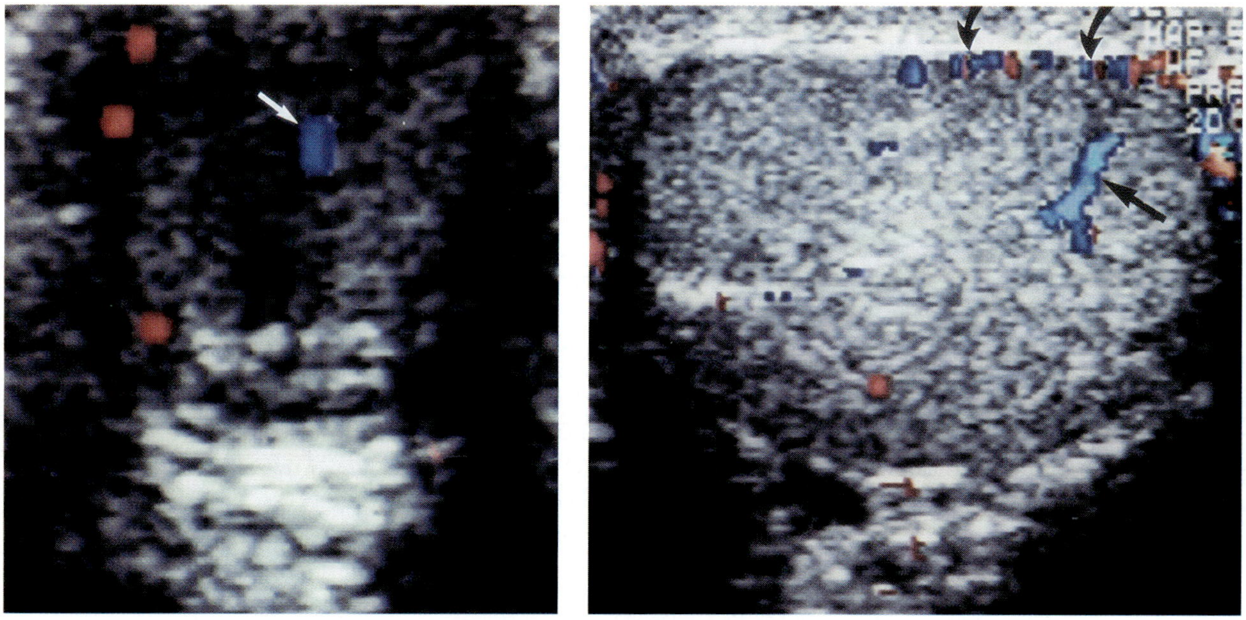

B

FIG. 61-41. A, Normal color flow Doppler imaging in prepubertal testis. Pulsatile focus of color within *(arrow)* and adjacent to the testis. **B, Normal color flow Doppler imaging in postpubertal testis.** Longitudinal view of the testis with color flow Doppler imaging reveals normal postpubertal blood flow in capsular *(curved arrows)* and centripetal *(straight arrow)* arteries.

ticular vessels reflects supply from the cremaster and deferential arteries and has a higher resistance pattern (low diastolic flow).[139]

The epididymis lies along the posterior lateral aspect of the testis. The triangular-shaped epididymal head is isoechoic with the testis or slightly hyperechoic whereas the echogenicity of the epididymal body is isoechoic or slightly hypoechoic in relationship to the testis, and the tail is usually not seen. Flow is not detected in the normal prepubertal epididymis, but may be seen on both color flow and power mode Doppler imaging in postpubertal epididymides.[137]

Congenital Abnormalities

Cryptorchidism. The testis descends via the inguinal canal into the scrotum between the seventh and eighth months of gestation. In most cases, the testes are located within the scrotum at birth or within 4 to 6 weeks after birth. Undescended testes are seen in 4% of full-term newborns. Only 0.7% of these infants have true cryptorchidism, and in 10% to 25% it is bilateral cryptorchidism.[35,140,141] Although the malpositioned testis may lie anywhere along its course from the retroperitoneum to the scrotum, most testes are located at or below the inguinal canal and thus are amenable to sonographic localization (Figs. 61-42 and 61-43). An MRI should be performed for localizing intraabdominal cryptorchid testes.[142] Localization of the undescended testis is important in disease prevention because cryptorchidism is associated with increased risks of malignancy, infertility, and torsion.

The number of testes may vary and range from anorchidism to polyorchidism, which normally presents in the older child as an asymptomatic scrotal mass. Usually, a single, small, accessory testis is demonstrated within the scrotum in addition to two normal testes.[143]

True Hermaphroditism. True hermaphroditism is an intersex condition in which the patient has both ovarian and testicular tissue, either in the form of separate structures or an ovotestis. Ultrasound can demonstrate the textural difference within an ovotestis in that the testicular portion is more homogeneous with medium-level echoes whereas the ovarian tissue is more heterogeneous with small, anechoic, cystic follicles interspersed with the low- to medium-level parenchymal echogenicity (Fig. 61-44).[144] These patients either present prepubertally with ambiguous genitalia or postpubertally with new gynecomastia, cyclic hematuria, or cryptorchidism in a patient reared as a boy, or amenorrhea in a patient reared as a girl.[145]

Cystic Dysplasia of the Testis. Cystic dysplasia of the testis is a rare congenital condition consisting of dilated rete testis and adjacent parenchymal atrophy.[146] The ultrasound appearance consists of multiple, small, anechoic, cystic structures seen predominantly in the region of the mediastinum testis. The defect may result from an embryologic defect pre-

A

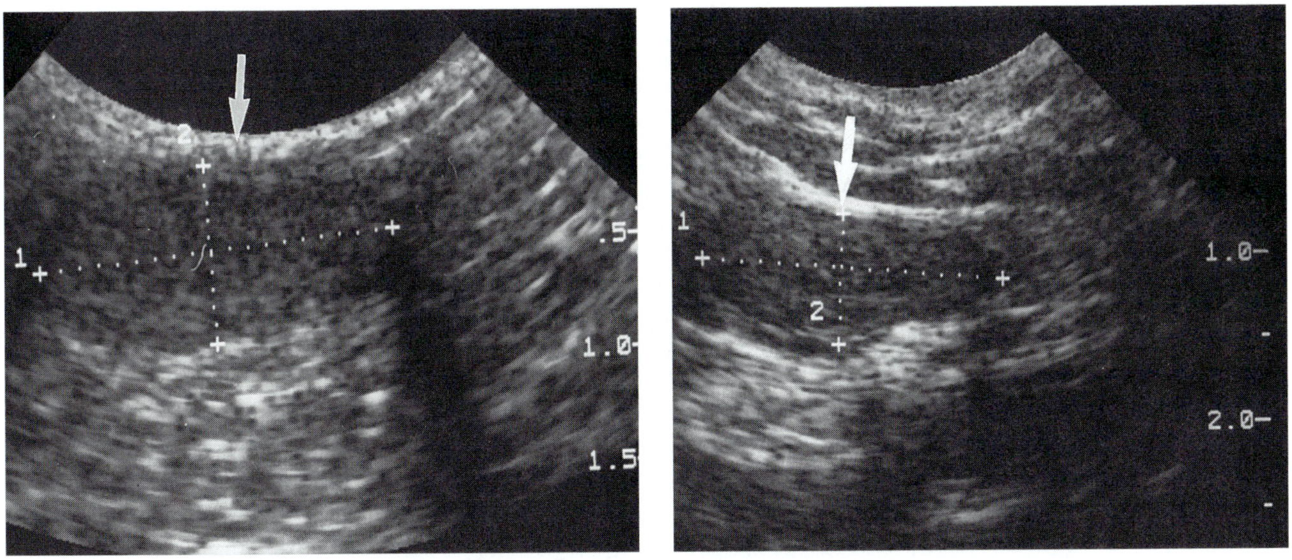

B

FIG. 61-42. Descended and undescended testicles *(arrows)*. **A,** Normal descended left testicle is imaged in sagittal plane. **B,** Smaller right undescended testicle is identified in right inguinal canal.

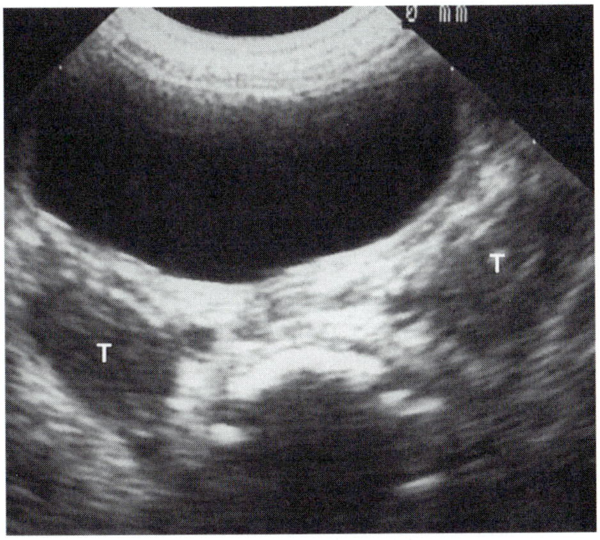

FIG. 61-43. Undescended pelvic testes. Transverse gray-scale imaging of the pelvis in this 36-week-old premature infant boy reveals bilateral undescended testes, *T*, in the pelvis.

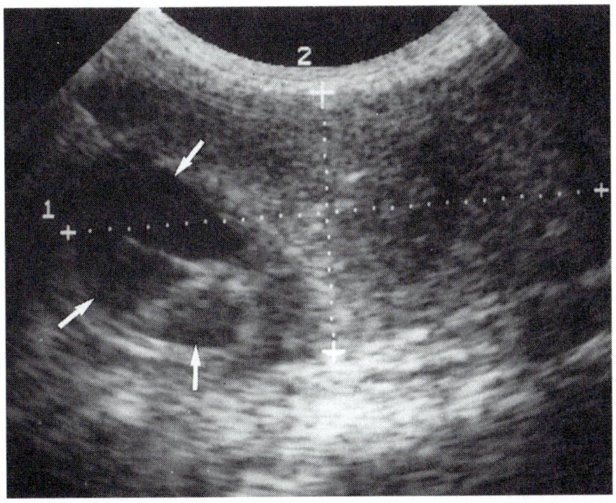

FIG. 61-44. Ovotestis in a 15-year-old phenotypic boy with bilateral gynecomastia, intermittent scrotal pain and swelling, and recent scrotal trauma. Sagittal sonogram of the right hemiscrotum reveals a heterogeneous right gonad *(calipers)* with focal cystic areas representing follicles in the upper pole *(arrows)*. This gonad contains pathologically proven ovarian and testicular tissue. (From Eberenz W, Rosenberg HK, Moshang T et al. True hermaphroditism: sonographic demonstration of ovotestes. *Radiology* 1991;179:429-431.)

venting connection between the rete testis tubule and efferent ductules.[146] Several reported cases in children were associated with ipsilateral renal agenesis or renal dysplasia.[146] The appearance in the scrotum is similar to the incidentally noted condition of tubular ectasia of the rete testis described in adults, which probably represents an acquired condition secondary to prior inflammation or trauma.[147] The lack of color flow within these cystic structures distinguishes tubular ectasia from **intratesticular varicocele,** which can have a similar gray-scale appearance but demonstrates venous flow on color flow Doppler imaging.[148]

The Acute Scrotum

The more common causes of acute pain and/or swelling in the pediatric scrotum include testicular tor-

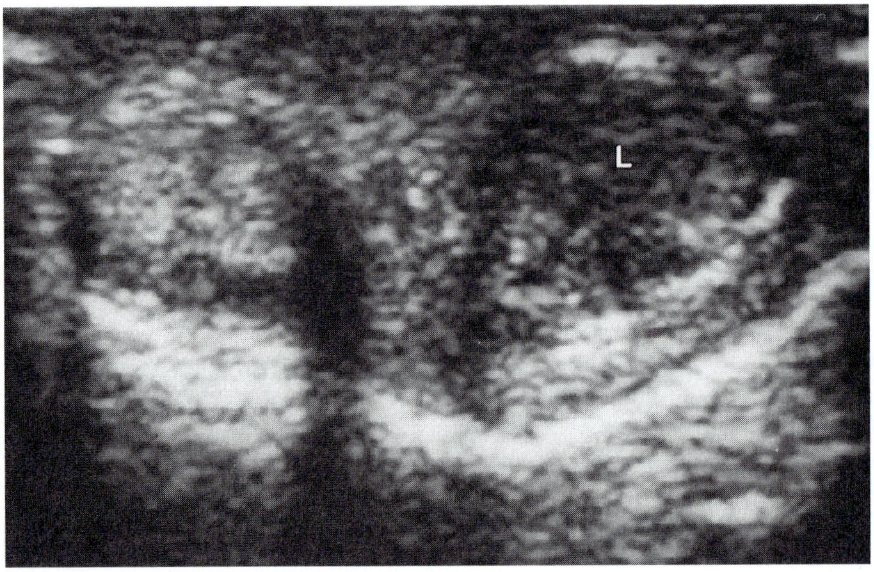

FIG. 61-45. Extravaginal torsion in a 1-day-old boy with a hard, nontender, left testis. Transverse image of the scrotum reveals a slightly enlarged, hypoechoic, left testis, *L*, with an echogenic rim representing an old "missed torsion." The right testis is normal. Note that no flow was detected in either testis on color flow Doppler imaging.

ACUTE SCROTUM IN CHILDREN

Common

Testicular torsion
Epididymitis with and without orchitis
Torsion of testicular appendages
Testicular trauma
Acute hydrocele
Incarcerated hernia

Uncommon

Idiopathic scrotal edema
Henoch-Schönlein purpura
Scrotal fat necrosis
Familial Mediterranean fever
Abdominal pathology

SONOGRAPHIC SIGNS OF TESTICULAR TORSION

Testes

Normal early
Hypoechoic after 4 to 6 hours from edema
Heterogeneous after 24 hours from hemorrhage and infarction (missed torsion)

Peritesticular

Hypoechoic epididymis
Reactive hydrocele
Skin thickening
Enlarged, twisted spermatic cord

sion, epididymitis with or without orchitis, torsion of the testicular appendages, testicular trauma, acute hydrocele, and incarcerated hernia. Less common causes are idiopathic scrotal edema, Henoch-Schönlein purpura, scrotal fat necrosis, familial Mediterranean fever, or secondary scrotal involvement from abdominal pathology[149-157] (see box in left column).

Testicular Torsion. Testicular torsion and **epididymitis** (with or without orchitis) are the two most frequently encountered causes of the acute scrotum in the pediatric population. High-resolution ultrasound with color flow Doppler imaging has become the method preferred for distinguishing between these two entities.[136,158] This is crucial because testicular torsion is treated surgically and epididymitis with or without orchitis is treated medically.

Testicular torsion has the highest prevalence during two age peaks: infancy and adolescence. The loose attachment of the spermatic cord and testes to surrounding structures may account for increased mobility and may predispose to the extravaginal type of torsion seen in neonates (Fig. 61-45). Torsion within the scrotal sac, or intravaginal torsion, is more commonly seen in adolescents, especially those with high attachment of the tunica vaginalis or the so-called "bell-and-clapper" deformity. Another less frequently

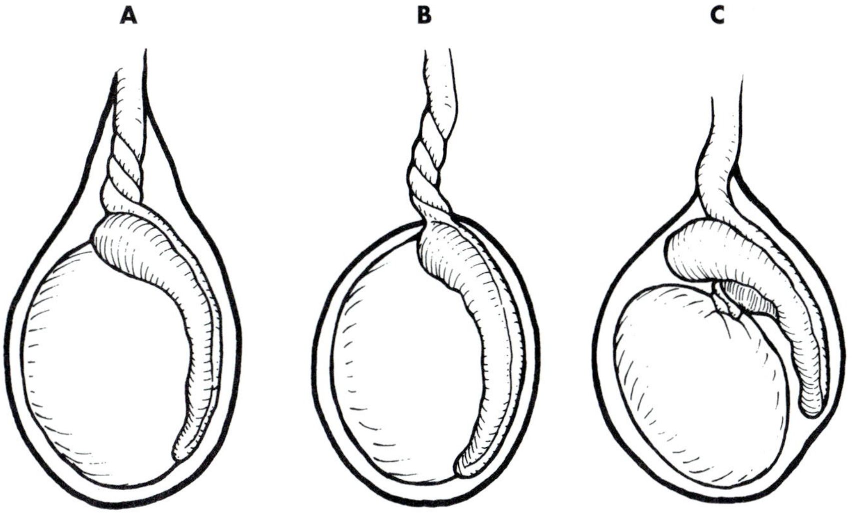

FIG. 61-46. Types of testicular torsion. **A,** Intravaginal torsion above the epididymis. **B,** Extravaginal torsion. **C,** Torsion of the testis below the epididymis. (From Leape LL. Torsion of the testis. In: Welch KJ, Randolph JG, Ravitch MM, eds. *Pediatric Surgery*. St Louis: Mosby-Year Book; 1986.)

encountered type of intravaginal torsion is torsion of the mesorchium, the tissue attachment between the testis and epididymis (Fig. 61-46).[136]

The ultrasound features encountered in testicular torsion depend on the duration and severity of the vascular compromise[159] (see box in right column on p. 1776). The gray-scale appearance of the torsed testis ranges from normal (early on) to enlarged and hypoechoic secondary to edema (usually after 4 to 6 hours) and then to a heterogeneous appearance with areas of increased echogenicity secondary to infarction and hemorrhage (usually after 24 hours) (Fig. 61-47).[136,160-162] The latter appearance is also known as **"missed torsion."** Associated findings include an enlarged, hypoechoic epididymis, reactive hydrocele, skin thickening, and sometimes an enlarged, twisted-appearing spermatic cord.[163]

Epididymitis. Although **epididymitis with or without orchitis** is a common cause of the acute, painful scrotum in postpubertal males, it is also frequently seen in prepubertal boys.[136,164] Sonographically, the inflamed epididymis is usually diffusely enlarged with coarse echoes. The overall echo pattern is usually decreased, but normal or increased echogenicity may be observed.[165] Associated orchitis is more often diffuse; however, when focal, is usually in close proximity to the inflamed epididymis. The involved portion of the testis is usually hypoechoic and enlarged. On color flow Doppler imaging, the inflamed epididymis and testis are typically hyperemic (Fig. 61-48), although occasionally normal flow may be seen in the involved organs.[164,165] Associated sonographic findings include reactive simple or complex hydrocele and skin thickening. Complications of severe epididymo-orchitis include abscess formation and ischemia leading to infarction. Testicular infarction secondary to severe epididymo-orchitis is indistinguishable from infarction secondary to torsion.

Because there is overlap in the gray-scale appearance of both testicular torsion and epididymo-orchitis, differentiation between these two entities is dependent on color flow Doppler imaging. **Torsion** is typically characterized on Doppler imaging by decreased or absent flow within the involved testis (see top box). The classic appearance of **epididymitis** is

TORSION ON COLOR FLOW DOPPLER ULTRASOUND

Decreased or absent flow
Spontaneous detorsion causes normal or increased flow
Incomplete torsion causes normal or decreased flow

EPIDIDYMITIS ON COLOR FLOW DOPPLER ULTRASOUND

Increased flow in epididymis
Increased flow in testes if also infected
Ischemia may cause decreased flow

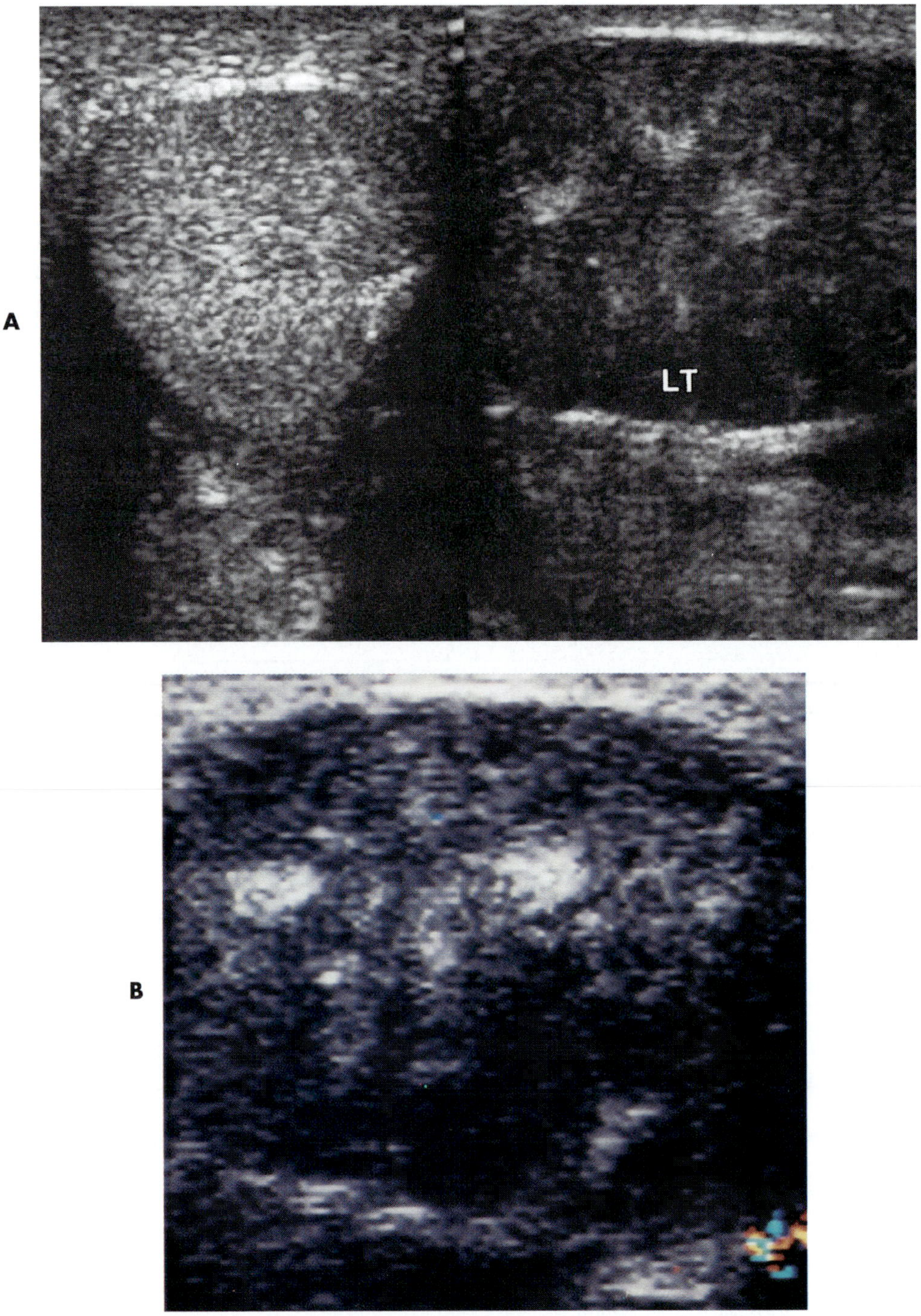

FIG. 61-47. Delayed torsion in a patient with 2 days of left scrotal pain and swelling. **A,** Transverse image of each testis reveals an enlarged, primarily hypoechoic, but heterogeneous left testis, *LT*, and a normal right testis for comparison. **B,** Color image of the left testis shows absence of flow in the surgically proven infarcted testis. A small amount of flow is seen in the paratesticular tissues.

A

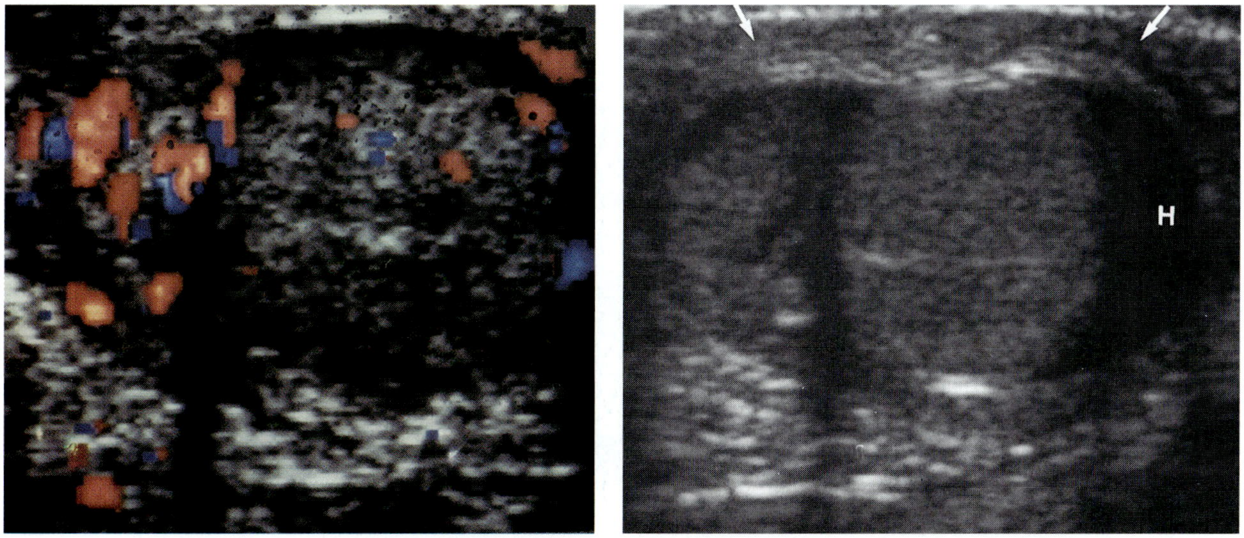

B

FIG. 61-48. Acute epididymitis in an 8-year-old boy with right scrotal pain. **A,** Longitudinal color flow Doppler image of the scrotum reveals increased flow in the epididymis with normal flow in the testis. **B,** Gray-scale longitudinal sonogram of the right hemiscrotum reveals findings associated with epididymo-orchitis, including a reactive hydrocele, *H,* and skin thickening *(arrows)*.

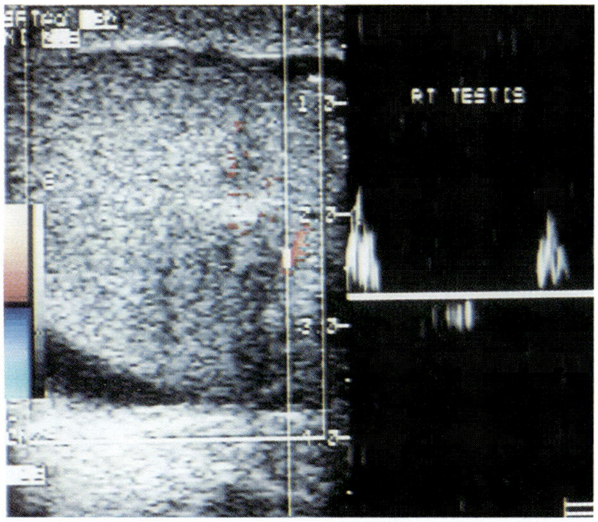

FIG. 61-49. Incomplete testicular torsion in a 14-year-old boy with 3 hours of right scrotal pain. Sagittal image of the right testis with color flow and pulsed wave Doppler imaging demonstrates decreased intraparenchymal testicular flow on color flow Doppler imaging and an abnormally high resistance pattern on pulsed wave Doppler imaging. (Note the color seen on and above the mediastinum testis is artifactual.)

increased flow within the epididymis and the involved testis if orchitis is present (bottom box on p. 1777). Of course, there is overlap between the two, which may lead to false-positive or false-negative diagnoses. These include hyperemic or normal color flow seen in testes with spontaneous detorsion, which may be confused for epididymitis. Incomplete torsion of the testis may reveal normal or decreased color flow (Fig. 61-49).[159,164,166] Ischemia and/or infarction may also be seen with severe epididymitis; however, this is usually less of a diagnostic dilemma because these patients also require surgery. Because Doppler imaging is limited in young patients with testes less than 1 cm^3, power and contrast agents may be helpful in distinguishing between torsed and normal testes.[167]

In patients whose clinical symptoms and signs strongly suggest testicular torsion, emergent surgery is recommended. Because testicular salvage rates are proportional to duration and severity of the torsion,[159] some authors believe that closed manual detorsion may improve salvage rates and convert an emergent situation to an elective surgical procedure for future orchiopexy (Fig. 61-50). This, however, is controversial.[168,169]

Torsion of a Testicular Appendage. **Torsion of a testicular appendage** (Fig. 61-51) may produce the same clinical signs and symptoms of testicular torsion or epididymitis. If the classic clinical finding of a small, round, mobile, tender mass in the superior aspect of the scrotum is not found, then ultrasound is recommended to avoid unnecessary surgery. The diagnostic sonographic appearance is that of a solid, ovoid mass with a variable-size hypoechoic center and hyperechoic rim adjacent to a testis with normal vascularity (Fig. 61-52).[170] Color flow Doppler imaging often reveals hypervascularity in the periphery of the mass.[170,171]

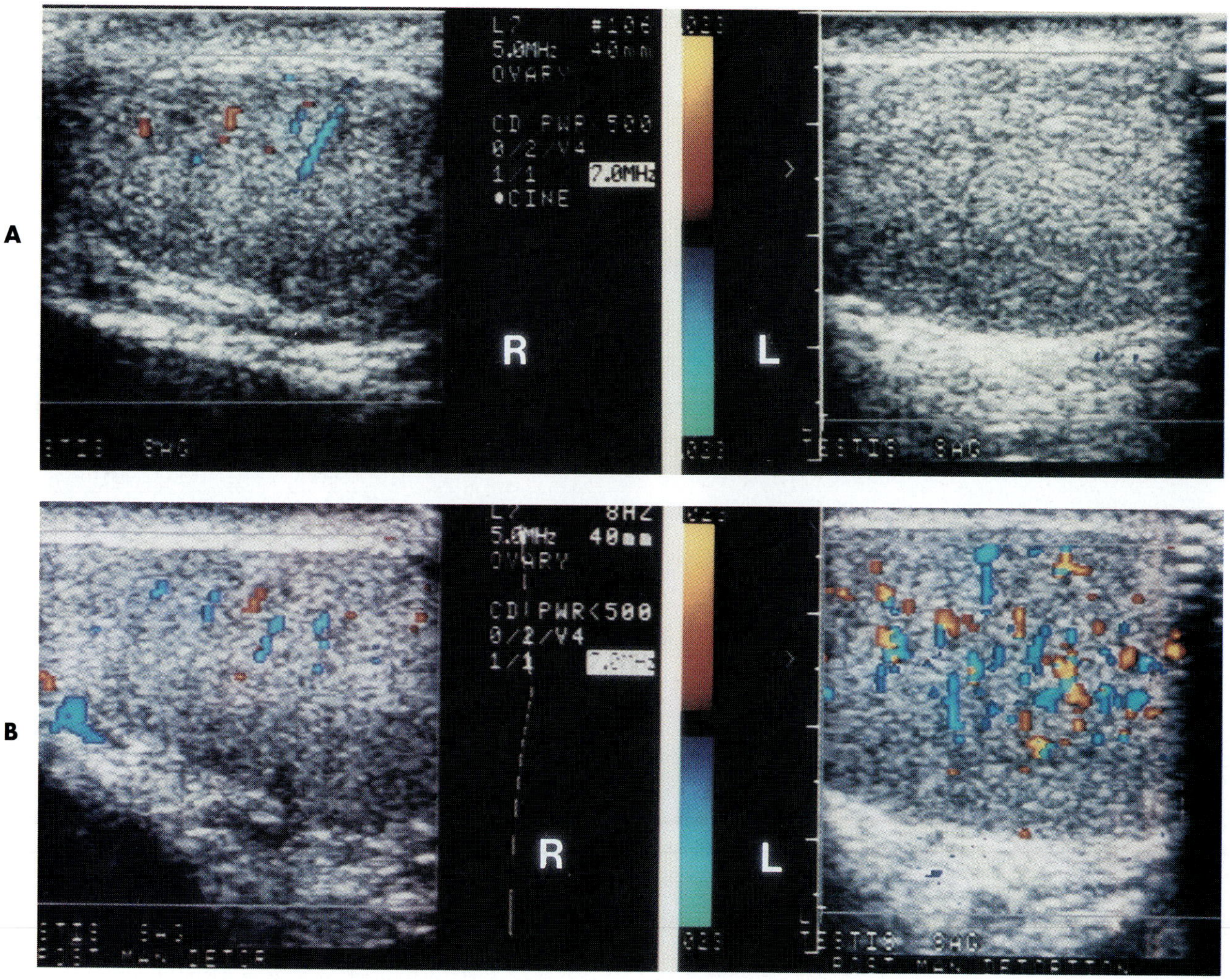

FIG. 61-50. Testicular torsion before and after closed manual detorsion in a 13-year-old boy with 7 hours of left scrotal pain. **A,** Color flow Doppler images of both testes reveal absent flow in the left, *L*, testis, representing testicular torsion. Normal flow in right, *R*, testis for comparison. **B,** Color flow Doppler images of both testes after 360-degree closed manual detorsion of the left testis shows new hyperemic flow in the left testis compared with normal flow in the right testis.

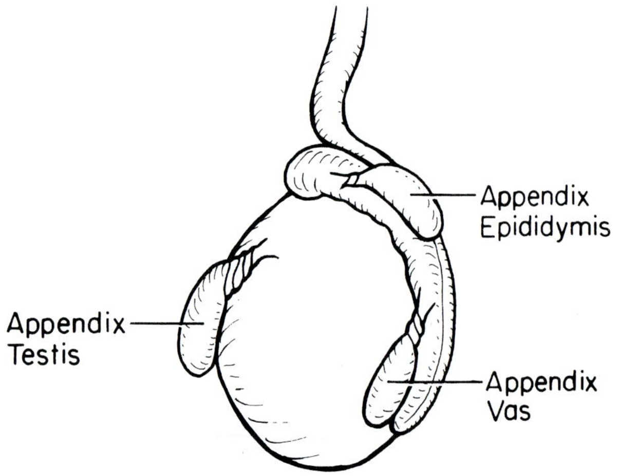

FIG. 61-51. Testicular appendages. Appendix testis, appendix epididymis, and appendix vas (vas aberrans of Haller). (From Leape LL. Torsion of the testis. In: Welch KJ, Randolph JG, Ravitch MM, eds. *Pediatric Surgery*. St Louis: Mosby-Year Book; 1986.)

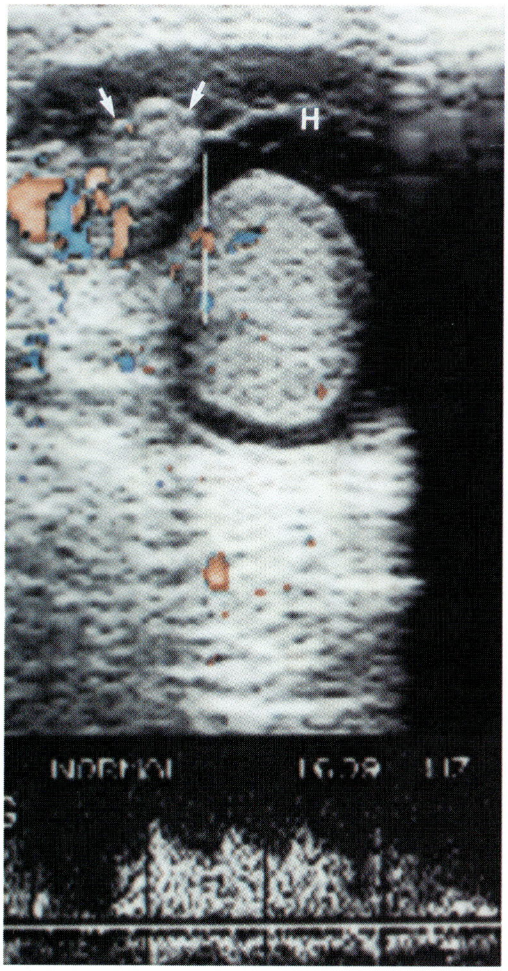

FIG. 61-52. Torsion of appendix epididymis in 12-year-old boy with 10 hours of scrotal pain. Sagittal color flow and pulsed wave Doppler image of the scrotum reveals an enlarged avascular paratesticular mass *(arrows)* with increased flow in the adjacent epididymis. Normal testicular flow detected, excluding testicular torsion. A reactive complex hydrocele, *H*, is seen. (Case courtesy of Heidi Patriquin, M.D.)

Trauma. Trauma to the scrotum most commonly results from sporting injuries but may be seen in straddle or handlebar injuries, motor vehicle accidents, child abuse, or birth trauma. Trauma can cause a testicular hematoma, fracture, or rupture. Testicular rupture is a surgical emergency. Improved salvage rates have been shown if surgery to repair a ruptured testis is performed within 72 hours of the traumatic event.[172] Sonographic findings of rupture (Fig. 61-53) include diffuse parenchymal heterogeneity with loss of a normal, smooth contour and disruption of the tunica albuginea, extrusion of seminiferous tubules, and nonvisualization of the testis. The presence of flow on color flow Doppler imaging in the traumatized testis is helpful in excluding testicular ischemia. Testicular

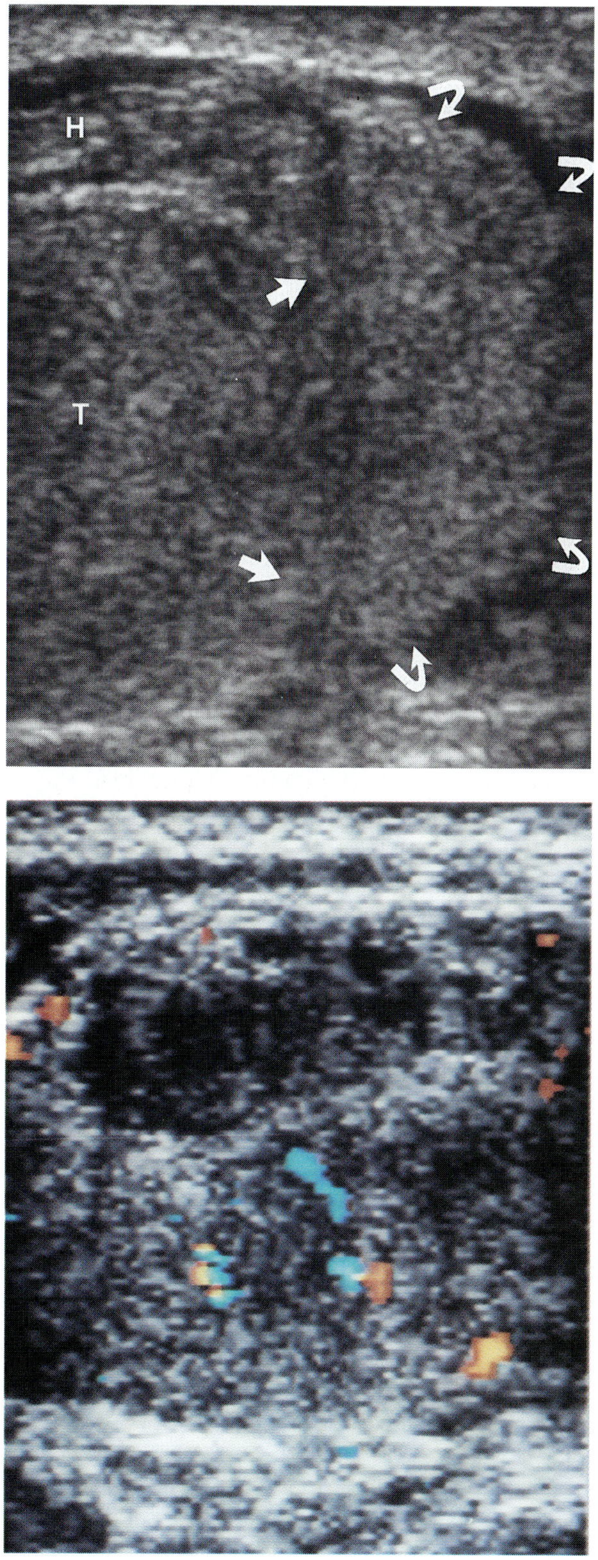

A

B

FIG. 61-53. Testicular rupture in a patient with scrotal pain after groin kick. A, Longitudinal view of the inferior aspect of the left testis shows disruption of the tunica albuginea *(straight arrows)* with extrusion of seminiferous tubules *(curved arrows)*. Associated hematocele, *H*, is present. *T*, Testis. **B,** Color flow Doppler image of the left testis reveals heterogeneity, representing contusion and hemorrhage within the testicular parenchyma. Intratesticular flow excludes infarction.

hematomas appear as avascular masses, the echogenicity of which varies depending on the age of the hematoma.[138] Associated findings include scrotal hematomas, hematoceles, and wall thickening. Complications of testicular rupture include infarction, chronic pain, abscess, and infertility.[173] Although ultrasound may aid in evaluating the traumatized scrotum, there is controversy as to its usefulness since some question its accuracy and recommend early surgical exploration even in the absence of testicular rupture.[174]

Idiopathic Scrotal Edema. **Acute idiopathic scrotal edema** is a less common cause of scrotal edema. This uncommon condition typically affects boys between 5 and 11 years of age and presents with scrotal swelling, erythema, and minimal pain (Fig. 61-54). Swelling may extend to the anterior abdominal wall and perineum. Sonographic findings include marked thickening of the scrotal wall with normal testes and epididymides. On color flow Doppler imaging there may be no to slightly increased flow to the scrotal wall with normal flow to the testes and epididymides.[138,175]

Henoch-Schönlein Purpura. Scrotal or testicular involvement is estimated in 15% to 38% of patients with **Henoch-Schönlein purpura.** Sonographic findings include diffuse swelling of the scrotum and contents with intact testicular flow, obviating the need for surgery in this entity, which usually resolves spontaneously and completely. Color flow Doppler imaging reveals hypervascularity, especially in the thickened scrotal wall.[138] Careful examination for the classic purpuric rash over the buttocks, lower extremities, and perineum aids in diagnosis.[176]

Intraabdominal Process. **Scrotal swelling and pain may also be secondary to an intraabdominal process,** especially in neonates with a patent processus vaginalis. Various fluids such as blood, chyle, pus, dialysis fluid, CSF from ventriculoperitoneal shunt, or other intraperitoneal fluids can drain into the scrotum. Blood from the abdomen can enter the scrotum through diapedesis into the tissue planes or through a patent processus vaginalis and can represent the presenting findings in patients with adrenal hemorrhage,[153] hepatic laceration, or delayed splenic rupture in a battered child.[151] Scrotal swelling has been reported in association with inflammatory or infectious conditions such as acute appendicitis, perforated appendicitis,[150] or Crohn's disease.[155] Another unusual cause for scrotal swelling includes testicular vein thrombosis from a femoral venous line during cardiac catheterization.[156] In the neonate with scrotal swelling or even older children in whom the cause of scrotal swelling is unclear, abdominal sonography may help diagnose a primary abdominal event as the cause for secondary scrotal pathology.[153]

Scrotal Masses

Intratesticular Causes. Benign and malignant testicular tumors are the seventh most common neoplasm in children. **Eighty percent of testicular tumors are malignant.** In the pediatric age group, there are two peak incidences of testicular neoplasms: in children less than $2^1/_2$ years (60%) and in late adolescence (40%). The incidence of malignancy in a cryptorchid (abdominal) testis is increased by a factor of 30 to 50. Both **seminomas** (malignant) and **gonadoblastomas** (benign) commonly develop in dysplastic gonads associated with undescended testes, testicular feminization syndrome, male pseudohermaphroditism, and true hermaphroditism.[177]

Primary testicular neoplasms are divided into those of germ cell and nongerm cell origin. In prepubertal children, 70% are of germ cell origin, and 40% of these are endodermal sinus tumors (yolk sac carcinoma).[178] **Endodermal sinus tumors** occur primarily as a painless scrotal mass in infants 12 to 24 months of age. There may be an associated ipsilateral hydrocele (25%) or inguinal hernia (21%). The tumor may metastasize to the lungs, especially in older children, but retroperitoneal lymph node metastasis is rare. **Embryonal carcinoma** usually occurs in adolescence or young adulthood (Fig. 61-55). It is highly malignant and commonly spreads to retroperitoneal and mediastinal lymph nodes with hematogenous metastases to the lung, liver, and brain.[177] The other germ cell tumors seen commonly in adults, including seminoma, teratocarcinoma, and choriocarcinoma, are rare in children.[178] Testicular teratomas in infants and young children are uncommon and usually benign.

The most common primary nongerm cell tumors of the testes are Sertoli's cell and Leydig's cell tumors. They are usually hormone-secreting tumors. The Leydig's cell tumor can synthesize testosterone and thus cause precocious puberty. Sertoli's cell tumors can secrete estrogen, causing feminization. Both of these nongerm cell tumors are slow growing and benign.[177]

The testes are a well-known sanctuary site for **leukemia** and **lymphoma** (Fig. 61-56).[179,180] **Neuroblastoma** can metastasize to the testicle.[181]

The sonographic findings in all of the above-mentioned testicular tumors are not specific. The involved testicle is usually enlarged with a globular or lobulated contour. Both primary and metastatic tumor may result in focal masses or diffuse involvement. The echotexture may be hypoechoic, heterogeneous, or even normal.[182] Gray-scale abnormalities may be seen more frequently in the testes of older postpubertal patients with testicular tumors. This may reflect the histologically different tumors affecting different age groups. Color flow Doppler imaging is helpful in the evaluation of pediatric testicular tumors. Disorganized hypervascular blood

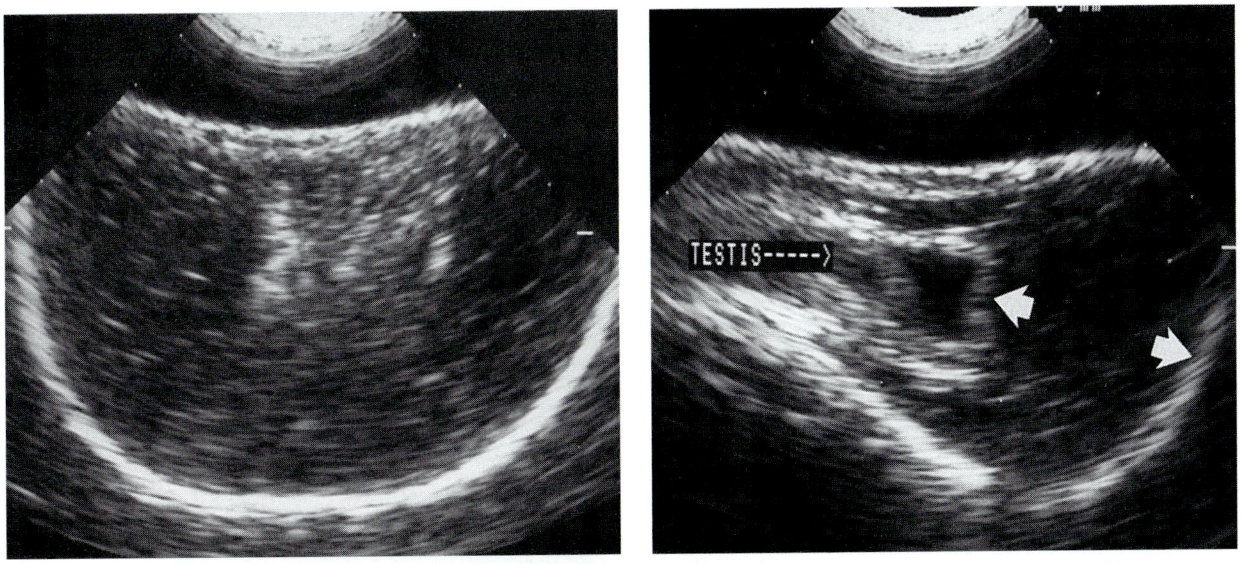

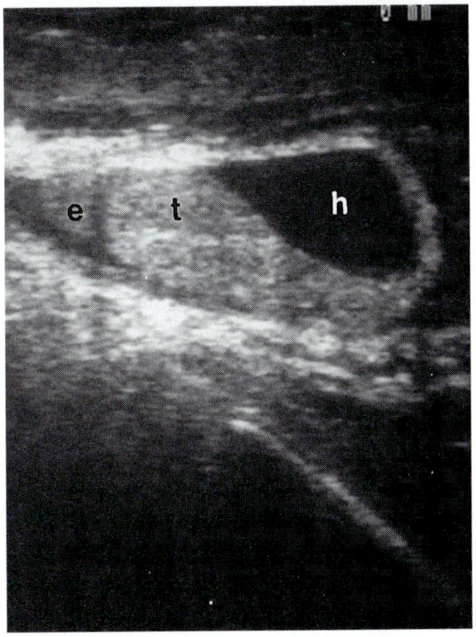

FIG. 61-54. Acute idiopathic scrotal edema in a 4-year-old boy with sudden, painless, scrotal swelling. **A,** Transverse and, **B,** sagittal images of the scrotum using a step-off pad reveal marked scrotal swelling *(arrows)*. **C,** Sagittal image of the right hemiscrotum reveals a normal right testis, *t*, and epididymis, *e*, with an adjacent hydrocele, *h*. The left testis and epididymis (not shown) were also normal.

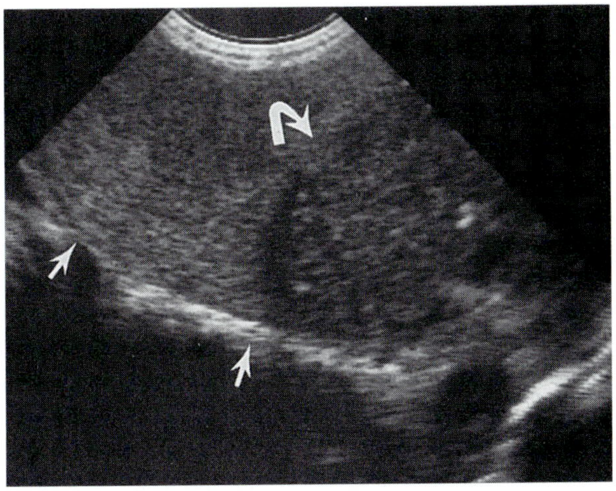

FIG. 61-55. Embryonal carcinoma of the testicle. This 20-year-old man presented with painless scrotal mass. Note complex mass *(curved arrow)* in lower pole of right testicle *(straight arrows)*. Multiple, echogenic foci seen within mass are consistent with calcifications.

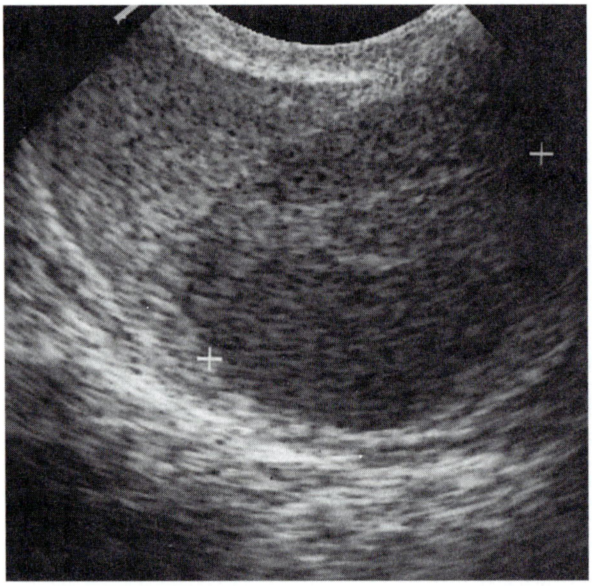

FIG. 61-56. Leukemic infiltration of the testis in a 20-year-old man with acute lymphocytic leukemia relapse. Sagittal image reveals an enlarged right testis with an oval, hypoechoic mass *(calipers)*, representing focal leukemic infiltration.

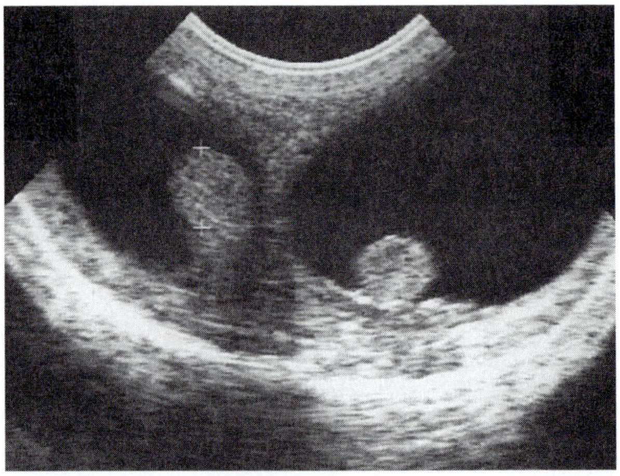

FIG. 61-57. Bilateral hydroceles in a newborn. Transverse view of the scrotum shows both testes outlined by large, anechoic fluid collections.

flow was seen in 6 (86%) of 7 patients in a study of pediatric patients with testicular tumors by Luker and Siegel.[182] Although all the patients had testicular enlargement, the testicular echotexture in 4 (57%) of 7 patients was normal, thus color flow Doppler was helpful in depicting the tumor in these patients. Hypervascularity with normal echogenicity may be seen in orchitis; however, orchitis without epididymitis is uncommon, especially in prepubertal children, and history helps in distinguishing the two entities since tumor frequently presents as an enlarged, nontender mass.[182]

Solitary simple cysts with preserved adjacent testicular parenchyma, although uncommon, have been described in the testes. These lesions are benign and thus may be followed with sonography. If there is growth of the cyst, then conservative surgery with removal of the cyst and preservation of the adjacent parenchyma may be performed.[183] The cysts differ from epidermoid cysts and other cystic neoplasms that contain internal echoes.

Extratesticular Causes. **Hydroceles** are the most common cause of scrotal enlargement in children. As the testis descends into the scrotum, it becomes invested with a portion of peritoneum, the processus vaginalis. At birth, the processus vaginalis normally closes off proximally and forms the tunica vaginalis. A variable amount of peritoneal fluid may be trapped within the tunica vaginalis, forming a stable hydrocele in the neonate. This fluid is resorbed slowly during the first 18 months of life. If the processus vaginalis fails to close, then an open communication exists between the peritoneal cavity and scrotum. This can result in a scrotal hernia or a communicating hydrocele in which the amount of fluid varies. Extension of the hydrocele into the pelvis can be seen in a communicating hydrocele. Surgical ligation is required to close the patent processus vaginalis.[143]

The usual sonographic appearance of a hydrocele is an anechoic, well-demarcated area with through transmission (Fig. 61-57). The presence of echoes or septations in the fluid suggests a reactive hydrocele caused by infection, torsion, trauma, or tumor. Other collections such as chronic hemorrhage or lymphoceles (associated with ipsilateral renal transplantation) may be seen and confused for a reactive hydrocele.

A **scrotal hernia** is usually evident clinically. Sonography may demonstrate fluid- or air-containing bowel loops in the scrotum, normal testes and epididymides, and/or an echogenic area representing herniated omentum. Lack of peristalsis within herniated bowel loops is worrisome for ischemia. Ischemia and incarceration (nonreducibility of bowel loops) convert an elective surgical procedure to an emergent one. Extratesticular pathology such as hematoceles and loculated hydroceles can mimic fluid-filled bowel loops, and herniated omentum can be confused for primary scrotal masses. Thus, examination of the inguinal canal and the region of Hesselbach's triangle is recommended to evaluate for a hernia sac and exclude a primary scrotal pathology.[184]

Other commonly identified scrotal masses in adolescent and postpubertal males are varicoceles, spermatoceles, and epididymal cysts. **Varicoceles** represent dilated veins in the pampiniform plexus

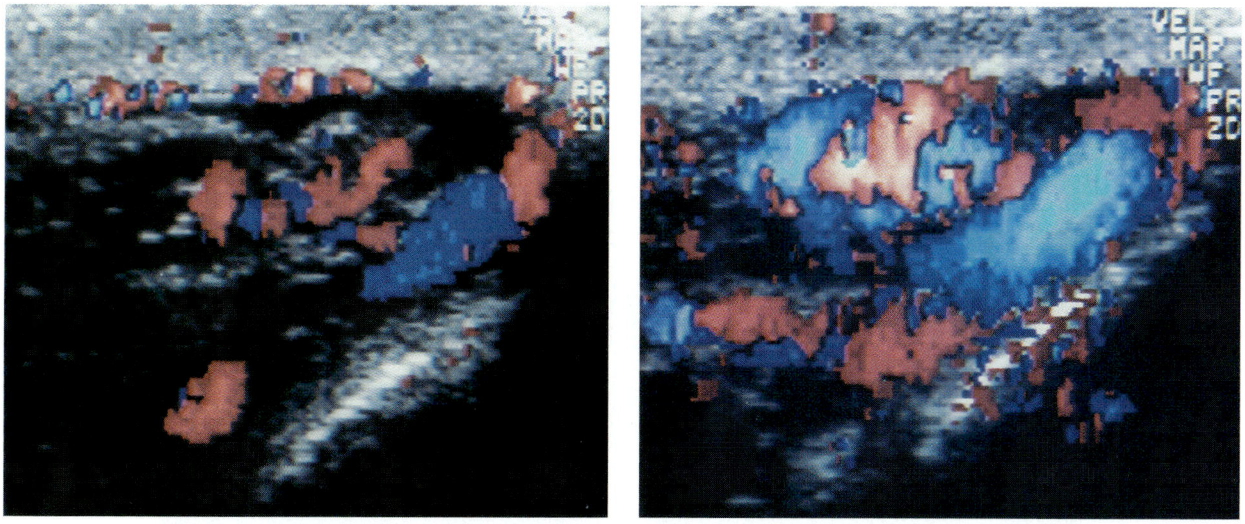

FIG. 61-58. Left varicocele in a postpubertal patient complaining of feeling "wormlike" structures in his scrotum. **A,** Longitudinal color flow Doppler image of the paratesticular tissues reveals multiple, prominent, anechoic, tubular structures, some of which demonstrate color flow. **B,** Longitudinal color flow Doppler image with Valsalva's maneuver reveals increased size and exuberant flow in these paratesticular veins.

positioned posterior to the testis. The majority (85% to 98%) of cases are on the left side.[132,138] The presence of varicoceles in young boys is uncommon and may result from compression of the spermatic cord by tumor. Gray-scale sonographic evaluation reveals small, serpentine, anechoic structures that display flow on color flow Doppler imaging and venous waveforms on pulsed wave Doppler imaging. Augmentation of Doppler flow occurs with Valsalva's maneuver and upright positioning (Fig. 61-58).

Spermatoceles occur in the epididymal head and consist of fluid, spermatozoa, and sediment. **Epididymal cysts** contain no spermatozoa and can occur in the epididymal head, body, or tail. Sonographically, these entities appear as round structures with through transmission, well-defined back walls, with and without debris. They range in size from a few millimeters to several centimeters.[132] Other cystic lesions include spermatic cord cysts and cysts of the tunica vaginalis.

Rhabdomyosarcoma is the most common paratesticular tumor in childhood (Fig. 61-59). Other malignant lesions include metastatic neuroblastoma, lymphoma, leiomyosarcoma, and fibrosarcoma. Benign paratesticular tumors include fibromas, hemangiomas, lipomas, leiomyomas, lymphangiomas, and neurofibromas.[185,186] Both benign and malignant paratesticular tumors may appear hypoechoic or hyperechoic, and heterogeneity may be evident. Ultrasound cannot clearly distinguish between benign and malignant lesions.[187] Increased vascularity on Doppler imaging in a paratesticular rhabdomyosarcoma may mimic that seen with epididymitis.[188] Thus clinical

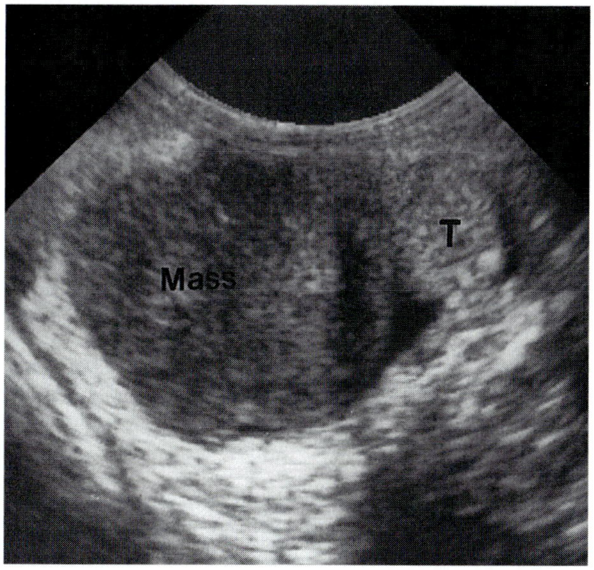

FIG. 61-59. Paratesticular rhabdomyosarcoma. Large, solid mass was identified medial to left testis, *T*, with small amount of free intrascrotal fluid in this 18-month-old boy.

and/or **sonographic follow-up should be performed in cases of suspected epididymitis in order to ensure resolution of a palpable mass or sonographic abnormality.**

Focal calcifications from meconium periorchitis may present as palpable scrotal masses (Fig. 61-60). These dystrophic calcifications result from *in utero* bowel perforation. Free meconium enters the scrotum via a patent processus vaginalis and elicits a

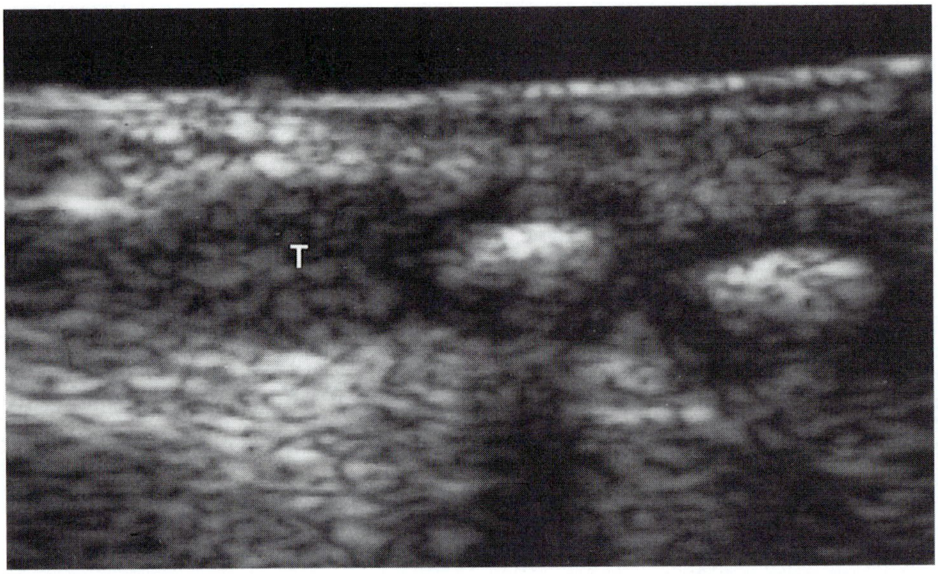

FIG. 61-60. Meconium periorchitis in a 5-year-old boy with painless scrotal masses. Sagittal view of the left hemiscrotum via a step-off pad shows two well-defined, oval, brightly echogenic masses with hypoechoic halos and acoustic shadows, which lie inferior to the normal left testis, *T*. (From Mene M, Rosenberg HK, Ginsberg PC. Meconium periorchitis presenting as scrotal nodules in a five year old boy. *J Ultrasound Med* 1994; 13:491-494.)

foreign body inflammatory response resulting in focal calcifications. Like calcification elsewhere, sonographically these areas appear echogenic with strong posterior shadows. There is eventual spontaneous regression of these calcifications and thus conservative management is recommended.[189] Differential diagnosis of scrotal or testicular calcifications in the pediatric patient includes teratoma, gonadoblastoma, Leydig's cell tumor, testicular microlithiasis, meconium peritonitis, and postinflammatory or infectious scrotal calculi.

Testicular microlithiasis is an asymptomatic condition that has a characteristic sonographic appearance and usually is discovered incidentally. Testicular microlithiasis represents calcified debris within the seminiferous tubules and correspondingly appears on ultrasound as tiny, 1 to 2 ml, hyperechoic, nonshadowing foci (Fig. 61-61). The number of echogenic foci within the testis can range from few to many. Although testicular microlithiasis represents pathologically benign disease, it is associated with conditions that have increased risk of malignancy such as cryptorchidism, infertility, and testicular atrophy. In addition, Backus et al. reported in a retrospective study the presence of germ cell neoplasms in 17 (40%) of 42 patients.[190] Until the association of testicular microlithiasis is better understood, clinical and/or sonographic monitoring of these patients is advised.[190]

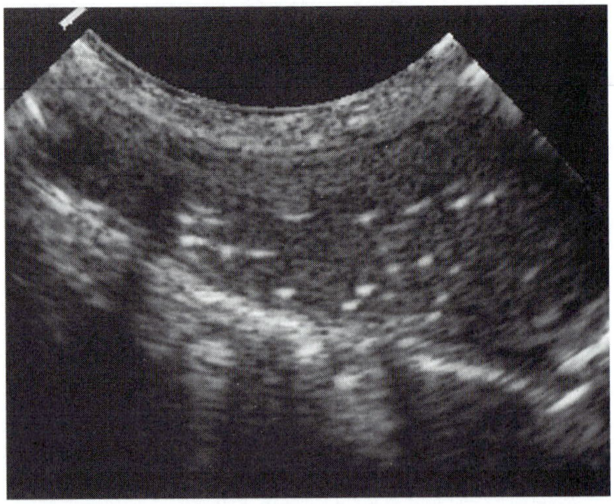

FIG. 61-61. Testicular microlithiasis in a 7-year-old boy with a history of left cryptorchidism and a possible right scrotal mass. Multiple, tiny, hyperechoic foci are seen scattered throughout the right testis. No scrotal mass was identified.

GASTROINTESTINAL TRACT

Obstruction

Sonography has become an important imaging modality in the evaluation of the pediatric gastrointestinal tract.[191,192] In the child with a distended abdomen, ultrasound is a useful diagnostic tool for the

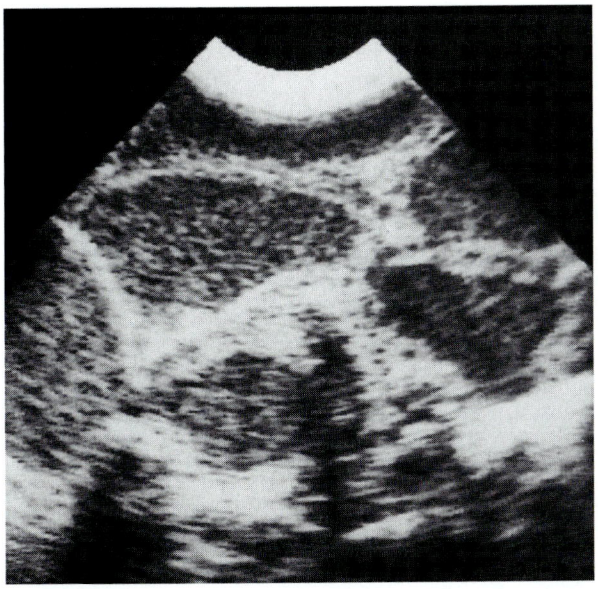

FIG. 61-62. Meconium ileus. Transverse sonogram of right lower quadrant shows distended, meconium-filled, small bowel loops. (From Sherman NH, Boyle GK, Rosenberg HK. Sonography in the neonate. *Ultrasound Q* 1988;6:91-150.)

detection of ascites, dilated fluid-filled bowel loops, masses, abscess collections, and closed-loop obstructions that may not be evident on the plain abdominal radiographs.[193] In a distal bowel obstruction, real-time ultrasound shows active peristalsis in dilated, fluid-filled, tubular-shaped proximal bowel loops. The small bowel mucosal pattern and colonic haustrations become obliterated as the bowel lumen distends. The normal gut wall is uniform and compliant, with an average thickness of 3 mm when distended. Acutely, the thickness of the bowel wall is normal, but as the obstruction persists, the bowel wall thickens as a result of edema. In a paralytic ileus, peristaltic activity is markedly diminished, but the valvulae conniventes can be appreciated within discrete tubular loops.[191]

Distal bowel obstruction in the neonate results in the retention of meconium proximal to the obstruction. The meconium appears as echogenic material within the bowel lumen (Fig. 61-62).[35] The most common causes of neonatal distal bowel obstruction include **ileal atresia, meconium ileus, meconium plug syndrome,** and **Hirschsprung's disease** (Fig. 61-63). Although contrast enemas usually provide the diagnosis, ultrasound has been helpful in difficult cases. In meconium ileus, the thick, tenacious meconium appears as brightly echogenic masses and little fluid within the small bowel lumen.[194] In contrast, the meconium in ileal atresia has a normal consistency, and therefore the echogenic meconium is admixed with fluid-filled loops.

Sonography has been used in the evaluation of **imperforate anus** to determine the level of the rectal pouch.[195,196] The position of the rectal pouch, in relation to the levator sling, determines the surgical approach. A direct perineal approach and pull-through technique is performed if the rectal pouch is low and passes through the levator sling. In high lesions above the puborectalis muscle, a decompressive colostomy is performed initially. There is also a high association of renal and vertebral anomalies and rectal fistulae with the genitourinary tract in high imperforate anus. Ultrasound has now been added to the radiologist's armamentarium for the evaluation of this difficult problem. High-resolution, real-time sonography with a 7.5-MHz transducer is performed in the sagittal plane through the anterior abdominal wall with the patient in the supine position. A longitudinal midline transperineal scan is also obtained (Fig. 61-64). The distance between the fluid-filled rectal pouch and the perineum is measured. A distance of 1.5 cm or less indicates a low imperforate anus. The authors advise gentle scanning pressure to avoid compression reduction of the area of interest. On transabdominal images, the rectal pouch does not pass below the base of the bladder in high imperforate anus.

Cloacal malformation is an uncommon anomaly in which the rectum, vagina, and urethra end in a common terminal channel as the only outlet for the three systems. There is no anus, at times the external genitalia may be ambiguous, the sacrum is frequently deformed, and there may be associated uterine, vaginal, gastrourinary tract (particularly vesicoureteral reflux), musculoskeletal, cardiovascular, gastrointestinal, and central nervous system anomalies.[197]

Inflammation

Acute appendicitis is the most common cause of emergency surgery in children. Perforation with acute appendicitis is more common in children than adults. In infants, appendiceal perforation may occur in 80% of cases. In addition, the progression of disease from the onset of symptoms to perforation is more rapid in infants than in older children and adults.[198]

Using the graded compression technique,[199,200] the inflamed appendix can be directly visualized with high-resolution ultrasound (see first box on p. 1789). The inflamed appendix appears as a tubular, blind-ending structure with a hypoechoic center that is surrounded by an inner echogenic and outer hypoechoic layer (Fig. 61-65).[201] The appendix is rigid, lacks peristalsis, has a maximum outer diameter greater than 6 mm, and does not compress when the examiner gently presses the abdominal wall with the transducer. Appendiceal wall thickening of greater than 2 mm is often asymmetric.[202] Sonography can also identify appendiceal calculi and surrounding periap-

A

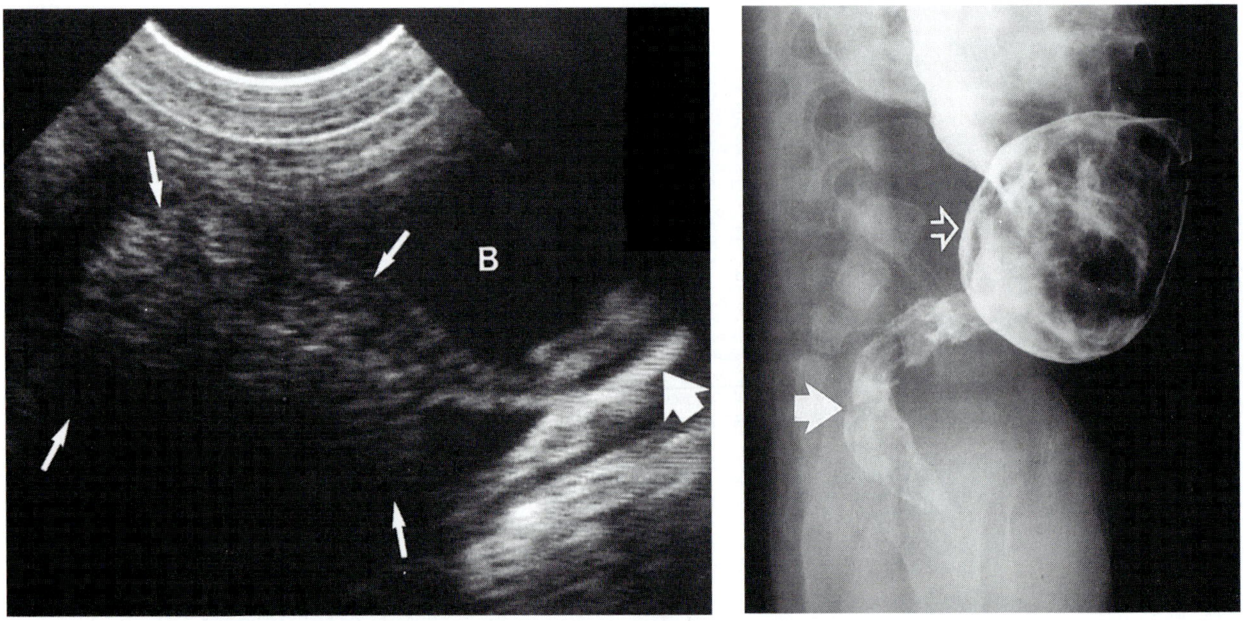

B

FIG. 61-63. Hirschsprung's disease; 9-month-old boy with hypotonia, weakness, normocytic anemia, and large abdomen. **A,** Sagittal sonogram of pelvis shows narrow, unfilled rectum *(large arrow)*. Above this area is massively distended sigmoid *(small arrows)* filled with tremendous fecal boluses, which shadow the ultrasound beam. **B,** Barium enema demonstrating collapsed aganglionic segment *(solid arrow)* and distended, feces-filled, sigmoid colon *(open arrow)*. (From Rosenberg HK, Goldberg BB. Pediatric radiology: sonography. In: Margulis AR, Burhenne HJ, eds. *Alimentary Tract Radiology*. 4th ed. St Louis: Mosby–Year Book; 1989.)

A

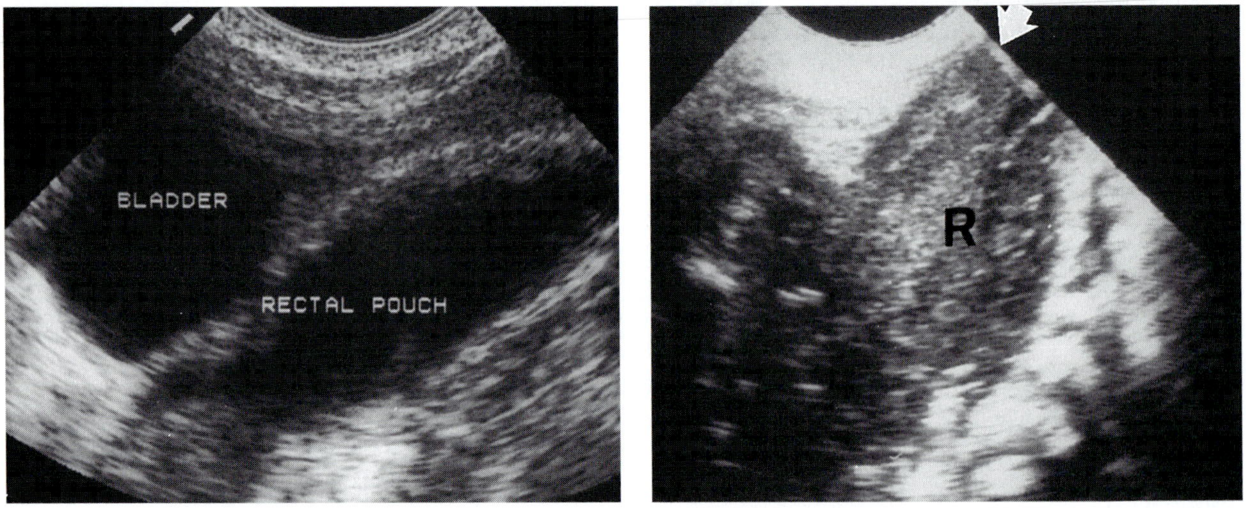

B

FIG. 61-64. Imperforate anus. **A,** Sonogram of the pelvis through a well-distended bladder demonstrates a fluid-filled rectal pouch extending inferiorly, implying a low, imperforate anus. **B,** Perineal scan of same newborn as in Fig. 61-64, *A*, shows that the rectal pouch is in fact a "covered anus" *(arrow)*. *R*, Rectum. (From Rosenberg HK, Goldberg BB. Pediatric radiology: sonography. In: Margulis AR, Burhenne HJ, eds. *Alimentary Tract Radiology*. 4th ed. St Louis: Mosby–Year Book; 1989.)

pendiceal edema and abscess (Fig. 61-66). Three sonographic findings have been reported to be associated with appendiceal perforation[203] (see second box on p. 1789). These include a loculated pericecal fluid collection, indicating abscess; prominent pericecal fat of more than 10 mm in thickness; and circumferential loss of the echogenic submucosal layer of the appendix. Sonography is also helpful in the detection and follow-up evaluation of postappendectomy fluid collections.[204]

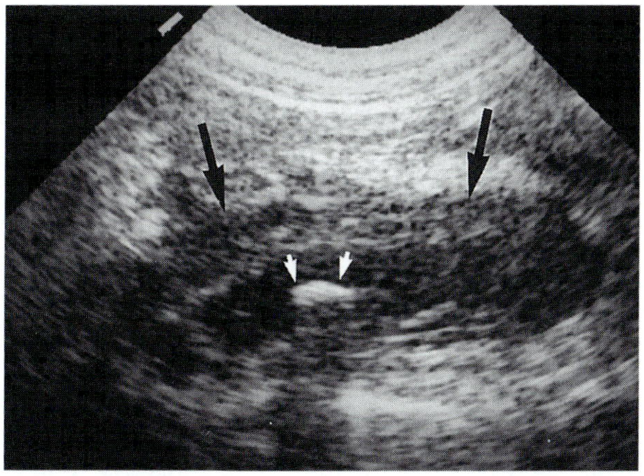

FIG. 61-65. Acute appendicitis with appendicolith in a 13-year-old girl with right lower quadrant pain and fever. Sagittal sonogram of the right lower quadrant/upper pelvis shows a thick-walled noncompressible, fluid-filled appendix *(black arrows)* with a bright, shadowing, echogenic focus representing an appendicolith *(white arrows)*.

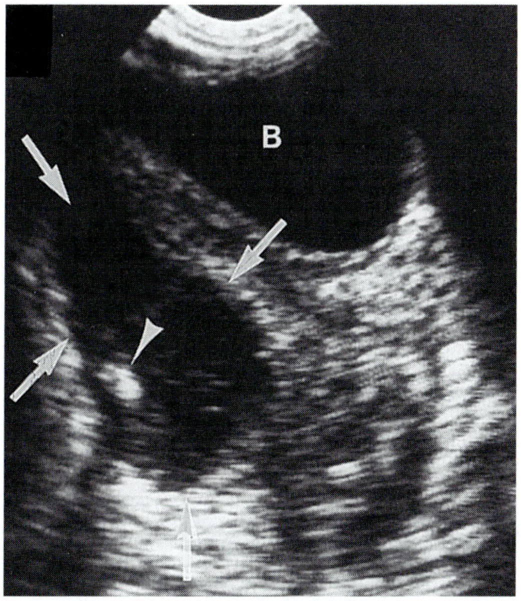

FIG. 61-66. Appendiceal abscess. Loculated fluid collection *(arrows)* was noted in right lower quadrant, containing scattered internal debris and calcified appendicolith *(arrowhead)*. *B*, Bladder. (From Fisher MR, Kricun ME. *Imaging of the Pelvis*. Gaithersburg, Md: Aspen Publishers; 1989.)

ULTRASOUND FINDINGS IN APPENDICITIS

Tubular, blind-ending mass
Noncompressible
Appendix >6 mm
Periappendiceal edema

ULTRASOUND FINDINGS IN APPENDICEAL PERFORATION

Loculated pericecal fluid or abscess
Prominent pericecal fat >10 mm thick
Loss of echogenic submucosa of appendix

COLOR FLOW DOPPLER ULTRASOUND IN APPENDICITIS

Hypervascularity of appendix
Hypervascularity of periappendix area
Hypervascularity around a fluid collection with perforation

Quillin and Siegel showed that the addition of color flow Doppler imaging to routine gray-scale imaging can increase the sensitivity of the ultrasound examination for detecting appendicitis to 95%[205] (see third box). The normal appendix and periappendiceal tissues have minimal to no flow on color flow Doppler imaging. The presence of hypervascularity in the appendix or periappendiceal tissues reflects an infectious or inflammatory process. This proved useful in identifying inflamed appendices in 9% of patients in Quillin and Siegel's study despite normal appendix size on gray-scale imaging.[205] Peripheral appendiceal hyperemia suggests the presence of nonperforated appendicitis.[206] The absence of appendiceal hyperemia, however, does not exclude appendicitis. Color flow Doppler predictors of appendiceal perforation include hyperemia in the periappendiceal soft tissues or around a periappendiceal or pelvic fluid collection. Bowel hyperemia may be seen in nonperforating appendicitis and in primary bowel disease and thus is not specific for perforation.[206]

Other causes of acute right lower quadrant and pelvic pain can also be diagnosed with pelvic sonography such as pelvic inflammatory disease and ovarian torsion. A **psoas abscess or hematoma** is usually confined to the psoas muscle, and the patient often presents with lower abdominal pain, pelvic pain, or both, which radiates to the groin and hip (Fig. 61-67). In **inflammatory bowel disease,** the involved bowel loops have a thickened, hypoechoic wall with dense central echoes. There is decreased mobility, compressibility, and peristalsis of the involved loop. The adjacent mesentery is thickened. Additional sonographic findings in **Crohn's disease** include associated adynamic ileus with distended, fluid-filled bowel loops; a complex heterogeneous mass caused by a conglomerate of matted, inflamed bowel loops; abscess; and secondary ureteral obstruction with hydronephrosis.[207]

Mesenteric adenitis and **acute terminal ileitis,** caused by *Yersinia enterocolitica* infection, often cause clinical symptoms identical to acute appendicitis. However, these entities are treated conservatively without surgical intervention. The graded compression technique can be used to differentiate these two diseases from appendicitis. The sonographic criteria of mesenteric adenitis and acute terminal ileitis are mural thickening (4 to 6 mm) of the terminal ileum and cecum with diminished peristalsis; multiple, round, enlarged, echolucent, mesenteric lymph nodes; and nonvisualization of an inflamed appendix (Fig. 61-68).[208]

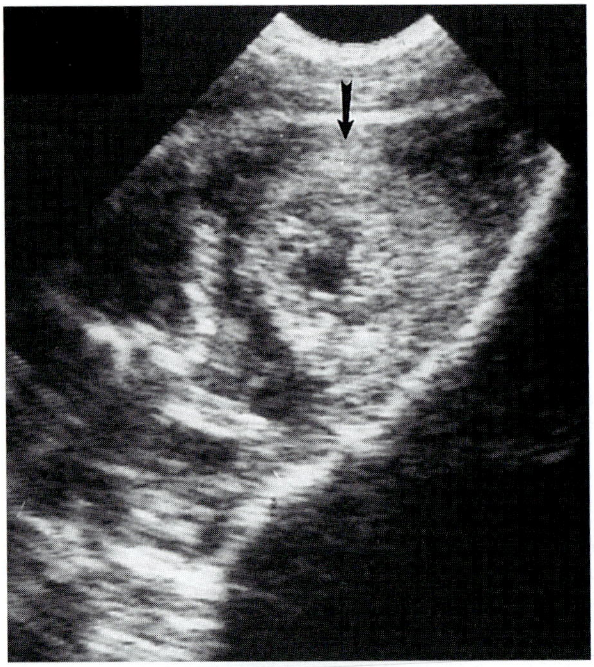

FIG. 61-67. Psoas hematoma. Transverse view of left psoas muscle shows rounded, complex, echogenic mass *(arrow)* within muscle consistent with psoas hematoma in this teenaged child with hemophilia.

PRESACRAL MASSES

The presacral space is a potential space between the perirectal fascia and the fibrous coverings of the anterior sacrum. A lesion in the presacral space can usually be identified on routine transabdominal sonograms through a distended bladder. To confirm the origin of the mass, a water enema can be performed to identify the rectosigmoid colon in relation to the lesion. Additional scans through the buttocks are often helpful to determine the true extent of the tumor (see box on p. 1792).

Sacrococcygeal teratoma is the most common presacral neoplasm in the pediatric age group. Fifty percent are noted at birth, with a 4:1 female-to-male incidence. Sacrococcygeal teratoma arises from multipotential cells in Hensen's nodes that migrate caudally and come to lie within the coccyx. Radiographic evidence of bony abnormalities of the sacrum or coccyx may be present. There is a 75% incidence of associated congenital anomalies, most commonly involving the musculoskeletal system.[209] These teratomas are most common in families with a high frequency of twins.[210]

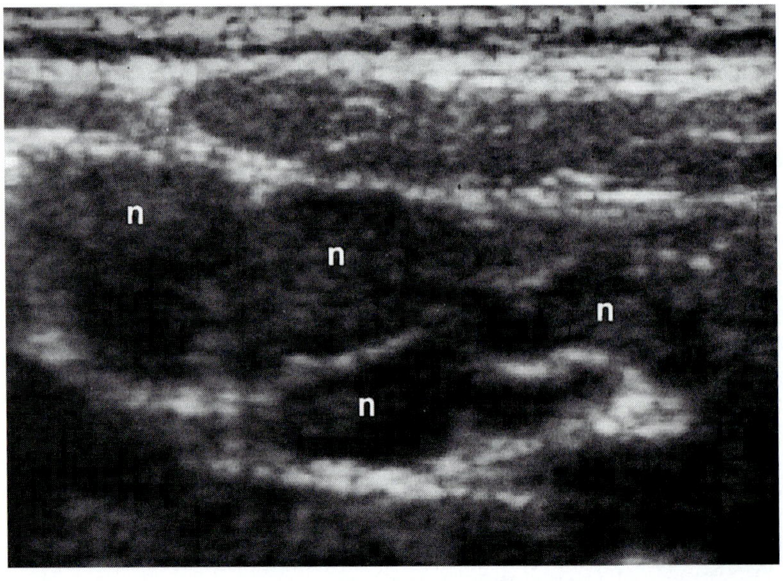

FIG. 61-68. Mesenteric adenitis in a 3-year-old boy with right lower quadrant pain and fever. Transverse ultrasound of the right lower quadrant and upper pelvis reveals multiple, ovoid, soft-tissue masses representing lymph nodes, *n*. The appendix was not visualized. The patient's symptoms resolved spontaneously.

Sacrococcygeal teratomas can be benign or malignant. Tumors detected before the age of 2 months are most likely benign. Those detected after 2 months of age have a 50% to 90% incidence of malignancy. Malignancy is more common in boys and in lesions that are predominantly solid on ultrasound and CT examinations. Cystic lesions are more likely benign. All teratomas have a malignant potential, regardless of their texture, location, or size. There is an increased risk of malignant transformation following recurrence of a benign teratoma after incomplete surgical extirpation. Therefore the coccyx must be removed in its entirely at surgery to prevent recurrence.[210]

Sacrococcygeal teratomas can be divided into four types, based on their location:

Type I: Predominantly external;
Type II: External with a significant intrapelvic component;
Type III: Small external mass with predominant intrapelvic portion; and
Type IV: Entirely presacral with no external component.

Type I lesions are usually benign and present at birth. Types II, III, and IV have a higher incidence of malignancy, probably because the large intrapelvic component goes unrecognized and undetected for longer periods than the large exophytic masses.[211,212] Malignant teratomas are usually endodermal sinus tumors.

There is a wide spectrum of ultrasound appearances of sacrococcygeal teratomas, ranging from purely cystic to mixed cystic and solid to purely solid (Figs. 61-69 and 61-70). Calcifications, seen in one third of

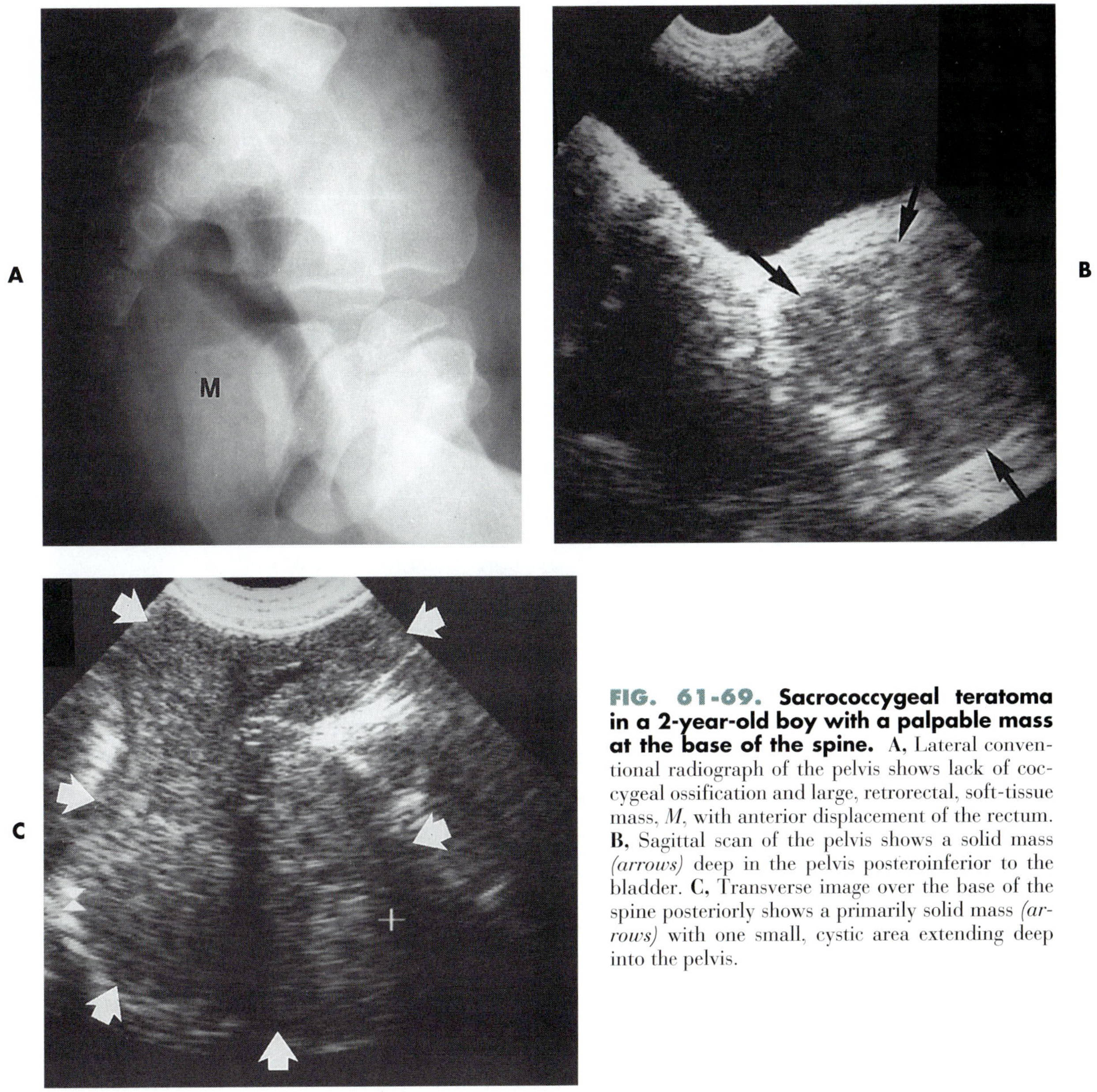

FIG. 61-69. Sacrococcygeal teratoma in a 2-year-old boy with a palpable mass at the base of the spine. **A,** Lateral conventional radiograph of the pelvis shows lack of coccygeal ossification and large, retrorectal, soft-tissue mass, *M*, with anterior displacement of the rectum. **B,** Sagittal scan of the pelvis shows a solid mass *(arrows)* deep in the pelvis posteroinferior to the bladder. **C,** Transverse image over the base of the spine posteriorly shows a primarily solid mass *(arrows)* with one small, cystic area extending deep into the pelvis.

A

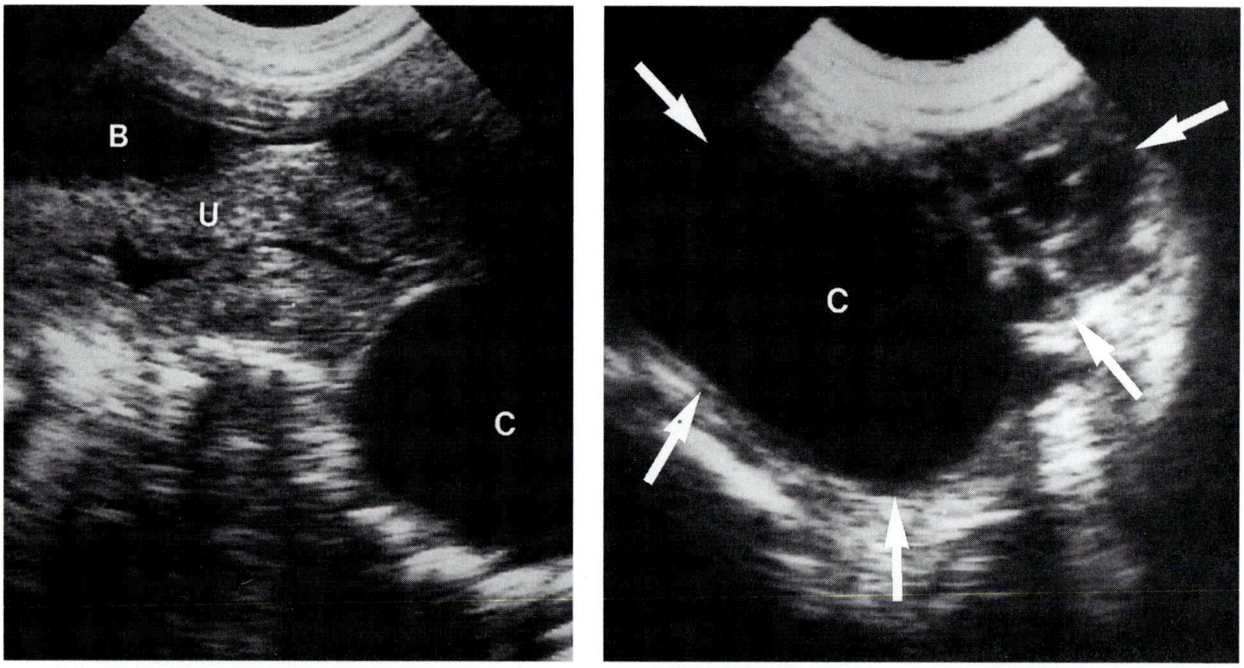

B

FIG. 61-70. Sacrococcygeal teratoma in a newborn girl with a buttock mass. **A,** Sagittal sonogram of the pelvis demonstrates a large, cystic mass, *C*, deep in the pelvis posteroinferior to the uterus, *U*. The small amount of fluid noted in the endometrial canal is secondary to residual material hormonal stimulation. *B*, Bladder. **B,** Transverse image over the base of the spine posteriorly demonstrates a complex mass *(arrows)* with a predominantly large cystic, *C*, component.

PRESACRAL MASSES IN CHILDREN

Solid

Sacrococcygeal teratoma
Neuroblastoma
Rhabdomyosarcoma
Fibroma
Lipoma
Leiomyoma
Lymphoma
Hemangioendothelioma
Sacral bone tumors

Cystic

Abscess
Rectal duplication
Hematoma
Lymphocele
Neurenteric cyst
Sacral osteomyelitis
Ulcerative colitis
Anterior meningocele

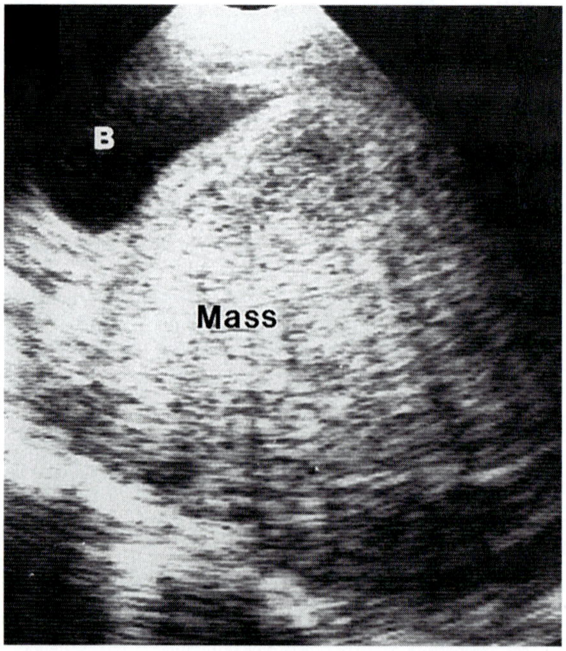

FIG. 61-71. Neuroblastoma. This large, solid, deep, pelvic mass causes anterior displacement and flattening of bladder, *B*, on a sagittal sonogram.

cases, can be amorphous, punctate, or spiculated. The presence of calcification suggests the lesion is benign. Fat within the tumor appears as bright areas of heterogeneous echogenicity.[213] Large tumors may displace and compress the bladder anteriorly and superiorly, causing urinary retention and hydronephrosis.

Neuroblastoma and other neurogenic tumors can arise in the presacral space in children. Five percent of neuroblastomas arise in the pelvis. Because of their midline location, they are considered stage III tumors. Pelvic neuroblastoma has a better prognosis than intraabdominal neuroblastoma. The pelvic lesions have a similar sonographic appearance to the adrenal lesions. They are solid, echogenic, heterogeneous masses with a 70% incidence of calcification. Areas of cystic necrosis and hemorrhage are uncommon (Fig. 61-71).[214,215]

Rhabdomyosarcoma arising from the pelvic musculature can present as a solid presacral mass. It is usually an infiltrating tumor with poorly defined margins. Anechoic spaces within a predominantly solid mass suggest areas of necrosis and hemorrhage. Calcification is rare.[53,216,217] Ultrasound is an excellent method for identifying and staging rhabdomyosarcoma arising from the genitourinary tract. However, CT provides more complete information for those tumors arising from the pelvic sidewalls.[51,53] Other predominantly **solid presacral masses** to be considered in the differential diagnosis include fibroma, lipoma, leiomyoma (and their malignant counterparts), lymphoma, hemangioendothelioma, and metastatic disease.[218] **Sacral bone tumors,** such as Ewing's sarcoma, osteosarcoma, chondrosarcoma, giant cell tumor, and aneurysmal bone cyst, may also present as presacral masses. Chordomas of the sacrococcygeal region are rare in children.[219]

Cystic presacral lesions, in addition to sacrococcygeal teratomas, can be detected on sonography. These include abscess, rectal duplication, hematoma, lymphocele, neurenteric cyst, sacral osteomyelitis, and ulcerative colitis.[218] An anterior sacral meningocele also presents as a cystic presacral mass. It represents herniation of the meninges through an anterior defect in the sacrum. The sacrum usually has a scimitar- or sickle-shaped configuration. A solid mural nodule within the cystic meningocele represents glial or lipomatous tissue.[216,219]

REFERENCES

Technique

1. Kangarloo H, Sarti DA, Sample WF. Ultrasound of the pediatric pelvis. *Semin Ultrasound* 1980;1:51-60.
2. Rosenberg HK. Sonography of pediatric urinary tract abnormalities. Pt I. *Am Urol Assoc Weekly Update Ser* 1986;35(5):1-8.
3. Rubin C, Kurtz AB, Goldberg BB. Water enema: a new ultrasound technique in defining pelvic anatomy. *J Clin Ultrasound* 1978;6:28-33.
4. Bellah RD, Rosenberg HK. Transvaginal ultrasound in a children's hospital: is it worthwhile? *Pediatr Radiol* 1991;21:570-574.
5. Jequier S, Rousseau O. Sonographic measurements of the normal bladder wall in children. *AJR* 1987;149:563-566.
6. Marchal GJ, Baert AL, Eeckels R, et al. Sonographic evaluation of the normal ureteral submucosal tunnel in infancy and childhood. *Pediatr Radiol* 1983;13:125-129.
7. Hennigan HW, DuBose TJ. Sonography of the normal female urethra. *AJR* 1985;145:839-841.
8. Cohen HL, Susman M, Haller JO et al. Posterior urethral valve: transperineal US for imaging and diagnosis in male infants. *Radiology* 1994;192:261-264.
9. McAninch JW, Laing FC, Jeffrey RB. Sonourethrography in the evaluation of urethral strictures: a preliminary report. *J Urol* 1988;139:294-297.

Normal Anatomy

10. Comstock CH, Boal DK. Pelvic sonography of the pediatric patient. *Semin Ultrasound* 1984;5:54-67.
11. Nussbaum AR, Sanders RC, Jones MD. Neonatal uterine morphology as seen on real-time ultrasound. *Radiology* 1986;160:641-643.

Lower Urinary Tract

12. Rosenberg HK. Sonography of the pediatric urinary tract. In: Bush WH, ed. *Urologic Imaging and Interventional Techniques.* Baltimore: Urban & Schwarzenberg; 1989:164-179.
13. Sample WF, Lippe BM, Gyepes MT. Gray-scale ultrasonography of the normal female pelvis. *Radiology* 1977;125:477-483.
14. Schiller VL, Grant EG. Doppler ultrasonography of the pelvis. *Radiol Clin North Am* 1992;30:735-742.
15. Nussbaum AR, Lebowitz RL. Interlabial masses in little girls: review and imaging recommendations. *AJR* 1983;141:65-71.
16. Siegel MJ. Pediatric gynecologic sonography. *Radiology* 1991;179:593-600.
17. Cohen HL, Shapiro MA, Mandel FS, Shapiro ML: Normal ovaries in neonates and infants: a sonographic study of 77 patients 1 day to 24 months old. *AJR* 1993;160:583-586.
18. Orsini LF, Salardi S, Pilu G, et al. Pelvic organs in premenarchal girls: real-time ultrasonography. *Radiology* 1984;153:113-116.
19. Cohen HL, Tice HM, Mandel FS. Ovarian volumes measured by US: bigger than we think. *Radiology* 1990;177:189-192.
20. Quillin SP, Siegel MJ. Transabdominal color Doppler ultrasonography of the painful adolescent ovary. *J Ultrasound Med* 1994;13:549-555.
21. Ingram S, Hollman AS, Azmy AFA. Ultrasound evaluation of the paediatric prostate. *Br J Urol* 1994;74:601-603.
22. Mascatello VJ, Smith EH, Carrera GF, et al. Ultrasonic evaluation of the obstructed duplex kidney. *AJR* 1977;129:113-120.
23. Geringer AM, Berdon WE, Seldin DW, et al. The diagnostic approach to ectopic ureterocele and the renal duplication complex. *J Urology* 1983;129:539-542.
24. Nussbaum AR, Dorst JP, Jeffs RD, et al. Ectopic ureter and ureterocele: their varied sonographic manifestations. *Radiology* 1986;159:227-235.
25. Gilsanz V, Miller JH, Reid BS. Ultrasonic characteristics of posterior urethral valves. *Radiology* 1982;145:143-145.
26. Cremin BJ, Aaronson IA. Ultrasonic diagnosis of posterior urethral valves in neonates. *Br J Radiol* 1983;56:435-438.
27. McAlister WH. Demonstration of the dilated prostatic urethra in posterior urethral valve patients. *J Ultrasound Med* 1984;3:189-190.
28. MacPherson RI, Leithiser RE, Gordon L, et al. Posterior urethral valves: an update and review. *RadioGraphics* 1986;6:753-791.

29. Hulbert WC, Rosenberg HK, Cartwright PC et al. The predictive value of ultrasonography in evaluation of infants with posterior urethral valves. *J Urol* 1992;148:122-124.
30. Garris J, Kangarloo H, Sarti D, et al. The ultrasound spectrum of prune-belly syndrome. *J Clin Ultrasound* 1980;8: 117-120.
31. Aaronson IA, Cremin BJ. *Clinical Pediatric Uroradiology*. Edinburgh: Churchill Livingstone; 1984:255-265.
32. Caro PA, Rosenberg HK, Snyder HM. Congenital urethral polyp. *AJR* 1986;147:1041-1042.
33. Kessler A, Rosenberg HK, Smoyer WE, Blyth B. Urethral stones: US for identification in boys with hematuria and dysuria. *Radiology* 1992;185:767-768.
34. Keller MS, Weiss RM, Rosenfeld NS. Sonographic evaluation of ureterectasis in children: the significance of peristalsis. *J Urol* 1993;149:553-555.
35. Sherman NH, Boyle GK, Rosenberg HK. Sonography in the neonate. *Ultrasound Q* 1988;6:91-150.
36. Marshall JL, Johnson ND, DeCampo MP. Vesicoureteric reflux in children: prediction with color Doppler imaging. *Radiology* 1990:175:355-358.
37. Jequier S, Paltiel H, Lafortune M. Ureterovesical jets in infants and children: duplex and color Doppler US studies. *Radiology* 1990;175:349-353.
38. Friedman AP, Haller JO, Schulze G, et al. Sonography of vesical and perivesical abnormalities in children. *J Ultrasound Med* 1983;2:385-390.
39. Erasmie V, Lidefelt KJ. Accuracy of ultrasonic assessment of residual urine in children. *Pediatr Radiol* 1989;19:388-390.
40. Cacciarelli AA, Kass EJ, Yang SS. Urachal remnants: sonographic demonstration in children. *Radiology* 1990;174:473-475.
41. Avni EF, Matos C, Diard F, et al. Midline omphalovesical anomalies in children: contribution of ultrasound imaging. *Urol Radiol* 1988;10:189-194.
42. Heaney JA, Pfister RC, Meares EM Jr. Giant cyst of the seminal vesicle with renal agenesis. *AJR* 1987;149:139-140.
43. Schukrke TD, Kaplan GW. Prostatic utricle cysts (Müllerian duct cysts). *J Urol* 1978;119:765-767.
44. Hayden CK, Swischuk LE, Fawcett HD, et al. Urinary tract infections in childhood: a current imaging approach. *RadioGraphics* 1986;6:1023-1038.
45. Rifkin MD, Kurtz AB, Pasto ME, et al. Unusual presentations of cystitis. *J Ultrasound Med* 1983;2:25-28.
46. Gooding GAW. Varied sonographic manifestations of cystitis. *J Ultrasound Med* 1986;5:61-64.
47. Hassel DR, Glasier CM, McConnell JR. Granulomatous cystitis in chronic granulomatous disease: ultrasound diagnosis. *Pediatr Radiol* 1987;17:254-255.
48. Lebowitz RL, Vargas B. Stones in the urinary bladder in children and young adults. *AJR* 1987;148:491-495.
49. Rosenberg HK, Zerin JM, Eggli KD, et al. Benign cystitis in children mimicking rhabdomyosarcoma. *J Ultrasound Med* 1994;13:921-932.
50. Sty JR, Wells RG. Other abdominal and pelvic masses in children. *Semin Roentgenol* 1988;23:216-231.
51. Tannous WN, Azous EM, Homsy YL, et al. CT and ultrasound imaging of pelvic rhabdomyosarcoma in children. *Pediatr Radiol* 1989;19:530-534.
52. McLeod AJ, Lewis E. Sonographic evaluation of pediatric rhabdomyosarcomas. *J Ultrasound Med* 1984;3:69-74.
53. Geoffray A, Couanet D, Montagne JP, et al. Ultrasonography and computed tomography for diagnosis and follow-up of pelvic rhabdomyosarcoma in children. *Pediatr Radiol* 1987; 17:132-136.
54. Williams JL, Cumming WA, Walker RD, et al. Transitional cell papilloma of the bladder. *Pediatr Radiol* 1986;16:322-323.
55. Bornstein I, Charboneau JM, Hartman GW. Leiomyoma of the bladder: sonographic and urographic findings. *J Ultrasound Med* 1986;5:407-408.
56. Shapeero LG, Vordermark JS. Bladder neurofibromatosis in childhood. *J Ultrasound Med* 1990;9:177-180.
57. Crecelius SA, Bellah R. Pheochromocytoma of the bladder in an adolescent: sonographic and MR imaging findings. *AJR* 1995;165:101-103.
58. Brereton RJ, Thillip N, Buyukpamukeu N. Rupture of the urinary bladder in children: the importance of the double lesion. *Br J Urol* 1980;52:15-20.
59. Zerin JM, Lebowitz RL. Spontaneous extraperitoneal rupture of the urinary bladder in children. *Radiology* 1989;170:487-488.
60. Mezzacappa PM, Price AP, Kassner EG, et al. Cohen ureteral reimplantation: sonographic appearance. *Radiology* 1987; 165: 851-852.
61. Hertzberg BS, Bowie JD, King LR, et al. Augmentation and replacement cystoplasty: sonographic findings. *Radiology* 1987;165:853-856.

Ovary

62. Nussbaum AR, Sanders RC, Benator RM, et al. Spontaneous resolution of neonatal ovarian cysts. *AJR* 1987;148:175-176.
63. Jafri SZH, Bree RL, Silver TM, et al. Fetal ovarian cysts: sonographic detection and association with hypothyroidism. *Radiology* 1984;150:809-812.
64. Kirkinen P, Jouppila P. Perinatal aspects of pregnancy complicated by fetal ovarian cysts. *J Perinatol Med* 1985;13:245-251.
65. Shawker TH, Hubbard VS, Reichert CM, et al. Cystic ovaries in cystic fibrosis: an ultrasound and autopsy study. *J Ultrasound Med* 1983;2:439-444.
66. Riddelsberger MM, Kuhn JP, Munschauer RW. The association of juvenile hypothyroidism and cystic ovaries. *Radiology* 1982;139:77-80.
67. Reith KG, Comite F, Shawker TH, et al. Pituitary and ovarian abnormalities demonstrated by CT and ultrasound in children with features of McCune-Albright syndrome. *Radiology* 1984;153:389-393.
68. Fakhy J, Khoury A, Kotval P, et al. Sonography of autonomous follicular ovarian cysts in precocious pseudopuberty. *J Ultrasound Med* 1988;7:597-603.
69. Haller JO, Friedman AP, Schaffer R, Lebensart DP. The normal and abnormal ovary in childhood and adolescence. *Semin US CT MR* 1983;4:206-225.
70. Ritchie WGM. Sonographic evaluation of normal and induced ovulation. *Radiology* 1986;161:1-10.
71. Alpern MB, Sandler MA, Madrazo BL. Sonographic features of parovarian cysts and their complications. *AJR* 1984; 143:157-160.
72. Grossman JA, Filtzer HS, Aliopoulios MA. Torsion and infarction of cystic ovaries in children. *AJDC* 1974;128:713-714.
73. Worthington-Kirsch RL, Raptopoulos V, Cohen IT. Sequential bilateral torsion of normal ovaries in a child. *J Ultrasound Med* 1986;5:663-664.
74. Farrell TP, Boal DK, Teele RL, et al. Acute torsion of normal uterine adnexa in children: sonographic demonstration. *AJR* 1982;139:1223-1225.
75. Rosado WM, Trambert MA, Gosink BB, Pretorius DH. Adnexal torsion: diagnosis by using Doppler sonography. *AJR* 1992;159:1251-1253.
76. Warner MA, Gleisher AC, Edell SL, et al. Uterine adnexal torsion: sonographic findings. *Radiology* 1985;154:773-775.
77. Graif M, Shalev J, Strauss S, et al. Torsion of the ovary: sonographic features. *AJR* 1984;143:1331-1334.

78. Graif M, Itzchak Y. Sonographic evaluation of ovarian torsion in childhood and adolescence. *AJR* 1988;150:647-649.
79. Baltarowich OH, Kurtz AB, Pasto ME, et al. The spectrum of sonographic findings in hemorrhagic ovarian cysts. *AJR* 1987;148:901-905.
80. Bass IS, Haller JO, Friedman AP, et al. The sonographic appearance of the hemorrhagic ovarian cyst in adolescents. *J Ultrasound Med* 1984;3:509-513.
81. Hann LE, Hall DA, McArdle CR, Seibel M. Polycystic ovarian disease: sonographic spectrum. *Radiology* 1984;150:531-534.
82. Kalstone CE, Jaffe RB, Abell MR. Massive edema of the ovary simulating fibroma. *Obstet Gynecol* 1969;34:564-571.
83. Young RH, Scully RE. Fibromatosis and massive edema of the ovary, possibly related entities: a report of 14 cases of fibromatosis and 11 cases of massive edema. *Interven Gynecol Pathol* 1984;3:153-178.
84. Lee AR, Kim KH, Lee BH, Chin SY. Massive edema of the ovary: imaging findings. *AJR* 1993;161:343-344.
85. Roth LM, Deaton RL, Sternberg WH. Massive edema of the ovary. *Am J Surg Pathol* 1979;3:11-21.
86. Miller JH, Ettinger LJ. Gonadal tumors and teratomas. In: Miller JH, ed. *Imaging in Pediatric Oncology*. Baltimore: Williams & Wilkins; 1985:295-304.
87. Golladay ES, Mollitt DL. Ovarian masses in the child and adolescent. *South Med J* 1983;76:954-957.
88. Sisler CL, Siegel MJ. Ovarian teratomas: a comparison of sonographic appearance in prepubertal and postpubertal girls. *AJR* 1990;154:139-141.
89. Laing FC, van Dalsen VF, Marks WM, et al. Dermoid cysts of the ovary: their ultrasonographic appearance. *Obstet Gynecol* 1981;57:99-104.
90. Quinn SF, Erickson S, Black WC. Cystic ovarian teratomas: the sonographic appearance of the dermoid plug. *Radiology* 1985;155:477-478.
91. Schaffer RM, Haller JO, Friedman AP, et al. Sonographic diagnosis of ovarian dysgerminoma in children. *Med Ultrasound* 1982;6:118-119.
92. Haller JO, Bass JS, Friedman AP. Pelvic masses in girls: an eight-year retrospective analysis stressing ultrasound as the prime imaging modality. *Pediatr Radiol* 1984;14:363-368.
93. Arger PH, Mulhern CB, Littman PS. Management of solid tumors in children: contribution of computed tomography. *AJR* 1981;137:251-255.
94. Siegel MJ, Glasier CM, Sagel SS. CT of pelvic disorders in children. *AJR* 1981;137:1139-1143.
95. Requard LK, Mettler FA, Wicks JD. Preoperative sonography of malignant ovarian neoplasms. *AJR* 1981;137:79-82.
96. Moyle JW, Rochester D, Seder L, et al. Sonography of ovarian tumors: predictability of tumor type. *AJR* 1983;141:985-991.
97. Walsh JW, Taylor KJW, Wasson JFM, et al. Gray-scale ultrasound in 204 proved gynecologic masses: accuracy and specific diagnostic criteria. *Radiology* 1979;130:391-397.
98. Yaghoobian J, Pinck RL. Ultrasound findings in thecoma of the ovary. *J Clin Ultrasound* 1983;11:91-93.
99. Sherman NH, Rosenberg HK. Pediatric pelvic sonography. In: Fisher MR, Kricun ME, eds. *Imaging of the Pelvis*. Rockville, Md: Aspen Publishers; 1989.
100. Bickers GH, Seibert JJ, Anderson JC, et al. Sonography of ovarian involvement in childhood acute lymphocytic leukemia. *AJR* 1981;137:399-401.
101. Shirkhode A, Eftekhari F, Frankel LS, et al. Diagnosis of leukemic relapse in the pelvic soft tissues of juvenile females. *J Clin Ultrasound* 1986;14:191-195.
102. Lane DM, Birdwell RL. Ovarian leukemia detected by pelvic sonography. *Cancer* 1986;58:2338-2342.

Uterus and Vagina

103. Deutsch AL, Gosink BB. Non-neoplastic gynecologic disorders. *Semin Roentgenol* 1982;17:269-283.
104. Rosenberg HK, Sherman NH, Tarry WF, et al. Mayer-Rokitansky-Küster-Hauser syndrome: ultrasound aid to diagnosis. *Radiology* 1986;161:815-819.
105. Grimes CK, Rosenbaum DM, Kirkpatrick JA. Pediatric gynecologic radiology. *Semin Roentgenol* 1982;17:284-301.
106. Haller JO, Fellows RA. The pelvis. *Clin Diagn Ultrasound* 1981;8:165-185.
107. Rosenberg HK. Sonography of pediatric urinary tract abnormalities. Pt II. *Am Urol Assoc Weekly Update Ser* 1986;(36)5:1-7.
108. Pedersen JH, Kuist N, Nielsen O. Hydrometrocolpos: current views on pathogenesis and management. *J Urol* 1984;132:537-540.
109. Swayne LC, Rubinstein JB, Mitchell B. The Mayer-Rokitansky-Küster-Hauser syndrome: sonographic aid to diagnosis. *J Ultrasound Med* 1986;5:287-289.
110. Jolly HE. The use of ultrasonography in elucidating the problem of imperforate vagina. *Aust NZ J Surg* 1983;53:49-51.
111. Malini S, Valdes C, Malinek LR. Sonographic diagnosis and classification of anomalies of the female genital tract. *J Ultrasound Med* 1984;3:397-404.
112. Kenney PJ, Spirt BA, Leeson MD. Genitourinary anomalies: radiologic correlations. *RadioGraphics* 1984;4:233-260.
113. Gilsanz V. Duplicated Mullerian duct remnants: unilateral occlusion and ipsilateral renal agenesis in a male. *AJR* 1981;137:174-175.
114. McCarthy S, Taylor KJW. Sonography of vaginal masses. *AJR* 1983;140:1005-1008.
115. Copeland LJ, Gershenson DM, Saul PB, et al. Sarcoma botryoides of the female genital tract. *Obstet Gynecol* 1985;66:262-265.
116. Hays DM. Pelvic rhabdomyosarcoma in childhood: diagnosis and concepts of management reviewed. *Cancer* 1980;45:1810-1814.
117. Schneider M, Grossman H. Sonography of the female child's reproductive system. *Pediatr Ann* 1980;9:180-186.
118. Hayden CK, Swischuk LE. *Pediatric Ultrasonography*. Baltimore: Williams & Wilkins; 1987:359-368.
119. Zwiebel WJ, Haning RV Jr. A rational approach to diagnosis and management in ectopic pregnancy. *Semin US CT MR* 1983;4:235-253.
120. Bulas DI, Ahlstrom PA, Sivit CJ et al. Pelvic inflammatory disease in the adolescent: comparison of transabdominal and transvaginal sonographic evaluation. *Radiology* 1992;183:435-439.
121. Swayne LC, Love MB, Karasick SR. Pelvic inflammatory disease: sonographic-pathologic correlation. *Radiology* 1984;151:751-755.
122. Cacciatore B, Leminen A, Ingman-Friberg S et al. Transvaginal sonographic findings in ambulatory patients with suspected pelvic inflammatory disease. *Obstet Gynecol* 1992;80:912-916.
123. Quillin SP, Siegel MJ. Transabdominal color Doppler ultrasonography of the painful adolescent ovary. *J Ultrasound Med* 1994;13:549-555.
124. Schoenfeld A, Fisch B, Cohen M et al. Ultrasound findings in perihepatitis associated with pelvic inflammatory disease. *J Clin Ultrasound* 1992;20:339-342.
125. Dinerman LM, Elfenbein DS, Cumming WA. Clinical Fitz-Hugh-Curtis syndrome in an adolescent: ultrasonographic findings. *Clin Pediatr* 1990;9:532-535.

Endocrine Abnormalities

126. Goske MJ, Emmens RW, Rabinowitz R. Inguinal ovaries in children demonstrated by high resolution real-time ultrasound. *Radiology* 1984;151:635-636.
127. Shawker TH, Garra BS, Lorianx DL, et al. Ultrasonography of Turner's syndrome. *J Ultrasound Med* 1986;5:125-129.
128. Shawker TH, Comite F, Rieth KG et al. Ultrasound evaluation of female isosexual precocious puberty. *J Ultrasound Med* 1984;3:309-316.
129. Haller JO, Schneider M, Kassner EG et al. Ultrasonography in pediatric gynecology and obstetrics. *AJR* 1977;128:423-429.

Scrotum

130. Zanganeth F, Limech GA, Brown BI et al. Hepatorenal glycogenosis (type 1 glycogenosis) and carcinoma of the liver. *J Pediatr* 1969;74:73-83.
131. Rubin JM, Bude RO, Carson PL et al. Power Doppler US: a potentially useful alternative to mean frequency-based color Doppler US. *Radiology* 1994;190:853-856.
132. Krone KD, Carroll BA. Scrotal ultrasound. *Radiol Clin North Am* 1985;23:121-139.
133. Daniel WA Jr, Reinstein RA, Howard-Peebles P, Baxley WD. Clinical and laboratory observations: testicular volumes of adolescents. *J Pediatr* 1982;101:1010-1012.
134. Cassorla RG, Golden SM, Johnsonbaugh RE et al. Testicular volume during early infancy. *J Pediatr* 1981;99:742-743.
135. Atkinson GO, Patrick LE, Ball TI Jr et al. The normal and abnormal scrotum in children: evaluation with color Doppler sonography. *AJR* 1992;158:613-617.
136. Patriquin HB, Yazbeck S, Trinh B et al. Testicular torsion in infants and children: diagnosis with Doppler sonography. *Radiology* 1993;188:781-785.
137. Luker GD, Siegel MJ. Scrotal US in pediatric patients: comparison of power and standard color Doppler US. *Radiology* 1996;198:381-385.
138. Luker GD, Siegel MJ. Color Doppler sonography of the scrotum in children. *AJR* 1994;163:649-655.
139. Middleton WD, Thorne DA, Melson GL. Color Doppler ultrasound of the normal testis. *AJR* 1989;152:293-297.

Congenital Abnormalities

140. Hill MC, Sanders RC. *Sonography of Benign Disease of the Scrotum.* New York: Raven Press; 1986:197-237.
141. Madrazo BL, Klogo RC, Parks JA et al. Ultrasonographic demonstration of undescended testes. *Radiology* 1979;133:181-183.
142. Maghnie M, Vanzulli A, Paesano P et al. The accuracy of magnetic resonance imaging and ultrasonography compared with surgical findings in the localization of the undescended testis. *Arch Pediatr Adol Med* 1994;148:699-703.
143. Finkelstein MS, Rosenberg HK, Snyder HM et al. Ultrasound evaluation of the scrotum in pediatrics. *Urology* 1986;27:1-9.
144. Eberenz W, Rosenberg HK, Moshang T et al. True hermaphroditism: sonographic demonstration of ovotestes. *Radiology* 1991;179:429-431.
145. Wilson JD, Griffin JE III. Disorders of sexual differentiation. In: Braunwald E, Isselbacher KJ, Petersdorf RG et al., eds. *Harrison's Principles of Internal Medicine.* 11th ed. New York: McGraw-Hill; 1987:1840-1853.
146. Cho CS, Kosek J. Cystic dysplasia of the testis: sonographic and pathologic findings. *Radiology* 1985;156:777-778.
147. Hamm B, Fobbe F, Loy V. Testicular cysts: differentiation with US and clinical findings. *Radiology* 1988;168:19-23.
148. Weiss AJ, Kellman GM, Middleton WD, Kirkemo A. Intratesticular varicocele: sonographic findings in two patients. *AJR* 1992;158:1061-1063.
149. Mueller DL, Amundson GM, Rubin SZ, Wesenberg RL. Acute scrotal abnormalities in children: diagnosis by combined sonography and scintigraphy. *AJR* 1988;150:643-646.
150. Friedman SC, Sheynkin YR. Acute scrotal symptoms due to perforated appendix in children: case report and review of literature. *Pediatr Emerg Care* 1995;11:181-182.
151. Sujka SK, Jewett TC Jr, Karp MP. Acute scrotal swelling as the first evidence of intraabdominal trauma in a battered child. *J Pediatr Surg* 1988;23:380.
152. Eshel G, Vinograd I, Barr J, Zemer D. Acute scrotal pain complicating familial Mediterranean fever in children. *Br J Surg* 1994;81:894-896.
153. Yang WT, Ku KW, Metreweli C. Case report: neonatal adrenal haemorrhage presenting as an acute right scrotal swelling (haematoma): value of ultrasound. *Clin Radiol* 1995;50:127-129.
154. Schroder CH, Rieu P, de Jong MCWJ. Peritoneal laceration: a rare cause of scrotal edema in a 2 year old boy. *Adv Peritoneal Dialysis* 1993;9:329-330.
155. Simoneaux SF, Ball TI, Atkinson GO Jr. Scrotal swelling: unusual first presentation of Crohn's disease. *Pediatr Radiol* 1995;25:375-376.
156. Chapman S. The acute scrotum: a complication of cardiac catheterization. *Br J Radiol* 1988;61:162-164.
157. Kilkenny TE. Acute scrotum in an infant: post-herniorraphy complication: sonographic evaluation. *Pediatr Radiol* 1993;23:481-482.
158. Middleton WD, Siegel BA, Melson GL et al. Acute scrotal disorders: prospective comparison of color Doppler US and testicular scintigraphy. *Radiology* 1990;177:177-181.
159. Meza MP, Amundson GM, Aquilina JW, Reitelman C. Color flow imaging in children with clinically suspected testicular torsion. *Pediatr Radiol* 1992;22:370-373.
160. Middleton WD. Scrotal sonography. *Ultrasound Q* 1991;9:61-87.
161. Middleton WD, Melson GL. Testicular ischemia: color Doppler sonographic findings in five patients. *AJR* 1989;152:1237-1239.
162. Hricak H, Lue T, Filly RA et al. Experimental study of the sonographic diagnosis of testicular torsion. *J Ultrasound Med* 1983;2:349-356.
163. van Dijk R, Karthaus HFM. Ultrasonography of the spermatic cord in testicular torsion. *Eur J Radiol* 1994;18:220-223.
164. Hollman AS, Ingram S, Carachi R, Davis C. Colour Doppler imaging of the acute paediatric scrotum. *Pediatr Radiol* 1993;23:83-87.
165. Horstman WG, Middleton WD, Melson GL. Scrotal inflammatory disease: color Doppler US findings. *Radiology* 1991;179:55-59.
166. Burks DD, Markey BJ, Burkhard TK, et al. Suspected testicular torsion and ischemia: evaluation with color Doppler sonography. *Radiology* 1990;175:815-821.
167. Coley BD, Frush DP, Babcock DS, et al. Acute testicular torsion: comparison of unenhanced and contrast-enhanced power Doppler US, color Doppler US, and radionuclide imaging. *Radiology* 1996;199:441-446.
168. Cattolica EV. Preoperative manual detorsion of the torsed spermatic cord. *J Urol* 1985;133:803-805.
169. Haynes BE, Haynes VE. Manipulative detorsion: beware the twist that does not turn. *J Urol* 1987;137:118-119.
170. Cohen HL, Shapiro MA, Haller JO, Glassberg K. Torsion of the testicular appendage: sonographic diagnosis. *J Ultrasound Med* 1992;11:81-83.
171. Lerner RM, Mevorach RA, Hulbert WC, Rabinowitz R. Color Doppler US in the evaluation of acute scrotal disease. *Radiology* 1990;176:355-358.
172. Schuster G. Traumatic rupture of the testicle and a review of the literature. *J Urol* 1982;127:1194-1196.
173. Jeffrey RB, Laing FC, Hricak H, McAninch JW. Sonography of testicular trauma. *AJR* 1983;141:993-995.

174. Corrales JG, Corbel L, Cipolla B et al. Accuracy of ultrasound diagnosis after blunt testicular trauma. *J Urol* 1993;150: 1834-1836.
175. Herman TE, Shackelford GD, McAlister WH. Acute idiopathic scrotal edema: role of scrotal sonography. *J Ultrasound Med* 1994;13:53-55.

Scrotal Masses

176. Laor T, Atala A, Teele RL. Scrotal ultrasonography in Henoch-Schönlein purpura. *Pediatr Radiol* 1992;22:505-506.
177. Miller JH, Ettinger LJ. Gonadal tumors and teratomas. In: Miller JH, ed. *Imaging in Pediatric Oncology*. Baltimore: Williams & Wilkins; 1985:289-295.
178. Barth RA, Teele RL, Colodny A, et al. Asymptomatic scrotal masses in children. *Radiology* 1984;152:65-68.
179. Lupetin AR, King W, Rich P, et al. Ultrasound diagnosis of testicular leukemia. *Radiology* 1983;146:171-172.
180. Phillips G, Kumari-Subaiya S, Sawitsky A. Ultrasonic evaluation of the scrotum in lymphoproliferative disease. *J Ultrasound Med* 1987;6:169-175.
181. Casola G, Scheible W, Leopold GR. Neuroblastoma metastatic to the testes: ultrasonographic screening as an aid to clinical staging. *Radiology* 1984;151:475-476.
182. Luker GD, Siegel MJ. Pediatric testicular tumors: evaluation with gray-scale and color Doppler US. *Radiology* 1994;191: 561-564.
183. Altadonna V, Snyder HM, Rosenberg HK, Duckett JW. Simple cysts of the testis in children: preoperative diagnosis by ultrasound and excision with testicular preservation. *J Urol* 1988;140:1505-1507.
184. Subramanyam BR, Balthazar EJ, Raghavendra BN et al. Sonographic diagnosis of scrotal hernia. *AJR* 1982;139:535-538.
185. McAlister WH, Sisler CL. Scrotal sonography in infants and children. *Curr Probl Radiol* 1990;6:201-251.
186. Zwanger-Mendelson S, Schneck EH, Doshi V. Burkitt lymphoma involving the epididymis and spermatic cord: sonographic and CT findings. *AJR* 1989:153:85-86.
187. Siegel MJ. Male genital tract. In: Siegel MJ, ed. *Pediatric Sonography*. 2nd ed. New York: Raven Press, Ltd; 1995:479-551.
188. Wood A, Dewbury KC. Case report: paratesticular rhabdomyosarcoma: colour Doppler appearances. *Clin Radiol* 1995; 50:130-131.
189. Mene M, Rosenberg HK, Ginsberg PC. Meconium periorchitis presenting as scrotal nodules in a five year old boy. *J Ultrasound Med* 1994;13:491-494.
190. Backus ML, Mack LA, Middleton WD et al. Testicular microlithiasis: imaging appearances and pathologic correlation. *Radiology* 1994;192:781-785.

Gastrointestinal Tract

191. Miller JH, Kemberling CR. Ultrasound of the pediatric gastrointestinal tract. *Semin US CT MR* 1987;8:349-365.
192. Carroll BA. Ultrasound of the gastrointestinal tract. *Radiology* 1989;172:605-608.
193. Seibert JJ, Williamson SI, Golladay ES, et al. The distended gasless abdomen: a fertile field for ultrasound. *J Ultrasound Med* 1986;5:301-308.
194. Barki Y, Bar-Ziv J. Meconium ileus: ultrasonic diagnosis of intraluminal inspissated meconium. *J Clin Ultrasound* 1985; 13:509-512.
195. Schuster SR, Teele RL. An analysis of ultrasound scanning as a guide in determination of high or low imperforate anus. *J Pediatr Surg* 1979;14:798-800.
196. Oppenheimer DA, Carroll BA, Shochat SJ. Sonography of imperforate anus. *Radiology* 1983;148:127-128.
197. Jaramillo D, Lebowitz RL, Hendren WH. The cloacal malformation: radiological findings and imaging recommendations. *Radiology* 1990;177:441-448.
198. Franken EA, Kao SCS, Smith WL, Sato Y. Imaging of the acute abdomen in infants and children. *AJR* 1989;153:921-928.
199. Puylaert JBCM. Acute appendicitis: ultrasound evaluation using graded compression. *Radiology* 1986;158:355-360.
200. Puylaert JBCM, Rutgers PH, Lalisang RI, et al. A prospective study of ultrasonography in the diagnosis of appendicitis. *N Engl J Med* 1987;317:666-669.
201. Rosenberg HK, Goldberg BB. Pediatric radiology: sonography. In: Margulis AR, Burhenne HJ, eds. *Alimentary Tract Radiology*. 4th ed St Louis: Mosby; 1989:1831-1857.
202. Jeffrey RB, Laing FC, Townsend RR. Acute appendicitis: sonographic criteria based on 250 cases. *Radiology* 1988; 167:327-329.
203. Borushok KF, Jeffrey RB, Laing FC, Townsend RR. Sonographic diagnosis of perforation in patients with acute appendicitis. *AJR* 1990;154:275-278.
204. Baker DE, Silver TM, Coran AG, et al. Post-appendectomy fluid collections in children: incidence, nature, and evaluation using ultrasound. *Radiology* 1986;161:341-344.
205. Quillin SP, Siegel MJ. Appendicitis: efficacy of color Doppler sonography. *Radiology* 1994;191:557-560.
206. Quillin SP, Siegel MJ. Diagnosis of appendiceal abscess in children with acute appendicitis: value of color Doppler sonography. *AJR* 1995;164:1251-1254.
207. Dinkel E, Dittrich M, Peters H, et al. Real-time ultrasound in Crohn's disease: characteristic features and clinical implications. *Pediatr Radiol* 1986;16:8-12.
208. Puylaert JBCM. Mesenteric adenitis and acute terminal ileitis: ultrasound evaluation using graded compression. *Radiology* 1986;161:691-695.

Presacral Masses

209. Altman RP, Randolph JG, Lilly JR. Sacrococcygeal teratoma: American Academy of Pediatrics Surgical Section Survey—1973. *J Pediatr Surg* 1974;9:389-398.
210. Schey WL, Shkolnik A, White H. Clinical and radiographic considerations of sacrococcygeal teratomas: an analysis of 26 new cases and review of the literature. *Radiology* 1977; 125: 189-195.
211. Ghazali S. Presacral teratomas in children. *J Pediatr Surg* 1973;8:915-918.
212. Valdiserri RO, Yunis EJ. Sacrococcygeal teratomas. *Cancer* 1981;48:217-221.
213. Siegel MJ. Computed tomography of the pediatric pelvis. *J Comput Assist Tomogr* 1983;7:77-83.
214. Miller JH, Sato JK. Adrenal origin tumors. In: Miller JH, ed. *Imaging in Pediatric Oncology*. Baltimore: Williams & Wilkins; 1985:305-340.
215. Kangarloo H, Fine RN. Sonographic evaluation of children with urinary retention caused by an extragonadal pelvic mass. *Int J Pediatr Nephrol* 1985;6:137-142.
216. King DR, Clatworthy HW. The pediatric patient with sarcoma. *Semin Oncol* 1981;8:215-221.
217. Neifeld JP, Godwin D, Berg JW, et al. Prognostic features of pediatric soft-tissue sarcomas. *J Surg* 1985;98:93-97.
218. Werner JL, Taybi H. Presacral masses in childhood. *AJR* 1970;109:403-409.
219. Richards AT, Stricke L, Spitz L. Sacrococcygeal chordomas in children. *J Pediatr Surg* 1973;8:911-913.

CHAPTER 62

The Pediatric Hip

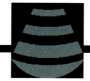

Leslie E. Grissom, M.D.
H. Theodore Harcke, M.D.

CHAPTER OUTLINE

The use of ultrasound to assess the hip is a relatively new application that has gained wide acceptance in the last few years. There are two specific instances in pediatrics in which hip sonography offers clear advantages over other imaging techniques. **Developmental dislocation and/or dysplasia of the hip** (DDH), formerly called congenital dislocation of the hip, is a problem that manifests in the first year of life. At that age, the femoral head and acetabulum consist of cartilage components that are clearly identified by ultrasound. Real-time sonography makes it possible to assess the hip in multiple planes, both at rest and with movement. Ultrasound can replace radiographic studies and thereby reduce radiation exposure to the young infant. **Hip pain** is a common presenting symptom throughout the pediatric age range, and it can be caused by a number of inflammatory and infectious conditions. Early in their course, radiographic findings are absent or limited to subtle soft-tissue changes. The presence of **fluid in the hip joint** is an important finding that may lead to diagnostic aspiration. In this chapter, we describe the use of sonography in DDH and in the detection of hip effusion. Techniques of examination are discussed, as are the normal and pathologic anatomy of the hip.

DEVELOPMENTAL DISLOCATION AND DYSPLASIA OF THE HIP

Clinical Overview

Early detection of an abnormality in the infant hip is the key to successful management. If treatment is begun at a young age, most of the sequelae that occur when DDH goes unrecognized until walking age can be prevented. Clinical screening programs have been instituted, and primary care physicians are taught to evaluate the hips as part of the newborn physical examination. Until recently, infants with abnormal clinical examinations were referred for plain radiographic film examinations. Ultrasound has now provided an alternative technique that is being selected with increasing frequency.

The **incidence of DDH** varies throughout the world. In Caucasian populations, overt dislocation is reported to be 1.5 to 1.7 per 1000 live births.[1,2] When lesser degrees of abnormality such as subluxation are included, as many as 10 infants per 1000 live births may show some features of the disorder.[3]

The **cause of DDH** is multifactorial, with both physiologic and mechanical factors playing a role. Maternal-fetal interaction influences the development of hip problems in both instances. Maternal estrogens and hormones that affect pelvic relaxation just before delivery are believed to lead to temporary laxity of the hip capsule in the perinatal period. Most fetuses are exposed to extrinsic forces in the later weeks of pregnancy because of their increasing size and the diminishing volume of amniotic fluid. It is theorized that these forces, although gentle, can lead to deformation if persistently applied.[4] There is an increased incidence of DDH in infants with a positive family history of DDH, in firstborns, and in pregnancy with oligohydramnios. Infants born in the breech position with skull-molding deformities, congenital torticollis, and foot deformities are also at increased **risk for DDH.**[5]

The **mechanism of a typical dislocation** is thought to be a gradual migration of the femoral head from the acetabulum because of the loose, elastic joint capsule. In the newborn period the head usually dislocates in a lateral and posterosuperior position relative to the acetabulum. The displaced femoral head can usually be reduced, and the joint components typically do not have any major deformity. When dislocation is not recognized in early infancy, the muscles tighten and limit movement. The acetabulum becomes dysplastic because it lacks the stimulus of the femoral head. Ligamentous structures stretch and fibrofatty tissue occupies the acetabulum. Thus it becomes impossible to return the femoral head to the acetabulum with simple manipulation; a pseudoacetabulum may form where the femoral head rests superolaterally.

There is some evidence of familial acetabular dysplasia,[6] although this is not considered to be a cause in the majority of cases. Another form of hip dislocation and dysplasia is the teratologic dislocation that occurs early in fetal life. In these cases, the infant exhibits advanced adaptive changes in the pelvis and femoral head. The clinical and radiographic findings are more obvious, and this uncommon form of hip dislocation has a poor prognosis.[7]

RISK FACTORS FOR DDH

- Family history of DDH
- Firstborn child
- Oligohydramnios
- Breech delivery
- Skull-molding deformities
- Congenital torticollis
- Foot deformities

Development of Hip Sonography

The first in-depth use of sonography was performed by Graf, an Austrian orthopedic surgeon.[8] He used an articulated arm B-scan unit and developed a technique of evaluation based on a coronal image of the hip. Scanning was performed from the lateral approach with the femur in its anatomic position. His method established ultrasound's ability to distinguish between the cartilage, bone, and soft-tissue structures that compose the immature hip joint.

With real-time sonographic equipment, sonographers[9,10] have experimented with different views, and this led to an alternative approach to hip sonography—one that emphasizes dynamic assessment of the hip in multiple positions. Although two basic philosophies, morphologic and dynamic, evolved, it is recognized that the two methods, in fact, have common features. Both approaches recognize the need for critical landmarks of the femur and acetabulum. The dynamic technique, in addition to stressing positional relations and stability, includes a limited assessment of critical acetabular landmarks.[11] The morphologic approach describes a limited dynamic assessment.[12] In 1993 the chief proponents of the two techniques proposed a minimum standard exam drawing on elements from both techniques (see "Minimum Standard Exam" section).

Dynamic Sonographic Technique: Normal and Pathologic Anatomy

Technical Factors. Sonographic examinations are presently performed with **real-time linear array transducers.** Although sector scanners were initially used with success,[13] current preference is for the linear configuration to cover a broader field of view. One should use the **highest-frequency transducer** that provides adequate penetration of the soft tissues to the depth required. For infants up to 3 months of age, the 7.5-MHz transducer is successful. A 5-MHz transducer is generally required between 3 and 7 months of age. With improvements in transducer design, the 5-MHz electronically focused transducers offered by some manufacturers have proved suitable for both the newborn and the older infant. It is only on rare occasions that we use a 3-MHz transducer to evaluate a large infant or to increase the field of view and include more of the iliac and femoral anatomy.

All scanning is performed from the lateral or posterolateral aspect of the hip, moving the hip from the neutral position at rest to one in which the hip is flexed.

With the hip flexed, the femur is moved through a range of abduction and adduction, with stress views performed in the flexed position. One aspect of hip sonography that is relevant to dynamic examinations is the shift of the transducer between the examiner's hands when examining the right and left hip. The infant is lying supine with the feet toward the sonographer. When examining the left hip, the sonographer grasps the infant's left leg with the left hand, and the transducer is held in the right hand. When the right hip is examined, we recommend that the sonographer hold the transducer in the left hand and use the right hand to manipulate the infant's right leg. Although sonographers find this awkward at first, ambidexterity is easily mastered. We found that this technique makes it possible to perform the stress maneuver more reliably and to better maintain the planes of interest.

To obtain a satisfactory examination, the infant should be relaxed. Infants can be fed before or during the examination. Toys and other devices to attract the infant's attention are helpful and can be used during the time sonography is being performed. A parent can hold the infant's arms or head and can talk to the infant. There is no need for sedation. The upper body may remain clothed. Our standard practice is to leave the infant diapered and expose only the side of the hip being examined (strongly recommended for boys).

For the sake of understanding, the **anatomy is considered in four different views.** It is our routine practice to record images in each of these views for permanent records. This standardizes the examination and, in our institution, provides a guideline for the technologist who performs the initial examination. In describing the four views, we use a **two-word combination** that indicates the plane of the transducer with respect to the body (transverse or coronal) and the position of the hips (neutral or flexed).

It is the objective of the dynamic hip assessment to determine the position and stability of the femoral head, as well as the development of the acetabulum. With a normally positioned hip, the femoral head is congruently positioned within the acetabulum. Mild displacement, such as when the head is either in contact with part of the acetabulum or is displaced but partly covered, is referred to as subluxation. The dislocated hip has no contact with or coverage by the acetabulum. A change in position of the femur may change the relationship of the femoral head and acetabulum. It is possible that a hip that is subluxated in the neutral or rest position will seat itself with flexion and abduction. This is, in fact, a principle of treatment.

The stability of the hip is determined through motion and the application of stress. The stress maneuvers are the imaging counterparts of the clinical Barlow and Ortolani maneuvers, which are the basis for the clinical detection of hip abnormality. The **Barlow test** determines whether the hip can be dislocated. The hip is flexed and the thigh is brought into the adducted position. The gentle push posteriorly can demonstrate instability by causing the femoral head to move out of the acetabulum.[1] The **Ortolani test** determines the opposite—if the dislocated hip can be reduced. As the flexed, dislocated hip is abducted into a frogleg position, the examiner feels a vibration or click that results when the femoral head returns to the acetabulum.[7] During dynamic hip sonography, stress maneuvers are performed in a manner analogous to the Barlow and Ortolani clinical maneuvers. The normal hip is always seated at rest, with motion, and during the application of stress. The lax hip is normally positioned at rest and shows abnormal movement with stress. It must, however, invariably remain within the confines of the acetabulum. The subluxable hip is displaced laterally at rest and is loose, but is not dislocatable. When a hip is able to be pushed out of the joint, it is considered to be dislocatable. A dislocated hip may be able to be returned to the acetabulum with traction and abduction. This hip is distinguished from the most severe form of DDH in which the femoral head is dislocated and cannot be reduced.

At birth, the proximal femur and much of the acetabulum are composed of cartilage. On sonographic examination, **cartilage is hypoechoic** compared with soft tissue so that it is easy to distinguish. A few scattered specular echoes can be visualized within the cartilage when high-frequency transducers are used and technique adjustments are optimally set. The acetabulum is composed of both bone and cartilage. At birth the bony ossification centers in the ilium, ischium, and pubis, which are separated by the triradiate cartilage, have a Y configuration. A cartilaginous acetabular rim (the labrum) extends outward from the acetabulum to form the cup that normally contains the femoral head. Most of the acetabular cartilage has an echogenicity similar to the femoral head. It is still possible to determine the joint line, which distinguishes the cartilaginous acetabulum from the femoral head, by simply rotating the femur. More pronounced movement of the hip often creates echoes within the joint space, probably as a result of the formation of microbubbles. At the lateral margin of the labrum, the hyaline cartilage changes to fibrocartilage, and this shows increased echogenicity. The echogenic hip capsule, which is composed of fibrous tissue, borders the femoral head laterally. The bony components of the hip reflect all of the sound beam from their surface. This creates a bright linear or curvilinear appearance on the sonogram, indicating the contour of the osseous surfaces in that plane.

Radiographically, the **ossification center of the femoral head** is recognized between the second and eighth months of life. It is typically seen earlier in females than in males, and there is a wide normal variation for the time of appearance. Although some asymmetry between the left and right hips both in time of appearance and size can be normal, delayed appearance and development are associated with DDH. Hip sonograms reflect the development of the ossification center and can be used to document the development of the center.[14] It is possible to find the ossification center by ultrasound several weeks before it is visible radiographically. Initially, a confluence of blood vessels produces increased echoes within the cartilage. This precedes actual ossification. As ossification begins, the calcium content is insufficient to produce a visible radiographic density; however, the sound waves are reflected. With maturation, the size of the ossification center increases. In early development, the echoes from the center have a more linear appearance whereas later in the first year of life the growth in size gives it a curvilinear margin. As the normal infant approaches 1 year of age, the size of the ossification center precludes accurate determination of medial acetabular landmarks. It is our belief that sonography of the hip is practical only up to 1 year of age, unless there is delayed ossification of the femoral head. The presence and size of the ossific nucleus can be evaluated in all four of the following views.

Coronal/Neutral View. This view, which forms the basis for the morphologic technique, is performed from the lateral aspect of the joint with the plane of the ultrasound beam oriented coronally with respect to the hip joint. The femur is maintained with a physiologic amount of flexion. Graf recommends the use of a special device that allows the infant to be maintained in a lateral decubitus position while the hip is being examined, but the view can also be performed with the patient supine (Fig. 62-1, *A*).[15] A linear, real-time, 5- or 7.5-MHz transducer is placed on the lateral aspect of the hip, and the hip is scanned until a standard plane of section is obtained (Fig. 62-1, *A* to *C*). The plane must precisely demonstrate the midportion of the acetabulum with the straight iliac line superiorly and the inferior tip of the os ilium seen medially within the acetabulum. The echogenic tip of the labrum should also be visualized. The **alpha and beta angles,** if measured, relate to fixed points on the bony and cartilaginous components of the acetabulum (Fig. 62-1, *D*),[15] and the exact plane must be obtained for the measurements to be reliable. The similarity can be noticed between the appearance of the acetabulum in this view and in the coronal/flexion view (see Fig. 62-2, *C*). The difference lies in the fact that the bony shaft (metaphysis) of the femoral neck is visualized below the femoral head in the coronal/neutral projection. In the coronal/flexion view, the femoral shaft is not in the plane of examination because the femur is flexed. A stability test can be performed in this view by gently pushing and pulling the infant's leg. This helps to verify deformity of the acetabulum and to identify craniodorsal movement of the femoral head under pressure. A further adaptation of this view has been proposed by Zieger et al., who advocate flexing and adducting the hip to identify lateral displacement when instability is present.[16]

In the **normal** coronal/neutral view, the femoral head is resting against the bony acetabulum. The ac-

A

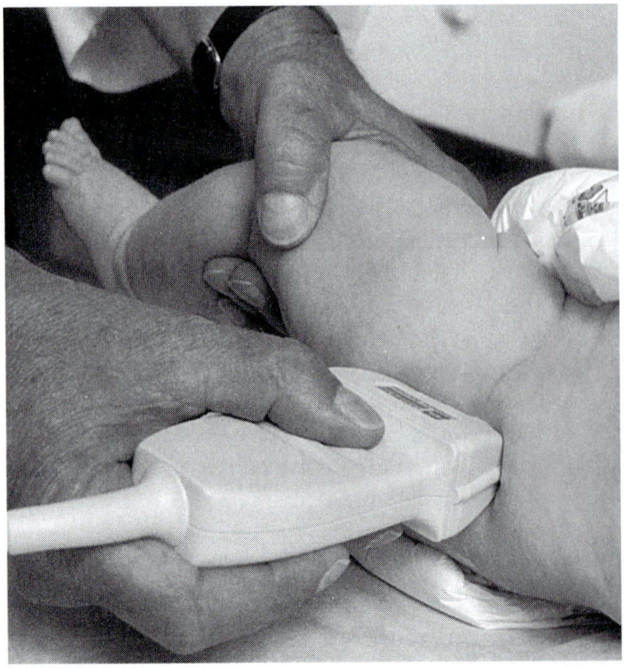

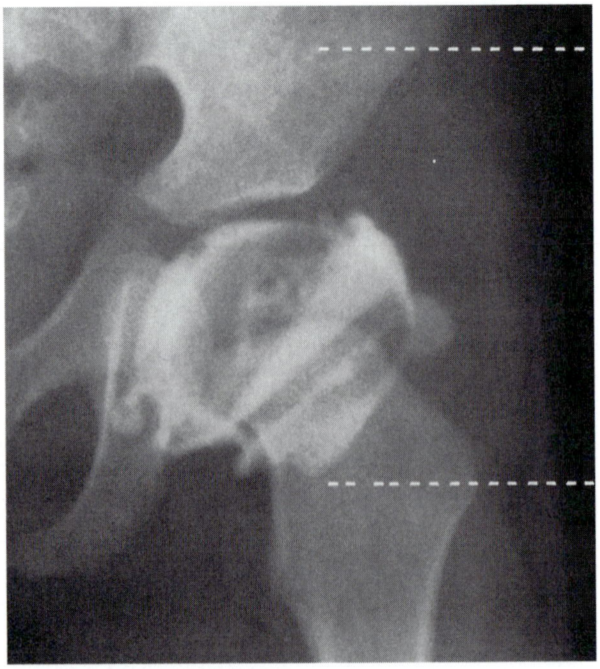

B

FIG. 62-1. Coronal/neutral view. A, Transducer is coronal with respect to the hip. The femur is in physiologic neutral for the infant (slight hip flexion). **B,** Scan area *(dotted lines)* on arthrogram.

Continued.

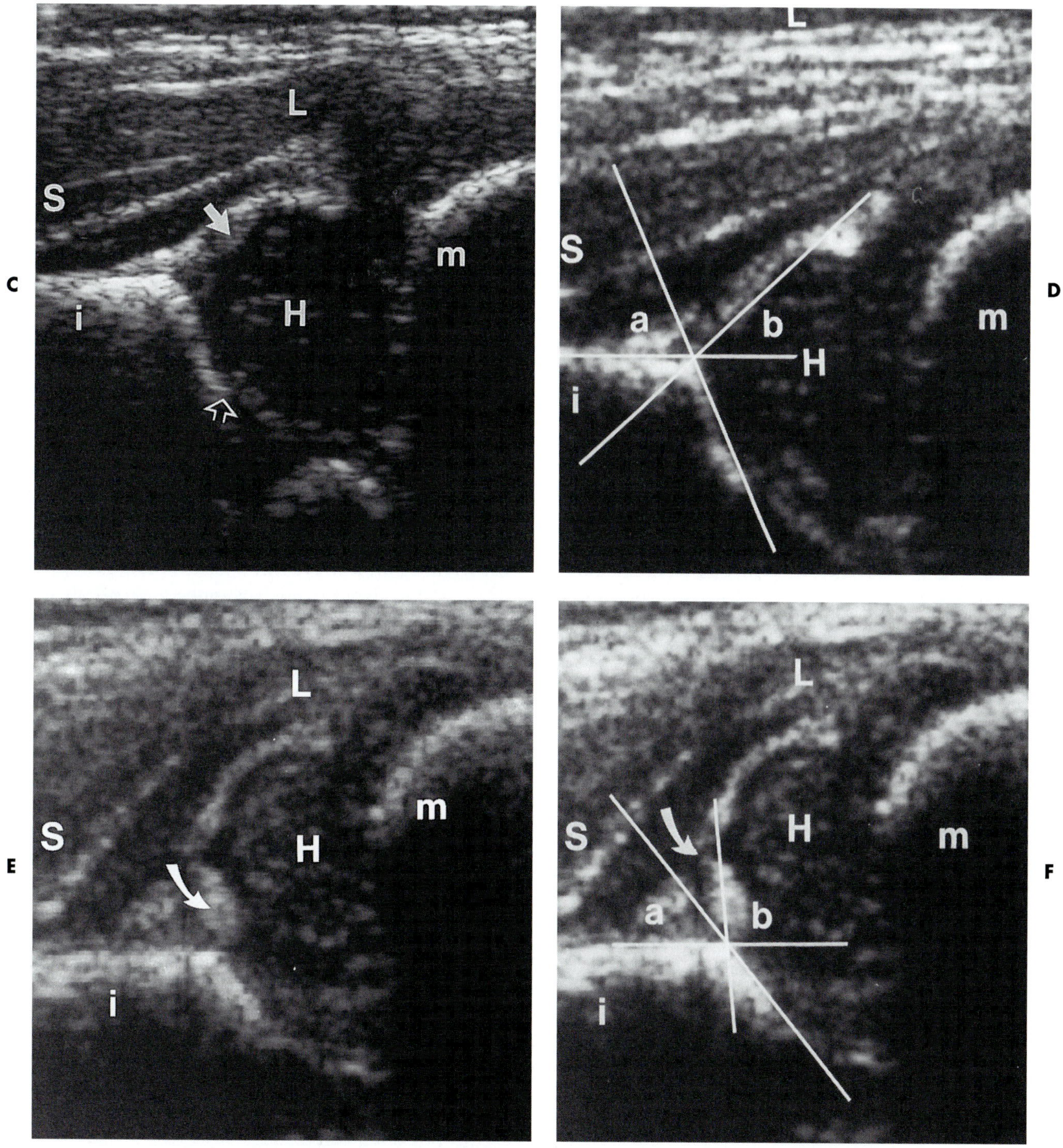

FIG. 62-1, cont'd. C, **Normal hip sonogram** shows sonolucent femoral head resting against the bony acetabulum. Note: Fibrocartilaginous tip of labrum *(solid arrow)* and junction of bony ilium and triradiate cartilage *(open arrow)*. **D, Normal hip sonogram** with alpha, *a*, and beta, *b*, angles used in measurement. **E, Dislocated hip sonogram** shows displacement of femoral head laterally with deformity of labrum *(curved arrow)*. **F, Dislocated hip sonogram** with abnormal alpha and beta angles. *H*, Femoral head; *L*, lateral; *S*, superior; *i*, iliac line; *m*, femoral metaphysis.

etabular roof should have a concave configuration and cover at least half of the femoral head. The cartilage of the acetabular roof is hypoechoic and extends lateral to the acetabular lip, terminating in the labrum, which is composed of fibrocartilage and is echogenic (Fig. 62-1, *C*). When a hip becomes **subluxed** or **dislocated,** the femoral head gradually migrates laterally and superiorly with progressively decreased coverage of the femoral head (Fig. 62-1, *E*). In hip **dysplasia,** the acetabular roof is irregular and angled, and the labrum is deflected superiorly and becomes echogenic and thickened. When the hip is frankly dislocated, the labrum may be deformed. Echogenic soft tissue is interposed between the femoral head and the bony acetabulum. A combination of deformed labrum and fibrofatty tissue (pulvinar) (Fig. 62-1, *E*) prevents the hip from being reduced.

The acetabulum can be assessed visually or with alpha and beta angles (Fig. 62-1, *F*), noting the depth and angulation of the acetabular roof as well as the appearance of the labrum. This can be seen in both coronal/neutral and coronal/flexion views and described verbally. In a previous report, we correlated coverage of the femoral head by the bony acetabulum with radiographic measurements of the acetabular angle.[17] This data showed normal radiographic measurements always had a femoral head coverage that exceeded 58% and that clearly abnormal radiographic measurements had coverage of less than 33%. This information is of limited use because there is a significant group of intermediate values for which sonographic and radiographic measurements do not correlate. We have also noted cases in which sonography showed the acetabulum to be better developed than it appeared radiographically, and on occasion, we have seen an acetabulum that looked more well developed radiographically than it did on ultrasound.[18]

Classification of hip joints may also be based on the measurement of the alpha and beta angles (Fig. 62-1, *D* and *F*). The alpha angle assesses the inclination of the superior osseous acetabular rim with respect to the lateral margin of the iliac bone (baseline). The beta angle is formed by the baseline ilial bone and the inclination of the cartilaginous acetabular roof, for which the tip of the labrum is its key landmark. Ultrasound units may contain software that facilitates measurement of these angles. Four basic hip types have been proposed on the basis of alpha and beta measurements.[15] Most of these subtypes have been subdivided, and small changes in angular measurements can result in a change in category. The reproducibility of angular measurements and subtypes has been a point of considerable discussion. In Europe, there is considerable experience with the classification by measurement. Large numbers of infants have been examined. Some examiners have experienced problems with the use of measurements.[16,17,19-21] On the other hand, those who adhere strictly to the technique find acceptable reproducibility.[22-24]

Coronal/Flexion View. The transducer is maintained in a coronal plane with respect to the acetabulum (Fig. 62-2, *A*) while the hip is moved to a

A

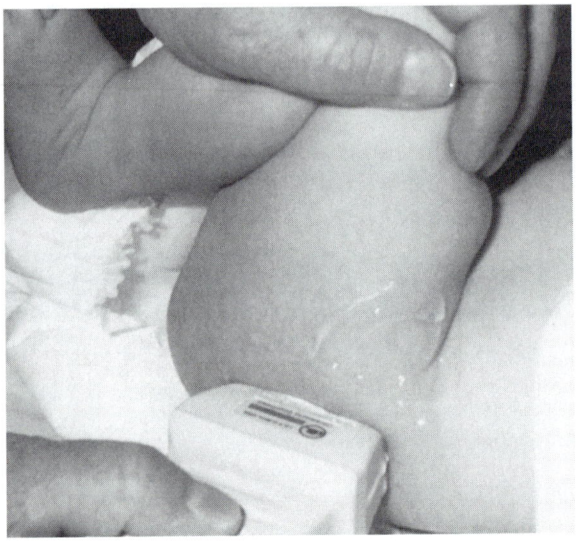

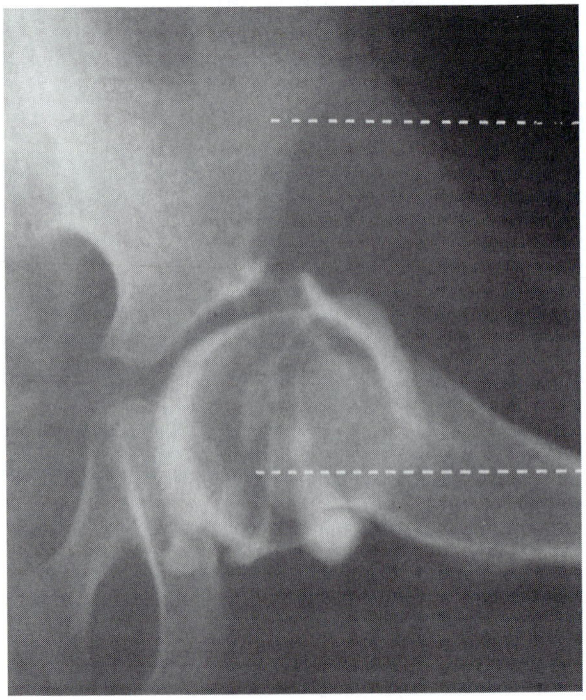

B

FIG. 62-2. Coronal/flexion view. **A,** Transducer is coronal to flexed femur. **B,** Scan area *(dotted lines)* on arthrogram.

Continued.

90-degree angle of flexion. During the assessment in this view, the transducer is moved in an anteroposterior direction with respect to the body to visualize the entire hip. Anterior to the femoral head, the curvilinear margin of the bony femoral shaft is identified. In the midportion of the acetabulum, the normally positioned femoral head is surrounded by echoes from the bony acetabular components (Fig. 62-2, *B* and *C*). Superiorly, the lateral margin of the iliac bone is seen, and the transducer position should be adjusted so that it becomes a straight horizontal line on the monitor. This landmark is a key to accurately visualizing the midacetabulum and to obtaining the maximum depth of the acetabulum. When the transducer is positioned too anteriorly, the iliac line is inclined laterally, and if too posteriorly, the iliac line exhibits some concavity. When the plane is not correctly selected, it could be falsely concluded that the acetabulum is maldevel-

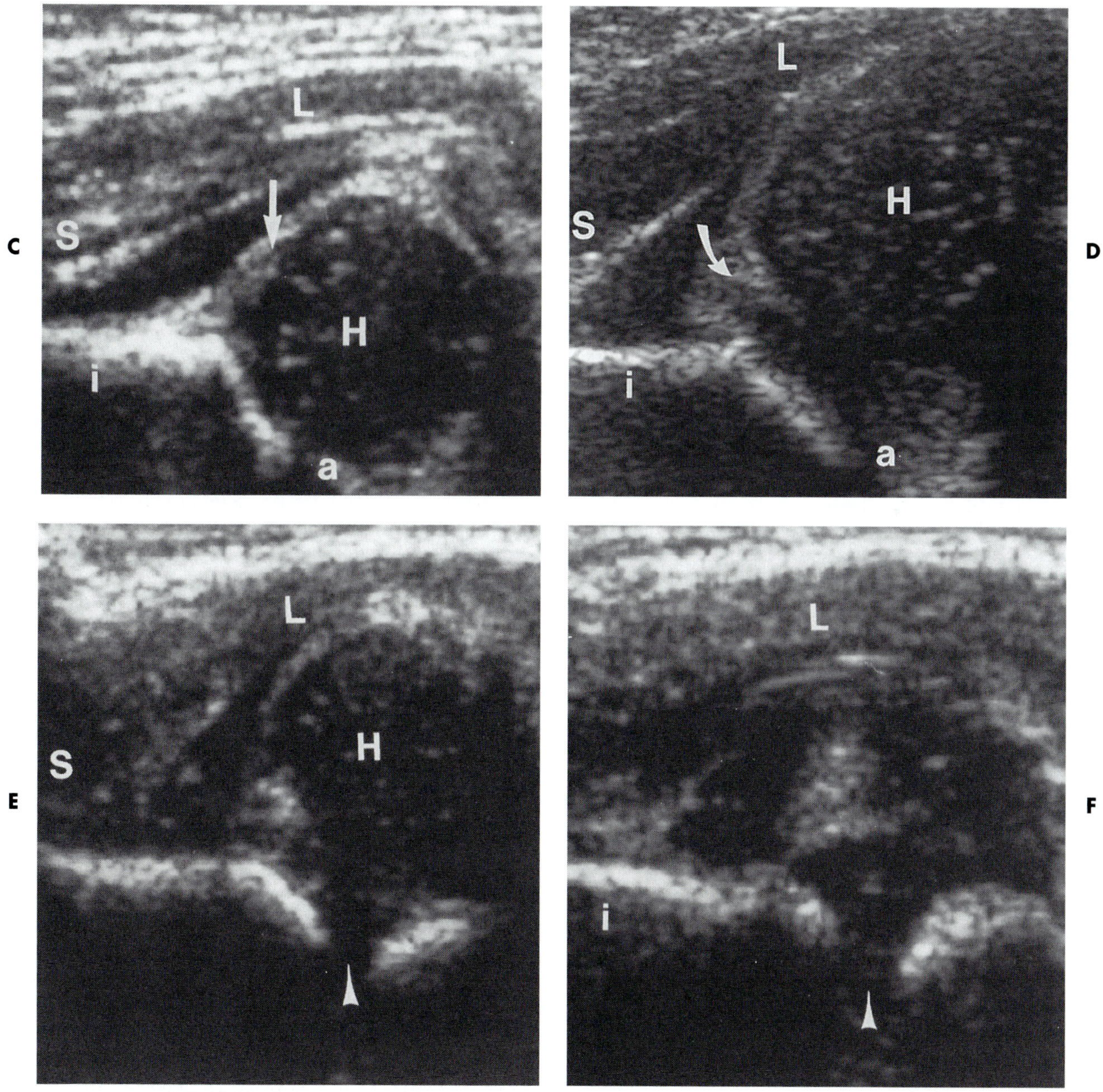

FIG. 62-2, cont'd. **C, Normal hip sonogram** shows sonolucent femoral head resting against bony acetabulum. Note fibrocartilaginous tip of labrum *(arrow)*. **D** to **F, Dislocated hip sonograms. D,** Displacement of sonolucent femoral head laterally and superiorly with deformity and increased echogenicity to labrum *(curved arrow)*. **E, Push maneuver** shows displacement of femoral head over posterior acetabular lip. **F, Pull maneuver** reveals head no longer positioned over triradiate cartilage *(arrowhead)* of posterior lip of acetabulum. *H*, Femoral head; *L*, lateral; *S*, superior line; *a*, acetabulum; *i*, iliac line.

oped. A **normal hip** gives the appearance of a "**ball on a spoon**" in the midacetabulum. The femoral head represents the ball; the acetabulum forms the bowl of the spoon; and the iliac line is the handle. When the transducer is moved posteriorly and the scan plane is over the posterior margin of the acetabulum, the posterior lip of the triradiate cartilage becomes an easily recognized landmark. The bone above and below the cartilage notch is flat, and the normally positioned femoral head is not visualized.

In **subluxation**, the femoral head is displaced laterally, posteriorly, or both, with respect to the acetabulum. Soft-tissue echoes are seen between the femoral head and the bony reflections from the medial acetabulum. In **dislocation,** the femoral head is completely out of the acetabulum (Fig. 62-2, *D*). With superior dislocations, the femoral head may rest against the iliac bone. In posterior dislocations, the femoral head is seen lateral to the posterior lip of the triradiate cartilage. The acetabulum is usually not visualized in a dislocation because the bony shaft of the femur blocks the view.

There are two components to the dynamic examination in the coronal/flexion view. The first is performed over the posterior lip using a "push-and-pull" maneuver (Fig. 62-2, *E* and *F*). In the normal hip, the femoral head is never seen over the posterior lip of the acetabulum. When there is instability, a portion of the femoral head appears over the posterior lip of the triradiate cartilage as the femur is pushed. With a pull, the head disappears from the plane. In a dislocated hip, the femoral head may be located over the posterior lip and may or may not move out of the plane with traction. The second component of the examination is performed over the midacetabulum. The Barlow-type maneuver is performed with adduction and gentle pushing against the knee. In the normal hip, the femoral head will remain in place against the acetabulum. With subluxation or dislocation, the head will migrate laterally and posteriorly, and there will be echogenic soft tissue between the femoral head and the acetabulum.

Transverse/Flexion View. Transition from the coronal/flexion view to the transverse/flexion view is accomplished by rotating the transducer 90 degrees and moving the transducer posteriorly so that it is in a posterolateral position over the hip joint. The horizontal orientation of the scan plane with respect to the body is maintained (Fig. 62-3, *A*). The plane of the transducer and the landmarks is demonstrated on a computed tomography (CT) scan of a patient in spica cast (Fig. 62-3, *B*). Sonographically, the bony shaft and metaphysis of the femur give bright reflected echoes anteriorly, adjacent to the sonolucent femoral head. The echoes from the bony acetabulum appear posterior to the femoral head, and in the **normal hip, a U configuration is produced** (Fig. 62-3, *C*). The relation of the femoral head and acetabulum is observed while the flexed hip is moved from maximum adduction to wide abduction. The sonogram changes its appearance in abduction and adduction. The deep U configuration is produced with maximum abduction whereas in adduction, a shallower V appearance is observed. It is important to have the transducer positioned posterolaterally over the hip to see the medial acetabulum. When the transducer is not posterior enough, the view of the acetabulum is blocked by the femoral metaphysis, and the hip can appear falsely displaced. In adduction, the hip is stressed with a gentle posterior push (a **Barlow** test). In the **normal** hip, the femoral head will remain deeply in the acetabulum in contact with the ischium with stress. In **subluxation,** the hip will be normally positioned or mildly displaced at rest and there will be further lateral displacement from the medial acetabulum with stress, but the femoral head will remain in contact with a portion of the ischium. With **frank dislocation,** the hip will be laterally and posteriorly displaced to the extent that the femoral head has no contact with the acetabulum, and the normal U configuration cannot be obtained (Fig. 62-3, *D*). The process of dislocation and reduction is able to be visualized in unstable hips in the transverse/flexion view. With abduction, the dislocated hip may be reduced, and this represents the sonographic counterpart of the **Ortolani** maneuver.

Transverse/Neutral View. The transition from the transverse/flexion view to the transverse/neutral view is accomplished by bringing the leg down into a physiologic neutral position. The transducer is directed horizontally into the acetabulum from the lateral aspect of the hip (Fig. 62-4, *A*). The plane of interest is one that passes through the femoral head into the acetabulum at the center of the triradiate cartilage (Fig. 62-4, *B*). This can be located by beginning the examination caudally over the bony shaft of the femur. Moving cephalad, the transition from bone to cartilage in the proximal femur becomes apparent, and the circular cross section of the spherical femoral head is identified. In the **normal hip** the sonolucent femoral head is positioned against the bony acetabulum over the triradiate cartilage (Fig. 62-4, *C*). The elements of the sonogram resemble the components of a **flower.** The femoral head represents the flower, and the echoes (from the ischium posteriorly and pubis anteriorly) form the **leaves** at its base. The **stem** is formed by echoes that pass through the triradiate cartilage into the area of acoustic shadowing created by the osseous structures. Since the cartilage over the pubis is thicker than over the ischium, the head appears slightly displaced from the bone echoes anteriorly. When an ossific nucleus is present, echoes appear within the femoral head. The examiner must angle the plane of the transducer above or below the nucleus to

A

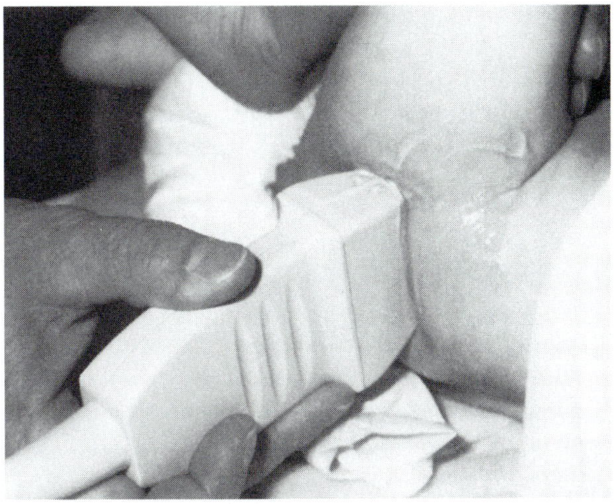

FIG. 62-3. Transverse/flexion view. **A,** Transducer is in the axial plane posterolaterally over the hip joint with the hip flexed. **B,** Scan area *(dotted lines)* on a prone CT scan. Scan demonstrates relationship of femoral head, metaphysis, and ischium in a normal (left) and a dislocated (right) hip. **C, Normal hip sonogram** shows echolucent femoral head surrounded by metaphysis (anterior) and ischium (posterior), forming a U around femoral head. **D, Dislocated hip sonogram** shows sonolucent femoral head displaced posterolaterally. The U configuration of normal metaphysis and ischium is not seen. *H,* Femoral head; *L,* lateral; *P,* posterior; *i,* ischium; *m,* metaphysis.

B

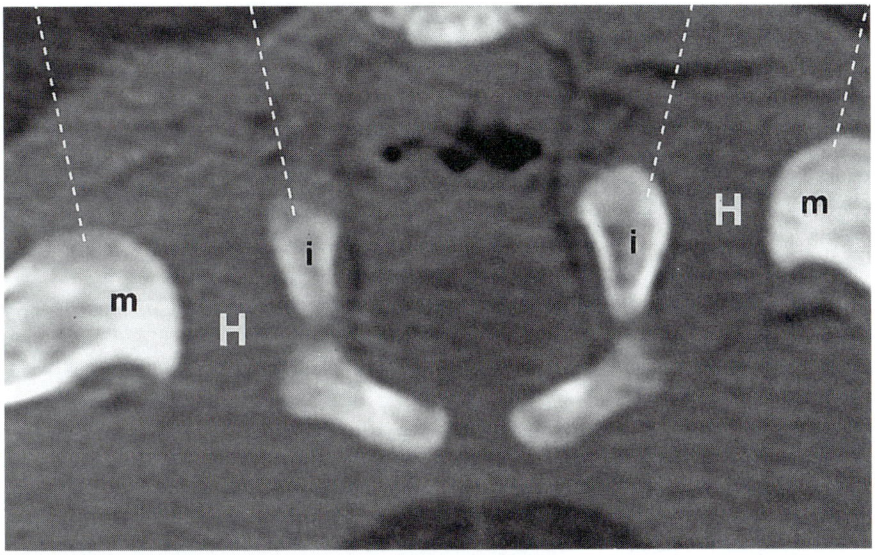

C

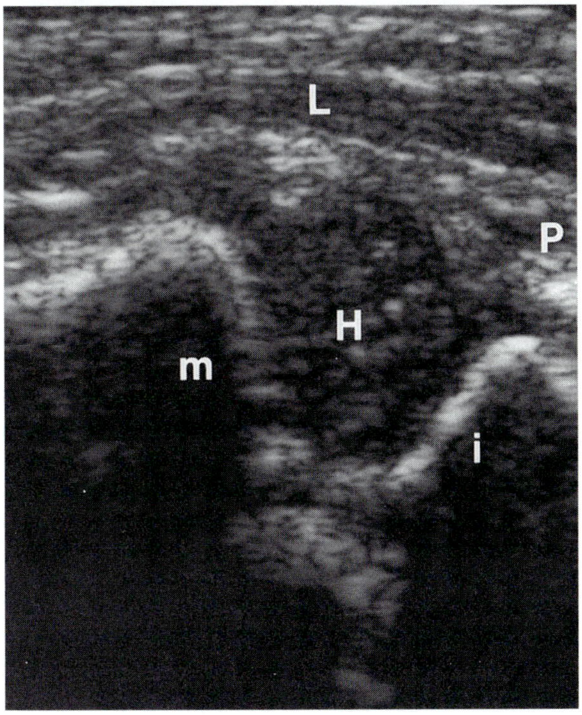

D

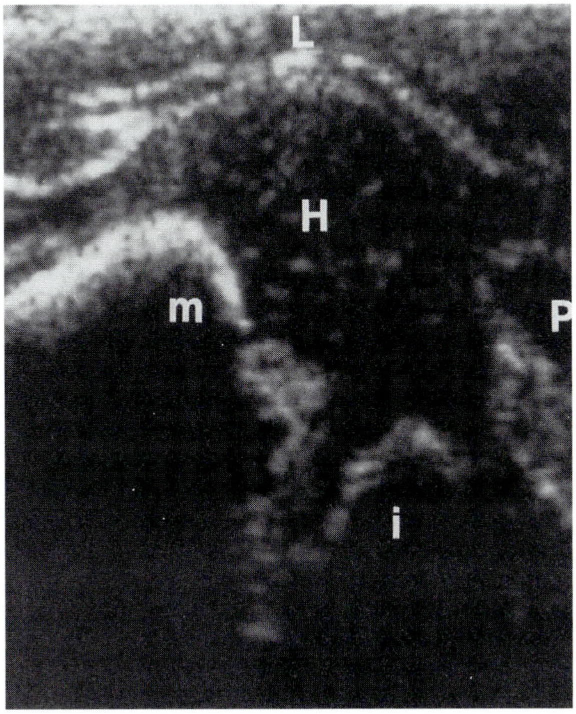

identify the triradiate cartilage. Acoustic shadowing by the ossification center should not be mistaken for the triradiate cartilage because there are no echoes in the gap. The presence and size of an ossific nucleus can be evaluated in this view. We do not use this view to assess acetabular development.

In the transverse/neutral view, **malpositioned hips** show soft-tissue echoes between the femoral head and acetabulum (Fig. 62-4, *D*). The width and configuration of the gap depend on the nature of the displacement. With **subluxation,** the femoral head usually moves posteriorly and, in mild cases, remains in contact with the posterior aspect of the acetabulum. With more severe subluxation, lateral displacement accompanies the posterior migration. Most **dislocations** are lateral, posterior, and superior. Often the dislocated head rests against some portion of the bony ilium. In this case, reflected echoes from the bone are apparent medially. Inability to find the hypoechoic gap of the triradiate cartilage distinguishes this hip from the normal hip. With some lateral dislocations, the femoral head does not rest against bone, and in these cases soft-tissue echoes completely surround the sonolucent head.

Minimum Standard Exam

Is it necessary to use all of the four views described for each hip examination? By consensus, experienced hip sonographers proposed the minimum exam should consist of two orthogonal views, one incorporating stress.[25] Measurements are optional. A typical examination consists of coronal/flexion or coronal/neutral and transverse flexion, with stress in either or both of the views.

Alternative Techniques: Anterior Views

A number of anterior views have been described, and those who take the time to learn them completely have indicated success with their use. In one of the first papers on real-time sonography, Novick et al. reported an anterior view performed with the hip flexed and abducted.[9] Gomes et al. modified this approach with an anterior view that is also done with flexion and abduction but evaluates the hip in a slightly different plane.[26] A dynamic stress test was incorporated to demonstrate the presence of instability. The anterior approach mentioned by Dahlstrom et al.[27] is executed with the patient supine and the hips flexed and abducted. The transducer is placed anterior to the hip joint and is centered over the femoral head with the plane of the sound beam parallel to the femoral neck. The image produced represents a transverse or horizontal section through the acetabulum and a longitudinal section through the femoral head and neck (Fig. 62-5, *A* and *B*).[27] With this view, a Barlow or push maneuver can be performed to detect instability. An attempt is made to displace the femur posteriorly. The criterion for subluxation is head displacement exceeding 20% of the diameter. Complete dislocation is considered to be present when head subluxation exceeds 50% of its diameter (Fig. 62-5, *C*). This view is particularly useful in rigid abduction splints and casts in which the posterior aspect of the hip is covered.

Clinical Applications and Experience

Evaluation of the Infant at Risk. Sonography is most commonly employed for evaluation of an infant with an **abnormal physical examination** or a **DDH risk factor** such as positive family history, breech delivery, foot deformity, or torticollis. In these situations, ultrasound replaces the radiograph of the pelvis, which was routinely obtained in the past when hip abnormality was suspected. When the abnormal physical exam is found shortly after birth, we suggest that sonography be done at 1 to 2 weeks of age. Hip instability may resolve on its own. Newborns with a risk factor for DDH can be checked at 4 to 6 weeks. This avoids multiple exams in cases of transient instability and immaturity. We examine each hip using the four dynamic sonographic views (see Figs. 62-1 to 62-4) and report our findings with an emphasis on position and stability (Table 62-1). Femoral head position is described as **normal, subluxed,** or **dislocated.** Dislocations are easy to determine, and we have had no difficulty with their identification. Sometimes it can be problematic to decide whether an abnormal hip, which is widely malpositioned, should be called subluxed or dislocated. Stability testing is reported as **normal, lax, subluxable, dislocatable** (for subluxed hips), and **reducible** or **irreducible** (for dislocated hips). When stress maneuvers are performed, it is important that the infant be relaxed; otherwise, inconsistency may be found between the sonographic and clinical examination findings and between serial ultrasound studies. The **acetabulum** is assessed visually and is described as **normal, immature,** or **dysplastic.** More important is the development of the cartilaginous labrum and its coverage of the femoral head. Situations in which the bony component is steeply angled but the cartilage is well developed and covers the femoral head should be noted. Deformity of the cartilage and increased echogenicity are indications of more severe acetabular dysplasia.

Irrespective of the technique used, many reports attest to the **efficacy of ultrasound** in comparison with the clinical and radiographic examination.[24,26-29] In young infants, ultrasound is able to detect hip laxity and malposition not apparent on the clinical and radiographic evaluations. Experience has indicated that most infants who are less than 30 days of age have hip laxity that becomes normal after a few weeks without treatment. This is not a new observation because the phenomenon was recognized clinically by Barlow.[1] It

A

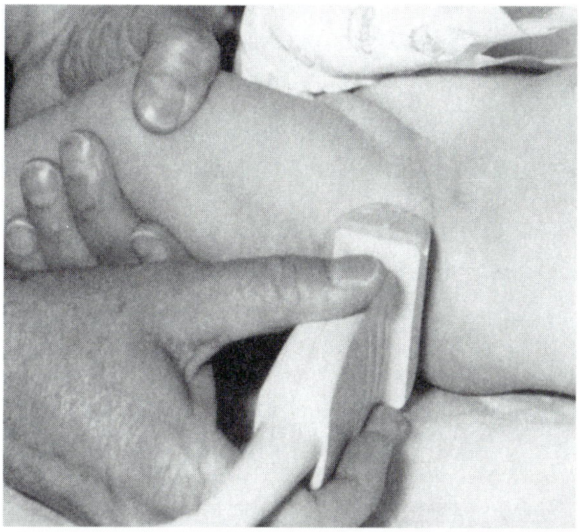

FIG. 62-4. Transverse/neutral view. **A,** Transducer is perpendicular to neutral femoral head in the plane of acetabulum. **B,** Scan area *(dotted lines)* on supine normal MRI. **C, Normal hip sonogram** shows sonolucent femoral head centered over triradiate cartilage with pubis (anterior) and ischium (posterior). **D, Subluxed hip sonogram** shows sonolucent femoral head displaced posterolaterally with gap between pubis and femoral head *(arrow)*. *H,* Femoral head; *L,* lateral; *P,* posterior; *i,* ischium; *arrowhead,* triradiate cartilage; *p,* pubis.

B

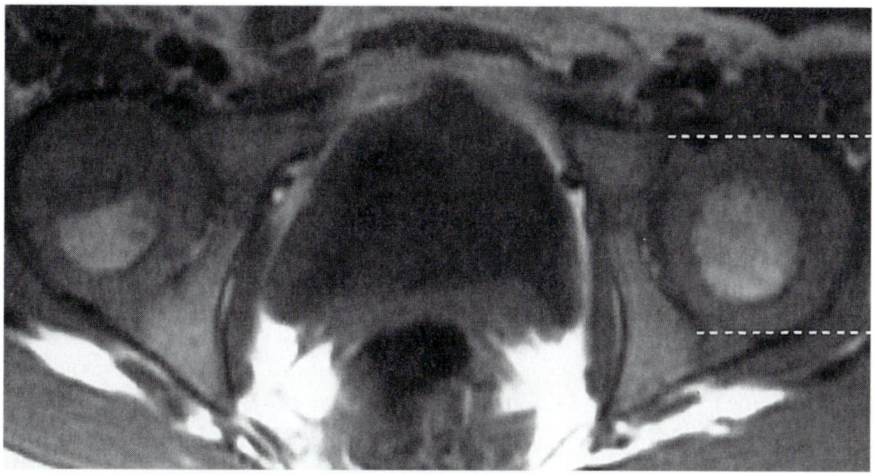

C

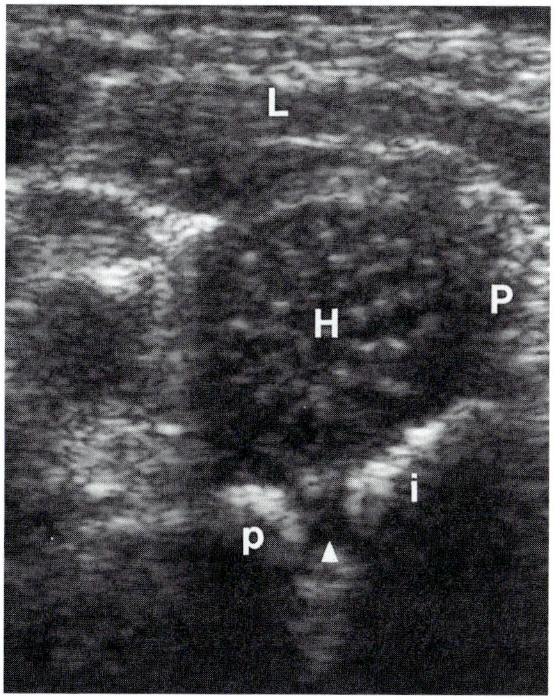

D

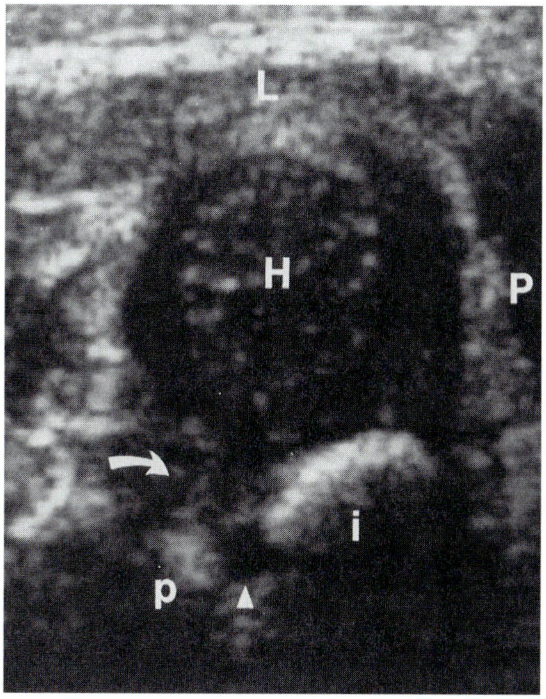

TABLE 62-1
DYNAMIC SONOGRAPHY CLASSIFICATION

View and Maneuver	Normal	Laxity w/Stress (Subluxable)	Subluxed	Dislocatable/Dislocated
Coronal/neutral* (standard plane)	N	N	A	A
Coronal/flexion (standard plane)	N	N	A	A
Coronal/flexion (posterior lip) No stress—piston stress	N	N—A	A	A
Transverse/flexion Abduction—adduction	N	N—A	N—A	A
Transverse/neutral	N	N	A	A

N, Normal; *A*, Abnormal.
*Measurement of acetabular landmarks (angles/coverage) is optional. If performed, either the coronal/neutral or coronal/flexion view in the standard plane can be used.

identifies, however, a group of infants who need follow-up. Not all infants become normal, and therefore continued observation is required.[24]

Evaluation During Treatment. The usefulness of ultrasound in the follow-up of infants with DDH—whether for observation of resolving abnormality or in conjunction with a defined treatment regimen—is widely accepted. Currently, sonography is routinely used to follow borderline cases, particularly in very young infants, before a commitment is made to a treatment regimen. When treatment is indicated, it is common to use ultrasound to monitor hip position during treatment. Dynamic splints, such as the Pavlik harness, hold the hip in a flexed/abducted position. These and similar devices are popular, and ultrasound has been tested as a way of monitoring hip position for infants in splint devices.[18,30,31] The sonographic examination in these patients is limited to the transverse/flexion and coronal/flexion views. The stress portion of the examination is not performed unless requested. Typically, stress is not used until the conclusion of treatment, when weaning from the harness is instituted.

One of the problems with follow-up sonography has been its reliability in morphologic assessment of the bony acetabulum. Reports of discrepancies between the sonographic appearance of the bony acetabulum and the radiographic appearance indicate that there is not always an exact correlation.[18] This may result from observer variation and the nature of the ultrasound measurements. We have chosen to include the pelvic radiograph as a baseline toward the end of the treatment protocol. The older the infant, the more we tend to consider radiography, particularly when the ossification centers get large.

At one time, in severe cases of DDH that required rigid casting, we removed a plug from the cast over the posterolateral aspect of the hip; this enabled us to evaluate the hip position using our standard views. Although this was successful for us and others,[13,32] there is a question of whether the reduction can be compromised by removal of the plaster plug. The use of anterior or groin views is possible; however, we have not been comfortable with those approaches. In our institution, infants in rigid casts are evaluated using CT. The localizer CT film enables the examiner to select one or two slices that are adequate to assess hip position. Magnetic resonance imaging (MRI) offers another alternative and gives no ionizing radiation, although its high cost and the necessity for sedating the infant are disadvantages.

Screening Program. The **routine screening** of all newborn infants with ultrasound is a controversial issue. Based on a comparison between clinical and sonographic screening with sonography, Tonnis et al. concluded that all newborns should be screened with ultrasound because it detects more pathologic joints than the clinical examination.[24] In some European countries, routine screening has been tried on a regional basis. Critics of newborn screening programs note the high number of infants undergoing treatment or requiring follow-up studies (whether for minor instability or immaturity in acetabular development). Studying only infants at risk will not eliminate late cases of DDH.[33,34] Presently, sonographic screening of all newborns is not considered practical in the United States because of the resources that would be required. Screening by clinical examination is recommended, and ultrasound is reserved for infants having an abnormal examination or risk factor.[35,36]

HIP JOINT EFFUSION

Clinical Overview

After 1 year of age, when sonography becomes unreliable for evaluation of DDH, it can be used to assess the

A

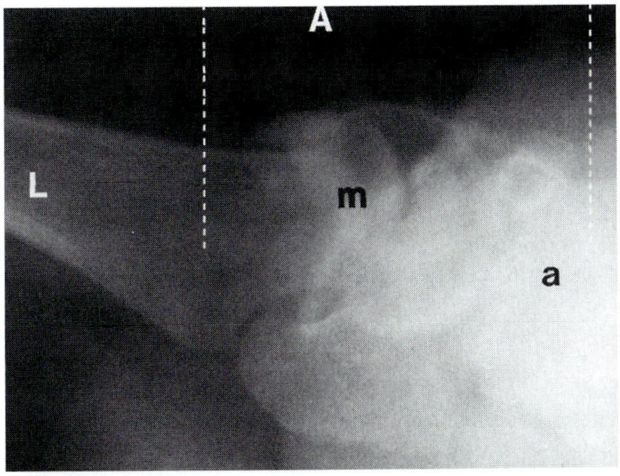

FIG. 62-5. Dahlstrom anterior views. **A,** Scan area *(dotted lines)* on true lateral view of hip arthrogram. **B, Normal hip sonogram** shows sonolucent femoral head, *H*, bordered by metaphysis, *m*, laterally, and acetabulum, *a*, medially. **C, Dislocated hip sonogram** shows posterior displacement of femoral head, *H*, and metaphysis, *m*. *A*, Anterior; *L*, lateral.

B

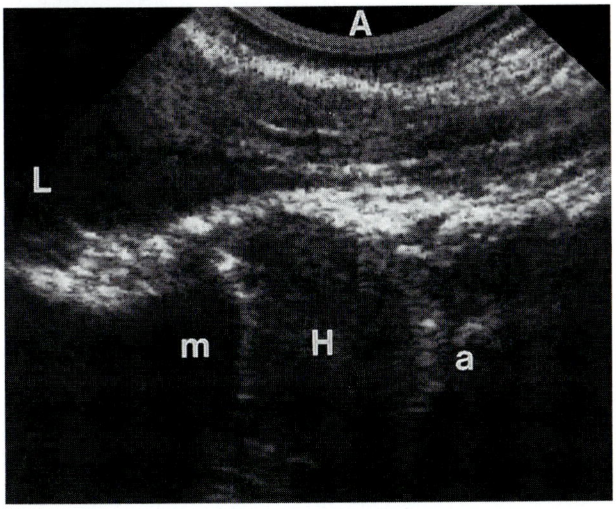

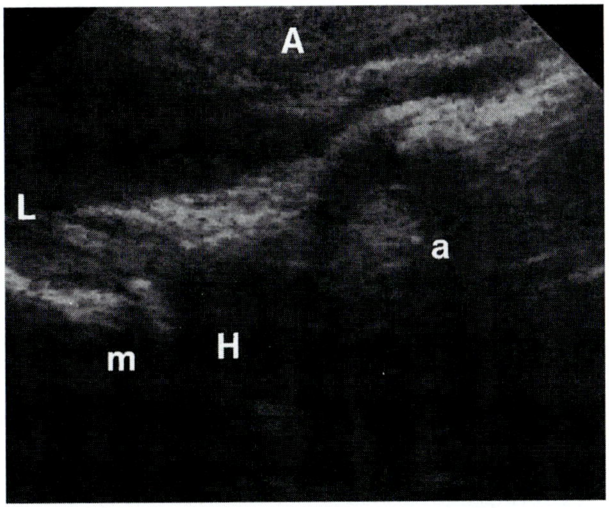

C

painful hip. A variety of conditions cause **hip pain** in pediatric patients, including transient synovitis, osteomyelitis, Perthes' disease, slipped capital femoral epiphysis, fracture, and arthritis. Although radiography is performed initially and is often diagnostic, there are frequent instances when the plain radiographic film is normal in the presence of small **joint effusions.** Sonography can be used to determine if an effusion is present and to guide arthrocentesis.

Sonographic Technique and Anatomy

The patient is examined in the supine position with the hips in the neutral position without flexion if possible. A high-frequency linear transducer is recommended. The hip is scanned in a ventral, oblique plane along the long axis of the femoral neck (Fig. 62-6, *A* and *B*). The brightly echogenic anterior cortex of the femoral head and neck with the intervening echolucent physis are seen; the anterior margin of the bony acetabulum is visualized superiorly. The **anterior recess of the joint capsule** parallels the femoral neck in this area, with the outer margin forming an echogenic line anterior to the cortex of the femoral neck and extending over the femoral head (Fig. 62-6, *C*). The iliopsoas muscle is superficial to the capsule.

In the normal hip, the joint capsule has a concave contour and the thickness of the capsule from the outer margin to the cortex of the femoral neck measures 2 to 5 mm. The hip capsules should be symmetric within 2 mm. When there is an effusion, the anterior recess of the capsule becomes distended with a convex outer margin, and there is greater than 2 mm increased thickness of the abnormal joint capsule (Fig. 62-6, *D*) compared with the normal contralateral capsule (see Fig. 62-6, *C*).[37-39] The use of measurements alone is more difficult when both hips are abnormal, yet that is an infrequent occurrence.

Fluid of varying echogenicity is seen within the capsule. The echoes are created by inflammatory debris or hemorrhage.[38] Some studies have indicated specificity with regard to the appearance of the fluid. Zeiger et al.[40] reported the fluid to be anechoic or hypoechoic in transient synovitis and more echogenic in septic arthritis, concluding that if the fluid is anechoic, the

A

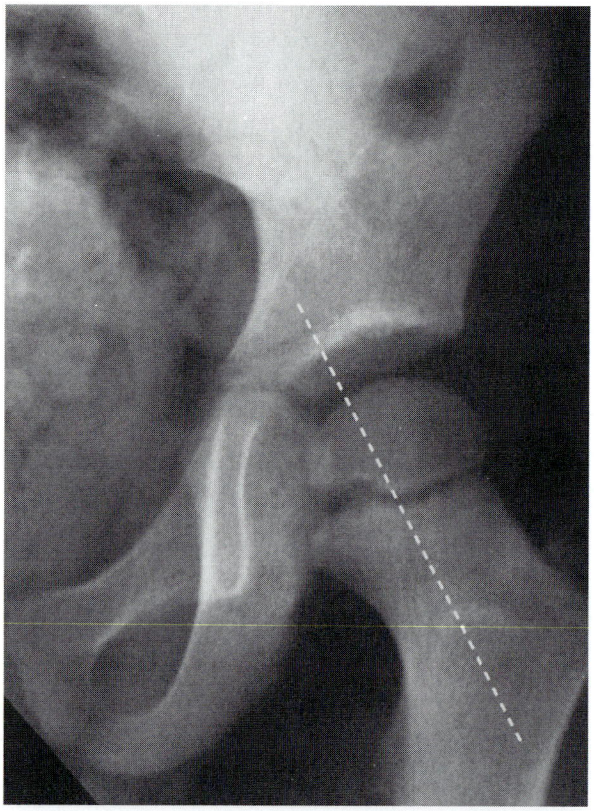

FIG. 62-6. Joint effusion. **A,** Transducer position parallels femoral neck. Scan plane *(dotted line)*. **B, Normal hip sonogram** shows joint capsule *(arrows)* following contours of femoral head, *H*, and neck, *N*. **C, Hip effusion sonogram** shows bulging joint capsule *(arrows)* with mixed echogenicity within capsule caused by hemorrhage or inflammatory debris. *A*, Anterior; *S*, superior.

B

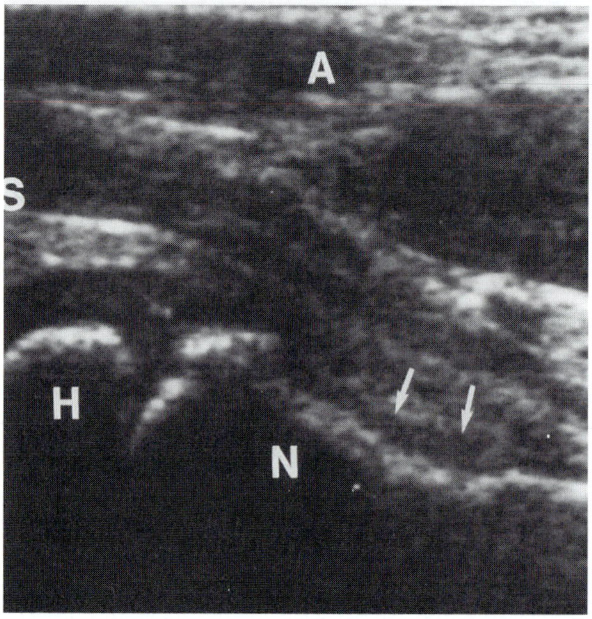

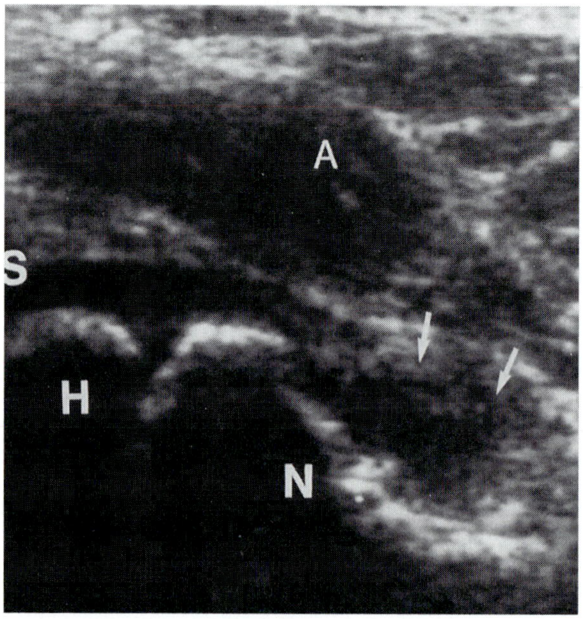

C

diagnosis of septic arthritis could be excluded. Other investigators have found the **character of the fluid to be nonspecific,**[37,41] describing echoes (probably representing hemorrhage) in the fluid in transient synovitis and anechoic fluid in cases of septic arthritis.

When fluid is detected, **arthrocentesis** can be performed and a saline lavage can be used if fluid cannot be withdrawn. Although the procedure requires patient cooperation, it is relatively easy to execute, and it avoids the ionizing radiation required in fluoroscopic arthrocentesis. Some clinicians use arthrocentesis therapeutically in Perthes' disease because it reduces pain and allows a more normal range of motion.[38]

Other sonographic observations include fragmentation of the femoral head in Perthes' disease, slippage of the head in slipped capital femoral epiphysis, and cortical disruption in fracture or osteomyelitis, yet these findings are better evaluated radiographically. Soft-tissue swelling and other soft-tissue abnormalities outside the joint capsule have also been diagnosed.

Clinical Applications and Experience

Several large studies of sonographic hip joint effusion detection have been reported. They show the technique to be easy to master and rapidly performed. The results have been highly sensitive in the detection of effusion, with as little as 1 mm of fluid recognized experimentally. False-negative examination results have been reported in infants who are less than 1 year of age,[40] probably for technical reasons related to the transducer shape and the configuration of the immature hip.

Although hip sonography is sensitive in the detection of effusion, its place in the work-up of the painful hip is not clearly defined. In one large series, although ultrasound facilitated early diagnosis or prompted further investigation in some patients, it altered the therapy or outcome in only 1% of the patients.[41] Another group[42] recommends the use of a protocol to evaluate the painful hip using radiography, hip ultrasound, and scintigraphy as follows: when the radiographic findings are negative, sonography is performed, to be followed by aspiration if there is an effusion or by bone scan if there is no effusion.

At our institution, **the work-up of the painful hip** is individualized, and we find hip sonography to be helpful in certain circumstances. When the clinical picture is unclear, the presence or absence of an effusion can guide the clinician in the diagnosis and need for further evaluation. For example, in the patient with clinical and laboratory signs of **transient synovitis,** hip sonography may be used to demonstrate an effusion; however, the patient does not usually undergo joint aspiration. In a patient with signs of sepsis and an effusion, a bone scan is performed regardless of the results of aspiration to exclude **osteomyelitis.** When the hip ultrasound is negative in a septic patient, it rapidly and accurately excludes the possibility of **septic arthritis** but not osteomyelitis, and a bone scan may be required. Finally, sonography can be used to guide arthrocentesis, and this avoids the ionizing radiation of fluoroscopic aspiration.

REFERENCES

Congenital Hip Dislocation and/or Dysplasia (DDH)

1. Barlow TG. Early diagnosis and treatment of congenital dislocation of the hip. *J Bone Joint Surg* 1962;44B:292-301.
2. VonRosen S. Prevention of congenital dislocation of the hip joint in Sweden. *Acta Orthop Scan* 1970;130(suppl):1-64.
3. Treadwell SJ, Bell HM. Efficacy of neonatal hip examination. *J Pediatr Orthop* 1981;1:61-65.
4. Dunn PM. Perinatal observations on the etiology of congenital dislocation of the hip. *Clin Orthop* 1976;119:11-22.
5. MacEwen GD, Bassett GS. Current trends in the management of congenital dislocation of the hip. *Int Orthop* 1984;8:103-111.
6. Wynn-Davies R. Acetabular dysplasia and familial joint laxity: two etiological factors in congenital dislocation of the hip. *J Bone Joint Surg* 1970;52B:704-716.
7. Hensinger RN. Congenital dislocation of the hip: treatment in infancy to walking age. *Orthop Clin North Am* 1987;18:597-616.
8. Graf R. The diagnosis of congenital hip-joint dislocation by the ultrasonic Combound treatment. *Arch Orthop Trauma Surg* 1980;97:117-133.
9. Novick G, Ghelman B, Schneider M. Sonography of the neonatal and infant hip. *AJR* 1983;141:639-645.
10. Harcke HT, Clarke NMP, Lee MS, et al. Examination of the hip with real-time ultrasound. *J Ultrasound Med* 1984;3:131-137.
11. Harcke HT, Grissom LE. Performing dynamic sonography of the infant hip. *AJR* 1990;155:837-844.
12. Graf R. Ultrasonography of the infantile hip. In: Sanders RC, Hill MC, eds. *Ultrasound Annual.* New York: Raven Press; 1985:177-186.
13. Harcke HT, Grissom LE. Sonographic evaluation of the infant hip. *Semin Ultrasound* 1986;7:331-338.
14. Harcke HT, Lee MS, Sinning L, et al. Ossification center of the infant hip: sonographic and radiographic correlation. *AJR* 1986;147:317-321.
15. Graf R. Classification of hip joint dysplasia by means of sonography. *Arch Orthop Trauma Surg* 1984;102:248-255.
16. Zieger M, Hilpert S, Schultz RD. Ultrasound of the infant hip. I. Basic principles. *Pediatr Radiol* 1986;16:483-487.
17. Morin C, Harcke HT, MacEwen GD. The infant hip: real-time ultrasound assessment of acetabular development. *Radiology* 1985;157:673-677.
18. Polaneur PA, Harcke HT, Bowen JR. Effective use of ultrasound in the management of congenital dislocation and/or dysplasia of the hip (DDH). *Clin Orthop* 1990;252:176-181.
19. Zieger M. Ultrasound of the infant hip. II. Validity of the method. *Pediatr Radiol* 1986;16:488-492.
20. Bialik V, Pery M, Kaftori JK, et al. The use of ultrasound scanning in the management of developmental disorders of the hip. *Int Orthop* 1988;12:75-78.
21. Engessaeter LB, Wilson DJ, Nag D, et al. Ultrasound and congenital dislocation of the hip: the importance of dynamic assessment. *J Bone Joint Surg* 1990;72B:197-201.
22. Langer R. Ultrasound investigation of the hip in newborns in the diagnosis of congenital hip dislocation: classification and results of a screening program. *Skeletal Radiol* 1987;16:275-279.
23. Szoke N, Kuhl L, Henrichs J. Ultrasound examination in the diagnosis of congenital hip dysplasia of newborns. *J Pediatr Orthop* 1988;8:12-16.
24. Tonnis D, Storch K, Ulbnrich H. Results of newborn screening for DDH with and without sonography and correlation of risk factors. *J Pediatr Orthop* 1990;10:145-152.
25. Harcke HT. Screening newborns for developmental dysplasia of the hip: the role of sonography. *AJR* 1994;162:395-397.
26. Gomes H, Menanteau B, Motte J, et al. Sonography of the neonatal hip: a dynamic approach. *Ann Radiol* 1987;30:503-510.
27. Dahlstrom H, Oberg L, Friberg S. Sonography in congenital dislocation of the hip. *Acta Orthop Scand* 1986;57:402-406.
28. Clarke NMP, Harcke HT, McHugh P, et al. Real-time ultrasound in the diagnosis of congenital dislocation and dysplasia of the hip. *J Bone Joint Surg* 1985;67B:406-412.
29. Berman L, Klenerman L. Ultrasound screening for hip abnormalities: preliminary findings in 1001 neonates. *Br Med J* 1986;293:719-722.

30. Grissom LE, Harcke HT, Kumar SJ, et al. Ultrasound evaluation of hip position in the Pavlik harness. *J Ultrasound Med* 1988;7:1-6.
31. Dahlstrom H. Stabilization and development of the hip after closed reduction of late DDH. *J Bone Joint Surg* 1990;72B:9-12.
32. Boal DKB, Schwentker EP. The infant hip: assessment of real-time ultrasound. *Radiology* 1985;157:667-672.
33. Clarke NMP, Clegg J, Al-Chalabi AN. Ultrasound screening of hips at risk for DDH. *J Bone Joint Surg* 1989;71B:9-12.
34. Rosendahl K, Markestad T, Lie RT. Ultrasound screening for developmental dysplasia of the hip in the neonate: the effect of treatment rate and prevalence of late cases. *Pediatrics* 1994; 94:47-52.
35. Boeree NR, Clark NAP. Ultrasound imaging and secondary screening for congenital dislocation of the hip. *J Bone Joint Surg* 1994;76B:525-533.
36. Harcke HT. The role of ultrasound in diagnosis and management of developmental dysplasia of the hip. *Pediatr Radiol* 1995;25:225-227.

Hip Joint Effusion

37. Marchal GJ, Val Holsbeeck MT, Raes M. Transient synovitis of the hip in children: role of ultrasound. *Radiology* 1985;56: 367-371.
38. Alexander JE, Seibert JJ, Glasier CM, et al. High-resolution hip ultrasound in the limping child. *J Clin Ultrasound* 1989; 17:19-24.
39. Kallio P, Ryoppy S, Jappinen S, et al. Ultrasonography in hip disease in children. *Acta Orthop Scand* 1985;56:367-371.
40. Zieger MM, Dorr U, Schulz RD. Ultrasonography of hip joint effusions. *Skeletal Radiol* 1987;16:607-611.
41. Miralles M, Gonzalez, Pulpeiro JR, et al. Sonography of the painful hip in children: 500 consecutive cases. *AJR* 1989; 152:579-582.
42. Alexander JE, Seibert JJ, Aronson J, et al. A protocol of plain radiographs, hip ultrasound, and triple phase bone scans in the evaluation of the painful pediatric hip. *Clin Pediatr* 1988; 27:175-181.

CHAPTER 63

Pediatric Interventional Sonography

Neil D. Johnson, M.B., B.S., F.R.A.C.R., M. Med.

CHAPTER OUTLINE

GENERAL PRINCIPLES

The Patient

Unlike the usual adult patient, most pediatric patients are medically robust and without superimposed coronary or cerebral disease. **The smaller the patient, the more appropriate is the use of ultrasound for guidance of at least the initial phase of an interventional procedure.** Most procedures can be accomplished with intravenous sedation and proper local anesthetic technique. Physicians whose training and experience have involved them solely with adults often regard a baby as a "fragile" patient, but on the contrary, children tolerate levels of pH, creatinine, and sedation that might cause major complications in adults. The pediatric patient is often quite unconcerned with the details of the disease and treatment, and all but the sickest patients simply want to get out of the imaging department with the maximum of play and the minimum of discomfort. The parent, on the other hand, is sometimes more difficult to manage—as if the procedure were to be performed on him or her. Attention to the needs and expectations of the dual "patients"—the parents and the child—is essential from the beginning of the interaction.

Personnel and Equipment

Adequate equipment and experienced assistants are essential for successful and safe pediatric intervention. Although most radiologists should be able to perform basic procedures on children, some cases are not for the faint-hearted, inexperienced, or occasional operator. A commitment to careful, graded learning, including the use of training phantoms, is needed as is a good knowledge of regional anatomy or the willingness to learn the anatomy before attempting difficult procedures.

By its nature, the timing of interventional practice is not always predictable, and it is common for the ultrasound department to resent calls for equipment on short notice. **Despite the inconvenience, the interventionist should aggressively insist on the best technical ultrasound equipment available.** The slightly out-of-date machine with the broken transducer is more appropriate for the routine, repeat renal ultrasound patient than for the difficult interventional case.

GUIDANCE METHODS

CT Versus Ultrasound

CT is necessary for some procedures, especially bone biopsy, but in most cases, ultrasound guidance with either ultrasound or fluoroscopic monitoring of wire and catheter placement is ideal (Table 63-1). MRI guidance is uncommon except in a few institutions and is unnecessary in most pediatric conditions.

Ultrasound Guidance and Fluoroscopic Monitoring

The addition of ultrasound guidance to a fluoroscopy or angiographic room is the ideal for most nonbone procedures. Ultrasound allows complex approach paths, especially around the diaphragm, and real-time visualization, while fluoroscopy allows monitoring of the guide wire and catheter insertion. Beginners often kink the guide wire as the dilator or catheter is being inserted through the capsule or fascia, and fluoroscopy allows quick recognition and remedy of this situation. Some procedures such as antegrade nephrostomy require contrast diagnostic studies following initial puncture.

ULTRASOUND TECHNIQUES

Equipment/Transducers

A selection of transducers is essential. Small babies require high-frequency transducers (**at least 5 MHz**), and procedures performed around ribs are best done with small-footprint-sector transducers. Color

TABLE 63-1
CT VS. ULTRASOUND

	CT	Ultrasound
Radiation	Used	None
Scan Plane	Limited to axial (especially difficult near the diaphragm)	Unlimited, except by bone or gas
Resolution	Excellent, although lack of fat in children can limit visualization	Excellent, especially for membranes in fluid collections
Convenience	More difficult to schedule	High
Cost	High	Intermediate
Monitoring	By repeat scan; no real-time ability; recovery from kinked wires difficult	Real time
Gas Bowel	Excellent, especially with contrast	Poor

Doppler is very useful for localization of major blood vessels. Transducers with good near-field resolution are used for superficial lesions and for initial accurate placement of local anesthetic on the peritoneum or organ capsule.

One Operator Versus Two

It is common for inexperienced operators to require the technologist or another radiologist to perform the scanning. This should be vigorously discouraged! Although large, simple fluid collections can be drained this way, the necessary skills for accurate needle and biopsy placement in small organs or near critical structures will never be learned. Communication between the eyes and hands of a single operator is achieved through the spinal cord (occasionally supervised by the cerebral cortex!), which is considerably more accurate than the verbal "Where's my needle now?" communication between two operators.

Freehand Versus Mechanical Guides

Most manufacturers supply well-designed mechanical guides that attach to a transducer and allow a predictable needle path to be visualized. These guides are useful for keeping the needle in the plane of the ultrasound beam and can be used for lesions with a simple approach path or a wide access window. Most devices require a disposable sterile kit when the device is used, adding to the cost of the procedure.

Freehand guidance is more difficult to learn, but it allows much more flexibility of approach, and when the needle can be positioned 90° to the beam, even fine needles are easily visible. Freehand guidance allows the operator to choose the most advantageous transducer geometry and to steer the needle or biopsy device around other structures on the way to the lesion. Placement of local anesthetic on the peritoneum and other sensitive structures is made easier by freehand technique.

Color Doppler

Color Doppler is used for localization of vascular structures so as to avoid them during most procedures or for guidance during PICC line or central line placement. Color Doppler has been advocated for visualization of the moving needle during interventional procedures, but our experience has been that the potential for better visualization of the needle is outweighed by the degradation of the gray scale image when color Doppler is active. Most needles, including 27-gauge local anesthetic needles, can be readily localized by choosing the optimal transducer, maintaining accurate transducer alignment, and using short, manual in-and-out movements of the needle being localized. Various devices are available to enhance the visualization of the needle, but these all add expense and are unnecessary if accurate ultrasound technique is learned.

FREEHAND TECHNIQUE

The essence of the freehand technique is that the operator never has a free hand! Instead, the user is free to choose the path of the needle without the restraint imposed by a mechanical guide. This is most useful around ribs and near the diaphragm but is applicable anywhere in the body.

The technique requires that the transducer be held in one hand and the needle or biopsy device in the other. The user needs to be able to use either hand as the needle, or operating, hand. Crossed hands invite crossed thinking and usually lead to difficulties in orientation. For example, a biopsy of the liver might be obtained by placing the transducer on the anterior abdominal wall using the right hand and making the needle approach from the lateral position, parallel to the table, using the left hand. A left-sided biopsy would suggest using the left hand for the transducer and the right hand for the needle approach from the left flank. With some practice and some simple rules, it is not difficult to use the nondominant hand as the needle hand.

Initial Needle Placement and Localization

The most important technique to learn in freehand sonography is needle localization. These rules work equally well for a needle entry site near the transducer or one at a distance (Fig. 63-1, *A*, *B*). The entry point is chosen after careful consideration of the anatomy and important structures such as ribs, large vessels, diaphragm, and bowel. Indentation of the entry site using a finger to compress the skin (Fig. 63-2, *A*, *B*) allows the exact entry site to be assessed, especially in the lateral entry position, and the site is marked on the skin. Once the entry site is chosen, I often do a last check by placing the transducer exactly over the marked spot for a last "needle's-eye view" to insure that there will be no surprises such as, for example, the internal mammary arteries during mediastinal biopsy, which may be overlooked unless specifically localized. Once the entry path has been chosen and after proper application of local anesthetic (see below), the needle or biopsy device is placed through the skin toward the target. **The needle and transducer need to be absolutely parallel on the skin surface.** This can be checked by looking directly down onto the top of the transducer and needle as the initial placement is made (Fig. 63-3). The depth of the target should be measured (and remembered) before needle placement.

A

B

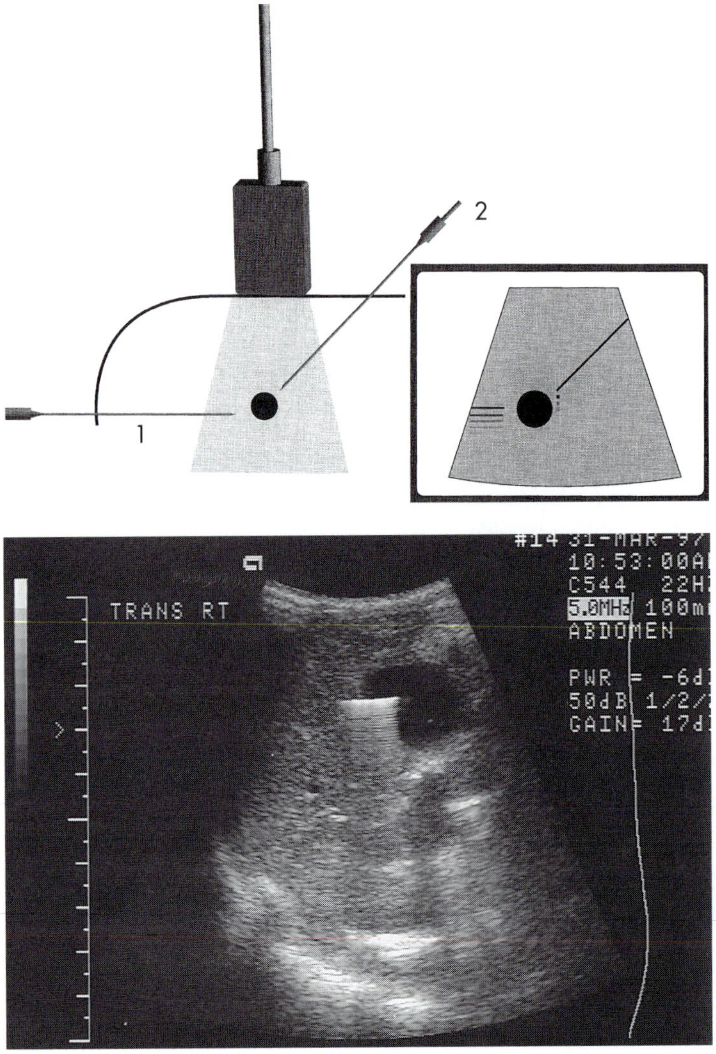

FIG. 63-1. Common approaches. A, The most common entry sites are either, 1, lateral (parallel to the transducer face) or, 2, adjacent to the transducer. When the needle is parallel to the transducer face, a prominent reverberation artifact is seen (Fig. 63-1, *B*), or a "comet-tail" artifact is seen when the needle is not parallel. The needle is more difficult to locate in position 2.

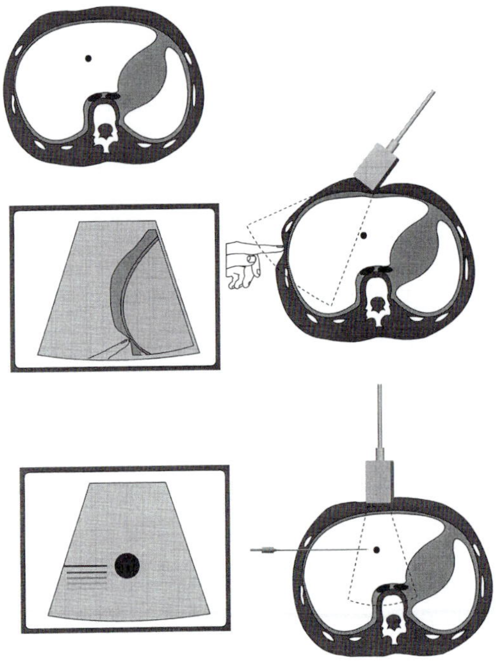

FIG. 63-2. Locating the entry site laterally. The exact point of entry can be tested by rotating the transducer toward the body wall and palpating potential entry sites with a finger which is readily visible on the ultrasound real-time images.

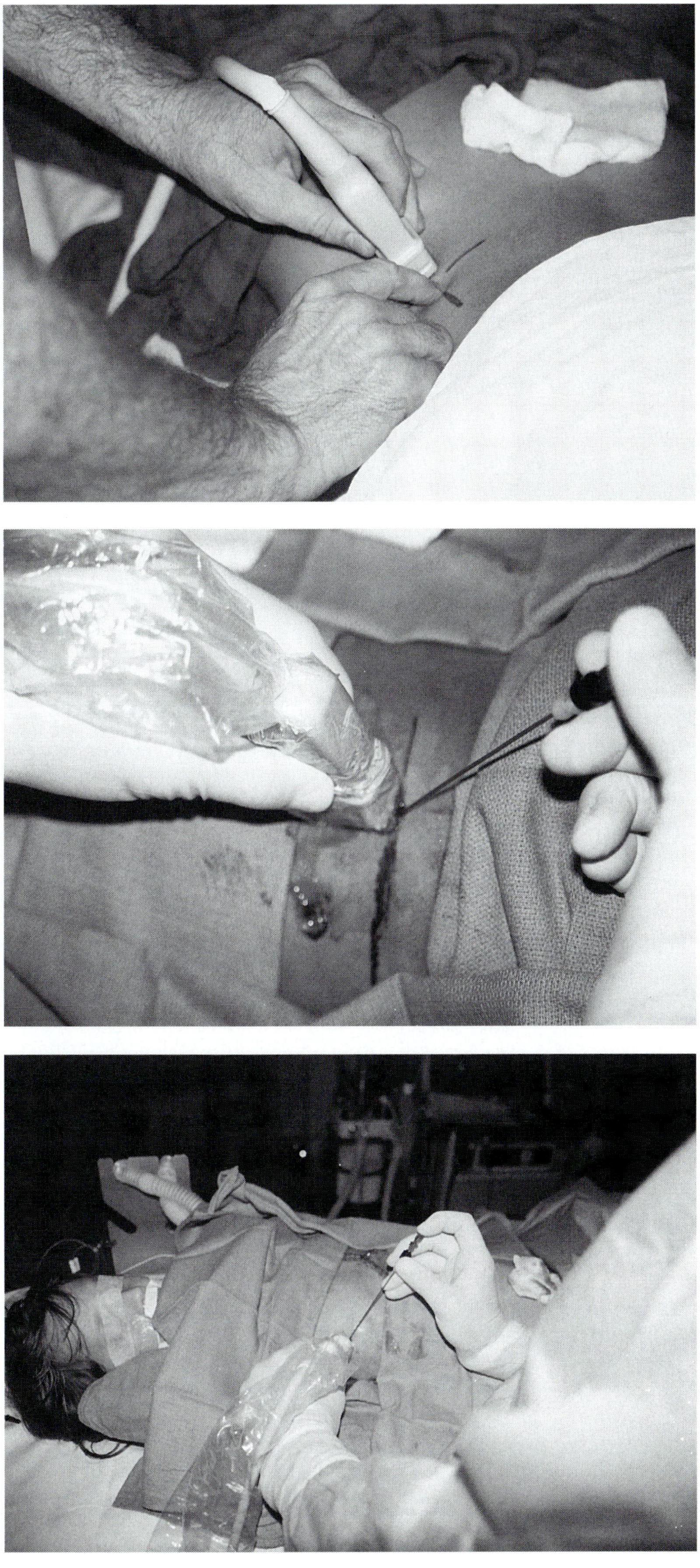

A

B

C

FIG. 63-3. Needle alignment. **A,** After locating the entry site, **B** and **C,** the needle is inserted in a plane strictly parallel with the transducer.

Providing there are no superficial vital structures in its path, the needle initially should be advanced about half of the distance to the target under direct ultrasound monitoring. If necessary, the preplanned distance of insertion can be marked on the needle with a steristrip. **Most beginners have an uncontrollable urge to keep pushing the needle** in the hope that it will magically make the needle visible. This is a mistake!

Radiologists who usually work with adults may not appreciate the short insertion distances required in small children and babies. I am aware of at least one instance in which the needle was placed right through the patient and into the table.

Locating the Needle after Insertion

With experience, it is possible to keep the needle visible starting from the moment of insertion, but if not, the needle must be localized before any further advancement is made. Check that the transducer and needle are parallel to each other by looking down the cable of the transducer with one eye closed. **If the two are not parallel, adjust the position of the transducer, not the needle.** Once the transducer and needle are parallel, keep the transducer in that plane and move it back and forth strictly in the plane of the needle (Fig. 63-4). It is often useful to anchor the transducer hand on the patient by placing the fourth and fifth digits or the hypothenar border of the transducer hand firmly on the patient's skin, using the thumb and the second and third digits to hold and move the transducer (Fig. 63-5). A slight (2 to 3 mm) in and out motion of the needle may help make the tip visible, but it is important not to jab the needle in and out aggressively or to try to move the needle and transducer in complex directions or angles in a hopeful and usually ineffective attempt to localize the needle.

If the whole length of the needle is not visible, it may be angled obliquely to the plane of the transducer, resulting in an erroneous understanding of the position of the needle's tip (Fig. 63-6, *A*, *B*, *C*). Usually, only a few degrees of rotation are required to obtain an image of the whole of the needle shaft. This is easier to achieve when the needle is parallel to the transducer face, but the same principle applies when the needle is inserted adjacent to the transducer.

The localization of the needle after initial placement must be a calm, thoughtful, and purposeful process that involves moving the transducer back and forth, adjusting and rotating its position in small increments until the whole length of the needle is visible.

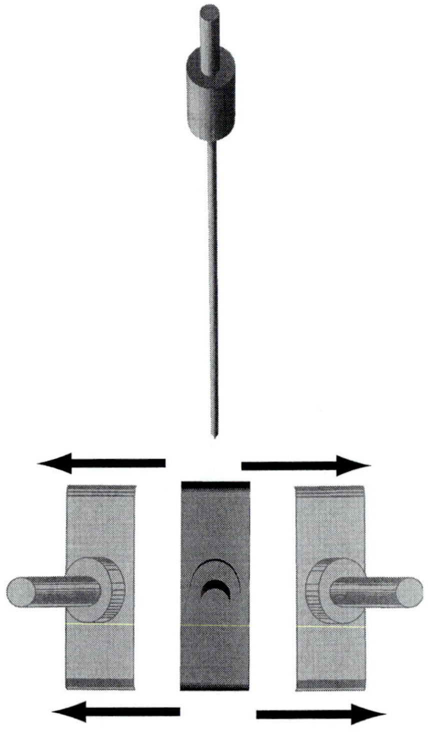

FIG. 63-4. Transducer motion. After inserting the needle, the transducer is translated backwards and forwards in the plane of the needle until the needle is localized. The actual amount of movement required is much less than in this diagram; typically, it is only a few millimeters.

If Everything Goes Well

If the needle is visible *and* the target is visible *and* the needle is pointing at the target, the needle can be advanced toward the target and it should remain visible during the advancement. The needle may need a short sharp jab to enter the target, particularly if the target is a normal structure such as the gallbladder, a calyx, or a bile duct. The organs of children are soft and compliant and can sometimes "float" away from the needle tip as it is advanced, but the short jab required to puncture such organs or structures must always be a kind jab, made under control and with a purpose, never an angry or frustrated jab!

If Everything Does Not Go Well

The most common problem is that either the needle is not pointing at the target or the target is no longer visible in the scan.

Correcting Needle Angle

If the needle and target are visible in the one image, but the needle angle is incorrect, do not attempt to radically change the angle of the needle while it is deep in an organ. Doing so, especially with a rigid biopsy needle, may result in a tear of the organ with acute hypotension in the patient and hypertension in the operator.

A

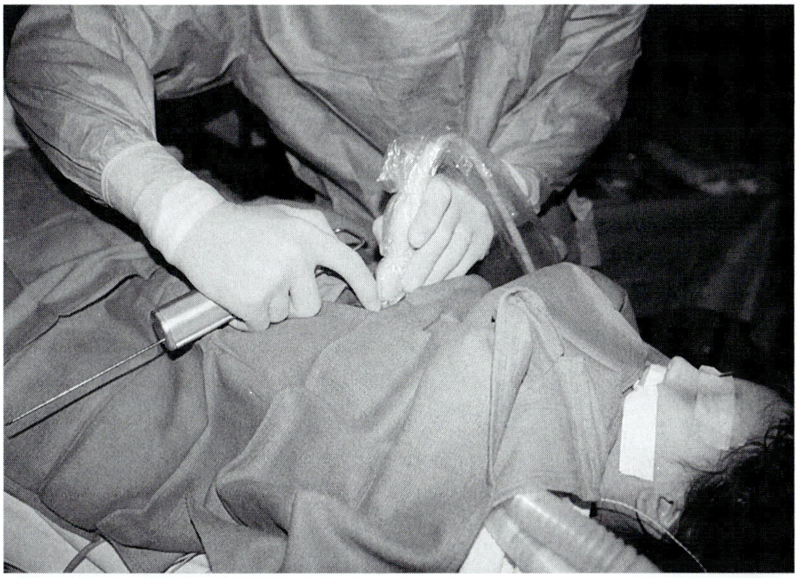

B

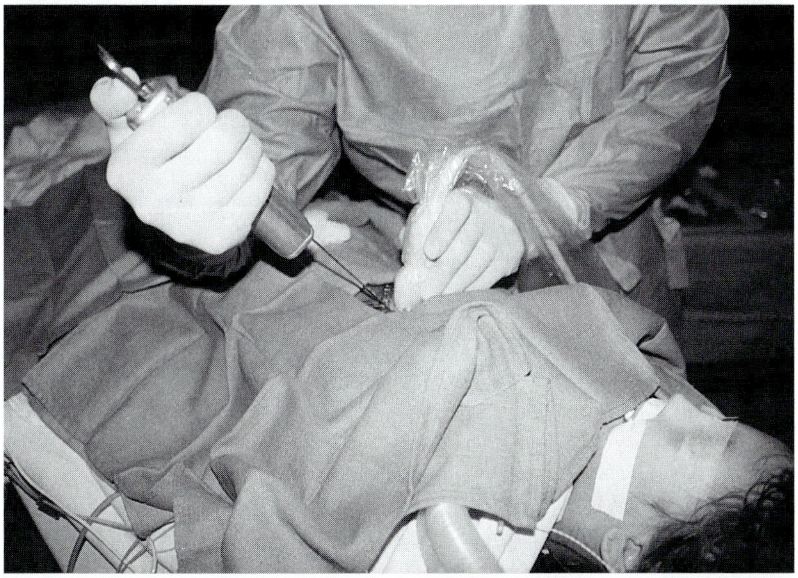

C

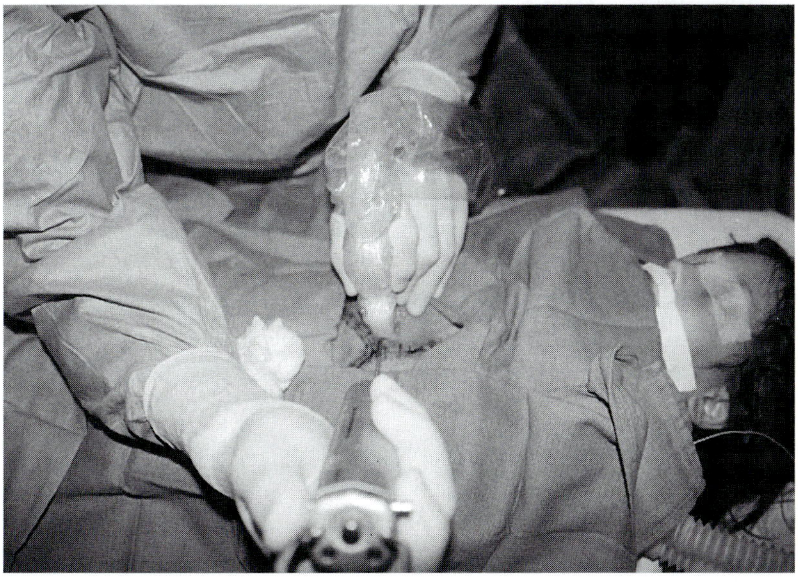

FIG. 63-5. Biopsy guidance. The usual principles apply: **A,** Check entry site; **B,** insert device parallel to transducer; **C,** check position by looking from above.

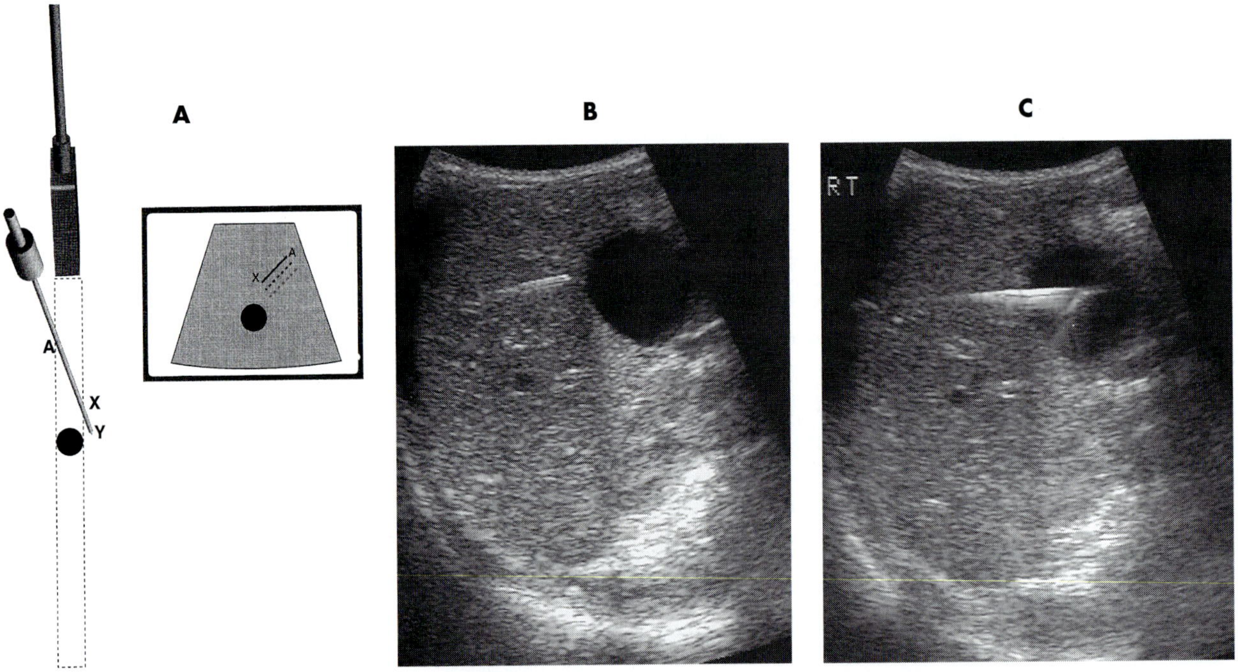

FIG. 63-6. Off-plane needle position results in a shortened view. **A, X** of the needle and a false sense of needle tip position at point X, whereas the real position of the tip is at point Y. **B,** Off-plane view of part of the shaft of the needle during gallbladder puncture. **C,** With slight rotation of the transducer, without moving the needle, it is now clear that the needle tip is actually in the gallbladder. (Normally, the tip would be accurately localized **before** puncture of the gallbladder.)

Instead, withdraw the needle until it is subcutaneous, adjust the angle, and reinsert it under direct ultrasound monitoring, as before (Fig. 63-7).

If the transducer is not vertical, it is sometimes difficult to decide which way to adjust the needle's angle. This simple rule will always work: **Consider the position of the transducer cable and move the needle in relation to it** (Fig. 63-7, *D, E*). It is important, however, to know which side of the transducer belongs to which side of the ultrasound monitor screen. One should always test the orientation of the image before beginning a procedure by running a finger over the transducer face and noting where the finger appears on the screen. It is always embarrassing when the image of the needle is expected on one side of the screen but is actually on the other side of the screen where it is not noticed and is well on its way toward the aorta or some other minor structure.

Correcting the Off-Target Needle

If the needle is visible, but the target is not, move the transducer parallel to the plane of the needle, first one way and then the other, until the target is reestablished. Remember which way the transducer needed to be moved to reimage the target, then withdraw the needle, move the skin entry site in the same direction by moving the needle tip in the subcutaneous tissues, and advance the needle once again into the patient.

Training Aids for Freehand Sonographic Intervention

These techniques can be practiced on various phantoms, which have been described.[1] The most readily available and practical practice phantom consists of a turkey breast and various materials, such as beef kidney, olives, cocktail onions, or artificial cysts made by tying off the finger of a surgical glove that has been filled with water. These materials are placed in the plane between the pectoralis major and minor muscles while the turkey breast is under water.[2, 2a, 2b]

NEEDLES, WIRES, CATHETERS, AND BIOPSY DEVICES

Many needles and devices are available on the market and each practitioner should select and become very familiar with a limited selection of these devices. Listed below are the basic categories of devices, some general comments, and our preferred choice of devices.

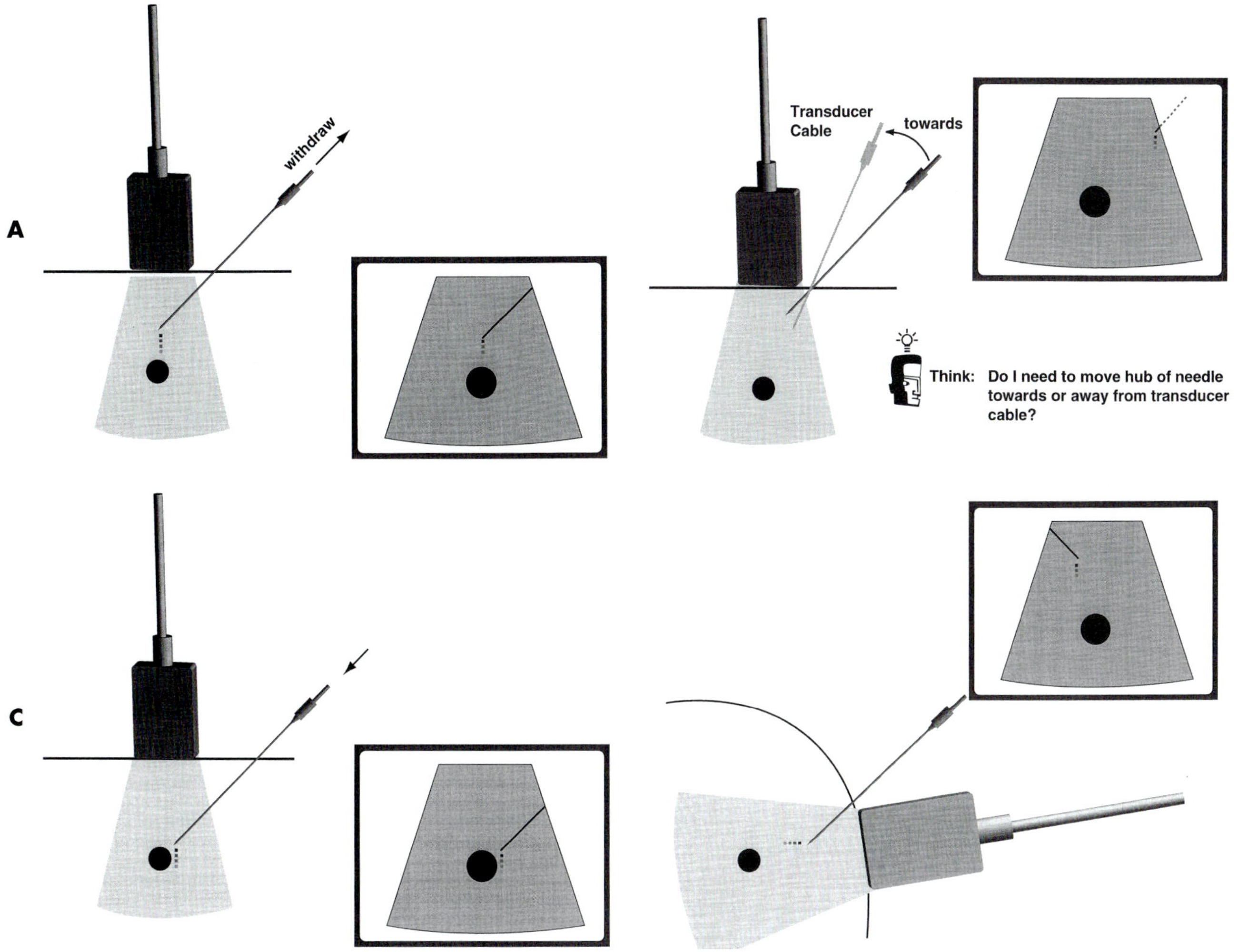

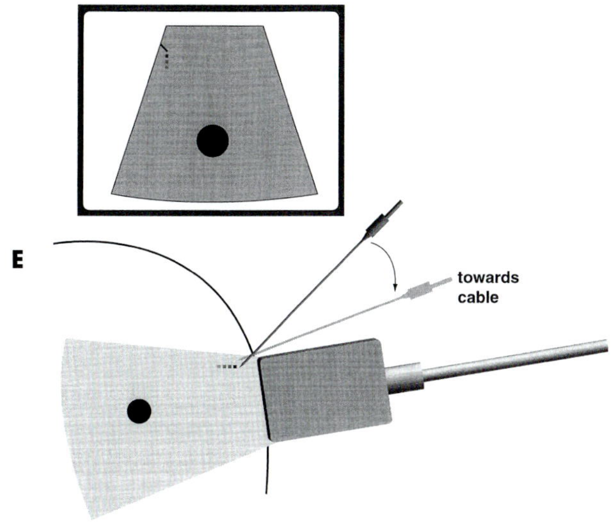

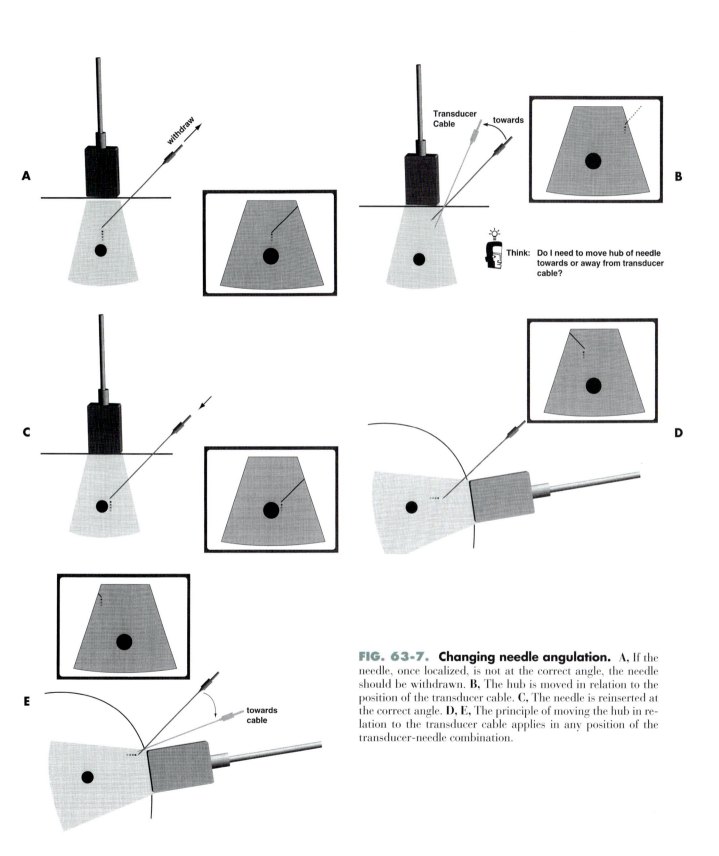

FIG. 63-7. Changing needle angulation. **A,** If the needle, once localized, is not at the correct angle, the needle should be withdrawn. **B,** The hub is moved in relation to the position of the transducer cable. **C,** The needle is reinserted at the correct angle. **D, E,** The principle of moving the hub in relation to the transducer cable applies in any position of the transducer-needle combination.

Chiba Needles

These are a class of relatively safe, very useful, flexible, small-diameter (usually 22-gauge) needles used for diagnostic contrast studies or for initial puncture of a target, especially if the target is near a vital structure. If the procedure involves subsequent placement of a guide wire or catheter, only a thin guide (typically 0.018 inches) can be placed through the needle. This is a relative disadvantage because a dilator will have to be placed over the 0.018 wire, and the thin wires are subject to kinking, especially when the dilator meets the deep fascia or capsule of an organ.

Drainage Catheters

Modern commercial catheters are of high quality, and usually, a general purpose or locking loop catheter will suffice. For thick pus or old blood, a large caliber catheter or even a chest tube may need to be placed. Sump-type catheters with separate flushing and aspiration channels were once popular but have not been demonstrated to be superior to a large-caliber, single-lumen catheter for most applications.

A Note on Catheter Sizes. Catheters are usually measured by the French scale. It is a common misconception that the French scale defines the diameter. The **French size** is actually the **outside circumference in millimeters.** The diameter of the catheter can easily be derived by elementary school arithmetic, but the primary measurement is the outside circumference. The French scale does not measure the internal diameter or necessarily define which wire can be used with a particular catheter.

Most drainage catheters need to be placed over a 0.035 wire, which necessitates an exchange maneuver, and each passage of a wire or dilator adds to the complexity of the procedure and the risk of losing position or kinking the wire.

Various prepackaged exchange sets are available commercially. Some sets have a dilator/sheath that is placed over the 0.018 wire and then the dilator is removed, leaving the larger sheath in place; this allows placement of the 0.035 wire in one step.

Lumbar Puncture Needles

These needles come in various lengths and sizes and are much more rigid than the Chiba needles. They are useful in the musculoskeletal system but should not generally be used in the abdomen.

Sheathed Needles

These consist of an integrated catheter/needle system, usually 19-gauge or larger. Initial puncture is made directly with the system. Once the system is properly located, the needle is removed, leaving the thin-walled sheath in place. The sheath accepts a 0.035 wire directly, minimizing the risk of kinking the wire inherent in the 0.018 systems. The larger diameter of the initial needle is not a problem, provided the system is accurately inserted under ultrasound guidance as previously described. The Cook (Bloomington, IN) TDCHN 3.5, 19, 14.0 CHILD-010494 system is our preferred device (Fig. 63-3, *A*, *B*).

Wires

Usually the standard 0.035 Teflon-coated guide wires are adequate for most procedures. A wire with a J-tip configuration is useful when entering fluid collections or the collecting system of the kidney. The wire should regain the J configuration as soon as it exits the placement sheath or needle. If it does not, it is not free in a fluid cavity and should be repositioned or withdrawn. **NEVER WITHDRAW A WIRE THROUGH A METAL NEEDLE.** The risk of severing the wire is too great.

Occasionally, a super stiff wire is needed, but that is unusual and when such a wire is used, it should be used with respect, and the tip position should be carefully monitored.

Use of the techniques described above allows a 0.035 wire to be placed initially, eliminating the need to place a less substantial 0.018 wire, but if it is necessary to place a 0.018 wire, the mandril-type wires, which consist of a solid "piano wire" shaft with a flexible, high-visibility tip, are safer than the regular 0.018 wire. The use of such a wire is often necessary when entering the bile ducts in a liver transplant patient, as the duct walls are often very hard. For drainage, it may be necessary to make a central puncture next to the hepatic artery which must not be damaged. In these cases, it is prudent to puncture the duct using a 22-gauge Chiba needle, with subsequent placement of a mandril 0.018 wire and graded dilatation and exchange for a 0.035 wire and appropriate catheter.

Biopsy Devices

Aspiration cytology is not widely used in children because there is a much more diverse group of potential lesions in children than in adults. Many of the pediatric tumors depend partly on cellular arrangement for diagnosis, and pediatric pathologists are generally uncomfortable making important diagnoses based on cytology specimens.

Cutting-slot or suction-core instruments are most often used. Although it may seem logical that small-diameter devices should be used in children, **in general, 14- or 15-gauge needles are used** by experienced practitioners in order to obtain sufficient material for pathology examination. The larger needles may seem more dangerous, but if they are placed and monitored under ultrasound guidance, the risk is minimized.

Automated slot-type biopsy devices come in short-throw (9 to 11 mm) and long-throw (22 to 23 mm) varieties. An excellent review[3] of many of the commercial devices revealed that the **short-throw devices provide a far inferior sample compared to that provided by the long-throw devices.** This is probably because these devices work by allowing the inner stilet to curve into the tissue aided by the single, steeply angled face of the inner needle. The stilet is then forced up into the tissue by the outer metal sheath which, at the same time, cuts off the sample in the slot. The short-throw devices do not allow the inner stilet to curve into the tissue, so the samples obtained by the short-throw devices are typically both short and very thin.

In a small organ or adjacent to a vital structure, it is better to use a long-throw device and start the biopsy farther away from the edge of the lesion than to use a short-throw device and obtain a non-diagnostic sample. A bewildering array of commercial devices exists, but with the exception of the short/long throw principle, whatever device works best for the individual practitioner is best for the patient. **What really matters is that ultrasound-guided biopsies be done under precise control and with real-time monitoring.**

ANATOMY

Diaphragm

A thorough knowledge of regional anatomy is essential. If a procedure is to take place in an unfamiliar area, there is always time to look up the anatomy in a text before proceeding. **The surface anatomy of the diaphragm must be thoroughly understood** (Fig. 63-8), and it is important to remember that even if the apex of the diaphragm is grossly elevated by a mass or a fluid collection, **it is still *attached* to the chest wall at the same place it was at birth.** If the pleural space is to be avoided, one must still enter a subphrenic collection below the peripheral attachment of the diaphragm. The diaphragm generally passes across the junction of the middle and outer thirds of the twelfth rib posteriorly. From this point, a line drawn around the chest to the xiphoid process of the sternum (xiphisternum) will trace out the peripheral attachment of the diaphragm. It is important to know that the pleural space extends ***below*** the inner third of the twelfth rib.

Colon/Bowel

The colon lies just anterior to the kidneys and may be inadvertently punctured during percutaneous nephrostomy. The nondistended colon may not be

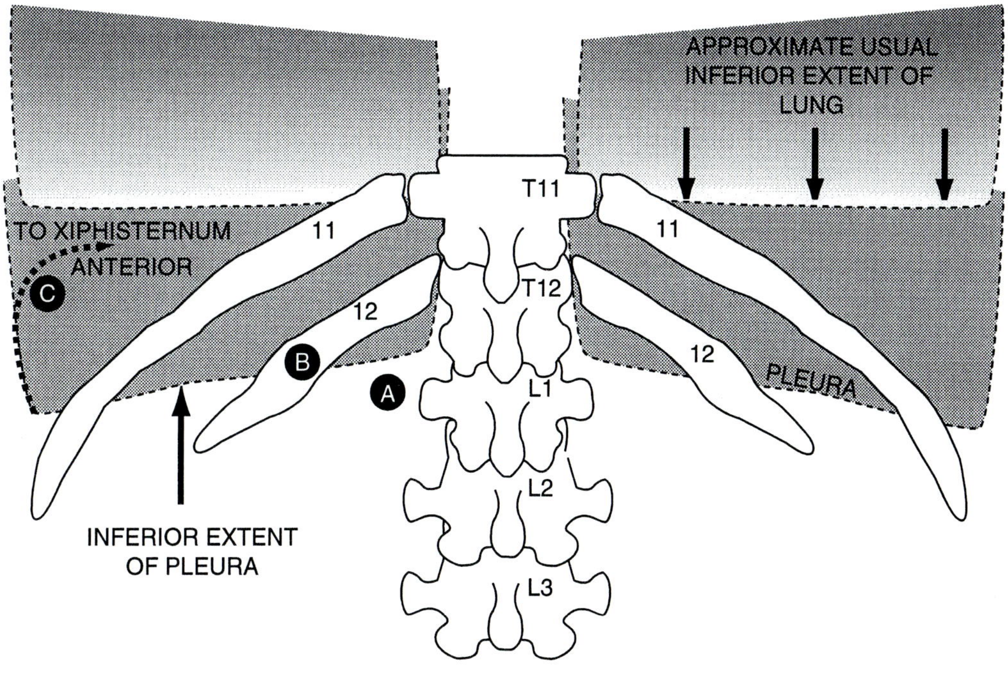

FIG. 63-8. The surface anatomy of the diaphragm. The pleural space extends inferior to the 12th rib medially (position A), and superior to the lateral third of the 12th rib (position B). A line drawn from position B to the xyphoid process of the sternum (the xiphisternum) (position C) will map out the surface markings of the peripheral attachment of both the **normal and the elevated** diaphragm.

easily detectable by ultrasound and one must be careful to avoid placing a nephrostomy too anterior. If there is any doubt, a contrast enema can be performed and the position of the colon localized by fluoroscopy before or during the procedure.

SEDATION

Few children under 12 years will cooperate during an invasive procedure, and a thorough familiarity with pediatric sedation is necessary, together with skilled personnel and adequate resuscitation facilities. It is better to do a procedure under general anesthetic than to attempt the procedure without adequate sedation. If the child is moving excessively, the sedation should be increased, help should be obtained, or the procedure should be terminated.

Our sedation protocol has been previously published.[4] In general, we prefer either IV Nembutal and fentanyl or IV Versed and fentanyl for children over 10 years. Details of sedation are beyond the scope of this chapter, and specific publications should be consulted or training acquired before performing deep sedation in children. **A well-organized and experienced team that performs sedation regularly, with appropriate guidelines and limits, is much more important than which particular drugs are used.**

LOCAL ANESTHETIC TECHNIQUE

The most commonly used agent is lidocaine (Abbott Labs, Chicago, IL) 1% solution. The usual maximum adult dose for local anesthesia is 4.5 mg/kg (0.45 ml/kg of 1% solution). A maximum dose of 3 to 4 mg/kg (0.3 to 0.4 ml/kg of 1% solution) for children over 3 years of age is noted in the product-insert dosage recommendations, but there is no recommendation for younger children. We routinely use the 3 to 4 mg/kg (0.3 to 0.4 ml/kg of 1% solution) for all but extremely premature babies. If the lidocaine is mixed with sodium bicarbonate 8.4% solution in a ratio of 10:1, the sensation of stinging as the local anesthetic is injected is reduced. Liberal use of topical agents such as EMLA cream (ASTRA, Westborough MA) is also useful, but these must be applied 20 minutes before the procedure, and the entry site for a procedure is not always known in advance.

It is a common error to inject the local anesthetic and then immediately commence the procedure. Local anesthetic needs 5 to 8 minutes to achieve full effect, so we often place the local anesthetic, at least in the skin and subcutaneous tissues, before gowning and gloving and preparing the tray. This allows time for the anesthetic to achieve maximal effect. (A drug company representative once suggested to me that doctors should recite the Hippocratic Oath forwards and backwards between giving local anesthetic and commencing the procedure. I have found this to be good advice.)

Use of 30-gauge or smaller needles for initial subcutaneous injection minimizes the discomfort and often allows initial injection without the patient's being aware of the skin puncture at all.

Care must be taken to exclude air from the needle before injecting the local anesthetic, as even the amount of air in a small needle may seriously degrade the ultrasound image over the insertion point.

Ultrasound-Guided Local Anesthetic Administration

One of the keys to successful percutaneous procedures in children is adequate local anesthetic control of ***deep*** sensation. Many practitioners anesthetize the skin and subcutaneous tissues only and are then surprised when the patient moves or complains vigorously as the dilator is passing through the peritoneum or the capsule of the organ. The solution is to place the majority of the local anesthetic on the peritoneum or capsule. **In general, it is the *external covering* of an organ, the peritoneum, or the deep fascia that registers pain sensation.** Placing local anesthetic equally throughout the subcutaneous fat and muscle layers is wasteful. It is better to place most of the local anesthetic directly on the sensitive layers. This is best achieved by using sonographic guidance (Fig. 63-9) during deep local anesthetic placement in a manner similar to the use of ultrasound guidance during the actual procedure. **Surprisingly, even 30-gauge needles can be identified close to the skin with high-quality 7 or 10 MHz transducers.** The focal zone must be adjusted appropriately, but with optimal conditions, the local anesthetic can be deposited where it will have the most effect. This reduces the depth of sedation required and allows some procedures to be completed faster and without general anesthesia when it would otherwise be required.

ANTIBIOTICS

Antibiotics are routinely needed only when draining an infected collection or when the patient is immunesuppressed. We usually use periprocedural antibiotics for liver and renal transplant patients. The choice of antibiotics is individualized after consultation with the referring service and they are usually given intravenously at the time of sedation or anesthesia induction.

A

B

C

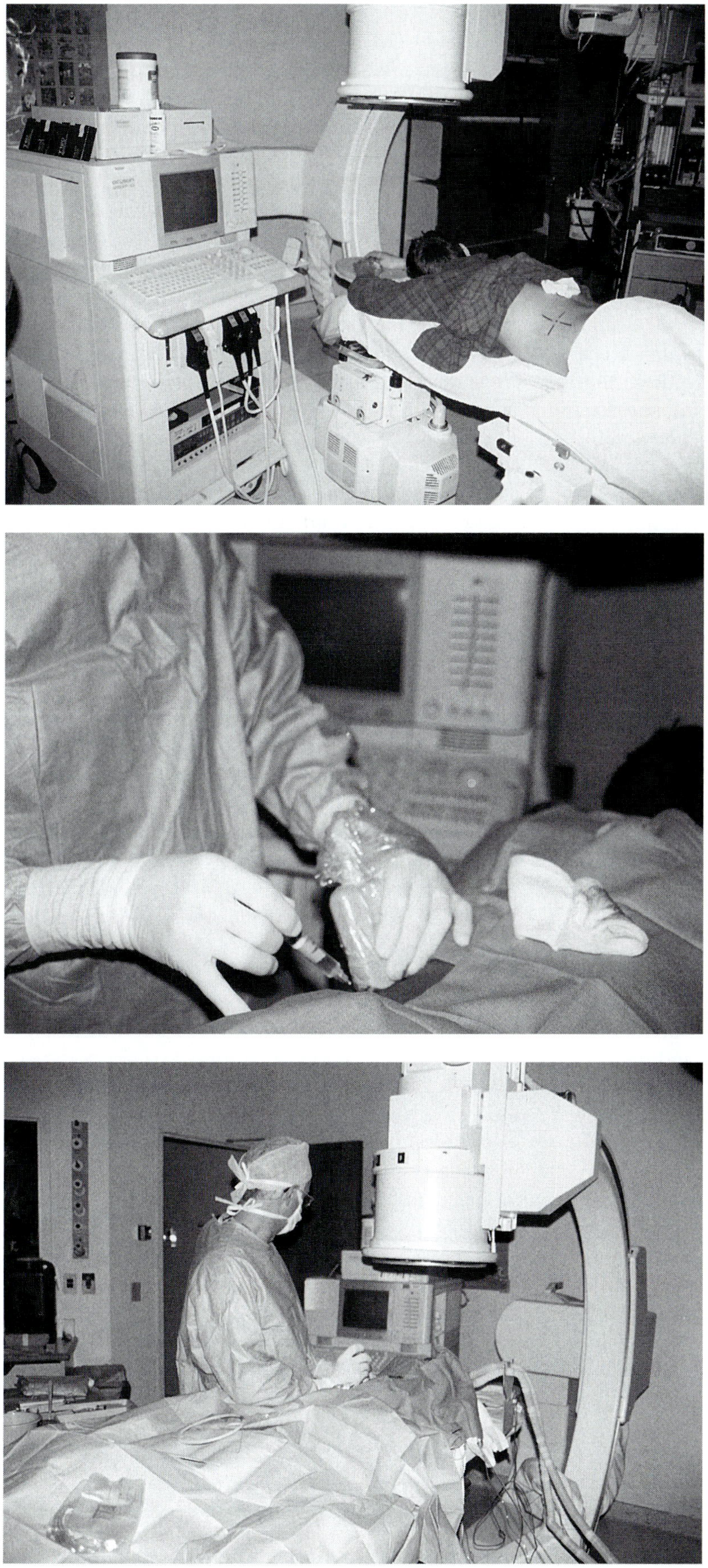

FIG. 63-9. A, Position of ultrasound equipment. The ultrasound and fluoroscopy equipment must be arranged in positions that are convenient and comfortable for the radiologist. **B,** Administering deep local anesthetic under ultrasound control. **C,** Typical working position.

THE TYPICAL PROCEDURE

Prior Consultation and Prior Studies

It is remarkable how many times interventional procedures are performed without complete knowledge of prior studies or procedures. One should know what difficulties were encountered the previous time or that there was a contrast reaction at a previous CT scan. The interventionist is responsible for having a clear idea of the clinical reasons for the procedure and the expected benefits. In large institutions it is easy for the interventionist to become the "meat in the sandwhich" between feuding clinical services, and if one simply accepts orders from a service without becoming knowledgeable about the case and the surrounding politics, the other services may not be supportive if a complication occurs. At times, it is the radiologist's duty to insist on a combined-care conference before undertaking a major procedure and this can be the greatest contribution a radiologist can make to a patient's welfare.

Clotting Studies

Clotting studies are indicated for most biopsies,[5] but they are generally not necessary for simple diagnostic procedures or drainage procedures unless there is a clear indication for them, as in liver transplant patients. A platelet count is usually obtained in oncology patients. Caution should be exercised when the platelet count is below 80,000, and it is important to remember that platelet function may be affected by some nonsteroidal anti-inflammatory agents, by uremia, and by other medical conditions. Patients with Wilms' tumor may rarely have an acquired von Willebrand's syndrome. Be cautious if the skin incision continues to bleed vigorously for more than a minute or so. It is better to cancel a procedure and do a full clotting workup than to continue and cause a major hemorrhage.

Even in normal patients, it is a rare radiologist (or a beginner) who has not encountered a substantial hemorrhage during routine nephrostomy. The kidney should always be regarded as a "sponge of blood." There is an old saying in the aviation industry: "There are two types of pilot—those who have landed with the wheels up and those who are going to." Likewise, **there are radiologists who have had a major complication during interventional procedures and those who are going to!** It is wise to approach each patient with confidence, modified by cautious optimism.

Consent

It is the responsibility of the radiologist performing the procedure to obtain consent from the responsible party. Allowing a junior surgical resident to have a piece of paper signed for you is inviting problems if a complication occurs. Parents are much less likely to be critical if genuine care and attention have been shown to them prior to the procedure than if the first time you talk to them is the time you come to discuss the complication.

Aims and Expectations

Anticipation of problems is a good idea, not a sign of weakness. No procedure should be undertaken without a clear understanding of the aims, the expected benefit, and a reasonably detailed plan for completing the task. If an abscess is difficult to see (for example, in the psoas muscle in a large adolescent), then a transfer to the CT suite should be considered. Often, however, after localization of a deep abscess by CT, we transfer the patient to the fluoroscopy suite and use ultrasound to guide needle placement. Once the abscess is entered, fluoroscopy can be used to monitor the guide-wire placement, and fluoroscopy allows early detection of guide-wire kinking during tract dilatation, the most common cause of difficulty encountered. Fluoroscopy allows the kinked wire to be withdrawn into the dilator and replaced or advanced into the abscess. The kinked wire is much more difficult to recognize by CT because the procedure is not monitored in real time and there is little room for recovery. CT is essential in some areas, notably pelvic abscesses requiring drainage through the greater sciatic notch.

A well-thought-out alternate plan is important, especially in complex procedures such as renal stone removal or ureteric stent placement. What happens if the patient moves or the wire is dislodged? A second safety wire tucked up in an upper-pole calyx is always good insurance in complex renal procedures. Expect the unexpected and the procedure will always go as planned!

Patient and Equipment Position

In most cases, it is ideal to perform ultrasound-guided procedures in the interventional or fluoroscopy room. A C-arm configuration (Fig. 63-9) allows wide access to the patient. Standard fluoroscopy tables, which typically have a large overhead film changer, can be used, and they result in a lower radiation dose to the operator, but they restrict access to the patient. The ultrasound equipment is arranged in the position most comfortable for the operator, usually toward the head of the patient and to the left. It is important for the operator to be comfortable and to be able to operate the table and the ultrasound equipment from the one position. Test the position of the patient under the fluoroscopy before beginning the procedure.

The equipment tray is positioned to the right. An experienced radiologist should be able to use the dominant or the nondominant hand for needle placement.

Initial Ultrasound Scan

Understand the individual patient's anatomy **before** sedation or general anesthesia. In preparation for a transcholecytstic cholangiogram, I once relied on an outside ultrasound report of a normal gallbladder without checking the images, only to find, once the patient was under general anesthesia, that there was no gallbladder visible. The patient was eventually diagnosed with biliary atresia. There are many variations on this mistake, and a **scan prior to sedation** will eliminate the problem.

Spending enough time to consider the most effective approach and the adjacent anatomy is as important as placing the needle well. It is less than perfect technique to pass a needle through the colon when a little time and care would have avoided the problem. The radiologist should have a good three-dimensional understanding of the patient's regional anatomy before commencing a procedure.

Pus. Pus is the liquefied product of inflammation. "Liquefied" is the most important word for the interventionist. Unlike CT, which generates a static image, real-time ultrasound allows exploration of the liquidity and therefore of the drainability of a lesion. Urinomas are notoriously echogenic when first examined, but if the operator vigorously prods the collection with the ultrasound probe, the free-flowing nature of the collection becomes apparent and it can be drained by a simple 8 French catheter, rather than by the large-caliber sump catheter you thought would be necessary.

Beware the "Pulsatile Red Abscess"! It is always prudent to check a potential lesion for blood flow using either color or pulsed Doppler. If a fast-flowing red "abscess" is inadvertently entered, leave the catheter in position and perform a contrast study to assess the flow characteristics. Although the natural reaction is to withdraw the needle immediately, leaving the needle in place will provide some tamponade of the track and provide time to consider the options. Abnormal cavities such as postbiopsy arteriovenous fistulas can sometimes be embolized, avoiding surgery. (To borrow another aviation aphorism, "Never panic when performing interventional procedures, but if you need to panic, panic constructively.")

Catheter Fixation

Catheters are objects of wonder for small children and babies and are great chewing material if left in the grasp of tiny hands. Often, when a catheter "just falls out by itself," there has been some lapse in care on the part of professional staff. Either the catheter was not properly secured in the first place or the nursing staff forgot to undo the safety pin when taking the child to the bathroom.

A Dislodged Catheter Is a Failed Procedure

To slightly overstate the position, a baby should be able to be suspended by the catheter without the catheter's being dislodged. (Don't try this at work—or at home!)

Some methods of fixation include standard sutures, sutures secured to the catheter by waterproof tape, or various skin fixation devices that are available. The fixation devices (Fig. 63-10) are convenient and robust and help avoid kinking of the catheter. Often all three methods are necessary, and in babies and infants, the catheter is hidden out of reach if possible, and secured with transparent plastic adhesive film.

Postprocedure Care and Follow-Up

The quickest way to destroy an interventional referral pattern is to ignore the patient once he or she has left

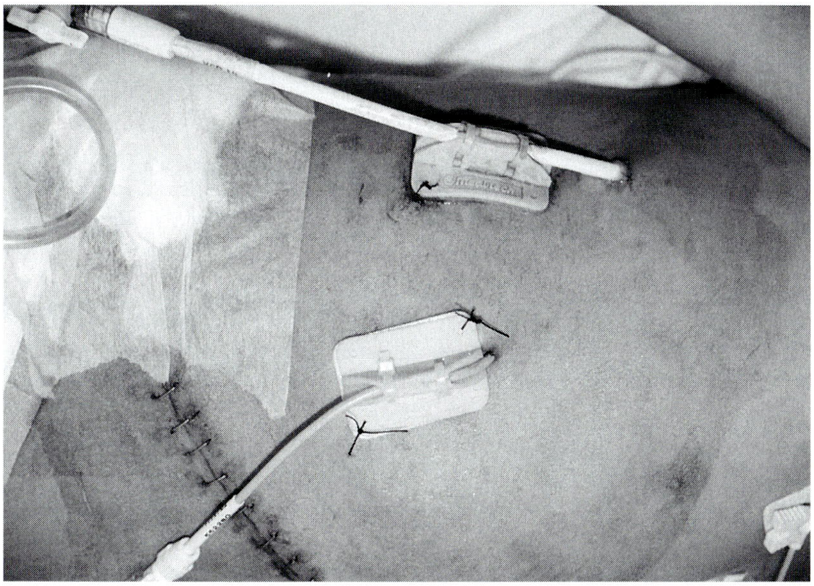

FIG. 63-10. Catheter fixation. The fixation devices are comfortable and minimize kinking of the catheters. In a younger or uncooperative patient, the catheters would also be firmly sutured, taped, and hidden from busy hands!

the radiology department. The interventionist is responsible for accepting the patient, for being satisfied that the procedure is justified and likely to be of significant benefit to the patient, and for follow-up, both in the immediate postprocedure period and for the long term. Leaving your pager number in the medical notes may result in a few trivial calls, but overall, it will benefit the patient and increase referrals and satisfaction. If a complication occurs, either deal with it or consult another service, but do the consultation personally, not through the intern messaging service.

A hematocrit before and 2 hours after biopsy is a prudent precaution. **Be cautious of blood loss in children after liver or other biopsy.** Blood loss is typically slow and self-limiting, but if bleeding persists, often the only objective sign is a rising pulse rate. **Children notoriously maintain blood pressure, tissue, and brain perfusion until very late and then suddenly deteriorate.**

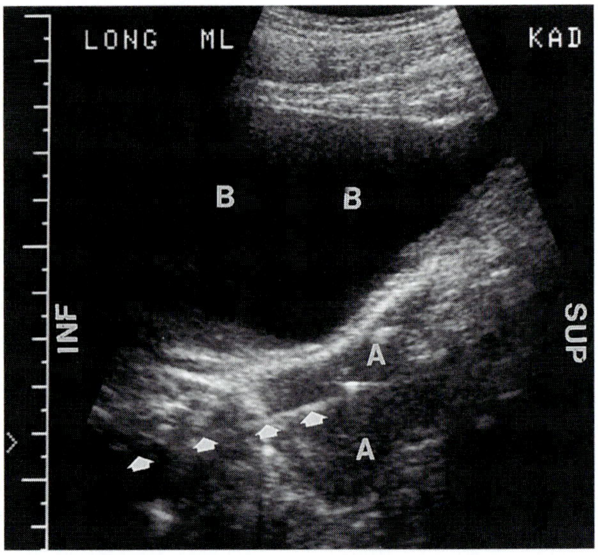

FIG. 63-11. Ultrasound-guided transrectal abscess drainage. The needle (*arrows*) has been inserted through the rectum and has punctured the high pelvic abscess (A) under ultrasound guidance. The bladder (B) is anterior to the abscess.

SPECIFIC PROCEDURES

Therapeutic Procedures

Abscess Drainage. This is one of the common procedures. When entering an abscess cavity, a sample is usually obtained for culture, but the cavity should not be aspirated completely before placement of the catheter. Once the catheter is in position, simple aspiration with ultrasound monitoring for completeness is all that is required. **Flushing with large volumes of saline or performing a contrast study will only result in intravasation of infected material** through the raw granulation tissue that always lines these abscesses. Contrast studies and flushing can be done later, once the cavity is healing. During initial aspiration, it is not uncommon to get dark blood return near the end of aspiration. This is probably blood arising from the granulation tissue and at times it can be alarming in amount. If active aspiration is ceased, the bleeding usually stops. The catheter should be left in place until the aspirate is straw-colored and less than a few ml per day.

Transrectal Drainage. Deep pelvic abscesses can be drained by means of surgery or by a catheter that has been inserted under ultrasound control.[6] The ultrasound-guided method is particularly appropriate for high collections that are beyond the reach of the surgical digit (Fig. 63-11). The catheter can be withdrawn after complete aspiration of the cavity or left in place and secured to the leg with tape. Usually the catheter is promptly dislodged by the patient, but the abscess rarely reaccumulates.

Pleural Drainage. Ultrasound-guided diagnostic aspiration of pleural fluid is a common and useful procedure. Drainage of empyema has been described and can result in complete cure if performed early enough, but the pleura has a remarkable ability to thicken and produce fibrin, and these infected collections often loculate and become incompletely drained. The administration of urokinase through the tube can be useful to change the physical characteristics of the thick fluid.[7] Any chest tube for empyema drainage must be of substantial caliber, and its position must be monitored frequently to insure that loculation has not occurred.

PICC Lines. Peripherally inserted central catheters (PICCs) are a useful way of obtaining safe central access for short- to medium-term use. The catheters are from 2 French to 5 French in size, and various commercial units are available with insertion sets containing either a peel-away canula similar to an IV catheter or a peel-away Seldinger-style sheath. After insertion of the sheath into a peripheral vein (arm, leg, or scalp), the premeasured catheter is placed through the sheath and positioned in the central veins. Access to the arm veins is often easy in the older individual, but the veins of babies and infants can be notoriously difficult to cannulate. Ultrasound can be used for localization of deeper arm veins. The technique of ultrasound guidance is different from previously described techniques in that it is best to **monitor the needle position by transverse position of the transducer** (Fig. 63-12). The veins are usually so small that monitoring position with the transducer in the plane of the needle results in malpositioning the needle because of the width of the ultrasound beam.

A

B

C

D

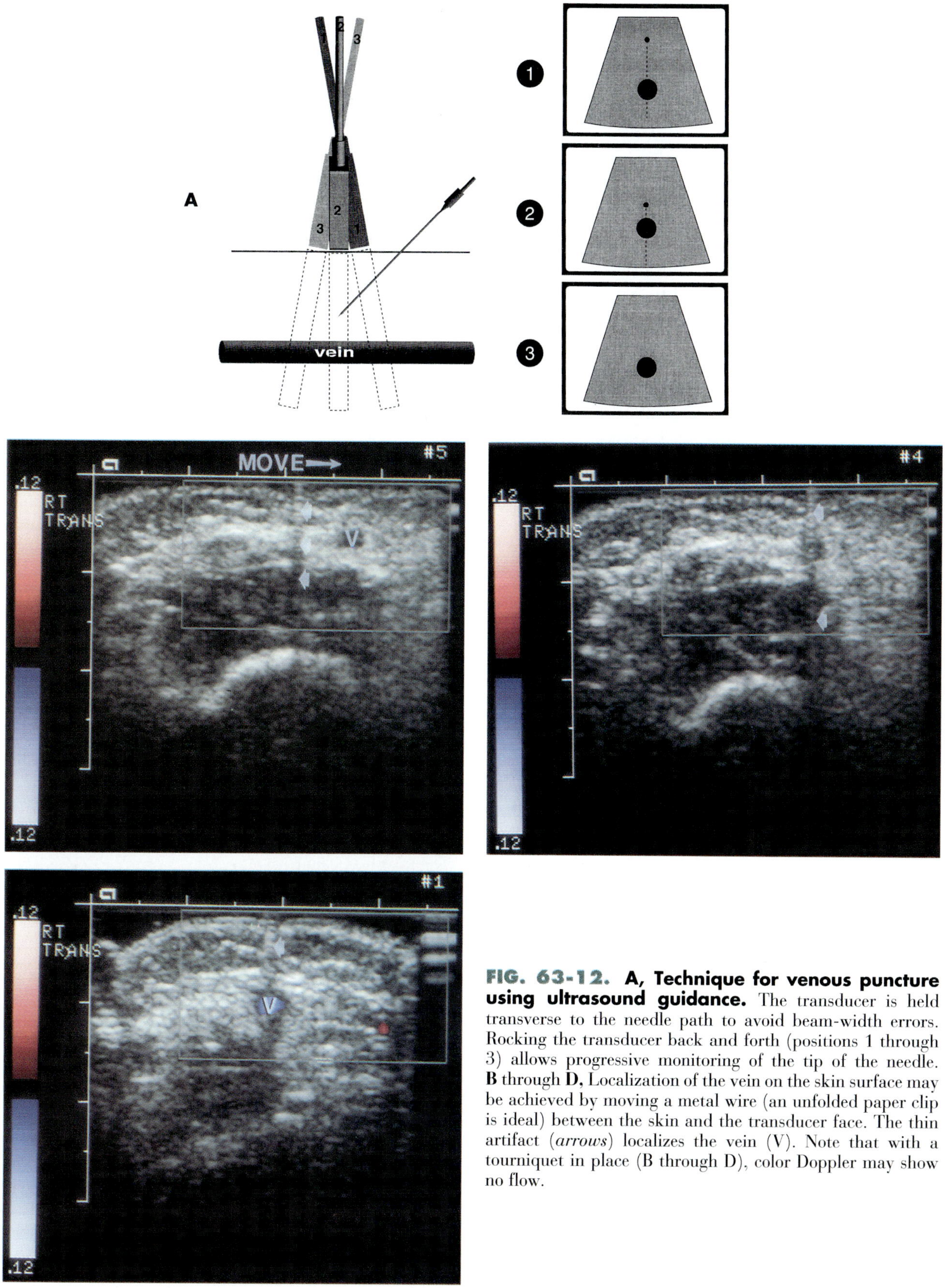

FIG. 63-12. A, Technique for venous puncture using ultrasound guidance. The transducer is held transverse to the needle path to avoid beam-width errors. Rocking the transducer back and forth (positions 1 through 3) allows progressive monitoring of the tip of the needle. **B** through **D,** Localization of the vein on the skin surface may be achieved by moving a metal wire (an unfolded paper clip is ideal) between the skin and the transducer face. The thin artifact (*arrows*) localizes the vein (V). Note that with a tourniquet in place (B through D), color Doppler may show no flow.

A B

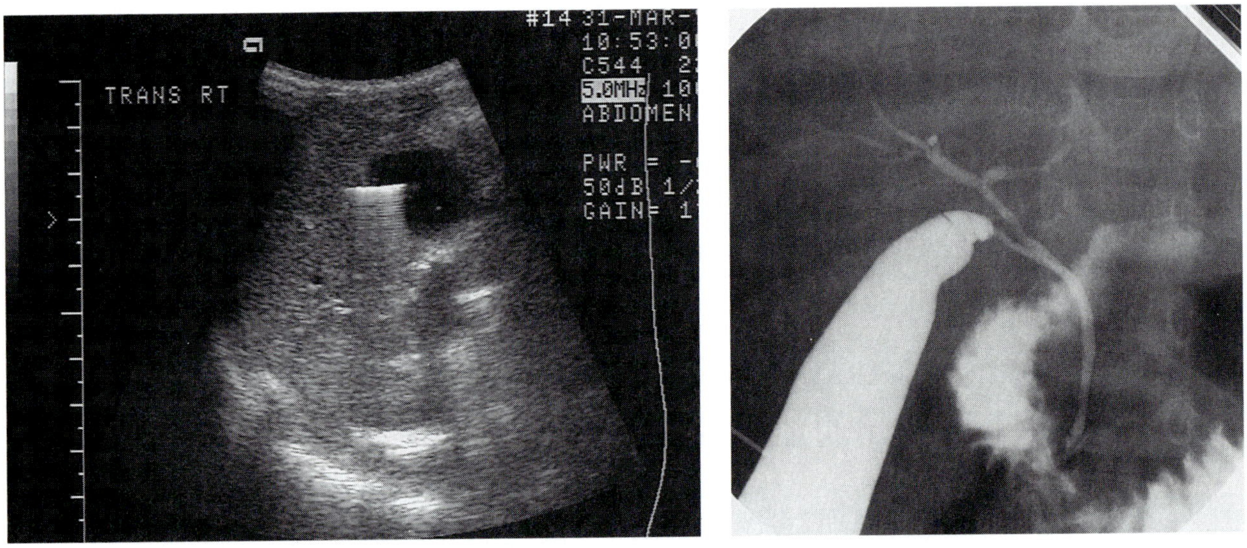

FIG. 63-13. Percutaneous cholecystic cholangiography. **A,** Needle puncture of the gallbladder. **B,** Resulting cholangiogram with excellent visualization of intrahepatic and extrahepatic ducts.

DIAGNOSTIC PROCEDURES

Percutaneous Transhepatic Cholangiography

Percutaneous transhepatic cholangiography (PTC) can be successfully performed in children with or without duct dilatation. Ultrasound is used to guide the Chiba needle toward the bile ducts, which lie in the portal tracts. The optimal diagnostic puncture site is at the junction of the middle and peripheral thirds of the duct. If the ducts are dilated, the needle can be guided directly into the ducts using the usual ultrasound techniques. Puncture should be made at a site and at an angle that will allow conversion of the track to a catheter drain, should the diagnostic study reveal complete obstruction, especially in liver transplants. These patients invariably have a degree of infective cholangitis, and catheter drainage allows time for control of the infection before interventional or surgical treatment of the stricture.

In patients with nondilated ducts, the easiest and safest way to image the ducts is by puncture of the gallbladder and retrograde contrast study, but if there is no gallbladder, a PTC can still be done by placing the Chiba needle in close proximity to the peripheral branches of the portal triads. Eventually, with contrast injection as the needle is withdrawn, a duct will be entered and a cholangiogram achieved. The procedure may require multiple passess, but there is little risk, providing the clotting function is normal and the punctures are under ultrasound control.

Percutaneous Cholecystic Cholangiography

Percutaneous cholecystic cholangiography (PCC) is a useful technique in which the gallbladder is punctured transhepatically and contrast is injected into the gallbladder. The contrast exits the gallbladder and gives an excellent cholangiogram (Fig. 63-13). In our experience, the procedure is much less traumatic than endoscopic retrograde cholangio pancreatography (ERCP) in small children.[8]

REFERENCES

1. Gibson RN, Gibson KI. A home-made phantom for learning ultrasound-guided invasive. *Australasian Radiology* 1995;39: 356-357.
2. This training system was developed by Dr. William Shiels and is available as a videotape at nominal cost from Radiology Department Children's Hospital Medical Center, Cincinnati, OH 45229; (513) 636-8574.
2a. Georgian Smith D, Shiels WE. Freehand interventional sonography in the breast: basic principles and clinical applications. *RadioGraphics* 1996;16:149-161.
2b. Harvey JA, Moran RE, Hamer MM, et al. Evaluation of a turkey-breast phantom for teaching freehand, US-guided coreneedle breast biopsy. *Acad Radiol* 1997;4:565-569.
3. Hopper KD, Abendroth CS, Sturtz KW et al. Automated biopsy devices: a blinded evaluation. *Radiology* 1993; 87:653-660.
4. Egelhoff JC, Ball Jr WS, Koch Bernadette, Parks TD. Safety and efficacy of sedation in children using a structured sedation program. *AJR* 1997;168:1259-1262.
5. Murphy TP, Dorfman GS, Becker J. Use of preprocedural tests by interventional radiologists. *Radiology* 1993;186:213-220.
6. Pereira JK, Chait PG, Miller SF. Deep pelvic abscesses in children: transrectal drainage under radiologic guidance. *Radiology* 1996;198:393-396.
7. Moulton JS, Moore T, Mencini, R. Treatment of loculated pleural effusions with trand catheter intracavity urokinase. *Am J Roentgenol* 153:941-945.
8. Brunelle F, Chaumont P. Percutaneous cholecystography in children. *Ann Radiology* 1984;27:111-116.

Index

A

D

E

F

H

M

N

O

Q

R

S